Dental Hygiene Theory and Practice

Dental Hygiene Theory and Practice

Michele Leonardi Darby, BSDH, MS
Eminent Scholar and Graduate Program Director
Gene W. Hirschfeld School of Dental Hygiene and Dental Assisting
College of Health Sciences
Old Dominion University
Norfolk, Virginia

Margaret M. Walsh, RDH, MS, MA, EdD
Professor
Department of Dental Public Health and Hygiene
University of California, San Francisco
School of Dentistry
San Francisco, California

W.B. Saunders Company
A Division of Harcourt Brace & Company
Philadelphia London Toronto Montreal Sydney Tokyo

W.B. SAUNDERS COMPANY
A Division of Harcourt Brace & Company

The Curtis Center
Independence Square West
Philadelphia, Pennsylvania 19106

Library of Congress Cataloging-in-Publication Data

Dental hygiene theory and practice / [edited by] Michele Leonardi Darby, Margaret M. Walsh. — 1st ed.
p. cm.
ISBN 0-7216-2966-0
1. Dental hygiene I. Walsh, Margaret M.
[DNLM: 1. Oral Health. 2. Dental Care. WU 113 D4133 1994]
RK60.5.D445 1995
617.6′01—dc20
DNLM/DLC 94-32189

DENTAL HYGIENE THEORY AND PRACTICE ISBN 0-7216-2966-0

Printed in the United States of America.

Last digit is the print number: 9 8 7 6 5 4 3

To my parents for their continued guidance and love.
To my husband, Dennis, and our children, Devan and Blake—for making everything worthwhile.

MLD

To the memory of my parents, who gave me so much love and support over the years,

and

To my husband, Jerry, and son, T.J., for their patience, love, and encouragement.

MMW

Contributors

Gerry J. Barker, RDH, BS, MA
Dental Hygiene Care for the Individual with Cancer
Assistant Professor and Coordinator of Oncology Education, Department of Diagnostic Sciences, University of Missouri–Kansas City School of Dentistry, Kansas City, Missouri

Deborah Blythe Bauman, BSDH, MS
Dental Hygiene Care for the Individual with Diabetes
Associate Professor, Gene W. Hirschfeld School of Dental Hygiene and Dental Assisting, College of Health Sciences, Old Dominion University, Norfolk, Virginia

Denise M. Bowen, RDH, MS
Personal Mechanical Oral Hygiene Care and Chemotherapeutic Plaque Control
Professor and Chair, Department of Dental Hygiene, Idaho State University, Pocatello, Idaho

Pamela Parker Brangan, BSDH, MS, MPH, EdS
Dental Hygiene Care for the Older Adult
Associate Professor, Gene W. Hirschfeld School of Dental Hygiene and Dental Assisting, College of Health Sciences, Old Dominion University, Norfolk, Virginia

Cheryl A. Cameron, RDH, PhD
Restorative Therapy and the Dental Hygiene Process
Associate Professor, Department of Dental Public Health Sciences, School of Dentistry, University of Washington, Seattle, Washington

Michele Leonardi Darby, BSDH, MS
The Evolving Profession of Dental Hygiene; Dental Hygiene Human Needs Conceptual Model and Its Application to the Dental Hygiene Process; Introduction to the Dental Hygiene Process; Cultural Diversity and the Dental Hygiene Process; Extraoral and Intraoral Clinical Assessment; Periodontal and Oral Hygiene Assessment; Dental Hygiene Diagnosis; Dental Hygiene Care Plan; Evaluation of Dental Hygiene Care; Dental Hygiene Management and Leadership
Eminent Scholar and Graduate Program Director, Gene W. Hirschfeld School of Dental Hygiene and Dental Assisting, College of Health Sciences, Old Dominion University, Norfolk, Virginia

Maureen E. Fannon, RDH, MS
Dental Hygiene Care: Caries Prevention and Control
Dental Hygiene Instructor, Foothill College, Los Altos Hills, California

Glenn E. Gordon, DDS, MS
Restorative Therapy and the Dental Hygiene Process
Senior Lecturer, University of Washington School of Dentistry; Attending Staff, Harborview Medical Center, Seattle, Washington

Renee Trepanier Hannebrink, RDH, MS
Local Anesthesia
Associate Clinical Professor, University of California, San Francisco, San Francisco, California

Barbara L. Heckman, RDH, MS
Current Concepts of Infection Control; Infection Control Protocols for the Dental Hygiene Process of Care; Instrument Recirculation: Containment, Decontamination, Packaging, Renewal (Sterilization), Maintenance, and Dispensing
Dental Hygiene Program Coordinator, Dental Hygiene Department, Diablo Valley College, Pleasant Hill, California; Adjunct Associate Clinical Professor, Department of Dental Public Health and Hygiene, University of California, San Francisco, School of Dentistry, San Francisco, California

Linda G. Kraemer, RDH, PhD
Research and Theory Development in Dental Hygiene
Professor, Department of Dental Hygiene, and Senior Associate Dean, College of Allied Health Sciences, Thomas Jefferson University, Philadelphia, Pennsylvania

Sandra Kramer, RDH, MA
Professional Mechanical Oral Hygiene Care for the Prevention and Control of Periodontal Diseases; Practice Management and Professional Development
Private Practice, Berkeley, California

Mari-Anne L. Low, RDH, BS
Dental Hygiene Care for the Edentulous Individual
Assistant Clinical Professor, Division of Dental Hygiene and Preventive Dentistry, University of California, San Francisco, School of Dentistry, San Francisco, California

Laura Lee MacDonald, DH, BScD(DH), MEd
Concepts of Health and Wellness
Assistant Professor, School of Dental Hygiene, University of Manitoba, Winnipeg, Manitoba, Canada

Ginger L. Byrd Mann, RDH, BS, MS
Dental Hygiene Care for the Individual with Mental Retardation
Clinical Assistant Professor, University of North Carolina School of Dentistry, Chapel Hill, North Carolina

Maria McKenzie, RDH, BA
Dental Hygiene Care: Caries Prevention and Control
Adjunct Faculty, Department of Dental Public Health and Hygiene–Restorative Dentistry, University of California, San Francisco, San Francisco, California

Beth E. McKinney, BSDH, MS
Quality Assurance in Dental Hygiene
Former Quality Assurance Coordinator, Randmark Management, Inc., Washington, District of Columbia

Cara Miyasaki-Ching, RDH, MS
Assessment of Client Health History Data and Vital Signs
Director, Dental Assisting Program, Foothill College, Los Altos Hills, California; Assistant Clinical Professor, University of California, San Francisco, School of Dentistry, San Francisco, California

Laura Mueller-Joseph, BSDH, MS
Dental Hygiene Care for the Individual with Cardiovascular Disease
Assistant Professor, State University of New York College of Technology at Farmingdale, Farmingdale, New York

Dorothy A. Perry, RDH, PhD
Dental Hygiene Care for Acute Gingival and Periodontal Conditions; Dental Hygiene Care for the Individual with HIV Infection
Assistant Professor and Chair, Division of Dental Hygiene and Preventive

Dentistry, University of California, San Francisco, School of Dentistry, San Francisco, California

Janice F. L. Pimlott, DipDH, BScD, MSc
Assessment of the Dentition
Associate Professor and Chair, Division of Dental Hygiene, University of Alberta, Edmonton, Alberta, Canada

Sandra K. Rich, RDH, MPH, PhD
Behavioral Foundations for the Dental Hygiene Process
Associate Professor and Chair, Department of Dental Hygiene, University of Southern California School of Dentistry, Los Angeles, California

Ann Flynn Scarff, RDH, MA
Periodontal and Oral Hygiene Assessment
Product Specialist, Johnson & Johnson Medical, Inc.; Private Practice, Burlingame, California

Deanne Shuman, BSDH, MS
Computer Applications in Dental Hygiene
Professor and Chair, Gene W. Hirschfeld School of Dental Hygiene and Dental Assisting, College of Health Sciences, Old Dominion University, Norfolk, Virginia

Ann Eshenaur Spolarich, RDH, MS
Basic Principles of Working with Clients with Special Dental Hygiene Care Needs
Former Assistant Professor and Senior Clinic Coordinator, Department of Dental Hygiene, College of Allied Health Sciences, Thomas Jefferson University; Research Dental Hygienist, Dental Service, Philadelphia Veterans Administration Medical Center, Philadelphia, Pennsylvania

Margaret M. Tan, BS, RDH
Extraoral and Intraoral Clinical Assessment
Assistant Clinical Professor, Department of Dental Public Health and Hygiene, University of California, San Francisco, School of Dentistry, San Francisco, California

Peggy T. Tsutsui, RDH, MS
Instrumentation Theory for Professional Mechanical Oral Hygiene Care
Associate Professor, University of Southern California School of Dentistry, Los Angeles, California

Margaret M. Walsh, RDH, MS, MA, EdD
The Evolving Profession of Dental Hygiene; Dental Hygiene Human Needs Conceptual Model and Its Application to the Dental Hygiene Process; Introduction to the Dental Hygiene Process; Cultural Diversity and the Dental Hygiene Process; Extraoral and Intraoral Clinical Assessment; Periodontal and Oral Hygiene Assessment; Dental Hygiene Diagnosis; Dental Hygiene Care Plan; Professional Mechanical Oral Hygiene Care for the Prevention and Control of Periodontal Diseases; Nitrous Oxide-Oxygen Analgesia; Evaluation of Dental Hygiene Care; Dental Hygiene Management and Leadership
Professor, Department of Dental Public Health and Hygiene, University of California, San Francisco, School of Dentistry, San Francisco, California

Karen B. Williams, RDH, MS
Dental Hygiene Care for Individuals with Eating Disorders
Associate Professor, University of Missouri–Kansas City School of Dentistry, Kansas City, Missouri

Merry Greig Wong, RDH, MS
Root Morphology
Program Director, Dental Health Programs, Chabot College, Hayward, California; Assistant Clinical Professor, University of California, San Francisco, School of Dentistry, San Francisco, California

Judy Yamamoto, RDH, MS
Dental Hygiene Care: Caries Prevention and Control
Assistant Clinical Professor, Department of Dental Public Health and Hygiene, University of California, San Francisco, School of Dentistry, San Francisco, California

Vivian L. Young-McDonald, RDH, BS
Dental Hygiene Care for the Individual with Osseointegrated Dental Implants
Implant Coordinator, oral and maxillofacial surgery private practice, Pinole, California

Pamela Zarkowski, BSDH, MPH, JD
Ethical and Legal Decision Making in Dental Hygiene
Associate Dean of Admissions and Community Relations, Chairperson, Dental Hygiene Department, Associate Professor, University of Detroit Mercy School of Dentistry, Detroit, Michigan

Preface

Dental Hygiene Theory and Practice is written for dental hygiene students and professionals who are interested in the development of the body of knowledge in dental hygiene and the use of that knowledge to guide practice, education, and research. The purpose of the book is to develop dental hygienists who view their profession with confidence and pride, understand its territory and scope of practice, and are able to influence the factors that affect professional advancement. The challenge for us was to design the book as a process of care that is guided by the human needs conceptual model, rather than as a series of chapters that present isolated tasks, and to have recognized in a textbook that contemporary dental hygiene practice requires professionals who function as practitioners, client advocates, managers, researchers, oral health promoters, and change agents. Therefore, we have attempted to develop these roles throughout the book.

In this age of wellness, the dental hygienist's expertise in oral disease prevention and health promotion is assuming more value to the public than ever before. The public also is holding the dental hygienist accountable for a defined scope of practice. Dental hygienists have been held legally accountable for judgments exercised and actions taken in the course of providing dental hygiene care.

Societal changes, values, and healthcare reforms clearly forecast the need for a theoretically based dental hygiene practitioner who is able to make decisions within the scope of dental hygiene practice and to collaborate with the dentist in providing the best possible oral healthcare to the public. *Dental Hygiene Theory and Practice* is a bold step into the future of dental hygiene care and is predicated on three key assumptions. First, dental hygienists are responsible for the services they provide and for the judgments and professional decisions they render. Second, accountability requires a systematic approach to practice, and this approach is the dental hygiene process. Third, both theory and research serve as the basis for all roles in dental hygiene. Given these assumptions, society has a right to expect ready access to care from individuals who possess a substantial theoretical foundation for making dental hygiene assessments, diagnoses, and care plans, and for providing interventions and evaluating the effects of those interventions on oral health outcomes. These behaviors, inherent in the dental hygiene process, provide the framework for delivering high quality dental hygiene care to all types of clients in a variety of settings and serve as the core of professional dental hygiene practice.

Throughout the book, the dental hygiene process is supported by dental hygiene theory, defined as interrelated concepts that can be used to systematically support acceptable approaches to dental hygiene care and to predict the outcomes of that care. In an emerging discipline such as dental hygiene, theory provides a body of knowledge that can be used to guide and direct practice. Theory provides a framework for decision making, problem solving, explaining phenomena, and predicting outcomes that enables the dental hygiene practitioner to continually reevaluate and advance the theories on which service to society is based.

Although the dental hygiene human needs conceptual model is used as the framework for this book, we believe that it is just one model, the first of many, that can be used to explore the full potential of dental hygiene. It is our hope that the book sets a new direction for future work with conceptual models of dental hygiene.

Many may ask why human needs theory was used to develop the conceptual model of dental hygiene that serves as the foundation of this book. The answer lies in the inherent nature of dental hygiene as we perceived it: to promote oral health and wellness through the fulfillment of human needs. Human needs are universal, transcend all cultures, and are applicable to both individuals and groups. Human need fulfillment contributes to the quality of life of the individual, community, nation, and world. These facts were recognized by the World Health Organization when, in 1984, it redefined health as "the extent to which an individual or group is able, on the one hand, to realize aspirations and satisfy needs and, on the other hand, to change and cope with the environment."

If dental hygiene care can assist individuals in their attainment of human needs, it will be recognized by society for its ability to enhance the quality of life. If dental hygiene is conceptualized from a human needs framework, then dental hygiene is viewed as an essential component of the healthcare system and as a valued entity in today's wellness-oriented society.

Progressing through the book, one quickly notices that the word "client" is used throughout instead of "patient." We are sensitive to the responses that the word "client" may evoke. However, we deliberately chose the word "client" because it is broader in scope than the term "patient" and can refer to a group as well as to an individual. Moreover, the term "client" connotes wellness rather than illness. Given that the focus of dental hygiene is to prevent oral disease and promote wellness, the term "client" emphasizes that not all those for whom we provide care are in need of "treatment" for a disease. Last, the term "client" emphasizes the self-determination of the recipient of dental hygiene care, since individuals who seek dental hygiene care generally choose to do so and are in a partnership with the dental hygienist to promote and maintain personal oral health and wellness.

Dental Hygiene Theory and Practice is organized into seven major sections comprising a total of 41 chapters. Integrated throughout the majority of chapters is risk management theory, teaching and learning theory, and principles of ethics and law, which, in our opinion, transcend all facets of dental hygiene. Each chapter also includes behavioral objectives to guide the teacher and the learner, a theoretical and pragmatic discussion of the subject based on current research findings, procedures outlined in a sequential format with accompanying rationales to ensure that the learner understands the reason underlying each step of certain dental hygiene techniques, and reference and supplemental reading lists for those who wish to pursue a topic further. The comprehensive glossary defines terms quickly and easily for the busy reader. Recognizing that this book may be used throughout North America, we have included, where appropriate, information that reflects the practice of dental hygiene in Canada.

Section I, Conceptual Framework for Dental Hygiene, describes the evolving profession of dental hygiene, introduces the dental hygiene human needs conceptual model and the dental hygiene process of care, and provides the behavioral science theory used by dental hygienists in a multiplicity of roles. Because dental hygiene's main focus is on oral disease prevention and health promotion, an entire chapter is devoted to concepts of health and wellness. Moreover, since the multicultural dimension of our society clearly underscores how culture influences one's concepts of health, disease, behavior, and lifestyle, a chapter on cultural diversity and the dental hygiene process also is included in this section.

Section II, Prevention of Disease Transmission, describes the current guidelines and practices for infection control and presents detailed infection control protocols separately for each major clinical intervention associated with dental hygiene care. An entire chapter is also devoted to instrument recirculation.

Although the dental hygiene process was introduced in Section I, it now provides the organizational framework for the majority of the remaining sections.

Section III, Dental Hygiene Assessments, contains four chapters that delineate the important role of the dental hygienist in the assessment of various aspects of a client's general and oral health.

Section IV, Dental Hygiene Diagnosis and Care Plan, details the second phase of the process of care by defining a dental hygiene diagnosis, distinguishing it from a dental diagnosis, and illustrating how a dental hygiene diagnosis is made within the human needs conceptual model.

This section also details the third phase of the process of care by describing how a care plan is developed from assessment data and the dental hygiene diagnosis. The value of including the client goals in the care plan is also discussed.

Section V, Implementation and Evaluation, presents some of the common interventions that compose dental hygiene care. Procedures have been prepared to facilitate mastery of a variety of dental hygiene techniques, including the administration of intraoral local anesthesia and nitrous oxide–oxygen analgesia. This section strongly advises the regular use of the last phase of the dental hygiene process, that of evaluation. It is this step in the process of care that requires documentation of outcomes of care. With evaluation, the dental hygienist can be confident that dental hygiene actions made a positive difference in the individual's general and oral health status.

Section VI, Dental Hygiene Care for Individuals with Special Needs, recognizes that in today's world, dental hygienists care for a growing number of individuals with diseases or disabilities that affect their daily living, self-care, and ability to access professional care. The more common conditions that a dental hygienist might find in clients are given chapter status for adequate coverage.

Section VII, Leadership and Management, provides the capstone for the book. In this section, important yet often ignored subject areas are developed for the dental hygienist. Of particular importance are management and leadership strategies, practice management, computer applications, ethical and legal decision making, quality assurance, and research and theory development.

We would like to express our sincere appreciation to all the contributors who helped make *Dental Hygiene Theory and Practice* a reality. Very special thanks are extended to the faculty and staff of the Gene W. Hirschfeld School of Dental Hygiene and Dental Assisting at Old Dominion University and to the faculty and staff of the Division of Dental Hygiene and Preventive Dentistry at the University of California, San Francisco, who made it possible for us to complete this book despite the demands of continuing responsibilities. Appreciation is extended to the American Dental Hygienists' Association, particularly Deborah McFall, 1992–93 President, and to the clients and staff at the Philadelphia Veterans Administration Medical Center Dental Service and the Media Department at Thomas Jefferson University for their cooperation and support. We also acknowledge the authors and publishers who granted permission to use concepts, quotes, photographs, figures, and tables. Several individuals who contributed content reviews of selected areas and/or photographs and diagrams should be acknowledged: Lynn Tolle-Watts, BSDH, MEd, Gregory Schrumpf, DDS, and Scott Sechrist, Old Dominion University; Mary Martha Stewart, RDH, PhD; Edward Green, DDS, Edward J. Taggart, DDS, and Margaret Ash, DDS, University of California, San Francisco, School of Dentistry; Connie Drisko, RDH, DDS, University of Louisville, Kentucky, School of Dentistry; Shari Center, MEd, College of Allied Health Sciences, Thomas Jefferson University; Thomas Flynn, DMD, University of Connecticut; Maureen and David Howes, Onondaga Community College; Bruce Barker, DDS, University of Missouri–Kansas City School of Dentistry; James R. Clark, University of Washington School of Dentistry, Department of Orthodontics; Ann Gabrick, MSW, LSCSW, Eating Disorders Unit, Baptist Medical Center, Kansas City, Missouri; Robert Cowan, DDS, Advanced Education General Dentistry, University of Missouri–Kansas City School of Dentistry; Greg Mann; Paul Hains, Down syndrome client, University of North Carolina School of Dentistry; Linda Ross Santiago, RDH, Diablo Valley College, Pleasant Hill, California; James R. Winkler, DDS, School of Dental Medicine, Clinic of Periodontology and Fixed Prosthodontics, University of Berne; Philip R. Melnick, University of California, Los Angeles, School of Dentistry; F. T. McIver, DDS, Department of Pediatric Dentistry, University of North Carolina School of Dentistry; Bob Perry from Oral-B Laboratories; Victoria Vick, RDH, from Procter & Gamble; Hewlett-Packard Company; Bausch and Lomb; Tech Poll Studios, Inc.; Singer Professional Services, Inc.; and the QUE Corporation. We gratefully acknowledge the technical assistance of Bryce Bawden, Joanna Hill, Tina Cancelliere, and Betty Grizzard in preparing manuscripts, and the skills of Laura Heisler, BSDH, Old Dominion University, in organizing the glossary.

We also acknowledge the staff at W.B. Saunders, particularly Selma Ozmat, Senior Editor for Health-Related Professions, and Shirley Kuhn, Senior Developmental Editor, for shepherding the manuscript throughout the publication process. We are indebted to Dr. Helen Yura Petro for her mentorship and generosity in sharing time and knowledge, without which the human needs conceptual model for dental hygiene would never have become a reality. Without the contributions of these outstanding individuals, the book would not have been possible.

As with any new text, we shall be grateful to readers who have suggestions for additions or revisions, or who are interested in sharing their responses with us.

Michele Leonardi Darby

Margaret M. Walsh

Contents

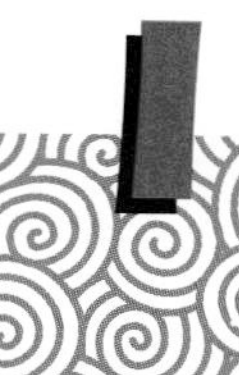

I CONCEPTUAL FRAMEWORK FOR DENTAL HYGIENE

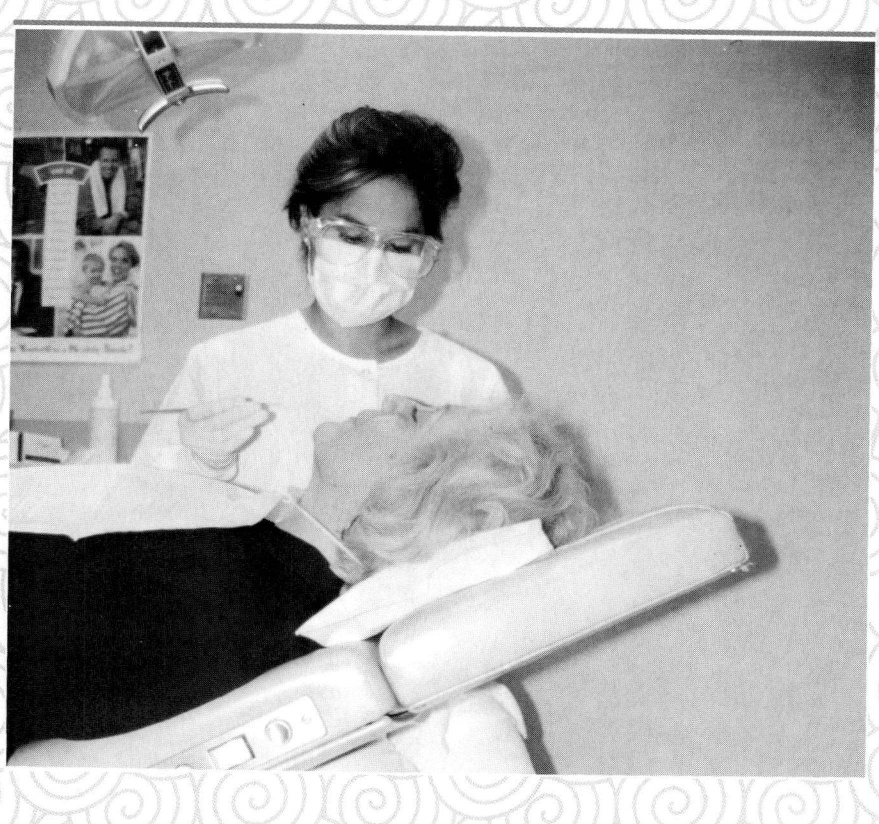

1 The Evolving Profession of Dental Hygiene

OBJECTIVES

Mastery of the content in this chapter will enable the reader to:

- Define the key terms used
- Discuss the historical development of professional dental hygiene
- Discuss some modern definitions and philosophies of dental hygiene
- Define a paradigm and distinguish it from a conceptual model
- Describe the different educational programs for becoming an entry-level dental hygienist and dental hygiene specialist
- Describe roles and functions of the dental hygienist
- Describe at least three career paths for the dental hygienist

INTRODUCTION

The **dental hygienist** is a licensed, professional member of the healthcare team who integrates the roles of educator, consumer advocate, practitioner, manager, change agent, and researcher to support total health through the promotion of oral health and wellness.

The purpose of dental hygiene is to promote and maintain oral wellness and, thereby, contribute to the quality of life. If the state of an individual's oral health changes, the dental hygienist, within the scope of dental hygiene practice, provides the highest quality of dental hygiene care to direct the person back to oral wellness. If oral wellness cannot be achieved, dental hygiene care helps maximize the degree of oral health. In addition, the dental hygienist assists individuals in seeking other healthcare services as needed.

Inherent in the fulfillment of the purpose of dental hygiene is the **dental hygiene process.** The identification of the dental hygiene problem, which can be actual or potential in nature, constitutes the focal point for establishing goals with behavioral outcomes in the dental hygiene care plan, implementing specific strategies, and evaluating their effectiveness. The dental hygienist's effort toward meeting the individual's oral hygiene needs takes into account such individual and environmental factors as

- The person's level of growth and maturity
- Psychomotor ability
- Age
- Gender
- Role
- Lifestyle
- Culture
- Attitudes
- Health beliefs and behaviors
- Level of knowledge

In addition, the dental hygienist evaluates critically the relevant scientific literature and applies appropriate research findings when providing client care. The dental hygiene process is applied more broadly in the roles of leader, educator, and scholar as the dental hygienist strives to effect change that leads to conditions favorable to the fulfillment of the oral health needs of the client—whether the client is the individual, family, organization, or community as a whole.

Society consists of a complex network of individuals, families, groups, communities, and nations that exist to facilitate the meeting of its members' human needs. Demographic changes that have been predicted for the United States include

- Growth in the elderly population
- A slow overall population growth with increases in Asian, Hispanic, and African-American groups
- A changing concept of the family
- Feminization of the workforce
- A rising proportion of poor
- Increased cultural diversity

Societal health needs have changed, and more alterations are anticipated with the advent of the twenty-first century. Predictions about health and the healthcare system have been made. (See Predictions about Health and the Healthcare System chart.) These predicted changes require the dental hygiene profession to reflect on the way it views

PREDICTIONS ABOUT HEALTH AND THE HEALTHCARE SYSTEM

- Increased demand for healthcare
- Alternative healthcare systems with emphasis on cost containment, access, quality, and accountability
- Competition for consumers and business
- Rising professional autonomy for healthcare providers other than the physician
- Access to care, the medically uninsured, and national health insurance emerging as major political issues
- Financial burdens on the healthcare system
- Philosophical and ethical issues will require resolution
- National standards of practice

itself, its societal responsibilities, its role in healthcare, and its clients. In this age of consumerism, wellness, and self-care, the preventive role of the dental hygienist is assuming more value to the public than ever before. The consumer's role in healthcare is changing. The healthcare consumer is demanding greater rights in the healthcare setting. Consumers expect to make healthcare decisions, have skeptical and questioning attitudes, view healthcare professionals as fallible, and challenge authority and the status quo.

The term "client" is used instead of "patient" with increasing frequency in some healthcare settings as a more accurate way to describe the contemporary healthcare consumer. This preference is because "patient" suggests a sick, dependent person who is in need of therapy, whereas "client" connotes wellness as well as illness and suggests a person who is an active participant in oral healthcare and who is responsible for personal choices and the consequences of those choices. Moreover, "patient" is limited in reference to an individual, whereas "client" is a broader term that may refer to an individual, family, group, community, or nation. Because of its versatility and meaning, "client" is used throughout this book to denote the recipient who is the central focus of dental hygiene care.

This chapter presents the emerging profession of dental hygiene; an overview of dental hygiene theories; an introduction to dental hygiene's paradigm and to a conceptual model for dental hygiene practice, education, and research; and a summary of educational and career opportunities for dental hygienists to create a picture of the profession as a whole.

HISTORY OF DENTAL HYGIENE

Nineteenth Century to the Twentieth Century[1]

In *A Practical Guide to the Management of the Teeth* published in 1819, Levi Spear Parmly emphasized the importance of daily preventive oral health behavior (toothbrushing, flossing, and use of a dentifrice) to preserve the teeth and gingiva from oral disease. At that time, some dentists were beginning to recognize the value of preventive therapies for the public. In 1845, the editors of the *American Journal of Dental Science* published an editorial criticizing dentistry's neglect of preventive oral healthcare and its focus on mechanical dentistry and surgery. By the twentieth century, more dentists wanted to provide preventive oral healthcare to patients but had time to perform only the dental procedures for which they were trained.

Dr. Alfred C. Fones, a leader in the oral hygiene movement, recognized that teaching children appropriate oral health behaviors was an element critical to the prevention of dental disease over the lifespan. Fones developed a plan to operationalize this concept in the Bridgeport, Connecticut, public schools by preparing women to implement the program.[2] The role of these women in the public schools was to provide children with prophylactic dental care and instruction in toothbrushing, flossing, nutrition, and general hygiene. Dr. Fones' concept of women working as preventive specialists was the root of the evolution of the dental hygiene profession of today. Fones used the term "dental hygienist" rather than the then commonly used phrase "dental nurse" to emphasize the importance of mouth cleanliness as a therapeutic regimen for the prevention and treatment of some oral diseases.[3]

Table 1–1 gives a chronology of some of the key events that shaped the evolution of the emerging profession of dental hygiene. Although the practice of dental hygiene has changed markedly over the century, the changes have been slow and have varied significantly throughout various geographical locations both nationally and internationally. The foundation of dental hygiene practice has been oral health promotion and disease prevention to facilitate consumers' self-care, arrest the disease process, and decrease the incidence of oral disease. These key elements have led dental hygienists to be recognized today as the preventive oral health specialists in the Western healthcare system.

CONTEMPORARY DENTAL HYGIENE

What Is Dental Hygiene?

Dental hygiene, like other sciences, is a synthesis of facts, ideas, concepts, and philosophies—a unique entity. It is not merely a summation of principles and theories from other fields dealing with different phenomena and rooted in different paradigms.

> Dental hygiene is the study of preventive oral healthcare and the management of behaviors required to prevent oral disease and promote health. The central concepts in dental hygiene include the client, the environment, health/oral health, dental hygiene actions, their relationship and the factors that affect them.[5]

> Dental hygiene involves assessment, diagnosis, planning of interventions, and evaluation, through oral disease prevention, treatment, oral health promotion, and collaboration.[6]

Preventive oral healthcare includes:

- Preventive oral health services delivered by dental health professionals
- Preventive oral health practices performed by the client
- Removal of barriers for access to preventive oral health services
- Promotion of client compliance with professional recommendations for oral healthcare
- Provision of oral health educational outreach to special populations
- Therapeutic oral hygiene interventions to prevent further gingival disease[5]

TABLE 1–1
HISTORICAL POINTS OF INTEREST IN THE EVOLUTION OF DENTAL HYGIENE

Date	Event
1819	Dr. Levi Spear Parmly recommended to the American Society of Dental Surgeons a daily oral hygiene regimen to promote among patients
1843	Beginning of the oral hygiene movement
1870	Professor Andrew McLain of the New Orleans Dental College published "Prophylaxis, or Prevention of Dental Decay," in which he advanced the concept of oral cleanliness, preventive measures, and diet. He was also the first to use the term "prophylaxis"
1871	Dental hygiene was advocated as a part of the practice of dentistry by Dr. A. Arthur of Baltimore, Maryland
1888	Southern Dental Association resolved that a person should be employed to visit public and private schools to instruct children in the proper care of the teeth
1898	Dr. M. L. Rhein employed a young woman whom he called a dental nurse to perform prophylactic and educational services in his office
1902	Dr. Cyrus Mansfield Wright of Cincinnati, Ohio, was probably the first to suggest that women be trained to clean teeth and that their profession be considered a subspecialty of dentistry; advocated 1 year of college study
1902	F. W. Low advocated a new profession of women who would go from house to house to clean and polish teeth; he called the profession odonticure
1903	Dr. Thaddeus P. Hyatt of New York City promoted the value of educating the public concerning mouth hygiene among his colleagues and encouraged the acceptance of the dental hygienist; known as the "father of preventive dentistry"
1903	M. L. Rhein proposed the education and legalization of dental nurses to the American Medical Association; he also suggested the institution of a state board examination and a scope of practice
1905	Dr. W. George Ebersole, founder of the Mouth Hygiene Association, began using a dental nurse in his office to perform prophylactic and educational services
1906	Dr. Alfred C. Fones trained his assistant, Mrs. Irene Newman, to provide prophylactic procedures in his practice; acknowledged that training would eventually occur in colleges; considered the founder of dental hygiene
1907	The first dental law to allow prophylactic treatment by a specially trained person, other than a dentist, was accepted in the state of Connecticut. With this law, it became illegal for Connecticut dentists to employ unlicensed assistants to perform prophylactic procedures in their offices
1910	The Ohio College of Dental Surgery began offering a course for dental nurses. The program was discontinued in 1914 because of the strong opposition by Ohio dentists
1913	Dymple B. Johnson of Fort Smith, Arkansas, claimed that she had been performing prophylactic procedures in a dental office since 1893; she advocated a course of study in a "School for Dental Nurses" with specific entrance requirements (e.g., 20 years of age, perfect health, high school diploma, and income sufficient to allow for 2 years of study)
1913	The term "dental hygienist" was coined
1913	Dr. Alfred C. Fones started the first courses for dental hygienists at his carriage house in Bridgeport, Connecticut
1914	Dr. H. S. Seip, president of the Pennsylvania Dental Association, advocated licensing of the dental nurse
1914	Twenty-seven women became the first graduates of Dr. Fones' program
1914	Fones' 5-year Bridgeport demonstration project in the public schools was initiated to have dental hygienists provide prophylactic treatment, classroom talks and lectures, and education for parents; the project proved the success of the dental hygienist in education and dental disease prevention
1914	Colorado College of Dental Surgery initiated a dental nurse program; this became a dental hygiene program in 1920
1915	Connecticut and Massachusetts dental laws outlined the scope of dental hygiene practice
1916	Rochester Dental Dispensary initiated a dental hygiene education program
1916	Forsyth Dental Infirmary initiated a dental hygiene education program
1916	New York State enacted legislation defining dental hygiene practice
1916	Columbia University became the first school of dental hygiene to develop specific educational requirements
1917	Emma Crabbe was employed by Yale and Towen Company of Stamford, Connecticut, to provide prophylactic treatment to the employees
1917	First dental hygiene license issued to Irene Newman in Connecticut
1918	University of California Dental School in San Francisco started a 1-year education program for dental hygienists; this was expanded to a 2-year program in 1924
1919	The University of Minnesota instituted the first 2-year education program in dental hygiene
1920–1925	Dental hygiene education programs started at the University of Michigan, Temple University, University of Pennsylvania, Northwestern University, and Marquette University
1922	American Dental Association adopted a model dental hygiene practice act to be used by the states
1923	First meeting of the American Dental Hygienists' Association held in Cleveland, Ohio; Winifred A. Hart elected as its first president
1925	American Dental Hygienists' Association adopted a Constitution and By-laws
1926	American Dental Hygienists' Association drafted the Code of Ethics; this was adopted in 1929 and revised in 1953, 1969, 1974, and 1994
1927	American Dental Hygienists' Association inaugurated the *Journal of the American Dental Hygienists' Association;* the name was changed to *Dental Hygiene* in 1972 and to *Journal of Dental Hygiene* in 1988
1931	Sixteen dental hygiene education programs were in existence
1932	American Dental Association established the Committee on Dental Hygiene to collect data on dental hygiene education and practice
1932	National Dental Hygienists' Association established by African-American dental hygienists
1937	American Dental Association established the Council on Dental Education to oversee education programs in dentistry and dental hygiene
1939	University of Michigan offered a baccalaureate degree program in dental hygiene
1940	American Dental Hygienists' Association recommended that dental hygiene education programs be 2 years in length

Table continued on following page

TABLE 1–1
HISTORICAL POINTS OF INTEREST IN THE EVOLUTION OF DENTAL HYGIENE *Continued*

Date	Event
1946–1953	United States Public Health Service initiated research studies to measure the effectiveness of the expanded use of dental assistants and dental hygienists; Forsyth Dental Clinic initiated a research project to evaluate the feasibility of dental hygienists restoring primary teeth
1947	American Dental Association Council on Dental Education required that all dental hygiene programs be *at least* 2 years in length and proposed curriculum standard
1947	Francis Stolle, in a paper presented at the third Congress of Dental Education and Licensure in Chicago, stated that dental hygiene education should be a university discipline with full credit toward a BS or BA degree
1950	Full-time dental hygienist hired by the Canadian Department of National Health and Welfare in Ottawa
1950	Establishment of an accreditation committee on dental hygiene education by the Canadian Dental Association
1951	American Dental Association Council on Dental Education recommended that dental hygienists receive expanded training ("expanded duties"); it also began accrediting dental hygiene education programs
1951	University of Toronto established the first dental hygiene education program in Canada
1954	By this time, dental hygiene licensure was available in all 50 states, the District of Columbia, and Puerto Rico
1958	The National Honor Society of Dental Hygiene, Sigma Phi Alpha, was established
1960–1965	Graduate education leading to the master's degree initiated at Columbia University, the University of Iowa, and the University of Michigan
1962	National Dental Hygiene Board Examination was developed and immediately recognized by 25 states
1963	University of Manitoba established the School of Dental Hygiene
1963	Vocational Education Act of 1963 contributed to the growth of dental hygiene programs in technical schools and community colleges
1965	15,400 dental hygienists employed in the United States
1965	Dental Hygiene Educators Conference held to establish student competencies, define responsibilities of dental hygienists, and develop an educator's network
1966	Allied Health Professions Personnel Training Act provided capitation grants to dental hygiene programs
1967	National Advisory Commission on Health Manpower identified need for additional allied health professionals
1967	American Dental Hygienists' Association studied the need for associate, baccalaureate, and master's degree dental hygiene programs
1968	Health Manpower Act provided funds for the education of health professionals
1968	National Institutes of Health, Research Training Grants provided funds to dental and dental hygiene faculty for research, teaching, and other related activities
1968	Administration of the first Northeast Regional Board Examination
1968	Canadian Department of National Health and Welfare convened the Ad Hoc Committee on Dental Auxiliaries; the report of this committee was significant in developing expanded services for dental hygienists in Canada
1968	University of British Columbia established the Program of Dental Hygiene; terminated the program in 1986; established baccalaureate degree completion program in 1992
1970	First International Symposium on Dental Hygiene, sponsored by the American Dental Hygienists' Association, held in Italy
1970	*Curriculum Essentials* document published by the American Dental Hygienists' Association
1970	Commissioning of baccalaureate-trained dental hygienists as officers in the United States Army
1970	Training in Expanded Auxiliary Management (TEAM) projects funded to study the feasibility of teaching registered dental hygienists to perform expanded services under dentist supervision
1970	International Liaison Committee on Dental Hygiene was founded and included representatives of national dental hygiene associations from the seven countries of Canada, Japan, the Netherlands, Norway, Sweden, the United Kingdom, and the United States
1970	Studies conducted at Forsyth Dental Clinic, the University of Pennsylvania, the University of Iowa, and Howard University reported that graduate dental hygienists could be trained to successfully perform expanded services; several projects were stopped because of local dentist opposition
1971	University of Montreal established the baccalaureate degree program in dental hygiene
1971	Second International Symposium on Dental Hygiene held in Switzerland
1971	Dental hygienists became involved in Dental Auxiliary Utilization (DAU) Demonstration Projects in North Carolina, Iowa, Alabama, Kentucky, Florida, Maryland, Missouri, and Ohio
1972	Third International Symposium held in the United Kingdom
1972	Dental hygiene education programs established at six colleges d'Enseignement general et professional in Quebec; another established at CEGEP John Abbot in 1973
1973	Fourth International Symposium on Dental Hygiene held in the Netherlands
1974	Canadian Dental Association sponsored the Conference on Dental Auxiliaries held at Banff, Alberta; issues discussed included the role of auxiliaries, implications for dentistry, guidelines for implementing change, and problems experienced by dental hygienists and dental assistants (e.g., lack of career mobility, levels of supervision, mechanisms for quality assurance, need for representation on policy-making bodies and continuing education)
1975	The Professional Corporation of Dental Hygienists of Quebec, with the endorsement of the Quebec government, transformed dental hygiene into an autonomous, self-regulating profession
1975	Fifth International Symposium on Dental Hygiene held in Japan
1976	*Educational Directions* became the second official publication of the American Dental Hygienists' Association
1976	Linda Krol, in California, became the first dental hygienist to own and manage a dental hygiene practice
1977	Sixth International Symposium on Dental Hygiene held in Sweden
1977	University of Toronto established a baccalaureate degree completion program in dental hygiene
1978	Hygienists Political Action Committee established
1979	Two decades of rapid expansion resulted in 201 dental hygiene programs in the United States
1979	University of Montreal established a baccalaureate degree completion program
1979	73,500 licensed dental hygienists in the United States

TABLE 1–1
HISTORICAL POINTS OF INTEREST IN THE EVOLUTION OF DENTAL HYGIENE *Continued*

Date	Event
1980	Canadian Dental Hygienists' Association presented 14 recommendations to the commission on the review of health services in Canada; recommendations addressed research in dental care delivery, the regulation and supervision of dental hygienists, the need for practice standards and quality assurance mechanisms, improvements in dental hygiene education and accreditation, and a larger role for dental hygienists
1980	By this time, 33 states had dental hygiene representation on boards of dental examiners
1980	Eleven states required mandatory continuing education for dental hygiene licensure
1980	Federal Trade Commission proposed that state restrictions requiring dentist supervision of dental hygienists be nullified
1980	American Dental Hygienists' Association adopted policy that a dental hygienist may own a dental hygiene practice
1981	American Dental Hygienists' Association membership exceeded 22,000
1981	*RDH* magazine established to address diverse issues that affect dental hygienists
1981	Eighth International Symposium on Dental Hygiene held in the United Kingdom
1982	First Conference on Dental Hygiene Research, sponsored by the Working Group on the Practice of Dental Hygiene's Subcommittee on Research and the University of Manitoba, held in Winnipeg, Manitoba
1982	Federal Trade Commission's authority over state-regulated health professions was challenged by the American Medical Association and American Dental Association; Congress reaffirmed the Federal Trade Commission's authority over the health professions in 1984
1983	The State of Washington established, via legislation, a Dental Hygiene Examining Committee to license dental hygienists, and a Dental Hygiene Practice Act to govern the practice of dental hygiene
1983	Ninth International Symposium on Dental Hygiene held in the United States (Philadelphia)
1984	Legislation permitting unsupervised dental hygiene practice in nursing homes, hospitals, institutional settings, and public health facilities was passed in the State of Washington
1985	American Dental Hygienists' Association published *Standards of Applied Dental Hygiene Practice*
1986	American Dental Hygienists' Association adopted policy supporting the baccalaureate degree as the minimum entry-level credential for practice
1986	Legislation was passed in Colorado permitting unsupervised dental hygiene practice (independent dental hygiene practice) in all settings; this excluded root planing and radiographic services
1986	Health Manpower Pilot Project (HMPP #139), sponsored by the University of California at Northridge and accepted by California Office of Statewide Health Planning and Development, was designed to study safety and access to dental hygiene care in unsupervised settings; California Dental Association attempted to stop the project with lawsuits
1986	International Dental Hygienists' Federation was founded during the Tenth International Symposium on Dental Hygiene in Oslo, Norway; founding countries of Canada, Japan, Norway, the Netherlands, Sweden, the United Kingdom, and the United States were joined by Australia, Denmark, and Switzerland
1986	Colleges d'Enseignement general et professionnel's (CEGEP) in Hull and Chicoutimi, Quebec, established dental hygiene programs
1987	American Dental Hygienists' Association published *ACCESS* as its monthly news magazine
1987	Ontario dental hygienists were granted self-governing status
1988	American Dental Hygienists' Association published *Prospectus on Dental Hygiene* to project a future course for the profession
1988	The Canadian Working Group on the Practice of Dental Hygiene published *Clinical Standards for Dental Hygienists in Canada*
1989	Eleventh International Symposium on Dental Hygiene held in Ottawa, Ontario
1990	Controversy between organized dentistry and organized dental hygiene regarding whether a dental hygiene manpower shortage exists
1990	State dental associations in Georgia, Montana, Pennsylvania, South Carolina, South Dakota, Tennessee, and Virginia considered preceptorship as a dental hygiene training option
1990	The Academy of General Dentistry's legislature rescinded its existing policy on formal accredited education as the only route for training dental hygienists
1991	The American Dental Hygienists' Association engaged in strategic planning aimed at the goal of professionalization of dental hygiene
1991	Legislatures of Ontario passed the Regulated Health Professions Act. This legislation established the College of Dental Hygienists of Ontario, the regulatory body for the provinces' dental hygienists. (Dental hygienists in the three Canadian provinces of Quebec, Alberta, and Ontario are now self-governing)
1992	Twelfth International Symposium on Dental Hygiene held in The Hague, the Netherlands
1992	The American Dental Hygienists' Association House of Delegates adopted a definition and theoretical paradigm for the professional discipline of dental hygiene
1993	The American Dental Hygienists' Association adopted framework for a new code of ethics

Adapted from Motley, W. History of the American Dental Hygienists' Association, 1923–1982. Chicago, IL: American Dental Hygienists' Association, 1986.

Thus, the study and management of the preventive oral health behaviors in which human beings engage are key features of dental hygiene and delineate its knowledge base from that of all other disciplines.

Dental hygienists use four main processes—the dental hygiene process, the communication process, the leadership process, and the research process—as a means of oral health promotion and oral disease prevention. Furthermore, dental hygienists carry out these processes as they function in the roles of clinician, manager, change agent, consumer advocate, educator, and researcher. A model of the roles and processes used by the dental hygienist is displayed in Figure 1–1.

History suggests that the dental hygienist's primary con-

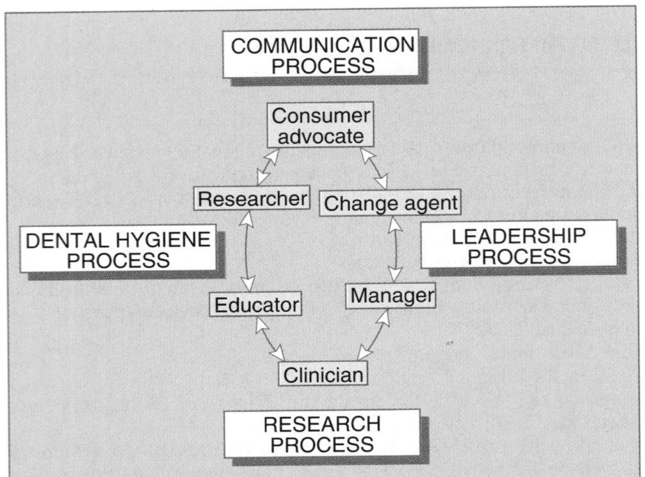

FIGURE 1-1
Model of the roles and processes used by the professional dental hygienist. (Courtesy of L. McDonald.)

cern has been for the whole person who either has oral disease or may develop it, rather than for the oral disease itself, and for the role of the environment and person in fostering or preventing oral disease. It is this emphasis on the individual's adjustments and adaptations to the environment, to personalized care, and to focus on client lifestyle and behavior patterns related to oral health that is unique to dental hygiene. It is the dental hygienist who primarily views the client as being actively involved in the process of care because it is ultimately the client who must use self-care to obtain and maintain oral wellness. Dental hygienists encourage clients to participate in and make choices about their oral healthcare rather than being passive subjects.[7] The profession of dental hygiene, since its inception, has emphasized client education, the prevention of oral disease, and the role of the client in controlling factors that cause disease.

Definitions and Conceptualizations of Dental Hygiene

Historically, the most widely held definition of a dental hygienist is by Wilkins, who states that "[t]he registered dental hygienist is a licensed, professional, oral health educator and clinician who, as a co-therapist with the dentist, uses preventive, educational, and therapeutic methods for the control of oral diseases to aid individuals and groups in attaining and maintaining optimum oral health."[8] The following sections describe, in chronological order, the general focus of several important theorists' conceptualizations of dental hygiene (Table 1-2).

Fones' Concept of Dental Hygiene

Alfred C. Fones, a dentist, opened the first school of dental hygiene in 1913. As the "father of dental hygiene," Fones presented a theory of dental hygiene that emphasized the role of the dental hygienist as a health educator of the public. In 1934, he wrote:

> It is primarily to this important work of public education that the dental hygienist is called. She must regard herself as the channel through which dentistry's knowledge of mouth hygiene is to be disseminated. The greatest service she can perform is the persistent education of the public in mouth hygiene and the allied branches of general health.[9]

Although Fones emphasized the educational and public health aspects of dental hygiene, he viewed dental hygiene as an appendage of dentistry rather than a separate profession unto itself.

Fones did not like the then commonly used term "dental nurse" because of its association with disease. He used the term "hygienist" to describe "one who is versed in the science of health and prevention of disease."[1,10] Eventually, the term "dental hygienist" took hold. Since that time, dental hygiene has been conceptualized and reconceptualized by a number of individuals from dental hygiene and dentistry.

Concept of the Preventive Dental Auxiliary

Many theorists since Fones have viewed the dental hygienist as an *auxiliary person* who implements treatment plans and carries out isolated duties as directed by the supervising dentist. This theory emphasizes the provision of oral prophylaxis in the dental office (defined as oral hygiene, home care instruction, thorough calculus removal, and coronal polishing), as the primary duty delegated to the dental hygienist by the dentist under the precept of direct supervision. Actual therapeutic aspects of dental hygiene care, such as initial periodontal therapy, evaluation of the effect of therapy on oral health and disease, and decision making, were not stressed.[11]

Under this approach, the focus of assessment is to gather data for the dentist to use in determining the dental diagnosis and treatment plan, part of which will be implemented by the auxiliary person. This occupational model, however, conveys the idea that the dental hygienist, as an auxiliary person, is responsible for the less complex, easier, and less valued aspects of oral healthcare, leaving the dentist time for the services perceived as being more complex. Under this concept, the dental hygienist is accountable to the supervising dentist, who is then accountable to the client. Table 1-3 compares some of the basic propositions from this occupational conceptualization of dental hygiene with those of a professional conceptualization of dental hygiene. This occupational model fails to recognize dental hygiene as an emerging profession. It perpetuates the attitude that dental hygiene is an auxiliary of dentistry.[12]

Periodontal Co-therapist Concept

Theories on periodontal co-therapy describe dental hygiene care as therapeutic and the dental hygienist as a periodontal co-therapist with the dentist.* The periodontal co-therapy theory describes a major role for the dental hygienist in assessment and evaluation of periodontal conditions and in the differentiation between periodontally healthy clients who require preventive or maintenance care and clients with periodontal disease who require special consideration for diagnosis and care planning by the general dentist or specialist. Dental hygiene periodontal co-therapists provide

* The periodontium is the supporting tissue of the teeth, such as the gum (gingiva) and the underlying bone.

TABLE 1–2
SUMMARY OF SELECTED CONCEPTUALIZATIONS OF DENTAL HYGIENE

Theorist	Goal of Dental Hygiene	Emphasis
Fones, 1934	To channel dentistry's knowledge of mouth hygiene to the public	The dental hygienist promotes oral disease prevention in children, within public health and school settings. Emphasizes the role of the dental hygienist as a public health educator
Wilkins and McCullough, 1959, 1964	To aid individuals and groups in attaining and maintaining optimum oral health	The clinical practice of the dental hygienist integrates specific care and instructional services as required by the individual patient. Emphasizes role of the dental hygienist as an auxiliary to the dentist
Woodall, 1980, 1985, 1989, 1993	To involve the client as a partner in care as a necessary condition for restoring and maintaining the client's oral health	Philosophy of client-centered care with client as a decision maker. Emphasizes the problem-solving and decision-making roles of the dental hygienist
Darby, 1983	To promote and maintain the client's oral health via collaboration between dental hygienists and dentists as directed by the oral health needs of the client	Collaborative practice model. Emphasizes the distinctiveness of the roles of dental hygienist and dentist and their ability to enter into a collegial relationship as healthcare providers
Walsh and Robertson, 1985	To promote and maintain oral health and to control oral disease through three distinct professional, mechanical oral hygiene interventions	Disregards the concept of the dental hygienist's carrying out the routine oral prophylaxis and substitutes the concept of multiple categories of dental hygiene care: preventive oral prophylaxis, therapeutic scaling and root planing, and periodontal maintenance care
Wilkins, 1989	To aid individuals and groups in attaining and maintaining optimal oral health, with the hygienist as a co-therapist with dentist	Emphasizes the preventive, educational, and therapeutic role of the dental hygienist as both an auxiliary and co-therapist with the dentist
Darby, 1990	To facilitate the client's attainment of total self-care	Client demonstrates a self-care deficit. Dental hygiene care is necessary when the client is unable to fulfill self-care needs because of developmental, social, psychological, financial, physical, or mental reasons
Darby and Walsh, 1991	To assist individuals in meeting their human needs through the use of interventions aimed at meeting deficits in the performance of those oral health behaviors and practices that will lead to optimal oral wellness over the lifespan	Human needs theory suggested as a conceptual framework for the dental hygiene process. Requires dental hygienists to be aware of basic human needs and identifies 11 human needs related to dental hygiene care; encourages dental hygiene diagnoses based upon deficits in these 11 human needs related to dental hygiene care; and aims dental hygiene interventions at eliminating these deficits

initial periodontal therapy consisting of bacterial plaque control instruction, soft tissue management, subgingival scaling and root planing, and follow-up supervision and documentation of the client's periodontal condition at continuous care appointments. When indicated, use of local anesthetics, nitrous oxide and oxygen analgesia for pain control, and subgingival irrigation and microbiological assessment of plaque also are provided. Unlike the hygienist confined to a traditional role—that of solely cleaning the teeth—the periodontal co-therapist prevents, treats, and monitors disease. Assessing signs of health and disease, and providing therapeutic as well as preventive care, distinguish this theory from those already presented.[8,13–15]

Collaborative Practice Model

Collaboration is the process of working together for the achievement of common goals. The collaborative practice model assumes that the provision of oral healthcare is a complex process that requires a full spectrum of professional knowledge, skills, and judgments; therefore, collaboration between dentists and dental hygienists, working together as colleagues, has the potential for offering quality, comprehensive oral healthcare to the public.[16] Darby defines **collaborative practice** as "dental hygienists and dentists cooperating as colleagues to integrate their respective care regimens into a single comprehensive approach to

TABLE 1–3
SAMPLE PROPOSITIONS FROM TWO CONCEPTUAL MODELS OF DENTAL HYGIENE

Occupational	Professional
Hygienist implements preventive treatment plans developed by dentist	Hygienist implements self-generated preventive care regimens
Secondary care providers	Primary care providers
Hygienist carries out isolated duties as indicated by supervising dentist	Hygienist uses process of care to assess needs, plan and implement care, and evaluate client
Hygienist is an auxiliary of dentistry	Hygienist is a professional who collaborates with dentist and other health professionals
Hygienist is responsible for less complex, easier oral healthcare services	Hygienist is responsible for services that include some of the more difficult techniques to master in oral healthcare
Hygiene care involves an oral prophylaxis every 6 months at a 30–45-min appointment	Hygiene care involves multiple interventions that may require multiple appointments and appointment lengths
Hygienist is responsible for less valued services, leaving dentist time for important services	Hygienist is responsible for preventive and oral maintenance care, which is highly valued by today's wellness-oriented consumer
Unsupervised dental hygiene practice reduces the quality of oral healthcare and increases client risks	Unsupervised dental hygiene practice increases public access to oral hygiene care and lowers healthcare costs
Dentistry is responsible for making decisions about dental hygienists	Dental hygiene is responsible for making decisions about dental hygienists
Dental hygienists are accountable to the dentist	Dental hygienists are accountable to the client (consumer)
Client is passive because the dentist is responsible for the client's oral health	Client is active because clients are responsible for their own oral health
Hygienist fulfills role through the function of a clinician	Hygienist fulfills role through functions of clinician, educator/health promoter, manager, change agent, consumer advocate, and researcher
Dental hygiene is technically based	Dental hygiene is knowledge-based

quality client care. Although both professions can and should work together to improve the dental health status of the public, each has a specific role that complements and augments the effectiveness of the other."[16] Darby's collaborative practice model emphasizes the distinctiveness of the roles of dental hygienist and dentist and their ability to enter into a collegial relationship as healthcare providers. In the collaborative model, the dentist and the dental hygienist are in a co-therapist relationship, and both are offering their professional expertise for the goal of optimal oral health for the client.

The collaboration between dentists and dental hygienists, as directed by the oral health needs of the individual, establishes the common basis for providing client-centered healthcare, without requiring either profession to give up its identity or autonomy. In a collaborative practice, dental hygienists are viewed as experts in their field, are consulted about appropriate dental hygiene interventions, are expected to make clinical dental hygiene decisions, and are given freedom in planning, implementing, and evaluating the dental hygiene component of the overall care plan. Other advantages of collaborative practice relate to the provision of recognition and respect for the expertise of all members of the healthcare team and the latitude for the dental hygienist to work in a variety of practice settings under established legal guidelines or protocols.

Roles of Dental Hygienists

In 1984 the American Dental Hygienists' Association sponsored a conference to articulate the evolving functional roles of dental hygienists in dental hygiene. Outcomes of that conference offered a more comprehensive view of the dental hygienist as a licensed, professional member of the healthcare team who serves as an oral health educator, consumer advocate, manager, clinician, change agent, and researcher (see Table 1–4). These roles are discussed in greater detail later in this chapter (see the section on roles and functions of the professional dental hygienist).

Theory on Levels of Dental Hygiene Care

This theory eliminates the single concept of a professional "tooth cleaning" as being the realm of professional mechanical oral hygiene care provided by the dental hygienist, and substitutes the concept of multiple categories of care that the dental hygienist may provide, depending on the client's level of periodontal health. According to this theory, professionally administered mechanical oral hygiene procedures performed by a dental hygienist are categorized into several levels of care described by Walsh and Robertson: preventive oral prophylaxis, therapeutic periodontal scaling and root planing, and periodontal maintenance care.[17] Although these three professional levels of care share a number of features, particularly instrumentation of the tooth surface and establishment of an effective personal oral hygiene program, the objective, rationale, and skill level required of the dental hygienist for each category of care are different. Like Darby's collaborative practice theory, this theory on levels of care views the provision of dental hygiene care as a complex process that requires a full spectrum of professional knowledge, skills, and judgments.

A Conceptual Model for Dental Hygiene

A **conceptual model** is defined as a set of concepts, and propositions that describe them, that are organized into a meaningful configuration of the domain of dental hygiene. Conceptual models are important for dental hygiene because they provide philosophical and practical perspectives on the care dental hygienists deliver.

As exemplified in the previous section on definitions and conceptualizations of dental hygiene, conceptual models explain dental hygiene from different perspectives. For example, one model might explain dental hygiene as a public health–oriented practice, another as an auxiliary occupation, still another as a co-therapeutic or collaborative profession, or another as an independent profession. One model builder may use terms such as "auxiliary," "dependence," "supervision," "dental care," and "duties," whereas another may stress professionalism, autonomy, and process of care. Terms, propositions, and belief systems are defined according to the focus of the particular model. The same terms may have different meanings in alternative conceptual models.

Dental Hygiene's Paradigm

A **paradigm** is a widely accepted worldview of a discipline that shapes the direction and methods of its practitioners, educators, administrators, and researchers.[18] A discipline's paradigm comprises major concepts selected for study by the discipline and statements about the concepts that identify its relevant phenomena in a global manner. A paradigm specifies the unique perspective of each discipline and is the first level of distinction between disciplines.[19–21] In a discipline, "the structural hierarchy of knowledge progresses from a single paradigm to multiple conceptual models and multiple theories derived from each model."[19]

The paradigm for the discipline of dental hygiene, as defined by the American Dental Hygienists' Association,[5] consists of the following four major concepts (Fig. 1–2):

Client: The potential or actual recipient of dental hygiene care; includes persons, families, groups, and communities of all ages, genders, and sociocultural and economic states.

Environment: Factors other than dental hygiene actions that affect the client's attainment of optimal oral health. These include economic, psychological, cultural, physical, legal, educational, ethical, and geographical factors.

Health and oral health: The client's state of being that exists on a continuum from optimal wellness to illness and fluctuates over time as the result of biological, psychological, spiritual, and development factors. Oral health and overall health are interrelated because each impacts the other.

Dental hygiene actions: Interventions that a dental hygienist can initiate to promote oral wellness and to prevent or control oral disease. These actions involve cognitive, affective, and psychomotor performances and may be provided in independent, interdependent, and collaborative relationships with the client and the healthcare team.

It is these four concepts that identify the phenomena central to the discipline of dental hygiene in an abstract global manner. These four paradigm concepts can be defined, developed, and expanded in numerous ways for conceptual models of dental hygiene to evolve.

In this book, the four paradigm concepts are expanded and used as the basis for the human needs conceptual model of dental hygiene. Briefly, within the human needs conceptual model of dental hygiene, basic human needs theory is used to explain the four major paradigm concepts and provide the theoretical framework for the dental hygiene process. This relationship of human needs theory to the dental hygiene process is detailed in Chapter 2. This conceptualization of dental hygiene draws heavily from the work of Yura and Walsh.[23]

EDUCATIONAL PREPARATION FOR THE PROFESSION OF DENTAL HYGIENE

Historically, dental hygiene education in the United States and Canada has involved multiple methods. The existence of a multiple-method educational system, failure to standardize entry-level education, and lack of specificity in defining roles of graduates from various educational levels have had a negative impact on the growth and credibility of the dental hygiene profession.

Behavioral and role expectations exist among individuals holding the associate, baccalaureate, master's, and doctoral degrees in other disciplines, and this holds true for dental hygiene. In 1992, outcomes for various types of degree programs in dental hygiene were formulated by the Task Force on Dental Hygiene Education of the American Association of Dental Schools, Committee of Dental Hygiene Directors.[24]

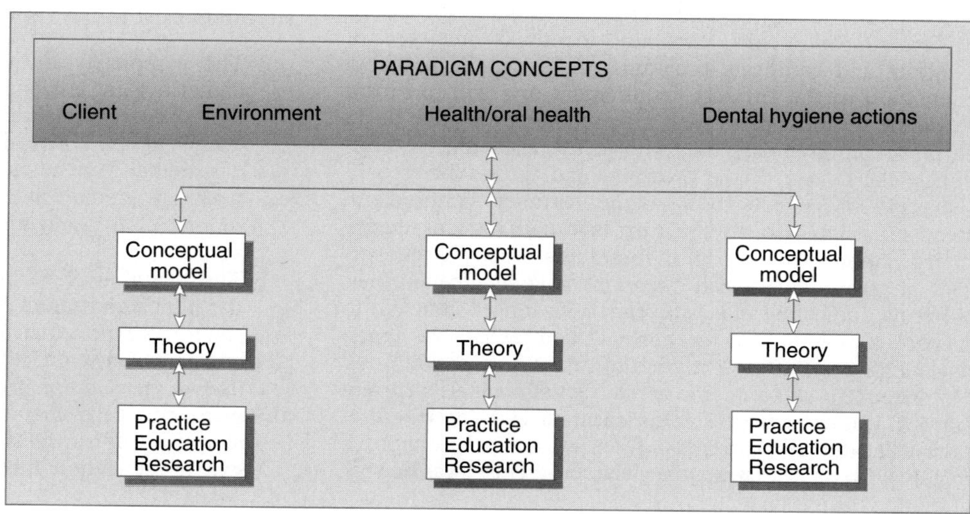

FIGURE 1–2
Dental hygiene theory development framework. (With permission from American Dental Hygienists Association. Proceedings of the 69th Annual Session, House of Delegates, Denver, CO, June 1993.)

This section reviews the various types of educational programs for preparing entry-level dental hygienists in the United States and Canada, as well as for graduate dental hygiene education. The Task Force on Dental Hygiene Education[24] indicated that the dental hygiene educational system is in transition and that in the future it will emphasize greater levels of advanced education. Many dental hygiene educators and practitioners maintain that in the future the **dental hygiene generalist** will be educated at a standard entry level, and **dental hygiene specialization** will occur at the master's and doctoral levels, consistent with educational models used in other disciplines.

Formal Dental Hygiene Education in Institutions of Higher Education

Basic premises exist about the formal educational system of any discipline. First, formal education exists for the purpose of effectively transmitting knowledge to later generations. Second, formal education provides a framework for generating new knowledge about the discipline. Third, formal education increases the likelihood that society's needs will be met by competent, educated individuals. Last, formal education enables society to establish standards, with expectations that standards have been met by those who complete the formal system of education.

The need for and value of formal education as a mechanism to protect society are widely documented in the annals of history of professions, such as medicine, dentistry, nursing, and dental hygiene, that started with the preceptorship model of training but quickly changed to the formal educational system.

Entry-level Dental Hygiene Education

Certificate and Associate Degrees in Dental Hygiene Certificate and associate degree programs in dental hygiene focus on practical courses related to the practice of dental hygiene and include some courses in basic sciences and the humanities. Although the associate degree is traditionally completed in two academic years, this is not the typical case in dental hygiene education. Many dental hygiene associate and certificate level programs have prerequisite and requisite curricula beyond the minimum 2-year time standard for curricular length established when the American Dental Association began accrediting programs in 1952. Despite the existence of accreditation standards, several different associate degree and certificate models for dental hygiene education exist. Wayman[25] identified three types of associate and certificate programs: those with high school graduation as the entrance requirement and with no extra academic sessions; those with high school completion as an entrance requirement, but with extra academic sessions during the course of the program; and those with 1 or 2 years of college education as the entrance requirement, some of which also require extra summer sessions during matriculation. Wayman also found that "sixty-seven percent of associate/certificate programs have lengthened their curricula, indicating that two years is no longer sufficient to prepare a practitioner for current, comprehensive dental hygiene practice under a myriad of supervisory conditions." Unfortunately, the outcome is that dental hygienists are not earning academic degrees commensurate with the length of their educational programs. Mescher found that approximately 70% of the dental hygiene programs awarding an associate degree require prerequisite and requisite courses equal to 2½ years or more of postsecondary education.[26] Of that 70%, one-third of these associate degree programs require more than 3 years for completion. Therefore, approximately 70% of the dental hygiene programs have found that 2 academic years' time is inadequate to prepare dental hygienists for today's healthcare environment.

Dental hygiene education may be beginning to outgrow the associate degree program format. It lies in transition between associate and baccalaureate education. Graduates of accredited programs are eligible to take national, regional, and clinical board examinations for licensure.

Baccalaureate Degree in Dental Hygiene The 1985 House of Delegates of the American Dental Association resolved that

> . . . the American Dental Association supports the education of dental hygienists in two-year training programs and believes that two academic years are adequate to prepare a dental hygienist to perform dental hygiene services.

Less than a year later, the American Dental Hygienists' Association (ADHA) House of Delegates passed a resolution to declare "its intent to establish the baccalaureate degree as the minimal entry level credential for future dental hygiene practice." The promotion of baccalaureate dental hygiene education has been a recurring theme of ADHA-sponsored Dental Hygiene Education and Practice Workshops I, II, and III[27–29] and its landmark publication of *Prospectus for Dental Hygiene.*[30] The *Prospectus* delineates societal trends and future needs and calls for dental hygiene to move from a technically based to a knowledge-based discipline.

According to the literature in higher education, baccalaureate degrees are designed to educate liberally.[31,32] Liberal education produces capable thinkers, communicators, problem solvers, and decision makers—people with a capacity for initiation, reflection, and review that enables them to respond to the changing issues they confront.[32] Liberal education distinctively fosters key competencies such as critical thinking skills, cause-and-effect reasoning, intellectual empathy (seeing all sides of an issue), maturity of social-emotional judgment, adaptation to the environment, and increased respect for diversity.[32] Moreover, liberal education outcomes, more than SAT scores and college honors, predict enhanced self-image and career attainment.[32]

Several different baccalaureate models for dental hygiene education exist in the United States:

- The completely integrated curriculum in which the dental hygiene major is distributed at all four levels of the college experience (e.g., Marquette University and West Virginia University)
- The dental hygiene curricular major built on 1 year of freshman prerequisites and then integrated at the sophomore, junior, and senior levels (e.g., Ohio State University)
- The dental hygiene curricular major concentrated at the junior and senior levels and built on freshman and sophomore prerequisites (e.g., University of Maryland and University of California at San Francisco)
- The degree completion program with the dental hygiene curricular major concentrated at the lower division, with upper division courses in dental hygiene and general education taken to complete the degree (e.g.,

Old Dominion University, and University of Minnesota)

Baccalaureate study includes theory and research as a basis for all functional roles and emphasizes the use of processes and theoretical frameworks. With this broad, generalist perspective provided by a baccalaureate degree, the dental hygiene practitioner is in an excellent position to move into entry-level managerial, research, and advocacy roles as well as to adapt to new roles necessitated by an ever-changing environment.

Graduate Education in Dental Hygiene In most disciplines, professional advancements depend on those with the highest academic credentials—the **terminal degree.** The terminal degree is the highest degree attainable within the discipline, and in most disciplines it is the doctoral degree. Although some dental hygienists have earned a doctoral degree, their doctoral major tends to be education, public health, urban services, psychology, economics, or other related areas, because doctoral programs in dental hygiene have yet to be developed. Graduate education prepares individuals to advance knowledge of the discipline and is critical to the profession.

Master's Degree Education in Dental Hygiene Currently, the master of science is the highest degree offered in dental hygiene. Five master's degree programs in dental hygiene exist in the United States (see Master of Science in Dental Hygiene Programs in the United States chart.) There is none in Canada. Most of these programs require approximately 30 to 40 graduate credit hours and may include both thesis and nonthesis course options. Master's degree programs provide a unique educational experience that includes advanced knowledge of the science and practice of dental hygiene based on the rationale that specialization in the discipline is a fundamental attribute of the master's level dental hygienist. Although master's degree programs vary in their course offerings and strengths, most build on the baccalaureate degree to prepare professional dental hygienists with specialized skills for various roles in academic, business, industry, research, and community health settings. Ultimately, master's degree programs prepare graduates to assume leadership roles and promote acquisition of skills in research, critical thinking, problem solving, planning, evaluation, and oral and written communication.[24]

Doctoral Education in Dental Hygiene Although the concept of doctoral education in dental hygiene is just beginning to evolve, its primary purpose will be to prepare individuals of superior ability for leadership roles in expanding the theoretical, scholarly, and scientific dimensions of dental hygiene. Doctoral education would prepare a cadre of scholars to develop and test theory, generate new dental hygiene knowledge, and bring knowledge from other disciplines to expand dental hygiene's body of knowledge. The evolution of dental hygiene education toward doctoral education would provide dental hygiene leaders, researchers, and scholars; strengthen dental hygiene's research and educational capabilities; develop dental hygiene theory; secure for dental hygiene credibility and strength as a valid professional discipline; and create academic legitimacy. The outcome will be the expansion of an organized body of dental hygiene knowledge that serves as the foundation for quality dental hygiene care for society.[24]

MASTER OF SCIENCE IN DENTAL HYGIENE PROGRAMS IN THE UNITED STATES

Graduate Dental Hygiene Education
School of Dentistry
University of Missouri, Kansas City
650 East 25th Street
Kansas City, Missouri 64108–2795

Department of Dental Hygiene
Baltimore College of Dental Surgery
Dental School
University of Maryland at Baltimore
666 West Baltimore Street
Baltimore, Maryland 21201

Department of Dental Hygiene
School of Dentistry
West Virginia University
Health Sciences Center
Morgantown, West Virginia 26506

Curriculum in Dental Hygiene
School of Dentistry
University of Michigan
1011 North University
Ann Arbor, Michigan 48109

School of Dental Hygiene
College of Health Sciences
Old Dominion University
Norfolk, Virginia 23529–0499

PROFESSIONAL REGULATION

In addition to formal education, accreditation, certification, and licensure are the major credentialing processes used to increase the likelihood that dental hygiene practitioners are adequately prepared and qualified to practice. In the United States, dental hygiene education, accreditation, certification (National Board), and licensure are regulated by the dental profession.

Accreditation

Accreditation is the process by which an external agency evaluates an institution or program of study according to predetermined, national standards. Associate degree, diploma, certificate, and baccalaureate degree programs focusing on entry-level dental hygiene education must meet certain national standards to remain accredited. These criteria are established by the American Dental Association, Commission on Dental Accreditation, and, in Canada, by the Canadian Dental Association, Council on Education and Accreditation.

Certification

Certification is the process by which a nongovernment agency or organization grants formal recognition to an individual for such accomplishments as completion of a specified amount of further training or coursework, acceptable performance on an examination or series of examinations, or graduation from a formal program. Granting a certificate is the tangible outcome of the certification process. Dental hygienists in the United States receive a certificate of acceptable performance after passing the National Dental Hygiene Board Examination.

Licensure

Licensure is the process by which a government agency certifies that individuals have met predetermined standards and are minimally qualified and are permitted to practice in its jurisdiction. The purpose of licensure is to ensure that the public health, safety, and welfare are protected from incompetent practitioners.

Dental hygiene licensure in states (except Alabama) and provinces requires that the dental hygienist complete a prescribed course of study in an accredited program. In the United States, registered dental hygienist candidates must pass the National Dental Hygiene Board Examination for Dental Hygiene, which is administered by the American Dental Association, prior to taking a licensure examination. In addition, most states have their own licensing examination and requirements based on unique dental and dental hygiene practice acts. Some states have agreed to accept regional examinations, such as the Northeast Regional Board Examination for Dental Hygiene, which is recognized for licensure by 14 states. In Canada, there is no national board examination. Instead of a standardized national, written examination, each provincial government establishes its own requirements for licensure and relicensure. Requirements for licensure vary from province to province and according to whether the individual graduated from an accredited or a nonaccredited program. Notably, in the Canadian provinces of Quebec, Alberta, and Ontario, dental hygienists regulate the dental hygiene licensing system. This means that in Canada the profession of dental hygiene regulates the practice of 75% of the dental hygienists.[34]

Reciprocity (or portability) is the act by which one licensing jurisdiction recognizes and accepts the license obtained from another jurisdiction. Reciprocity continues to be an issue for both Canadian and United States dental hygienists.

Continuing Education

Changes are occurring continually in the sciences, in technology, and in dental hygiene. Accreditation, certification, and licensure, although valuable, do not prevent educational obsolescence. After several years in practice, minimal standards of safety may no longer be met by some practitioners. **Continuing education** (CE) is the term used to describe the educational or informational renewal that takes place after the degree-earning education has been completed. Continuing education programs have been developed to help dental hygienists remain current in skills, knowledge, and theory related to their roles as clinician, educator, researcher, manager, change agent, and consumer advocate.

Continuing education involves formal, organized short-term educational programs offered by educational and healthcare institutions as well as private companies. During the 1970s, the ADHA discarded its role as the one national accreditation body for CE programs for dental hygienists.

Today, the state boards of dentistry and universities serve as accrediting agencies for CE programs. The ADHA also awards continuing education units on completion of specific courses. Continuing education may be mandatory for dental hygiene licensure (i.e., most licensing jurisdictions require dental hygienists to take specific types of CE courses and earn CE units for license renewal).

ROLES AND FUNCTIONS OF THE PROFESSIONAL DENTAL HYGIENIST

Contemporary dental hygiene practice requires that dental hygienists possess a breadth of knowledge and skills in a variety of areas. In the past, the principal services of dental hygienists were oral health education and professional removal of calculus, bacterial plaque, and other exogenous accretions from the tooth surface. Changes in healthcare knowledge and practice have expanded the philosophy of dental hygiene to include interrelated roles of clinician, educator/oral health promoter, administrator/manager, change agent, consumer advocate, and researcher for the dental hygienist.[27,28] These roles possess a common denominator of improved oral health for society. The profession now recognizes that these six roles articulate to create the model for the professional dental hygienist (see Fig. 1–1). The dental hygienist is most effective when skilled in all six roles and applying these skills in the workplace. Table 1–4 outlines these roles, their characteristics and common responsibilities, and the settings where these roles are most likely to be performed. The reader is challenged to expand the outline further.

Dental Hygiene Clinician

The contemporary role of the **dental hygiene clinician** includes the assessment of signs of health and disease in the oral cavity; identification of the dental hygiene problem (dental hygiene diagnosis); and planning, implementing, and evaluating dental hygiene care. In the prevention and control of periodontal disease, the dental hygienist provides bacterial plaque control instructions and the appropriate nonsurgical treatment via preventive oral prophylaxis, nonsurgical periodontal therapy, or periodontal maintenance care. Moreover, evaluation of care has emerged as both a legal and an ethical responsibility. Although scaling and root planing skills to promote physical healing are important to the dental hygienist in this role, appropriate skills for assessment of human needs and related psychosocial, cultural, and behavioral practices are also necessary to reach diverse clients and achieve adherence to recommended dental hygiene care.

As a clinician, the contemporary dental hygienist helps the client set oral health goals and collaborates with the client to meet those goals with a minimal cost of time and energy. In addition to addressing periodontal health, the clinical role of the dental hygienist also has become more involved with dental caries prevention through increased emphasis on fluoride therapy and dental sealants and on preventive counseling to control dietary sucrose.

To provide effective dental hygiene care, dental hygienists apply decision-making theory throughout the dental hygiene process. Before undertaking any dental hygiene action, whether it is to assess the client, provide care, or evaluate the results of care, the dental hygienist plans the action by deciding the best interventions within the scope of dental hygiene practice, given the client's unique situation. The dental hygienist makes decisions independently or in collaboration with the client and family, the dentist, or other healthcare professionals.

TABLE 1–4

SIX INTERRELATED ROLES OF THE PROFESSIONAL DENTAL HYGIENIST (GENERALIST)

The professional dental hygienist is the point of first contact for many clients; assesses client conditions; identifies disease risk factors, client priorities, and the social, cultural and economic factors which affect the individual; develops modalities to manage oral disease prevention and health maintenance; refers to appropriate healthcare professionals as needed; prioritizes care; implements self-generated preventive care regimens; and is primary preventive therapist. This practitioner must, therefore, be skilled in combining the following six interrelated roles:

Roles/Settings	Responsibilities Include But Are Not Limited To
Administrator/Manager Health promotion programs Disease prevention programs Educational institutions Clinical practices Managed care programs Community health agencies Armed forces Oral healthcare industry	Evaluates and modifies programs of oral health education or oral healthcare Utilizes data collection, persuasion, and protocol skills to justify initiation and development of health promotion or healthcare Organizes services for consumers Communicates objectives of the program to consumers, health professionals, and agency personnel Identifies, gathers, and procures necessary resources for program operation Applies organizational skills in formulating policies and procedures and in carrying out operational aspects of the program Manages human and material resources effectively Evaluates program quality in relation to predetermined goals, perceived needs of the population served, and cost-effectiveness to meet national standards Modifies the program on the basis of evaluation results Delegates some responsibility and supervises other personnel Coordinates activities of others in the healthcare team Provides staff development training
Change Agent Lobbyist for legislative changes in healthcare Hospitals Community health agencies Client care coordinator in healthcare facility Entrepreneur Coordinator of oral healthcare services for persons with disabilities Nursing home services director State dental health program administration Community project coordinator	Implements processes and evaluates the success of programs that promote (change) health for clients Promotes the need for innovation and change in healthcare Uses current knowledge and interpersonal skills Works with individuals, organizations, agencies, and social institutions that have authority for, or influence on, dental hygiene education, health, and practice Creates an atmosphere conducive to the dynamics of change and selects mechanisms that are compatible with the target of change Promotes public's well-being and attainment of dental hygiene's oral health goals for society Uses appropriate areas of influence to promote health for individuals, families, or communities Systematically develops career alternatives and develops roles for hygienists, including these activities to fulfill this responsibility: ■ Analysis of barriers to gaining employment ■ Removing resistance ■ Changing attitudes, beliefs, and values of dental hygienists and potential employers ■ Instructing students in essential knowledge and skills ■ Placing graduates in a variety of career settings ■ Creating change through the legislative process Utilizes the steps in the process of change Influences legislators, health agencies, and other organizations to solve existing health problems
Clinician Managed care programs Hospitals Community health projects Extended care facilities Clinical practice (e.g., private practice, group practice, independent practice, armed forces)	Uses the dental hygiene process of care (assesses, diagnoses, plans, implements and evaluates) to intervene in, and for the prevention, or control of, oral diseases Integrates all other roles to promote wellness, prevent illness, maintain health, and facilitate coping Provides care to clients based on knowledge and skill with consideration for human needs Accepts the consumer as a partner in providing preventive and therapeutic oral healthcare, which includes: Assessing the consumer's oral health status ■ Develops comprehensive oral health profiles based on health histories; clinical examination and the individual's knowledge, attitudinal, and behavioral characteristics that serve as the basis for referral; provision and evaluation of therapeutic and preventive professional services Planning for care and disease prevention, intervention, or control ■ Prioritizes oral health needs of consumers and makes referrals to appropriate treatment centers ■ Performs dental hygiene diagnoses and makes appropriate referrals ■ Determines which treatment needs are within scope of training and abilities, provides care, and assesses client responses and care outcomes Implementing appropriate clinical services ■ Adapts oral health prevention, care, and education programs to the existing knowledge, values, and behaviors of diverse consumers

Table continued on following page

TABLE 1–4
SIX INTERRELATED ROLES OF THE PROFESSIONAL DENTAL HYGIENIST (GENERALIST) *Continued*

Roles/Settings	Responsibilities Include But Are Not Limited To
	■ Designs systems to monitor oral health prevention, care, and education programs to ensure that services are effective ■ Evaluates the effectiveness of the consumer's self-care and dental hygiene care in attaining or maintaining oral health ■ Interprets current theory and research and applies research to oral healthcare ■ Identifies group dynamics and communication patterns and, where necessary, develops behavior intervention strategies to promote effective healthcare delivery Works in collaboration with other healthcare professionals to provide dental hygiene care to a general or specific group of people for the purpose of promoting health and preventing disease Provides care with full knowledge of and adherence to moral, ethical, and legal responsibilities
Client Advocate Public dental programs Consumer groups Dental referral systems Periodontal disease screening centers Individual and group self-care programs Clinical practice settings	Influences legislators, health agencies, and other organizations on existing health problems and available resources to resolve problems Protects human and legal rights based on the belief that clients have the right to make their own decisions about health and life Uses strategies to influence those who control access to oral healthcare (e.g., legislators, health agency personnel, organizations, general public) for the purpose of obtaining health services for individuals and groups Represents individuals or groups in procurement of needed oral health services and assists them in obtaining services Develops networking systems to bring existing health problems and available resources together to resolve problems Monitors the quality of professional services and consumer self-care programs Addresses the growing concern for quality of care while assuring cost containment Advises consumers on the relative worth of payment mechanisms, commercial products, political issues affecting oral health, and criteria for evaluating professional services Uses screening, referral, and persuasive skills to bring people into healthcare delivery systems Applies legal, financial and informational leverage to protect oral healthcare for consumers Assists clients in obtaining the best possible care in the situation with informed consent and knowledge of alternatives Supports clients in the decisions they make (e.g., actively reassures clients that it is their decision and they have a right to make it without giving in to outside pressures)
Educator/Oral Health Promoter Public health programs Public school programs Faculty in dental schools and dental hygiene schools Clinical and managed care programs Staff development in healthcare agencies	Utilizes educational theory and methods to analyze oral health needs Develops oral health promotion strategies Promotes concepts of prevention in community-based programs designed for specific population groups Designs and produces instructional materials and media for the consumer Use communication theory, marketing strategies, and computer skills Conducts research Conducts health promotion (e.g., health screenings, risk appraisal, behavior modification classes, educational programs, and wellness programs) Has a clinical dental hygiene background exhibiting practice skills and theoretical knowledge Applies educational theory and the teaching-learning process (e.g., assessing the health knowledge and oral health status of individuals and groups; planning health education; transmitting current concepts, facts, and theories of health promotion and disease prevention to individuals and groups; and evaluating educational outcomes) Analyzes health needs and behavioral characteristics of specific population groups Marshals political, organizational, and economic support to make health plans and policies operational Develops health promotion strategies and healthcare programs which are attractive and relevant to the social and cultural values of the targeted population and which are based on scientifically accurate information Manages resources and delivers programs that are cost-effective and utilized by the targeted population Works independently or in collaboration with other health professionals to provide health education for the purpose of influencing behavior in a manner that promotes health Evaluates health education and health promotion strategies in healthcare programs through appropriate methods Uses communication and interpersonal skills to meet learning needs of clients Promotes, and recruits for, the profession of dental hygiene

TABLE 1–4
SIX INTERRELATED ROLES OF THE PROFESSIONAL DENTAL HYGIENIST (GENERALIST) *Continued*

Roles/Settings	Responsibilities Include But Are Not Limited To
Researcher	
Research institutions, higher education, oral healthcare industry, clinical practice	Interprets and applies findings and solves problems Develops a knowledge base for dental hygiene to extend the boundaries of the profession's body of knowledge Contributes to creation of new knowledge to benefit society Data collection and evaluation to develop new modalities of service Conducts research for the purpose of improving client care Applies the scientific method in: ■ Selecting therapeutic and preventive modalities and educational concepts and methods ■ Evaluating the effectiveness of selected procedures, materials, and methods ■ Modifying oral healthcare or education on the basis of findings Interprets and evaluates research findings and applies findings to practice Uses principles of problem solving in clinical and nonclinical work efforts Participates in studies to determine the validity of procedures, materials, or education Contributes to the theoretical and scientific knowledge base for dental hygiene practice, through communication of findings

In the United States and Canada, clinical dental hygienists usually provide dental hygiene care in collaboration with a general dentist or a dental specialist in a private dental practice. Other clinical hygienists have chosen to provide dental hygiene care in public health facilities, the armed forces, corporate dental clinics, research institutions, and extended care facilities. Dental hygienists in the state of Colorado can practice autonomously as independent dental hygiene practitioners. Currently, only the state of Colorado legally permits independent practice for dental hygienists in the United States.

Dental Hygiene Educator/Oral Health Promoter

Trends in society have underscored the importance of the role of the **dental hygiene educator** and **oral health promoter.** Trends toward consumerism, self-care, disease prevention, and healthy lifestyles mean that clients want and need extensive information on oral health and disease. Dental hygienists assume the role of educator when clients have learning needs.

In the teacher-client relationship, the dental hygienist explains concepts and facts concerning oral health and disease, demonstrates self-care procedures, determines client understanding, reinforces learning or desired behavior, evaluates the client's progress in learning, and so on. All these actions within the scope of dental hygiene practice, in addition to the direct presentation of information, are considered teaching. If a client has good oral health, teaching focuses on the continuation of present oral health practices. In contrast, a client with active disease is taught about the disease process, the dental and dental hygiene care required to control the disease, and the client behaviors required to restore health. Sometimes teaching is unplanned and informal, as when the dental hygienist responds to a client's question about an oral health issue in casual conversation. Other educational activities may be planned and more formal, as when the dental hygienist teaches an oral cancer patient to use high-concentration fluoride gel on a daily basis at home, or is called on to provide continuing education for office staff development.

Teaching is involved in the full range of dental hygiene activities directed toward helping the client achieve oral wellness. To help the client learn, the dental hygienist uses educational theory and methods that match the client's unique characteristics and capabilities and draws on other teaching and learning resources, such as the family, instructional aids, and reading materials.[35] The dental hygienist, as an educator, uses the teaching-learning process. The role of the dental hygiene educator/oral health promoter involves effective use of the communication process with clients, dentists, and other healthcare professionals. This educator role is critical in meeting the oral health and human needs of individuals, families, and communities. Practice acts in most legal jurisdictions specify oral health education as a responsibility of the dental hygienist. The ADHA Standards of Applied Dental Hygiene Practice identify oral health education within one of its six standards for acceptable dental hygiene care.

Dental hygiene educators teaching in settings other than private practice work primarily in four areas: schools of dental hygiene and of dentistry, public health departments, and the public school system. Dental hygiene educators generally possess advanced knowledge in dental hygiene practice, which provides them with practical skills as well as theoretical knowledge. A faculty member in a school of dental hygiene prepares students for careers as dental hygiene generalists or specialists. Dental hygiene faculty members are responsible for teaching current dental hygiene theory and practice, advancing dental hygiene knowledge through research, and providing public service. Often, schools of dentistry employ a dental hygienist to teach periodontal and preventive oral health concepts and skills to predoctoral dental students in classroom, laboratory, and clinical settings.

Dental hygiene educators in public health departments develop oral health educational materials and protocols for service programs, such as fluoride rinse programs for elementary school children and special programs for Native Americans. In addition, these educators also work to assess community oral health needs and analyze and develop policies related to oral health at the local, state, and national levels. Moreover, public school systems employ dental hygiene educators to implement dental screening programs; educators also provide classroom oral health education instruction to students, parents, and teachers. Dental hygiene educator positions require at least a baccalaureate degree, and usually they require a graduate degree in dental hygiene, public health, education, or some related basic or behavioral science discipline. Elaboration of the dental hygienist's role as educator/oral health promoter is included in Table 1–4.

Dental Hygiene Administrator/Manager

In various settings in which dental hygiene care is provided, the dental hygienist acts as **manager** or **administrator.** A manager is a person whose official position is to guide and direct the work of others. Interrelated responsibilities commonly associated with the manager include planning, decision making, organizing, staffing, directing, and controlling. Dental hygienists use management skills when they understand the administrative structure of the employment setting and use this structure to achieve organizational goals. Using the knowledge of a manager, the dental hygienist is knowledgeable about the line of authority, responsibilities of various co-workers, and channels of communication; is able to use and contribute to organizational policies and procedures; and values human and material resources. Other managerial strategies are used in the management of client periodontal care, for example, setting care priorities, eliminating causative factors, deciding appropriate continuing care intervals and self-care measures, and providing general client management.

Dental hygiene administrators may direct professional educational programs for dental hygienists and other related health professions, serve as deans and associate deans of schools of allied health, serve as associate deans of schools of dentistry, or administer statewide dental programs. These dental hygiene administrators also are employed in upper level and middle management positions in federal, state, and local health departments, and in private companies that market oral healthcare products. The minimum educational requirement is a graduate degree in dental hygiene or a related field. Many academic administrative positions require that the dental hygienist have a doctoral degree. The dental hygienist's role of administrator/manager is described in detail in Table 1–4.

Dental Hygiene Client Advocate

Advocacy refers to the dental hygienist's role in protecting and supporting clients' rights and well-being. Historically, the patient was kept in a subordinate position within the healthcare setting. The issuance of such landmark legislation as the 1967 Freedom of Information Act and the 1974 Privacy Act has led to an attitude of openness and broadened expectations about the rights of the consumer. Consumers demand their right to participate actively in their own healthcare and seek ways of exercising this right.

As an advocate, the dental hygienist believes that clients have the right to make their own decisions about healthcare after they have been provided with information to make an informed choice. The dental hygienist facilitates client decision making by providing clients with the information they need and by interpreting what the client's rights are in a given situation. Dental hygienists may interpret findings for the client, identify other variables and alternatives to consider, involve others in the decision-making process (dentist, physician, family), and help the client assess the options. Moreover, the dental hygienist helps maintain a safe environment for the client and takes steps to prevent injury and to protect the person from possible adverse effects of treatment measures. Confirming that a client does not have an allergy to a local anesthetic and checking to see whether a client has taken prescribed prophylactic antibiotics prior to dental hygiene care are examples of the dental hygienist's client advocacy role. Clients frequently need information and assistance in negotiating the many complexities in today's healthcare system. The dental hygienist, serving in the role of advocate, can provide clients with the information they need to make intelligent choices about their oral healthcare. Once a client has arrived at a healthcare decision, the dental hygienist demonstrates respect for the client's decision. Table 1–4 further describes the dental hygienist's advocacy role.

Dental Hygiene Researcher

The education that students receive today is not expected to sustain a lifelong career. Throughout a professional career, the dental hygienist uses research skills to remain current in the art and science of dental hygiene. New knowledge, generated from research, is necessary to support decision making in all aspects of dental hygiene. Research provides the knowledge base for all dental hygiene actions. In any employment setting and role, the contemporary dental hygienist must be able to question, be creative, and think analytically to systematically solve problems and improve oral health. In reality, the dental hygienist is a critical consumer of research findings. The dental hygiene process (assessing, diagnosing, planning, implementing, and evaluating) reflects the basic framework of the research process. Whether the goal is evaluating a new therapeutic intervention or evaluating client progress, all professional behaviors require the analytical skills of a researcher.

A profession's research efforts are closely linked with its service role, responsibility, and accountability to the public; therefore, practice can be only as good as the research and theory that support it. The **dental hygiene researcher** tests assumptions underlying dental hygiene practice and investigates dental hygiene problems to improve oral healthcare and the practice of dental hygiene. The dental hygiene researcher may be employed in an academic setting; in a federal, state, or local health agency; in a research institution (e.g., National Institute of Dental Research); or in private industry. The minimal educational requirement is a graduate degree in dental hygiene or a related field, with a doctoral degree preferred. In summary, the contemporary dental hygienist ensures that actions taken are grounded in theory and research (see Table 1–4).

Dental Hygiene Change Agent

Change is the process of altering, modifying, or transforming an idea, event, individual, family, group, or community. The rapidity of societal, scientific, and technological change has created a need for dental hygienists who can manage change. The change process can be compared to the dental hygiene process because both can be used to facilitate change through assessment, diagnosis, planning, implementation, and evaluation.

A **change agent** is an individual who applies a theoretical body of knowledge that focuses on a systematic approach to change. Parker examined the actual role of the **dental hygiene change agent** in the change process and suggests that the dental hygienist can act in four change agent roles:

- Catalyst
- Solution giver
- Resource linker
- Process helper

The *catalyst* is the energizing force to get things started. The *solution-giver* has definite ideas for solving a problem; however, it is a challenge for the solution giver to know when and how to offer that change so that it is adopted. Solution givers should not be married to their own ideas but should adopt the objective stance that the idea and not the person is subject to rejection. This objective posture gives ideas a greater chance for survival as the seed for change is planted. In the role of *resource linker* the dental hygienist can help individuals and groups find and make the best use of resources, which may be people with the time, expertise, money, or motivation to help solve a particular problem.[37]

The role of *process helper* involves understanding the change process. As in the dental hygiene process, the first phase of planned change is the *assessment phase,* when dissatisfaction is identified. The next stage is the *planning phase,* when an accurate diagnosis of the problem is made and objectives are formulated. Included in the planning stage of the change process are examining alternative strategies and goals, establishing specific goals, and agreeing to act. At this point, there may be a question regarding what might have to be given up by those involved in the proposed change in order to accomplish ultimate aims. As a result, anxiety and resistance may surface when contemplating the change. During the planning phase, it is very important that the dental hygiene change agent have the support of the group and identify sources of power within the group to support the change. Such support is essential if change is to occur.[36,38–40]

Implementation of the actual change effort occurs in the *implementation phase.* The *evaluation phase* should be an ongoing process to determine the success or failure of the change. Success of the change should be measured by how well the original ineffectiveness is relieved and functional efficiency is achieved or restored.[36]

The final stage of the change process is the *termination phase,* which occurs once the change has been accepted and is an integral part of the operation. It is during this phase hygienists gradually reduce their role, remaining available for support in emergencies.[36,39,40]

Parker maintains that if change agents view change as being evolutionary rather than revolutionary, the chances of a successful change will be greater and the effects longer lasting. Incremental changes, guided by a master plan, are more likely to be achieved.[36,41,42] Table 1–4 identifies specific activities that dental hygienists perform when functioning in the role of change agent.

CAREER ROLES

The preceding roles and functions of the dental hygienist are inherent to most professional dental hygienists in most practice settings. Although most registered dental hygienists are clinical practitioners working in collaboration with dentists in private dental practices, many dental hygienists have gone into business for themselves in areas related to oral healthcare other than direct patient care. For example, dental hygienists have started dental assisting and dental hygiene programs, dental staff permanent and temporary placement agencies, private continuing education companies, and consulting firms. Some have invented new products, designed new instruments, and independently published books, games, computer programs, and instructional media.

GUIDELINES FOR DENTAL HYGIENE PRACTICE

Because of the complex interrelationship of roles and an ever-changing knowledge base, dental hygiene practice is viewed as a process rather than as a series of tasks or duties.

Dental Hygiene Process

The dental hygiene process is described in detail in Chapter 3. The concept of the **dental hygiene process** is the foundation of professional dental hygiene practice and provides a model for organizing and providing dental hygiene care in a variety of settings. The steps of the dental hygiene process are briefly defined as:

Assessing: the act of systematically collecting and validating data in order to identify client problems, needs, and strengths

Diagnosing: the act of identifying client strengths and oral health problems that dental hygiene interventions can improve

Planning: the act of establishing goals and selecting dental hygiene interventions that can move the client closer to optimal oral health

Implementing: the act of carrying out the dental hygiene care plan designed to meet the assessed needs of the client

Evaluating: the act of measuring the extent to which the client has achieved the goals specified in the plan of care

Standards of Dental Hygiene Practice

Standards in the United States

In 1979, the ADHA created the Commission for Assurance of Competence and, in 1980, established the Task Force to Develop Standards of Practice. These actions demonstrated the profession's willingness to assume responsibility for the quality of care that its members provide. By 1982, these groups presented the Competence Assurance Program, a detailed plan that included components of assessment, postgraduate education, study, and recognition of achievement.

The baseline components of the Competence Assurance Program are the **Standards of Applied Dental Hygiene Practice.** The Standards serve the profession and society in a number of ways. The Standards:

- Define the activities of dental hygienists that are unique to dental hygiene
- Provide consumers, employers and colleagues with

guidelines as to what constitutes quality dental hygiene care
- Provide guidelines for establishing goals for clinical dental hygiene education
- Serve as the foundation for competence assurance and continued professional development

The development of practice standards evolved somewhat differently in Canada. In 1981, the Working Group on the Practice of Dental Hygiene was established by the Department of National Health and Welfare. As part of their charge to undertake a comprehensive review of dental hygiene in Canada, the Working Group recommended to the Department of National Health and Welfare to establish the Advisory Committee on the Development of Clinical Practice Standards for Dental Hygienists. In 1983, a project to develop clinical dental hygiene practice criteria and standards that have been evaluated for content validity by practitioners was initiated. These criteria were modeled after the methodology used by the Manitoba Association of Registered Nurses in the Standards of Nursing Care.[43,44] Also highly involved were the Canadian Dental Hygienists' Association and the Professional Corporation of Dental Hygienists of Quebec.

The result of these efforts is outlined in the **Clinical Practice Standards for Dental Hygienists in Canada.** It serves as a landmark event in dental hygiene's professional growth and development in Canada. According to the Canadian Dental Hygienists' Association, the Standards "ensure that the highest level of dental hygiene care possible is provided to the Canadian public (quality of care) and that dental hygiene practitioners are capable of performing their roles in a competent manner. . . . dental hygienists have the professional responsibility to read and employ the published clinical practice standards in their work setting.[45]

Interestingly, United States and Canadian dental hygienists have used the dental hygiene process as the underlying structure in their standards of practice. The intent of and rationale for the standards used in both countries have obvious parallels.

Practice Acts and Licensure

Dental practice acts are laws established in each state (United States) or province (Canada) to regulate the practice of dentistry and dental hygiene. Locales such as Washington State, Alberta, Ontario, and Quebec have separate practice acts for dental hygiene. Although the laws that regulate dental hygiene practice vary with each licensing jurisdiction, each reflects common elements. In general, the practice act does the following:

- Establishes criteria for the education, licensure, and relicensure of dental hygienists
- Defines the legal scope of dental hygiene practice
- Protects the public by making the practice of dental hygiene by uncredentialed and unlicensed persons illegal
- Creates a board empowered with legal authority, to oversee the policies and procedures affecting the practice of dental hygiene in that jurisdiction

The board in each jurisdiction is given legal authority to design and administer licensing examinations to graduates of approved schools of dental hygiene. Individuals who pass the licensing examination earn a license to practice dental hygiene as it is defined in that jurisdiction. The liscense can be denied, revoked, or suspended for a variety of reasons, such as incompetence, negligence, chemical dependency, illegal practice, and criminal misconduct.

PROFESSIONAL DENTAL HYGIENE ORGANIZATIONS

Professional organizations exist to collectively represent the views of a profession and to influence resolution of issues relevant to education, practice, and research in that profession. Professional organizations have an enormous effect on dental hygiene as they address issues of professional growth, education, access to care, research and theory development, quality assurance, manpower, legislation, and collaboration with other professionals. Although many organizations exist, only the major ones are discussed in this chapter.

American Dental Hygienists' Association

The **American Dental Hygienists' Association (ADHA)** is a national organization of approximately 35,000 dental hygienists. To improve the public's total health, the mission of the ADHA is to advance the art and science of dental hygiene by increasing the awareness of and ensuring access to quality oral healthcare, promoting the highest standard of dental hygiene education, licensure, and practice, and representing and promoting the interests of dental hygienists.

The goals of the ADHA are to:

- Maximize the utilization of the services of dental hygienists and to continue consumer advocacy in the healthcare delivery system
- Promote the dental hygienist as a primary care provider of preventive and therapeutic services
- Promote the self-regulation of dental hygiene education, licensure, and practice
- Serve as the authoritative resource on all issues related to dental hygiene
- Promote research relevant to dental hygiene
- Increase membership and participation in the ADHA
- Provide for a viable financial base

Founded in 1923, the ADHA has a tri-level structure by which individual members are automatically part of local (component), state (constituent), and national levels of governance. The official publications of the ADHA include the *Journal of Dental Hygiene, Access,* and *Education Update.* The House of Delegates is its legislative body, which is composed of voting members who represent each constituent based on a proportional formula. The Board of Trustees, presided over by the organization's elected president, consists of voting members (president, president-elect, vice-president, treasurer, immediate past president, and thirteen district trustees) and nonvoting, ex officio members (executive director and editorial director). The ADHA plays a major role in issues that deal with legislation, access to care, education, practice, research, public relations, and health policy. The ADHA offers a variety of both tangible and intangible benefits and should be supported by professional and student dental hygienists in the United States.

National Dental Hygienists' Association

In 1932, the **National Dental Hygienists' Association (NDHA)** was founded by African-American dental hygienists to address the needs and special problems of the minority dental hygienist. The purposes of the NDHA are to:

- Cultivate and promote the art and science of dental hygiene
- Improve individual and community dental health
- Maintain the professional status of dental hygienists
- Encourage mutual support and goodwill among minority professionals
- Expand continuing education and employment opportunities
- Facilitate student recruitment and scholarship

Although the NDHA has members in most states, it also has constituents in Atlanta, Boston, Baltimore, Cleveland, Detroit, Houston, Los Angeles, Miami, Oakland, New Orleans, and Washington, DC. The NDHA offers annual scholarships to minority students and a courtesy membership to new graduates for 1 year. It holds an annual convention in conjunction with the National Dental Association and publishes a newsletter.

The Canadian Dental Hygienists' Association

The **Canadian Dental Hygienists' Association (CDHA),** officially founded in 1965, is the national association for registered dental hygienists in Canada. With a structure similar to that of the ADHA, the CDHA has provincial organizations supported by local components. The CDHA publishes *Probe,* the journal of the Canadian Dental Hygienists' Association, and has played a prominent role in developing the full potential of dental hygiene, continuing education, formal dental hygiene education, portability of licensure, and dental hygiene research and theory. The ADHA and CDHA have worked together to achieve many common goals. It should be supported by professional and student dental hygienists in Canada.

International Dental Hygienists' Federation

As the dental hygiene profession grew worldwide, forward-thinking representatives of national dental hygiene organizations from seven countries (Canada, Japan, the Netherlands, Norway, Sweden, the United Kingdom, and the United States) met for the first time in 1970 to form the International Liaison Committee on Dental Hygiene. From its inception, the committee organized several international symposia on dental hygiene to focus on issues that affect dental hygiene worldwide, and worked for many years toward the formation of an international organization of dental hygienists.

On June 28, 1986, during the Tenth International Symposium on Dental Hygiene in Oslo, Norway, dental hygiene representatives from the original seven countries were joined by the new member countries of Australia, Denmark, and Switzerland to charter the **International Dental Hygienists' Federation (IDHF).** The IDHF objectives are to:

- Represent and advance the profession of dental hygiene on a nongovernmental, worldwide basis
- Promote and coordinate the exchange of knowledge and information about the profession and its education and practice
- Raise the level of awareness of the public that oral disease can be prevented through proven regimens
- Foster the exchange of dental hygiene human resources

The IDHF recognizes that the need for dental hygiene is universal and that dental hygiene services should be unrestricted by consideration of nationality, sex, race, creed, color, politics, or social status. The IDHF provides a formal network by which dental hygienists worldwide can promote collegiality among nations, commitment to maintaining universal standards of dental hygiene care and education, and access to quality oral healthcare.

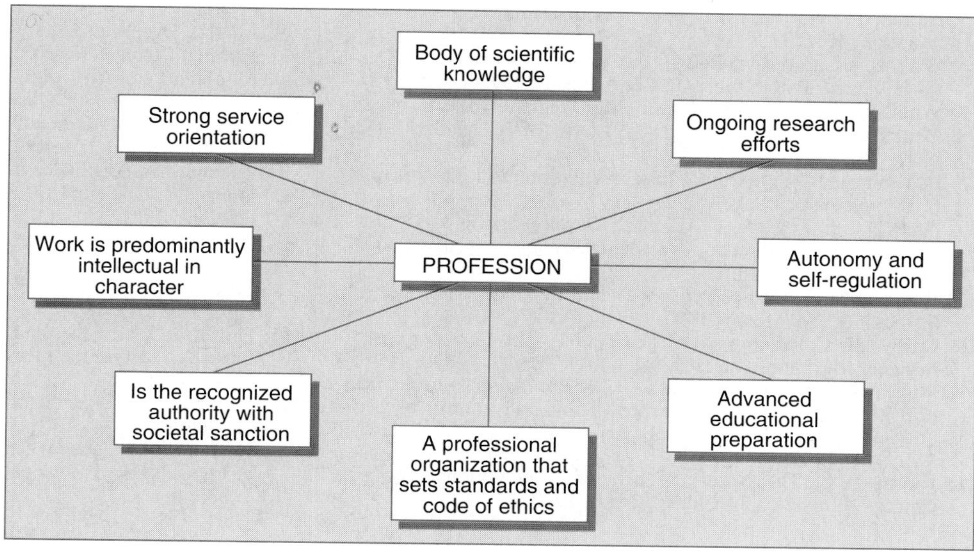

FIGURE 1–3
Characteristics of a true profession.

DENTAL HYGIENE IN TRANSITION

Dental hygiene continues to change in response to the needs and demands of a global society. The world at large is in transition. Political and economic systems are being redefined, demographics are changing, and science and technology are extending the parameters of human life. The changing world exerts social, political, cultural, and economic influences on the emerging profession of dental hygiene.

Dental hygiene continues to evolve as society in general and healthcare in particular continue to change. Since its inception in the early twentieth century, the dental hygiene profession has evolved from satisfaction with an auxiliary status to expectation of self-regulation, professional autonomy, and decision making in dental hygiene practice in order to increase access to quality care for the public and to take its place within the context of a true profession (Fig. 1–3).

References

1. Motley, W. History of the American Dental Hygienists' Association 1923–1982. Chicago, IL: American Dental Hygienists' Association, 1986.
2. McCarthy, M. C. Alfred C. Fones: The father of dental hygiene. Journal of the American Dental Hygiene Association 13(1):1, 1939.
3. Fones, A. C. Origin and history of the dental hygienists movement. Journal of the American Dental Hygiene Association 3(3):7, 1929.
4. Barrett, E. A. M. Visions of Rogers' Science-Based Nursing. New York: National League for Nursing, 1990, p. 6.
5. American Dental Hygienists' Association. Proceedings of the 68th Annual Session, House of Delegates. Louisville, KY: June, 1992, and 69th Annual Session, House of Delegates, Denver, CO, June 1993.
6. Darby, M. Theory development and basic research in dental hygiene: Review of the literature and recommendations (technical report). Chicago, IL: American Dental Hygienists' Association, June, 1990.
7. Cmich, D. E. Theoretical perspectives of holistic health. Journal of School Health 54(1):30–32, 1984.
8. Wilkins, E. M. Clinical Practice of the Dental Hygienist, 6th ed. Philadelphia: Lea & Febiger, 1989.
9. Fones, A. C. Mouth Hygiene, 4th ed. Philadelphia: Lea & Febiger, 1934, p. 248.
10. Motley, W. History of the American Dental Hygienists' Association, 1923–1982. Chicago: American Dental Hygienists' Association, 1986.
11. Wilkins, E., and McCullough, P. Clinical Practice of the Dental Hygienist. Philadelphia: Lea & Febiger, 1959.
12. Woodall, I. Legal, Ethical, and Management Aspects of the Dental Care System, 2nd ed. St. Louis: C. V. Mosby, 1983, p. 1.
13. Pattison, A. M. Periodontal Instrumentation, 2nd ed. Norwalk, CT: Appleton & Lange, 1992.
14. Hicks, M. J., DeVore, C. H., et al. Developing the periodontal cotherapist: New directions for dental hygiene education. Dental Hygiene 61(3):126, 1987.
15. Woodall, I. R. Comprehensive Dental Hygiene Care, 4th ed. St. Louis: C. V. Mosby, 1993.
16. Darby, M. Collaborative practice model—the future of dental hygiene. Journal of Dental Education 47(9):589, 1983.
17. Walsh, M. M., and Robertson, P. B. Professional mechanical oral hygiene practices in the prevention and control of periodontal diseases. Journal of the California Dental Association 13(12):58, 1985.
18. Kuhn, T. S. The Nature of Scientific Revolutions, 2nd ed. Chicago: University of Chicago Press, 1970.
19. Fawcett, J. Analysis and Evaluation of Conceptual Models of Nursing, 2nd ed. Philadelphia: F. A. Davis, 1989.
20. Eckberg, D. L., and Hill, L., Jr. The paradigm concept and sociology. American Sociological Review 44:925, 1979.
21. Conway, M. E. Toward greater specificity in defining nursing's metaparadigm. Advances in Nursing Science 7:73, 1985.
22. Johnson, D. E. Guest Editorial: Evaluating conceptual models for use in critical care nursing practice. Dimensions of Critical Care Nursing 6:195, 1987.
23. Yura, H., and Walsh, M. B. The Nursing Process, 5th ed. Norwalk, CT: Appleton & Lange, 1988, pp. 85–100.
24. American Association of Dental Schools, Standing Committee of Dental Hygiene Directors. Report of the Task Force on Dental Hygiene Education, 1988–1992. Washington, DC: American Association of Dental Schools, 1992.
25. Wayman, D. Issues arising from growth patterns in dental hygiene education (unpublished paper). Standing Committee of Dental Hygiene Directors, American Association of Dental Schools, 1986.
26. Mescher, K. A new look at the educational preparation of dental hygienists: Exploding the myth. Dental Hygiene 58:69, 1984.
27. American Dental Hygienists' Association. Dental Hygiene Education and Practice Workshop I Proceedings. Chicago: American Dental Hygienists' Association, 1984.
28. American Dental Hygienists' Association. Dental Hygiene Education and Practice Workshop II Proceedings. Chicago: American Dental Hygienists' Association, 1985.
29. American Dental Hygienists' Association. Dental Hygiene Education and Practice Workshop III Proceedings. Chicago: American Dental Hygienists' Association, 1986.
30. American Dental Hygienists' Association. Prospectus for Dental Hygiene. Chicago, IL: American Dental Hygienist's Association, 1988.
31. Lockwood, T. What should the baccalaureate degree mean? Change, November/December 1982, pp. 38–44.
32. Woditsch, G. A., Schlesinger, M. A., and Giardina, R. C. The skillful baccalaureate doing what liberal education does best. Change, November/December 1987, pp. 48–57.
33. Darby, M. Value of the terminal degree in dental hygiene—one educator's position. Educational Directions 7:25, 1982.
34. Wood, A. 4500 dental hygienists in Ontario will be self-regulated. Contact International, Journal of the International Dental Hygienists' Federation 11(1):1, 1992.
35. Potter, P. A., and Perry, A. G. Fundamentals of Nursing, 3rd ed. St. Louis: Mosby–Year Book, 1993.
36. Parker, E. The dental hygienist: Change agent for the future. Dental Hygiene 58(8):362, 1984.
37. Rogers, E. Shoemaker, M., and Floyd, F. Communications of Innovation, 2nd ed. New York: The Free Press, 1971.
38. Brooten, D., Hayman, L., and Naylor, M. Leadership for change: a guide for the frustrated nurse. Philadelphia: J. B. Lippincott, 1978.
39. Lippett, R., Watson, J., and Westley, B. The Dynamics of Planned Change. New York: Harcourt, Brace & Co., 1958.
40. Reinkemeyer, A. Commitment to an ideology of change. Nursing Forum 9(4):341, 1970.
41. Greiner, L. Fundamentals of management. In Donnelly, J., Gibson, J., and Ivancevich, J. (eds.). Fundamentals of Management. Dallas: Business Publications, 1975.
42. Dluhy, M. Changing the System. Beverly Hills, CA: Sage Publications, 1981.
43. Scherer, K. Content validation of the standards of nursing care, Manitoba Association of Registered Nurses. Victoria, BC: Proceedings of the National Nursing Research Conference, April 1982.
44. Farrell, P., and Scherer, K. The delphi technique as a method for selecting criteria to evaluate nursing care. Nursing Papers 15(1):51, 1983.
45. Brownstone, E. Report of the Working Group on the Practice of Dental Hygiene. In Clinical Practice Standards for Dental Hygienists in Canada, part two. Minister of Supply and Services, Canada, The Canadian Dental Hygienists' Association, 1988.

Suggested Readings

Ayers, C., Williams, D., and Lausten, L. A survey of prevention in dental education. Journal of Dental Education, 43:515, 1979.

Bailit, H. Changing patterns of oral health and implications for oral health manpower: Responsibility to the public. International Dental Journal 58:56, 1988.

Byrd, G. L. A comparison of associate and baccalaureate dental hygiene education. Norfolk, VA: Old Dominion University, School of Dental Hygiene, 1991 (unpublished report).

Clinical Practice Standards for Dental Hygienists in Canada, part two. Report of the Working Group on the Practice of Dental Hygiene. Minister of Supply and Services, Canada, the Canadian Dental Hygienists' Association, 1988.

Editorial. Dental hygiene. American Journal of Dental Science 5:244, 1945.

Eslami, J. G. Humanistic approach and its relevance to dental hygiene education and practice. Norfolk, VA: Old Dominion University, School of Dental Hygiene, 1991 (unpublished literature review).

Leverett, D. A critical examination of the barriers to the receipt of dental care. Journal of Public Health Dentistry 35(1):28, 1975.

Motley, W. Dental hygiene at 75. Dental Hygiene 62(10):458, 1988.

Ottofy, L. The origin of the dental hygiene movement. Journal of the American Dental Hygiene Association 7(7):11, 1933.

Parmly, L. S. A Practical Guide to the Management of the Teeth. Philadelphia: Collins and Croft, 1819, p. 119.

Pew Health Professions Commission. Final Draft Report of the Advisory Panel for Allied Health to the Pew Health Professions Commission. Journal of Allied Health 21(4):1–74, Fall 1992.

Pollack, B. Handbook of Dental Malpractice Risk Management. Littleton, MA: PSG Publishing, 1987.

Wright, C. A plea for a subspecialty in dentistry. International Dental Journal 23:235, 1902.

2 Dental Hygiene Human Needs Conceptual Model and Its Application to the Dental Hygiene Process

OBJECTIVES

Mastery of the content in this chapter will enable the reader to:

- Compare Maslow's hierarchy of needs theory with nursing's human needs theory
- Identify and define the four central paradigm concepts for the dental hygiene human needs conceptual model
- Define the 11 human needs related to dental hygiene care and describe their implications for dental hygienists
- For each of the 11 human needs, identify at least one related deficit and plan a dental hygiene intervention to meet the unmet need
- Discuss the relationship of human need theory to the dental hygiene process

INTRODUCTION

Dental hygiene care focuses on the promotion of oral health and the prevention of oral disease over the human lifespan. To this end, the dental hygienist is concerned with the whole person, applying specific knowledge about the client's emotions, values, family, culture, and environment as well as general knowledge about the body systems. Clients are viewed as being actively involved in the process of dental hygiene care, because ultimately it is they who must use self-care and seek professional care to obtain and maintain oral wellness. Thus, dental hygiene care focuses on the individual's adjustments to the environment in order to promote oral health and prevent oral diseases.

Human needs theory can assist dental hygienists to understand the relationship between human need fulfillment and human behavior when providing dental hygiene care. A **human need** is defined as a tension that results from an alteration in a person's system. This tension may express itself in some goal-directed behavior that continues until the goal is reached. Human needs theory explains that need fulfillment dominates human activity, and behavior is organized in relation to unsatisfied needs. Moreover, unsatisfied needs serve as motivators that can be used to guide the client toward optimal oral wellness.

Dental hygiene theorists have proposed human needs theory as a theoretical framework for the dental hygiene process.[1,2] Before discussing the human needs conceptual model for dental hygiene, it is necessary to review basic human need theory. Although many human need theorists have provided the theoretical substance for the understanding of human needs and the motivation inherent in meeting these needs, the work of Maslow and of nursing theorists is highlighted here as a basis for discussing dental hygiene's human needs theory.

MASLOW'S HIERARCHY OF NEEDS

Abraham Maslow identified and assigned priorities to basic human needs. According to his theory, certain human needs are more basic than others; that is, some needs must be met before one turns one's attention to meeting others.[3,4] Maslow prioritized human needs in a hierarchy of five categories, based on their power and strength to motivate behavior (Fig. 2–1). The hierarchy is arranged with the most imperative needs at the bottom and the least imperative at the top. On the most basic, or first, level of human needs are **physiological needs,** such as the need for food, fluids, sleep, and exercise. According to Maslow's theory, a person is dominated by physiological needs; if these needs are not reasonably satisfied, all other categories of needs in the hierarchy may seem irrelevant or are relegated to low priority.

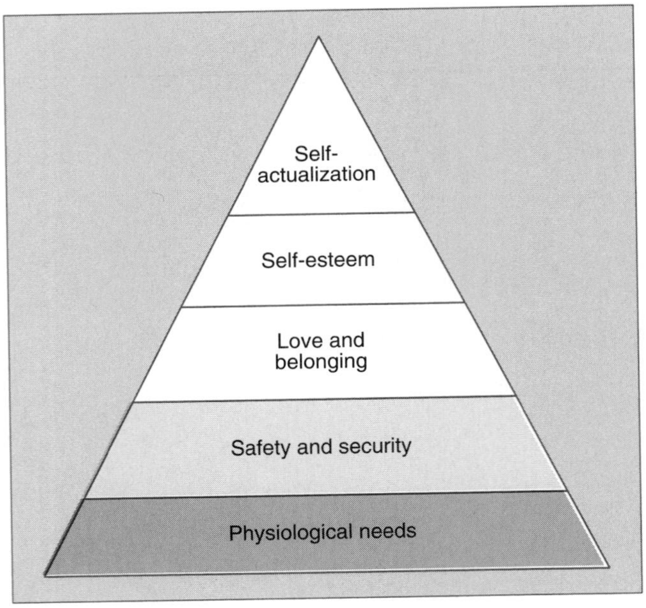

FIGURE 2–1
Maslow's hierarchy of needs. (Redrawn from Potter, P.A., and Perry, A.G. Fundamentals of Nursing, 3rd ed. St Louis: C. V. Mosby, 1993.)

On the second level are **safety needs,** including the need for both physical and psychological security. Safety needs include the need for stability, protection, structure, and freedom from fear and anxiety. In times of danger, the need to ensure safety and protection becomes paramount. Every other need becomes less important. Loss of parental protection, war, and being confronted with new tasks, strangers, or illness all are threats to the need for safety.[5]

On the third level are **needs for love and a sense of belonging.** They include the need for affectionate relationships and the need for a place within one's culture, group, or family. Love and belonging needs are expressed in one's desire for tenderness, affection, contact, intimacy, togetherness, and face-to-face encounters. Love needs involve both giving and receiving love. Love and belonging needs also are expressed in the need to overcome feelings of alienation, aloneness, or strangeness brought on by the scattering of family, friends, and significant others.[5]

On the fourth level of Maslow's hierarchy is the **need for self-esteem,** the feeling of confidence, usefulness, achievement, and self-worth. Esteem needs include the need for a stable, firmly based, wholesome self-evaluation; the need for respect and esteem of self as well as esteem from others; a desire for strength, mastery, and competitiveness; and a need for feeling confident in the face of the world, for independence, and for freedom. Deprivation of these needs results in feelings of inferiority, helplessness, and discouragement. Fulfillment of esteem needs results in feelings of capability and a willingness to be a contributor to society.[5]

The final level of the hierarchy is the need for what Maslow calls **self-actualization,** a state in which one is fully achieving one's potential and is able to solve problems and cope realistically with life's situations.[5]

Maslow points out that it is precisely those persons in whom a certain need has always been met or satisfied who are best equipped to withstand deprivation of that need at some future time. Persons who have been deprived in the past respond differently to current need deprivation than the person who has never been deprived.[5]

Implications for Dental Hygiene Care

Maslow's hierarchy of needs is a theoretical model; that is, the priorities given human needs generally are true of people but not necessarily of all individuals. For example, a woman who attempts to meet her self-esteem needs by working 18 hours at a time may ignore physiological needs for adequate sleep and nutrition because her need for self-esteem takes priority. Eventually, however, this woman may be forced to give more attention to her physiological needs if she can no longer function as usual because she has been weakened by inadequate nutrition and rest. Thus, the hierarchy of needs can still be applied to individuals who seem to have different priorities. In providing care to those with human need deficits, the dental hygienist takes into account the priorities of individual clients, as well as other factors, such as their environment and social interactions, that influence how well they can meet their needs.[6]

HUMAN NEEDS THEORY OF YURA AND WALSH

Nursing theorists Yura and Walsh postulated a human needs theory of nursing that includes all the human need categories articulated by Maslow but arranged differently. These nursing scholars identified additional human needs and defined them in detail to facilitate their clinical assessment.[5] Specifically, this human needs theory encompasses 35 human needs, arranged according to survival, closeness, and freedom groups.

Nursing uses **subjective** and **objective data** to evaluate the degree of human need fulfillment in clients. Objective data are more likely to be obtained for human needs that are concrete, and subjective data are more likely to be obtained for abstract human needs. Nursing postulates that reasons why human needs may be unmet include personal and situational occurrences; environmental affronts; illness-related therapies; pathophysiological states; congenital alterations; philosophical, ethical, cultural, and religious impositions; educational and informational deficits; social and economic affronts; and growth and development alterations.[5]

A HUMAN NEEDS CONCEPTUAL MODEL FOR DENTAL HYGIENE

One conceptual model recently proposed for dental hygiene is the human needs conceptual model.[1] Human needs theory was selected as the theoretical framework for this dental hygiene conceptual model because of the characteristic client-centered approach of dental hygienists and because of the essential contributions of oral health and wellness to overall quality of life. History suggests that the dental hygienist's primary concern has been for the whole person who either has oral disease or is at risk for having oral disease, rather than on the oral disease itself, and for the role of the environment and the individual in fostering or preventing oral disease. It is dental hygiene that primarily views the client as being actively involved in the process of care because it is ultimately the client who must use self-care to obtain and maintain oral wellness. It is the dental hygienist who focuses on client lifestyle and behavioral patterns as they relate to oral health. It is the dental hygienist who attempts to motivate the client toward oral health behaviors. Because of all these client-centered concerns, human needs theory was deemed an appropriate theoretical framework for a conceptual model of dental hygiene. In this model, basic human needs theory is utilized to explain the four major concepts of the dental hygiene paradigm: client, environment, health and oral health, and dental hygiene actions. The resultant definitions of the four major concepts and the set of propositions or statements that define each provide the theoretical framework for the dental hygiene process and the context within which dental hygiene care is provided. The relationship of human needs theories to the four major paradigm concepts is described below and is adapted from the work of Yura and Walsh.[5]

Concept 1: Client

Based on human needs theory, a **client** is viewed as a biological, psychological, spiritual, social, cultural, and intellectual human being who is an integrated, organized whole and whose behavior is motivated by fulfillment of his human needs. Figure 2–2 shows a model for this concept. This model further indicates that to meet their human needs and thereby to restore their sense of wholeness as human beings, individuals respond holistically as integrated beings to life situations. Individuals are also unique beings in that the nature of their experience is theirs alone. In many circumstances they have the power to choose their way of life, and their choices give meaning to their existence.[2,5,7] The client can be an individual, a family, or a group and is viewed as having 11 human needs that are especially related to dental hygiene care. Additional propositions associated with this concept of client are listed in the Propositions Associated with the Concept of Clients chart.

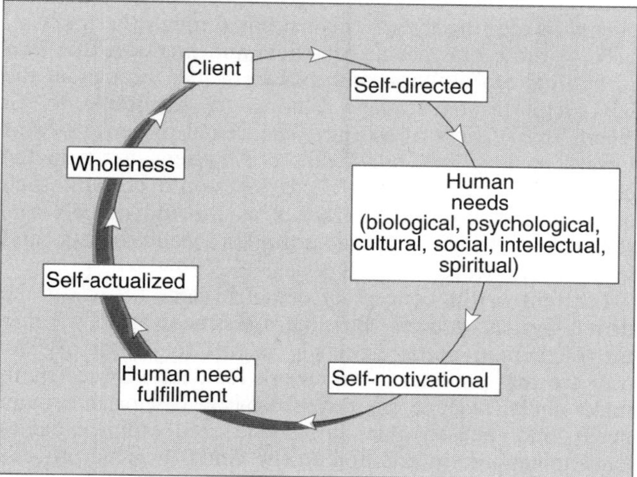

FIGURE 2–2
The concept of client in the human needs conceptual model of dental hygiene. (Redrawn from Yura, H., and Walsh, M. B. The Nursing Process, 5th ed. Norwalk, CT: Appleton & Lange, 1988, p. 95.)

PROPOSITIONS ASSOCIATED WITH THE CONCEPT OF CLIENTS

- Biopsychosocial beings
- Holistic and respond holistically
- Responsible for the fulfillment of their human needs
- Motivated toward meeting their human needs
- Self-directed in determining the priority of their human needs fulfillment
- Unique, which requires modification to accommodate variables such as attitude, beliefs, culture, growth and development, age, roles, gender, lifestyle, knowledge level
- Capable of controlling their environment to various degrees
- Capable to varying degrees in using self-care to obtain and maintain oral wellness
- Nature of clients' human experience is unique
- Clients have 11 human needs especially related to dental hygiene care

Adapted from Yura, H., and Walsh, M. B. The Nursing Process, 5th ed. Norwalk, CT: Appleton & Lange, 1988, p. 95.

Concept 2: Environment

Environment is the milieu in which the client and dental hygienist find themselves. The environment affects the client and the dental hygienist, and the client and dental hygienist are capable of influencing the environment. In the human needs conceptual model, the concept of environment is defined to include dimensions such as society, climate, geography, politics, economics, education, socioethnocultural factors, significant others, the family, the community, the state, the nation, and the world (Fig 2–3). These dimensions are viewed as influencing the manner, mode, and level of human need fulfillment for the person, family, and community. Society, a major environmental factor, is in constant change, and most human beings attempt to adapt to its changing nature in order to fulfill their human needs.[2,5,7] Society is composed of human beings interacting in a complex network of individuals, families, groups, and communities. Society exists to facilitate meeting the human needs of its membership, with the family as the primary unit responsible for the fulfillment of its members' human needs. Human needs that cannot be met within the family structure are assumed by the community, state, and nation. The model for the concept of environment is shown in Figure 2–3. Propositions associated with the concept of environment are listed in the Propositions Associated with the Concept of Environment chart.

Concept 3: Health and Oral Health

In the human needs conceptual model, the concept of **health** is viewed as a relative condition—a state of well-being with both objective and subjective aspects that exists on a continuum from maximal wellness to maximal illness (Fig. 2–4). The higher the level of human need fulfillment, the higher the state of wellness for the individual. An indi-

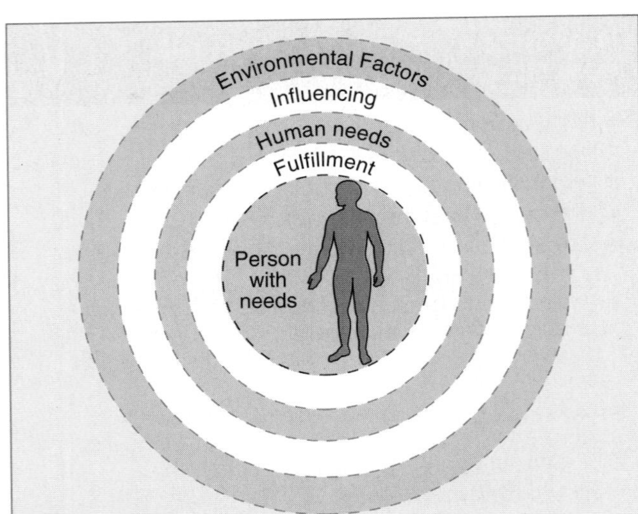

FIGURE 2–3
The concept of environment in the human needs conceptual model of dental hygiene. (Redrawn from Yura, H., and Walsh, M. B. The Nursing Process, 5th ed. Norwalk, CT: Appleton & Lange, 1988, p. 96.)

+	HEALTH/ORAL HEALTH CONTINUUM	-
Wellness	health/oral health ...... Illness	Death
Oral wellness	....	Oral disease
Human need fulfillment	....	Alterations in human need fulfillment

FIGURE 2–4
The concept of health and oral health in the human needs conceptual model of dental hygiene. (Redrawn from Yura, H., and Walsh, M. B. The Nursing Process, 5th ed. Norwalk, CT: Appleton & Lange, 1988, p. 97.)

vidual's health may change along this continuum under the influence of biological, psychological, spiritual, social, and cultural factors that are interrelated and fluctuate over time.[2,5,7–9] Maximal wellness is achieved with maximal fulfillment of human needs; maximal illness occurs with minimal or absent human need fulfillment. Along the health continuum, there are degrees of wellness and illness that are associated with varying levels of human need fulfillment.

Although oral health per se involves the orofacial complex, it exists in a biological interrelationship with the entire body and is therefore influenced by the same factors as general health. Oral health can affect general health through oral infections and impaired masticatory function; conversely, the oral tissues are often sensitive indicators of the general health of the individual.[10] Many systemic diseases produce oral changes that may be part of the primary disease process or a complication of it. Because the oral cavity is analogous to other body cavities, its health status is governed by the same physical and chemical laws and physiological principles, and affected by the same social, cultural, psychological, and spiritual factors as other body cavities.[11,12] For that reason, oral health as well as general health is associated with human need fulfillment. Viewed through the conceptual framework of human needs theory, **oral health** is defined as the oral condition that results from the interaction of individuals with their environment, under varying levels of human need fulfillment. This concept is described in the Propositions Associated with the Concepts of Health and Oral Health chart.

PROPOSITIONS ASSOCIATED WITH THE CONCEPT OF ENVIRONMENT

- Dimensions include society, climate, geography, politics, economics, education, culture, and socioethnocultural factors
- Significant others, the family, the community, the state, the nation, and the community of nations facilitate human needs fulfillment in its members
- The family usually is the basic unit of human needs fulfillment of the person
- Environmental factors such as climate, geography, politics, economics, education, architectural barriers, heredity, society, and socioethnocultural factors influence the human needs fulfillment of the person, family, community, and world
- Environment is in constant change, and clients attempt to adapt to its change in order to fulfill their human needs
- Change in the environment, or adaptation of the person to the environment, can improve oral health and facilitate human needs fulfillment

Adapted from Yura, H., and Walsh, M. B. The Nursing Process, 5th ed. Norwalk, CT: Appleton & Lange, 1988, p. 96

Concept 4: Dental Hygiene Actions

In the human needs conceptual model, **dental hygiene actions** are defined as those interventions aimed at assisting clients in meeting their human needs through the performance of those oral health behaviors and practices that lead to optimal oral wellness and quality of life, throughout the life cycle. Dental hygiene actions are applicable to all clients in a variety of settings. The dental hygienist's effort toward meeting the individual's oral hygiene needs in the context of related human needs takes into account such client and environmental factors as the individual's age, sex, roles, lifestyle, culture, attitudes, health beliefs, and level of knowledge.

Inherent in the concept of dental hygiene actions is the dental hygiene process. Baseline assessment as to whether the 11 human needs especially related to dental hygiene care are met provides a framework for dental hygienists to make dental hygiene diagnoses based on deficits in human needs, and then to plan, implement, and evaluate dental hygiene actions. In addition to the dental hygiene process, dental hygienists use the communication process, the leadership process, and the research process as means of oral health promotion and maintenance and oral disease prevention. Dental hygienists carry out these four main processes as they function in the roles of clinician, manager,

PROPOSITIONS ASSOCIATED WITH THE CONCEPTS OF HEALTH AND ORAL HEALTH

- Health and oral health are viewed as an everchanging continuum between the dimensions of optimal wellness and illness
- Health is defined as subjective and objective states of well-being that exist on a continuum from maximal wellness to maximal illness; the higher the level of human need fulfillment, the higher the state of wellness
- Oral health is defined as the oral condition that results from the dynamic state of person-environment interaction associated with varying levels of human need fulfillment
- Human need fulfillment leads to maximal wellness for the client
- Optimal wellness is unique for each client
- Deficits in human need fulfillment lead to diminished wellness
- Health and oral health contribute to human need fulfillment
- Oral wellness is achieved through fulfillment of human needs of the client

Adapted from Yura, H., and Walsh, M. B. The Nursing Process, 5th ed. Norwalk, CT: Appleton & Lange, 1988, pp. 97–98.

PROPOSITIONS ASSOCIATED WITH THE CONCEPT OF DENTAL HYGIENE ACTIONS

- Dental hygiene is interpersonal in nature
- The goal of dental hygiene is the achievement of optimal oral wellness for the client
- Oral wellness is achieved by facilitating the integrity of human need fulfillment of the client
- Oral wellness, the goal of dental hygiene, is achieved through the use of the dental hygiene process
- Dental hygiene actions effect changes in the client-environment interaction that enable the client to achieve greater human need fulfillment
- The dental hygienist and client are co-participants in the application of the dental hygiene process
- Dental hygiene outcomes depend on the client's active involvement in the process of care
- Human needs theory is the framework for using the dental hygiene process, research process, communication process, and leadership process to enable the client to achieve greater human need fulfillment
- Dental hygiene interventions facilitate fulfillment of human needs over the lifespan

Adapted from Yura, H., and Walsh, M. B. The Nursing Process, 5th ed. Norwalk, CT: Appleton & Lange, 1988, pp. 99–100.

change agent, consumer advocate, educator, and researcher. Figure 1–1 (see Chapter 1), developed by MacDonald, emphasizes this latter point. The model for the concept of dental hygiene actions is shown in Figure 2–5. This concept is described in the Propositions Associated with the Concept of Dental Hygiene Actions chart.

The Human Needs Conceptual Model and the Dental Hygiene Process

Having defined the four major paradigm concepts of client, environment, health and oral health, and dental hygiene actions in terms of human needs theory, the human needs conceptual model proposed by Darby and Walsh identifies 11 human needs as being particularly relevant to dental hygiene care.[1,2,7] The four major concepts, the propositions that define them, and the 11 human needs related to dental hygiene care provide a theoretical framework for the application of the dental hygiene process (Fig. 2–6). Baseline assessment to determine whether the 11 human needs are met provides a framework for planning, implementing, and

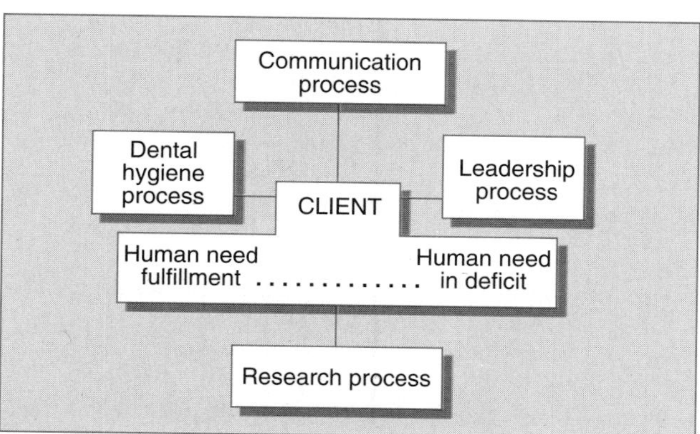

FIGURE 2–5
The concept of dental hygiene actions in the human needs conceptual model of dental hygiene. (Redrawn from Yura, H., and Walsh, M. B. The Nursing Process, 5th ed. Norwalk, CT: Appleton & Lange, 1988, p. 99.)

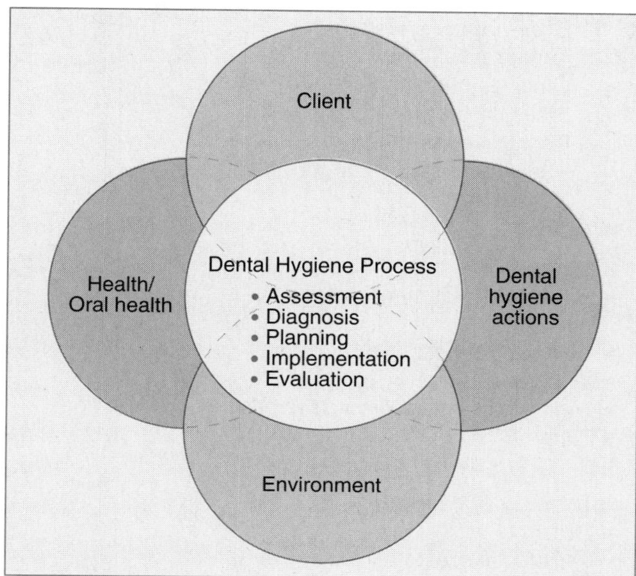

FIGURE 2–6
Relationship of human need theory to the dental hygiene process. (Redrawn from Yura, H., and Walsh, M. B. The Nursing Process, 5th ed. Norwalk, CT: Appleton & Lange, 1988, p. 98.)

Below are 11 human needs related to dental hygiene care. Please indicate whether the need is *unmet* by circling "yes" or "no" in the space provided. If the need is unmet, circle in red the specific deficit listed under each need, and note salient comments.

Human Needs/Deficits	Unmet?	Comments
Safety ■ BP outside of normal limits ■ Current serious illness ■ Need for prophylactic antibiotics ■ Concern about: Infection control Radiography Fluoride therapy Fluoridation Mercury toxicity Dental hygiene care planned Previous dental experience ■ Potential for injury ■ *Other*	Yes/No	
Freedom from Pain/Stress ■ Reports or displays: Fear/anxiety Extra-/intraoral pain or sensitivity Discomfort during dental hygiene care Oral habits Substance abuse ■ *Other*	Yes/No	
Wholesome Body Image ■ Dissatisfaction with appearance of: Teeth Gingiva Facial profile ■ *Other*	Yes/No	
Skin and Mucous Membrane Integrity of Head and Neck ■ Presence of: Extra-/intraoral lesion Tenderness, swelling Gingival inflammation Bleeding on probing Pockets > 4 mm Attachment loss > 4 mm Xerostomia ■ *Other*	Yes/No	
Nutrition ■ Extra-/intraoral manifestations of malnutrition ■ Rampant caries ■ Unbalanced diet ■ High sugar intake on a daily basis ■ *Other*	Yes/No	
Biologically Sound Dentition ■ Difficulty in chewing ■ Presents with: Defective restorations Teeth with signs of disease	Yes/No	

FIGURE 2–7
Baseline assessment of 11 human needs related to dental hygiene care.

Human Needs/Deficits	Unmet?	Comments
Biologically Sound Dentition Missing teeth Ill-fitting dentures, appliances Calculus, plaque, or stain Abrasion, erosion ■ No dental examination within the last 2 years ■ *Other*		
Conceptualization and Problem Solving ■ Has questions or misconceptions associated with dental hygiene care ■ Does not understand: What plaque is, its relationship to oral disease, and/or the importance of daily plaque control ■ *Other*	Yes/No	
Appreciation and Respect ■ Expresses dissatisfaction with clinician and/or dental hygiene care ■ Reports disapproval from others about oral hygiene status ■ *Other*	Yes/No	
Self-Determination and Responsibility ■ Does not verbalize awareness of own role in oral hygiene care ■ Inadequate oral health behaviors ■ Does not participate in setting goals for dental hygiene care ■ Inadequate parental supervision ■ *Other*	Yes/No	
Territoriality ■ Verbally or nonverbally expresses discomfort with the proximity of the operator during conversation or dental hygiene care ■ Expresses a need for confidentiality ■ *Other*	Yes/No	
Value System ■ Indicates oral health and hygiene is a low priority ■ Has history of failing appointments ■ *Other*	Yes/No	

FIGURE 2–7 *Continued*

evaluating comprehensive dental hygiene care with diverse clients in a variety of environments. Figure 2–7 provides a tool for the baseline assessment of the 11 human needs related to dental hygiene care. Using this framework, dental hygienists can make dental hygiene diagnoses based upon deficits in these 11 human needs, and then plan, implement, and evaluate dental hygiene interventions designed to meet the identified unmet needs. Grounded in the theory of Maslow, the nursing profession, and others, this human needs conceptual model for dental hygiene care provides a guide for comprehensive and humanistic client care and defines the territory for the practice of dental hygiene.

DENTAL HYGIENE'S 11 HUMAN NEEDS

The 11 human needs listed in Table 2–1 relate to physical, emotional, intellectual, social, and cultural dimensions of the client that are inherent in dental hygiene care. Through the dental hygiene process, the dental hygienist contributes to the fulfillment of these human needs in the client. A discussion of the 11 human needs follows.

Safety

Safety is the need to experience freedom from harm or danger involving the integrity of the body structure and

TABLE 2–1
HUMAN NEEDS RELATED TO DENTAL HYGIENE CARE

Human Needs	Some Dental Hygiene Actions/Implications
1. Safety The need to experience freedom from harm or danger involving the integrity of the body structure and environment around the person	Ensure safety and protection; use current standards for infection control, radiation safety, fluoride therapy, etc. Discuss previous negative experiences related to dental or dental hygiene care Discuss dental hygiene care plan and address safety factors as deemed by client
2. Freedom from Pain/Stress The need for freedom from pain and stress is the human need for exemption from physical and emotional discomforts	If oral pain is reported, initiate pain control immediately, if appropriate, refer client to dentist for immediate care Initiate pain control strategies (i.e., reassurance, utilization of desensitizing agents, instrumentation techniques with care and gentleness, administration of topical anesthesia, local anesthetics and nitrous oxide–oxygen analgesia) Utilize appropriate supra- and subgingival instrumentation procedures and techniques Initiate and/or refer to a program for control of oral habits, substance abuse, chemical dependency, stress
3. Wholesome Body Image The need for a wholesome body image is the need for a positive mental representation of one's own body boundary and how it looks to others	Understand and possess knowledge of how one's body image can affect one's self-concept and motivate behaviors Accept a client's body image, acceptance of the client as a human being who has ideas, feelings, and values Listen to doubts and provide information on outcomes to help meet the client's need for a wholesome body image Focus on positive attributes and features (i.e., compliment client on some aspect of his appearance) Encourage the client to seek other support systems to share feelings about body changes Sensitivity to the client's feelings of insecurity, fears of rejection, or loss of self-worth Awareness of one's own feelings, self-confidence, self-awareness Refer to general dentist or dental specialist, e.g., orthodontist
4. Skin and Mucous Membrane Integrity of Head and Neck The need to have an intact and functioning covering of the person's head and neck area, including the oral mucous membranes and gingivae, which defend against harmful microbes, provide sensory information, and resist injurious substances and trauma	Observe and record finding about all skin and mucous membranes in and about the oral cavity Recognition, care, and follow-up of specific lesions significant to the general and oral health of the client Dental hygiene strategies Plaque control instruction Performing therapeutic scaling and root planing Referral to other healthcare providers Subgingival irrigation with antimicrobial Oral cancer examination Measure outcomes of dental hygiene care
5. Nutrition The need to ingest and assimilate sufficient amounts of carbohydrates, proteins, fats, vitamins, minerals, trace elements, and fiber required for growth, repair, and maintenance of structurally and functionally competent bodily parts	Intra- and extraoral examination, assessment, and interviewing skills may be used to identify nutritional problems and provide sound counseling and appropriate referral Recognition of signs of inadequate nutrition and initiate change Referral to other healthcare providers
6. A Biologically Sound Dentition The need for intact teeth and restorations that defend against harmful microbes and provide for adequate function and esthetics	Continuous evaluation of client's dentition and its condition specific to dental hygiene care Advocacy for sound and functioning dentition Referral to general dentist or specialist
7. Conceptualization and Problem Solving The need to grasp ideas and abstractions, to make sound judgments about one's life and circumstances	Explain rationale and details of methods recommended for the prevention and control of oral diseases Measure the client's oral health knowledge Appeal to the client's need for conceptualization and problem solving Promote self-evaluation of oral cavity and head and neck by the client
8. Appreciation and Respect The need to be acknowledged for achievement, worth, service or merit, and to be regarded favorably, with admiration and approval by others	Incorporate attributes for a good clinician-client relationship Verbal and nonverbal cues Empathy and empathic communication skills Understand and accept the client's feelings, emotions, and attitudes Foster acceptance of self (client) as a human being Facilitate acceptance of his oral health status and treatment needs Serve as a client advocate

TABLE 2–1
HUMAN NEEDS RELATED TO DENTAL HYGIENE CARE *Continued*

Human Needs	Some Dental Hygiene Actions/Implications
9. Self-Determination and Responsibility The need to exercise firmness of purpose about one's self and accountability for one's behavior	Initiate behavior patterns to maintain oral wellness and measure the client's oral health behaviors Appeal to the client's sense of self-care and the client's active participation in formulating objectives for dental hygiene care Facilitate decision making by the client
10. Territoriality The need to possess a prescribed area of space or knowledge that a person denotes as one's own, maintains control over, and defends if necessary, and is acknowledged by others as owning	Respect the client's personal space by awareness of verbal and nonverbal cues Recognize the need for territoriality as a significant factor when interacting with clients from diverse cultures
11. Value System The need to have the freedom to develop one's own sense of the importance of people, institutions, things, activities, and experiences in one's life	Influence client's value of oral hygiene care, oral disease prevention, and oral health maintenance Advocate optimal oral wellness as one of the client's priorities Recognize cultural diversity and the values associated with health and disease within a defined culture or subculture Serve as a client advocate

Adapted from Yura, H., and Walsh, M. B. The Nursing Process, 5th ed. Norwalk, CT: Appleton & Lange, 1988.

environment around the person. Generally, the safety need also includes the need for security, stability, dependency, protection, and freedom from fear and anxiety.[5] It also encompasses the need to be in a state of good general health through efficient functioning of body organs and systems, or under the active care of a physician in a controlled state of general health that provides for adequate function of body organs and systems.

Assessment

This need is assessed by careful evaluation of the client's verbal and nonverbal behavior during the history taking, and by direct observation of the client's techniques and dexterity in using oral hygiene devices for personal bacterial plaque control to ensure that no self-harm can occur. Information related to the client's general health is obtained by the dental hygienist through interview and questionnaire methods as well as by clinical and radiographic examination techniques. Indications that the client's need for safety is *unmet* include, but are not limited to, the following:

- Indication on the health history of the need for immediate referral to or consultation with a physician regarding uncontrolled disease (e.g., signs of a cardiac problem or of a blood pressure reading outside of normal limits) or of the need for prophylactic antibiotic premedication
- Evidence that the client is at risk for oral injury
- Evidence of the client's anxiety over such issues as previous negative dental experiences, current care to be provided, infection control, having radiographs made, and recommended fluoride therapy

Implications for Dental Hygiene Care

The need for stable general health significantly affects all dental hygiene care provided and its expected outcomes. Oral health exists in a biological relationship with the entire body. Oral tissues are often sensitive indicators of the general health or disease state of the client. Many systemic diseases produce oral changes that may be part of the primary disease process (e.g., oral cancer) or a complication of it (e.g., candidiasis resulting from antibiotic therapy for a systemic problem). Thorough monitoring of health histories, vital signs, and extra- and intraoral tissues can assist in the recognition of undiagnosed conditions for which the client should be referred to a physician.

Deficits related to the client's need for stable general health greatly affect the dental hygiene care that is planned and implemented. Such deficits also influence the client's response to care, such as tissue healing or compliance with recommended personal oral hygiene care. For example, before assessing oral hygiene and periodontal status with an explorer or periodontal probe, it is essential that the dental hygienist assess the client's general health status by taking a complete health history. This is done to determine whether there are medical conditions that require modification of dental hygiene care so that the client is not put at risk for life-threatening disease. In fact, before performing *any* dental hygiene procedure that involves using an instrument that may impinge on oral soft tissues, the dental hygienist must be certain that the client has no medical condition that requires additional protective measures before treatment (e.g., antibiotic premedication for a client susceptible to infectious [bacterial] endocarditis, or immediate physician referral for a client with malignant hypertension). In addition, using information about the client's general health, the dental hygienist should assess the need for precautions *during* the dental hygiene appointment (e.g., the need to place a client's nitroglycerin tablets within easy reach, or the avoidance of radiation with a pregnant woman) to meet the client's need for safety and to prevent possible emergencies.

If the dental hygienist has any questions regarding the client's general health status and its influence on dental hygiene care, the client's physician should be consulted before dental hygiene care is provided, or clients with no physician of record should be referred to one for examination. Initially obtaining information about the client's general health and updating it at each dental hygiene care appointment is essential to ensuring that the client's need for safety is met.

To some clients, the dental hygiene appointment itself may signal threat or danger and may trigger the need to ensure safety and protection. Being confronted with strangers, uncontrollable objects (e.g., dental hygiene instruments), loss of parental protection (for children), and the risk (however minute) of contracting an infectious or life-threatening disease such as acquired immunodeficiency syndrome (AIDS) all are threats to the need for safety.

The dental hygienist should discuss with the client previous negative experiences related to dental or dental hygiene care and should reassure the client that every effort will be made to provide care in as comfortable and safe a manner as possible. Planned care and its rationale should be discussed in detail, as should the methods taken to ensure the client's safety. Clients also may reveal lifestyle practices that place them at risk for oral injury, oral infection, or oral cancer. For example, the potential for oral injury may exist in an adolescent who plays contact sports without the benefit of an athletic mouth protector. A client taking an immunosuppressant drug may be at risk for oral infection, and the person who uses spit tobacco (smokeless tobacco) has a risk for oral cancer. All of these individuals have an unmet human need for safety that can be met through comprehensive dental hygiene care.

To help satisfy the client's human need for safety, the hygienist should answer all questions as completely as possible. For example, clients often ask about safety factors associated with radiation, infection control, mercury-containing dental restorations (amalgam), fluoridation, and fluoride therapy. The client must be reassured with confidence about the safety of these procedures and provided with factual knowledge about the rationales for their use. Informing the client about current research findings is frequently a strategy for meeting the client's safety needs in the oral healthcare environment. Of course, current standards of care to ensure the client's safety and protection always should be followed.

Freedom From Pain and Stress

The need for **freedom from pain and stress** is the human need for exemption from physical and emotional discomforts.[5] This human need is a strong motivator for clients to perform behavior that will lead to its fulfillment.

Assessment

Whether this need is fulfilled can be assessed by evaluating the client's verbal and nonverbal behavior, as well as by careful examination of the face and oral cavity for signs of stress. Verbal behavior is evaluated by inquiring about the client's reason for seeking dental hygiene care and in collecting data during history taking and during the intra- and extraoral examinations. Nonverbal behavior is evaluated by careful observation of the client upon reception, during history taking, and throughout the provision of dental hygiene care. For example, when the need for freedom from pain and stress is fulfilled, the client:

- Reports comfort and no emotional distress or systemic pain, no medication being taken for pain, and no extra- or intraoral pain or sensitivity is found upon examination
- Displays ease of movement, relaxed face, hands, and legs
- Speaks without hesitation or breaks in sentences
- Evidences no excessive perspiration (no sweaty palms or beads of perspiration on forehead) and no tears from crying

Specifically, with regard to dental hygiene care, indications that the client's need for freedom from pain and stress is *unmet* include, but are not limited to, the client's self-report or display of at least one of the following:

- Fear or anxiety
- Extra- or intraoral pain or sensitivity
- Discomfort or pain during dental hygiene care
- Oral habits related to stress (e.g., bruxism, nailbiting, thumbsucking)
- Substance abuse

Table 2–2 lists some oral habits associated with stress, their clinical manifestations, and suggested dental hygiene interventions.

TABLE 2–2
SELECTED ORAL HABITS ASSOCIATED WITH STRESS

Oral Habits	Clinical Manifestations	Suggested Interventions
Bruxism	Decrease in canine height and flattening of occlusal plane and/or incisal edge	Night guard Stress management
Thumb- and fingersucking	Altered facial appearance Crossbite Anterior overjet Lips irreversibly stretched by protruding teeth Deep, narrow palate Callous on finger or thumb	Build a cooperative alliance with the child Increase child's awareness of problems related to sucking Block hand-to-mouth movement Add incentives for success (see chart Interventions To Break The Thumb- or Fingersucking Habit)
Smoking	Nicotine stomatitis Bad breath Black hairy tongue Discoloration of teeth Oral leukoplakia Oral cancer	Advise to quit Set quit date Cut down use prior to quit date Self-help techniques for coping with withdrawal Nicotine gum or patch prescription
Spit*(smokeless) tobacco use	Oral leukoplakia Localized gingival recession Tooth abrasion and erosion Oral cancer	See above (smoking)

*The term "spit" is preferred over "smokeless" by the Surgeon General because smokeless conveys a sense of safety and acceptability.

Implications for Dental Hygiene Care

If stress or pain is apparent at the beginning of or during the dental hygiene appointment, the dental hygienist should initiate pain or stress control interventions immediately, if appropriate, or should refer the client to the dentist for immediate care. Ways in which the dental hygienist can provide pain control and stress control for clients are listed in the Pain Control Interventions chart and the Stress and Anxiety Control Interventions chart. Because the mouth is a very sensitive area of the body, dental hygienists need to provide supra- and subgingival instrumentation as carefully and as gently as possible, especially when treating a client who is not anesthetized.

When indicated, the dental hygienist should initiate, or refer clients to, a program for control of oral habits, substance abuse, chemical dependency, and stress. If evidence of chemical dependency on tobacco or other substances is noted, the dental hygienist should advise clients to quit using it and provide information on the associated negative health effects and on strategies and resources available to help them quit. For example, with regard to tobacco, research suggests that advice to quit from a health professional may be an effective intervention for promoting cessation of tobacco use.[15] Clients who evidence oral habits associated with stress, such as bruxism or thumbsucking, also should be informed of the risks for negative effects and provided with strategies and resources to help them modify their behavior. (See Interventions to Break the Thumb- or Fingersucking Habit chart.)

STRESS AND ANXIETY CONTROL INTERVENTIONS

- Demonstrating humanistic behaviors such as compassion, warmth, empathy, acceptance of feelings, sensitivity, respect for privacy, listening, helping, demonstrating, and touching
- Providing the client with a sense of control (e.g., always ask permission, explain procedures, make care predictable, and stop when the client requests a break)
- Encouraging client involvement and participation in care
- Obtaining informed consent
- Using open and honest communication
- Planning short appointments and scheduling them in the early morning
- Using nitrous oxide–oxygen analgesia unless contraindicated
- Conversing with the client throughout the appointment; regularly asking how the client is doing
- Using the "tell-show-do" approach
- Reinforcing client successes in treatment

PAIN CONTROL INTERVENTIONS

- Providing the client with a sense of control (e.g., always ask permission, explain procedures, and make care predictable)
- Reassuring the client that the dental hygiene care procedure will be made as comfortable as possible
- Adjusting the chair so that the client with back trouble is comfortable
- Applying topical desensitizing agents to sensitive roots
- Performing instrumentation techniques with as much care and gentleness as possible
- Administering, if indicated, topical and local anesthetic agents to block the transmission of painful stimuli during dental hygiene care
- Depositing a few drops of anesthetic solution and waiting for 5 seconds before advancing the needle during intraoral administration of local anesthetic agent
- Administering nitrous oxide–oxygen analgesia to control clients' apprehension and to help them relax, if indicated
- Taking the client seriously when concern is expressed

With regard to supra- and subgingival instrumentation, the dental hygienist should:

- Adapt instrument blades to the tooth to prevent tissue laceration
- Keep the working-end tip of the instrument in contact with the tooth so that it is not in soft tissue
- Refrain from resting the mouth mirror on the floor of the client's mouth
- Run the hand piece at moderate speed
- Keep the tip of the ultrasonic scaler and the rubber cup in constant and gentle motion when using them to prevent heat from building up on the tooth

Another element of dental hygiene care that should be discussed in terms of the need for freedom from pain and stress is the manner in which the dental hygienist conveys "hurtful" news to the client. (This situation was discussed earlier in conjunction with the need for safety.) Generally speaking, before conveying anxiety-arousing information to a client about an oral condition, dental hygienists should attempt to lessen the client's anxiety by commenting on something favorable about her condition and offering reassurance by stressing positive aspects of her oral health status. For example, instead of saying "You have periodontal disease throughout your mouth," one might say "You were wise to come in for this examination, so that we could begin treatment of your periodontal problem while it's still in the early stages." Other ways of stressing the positive when transmitting "bad news" are listed in the chart Examples of Stressing the Positive and Offering Reassurances When Conveying Anxiety-Arousing Information.

Wholesome Body Image

The **need for a wholesome body image** is the need for a positive mental representation of one's own body boundary and how it looks to others. Body image is determined by one's perception of one's physical characteristics and interpretation of how that image is perceived by others. A person's self-concept is influenced by his view of his physical characteristics and physical abilities. The reverse is also true: a person's self-concept influences how he views his body.[5,6]

Body image is influenced by normal and abnormal physical changes, and by cultural and societal attitudes and values as well. Normal developmental changes, such as growth and aging, affect a person's body image. For example, a 2-year-old's body image is very different from an infant's, because of the ability to walk. This physical change, walking, depends on physical maturation. In addition, hormonal changes produce physical changes during adolescence, pregnancy, menopause, and middle and old

INTERVENTIONS TO BREAK THE THUMB/FINGERSUCKING HABIT

Build a cooperative alliance with the child. At age 5 generally, children are ready to stop.

Parental Intervention

1. Select a quiet time to initiate a thumbsucking discussion. "Maybe it's time to stop thumbsucking." Begin by making the child aware of the problems thumbsucking can cause. Child must be motivated to decide to end the habit. Reading a book like *David Decides** to a child provides a relaxed and effective way to launch the information and motivation process
2. Select a follow-up program of behavior modification through concrete rewards
   - For example, offer a longed-for toy, special privileges, or a desirable outing
   - Use a chart to keep count of successful thumbless days and nights with stars. Give a reward after the first day or night and again after five stars
3. Help the child become aware of habitual sucking by covering the thumb or finger with a bandage, taping a tongue depressor to the inside of the child's elbow, putting socks around each hand at night and taping them to the wrist so they cannot be pulled off while sleeping; thumb-coating solutions can be painful if they are rubbed into the eye and therefore are not recommended
4. Praise success; do not dwell on failures
5. Can take 2 weeks to 2 months of client-focused parent support

Dental Hygienist Intervention

1. Speak directly to the child about problems associated with thumb- or fingersucking; give practical suggestions that will help to end the habit (see above); dispense thumb bandages, tongue depressors, or tape for socks over the hand at night
2. Do not involve the parent in the follow-up plan (e.g., instruct the child to phone back after a week, and after a month, or to return when the habit has been conquered). In bypassing the parents, the dental hygienist places responsibility directly on the child for breaking the habit and communicates a vital message of confidence that the child can overcome the impulse to suck

* Heitler, S. M. David Decides About Thumb Sucking, A Motivating Story for Children and An Informative Guide for Parents. Reading Matters. Box 300309, Denver, CO 80203.

age that influence a person's body image. Aging involves a decrease in visual acuity, hearing, mobility, and perception, all of which may affect body image.[6]

Cultural and societal attitudes and values also influence a person's body image. For example, Surma women in Ethiopia wear lip plates as a sign of physical beauty. In the United States, society emphasizes youth, beauty, and wholeness, a fact that is apparent in television programs, movies, and advertisements. Thus, these cultural attitudes and values affect how people perceive their physical bodies, because body image is a combination of the ideal and the real.[6]

People generally do not adapt quickly to changes in the physical body. Studies have shown, for example, that people who have experienced significant weight loss do not readily perceive themselves as thin; in some cases such people continue dieting to an extreme degree in an effort to become thinner, because they still retain their old body images. Another example is normal aging. People often report that they do not feel different, but when they look in the mirror they are surprised by their aged facial characteristics.[6]

Changes in the appearance or function of a body part or feature are **body image stressors** because they may bring about change in a person's body image. For example, facial disfigurement due to disease, trauma, or surgery is an obvious stressor affecting body image. Stressors that affect body image through a change in function include but are not limited to arthritis, diabetes, renal disease, cardiac disease, and tooth loss. With such changes, the body no longer functions at an optimal level and the person is physically limited. Even the normal changes resulting from aging are stressors that can affect a person's body image.[6]

The importance of a loss of function or a change in appearance is partly determined by individual perceptions of the alteration and personal estimations of how others perceive that alteration. For example, if one associates possession of natural teeth with femininity or masculinity, loss of teeth may be a very significant alteration, one that may threaten the person's sexuality or sense of self. Similarly, clients with dentures, a cleft lip, or facial disfigurement after surgical treatment of oral cancer may reduce social contacts out of fear of people's reactions to them.[13] Such clients may feel isolated, excluded, stigmatized, or helpless. Their feeling of social isolation may be based in reality, because people may avoid contact with them for fear of causing embarrassment or offense. Thus, body image stressors can negatively alter one's body image, which in turn may negatively alter one's self-concept and behavior.[14]

Indications that the client's need for a wholesome body image is fulfilled include such evidence as clients' stating

EXAMPLES OF STRESSING THE POSITIVE AND OFFERING REASSURANCES WHEN CONVEYING ANXIETY-AROUSING INFORMATION

"It's a good thing this problem was discovered in time, this gives us a chance to do something about it."

"Most of your mouth is in good health. . . . "

"No problem with your toothbrushing, but we could do something about. . . . "

"Fortunately it's in its early stages. . . . "

"There's a lot you can do to save your teeth. . . . "

From Department of Periodontology, School of Dentistry, University of California at San Francisco. Plaque Control Instruction. Berkeley, CA: Praxis Publishing Co., 1978.

they are actively engaged in exercise to maintain body health; expressing satisfaction with their appearance; being neatly groomed, making an effort to bring out the best of bodily assets—clothing, makeup, hairstyle—and having good posture and weight congruent with height. The dental hygienist must be careful to assess wholesome body image in terms of the client's culture and not from an ethnocentric perspective (see Chapter 6).

In relation to dental hygiene care, the satisfaction one has with the general appearance of one's teeth, gingivae, mouth, and facial profile is intimately related to whether one's need for a wholesome body image is satisfied.

Assessment

The dental hygienist bases the assessment of the client's need for a wholesome body image on information obtained from the health, dental, personal, and cultural histories; perceptions resulting from direct observation of the client; and inferences from casual conversation with the client. For example, the satisfaction a client has with the general appearance of the teeth, mouth, and facial profile can be determined by asking specific questions such as, "Is anything about your teeth bothering you?" or "Is there anything about your mouth that concerns you?" Similar questions may elicit responses indicating dissatisfaction with such conditions as extrinsic stain, calculus, receding gums, bleeding gums, a discolored restoration, or malaligned teeth. Specifically with regard to dental hygiene care, indications that the client's need for a wholesome body image is *unmet* or *in deficit* include, but are not limited to, the client's self-report of dissatisfaction with the appearance of the teeth, gingivae, or facial profile. Such need deficits have implications for dental hygiene care and for referral to other health professionals for additional care.

Implications for Dental Hygiene Care

Tooth loss, malaligned teeth, oral cancer, and facial disfigurement are examples of body image stressors related to the oral cavity that dental hygiene clients may experience. For clients undergoing treatment related to these stressors, the dental hygienist should listen to their doubts about treatment outcomes and provide information and reassurance as needed. Complimenting such clients on some aspect of their appearance assists them to focus on positive attributes and features. For some clients, encouragement to seek other support systems to share feelings about body changes may be helpful in assisting them to reinforce accomplishments, strengths, and positive attributes.[14]

Body image stressors affect self-concept and motivate behavior, including oral health behavior. The dental hygienist's acceptance of a client with an altered self-concept due to body image stressors may be the factor that stimulates positive rehabilitative results. For example, for clients whose physical appearance has changed drastically from head and neck cancer surgery and who must adapt to a new body image, being accepted by the dental hygienist as a human being who has ideas, feelings, and values and who is worthy and whole despite illness or physical alterations is important and can provide an example for the client and his family that affirms the client's self-worth. The client's feelings of insecurity, fears of rejection, or loss of self-worth can be lessened through sensitive, knowledgeable dental hygiene care. Being in touch with one's own feelings and expectations about clients undergoing such body image stressors is extremely important, because a dental hygienist's reaction to a client's illness or physical alteration can have a significant impact on the client's self-concept and the outcome of care. A client with low self-esteem because of altered body image may be particularly sensitive to the way in which the dental hygienist involves him in his own care. A dental hygienist who lacks self-confidence regarding her own feelings about the client's physical alteration may be hesitant in making suggestions, thus inadvertently implying that the client might be unable to follow suggestions. Or the dental hygienist may insist that the client assume too much responsibility for his own care, thus causing anxiety and frustration. In either case the client's self-esteem and body image may be additionally threatened rather than strengthened. If, however, the dental hygienist demonstrates confidence in the client's abilities and is self-confident with regard to her personal feelings about and expectations of the client, then the client's sense of wholesome body image, as well as self-worth, will be reinforced.[6]

Skin and Mucous Membrane Integrity of the Head and Neck

This human need is defined as the need for an intact and functioning covering of the person's head and neck area, including the oral mucous membranes and gingivae, which defend against harmful microbes, provide sensory information, and resist injurious substances and trauma.

Assessment

Assessment of this human need occurs initially by careful observation of the client's face, head, and neck area as part of an overall appraisal of a client upon reception and seating, and by careful examination of the oral cavity and adjacent structures prior to planning and implementing dental hygiene care.

With regard to dental hygiene care, indications that this human need is *unmet* include, but are not limited to, the following:

- The presence of extra- and intraoral lesions, tenderness, or swelling
- Gingival inflammation
- Bleeding on probing
- Probing depths or attachment loss greater than 4 mm
- Presence of xerostomia, with accompanying oral mucous membranes that are not uniform in color

Implications for Dental Hygiene Care

The dental hygienist should chart existing conditions of the periodontium and oral mucosa, including all deviations from normal. Basic periodontal assessments that should be charted are recession, pocket depth measurements, attachment loss, possible food impaction areas, areas of suspected mucogingival involvement, furcation involvement, abnormal frenal attachments, inadequate zones of attached gingivae, and mobility and fremitus of teeth. Degree of severity of periodontal disease (slight, moderate, severe), extent of bleeding on probing, and areas where exudate can be expressed from the pockets should also be recorded. Moreover, distribution of gingival changes such as inflammation and recession should be documented as being localized or generalized, and the areas of most severe disease involvement should be specified (see Chapter 13).

The dental hygienist has the responsibility to observe all skin and mucous membranes in and about the oral cavity, and to record and call to the attention of the dentist and the client those areas that evidence disease. A variety of skin and oral mucosal lesions may be observed that may or may not be symptomatic. Recognition, treatment, and follow-up of specific lesions may be of great significance to the general and oral health of the client. Routine extra- and intraoral examination of clients at the initial and each maintenance care appointment provides an excellent opportunity to control oral disease by early recognition of lesions that can then receive treatment and follow-up care. At least annually, clients should be screened to detect potentially cancerous lesions. Moreover, it may be necessary for the dental hygienist to postpone a current appointment because of a client's need for urgent medical consultation or because of evidence of infectious lesions, such as herpes labialis or chancre.

Because periodontal disease is epidemic in the United States and elsewhere, the human need for skin and mucous membrane integrity of the head and neck is usually *unmet* in clients seeking dental hygiene care. In periodontal disease, the sulcular, or pocket, epithelium becomes ulcerated and bleeds readily on gentle probing. Because the epithelium is not intact, harmful microbes enter the periodontal tissues. Exudate may appear at the entrance to the pocket or may be expressed from the pocket. Under these circumstances, dental hygiene strategies to meet the human need for skin and mucous membrane integrity of the head and neck include the following:

- Providing bacterial plaque control instruction
- Performing scaling with or without a coronal polish
- Performing root planing, and possibly subgingival irrigation with antimicrobial agents
- Referral to the general dentist or the periodontist for specialty care

Nutrition

Nutrition is the need to ingest and assimilate sufficient amounts of carbohydrates, proteins, fats, vitamins, minerals, trace elements, and fiber required for growth, repair, and maintenance of structurally and functionally competent body parts.[5] That this need is met is indicated when the client reports normal healing patterns within the confines of the health history; reports eating a variety of foods, including those in the four main food groups and food pyramid; reports low daily sugar intake and having access to food sources and financial resources for food purchases; and maintains weight within 15% of ideal as listed in height and weight standards of Metropolitan Life Insurance Tables.

Assessment

Dental hygienists committed to health maintenance and promotion make nutritional assessment part of the dental hygienist-client relationship. Because food and fluid intake are basic biological needs of all human beings, a nutritional assessment is an essential part of an overall dental hygiene assessment. Nutritional assessment is particularly important for clients who may be at risk for nutritional problems related to tooth loss, ill-fitting dentures, dental caries, and periodontal diseases. A complete nutritional assessment includes collecting data from observation and from a dietary history. When malnutrition or a serious eating disorder such as anorexia nervosa or bulimia nervosa is suspected, referral of the client for medical evaluation is a priority.

Within the scope of dental hygiene, indications that the human need for nutrition is *unmet* include, but are not limited to, the following deficits:

- Presence of extra- or intraoral manifestations of malnutrition
- Rampant caries
- Report of an unbalanced diet or high daily sugar intake
- Evidence of an eating disorder (e.g., trauma around the mouth from implements used to induce vomiting; erosion of teeth, particularly on the lingual and incisal surfaces of maxillary anterior teeth and the occlusal and palatal surfaces of maxillary molars)

Implications for Dental Hygiene Care

Dental hygienists can use their extra- and intraoral examination and interviewing skills to identify nutritional problems and provide sound counseling or appropriate referral. Dental hygienists are in an excellent position to recognize signs of poor nutrition and to take steps to initiate change. Regular contact with continued-care clients at 3-, 4-, or 6-month intervals enables dental hygienists to make observations of the clients' physical status, food intake, and response to dental hygiene care. Dental hygienists should inform dentists of observations that indicate nutritional problems and should incorporate approaches to solving the problem in their care plans.

Clients with rampant dental caries or acute gingival disease, as well as most clients undergoing periodontal therapy, need specific instruction in diet conducive to oral health. (See Diet Instructions Related to Dental Caries and Periodontal Disease chart.) A dietary survey and analysis is necessary to obtain an accurate assessment of the client's diet for study and counseling (see Chapter 21).

A Biologically Sound Dentition

This human need refers to the need for intact teeth and restorations that defend against harmful microbes and provide for adequate function and esthetics.

Assessment

Assessment of a **biologically sound dentition** is ongoing throughout the dental hygiene care appointment, but initially it occurs while the hygienist is taking a careful dental history and carefully observing the client's dentition as part of a thorough examination of the oral cavity and adjacent structures preliminary to dental hygiene care. Indications that the client's need for a biologically sound dentition is *unmet* include, but are not limited to, the following:

- Difficulty in chewing
- Defective restorations
- Teeth with signs of dental caries, abrasion, or erosion
- Missing teeth
- Ill-fitting prosthetic appliances
- Teeth with calculus, bacterial plaque, or extrinsic stain

DIET INSTRUCTIONS RELATED TO DENTAL CARIES AND PERIODONTAL DISEASE

Dental Caries

- Decrease sugar content of diet
- Eat sugar snacks with meals rather than in between meals to reduce acid attacks on the tooth

Periodontal Disease

- Recommended daily allowance of the four food groups; Adequate amounts of protein, ascorbic acid, B-complex vitamins, vitamin A, and mineralizing nutrients such as calcium, phosphorus, and vitamin D
- Avoid eating soft, sticky foods to help minimize plaque build-up
- Before periodontal surgery, ingest adequate amounts of calories, proteins, and vitamins such as folic acid, ascorbic acid, pyridoxine, and pantothenic acid to promote rapid wound healing
- High-energy and high-protein proprietary supplements such as Sustercal or Carnation Instant Breakfast may also be recommended preoperatively and postoperatively
- For clients with acute necrotizing ulcerative gingivitis (ANUG), fulfill the daily food intake requirements by six to eight small meals. Only one or two foods need to be eaten at each meal, but a large enough variety of foods should be selected to satisfy the recommended daily allowance of each food group as reflected in the Food Pyramid

In order to improve the usual deficit in protein intake, foods from the milk, meat, and legumes categories should be especially recommended. The client should make a special effort to eat foods that are rich in vitamin C but not irritating to the sensitive gingivae, such as cooked broccoli, turnip greens, green peppers, and baked potatoes.

Implications for Dental Hygiene Care

Complete examinations with accurate documentation by records and chartings are basic to all healthcare. The dental hygienist is an advocate for a sound, functional dentition. Therefore, the dental hygienist documents existing conditions of the teeth, including restorations, all deviations from normal, and missing teeth.

Preparation of oral radiographs in advance facilitates coordination of clinical and radiographic findings. A bitewing survey is sufficient for charting signs of posterior interproximal dental caries. All teeth with signs of disease and all functional problems should be called to the immediate attention of the dentist. Referral to the dentist and application of topical fluoride and sealants are the interventions most frequently used by dental hygienists to ensure that the client's need for a biologically sound dentition is met.

Conceptualization and Problem Solving

This human need refers to the ability to grasp ideas and abstractions, to make sound judgments about one's life and circumstances.[5] The need for conceptualization related to dental hygiene care is considered to be met if the client understands the rationale for recommended oral hygiene interventions; participates in setting goals for oral healthcare; has no questions about professional dental hygiene care or dental treatment; and has no questions about the etiology of his oral problem, its relationship to oral diseases, and the importance of the solution suggested to solve the problem.

Assessment

The need for **conceptualization** is assessed by listening to clients' responses while counseling them about the causes of oral diseases, ways to prevent and control disease, and contraindications to care.

Indications in the dental hygiene care setting that this need is *unmet* include, but are not limited to, the following:

- Evidence that the client does not understand what bacterial plaque is, its relationship to oral disease, or the importance of daily plaque control
- Evidence that the client has questions, misconceptions, or a lack of knowledge about salient issues related to recommended dental hygiene care

Implications for Dental Hygiene Care

In counseling clients, dental hygienists need to present the rationale and details of methods recommended for the prevention and control of oral diseases. For example, rather than merely telling a client she should floss once a day "to clean her teeth," it is important to explain to her what bacterial plaque is, its relationship to oral disease, and the importance of plaque control in preventing and controlling disease. For example, we know that to promote and maintain periodontal health, one does not have to remove subgingival bacterial plaque completely but need only disturb it mechanically once a day in order to cause a shift in the subgingival flora toward a greater proportion of aerobic microorganisms (those that live in the presence of oxygen), which are associated with health. To help the client understand this concept, the dental hygienist might use an analogy such as the following and say:

> Conceptually, the bacterial plaque on the surface of your teeth below the gum line can be compared to the bacteria found in a pool of water. If you regularly disturb a pool of water, the bacteria growing in it tend to live in the presence of oxygen and in turn are associated with health. However, if you have a pool of water that is not regularly disturbed, the water stagnates and the type of bacteria growing in it shifts to greater proportions of bacteria that live in the absence of oxygen and are associated with disease. Similarly, mechanically disturbing the bacterial plaque on the part of the tooth below the gum once a day creates an environment conducive to the growth of bacteria that grow in the presence of oxygen and are associated with periodontal health. If, however, the plaque below the gum is not disturbed daily, it stagnates and promotes the growth of bacteria that live in the absence of oxygen and cause periodontal disease. The mechanical disturbance of the bacterial plaque on the part of the tooth below the gum oxygenates the plaque and promotes an environment conducive to the growth of "healthy" bacteria.

To help the client conceptualize what bacterial plaque is, where it needs to be disturbed, and its relationship to periodontal disease, the dental hygienist may sketch on a pad of paper, or use already prepared materials, to show where plaque accumulates around the neck of the tooth and in the sulcus; may relate this plaque to inflammation and destruction of the supporting tissues of the teeth; and may explain to the client the use of a disclosing agent to aid in plaque detection and removal. Then, while the client watches in a hand mirror, the dental hygienist should use a disclosant in the client's mouth to clearly demarcate the location and distribution of plaque, have the client point out areas of disclosed plaque, and relate these areas of plaque to the health of the supporting structures of the teeth. To further address the client's need for conceptualization and problem solving, the hygienist should point out signs of gingival and periodontal infection in the client's mouth and should provide the client with skills to self-evaluate plaque removal and gingival health status. For example, while the client observes in a hand mirror, a healthy area of gingivae should be compared with an inflamed area by the dental hygienist. In addition, the value of the periodontal probe should be explained and the probe used to differentiate between a healthy and a pathologically deepened sulcus in the client's mouth. Techniques for toothbrushing and interdental cleaning should be demonstrated in the client's mouth, first by the dental hygienist and then by the client. The client should practice the oral hygiene techniques under the direction of the dental hygienist, and corrections should be made when necessary. In follow-up counseling sessions, the dental hygienist should review basic concepts and goals of care, evaluate the client's success in attaining the goals, and expand the knowledge content of previous sessions.

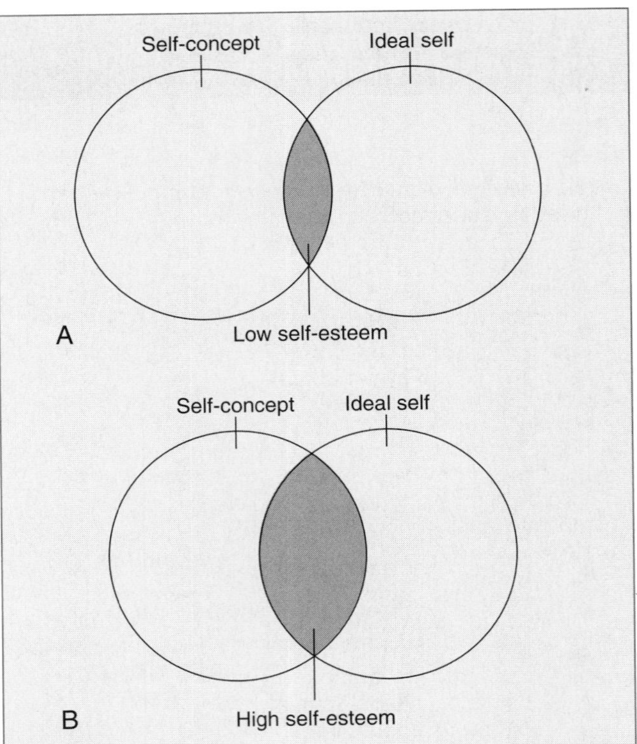

FIGURE 2–8
A, Individual with a low level of self-esteem owing to a large discrepancy between self-concept and ideal self. *B*, Person with a greater conformity of self-concept and ideal self and therefore a high level of self-esteem. (Redrawn from Potter, P.A., and Perry, A.G. Fundamentals of Nursing, 3rd ed. St Louis: C. V. Mosby, 1993.)

Appreciation and Respect

The need for **appreciation and respect** refers to the need to be acknowledged for achievement, worth, service, or merit, and to be regarded favorably, with admiration and approval, by others. Society, culture, and the family generally set the standards by which individuals evaluate themselves.[5,14]

A person has an imperative need to feel competent and worthy of living. Self-esteem is an individual's evaluation of self-worth. Self-esteem begins to develop in infancy, when perceived acceptance or rejection by parents is an important factor. According to Erikson, young children begin to develop a sense of usefulness by learning to act on their own initiative.[16] Self-esteem is often related to one's evaluation of personal effectiveness at school, at work, within the family, and in other social situations.[6]

Although self-esteem depends on many factors, it can be understood in terms of the relationship of a person's self-concept to his or her ideal self. The ideal self consists of the aspirations, goals, values, and standards of behavior that the person considers ideal and strives to attain. The ideal self originates in early childhood and develops throughout life; it is influenced by societal norms, culture, and the expectations and demands of parents and significant others. In general, people whose self-concept comes close to matching their ideal self have a high level of self-esteem, whereas people whose self-concept varies widely from their ideal self have a low level of self-esteem (Fig. 2–8). Extreme disparity between ideal self and self-concept is characteristic of many persons with mental illness.[14]

People with high self-esteem are generally happier and better able to cope with demands and stressors than people with low self-esteem.[17] People with low self-esteem tend to feel unloved and often experience depression and anxiety. Like body image, self-esteem is involved in the enhancement and maintenance of self-concept.[6]

Many stressors may affect the self-esteem of the infant, toddler, preschooler, or adolescent. Inability to meet parental expectations, harsh criticism, inconsistent punishment, sibling rivalry, inability to emulate a successful sibling or parent, or repeated defeats may reduce the level of self-worth. Stressors affecting the self-esteem of adults include failures in relationships, divorce, and loss of a job.[14]

Illness, surgery, or accidents that interrupt or change one's life patterns may also decrease one's feeling of self-worth. Chronic illnesses such as diabetes, arthritis, cerebral palsy, spinal cord injuries, and cardiac dysfunction require changes in a person's accepted and long-assumed behavioral patterns. When a change is slow and progressive, one sometimes has an opportunity for anticipatory mourning, and adaptation occurs along with the change. However, the more a chronic illness interferes with one's ability to engage in activities that make one feel worthy or successful, the more it affects one's self-esteem.[14]

Individuals base their evaluation of self on their relationships with others and on their activities. How an individual defines success or failure influences whether a change is a stressor in terms of self-concept. Societal standards and the responses of significant others also affect the significance of a stressor and its impact on self-esteem.[14] Many people, for example, consider success at work to be important to a sense of achievement and worth. Chronic illness, disability, surgery, or severe trauma may necessitate a change in a person's life work and thus may be self-esteem stressors.

Assessment

In the context of dental hygiene care, the human need for appreciation and respect is assessed by noting clients' responses while taking their health, dental, and personal and cultural histories and while counseling them about the causes of oral diseases and ways to prevent and control them. Possible indications that this need is *unmet* include, but are not limited to, the client's expression of dissatisfaction with the dental hygienist throughout any phase of the dental hygiene process of care.

Implications for Dental Hygiene Care

Appreciation and respect for the client contribute to a good clinician-client relationship, fostering trust and self-acceptance in the client and making adherence to recommended oral care regimens more likely. In general, to meet the client's need for appreciation and respect, the dental hygienist must be sensitive to the client's verbal and nonverbal cues, must practice humanistic behavior during professional interactions, must communicate with empathy and must provide positive reinforcement of desired behavior. At all times, the dental hygienist must demonstrate, through behavior, the unique worth of each client as a human being and ensure that the client's dignity is supported. It is particularly critical for the dental hygienist to be aware of and to exhibit respect for diversity in cultural and ethnic groups and the health beliefs, values, and behaviors associated with them. Moreover, as discussed previously with regard to the need for a wholesome body image, the dental hygienist's acceptance of clients as human beings who are worthy and whole despite physical alterations can lessen their feelings of insecurity, fear of rejection, and loss of self-worth, and stimulate positive rehabilitative results.

Appreciation is primarily communicated by verbal praise of the client and, more powerfully, through nonverbal behaviors, such as head-nodding, eye contact, appropriate facial expression, and other signs of interest and attention. Eye contact is an especially important means of conveying appreciation, and respect. Lack of eye contact is most often interpreted as lack of interest. If the dental hygienist asks the client "How are you today?" while standing with back turned washing hands, or checking the instrument tray, the hygienist may convey indifference about the answer to the question. A good rule of thumb for the dental hygienist is to address the client only when prepared to devote full attention to the client's reply. If clients are made to feel merely like bodies being manipulated by healthcare professionals, they may suffer a loss of self-esteem and avoid dental hygiene care altogether.

Empathy is the attempt to perceive and understand a situation from the point of view of another person and also is a very important component of showing appreciation for and respect to the client. The empathetic clinician conveys the message "I care enough about you to try to understand your feelings, values, and point of view even when they are very different from my own." Empathetic communication requires active listening and an open mind that avoids quick judgments or premature responses, such as finishing the client's sentences. Empathic communication builds up the other person's self-esteem and sense of self-worth, and therefore is an essential communication element related to satisfying the human need for appreciation, attention, and respect.[18]

A powerful and direct means of communicating empathy for the client's situation is a method known as **reflective responding.** In using reflective responding, the listener serves as a mirror to reflect back to the client the attitudes and feelings he or she has expressed. This method was originally developed for use in psychotherapy to communicate the therapist's understanding and acceptance of the client's feelings, emotions, and attitudes. The primary purpose of reflective responding is to communicate the message "I am listening, and I understand." This message is perhaps the single most important ingredient for a good clinician-client relationship. The process of reflective responding can be described very simply. First the dental hygienist must listen and observe to identify the feeling expressed, usually nonverbally, by the client, then restate in her own words the emotion and the situation causing these feelings. The formula "You feel A (describe emotion) because B (describe situation)" may be helpful to remember the components of a reflective response (Fig. 2–9). If, for example, a client's tone of voice and facial expression indicate that he is angry, the hygienist might say "You're pretty angry about losing this tooth" or "You're pretty angry that I didn't spend enough time teaching you to floss last visit." In doing this, the hygienist builds up the client's self-esteem by acknowledging the client's perspective and communicating the message "I care enough about you to listen and to try to understand why you feel the way you do."[18]

Among other nonverbal behaviors that communicate appreciation is the way in which the clinician touches the client. For instance, during the extra- and intraoral examination and in moving the client's head from one side to the other, a gentle touch as opposed to a rough touch communicates concern. Also, alerting the client before adjusting the chair shows the client important consideration.[18]

Respect means an awareness that others are entitled to have feelings and perceptions that are different from one's own. Respect implies the realization that no one holds a monopoly on absolute truth; that others have a right to view things differently from the way in which we do. Note that respect does not necessarily imply agreement. To respect the right of another person to view the world differently is merely to acknowledge that he or she does have that right. One of the most common ways in which lack of respect is communicated is by giving judgmental advice. It is very important to distinguish between giving advice that attempts to make a decision for the client, and giving information. The statement "If you do not brush and floss your teeth daily and seek professional dental hygiene care regularly, you will probably lose that tooth" is information. The hygienist draws on special knowledge and provides the client with facts to which the hygienist has access but the client does not. On the other hand, if the hygienist says "If

**"You feel A [DESCRIBE THE EMOTION]
because of B [DESCRIBE THE SITUATION]"**

FIGURE 2–9
Formula for a reflective response.

I were you I would certainly get up a few minutes earlier in the morning so I could brush and floss my teeth—surely keeping your teeth must be that important to you," the statement constitutes an attempt to make a decision for the client that only she can make. Giving this type of advice may trigger counterproductive responses in the client, which work against a positive clinician-client relationship and against meeting the client's need for appreciation, and respect.[18]

Discussing all procedures with clients, obtaining informed consent, and encouraging their participation in the dental hygiene care plan are examples of ways in which dental hygienists can respect their clients' identities as people who are capable of making decisions for themselves.

Last, the dental hygienist helps fulfill the client's need for appreciation, and respect by assuming the advocacy role. The dental hygienist, acting as a client advocate, recognizes that the client is responsible for the decisions made about his personal oral health. Once that decision is made by the client, the dental hygienist respects the client's decision. Additional information on effective client-dental hygiene interactions is found in Chapter 5 on behavioral science foundations for the dental hygiene process.

Self-Determination and Responsibility

Self-determination and responsibility refer to the need to exercise firmness of purpose about one's self and accountability for one's behavior.[5]

Assessment

This need is assessed from data collected in the client's health, dental, personal, and cultural histories and from direct observation of whether the client is capable of acquiring the skill and know-how for adequate daily oral self-care and interested in accepting the responsibility for performing such care to prevent and control oral diseases.

Indications that this need is *unmet* include, but are not limited to, the following deficits related to the client:

- Inadequate oral health behavior
- Lack of awareness of one's role in oral hygiene care
- Inadequate self-monitoring of active oral disease
- In the case of small children, inadequate parental supervision of daily oral hygiene practices

Implications for Dental Hygiene Care

The dental hygienist should assess the client's oral health behaviors and suggest behavior patterns to the client (or to the parent, when the client is a child) that need to be initiated to obtain and maintain oral wellness. In so doing, the dental hygienist should appeal to the client's sense of self-care and try to evoke the client's need for self-determination and responsibility. The dental hygienist should encourage the client to participate in setting goals and objectives for dental hygiene care, and thus facilitate decision making by the client. Deficits in psychomotor skill development necessary for the client to properly manipulate the toothbrush, floss, or other oral hygiene tools for personal oral hygiene care need to be addressed by the dental hygienist and the client. Recommendations for compensating for psychomotor skill deficits that might be related to degenerative disabilities also should be addressed.

A primary role of the dental hygienist is to motivate clients to adopt and maintain behavior patterns related to oral health. In this effort, the dental hygienist should view the client as being actively involved in the process of care. Using information from the client's history, oral examination, radiographs, and all other data collected during the initial assessment, the dental hygienist in collaboration with the client establishes goals for dental hygiene care. These goals must be related realistically to the client's individual needs, values, and ability level. Because each client has personal requirements for self-care, clients must participate in setting goals and must personally commit themselves to achieving them if oral disease control and prevention are to be successful over the lifespan.

Territoriality

Territoriality is a need to possess a prescribed area of space or knowledge that a person denotes as his own, maintains control over, and defends if necessary, and is acknowledged by others as owning.[5]

Territoriality, the tendency to lay claim to and defend a territory, has been extensively studied in animals. It is not uncommon for animals to risk injury or even death in defending their territory against invasion. Human beings also engage in territorial behavior. Territory usually refers to a specific geographic area, but there is also a kind of portable territory one carries around like an invisible bubble. This zone of distance between the self and others is called personal space, and it is an important but often overlooked variable in interpersonal relations.

Social norms govern the use of personal space. These norms vary with different cultures and within a culture with age, sex, and status. (See Chapter 6 on cultural diversity and the dental hygiene process.) Women, for example, generally stand closer together than do men, children closer than adults, and friends closer than strangers. Distinct zones in which different kinds of social interactions occur have been identified within the mainstream culture of North America. The public zone is approximately 12 to 25 feet and is the distance used to separate public speakers from their audiences. The social zone spans from approximately 2 feet to 11 feet and is the distance used for social interaction between friends or individuals discussing business. The intimate zone spans from touch to 1½ feet, and it is the distance reserved in most cultures for interaction between lovers and between parents and children. When these norms are violated, people react with discomfort and sometimes even with violence. Consider what the reaction of an individual standing alone in an elevator would be if another individual entered the elevator and stood in the intimate zone. Most likely the reaction would be one of such discomfort that the first person would move away immediately, and if the second person followed, angry words and violence might ensue.

Territoriality can also imply the client's need for confidentiality and the dental hygienist's respect for the client's desire for privacy. Failure to meet a client's need for territoriality via a breach of confidentiality may lead to a lawsuit.

Assessment

The human need for territoriality is assessed by directly observing and actively listening to the client during the delivery of dental hygiene care. If the client verbally or nonverbally (by pulling away from the clinician) expresses discomfort with the proximity of the clinician during conversation or dental hygiene care that indicates or suggests a need for personal space, or if the client seems uncomfortable when asked questions on the health history, suggesting a need for privacy with regard to the content of the answers, the human need for territoriality in the dental hygiene care setting is said to be *unmet.*

Implications for Dental Hygiene Care

By its nature, dental hygiene care involves violation of the client's personal space and privacy. For example, it is usually within the intimate zone that dental hygiene care is delivered. In addition, to ensure that the client has no health condition that requires additional protective measures before treatment, the dental hygienist initially must obtain information related to the client's general health and update it at each appointment. The invasion of the client's "personal territory" can be an inherent handicap to communication, and it is critical that the dental hygienist respect personal space and privacy when possible. For example, dental hygienists should keep at least 12 inches between them and the client during intraoral instrumentation, and should back up to at least 2 feet from the client when interviewing or counseling so as not to be threatening. Clients should be reassured that all health history information is confidential. In addition, the dental hygienist should interview clients about their health history in a private area so that answers to sensitive questions (such as "Have you ever had venereal disease?" or, "Are you HIV positive?") can be relayed in a confidential manner. A low tone of voice easily audible to the client, but not to individuals in surrounding treatment areas, should be used when asking questions of a personal and confidential nature. The need for territoriality significantly affects all dental hygiene care provided and may be especially important in interactions with disabled clients and clients from diverse cultures. It is essential for the dental hygienist to be aware of verbal and nonverbal cues related to personal space and invasion of privacy.

Value System

The need for a **value system** refers to the need to have the freedom to develop one's own sense of the importance of people, institutions, things, activities, and experiences in one's life.[5] A **value** is "a personal belief about the worth of a given idea or behavior."[14] If one values a particular idea or behavior, one considers it preferable to others. One then makes decisions based on one's values. Values reflect an individual's human needs, culture, community, and significant relationships. Values differ from individual to individual, and change as individuals grow and mature.[6]

Values provide goals that motivate behavior and are part of a person's identity. For example, the dental hygienist who values compassion interacts with clients in a manner that displays sensitivity and a genuine interest in their comfort. During a conversation or while providing care, such a dental hygienist is aware of the behaviors that exhibit compassion. Such a dental hygienist may also strive to learn new communication techniques that allow for the expression of compassion more effectively.[14]

Related values are organized into a value system, such as those related to religion, freedom, and health. A person's value system provides practical guidance in life.[6] For example, the client who values oral health is motivated to act to achieve and maintain it.

Two types of values, terminal and instrumental, have been identified. **Terminal values** are an individual's ultimate goals, such as a high quality of life or happiness; **instrumental values** involve behaviors deployed in order to reach ultimate goals. Instrumental values are subject to change as a result of life experience. For example, clients whose terminal value is a high quality of life may decide they need to practice good oral health habits in order to reach their ultimate goal.[6] The frequency and intensity with which clients practice oral health–promoting behaviors depend on the value they place on reducing the threat of tooth loss and on achieving the benefit of oral health.

Assessment

In the context of dental hygiene care, a client's values regarding the importance of oral health and hygiene are assessed by evaluating verbal and nonverbal responses about personal oral health and hygiene behaviors, and by evaluating clinical evidence of the client's oral health and hygiene status. Indications that the client's value system is in deficit with regard to dental hygiene behaviors and care include, but are not limited to, the following indications that oral health and hygiene are low priorities:

- Evidence of poor oral health and hygiene despite the possession of accurate oral health knowledge
- A pattern of infrequent or broken oral healthcare appointments
- Failure to adhere to recommended oral care regimens

When evaluating the client's value system, the dental hygienist must rule out the influence of temporary life stressors, such as recent illness, death in family, and financial problems, that may contribute to poor oral health behaviors or lack of compliance in a client. Inadequate oral health behaviors under such circumstances should not lead the dental hygienist to conclude there is a deficit in the client's value system.

Implications for Dental Hygiene

As individuals gain life experience, their values are subject to change. They may reprioritize old values or substitute new ones. When values change, an individual modifies his attitudes and behaviors.[6] The threats posed by disease motivate an individual to reassess health-related values.

A dental hygienist has the responsibility to educate the client about the threats of oral disease and the benefits of oral health–promoting behaviors. Often a client is taught facts and concepts about his oral health status, but his oral health behavior remains unchanged. The dental hygienist who can identify what the client values and wants to know is more likely to develop a successful educational program for the client.

When providing care, the dental hygienist enters into a relationship with a client while possessing a personal and professional set of values. Each client has a value system unique to his own needs. Dental hygienists should not allow their values to conflict with those of clients. Remaining objective enhances the dental hygienist's ability to assist clients in identifying values that influence their own atti-

VALUE SCALE

Below you will find 10 values listed in alphabetical order. Arrange the values in order of their importance as guiding principles in your life. Study the list carefully and choose the one value that is most important to you. Write the number "1" in the space to the left of that value. Write the number "2" for the value that ranks second in importance. Continue in the same manner for the remaining values until you have included all ranks from 1 to 10. Each value will have a different rank.

- A comfortable life (a prosperous life)
- An exciting life (a stimulating, active life)
- A sense of accomplishment (lasting contribution)
- Freedom (independence, free choice)
- Happiness (contentedness)
- Health (physical and mental well-being)
- Inner harmony (freedom from inner conflict)
- Pleasure (an enjoyable, leisurely life)
- Self-respect (self-esteem)
- Social recognition (respect, admiration)

Adapted from Potter, P. A., and Perry, A. G. Fundamentals of Nursing, 3rd ed. St. Louis, C. V. Mosby, 1993, p. 266; and data from Uustal, D. D. Values clarification in nursing: Application to practice. American Journal of Nursing 78:2058, 1978.

tudes and behavior related to oral health. For example, a client threatened by early-to-moderate periodontitis may need to resolve his conflicting attitudes over whether tooth loss is simply a part of living, a punishment from God, or a threat to his overall well-being. The dental hygienist who is able to identify the client's values and incorporate them into the process of care can help the client clarify personal values related to oral health, reorder value priorities, minimize conflict, and achieve harmony among values.

The value scale is a method dental hygienists can use with clients to identify their value priorities. (See Value Scale chart.) When using the value scale, clients rank 10 values in order of importance to them personally. If health is ranked 1, 2, 3, or 4, a client is judged to place a high value on health. If a client ranks health 5, 6, or 7, the value placed on health is moderate, and low if ranked 8, 9, or 10. The information obtained from completing this exercise can help the dental hygienist plan teaching and motivational strategies. Giving clients meaningful and practical information congruent with their lifestyle increases the likelihood that they will assume behaviors that promote oral health.

SIMULTANEOUS MEETING OF NEEDS

Identification of the 11 human needs related to dental hygiene care is a useful way for dental hygienists to evaluate and understand the needs of all clients and to achieve a client-centered practice. A client entering the oral healthcare environment may have one or more unmet needs, and dental hygiene care delivered within a human needs conceptual framework may address all of them simultaneously. Human needs theory provides dental hygiene a holistic and humanistic perspective by addressing the client's needs in the physical, emotional, intellectual, and social dimensions, and defines the territory for the practice of client-centered dental hygiene. Applying this theory when interacting with clients, whether the client be an individual, family, or community, enhances the dental hygienist's relationship with the client and promotes the client's adoption of, and adherence to, the dental hygienist's professional recommendations.

Oral disease disrupts the client's ability to meet his human needs not simply in the physical dimension but also in the emotional, intellectual, social, and cultural dimensions. Therefore, the dental hygienist plans and provides interventions for clients with diverse needs. The dental hygienist first assesses the client's needs and then considers how dental hygiene care can best help meet those needs. After identifying which of the client's human needs are specifically related to dental hygiene care, the dental hygienist, in collaboration with the client, must set goals and establish priorities for providing care to fulfill these needs. Setting goals and establishing priorities, however, does not mean that the dental hygienist provides care for only one need at a time. In emergency situations, of course, physiological needs take precedence, but even then the dental hygienist is aware of the client's other psychosocial needs. For example, when providing care for a client with acute necrotizing ulcerative gingivitis, whose human needs for skin and mucous membrane integrity of the head and neck and for freedom from pain require immediate attention, the dental hygienist also takes into consideration the client's need for appreciation, and respect as well as for safety and territoriality. Although one need may take priority and the dental hygienist often must first be concerned with the highest priority need (such as helping the client cope with her fear of having her teeth scaled before helping the client restore the integrity of the gingival tissues), often the dental hygienist simultaneously addresses needs such as assisting a client in meeting the need for self-determination and responsibility while also helping her achieve adequate nutrition.

References

1. Darby, M. L. Theory development and basic research in dental hygiene: review of the literature and recommendations. Paper presented at the 67th Annual Session of ADHA in San Antonio, Texas, 1990.
2. Walsh, M. M. Theory development in dental hygiene. Probe 25:12–18, 1991.
3. Maslow, A. H. Toward a Psychology of Being, 2nd ed. New York: Van Nostrand Reinhold, 1968.
4. Maslow, A. H. Motivation and Personality, 2nd ed. New York: Harper & Row, 1970.
5. Yura, H., and Walsh, M. B. The Nursing Process, 5th ed. Norwalk, CT: Appleton & Lange, 1988.
6. Potter, P. A., and Perry, A. G. Fundamentals of Nursing, 5th ed. St. Louis: Mosby Year Book, 1993.
7. Walsh, M., Heckman, B., et al. Conceptual Framework for UCSF Dental Hygiene Curriculum. 1988.
8. Fodor, J. T. and Dalis, G. T. Health Instruction Theory and Application, 4th ed. Philadelphia: Lea & Febiger, 1989, pp. 1–163.
9. Bonheur, B., Coots, P., and Kozak, G. Centennial State University, Futyura College of Nursing Curriculum Development Project (unpublished paper). Norfolk, VA: Old Dominion University School of Nursing, 1986.
10. American Dental Association Accreditation Standards for Dental Hygiene Education Programs. Chicago: American Dental Association, 1993.
11. Burket, L. W. Oral Medicine: Diagnosis and Treatment, 6th ed. Philadelphia: J. B. Lippincott, 1971.

12. Jonas, H. J. Oral mucosa membrane markers of internal disease: Part 1. In Dolby, A. E. (ed.). Oral Mucosa in Health and Disease. London: Blackwell, 1975.
13. Dropkin, N. J. Compliance in postoperative head and neck patients. Cancer Nursing 2(5):379, 1979.
14. Potter, P. A. and Perry, A. G. Fundamentals of Nursing, 3rd ed. St. Louis: Mosby Year Book, 1993.
15. Cummings, S. R., Coates, T. J., et al. Training physicians in counseling about smoking cessation. Annals of Internal Medicine 110:640, 1989.
16. Erikson, E. H. Childhood and Society, 2nd ed. New York: W. W. Norton, 1963.
17. Gibson, D. E. Reminiscence, self-esteem, and self-other satisfaction in adult male alcoholics. Journal of Psychiatric Nursing, March 1980.
18. Ingersoll, B. D. Behavioral Aspects in Dentistry. New York: Appleton-Century-Crofts, 1982.

Suggested Readings

Brundage, D. J., and Broadwell, D. C. Altered body image. In Phipps, W. J., Long, B. C., and Woods, N. F. (eds.). Medical-Surgical Nursing: Concepts and Clinical Practice, 2nd ed. St. Louis: C. V. Mosby, 1983.

Combs, A., Richards, A. C., and Richards, F. Perceptual Psychology: A Humanistic Approach to the Study of Persons. New York: Harper & Row, 1976.

Maslow, A. H. Toward a humanistic biology. American Psychology, 24:724, 1969.

McHale, J., and McHale, M. Basic Human Needs: A Framework For Action. New Brunswick, NJ: Transaction Books, 1978.

Molla, P. M. Self-concept in children with and without physical disability. Journal of Psychiatric Nursing 19(6):22, 1981.

Montagu, A. On Being Human. New York: Hawthorn, 1966.

Montagu, A. The Direction of Human Development. New York: Hawthorn, 1970.

Nizel, A. E. Nutrition in Preventive Dentistry: Science and Practice. Philadelphia: W. B. Saunders, 1981.

Piaget, J., and Inhelder, B. The Psychology of the Child. New York: Basic Books, 1969.

Rogers, C. On Becoming a Person. Boston: Houghton Mifflin, 1961.

Sultenfuss, S. R. Psychological issues and therapeutic intervention. In Broadwell, D. C., and Jackson, B. S. (eds.). Principles of Ostomy Care. St. Louis: C. V. Mosby, 1982.

Wilkins, E. M. Clinical Practice of the Dental Hygienist. Philadelphia: Lea & Febiger, 1989.

Yamamoto, K. The Child and His Image. Boston: Houghton Mifflin, 1972.

3 Introduction to the Dental Hygiene Process

OBJECTIVES

Mastery of the content in this chapter will enable the reader to:

- Define the key terms used
- Describe the five stages of the dental hygiene process: assessment, diagnosis, planning, implementation, and evaluation
- Discuss the benefits of using the dental hygiene process as the core of professional practice
- Explain the relationship between human need theory and the dental hygiene process
- Explain the importance of decision making in the dental hygiene process of care
- Note the similarities among processes such as the dental hygiene process, decision making, problem solving, and the scientific method

INTRODUCTION

The **dental hygiene process** is a systematic approach to dental hygiene care. The key behaviors in the dental hygiene process include:

- Assessment
- Dental hygiene diagnosis
- Planning
- Implementation
- Evaluation

These behaviors (Fig. 3-1), inherent to the dental hygiene process, provide the framework for delivering quality dental hygiene care to all types of clients in any environment. Since the term "dental hygiene process" first appeared in the dental hygiene literature,[1] dental hygienists have worked to apply this process in practice. The steps in the process were formally recognized in 1985, when the American Dental Hygienists' Association published Standards of Applied Dental Hygiene Practice (Table 3-1).

The dental hygiene process, with its expectations of decision making and clinical judgment, assumes that dental hygienists are responsible for identifying and resolving client problems within the scope of dental hygiene practice. The process is similar to traditional problem solving, decision making, and the scientific method (Table 3-2).

The process provides a guide for individualizing dental hygiene care. In each step of the process, the dental hygienist and client work collaboratively as co-therapists or partners. When the client's health state or developmental stage restricts client participation, the process is conducted with the help of a primary caregiver, parent, or other support person. The dental hygiene process, with its emphasis on client participation, has transformed dental hygiene so that client values also influence therapeutic strategies and interventions.

Some educational programs have adopted the dental hygiene process as the core of professional dental hygiene practice. They not only teach but also evaluate dental hygiene student performance based on the process of care.

HUMAN NEED THEORY AND THE DENTAL HYGIENE PROCESS

When human need theory is applied to the dental hygiene process, dental hygienists make clinical decisions regarding the need for dental hygiene interventions that, when implemented, satisfy human need deficits and improve the quality of life for individuals, families, communities, and other groups. Human need theory affords the dental hygiene process a theory and philosophy. Human need theory provides a theoretical framework for carrying out the dental hygiene process of care and for exercising clinical decision making, problem solving, and judgment.

In applying human need theory, the professional dental hygienist uses a scientific knowledge base to *assess* the clients' human need deficits related to dental hygiene care, formulate dental hygiene diagnoses, plan and implement dental hygiene care, and evaluate the outcomes of care. The primary purpose of using a human needs framework

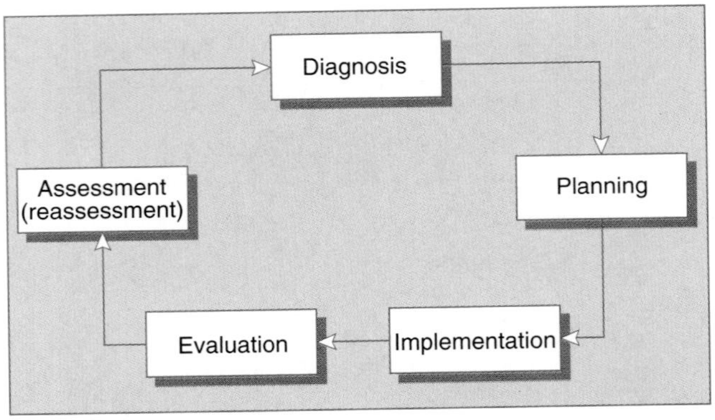

FIGURE 3–1
The dental hygiene process.

for the dental hygiene process is to allow the dental hygienist to manage client care scientifically, humanistically, and holistically and *to ensure that care is client-centered rather than task-oriented.* The five steps of the dental hygiene process are illustrated in Figure 3–1 and defined in Table 3–3. Throughout the process of care, application of human need theory helps the dental hygienist initiate a trusting relationship so that the client feels that individuality is recognized, validated, and respected. The incorporation of human need theory into the five steps of the dental hygiene process is described below and summarized in Table 3–3.

Assessment and Diagnosis

The **assessment** phase is the foundation of the dental hygiene process. It is the art of collecting and analyzing sub-

TABLE 3–1
CORRELATION OF THE ADHA STANDARDS OF APPLIED DENTAL HYGIENE PRACTICE AND THE DENTAL HYGIENE PROCESS

Phases of the Dental Hygiene Process	Standards	Components of the Standards (Assist in Measuring the Quality of Care)
Assessment and diagnosis	**Standard 1** Data on the general and oral health status of the patient are collected systematically, recorded accurately, and communicated and updated continuously using methods consistent with medicolegal principles **Standard 2** The patient data are analyzed, and a dental hygiene diagnosis is formulated	**Standard 1** 1. Data on health status are comprehensive and include information on the patient's general health, oral health, behavioral patterns, environment, and cultural, religious, and socioeconomic background 2. Data are collected from the patient and/or family 3. Health professionals are consulted as indicated **Standard 2** 1. The patient's general health status is analyzed to assess its relationship to oral health status and dental hygiene care 2. The patient's oral health status is analyzed in relation to accepted standards of practice and the degree of deviation is identified 3. Limitations to achieving optimal oral health are identified 4. The dental hygiene diagnosis is related to and congruent with the diagnoses of dentists and other health professionals
Planning	**Standard 3** The dental hygiene care plan is derived from the dental hygiene diagnosis and includes goals, priorities, dental hygiene procedures, and patient action	**Standard 3** 1. Goals are set with the patient and/or family to maximize potential and are congruent with other planned dental treatment and oral and general health status 2. The dental hygiene treatment plan is (a) a sequence of procedures; (b) consultation and referral of treatment when indicated; (c) the optimal type and amount of treatment included at each appointment; and (d) measures to present or control specific patient problems 3. The dental hygiene treatment plan is based on current scientific information, requirements for a functional healthy oral cavity, oral health goals of the patient, patient's responsibility for self-care, and the integration of dental hygiene care with other dental care 4. Priorities are formulated on the basis of the extent and severity of patient needs and are congruent with other planned dental and general health care 5. An explanation to the patient and/or significant others includes the rationale, nature, and prognosis of the recommended dental hygiene care; alternative treatment plans, potential results of nontreatment, and potential risks involved in treatment are discussed

TABLE 3–1

CORRELATION OF THE ADHA STANDARDS OF APPLIED DENTAL HYGIENE PRACTICE AND THE DENTAL HYGIENE PROCESS *Continued*

Phases of the Dental Hygiene Process	Standards	Components of the Standards (Assist in Measuring the Quality of Care)
Implementation	**Standard 4** The dental hygiene treatment includes preventive and therapeutic procedures to promote and maintain oral health, and procedures to prevent or control disease or patient problems and assist the patient in achieving oral health goals **Standard 5** Oral health education assists dental hygiene patients in assuming responsibility for their oral health and in attaining oral health goals	**Standard 4** 1. The patient's general and oral health data are used throughout dental hygiene care to aid in selecting and modifying procedures 2. Consideration is given to the effect of specific procedures on contiguous tissues and the patient's general health and well-being through dental hygiene care. 3. The patient, and family if appropriate, in addition to relevant health professionals are informed of the progress and results of dental hygiene care and self-care 4. The patient, and family if appropriate, are provided with information regarding promoting, maintaining or restoring oral health **Standard 5** 1. An oral health education plan: Is developed on the basis of the dental hygiene diagnosis Is related to the patient's motivational needs, physical limitations, environment, lifestyle, and culture Is comprehensive and an integral part of the dental hygiene care plan and reflects a total body wellness philosophy Reinforces the patient's responsibility for his oral health Involves the patient in establishing goals for self-care, and assessing their attainment 2. The effectiveness of oral health education is evaluated; educational methods and self-care goals and techniques are revised as indicated
Evaluation	**Standard 6** The patient's attainment of oral health goals is evaluated by the dental hygienist and patient. Based on this mutual evaluation, the plan for dental hygiene care is implemented	**Standard 6** 1. Patient data related to the attainment of oral health goals are continuously evaluated by the dental hygienist and the patient 2. Dental hygiene care is analyzed for its effectiveness in attaining treament and educational goals 3. New priorities and goals are established, and additional dental hygiene care and patient self-care are identified and carried out when indicated

Adapted with permission from American Dental Hygienists' Association. Standards of Applied Dental Hygiene Practice. Chicago: American Dental Hygienists' Association, 1985.

TABLE 3–2

SIMILARITIES AMONG THE VARIOUS PROBLEM-SOLVING PROCESSES

Traditional Problem Solving	Decision Making	Scientific Method	Dental Hygiene Process
Problem found or given	Problem in need of action	Statement of the problem	Assessing
Clarification of the problem	Clarification of the problem	Hypothesis formulation	Diagnosing
Finding, creating solutions to the problem	Finding creative alternatives	Plan of action to test hypothesis (data collection)	Planning
Weighing alternatives	Weighing alternatives	Analysis and interpretation of the data collected	
Choosing action to be taken and implementing it	Choosing action to be taken and implementing it	Formulation of conclusions	Implementing
Evaluation outcome	Evaluation of outcome	Verification, rejection, or modification of the hypothesis (repeat cycle if necessary)	Evaluating (repeat cycle if necessary

TABLE 3–3
OVERVIEW OF THE DENTAL HYGIENE PROCESS IN ACTION

Component	Description	Purpose	Activities
Assessing	Collection, validation, and documentation of client data	To make a judgment about the client's oral health status within a human needs framework To determine the client's ability to participate in care	Develop a data base about the client, e.g., health, dental, and socioethnocultural history; intra- and extraoral examinations, dental and periodontal charting, oral radiographs, vital signs, etc. Continuously update and validate the data base Communicate data
Diagnosing	Analysis of client data to identify human need deficits that can be fulfilled through dental hygiene care	To identify human need deficits related to the client's oral health or diseases To identify factors contributing to or causing human need deficits related to oral health To make a dental hygiene diagnosis that will focus on subsequent care To prioritize dental hygiene diagnoses	Analyze and interpret client data Cluster data according to the human needs framework Formulate and validate dental hygiene diagnoses Prioritize list of dental hygiene diagnoses
Planning	Formulation of client goals that, if achieved, will fulfill the client's diagnosed human needs related to oral health	To develop a dental hygiene care plan	Identify dental hygiene interventions and strategies to achieve goals Establish priorities Write dental hygiene care plan
Implementing	Carrying out of the dental hygiene care plan	To work collaboratively with the client and other health professionals to facilitate achievement of goals	Implement strategies Document care provided for continuity, quality assurance, and risk management
Evaluating	Determining if the client's human needs related to oral health have been met as evidenced by the achievement of the established goals	To judge whether the dental hygiene care plan should be continued, modified, or terminated	Measure how well the client has achieved goals Formulate evaluative statement to document client status Identify factors related to success or failure Continue, modify, or terminate the plan

jective and objective data about the client and arriving at a judgment about the client's human needs and barriers to need fulfillment related to dental hygiene care. Client assessment includes obtaining complete health, personal, and socioethnocultural histories, conducting the preliminary intraoral and extraoral examinations, analyzing, and making decisions regarding the findings. Data are derived using both objective and subjective means (Table 3–4). Subjective data are obtained from the client, the client's primary caregiver, or the community or agency of interest. Subjective data, by nature, are less likely to be measurable than objective data and include the reported symptoms, feelings, and beliefs related to oral health and disease. Objective data are measurable by nature because they are signs that can be directly observed. Objective data include physical assessment and oral examination data, the client's record, and observations made by members of the healthcare team. The main focus of data collection is the client's oral health, oral health beliefs and practices, and behaviors as they are affected by his level of human needs fulfillment. During assessment, data are collected and systematically recorded and serve as the basis for decision making throughout the dental hygiene process using the human needs conceptual model. (See Guidelines for Data Collection During the Dental Hygiene Process chart).

The dental hygiene **diagnosis** is the natural conclusion to assessment and focuses on those human needs that can be fulfilled through dental hygiene care. When client human needs are beyond the scope of dental hygiene care, referral to other healthcare professionals is indicated. Dental hygiene diagnoses must be prioritized to provide direction for the dental hygiene actions that follow. The dental hygiene diagnosis increases the likelihood that dental hygiene care is individualized and focused rather than ritualistic and routine.

Dental hygiene diagnoses must be validated to ensure that the client's human needs are the focus of the care plan. A dental hygiene diagnosis is valid when:

- It is based on accurate and complete data
- Both subjective and objective data describe a pattern characteristic of a deficit in a human need related to oral health and disease
- It is based on scientific dental hygiene knowledge
- It can be prevented, reduced, or resolved by dental hygiene care

TABLE 3–4
TOOLS USED DURING ASSESSMENT TO COLLECT OBJECTIVE AND SUBJECTIVE CLIENT DATA

Tool	Purpose	Example
Interaction Data obtained through verbal communication with the client, the primary caregiver, significant other, or healthcare personnel	To gain information To establish a quality dental hygienist–client relationship	Health and dental history taking Discussing Interviewing Socioethnocultural history taking
Observation Data obtained using one's senses (sight, touch, hearing, smell, taste)	*Sight* To gain information about the client's physical characteristics, environmental factors, and nonverbal cues	Reading data from written records
	Touch To gain data from palpation	Intraoral and extraoral examinations; pulse
	Hearing To gain data from the client's verbal messages, as well as percussion and auscultation and environmental factors	Evaluating the opening and closing of the mandible; listening for heartbeat during blood pressure measurement
	Smell To gain data about the odors of the client and environment	Observing the client's breath
Measurement Data obtained using more precise methods than observation	To gain data that is quantifiable	Vital signs Epidemiological data Dental indices Periodontal probe and attachment levels Video and computer technology Photography

Once dental hygiene diagnoses are validated, they provide the major focus for assisting the client in meeting his human need for oral wellness through appropriate dental hygiene interventions. (See Chapter 14 for a more complete discussion of the dental hygiene diagnosis.)

Planning

Planning is the act of determining the types of dental hygiene interventions that can be implemented to solve the client's problem and assist the client in meeting his human needs related to oral health. Planning provides the framework for making decisions and exercising clinical judgments in implementing care. In essence, the plan provides an opportunity to integrate decisions that support a well-focused goal. Furthermore, it focuses the attention of both the client and the clinician and, together with assessment data, establishes the basis on which success is judged during the evaluation phase of the process of care. The tangible outcome of the planning phase is the **dental hygiene care plan.** Sample dental hygiene care plans are found in Chapters 14, 15, and 25.

Dental hygiene diagnoses guide the dental hygiene practitioner's development of the plan of care. Planning involves judging priorities, establishing client goals collaboratively by the dental hygienist and client, based on the dental hygiene diagnosis, and identifying interventions. (See Guidelines for Planning During the Dental Hygiene Process chart). Each

GUIDELINES FOR DATA COLLECTION DURING THE DENTAL HYGIENE PROCESS

- Data are collected using a systematic format
- Data must be focused on the client's oral health status and clustered within a human needs framework
- Data are collected using interaction, observation, and measurement
- Data are both subjective and objective, with attempts to validate both types of information
- Data collection occurs continuously throughout the dental hygiene process
- Data are updated continuously throughout the dental hygiene process
- Data are recorded and discussed with the client and other healthcare professionals responsible for client care
- Data are permanently recorded in a retrievable recordkeeping system for continuity and quality assurance

GUIDELINES FOR PLANNING DURING THE DENTAL HYGIENE PROCESS

- Life-threatening concerns supersede actual or potential human need deficits related to oral health
- Human and material resources available to the dental hygienist and client influence the priorities
- The client's priorities strongly influence the care plan
- Priorities are strongly influenced by the theory and knowledge base of practice
- Planning is influenced by the rules and regulations governing practice and standards of care
- The client's level of human need fulfillment guides the plan of care

goal is related to a specific human need deficit (dental hygiene diagnosis), reflects the expected client outcomes, and guides the dental hygiene and client interventions required to achieve the desired outcome. The goals are client focused and reflect mutual planning with the client. Goals identify specific indicators to measure client performance and a realistic time reference for goal attainment. Goals also facilitate communication among the members of the healthcare team. Although goals vary with the needs of the client, examples of goals might include:

By 9/9, the client verbalizes the importance of interdental bacterial plaque removal
By 10/15, the client reports a decrease in sugar exposures from 12 to four per day
By 12/5, the client reports no gingival bleeding points during daily flossing
By 1/5, the client reports that she regularly wears the athletic mouth protector during all soccer games and practice sessions
By 5/6, the client's pseudopocket on #11 will be reduced by 2 mm

When the client and healthcare providers are aware of the goals being pursued, they are more likely to collaborate successfully to meet the client's needs. This averts the problem of redundancy and omission in rendering care.

Once client goals are identified, the final step in planning is to determine strategies to accomplish the goals. Strategies or dental hygiene interventions should balance ideal and alternative therapies, client capabilities and resources, and client preferences. Although the recommended plan with rationale is shared with the client, the dental hygienist as an advocate supports the ultimate decision of the client. The agreed-on plan is recorded in the client's record.

The dental hygienist collaborates with others while developing the plan (e.g., the client, family, dentist, physician, speech therapist, physical therapist, occupational therapist). Collaboration with other professionals is directed by the client's human needs.

During the planning process, priorities must be established. Judgments are made concerning the relative importance of one diagnosis over another based on risks to life and health, human and material resources, the client's priorities, standards of care, and rules and regulations governing dental hygiene practice. For example, a dental hygienist may analyze client assessment data and determine that the client has human need deficits related to nutrition, wholesome body image, freedom from pain, and a biologically sound dentition. Based on these human need deficits (dental hygiene diagnoses), dental hygiene interventions are planned and prioritized. With top priority attached to freedom from pain, the client in pain is immediately referred to the dentist so the dentist can treat the oral problem causing the pain and restore the oral cavity to function.

Another client may have human need deficits in skin and mucous membrane integrity of the head and neck, wholesome body image, and self-determination and responsibility. The client's priorities and underlying motivations may suggest that the dental hygiene interventions that meet his human need for a wholesome body image supersede other dental hygiene interventions.

Whenever possible, the client is encouraged to engage in the process of care. At one time, planning for client care was done by the dentist for the client based on the dental diagnosis. The client was passive and the dentist and dental hygienist assumed that the client would readily follow "doctor's orders." In today's healthcare environment, the consumer is knowledgeable about health and disease and expects to have an active role in the decisions that affect his oral health, wellness, lifestyle, and quality of life. Therefore, dental hygienists formulate dental hygiene care plans *with* the client. Some clients, by virtue of their age, health status, or limitations, are not capable of being completely involved in the planning process; nevertheless, these clients should be involved as much as possible to meet their human needs for respect, self-determination, and responsibility.

Implementation

Implementing is the act of carrying out the dental hygiene care plan that has been specifically designed to meet the assessed human needs of the client. Implementation includes those actions carried out by the dental hygienist, client, or designated other in order to meet client goals. Each action is performed, and the results are documented in the client's record. The hygienist succinctly records what was done and the client's response to that care.

Evaluation

After dental hygiene care is completed, final evaluation occurs. **Evaluating** is comparing client data at the completion of care with data collected during the initial assessment phase in order to determine the client's progress or lack of progress toward goal attainment. The evaluation phase should produce information about client goals that have been achieved, or that need to be modified. Without evaluation, the dental hygienist can only assume that the interventions were effective. Without evaluation, the client may be dismissed from dental hygiene care prematurely with unmet needs and ongoing risk factors still affecting his oral health status. Each phase of the dental hygiene process is described further and applied in subsequent chapters.

DECISION MAKING AND THE PROCESS OF CARE

Decisions are made by the dental hygienist throughout the process of care. Decision making is the result of deliberate, logical judgment that is guided by human need theory, the dental hygiene process, education, and experience. Dental hygienists use a combination of rational and irrational thought processes as they make decisions required in their many roles. "Rational" and "irrational" are used as descriptors because in reality, decisions are composed of a mixture of approaches to decision making, (e.g., intuition, emotion, trial and error, past experience, acquiescence to others, and using a systematic approach). However, good decision-making skills are essential when a person faces professional, moral, and legal accountability for action taken and judgments made, such as those made in the dental hygiene process. Although the decision-making process is discussed here in terms of the clinician, the principles involved are applicable to the dental hygienist educator, manager, researcher, change agent, and consumer advocate.

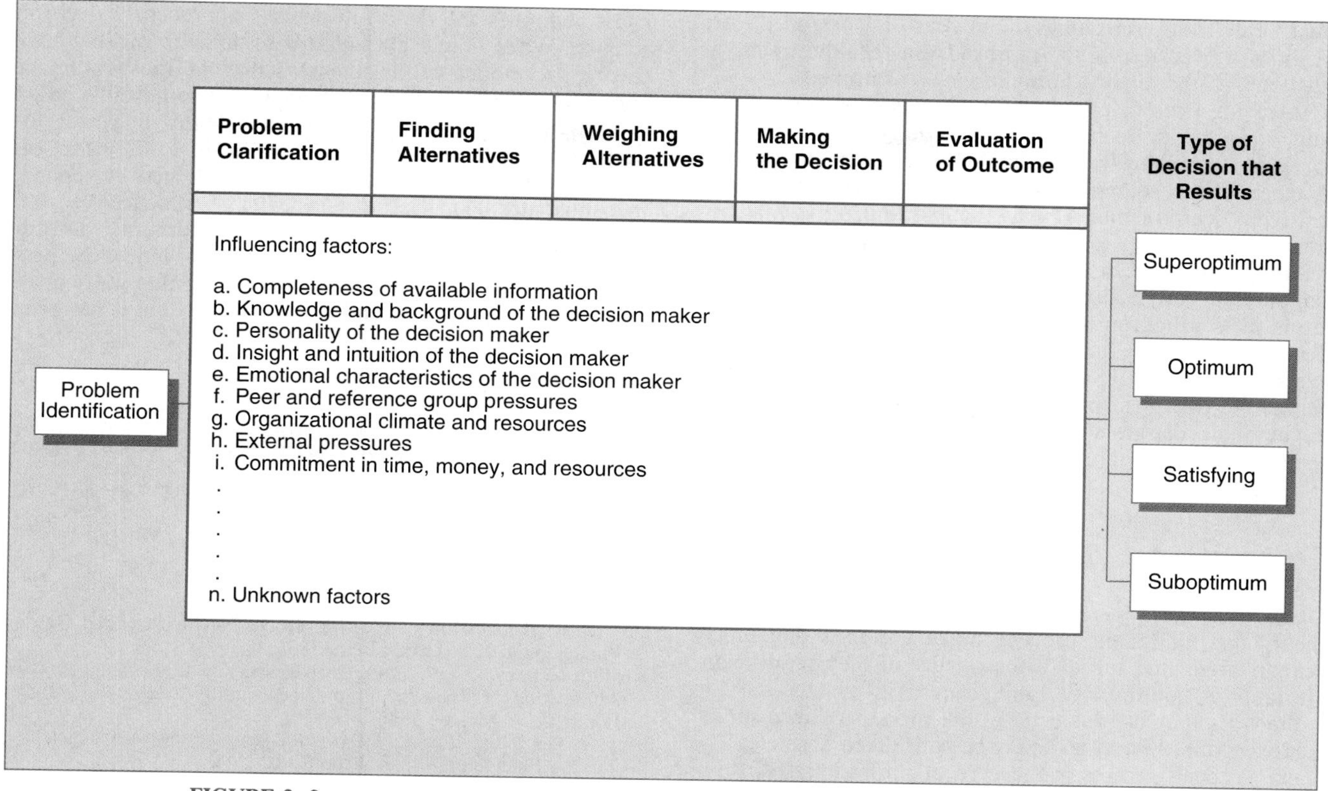

FIGURE 3–2
Decision-making model. (Adapted from DuBrin, A. F. Fundamentals of Organizational Behavior, 2nd ed. New York: Pergamon Press, 1978, p. 78.)

There are various conceptions of decision making. The decision-making model, shown in Figure 3–2, represents the approach to decision making suggested. Following the decision-making scheme, the process is initiated when a problem is identified by the dental hygienist. The dental hygienist may be successful, to varying degrees, depending on the factors that can affect the decision made, e.g., knowledge and personality of the decision maker, peer group influences. It is these intervening factors that account for individual differences in decision-making ability[2] and that make decision making both a rational and an irrational process.

Stages of Decision Making

The stages of decision making include:

- Clarification of the problem
- Finding alternatives
- Weighing alternatives
- Making the decision
- Evaluating the outcome

Clarification of the problem requires the decision maker to explore the problem in greater depth. What are its causes, parameters, and implications if it goes unresolved? Finding creative alternatives enables the decision maker to expand and develop a wide array of possible actions that, if implemented, would improve or resolve the problem. Once problem-solving strategies are identified, they are analyzed (weighing alternatives) according to their relative merits and potential for resolving the problem. The most desirable strategy surfaces, and the choice or action to be taken is made and implemented. The final stage of decision making requires the dental hygienist to evaluate the outcome of the decision. The quality of the decision can be determined only after the result is observed in terms of its ability to move the decision maker or organization closer to the established goal. Hence, evaluation always occurs in terms of the preestablished goal.

Consequences of Decisions

Every decision made by a dental hygienist has some kind of consequence and can be characterized along a continuum from the best to the worst possible outcome. "Superoptimum," "optimum," "satisfying," and "suboptimum" are the terms that have been used to denote the relative quality or adequacy of decisions.

"Superoptimum" refers to a decision that leads to the achievement of goals and beyond. A superoptimum decision might create new directions, philosophies, or constituencies; achieve higher states of client wellness; or meet human needs beyond those originally planned for. For example, the dental hygienist's and dentist's decision to conduct oral health screenings in at least 10 extended-care facilities a year resulted in a 135% unexpected increase in new private practice clients, primarily from the extended families of the nursing home residents. This decision proved to be a superoptimum one.

Optimum decisions are those that result in favorable outcomes as defined by the achievement of the goals established. The dental hygienist's and dentist's decision to conduct oral health screenings in at least 10 extended care facilities a year results in improved oral healthcare for at least 50% of the nursing home residents examined.

Satisfying decisions result in outcomes that are satisfactory, adequate, or acceptable. Conducting oral screenings in at least 10 nursing homes annually in order to provide emergency care to residents in pain might be viewed as a satisfying decision made by the dentist and the dental hygienist.

Suboptimum decisions result in undesirable outcomes. Conducting oral health screenings in nursing homes may result in a suboptimum decision for the dentist and the dental hygienist if time lost from the practice decreases overall office income, if other nursing homes refuse to facilitate the treatment of oral problems in their residents, or if guardians choose to ignore the clients' need for oral healthcare.

CONCLUSION

Dental hygienists, via the dental hygiene process and the theory that guides the process, make decisions that satisfy human needs and improve the quality of life for individuals, families, communities, and groups.

Practices that do not employ the process of care model guided by theory may someday be considered obsolete. The dental hygiene process is the core of professional care because it unifies the dental hygienist's approach to decision making. When dental hygienists base decision making on a theoretical model within the structure of the process of care, they accept dental hygiene as a scientifically based profession. This approach keeps the dental hygienist focused on the unique needs of the client, rather than on tasks (duties). When the dental hygiene process is applied, it contributes to effective and efficient practice because clients can be treated in an individualized manner according to their expressed and observed needs. Hence, the process makes dental hygiene care more deliberate, more goal-oriented, more effective, and less ritualistic than it has been in the past.

References

1. Darby, M. L. The Dental Hygiene Process. Dental Hygiene 55:10, 6, 1981.
2. DuBrin, A. F. Fundamentals of Organizational Behavior, 2nd ed. New York: Pergamon Press, 1978, p. 78.

Suggested Readings

Alfaro, R. Application of Nursing Process: A Step-by-Step Guide. Philadelphia: J. B. Lippincott, 1986.

Griffith-Kenney, J. W., and Christensen, P. J. Nursing Process Application of Theories, Frameworks, and Models, 2nd ed. St. Louis: C. V. Mosby, 1986.

Taylor, C., Lillis, C., and LeMone, P. Fundamentals of Nursing, 2nd ed. Philadelphia: J. B. Lippincott, 1990.

4 Concepts of Health and Wellness

OBJECTIVES

Mastery of the content of this chapter will enable the reader to:

- Discuss the differences between the World Health Organization's 1947 and 1984 definitions of health and others' definitions, as well
- Discuss the concepts of wellness and high-level wellness in relation to health
- Discuss the models of health and health behavior associated with the treatment-orientation and prevention-orientation paradigms of healthcare leading to the current health promotion paradigm
- Differentiate between the three levels of prevention: primary, secondary, and tertiary, and provide an oral health example for each
- Differentiate between health education, health prevention, and health promotion
- Describe health promotion strategies of social marketing, health education, mass media, community organization, advocacy, and legislation
- Discuss the role of the dental hygienist as change agent, manager, consumer advocate, researcher, and educator in health promotion

INTRODUCTION

He is 30 years old and just diagnosed with multiple sclerosis. He is actively involved in his profession (computer programming for the high school curriculum), is committed to fitness, and leads a generally healthy lifestyle. He feels a spiritual awareness that he nurtures through religious activity. Despite the prognosis associated with multiple sclerosis, he does not feel impending doom in his life, but rather a challenge, a learning experience, an opportunity to offer himself to those around him. This person is healthy and well. He is able to meet his human needs.

She has two children, a toddler and a preschooler. They are good youngsters. She is staying home to raise the children while her husband pursues his career. Over the last 2 years, she had been going to school part-time to complete her baccalaureate degree in animal science. Recently, she registered as a full-time student in an effort to complete the program. Her husband would rather she not do this, stating that he would not be prepared to support such an endeavor. Physically, she is in good shape, but emotionally she is very unhappy and in long-standing turmoil. She is not healthy or well. Her human needs are going unmet.

Do you agree with the concluding statements of these two fictional case studies? What constitutes a healthy state? What does it mean to be well? What do these two case studies have to do with being a dental hygienist?

Dental hygienists have a responsibility as advocates and promoters of oral and general health and wellness, change agents, and leaders in achieving health for all (see Fig. 1–1). This chapter conceptualizes the dental hygienist's role in health and wellness promotion, which encompasses the functions of clinician, educator, researcher, manager, client advocate, and change agent.

Dental hygienists view themselves as advocates of personal and professional oral hygiene care for the prevention of dental caries and oral soft tissue diseases. However, to strictly focus on oral health would be narrowly defining the role of the dental hygienist in providing comprehensive dental hygiene care. The scope of responsibility for dental hygienists and all health professionals is to serve the community as resource, as facilitator, and sometimes as mover and shaker to ensure healthy environments. Successful dental hygienists think holistically, envisioning the totality of the body, the mind, and the spirit of the client, perceive how the person relates to the community, and understand which factors influence personal and community health.

Health Defined

Two philosophical trends emerge when one reviews the numerous definitions of health found in the literature. The first has negative implications in that disease is referenced in the definition. Disease is inclusive of all forms of conditions that put humans and their environment at "dis-ease." The second and more contemporary trend is a positive orientation whereby health is an investment toward quality living—the achievement of individual and community wellness. These trends are reflections of the current attitudes and beliefs of society toward the value of health.

In 1947 the World Health Organization (WHO) described **health** as "a state of complete physical, mental and social well-being, not merely the absence of disease or infirmity."[1] Although this definition was very popular in its time, WHO redefined health in 1984 as "the extent to which an individual or group is able, on the one hand, to realize aspirations and satisfy needs, and on the other hand, to change and cope with the environment."[2] This definition recognizes the role of human need fulfillment in the attainment of health and wellness.

In an attempt to define health, and in consideration of the fact that health has historically been measured by the absence of disease, health and disease are viewed as a continuum, with each existing in a dynamic state of flux and in varying degrees, rather than as an either/or state.[3–7]

Health has come to mean the "possessed resource" that enables individuals and the community to achieve their aspirations and adapt to and manage the environment. In defining health, it is essential to consider the cultural reference and the norms of society, so as to avoid imposing biases often associated with the construct of health. For example, Meyerson, in her cultural considerations of Latinos, reported that to many Latinos illness is caused by both chance and a divine plan to test an individual through suffering.[8] She summarizes one study involving several hundred women in Mexico City who were asked what they thought caused their child's cleft lip and palate.[9] The most frequently reported etiologies they cited were paternal alcoholism (71%), lunar eclipse (63%), and God's punishment for sins (52%). Another study was the belief that if a woman did not satisfy her food craving during pregnancy, the fetus would become damaged.[10] Some Latino groups believed that a child with a defect was a gift from God to a chosen family, that is, the defect was not seen as unhealthy.[11] Healthcare professionals must avoid imposing their own definition of health on their clients because successful healthcare intervention requires knowledge and appreciation of cultural attitudes.[8,12–14]

Wellness Defined

The wellness concept emerged in the mid-twentieth century when Dunn presented a philosophy of life that went beyond the possession of health and the absence of disease as measures of good productive lives.[15] Dunn differentiated health from wellness, defining the former as "a relatively passive state in which an individual is at peace with the environment—achieving a condition of relative homeostasis.[16] **Wellness** is a dynamic method of functioning—a condition of change in which the individual moves forward, climbing toward a higher potential of functioning."[16] Well-

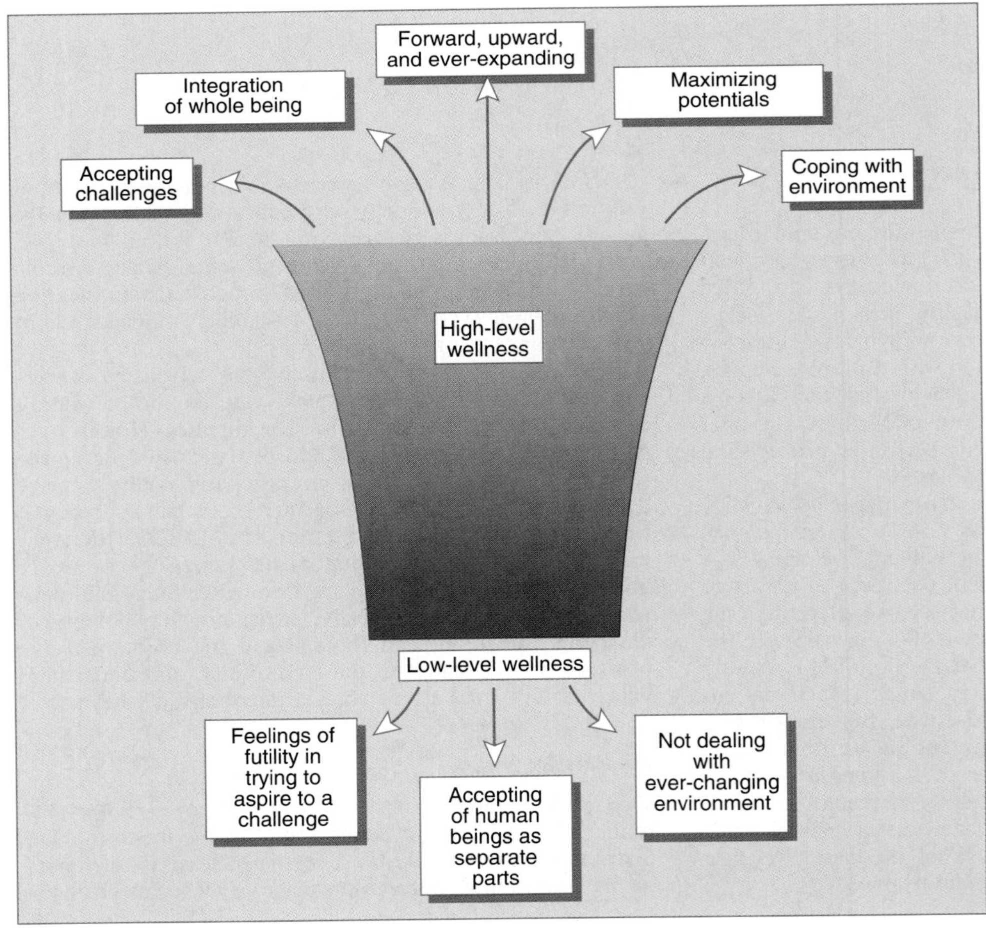

FIGURE 4–1
High-level wellness continuum.

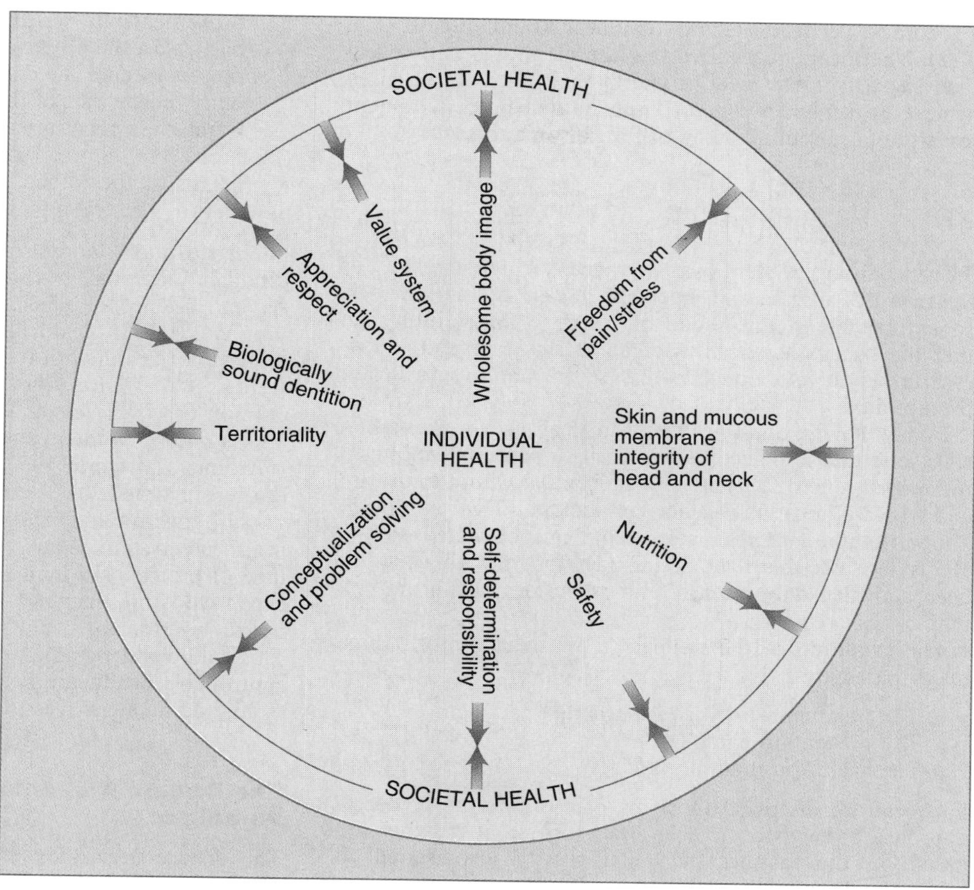

FIGURE 4–2
Human need theory applied to oral health of individual and society.

ness is a "direction" in progress, an approach to living; health is a state of being. There is no optimal level of wellness and no limitation on facets of the individual (physical, intellectual, spiritual, etc.), but rather a continual forward direction of being all that one can be.

Dunn believed that people needed to know themselves, to be encouraged to express themselves and to venture into the unknown "in search for universal truth, thus satisfying deep psychological and emotional needs of their own worlds and simultaneously radiating that outwards."[15] He coined a term for the successful quest for this state; he introduced "high level wellness," an "integrated method of functioning which is oriented toward maximizing the potential of which the individual is capable, within the environment where he is functioning" (Fig. 4–1).[16,17] High-level wellness is:

- A direction in progress forward and upward toward a higher potential of functioning
- An open-ended and ever-expanding tomorrow with its challenge to live at a fuller potential
- The integration of the whole being of the total individual—body, mind, and spirit—in the functioning process

Dunn's thesis of high-level wellness is based on the nature of humans and human needs.[16] The five major factors in human nature are:

- Humans' totality
- Humans' individual uniqueness
- Humans as manifestations of organized energy with the capacity to extract energy for own use
- Humans who possess both an outer and an inner world (perception and insight)
- Humans' self-integration and energy use

For Dunn, the 5 factors are interrelated with 12 basic human needs: survival, communication, fellowship, growth, imagination, love, balance, environment, communion with the universe, way of life, dignity, and freedom and space. Dunn theorized that "needs must be met to prevent the breakdown of the mind and that cultivation of activity pursuing the satisfaction of needs orients the individual toward maximizing the potential of which she/he is capable."[16]

Wellness is inclusive of health, but health is not inclusive of wellness. Health is an element that contributes to wellness in that it provides a foundation for relative homeostasis versus confusion and unrest, leading to lack of peace with the environment (social, political, physical). For example, an individual living in a favorable environment (job security, family support, healthcare) can exist passively at that level of existence, or he can continue to strive for improvements in life, aiming for self-actualization and self-integration (high-level wellness). A person whose environment is poor (political unrest, family breakdown, residential deterioration) but who maintains an optimistic attitude for a better tomorrow and continues to expend personal energy toward this quest is a person with emergent high-level wellness. Such persons do not fall victim to accepting their existence as being beyond their personal influence and control.

As a theoretical foundation, the human needs conceptual model of dental hygiene (see Chapter 2) directs the dental hygienist to view oral health by assessing the fulfillment of

11 human needs related to oral health and disease (Fig. 4–2). The theory recognizes that the individual and collectively, society must meet or satisfy their needs in order to achieve health and wellness. Thus, human need fulfillment leads to optimal functioning of the person and society.

THE WELLNESS EVOLUTION

The healthcare system was founded on the concept of treatment of disease and, later, on disease prevention. It is so entrenched in this mode of response that critics state that the system has been oriented to sick care and to disease rather than oriented to disease prevention and health promotion.[18]

Today, having one's health means leading a wellness lifestyle, one that is reflective of a positive proactive approach rather than one of a reactive or preventive nature to disease and disease-inducing agents or factors. This approach, known as the **wellness movement,** can be dated to the 1950s. Despite this date of introduction, the concept has been activated only recently in the Western healthcare system.

The evolution of the wellness movement involves three major paradigms:

- The treatment- and disease-oriented paradigm
- The prevention paradigm
- The health promotion paradigm

Each can be discussed in terms of the patterns of health and health behavior (Table 4–1). These paradigms are based on the manner in which society has aspired to achieve and maintain health and wellness.

The Treatment- and Disease-Oriented Paradigm

As early as the turn of the nineteenth century, the stage had been set for the foundations of societal response to health conditions. The reaction was heavily laden with treatment-oriented medical services in response to the great need and demand for healthcare. The treatment- and disease-oriented paradigm reflects passive treatment-based healthcare and was characterized by at least three descriptors:

- Little is done in terms of identifying the cause of the disease and thwarting its occurrence through prevention
- There is heavy reliance on medical care for the improvements in health, that is, medical manpower (in particular, the physician is worshipped as having heroic powers to cure the disease with little effort or responsibility on the part of the diseased person)
- It removes accountability from sectors other than the healthcare system; these sectors also influence the health of the public (industry, housing, environment, culture, lifestyle)

The treatment- and disease-oriented paradigm, or the traditionally accepted view of "healthcare" purports that the art and science of medicine is the fount from which all improvements in health flow, with popular belief equating the level of health with the quality of medicine.[19] Disease is seen as a deviance from normal where normalcy is the opinion of the professional and the public.[20] This paradigm also is known as the medical model of healthcare.

Around the world the disease-oriented, treatment-based healthcare system has received criticism from some professionals, governments, and organizations. A treatment-based healthcare system incurs escalating costs, requires a multitude of professional manpower (with emphasis on the most expensive kind; namely, the physician), and is passively based, not solving health problems but reacting to them. This traditional paradigm for healthcare makes for an uncontrollable healthcare system, one that finite human, material, and financial resources cannot support.

TABLE 4–1
PARADIGMS OF THE WELLNESS MOVEMENT AND MODELS OF HEALTH OR HEALTH BEHAVIOR

Paradigm	Model of Health or Health Behavior
Treatment-oriented	Medical model
Prevention-oriented	Agent-host-environment model[22]
	Health belief model[83]
	Health field concept[19]
Health promotion–oriented	Mandala of health[42]
	Health promotion framework[43]

The Disease Prevention–Oriented Paradigm

The disease **prevention** paradigm asserts that response to disease is such that it could be better treated by identifying the causative agent and avoiding it. Numerous models have been presented to operationalize this paradigm, a few of which will be discussed in this chapter.[19,21]

The Agent-Host-Environment Model

The agent-host-environment model, described by Leavell and Clark in 1965, conceptualizes disease as the result of disequilibrium occurring in one or all of three factors—the agent, the host, and the environment.[22] The model is based on four principles:

- Any disease or condition in man is a result of a dynamic process of achieving a state of equilibrium among the agent, the host, and the environment
- Disease is not a static condition, but a process that follows a more or less natural history
- Effective preventive measures require that the process be interrupted as early as possible
- "Normality" and "health" are relative attributes and require careful statistically controlled studies for definition.

The agent-host-environment model employs a multiple cause–multiple effect concept. The multiple cause–multiple effect concept is exemplified in Figure 4–3. It illustrates the "web of causation" for myocardial infarction, which depicts that predisposing factors to a disease, such as heart disease, have complex intricate relations with each other.[23] To prevent a myocardial infarction, it would be necessary to intervene at one of the web strings, such as dietary modification (agent), cessation of smoking tobacco (host), or industrial society (i.e., fast-pace, fast foods, high-stress

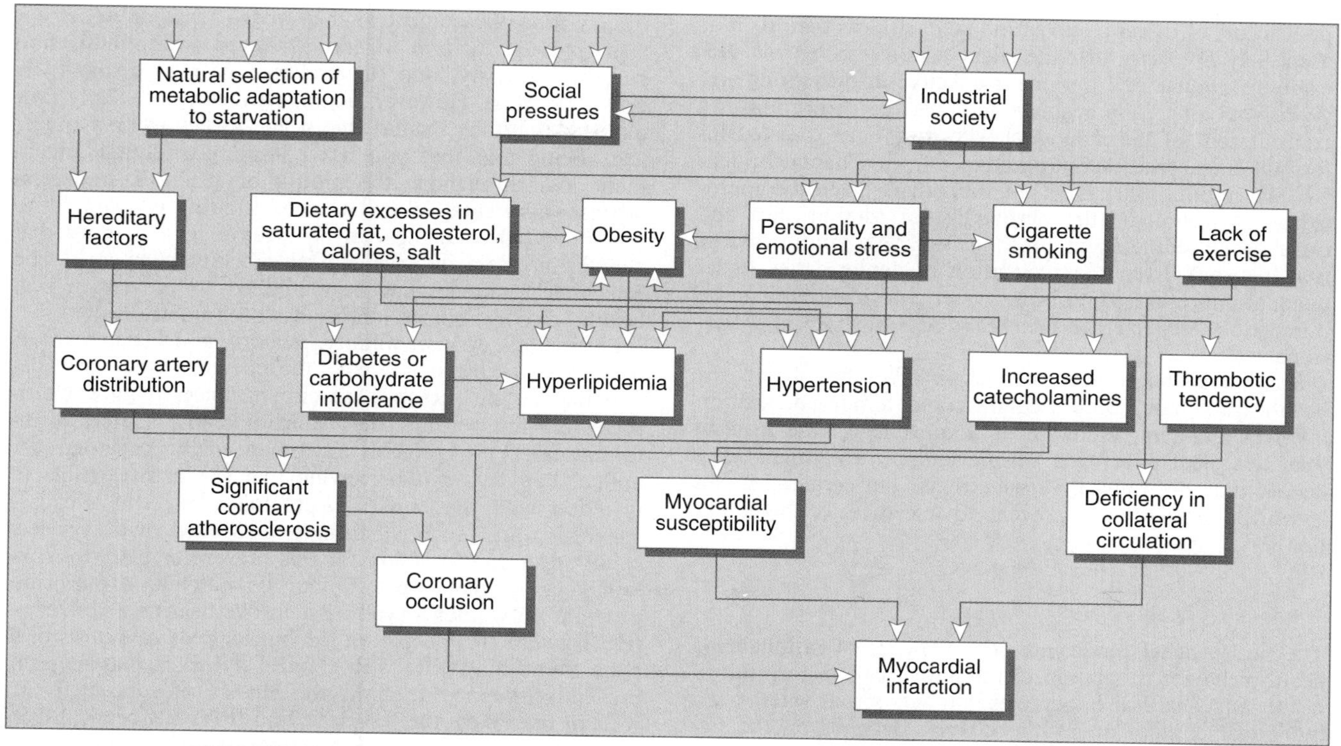

FIGURE 4–3
Web of causation. (Adapted and reproduced with permission from Friedman, G. Primer of Epidemiology, 3rd ed. New York: McGraw-Hill, 1987.)

working environments). The earlier the interception in the flow of the web, the better the prognosis. When using this theory, the ultimate goal is the prevention of the start of the web.

Levels of Prevention

The agent-host-environment model identifies three levels of application of preventive measures: primary, secondary, and tertiary. Primary prevention consists of interventions to prevent the onset of disease or injury. Secondary prevention consists of intervention designed to stop or minimize the progression of early disease while the person is generally asymptomatic. Tertiary prevention consists of intervention to prevent disability and to improve or restore residual function. The goal is to prevent further deterioration.[24] Table 4–2 provides oral health examples of the application of the three levels of prevention and the corresponding modes of intervention and activities.

The Health Professional's Responsibility Toward Prevention Primary prevention requires more than healthcare services provided by a health professional. Because primary

TABLE 4–2
EXAMPLES OF THE MODES OF ORAL HEALTH INTERVENTION FOR THE THREE LEVELS OF PREVENTION

Level of Prevention	Modes of Intervention	Activities
Primary	Health promotion	Chairside oral hygiene instruction
		Classroom education
		Workshops for caregivers
	Specific protection	Athletic mouth protectors
		Water fluoridation, self-applied and professionally applied oral health products
		Pit-and-fissure sealants (no caries activity)
Secondary	Early detection and early treatment	Oral health screening programs
		Self-examination and/or professional examinations
		Pit-and-fissure sealants (given incipient caries)
		Oral-physiotherapeutic aids for periodontal pockets
		Comprehensive oral antimicrobial therapy
Tertiary	Rehabilitation and treatment	Prosthodontic treatment
		Periodontal therapy, such as scaling, root planing, debridement, and surgery
		Restorative and reconstructive therapy
		Comprehensive oral antimicrobial therapy

prevention is disease prevention and risk reduction, it is absolutely necessary that the client take a leading role. For example, regular oral hygiene is effective in preventing gingivitis, but this daily regimen requires the dedication and commitment of the individual who may have received information, motivation, and guidance from a dental hygienist. The responsibility is on the individual, given the appropriate environment (the availability of toothbrushes and other orophysiotherapeutic aids, as well as a family valuing oral hygiene). Even the prevention of dental caries is dependent more on community water fluoridation than on interaction between the client and the healthcare professional.

Secondary and tertiary prevention relies heavily on the healthcare system. Both secondary and tertiary prevention involve treatment; therefore, it is quite legitimate to state that treatment is a type of prevention. Treatment of a disease may not prevent its occurrence, but certainly it can lessen the disability and prevent advancement of the condition.

The Health Belief Model

The health belief model presents a means of rationalizing health behavior in relation to the individual's perception of health and healthcare therapies.[21] It views that whether an individual engages in health behavior depends on the following three components of the health belief model (Fig. 4–4). The people must perceive that (1) they are susceptible to the disease or condition; (2) the occurrence of the disease or condition will have an impact on some component of their life of at least moderate severity; and (3) the benefits of taking action outweigh the barriers to that action. Within the context of this model, these three perceptions provide the will to act (perceived susceptibility and perceived severity) and the preferred path of action (perceived benefits). However, action need not necessarily take place. Rosenstock[21] states that a cue to action or a trigger (e.g., being told that you have 5-mm periodontal attachment loss throughout the mouth or seeing a smokeless tobacco–associated lesion in your mouth) is required to spark the individual to actively behave in a manner that denotes disease avoidance or health-seeking behavior.[21] The health belief model has been applied to preventive oral health behavior, but its validity has been questioned.[25]

Perceptions of susceptibility, severity, and benefits versus barriers to taking action and the cue to action vary, depending on the person's life circumstances (e.g., environment, practices, values, beliefs, attitude, and sources of information). For example, a woman might postpone her annual Pap test, not perceiving that she is susceptible to infection with the human papilloma virus, which causes venereal warts and is strongly associated with cervical cancer. Her cue to action for this preventive behavior (obtaining an annual Pap test) may be watching a television program on women's health issues, overhearing a conversation between two people on the bus, or receiving news of a close friend diagnosed with cervical dysplasia that requires preventive therapy to limit the chance of cancer. If the woman does have the test done and it reveals cervical dysplasia, she may choose no treatment, perceiving the condition as not serious. Perhaps she is fearful of the treatment (cone biopsy, cryotherapy, or laser surgery) and her fear greatly outweighs the benefits of therapy.

For the person with periodontal disease, the most important factor in successful resolution is diligent daily mainte-

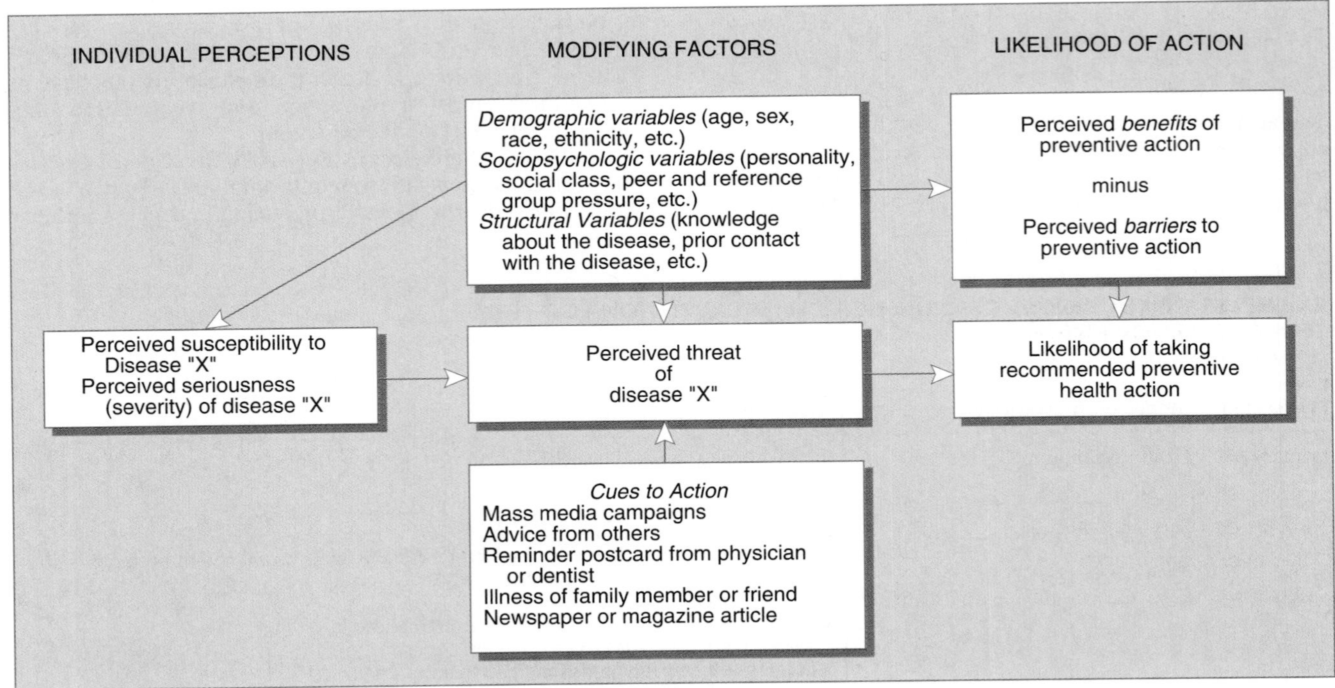

FIGURE 4–4
Health belief model. (Adapted from Rosenstock, I. Historical origins of the health belief model. In Becker, M., and Marshall H. [eds.]. The Health Belief Model and Personal Health Behavior. Thorofare, NJ: Slack, 1974.)

nance care.[26] The client must agree to professional therapy as well as to a careful home oral hygiene regimen to prevent progression of the disease and maintain tissue health. The agreement to proceed with treatment relies on the individual's perception of periodontal disease as a health threat (periodontal disease can lead to tooth loss, which can affect a person's dietary habits, body image, and verbal communication). If the client does not perceive periodontitis as a health threat, she is unlikely to proceed with professional intervention and diligent daily home care.

Health Field Concept

The health field concept attributes the health status of the individual and community to the outcome of an interaction between four elements:

- Human biology
- Environment
- Lifestyle
- The healthcare organization (Fig. 4–5)[19]

The element of human biology includes physical and mental aspects of health, which develop within the human body as a consequence of the basic biology of man and the organic makeup of the individual.

The environmental element consists of everything external to the body and over which the individual has little or no control, such as neighborhood pesticide spraying and industrial pollution. The lifestyle element includes all decisions made by individuals that affect their health and over which they do, more or less, have control, such as smoking, diet, excessive alcohol consumption, and wearing seatbelts. The healthcare organization element corresponds to the quantity and quality of the healthcare system, such as the availability of hospital beds, oral health services provided to rural areas, the purchase of magnetic resonance imaging (MRI) technology, and the monies to finance research. These elements reflect the orientation of the healthcare system toward health.

The four elements of the health field concept were identified from an assessment of the causes and underlying factors of morbidity and mortality in Canada, and by an examination of the roles these elements play in the health of Canadians. Results of the assessment indicated a change in the 10 leading causes of death in North Americans from 1900 to 1979. In the beginning of the century, people died of infectious diseases (influenza, pneumonia, tuberculosis), whereas the main killers in the latter half of the century are lifestyle disease (heart disease, cancer, and cerebrovascular disease).[27]

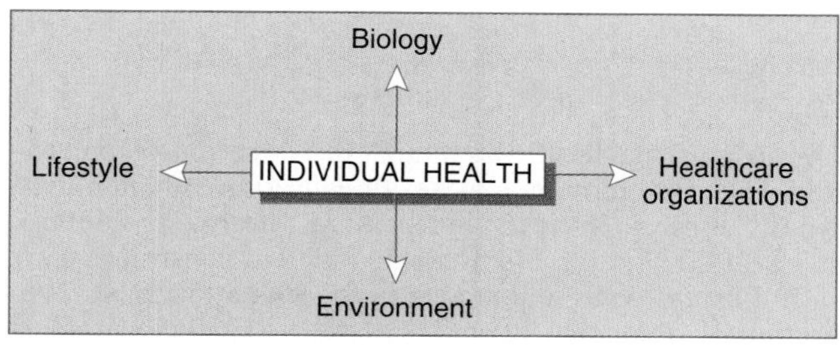

FIGURE 4–5
Health field concept.

The risk factors for morbidity and mortality at the start and end of the century were preventable, modifiable, and controllable. The communicable diseases that plagued North Americans in the early 1900s were controlled eventually through improved environmental conditions and, to a much lesser extent, through vaccinations. The risk factors associated with contemporary diseases are less easily modified (attitudes, beliefs, behaviors) because there is a strong relationship between lifestyle and the diseases of cancer, cardiovascular disease, and others.[28]

The health field concept provides a comprehensive, systematic framework to analyze the cause of disease; it presents a new perspective on health. It maps out the underlying factors identifying the elements of lifestyle, environment, and biology as having significant influence on health and demands unification of all participants in decisions that affect health (health professionals, the scientific community, governments, the business sector, and the people themselves).

Tobacco smoking provides a good example for application of the health field concept. It is physically and psychologically addicting and strongly associated with cancer, cardiovascular disease, and lung disease. Hence, there is a human biological element. However, it was not until the 1960s that society began to be informed that smoking has negative health effects. By this time, it was the socially acceptable thing to do. Smoking was the norm; the nonsmoker was in the minority. Hence, there is also a lifestyle element.

Tobacco companies present appealing and tantalizing advertisements in household magazines, on billboards, and through other media. Brand products are associated with personality types, lending a person class and elegance or a rugged masculinity. The imagery presented is designed to entice people to adopt the habit, to switch brands, and to continue to smoke.

There is also a healthcare organization element. Only recently the Surgeon General has claimed smoking to be hazardous to one's health. In addition, environmental elements have played influential roles in the sale of tobacco.[29] The tobacco industry employs a large number of people, thus contributing to the economy of the country, and the government receives revenue from the sales of tobacco products.

To blame the victim of lung cancer for the development of his condition is an erroneous oversimplification. The four elements of human biology, environment, lifestyle, and healthcare organization influence a person's decision to smoke in the first place.

The health field concept led to the reordering of public health policies in the United States with the publication of *Healthy People, The Surgeon General's Report on Health Promotion and Disease Prevention.*[30] This report presents five national goals and relates objectives aimed at improving the health of infants, children, adolescents, and adults by the year 1990. The strategies outlined to accomplish these goals are preventive health services (which can be delivered to individuals by health professionals), health protection (measures that can be used by governmental and other agencies, as well as by industry, to protect people from harm), and **health promotion** (activities in which individuals and communities can engage to promote healthy lifestyles) (Table 4–3).

Prevention and promotion measures pertaining to oral

TABLE 4–3
SELECTED HEALTH STRATEGIES FOR THE NATION*

Category	Strategy
Preventive services	High blood pressure control Family planning Pregnancy and infant health Immunization Sexually transmitted disease control
Health protection	Toxic agent control Occupational safety and health Accident and injury prevention Fluoridation and oral health Surveillance and control of infectious diseases
Health promotion	Tobacco cessation programs Misuse of alcohol and drug programs Nutrition Physical fitness and exercise Control of stress and violent behavior

*A selection drawn from 22 priority areas.
Source: U.S. Department of Health and Human Services. The 1990 Health Objectives for the Nation: A Midcourse Review. 1986.

health, as outlined in the *Health Objectives for the Nation,* are directed at the three principal contributing factors to oral disease:

- Host susceptibility
- Presence of bacterial plaque
- Dietary environment
- Time (Fig. 4–6)[31]

Strategies include:

- Water fluoridation
- Public education efforts regarding dental caries and periodontal diseases (school-based and otherwise)
- Developing local advocacy groups to encourage community fluoridation and alternative measures

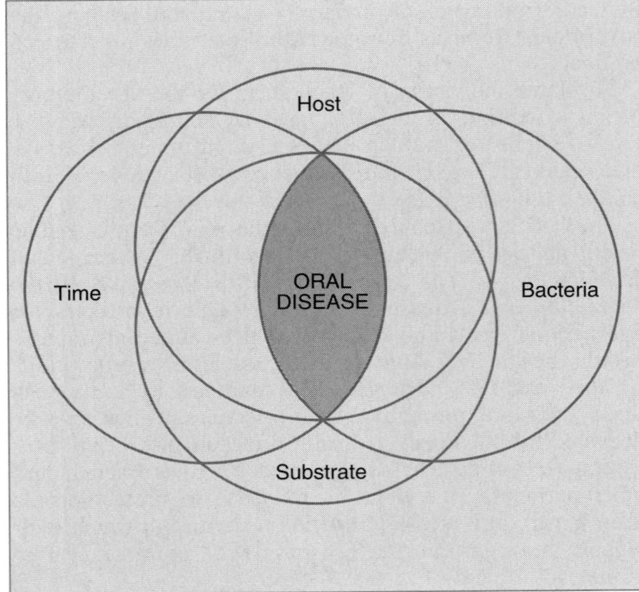

FIGURE 4–6
Principal factors necessary for oral disease.

- Elimination of high cariogenic foods in vending machines or in school breakfast and lunch programs[31,32]

Health protection measures for oral health involve mainly legislative support of community water fluoridation.

The Health Promotion–Oriented Paradigm

The health promotion paradigm focuses on creating environments that enable people to increase control over and improve their current and future health.[33] This concept is based on health being defined as "the extent to which an individual or group is able, on the one hand, to realize aspirations and satisfy needs, and on the other hand, to change and cope with the environment."[2] Health is perceived as a resource for everyday life, not the objective of living. Health promotion represents a mediating strategy between people and their environment, synthesizing personal choice and social responsibility in health to create a healthier future (see Definitions of Health Promotion chart).[34–36]

Health promotion calls for the building of public policy, strengthening community action (through empowerment of the community, ownership and control of their own endeavors and destinies), development of personal skills, and reorientation of health services. It is an invitation to partnership between all sectors of society, a call for action.[37] Although the disease prevention paradigm recognized this, much effort was devoted to changing the client's lifestyle behaviors that were not conducive to health, by augmenting physical activity and reducing tobacco use and high-fat diets. These efforts, "victim blaming," were expended on the individual as opposed to a collaboration of all sectors of society toward environmental factors that influence the health of the people.[29]

WHO responded by producing a series of documents called *Achieving Health for All by the Year 2000,* which challenges all countries to operationalize strategies for disease prevention and health promotion.[38,39] Specific to oral health, WHO produced guidelines for *Self-care in Oral Health for All by the Year 2000* (Fig. 4–7).[40] The publication provides an elaborate framework identifying the tasks of content, process, development and dissemination, and evaluation. The tasks are accomplished by the developers (planners, researchers, educators), enablers (legislators, family), carers (health workers, family, teachers), and individuals in order to achieve oral health. For example, legislators are enablers of the self-care model for oral health because they are the individuals who, on behalf of the community, discuss (process) issues such as water fluoridation (content) and pass legislation for or against the issue (dissemination and development).

Differentiating Among Disease Prevention, Health Promotion, and Health Education

Throughout the health literature, the concepts of prevention, health promotion, and health education are often used synonymously. However, prevention, health promotion, and health education are uniquely different constructs, each with different goals and strategies for goal attainment. Prevention is negatively oriented in that it is disease that is being prevented to achieve or maintain health; health promotion is positively oriented in that it is health and wellness that is being promoted; and health education, depend-

DEFINITIONS OF HEALTH PROMOTION

Source	Definition
Dwore and Kreuter[34]	"Health promotion is the process of advocating health in order to enhance the probability that personal (individual, family and community), private (professional and business) and public (federal, state and local government) support positive health practices as a societal norm. The process of advocating health may be conducted by a variety of modalities, including, but not limited to, health education."
Green[35]	"Health promotion is any combination of health education and related organizational, economic and environmental supports for behavior conducive to health in individuals, groups or communities."
World Health Organization (EUROPE)[36]	"Health promotion is the process of enabling individuals and communities to increase control over the determinants of health and thereby improve their health."

ing on its intent and context (disease prevention or health promotion), can be either negative or positive in its orientation.

To distinguish preventive activities from those of health promotion in your own life ask yourself this question: Do you do what you do to avoid disease and disability, or do you do what you do because it makes you feel great and enables you to achieve your aspirations? Do you participate in a physical activity at least three times a week, sustaining a cardiovascular output for at least 20 minutes per session, because you want to avoid getting fat or avoid the risk of a myocardial infarction, or do you do it because of a natural high and inner glow you achieve from having participated in the activity? One may initially start a physical fitness program with disease prevention in mind but may become addicted to the natural high that comes from keeping the physical body in good shape. This vignette exemplifies the semantic problem with differentiating between disease prevention and health promotion: If exercise is done to avoid putting on weight, the aim is prevention; if exercise is done because it enables one to strive toward personal goals and aspirations, it is health promotion.

Prevention entails providing specific services or procedures as well as education. Prenatal classes for parents, radio announcements, guidebooks for caregivers, and toothbrush demonstrations in classroom settings and tobacco cessation programs all are examples of health education for disease prevention. The distribution of prenatal multivitamin tablets with iron and school-based fluoride mouth rinse programs, and community-wide pit-and-fissure sealant programs, are prevention strategies without educational components.

Prevention and education are firmly linked and should be integrated for two reasons:

- An educational component incorporated into a prevention program offers the opportunity to impart knowledge and influence attitudes and behaviors

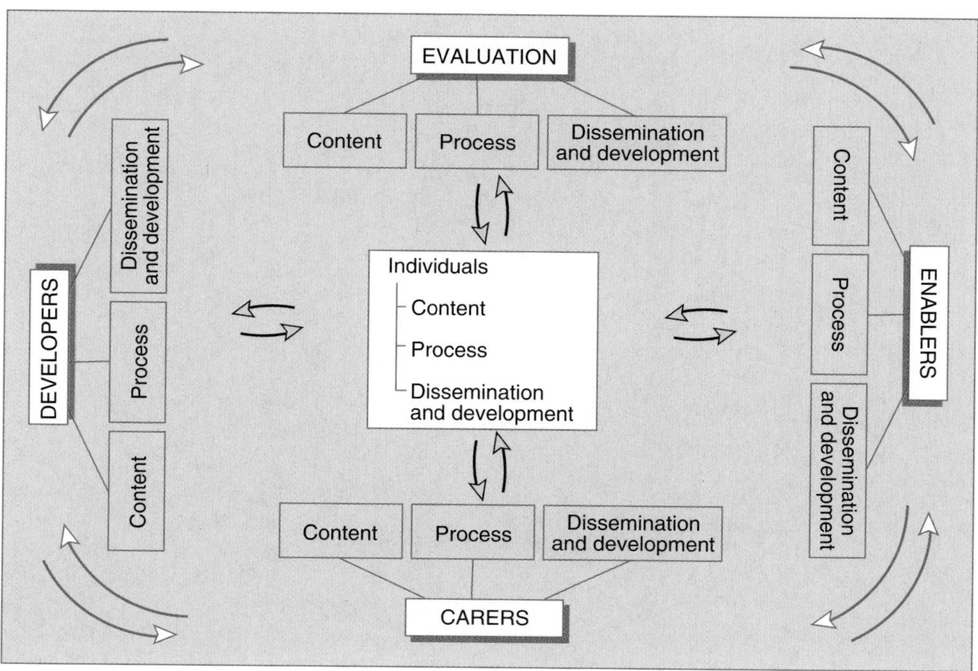

FIGURE 4–7
The self-care model for oral health. (Adapted from Oral Health for All by the Year 2000: Guidelines for Self-Care in Oral Health. WHO Regional Office for Europe, Copenhagen, 1988.)

> Preventive elements in an educational program can provide the means for applying the knowledge and desired behavior[41]

Prescribing fluoride tablets for children not exposed to optimal water fluoridation levels is a preventive measure that is available to parents interested in protecting their children's dentition from decay. However, such measures rely on adherence to the regimen; hence, there must be some belief attached to the behavior that ensures its action—thus the importance of the educational factor.

Models of Health Promotion

Two models of health that support and operationalize the philosophy of health promotion are the mandala of health and the health promotion framework.[42,43] The common focus of these models is the holistic conceptualization of health and the emphasis on community responsibility for health stemming from legislative action to individual choices.

Mandala of Health The mandala of health is a redesign of the health field concept.[18,42] Hancock's choice of title for the model provides an immediate graphic or visual aid in conceptualizing the foundation of health promotion. A mandala is a circle (the wholeness) enclosing a square usually divided into separate sections (elements of the whole). This model is an integrative concept that views health (mind, body, and spirit) as the nucleus, stressing the importance of the interrelationship of the psychosocioeconomic and physical environment, human biology, and personal behavior (Fig. 4–8). A key determinant of health in the individual is the family, because this is the source of many learned values, beliefs, and behaviors. The "sick care" system is relatively unimportant in the model, except in that it treats disease. Workplace is important to individual and family health, as it relates to both the psychosocioeconomic environment and the physical environment. All of these influences on individual and family health are derived from the community, which has its own set of values, standards, support systems, and community lifestyle. The community is an important mediating structure that exists within human-made environments (urban and rural). The outer level of the model consists of culture and biosphere. Cultural values and beliefs are of great importance to individual and community perceptions of health and well-being, as well as how disease is treated. Humans exist in the biosphere of the planet Earth, and hence health and wellness are dependent on the world ecosystem. How we use our resources, whether we are a consumer society or a conserving one, will map the future of our life-giving Earth and its humanity.

The Health Promotion Framework The health promotion framework is aimed at achieving health for all by accepting specific challenges, identifying mechanisms, and implementing health promotion strategies to meet these

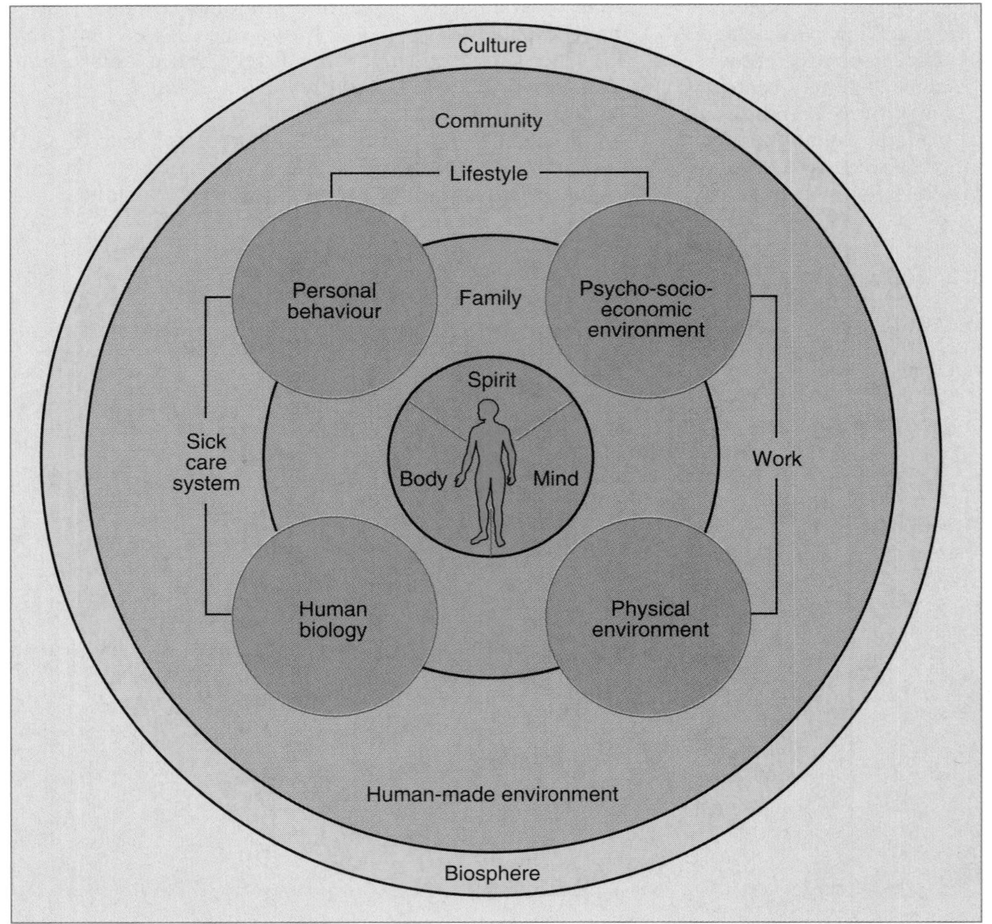

FIGURE 4–8
Mandala of health: A model of the human ecosystem. (Adapted from Hancock, T. The mandala of health; A model of the human ecosystem. Family and Community Health 8:1, 1985. Permission of Trevor Hancock and Fran Perkins, City of Toronto Department of Public Health.)

challenges (Fig. 4–9).[43] The challenges are:

- Reducing the inequities in access to health promotion activities
- Increasing the prevention effort against disease
- Enhancing people's capacity to cope with an ever-changing environment

The mechanisms of health promotion are self-care, mutual aid (lending support and assistance to others), and the creation of healthy environments. Health promotion strategies include fostering public participation, strengthening community health service, and coordinating healthy public policy.

THE WELLNESS MOVEMENT

In the days of kings and queens, the kingdom crier would announce "All is well" at hourly intervals, which told the people the castle was secure, the fields were productive, and the people were well fed and thought to be happy and healthy. In the twentieth century, if the town crier decreed "All is well," the proclamation would be denounced as erroneous because all is not well. The castle (Earth) suffers from many problems, such as the greenhouse effect, acid rain, destructive mining, groundwater contamination, waste of natural resources, unemployment, social inequities, and chronic disease.

All may not be well, but there is a distinct movement by government, agencies, organizations, and communities to change this state. This movement is called the **wellness movement.** Ardell[43a] in 1985 proposed several forces or trends that initiated the wellness movement, some of which are consumer consciousness regarding health, the healthcare cost crisis, mind and body awareness, industry's responsiveness and initiatives (worksite health promotion and wellness to reduce absenteeism and high turnover rates and to improve employee morale), and powerful individual voices (Ivan Illich's *Medical Nemesis* or Covert Bailey's *Fit or Fat*).

Oral Health and Wellness and Human Need Theory

Oral Health as Integral to Health and Wellness

Dental caries and periodontal disease, although not life-threatening diseases, are integral to health and wellness and thus affect the quality of life. It is not easy to assess how oral disease influences a person's wellness because of the difficulty in developing reliable and valid measurement tools. For the most part, behavioral indicators such as disability days, work loss, and dental care utilization have been used to measure the extent of dental disability and the quality of life.[44,45] However, these factors are underestimates of the true state of oral health because they describe acute conditions and neglect chronic problems. Investigators have relied on measurement tools, such as various dental and periodontal indices, rather than developing indices that indicate a person's oral health status (through the existence of health, not disease). Recently, psychological and affective indices have been used to measure the effect that oral disability has on an individual's lifestyle.[46–50] A notably good measurement is the human need theory to the practice of dental hygiene, which provides a tool for assessing oral health factors as they relate to quality of life of the individual and society over the lifespan.

Three orally related factors measured by researchers that affect quality of life are:

- Pain
- Acceptance of prosthetic appliances
- Aesthetics

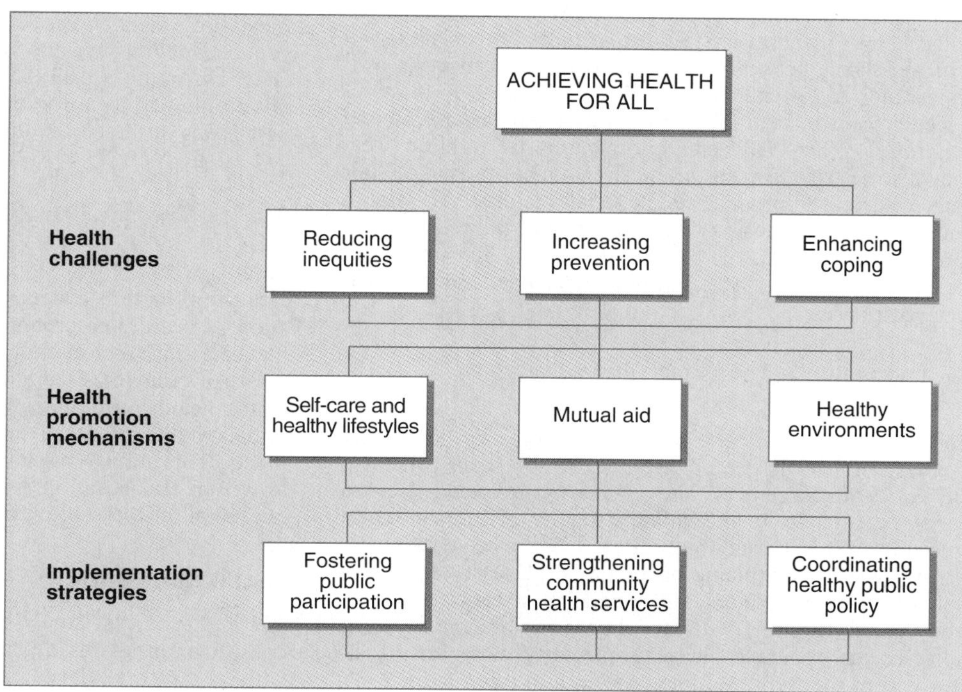

FIGURE 4–9
Health promotion framework. (Adapted from Epp, J. Achieving Health for All: A Framework for Health Promotion. Ottawa, Canada, Health Canada, 1986. With permission of the Minister of Supply and Services Canada 1994.)

Pain

Whether orofacial pain originates from dental caries, temporomandibular joint (TMJ) dysfunction, or muscles of the masticatory system, the outcome within the client is a resultant loss of work,[44] sleep disturbance,[46,51] change in eating behavior because of discomfort,[52] and social incapacity.[49,50] People suffering from chronic dental disability, such as that related to TMJ dysfunction, have reported poor ratings of well-being.[50]

Acceptance of Prosthetic Appliances

Ill-fitting prosthetic appliances can create human need deficits in wholesome body image, freedom from pain and stress, and nutrition. Smith reported that among 254 adults aged 64 years or older, 20% were embarrassed by their dentures falling out during social contact.[52] This made them less likely to become involved socially. Straus, Sandifer, Hall, and Haley stated that subjects who initially had ill-fitting dentures replaced by well-fitting ones found that once their dentures were fitted, they enjoyed their food more, their diet improved, and they felt more secure and confident speaking (no longer hiding their faces). They were less stressed and felt better emotionally, generally experiencing an overall increase in their sense of well-being.[53] Ekelund reported that edentulous individuals avoided foods more often than those persons wearing dentures.[54] He commented that the lack of appetite was related to poor oral health status resulting from ineffective chewing ability.

Aesthetics

The appearance of the face and oral cavity influences a person's sense of body image. Sticker indicated that unaesthetic occlusal traits may affect the well-being of an individual by resulting in an unfavorable social response and poor self-esteem.[55] Shaw, Addy, and Ray reported considerable evidence citing one's individual level of satisfaction with facial appearance having important implications for self-esteem. Further, they found that there probably exists a critical balance between individual perception of one's own appearance and social feedback.[56]

Teeth seem to be a target for teasing and ridicule among children.[57] When 12 facial photographs of children were shown to 82 children, teeth and eyes ranked second to hair with respect to importance of facial features. The more deviant the malocclusion, the more salient became the feature. Further research is needed to identify the impact of malocclusion on societal, cultural, personal, and interpersonal response.

An Application of the Human Need Theory to Oral Health and Wellness

The existence of oral diseases has an impact on health and wellness. Although dental diseases do not often present a life or death prognosis, they certainly influence human needs essential to an individual's quality of life. A person ignorant of his periodontal disease but who continually strives toward maximizing his potential possesses a sense of wellness. The individual with malaligned central incisors who refuses to smile with an open grin for fear of being ridiculed may consider herself somewhere closer to the illness end of the wellness-illness continuum (see Figure 2–4).

TABLE 4–4
HUMAN NEED THEORY APPLIED TO COMMUNITY HEALTH AND THE ROLE OF THE DENTAL HYGIENIST

Human Needs	Role of the Dental Hygienist
Nutrition	Advocacy for nutritious and noncariogenic school lunch programs and food choices in vending machines Advocacy for policy statements regarding the prohibition of placing confectioneries at children's eye level in stores
Safety	Advocacy for policy statements regarding mandatory headguards and mouth protectors for all contact sports Promotion of universal use of seatbelts and airbags in motor vehicles Educating consumers regarding infection control standards
Conceptualization and problem solving	Initiating community water fluoridation Promoting the acceptability of universal access to dental hygiene care

Human need theory also is applicable to community health outreach. The role of the dental hygienist as a health professional does not stop at the oral healthcare setting. The dental hygienist has the responsibility to reach those who do not seek healthcare. Table 4–4 outlines activities that the dental hygienist can initiate to promote community oral health so that residents can achieve maximal human need fulfillment. For example, to meet the human need for nutrition, the dental hygienist can advocate nutritious lunch programs and vendor food selection in school settings, or participate in institutional meal planning. To meet the human need for safety on a community level, the dental hygienist can advocate athletic mouth protectors for all age levels involved in contact sports. To meet the need for conceptualization and problem solving, the dental hygienist can work in the community to ensure that people make informed choices about water fluoridation. In this context, dental hygiene strategies include providing the facts, becoming a spokesperson, and facilitating the efforts of community organizations that raise the health and wellness levels of the community.

STRATEGIES OF HEALTH PROMOTION

Health promotion fosters self-care, mutual aid, and the creation of healthy environments. Its goal is to achieve health for all despite socioeconomic status, geographical residence, or other variables. Figure 4–10 illustrates how the strategies of the health promotion framework can be further divided into activities of social marketing, health education, mass media, community organization, advocacy, and legislation as well as collaboration.[58] The dental hygienist has a role to play in all of these activities.

Social Marketing

Marketing is the "analysis, planning, implementation and control of programs designed to bring about an exchange with a target audience for the purpose of personal and

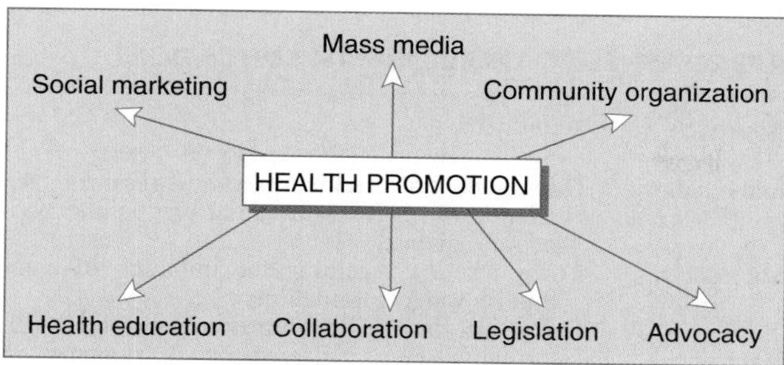

FIGURE 4-10
Strategies for health promotion.

mutual gain."[59] The success formula is "the development of the right product backed by the right promotion and put in the right place at the right price."[59] Figure 4-11 illustrates the relationship between these four Ps:

- Product—the actual item being marketed
- Promotion—communication-persuasion strategies that attempt to make the product familiar, acceptable, and desirable
- Place—the provision of adequate and compatible distribution and response channels
- Price—the cost the buyer must accept to obtain the product (including financial cost, opportunity costs, energy costs)

Marketing a concept to society is termed **social marketing.** Kotler and Zaltman define it as "the design, implementation and control of programs calculated to influence the acceptability of social ideas. . . ."[59] Social marketing involves the sale of intangibles. Health and wellness are intangibles; therefore, both are marketable via the application of the creative social marketing principles.

Generally, nonprofit organizations like health associations tackle social marketing to change behavior regarding social practices not conducive to health. Examples of such marketing include campaigning against spouse, child, and elder abuse; drinking and driving; and tobacco and substance abuse. For successful social marketing, the organization must have a good public image consisting of credibility, integrity, accountability, and recognized goodwill for the public.

For example, the Heart and Stroke Foundation of Manitoba, in collaboration with numerous Manitoba restaurants, developed "Heart Smart," a program that enabled people to enjoy the pleasures of dining out while avoiding meals laden with cholesterol and calories. Heart-healthy cuisines were offered in many restaurants that voluntarily joined the campaign. Restaurateurs welcomed the nutritional analysis of their menus. Those menu items that met heart-healthy standards were signified with a heart symbol. Restaurants could profitably offer a menu to health-conscious clients, adding new patrons from those who previously had limited healthy food selection. This social marketing campaign identified a tangible product, heart-healthy menu choices, and facilitated the making of informed choices by people regarding their dietary intake.

For-profit organizations (business and industry) are recognizing the benefit of associating themselves with health and wellness consciousness, and creating a public image of caring for health. Consider the intent of a doughnut shop's portrayal of a health consciousness image by publicizing the variety of cholesterol-free doughnuts available at the shop.

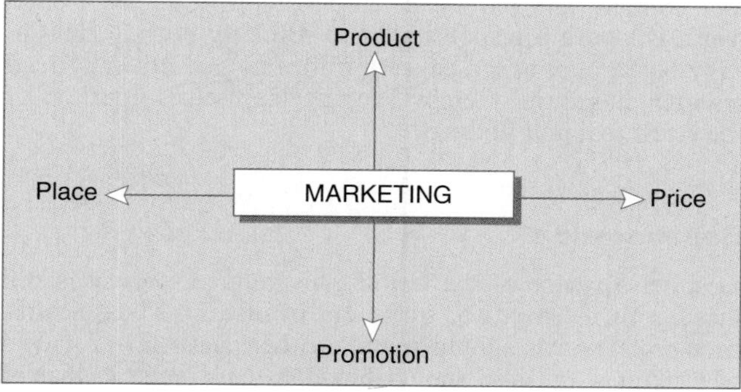

FIGURE 4-11
The four Ps of marketing.

The Social Marketing of Oral Health

Social marketing is essential for promoting health and wellness. It persuades people, through exposure, awareness, and provision of knowledge and skills, to accept responsibility for their health and that of the community. When implementing a social marketing strategy it is essential to know the target population—what they like, desire, need; what they would be receptive to; where you would most likely find the target; where and when they would most likely be receptive to the product; and what would entice them to buy the product. An example of a marketing strategy for the promotion of oral health and well being that illustrates the relationship of product, promotion, place, and price follows (Table 4-5).

Product How can this product, "oral health as part of total health," be marketed? As examples it can be marketed in the context of:

- Fear, pain, and tooth loss
- Preventing dental caries and periodontal disease

TABLE 4-5
SOCIAL MARKETING THEORY APPLIED TO ORAL HEALTH

Elements of Social Marketing	Oral Health Example
Product	Oral health as part of total health
	Name of campaign, e.g., "Smile"
	Make "Smile" a tangible product, e.g., with photographs
Promotion	Radio and television announcements
	Free preventive oral health services offered during National Dental Hygiene Campaign
	Bus poster announcements
Place	Workplace and public school locations
	Information telephone hotlines
	Booth display at local mall
Price	Psychic costs (client's fear and anxiety)
	Monetary considerations
	Resource costs (babysitting while parent attends oral healthcare appointment, business of household leaving no perceived time for parental supervision of children's oral health behaviors)

- Physical fitness
- Sex appeal
- In reference to the pursuit of health, wellness, and quality of life

The context selected establishes the foundation for developing the social marketing strategy. The product needs an appealing, easy-to-remember name, such as "Smile." "Smile" is short, a smile is contagious, and when one smiles, teeth are visible.

Place The organization must identify locations to promote "Smile." For example, the Canadian Dental Hygienists' Association established a toll-free information hotline co-sponsored with a dental corporation. The telephone number was advertised during a television commercial and in numerous popular magazines. People needed only to pick up their phone and receive either prerecorded information or speak directly with a dental hygienist—the choice was theirs. Another example of good marketing for "Smile" is workplace seminars or workshops that make it easy for employees to participate in oral health education programs, from prenatal information to the care of dentures. The attractive feature of a workplace site is that it offers educational opportunities during work hours and hence does not impinge on nonworking hours.

Price The organization must identify the price of "Smile" to the public. There may be psychic costs in that many people claim fear and anxious feelings related to dental care. There may be financial hardships associated with oral healthcare and products. There may even be energy costs in that it is quite common to hear people claim that they do not have time to floss, brush, or irrigate their teeth and gums.

Health Education

Health education is "any combination of learning opportunities designed to facilitate voluntary adoption of behaviors which are conducive to health."[60] Historically, dental hygiene employed oral health education as a means of informing the public about oral disease and its prevention and treatment. This provision of information was based mainly on avoidance behavior with respect to oral diseases, such as periodontal disease and dental caries. Health education, as it is used as a health promotion strategy, includes disease prevention, but its main emphasis is health achievement via a wellness approach. Health education entails the education of the individual and the community as well as the political sector of the community.

Locker describes three approaches to oral health education that focus on the individual and the microsocial and macrosocial levels of the community.[61] Table 4–6 outlines working examples of each of these approaches.

TABLE 4–6
APPROACHES TO ORAL HEALTH EDUCATION

Approach	Activity
Individualistic	One-to-one oral health instruction regarding the relationship between bacterial plaque and periodontal diseases
Microsocial	Town meeting regarding the initiation of community water fluroidation
	Caregivers' oral health education workshop
Macrosocial	Informative letters to legislators or ministers of parliament or congress regarding need for universal oral healthcare coverage
	Lobbying for self-regulation of dental hygiene to achieve universal access to quality dental hygiene care

The traditional approach focusing on the person uses behavior modification to stimulate changes in knowledge, attitudes, or belief. The strategies employed are information provision, skill development and repetitive learning, behavior modification, and cognitive awareness (e.g., chairside oral hygiene instruction).

The microsocial approach tries to achieve behavioral change in the client by using individual and small group strategies, such as peer group influences and counseling in the oral healthcare setting. Locker, in his review of the vast literature on health education, believes that client nonadherence to health behavior should not be viewed as the client's failure to become motivated, but rather as a fault in the communication between client and practitioner.[61] Furthermore, he states that "information given in the context of healthcare seeking encounters may be less retained than information given during group instructions."

The macrosocial approach focuses on the impact of economic, political, sociocultural, and environmental factors on oral health behavior. For example, the fact that oral healthcare is not covered by national health insurance, with the exception of certain groups of people (members of the armed forces in the United States and Canada and social security recipients in Canada), is indicative of the low priority oral healthcare has in the overall healthcare system. Regulatory requirements for dental hygienists confine their practice to healthcare settings supervised by dentists. This limitation restricts access to dental hygiene care for a large portion of society, such as the homebound and institutionalized. To address such issues, dental hygienists are applying macrosocial health education approaches to effect favorable changes in society. Health education efforts need to be broadened to include decision makers, such as governmental bodies, consumers, and public interest groups.

All three approaches to health education support the concept of health promotion. The individualistic approach enhances self-help, the microsocial approach identifies with people helping people, and the macrosocial approach considers the creation of public policy.

Dental hygienists as oral disease prevention specialists should play a role in information transfer. For example, dental hygienists can ensure that school health curricula are based on scientifically valid material, develop curricula, provide in-service training for teachers to explain the curricular content, and participate in classroom teaching. Dental hygienists have a responsibility to regularly attend scientifically based continuing education forums and critically read research literature, thereby keeping themselves apprised of the latest research findings.

Collaboration

Despite existence of the wellness movement, society is still faced with the need for treatment of disease. Thus, healthcare professionals should maintain their status as providers of treatment but also should broaden their scope to that of resource persons or facilitators of health and wellness. To achieve this end, the healthcare system must move away from fragmentation into various disciplines and move toward a holistic and humanistic system.

Health professionals should be collaborating with each other. **Collaboration** includes:

- Being aware of a client's health holistically to enhance the person's capacity to adopt preventive and promotional practices
- Interacting with other disciplines to avoid territorial boundaries over disease, which limit the opportunity to enhance client's self-care, mutual aid, and coping ability (Fig. 4–12)

Collaboration among professionals can exist by offering comprehensive health services to the public within traditional and nontraditional settings, thereby promoting interaction among healthcare providers and others (e.g., social workers). Examples of a holistic approach to healthcare services in the oral care environment include nutritional counseling, physical abuse detection, and blood pressure screening.

Diet affects major health problems, such as cardiovascular disease, stroke, and diabetes. Elbon and Karp reported on the effectiveness and acceptance, as well as cost implications, of the dietitian as a member of the oral health team, stating that the need for nutritional education and skill development is not being met but could be met if a dietitian was employed.[62]

Health professionals should be able to provide clients with information on other health-promoting resources and programs in the community, such as smoking cessation programs, cardiovascular fitness programs, fat-free cooking programs, and various support groups. For example, the oral health practitioner, when performing an intra- and extraoral examination, may be the initial professional who identifies the symptoms of physical abuse. In order to meet the client's human need for safety, the dental hygienist could recommend community-based domestic violence prevention programs, crisis telephone numbers, or safe houses. For victims, knowing that others care for their welfare and offering the means of seeking assistance may facilitate positive action and human need fulfillment.

Blood pressure screening in the dental office not only facilitates quality assurance to the client but also supports national goals pertaining to this condition.[63] Clients benefit in that they become aware of the blood pressure reading and are better informed regarding their health status. Moreover, assessing blood pressure in the oral healthcare environment serves as both a screening mechanism for people who are at high risk for cardiovascular disease and a referral point of entry for medical intervention. The hygienist can act as an advocate and change agent for ensuring that blood pressure assessment is a service to clients. This advocacy may require conducting staff meetings or continuing education sessions, selecting blood pressure equipment, and developing a blood pressure policy for the office.

Mass Media

Mass media primarily are used to increase public awareness and knowledge and are much less efficient in actually

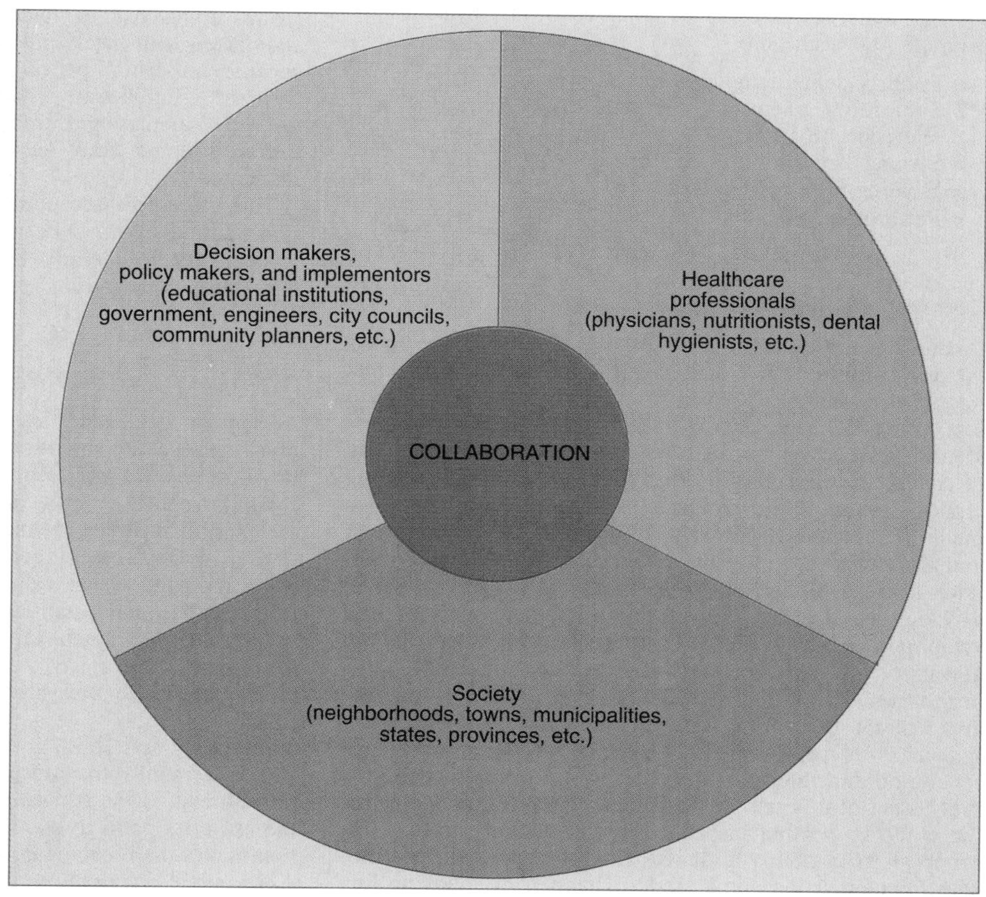

FIGURE 4–12
Collaboration: Awareness and interaction.

changing behavior,[64–71] although behavior change may be achieved.[72] Increased awareness and knowledge made possible through mass media are enabling factors that prepare the individual for lifestyle changes that influence health and wellness.

Nonprofit organizations, such as the American Dental Hygienists' Association and Canadian Dental Hygienists' Association, and local professional associations collaborate with corporate sponsors to promote oral health via mass media. This collaboration is mutually beneficial to both groups.[73] Nonprofit organizations can use mass media such as commercial television and radio rather than relying on public service announcements (usually used as fillers), which have smaller audiences and are often less flashy and attractive because of smaller budgets.[74] The corporate sponsor benefits in that it becomes linked with a credible source, and hence its own credibility is increased.

In seeking corporate sponsorship for mass media messages on health promotion, it is necessary to deal creatively with business. Potential corporate sponsors may include oral product companies, the baby food industry, or even insurance companies. What do companies have to gain from corporate sponsorship of an oral health promotion campaign? Parents buy baby food for their infants and also seek oral healthcare and advice from the dental hygienist regarding their infants, thus forming a mutually beneficial arrangement. Insurance companies have profits to gain if people engage in health-promoting behaviors, which are exactly what the dental hygienist promotes. Mutually beneficial partnerships among organized dental hygiene, business, and the public can lead to successful health outcomes for society.

Other activities that can be assumed by the hygienist to promote oral health are:

- Publicly denouncing incorrect information
- Submitting scientifically based scripts to radio and television programs
- Serving as contributing editors
- Holding press conferences
- Performing radio and television spots

Community Organization

Community organization is the process aimed at developing the skills, abilities, and understandings of groups of people for the purpose of self-led improvement. It is a group process, using the group as a medium for change. Cartwright[75] identifies five principles of group dynamics used as a force of change: belongingness, attractiveness, relevance, prestige, and resistance. If the group is to be used effectively as a medium for change, those people who are to be changed, and those who are exerting influence for the change, must have a sense of belongingness to the same group. Table 4–7 outlines the five principles with application to the development of a community-based health clinic that offered a variety of health-related services not including oral healthcare. The clinic served clients from a low-income area, many of whom were unemployed and otherwise known as "street people." The clinic, having an excellent reputation and referral system, both on a formal and informal basis (local hotel bar managers often referred people to the clinic by writing the address on a napkin), initiated a proposal to establish a dental clinic on-site. The people who frequented the clinic made it happen by lobbying for public funds and manpower resources to operate it.

TABLE 4–7
COMMUNITY-BASED HEALTH CENTERS IN LOW-INCOME AREAS EMPLOYING GROUP DYNAMIC PRINCIPLES

Principle	Consideration
Belongingness	Employment of community people Avoiding the professional appearance Community ownership Professional as resource, not implementor or planner
Attractiveness	Centered in community Open house policy Removal of stereotypes Low cost
Relevance	Health needs and demands assessed by the community people, not by experts Services are required and demanded
Prestige	Established success rate Significant persons recommend it
Resistance	Competition Lack of knowledge and awareness Cost factor

Social learning theory is integral to community organization because it explains human behavior as a socially learned construct.[76] Behavior is believed to be learned observationally through modeling and is reinforced either positively or negatively by personal and societal response to the behavior. For example, athletic head and neck protective shields are much more commonly worn in all age groups involved in contact sports than they were 10 years ago. Head and neck protective shields became accepted because important persons (renowned athletes) advocated their use, significant persons (coaches) encouraged their use, and increasing numbers of persons playing contact sports accepted their use (and eventually their use was mandated).

The process of acceptance reflects the concept of diffusion of innovation. Diffusion of innovation suggests that it is necessary to identify the opinion leadership and gain their support regarding proposed change or new experience.[77]

Advocacy, Legislation, and Public Policy

A dog defecates and his owner, carrying a poop-scoop, must remove the deposit from the sidewalk for later disposal in the garbage can. Smokers must extinguish their cigarettes before entering a public place. Traffic stop signs are placed at street intersections. Schoolchildren must be immunized against numerous childhood diseases prior to attending school. All children's sleepwear must be made from nonflammable fabrics. Children 6 to 13 years of age in Manitoba, Canada, receive comprehensive oral care from dental therapists. All these are examples of public policy for health instigated through advocacy and legislation.

Advocacy and legislation go hand in hand in that advocacy is generally the precursor to legislation. **Advocacy,** in this context, is the education of decision makers to provide the essential political support for changes, whereas **legislation** makes these behaviors mandatory.

All public policy must consider the health implications of that policy, otherwise known as proactively creating

"healthy public policy."[33] It means that the health impact of any endeavor is considered an outcome equally important as the goal of that policy.[78] Health policy emphasizes economics, social programs, agriculture, sports and leisure, mining, and transportation.

THE ROLE OF THE DENTAL HYGIENIST IN HEALTH PROMOTION

The dental hygienist has a role in health promotion. A framework for health promotion (see Fig. 4–9)[43] enables dental hygienists to place into perspective their role in creating healthy environments for the nation.[79,80] Dental hygienists have the responsibility to:

- Promote oral health as being integral to overall health
- Increase oral disease prevention and oral health promotion
- Reduce inequities among population groups (increasing access to dental hygiene care, for example)

These responsibilities can be achieved by employing the strategies of fostering public participation, strengthening community health service, and coordinating "healthy public policy."

Fostering public participation requires helping people assert control over factors that affect their health and enabling people to act in ways that preserve or improve their health. For example, oral health should always be a component of prenatal education, tobacco cessation programs, workshops for caregivers and nurses' aides, and certainly a part of the school health curriculum. Dental hygienists should be assuming primary activist roles for ensuring that these programs take place. Whether on an individual leadership basis or collectively through dental hygiene associations, dental hygienists have a responsibility to foster public participation in influencing public policy to promote health.

Dental hygienists, as change agents and consumer advocates, can lead the public in their demands for access to quality community oral healthcare. Numerous homes and daycare centers for the elderly, facilities for individuals with mental and physical impairments, as well as disadvantaged groups (immigrants, Native Americans/Inuit) have limited access to oral disease prevention and oral health promotion. The advocacy powers of the dental hygienist are required to ensure the provision of oral healthcare to persons of disadvantaged groups.

When oral healthcare is provided to disadvantaged groups, it is generally treatment oriented, possibly with an oral disease educational component at chairside. Dental hygienists should be in the forefront organizing public forums to provide the rationale and incentive for the public to lobby with community councils, legislators, and higher government for the establishment of facilities aimed solely at health promotion.

On an interprofessional basis, dental hygienists have an important challenge in educating allied health professionals, community workers, employers, and others regarding the significance of oral health to quality of life. Dental hygienists should serve on school boards, parent-teacher associations, curriculum committees, boards of institutional facilities, and governmental health promotion task forces, among many others. As people are made aware of the oral health needs and demands of the public, the likelihood of expanding community oral healthcare services is increased.

Public policies that promote oral health must involve the leadership of the dental hygienist and be supported by valid and reliable research. For example, a Canadian health survey involving a random selection of citizens throughout the nation failed to recognize and address oral health as a component of the survey. Dental hygienists should have become involved in the survey, ensuring that oral health was assessed. Dental hygienists should be involved in research that directly influences their field of study (oral health behavior or practice, attitudes and beliefs regarding oral health).[81] A framework for promoting oral health should apply the dental hygiene process in the assessment of community need, public policy formation, program planning, implementation, and evaluation. Such a framework enables oral health professionals to assume leadership roles in oral health promotion.[82]

Dental hygienists need to be consumer advocates and change agents, convincing decision makers to support oral health promotion policy. Advocacy factors the dental hygienist may advocate include:

- Cost-effectiveness of having dental hygienists employed in a variety of nontraditional settings (e.g., schools, institutions, work sites)
- Inclusion of oral health education in school curricula
- Elimination of nutritionally unsound foods in school cafeterias
- Benefits of community water fluoridation

References

1. World Health Organization. Chronicle of World Health Organization, The Organization, Interim Commission. Geneva, Switzerland, 1974.
2. World Health Organization. Regional Office for Europe. Copenhagen, Denmark, 1985.
3. Whitbeck, C. A theory of health. In Caplan, A., Englehart, T., and McCartney, J. Concepts of Health and Disease. Redding, MA: Addison-Wesley, 1981, pp. 611–626.
4. Balog, J. The concepts of health and diseases: A relativistic perspective. Health Values 6:7, 1982.
5. Walsh, M., Heckman, B., et al. Conceptual Framework for UCSF Dental Hygiene Curriculum (unpublished paper). San Francisco: University of California at San Francisco, Division of Dental Public Heath and Hygiene, 1988.
6. Darby, M. Theory development and basic research in dental hygiene: Review of the literature and recommendations. Paper presented at the 67th Annual Session of ADHA, San Antonio, Texas, 1990.
7. Walsh, M. Theory development in dental hygiene. Probe, The Canadian Dental Hygienists' Journal 25:12, 1990.
8. Meyerson, M. Cultural considerations in the treatment of Latinos with craniofacial malformations. Cleft Palate Journal 27:279, 1990.
9. Gorlin, R. (1983) Facial folklore: Developmental medicine and neonatal genetics. Cited in Meyerson, M. Cultural considerations in the treatment of Latinos with Craniofacial Malformations. Cleft Palate Journal 27:279, 1990.
10. Poma, P. Pregnancy in Hispanic women (1987). Cited in Meyerson, M. Cultural considerations in the treatment of Latinos with craniofacial malformations. Cleft Palate Journal 27:279, 1990.
11. Diaz, V. Caribbean Hispanics (1987). Cited in Meyerson, M. Cultural considerations in the treatment of Latinos with craniofacial malformations. Cleft Palate Journal 27:279, 1990.
12. Toliver-Weddington, G. Cultural considerations in the treatment of craniofacial malformations in African-Americans. Cleft Palate Journal 27:289, 1990.
13. Cheung, L. Asian-American cultural perspectives on birth defects: Focus on cleft palate. Cleft Palate Journal 27:294, 1990.
14. Scheper-Hughes, N. Difference and danger: The cultural dynamics of childhood stigma, rejection, and rescue. Cleft Palate Journal 27:301, 1990.

15. Dunn, H. High-level wellness for man and society. American Journal of Public Health 49:786, 1959.
16. Dunn, H. What high-level wellness means. Canadian Journal of Public Health 50:447, 1959.
17. Dunn, H. What high-level wellness means. Health Values 1:9, 1977.
18. deLeeuw, E. The Sane Revolution: Health Promotion: Background, Scope, Prospects. Assen, The Netherlands: Van Gorcum & Company B.V., 1989.
19. Lalonde, M. A New Perspective on the Health of Canadians: A Working Document. National Health and Welfare Canada, 1974.
20. Carolyn, W. Myths, mindsets, and the Medical Model: Misunderstandings in school health instruction. Health Values 5:207, 1981.
21. Rosenstock, I. Historical origins of the Health Belief Model. In Becker, M., and Marshall, H. (eds.). The Health Belief Model and Personal Behavior. Thorofare, NJ: Slack, 1974, pp. 1–8.
22. Leavell, H., and Clark, E. Preventive Medicine for the Doctor in His Community, 3rd ed. New York: McGraw-Hill, 1965, pp. 28–64.
23. Friedman, G. Primer of Epidemiology, 3rd ed. New York: McGraw-Hill, 1987.
24. Kligman, E. W., Feldhauser, J. K., and Hale, F. A. Manual of Clinical Preventive Medicine. Proposed under contract no. 240–84–0093 from Health Resources and Services Administration. Washington D.C.: Bureau of Health Professions, Divisions of Medicine. Department of Health and Human Services, 1986.
25. Haefner, D. The Health Belief Model and preventive dental behavior. In Becker, M. (ed.). The Health Belief Model and Personal Health Behavior. Thorofare, NJ: Slack, 1974, pp. 93–105.
26. Dental Products Reports, Periodontal Care 1992. January, 1992, pp. 58–58a.
27. Taylor, R., Ureda, J., and Denham, J. Health Promotion: Principles and Clinical Application. Norwalk, CT: Appleton-Century-Crofts, 1982.
28. Manitoba Health. Partners for Health: A New Direction for the Promotion of Health in Manitoba. A Manitoba "Partners in Health" policy paper, 1989.
29. Labonte, R., and Penfold, S. Health Promotion Philosophy from Victim-Blaming to Social Responsibility. Health Promotion Directorate, Health and Welfare, Canada, 1981.
30. United States Department of Health, Education and Welfare. Public Health Service. Healthy People: The Surgeon General's Report on Health Promotion and Disease Prevention. Washington, DC, DHEW, 1979.
31. United States Department of Health and Human Services. Public Health Service. The 1990 Health Objectives for the Nation: A Midcourse Review. Washington, DC, DHHS, 1986.
32. United States Department of Health and Human Services. Public Health Service. Promoting Health, Preventing Disease: Objectives for the Nation. Washington, DC, DHHS, 1980.
33. Ottawa Charter for Health Promotion. An International Conference on Health Promotion. The Move towards a New Public Health. Ottawa, 1986.
34. Dwore, R., and Kreuter, M. Update: Reinforcing the case for health promotion. Family and Community Health 2:103, 1980.
35. Green, L. Measurement and evaluation in health education and health promotion. Palo Alto, CA: Mayfield, 1986.
36. World Health Organization. Regional Office for Europe. Health Promotion: Concepts and Principles in Action: A Policy Framework. Copenhagen, Denmark, 1986.
37. Rootman, I. Knowledge development: A challenge for health promotion. Health Promotion 27:2, 1988.
38. World Health Organization. Achieving Health for All by the Year 2000, 1981.
39. World Health Organization. Advisory Committee on Health Research. Health Research Strategy. Geneva, Switzerland, 1986.
40. World Health Organization. Regional Office for Europe. Oral Health for All by the Year 2000. Guidelines for Self-Care in Oral Health. Copenhagen, Denmark, 1988.
41. Burt, B. The prevention connection: Linking dental health education and prevention. International Dental Journal 33:188, 1983.
42. Hancock, T. The mandala of health: A model of the human ecosystem. Family and Community Health 8:1, 1985.
43. Epp, J. Achieving Health for All: A Framework for Health Promotion. Ottawa, Canada: National Health and Welfare, 1986.
43a. Ardell, D. The history and future of wellness. Health Values 9:37, 1985.
44. Reisine, S. Dental disease and work loss. Journal of Dental Research 63:1158, 1984.
45. Reisine, S. Dental health and public policy: The social impact of dental disease. American Journal of Public Health 75:27, 1985.
46. Locker, D., and Grushka, M. Prevalence of oral pain and discomfort: Preliminary results of a mail survey. Community Dental and Oral Epidemiology 15:169, 1987.
47. Oosterhaven, S., Westert, G., and Schaub, R. Perception and significance of dental appearance: The case of missing teeth. Community Dental and Oral Epidemiology 17:123, 1989.
48. Westert, P., Osterhaven, S., and Schaub, R. Spontaneous recall as an indicator of the impact of dental complaints. Community Dentistry and Oral Epidemiology 15(16):306–308, 1987.
49. Reisine, S., Fertig, J., Weber, J., and Leder, S. Impact of dental condition on patients' quality of life. Community Dentistry and Oral Epidemiology 17:7, 1989.
50. Reisine, S., and Weber, J. The effects of temporomandibular disorders on patients' quality of life. Community Dental Health 6:357, 1989.
51. Locker, D., and Slade, G. The prevalence of symptoms of temporomandibular joint disorders in a Canadian population. Community Dentistry and Oral Epidemiology 16:310, 1988.
52. Smith, J. Oral and dental discomfort—a necessary feature of old age? Age and Aging 8:25, 1979.
53. Straus, R., Sandifer, J., Hall, D., and Haley, J. Behavioral factors and denture status. Journal of Prosthetic Dentistry 37:264, 1977.
54. Ekelund, R. Dental state and subjective chewing ability of institutionalized elderly people. Community Dental and Oral Epidemiology 17:24, 1989.
55. Sticker, G. Psychological issues pertaining to malocclusion. American Journal of Orthodontics 58:276, 1970.
56. Shaw, W., Addy, M., and Ray, C. Dental and social effects of malocclusion and effectiveness of orthodontic treatment: A review. Community Dentistry and Oral Epidemiology 8:36, 1980.
57. Shaw, W., Meek, S., and Jones, D. Nicknames, teasing and harassment and the salience of dental features among schoolchildren. British Journal of Orthodontics 7:75, 1980.
58. Dexter, H. Directions for dental health promotion research. A paper presented at the Conference on Dental Hygiene Research, Winnipeg, 1982.
59. Kotler, P., and Zaltman, G. Social marketing: An approach to planned social change. In Zaltman, G., Kotler, P., and Kaufman, I. (eds.). Creating Social Change. New York: Holt, Rinehart, & Winston, 1972.
60. Green, L. National policy in the promotion of health. International Journal of Health Education 22:161, 1979.
61. Locker, D. Approaches to dental health education. In Preventative Dental Services, 2nd ed. Health and Welfare, Canada, 1988, pp. 144–146.
62. Elbon, S., and Karp, W. The dietitian as a member of the dental health care team. Journal of American Dietetic Association 87:1062, 1987.
63. Ramprasad, R., Carson, P., et al. Dentists and blood pressure measurement: A survey of attitudes and practices. Journal of American Dental Association 108:767, 1984.
64. Epstein, J., Magrowski, W., and McPhail, C. The role of radio and television spot announcements in public health education. Canadian Journal of Public Health 66:396, 1975.
65. Weiss, R., Lee, E., and Williams, L. Mass communication media and local participation—community dental health education. Journal of American Dental Association 84:345, 1972.
66. Bakdash, M., Lange, A., and McMillan, D. Impact of peri-

odontal public service announcements (abstract). Journal of Dental Research 61:242, 1982.
67. Bakdash, M., Lange, A., and McMillan, D. The effect of a televised periodontal campaign on public periodontal awareness. Journal of Periodontology 54:666, 1983.
68. Schou, L. Use of mass media and active involvement in national dental health campaign in Scotland. Community Dental and Oral Epidemiology 15:14, 1987.
69. Rise, J., and Sogaard, A. Effect of a mass media periodontal and behavioral campaign upon knowledge and behavior in Norway. Community Dental and Oral Epidemiology 16:1, 1988.
70. Horstter, G., and Hoogstraten, J. Immediate and delayed effects of dental health education films on periodontal knowledge, attitude, and reported behavior of Dutch adolescents. Community Dental and Oral Epidemiology 17:183, 1989.
71. Folke, E., Johannson, L., and Stromberg, L. Campaign to promote periodontal disease awareness (abstract). Probe, Canadian Dental Hygienists' Association Journal 25:44, 1990.
72. Pucka, P., Wiio, J., et al. Planned use of mass media in national health promotion: The "keys to health" television program in 1982 in Finland. Canadian Journal of Public Health 76:336, 1985.
73. Thornton, A. Mass communication and dental health behavior. Health Education Monographs 2:201, 1974.
74. Newman, I., Martin, G., and Farrell, K. Changing health values through public television. Health Values 2:92, 1978.
75. Cartwright, D. Achieving change in people: Some application of group dynamics theory. In Zaltman, G., Kotler, P., and Kaufman, I. (eds.). Creating Social Change. New York: Holt, Rinehart, & Winston, 1972, pp. 74–82.
76. Bandura, A. Social Learning Theory. Englewood Cliffs, NJ: Prentice-Hall, 1977.
77. Rogers, E., and Shoemaker, F. Communication of Innovation: A Cross Cultural Approach, 2nd ed. New York: The Free Press, 1971, pp. 180–191.
78. Fulton, J. Sinking our teeth into public policy. Probe, Canadian Dental Hygienists' Association Journal 24:129, 1990.
79. Brownstone, E. The role of the dental hygienist in health promotion. Probe, Canadian Dental Hygienists' Association Journal 21:164, 1987.
80. Gallagher, D. The role of dental hygiene in achieving health for all. Probe, Canadian Dental Hygienists' Association Journal 21:119, 1987.
81. Fooks, C. Policies, politics, and economic priorities: Issues for dental hygienists. Probe, Canadian Dental Hygienists' Association Journal 24:138, 1990.
82. Cohen, L. Leadership role of dental associations: Oral health promotion. International Dental Journal 40:48, 1990.
83. Becker, M., and Marshall, H. (eds.). The Health Belief Model and Personal Behavior. Thorofare, N. J.: C. B. Slack, 1974.

Suggested Readings

Blum, H. Planning for Health: Development and Application of Social Change Theory. New York: Human Science Press, 1974.
Clovis, J. The Active Health Report—perspectives on Canada's Health Promotion Survey 1985. Probe, Canadian Dental Hygienists' Association Journal 21:161, 1987.
Promoting oral health: Guidelines for dental associations. International Dental Journal 40:79, 1990.
Vickers, G. Through the centuries. In Greene, L., and Anderson, C. (eds.). Community Health. St. Louis: C. V. Mosby, 1982, pp. 3–21.
Walker, S., Seichrist, K., and Pender, N. The health-promoting lifestyle profile: Development and psychometric characteristics. Nursing Research 36:76, 1987.

5 Behavioral Foundations for the Dental Hygiene Process

OBJECTIVES

Mastery of the content of this chapter will enable the reader to:

- Define the key terms used
- Relate the importance of communication to the profession of dental hygiene
- List the basic components of the communication process
- Describe verbal and nonverbal communication
- Discuss therapeutic communication techniques
- Discuss nontherapeutic communication techniques
- Describe the domains of learning
- Identify major theories of motivation
- Describe how teaching, learning, and communication are interwoven
- Describe the application of learning theory in behavioristic, cognitive, and humanistic psychology
- Identify communication, teaching, and learning techniques appropriate throughout the lifespan

INTRODUCTION

Behavioral science theory provides the knowledge base for effective client communication, health education and promotion, and interpersonal interactions during the dental hygiene process (Table 5–1). Principles drawn from the behavioral sciences guide the dental hygienist's client interactions in a manner that can facilitate human need fulfillment via the achievement of optimal oral health. Human need theory can provide the framework for understanding motivation and learning. Although human behavior can be conceptualized in an infinite number of ways, human need theory is highlighted throughout this chapter.

Dental hygienists perceive their role as one of "caregiver," but often the psychological support offered in that capacity is based more on personal intuition and "doing what comes naturally" than on scientific theory and research. Although it is valuable to follow one's own moral and ethical feelings of kindness and empathy toward clients, it also is expected that educated professionals look to theory for guidance in the complex area of human communication.

The behavioral sciences theory supports a humanistic approach to client care that emphasizes empathy and respect. It has been suggested that if dental hygienists possess technical skills and knowledge but are unable to understand human behavior or perceive human needs, they may fail to reach important goals related to client comfort, pain and anxiety reduction, long-term behavior change, oral health maintenance, and oral health promotion.[1] Furthermore, oral health needs cannot be separated from other human needs. Thus, the client must be viewed and accepted holistically, that is, as a "whole person."

The benefits of effective communication for dental hygienists are twofold. First, during the assessment phase the hygienist obtains and validates information from the client concerning health history, dental/sociocultural history, and oral health behaviors. This information, if gathered and assessed properly, provides the basis for the dental hygiene diagnosis and care plan. The second benefit is the obvious value of communication skills in influencing client adherence to preventive and other therapeutic recommendations. When rapport, confidence, and trust are present, a client can respond to the dental hygienist's advice, learn the nature of oral disease processes and adhere to specific recommendations.

CHANGE AGENT ROLE AND COMMUNICATION

The roles of the dental hygienist have been delineated and defined by the American Dental Hygienists' Association in 1984, 1985, and 1986:

TABLE 5-1
MODES OF COMMUNICATION IN THE DENTAL HYGIENE PROCESS

Dental Hygiene Process	Modes of Communication
Assessment	
Gathering information related to the current status of client	Interviewing for health, dental, and sociocultural histories, details of oral hygiene behaviors Intra- and extraoral examinations (using visual, tactile, olfactory, and auditory methods) Observing nonverbal behavior Reviewing client record for previous care
Dental Hygiene Diagnosis	
Identification of human need deficits that require dental hygiene care	Written analysis and assessment of findings Discussion with collaborating dentist Discussion with other healthcare providers, e.g., physician of record Discussion of oral health findings with client
Planning	
Determining appropriate dental hygiene interventions and referrals	Discussion with client to set goals, determine methods of implementing dental hygiene care, and an oral hygiene regimen Discussion with collaborating dentist and other members of the health team Written documentation of plan; obtaining informed consent
Implementation	
Providing dental hygiene care	Interaction with client during the delivery of dental hygiene interventions Oral health teaching Written documentation of services rendered
Evaluation	
Evaluating outcomes of dental hygiene care	Obtaining verbal and nonverbal feedback from client Recording results of previous dental hygiene care including oral health education Documentation of treatment outcomes

Adapted with permission from Potter, P. A., and Perry, A. G. Fundamentals of Nursing: Concepts, Process, and Practice, 3rd ed. St. Louis: C. V. Mosby, 1993.

- Clinician
- Educator and health promoter
- Change agent
- Administrator and manager
- Client advocate
- Researcher

All roles require use of effective communication skills. A dental hygienist in the clinician and educator and health promoter roles also serves as a change agent in daily interactions with clients and other health professionals. The dental hygienist has the responsibility of introducing new oral hygiene regimens, providing new information, and helping clients to clarify values regarding their health. Communication is essential in creating an environment conducive to making changes in psychomotor skills, level of knowledge, values, attitudes, and lifestyles. As an administrator and manager, the dental hygienist uses communication skills in relationships with other health professionals and may be able to effect changes in organizational policy and procedures, infection control, or personnel relations that can improve the work environment for all. The client advocate role demands that the hygienist possess communication skills necessary for influencing legislators, health agencies, and other organizations in resolving issues that may be affecting the quality of community oral health. The researcher role requires that, in order to contribute to the theoretical and scientific knowledge base, the dental hygienist communicate clearly with co-investigators, students, colleagues, and the general public to effect change based on research findings. Healthcare is communication-centered, and hygienists who learn to communicate effectively and efficiently are satisfied, rewarded, and fulfilled in their healthcare role.

DEFINITION OF COMMUNICATION

Communication is the process by which a person sends a message to another person with the intention of evoking a response. A basic communication model might simply be depicted as shown in Figure 5-1.

Communication is never static but rather is a dynamic, ongoing process that has no specific beginning or end. Messages may be verbal or nonverbal, and the entire process involves a complex set of interrelated, constantly changing components. A closer examination of the components inherent in the communication process assists in understanding the concept more clearly.

The **sender** is the person who constructs a message to initiate the interpersonal communication. The message construction process is known as **encoding.** The role of sender changes as the communication process progresses.

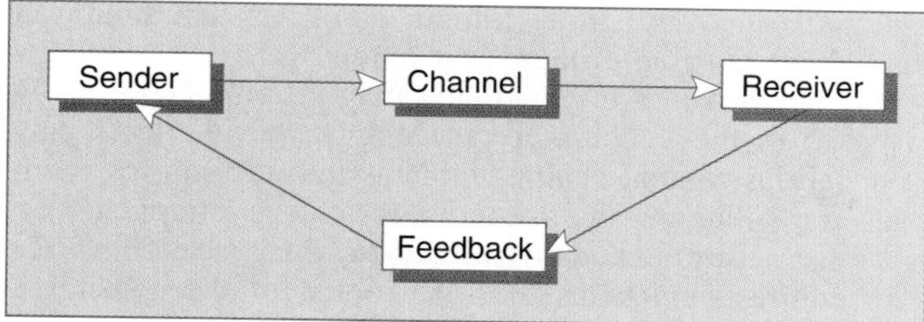

FIGURE 5-1
Basic communication model.

The **message** itself contains information the sender wishes to transmit. It must be in a format of symbols that are understandable to the other person. It should be clearly organized and well expressed and may be comprised of both verbal and nonverbal content.

The message is sent via a channel or medium. In education the channel may be a chalkboard, an overhead projector, a videotape, or television. Between hygienist and client, the channel may simply be a voice. The channel may involve any of the five senses but is likely to be visual, auditory, or tactile.

The **receiver** is the person who accepts the message and deciphers its meaning, a process known as **decoding.** The receiver must share a common language and a common set of definitions with the sender to decode the message accurately. When the sender is able to communicate accurately the message he wishes to convey, then the receiver has decoded the message just as the sender meant it to be. In such an instance, effective communication has taken place.

The dynamic process does not generally stop with one encoded and decoded message. The receiver is prompted to respond and provides a feedback message. He then becomes the sender and the cycle repeats itself. The feedback model of communications illustrates how each person has an encoding and a decoding role in the communication (Fig. 5-2).[2]

People are more likely to communicate effectively in an environment that is comfortable. Factors such as lighting, heating, ventilation, and acoustics may affect the process. In the oral healthcare setting, privacy (human need for

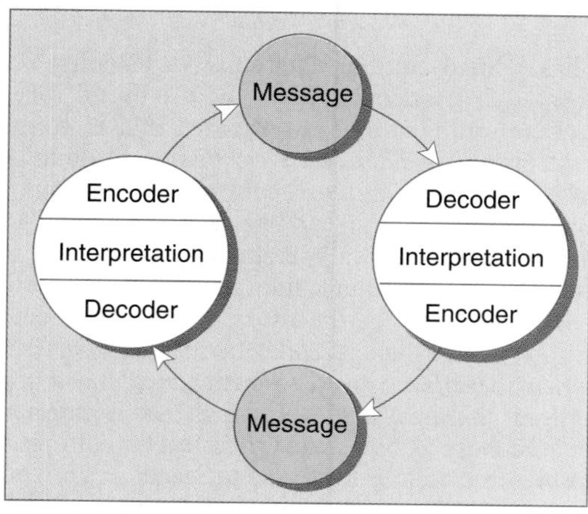

FIGURE 5-2
Wilbur Schramm feedback model. (Adapted with permission from Schramm, W. How communication works. In Schramm, W. (ed.). The Process and Effects of Mass Communication. Urbana, IL: University of Illinois Press, 1955. Copyright 1954 Board of Trustees of the University of Illinois.)

territoriality) may be important if clients are revealing sensitive information about their health. A bustling environment may pose annoying distractions that could block communication.

LEVELS OF COMMUNICATION

The three levels of communication are

- Intrapersonal
- Interpersonal
- Public

Intrapersonal communication refers to communication within oneself. When a dental hygienist notices a client with a careful step and slightly bent posture, she thinks, "His back seems to be hurting him. I'd better ask him if reclining the chair back too far today will bother him." The dental hygienist is "talking to herself" or communicating intrapersonally.

Corno and Mandinach delineated some metacognitive skills or "thinking about thinking" skills, which are essential in learning and in intrapersonal communication.[3] Self-rehearsing is conducted as one thinks about how to proceed with speech or actions. Self-checking occurs as one judges oneself and makes adjustments in behavior. Connecting takes place as one searches memory to link new information with that previously learned. Attention to these internal skills can enhance communication by helping us to better express ourselves to others.

Interpersonal communication refers to that which occurs between two people or in small group sessions. An essential part of living is social interaction between people who come together to share ideas and solve problems. Dental hygienists' communication skills are constantly being challenged as they meet daily with clients and other professionals. Interpersonal communication truly is central to the dental hygiene process.

Public communication is communication within large groups. Lecturing to groups of parents, schoolchildren, or teachers is an example of public communication. Public speaking skills are of importance to the hygienist in such roles.

FACTORS THAT AFFECT COMMUNICATION

Potter and Perry point out that a person's perceptions, values, emotions, sociocultural background, and level of knowledge influence the way messages are sent and received.[4] These factors provide insight into the communication process in dental hygiene.

Perceptions

Perceptions can vary greatly from person to person. One individual's analysis of a situation may differ entirely from another's, even though all basic elements are the same. As an example, it is possible for a dental hygienist to take a very aggressive approach to oral health education. The hygienist may communicate strong demands for client response and loud, clear warnings about the progression of disease if recommendations are not followed. Some clients may perceive the dental hygienist as an authority figure whom they can respect and respond to very favorably. Others may be offended and perceive the dental hygienist as "pushy" and judgmental with a generally adverse reaction to attempts to influence their behavior or health.

Perceptions are formed based on past experience and are difficult to change. If the client had previous contact with a dental hygienist who communicated respect and warmth, he would be more likely to respond well to the hygienist's attempt to resolve a health issue that has become more pressing. When a hygienist takes an aggressive stance with a new client, the risk of blocked communication from the client's negative perception of the dental hygienist is great.

In contrast, the hygienist should be aware of personal perceptions of the client. Initial impressions that the client is rude or egotistical may be difficult to overcome. For client-centered healthcare to occur, the hygienist must demonstrate humanistic behaviors throughout the process of care. This approach is likely to work well with clients who universally desire to be treated kindly in healthcare settings and who may be projecting a misleading image of themselves because of their anxiety about the unknown.

Values

Values are personal beliefs that may have moral and ethical implications. Whatever we consider important in our lives influences the way we communicate our ideas and feelings. Each individual has a unique set of values that has been shaped by personal experiences. The hygienist can influence the communication process by exercising tolerance and understanding for the wide differences of opinion that exist.

Not all clients value oral health. Individuals have reasons, both known and unknown, for holding their respective values. A person from an impoverished background may have had to prioritize values to survive. Oral health and education may not be highly valued when food, shelter, and clothing have not been readily available. On high school campuses, a sugar-free diet may not be valued when candy and soft-drink machines beckon. Water fluoridation may not be valued by people who have been deluged with information from antifluoridationists.

Values can be changed but the experts have suggested that they are slow to form and change. Christen and Katz suggested that certain conditions must exist for value change to occur in the oral healthcare environment.[5] Oral healthcare professionals must:

- *Be aware of their own values* and how they affect the choices they make in planning and implementing oral health behavior change programs
- *Understand the values held by the client* through careful observation and analysis of behavior
- *Avoid imposing their values on a client* who has a different set of values

Sometimes client values related to oral health and disease can be changed by education. The methods used to obtain change and the degree of success are dependent on how wide the gap is between the desired value and the client's current value.

Emotions

One cannot underestimate the influence of emotions in everyday communication. Emotions are strong feelings people have about other people, places, and things in their environment. Fear, wonder, love, sorrow, and shame are examples of a few strong human emotions that touch all individuals at some time in their lives.

Hygienists who are empathetic may become emotionally involved in their clients' lives. Dental hygiene clients may have serious general health problems that are causing them grief and suffering. The hygienist should be compassionate but must act professionally throughout the process of care.

In contrast, emotions that are rooted in the hygienist's own personal life should not interfere with client care. Potter and Perry discuss an interesting hypothetical situation:[4]

> A young nurse has had an argument with her husband before coming to work. Her husband is just out of law school and establishing his practice. The nurse's income is needed for the family's survival. Her husband has proposed that they begin having children. The nurse knows that she and her husband would have difficulty rearing a family now, particularly since she would soon have to take a leave from work. The nurse goes to work angered by her husband's lack of understanding. The first client she sees is a 24-year-old mother of three who is divorced and living on welfare. The nurse cannot allow herself to transfer her anger at her husband to the client's situation. This would prevent her from understanding this client as an individual. If the nurse is to communicate effectively with the client, she must be aware of her emotions.

Sociocultural Background

Sociocultural differences are important in social interaction and communication. A dental hygienist who has a broad understanding of cultural diversity is better prepared to communicate with clients from varying backgrounds (see Chapter 6). Cultural origins are reflected in both verbal and nonverbal behaviors. It is natural for an individual to identify with and learn from those persons who are closest to him. One's own sociocultural group provides a frame of reference for the rest of one's activities, including communication.

A person's cultural background may cause him to question certain health values. This can be frustrating for the oral health educator who must be understanding of the client's perspective in order to engage his trust and cooperation.

Hall has studied cultural differences in listening behavior and provided a good example of how cultural differences can affect communication.[6] He reported that in certain cultures, communicative use of eyes, hands, orientation and position of the body, and tone of voice are unique to the particular group. Consequently, he feels that many gestures are frequently misread by members of the larger society. He states that an informal rule in a particular minority culture is, "If you are in the room with another person or in a context where he has ready access to you, there are times when there is no need to go through the motions of showing him you are listening because that is automatically implied." Because people from most other cultures generally expect some visible feedback to signal attentiveness in conversation, this behavior can cause problems in communication attempts between members of different groups. Misinterpretation on the part of individuals outside of the minority culture is unfortunate when no discourtesy is intended. Further study in the area of sociocultural differences may create a greater awareness for health professionals interacting with culturally diverse clients.

Knowledge

Communication can be hindered when levels of knowledge differ between those interacting. Recipients of oral healthcare may be highly educated but have an area of expertise quite outside the realm of oral health. A highly technical vocabulary is inappropriate with a client unless terms are carefully explained. Most people have no need to distinguish between the "mesials" and "distals" of their teeth, but this terminology, which is essential in professional communication, is commonplace for members of the oral healthcare team. If the dental hygienist uses language the client cannot understand, she loses attention and cooperation and lessens the chances that goals will be achieved. The effective dental hygienist avoids "talking down" to clients and monitors client feedback to guide the appropriate level of language usage.

VERBAL COMMUNICATION

Myerscough has used the word CARE as a simple mnemonic or memory-assisting technique to identify the skills a health professional should develop:[7]

CARE
C = Comfort A = Acceptance R = Responsiveness E = Empathy

Comfort

Comfort in the mnemonic denotes the ability to deal with embarrassing or emotionally painful topics related to a person's health. In dental hygiene practice this could be loss of teeth and wearing of prosthetic appliances, inability to seek oral healthcare because of financial difficulties, or another personal or medical reason that may interfere with an ability to develop an oral hygiene regimen. Comfort also includes the verbal support extended to a client who fears injections or other dental procedures. It could also refer to an awareness of the client's physical comfort during dental hygiene care (for example, client positioning or emotional comfort, territorial distance between client and practitioner). To meet the client's human need for freedom from pain or stress, the hygienist strives to keep the client's comfort a top priority.

Acceptance

Acceptance refers to the ability to accept a client as the person he is without allowing any judgment of that person's attitudes or feelings to interfere with communication. Acceptance of others is necessary if the hygienist is to meet the client's human need for appreciation and respect. A client may appear unwilling to assume responsibility for his own health; he may be critical or untrusting. His poor oral health may seem to be self-imposed and related to an unhealthy lifestyle. The client's appearance and attitudes may have deep cultural roots that are unfamilar to the hygienist. As discussed previously, cultural values are factors that may affect communication. The dental hygienist must develop an attitude of acceptance toward individuals whose values and sociocultural backgrounds seem unusual or foreign. The fact that the client senses that the hygienist is accepting of him can greatly facilitate understanding and a therapeutic, professional relationship.

Responsiveness

Responsiveness in a healthcare provider is the ability to reply to messages at the very moment they are sent. It requires sensitive alertness to cues that something more needs to be said. When a client arrives for a scaling appointment and mentions oral discomfort, indicating an unmet human need for freedom from pain, the comment should be pursued immediately. Scaling and root planing might have been scheduled, but other problems may be an immediate priority and supersede the planned care.

Empathy

Empathy is said to result when we place ourselves in another's "shoes." It is a type of intellectual role-playing in which one attempts to experience the emotional state of another individual. Carl Rogers, the psychologist who developed client-centered therapy, describes the state of being empathetic as "perceiving the internal frame of reference" of another with accuracy.[8] He states that empathy means to perceive the client "himself as he is seen by himself"—to sense his hurt or pleasure as he senses it. This perception of a client's viewpoint should help the dental hygienist better understand him, his reaction to dental hygiene care, and his capabilities for taking responsibility for his own health.

NONVERBAL COMMUNICATION

Communication in accordance with the CARE principle can be exhibited by both verbal and nonverbal behaviors. The following is a categorization of types of nonverbal messages.[9]

Kinesic Behavior

Kinesic behavior, or body motion, includes posture, gestures, facial expressions, eye behavior, and body movement. Because of all the different combinations of movement, the message can be extremely complex. The movement patterns a person develops set him apart from others. How many times have you recognized someone from afar because of his walk or some other gesture? To facilitate communication in the healthcare setting, different aspects of kinesic behavior are considered.

Eye Behavior

Eye behavior can be discussed separately from facial features and body movements, but, obviously, the messages being sent depend on all behaviors collectively. Generally, we are told to make eye contact with people as we speak to them. Eye contact is often made before the first spoken word. Thus, it is the first message sent when two people meet. The eye can convey trust, interest, or attention. Eye contact is avoided when we feel uncomfortable and maintained steadily when we are taking an offensive as opposed to a defensive approach to someone.

Along with the muscles of the forehead and the eyebrows, the eyes are extremely expressive. Raising an eyebrow can imply a question. Raising both eyebrows may indicate shock or surprise. Narrowed eyes may suggest skepticism, whereas wide open eyes show amazement.

A dental hygienist works in close proximity to a client's eyes and should always be monitoring them for nonverbal messages that convey pain or discomfort. Additionally, the dental hygienist's eyes are likely to be watched by the client for signs of approval, disapproval, kindness, or displeasure. A face mask hides most of the hygienist's face; therefore, eyes become an even more important source of expression.

Mouth Movement

Movements of the lips and mandible are closely related to eye behavior. Smiles come in many different varieties. Three types of smiles that have been identified are the "simple" smile, "upper" smile, and "broad" smile.[10] The simple smile can occur in solitude as well as in social settings and is distinguished by a slight upward curve of the lips. It is often shown when a person is meditative or contemplative. The upper smile is so named because it emphasizes the upper part of the face. It exposes the upper teeth and is used to greet relatives or friends. Laughter produces the broad smile and exposes both the maxillary and mandibular teeth. The lip muscles also can be inverted to form a grimace that may convey pain, fear, disapproval, or indifference.

Gestures

"Gesture" usually refers to movement by the arms, hands, head or, possibly, the whole body. These movements may reveal much about a person's feelings. Intense gesturing suggests excitement and pleasure, whereas a lack of gesturing may indicate weariness or demoralization. Actors learn to use their hands and arms for emphasis of feelings, moods, attitudes, or physical states. An observation of a client's hands clenching the arm of the dental unit is a cue to his human need deficits in safety and freedom from pain or stress.

Posture and Body Movement

Posture and body movement may be considered another category of gesture. The way a person moves can tell us whether he is comfortable or uncomfortable, bold or timid. A shift in posture can be an indication of a changing emotional state. Movement toward someone suggests trust and liking. Movement away sends a negative message. The speed at which people move can mean something definite. A slow movement suggests uncertainty; a rapid movement can indicate eagerness, playfulness, or possibly impatience. Posture is affected by size and overall physical appearance. An erect posture and a sharp, snappy step can do much to draw respect to a person of any size.

Touch

Touching is one of the most sensitive means of communication and is most closely related to the human need for territoriality, the human need for appreciation and respect, and the human need for safety. Touch can be reassuring in some contexts. A hand gently placed upon a shoulder may mean more to a client than any verbal expression of support. It is important to note, however, that people have different attitudes toward being touched. Some are not accustomed to it and may cringe or pull away as the hygienist attempts to comfort them. Touch should be used discriminately so it is not misinterpreted.

The nature of the dental hygiene process of care requires touching clients. The way in which the hygienist touches the client can communicate feelings about the client and the practice of dental hygiene. Rough jerking movements may send a message of careless indifference, resulting in uncooperative behavior from a client. Accidental touching, such as bumping a person's nose or poking him with an elbow, also can carry a negative message, such as carelessness or haste. A professional, careful approach to touching is appreciated and respected by recipients of healthcare.[11]

Paralanguage

Vocal sounds other than words themselves can form messages in communication. Characteristics such as intonation, rate, pitch, volume, and vocal patterns make up what is known as paralanguage. It refers to the vocal rather than the verbal aspects of speech.

Intonation is the modulation of the voice. The whisper of confidentiality, the rising crescendo of anger, and the dull tones of despair are examples of how intonation is used to communicate.[7] Rate refers to the cadence of speech or the speed and rhythms with which we speak. The drawl of a Southerner is contrasted against the fast-paced speech of a New Englander. Pitch is the frequency and range of a voice. Women's voices are pitched higher than men's voices. A shift in pitch may indicate a change in emotion. A high pitch may mean fear or excitement, whereas a low pitch may sound sinister or indicate that the speaker is suspicious of another. Volume is determined by the intensity of the sound waves produced. Loudness or softness of voice can affect the interpretation of a message. "Vocal patterns of speech" refer to variations in dialect or inflection that are characteristic of geographic or cultural inflences on language. The friendly sounding language of the Southerners has not only a slow rate but also a pattern of inflections that makes it sound unlike English spoken in other parts of the world.

THERAPEUTIC COMMUNICATION TECHNIQUES

No single communication technique works with all clients. One individual may be encouraged to express his feelings when the dental hygienist is silent whereas another may need coaxing with active questioning. Practice and experience, based upon a strong theoretical foundation, are required for choosing communication techniques to use in different situations. The following are communication techniques suggested by Potter and Perry that can be adapted by the dental hygienist.[4]

Maintaining Silence

Silence can be used effectively in communication because it provides an opportunity for the senders and receivers of messages to gather and reorganize their thoughts and feelings. During silent moments, nonverbal messages such as loss of eye contact or a wrinkled brow can be sent. Remaining silent may be uncomfortable, but adhering patiently to silence demonstrates the hygienist's willingness to listen and encourages the client to share his thoughts.

The nature of dental hygiene care often precludes talking by the client. A common complaint, usually shared good-naturedly among clients, is that their dental hygienist asks them questions when their hands are in clients' mouths! This typical scenario is unfair to a client and dental hygienists should guard against it. Common courtesy dictates that immediately upon asking a question, the hygienist remove hands, instruments, and saliva ejectors from the client's mouth to allow him an opportunity to respond through speaking, not just grunting. Also, hygienists sometimes find themselves engaged in a one-way conversation with clients if they talk during intraoral procedures. The client must be given a chance to respond. Silence should not be imposed upon recipients of dental hygiene care but rather observed at appropriate times.

Skill and timing are required to use silence effectively. The tendency for some is to want to break the silence too soon. Poor timing can prematurely interrupt the client's effort in choosing words and frustrate his attempts to communicate.

Listening Attentively

Being attentive to verbal and nonverbal messages by listening carefully is necessary for good communication. The dental hygienist indicates interest by appearing natural and relaxed and facing the client with good eye contact. Whatever the services being rendered, the client should remain the center of attention, with the hygienist's ears available to evaluate and respond. Geboy provided a list of interpersonal attending skills shown in Table 5–2 which, when applied, indicate involvement with the client and facilitate communication.[12] He has specific suggestions for eye contact, body orientation, posture, silence, following cues, distance, and distractions, which all add up to improving listening skills with dental hygiene clients.

TABLE 5–2
CHECKLIST OF INTERPERSONAL ATTENDING SKILLS

Skill Area	Criteria
Eye contact	Listener consistently focuses on the face and eyes of the speaker
Body orientation	Listener orients shoulders and legs toward the speaker
Posture	Listener maintains slight forward lean, arms maintained in a relaxed position
Silence	Listener avoids interrupting the speaker, uses periods of silence to facilitate continued communication
Following cues	Listener uses verbal and nonverbal cues to facilitate communication and indicate interest and attention
Distance	Listener maintains distance of 3–4 feet from speaker
Distractions	Listener avoids distracting behaviors such as pencil tapping, looking at a clock, and extraneous movements

Reprinted with permission from Geboy, M. J. Communication and Behavior Management in Dentistry. © 1985, The Williams & Wilkins Co., Baltimore.

Conveying Acceptance

It is certain that every hygienist comes in contact with people from culturally diverse backgrounds, lifestyles, values, and interests (see Chapter 6). Conveying acceptance requires a tolerant, nonjudgmental attitude toward clients. An open, accepting approach is needed to foster a helping relationship between hygienist and client. Care should be taken to avoid nonverbal behavior that may be offensive or that may prevent free-flowing communication. Gestures such as frowning, rolling eyes upward, or shaking the head may communicate disagreement or disapproval to the client. The dental hygienist should show willingness to listen to the client's viewpoint while providing feedback that indicates understanding and acceptance of the person.

Asking Related Questions

Questioning is an essential part of communicating with clients in the oral healthcare environment. The purpose of questioning is to obtain specific information from clients about their health status. Well-directed questions can set the professional tone and pace of the conversation and help the dental hygienist to elicit essential information in a logical and timely manner.

Open-ended questions are usually more effective than questions that require a simple "yes" or "no" answer. This allows the client to elaborate and show his genuine feelings by bringing up whatever he thinks is important. For example, the dental hygienist might say, "What are you currently doing each day to care for your mouth?" rather than "Do you floss every day?" or "Do you brush in the morning?" or "Do you brush at bedtime?"

When attempting to gain specific information about an oral or general health condition, questions that are directly related to the topic being discussed keep the client focused and lead logically to the point where the hygienist can make an accurate assessment.

Paraphrasing

Paraphrasing means restating or summarizing what the client has just said. Through paraphrasing, the client receives a signal that his message has been received and understood and he is prompted to continue a communication effort by providing further information. The client may say, "I don't understand how I could have periodontal disease. My teeth and gums feel fine. I have absolutely no pain." The hygienist could paraphrase the statement by saying, "You're not convinced that you have periodontal disease or any gum problems because you have no discomfort?" The client may respond, "Right, I just can't believe anything is wrong with my mouth."

The dental hygienist must carefully listen and analyze messages received so that the paraphrase is an accurate account of what the client actually said or feels. If the paraphrase misses the mark widely, the person may feel frustrated or offended at the misinterpretation, and communication will be blocked.

Clarifying

At times the message sent by the client may be so vague that the dental hygienist is unable to paraphrase it without clarification. When clarification is needed, the discussion should be temporarily stopped until confusing or conflicting statements have been understood. In the following scenario, a client has come to the oral care environment for a preventive oral prophylaxis:

Client: My mother had pyorrhea and lost all her teeth at a young age. I'm sure it's hereditary. I can only hope to stall it off.
Hygienist: I'm sorry, Mrs. Thompson. Can you tell me if you're having some problem with your teeth or gums?

In responding this way, the hygienist is trying to get clarification. The client's rush of words seems to be related to her own problems, but the hygienist cannot be sure until the client states so in a clear manner.

In addition, the hygienist should be aware that statements made to the client may need clarification. In order to fulfill their human need for conceptualization and problem solving, recipients of dental hygiene care need to understand why they are asked to comply with a specific home care regimen. In the following example, the dental hygienist has completed therapeutic scaling and root planing on the mandibular left quadrant that has been anesthetized.

Hygienist: Mr. Johnson, after you leave, try not to chew on your left side for awhile.
Client: Do you mean today or for several days?
Hygienist: Oh no, I just mean for a few hours.
Client: What might happen if I do chew on that side? Will it hurt my teeth or gums?
Hygienist: Oh no, I was referring to your anesthesia. I'm afraid you might bite your cheeks or tongue if you chew on that side since everything is numb. The numbness should be completely gone by about 5:00 P.M.

The more specific the hygienist can be, the clearer the message to the client. In the case above, the client's human need for safety is in potential deficit because injury could result if postoperative instructions are not followed.

Focusing

When a client is discussing health-related issues, there are times when messages become redundant or rambling. Important information may not surface because the client is "on a tangent." In clarifying, the dental hygienist is unsure of what the individual is talking about; in focusing, the hygienist knows what the person is talking about but is having trouble keeping him on the subject so that data gathering and assessment can be completed.

The dental hygienist should encourage verbalization but steer the discussion back on track as a technique to improve communication. Rather than asking a question, a gentle command may be in order, such as "Please point to the tooth that seems to be causing your discomfort," or "Show me exactly what you do when you floss your back teeth."

Stating Observations

A client may be unaware of the nonverbal messages she is sending. When a client is asked, "How are you, Mrs. Jones?" as a friendly greeting, she may respond, "Oh, just fine." Her appearance, gait, and mannerisms may indicate something different. She may look slightly unkempt, walk with a slow shuffle, and display generally unenthusiastic gestures and facial expressions. When nonverbal cues conflict with the verbal message, stating a simple straightforward observation may open the lines of communication. The hygienist may say, "You appear very tired, Mrs. Jones." This is likely to cause the person to volunteer more information about how she feels without need for further questioning, focusing, or clarifying.

The client may feel sensitive about how observations are worded. Saying you look "tired" is different from saying you look "haggard," which could embarrass or anger a person. Other observations that can soften a client's response are stating that teeth are "crowded" rather than "crooked," that a troublesome tongue is "muscular" not "fat," that gingiva is "pigmented" not "discolored."

Offering Information

When clients are provided with detailed information, communication is facilitated. Although providing information may not be enough to motivate people to change health behaviors, clients have a right to receive information based on the hygienist's expertise so that they can make health-related decisions based on that information. Because persons are motivated by their human needs, an individual is likely to act (carry out appropriate oral health behaviors) if he has information that facilitates human need fulfillment.

In any setting, a dental hygienist maintains a professional obligation to provide health information to all clients, not just individuals who request information. A commitment to health promotion requires a sustained effort to be forthcoming with complete, scientifically based information for clients, even though one may feel like a "broken record" or may be too tired or busy to talk.

Summarizing

Summarizing points discussed at a regularly scheduled appointment focuses attention on the major points of the communicative interaction. For example, the dental hygienist may conclude the appointment with, "Today we discussed the purpose of therapeutic scaling and root planing and the periodontal disease process, and we practiced flossing technique. Remember, you decided to floss daily and to try to slip the floss carefully down below the gumline." If the client is coming in for multiple appointments to receive quadrant or sextant scaling and root planing, the discussion from the previous appointment should be summarized in a similar manner before proceeding with new information. Documentation within the client's chart at each appointment should reflect topics discussed at each appointment as related to the client's goals.

The summary serves as a review of the key aspects of the information presented so that the client can ask for clarification. Adding new information in the summary may confuse the person; however, a comment about what will be discussed at the next appointment is appropriate. Such a statement might be, "At your next appointment, we will talk about use of the Perio Aid and continue discussion of the periodontal disease process."

Reflective Responding and Active Listening

Reflective responding or active listening integrates the therapeutic communication technique of listening attentively, but also emphasizes maintaining silence, conveying acceptance, paraphrasing, clarifying, and summarizing. Carl Rogers has been credited as the original inspiration for this technique, which grew out of his "nondirective" or "client-centered" counseling methods.[8] The idea is to let the client take the therapy session where he wants it to go with only gentle guidance from the therapist. The opposite is a more authoritarian, directive type of counseling led by the therapist's notions of what should be accomplished.

Gordon used the nondirective communication technique in teaching parents how to communicate with their children and called it "active listening."[13] The active listener carefully assesses the feelings expressed by the client and responds in a manner that restates, rewords, or reflects what the client has said back to him again. For example, if a client is sending verbal or nonverbal messages that he is angry or frustrated about being told that he needs to floss more, the dental hygienist could say, "It sounds like this situation has really upset you and that you are frustrated with me for not recognizing your efforts." The client generally responds by affirming the analysis and by expanding on it. He may say, "Yes, I am frustrated, but not with you, only with myself," or some other clarification of his feelings. By responding reflectively (in a mirror-like manner), the dental hygienist can encourage clients to communicate further about health problems. Passive listening or silence on the part of the receiver with no attempt to decode the message would have resulted in an uncomfortable impasse in the communication process. The dental hygienist's reflective response allows further analysis of the problem and opens the conversation for true communication and problem solving.

NONTHERAPEUTIC COMMUNICATION OR FACTORS THAT INHIBIT COMMUNICATION

The dental hygienist may unintentionally impede communication. The following discussion focuses on "factors that inhibit communication."[4]

Giving an Opinion

A helping relationship should foster the client's ability to make his own decisions about health. A hygienist may be tempted to offer an opinion, which may weaken the client's autonomy and jeopardize his need for self-determination. Clients may volunteer personal information about themselves and may ask for the hygienist's opinion. It is best in such a situation to acknowledge the individual's feelings but to avoid the transfer of decision making from client to hygienist. The following is a hypothetical situation presenting two possible responses by the dental hygienist in an interaction with a client:

Hygienist: Mrs. Smith, you look troubled today.
Client: Well, actually, I'm feeling quite down in the dumps. Yesterday was my birthday and I didn't hear a word from my daughter. I'm sure you wouldn't do such a thing to your mother!
Hygienist (Response #1): Heavens, no! How terribly inconsiderate of her.

The hygienist might have answered differently.

Hygienist (Response #2): You seem to feel really disappointed. I'm sorry you're so distressed.

The latter response by the dental hygienist recognizes feelings without expressing an opinion that could make the client feel worse by confirming a doubt that she has about her daughter, as in the first response.

Offering False Reassurance

Hygienists may at times offer reassurance when it is not well grounded. It is natural to want to alleviate the client's anxiety and fear, but reassurance may promise something that cannot occur. For example, the dental hygienist should not promise the client that he will experience no discomfort in an anticipated dental treatment. Although the dental hygienist may feel confident that the oral surgeon or periodontist is competent and kind, discomfort may be unavoidable. A person who is distraught about his periodontal disease should not be told, "There's nothing to worry about. You'll be fine." Indeed, depending on the amount of bone loss present and disease susceptibility of the client, the periodontist may not be able to control the disease, even with extensive therapy.

The following example illustrates how the dental hygienist can listen and acknowledge a client's feelings *without* falsely assuring her that the problem is a simple one.

Mrs. Frank, a 75-year-old woman, has been told by the dentist that her remaining teeth are hopeless and must be extracted for a full denture placement. The hygienist enters the room as the dentist leaves.

Mrs. Frank: I can't believe this is happening to me. I don't deserve it. I've tried to take good care of my teeth. I'm so distressed. Oh, I'm sorry, I know you don't want to hear about my problems.
Hygienist: Mrs. Frank, I am interested in your feelings about this.

Being Defensive

When clients criticize services or personnel, it is easy for the hygienist to become defensive. A defensive posture may threaten the relationship between dental hygienist and client by communicating to the client that he does not have a right to express his opinion. For example:

Mr. Tucker has been a regular client in the dental practice for many years. At the last appointment, the dental hygienist noted a 2-mm circumscribed white lesion in the retromolar area. Mr. Tucker was a former smoker and the dentist referred him to an oral surgeon for consultation and possible biopsy of the lesion. The following describes the hygienist-client interaction when Mr. Tucker is now returning for his periodontal maintenance appointment.

Client: I hope I don't have to see Dr. Herman today.
Hygienist: What's wrong, Mr. Tucker? Dr. Herman usually sees you after your periodontal maintenance care.
Client: He sent me to the oral surgeon and it was a complete waste of my time.
Hygienist: Of course, it wasn't. Dr. Herman is an excellent dentist.
Client: You may think so but he didn't send you for a biopsy for no reason.
Hygienist: Mr. Tucker, that lesion looked very unusual. I'm sure Dr. Herman made a good decision in sending you.

In the preceding scenario, the dental hygienist's response ignores the client's real feelings and hurts future rapport and communication with him. The hygienist should use the therapeutic communication techniques of active listening to verify what the client has to say and to learn why he is upset or angry. Active listening does not mean that the dental hygienist agrees with what is being said, but rather conveys interest in what the client is saying. This latter approach is illustrated in the following scenario:

Client: I hope I don't have to see Dr. Herman today.
Hygienist: You sound upset. Can you tell me something about it?
Client: I just don't think he should have sent me to that oral surgeon.
Hygienist: You think the visit there was unnecessary?
Client: Yes, I didn't mind the biopsy, the results were negative, but first, I got lost trying to find the place, then I couldn't find a parking place, then they made me wait for 2 hours and, finally, they charged me a fortune for the procedure. Actually, I didn't mind the cost as much as the inconvenience.

Some care in listening led to discovery of the source of the client's anger, which was the inconvenience of a particular oral surgeon's location, parking, and office procedures. By avoiding defensiveness and applying active listening and reflective responding, the hygienist allowed Mr. Tucker to vent his anger. Therefore, communication was facilitated, not blocked.

Showing Approval or Disapproval

Showing either approval or disapproval in certain situations can be detrimental to the communication process. Excessive praise may imply to the client that the hygienist thinks the behavior being praised is the only acceptable one. Often, clients may reveal information about themselves because they are seeking a way to express their feelings. They are not necessarily looking for approval or disapproval from the dental hygienist. In the following scenario, the hygienist's response cannot be interpreted as neutral:

Client: I've been walking to my dental appointments for years. My daughter offered to drive me today and I accepted. She feels the walk has become too much for me.
Hygienist: I'm so glad you didn't walk over. You definitely made the right decision. Your daughter should drive you to your appointments from now on.

The above discussion is likely to stop with the dental hygienist's statements. The client probably sees the hygienist's viewpoint as supportive of her daughter's. Perhaps the woman is better off having her daughter drive her. It is also possible that she is capable of walking, likes the exercise, and enjoys the independence of getting to her own appointments. The dental hygienist's strong statements of approval may inhibit the client's self-determination by not allowing her to think or act freely.

Behaviors that communicate disapproval cause the client to feel rejected, and her desire to interact further with the dental hygienist may be weakened. Disapproving statements may be issued by a dental hygienist who is not thinking carefully about how the client may react. The following scenario exemplifies a dental hygienist's response that communicates hasty disapproval:

Client: I've been working so hard at flossing! I only missed two or three times last week.
Hygienist: Two or 3 days without flossing! You'll have to do better than that. Your inflammation will not improve at that rate.

Instead of the above response, the dental hygienist might have said, "You're making progress. Tell me more about your activities on those 3 days when you weren't able to floss. Perhaps, together, we could find a better way of integrating flossing into your lifestyle."

Asking Why

When one is puzzled by another's behavior, the natural reaction is to ask "why?" When the dental hygienist discovers that a client has not been following recommendations, she may feel a natural inclination to ask "why" this has occurred. A client may interpret such a question as an accusation. He may feel resentment, leading to withdrawal and a lack of motivation to communicate further with the dental hygienist.

Efforts to search for the reasons the client has not practiced the oral healthcare behaviors as recommended can be facilitated by simply rephrasing a probing "why" question. For example, rather than saying, "Why haven't you used the oral irrigator?" the hygienist might say, "You haven't used the oral irrigator. Is something wrong?" For anxious clients, rather than asking, "Why are you upset?" the hygienist might say, "You seem upset. Would you like to talk about it?"

Changing the Subject Inappropriately

Changing the subject abruptly shows a lack of empathy, could be interpreted as rude, and prevents the client from discussing an issue with important implications for care. The following is a sample client–dental hygienist interaction:

Hygienist: Hello, Mrs. Johnson. How are you today?
Client: Not too well. My gums are really sore.
Hygienist: Well, let's get you going. We have a lot to do today.

The dental hygienist's response shows insensitivity and an unwillingness to discuss Mrs. Johnson's complaint. It is possible that the client has a periodontal or periapical abscess or some other serious problem. The dental hygienist is remiss in ignoring the client's attempt to communicate a problem. Communication has been stalled and the client's oral health jeopardized. The client should be given an opportunity to elaborate on the message she is trying to send.

MOTIVATION TO PERFORM HEALTH BEHAVIOR

Influencing people to comply with or adhere to regimens for oral hygiene care is one of the major challenges facing a dental hygienist. Compliance, or adherence, as it is often referred to, can be interrupted by lapses or temporary slips back to one's former behavior. Weinstein and colleagues maintain that occasional lapses are normal and may not necessarily threaten oral health or gains made.[14] The situation to avoid is the complete breakdown of an individual's bacterial plaque control program. The possibility of lapsing should be discussed with the client so that he understands that occasional slips do not have to result in total relapse to one's previous status.

In the communication process a dental hygienist is constantly striving to influence the client's motivation to perform oral health behaviors. **Motivation** can be defined as "the impulse that leads an individual to action." Within the framework of human need theory, a person's attempt to satisfy a need could be viewed as the "impulse that leads an individual to action" or, in the context of other theories, different thoughts or events could provide the impulse. Many theories of motivation have been formulated and can be appropriately applied to client motivation in the healthcare environment.

Self-efficacy Theory

Self-efficacy is the strength of belief in one's ability to perform specific behaviors.[15] Research has shown that self-efficacy has a strong influence on initial attempts at performance of difficult tasks as well as on persistence in following through.

Based on the self-efficacy theory, motivation to floss should be stronger when a client has a past history of having successfully incorporated other health behaviors into a daily regimen. For instance, a client who has already disciplined himself with a daily exercise routine might be expected to exhibit a highly positive attitude toward self-efficacy when presented with a plan to improve and maintain periodontal health with a new flossing routine.

Self-efficacy is judged on the background of one's observation of her own environment. When others, especially those seen as similar to oneself, have performed well and attested to their own successes, one is led to the thought, "If she can do it, I can, too." Knowledge of the successes of peers in their endeavors to improve health behavior can strongly influence the client's motivation to accomplish tasks.

Anxiety is a physiological state that can result in negative self-appraisal. Repeated failure creates anxiety and can result in a disintegration of motivation. Past learning experiences that have been negative and resulted in failure yield feelings of inadequacy and fear of future failure. This can cause a person to avoid activities that they believe will result in failure. This need to avoid failure may prevent a client from any attempt to incorporate new oral health behaviors into a daily effort.

Attribution Theory

According to Weiner, *attributions* are the explanations students give for their performance.[16] Although Weiner's attribution theory applies to academic success or failure, it can be extended to fit chairside teaching as well as classroom instruction in oral health education.[16] The basic framework of the theory is that people attribute their successes and failures to effort, luck, ability, or task difficulty. These "attributions" can determine motivation to perform new tasks or to persist with previously exhibited behaviors.

This theory is a cognitive theory that emphasizes the importance of content of thoughts. What people attribute to their success or failure determines their feelings about themselves, their predictions of success at accomplishing the task, and the probability that they will try harder or less hard at a task in the future. For example, when a person attributes her failure to low ability, she feels depressed, predicts that she will fail again, and uses less effort in the future. Therefore, attributions affect (1) expectations of success; (2) emotional (affective) reactions; and (3) persistence at future tasks.

If a person attributes her success at performing a task to effort, she may feel pleased because effort is something she can control. She will predict that she can succeed in the future if she continues to exert effort and, in fact, will exert more effort in the future.

Gagne has suggested that when people perceive effort to be stable they are more likely to feel positive about their successes and realize their expectations for future success.[17] We should encourage students to view their effort-making as a stable characteristic that will likely result in an increase in effort and persistence in the future. For example, educators can do this by saying to a student, "You are a hardworking person," rather than, "You really worked hard that time." Likewise, clients can be encouraged to think of themselves as "conscientious" individuals who are concerned about their health on a long-term basis.

The most problematic cycle in education is when learners attribute their lack of success to low ability. This leads to disillusionment with oneself and lack of effort toward future tasks. Ability is not within the control of a person. Unlike effort, it is not something that can be manipulated at will.

In addition, consistent with self-efficacy theory, Ames and colleagues found that in academic settings with children, those students with low self-concepts and little confidence in their ability do not easily change their view of themselves.[18] If the student does succeed at a task, the success is a surprise and the student tends to attribute it to luck or task ease.[19,20] Only with extreme patience and persistence can a teacher help students change effort attributions to change a negative self-concept to a positive one. It is wise for a dental hygienist to remember the value placed on patience and persistence when attempting to work with persons who may have low self-concepts and little confidence in their abilities.

Locus of Control

Some clients may blame someone or something else for their poor performance in maintaining oral health. These people believe that external aspects of their environment have control over their failure (or their successes). The counterpart to this individual is one who believes he holds his fate in his own hands and is responsible for his own actions. He is focused on the internal aspects of himself and how he can influence his environment.

Psychologists categorize such internal and external personality dispositions under the construct "locus of control." Much of the research in this area stems from the social learning theory of Rotter.[21] He developed a 23-item internal-external locus of control scale for classification of individuals. Three examples of items on Rotter's scale follow. The respondent reads each statement and selects the statement he most agrees with:

1a. Many times I feel that I have little influence over the things that happen to me. (external)

1b. It is impossible for me to believe that chance or luck plays an important role in my life. (internal)

2a. Getting a good job depends mainly on being in the right place at the right time. (external)

2b. Becoming a success is a matter of hard work; luck has little or nothing to do with it. (internal)

3a. Without the right breaks one cannot be an effective leader. (external)

3b. Capable people who fail to become leaders have not taken advantage of their opportunities. (internal)

The individual classified as having an external locus of control believes that events are caused by factors beyond his control. He may believe that luck, task difficulty, or powerful others determine his future. The individual classified as having an internal locus of control believes that an outcome is contingent upon his own behavior or relatively permanent characteristics such as ability.

Table 5–3 indicates how locus of control can be used to understand client oral health behavior. It suggests some helpful strategies for communicating with clients who fit the locus of control descriptions.[22] Comments by clients that are similar to those suggested in the table can help the health provider determine the client's orientation. Woodall contends that clients who function from an external locus of control often appear willing and agreeable but are unlikely to adhere to recommendations. They may ultimately blame the clinician when their oral hygiene regimen fails. The challenge is for the clinician to redirect the client's perceptions of how effective he can be in achieving health goals by providing feedback that affirms the client's efficacy.

Those individuals who are internally controlled are autonomous people who may follow good oral hygiene practices regardless of the clinician's influence. Some research has shown, however, the clients who are strongly internally controlled may sometimes comply less with professional recommendations.[23] This lack of compliance can be attributed to their often sharp consumer sense; they consider the health professional's advice as just another opinion in the broad range of information they constantly seek. They may challenge advice, listen silently, ignore recommendations, or try popular home remedies. They are skeptical but, on the whole, are highly desirable as clients because they are generally responsible, self-motivated individuals who will likely practice preventive measures.

TABLE 5–3
INDICATORS OF INTERNAL AND EXTERNAL LOCI OF CONTROL

Internal Locus of Control	External Locus of Control
Ownership of Situation	
"My teeth are bad because I never took very good care of them."	"I've always had soft teeth."
"I should have found a dentist who could really help me."	"The dentist I went to didn't care."
"What can I do to keep my teeth?"	"Just take them all out. I know they'll go sooner or later."
Need for Involvement in Treatment	
"Now, what will this series of treatments do for me in the long run? And let me see if I have the reasoning clearly understood?"	"Just do what you need to do to fix me up."
Reaction to Professional Recommendation	
"I'll try it out and see how it works."	"I'll do whatever you say. My teeth will be clean whenever you see me."

Reprinted from Woodall, I. R. Patient motivation and locus of control. Compendium of Continuing Education in Dentistry, 6:147–151, 1985.

Health Belief Model

See Chapter 4, pages 60 to 61.

TEACHING-LEARNING PROCESS

Teaching and dental hygiene care are firmly linked. By helping persons learn, the hygienist helps them fulfill human needs for conceptualization and assume responsibility for their oral healthcare. The teaching-learning process in dental hygiene leads to better understanding of etiology of oral diseases and to improved adherence to recommended therapies. The following sections provide an overview of learning theory highlighted with oral health education examples.

Learning Objectives and Domains

The objectives of an oral health educational plan may be formally stated or informally conceptualized by the dental hygienist. An objective is a statement of what is to be accomplished or the aim of the education. An *objective* can be defined as a "precise statement of what the student will be able to do as a result of the instruction."[23] Each statement should have content dimension and a behavioral dimension and the performance expected should be measurable.[24] For example, the dental hygienist may contend that at the end of the educational session the client will

- Demonstrate the modified Bass toothbrushing technique using a toothbrush in her own mouth
- Verbally describe the composition of bacterial plaque
- Verbally summarize the etiology of dental caries

These objectives are developed for the client in the same manner that objectives are prepared for a textbook or lesson plan.

Learning behaviors can be classified in three domains and all have application to the teaching-learning process used by the dental hygienist. The domains are known as cognitive, affective, and psychomotor. The three classes tend to overlap because behavior to be learned may be complex and may fit into more than one category. For example, both psychomotor skills and cognitive skills are required if the client is to acquire oral hygiene behaviors.

Cognitive Domain

The **cognitive learning domain** classifies learning objectives involving intellectual tasks. The most widely recognized cognitive or knowledge taxonomy was developed by Bloom and colleagues[25] (see Major Categories in the Cognitive Domain of the Taxonomy of Educational Objectives and Examples of General Instructional Objectives and Behavioral

MAJOR CATEGORIES IN THE COGNITIVE DOMAIN OF THE TAXONOMY OF EDUCATIONAL OBJECTIVES[25]

Descriptions of the Major Categories in the Cognitive Domain

1. *Knowledge.* Knowledge is defined as the remembering of previously learned material. This may involve the recall of a wide range of material, from specific facts to complete theories, but all that is required is the bringing to mind of the appropriate information. Knowledge represents the lowest level of learning outcomes in the cognitive domain.

2. *Comprehension.* Comprehension is defined as the ability to grasp the meaning of material. This may be shown by translating material from one form to another (words to numbers), by interpreting material (explaining or summarizing), and by estimating future trends (predicting consequences or effects). These learning outcomes go one step beyond the simple remembering of material, and represent the lowest level of understanding.

3. *Application.* Application refers to the ability to use learned material in new and concrete situations. This may include the application of such things as rules, methods, concepts, principles, laws, and theories. Learning outcomes in this area require a higher level of understanding than those under comprehension.

4. *Analysis.* Analysis refers to the ability to break down material into its component parts so that its organizational structure may be understood. This may include the identification of the parts, analysis of the relationships between parts, and recognition of the organizational principles involved. Learning outcomes here represent a higher intellectual level than comprehension and application because they require an understanding of both the content and the structural form of the material.

5. *Synthesis.* Synthesis refers to the ability to put parts together to form a new whole. This may involve the production of a unique communication (theme or speech), a plan of operations (research proposal), or a set of abstract relations (scheme for classifying information). Learning outcomes in this area stress creative behaviors, with major emphasis on the formulation of new patterns or structures.

6. *Evaluation.* Evaluation is concerned with the ability to judge the value of material (statement, novel, poem, research report) for a given purpose. The judgments are to be based on definite criteria. These may be internal criteria (organization) or external criteria (relevance to the purpose) and the student may determine the criteria or be given them. Learning outcomes in this area are highest in the cognitive hierarchy because they contain elements of all of the other categories, plus conscious value judgments based on clearly defined criteria.

EXAMPLES OF GENERAL INSTRUCTIONAL OBJECTIVES AND BEHAVIORAL TERMS FOR THE COGNITIVE DOMAIN OF THE TAXONOMY

Illustrative General Instructional Objectives	**Illustrative Behavioral Terms for Stating Specific Learning Outcomes**
Knows common terms, knows specific facts, knows methods and procedures, knows basic concepts, knows principles	Defines, describes, identifies, labels, lists, matches, names, outlines, reproduces, selects, states
Understands facts and principles, interprets verbal material, interprets charts and graphs, translates verbal material into mathematical formulas, estimates future consequences implied in data, justifies methods and procedures	Converts, defends, distinguishes, estimates, explains, extends, generalizes, gives examples, infers, paraphrases, predicts, rewrites, summarizes
Applies concept and principles to new situations, applies laws and theories to practical situations, solves mathematical problems, constructs charts and graphs, demonstrates correct usage of a method or procedure	Changes, computes, demonstrates, discovers, manipulates, modifies, operates, predicts, prepares, produces, relates, shows, solves, uses
Recognizes unstated assumptions, recognizes logical fallacies in reasoning, distinguishes between facts and inferences, evaluates the relevancy of data, analyzes the organizational structure of a work (art, music, writing)	Breaks down, diagrams, differentiates, discriminates, distinguishes, identifies, illustrates, infers, outlines, points out, relates, selects, separates, subdivides
Writes a well-organized theme, gives a well-organized speech, writes a creative short story (or poem, or music), proposes a plan for an experiment, integrates learning from different areas into a plan for solving a problem, formulates a new scheme for classifying objects (or events, or ideas)	Categorizes, combines, compiles, composes, creates, devises, designs, explains, generates, modifies, organizes, plans, rearranges, reconstructs, relates, reorganizes, revises, rewrites, summarizes, tells, writes
Judges the logical consistency of written material, judges the adequacy with which conclusions are supported by data, judges the value of a work (art, music, writing) by use of internal criteria, judges the value of a work (art, music, writing) by use of external standards of excellence	Appraises, compares, concludes, contrasts, criticizes, describes, discriminates, explains, justifies, interprets, relates, summarizes, supports

Terms for the Cognitive Domain of the Taxonomy charts). Dental hygienists find these categories useful for care planning when a deficit in the client's human need related to oral health and disease is identified.

Consider the following example:

A dental hygienist, Ms. Forman, sees her client, Mr. Warner, at a regular continued care appointment. Mr. Warner has recently been to the periodontist for full-mouth periodontal surgery. Ms. Forman provides Mr. Warner with the information he needs about the disease process and the purpose of his surgery to help expand upon and clarify what was previously presented by his periodontist (knowledge). Mr. Warner understands what led to his periodontal condition and the reasons for his surgery (comprehension). Ms. Forman cautions Mr. Warner that his level of periodontal health could deteriorate if he does not follow through with regular professional maintenance care and conscientious home care. Mr. Warner agrees that he will follow all instructions and recommendations (application). Mr. Warner also learns the signs of worsening periodontal health including bleeding, inflammation, and increased loss of periodontal attachment, and describes how he will watch for these signs and use his knowledge of proper maintenance care to avoid relapse (analysis and synthesis). Finally, Ms. Forman helps Mr. Warner consider the value of all information provided and whether it is sufficient to achieve an optimal periodontal status in his case (evaluation).[4]

Affective Domain

The **affective learning domain** of Krathwohl and colleagues classifies objectives involving attitudes, values, and interests.[26] Again, each taxonomy organizes objectives into a hierarchical framework of behaviors with each being more complex than the previous category (see Major Categories in the Affective Domain of the Taxonomy of Educational Objectives and Examples of General Objectives and Behavioral Terms for the Affective Domain of the Taxonomy charts).

The dental hygienist will find the affective taxonomy valuable for planning dental hygiene interventions aimed at meeting a deficit in the client's value system related to oral health. The affective classification begins with an attitude or value at a level of mere awareness and proceeds to the point where it totally guides a person's actions. For example, a person's value regarding the health and oral health of society can develop from

- An awareness of the need of a particular group of people for better health care, such as pregnant teenagers (receiving)
- A financial contribution to an agency providing prenatal care to teenagers (responding)
- A commitment to work in a local program for teenagers who are pregnant (valuing)
- Internalizing the ideal of the "greatest good for the greatest number" into political, religious, and economic value system (organization)

MAJOR CATEGORIES IN THE AFFECTIVE DOMAIN OF THE TAXONOMY OF EDUCATIONAL OBJECTIVES[26]

Descriptions of the Major Categories in the Affective Domain

1. *Receiving.* Receiving refers to the student's willingness to attend to particular phenomena or stimuli (classroom activities, textbook, music, etc.). From a teaching standpoint, it is concerned with getting, holding, and directing the student's attention. Learning outcomes in this area range from the simple awareness that a thing exists to selective attention on the part of the learner. Receiving represents the lowest level of learning outcomes in the affective domain.

2. *Responding.* Responding refers to active participation on the part of the student. At this level he not only attends to a particular phenomenon but also reacts to it in some way. Learning outcomes in this area may emphasize acquiescence in responding (reads assigned material), willingness to respond (voluntarily reads beyond assignment), or satisfaction in responding (reads for pleasure or enjoyment). The higher levels of this category include those instructional objectives that are commonly classified under "interests;" that is, those that stress the seeking out and enjoyment of particular activities.

3. *Valuing.* Valuing is concerned with the worth or value a student attaches to a particular object, phenomenon, or behavior. This ranges in degree from the more simple acceptance of a value (desires to improve group skills) to the more complex level of commitment (assumes responsibility for the effective functioning of the group). Valuing is based on the internalization of a set of specified values, but clues to these values are expressed in the student's overt behavior. Learning outcomes in this area are concerned with behavior that is consistent and stable enough to make the value clearly identifiable. Instructional objectives that are commonly classified under "attitudes" and "appreciation" would fall into this category.

4. *Organization.* Organization is concerned with bringing together different values, resolving conflicts between them, and beginning the building of an internally consistent value system. Thus the emphasis is on comparing, relating, and synthesizing values. Learning outcomes may be concerned with the conceptualization of a value (recognizes the responsibility of each individual for improving human relations) or with the organization of a value system (develops a vocational plan that satisfies his need for both economic security and social service). Instructional objectives relating to the development of a philosophy of life would fall into this category.

5. *Characterization by a Value or Value Complex.* At this level of the affective domain, the individual has a value system that has controlled his behavior for a sufficiently long time for him to have developed a characteristic "life style." Thus the behavior is pervasive, consistent, and predictable. Learning outcomes at this level cover a broad range of activities, but the major emphasis is on the fact that the behavior is typical or characteristic of the student. Instructional objectives that are concerned with the student's general patterns of adjustment (personal, social, emotional) would be appropriate here.

EXAMPLES OF GENERAL INSTRUCTIONAL OBJECTIVES AND BEHAVIORAL TERMS FOR THE AFFECTIVE DOMAIN OF THE TAXONOMY

Illustrative General Instructional Objectives	Illustrative Behavioral Terms for Stating Specific Learning Outcomes
Listens attentively, shows awareness of the importance of learning, shows sensitivity to human needs and social problems, accepts differences of race and culture, attends closely to the classroom activities	Asks, chooses, describes, follows, gives, holds, identifies, locates, names, points to, selects, sits erect, replies, uses
Completes assigned homework, obeys school rules, participates in class discussion, completes laboratory work, volunteers for special tasks, shows interest in subject, enjoys helping others	Answers, assists, complies, conforms, discusses, greets, helps, labels, performs, practices, presents, reads, recites, reports, selects, tells, writes
Demonstrates belief in the democratic process, appreciates good literature (art or music), appreciates the role of science (or other subjects) in everyday life, shows concern for the welfare of others, demonstrates problem-solving attitude, demonstrates commitment to social improvement	Completes, describes, differentiates, explains, follows, forms, initiates, invites, joins, justifies, proposes, reads, reports, selects, shares, studies, works
Recognizes the need for balance between freedom and responsibility in a democracy, recognizes the role of systematic planning in solving problems, accepts responsibility for his own behavior, understands and accepts his own strengths and limitations, formulates a life plan in harmony with his abilities, interests, and beliefs	Adheres, alters, arranges, combines, compares, completes, defends, explains, generalizes, identifies, integrates, modifies, orders, organizes, prepares, relates, synthesizes
Displays safety consciousness, demonstrates self-reliance in working independently, practices cooperation in group activities, uses objective approach in problem solving, demonstrates industry, punctuality, and self-discipline, maintains good health habits	Acts, discriminates, displays, influences, listens, modifies, performs, practices, proposes, qualifies, questions, revises, serves, solves, uses, verifies

- Entering a career in public health dental hygiene and specializing in the oral health education and care of pregnant teenagers (characterization of a value)

Psychomotor Domain

Other instructional objectives relate to the acquisition of skills that require muscle development and coordination. They are arranged in what is known as the **psychomotor learning domain.** Personal oral hygiene behaviors such as brushing, flossing, using a Perio Aid or rubber tip fall into this learning domain. A psychomotor taxonomy was developed by Harrow and patterned after those developed by Bloom, Krathwohl, and colleagues.[25–27] In brief, the psychomotor hierarchy involves objectives starting with awareness, readiness to learn, guided instruction in the skill, establishing the motor skill as a habit, and achieving the level of adopting and modifying performance as conditions change. The pattern described by the taxonomy is familiar to dental hygienists who use a large number of psychomotor skills themselves in their daily work and are focused on client psychomotor skill acquisition.

The professional dental hygienist draws from all three learning domains when educating clients in the practice and value of personal oral healthcare. The client must

1. Understand the reason for a strict oral hygiene regimen (cognitive)
2. Learn the proper manipulation of the required oral devices (psychomotor)
3. Personally commit to practice behaviors as appropriate for health maintenance (affective)

Knowledge of each learning domain prepares the hygienist to assess the client's educational needs, set client goals, select proper educational strategies and interventions, evaluate learning outcomes, and be successful in the role of health educator and oral health promoter.

LEARNING THEORY AND APPLICATION

A professional dental hygienist must understand and apply learning theories from behavioristic, cognitive, and humanistic psychology.[23]

Behavioristic Psychology

B. F. Skinner's research in human behavior resulted in the development of reinforcement theory, based on the idea that the purpose of psychology is to predict and control behavior **(behavioristic psychology).**[28,29] Reinforcement theory emphasizes the importance of feedback and rewards in changing human behavior. Positive reinforcement operates by consistently pairing desirable behaviors with rewards or feedback. Through the reward system the behavior is "shaped" by being encouraged to recur in its most desirable form. As an example, in oral health education, when a plaque index shows that the client exhibits a reduction in plaque, the client then receives feedback (praise) from the hygienist, which encourages recurrence of the plaque control behavior.

Weinstein and colleagues developed a program for preventive dentistry based on behavioral theory for changing behavior.[14] The educational intervention they recommend uses strategies and techniques based upon the behaviorist theory of reinforcement. Reinforcers are categorized as material, activity, and social. *Material reinforcers* are tangible items a person could receive to strengthen a desirable oral health behavior. Depending on the age, needs, interests, and values of a client, these rewards can include toys, clothes, money, food, or recreational equipment. An adult client, for example, can agree to set aside a certain amount of money for each performance of the target behavior (e.g., one dollar for each day in which he flosses). The client can be encouraged to physically place the money in a "cookie jar" following flossing, which makes the reward immediate and tangible.

An *activity reinforcer* is whatever a person likes to do. The activity may include watching television, playing computer games, or taking a walk. Obviously, the activity must be valued by the client for the activity to serve as a reinforcer. Activities have the advantage of minimal cost and ready availability. The disadvantage is that often the individual may be unwilling to withhold these activities from himself if he has not performed his target behavior.

Verbal praise is the best example of a *social reinforcer.* It could also consist of anything done or said to make a person feel appreciated, accepted, or important (meeting the client's need for appreciation and respect). Attention and respect are both reinforcing. Feedback, or simply letting a person know how he is doing, is also a good form of social reinforcement. A mouth mirror or disclosing tablet facilitate providing feedback to a person on effectiveness of his brushing.

Material, activity, and social reinforcers are aimed at the goal of establishing effective oral health behaviors in clients. The difference between the modern-day behavioristic programs developed by psychologists like Weinstein and colleagues and the early Skinnerian approach is the emphasis on cognitive aspects of behavior, that is, thoughts, feelings, and values that Skinner ignored. Activity or social reinforcers, in particular, acknowledge the importance of thoughts, feelings, and values in causing behavior change. Figure 5–3 shows how thoughts enter into the chain of events that lead to establishing a habit. A cognitive view as opposed to a behaviorist view of learning places emphasis on the internal events of thoughts and feelings. Learning theories in **cognitive psychology** focus on the notion that a person's behavior is determined by an act of knowing or thinking (cognition) about the situation in which behavior occurs. For example, the way children think and thus behave depend on their stage of development. Adults may have "inspirations" or "insights" that cause them to behave in certain ways or they may simply make rational decisions to behave in a particular manner because of some specific information that has been presented to them. In contrast, the behavioristic view emphasizes the role of external events, usually tangible material rewards, in determining the direction and intensity of behavior.

Behavioristic techniques can be successfully applied by the dental hygienist to change client behavior. In *operant conditioning,* described by Skinner, learning takes place in a situation in which a response is more likely to occur in the future as a result of immediate reward or reinforcement. In the classroom, teachers strive to reinforce (praise or some other reward) desirable behavior to increase the probability that it will happen again. Dental hygienists can do the same as they work with their patients individually or in groups. Thorndike believed that reinforcement merely strengthened the connection between stimulus and response.[29a,29b] Skinner viewed the situation not as a strengthening of the stimulus-response bond, but of the consequences of the behavior increasing the probability that the same response will be chosen.

In oral health education a dental hygienist can develop a behavior modification program for a client using material or activity reinforcers to encourage toothbrushing, flossing, or other oral hygiene behaviors. The response (the oral hygiene behavior) becomes "reinforced" in the manner described by Skinner. Social reinforcers (anything said or done to meet the client's need for appreciation and respect, such as praise) cause changes in thoughts and feelings that can lead to behavior change.

Early in the twentieth century behaviorism emerged strongly as the science of human behavior.[30] The behaviorists maintained that in order to be a science, the discipline must restrict itself to public methods of observation that could be quantified and focus exclusively on behavior. According to the behaviorists, all psychological activity, introspection, and self-reflection could be adequately explained without resorting to study of mysterious mental entities. A strong component of the behaviorist view was a belief in the supremacy and determining power of the environment —that events, objects, and situations outside of oneself were responsible for guiding and determining one's behavior.[30]

Gardner describes how a narrowly defined behaviorism made its important impact on learning theory in the early part of this century but began to change the strict stance on eliminating thoughts and feelings from the science by the 1950s.[30] He states that in the opening decades of the century "behaviorism seemed like a breath of fresh air, caught on quickly and captured the attention of the best minds in psychology."[30] As time wore on, however, it became clear that the simple associative chains between a stimulus and a response could not possibly account for complex, organized behaviors involving planning, problem solving, creativity, intentions, or imagination. Dental hygienists who use behavioristic techniques like behavior modification must remember that behavior is complex and feelings, thoughts and values of the client enter into its determination.

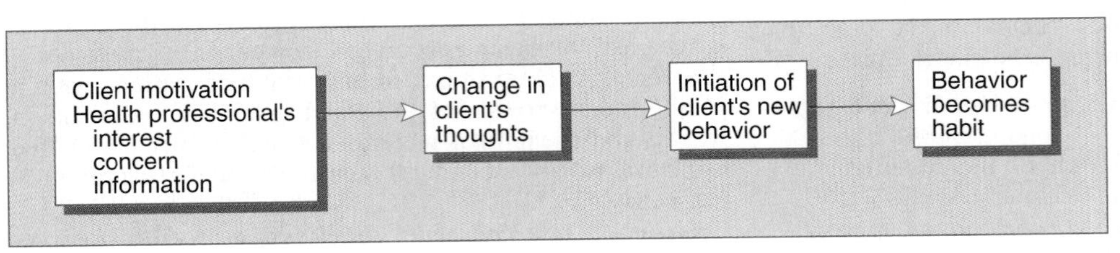

FIGURE 5–3
Behavior change. (Adapted with permission from Weinstein, P., Getz, T., and Milgrom, P. Oral Self Care: Strategies for Preventive Dentistry, 3rd ed. Seattle, WA: University of Washington Continuing Dental Education, 1991.)

Cognitive Psychology

A basic assumption of cognitive psychologists is that a person's behavior is based on cognition or thinking. An act of knowing or thinking about a situation determines what behavior will occur. Their position is that stimulus, response, and reinforcement cannot adequately explain the learning process. Cognitive psychologists focus on aspects of the cognitive realm such as organization of knowledge, information processing, and decision making.

As behavioristic theories were being criticized more frequently in the 1920s and 1930s, a group of German psychologists rejected the position that learning was simply the formation of associations between stimuli and responses. Wertheimer studied perception and problem solving and proposed the basic concepts of gestalt psychology.[31] The word "gestalt" translates into English as "form," "pattern," or "configuration." Insight as a sudden perception is often referred to as the "aha!" or "now-I-see!" phenomenon and is the key meaning of the word "gestalt." It is contrasted to learning by trial and error, which is characteristic of behavioral learning models.

Gestalt psychology views learning as dependent on patterns as opposed to parts. In teaching strategy, this implies that an educator should provide a student with a good overview of material to be covered and emphasize the relationships between various topics. It is a general rather than specific approach, more abstract than concrete. Step-by-step instruction, drill, or arbitrary explanations (techniques based on behavioristic theory) are not advocated by gestalt theory. In oral health education the method can be utilized by presenting a hypothetical problem to a classroom of students and encouraging them to solve it. The problem can be that of a complex community oral health issue, such as whether to institute community water fluoridation or whether an oral health education curriculum should be developed and implemented in the public school, grades K to 12. The hypothetical problem involves facts, values, opinions, emotions, and the need for change. It was intended that the students would determine solutions by making associations and seeing patterns of behavior that could lead to improved oral health for an entire community.

A Swiss psychologist, Jean Piaget, is well known for his contributions to cognitive theories of learning and particularily his application of the theories to child development. He has theorized that the thinking process gradually shifts from concrete to abstract as the child grows and develops.

The stages of development that have been explored by Piaget are[32]:

- Sensorimotor stage (0 to 2 years)
- Preoperational stage (2 to 7 years)
- Concrete operations stage (7 to 11 years)
- Formal operations stage (11 years and above)

The age ranges are only approximations and children may proceed through the stages at different rates. Each stage is built, however, on the preceding stage.

Sensorimotor Stage

The sensorimotor stage (0 to 2 years) covers approximately the first 2 years of life and is dominated by innate reflexes such as sucking and grasping. Some basic behaviors such as hearing and looking are explored and combined to form more complex behaviors. The infant begins to look toward sounds, smiles in response to voices, mimics facial expressions, and performs other behaviors. Gradually, he becomes more active within his environment. He is driven by curiosity to interact with his surroundings. He begins systematic trial and error behavior. Concepts of space, time, and causality develop and begin to influence behavior.

An infant does not understand the concept of object permanence. When his parents hide an object from view, he does not attempt to look for it. As he nears the end of the sensorimotor stage, he will show evidence that he realizes an object still exists when it is hidden from him, and he will begin to look for it when it is hidden.

When a child younger than 2 years of age is introduced to a toothbrush, she regards the object with curiosity. It is good to familiarize an infant child with a toothbrush even though cleaning the mouth and newly erupted primary teeth is, of course, a task for the parents. The infant can respond positively to sounds and smiles, and parents who make first oral hygiene experiences pleasant have laid the foundation for a positive attitude toward future oral health behavior.

Preoperational Stage

In the preoperational stage (2 to 7 years), the child begins to use symbols and language to represent her environment. During this stage the child tends to "center" on the most salient attributes of an object. Height has a dominating perceptual quality that overrides all other considerations. For example, if a child is shown two equal mounds of clay, she sees them as equivalent. If one is then flattened to a pancake form and the other is left alone, the child of 4 or 5 typically believes that the taller one contains more clay. Later on, she realizes that both masses of clay remain identical in this situation. The child does not have the ability to think of the reverse of what has happened or to go in one direction and compensate for it in another. This is Piaget's concept of conservation, which is important in the development of mathematics skills. It is also related to the characteristic of centering or focusing on only one dimension and neglecting other important aspects.

In the preoperational stage, the child is capable of the abstract process of manipulating symbols but remains concrete in her thinking compared to the adolescent or adult. The child is capable of some generalization in reasoning but still moves mostly from particular to particular without seeing complex relationships between objects or events.

In the oral healthcare setting, children at the preoperational stage should be allowed to explore the environment through smell, taste, touch, sight, and sound, perhaps to handle a mouth mirror and rubber cup, smell the cleansing agent and fluoride, hear the compressed air and dental engine. They are capable of focusing on and understanding the important features of objects. Simple language, involvement of their five senses, and basic explanations are appropriate to meet their concrete (versus abstract) manner of thinking (Table 5–4).

Concrete Operations Stage

In the concrete operations stage (age 7 to 11 years), the child becomes more evaluative in her thought processes (operations) and can apply them to concrete problems. When there is a discrepancy between thought and perception, as in the conservation problem with the clay mounds,

TABLE 5–4
TECHNIQUES FOR COMMUNICATING WITH CLIENTS THROUGH THE LIFESPAN

Level	Developmental Characteristics	Communication Techniques
Preschoolers	Beginning use of symbols and language; egocentric, focused on self; concrete in thinking and language	Allow child to use his five senses to explore oral healthcare environment (handle a mirror, feel a prophy cup, taste and smell fluoride, etc.) Use simple language and concrete, thorough explanations of exactly what is going to happen Let child see and feel cup "going around" or compressed air before putting in his mouth
School-age children	Less egocentric; shift to abstract; abstract thought emerges, but much thought still concrete	Demonstrate equipment, allow child to question, give simple explanations of procedures
Adolescents	Concrete thinking evolves to more complex abstraction; can formulate alternative hypotheses in problem solving; may revert to childish manner at times; usually enjoy adult attention	Allow self-expression and avoid being judgmental Give thorough, detailed answers to questions Be attentive
Adults	Broad individual differences in values, experiences and attitudes; self-directed and independent in comparison to children; have assumed certain family and social roles, periods of stability and change	Appropriately applied therapeutic communication techniques: maintaining silence, listening attentively, conveying acceptance, asking related questions, paraphrasing, clarifying, focusing, stating observations, offering information, summarizing, reflective responding
Older adults	May have sensory loss of hearing, vision; may have high level of anxiety; may be willing to comply with recommendations, but forgetful	Approach with respect, speak clearly and slowly Give time to formulate answers to answer questions and to elaborate Be attentive to nonverbal communication

Adapted with permission from Potter, P. A., and Perry, A. G. Fundamentals of Nursing: Concepts, Process & Practice 3rd ed. St. Louis: C. V. Mosby, 1993.

the child makes logical decisions instead of perceptual decisions. Her thinking shows increased flexibility and she grows less egocentric, showing a willingness to consider others' viewpoints. Reversibility in problem solving is present, but the child remains fixed on the concrete qualities and events in her surroundings.

Children in the concrete operations stage can begin to make evaluations and judgments concerning their oral health and self-care procedures. Equipment can be demonstrated and questions encouraged. The value of oral health can be discussed. Children are still focused mainly on the concrete aspects of their environment at this age, but are beginning to show greater capability for complex thinking (see Table 5–4).

Formal Operations Stage

The formal operations stage (11 years and above) is characterized by thought based on reasoning and judgment. The shift to abstraction and detailed logical analysis emerges in this period. The child can analyze a problem in the abstract and does not need the problem to be concretely represented to her. She searches for alternative hypotheses to solve problems and rejects those that seem inappropriate.

Children in this category of formal operations are capable of abstract thinking and can be given detailed instructions and explanations. The dental hygienist should provide them with a nonjudgmental invitation to demonstrate and discuss exactly what they are currently doing for oral self-care and allow them to participate in dialogue about what is needed to improve their oral health. Self-expression of the child should be respected (see Table 5–4).

If the dental hygienist understands the nature of the development of the thinking processes, he is more likely to be effective as an oral health educator of children. Piaget's development stage observations can assist in structuring and sequencing subject matter when planning and delivering oral health education to individuals and groups.

Piaget's theory advances the belief that children should be given an active role in their learning processes. His view finds favor with many cognitive psychologists who believe in learning by discovery. John Dewey is often credited as the first advocate of discovery learning.[33,34] His writings, which have made a significant impact on public education in America, encourage an active problem solving approach to education. Rather than a logical and ordered presentation of material, Dewey recommended that students be offered only gentle and minimal guidance to give them a basic framework in which they can learn by experience. This participatory type of learning has a special relevance for a child. By engaging her in the process rather than forcing her to be a passive receptor of information, the experience is exciting and meaningful.

Although much of Dewey's philosophy was related to social consciousness and the true meaning of the school as a social institution, many of his thoughts can be applied within the realm of oral health education. He believed that a good educator takes the subject matter, whatever it may be, and makes it interesting. He felt that the potential of the child to learn was unlimited if properly unleashed. If the child's attention is aroused and she is involved in activities related to the subject at hand, learning naturally occurs.

Teachers use techniques to create arousal or curiosity to get the attention of their students. A science experiment with unexpected results motivates students to understand why the results were different than expected. The dental hygienist in a third-grade classroom can place one hard-boiled egg in a soft drink and one in water and have the class record their observations over several days. The experiment can be said to imitate the effect of an acid on tooth enamel. The changes in the egg in the soft-drink solution will likely surprise and impress the children, motivating them to understand the dental caries process and the relationship of sugary soft drinks to tooth decay formation. Although this type of approach in oral health education requires planning and preparation, a creative presentation can result in a motivated client.

Humanistic Psychology

Like cognitive educational psychology, **humanistic psychology** places emphasis on the personal meaning that the educational material has for a student. Humanistic psychologists believe that learning is more likely to take place if students can attach personal meaning, feelings, or needs to their learning experiences. This line of thought is not represented by a particular psychologist. The positions of Abraham Maslow, Clayton Alderfer, Carl Rogers, and A. S. Neill are discussed here as representing this viewpoint.

"Humanistic psychology focuses primarily on the concerns of how individuals are influenced and guided by the personal meanings they attach to their experiences."[23] The emphasis for the humanistic psychologist is on the unique perceptions and needs of each individual and on the depth of meaning the learning experience holds for that individual at any point in the development of his life.

The humanistic and behavioristic psychologists have clear ideological differences. The behaviorists view people as respondents in their environment who have all their behavior shaped and conditioned by past experiences. The humanistic view sees people as free beings who determine their own behavior.

Historically, the concept of free will versus determinism has been a much-debated philosophical issue. In modern times it has been addressed by psychologists like Carl Rogers (humanistic view) and B. F. Skinner (behaviorist view). Their ideas and arguments are examined here in an attempt to understand the thinking that has influenced the evolution of learning theory.

Rogers was a strong proponent of allowing an individual unbridled freedom in learning experiences.[34a] He believed that self-initiated learning occurs in situations that have meaning and relevance for a student. If trusted, respected, and accepted, a student who is given a facilitative climate and plentiful resources seeks knowledge independently. According to Rogers, students should not be bound by strict formal education or rigid teachers who select learning content. When given freedom in a flexible environment, students spontaneously direct their energies to learn what they need to know to function in society and to pursue what is self-fulfilling. In this way education is not forced upon a person who freely chooses to learn, seizes opportunity to gain knowledge, and performs beyond traditional expectations. By establishing the right educational conditions, flexible, adaptive, and creative individuals are developed.

Perhaps the best example of an educational institution adhering to such a philosophy is that of Summerhill, the well known private, co-educational boarding school founded in England by A. S. Neill.[35] At this "free school," students choose what they want to learn, when to learn it, and how to learn it. Lessons are optional and children may play all day if they choose. There are no special teaching methods because it is believed that teaching in itself does not matter very much. Neill's position is that if children want to learn long division, they learn it no matter how it is taught. Teachers offer students trust, approval, and understanding and the result, according to Neill, is a student who develops the ability to work joyfully and live positively.

B. F. Skinner, the best known proponent of operant conditioning, has published strong reaction against the humanistic approaches of educators like Carl Rogers and A. S. Neill. Skinner expresses skepticism that many students flourish under such liberal teaching policy. He feels that most people possess very little natural curiosity or drive to learn and, furthermore, what they want to learn is only what will serve them most immediately.[36] Formal and structured education is necessary to prepare students for their future. This means acquiring skills and knowledge that may not particularly interest the student or seem relevant and meaningful at the moment. The approach to follow is clearly based on the scientific methods known to work, that is, positive reinforcement that emphasizes success rather than failure. The result, according to Skinner, is a happy and satisfied student who is carefully molded into a contributing member of society.

Another individual who is considered representative of the humanistic viewpoint deserves attention here. Abraham Maslow's work (1970) on gratification of human needs is helpful in understanding motivation to learn. As described in Chapter 2, Maslow believed that the most basic human needs must be satisfied before higher level needs can be addressed.

Maslow's hierarchy of human needs has important implications for the dental hygienist as an educator and health promoter in a variety of settings. A hygienist in a classroom setting may have difficulty understanding why a child is restless or uninterested in oral health education activities. Maslow has suggested that motivation or interest to learn may not be manifested until other basic needs have been met. A child who comes to school anxious because of personal family problems, or one who has not had breakfast or sufficient sleep, may not be interested in fulfilling higher order human needs. Educators must recognize that motivation to learn is a higher order need and that a failure of students (or clients) to respond may be related to deficits in basic human needs.

Clayton Alderfer reorganized Maslow's hierarchy into just three needs:[37] (1) existence, which combines physiological and safety needs; (2) relatedness, which refers to love and belonging needs; and (3) growth, which includes all higher level needs. Alderfer agreed with Maslow that needs on the lower level of the hierarchy must be met before the upper level needs can be attended to. However, he also theorized that when a person is frustrated in meeting a need, he may regress to a lower level need that can be satisfied more easily.

An example, according to Alderfer, may be a person who is attempting to incorporate a special dental aid into her daily oral hygiene regimen and is trying to understand the rationale and necessity of the task ("growth need" according to Alderfer or the "need for self-esteem or self-actualization that motivates a desire to know and understand," according to Maslow). For various physical or emotional reasons, she may become frustrated at performing this new task and stop doing it until she gets further advice and support from her hygienist, dentist, or friends who have experienced a similar situation. Alderfer would maintain that, in her frustration, she reverts back to a lower level on the hierarchy (back to the "relatedness need" according to Alderfer and back to the "love and belongingness need" in

Maslow's view). Therefore, she reverts back to a lower level on the hierarchy until the need there is more solidly fulfilled.

Additionally, Alderfer attributed need differences in individuals to variation in developmental level as well as to differences individuals experience environmentally. This indicates that both stage of development and environment play a role in determining needs and motivating a person to act.

Gordon has posed a number of questions one might ask when using human need theories to describe, predict, or explain motivational problems.[38] These questions may be helpful in dental hygiene client education.

- What human needs do individuals involved in the situation have?
- What human needs have been satisfied? How?
- Which unsatisfied human need is the lowest in the hierarchy?
- Have some higher order human needs been frustrated? Why?
- Has the person refocused to a lower level?
- How can the unsatisfied human needs be met?

With regard to the dental hygienist and oral health education, we need not be thrown into an indecisive mode based on educational theories that are contradictory. Rather, it is best that we take from each theory what is helpful and useful in achieving educational goals with clients. Positive reinforcement should be a highly valued tool for changing behavior. Consideration of thoughts and feelings involving the client in the teaching and learning process and careful consideration of a person's particular stage of development also are important. Integrating various theories and methods is acceptable and desirable in oral health education.

COMMUNICATION, TEACHING, AND LEARNING THROUGH THE LIFESPAN

The communication and the teaching and learning processes can be integrated and applied through the lifespan. **Andragogy** is the term applied to the art and science of helping the older person learn, whereas **pedagogy** is the art and science of teaching children. Pedagogy assumes that the learners are young, dependent recipients of knowledge and that subject matter has been arbitrarily decided upon by a teacher who is preparing them for their future. The teacher is the authority in this model and little regard is given to how the learner feels about the material or to his contribution in the process. Andragogy, on the other hand, assumes that the initiative to learn comes from the learner who is viewed as entering the learning process with a background of prior knowledge and experience. The teacher is a facilitator who learns along with the student, who in turn benefits from the teacher's contribution. The adult learner has a diverse history of experiences and is, in general, independent and self-directed. Pedagogy assumes that the child learner is moving toward becoming a fully matured human being, whereas andragogy assumes that the learner has arrived at this point. The purpose of this section is to address considerations for communication with persons throughout the lifespan.

Table 5–4 summarizes the key developmental characteristics at different age levels over the lifespan with those communication techniques appropriate at each level.

Preschool and Younger School-age Children

Communicating with children requires an understanding of the influence of growth and development of language, thought processes, and motor skills. Children begin development with simple, concrete language and thinking and move toward the more complex and abstract. Likewise, communication techniques and teaching methods can increase in complexity as the child grows older.

With preschoolers, nonverbal communication is more important than it is with the school-age child whose communication is better developed. The preschooler learns through play and enjoys a game-like atmosphere. Dentists have often called the dental engine the "Buzzy Bee," and hygienists refer to their polishing cup as the "Whirly Bird" and the saliva ejector as "Mr. Thirsty." Imaginary names help lighten the healthcare experience for small children. Oral health professionals are advised to use simple, short sentences, familiar words, and concrete explanations.

Weinstein and colleagues suggested five principles for what they call the "guidance-cooperation" model.[14] They believe that because the model is neither permissive or coercive, it is ideally suited for the preschool or young school-age child. Under this model, the health professional is placed in a parental role whereby the child is expected to respect her and cooperate with her. The principles inherent to the guidance-cooperative model are:

Tell the Child the Ground Rules Before and During Treatment Let the child know exactly what is expected of him. A comment such as, "You must do exactly as I ask and please keep your hands in your lap like my other helpers," will prepare the child to meet expectations. Structuring time so the child also knows what to expect may be useful. For fluoride treatments, a timer should be set and made visible to the child so he knows how long it will be before the trays will come out of his mouth.

Praise All Cooperative Behavior When the child responds to a directive like, "open wide," praise him with, "That's good! Thank you!" When he is sitting quietly, remember to praise him for cooperation. It is a mistake to ignore his behavior until it is a problem.

Keep Your Cool Ignore negative behavior like whining if it is not interfering with the healthcare. Showing anger will only make matters worse. Showing displeasure and using a calm voice for statements such as "I get upset (or unhappy, etc.) when you . . . ," is likely to get the point across more successfully.

Use Voice Control A sudden change in volume can gain attention from a child who is being uncooperative. Modulate voice tone and volume as soon as the child begins to respond.

Allow the Child to Play a Role Let the child make some structured choices. For example, "Would you like strawberry or grape-flavored fluoride today?" Most younger children enjoy the role of "helper" and are happy to hold mirrors, papers and pencils, and to receive praise for their good work.

Avoid Attempting to Talk a Child Into Cooperation Do not give lengthy rationales for the necessity of procedures. Rather, acknowledge the child's feelings, as in the statements "I understand you don't like the fluoride treatment; however, we must do it to make your teeth stronger. I understand that you would rather be outside playing, but we need to polish your teeth now." Then, firmly request his attention and cooperation and proceed with the service.

Both the preschool and school-age child are eager to learn and explore but may have fears about the oral healthcare environment, personnel, and treatment. Studies have shown that dental fears begin in childhood, and making early oral care a positive experience is necessary if the dental hygienist is interested in the client's long-term attitude toward oral health.[41,42] Rapport must be established as a foundation for cooperation and trust. The best teaching approaches for younger children follow behavioral rather than cognitive theory. Positive reinforcement used as immediate feedback, short instructional segments with simplified language and content that is concrete rather than abstract, close monitoring of progress, and encouragement for independence in the practice of oral hygiene skills are all indicated.

Older School-age Children and Adolescents

Adolescence is not a single stage of development. The rate at which children progress through adolescence and the psychological states that accompany the change can vary considerably from one child to another.[43] In early adolescence (about 13 to 15 years old), children may rather suddenly demonstrate an ambivalence toward parents and other adults, manifested by questioning of adult values and authority. By late adolescence (18 years and older) much of the ambivalence is gone and values that characterize the adult years have fully emerged. Friendship patterns in early and midadolescence are usually intense as the child begins to explore companionship outside the family and to establish himself as an independent person.

Some common complaints from the adolescent's point of view can sensitize health professionals for positive interactions with this group of young people.[43] First, a frequently voiced complaint of adolescents is that adults do not listen to them. They seem to feel that adults are in too much of a hurry, appear to be looking for certain answers, or listen only to what they want to hear. A second complaint is that too often a conversation turns into unsolicited advice or a mini-lecture. A testimonial of such an incident was reported in a study by Kleinknecht and Bernstein.[44] A young person, asked to describe specific experiences in dentistry, related the following:

> My dentist bugged me a lot. He would become angry if I felt pain. He pushed my hair around and lectured constantly about young people and their hair.

Other less common complaints from adolescents are that they are patronized, that they do not understand questions being asked, and finally that adults lack humor.

Dental hygienists should consider carefully these complaints and practice behaviors that enhance communication with adolescents. Being attentive and allowing the adolescent time to talk enhance rapport and communication. Some rapport-building questions at the beginning of the appointment may relate to family, school, personal interests, or career intentions. It is useful to have some knowledge of the contemporary interests of adolescents, which may include trends in music, sports, and fashion. They want a sense of being understood and do not want to be judged or lectured.

Adolescents have a strong human need for self-determination and responsibility. An astute dental hygienist can use these unfulfilled needs to motivate the adolescent client to adopt oral self-care behaviors. This educational approach, based upon human need theory, can enhance the adolescent's sense of personal responsibility toward the care of his mouth. In order that adolescents do not feel singled out, a dental hygienist might say, "We encourage all of our adult clients to floss daily. This is because we know it works. We've seen the results." In addition, the teenagers do not feel patronized or confused if questions and advice are offered in a sincere, straightforward manner.

The adolescent complaint that adults lack humor bears consideration in dental hygienist-client interactions. Humor is a communication technique that should be used comfortably and naturally with clients of all ages and stages of development. The therapeutic advantages of humor and laughter have been documented.[45] For example, Cousins has described the role of recovery from two life-threatening illnesses, which seems to prove that laughter and positive emotions are vital to the success of any medical treatment as well as to life in general.

Healthcare personnel and facilities can be perceived as frightening for clients of all ages. Humor as a technique of communication can put people at ease and thereby meet their human need for freedom from stress. Even a simple smile can help establish a warm social bond. In her book *Communication in Health Care,* Collins states, "humor has childlike qualities of playfulness. If one can be playful, one still has vestiges of youth and vigor."[46] The unexpected, the incongruous, the pun, the exaggeration or understatement are examples of humor that can be effective with both younger and older clients.[47]

Teaching approaches for older school-age children and adolescents may follow cognitive as well as behavioristic theories. Instructional materials can be detailed and abstract with use of analogies that assume previously acquired knowledge, for example, presenting the complexities of the etiology of dental caries and periodontal diseases. Humanistic theories such as those inspired by the human needs hierarchies of Maslow and Alderfer are appropriate for children of all ages. Adolescent clients can be enlisted to help identify deficiencies related to the need for a sound dentition and the need for skin and mucous membrane integrity of the head and neck. Once needs are identified, the client's thoughts and feelings regarding personal priorities and motivation to meet these needs through self-care can be explored.

Adults

Havighurst delineated three developmental stages for adults and listed common adult concerns at each stage.[48] Although communication techniques may not differ greatly for the adult stages, knowledge of general differences in characteristics between age groups can enlighten the hygienist about typical concerns of clients at different periods of adulthood. An awareness of how priorities in life change for adults as they develop can help the hygienist identify learning needs and "teachable moments" for different clients. The Havighurst adult stages have been summarized according to early adulthood, middle age, and late maturity in Table 5–5.[47] The dental hygienist should be aware, without asking personal questions, that young adults may be trying to institute oral hygiene self-care behaviors while adjusting to major life stresses such as bringing up young children, managing a home, or starting a demanding career. Adults in the middle years may be more settled in careers and have less responsibility for child care, but may be heavily involved in social responsibilities, adjusting to their

TABLE 5–5
HAVINGHURT'S DESCRIPTION OF THE ADULT DEVELOPMENTAL STAGES

Early Adulthood	Middle Age	Late Maturity
Selecting a mate Learning to live with a marriage partner Starting a family Bringing up young children Managing a home Getting started in an occupation Taking on civic responsibilities Finding a congenial social group	Achieving adulthood and social responsibilities Establishing and maintaining an economic standard of living Assisting one's children to become adults Developing durable leisure-time activities Relating to one's marriage partner as a person Accepting and adjusting to physical change Adjusting to one's aging parent	Adjusting to decreasing physical strength and to death Adjusting to retirement and to reduced income Adjusting to death of one's marriage partner Establishing an explicit affiliation with one's age group Meeting social and civic obligations Establishing satisfactory physical living arrangements in light of physical infirmities

Reprinted with permission from Darkenwald, G. G., and Merriam, S. B. Adult Education: Foundations of Practice. New York: Harper & Row, 1982, pp. 90–91.

personal physical changes or the demands of caring for aging parents. Older adults may be adjusting to decreasing physical strength, a chronic health problem, retirement, or death of a spouse.

Communication approaches appropriate for adults are the therapeutic communication techniques discussed previously in this chapter. In utilizing the techniques, it is important for the dental hygienist to be familiar with the adult developmental stages and aware of what demands may be preventing adults of the different stages from easily making oral healthcare behavior changes.

Modern adult learning theory has been supported by some basic assumptions expressed by Lindeman in the early part of this century.[50] The assumptions have been aptly paraphrased by Malcolm Knowles in his book, *The Adult Learner: A Neglected Species*.[51] Keeping these assumptions in mind facilitates communication with adults who become "learners" as dental hygienists become "teachers" in the healthcare setting. These assumptions can enhance the dental hygiene educator's approach to teaching adults:

- **Adults are motivated to learn as they experience needs and interests that learning will satisfy; therefore, these are the appropriate starting points for organizing adult learning activities.** Adults are more likely than children or adolescents to acknowledge their needs readily. Well before Maslow developed his human needs hierarchy, Lindeman recognized the role that human needs play in motivating adult behavior. He applied needs identification to learning with the understanding that mature adults know from past experience how to recognize needs and are motivated to seek information (education) to satisfy these needs. The dental hygiene educator can help the adult identify human needs related to oral health and disease, and can expect to find most adults willing to recognize the needs and act to satisfy them.
- **Adults' orientation to learning is life-centered; therefore, the appropriate units for organizing adult learning are life situations, not subjects.** Adults are used to learning from everyday events rather than from books and formal lectures. They respond well to anecdotes about other clients' experiences with oral hygiene regimens because they identify with those individuals and their experiences. The dental hygienist may remark, "I have heard such good testimonials from my clients who have begun to floss regularly. They say their mouths feel so much healthier and do not feel really clean unless they floss every day." This statement is likely to have more impact on the client than simply providing information on the subject of flossing.
- **Experience is the richest resource for adults' learning; therefore, the core methodology of adult education is the analysis of experience.** When adults return for their maintenance care, the dental hygienist should help them analyze their experiences in trying to institute new self-care procedures. For example, if clients are experiencing difficulty in flossing technique or in incorporating flossing into a busy schedule, they should be encouraged to discuss the problems and receive help from the dental hygienist in developing solutions. This approach is likely to meet the person's human need for conceptualization.
- **Adults have a deep need to be self-directing; therefore, the role of the teacher is to engage in a process of mutual inquiry with them rather than to transmit his or her knowledge to them and then evaluate their conformity to it.** The human need for self-determination and responsibility is strong in adults. The dental hygienist should engage adults in discussions that lead to problem solving with their participation. The hygienist should not dictate solutions or expect adults to follow rules of oral hygiene that they have had no part in developing.
- **Individual differences among people increase with age; therefore, adult education must make optimal provision for differences in style, time, place, and pace of learning.** The dental hygienist should expect people to differ widely in their responses to a particular educational methodology. Although adults are similar in that learning for them is life-centered, their individual histories of life experiences differ greatly. Individual differences increase with age, and the next section describes teaching and learning with the older adult.

Older Adults

The elderly population is a highly diversified group. Weinstein and colleagues caution against regarding the elderly as a homogeneous group and suggest that the wide variations in health and psychological states dictate the necessity of careful assessment of each individual.[14] (For more information, see Chapter 30 on dental hygiene care for the older adult.)

Weinstein and colleagues recommend the following in communicating with older adult clients:[14]

Establish Rapport Elderly clients may be suspicious of professionals so it is best to spend a little extra time earning their confidence. Good eye contact and a comfortable physical proximity to the client help convey personal interest.

Treat Clients with Dignity Older adults may have diminished self-images because of losses they have sustained in death of loved ones, work roles, financial security, and personal health. Their human needs for appreciation, respect, self-determination, and responsibility can be increased by encouraging participation in dental hygiene care plan decisions and by expecting active participation in oral hygiene regimens. Expressing confidence in their opinions and ability helps give them a renewed sense of control over their lives.

Assess Psychological Factors Through careful observation of the client's verbal and nonverbal behavior and interaction with others, the dental hygienist can make some assessment of the client's psychological state. This includes the person's attitude toward his overall health, oral health, mobility, general disposition, and approach to life. This assessment enables the hygienist to estimate how well the client may perform daily self-care behaviors. Recommendations to the client, communication and teaching approaches must be adjusted to fit the individual.

Keep a Slow Pace Although older adults display a slowing down of reaction time, no decline in knowledge or reasoning ability has been determined.[52] Impaired vision or hearing, not reduced mental abilities, means more time is needed to absorb information. Recommendations should be presented clearly and slowly so that the elderly client can accurately interpret and assimilate the information. Written instructions and reading materials may be an appreciated follow-up.

COMMUNICATING WITH THE ANXIOUS CLIENT

Achieving effective communication with the client who has generalized anxiety or fear (an unmet need for freedom from stress or pain) is inevitably a problem for every oral health practitioner. The word "anxiety" usually refers to a vague uneasiness about something. In its more intense form, anxiety is known as "fear." Some psychologists do not distinguish between anxiety about, and fear of, the oral healthcare situation.[53]

A *phobia* is a fear that is extreme and often described as irrational or unreasonable. Estimates of the level of dental phobia in the population range from 6% to 20%.[53] The level of extreme fear may be low, but it is commonly understood that almost every client experiences some stress. This fear is often responsible for canceled appointments. Therefore, the dental hygienist is likely to encounter dental fear and anxiety on a daily basis in her work.

Developing an understanding of the origins, assessment, and management of dental fear is a necessity for the professional dental hygienist. Although the dental hygienist cannot be expected to control fear with the same sophisticated techniques used by professional psychologists, the dental hygienist should recognize a client's fearful emotional state and demonstrate behaviors that relax the client. Hygienists must use appropriate therapeutic communication skills with fearful clients to facilitate quality dental hygiene care and meet the client's human need for freedom from stress and pain.

Origins of Dental Fear

Dental fears can be learned through a variety of personal and nonpersonal experiences. Both children and adults may have had negative medical experiences that caused them to fear the dental setting. For example, a history of hospitalization may lead a client to associate injury, pain, and fear with white walls and uniforms.[54] When the phobic child or adult enters the oral healthcare environment and finds white walls and a staff dressed in white, the tendency is to recall the hospital experience, and the fearful response to professional oral care is intensified.

Other dental or medical incidents that may precipitate dental fear include various negative experiences with injections. For example, rough, uncomfortable injections performed during childhood immunizations may be remembered. Inadequate anesthesia with previous dental care causing pain or discomfort may be associated with all oral care in the client's mind. An incident of adverse reactions to local anesthetics (pallor, dizziness, nausea, sweating, and fainting) may lead to adverse psychological reactions when the client is confronted with the thought of future appointments.

Many fearful clients have deteriorating oral conditions that can be part of a "snowballing" effect.[54] The person's fear prevents him from seeking treatment; therefore, his oral condition continues to worsen. As his teeth and periodontal structures cause more discomfort and embarrassment, his fear escalates. The individual fears the pain, criticism, embarrassment, and also the cost he imagines is awaiting him at the healthcare facility.

The influence of family, friends, and the general media on the development of attitudes is well known. The family is an early source of information for children who learn from observing the behavior of others. Mothers anxious about dental care are suspected of transmitting that fear to their children.[55] In later childhood, peer pressure affects beliefs and behavior related to dental fear. Finally, the media is known for depicting the dental setting as a "torture chamber." Cartoons, movies, and jokes circulated worldwide portray negative images that are difficult to overcome.

Dental hygiene care does not fall outside the realm of client fear because a number of specific dental hygiene procedures can cause anxiety or discomfort. For example, use of a local anesthetic, an important method of pain control in dental hygiene care of clients with advanced periodontal disease, has been shown to cause fear.[42] Moreover, therapeutic scaling and root planing without local anesthesia also can cause discomfort for a client. A partial list of potential sources of pain or discomfort during the dental hygiene process of care includes heavy-handed probing or exploring, excessive palpating of the tissue during intraoral and extraoral examinations, unnecessary soft tissue laceration, allowing the polishing cup to "heat up" on the tooth or polishing carelessly onto the gingiva, allowing build-up of too much saliva during fluoride treatments, inadvertently pinching the client's lip or pressing on the gingiva with the mirror or other instruments during scaling, and improper handling of the ultrasonic scaler leading to heating of the instrument tip. In addition, the client may experience fatigued orofacial and temporomandibular joint, restlessness, muscular stiffness, or back pain due to long confinement in the dental chair. Discomfort in many of these incidents may be unavoidable, but the dental hygienist who is sensitive to the client's human needs for safety and for freedom from pain and stress and who uses the CARE principle (Comfort, Acceptance, Responsiveness, and Empathy) will, through deliberate intervention, prevent or control these possible sources of anxiety.

Assessment of Dental Fear

To control fear in clients, the dental hygienist must be able to identify when the client's needs for safety and freedom from stress and pain are unmet. Measurement of fear can be physiological, psychological, or made by observation of behavior. Physiological changes attributed to fear, such as increased heart rate and sweat gland activity, decreased peripheral blood flow, altered gastric activity and respiration, are known to exist.[44] Precision in this type of measurement is more or less reserved for researchers, but the hygienist is able to identify a fast pulse rate, perspiration, or changes in respiration that may be related to anxiety. Some physiological indicators are subtle but the hygienist may notice white knuckles, perspiration on hands, forehead, and upper lip, or xerostomia.

Two commonly used questionnaires to assess dental fears are the Corah Dental Anxiety Scale and the Dental Fear Survey.[42,56] Both of these instruments are self-report measures based on the concept that the best way to determine a person's anxiety about professional oral care is to ask him.

Informal methods of fear assessment include verbal and behavioral indicators of a client's nervousness and anxiety.[14] Verbal indicators are talking too much or not at all, talking too loudly or too quietly, making inappropriate jokes, or jumping from subject to subject. Behavioral indicators can never be completely anticipated because the possibilities are limitless. With children, indicators may be overt such as crying, random movements, or running away. Signs of adult anxiety include excessive random movement, trembling hands, rubbing hands together, gripping the chair arms tightly, constantly canceling or breaking appointments, or being late for appointments. When some indicators of fear have been noted, communication is the key to determining whether hunches or intuitions are right. Communication is, in fact, the most fundamental process available for helping the client cope with fear.

Treatment of Dental Fear

Psychologists have developed a variety of techniques to reduce fear in their clients, and many of these have been adapted for use in the oral healthcare setting. The best known are systematic *desensitization,*[57] *flooding* or *implosion,*[58] and *modeling.*[59] The purpose of all techniques is to expose the person to the feared object until the fear is desensitized or extinguished or the person learns to control it.[53] With *desensitization,* gradual exposure to the least fear-arousing aspects of an object or behavior is advanced to exposure to the most fear-arousing situation. A sample hierarchy to desensitize for fear of the dental drill has been suggested.[60] A client is instructed to substitute relaxation for anxiety response at each level of the hierarchy, which can be either experienced or imagined. The hierarchy is listed as making an appointment, going to the dental office, sitting in the reception area, entering the treatment area, sitting in the chair, seeing the dentist, hearing noises, receiving an injection, receiving the drilling.

With flooding or implosion, the exposure to the feared situation is sudden or "all at once." Subjects are required to imagine the most fear-arousing situations they can think of and are trained to relax while imagining them. This treatment has been of some value in helping phobic clients accept dental treatment.[61]

With modeling, the exposure is vicarious because the fearful person is required to observe another person being exposed to the feared situation. This technique has been particularly useful with children.[62] When children observe other children successfully undergoing dental treatment it appears to quiet their own fear and they tend to model their own behavior after the cooperative child.

Chambers and colleague have offered assurance that anxiety can almost always be handled by talking about it.[63] The average dental hygienist may not have the knowledge base to formally employ the techniques of desensitization, flooding, or modeling; however, talking about fear and applying therapeutic communication techniques are well within the dental hygiene scope of practice. Discussing the anxiety and possible sources of it help both the dental hygienist and client to understand it in perspective. The CARE principle, reflective responding, and all the therapeutic communication techniques discussed in this chapter provide sensible and humanistic strategies for the dental hygienist to control client fear.

Relaxation Techniques for the Anxious Client

Relaxation and *attention diversion* techniques are strategies that can be used by the dental hygienist with fearful clients.

Relaxation The professional psychology treatments of desensitization, flooding, and modeling all use imagery and a relaxation procedure with deep breathing. The list below describes a typical, self-directed, step-by-step progressive relaxation procedure that can be used during the dental hygiene process.

1. Lie down on your back on a comfortable couch, bed or mat.
2. Place your hands at your sides.
3. Close your eyes.
4. Breathe deeply and slowly. Be aware of your breathing, the feeling and the sound of it.
5. Take a deep breath and hold it briefly, then, exhale.
6. Repeat two more times.
7. Continue to breathe deeply and quietly while you concentrate on your feet. Imagine your feet and toes becoming very relaxed.
8. After a few moments, concentrate on your lower legs, imagine them feeling very relaxed along with your feet.
9. After a few moments, concentrate on your upper legs, imagine them feeling very relaxed along with your lower legs and feet. Imagine that all tension is flowing away from these parts of your body.
10. Continue to breathe deeply, slowly, and quietly as you continue up the rest of your body, concentrating on each section and imagining all tension flowing away.
11. When you have relaxed all parts of your body, begin

to imagine the event or sequence of events you have chosen to focus on today.

12. Continue to breathe deeply, slowly, and quietly while you are imaging these events with as much detail as possible.

13. If you feel anxiety when imagining the situation, open your eyes briefly to "clear the image," tell yourself to relax, and try it again.

14. Try to imagine the situation at least three times before ceasing your effort.

15. After this imagery attempt, allow yourself to think of something pleasant, remain in position a few more moments.*

The concept of reduction of anxiety by relaxation is based on research findings that a person cannot be simultaneously relaxed and tense.[57] This relaxation procedure does not have to be formally introduced. A simple explanation to either children or adults of the value of taking deep, slow breaths and encouraging them to do so can manage the situation. A rich supply of oxygen helps the client relax; keeping her focused on her breathing can help distract her from the procedure being performed.

Attention Diversion Directing attention away from an anxiety-provoking object or event to something that is neutral or gives pleasure is known as attention diversion. Examples of diverting attention to facilitate client management are:

- Talking to a child about his favorite toy during an intraoral procedure
- Decorating treatment areas with plants and paintings to look at and enjoy
- Playing soothing music for a calming effect

Distraction and diversion must be carefully balanced against informing clients of exactly what is going to happen next in a tell-show-do manner.[64] An anxious client needs an introduction to office equipment and explanation of dental and dental hygiene procedures. Relaxation and distraction strategies can be used together, for example, by stating to a client during an injection, "Breathe deeply and slowly through your nose. Think about your finger and toes right now." Distraction does not mean deceiving the client or hiding information and can be used on many occasions with great success (see Guidelines for Providing Dental Hygiene Care to the Fearful Client chart).

GUIDELINES FOR PROVIDING DENTAL HYGIENE CARE TO THE FEARFUL CLIENT

- **Avoid inflicting pain if possible.** If pain or discomfort can be minimized or eliminated, all means to do so should be employed.
- **Pain inflicted accidentally should be identified and the cause stopped immediately.** If the client sends a signal in some way that he is in pain, treatment should stop immediately and all temptation to continue with the procedure to "get it over with" should be abandoned. For example, additional anesthetic may be indicated before scaling in a deep pocket can be continued.
- **If there is any possibility that the client will feel pain, communicate this possibility.** The client can cope more effectively with an impending painful event if he is prepared for it in advance. Right before the needle enters the tissue, the hygienist might say, "You're going to feel just a little pinch at first."
- **Avoid using emotion-charged words like "pain" and "hurt."** It is better to use words like "discomfort" and "tenderness."
- **If you say, "This will not be uncomfortable," be absolutely sure you are correct.** You will lose credibility and the client's trust if such a statement is followed by careless or heavy-handed instrumentation.
- **Tell the client that he can signal you to stop by raising his hand.** If he signals, stop immediately. This gives the client a feeling of control and reduces the stress he may be experiencing.
- **Introduce new procedures slowly and gently.** This rule goes along with the obligation to thoroughly inform the client.
- **Praise desirable behaviors but never chastise for undesirable behaviors.** The client should be praised for merely coming to his appointment and never criticized for having stayed away so long. His presentation in the oral healthcare setting is strong positive evidence of his desire to attend to his oral health and to seek professional care and should be recognized as such.
- **The dental hygiene environment should be as quiet and relaxed as possible.** A noisy disorganized atmosphere can increase client anxiety. Clients should be approached in a slow, quiet, relaxed manner that can cue them to a similar response with their own behavior.

Adapted from Jackson, E. Managing dental fear: A tentative code of practice. Journal of Oral Medicine 20:96, 1974.

References

1. Ghazizadeh-Eslami, J. Humanistic approach and its relevance to dental hygiene education and practice. A literature review (unpublished). Norfolk, Virginia: Old Dominion University, 1991.
2. Schramm, W. How communication works. In Schramm, W. (ed.). The Process and Effects of Mass Communication. Urbana, IL: University of Illinois Press, 1955, pp. 4–8.
3. Corno, L., and Mandinach, E. B. The role of cognitive engagement in classroom learning and motivation. Educational Psychologist 18(2):88, 1983.
4. Potter, P. A., and Perry, A. G. Fundamentals of Nursing: Concepts, Applications, and Practice, 3rd ed. St. Louis: C. V. Mosby, 1993.
5. Christen, A. G., and Katz, C. A. Understanding human motivation. In Harris, N. O., and Christen, A. G. (eds.). Primary Preventive Dentistry, 3rd ed. Norwalk, CT: Appleton & Lange, 1991, pp. 373–395.
6. Hall, E. T. Listening behavior: Some cultural differences. Phi Delta Kappa 50:379, 1969.
7. Myerscough, P. R. Talking with Patients: A Basic Clinical Skill. Oxford: Oxford University Press, 1989.
8. Rogers, C. R. Client-Centered Therapy. Boston: Houghton-Mifflin, 1951.
9. Smith, V. M., and Bass, T. A. Communication for Health Professionals, 2nd ed. Philadelphia: J. B. Lippincott, 1979.
10. Sathre, F. S., Olson, R. W., and Whitney, C. I. Let's Talk. Glenview, IL: Scott Foresman, 1973.
11. Wiles, C. B., and Ryan, J. Communication for Dental Auxiliaries. Reston, Virginia: Reston Publishing Company, 1982.

*Adapted with permission from: Rich, S. K., and Tsutsui, P. T. Densensitization for fear of administering intraoral local anesthesia: Four case reports. Educational Directions 3:24–27, 1985. Copyrighted 1985 by the American Dental Hygienists' Association.

12. Geboy, M. J. Communication and Behavior Management in dentistry. Baltimore: Williams & Wilkins, 1985.
13. Gordon, T. Parent Effectiveness Training. New York, Peter H. Wyden, Inc., 1972.
14. Weinstein, P., Getz, T., and Milgrom, P. Oral Self-care: Strategies for Preventive Dentistry. Reston, VA: Reston, 1991.
15. Bandura, A. Self-efficacy: Toward a unifying theory of behavior change. Psychological Review 84:191, 1977.
16. Weiner, B., Nierenberg, R., and Goldstein, M. Social learning (locus of control) versus attributional (causes stability) interpretations of expectancy of success. Journal of Personality 44:52, 1976.
17. Gagne, E. The Cognitive Psychology of School Learning. Boston: Little, Brown 1985.
18. Ames, R., Ames, C., and Garrison, W. Children's causal ascriptions for positive and negative interpersonal outcomes. Psychological Reports 41:595, 1977.
19. Simon, J. G., and Feather, N. T. Causal attributions for success and failure at university examinations. Journal of Educational Psychology 64:46, 1973.
20. Valle, V. A., and Frieze, I. H. Stability of causal attributions as a mediator in changing expectations for success. Journal of Personality and Social Psychology 33:579, 1976.
21. Rotter, J. Generalized expectancies, for internal versus external control of reinforcement. Psychological Monographs 80:1, 1966.
22. Woodall, I. R. Patient motivation and locus of control. Compendium of Continuing Education in Dentistry 6:147, 1985.
23. Dembo, M. H. Teaching for Learning; Applying Educational Psychology in the Classroom, 4th ed. New York: Longmans, 1991.
24. Fodor, J. T., and Dalis, G. T. Health Instruction: Theory and Application, 4th ed. Philadelphia: Lea & Febiger, 1989.
25. Bloom, B. S., Englehart, N. D., et al. Taxonomy of the Educational Objectives. Handbook I. Cognitive Domain. New York: McKay, 1956.
26. Krathwohl, D. R., Bloom, B. S., and Masia, B. Taxonomy of Educational Objectives. Handbook II. Affective Domain. New York: McKay, 1964.
27. Harrow, A. J. A Taxonomy of the Psychomotor Domain: A Guide for Developing Behavioral Objectives. New York: McKay, 1972.
28. Skinner, B. F. Science of Human Behavior. New York: Macmillan, 1953.
29. Skinner, B. F. The science of learning and the art of teaching. Harvard Education Review 24:86, 1954.
29a. Thorndike, E. L. Educational Psychology. New York: Columbia University Teachers College, 1913.
29b. Thorndike, E. L. Measurement of Intelligence. New York: Columbia University Teachers College, 1927.
30. Gardner, H. The Mind's New Science: A History of the Cognitive Revolution. New York: Basic Books, 1987.
31. Wertheimer, M. Productive Thinking. New York: Harper, 1945.
32. Piaget, J. Development and learning. In Ripple, R. E., and Rockcastle, V. N. (eds.). Piaget Rediscovered: A Report of the Conference on Cognitive Skills and Curriculum Development. Ithaca, NY: Cornell University School of Education, 1964.
33. Dewey, J. Democracy and Education. New York: Macmillan, 1916.
34. Dewey, J. Experience and Nature. Chicago: Open Court, 1925.
34a. Rogers, C. R. Freedom to Learn. Columbus, Ohio: Charles E. Merrill, 1969.
35. Neill, A. S. Summerhill. New York: Hart, 1960.
36. Skinner, B. F. The Free and Happy Student. Phi Delta Kappa 55:13, 1973.
37. Alderfer, C. P. Existence, Relatedness, and Growth: Human Needs in Organizational Settings. New York: Free Press, 1972.
38. Gordon, J. R. A Diagnostic Approach to Organizational Behavior. Boston: Allyn and Bacon, 1983.
39. Meyer, S. L. Andragogy and the aging adult learner. Educational Gerontology: an International Quarterly 2:115, 1977.
40. Weinstein, P., Gretz, T., and Milgram, P. Oral Self-care: Strategies for Preventive Dentistry. Reston, VA: Reston, 1985.
41. Forigone, A., and Clark, E. Comments on an empirical study of the cause of dental fears. Journal of Dental Research 53:496, 1974.
42. Kleinknecht, R. A., Klepac, R., and Alexander, L. Origins and characteristics of fear of dentistry. Journal of the American Dental Association 86:842, 1973.
43. Wrate, R. E. Talking to adolescents. In Meyerscough, P. R. (ed.). Talking with Patients: A Basic Skill. Oxford: Oxford University Press, 1989, pp. 82–98.
44. Kleinknecht, R. A., and Bernstein, D. A. Fear assessment in the dental office. In Ingersoll, B. D., and McCutcheon, W. R. (eds.). Clinical Research in Behavioral Dentistry: Proceedings of the Second National Conference on Behavioral Dentistry. Morgantown, WV: West Virginia University, 1979.
45. Cousins, N. The Healing Heart. New York, Avon Books, 1984.
46. Collins, M. Communication in Health Care: Understanding and Implementing Effective Human Relationships. St. Louis: C. V. Mosby, 1977.
47. Smith, V. M., and Bass, T. A. Communication for Health Professionals. Philadelphia, J. B. Lippincott, 1979.
48. Havighurst, R. J. Developmental Tasks and Education. New York: McKay, 1952.
49. Darkenwald, G. G., and Merriam, S. B. Adult Education: Foundations of Practice. New York: Harper & Row, 1982 pp. 90–91.
50. Lindeman, E. C. The Meaning of Adult Education. New York: New Republic, 1926.
51. Knowles, M. The Adult Learner: A Neglected Species, 3rd ed. Houston: Gulf, 1984.
52. Lenz, E. The Art of Teaching Adults. New York: Holt, Rinehart, Winston, 1982.
53. Bochner, S. The Psychology of the Dentist-patient Relationship. New York: Springer-Verlag, 1988.
54. Kroeger, R. F. Managing the Apprehensive Dental Patient: A Management-guide for the Dentist and Staff for Effective Practice Building and Internal Marketing. Cincinnati: Heritage Communications, 1987.
55. Wright, G. Z., Alpern, G. D., and Leake, J. L. The modifiability of maternal anxiety as it related to children's cooperative behavior. Journal of Dentistry for Children 40:265, 1973.
56. Corah, N. L. Development of a dental anxiety scale. Journal of Dental Research 48:596, 1969.
57. Wolpe, J. The Practice of Behavior Therapy. New York: Pergamon Press, 1969.
58. Boulegouris, J. C., and Marks, I. M. Implosion (flooding)—a new treatment for phobias. British Medical Journal 2:721, 1969.
59. Bandura, A., Blanchard, E. B., and Ritter, B. Relative efficacy of desensitization and modeling approaches for inducing behavioral, effective, and attitudinal changes. Journal of Personality and Social Psychology 13:173, 1969.
60. Milgrom, P., Weinstein, P., et al. Treating Fearful Dental Patients: A Patient Management Handbook. Reston, VA: Reston, 1985.
61. Matthews, A., and Rezin, V. Treatment of dental fears by imaginal flooding and rehearsing of coping behavior. Behavior Research and Therapy 15:321, 1977.
62. White, W. C., Akers, J., Green, J., and Yates, D. Use of imitation in the treatment of dental phobia in early childhood: A preliminary report. Journal of Dentistry for Children 41:26, 1974.
63. Chambers, D. W., and Abrams, R. G. Dental Communication. Norwalk, CT: Appleton & Lange, 1991, pp. 373–395.
64. Addelston, H. K. Child patient training. Fortnightly Review of the Chicago Dental Society 38:7–9, 27–29, 1959.

Suggested Readings

Berlyne, D. E. Conflict, Arousal, and Curiosity. New York: McKay, 1956.

Calman, J. Talking with Patients: A Guide to Good Practice. London: William Heinemann, 1984.

Dummett, C. O. Minority elderly: Essential curricula content in dentistry. In Minority Aging, Essential Curricula Content for Selected Health and Allied Health Professions. Washington, DC:

U.S. Department of Health and Human Services, Public Health Service, Health Resources and Services Administration, DHHS Publication No. HRS (P-DV-90-4), 1990.

Jackson, E. Managing dental fear: A tentative code of practice. Journal of Oral Medicine 29:96, 1974.

Janz, N. K., and Becker, M. H. The health belief model: A decade later. Health Education Quarterly 11(1):1, 1984.

Kegeles, S. S. Some motives for seeking preventive dental care. Journal of the American Dental Association 67:90, 1963.

Ley, P. Communication with Patients: Improving Communication, Satisfaction, and Compliance. London: Croom Helm, 1988.

Rosenstock, I. M. Historical origins of the health belief model. Health Education Monographs 2:328, 1974.

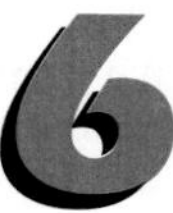

Cultural Diversity and the Dental Hygiene Process

OBJECTIVES

Mastery of the content in this chapter will enable the reader to:

- Define the key terms used
- Differentiate among the concepts of race, ethnicity, ethnic group, culture, and subculture
- Explain how an understanding of a client's cultural frame-of-reference improves the quality of dental hygiene care
- Describe the importance of cultural health beliefs as related to dental hygiene care
- Describe several cultural barriers to dental hygiene care
- Identify some traditional health-related beliefs and practices of various ethnic groups
- Discuss cultural diversity
- Identify cultural aspects of cross-cultural client care

INTRODUCTION

In a recent book entitled *The Borderless World,*[1] Ohmal contends that national borders increasingly are disappearing in international trade, culture, health, and communication. The nations of the world have been grouped according to their level of economic development. Countries in the **First World** are economically developed and capitalistic; the **Second World** includes the economically developed socialist countries; and the **Third World** refers to those countries that are still developing, for example, some countries in Africa, Asia, Central America, and South America. North America continues to experience an influx of immigrants from all over the world; American entities such as McDonald's and Burger King continue their global expansion. "American-made" automobiles may be assembled in the United States by a Japanese-owned company using parts manufactured in a number of other countries; students from other countries compete to study in American centers of higher education; and Tiffany's in New York now requires basic instruction in Japanese as part of its training for new employees. Daily, people read articles and watch TV programs about the impact of rain forest destruction; pollution of the groundwater, bays, and oceans; the global problems of toxic waste, acid rain, and the greenhouse effect; and the production and sale of illegal drugs. When one considers these major global issues, it becomes clear that the policies of each nation articulate with the lifestyle and future of all the others. In the United States, demographic changes will alter the racial and ethnic composition of our cities, institutions, workplaces, and clients. Women and minorities will represent the largest share of new entrants into the labor force, while immigrants will be responsible for the largest increase in the population since World War I.[2] The demographic characteristics of the United States population are displayed in Table 6–1. As the nations of the world become more racially and ethnically diverse, human efforts to find a common ground among all of mankind must be escalated. The profession of dental hygiene can achieve its full potential only in the context of a global society.

The message is clear. To be successful in our global society, dental hygienists must develop an international perspective. The dental hygienist must be internationalist, that is, be able to integrate current knowledge of oral healthcare with the ways of multiple cultures. Frequently, it is the dental hygienist who faces the challenge of meshing diverse cultural systems when the client appears for care. Dental hygiene can affect the quality of the lives of the people of the world and meet human needs related to oral health and disease if the challenge of blending an international perspective into the dental hygiene process is met.

The purpose of this chapter is to help the professional dental hygienist interact effectively with people from various cultures and function in cross-cultural care settings. In multicultural environments, knowledge about and practical attention to cultural diversity is essential for applying the dental hygiene process within the context of the human needs conceptual model. For the dental hygienist interested in further developing cross-cultural perspectives, *A Practitioner's Guide to Understanding Indigenous and Foreign Cultures,* by Henderson,[3] is recommended.

TABLE 6–1
CULTURAL DIVERSITY OF THE POPULATION OF THE UNITED STATES AS OF 1990

White	199,686,070	80.3%
African American	29,986,060	12.1%
Hispanic	22,354,059	9.0%
American Indian, Eskimo, Aleut	1,959,234	0.8%
Asian or Pacific Islander	7,273,662	2.9%
Other Races	9,804,847	3.9%
TOTAL*	248,709,873	100%

*Data exceed total and 100% owing to rounding.
From U.S. Bureau of the Census. Commerce News. Washington, D.C., March 11, 1991, CB 91-100.

CROSS-CULTURAL DENTAL HYGIENE

Cross-cultural dental hygiene is defined as the effective integration of the client's socioethnocultural background into the dental hygiene process of care. Cross-cultural dental hygiene encompasses the social, political, ethnic, religious, and economic realities that people experience in culturally diverse human interactions and environments. In North America and abroad, cultural diversity is evident in different languages, foods, dress, daily cultural practices, motivational factors, cultural beliefs and values, and cultural influences on disease and health behaviors. All these factors influence human need fulfillment of the client. Therefore, they must be recognized and integrated into dental hygiene care if preventive and therapeutic goals are to be achieved.

Culture plays an integral role in dental hygiene care because oral wellness, disease, and illness are culturally determined. In different cultures, conceptual differences exist between the client and the healthcare provider. The dental hygiene human needs conceptual model provides a framework for implementing the dental hygiene process with culturally diverse clients. Human needs transcend all cultures; culture pervades all human interactions; and human needs may have a culturally based etiology. Dental hygienists know how to assess clients but may not know what to assess and how to interpret data when the client comes from a different culture. Furthermore, planning of interventions and the implementation of the dental hygiene care plan are further complicated by cultural diversity. Oral health therapy and promotion strategies used by the dental hygienist must be delivered in relation to the cultural environment of the client. For example, a client's food preferences may result in an erroneous dental hygiene diagnosis of a deficit in the human need for nutrition, or language differences may be interpreted as an unmet need for conceptualization. The client's homecare products used (or preferred) may result in a dental hygiene diagnosis of a deficit in the need for safety because of the practitioner's belief that the product may cause oral harm or injury.

Dental hygiene care is culturally determined. Although most contemporary therapies are based on Western practices and research, the vast majority of the world populations are non-Western.[3] The techniques that we use and the behaviors that we promote in clients may be interpreted as good, bad, or indifferent, according to the cultural values and needs of the client. Likewise, a dental hygienist may fail to recognize the cultural frame of reference in the client and erroneously label the client as bad, difficult, unmotivated, uncooperative, noncommunicative, or noncompliant. Western, non-Western, and Third World healthcare practices may be viewed as functional or dysfunctional, depending on the cultural system of origin. For example, the practice of putting a loved one in a nursing home may be viewed by some cultures as an appropriate action for providing the best possible care on a 24-hour basis, while others would perceive this practice to be barbaric or inhumane.

Basic Concepts in Cross-Cultural Dental Hygiene

"Consideration of individual value systems and lifestyles should be included in the planning and health care for each client."[4] For a dental hygienist to provide quality care to a client of different ethnic or cultural background, effective intercultural communication must take place. Effective intercultural communication means that each person involved in the transaction is able to understand the other from his unique cultural perspective. For the dental hygienist, the cultural perspectives of the client are reflected throughout the dental hygiene process when it is used in a human needs conceptual framework.

Humanism and Holism

Dental hygienists work with a variety of people and must understand the basic dimensions of culture and its influence on human need, client motivation, health promotion, and oral disease and healthcare. The dental hygienist, as a therapist, is at a distinct disadvantage when the client is from a different race or ethnic group, speaks a different language, or is of a different socioeconomic status. Such cultural differences create barriers to communication, decrease trust, and raise anxiety levels for both the dental hygienist and the client. Dental hygienists who are able to incorporate cultural perspectives into practice may find their effectiveness augmented.

"**Humanism** attests to the dignity and worth of all individuals through concern for and understanding of their network of attitudes, values, behavior patterns, and way of life."[5] All humans have basic human needs. Humanism recognizes the right of all humans to meet their needs. All cultures do not recognize humanism or human rights. Although U.S. President Carter made human rights a thematic issue during his presidency (1977–1981), other governments and cultures may value country, religion, dictators, pride, or family over individual human rights.

"**Holism** views an individual as more than the total sum of parts and shows concern and interest in all aspects of the individual."[5] An individual is more than the sum of the bodily parts that make up a human being. An individual is a biopsychosocial and spiritual being who brings uniqueness in race, culture, ethnicity, attitudes, beliefs, knowledge, and experience. These factors interact to constitute the individual. This interaction of factors causes clients and dental hygienists to have differing worldviews and interpretations about health, oral health, and oral disease. A comparison of Western and non-Western views of the individual (Table 6–2) provides some insight into how culture can influence human attitudes and behaviors. Contemporary dental hygiene care is based on the beliefs of humanism and holism. The holistic philosophy as applied to healthcare has particular relevance in a multicultural envi-

TABLE 6–2
MAJOR DIFFERENCES BETWEEN WESTERN AND NON-WESTERN VIEWS OF THE INDIVIDUAL OR SOCIETY

Western Values	Non-Western Values
Freedom of choice	Group decision-making
Uniqueness of the individual	Group commonality
Independence	Compliance
Interdependence	Harmony
Competition	Cooperation
Nonconformity	Conformity
Expression of feelings	Control of one's feelings
Fulfillment of individual needs	Fulfillment of the needs of the group

With permission from Ho, D. Psychological implications of collectivism: With special references to the Chinese case and Maoist dialects. *In* Eckensberber, L., Lonner, W., and Poortinga, Y. (eds.). Cross-Cultural Contributions to Psychology. Amsterdam: Swets and Zeitlinger, 1979.

ronment. The distinguishing characteristics of holistic healthcare, if applied, can make the dental hygiene care setting a welcome place for individuals who might otherwise feel disconnected or disenfranchised (see the Characteristics and Beliefs Inherent to Holistic Healthcare chart).

Race and Ethnicity

Race refers to one of three classifications of human beings based on physical characteristics, such as skin color, stature, eye color, hair color and texture, facial characteristics, and general body characteristics, all of which are hereditary. Most people recognize three races

white (Caucasian)
black (Negroid)
yellow (Mongoloid)

which overlap each other. The concept of race is a dangerous myth because there are more similarities than differences among the racial groups.

Ethnicity refers to the unique cultural and social heritage and traditions of minority groups within the primary racial divisions that reflect distinct customs, language, and social values. People who share similarities in heritage and tradition, passed on from generation to generation, are said to be members of the same **ethnic group.** Ethnic groups share common factors such as language, dialect, nationality, music, folklore, food preferences, geographical location, and a sense of uniqueness. Examples of some ethnic groups include Japanese, Italian, Polish, Haitian, and Hispanic, just to name a few. Religious beliefs also constitute an important component of ethnicity. *Religion* is one's belief in a supernatural power who is the creator and ruler of the universe. Religious beliefs shape one's values, ethics, morals, and behaviors. Some religious beliefs influence health beliefs and practices. For example, some religions teach practices related to hygiene and cleanliness, eating habits, dressing habits, and food preparation requirements. Table 6–3 is an overview of how some religious beliefs influence health beliefs and practices.

Ethnic values are retained for generations[6,7] and are central in development throughout the lifespan.[8] Traditional values, lifestyles, and behaviors are retained even in fourth-generation immigrants. Ethnicity is a key determinant of an individual's diet, work habits, religious beliefs, philosophy, and methods of dealing with illness and death.[9,10]

Culture and Subculture

Culture is defined as "the sum total of human behavior or social characteristics peculiar to a specific group and passed from generation to generation or from one to another within the group."[5] Culture may also be defined as the rules of behavior learned in order for a person to adapt successfully to life within a particular group. Culture includes beliefs, values, traditions, experiences, customs, rituals, and language.

For example, dental hygienists should be aware that people who speak different languages perceive the world differently. Language systems that are different should not be viewed as deficient. In fact, dental hygienists who speak standard English should know that other cultures may find it difficult to comprehend because standard English:

- Lacks certain language sounds
- Has language sounds for which others may serve as substitutes
- Doubles and drawls some of its vowel sounds in sequences that are difficult for non-Americans to imitate
- Lacks a method for forming an important tense
- Requires several ways to indicate tense, gender, and plurality
- Does not mark negatives sufficiently for words to make optimally strong negative statements[3]

Although cultures may share commonalities in lifestyles and basic beliefs, there are significant differences in subcultural attitudes, interests, goals, and dialects.[3] "A **subculture** is formed by a group of persons who have developed interests or goals different from the primary culture, based on such things as occupation (Hollywood culture), sex (gay culture), age (youth culture), social class (middle class), or religion (fundamentalism)."[5] Dental hygienists can be

CHARACTERISTICS AND BELIEFS INHERENT TO HOLISTIC HEALTHCARE

- Search for patterns and causes as well as symptoms
- Emphasis is on the integrated whole person
- Concern with human values
- Caring is a component of healing
- Pain is an indicator of disharmony
- Mind is a co-equal factor in all illness
- Prevention is synonymous with wholeness
- Minimal intervention is advocated
- Body is a dynamic system and field of energy
- Client is autonomous
- The professional is the therapeutic partner
- Body and mind are interrelated
- Value on qualitative information

Adapted from Ferguson, M. The Aquarian Conspiracy: Personal and Social Transformation in the 1980s. Los Angeles: The Putnam Publishing Group, 1980.

TABLE 6–3
GUIDE TO WORKING WITH PEOPLE OF VARIOUS RELIGIOUS GROUPS*

Religious Group	Basic Beliefs and Concepts	Healthcare Practices and Beliefs
Christian Scientists	Metaphysical approach to religion, sickness, and healing Prayer and religious counsel with sick will make them well Sickness is mentally originated and can be cured through proper mental processes Body is its own laboratory Healing is private, abstract, and highly intellectual	Healing done by certified practitioner employing three dimensions of therapeutic treatment: 1) "Affirmation/Denial/Argument" tries to destroy sick person's belief in suffering 2) "Absolute Consciousness of Good" convincing sick person that he is well and knows it 3) "Impersonal Treatment" practitioner focuses on own thoughts to free afflicted person in belief of illness Accept drugless practices, i.e., osteopaths and chiropractics and natural methods, such as dietary regulation and manipulation of the body
Eastern Orthodox	God did not create humans in his own image; however, we have the potential to become like God in terms of goodness Do not believe in original sin of Adam —we choose to imitate Adam	Humans need the spirit of God for healing to occur Caring for the sick has a special place in the church Praying for the sick is a very involved process Sick are encouraged to seek scientific medical cures
Evangelists	Belief in: 1) Authentic and authoritative Holy Scriptures 2) The life, teachings, death, and resurrection of Christ and eternal life *Deliverance Evangelists:* Claim Holy Spirit has given them power of divine healing	Healing occurs by God in only some situations, God heals all *through* different people, modalities, and techniques
Jews	Ten commandments are a holy contract Modern contracts govern areas of personal and human behavior in an attempt to embody the spirit of ten commandments Reverence for life Emphasis on the family Emphasis on learning	Traditional Jewish kosher Emphasis on cleanliness Circumcision is a practice used to prevent disease
Mormons (similar to conservative Protestants)	Two personages of God, Father and Son, have flesh and bone bodies; Holy Spirit does not Salvation will come through atonement of Christ and obedience of laws of Gospel	Holy handkerchief (faith healing method) and laying on of hands Seek scientific relief for illness and poverty
Native American Church or Peyotists (American Indians)	Believe in Great Spirit and Christian Trinity Earth is our mother to be treated with respect All people are brothers and sisters Abstinence from alcohol Peyote service includes audience participation. Peyote is consumed to have closer contact with God. Ritual is performed under guidance of "road chief"	Peyote is medicine (cactus found in Indian territory) Through prayer and communion with God, sins are forgiven and illness is cured
Pentecostalism (composed of Evangelists and Fundamentalists)	Concerned with holiness (state of mind and spiritual purity), literal interpretation of the Bible, and renewal of Pentecostal experiences	Belief in divine healing, prophecy, "speaking in tongues," and working miracles

TABLE 6–3
GUIDE TO WORKING WITH PEOPLE OF VARIOUS RELIGIOUS GROUPS* *Continued*

Religious Group	Basic Beliefs and Concepts	Healthcare Practices and Beliefs
Protestantism	Four Principles of Protestantism 1) Resolution to live by faith 2) Freedom to initiate new life 3) Openness to truth revealed in scientific and nonscientific ways 4) Vocation in the world (caring for sick and poor)	Four Principles lend themselves to Faith Healing

*Religion affects healthcare practices, beliefs, and interactions with healthcare providers.
Data from Henderson, G. Understanding Indigenous and Foreign Cultures. Springfield, IL: Charles C Thomas, 1989.

viewed as members of a subculture (dental hygiene) with unique philosophical attitudes, practices, beliefs, and values. Within American society, we are familiar with the culture of poverty, the drug culture, Yuppie culture, "flower children," and "bag people" (street people). Members of subcultures have lifestyles, behaviors, and language significantly different from those of the general population. Some would consider these lifestyles to be unusual, different, or deviant from the predominant culture. For example, there may be people from the Polish ethnic group who are Catholic or Jewish, with subcultures that span high socioeconomic levels to the culture of poverty, gay culture, or the drug culture.

Stereotyping

Stereotyping refers to the common but erroneous behavior of assuming that people possess certain characteristics or traits simply because they are members of a particular group. Stereotyping is problematic because it fails to recognize the uniqueness of the individual and prevents the person from perceiving the situation accurately and without bias. Stereotyping clouds our perceptions and makes us less effective as professionals and human beings. Although stereotyping can provide a comfortable foundation for an individual in a strange environment with new people, an accurate assessment should always be made of another human being.

Fortunately, stereotypical behaviors can be unlearned. Taking the time to learn about people is an important step toward eliminating old stereotypical thinking. Learning about other cultures, languages, customs, religions, and practices also enables the dental hygienist to accept cultural diversity and to value people as individuals with unique human needs. Getting in touch with our own cultural base is important if change is to occur in the way one relates to people. Periodically, it is good to participate in a little self-assessment to monitor stereotypical thinking. For example, one can observe people in a restaurant, in a reception area, or at a party and think about the assumptions you make about these people given the way they look, dress, behave, or speak. Assumptions can then be compared to who they are and what they are like once you have had a chance to get to know them.

Ethnocentrism

Ethnocentrism refers to the natural belief that one's culture is superior to that of others. People who are ethnocentric use their own cultures as the standard of excellence against which people from other cultures are judged. Ethnocentric behavior is characterized as judgmental, condescending, insulting, and narrow-minded. Dental hygienists who are ethnocentric may belittle clients whose oral health practices may be rooted in culture rather than in scientific fact. They may convey the feeling that their way is the right way and that the client is ignorant or uneducated. It is easy to fall prey to this type of thinking if we are blind to ethnocentrism in our own behavior. Ethnocentrism makes it difficult for many healthcare providers to assess, plan, or implement quality care with clients from minority groups. For the dental hygiene manager, it may lead to subtle discrimination in the workplace, employee turnover, and loss of clients.

The Melting Pot Versus the Salad Bowl

Some social theorists advanced the proposition that people of different cultures in the United States assimilate into the mainstream white Anglo-Saxon Protestant culture. The theory of the melting pot explained that people give up their previous cultural identity in favor of the predominant culture of the society in which they find themselves. Such intermingling of cultural diversity was thought to result in a blended culture with liberty, equality, and justice for everyone.

The melting pot theory has slowly given way to the salad bowl approach to explaining cultural assimilation in a society. The salad bowl theory recognizes cultural diversity as separate and unique components that remain heterogeneous within society. Related to health, the salad bowl theory recognizes that culture influences the health status, beliefs, and behaviors of individuals, and that healthcare providers and managers thus must be prepared to accommodate these differences. Treatment, educational programs, and client-provider interactions must be designed so that they are culturally appropriate. Some work settings proactively encourage cultural awareness through employee-training programs that identify cultural biases and facilitate positive attitudes and behaviors, such as valuing diversity and team building.

INCOME AS A DETERMINANT OF HEALTH

The Culture of Poverty and Its Relationship to Health

Socioeconomic status is defined by income, occupation, and level of education. In the United States and Canada, society is made up of a large middle socioeconomic group, and smaller upper and lower socioeconomic groups. Socioeconomic status permeates every aspect of a person's life. It affects where one lives, how one spends money, how one uses free time, where one receives healthcare, how one pays for that healthcare, and, ultimately, one's general and oral health status.

Although poverty is universal, the definition of poverty is culturally determined. **Poverty** is "a relative term that reflects a judgment made on the basis of standards prevailing in the community. The standards change in time and place; what is judged poverty in one community might be regarded as wealth in another."[12] The U.S. Bureau of the Census[13] reported that 31.5 million persons, or 12.8% of the population, live below the official government poverty level as defined by financial income. The poverty definition used here is from the Office of Management and Budget and consists of a set of money income thresholds that vary by family size and composition. Families or individuals with income below their appropriate thresholds are classified below the poverty level (Table 6–4). Of the people living in poverty in the United States, the majority are children in female-headed households, hence the phrase the "feminization of poverty." Moreover, many of the homeless are single-mother family units. Factors contributing to the feminization of poverty include teenage pregnancy, pregnancy out of marriage, divorce, abandonment, and female longevity. African-Americans and Hispanics also are overrepresented in the segment of the population classified as poor, making up 36% and 30%, respectively, of those in poverty.

Poverty has been described as a culture, and as a culture it is passed on from generation to generation. This can be observed in people on the welfare rolls, in the urban and rural poor, and in migrant workers who seem to be in an ongoing cycle of poverty. The culture of poverty manifests the following characteristics in its members:

- Unemployment
- Dependence on government assistance for survival
- External locus of control (e.g., fatalism, lack of control)
- Abuse of drugs, alcohol
- A live-for-today mentality
- Inability to set, or work toward, future goals
- Feelings of despair
- Loss of self-esteem and self-respect
- Lack of respect for others

These characteristics manifest themselves in the healthcare setting and affect the dental hygiene process of care. For example, the unemployed may need care but choose not to enter the healthcare setting because of financial barriers and no health insurance. Those who are eligible for government-funded healthcare may find that oral healthcare is not covered. In some cultures, a fatalistic attitude might translate into a "no matter what I do, I'll lose my teeth anyway" attitude. Those who are chemically dependent have difficulty seeing other human needs as a priority. Those with a present-oriented philosophy may not seek care until the need has become an emergency—they find the future benefits derived from preventive behavior irrelevant. In addition, feelings of despair and loss of self-worth mean that personal healthcare is of little consequence.

In this manner, poverty continues to be a major barrier to healthcare that prevents individuals from meeting their basic human need for general and oral health. Other barriers associated with the culture of poverty include feelings of disenfranchisement, lack of transportation, no health insurance, homelessness, seasonal work occupations, prejudice, language difficulties, inadequate levels of education, general lack of understanding of the healthcare system and how it works (the subculture of healthcare), and a lack of healthcare personnel from the individual's own culture. Given these barriers, it is easier to understand why poor people might resort to self-therapy, home remedies, or the services of a folk or faith healer, all of which are more accessible, less expensive, and more familiar than the modern healthcare system.

The environment of poverty directly influences the health status of the client. Low-income housing is usually associated with isolation from the community; poor maintenance; inadequate heat, light, water, electricity, and ventilation; crowded living conditions; infestation; and lead poisoning. The frustrations experienced from inadequate housing and high-density living translate into high rates of crime, physical and emotional abuse, stress, psychological problems, alienation, and transmission of infectious diseases. According to Kotelchuck,[14] poor people get sick more often, experience greater complications with their illness, take longer to recover, and are less likely to regain their previous level of functioning, as compared with people from higher income groups. Individuals locked in the vicious cycle of poverty do not readily take advantage of preventive health services, nor do they perceive the future benefits of these services.

Canada's experience with making healthcare accessible to all people presents an interesting model of the effects of poverty on health. In 1968, Canada initiated a national health insurance program to provide healthcare to the Canadian people without regard to financial resources, age, ethnic origin, or creed. More than two decades later, health remains directly related to people's economic status.

TABLE 6–4
WEIGHTED AVERAGE POVERTY THRESHOLDS IN 1989

Size of Family Unit	Threshold
One person (unrelated individual)	$6,311
15 to 64 years	6,452
65 years and over	5,947
Two persons	8,076
Householder 15 to 64 years	8,343
Householder 65 years and over	7,501
Three persons	9,885
Four persons	12,675
Five persons	14,990
Six persons	16,921
Seven persons	19,162
Eight persons	21,328
Nine persons or more	25,480

From U.S. Bureau of the Census. Current Populations Reports, Series P-60, No. 168, Money Income and Poverty Status in the United States: 1989 (Advance Data from the March 1990 Current Population Survey). Washington, DC: U.S. Government Printing Office, 1990, p. 86.

Wealth and Its Relationship to Health

Wealth is usually associated with high levels of education, prestige, self-esteem, power, and internal locus of control.

The wealthy are able to afford clean comfortable housing, recreational activities, quality diets, and, of course, use of the healthcare system. Because of their higher levels of education, individuals who are financially secure are not intimidated by healthcare professionals and the system. They are able to verbalize their concerns, assert their needs, determine their level of participation in care, be critical healthcare consumers, and seek second opinions. Because the wealthy are typically employed, they benefit from third-party payment systems to finance large portions of their healthcare bills. People in the upper socioeconomic levels of society live longer and experience less disability than those from low-income groups.[15]

COMMUNICATION IN A CROSS-CULTURAL ENVIRONMENT

Cultural preferences, stereotypes, and prejudice are major barriers in the communication process. Members of different cultures actually live in different worlds. Lack of sensitivity to a client's cultural needs, preferences, and beliefs often creates barriers that lead to termination of the client-provider relationship. Communication with persons from one's culture is at best uncertain; communication with persons from a different culture is a complex and arduous task. A dental hygienist can initiate communication by exhibiting a positive and empathetic attitude while attempting to establish some initial areas of commonality (e.g., parenthood, children, marriage). Some common customs and courtesies indigenous to various cultures are presented in Table 6–5. These customs should be used to enhance the communication process.

Verbal Communication

A healthcare provider's ability to understand and communicate with culturally diverse people facilitates effective client care. Variations exist in the typical way members of diverse cultures think and communicate thoughts. The term *polychronic* is used to describe individuals who do many things at the same time, who are repetitive in their speech, and who place a low value on time. Latino, African, Arab, and Asian cultures are polychronic. Dental hygiene interventions that require action on the part of the client at specific time intervals may be difficult for individuals from these cultures. Western European cultures are characterized as being *monochronic.* They are linear in thinking, sequential in behavior, and clock- and work-oriented.[3]

The language of a culture portrays the identity of the individual within that culture.[16] The view of the individual in a society can be gleaned from the language used in the culture. European languages (and English) denote the individual as a private, singular entity who has importance as exemplified by the pronoun "I." In Asian or African culture, the self has a strong group identity. In Japanese, the first person pronoun is expressed differently, depending on the situation (e.g., whether the interaction is with a male or female, private or public, or written or oral).

Manner of Speaking

According to Western culture, an emotional speaker is viewed as assertive, self-assured, and tough-minded; a calm, objective speaker is seen as trustworthy, honest, and people oriented.[17,18] Intensity of expression varies among different groups. For example, Asians respect silence and hesitate toward spontaneity. Culturally sensitive dental hygienists intentionally modify their manner of speaking to facilitate positive interactions.

Nonverbal Communication

Culture is a source of meaning and interpretation of nonverbal communication.[3] Various ethnic groups possess culturally acceptable gestures, etiquette, eye contact, physical contact, and methods of effective listening.

Gesticulation

Gesticulations are signals made with the body that communicate emotions. Facial expressions can be used to communicate with or deceive other people.[19–21] Culturally, a smile can mean very different things. The Japanese may smile when they are embarrassed, not when they are happy.

Facial expressions of emotion are universal.[20,22] There is cultural variability, however, in the rules for displaying these gestures. In most parts of the world, shaking the head from left to right means "no," but tossing the head to the side means "no" to some Arabs and in parts of Bulgaria, Greece, Turkey, and Bosnia-Herzegovina. A slap on the back might denote friendliness among Anglo-Saxon whites but is considered insulting to Asians.

Zones of Territory

Each culture teaches its members that there are appropriate distances that one keeps between people in various situations. In other words, custom "determines intimate, personal, social and public distances."[3] Therefore, the human need for territoriality is culturally influenced, and a dental hygienist interested in meeting this human need for clients must do so in a multicultural context. For example, depending on the culture, the appropriate zone of territory may be based on the degree of respect, authority, and friendship between the individuals communicating. People of high status in European cultures maintain a larger social distance than those in the United States. When a person invades the prescribed territory, she communicates her discomfort, apologizes for the invasion, and actively attempts to readjust to more comfortable territory.

In the role of educator and clinician, dental hygienists invade the spatial zones of clients. This spatial closeness can be uncomfortable for people of any culture. Research findings suggest that middleclass whites stand farther apart than lowerclass Africans or Puerto Ricans during interactions.[23] In general, people from Anglo countries require larger zones of territory than those from non-Anglo countries. Americans tend to readjust their zones during interactions with people from countries that accept closer contact (contact culture), for example, Latin Americans, Africans, Arabs, and southern Europeans. Noncontact cultures include Americans, Asians, Pakistanis, Indians, and northern Europeans. For example, Germanic and Russian people tend to keep a distance and smile conservatively; Asians would keep a proper distance and smile frequently. A dental hygienist must consider the client's culturally determined need for territoriality and attempt to explain procedures in detail to alert the person to necessary close encounters.

TABLE 6–5
GUIDE TO WORKING WITH SOME FOREIGN PEOPLE: CUSTOMS AND COURTESIES

Country	Customs	Courtesies	Behavior to Avoid	Customary Behaviors
AFRICAN Ghana	Greet with "Hello" and a firm handshake Children are taught to be quiet and will not look in elder's eyes	Expect Westerners to be on time, but they can be late	Do not refer to ethnic group as "tribe"; has offensive meaning Superior attitudes are offensive	Western etiquette is proper when eating
Kenya	Warm and friendly Greet with "Greetings, how are you?" and a firm handshake	When invited to someone's house, bring a small gift (candy, cookies) Bring flowers to someone in the hospital Visitors dress conservatively and modestly Punctuality is appreciated	Women should not wear shorts in cities	Personal visits rather than phone calls or letters are appreciated Appointments are made in advance
Nigeria	Dress varies throughout the country, but during business all dress well Respect for elders and tradition Men can practice polygamy	Titles should be used before names	"Tribe" is an offensive word, use "ethnic group" Avoid using colloquial greetings such as "Hi" or "What's happening?"	All business is discussed face to face Respect for older adults is valued Value hard work and responsibility
ANGLO United Kingdom	Nonaggressive handshake Use hand gesture judiciously Cross legs with one knee directly over the other When discussing something of importance, it is better to underestimate than exaggerate	Use titles and last names to show respect Use a handkerchief when sneezing Cover mouth when yawning and ask to be excused	Backslapping and touching new acquaintances Public displays of emotion Avoid the words "England" and "English" as UK is made up of four different states; when in doubt, say "British"	Adults dress conservatively Men will hold open doors and stand when women enter a room People tend to be reserved and formal Relationships are developed slowly Use last names until comfortable Value privacy—a new friend may not invite you to his house—highly selective with whom they invite over
Australia	Dress is relaxed due to climate Conversations are made while standing straight and using modest gestures After-hours socializing is part of business and represents Aussie warm hospitality	Punctuality is mandatory as is eye contact when speaking Shake a woman's hand only if it is offered Business appointments are made far in advance In business, use personal titles when addressing someone Cover mouth when yawning and say, "Excuse me"	Public hugging American hitchhiking sign is considered vulgar Avoid conversational topics of politics and religion	Usually friendly, gregarious and easy-going Men keep emotions to themselves Prefer to be called by first names and greeted with a handshake (men) It is acceptable to greet someone at a distance with a wave
Canada	Composed of many different cultures Handshake is a common greeting	Man will give his seat to a woman and open doors Use last names with older people unless told otherwise Maintain eye contact	Avoid speaking to only one person when in a group Never use first names of older persons	Very friendly, *BUT* adhere to rules of etiquette when dealing with French and English Canadians Men may be overly friendly to women they don't know Western Canadians and Quebecers will be the most friendly; Ontarians the least Maintain eye contact

TABLE 6–5

GUIDE TO WORKING WITH SOME FOREIGN PEOPLE: CUSTOMS AND COURTESIES *Continued*

Country	Customs	Courtesies	Behavior to Avoid	Customary Behaviors
India	Women cover heads in sacred places Use *right* hand for salaam gesture Hindus do not eat beef; alcohol consumed in moderation Moslems do not eat pork or consume alcohol at all Women are taught to be modest and humble NAMASTE: common Indian greeting; gently bending with palms together below chin; also done with palms down	Ask permission before leaving a group	Public displays of affection Backslapping Men do not touch women at formal gatherings Males do not whistle in public, nor should females	Couples express affection privately Educated women will shake Westerners' hands Pointing is done with the chin
GERMANIC Germany	Dress-conscious, formal, obsessed with etiquette Regional customs survived by local people	Respect their laws and order, as they do Titles are important Let host make first move—wave if he waves, shake if he shakes	Do not use first names, rather use titles	Shake hands when first introduced; if female, wait until she extends her hand
Austria	Tend to be conscious of tradition	When making an appointment ask for convenient time for person Make appointments well in advance	Do not use first names, rather use titles	Closer to American manners than Germans
Switzerland	Greetings are exchanged even among strangers (acceptable to wave across street) Men will tip hats Handshakes appropriate for men and women Appreciate punctuality, thrift, independence, and hard work Value family privacy	When invited to a home, bring impersonal gift (candy, flowers) When being introduced, say, "My pleasure/pleased to meet you"	Do not use first names unless with close friends Do not stretch out legs Rude for men to put hands in pocket during a conversation No gum chewing in public	Relaxed, composed posture is best
MIDDLE EAST COUNTRIES Saudi Arabia	Greeting is soft handshake with right hand and "salaam alekum," followed by touching right shoulder with left hand and kissing both cheeks Men can have four wives The third cup of tea signifies the end of a meeting	Women are to be accompanied by men wherever they go Give gifts to husband with your right hand Do not smoke unless host gives permission Put your hand over your cup to indicate you've had enough Maintain strong eye contact Left hand is "toilet" hand	Not every one who is Arab is Muslim, nor are all Middle Easterners Arab women should avoid short skirts and sleeveless blouses Impolite to remove head coverings Impolite to ask a man about his female family members Impolite to refuse drinks and drink more than three cups Never enter a Mosque Never show Saudi the soles of your feet Never cross your legs	Men may not introduce veiled women accompanying them Saudi men will walk hand in hand Women dress *very* modestly If a man and woman are invited to Saudi home, she will be expected to eat with the other women
Egypt	Predominantly Muslim Greetings are expressive and lengthy	New acquaintances should be addressed by titles; do not use first names until friendship is established	Resistance to socialize is considered rude	Philosophy is "don't worry, it will get done" Like to establish friendship before they'll trust with business

Table continued on following page

TABLE 6–5
GUIDE TO WORKING WITH SOME FOREIGN PEOPLE: CUSTOMS AND COURTESIES *Continued*

Country	Customs	Courtesies	Behavior to Avoid	Customary Behaviors
Israel	Land of informality Titles are unimportant "Shalom": hello and goodbye followed by handshake Parents take large role in providing children with good education	Back all statements up with fact Strictly observe Jewish holidays	Do not act proud; consider pridefulness an insult	Close friends will pat each other on the back or shoulder Israelis are eager readers and inquisitive listeners Dress is casual
Russia And previous "Communist" countries: Poland, Albania, Bulgaria, and Hungary	Shake hands when meeting and leaving Summon wait-people in restaurants with a nod Tipping is not allowed but change will be kept if not asked for Toasts are common and guests should reciprocate Fork in left hand, knife in right hand	When invited to a home, bring a gift (books, liquor) If a gift is selected from your country, choose modestly and do not reflect superior industry Compliment cook on food	Shaking a raised fist and American "OK" sign are offensive Men: avoid sitting with ankle on knees or with legs spread open Do not wave or beckon with a finger	Very generous, honest, and frank Keep hands above table, not in lap Men will embrace each other, kiss on lips, and cry publicly Will just say last name when meeting you Greetings and goodbyes between friends include hugging and three kisses on the cheek
FAR EAST COUNTRIES Japan	A bow is the traditional greeting Handshakes can also be used as a greeting	Deny all compliments graciously	Avoid yawning, gum chewing	Remove shoes before entering a Japanese home Obligated to return gifts and favors
China	Emphasis on good manners, hospitality, and humility Nod or slight bow is an appropriate greeting Married women retain their maiden names	Offer small gift to host	Avoid touching behaviors Impolite to exhibit physical familiarity Avoid boisterous behavior Tipping is forbidden Offering valuable gifts	Surname is always said first Strict punctuality Use business cards
NEAR EAST COUNTRIES Greece	Greeks are not clock watchers; will arrive when they feel like it Men possess a string of beads and hold them to relieve tension "Family" is center of social life Greek sense of family honor (philotimo); very protective of family members	Shake hands frequently	Be careful who you insult; their whole family will take offense	Greet one another cheerfully Will ask very personal questions, do not be offended Believe a stranger might be a "god in disguise;" they are treated with kindness
Turkey	Handshake is common greeting, as is a kiss on each cheek Women will not bare upper arms	Ask permission before smoking Do not refer to Turks as Arabs	Women should not cross legs when facing someone Rude to ask personal questions and talk about controversial topics Insult to direct sole of foot toward a Turk	Highly structured society—best to deal with individual with most power

Data from Henderson, G. Understanding Indigenous and Foreign Cultures. Springfield, IL: Charles C Thomas, 1989.

Eye Contact

In North America and in Third World countries, staring or continuously looking at another person is considered rude. Culture dictates looking at a person to establish eye contact, but then looking away so as not to stare. Indirect eye contact is acceptable and preferable within the Native American culture. Lack of eye contact may be interpreted as disinterest in England and polite behavior in some Far East countries.

Physical Contact

The dental hygienist's roles of clinician and educator require physical contact and touching of the client. Touch can convey acceptance or rejection, warmth or coldness, or positive or negative feelings.[24–27] Touching can communicate pleasure, empathy, closeness, and a desire to help. A sensitive touch can relieve tension and anxiety and instill confidence and courage. However, ethnicity, race, age, and gender affect how touch is interpreted as well as its effects. Physical contact is acceptable when greeting members of the same sex in Asian, Arab, Latin American, and Mediterranean countries. In the Far East, touching an older person is a sign of disrespect unless the person initiates the touching. Think about the custom of Iranian men and women kissing both sides of each other's faces as a gesture of friendship and greeting. When working with Hispanic, African, or African-American clients, the dental hygienist should:

- avoid forcing eye contact, since it may be interpreted as disrespect
- maintain close physical proximity
- avoid unnecessary bodily touching

In Third World countries, people of the same sex maintain close contact, but people of the opposite sex rarely touch. Traditional Japanese and Chinese men and women seldom touch in public. Yet in China, it is common to see two women walking along the street arm-in-arm.

USING THE DENTAL HYGIENE PROCESS IN A CROSS-CULTURAL ENVIRONMENT

The dental hygienist in a cross-cultural environment is faced with a true professional challenge. It is unlikely that a dental hygienist of one culture will be able to perceive, understand, and evaluate all the factors influencing the client from another culture unless she develops some degree of cultural sensitivity. In pluralistic, Western societies like the United States and Canada, dental hygienists cannot afford to function under the mirage of ethnocentrism.

The dental hygiene human needs model offers a conceptual approach to providing dental hygiene services in a cross-cultural environment. The client-centered focus of the model and the universality of human needs enable the dental hygienist to use the model during all phases of the dental hygiene process, recognizing that culture is a significant variable affecting and defining human needs. The central concepts of the model (client, environment, health and oral health, and dental hygiene actions) can be considered from the viewpoint of the client, that is, how does the client see himself, view his environment, define health and oral health, approach dental hygiene care, or value oral health. Knowledge of the client's own perceptions of reality influences the overall goals of dental hygiene care. The dental hygiene practitioner must recognize that the process of care with clients from different cultures or ethnic groups takes more time than that for clients from similar cultures. Longer time should be scheduled to accommodate the need for translation, repetition, clarification, and socialization to dental hygiene care.[27a] Additional guidelines for cross-cultural dental hygiene are listed in the chart below.

Assessment, Diagnosis, and Care Planning

The dental hygienist practicing cross-cultural dental hygiene understands that cultural values and experiences shape everyone's perceptions, beliefs, and attitudes. Assessment enables the dental hygienist to collect relevant data to develop dental hygiene diagnoses related to the human needs of the client. Most dental hygiene data collection tools direct the

GUIDELINES FOR CROSS-CULTURAL DENTAL HYGIENE

- Approach each client (individual, family, community) as an individual with unique characteristics and life experiences
- Try to get in touch with your own unique characteristics and life experiences. Sensitize yourself on how cultural factors have influenced your personal beliefs, attitudes, behaviors, practices, and values
- Try to identify biases and prejudices in your own life; their origins; their impact on interpersonal communication; their impact on your effectiveness as a healthcare provider, educator, manager, researcher, consumer advocate, and agent of change
- Become a lifelong student of other cultures, particularly the cultures unique to your community
- Assess the culturally related practices, attitudes, values, and beliefs of your clients as part of the dental hygiene process
- Display an accepting, nonjudgmental demeanor when presented with cultural diversity
- Reflect knowledge and recognition of the client's various cultural practices throughout the interaction
- Incorporate culturally relevant variables into the dental hygiene services that will be provided to the client
- Encourage the client to continue cultural health practices that can bring no harm; provide support, understanding, and time when trying to change potentially harmful oral health practice that is culturally determined
- Determine whether the dental hygiene plan of care is in harmony with the client's cultural values; modify dental hygiene plan of care that conflicts with the client's culture
- Recognize special dietary practices of the client; provide nutritional counseling within the framework of the client's culture
- Develop collegial relationships with health professionals from various ethnic and minority groups as a way of promoting cultural exchange that ultimately improves dental hygiene care

TABLE 6–6
DENTAL HYGIENE CULTURAL ASSESSMENT GUIDE

Culturally Relevant Categories	Key Questions to Ask the Client or to Consider	Data Collected/Comments
Ethnic Origin	Ethnic identification of the client? Place of birth?	
Race	Racial background?	
Domiciliary History	Where the client lived and where does the client now live?	
Valued Habits, Customs, Behavior	Describe habits, customs, values, and beliefs of the client about health, oral health, healthcare providers, and the healthcare system Client's value of courtesy, family, work, sex roles Client's expression of emotion, stress, pain, spirituality, fear	
Communication	Client's communication style, manner of speaking, language spoken, need for interpreter, reading skill, method of showing respect or deference, topic restrictions, eye contact, gesticulations	
Health Beliefs and Practices	What healing system and practices does the client believe in? (Wearing of chains, imbibing certain herbs or potions, voodoo, prayer, curandero, herbalist, etc.) How is disease and illness explained in the client's culture? (fatalism, punishment from God, germ theory, evil spirits, imbalance between yin and yang, etc.)	
Nutritional Factors	What are the culturally/religiously determined food preferences and restrictions?	
Sociological Factors	What impact does economic status have on health and disease, living conditions, lifestyle, ability to obtain healthcare?	

Table continued on following page

hygienist to gather basic information about the client's health, but only perceptive understanding of the values and beliefs of the culture, ethnic group, or subculture yields a true measure of the realities of the client. Therefore, assessing clients to produce culture-specific information is essential. A modification of Bloch's Ethnic/Cultural Assessment Guide is presented in Table 6–6. This guide need not be a separate form but rather should be incorporated into existing dental hygiene data collection documents and procedures. The dental hygiene diagnosis should identify the client's human need(s) that can be fulfilled through dental hygiene care, the cause (due to or related to), the evidence for the diagnosis, and cultural factors that are related. (See Chapter 14 for more information about the dental hygiene diagnosis.) With this detailed focus, an individualized dental hygiene care plan can be developed, and appropriate interventions selected. Using a nonjudgmental approach, the dental hygienist can assess the client's level of acculturation, English language skills, cultural health practices, and home remedies. Factors such as language comprehension, number of years in the country, dietary preferences, and attitudes about the predominant culture can provide important cues for assessing the influence of the client's culture. A client may be consistently late for an appointment because he is less future oriented and more interested in the activity in which he was previously engaged. A dental hygienist who is insensitive to the time orientation of this person's culture may erroneously attribute this action to a low value placed on oral health or anxiety about obtaining dental hygiene care. The dental hygienist who is able to demonstrate acceptance of diversity during client interactions will be able to establish a level of trust with the client and provide effective oral health care.

Implementation

Dental hygiene interventions, whether educational, technical, or interpersonal, must be congruent with local cultural values. The client's values and needs guide the selection of preventive and therapeutic strategies and interventions. In an unpublished paper, McKinney[28] related an experience of a dental hygienist that occurred in Liberia, Africa, in 1989. *A Liberian girl was brought by her family for oral care. The dental hygienist found that the child's oral and systemic health were poor. Surprisingly, the dental hygienist's oral hygiene recommendations (i.e., cleaning the teeth, gums, and tongue with a toothbrush, sponge, or gauze) were met with refusal. The young girl's family believed that she was*

TABLE 6–6
DENTAL HYGIENE CULTURAL ASSESSMENT GUIDE *Continued*

Culturally Relevant Categories	Key Questions to Ask the Client or to Consider	Data Collected/Comments
Sociological Factors *Continued*	What effect does level of education have on health status and ability to obtain health-care? Does the family (or significant others) participate in the dental hygiene process of care? Does the family or significant others participate in preventive health behaviors? Are there key institutions in the client's life that can influence health behavior, e.g., family, school, church, NAACP, Tribal Council, etc.?	
Psychological Factors	How does the client respond to the health-care system, e.g., anxiety, distrust, fear, loss of dignity, nonadherence, avoidance? How does the culture define a wholesome body image or perceive attractiveness? How does the client relate to people/institutions/environments that are outside of his culture?	
Physical Characteristics	What is within normal limits for individuals within this ethnic group, e.g., skin color, gingival color, facial characteristics? How are skin and mucous membrane color changes assessed between different ethnic groups? What variations in growth and development patterns exist within the cultural groups? What systemic problems or diseases are more prevalent within this culture? What socioenvironmental diseases may be common in this ethnic/cultural group? Are there any diseases to which individuals in this cultural group are resistant?	

Modified from Bloch, B. Bloch's ethnic/cultural assessment guide. In Orgue, M. S., Bloch, B., and Monroy, L. A. [eds.]. Ethnic Nursing Care: A Multicultural Approach. St. Louis: C. V. Mosby, 1983, pp. 63–69.)

cursed and that any items placed in her mouth would become a danger to the other family members who may touch them. Even the dental hygienist's suggestion to bury the used gauze was unacceptable because the ground would also become cursed. The family wanted the dental hygienist to cure the girl, that is, eliminate the curse. Within the cultural context, the only acceptable dental hygiene intervention was for the girl to use her own finger to clean her mouth. The family graciously accepted several bottles of a commercial mouth rinse, as if these bottles contained a magical potion.

Saparamadu[29] reported that in Sri Lanka, *"[o]ral hygiene exercises are performed in Sunday schools run by the monks to propagate the teachings of Buddha. The religious leadership provided in the village gives the needed credibility to the programme, and the villagers adhere strictly to the oral hygiene practices taught by the monks because of the respect they command in the villages."*

These vignettes underscore the need for dental hygienists to possess cross-cultural perspectives if client oral health is to be achieved. As long as cultural beliefs or practices cause no harm, the dental hygienist can determine their importance to the client and recognize that their continued practice might assist in maintaining an effective client-provider relationship. Even when the behavior is ineffective, the client's comfort with and belief in its effectiveness can lend strength and support in a situation where the person might otherwise feel alienated and out of touch. Table 6–7 provides an overview of some global beliefs held by some people within various cultures. This can serve as a starting point for understanding peoples of diverse cultures.

Evaluation

In the cross-cultural situation, the evaluation phase of the dental hygiene process calls for an awareness of the client's cultural perspectives of what constitutes success. "Those who are conscious of the importance of culture in forming values and of the fact that human responses are based on values and human needs, are able to approach clients from an ethnic perspective, the perspective of the client and the client's culture, rather than relying on their own ethnic (objective or external) perspective."[30]

In a cross-cultural situation, evaluation should take place throughout the dental hygiene process. Frequent solicitation of the client's perspectives, level of understanding, psychomotor skill development, and home care practices is particularly important. Evaluation should determine whether dental hygiene services are meeting the client's human need

TABLE 6–7
GUIDE TO WORKING WITH PEOPLE OF VARIOUS CULTURAL GROUPS

Cultural Group	Basic Beliefs and Concepts	Health Care Practice and Beliefs
African-Americans	Life is a process rather than a state Health occurs when there is harmony with nature; illness is disharmony No division between physical, emotional, and spiritual needs Present oriented Frequently very religious	Belief in both white magic and black magic Living and dead things influence health Employ faith healers, root doctors, and spiritualists to cast out evil spirits and demons Voodoo can cause or prevent malevolent forces Illness can be prevented by avoiding people who carry evil spirits, eating a good diet, and prayer *Common health problems:* Hypertension, sickle cell disease, lactose enzyme deficiency, diabetes, chemical abuse Religious and community group support networks May be using home remedies or folk healing for an oral problem *Remedies:* Bangles—thin silver bracelets that let evil out and prevent it from entering the body; sound of bangles frightens evil spirits Talismans—a drawn symbol that is worn or carried to ward off sickness Asafoetida—known as "incense of the devil" rubbed on to ward off colds and evil Snake—dehydrated, ground to a powder, and mixed with water; applied to skin lesions
Hispanic/Latin American	Health is the result of good luck or a reward from God Can maintain health and avoid disease via a balance among four humors *Curanderos*—folk healers who use the premise of humoral pathology *Humoral pathology:* Basic functions of body are regulated by body fluids (humors) defined by temperature and wetness: Blood (hot and wet) Phlegm (cold and wet) Black bile (cold and dry) Yellow bile (hot and dry) "Evil eye" is harmful magic Strong influence of the Catholic Church and the family Flexible sense of time Respect for tradition Taboos are methods of etiquette, custom, or conventions Believe in bad magic, spells, and other harmful magic Illness is the result of bad luck, punishment from God, or an imbalance among four humors	Good health means balance among four humors Foods are classified as hot or cold unrelated to their temperature; hot and cold food must be eaten or avoided at certain times Illness is caused by an improper diet of "hot and cold foods," dislocation of body parts, the supernatural, or envy (envidia) from others Illness and disease may be perceived as a punishment from God Illness can be prevented by proper diet, wearing of amulets, use of candles, prayer, avoiding too much success and harmful people *Common health problems:* Diabetes, poor nutrition, lactose enzyme deficiency Expectations of the family to care for the young and the elderly *Remedies:* Burning candles—to ward off evil spirits Amulets—worn to ward off evil and as a protection against the evil eye *Manzanilla* (chamomile) an herb used to treat stomach disorders, anxiety, and insomnia
Asian/Pacific Islander	Health is a state of harmony among body, mind, spirit, and nature (Taoism) The body is a gift that must be cared for and maintained Illness is caused by an upset in the balance (among body, mind, spirit, and nature) or by the weather, overexerting, or prolonged sitting Illness can be prevented by proper diet, exercise, avoiding temperature changes, and taking certain remedies	May be upset by loss of blood, since they consider it to be body's life force May refuse surgery because they believe the body should remain intact Common health problems include tuberculosis, lactose enzyme deficiency, malnutrition, communicable diseases, and suicide May use acumassage, acupressure, and acupuncture Use of soy sauce may be a concern during nutritional counseling for individuals with high blood pressure

TABLE 6–7
GUIDE TO WORKING WITH PEOPLE OF VARIOUS CULTURAL GROUPS *Continued*

Cultural Group	Basic Beliefs and Concepts	Health Care Practice and Beliefs
Asian/Pacific Islander *Continued*	Seldom complain about pain Strong family ties Preference for humility, modesty, self-control Respect for authority and tradition	*Remedies:* Jen Shen Lu Jung Wan—a tonic taken to strengthen the entire system Thousand Year Eggs—old, uncooked eggs eaten daily for good health Huo Li Jian Mei Su—pills taken to maintain youth, health, and beauty Tiger Balm—all purpose salve to relieve minor aches and pain Ginseng root—most famous all-purpose Chinese medicine Acupuncture—use of metal needles at certain points in the body to treat disease and control pain
Native Americans	Health is the result of total harmony with nature Both nature and the body must be treated with respect Illness is the result of disharmony among the body, mind, spirit, and nature Illness can be associated with evil spirits Large extended families who expect to be included in the healthcare process Great respect for elders Value placed on working together Present oriented Accumulation of wealth and goods is frowned on	Medicine man Prevention of illness is achieved through harmony of the body, mind, and spirit Illness can be associated with evil spirits, displeasing the holy people, disturbing nature, misusing a sacred ceremony *Common health problems:* Alcoholism, suicide, tuberculosis, poor nutrition, diabetes, hypertension, and gallbladder disease *Remedies:* Sandpainting by the medicine man Mask—to hide from evil spirits Sweet grass—burned as a rite of purification Thunderbird—a charm worn for protection and good luck Estafiata—leaves used to treat stomach ailments Use of herbs, ceremonies, fasting, meditation, heat, and massage
Whites	Health is viewed as freedom from illness and disease Illness is the presence of disease symptoms, pain, disability, malformations Youth valued over age Punctuality, physical attractiveness, competitiveness, cleanliness, achievement valued Control of emotion Emphasis on the nuclear family versus the extended family	Illness may be the result of punishment from God, breaking religious rules, drafts, climate *Common health problems:* Cardiovascular disease, gastrointestinal disease, cancer, suicide, chemical abuse *Remedies:* Varied because of the influence of multiple European cultures, e.g., Malocchio—horn-shaped amulet used by Italians to ward off the "Evil eye"
Third World	Use of "magic" for good and evil throughout culture Believe in the "here" world and "nether" world Avoid certain people, cold air, and evil eyes Distrust in nature Faithful to punitive god Suspicious of other people Distrust friends, relatives, and strangers *Major Themes:* 1) World is hostile and dangerous 2) Individuals are vulnerable to attack from external sources 3) Must depend on outside help to stay alive	Protective and evil magic determine illness, come from supernatural Spells and sacrifices will bring back health Will use curers from more than one healthcare system Good health centers on personal rather than scientific behaviors Explain emotional and physical illness in terms of imbalance between individual and physical, social, and spiritual life *Common health problems:* Malnutrition, high maternal and infant mortality, parasitic diseases
West Indies	Little value placed on time Present oriented	Obeah (witchcraft, black magic); power is very strong: scientific proof of sticking needles into people without bleeding or pain and frightening victims to death

Table continued on following page

TABLE 6–7
GUIDE TO WORKING WITH PEOPLE OF VARIOUS CULTURAL GROUPS *Continued*

Cultural Group	Basic Beliefs and Concepts	Health Care Practice and Beliefs
West Indies *Continued*		*Common health problems:* Malnutrition, high maternal and infant mortality, parasitic diseases
Spiritualism Hispanics Africans African-Americans American Indians	The visible world includes an invisible world inhabited by good and evil spirits who influence human behaviors Spirits become visible through mediums	Mediums treat emotional and physical illness, whole person concept Mediums share same ethnic, cultural language and social class as their followers Powers of mediums derived from supernatural

Data from Henderson, G. Understanding Indigenous and Foreign Cultures. Springfield, IL: Charles C Thomas, 1989; and Spector, R. E. Cultural Diversity in Health and Illness, 2nd ed. Norwalk, CT: Appleton-Century-Crofts, 1985.

deficits related to oral health and disease. Urging clients to talk about their oral health practices and status helps with cross-cultural communication. Client feedback and response is the basis for reassessment and continuing with the dental hygiene process of care. Validation occurs from feedback from the client and family (significant others) that her needs are being met.

THE FUTURE OF CROSS-CULTURAL DENTAL HYGIENE

Changes must take place if dental hygienists are to have a global perspective and a multicultural perspective. Dental hygiene educational programs (undergraduate, graduate, and continuing education) must create opportunities for international experiences for practitioners, students, and faculty and expand practice and internships that enable practitioners to practice cross-cultural dental hygiene. Programs leading to the baccalaureate degree and beyond could increase foreign language requirements, so dental hygienists can more effectively communicate outside the English language. Of course, faculty development activities that enable faculty to add international and multicultural content to dental hygiene courses would also be of benefit. Dental hygiene student organizations also might be encouraged to sponsor and promote activities that raise awareness about the cultural diversity of the population while simultaneously developing in their members competence in cross-cultural dental hygiene environments.

Professionals in all aspects of dental hygiene should consider the international element in healthcare delivery. Dental hygienists should recognize the available opportunities to work for employers abroad or for multinational companies in the United States and Canada involved in international markets. Opportunities in international dental hygiene encompass both the profit and the nonprofit sectors, for example, private practice, oral health products industry, higher education, the World Health Organization, Operation Smile International, and other international service agencies. Preparation should include skill development in second and third languages, experience in travel abroad, specialized study of the culture of another country, and even living in another country.

Dental hygienists might also try to talk with people from their own culture who have experienced foreign cultures. Hygienists can obtain books from the local library to learn about the history, politics, and geography of the culture that they will soon face and then develop acceptance of cultural differences and human diversity.

The expanding international involvement of both public and private organizations means that employers are placing greater emphasis on foreign language competencies. Knowledge of a foreign language not only allows for direct communication with a client but also provides the mechanism for understanding a people and how they think. Being able to speak another person's language communicates a sincere interest in the person. One cannot establish rapport easily through an interpreter.

References

1. Ohmal, K. The Borderless World. New York: Harper Business, 1990.
2. C & W Associates. A Sensitivity Seminar for Old Dominion University—Participant Manual. Newport News, VA: 1991.
3. Henderson, G. A Practitioner's Guide to Understanding Indigenous and Foreign Cultures. Springfield, IL: Charles C Thomas, 1989.
4. American Nurses' Association: Code for Nurses with Interpretive Statements. Kansas City, MO: American Nurses' Association, 1976.
5. Taylor, C., Lillis, C., and LeMone, P. Fundamentals of Nursing, 2nd ed. Philadelphia: J. B. Lippincott, 1993.
6. Greeley, A. M. Why Can't They Be Like Us? New York: Institute of Human Relations Press, 1969.
7. Staples, R., and Miranda, A. Racial and cultural variations among American families: A decennial review of the literature on minority families. Journal of Marriage and Family 42:887, 1980.
8. Gelfand, D. E., and Kutzik, A. J. (eds.). Ethnicity and Aging. New York: Springer, 1979.
9. Blalock, H. M., Jr. Race and Ethnic Relations. Englewood Cliffs, NJ: Prentice-Hall, 1982.
10. Feagin, J. R. (ed.). Racial and Ethnic Relations. Englewood Cliffs, NJ: Prentice-Hall, 1984.
11. Seymour, D. L. Black English. Intellectual Digest 2:72, 1972.
12. Spector, E. Cultural Diversity in Health and Illness. New York: Appleton-Century-Crofts, 1979.
13. U.S. Bureau of the Census. Current Population Reports, Series P-60, No. 168, Money Income and Poverty Status in the United States: 1989 (Advance Data from the March 1990 Current Population Survey). Washington, D.C.: U.S. Government Printing Office, 1990.
14. Kotelchuck, R. Poor diagnosis, poor treatment. Health PAC Bulletin 16(1):8, 1985.

15. Storch, J. Patient's Rights: Ethical and Legal Issues in Health Care and Nursing. Toronto: McGraw-Hill Ryerson, 1982.
16. Giles, H., and Edwards, J. R. Language and attitude in multicultural settings [symposium]. Journal of Multilingual and Multicultural Development 4, 1983.
17. Pearce, W. B., and Conklin, F. Nonverbal vocalic communication and perceptions of a speaker. Speech Monographs 30:235, 1971.
18 Scherer, K. R., London, H., and Wolf, J. J. The voice of confidence: Paralinguistic cues and audience evaluation. Journal of Research in Personality 7:31, 1973.
19. Mehrabian, A. Nonverbal Communication. Chicago: Aldine, 1972.
20. Ekman, P., and Friesen, W. V. A new pan-cultural expression of emotion. Motivation and Emotion 20:159, 1986.
21. Schulz, R., and Barefoot, J. Nonverbal responses and affiliative conflict theory. British Journal of Social and Clinical Psychology 13:237, 1974.
22. Ekman, P., and Friesen, W. V. Universals and cultural differences in judgment of facial expression of emotion. Journal of Personality and Social Psychology 43:712, 1987.
23. Aiello, J. R., and Jones, S. E. Field study of the proxemic behavior of young school children in three subcultural groups. Journal of Personality and Social Psychology 27:351, 1971.
24. Ingham, A. A review of the literature relating to touch and its use in intensive care. Intensive Care Nursing 5(2):65, 1989.
25. Suiter, R. L., and Goodyear, R. K. Male and female counselor and client perceptions of four levels of counselor touch. Journal of Counseling Psychology 32:645, 1985.
26. Fisher, L., and Joseph, D. H. A scale to measure attitude about nonprocedural touch. Canadian Journal of Nursing Research 21(2):5, 1989.
27. Willison, B. G., and Masson, R. L. The role of touch in therapy: An adjunct to communication. Journal of Counseling and Development 64:479, 1988.
27a. Harwood, A. Guidelines for culturally appropriate health care. In Harwood, A. (ed.). Ethnicity and Medical Care. Cambridge: Harvard University Press, 1981, pp. 482–507.
28. McKinney, B. Keep it Simple and Smile: the Role of the Dental Hygienist in International Health. Norfolk, VA: Old Dominion University, School of Dental Hygiene, November 1989 (unpublished).
29. Saparamadu, K. D. G. The provision of dental services in the Third World. International Dental Journal 36:194, 1986.
30. Sohier, R. Nursing care for the people of a small planet: Culture and the Neuman systems model. In Leininger, M. M. (ed.). Transcultural Nursing Care: Teaching, Practice, Research. Salt Lake City: University of Utah Press, 1980.

Suggested Readings

Birdwhistell, R. L. Kinesics and Content. Philadelphia: University of Pennsylvania Press, 1970.

Braithwaite, R. L., and Taylor, S. E. (eds.). Health Issues in the Black Community. San Francisco: Jossey-Bass Publishers, 1992.

Henderson, G., and Primeaux, M. Transcultural Heath Care. Menlo Park, CA: Addison-Wesley Publ. Co., 1981.

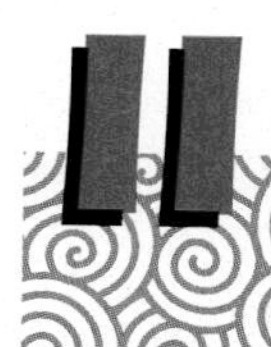

II PREVENTION OF DISEASE TRANSMISSION

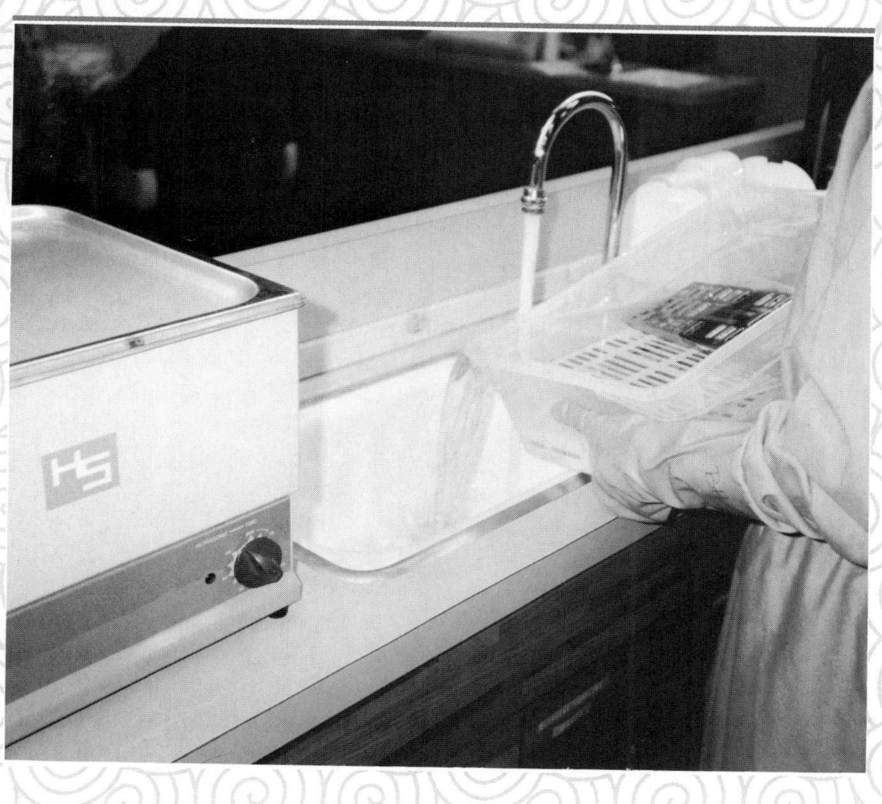

7 Current Concepts of Infection Control

OBJECTIVES

Mastery of the content in this chapter will enable the reader to:

- Define the terms used
- Describe the principal pathogenic organisms associated with oral transmission
- Explain the rationale for universal blood and body fluid precautions
- Explain the theory of disease transmission
- Describe the risks and modes of occupational transmission of human immunodeficiency virus (HIV) and hepatitis B virus (HBV)
- Identify the benefits and limitations of client assessments (health histories, extra- and intraoral examinations, periodontal evaluations, and laboratory tests) in identifying potential sources of infection
- Explain the ethical obligations to maintain standards of dental hygiene care that adhere to infection control protocols consistent with current federal, state, and local guidelines
- Describe the legal issues associated with the potential for disease transmission related to discrimination, rights of privacy and confidentiality, and HBV- and HIV-infected practitioners
- Describe the application of risk management theory to dental hygiene care infection control protocols
- Explain methods of preventing malpractice lawsuits with regard to infection control through written protocols, documentation of implementation, and monitoring of compliance and effectiveness of procedures
- Explain the role of the Occupational Safety and Health Administration's standard for protection of healthcare providers from bloodborne disease, including task analysis, infection control plan, training, protective equipment, waste, hepatitis B vaccine, and postexposure protocol
- Identify personal barriers and protocols routinely used to ensure protection against exposure to bloodborne infectious diseases

INTRODUCTION

Dental hygienists have been cited frequently as the role models in the oral healthcare arena with respect to prevention of disease transmission. In the preface to their textbook entitled *Practical Infection Control in Dentistry,* Cottone and colleagues identify the dental hygienist as traditionally the most knowledgeable source of basic information for the dental practitioner for infection-control information, but they add a note that dental hygienists have been discouraged once they are in clinical practice by some dentists' statements such as "We don't do it that way here."[1] Recent changes in **epidemiology** and biomedical information regarding infectious diseases, such as hepatitis, herpes, human immunodeficiency virus (HIV) infection, and acquired immunodeficiency syndrome (AIDS), have been the catalysts for increased interest in and careful review, evaluation, and expansion of existing infection-control procedures. Additionally, attention has been focused on the prevention of disease transmission because of the impact of standards from governmental agencies, such as the Occupational Safety and Health Administration (OSHA) of the Department of Labor and the Environmental Protection Agency (EPA).

Application of infection control principles to protect clients benefits, in turn, team members and their families and offers the dental hygienist minimal risk of disease transmission. The control of infection is an integral part of every aspect of dental hygiene care delivery. Client education should also be a vital part of dental hygiene care.

Informing clients of changes regarding infection-control practices, with an emphasis on the client, helps meet the individual's human needs for safety and freedom from stress associated with the perceived risks of disease transmission. Consistently and meticulously following infection-control protocols may be the most important preventive measure that dental hygienists and other oral healthcare providers perform to ensure their health and that of their staff, family, and clients.[2] Although infection control, when scrupulously maintained, greatly decreases the occupational risk of disease transmission, it does not eliminate it entirely.[3]

The federal government, through OSHA, has mandated that all workplaces that pose a potential for transmission of bloodborne diseases establish a written infection-control plan designed to minimize or eliminate employee exposure.[4] To accomplish this, infection-control programs should:[5]

- Reduce the number of pathogens in the dental hygiene environment so that normal resistance can prevent infections
- Break the cycle of disease transmission and eliminate cross-infection
- Apply universal precautions, treating every client, instrument, or contaminated surface as infectious
- Protect the client and personnel from infection

OVERVIEW OF INFECTIOUS DISEASES SIGNIFICANT FOR THE DENTAL HYGIENIST

Respiratory Infections

- Common cold
- Acute or chronic sinusitis
- Pneumonia
- Tuberculosis
- Tuberculous infection

Sexually Transmitted Diseases

- Herpetic infections
- Acute herpetic gingivostomatitis
- Herpes labialis
- Recurrent intraoral infections
- Herpetic whitlow
- Gonococcal infections
- Chlamydial infections
- Trichomonal infections
- Condyloma acuminatum
- Primary syphilis
- Secondary syphilis
- Late syphilis
- Congenital syphilis
- Infectious mononucleosis
- Hepatitis
- Acquired immunodeficiency syndrome (AIDS)

Childhood Diseases

- Chickenpox
- Herpangina
- Hand-foot-and-mouth disease
- Rubella (German measles)
- Rubeola (measles)
- Mumps
- Cytomegalovirus

Modified from Cottone, J. A., Terezhalmy, G. T., and Molinari, J. A. Practical Infection Control in Dentistry. Philadelphia: Lea & Febiger, 1991, p. 623.

INFECTIOUS HAZARDS FOR THE ORAL HEALTHCARE TEAM

The repeated exposure of dental hygiene practitioners to blood, saliva, and gingival fluid puts them at significantly high risk for a wide range of **communicable diseases,** including numerous respiratory infections, childhood diseases, and sexually transmitted diseases (see Overview of Infectious Diseases Significant for the Dental Hygienist chart).

Table 7–1 lists the specific infectious organisms, habitats, transmission vehicles, potential pathologies, and availability of vaccines. It is well documented that most human microbial pathogens have been isolated from oral secretions, and the incidence of hepatitis B virus (HBV) infection, tuberculosis (TB), and herpesvirus hominis (HVH-1 and HVH-2) infection is higher among oral healthcare professionals than in the general population.[1,6]

Among the three infectious occupational hazards with the highest incidence for the dental hygienist, HBV is the most important. Hepatitis, or inflammation of the liver, can be caused by various disease states, alcoholism, drug reactions, and *viruses.* The last etiological factor produces viral hepatitis, a complex of infections caused by viruses that are continuing to be discovered and investigated. Table 7–2 presents each of the four hepatitis-associated viruses and **immune globulins** associated with fighting the viral infection.

Hepatitis A virus (HAV), or infectious hepatitis, cannot be transmitted in the healthcare setting. It is HBV, "serum" or "long-incubation" hepatitis, that has the most serious implications for the dental hygienist[1,6] (see Six Possible Outcomes of Hepatitis B Infection chart).

Four of five individuals who contract HBV have subclin-

SIX POSSIBLE OUTCOMES OF HEPATITIS B INFECTION

- Cure
  Client develops immunity
- Chronic hepatitis
  3% of hepatitis clients
- Chronic carrier
  5–10% of hepatitis clients
- Cirrhosis
  30–50% of chronic hepatitis clients
- Liver cancer
  Hepatocarcinoma—risk of development 12–300 times greater than for uninfected individuals[6]
- Death
  1% of hepatitis clients die during acute phase

From "'A Few Seconds Was All It Took': Hepatitis Infection Changes Dentist's Life." ADA News, March 7, 1988, p. 11.

TABLE 7–1

INFECTIOUS HAZARDS FOR ORAL HEALTHCARE WORKERS AND CLIENTS IN THE HEALTHCARE SETTING

Infectious Organism	Habitat	Transmission	Potential Pathology	Vaccine
Bacteria				
Bordetella pertussis (B)	Nasopharynx	Nasopharyngeal secretions[1]	Whooping cough	Yes
Cardiobacterium hominis (A)	Nasopharynx	Nasopharyngeal secretions[1]	Endocarditis	No
Corynebacterium diphtheriae	Nasopharynx	Nasopharyngeal secretions[1]	Diphtheria	Yes
Enterobacteriaceae (A) *Escherichia coli* *Proteus vulgaris* *Klebsiella pneumoniae*	Mouth, gastrointestinal (GI) tract	Blood, lesion exudate[2]	Pneumonia, bacteremia, abscesses, wound infections	No
Haemophilus				
influenzae (C)	Mouth, nasopharynx	Blood, nasopharyngeal secretions[1]	Pneumonia, meningitis, otitis	Yes
parainfluenzae (A)	Mouth, nasopharynx	Blood, nasopharyngeal secretions[1]	Conjunctivitis, endocarditis	No
paraphrophilus (A)	Mouth, nasopharynx	Blood, nasopharyngeal secretions[1]	Endocarditis	No
Mycobacterium tuberculosis (D)	Pharynx	Pharyngeal secretions[1]	Tuberculosis	No
Mycoplasma pneumoniae (A)	Pharynx	Pharyngeal secretions[1]	Primary atypical pneumonia	No
Neisseria				
meningitidis (C)	Mouth, nasopharynx	Blood, nasopharyngeal secretions[1]	Cerebrospinal meningitis	Yes
gonorrhoeae (D)	Mouth, nasopharynx	Blood, lesion exudate, nasopharyngeal secretions[2]	Oral lesions, conjunctivitis	No
Pseudomonas aeruginosa (A)	Ubiquitous, sink and drain contaminant	Lesion exudate[1]	Pneumonia, wound infections	No
Staphylococcus				
aureus (A)	Mouth, skin, nasopharynx	Lesion exudate[1]	Suppurative lesions, bacteremia	No
epidermidis (A)	Mouth, skin, nasopharynx	Lesion exudate[1]	Endocarditis	No
Streptococcus				
pyogenes (A)	Nasopharynx	Blood, nasopharyngeal secretions[2]	Rheumatic and scarlet fever, otitis media, cervical adenitis, mastoiditis, peritonsillar abscesses, meningitis, pneumonia, acute glomerulonephritis	No
pneumoniae (A)	Nasopharynx	Blood, nasopharyngeal secretions[2]	Pneumonia, endocarditis	Yes
viridans group (A)	Nasopharynx	Blood, nasopharyngeal secretions[2]	Endocarditis	No
Treponema pallidum (D)	Blood, oral mucosa	Exudate from oral lesions[2]	Syphilis	No
Actinomyces species (sp) *Bacteroides* sp *Eubacterium* sp *Fusobacterium* sp (A) *Peptococcus* sp *Peptostreptococcus* sp *Propionibacterium* sp	Gingival crevice (normal oral flora)	Crevicular exudate[2]	Abscesses	No
Viruses				
Coxsackievirus (A)	Oropharyngeal mucosa	Ingestion	Hand-foot-and-mouth disease, vesicular pharyngitis	No
Cytomegalovirus (A)	Salivary gland	Saliva, blood[2]	Cellular enlargement and degeneration in immunocompromised individuals	No
Epstein-Barr virus (A)	Parotid gland	Saliva, blood[2]	Infectious mononucleosis	No
Hepatitis				
A (D)	Liver, GI tract	Blood (rare), ingestion	Liver inflammation, jaundice	Yes*
B (D)	Liver	Blood, saliva, tears, semen[3]	Eventual hepatocellular carcinoma in chronic antigen carriers	Yes

Continued on following page

TABLE 7–1
INFECTIOUS HAZARDS FOR ORAL HEALTHCARE WORKERS AND CLIENTS IN THE HEALTHCARE SETTING *Continued*

Infectious Organism	Habitat	Transmission	Potential Pathology	Vaccine
Viruses				
C (parenterally transmitted, formerly non-A, non-B)	Liver	Blood[3]	Acute viral hepatitis (~ 50% become chronic carriers)†	No
D (formerly delta) (A)	Liver	Blood[3]	Coinfection with hepatitis B virus (HBV) required	Yes (HBV vac)
E‡	Liver	Ingestion	Liver inflammation caused by a virus that resembles hepatitis A	?
Herpes simplex virus types 1 and 2 (A)	Nasopharynx	Lesion exudate, saliva[2]	Oral lesions, herpetic whitlow, conjunctivitis	No
Human immunodeficiency virus (HIV) (D)	T4 lymphocyte	Blood[3]	Acquired immunodeficiency syndrome (AIDS)	No
Measles rubeola (C) rubella (B)	Nasopharynx	Nasopharyngeal secretions, blood, saliva, vesicle exudate[1]	Generalized vesicular rash	Yes
Mumps virus (D)	Parotid gland	Saliva, ingestion	Parotitis, meningitis	Yes
Poliovirus (B)	Oropharyngeal mucosa, GI tract	Ingestion	Central nervous system paralysis	Yes
Respiratory Viruses (A)	Nasopharynx	Nasopharyngeal secretions[1]	Flu, common cold	
Influenza virus A and B				Yes
Parainfluenza virus				No
Rhinovirus				No
Adenovirus				Yes
Coronavirus				No
Varicella (A)	Skin	Vesicle exudate[1]	Chickenpox	No
Fungi				
Candida albicans (A)	Mouth, skin	Nasopharyngeal secretions[1]	(Opportunistic) candidiasis, cutaneous infections	No
Protozoa				
Pneumocystis carinii (A)	Mouth	Nasopharyngeal secretions[1]	(Opportunistic) interstitial pneumonia in immunocompromised individuals	No

* Control, The Infectious Disease Newsletter. Hepatitis A: A vaccine at last. 7(6), 1992.
† Data from Miller, C. H., Palenik, C. J. Infection Control and Management of Hazardous Materials for the Dental Team. St. Louis: Mosby, 1994, p. 66.
‡ American Liver Institute.
[1] Infected droplet contact: inhalation, ingestion, direct inoculation.
[2] Direct inoculation to tissue surface.
[3] Inoculation into circulatory system.
Inactivation: always use heat sterilization when possible. All of the above organisms can be killed by autoclaving at 121 °C, 15 minutes, 15 psi. Dry-heat sterilization: 170°C, 60 minutes. Heat-sensitive instruments and surfaces may be disinfected using phenolic or glutaraldehyde-based solutions.
References: Jawetz, E., Melnick, J. L., and Adelberg, E. A. Review of Medical Microbiology, 17th ed. Norwalk, CT: Appleton & Lange, 1987.
Centers for Disease Control reported new U.S. cases for 1987.
Key
A = nonreportable.
B = less than 1,000.
C = 1,000–9,999.
D = greater than 9,999.
Adapted from American Dental Association Research Institute, Department of Toxicology. Journal of the American Dental Association 117:374, 1988. Reprinted by permission of ADA Publishing Co., Inc. Copyright © 1988.

TABLE 7–2
TYPES OF VIRAL HEPATITIS

Abbreviation	Term	Signs and Symptoms	Transmission	Incubation	Communicability	Immunity
Hepatitis A						
HAV	Hepatitis A virus	Influenza-like illness with fever, headache, fatigue, nausea, vomiting, and abdominal pain; may have jaundice; lasts 4–6 weeks	Fecal-oral route (e.g., unsanitary water and food); blood route rare and only during the early days of the disease	2–6 weeks	2- to 3-week period before the onset of jaundice	Anti-HAV (antibody to HAV virus) detected in serum within 2 weeks of disease onset; immunity persists for lifetime (active immunity*); if exposed, obtain standard immune globulin (IG) within the first few days following exposure to achieve passive immunity†
Hepatitis B						
HBV	Hepatitis B virus	Influenza-like illness; may include itching, joint pains, and jaundice; usually lasts longer than 6 weeks	Blood, saliva, and other body fluids; perinatal transmission from mother to child	2–6 months	The presence of serum HBsAg (hepatitis B surface antigen) indicates communicability; HBsAg may be detected in the blood from a few days to 3 months after jaundice; a chronic carrier of HBV is anyone with HBsAg in the blood for more than 6 months (5–10% of infected persons)	Active immunity* from HB vaccine (plasma-derived or recombinant DNA HV vaccines) or from having the disease. If exposed, obtain hepatitis B immune globulin (HBIG) that contains high-titer antibodies to HBV to achieve passive immunity†

Continued on following page

TABLE 7–2
TYPES OF VIRAL HEPATITIS *Continued*

Abbreviation	Term	Signs and Symptoms	Transmission	Incubation	Communicability	Immunity
Hepatitis C (formerly non-A, non-B)						
PT-NANB	Parentally transmitted non-A, non-B hepatitis	Similar to all viral hepatitis	Parenteral route (e.g., piercing the skin barrier with a contaminated needle or instrument)	2 weeks to 6 months	Similar to that of HAV and HAB hepatitis	Varies, but similar to that of HAV and HAB hepatitis
HCV	Hepatitis C virus	Similar to all viral hepatitis	Parenteral route (e.g., piercing the skin barrier with a contaminated needle or instrument)	2 weeks to 6 months	Similar to that of HAV and HAB hepatitis	Varies, but similar to that of HAV and HAB hepatitis
ET-NANB	Enterically transmitted non-A, non-B hepatitis	Similar to all viral hepatitis	Enteric route (e.g., oral-fecal transmission)	2 weeks to 6 months	Similar to that of HAV and HAB hepatitis	Varies, but similar to that of HAV and HAB hepatitis
HEV	Hepatitis E virus	Similar to all viral hepatitis	Enteric route (e.g., oral-fecal transmission)	2 weeks to 6 months	Similar to that of HAV and HAB hepatitis	Varies, but similar to that of HAV and HAB hepatitis
Delta Hepatitis						
HDV	Delta virus	Etiological agent of delta hepatitis; causes infection only in presence of HBV	Same as that of HBV hepatitis	Same as HBV hepatitis	Occurs primarily in persons who have multiple exposures to HBV (causes infection only in presence of HBV)	Same as HBV
HDAg	Delta antigen	Detectable in early acute delta infection	Same as that of HBV hepatitis	Same as HBV hepatitis	Occurs primarily in persons who have multiple exposures to HBV (causes infection only in presence of HBV)	Same as HBV
Anti-HDV	Antibody to delta antigen	Indicates past or present infection with delta virus	Same as that of HBV hepatitis	Same as HBV hepatitis	Occurs primarily in persons who have multiple exposures to HBV (causes infection only in presence of HBV)	Same as HBV

* Active immunity: immunity that is produced by the development of antibodies in the body resulting from having the disease or from the injection of the infectious organism, usually attenuated, or products produced by the organism.

† Passive immunity: immunity that results from the actual injection of antibodies for the prevention of disease.

Adapted from Centers for Disease Control (ACIP): Protection against viral hepatitis. MMWR 39(RF 2):6–7, 1990; and Cottone, J. A., Terezhalmy, G. T., and Molinari, J. A. Practical Infection Control in Dentistry. Philadelphia: Lea & Febiger, 1991.

ical cases and therefore remain undiagnosed. Ten percent of individuals infected with HBV carry the virus for 1 year. Five percent remain potentially infectious for several years or throughout the remainder of their lives. Most HBV carriers do not know of their carrier state because the carrier state develops more commonly for those infected with asymptomatic HBV.[6]

Parenterally transmitted (exposure due to piercing skin) hepatitis C virus (HCV) (formerly non-A, non-B) is most commonly acquired after blood transfusion and parenteral drug abuse in the United States. Enterically (pertaining to the small intestine) transmitted HCV appears to be acquired by way of the fecal-oral route, as noted in documented outbreaks in India, the former Soviet Union, North Africa, Mexico, and Southeast Asia.[6]

Delta hepatitis virus (HDV) is dependent on HBV for clinical expression. The associated nonpercutaneous (other than through a break in the skin) mode of transmission of HDV and HBV is intimate contact and transmucosal exchange of body fluids. In North America and western Europe the transmission of HDV is confined to intravenous drug users and hemophiliacs who receive frequent percutaneous (through a break in the skin) exposures.[6]

All forms of hepatitis represent a serious threat to the dental hygienist. Although HCV has the highest carrier state after infection, HBV and HDV are the most *life-threatening*. It should be noted that immunization is available against HBV (see section on protection for the dental hygiene provider—immunizations, later in this chapter), which also provides protection against HDV infection.[6]

The significant risk posed by hepatitis viruses has been established, but the real challenge in relation to infection control with this potentially hazardous occupational infection is the ability of HBV to *survive* in the environment. It has been shown to survive on contaminated client charts for as long as 8 days. In addition, HBV produces very high titers, or counts, in the blood. These characteristics enhance the chances for disease transmission. The hepatitis B surface antigen (HBsAg), the agent of infectivity, has been detected in 76% of the salivary samples of known carriers. Even though the risk is greater with exposure to blood than it is with general client contact, the greatest concentration of HBV is at the gingival sulcus.[7,8] In most clients' mouths the sulcular area is routinely inflamed and bleeds easily. Blood then mixes with the saliva, thus making the saliva infectious with HBV. The dental hygienist, by virtue of contact with the crevicular area of the periodontium, is as much at risk occupationally as is the dentist, followed closely by the dental assistant and the laboratory technician.[9]

Although HIV has affected interest in infection control and regulation of practices related to prevention of disease transmission and has also raised anxiety levels and fear among clients and healthcare professionals (Table 7–3), HIV-1 is a more fragile virus than HBV. There have been no reported cases of HIV infection involving *documented* occupational exposures among dental workers, including dentists.[10] Documented occupationally acquired HIV infection requires evidence of HIV seroconversion (i.e., a negative HIV-antibody test at the time of the exposure that is subsequently positive) following a discrete percutaneous or mucocutaneous occupational exposure to blood, body fluids, or other clinical or laboratory specimens.[10] Six dental healthcare workers have *possible* occupationally acquired HIV infection with no behavioral or transfusion risks for HIV infection.

TABLE 7–3
INFECTIOUS AGENTS OF CONCERN TO HEALTHCARE WORKERS

	Transmissibility	Anxiety
Influenza	↑ (High)	(Low)
Tuberculosis		
Respiratory syncytial virus		
Varicella-zoster virus		
Hepatitis B		
Cytomegalovirus		
Human immunodeficiency virus	(Low)	↓ (High)

Adapted from Valenti, W. M. Infection control and the pregnant healthcare worker. AIDS Patient Care 3(3):14, 1989.

Despite the knowledge of oral infectious hazards, there often is a failure on the part of oral healthcare providers to comprehend or appreciate the infectious potential of saliva, gingival crevicular fluid, and blood. A lack of concern is most likely related to the fact that the client's spatter **(organic debris)** is not readily apparent, since it is transparent or translucent and dries as a clear film on skin or clothing and other surfaces such as paper **(fomites).** An analogy could be made with bacterial plaque, in that plaque is not readily apparent on clients' teeth unless it is disclosed or a sample is viewed under a microscope. Only then is the real impact of disease potential realized.[6] Figures 7–1 and 7–2 dramatically portray contamination from oral fluids by using a red dye for saliva so that the contamination can be visualized.[12] Even the most experienced dental hygienist is impressed by viewing videotapes or a slide series based on the premise "if saliva were red," which reveals the extent to which **microbial cross-infection** may occur during oral healthcare from the practitioner's "saliva-covered fingers."[11,12]

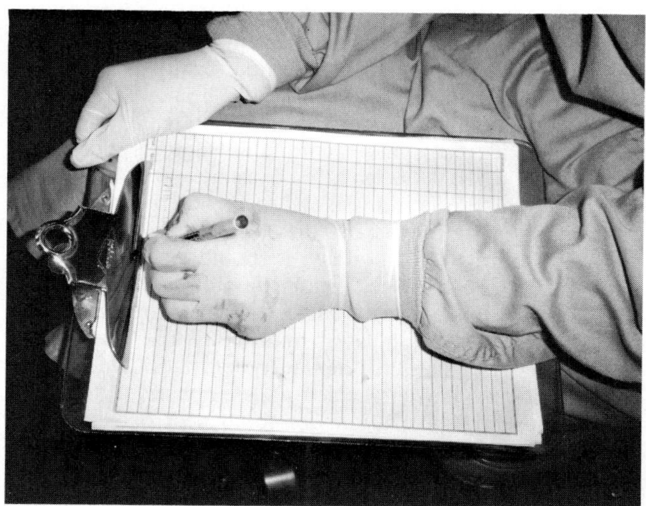

FIGURE 7–1
Cross-contamination.

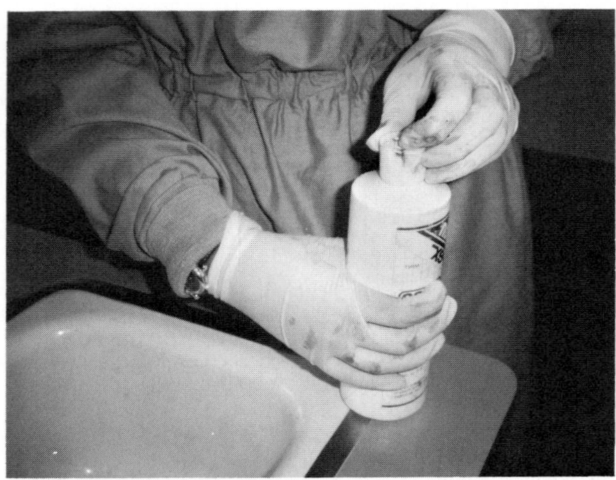

FIGURE 7-2
Cross-contamination.

UNIVERSAL PRECAUTIONS FOR BLOOD AND BODY FLUIDS IN THE PREVENTION OF DISEASE TRANSMISSION

Until the mid 1980s the primary occupational concerns for the dental hygienist in terms of disease transmission were HBV, TB, and herpes. The significant outcomes, potential for a carrier state, and ability of HBV to survive in the oral healthcare environment had warranted a separate protocol for caring for a client with a history of HBV. Additional knowledge about the potential of asymptomatic carriers of HBV and HIV with the advent of AIDS caused a reevaluation of the concept of a separate protocol or procedures for handling clients infected with HBV or HIV. In 1987 there was a significant change in philosophy for infection control protocol. The new philosophy and protocol called for a *uniform approach* for infection control requiring elimination of a separate protocol for clients considered to be carriers of HBV or at high risk for other transmissible diseases.[13] The new emphasis was on the need for healthcare providers to treat blood and other body fluids from *all* clients as potentially infective. Hepatitis B is the most important infectious occupational hazard for oral healthcare providers. The rationale for a separate protocol for clients with a history of hepatitis B was flawed because most HBV carriers do not know of their carrier state since the HBV carrier state develops more commonly among those with asymptomatic HBV.[6] Currently all clients must be considered potential carriers of HBV, because of the number of undiagnosed HBV clients and the associated unreliability of the health history. Additionally, it should be noted that an estimated 3,000 oral healthcare providers are persistent HBV carriers. Dental team members have three times the risk of the general population to acquire the disease and develop a carrier state. All dental hygienists should be considered potential carriers, which adds emphasis to the need for using optimal precautions for the benefit of both client and dental hygienist.

Although microbial-laden secretions have varying degrees of infection potential, universal precautions have been recommended by the **Centers for Disease Control** (CDC) for a number of years, and numerous governmental and professional organizations have joined the CDC in urging the incorporation of this concept as the guiding tenet of a healthcare approach to infection control. During the course of dental hygiene care, contact with blood and saliva is predictable; therefore, use of universal precautions for all clients regardless of the bloodborne infectious status prevents exposures for the dental hygienist and also protects the client from exposures to blood that may occur from breaks in the skin of the dental hygienists' hands.[14] Compliance with this principle is at the heart of the OSHA standard (see the section on policies of the Occupational Safety and Health Administration later in this chapter.) Therefore, the dental hygienist must consider *all* clients, instruments, and oral healthcare settings as potentially infected with HIV and/or other bloodborne pathogens and adhere rigorously to the same appropriate infection control procedures for minimizing the risk of exposure to blood and body fluids of all clients.

SOURCES OF CROSS-INFECTION WHILE PROVIDING DENTAL HYGIENE CARE

It has been estimated that in a dental practice that sees 20 clients a day, an average of at least two clients with oral herpes, one carrier of HBV, and an unknown number of clients infected with the HIV-1 virus associated with AIDS are treated in 7 working days.[15] Considering the number of clients for which the dental hygienist provides care in the course of a day, week, month, or year of clinical practice and the fact that most human microbial **pathogens** have been isolated from oral secretions, the sources of contamination and potential for disease transmission in the dental setting are enormous. The dental hygienist's knowledge of microbiology provides the background for an understanding of how microorganisms survive and proliferate. Although the specific characteristics of each **microorganism** are beyond the scope of this text, an overview of the chain of infection, including modes of disease transmission, will be presented. By understanding components of the infection chain, the dental hygienist can intervene to prevent infections from developing.[16]

Theory of Disease Transmission

Chain of Infection

The fact that pathogenic microorganisms are present in the oral cavity in great numbers and variety does not automatically mean that they will cause disease. The development of an infection occurs in a cyclical process that depends on six elements (Fig. 7-3). An infection develops if this cycle is uninterrupted. The dental hygienist's efforts to control infection are directed toward breaking the chain of infection.

Infectious Agent

Pathogenic organisms include bacteria, viruses, fungi, and protozoa. Food and the proper environment are essential for all organisms to grow. A dark, warm, moist habitat such as the oral cavity is ideal.[16] Hands present an environment that is quite different from the oral cavity, yet firmly

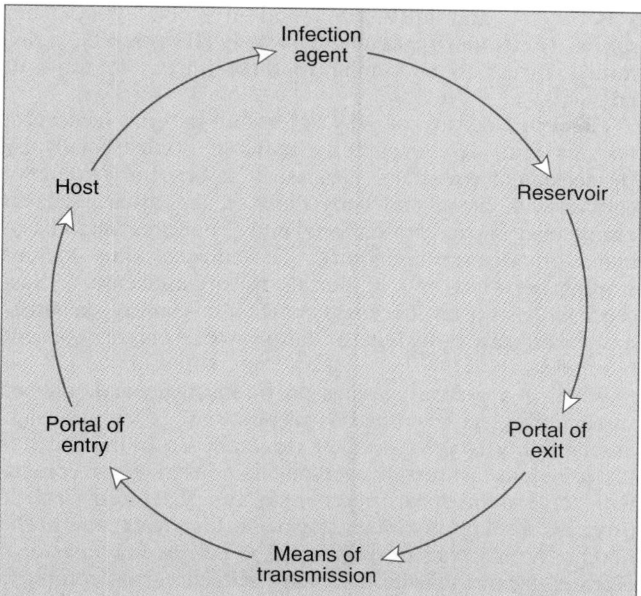

FIGURE 7-3
Six elements of cyclical infection process. (Adapted from Potter, P. A., and Perry, A. G. Fundamentals of Nursing, 3rd ed. St. Louis: C. V. Mosby, 1993, p. 398.)

adherent resident pathogens are always present in the creases and crevices of the skin (Fig. 7-4). Transient pathogens, in contrast, are more loosely adherent, temporary residents on the hands that are picked up during the course of daily activities and are easily removed with thorough handwashing (see the section on protection for the dental hygiene care provider—handwashing later in this chapter). Other areas of the body serve as environments for microorganisms to flourish as well, although the oral cavity and hands are the key environments of concern for the dental hygienist. Factors such as number and virulence of pathogenic organisms affect their ability to elude the body's defenses and cause disease.[16]

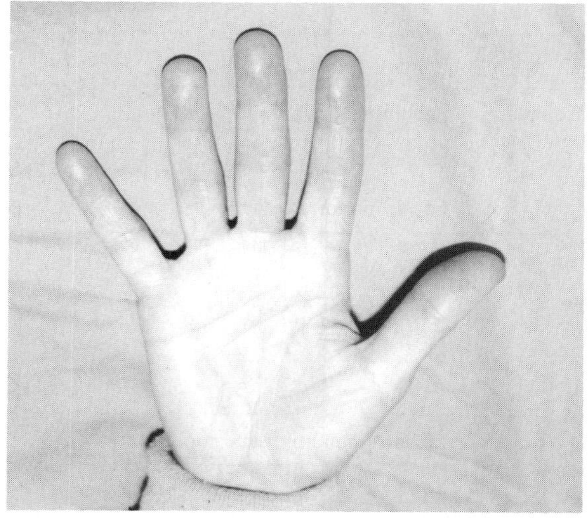

FIGURE 7-4
Palm view of hands, key environment of concern for the dental hygienist.

Reservoir

The most significant sources for pathogenic growth or *reservoirs* for microorganisms within the body are the mouth, skin, respiratory tract, vagina, colon, and lower urethra. Pathogenic organisms may be found on the skin and within body cavities and in fluids and discharges such as saliva, gingival crevicular fluids, blood, semen, vaginal secretions, tears, nasopharyngeal and pharyngeal secretions, lesion exudate, and possibly breast milk. The few areas within the body considered **sterile**—without organism growth—are the blood stream, spinal fluid, peritoneal cavity, urinary tract, muscles, bones, and chambers of the eye. Any entry of a foreign object into a sterile site (e.g., contaminated needle into the blood stream) leads to a high risk of infection. The presence of microorganisms does not always cause a person to be ill. **Carriers** are persons who show no symptoms of illness but have pathogens on or in their bodies that can be transferred to others. For example, a person can be a carrier of HIV, HBV, and tuberculosis without having manifestations of the disease. Exposure to HIV may result in infection and development of antibodies to HIV (anti-HIV), the marker used to determine HIV status through laboratory testing. It usually takes 6 to 12 weeks for the antibodies to develop after infection. During these 6 to 12 weeks, there may be a window of seronegativity when a laboratory test appears to be negative for antibodies to HIV, and even after the antibodies develop there may be no other indications of infection for 2 to 10 years. Throughout the entire asymptomatic period, from the time of exposure and initial infection until symptoms of HIV infection appear years later, the infected person can still transmit the virus to others.

The HIV-infected person is the reservoir, but transmission of the virus is dependent on the chain of infection and the necessary portal of exit, means of transmission, portal of entry, and a susceptible host, as will be explained below.

Environment of Microorganisms

Environmental factors within the reservoir and during the transmission process are key for pathogen survival. The conditions supportive of microorganism growth include food for nourishment and may include oxygen, water, temperature, limited light, and pH range. Most microorganisms require oxygen for survival and multiplication. Many need water for survival, certain temperature ranges, and limited light, and most prefer an alkaline environment with a pH range of 5 to 8.[16] These environmental characteristics must be considered when selecting methods of sterilization. For example, boiling water may be bactericidal for selected organisms, yet higher temperatures are required to kill HBV and certain spores.

Portal of Exit/Portal of Entry

Once microorganisms find a site to grow and multiply, they must find a portal of exit if they are to enter another host and cause disease. When the human is the reservoir, microorganisms can exit through a variety of sites.[16] Just as the chain of infection involves the necessary route of exit for the microorganisms to be able to enter another host, an equally important link is the route, or portal, of entry for the subsequent cross-infection to occur in another host. Pathogens can enter a person's body through the same routes they use for exiting (Fig. 7-5).

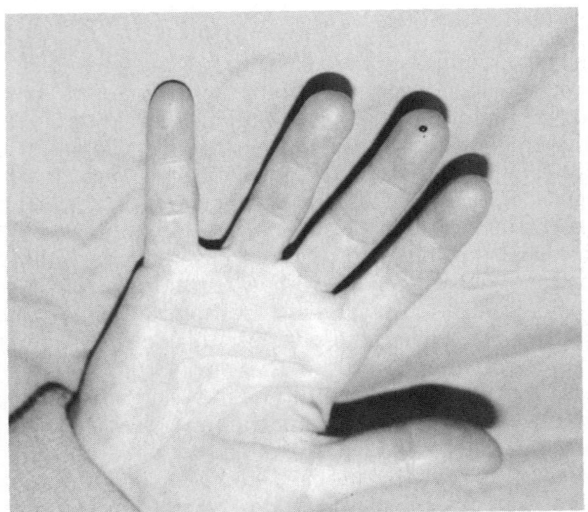

FIGURE 7-5
Portal of entry/exit: hand with bleeding after stick injury.

Common routes of exit and entry are skin and mucous membranes, oral cavity, gastrointestinal tract, respiratory tract, genitourinary system, and blood via transfusion of blood derivatives (Table 7-4).

The blood is normally sterile, but in the case of HIV, hepatitis, and septicemia (presence of bacteria in the circulating blood), it becomes a reservoir for infectious organisms. A break in the skin by needle puncture or a traumatic wound allows pathogens to exit the body in blood.

Both HIV and HBV are found in blood, semen, and saliva. Therefore, the routes by which HIV may be transmitted appear to be similar to those known to transmit HBV.[17]

There are reports of HIV infections in nine healthcare workers that were apparently acquired occupationally by (1) accidental parenteral needlestick injuries; (2) extensive contact with blood and body fluids in the absence of recommended barrier precautions; and (3) accidental spills of blood on mucous membranes or abnormal skin demonstrating both concepts of portals of exit and entry.[17] Susceptible hosts may be clients, dental hygienists, or other oral healthcare providers, or family members as innocent bystanders.

Whether a person acquires an infection depends on her susceptibility to microbial virulence and disease transfer. Susceptibility is the degree of resistance an individual has to pathogens. Although everyone is constantly in contact with large numbers of microorganisms, the more virulent (invasive, prolific, toxic) an organism, the greater the likelihood of a person's susceptibility. The integrity of a person's defenses against infection directly influences susceptibility. Factors such as increasing age, poor nutritional status, and stress impair an individual's immunological defenses.[16] When an individual's immune system is unable to recognize and destroy that which is foreign, the result is an increased susceptibility to infection. In addition, significant immunodeficiency occurs with autoimmune diseases, such as rheumatoid arthritis and systemic lupus erythematosus, and with drug therapies for immunological disease and organ transplants such as corticosteroids, which commonly result in complications with infection. Most notably, AIDS

TABLE 7-4
PORTALS OF EXIT/ENTRY, MODES OF TRANSMISSION, AND POTENTIAL PATHOLOGY

Portals of Exit/Entry	Mode of Transmission	Potential Pathology
Skin and Mucous Membranes	Direct Inoculation to Tissue Surface	
Any break in the integrity of the skin and mucous membranes (ocular mucosa) can lead to an infection	Infectious blood or serum onto mucosal surfaces/break in skin Blood, saliva, tears, semen Lesion exudate, saliva	HIV HBV Herpes
Oral Cavity	Direct Inoculation to Tissue Surface	
Mucous membranes of the oral cavity are susceptible to infection; portal for ingestion	Pharyngeal secretions (infected droplet contact) Exudate from oral lesion Crevicular exudate Saliva and blood	Pneumonia, TB Herpes, syphilis Abscesses CMV, mononucleosis
	Inoculation into Circulatory System	
	Blood Blood, saliva, tears, semen	HIV, HDV, HCV HBV
	Ingestion of Pathogens	
	Saliva	Mumps, hand-foot-and-mouth disease
Gastrointestinal Tract		
Bowel elimination and vomiting are portals of exit for pathogens	Fecal-oral	HIV

TABLE 7-4
PORTALS OF EXIT/ENTRY, MODES OF TRANSMISSION, AND POTENTIAL PATHOLOGY *Continued*

Portals of Exit/Entry	Mode of Transmission	Potential Pathology
Respiratory Tract	Infected Droplet Contact: Inhalation, Ingestion, Direct Inoculation	
Pathogens residing in the respiratory tract can be released from the body when the person sneezes, coughs, talks, or even breathes. The microorganisms exit via the mouth and nose	Nasopharyngeal secretions	Flu, common cold, whooping cough, candidiasis, opportunistic *Pneumocystis carinii*
	Pharyngeal secretions	TB
	Nasopharyngeal secretions, blood, saliva, vesicle exudate	Measles, rubeola, rubella
Genitourinary System	Direct Inoculation to Tissue Surface	
Pathogens exit via male's urethral meatus or female's vaginal canal or enter through surface breaks in the skin and mucosa	Lesion exudate, saliva	Herpes
	Lesion exudate, blood, pharyngeal secretions	Gonococcal infections
	Lesion exudate	Syphilis
	Inoculation into Circulatory System	
	Blood, semen, vaginal secretions and breast milk	HIV
	Blood, semen, saliva, tears	HBV, HDV, HCV
Blood	Inoculation into Circulatory System	
A break in the skin by needle, instrument or traumatic wound, burn or dermatitis; nonintact skin provides portals of exit/entry	Blood (also transmitted by semen, vaginal secretions, breast milk)	HIV
	Blood (also transmitted by saliva, semen, tears)	HBV, HDV, HCV
	Direct Inoculation to Tissue Surface	
	Blood, saliva	CMV, infectious mononucleosis

results in profound suppression of cellular immunity because of a defect in the cell-mediated immunity of the host, allowing development of opportunistic infections and cancers.[14] The nature of a particular disease process, a person's health status and lifestyle, and the ability of the body's normal defense mechanisms to fight infection affect the susceptibility of the host as the critical link in the chain of infection.

Modes of Disease Transmission

Although there are many vehicles of transmission of pathogens from the source (reservoir) to the host, the most common routes are summarized in Figure 7-6. The hosts in the oral healthcare environment and the three basic types of disease transmission include:

- Client to dental hygienist
- Dental hygienist to client
- Client to client

The last, although highly probable, has not been documented. Families of oral healthcare providers are susceptible to the hazard of transmission of pathogens as well.[2,16]

The oral cavity is one of the more bacterially contaminated sites of the body (Fig. 7-7), even though most of the organisms may be normal flora. Indigenous oral flora include bacteria, yeasts, certain fungi, mycoplasmas, protozoa, and viruses. Within the sulcus alone there are an estimated 200 billion cells per gram of crevicular fluid. However, organisms that are normal flora in one person can be pathogens in another. Organisms exit when a person expectorates saliva. Kissing also can provide a means of exit from the oral cavity.

Client to Oral Healthcare Provider

A New York dentist who denied risk factors other than occupational ones tested seropositive for HIV antibodies. He was the only oral healthcare provider of 1,309 dentists, dental hygienists, and dental assistants tested at a professional meeting who tested seropositive. The dentist reported that he had been practicing for 14 years in Manhattan, his only sexual contact had been his wife, and he had not had sexual relations with men, had not used illicit drugs, and had not received a blood transfusion. He had treated clients known to be at increased risk for AIDS, although to his knowledge he had never treated a client known to have AIDS. He reported that he frequently practiced without the use of personal barriers such as gloves, even though he often had obvious breaks in his skin. He estimated that he had received two accidental needlesticks (parenteral inoculations) within the previous year and 10 within the previous 5 years. He had no history of an HVB vaccine and a negative test result for HBsAg. The absence of other risk factors suggests that occupational exposure (client to oral healthcare provider) was the likely mode of acquisition of HIV infection.[17]

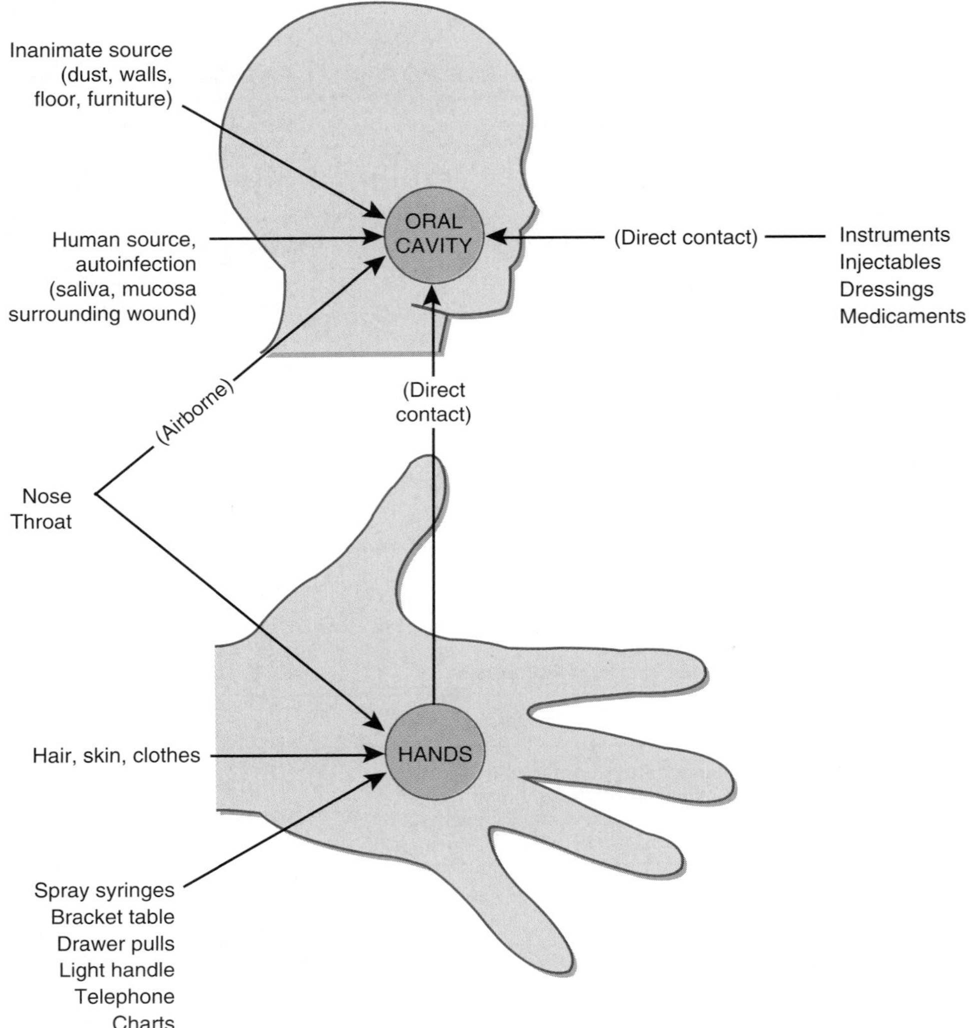

FIGURE 7–6
Vehicles of transmission of pathogens. (Courtesy of Johnson & Johnson.)

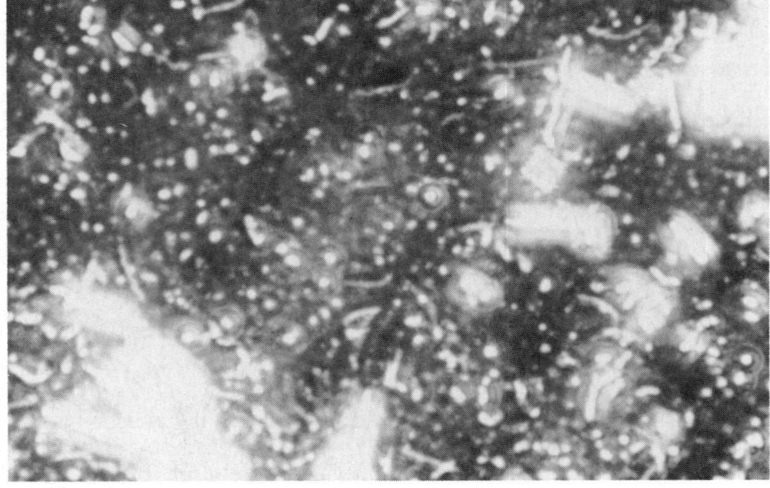

FIGURE 7–7
Microscopic view of microorganisms from the oral cavity.

Oral Healthcare Provider to Client

There have been 20 documented cases of herpes simplex virus type 1 (HSV-1) transmission to clients from an ungloved dental hygienist with herpetic lesions on the fingers.[18]

There have been 12 outbreaks of HVB infection in the United States linked to healthcare workers who transmitted the organism to their clients. The largest outbreak was from a dentist who infected 55 clients, resulting in two deaths, attributed to the dentist not using gloves.[19]

The risk of HIV transmission from an infected healthcare provider to a client is significantly less than the risk of HBV transmission from a hepatitis B e antigen (HBeAg)-positive healthcare provider to a client. The only known case of HIV transmission from a healthcare provider to a client has been revealed by a CDC investigation of a cluster of HIV infections among clients of one dentist with AIDS. Six clients of approximately 850 evaluated clients of the dentist were HIV infected. The investigation indicated that HIV transmission occurred during dental care, although the exact mechanisms of transmission have not been determined.[20,21]

Client to Client

Although not documented, indirect contact transmission of infection by contaminated instruments is possible. Infection control precautions should be taken routinely in the care of all clients.[13]

Autogenous Infection

Autogenous infection is a local or systemic posttreatment infection caused by clinicians introducing the microbial agents of the client into other tissues of the client during procedures ranging from probing to surgery. Subsequent infection is dependent on the host's immune system or compromised health status. For example, a client with cardiac valve damage might be at risk for infective endocarditis resulting from a bacteremia (presence of bacteria in the blood stream) initiated by instrumentation as basic as probing during periodontal assessments.[14]

Considering the presence of pathogens in the mouth and the documentation of disease transmission among individuals associated with oral healthcare providers, it is critical to have knowledge of the specific routes of disease transmission in order to appreciate the rationale and value of infection control protocols designed to break the chain of infection. The general routes of transmission of microbial agents associated with dental hygiene care and dentistry in general are:[1]

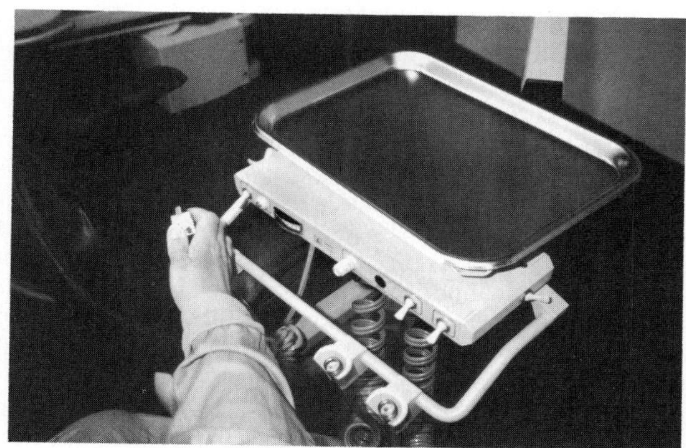

FIGURE 7–9
Hand touching equipment.

- **Direct contact** with infectious lesions or infected blood and saliva
  Percutaneous inoculation by a contaminated needle, instrument, or sharp object, also referred to as **parenteral exposure,** occurring as a result of piercing the skin barrier (with a needle or instrument) (Fig. 7–8)
  Nonneedle inoculation such as nicks, cuts, abrasions, scratches or burns, dermatitis, or nonintact skin, especially on hands (nonintact skin also considered percutaneous)
  Infectious blood or serum, or saliva in contact with mucosal surfaces (intraoral, nasal, and ocular mucosa)
- **Indirect transmission** of microorganisms via a contaminated intermediate object
  Transfer of infectious serum **(spatter)** by way of hands touching equipment (Fig. 7–9), instruments, environmental surfaces, and records (pulling drawers, picking up telephones)
  Aerosolization, the **airborne** transfer (Fig. 7–10) of microorganisms or infectious serum from the oral cavity into the air of the treatment area

Although the ***aerosol*** *mode* of disease transmission is more theoretical than documented, the potential for disease transmission occurs when debris is atomized and expelled

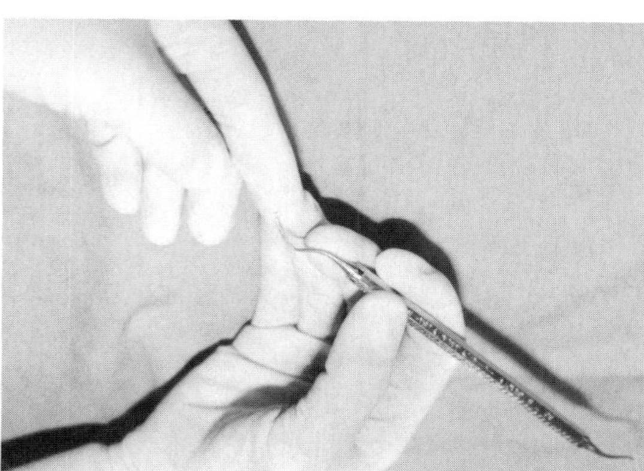

FIGURE 7–8
Instrument tip (reusable sharp) piercing glove.

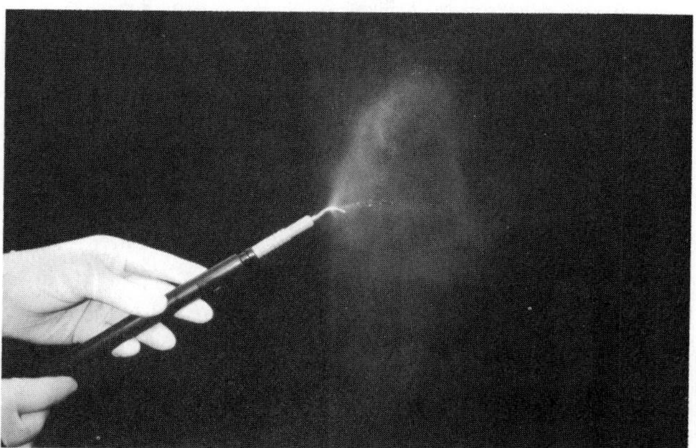

FIGURE 7–10
Creation of aerosols by ultrasonic scaling equipment.

from the mouth, creating a source of microorganisms capable of infection. Dental aerosols may be solid and/or liquid airborne particles. When the droplets evaporate, the residual droplet nuclei form and remain airborne in the operatory. These aerosol particles are usually less than 50 μm and cannot be seen but are subject to inhalation.[1] Spatter is described as having particle size greater than 50 μm in diameter, having inertial force greater than the frictional force of the air, and being ballistic in nature. The highest concentration is found 2 feet in front of the client, which is where the dental hygienist is usually positioned, and may be visible on eyewear (Fig. 7–11), lights, environmental surfaces, and clothing.[22]

Sources of contamination in the dental treatment area other than those transferred or expelled from the oral cavity during a procedure are the following:

- Dustborne organisms, inanimate source: dust, walls, floor, furniture
- Aerosols created by breathing, speaking, coughing, and sneezing **(droplet spread)**
- Dental equipment (unit) water lines have been shown to contain aquatic bacteria, microorganisms normally associated with water (e.g., *Pseudomonas aeruginosa*). High concentrations of bacteria, including microorganisms from saliva, have been found in the water from handpieces, air-water syringes (Fig. 7–12), and ultrasonic scalers.[23,24] Microorganisms enter the water lines by retraction up into the handpiece or water-spray syringe as a result of a mechanism in the equipment (retraction valve) designed to prevent dripping. An awareness of the related microbiological research and the potential for **microbial cross-contamination** via the water lines in equipment led to the creation of the American National Standard–American Dental Association Specification No. 47 (April 21, 1984), which states that the water should not retract more than 2.032 cm back into the handpiece. There are antiretraction valves that are inserted into the water hose that meet or exceed this standard. Although the antiretraction mechanisms lessen the potential for cross-contamination, the possibility of cross-contamination still exists, and other steps need to be taken to further minimize this source of contamination within the dental operatory.[1]
- Although not as significant as the aforementioned reservoirs of potential pathogens, the high- and low-volume evacuation (suction) devices (Fig. 7–13) harbor residues of infected material, leading to permanent bacterial growth on the inside of the tubes. Contact with the interior of the evacuation tubing is limited, and the potential for cross-contamination that involves the client is relatively nonexistent, yet the dental hygienist who is responsible for insertion and removal of attachments or maintenance that involves clearing, sanitization, and disinfection of the lines needs to follow infection control protocols to prevent the risk of self-contamination.

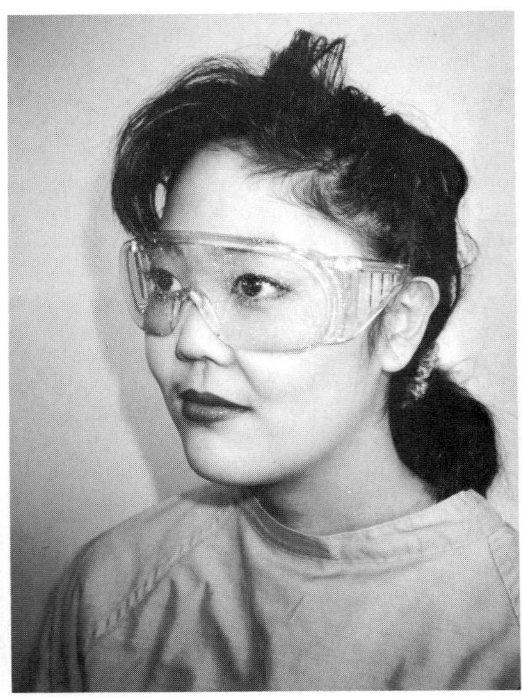

FIGURE 7–11
Spatter visible on surface of protective eyewear.

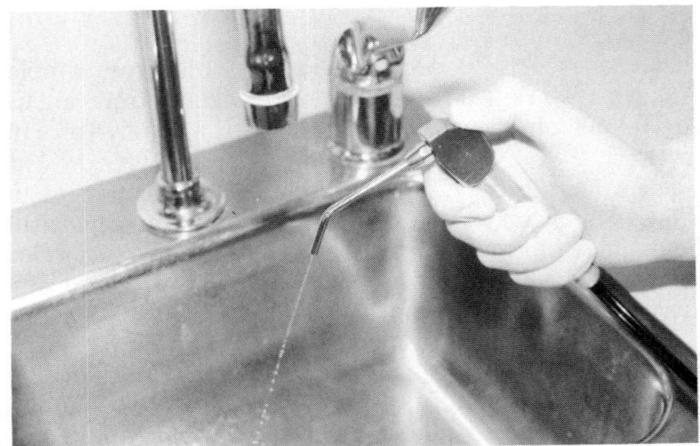

FIGURE 7–12
Water line associated with air-water syringe.

ROLE OF CLIENT ASSESSMENTS AS PART OF AN INFECTION CONTROL PROGRAM

The assessment phase of the dental hygiene process of care is composed of data-collection techniques that include

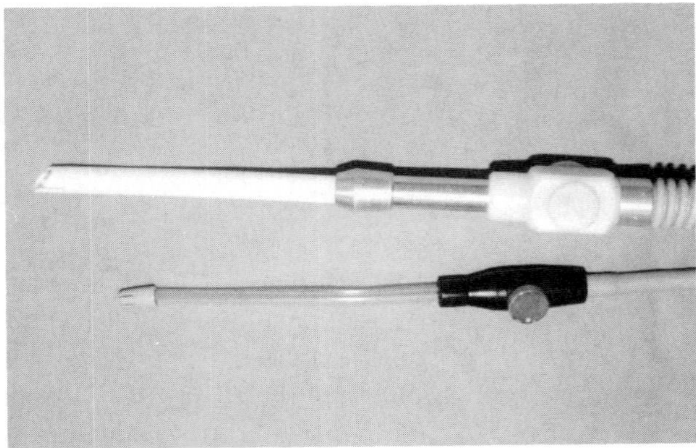

FIGURE 7–13
High- and low-volume suction lines.

questionnaires, interviews, clinical measurements, and/or examinations. The assessment procedures include a comprehensive health history and a general physical evaluation, including vital signs and health risk appraisal. Additionally, data collection may include human needs assessment related to dental hygiene, health behavior evaluation, extraoral and intraoral examination, examination of the teeth and periodontium, exposure and interpretation of radiographs, bacterial evaluation, impressions for study models, oral exfoliative cytology, pupal vitality testing, and intraoral photography.[25]

The primary assessments that come to mind when developing and implementing an infection-control program are the health history, extraoral and intraoral examination, and periodontal evaluation. Additional information on assessment can be found in Chapters 10 to 13.

Dental Hygiene Assessments: Health History and Extraoral, Intraoral, and Periodontal Assessments

Health History

The standard of care requires obtaining an accurate health history, which is reviewed and updated at subsequent visits. The health history provides some information on the presence or absence of transmissible disease (Fig. 7–14) and identifies the clients who are at risk for harboring potentially infectious organisms and those who may have increased susceptibility to infections. Although the health history is an important screening tool, it is not suitable for selecting a specific approach to infection control. The essential components of a health history include the chief complaint; the current health status; major hospitalizations; a history of childhood and adult diseases; allergies; a list of medications; pertinent family, social, or experiential history; and a review of major organ systems.[1] These elements are designed to elicit information on the presence or absence of transmissible disease, yet clients may suppress some information purposely or unknowingly (e.g., being HIV positive or a subclinical HBV carrier). Furthermore, questions related to current or recurrent illnesses, unintentional weight loss, lymphadenopathy, oral soft tissue lesions, or history of hepatitis or other infections should be included. Medical consultation may be indicated when a history of active infection or systemic infection is elicited.[13] Additionally, questions regarding hemophilia or other coagulopathies, earlier surgeries, injuries, accidents or hospitalizations, and comments about anesthesia and drug reactions should be included. These experiences may have been associated with blood transfusion(s) and may have predisposed the client to transmissible diseases. Also a client undergoing immunosuppressant therapy may be at risk for many viral, fungal, and bacterial infections, may have repeated hospitalizations for the same condition, may fail to respond normally to therapy for infection, or may have recurrent infection with the same pathogen or infection with unusual organisms.[1]

It is important to remember that the health history and examination cannot reliably identify all clients infected with HIV or other bloodborne pathogens. Therefore each client must be considered potentially infectious.[13,22,26] The health

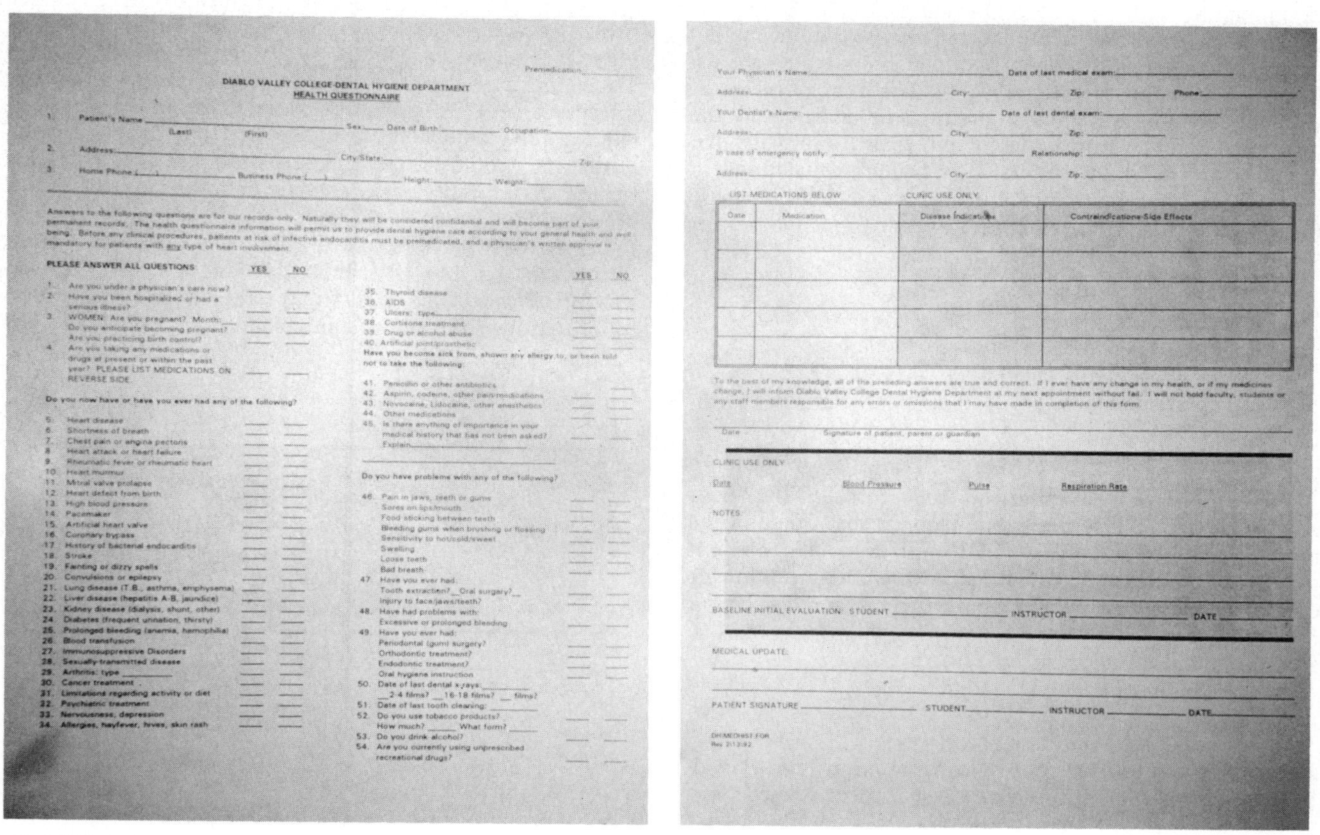
Premedication ____

DIABLO VALLEY COLLEGE DENTAL HYGIENE DEPARTMENT
HEALTH QUESTIONNAIRE

1. Patient's Name ____ (Last) (First) Sex ____ Date of Birth ____ Occupation ____
2. Address ____ City/State ____ Zip ____
3. Home Phone (   ) ____ Business Phone (   ) ____ Height ____ Weight ____

Answers to the following questions are for our records only. Naturally they will be considered confidential and will become part of your permanent records. The health questionnaire information will permit us to provide dental hygiene care according to your general health and well being. Before any clinical procedures, patients at risk of infective endocarditis must be premedicated, and a physician's written approval is mandatory for patients with any type of heart involvement.

PLEASE ANSWER ALL QUESTIONS YES NO

1. Are you under a physician's care now?
2. Have you been hospitalized or had a serious illness?
3. WOMEN: Are you pregnant? Month: ____ Do you anticipate becoming pregnant? Are you practicing birth control?
4. Are you taking any medications or drugs at present or within the past year? PLEASE LIST MEDICATIONS ON REVERSE SIDE.

Do you now have or have you ever had any of the following?

5. Heart disease
6. Shortness of breath
7. Chest pain or angina pectoris
8. Heart attack or heart failure
9. Rheumatic fever or rheumatic heart
10. Heart murmur
11. Mitral valve prolapse
12. Heart defect from birth
13. High blood pressure
14. Pacemaker
15. Artificial heart valve
16. Coronary bypass
17. History of bacterial endocarditis
18. Stroke
19. Fainting or dizzy spells
20. Convulsions or epilepsy
21. Lung disease (T.B., asthma, emphysema)
22. Liver disease (hepatitis A-B, jaundice)
23. Kidney disease (dialysis, shunt, other)
24. Diabetes (frequent urination, thirsty)
25. Prolonged bleeding (anemia, hemophilia)
26. Blood transfusion
27. Immunosuppressive Disorders
28. Sexually transmitted disease
29. Arthritis: type ____
30. Cancer treatment
31. Limitations regarding activity or diet
32. Psychiatric treatment
33. Nervousness, depression
34. Allergies, hayfever, hives, skin rash

YES NO

35. Thyroid disease
36. AIDS
37. Ulcers: type ____
38. Cortisone treatment
39. Drug or alcohol abuse
40. Artificial joint/prosthetic

Have you become sick from, shown any allergy to, or been told not to take the following:

41. Penicillin or other antibiotics
42. Aspirin, codeine, other pain medications
43. Novocaine, Lidocaine, other anesthetics
44. Other medications
45. Is there anything of importance in your medical history that has not been asked? Explain ____

Do you have problems with any of the following?

46. Pain in jaws, teeth or gums
Sores on lips/mouth
Food sticking between teeth
Bleeding gums when brushing or flossing
Sensitivity to hot/cold/sweet
Swelling
Loose teeth
Bad breath
47. Have you ever had:
Tooth extraction? ___ Oral surgery? ___
Injury to face/jaws/teeth?
48. Have had problems with:
Excessive or prolonged bleeding
49. Have you ever had:
Periodontal (gum) surgery?
Orthodontic treatment?
Endodontic treatment?
Oral hygiene instruction
50. Date of last dental x-rays: ____
___ 2-4 films? ___ 16-18 films? ___ films?
51. Date of last tooth cleaning: ____
52. Do you use tobacco products?
How much? ____ What form? ____
53. Do you drink alcohol?
54. Are you currently using unprescribed recreational drugs?

Your Physician's Name: ____ Date of last medical exam: ____
Address: ____ City: ____ Zip: ____ Phone: ____
Your Dentist's Name: ____ Date of last dental exam: ____
Address: ____ City: ____ Zip: ____
In case of emergency notify: ____ Relationship: ____
Address: ____ City: ____ Zip: ____

LIST MEDICATIONS BELOW CLINIC USE ONLY

Date	Medication	Disease Indications	Contraindications-Side Effects

To the best of my knowledge, all of the preceding answers are true and correct. If I ever have any change in my health, or if my medicines change, I will inform Diablo Valley College Dental Hygiene Department at my next appointment without fail. I will not hold faculty, students or any staff members responsible for any errors or omissions that I may have made in completion of this form.

Date ____ Signature of patient, parent or guardian ____

CLINIC USE ONLY

Date Blood Pressure Pulse Respiration Rate

NOTES:

BASELINE INITIAL EVALUATION: STUDENT ____ INSTRUCTOR ____ DATE ____

MEDICAL UPDATE:

PATIENT SIGNATURE ____ STUDENT ____ INSTRUCTOR ____ DATE ____

DH/MEDHIST.FOR
Rev 2/12/92

FIGURE 7–14
Health history questionnaire.

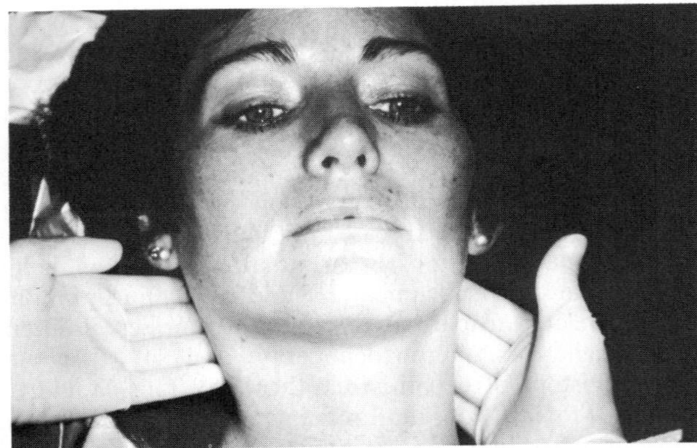

FIGURE 7-15
Palpation of the occipital lymph nodes as a component of the extraoral examination.

history assessment is not meant to be a mechanism for determining a specific approach to infection control, yet the data collected may be useful in guiding the course of treatment and indicating the possible need for consultation and premedication. When significant findings are observed on the health history, the dental hygienist's responsibility is to make the appropriate dental hygiene care modifications or to direct the client to an alternative source of care when necessary.

Extraoral and Intraoral Assessment

Another important assessment related to infection control is the performance of a thorough extraoral and intraoral examination. With the extraoral evaluation (Fig. 7-15), the recognition of chronic lymphadenopathy is significant because this precedes a diagnosis of AIDS in many clients. Lymphadenopathy is defined as swollen lymph nodes at two extrainguinal sites for 3 months, in addition to the inguinal glands (lymph nodes of the groin), especially the posterior cervical and occipital lymphadenopathy found in the absence of any current illness or drug known to cause lymphadenopathy.[27] The intraoral examination findings associated with HIV disease are:

- Candidiasis
- Herpes simplex ulceration
- Other infectious ulcers
- Recurrent aphthous ulcers
- Hairy leukoplakia
- Herpes zoster
- Kaposi's sarcoma

The extra/intraoral examination has been called the "poor man's HIV test," since this examination reveals some of the most significant early signs of HIV infection, and preliminary assessments can be performed with gauze and a tongue depressor. Early detection of clinical signs and symptoms may allow for early treatment, increased longevity of life, and prevention of the spread of HIV disease.[24]

Periodontal Assessment

Among the earliest signs of HIV infection are HIV gingivitis and HIV periodontitis (now termed linear gingival erythema and necrotizing [ulcerative] periodontitis, respectively). The characteristics of HIV gingivitis (linear gingival erythema) are:

- Spontaneous bleeding
- Petechiae-like lesions
- Lack of response to therapy or traditional treatment

HIV gingivitis may be either localized or generalized. The characteristics of HIV periodontitis (necrotizing [ulcerative] periodontitis) are:

- Pain and spontaneous bleeding
- Interproximal bleeding and cratering
- Edema and intense erythema
- Extremely rapid bone loss (Fig. 7-16)
- Soft tissue and bone necrotizing at the same time in a localized site (anterior and posterior) right next to a healthy area[29]

For more information see Chapter 33.

When some of the aforementioned signs or symptoms are observed in the absence of hard signs or diagnosis of any other condition associated with an immunocompromised state, the client should be considered at risk for immune deficiency and possibly HIV disease.

Laboratory Tests

Laboratory tests have limitations when it comes to assessment of bloodborne pathogens such as HIV and HBV and, therefore, have not been considered an appropriate protocol as a routine part of client evaluation prior to dental or dental hygiene care. If a client should report a history of HBV infection, it would be in his best interest, if he has not been tested, to determine his HBsAg status. If he is HBsAg positive, evaluation of his **hepatitis B e antigen** (HBeAg) status should be determined. The presence of HBeAg in serum is significant because it is associated with higher levels of circulating virus and therefore with greater infectivity of HBsAg-positive individuals.[20,21] Clients with chronic HBV infection are at greater risk of hepatic carcinoma and should be more closely monitored by their physician.[6] A limitation associated with testing of clients for HIV **antibody** status is the period of time between the initial infection with HIV and the time when tests can detect the presence of the HIV antibody. This is called the *window of seronegativity,* and it may range from 6 weeks to 6 months from the time of initial infection or contact. The

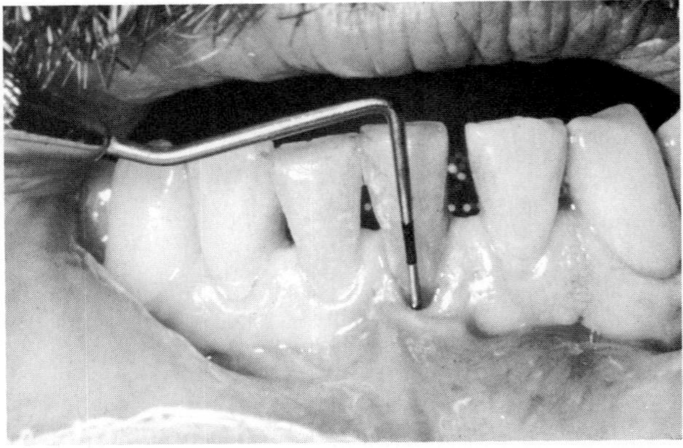

FIGURE 7-16
Close-up of periodontal probe inserted in pocket.

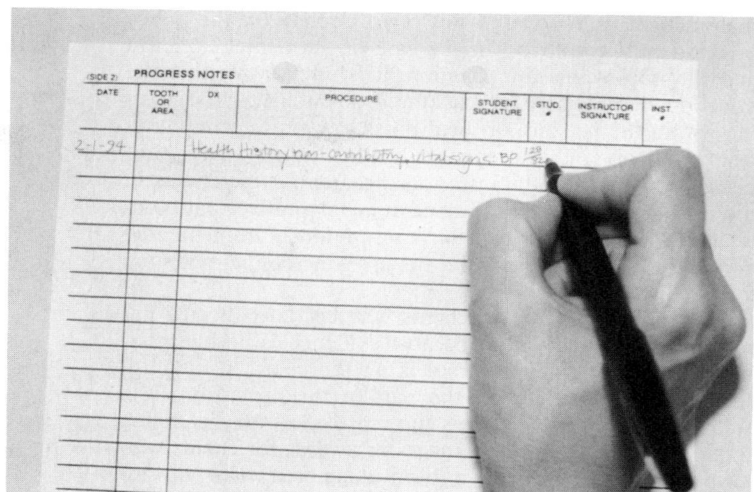

FIGURE 7–17
Close-up of handwriting documentation of dental hygiene care in client record.

client may test negative but still be infectious.[22] Also a client may remain HIV positive for as long as 7 to 10 years before developing AIDS.

Client Records

Performance and documentation (Fig. 7–17) of the previously mentioned client assessments require a professional and caring approach to ensure that the client understands the questions, is certain of the answers, appreciates the importance of the questions and the answers in the context of the care provided, understands the necessity of record keeping, and knows that the information provided will be kept confidential.[1] The interview and examination must be conducted with the intention of not isolating any single disease and keeping the responses confidential, with release only to necessarily interested parties not precluded by law. The health history of the clients may be disclosed to persons who require such information for the treatment of the client or for other necessary purposes, such as referral to an oral surgeon or oral pathologist. Every effort should be made to keep records confidential (see the section on the legal implications and prevention of malpractice later in this chapter).

ETHICAL, LEGAL, AND RISK MANAGEMENT CONSIDERATIONS RELATED TO INFECTION CONTROL

Prevention of disease transmission is a critical component in the provision of dental hygiene care. Ethical and legal considerations in this era of AIDS are evolving as issues are debated, such as the constitutional rights of the HIV-infected client, employment rights of HIV-infected healthcare providers, liability for disease transmission, admission and retention of HIV-positive student healthcare providers, and mandatory AIDS screening. Flexibility is a necessity as we move through this dynamic medical, legal, and ethical decision-making process. An overview of the ethical, legal, and risk management issues related to infection control is presented. A broader discussion of the legal and ethical issues related to dental hygiene practice is found in Chapter 39. Keeping abreast of the current related topics is required, through professional publications regarding research and public policy.[30]

Legal Implications and Prevention of Malpractice

Dental hygienists are responsible for their own actions. However, most malpractice actions target the dentist-employer or the employer's corporation even if it is the dental hygienist who is at fault. If the suit filed against the dentist's corporation is believed to have been caused by an action taken by the dental hygienist, the dentist's professional liability insurance may protect the dental hygienist under insurance coverage (see Factors Affecting Quality of Service chart). Even in this case, however, the policy may have a subrogation clause that allows the insurance company to sue the dental hygienist directly. One claim against a dental hygienist involved the issue of a purported infection caused when the dental hygienist cut the client's gingiva while taking an impression and the resultant postimpression intraoral infection required costly medical care. The claim against the dental hygienist was for $10,000 in medical costs incurred by the client.[31] This example underscores the importance of dental hygienists having their own

FACTORS AFFECTING QUALITY OF SERVICE

- Time Limitation
  (Imposed time constraints may affect compliance with standards for infection-control protocols)
- Supplies
  (Protective personal and surface barriers)
- Equipment for Sterilization and Disinfection
  (Heat sterilization and EPA approved disinfectants)
- Quality Assurance Aspects of Instrument Recirculation
  (Process indicators and biologic monitors)
- Client Care
  (Thoroughness of assessments, consultations, and evaluations)

Reprinted from Reveal, M. ADHA perspective. Journal of Dental Hygiene 64(1):18–19, copyrighted 1990 by the American Dental Hygienists' Association.

malpractice insurance and not relying solely on the policy of the dentist-employer. In the case of the dental hygienist and the impression complication, it is unclear whether the infection that resulted was acquired or autogenic (originating within the person), or what possible roles infection control protocols or the client's health history may have played. Considering the infectious hazards for the clients in the oral healthcare environment, it is imperative that compliance with infection control is scrupulously implemented and monitored to minimize the ever-increasing potential for liability.

Practitioner liability for clients who become infected has not been particularly clear because evidence of negligence is required. The burden of proof is on the client to establish that a breach of duty on the part of the professional resulted in the injury.[32] At this time, providers are beginning to see an increase in the damages or awards for clients who have contracted and have been diagnosed with an infectious disease when it should have been prevented with infection-control protocols established as the standard of care. After a malpractice suit becomes a matter of public record, succeeding similar suits become easier to prove or disprove. Once a precedent has been set, it may act to increasingly encourage lawsuits involving oral healthcare practitioners and staff persons.[33]

A case in point is *Acer* v. *Bergalis,* for HIV-1 transmission from dentist to client (one of six clients). The Acer estate settled the maximum amount on malpractice at $1,000,000, and the Cigna Insurance Corporation was involved in the lawsuits.[34] As a direct result of the cluster of HIV infections among clients in the Acer practice, the CDC has issued guidelines entitled "Recommendations for Preventing Transmission of Human Immunodeficiency Virus and Hepatitis B Virus to Clients During Exposure-Prone Invasive Procedures." Previous guidelines did not include specific recommendations on testing healthcare workers for HIV or HBV infection, and they did not provide guidance on which **invasive** procedures may represent increased risk to the client.[20,21] The guidelines that resulted from substantial public and professional input set the standard for additional precautions that are prudent in preventing HIV and HBV transmission from healthcare workers to clients until further data are available.

Malpractice associated with HIV and HBV transmission from the dental hygienist may be prevented if, as the CDC recommends, healthcare workers who perform exposure-prone procedures know their HIV antibody status and HBsAg/HBeAg status (in the absence of immunity to HVB) and, if they are infected with HIV or HBV (HBeAg positive), do not perform exposure-prone invasive procedures unless they have sought counsel from an expert review panel and have been advised as to the circumstances, if any, under which they may continue to perform these procedures. The circumstances also require that prospective clients be notified of healthcare workers' seropositivity before they undergo exposure-prone invasive procedures. Mandatory testing for all healthcare professionals is not recommended, because the current assessment of risk for transmission does not support the diversion of resources that would be required to implement mandatory testing programs.[20,21]

Another precedent-setting case, *McDonald* v. *Beaver State,* was filed by a dental client against a general dentist and a dental supplier, the client contending that the defendants had been negligent by allowing the use of a dental

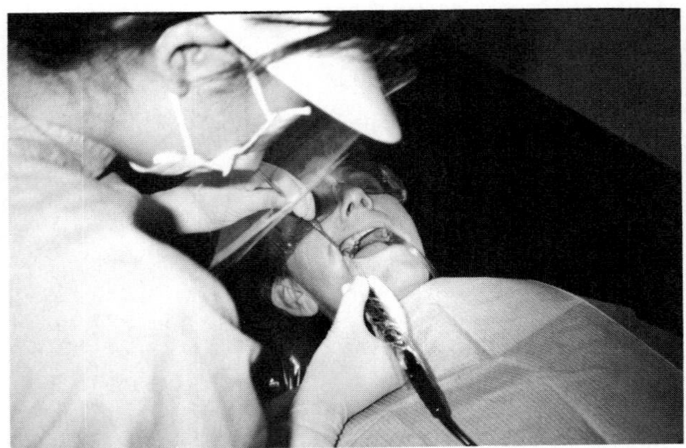

FIGURE 7–18
Ultrasonic scaling device with water spray.

unit lacking "check valves and still retaining a water retraction valve to create a classic suck-back phenomenon." The resulting infection in this case was bacterial endocarditis, which the client developed following ultrasonic curettage (Fig. 7–18), which subsequently was linked to the suck-back phenomenon. The client's attorney had a water sample drawn from the defendant general dentist's ultrasonic unit, which revealed a contamination of *Moraxella* CDC-6 in concentrations of more than 100,000 contaminants per unit measure (colony-forming units [CFU]). The infectious disease experts called to testify in this case by the client's (plaintiff's) attorney testified that there was a probable linkage between the infective endocarditis and the contaminated dental unit. The case resulted in an out-of-court settlement for an undisclosed amount of money.[33]

Contractual Responsibilities

The legal obligations associated with dental hygiene care assume the contractual responsibility of reasonable skill, care, and judgment and a current level of knowledge.[35] Meeting the standard of care for prevention of disease transmission requires monitoring the professional journals for the latest research, recommendations, and CDC, ADA, and OSHA guidelines for prevention of HIV and HBV transmission in healthcare settings.

Confidentiality and Documentation

The right to privacy applies to client records, health and dental histories, and other assessments. It also includes communication between the professional and the client, and documentation of all contacts with a client including warnings, advice, or instructions to the client, and any negative or positive comments made by the client concerning care. Inquiries regarding the sterilization and prevention of disease transmission protocols, barriers, or health status of other clients seen in the practice should be documented along with the dental hygienist response.

In general, information obtained must remain confidential unless otherwise specifically authorized by the client or, in the event of a legal action, it is requested by court order or subpoena or otherwise allowed or required by law.[32] The client's right of confidentiality and client's consent are inextricably linked together. The healthcare provider's duty to the client not to disclose confidential information obtained in the course of providing treatment is intended to encourage clients to make full disclosure, which facilitates proper diagnosis and treatment. While this certainly applies to information related to HIV infection, it is not limited to information concerning AIDS. Divulgence of confidential information without the client's consent is commission of an actionable wrong.[32] Breach of confidentiality associated with HIV disease inside and outside healthcare settings has resulted in litigation. There are many states with statutes mandating confidentiality regarding a client's HIV status. Some confidentiality laws have exceptions, so it is important to be familiar with specific state laws before sharing such confidential information. For example, Georgia law allows a breach of confidentiality when someone is at risk for contracting the AIDS virus in institutional care settings. When a healthcare provider knows that others are subject to harm by the client's medical condition, the provider has a duty to warn foreseeable victims of that harm.[36]

Discrimination

The duty to provide access to dental hygiene care for clients with AIDS or with an HIV-seropositive status is an ethical and moral responsibility.[37] Provision of care to all clients, including those who are HIV seropositive or are suffering with AIDS, is clearly a legal responsibility as well. Cases of HIV discrimination have been successfully won in the courts. The HIV-seropositive client has rights as a legally handicapped individual.[38] The equal rights protection provision of the Constitution grants specific benefits to handicapped individuals. The right to access to healthcare should be afforded to all persons, regardless of the label attached to their physical condition. Any imposed barrier to care would be an obvious act of discrimination.[30]

Informed Consent

Informed consent as a legal principle can be applied to the scenario of the HIV-infected dental hygienist, since before a health professional may proceed with treatment, the client must be adequately informed about proposed therapy, available treatment choices, and the associated dangers or risks inherently involved. The client must freely consent to being treated. This tenet is the basis for the client–dental hygienist relationship. The duty of the HIV-infected healthcare worker to disclose his condition has been addressed in the CDC's July 12, 1991, recommendations.[21]

Any healthcare worker who performs exposure-prone procedures should know her HIV antibody status and HBV immunity status or HBeAg status if she is positive for HBsAg.[21]

Healthcare workers who are infected with HIV or HBV (and are HBeAg positive) should not perform exposure-prone procedures unless they have sought counsel from an expert review panel and have been advised as to the circumstances, if any, under which they may continue to perform these procedures. Such circumstances include *notifying prospective clients of the healthcare worker's seropositivity before they undergo exposure-prone invasive procedures.*[20,21]

The client's right to make an informed decision about treatment requires that the dental hygienist reveal *all* information that is "material" to the client's decision to undergo treatment. Risks that are material usually depend on two factors:

- The probability that the risk will occur
- The seriousness of the harm that may result

The greater the potential harm, the greater the need to disclose.[38] The client must weigh the probability and seriousness of the risk against the potential health benefits.

If a dental hygienist is HBV infected and the proposed treatment (adhering to universal precautions) is an exposure-prone invasive procedure, the treatment poses a small risk of transmission of HBV to the client. Consider that an HIV-infected dental hygienist under the same circumstances presents less risk of transmission than the dental hygienist with HBV, since HIV is transmitted less readily than HBV.[20,21] Given the knowledge of the healthcare worker's HIV seropositivity, the client has information that is material to the decision to undergo treatment. In the case of the HIV-infected healthcare professional, the risk of transmission is low, but the potential harm is great. The client can avoid the risk entirely without adverse effects by choosing another dental hygienist.[32,39]

The CDC, after evaluation of currently available data, sees no basis for recommendations to restrict the practice of healthcare workers infected with HIV or HBV who perform invasive procedures *not identified as exposure-prone,* provided that the infected healthcare provider's techniques comply with universal precautions and current recommendations for sterilization and disinfection.[20,21]

The CDC recommendations are guidelines that greatly influence regulatory agencies, organizations, and the United States Congress. Federal legislation is pending addressing HIV-1 testing of healthcare workers and the disclosure of the healthcare worker's HIV-1–seropositive status to clients. Both federal and state governments are currently debating and will most likely enact legislation dealing with HIV-1 testing and disclosure laws that may include licensure revocation, imprisonment, and fines for violations.[21]

Prior to the recent concerns regarding the HIV-infected dentist transmitting the virus to six clients, the American Dental Association (ADA) had the following policy for professional conduct related to illness and impairment. The ADA Code of Professional Conduct includes this passage:

> A dentist who becomes ill from any disease or impaired in any way, shall, with consultation and advice from a qualified physician or other authority, limit the activities of practice to those areas that do not endanger the clients or members of the staff.[38,40]

While awaiting the CDC recommendations regarding preventing transmission of HIV to clients during exposure-prone invasive procedures, two dental professional organizations prepared policy statements to provide interim guidance. The interim policy of the ADA Board of Trustees adopted after considering the case of the Florida dentist is the following:

> [The ADA Board of Trustees is] calling on HIV-infected healthcare professionals to refrain from performing invasive procedures or to disclose their seropositive status to clients until the uncertainty about transmission is resolved.[39]

The American Association of Dental Schools policy is as follows:

> Dental personnel who pose a risk of transmitting an infectious agent should consult with appropriate health care professionals to determine whether continuing to

provide professional service represents any material risk to the client, and if so, should not engage in any professional activity that would create a risk of transmission of the disease to others.[41]

Liability for Occupationally Acquired HIV

Epidemiological trends in the number of new cases of hepatitis B and AIDS in 1992 (January 1–December 12), compared to the same period in 1991, show an 11% decrease in new cases of HBV infection and a 4.3% increase in the number of new cases of AIDS.[42] The impact from immunization for HBV is having an effect. The availability of the HBV vaccine and the mandate from OSHA that dental employers must offer employees the HBV vaccine, in addition to the CDC recommendation that all healthcare workers with potential for occupational blood exposure should have the hepatitis vaccine during their period of professional education, continue to reduce the number of new cases.[20,21] The concerns about the potential for occupationally acquired HIV continue as the number of new HIV cases increase. To date, there is no proven case of dental occupational transmission of HIV when adequate precautions have been utilized. The occupational risk of HIV infection is still unclear, and until more is known, universal precautions and prevention must be part of the dental hygiene protocol.[32]

If the dental hygienist is infected within the scope of employment, the dental employer is liable under worker's compensation laws.[32] State worker's compensation may be the only method of recovery for the injured employee. Since state worker's compensation laws set fixed amounts for recovery by the injured employees and prohibit the employees from filing lawsuits against their employers, the opportunity for recovery in an occupationally acquired infection may be limited. Exceptions to the constraints of the worker's compensation laws on the amount of an injured employee's recovery may be found if the employer's responsibility in the injury was a deliberate or an intentional act.[1] If OSHA standards are not met, especially those regarding the employer's responsibility to enforce employee observance of universal precautions, the employer is exposed to the risk of legal liability.[1] Also it must be remembered that the employee will need to prove that the disease contracted is an "occupational disease" or that an accidental injury occurred, and that the transmission or infection occurred in the dental workplace while the worker was on the job.[1]

Risk Management Theory: Protection for the Practitioner and the Client

Methods designed to control or eliminate situations that can lead to a malpractice claim or OSHA citation and fine are considered to be risk management. These methods include identification and evaluation of areas of vulnerability, implementing preventive measures, providing quality care, and purchasing liability insurance.[43] On a theoretical level, risk management is the monitoring of factors that can affect the probability of facing a lawsuit.[31] To appreciate the significance of risk management as it relates to prevention of disease transmission, consideration will be given to the role of consultants, the major reasons for dental lawsuits, risk management techniques applicable to infection control, and the dental hygienist's role in risk management as a clinician, an administrator, or a manager associated with an infection-control program.

Consultants

An outcome of consumer and client protection concerns has been a new group of consultants or collaborators, the *risk management team,* which is made up of medicolegal professionals whose primary objective is to educate healthcare providers about implementing risk management practices that protect not only the practitioners but also the clients. Dental hygienists and members of the oral health team with whom they work are not immune to the risks of malpractice that threaten all healthcare providers. The concept of an ongoing safety net in place with respect to each phase of the dental hygiene care process ensures client protection and malpractice prevention.[32,35]

A new type of consultant on the dental scene working to control the risk for the dental employer specifically related to disease transmission is found in the *infection-control training team,* whose objective is to prevent OSHA citations and fines by assuring compliance with the standard by employers and employees. The consultants may provide training manuals, videotapes, compliance forms, labels for hazardous chemicals, telephone support, in-office consultations, and even a mock OSHA inspection. The methods associated with this type of consultation or in-house development of the infection control program, compliance monitoring, and related procedures also fit the description of risk management. The same methods designed to prevent OSHA citations and fines will prevent malpractice claims as well as protect the employees and the clients from disease transmission and other hazards in the workplace.

Reasons for Lawsuits

Some of the reasons for lawsuits associated with actions of the dental team in a general practice setting are listed in the Reasons for Lawsuits in General Dental Practice Settings chart, with the factors most closely associated with infection control risks specifically identified. The malpractice examples cited in the previous section concerned legal issues related to the failure to utilize universal precautions for preventing transmission of bloodborne pathogens, the failure to provide adequate client health evaluation resulting in infection, and the failure to use appropriate standards of care in prevention of autogenous or cross-infection with medically compromised clients.

Another reason for malpractice claims associated with disease transmission relates to informed consent, the legal principle associated with the client's right to make an informed decision before proceeding with treatment. The client is entitled to know the risks associated with the proposed care and the seriousness of any harm that might result. If circumstances were such that an HIV-seropositive oral healthcare provider was permitted by a review panel to proceed with an exposure-prone invasive procedure, the client would need to be notified of the provider's seropositivity in order to make an informed decision.[20,21]

Risk Management Techniques Associated with Infection Control

The dental hygienist who is responsible for the implementation of risk management techniques and tools associated

REASONS FOR LAWSUITS IN GENERAL DENTAL PRACTICE SETTINGS

- Patient's expectations are different from services delivered
- Nonsupportive behavior of oral healthcare personnel
- Failure to treat
- Failure to diagnose
- Failure to take necessary precautions to prevent injury*
- Failure to identify medically compromised patients*
- Failure to take precautions to protect a medically compromised patient*
- Performing a service that is not in the best interest of the client, or failure to perform a service that is necessary
- Failure of treatment (e.g., dental implants)
- Failure to obtain informed consent*

*Most closely associated with risks surrounding issues of infection control.

Adapted from Kramer, S. Practice management and career development strategies. In Darby, M. L. (ed.). Mosby's Comprehensive Review of Dental Hygiene, 3rd ed. St. Louis: C. V. Mosby, 1994, p. 660.

with the prevention of disease transmission should address the following points with staff members:

Good Communication. All oral healthcare professionals involved should have input in the development of a comprehensive infection-control program. Communication of infection-control measures for newly employed or temporary team members is essential. Informing clients about infection-control measures also has positive benefits. The OSHA poster entitled "Job Safety and Health Protection" (OSHA form 2203) must be displayed to inform employees of their right to a safe workplace

Proper Protocol. The infection-control program and specific protocols must be based on the ADA recommendations, CDC guidelines, and OSHA standards and should be routinely incorporated into every aspect of dental hygiene care

Staff Training and Credentialing. Training programs on the prevention of transmission of bloodborne pathogens should include epidemiology, clinical presentation, modes of transmission, and prevention of HBV and HIV infection as well as protective measures to be taken to prevent exposure. If oral healthcare team members have not had the hepatitis B vaccine during their professional education, the employer needs to provide hepatitis B antibody testing if desired; the employer is required to assume the costs associated with the hepatitis B vaccine. Instruction should also include emergency procedures, protocol to follow in the event of an occupational exposure to blood or body fluids, and waste management and hazard communication. Training for staff should be updated annually, with notification of any changes in the guidelines as they are announced

Record Keeping and Documentation. Employee positions that require exposure to blood and other infectious material one or more times a month must be documented, as well as those positions that do not include exposure risks. Specific sources of exposure should be cited also. A record-keeping system should include a confidential file for each employee that includes name, social security number, hepatitis B serostatus and vaccination records, the employee's exposure incidents, and a listing of infection-control training programs and continuing education courses attended by the employee. Demonstration of efficacy of sterilization procedures with biological monitors should be documented as part of an ongoing quality assurance program

Informed Consent. The CDC has recommended that healthcare workers who perform exposure-prone invasive procedures be tested to determine HBV (HBeAG) and HIV status. If laboratory test results are positive, the dental hygienist may continue to perform exposure-prone procedures only if permitted by an expert review panel that would require notifying prospective clients of the dental hygienist's seropositivity before undergoing the exposure-prone invasive procedure. The client's right to make an informed decision about treatment requires that the dental hygienist reveal all information that is material to the client's decision to proceed with care[20,21]

Accepted Standard of Care. "Standard of care" means consistent adherence to universal precautions for contact with all clients' blood and body fluids, which are to be handled as if they contained bloodborne pathogens. It also means appropriate use of handwashing and protective barriers, complying with current guidelines for disinfection and sterilization of reusable instruments, and care in the use and disposal of needles and other sharp instruments. In order to continue to meet the standard of care, it is essential to remain current with infection control information, since modifications in the ADA, CDC, and OSHA guidelines are to be expected.

Commitment to a risk management program associated with the prevention of disease transmission requires application of the previously mentioned risk management techniques for infection-control practices. The greatest challenge is gaining consistent compliance from all members of the oral healthcare team to universal precautions and recommendations for disinfection and sterilization of instruments and equipment. Assessment of compliance requires scrupulously monitoring infection-control practices. The entire team faces risk when one member departs from the standard of care to save time or expense. The initial professional education and specific infection-control training programs in the clinical setting are critical preparation for infection-control practices and personnel safety. Procedures must be established within the clinical environment for monitoring compliance with the infection-control policies.[20,21] Dental hygienists may be involved in the development of compliance procedures or implementation of systems to evaluate compliance because of their educational preparation and interest in the prevention of disease transmission. Monitoring compliance, keeping meticulous records, and ensuring ongoing in-service education about infection control may be the most important techniques for effective risk management in the prevention of disease transmission. Practicing risk management not only prevents malpractice claims but also, and even more important, facilitates the provision of safe dental hygiene care to consumers.[32]

POLICIES OF OSHA ASSOCIATED WITH OCCUPATIONAL EXPOSURE TO BLOODBORNE PATHOGENS AND HAZARDOUS CHEMICALS

Background and Goal of OSHA Regulations

The federal agency called OSHA is under the umbrella of the United States Department of Labor and has had as its charge or goal the responsibility of ensuring the safety and health of all employees in many work settings. The federal agency perceived a need to respond to complaints of oral healthcare personnel against dental employers for not complying with the standing infection-control recommendations and guidelines of the ADA and the CDC. The concerns of the dental employees regarding the lack of provision of a safe work environment led the administration to develop OSHA regulations as specific guidelines for dentistry. These regulations were initially developed in 1987[44] and subsequently have evolved through a series of proposals and hearings for the response of all parties concerned, resulting in the Final Rule for Occupational Exposure to Bloodborne Pathogens, published on December 6, 1991. The standard became effective on March 6, 1992. The goal remains to provide a safe oral healthcare environment for clients, staff, and providers. OSHA's specific regulations for dentistry (developed in 1988, based on the CDC and ADA guidelines) have obligated dental employers to provide a safe working environment for all employees.

Although the emphasis on the safety of oral healthcare providers has been to reduce occupational exposure to HBV, HIV, and other bloodborne pathogens, OSHA's regulations also include the right of employees to know the potential dangers and to understand how to deal with chemical hazards to which they may be exposed during the course of their employment (see OSHA Hazard Communication Regulation in this section). The very procedures that are key components of infection control, primarily sterilization and disinfection, require the oral healthcare provider to encounter hazardous chemicals, such as sterilizing agents and disinfectants.

Dental hygienists must be well versed in the regulations that relate to the practice of dental hygiene and the prevention of disease transmission. The final rule for occupational exposure to bloodborne pathogens is the most significant legal development in infection control. It is imperative that the dental hygienist be prepared to facilitate implementation of effective infection control protocols that meet the OSHA standard.

The degree of responsibility that the dental hygienist is given in the area of infection control varies, depending on the specific dental hygienist role, whether it be that of clinician, health promoter or educator, consumer advocate, administrator or manager, change agent, or researcher. For example, as administrator or manager, the dental hygienist's responsibilities include evaluation of each employee's tasks that put them at occupational risk for bloodborne pathogens, implementation of an orientation or educational program, updating such a program, and monitoring for compliance. Additionally, as alternative methods of practice are explored and instituted in a variety of settings that feature the dental hygienist as a primary care provider of preventive services, the dental hygienist would assume the responsibility of employer and would ultimately be charged

OSHA RULES AND RESPONSIBILITIES OF EMPLOYER

- The dental employer is to identify each employee's tasks and procedures where occupational exposure such as reasonably anticipated skin, eye, mucous membrane, or pierced skin (parenteral) contact with blood or other potentially infectious materials may occur (exposure determination)
- The dental employer is responsible for the development of an infection-control plan (exposure-control plan) which includes at its core universal precautions and specific controls and procedures which remove the hazards through implementation of each specific regulation of the standard
- The dental employer is to ensure that all employees with occupational exposure participate in a training program which is designed to include content and vocabulary appropriate to the educational level, literacy, and language background of employees
- The dental employer is to provide accessible, appropriate personal protective equipment (such as gloves, masks, eye protection, and gowns) and, as indicated, disposal, cleaning, repair, and replacement of such equipment
- The dental employer is to assure that the worksite is maintained in a clean and sanitary condition, with special emphasis on cleaning and disinfection of surfaces contaminated by blood and other potentially infectious materials and protocol for laundry handling. Additionally, provision of infectious waste disposal in accordance with federal, state, and local regulations is mandated
- The dental employer is to offer and assume costs for hepatitis B antibody testing, hepatitis B vaccination if indicated, and postexposure evaluation and follow-up for all employees with an occupational exposure incident involving blood or other potentially infectious materials
- The dental employer is to maintain records to include confidential medical records regarding each employee's HBV immunization status and information associated with postexposure evaluation following an occupational exposure incident; records of training session dates, participants, trainers, and summary of the contents. The employer must transfer records if the employer ceases to do business
- The dental employer is to post signs, labels, and/or red bags and red containers which indicate infectious materials or waste as biohazardous.

Biohazard

From Department of Labor, Occupational Safety and Health Administration. Occupational exposure to bloodborne pathogens: Final rule. Federal Register 56(235):64004–64182, 1991.

with meeting the OSHA standards in their entirety even if the dental hygienist has only one employee (see OSHA Rules and Responsibilities of Employer chart.)

Overview of Standard

An overview of the final rule standard to reduce occupational exposure to bloodborne pathogens and the hazard communication regulations will be presented here; specific OSHA guidelines will be included following each topic as they pertain. The standard defines bloodborne pathogens as "pathogenic microorganisms that are present in human blood and can cause disease in humans; these pathogens include, but are not limited to, hepatitis B virus (HBV) and human immunodeficiency virus (HIV)."[4]

Once the standard became final, the following timetable went into effect 90 days after publication of the rules and regulations:

- Exposure determination—90 days to implement
- Infection control plan—120 days to implement
- All other regulations—150 days to implement (Hepatitis B immunization, postexposure follow-up, controls that remove occupational hazards, personal protective equipment, housekeeping, communication of hazards, and record keeping)

For the dental hygienist who pursues the role of researcher, it should be noted that the OSHA standard includes a number of regulations directed toward HIV and HBV research laboratories and production facilities. These regulations address microbiological practices, biosafety manuals, training, protective clothing, containment equipment, ventilation, sinks, and access doors.

The OSHA Hazard Communication Regulation that has been enforced since May 23, 1988, requires:

- Dental employers to provide employee training and information regarding the dangers of hazardous chemicals present in the workplace
- Dental employers to ensure that containers with hazardous chemicals are labeled properly
- Dental employers to obtain and maintain material safety data sheets for products with hazardous chemicals

Inspections: Types, Process and Procedures, and Violation Consequences

Healthcare employers who fail to comply with the OSHA regulations could face citations and stiff fines for each infraction. Even before the standard became law (on December 6, 1991) OSHA had cited healthcare employers for violating a section of the Occupational Safety and Health Act known as the General Duty Clause, which "requires an employer to maintain a work place free from recognized hazards that are causing or likely to cause death or serious physical harm."[44] The requirement to protect healthcare workers from bloodborne disease exposure covered under the General Duty Clause has enabled the agency to inspect healthcare facilities and enforce guidelines on worker safety and personal protective equipment. After more than 150 inspections of healthcare facilities, some employers have been cited for failure to provide safe work areas, proper protective equipment, and employee training regarding infection-control procedures, and to properly dispose of waste, especially needles.[45,46]

Inspections

Of the five basic types of OSHA inspections, the two that most apply to the oral healthcare settings are the employee complaint inspections and programmed (random) inspections, the greatest scrutiny being directed toward oral healthcare settings with 11 or more employees.[47] The other three types of inspections remotely applicable to the oral healthcare setting are inspections when imminent danger to employees is perceived, inspections when catastrophes and fatal accidents occur, and follow-up inspections. The inspection process for both employee complaint and random inspections that could occur based on the final bloodborne infectious disease standards is depicted in Figure 7–19. In either situation the OSHA inspector would do the following:

- Request infection control records from the employer
- Interview employees
- Inspect the workplace (primarily direct client care areas, secondarily laundry and general housekeeping procedures and the hazard communication program)

When an inspection is generated by a complaint, the area of complaint also is inspected.

Consequences

When a violation is found during the inspection, the employer is issued a citation that could result in a fine. The written citation includes any penalties incurred and an abatement (mitigation) date, the deadline by which recommended changes must be made and fines paid. The employer then has 15 working days to reply to the citation. The options open to the employer are:

- To respond by requesting an informal conference with OSHA representatives
- To contest the citation or
- To comply with the recommended changes and pay possible fines[47]

Prevention of both random inspections and inspections generated by employee complaint may be achieved by taking advantage of the consultation service OSHA provides, which exempts the healthcare setting from random inspections. Employers may also minimize the chance of an OSHA inspection by:[47]

- Following the recommended infection-control guidelines published by the CDC and ADA
- Informing and educating employees and providing personal protective equipment
- Offering employees HBV immunization
- Facilitating open communication among employees regarding the ongoing process of infection control
- Documenting infection-control practices
- Consulting with OSHA

Although a great deal of interest has been expressed regarding the OSHA rules and regulations, practicing proper infection control is an ethical responsibility of the professional, and failure to comply can lead to much more serious consequences than a citation and fine from OSHA.

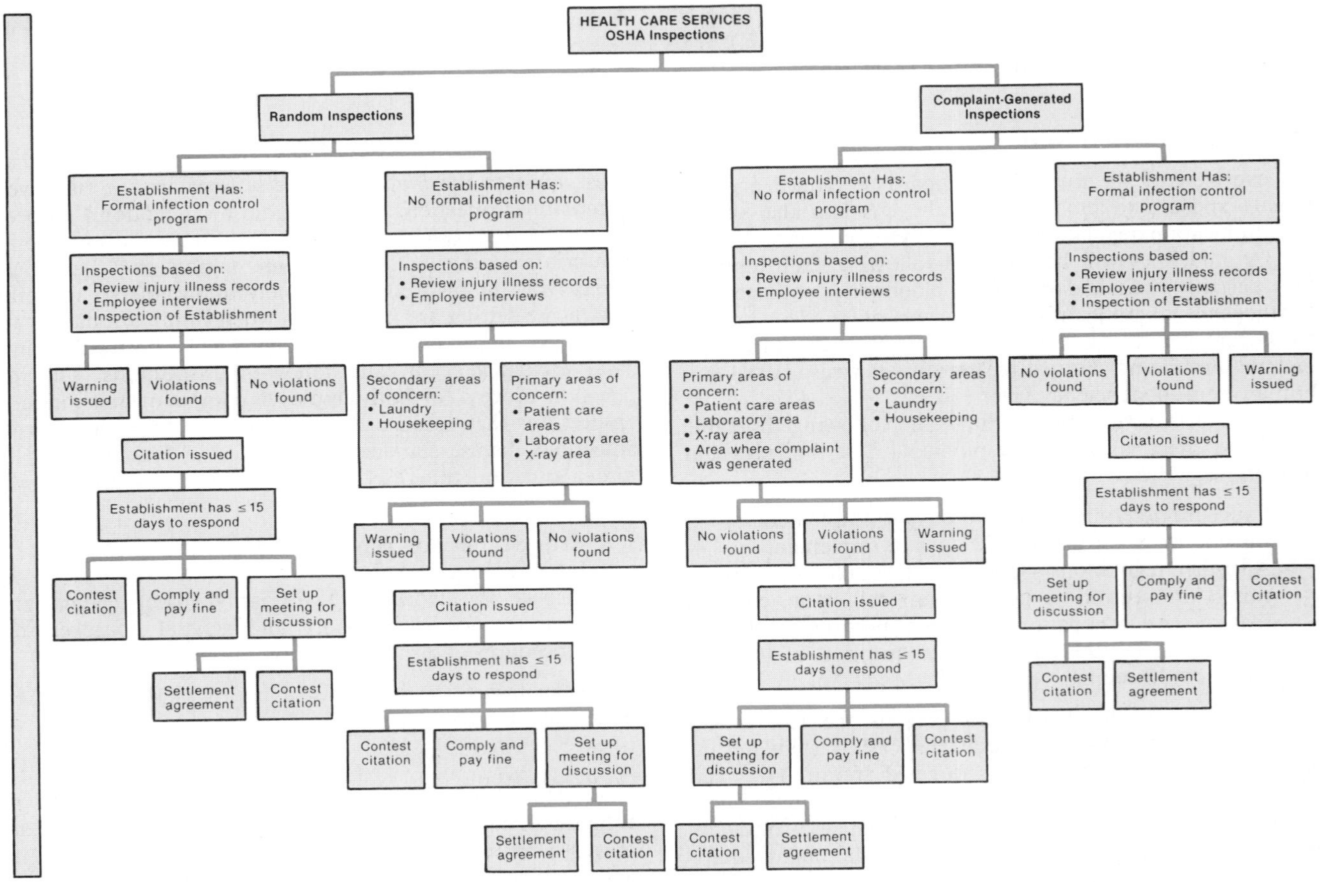

- HEALTH CARE SERVICES OSHA Inspections
  - Random Inspections
    - Establishment Has: Formal infection control program
      - Inspections based on: • Review injury illness records • Employee interviews • Inspection of Establishment
        - Warning issued
        - Violations found
          - Citation issued
            - Establishment has ≤ 15 days to respond
              - Contest citation
              - Comply and pay fine
              - Set up meeting for discussion
                - Settlement agreement
                - Contest citation
        - No violations found
    - Establishment Has: No formal infection control program
      - Inspections based on: • Review injury illness records • Employee interviews
        - Secondary areas of concern: • Laundry • Housekeeping
        - Primary areas of concern: • Patient care areas • Laboratory area • X-ray area
          - Warning issued
          - Violations found
            - Citation issued
              - Establishment has ≤ 15 days to respond
                - Contest citation
                - Comply and pay fine
                - Set up meeting for discussion
                  - Settlement agreement
                  - Contest citation
          - No violations found
  - Complaint-Generated Inspections
    - Establishment Has: No formal infection control program
      - Inspections based on: • Review injury illness records • Employee interviews
        - Primary areas of concern: • Patient care areas • Laboratory area • X-ray area • Area where complaint was generated
          - No violations found
          - Violations found
            - Citation issued
              - Establishment has ≤ 15 days to respond
                - Set up meeting for discussion
                  - Contest citation
                  - Settlement agreement
                - Comply and pay fine
                - Contest citation
          - Warning issued
        - Secondary areas of concern: • Laundry • Housekeeping
    - Establishment Has: Formal infection control program
      - Inspections based on: • Review injury illness records • Employee interviews • Inspection of Establishment
        - No violations found
        - Violations found
          - Citation issued
            - Establishment has ≤ 15 days to respond
              - Set up meeting for discussion
                - Contest citation
                - Settlement agreement
              - Comply and pay fine
              - Contest citation
        - Warning issued

FIGURE 7-19
OSHA inspection process. (Redrawn with permission from Miyasaki, C. M., Fowle, M., et al. Demystifying OSHA inspection guidelines. Journal of the California Dental Association 17[12]:28, 1989.)

PROTECTION FOR THE DENTAL HYGIENE CARE PROVIDER

Immunizations

The most important precaution for prevention of disease transmission for dental care professionals who are at documented increased occupational risk for exposure, as well as for their contacts (clients, other healthcare workers, and their families), is to be immunized (develop protective immunity for diseases they have not had or against which they have not been immunized). Even though vaccines are not available at this time for AIDS or herpes, a number of vaccines are readily available for mumps, measles, rubella, tetanus, diphtheria, pneumococcal infections, influenza, poliomyelitis, and hepatitis B (Fig. 7-20).

The protection offered to oral healthcare professionals by immunization is paramount. However, vaccines alone do not offer total protection. Therefore, additional mechanisms for minimizing the risk of disease transmission for the dental hygiene care provider are addressed in this section, including handwashing, gloves, masks, eyewear, faceshields, and gowns.[1,48]

There are three stages of immunizations:[1,21]

- Immunization that is recommended at the time of professional education for susceptible oral healthcare providers prior to any occupational exposure
- Immunization regimens that require booster doses to maintain protection
- Immunization and chemotherapeutic agents that are administered only in the event of inadvertent exposure to communicable disease

Immunization and other prophylaxis against preventable disease should be made available to all oral healthcare pro-

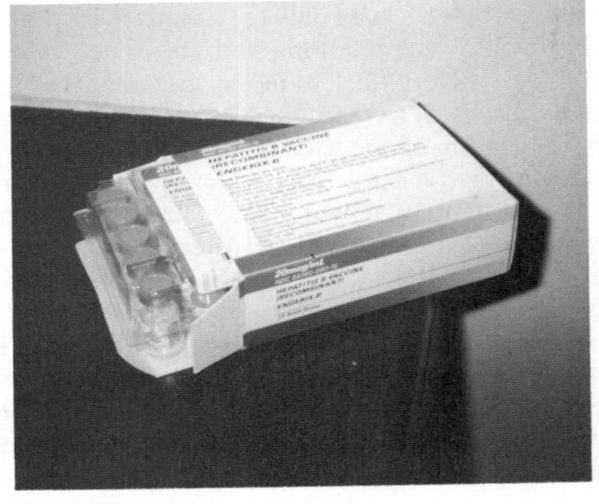

FIGURE 7-20
HBV vaccine.

viders. This saves valuable time and also averts emotional stress in the event of an exposure occurring on the job. Employers of oral healthcare personnel should request that each employee provide documentation of previous immunizations. From this history an assessment of need for additional immunizations may be made by the employer. There should be acute interest in the immunization status of oral healthcare providers in order to achieve optimal levels of protection against infectious diseases. This benefits the healthcare provider and reduces the risk of transmission to clients and family members.[1] Table 7–5 presents the recommended immunizations for healthcare providers other than the hepatitis B vaccine. Because of the significance of the hepatitis B vaccine, a more in-depth review is required.

The risk of HBV infection among healthcare workers is well established and correlates directly with the degree of exposure to blood or blood products. Consequently, HBV vaccine is recommended for all healthcare providers.[1]

There has been an estimated rise in the infection rate of HBV from 200,000 to 300,000 cases each year, and there has been a subsequent increase in the number of active hepatitis B carriers in the United States to more than 1 million.[49,50]

Association/Agency Recommendations

The ADHA advocates hepatitis B immunization for all dental hygiene students and licensed dental hygienists.[52] Hepatitis vaccine has been recommended by the ADA for all dental personnel since 1982. The ADA recommends hepatitis vaccine for dentists, students, dental hygienists, dental assistants, dental technicians, and office support personnel.[52]

The final OSHA standard requires that employers of endangered healthcare workers provide the hepatitis B vaccine (see OSHA Guidelines for Hepatitis B Vaccine chart).

Development of the Vaccine

Development of an effective vaccine to protect against hepatitis B began with identification of the hepatitis B surface antigen in the 1960s. As a result of encouraging clinical trials performed in more than 19,000 individuals since 1975, the plasma-derived vaccine (Heptavax-B) was licensed and introduced in the United States in 1982. This vaccine was the first clinically available vaccine derived from human sources. By the fall of 1982, however, concerns about the possibility of HIV infection from the vaccine were raised. Since that time numerous investigations and scientific publications have clearly demonstrated that the hepatitis B vaccine does not pose any risk for acquiring HIV infection, AIDS, or viral hepatitis.[49]

A recombinant DNA vaccine (Recombivax HB), licensed in July 1986, provided another clinically useful preparation as the first vaccine using recombinant DNA technology, creating an alternative to the plasma-derived vaccine. "Recombivax HB is produced in cultures of *Saccharomyces cerevisiae* (common baker's yeast) into which a plasmid containing the gene for HBsAg has been inserted. HBsAg is subsequently harvested after lysis of cultured yeast cells. Purified HBsAg protein then undergoes sterile filtration and treatment with formalin before packaging."[6] The recombinant DNA vaccine has undergone three approved modifications that have made definite improvements in the vaccine's immunogenicity. The immunogenicity of the Recombivax HB vaccine is comparable to the plasma-derived preparation, inducing protective antibody production (anti-HBs) in more than 99% of healthy adults aged 20 to 39 years. A similar recombinant DNA vaccine preparation, Energix-B, has been marketed as another alternative to the plasma-derived vaccine. In 1988, studies reported differences in immunogenicity between administration of Recombivax HB and the same regimen of Energix-B. More extensive studies are needed to verify these results. Recombinant hepatitis B vaccine should not be considered a generic vaccine at this time, as the effect of 1 μg of antigen can differ greatly from product to product.[6,49,53]

Serological Testing

Hepatitis B is well established as a critical occupational hazard for oral healthcare providers, and serological testing to look for HBV markers such as antibodies to HBsAg, which indicate past infection with and immunity to HBV, has been evaluated. One study revealed that 24% of oral surgeons, 17% of prosthodontists, 16% of general dentists, and 13% of allied dental professionals had HBV markers, indicating previous exposure and immunity, which in turn will not require the recipient to be vaccinated for the HBV.[14]

Prevaccine Testing for the Antibody to HBsAg

There has been a question about whether to pretest an individual for antibodies to the HBsAg based on the issues of cost-effectiveness and false-positive results. A survey has shown that only 6.7% of vaccine recipients in dentistry were already immune.[54] Cottone[6] points out that pretesting is not cost-effective in the average dental office. Also a significant number of false-positive reports for anti-HBs individuals have been documented, particularly in a pretesting situation, which would make it appear that immunization is not warranted when, in fact, it is needed for hepatitis B prevention.[55] The OSHA standard states that an employer is not permitted to require prevaccine testing prior to hepatitis B vaccination.[4]

Vaccine Administration

The injection regimen for all the vaccines requires three separate intramuscular injections: the first two doses 1 month apart and the third dose at 6 months (0, 1, 6 months). The site of injection should be the deltoid muscle of the arm, because studies indicate that anti-HBs seroconversion discrepancies occur when the buttocks is the site of the hepatitis B vaccine injection.[56] Oral healthcare providers who received the vaccine series in the buttocks for any or all of the injections should have serological testing for anti-HBs.[6]

Contraindications

The recombinant DNA vaccines (Recombivax HB and Energix-B) are contraindicated for use when individuals are hypersensitive to yeast or any component of the vaccine. The alternative immunization would be the plasma-derived vaccine (Heptavax-B).[6,53]

While immunizations during pregnancy have not been routinely recommended, pregnancy should *not* be consid-

TABLE 7–5
ADDITIONAL RECOMMENDED IMMUNIZATIONS FOR HEALTHCARE PROVIDERS

Vaccine Preventable Diseases	Immune Status Determination Prior to Vaccination	Vaccine of Choice	Contraindications	Postvaccination Side Effects/Complications	Boosters
Mumps	Persons born before 1956 are generally considered to be immune	Measles, mumps, and rubella (MMR) (live virus). One-time immunization, any time from 15 months of age	Immunocompromised persons; persons with anaphylactic hypersensitivity to neomycin or eggs; pregnant persons (pregnancy should be prevented for 3 months after vaccination)	Adverse clinical reactions are rare. Other than reports of burning and/or stinging of short duration at the injection site, infrequent reactions are malaise, sore throat, headache, fever, and rash	No booster required
Measles (rubeola)	Persons born before 1956 are generally considered to be immune	MMR combined or measles vaccine (live virus vaccine); if person was vaccinated between 1963 and 1967 with killed measles vaccine, should be reimmunized with live virus vaccine; if susceptible, nonpregnant, and exposed, may be protected if immunized within 72 hours of exposure	Live attenuated virus vaccine should not be given to immunocompromised or pregnant persons	5–15% of the vaccine recipients develop symptoms of attenuated measles; a transient rash may occur with about 5% of vaccines	No booster required
German measles (rubella)	Univeral immunization, especially for unimmunized women of child-bearing age if no laboratory evidence of immunity. If not immunized, provider could transmit rubella to associates and clients, some of whom might be pregnant (rubella is associated with serious birth defects)	Live attenuated rubella virus prepared in human cell cultures. Rubella vaccine may be given at any age. MMR combination may be used, since administration of vaccine to persons already immune is not deleterious	Immunocompromised persons; persons with anaphylactic hypersensitivity to neomycin or eggs; pregnant persons (pregnancy must be prevented for 3 months after vaccination because of risk of infecting fetus)	Infrequent complications in healthy persons; may experience joint pain (40%); rarely will arthralgias persist for up to 10 days	No booster required

Tetanus and diphtheria (Td)	Essentially no natural immunity to tetanus toxoid; even individuals with a previous history of tetanus should receive immunization	Tetanus-diphtheria (adult); vaccine series requires 2 doses of Td toxoids 4–8 weeks apart, followed by a third dose 6–12 months after the second	Individuals with a history of neurological or hypersensitivity reaction after previous dose	Some individuals have had neurological or hypersensitivity reactions; if boosters are given at a greater frequency than the recommended 10-year interval, tetanus toxid can cause severe local pain and swelling	Td booster every 10 years
Poliomyelitis	Immunization recommended for all—oral poliovirus vaccine (OPV) if younger than 18 years of age, or *any age* if direct contact with a case of polio; otherwise inactivated poliovaccine (IPV) for persons older than 18 years of age	Oral, attenuated OPV (live attenuated virus) requires two doses 2–8 weeks apart, followed by a third dose 6–12 months after the second; IPV requires three doses 3–4 weeks apart, followed by a fourth dose 6–12 months after the third	OPV: immunocompromised persons or those with immunocompromised family members; persons with hypersensitivity to neomycin	OPV: persons older than 18 years of age are at slightly increased risk for vaccine-associated paralysis; virus may be shed after OPV, inadvertently exposing immunocompromised contacts to live vaccine virus	OPV or IPV boosters are recommended only for persons who have had direct contact exposure with oral secretions or feces of a person with poliomyelitis
Influenza	Virus content of vaccine is revised annually to include the new strains expected to be prevalent; the multitude of influenza viruses precludes attaining immunity to all	Influenza vaccine formulated annually after season's particular virus identified; yearly fall immunization recommended	Anaphylactic hypersensitivity to eggs	Local tenderness at injection site for 1 or 2 days (33%); malaise and low-grade fever for up to 2 days (infrequent) (viruses in vaccine not infectious, will not cause influenza); hypersensitivity (rare)	Temporary immunity requires annual reimmunization with vaccine incorporating new strains of virus

Data from Cottone et al.[1]; Knoben et al., 1988; MacDonald[53]; PDR, 1990.

ered a contraindication for hepatitis B vaccination. The CDC report that the vaccination should pose no risk to either the woman or the fetus, based on the fact that both forms of the vaccine contain only noninfectious HBsAg particles.[57] The final decision regarding vaccination during pregnancy should be made in consultation with the woman's obstetrician.

Postimmunization Serological Testing

Posttesting following the hepatitis vaccine to ensure a positive response to the vaccine should be done soon after the last inoculation to determine the presence of appropriate antibody levels to be sure the individual is no longer susceptible to the disease. Specific posttesting recommendations vary from 6 weeks,[53] to 1 to 3 months,[14] and to within 6 months.[6] When too much time has lapsed after the vaccine administration, the results of the serological testing are difficult to interpret. If the individual's antibody levels are below the level for protection against the clinical disease, a fourth dose should be administered, with retesting after 1 month. Should the antibodies continue to be deficient, the three-dose series should be repeated.[58]

Boosters

The question of antibody persistence or continued protection from the vaccine's maintaining a detectable antibody titer is still being reviewed. Currently the CDC state that protection lasts for at least 7 years; therefore, the CDC do not promote routine yearly testing for anti-HBs following vaccination. The issue of recommendations for, and associated time intervals of, a hepatitis vaccine booster needs to be assessed as additional information becomes available. Currently the CDC Advisory Committee on Immunization Practices is not advocating a booster dose but is reviewing data as time passes and as the length of the postvaccine interval increases. To date, no one who has received either the plasma-derived or the recombinant vaccine licensed in the United States and who was immunocompetent has developed clinical hepatitis.

Universal Immunization

Consideration is being given to broadening recommendations for the hepatitis B vaccine to include adolescents before high-risk behaviors put them at risk for HIV infection. Individuals who are HIV positive do not respond as effectively to the hepatitis B vaccine, have a higher prevalence of chronic hepatitis, and are more frequently hepatitis carriers. Therefore, the CDC are considering a more extensive immunization strategy, and perhaps there should be a universal program for immunization for all children in the United States.[6] While this issue is being debated and evaluated, it is essential for the dental hygienist to appreciate the significance of the occupational hazard HBV presents and the efficacy of the various vaccines for preventing hepatitis B and to make use of the hepatitis B vaccine. Because of the low risks involved and the efficacy of the vaccines, the final OSHA standard for occupational exposure to bloodborne pathogens requires that employers provide HB vaccine at no cost to all at-risk employees (see OSHA Standard on Hepatitis B Vaccine chart.)

OSHA STANDARD ON HEPATITIS B VACCINE

The employer shall make available hepatitis B vaccine for all employees who have occupational exposure unless the employee has previously received the HBV vaccination series or unless antibody testing has revealed that the employee is immune or the vaccine is contraindicated for medical reasons. If the employee initially declines HBV vaccination but at a later date while still covered under the standard decides to accept the HBV vaccine, the employer shall provide the vaccine at that time. Employees who decline to accept the vaccination offered must sign a declination statement in Appendix A of the standard presented.

From Department of Labor, Occupational Safety and Health Administration. Occupational exposure to bloodborne pathogens: Final rule. Federal Register 56(235):64004–64182, 1991.

Personal Barrier Protection

After the immunization of the healthcare provider, the most significant precaution for the prevention of disease transmission related to occupational risks is the use of barrier techniques (personal protective equipment). The use of gloves (combined with handwashing before and after donning of gloves), masks, protective eyewear, faceshields, gowns, and protective clothing provides barriers to protect the easily infected sites of the hands, nasal mucosa, oral cavity, and mucous membranes of the eyes.[13,59] Information presented here on barriers includes the objective, risks, protocol for use, types, and regulations (Fig. 7–21).

Although initially the dental hygienist may consider the significance of the barriers to be predominantly occupational protection, their importance in meeting the client's

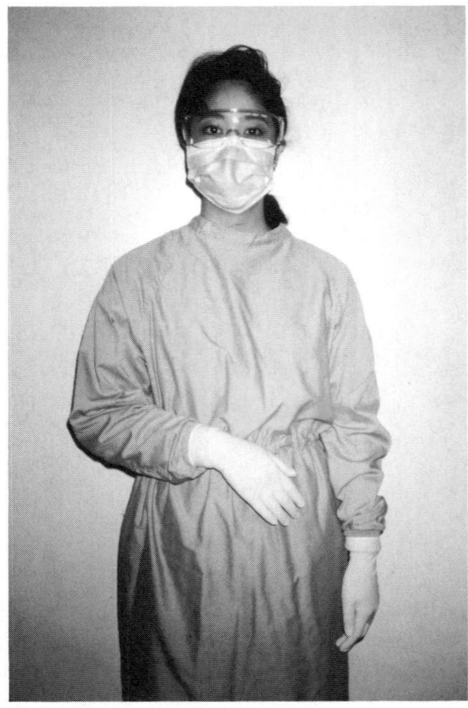

FIGURE 7–21
Protective barriers (gloves, protective eyewear, gown, and mask).

human need for safety and protection cannot be overemphasized. As a result of concerns about the potential for transmission of HIV infection from healthcare provider to client **(iatrogenic disease)** (e.g., the Acer-Bergalis case),[20,21] clients as consumers are generally sophisticated and appreciate the importance of these infection-control measures. Most clients are aware that the standard of care for all client treatment requires the wearing of gloves, masks, and protective eyewear regardless of the nature of the procedure or client care.

Handwashing

Objective Handwashing is an important adjunct to the use of gloves and can enhance the quality of protection for both client and dental hygienist by reducing microorganisms in the folds and crevices of the skin (Fig. 7–22). The action of lifting and rinsing microorganisms from the skin can prevent transfer of potential pathogens from one person to another [see Handwashing (OSHA Final Rule for Occupational Exposure to Bloodborne Pathogens] chart).

There are two categories of microorganisms present on the hands—resident and transient microbiota. The resident microbes are those that survive and multiply on the skin and may be found in the deeper areas of the surface epithelium. Some of the resident microbes that may be cultured repeatedly from the hands are *Staphylococcus epidermidis,* diphtheroids, and micrococci. In contrast, the transient microorganisms are recent contaminants that can survive or remain on the skin only for a limited period of time.[1]

Risks While the skin itself is a natural protective barrier and may, on examination, appear to be intact, there are microscopic breaks in the epidermis that originate from day-to-day minor trauma and provide a receptive portal of entry for a variety of viral and bacterial organisms. When there is a break in the skin, transient microorganisms may cause an autogenous infection. Occupationally, the chances of infection for the dental hygienist increase with the number and variety of microorganisms present in the bacterial plaque, saliva, and blood that are routinely associated with most dental hygiene procedures.[1,16,22,59]

Although gloves play a critical role in preventing transmission of pathogens by direct and indirect contact, they do not preclude the need for routine handwashing. Washing hands prior to donning gloves minimizes the number of microorganisms that will be enclosed in the warm, moist gloved environment, which is conducive to the rapid multiplication of bacteria and yeast (incubator effect). The preparation for gloving by suggested handwashing procedures helps protect the client from the dental hygienist's endogenous (resident) and transient flora being transmitted to the client should there be a defect or break (tear or puncture) in a glove during dental hygiene care (Fig. 7–23). The perforation or tear would also permit microorganisms to be transferred from the client to the dental hygienist; thus, handwashing after careful removal of gloves is imperative. Generally, the defects previously mentioned are not obvious on inspection but will be present in 1.5 to 9% of unused gloves.[60] Should a visible tear, cut, or puncture of a glove occur during care, the gloves should be removed as soon as possible, followed by thorough handwashing and donning of a new pair of gloves prior to completing the procedure.[1,13,16,22,59]

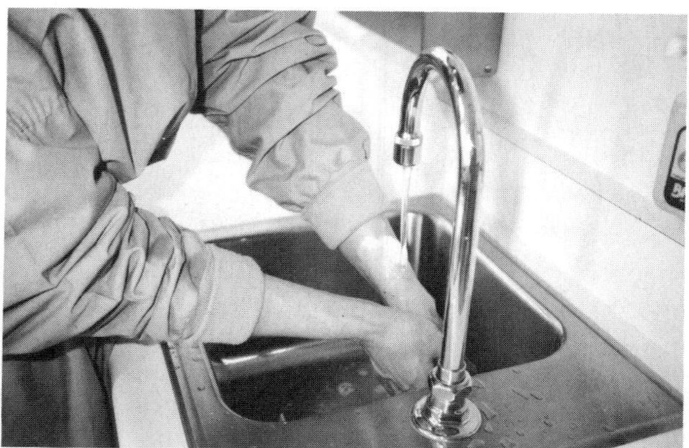

FIGURE 7–22
Handwashing at sink with antimicrobial soap.

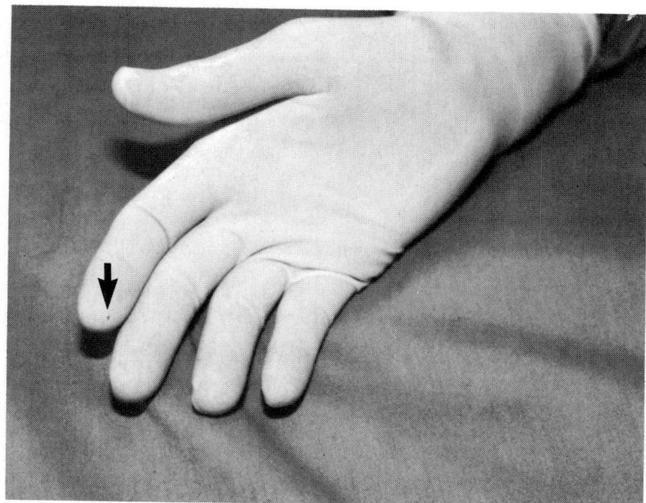

FIGURE 7–23
Tear in glove compromising protective barrier.

Protocol There are a variety of handwashing techniques, the two major techniques most frequently described in the literature being the surgical hand scrub and a shortened version or method for pre- and postdonning of gloves when client care does not involve surgery.[1,16,22] Procedure 7–1 describes the steps and associated rationale for the shortened version of the handwashing technique recommended for use prior to delivery of clinical dental hygiene care. This is the technique felt to be most effective in preparation for the work day for nonsurgical clients. It should be noted that other references may vary in the specifics of time spent lathering and the number of recommended lather-and-rinse repetitions. At the very minimum, two consecutive lather-and-rinse cycles of 15 seconds each may provide adequate handwashing according to a consensus of the Department of Veteran's Affairs, the American Dental Association, and the Department of Health and Human Services in their jointly developed instructional program "Infection Control in the Dental Environment."[22]

Additional variations are found from different sources in regard to handwashing techniques performed between clients or before and after lunch or any time hands become contaminated during the course of the day. For example, the minimal recommendation is a one-time lather-and-rinse cycle of 15 seconds,[22] with the maximum being three 10-second lather-and-rinse cycles.[1]

PROCEDURE 7–1

HANDWASHING

Equipment

Liquid antimicrobial soap
Sink with running water
Protective gloves
Orangewood stick

Steps	Rationale
1. Use a sink with cool to lukewarm running water equipped with liquid antimicrobial soap (Table 7–6) and paper towels	Running water facilitates removal of organisms. Paper towels are one-time-used disposable item
2. Remove jewelry from hands and forearms	Provides complete access to hands and wrists. Jewelry may harbor microorganisms, perforate gloves, thereby compromising glove protection. Even a smooth band may harbor microorganisms

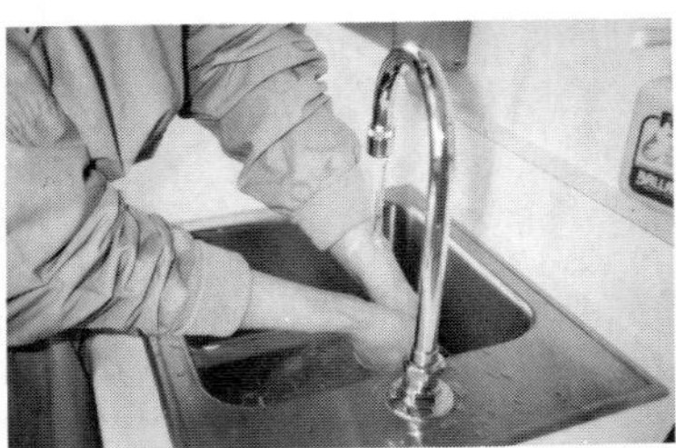

Steps	Rationale
3. Keep fingernails short and filed	Fingernails are common areas for dirt, sediment, secretions, and associated microorganisms to be harbored. Long fingernails can perforate gloves and impinge on the client's sensitive mucosa
4. Inspect the surface of the hands for any cuts or abrasions, sores, or hangnails in the skin or cuticles	Cuts or wounds can harbor high concentrations of microorganisms. Such lesions may serve as portals of exit, increasing a client's exposure to infection, or as portals of entry, increasing the dental hygienist's risk of acquiring an infection. If hands exhibit exudative lesions or weeping dermatitis, the CDC recommend refraining from direct or indirect contact with blood and saliva

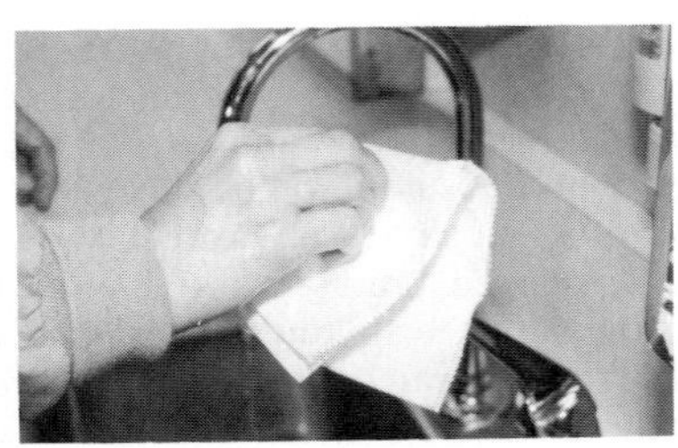

Steps	Rationale
5. Stand in front of the sink, keeping hands and protective clothing away from the sink surface. (If hands touch the sink during handwashing, repeat the process)	The benefits of handwashing can be negated by touching the inside of the sink, which is a contaminated area. Reaching over a sink increases the risk of touching the contaminated edge with hands or clothing
6. Turn on the water and regulate flow and temperature, depending on the sink design, by pressing foot pedals with foot, pushing knee pedals laterally, or turning on hand-operated faucets by covering the faucets with a paper towel or by using the elbow	When the hands come in contact with a faucet, they are considered contaminated. Organisms spread easily from the hands to the faucet

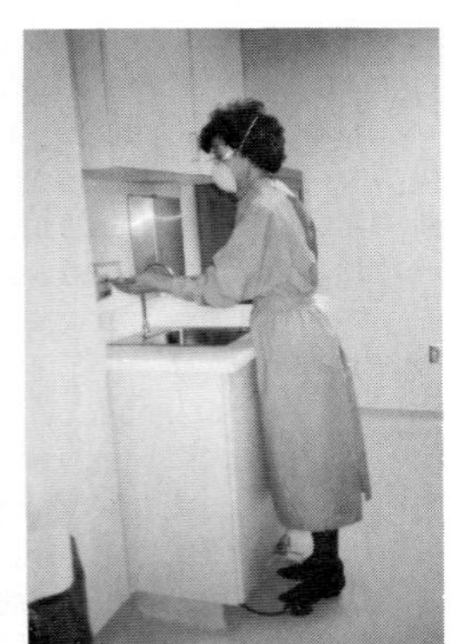

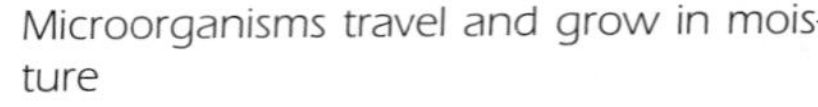

Steps	Rationale
7. Avoid splashing water against protective clothing	Microorganisms travel and grow in moisture
8. Regulate temperature of water so it is cool to lukewarm	Warm water is more comfortable. Hot water opens pores of skin, causing irritation by removing protective oils from skin, which increases the skin's sensitivity to soap. Cool water closes pores
9. Wet hands and lower arms thoroughly under running water. Keep hands and forearms lower than elbows during washing	The hands are the most contaminated parts to be washed. Water should flow from the least to the most contaminated area

CONTINUED ON FOLLOWING PAGE

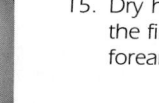

	Steps	Rationale
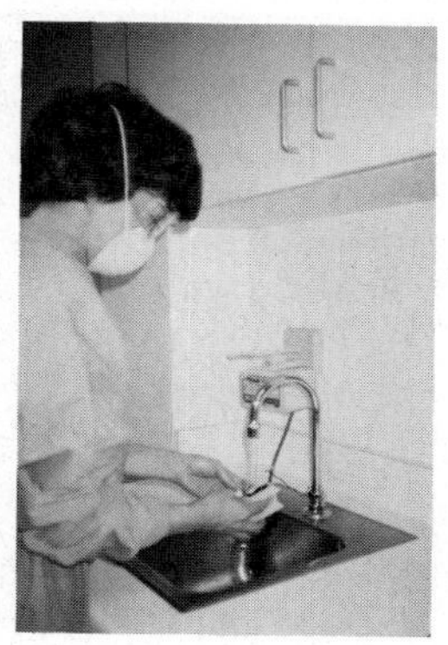	10. Apply liquid germicidal agent to hands, nails, and forearms and carefully scrub with a sterile brush for 2 minutes. Use a foot-controlled soap dispenser or a barrier such as a paper towel between hand and soap container for dispensing liquid germicide	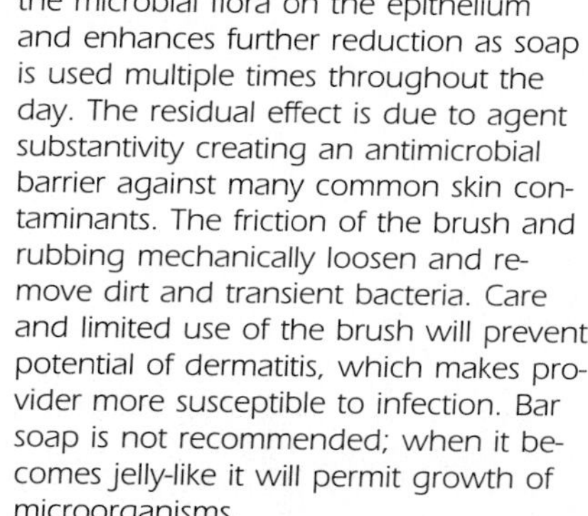 The use of germicidal soap minimizes the microbial flora on the epithelium and enhances further reduction as soap is used multiple times throughout the day. The residual effect is due to agent substantivity creating an antimicrobial barrier against many common skin contaminants. The friction of the brush and rubbing mechanically loosen and remove dirt and transient bacteria. Care and limited use of the brush will prevent potential of dermatitis, which makes provider more susceptible to infection. Bar soap is not recommended; when it becomes jelly-like it will permit growth of microorganisms.
	11. Wash hands using plenty of lather and friction for 2 minutes. Interlace the fingers and thumbs and rub the palms and back of hands with a circular motion	Friction is essential to loosening dirt and bacteria. Tests to evaluate nurses' handwashing found that the thumb and areas of the fingertips were frequently missed. Interlacing fingers and thumbs helps ensure that all surfaces are cleaned
	12. If areas underlying fingernails are soiled, clean them with the fingernails of the other hand and additional soap or a plastic or wood (orangewood) stick. Do not tear or cut the skin under or around the nail. An alternative is to use a sterile scrub brush but not more frequently than once a day	Mechanical removal of dirt and sediment under nails reduces microorganisms on hands. Blood, saliva, and plaque can contaminate the dental hygienist's hands. Fingernails are a common area for blood impaction if a glove is compromised. Blood under the fingernails is not easily removed by handwashing techniques. Skin is a natural barrier to be preserved; a minimum of brush use on hands will help prevent dermatitis
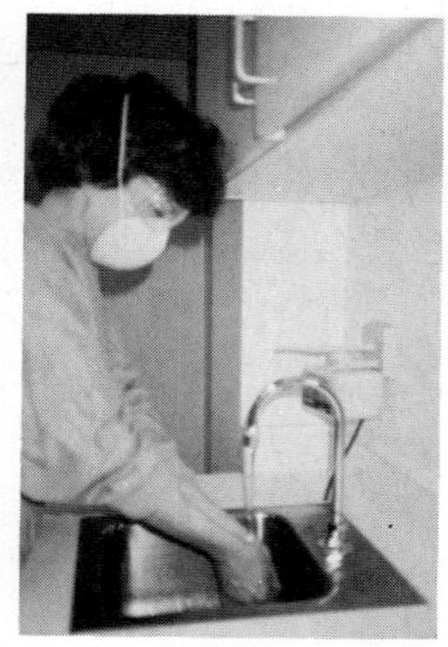	13. Rinse hands and wrists thoroughly for 10 seconds, keeping hands down and elbows up	Rinsing mechanically washes away dirt and microorganisms
	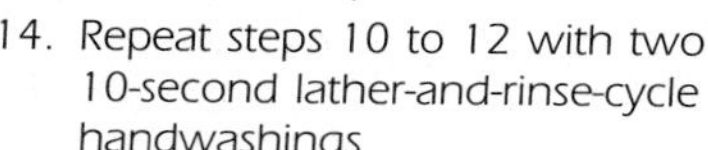 14. Repeat steps 10 to 12 with two 10-second lather-and-rinse-cycle handwashings	The greater the likelihood of hands being contaminated, the greater the need for thorough handwashing
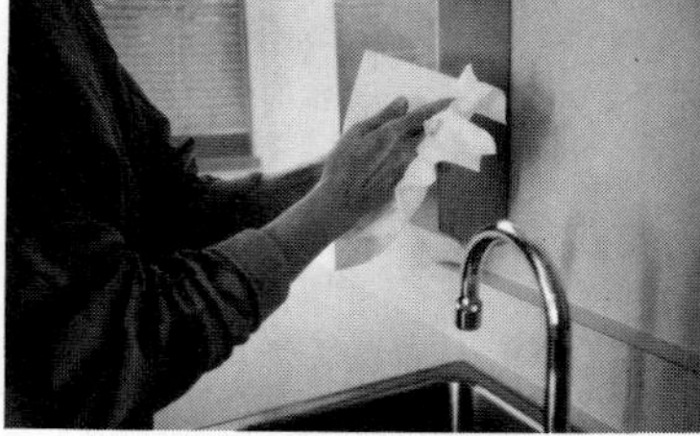	15. Dry hands thoroughly, wiping from the fingers down to the wrists and forearms	Dry from the cleanest area (fingertips) to the least clean (wrists) to avoid contamination. Drying hands prevents chapping and roughened skin. Dry, chapped hands are more susceptible to infection. Also thorough drying facilitates donning of gloves

CONTINUED ON FOLLOWING PAGE

PROCEDURE 7–1

HANDWASHING *Continued*

Steps	Rationale
16. Carefully discard paper towel in proper receptacle	Proper disposal of contaminated objects prevents transfer of microorganisms. Care must be used to avoid contaminating clean hands by touching waste bin lid or bag
17. Turn off water with foot control or knee pedals. To turn off a hand-operated faucet (hand-controlled sinks), use a clean, dry paper towel. If cloth towels are preferred, a new one must be used for each client, and it should be replaced if it becomes wet	A wet towel and wet hands allow the transfer of pathogens by capillary action
18. Keep hands and cuticles well lubricated with hand lotion or moisturizer	Dry, chapped skin cracks easily, creating a portal of entry for infection

Adapted from Potter, P. A., and Perry, A. G. Fundamentals of Nursing, 3rd ed. St. Louis: C. V. Mosby, 1993, pp. 876–877.

TABLE 7–6
ANTISEPTIC HANDWASHING AGENTS

Agents	Substantivity*	Seal of Acceptance ADA Council on Dental Therapeutics	Product Example	OSHA Identified Hazardous Chemical
Chlorhexidine Gluconate (CHX)				
Preparations:				
CHX 2%, isopropyl alcohol 2%	Yes	Yes	Bacto Shield 2	No
CHX 2%, isopropyl alcohol 4%	Yes	Yes	Cida-Stat	No
CHX 4%, isopropyl alcohol 4%	Yes	Yes	Hibiclens	No
Parachlorometaxylenol (PCMX)				
Preparation:				
0.5% PCMX	Yes	—	Vivorox-9	No
Povidone Iodine				
7.5–10.0%	Yes	Yes	Betadine	Yes†
Hexachlorophene				
3%	Yes	Yes	pHisoHex	No‡

* The ability to remain in the epithelial tissues for extended periods, creating residual antimicrobial benefit especially with CHX (Miller, C. H., and Palenik, C. J. Infection Control and Management of Hazardous Materials for the Dental Team. St. Louis: C. V. Mosby, 1994, p. 124.).

† Iodine, chemical named as one of the many potentially dangerous substances in the oral healthcare environment (iodophors are effective and usually do not irritate the skin).[1]

‡ FDA removed from the market as over-the-counter product; available by prescription only.

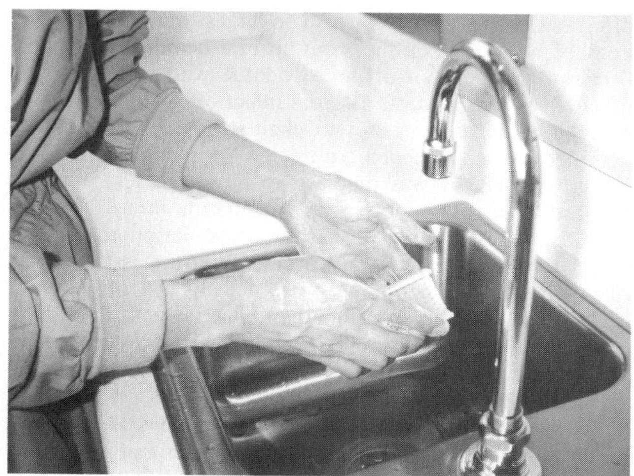

FIGURE 7-24
Surgical scrub handwashing.

Surgical handwashing obviously involves increased length of time and a more involved protocol, such as two sterile brushes for a two-step scrub coverage of hands to 5 cm above the elbow and two sterile towels, one for each hand and arm (Fig. 7-24). Cottone and associates[1] and Potter and Perry[16] recommend 7 minutes for the surgical handwashing, while the Department of Veteran's Affairs and other federal agencies recommend the 5-minute surgical scrub. The CDC do not specify an ideal time period for a surgical scrub, but they do report that 5 minutes appears to be adequate.[61] Since this technique is used less frequently, specific instructions for a surgical scrub should be posted in the appropriate sink area.

Effective handwashing before and after gloving, and prevention of contamination of washed hands by touching only sterile instruments or disinfected surfaces, maximize the benefit of gloving for the dental hygiene care provider and minimize cross-contamination (see Handwashing [OSHA Final Rule for Occupational Exposure to Bloodborne Pathogens] chart).

HANDWASHING (OSHA Final Rule for Occupational Exposure to Bloodborne Pathogens)

Methods of Compliance—Engineering and Work Practice Controls

"Employees shall wash their hands immediately or as soon as feasible after removal of gloves or other personal protective equipment and . . . wash or flush hands or any other skin following contact with blood or other potentially infectious materials."

HIV and HBV Research Laboratories and Production Facilities

HIV and HBV production facilities shall meet the following criterion: "Each work area shall contain a sink for washing hands. The sink shall be foot, elbow, or automatically operated and shall be located near the exit door of the work area."

From Department of Labor, Occupational Safety and Health Administration. Occupational exposure to bloodborne pathogens: Final rule. Federal Register 56(235):64004–64182, 1991.

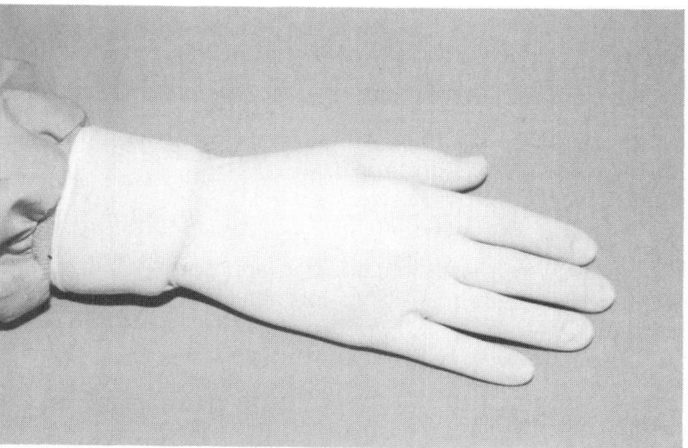

FIGURE 7-25
Well-fitted gloved hand with complete wrist coverage.

Gloves

Objective The use of gloves is an extremely effective infection-control procedure that prevents the transmission of pathogens by direct and indirect contact (Fig. 7-25). The rationale for wearing disposable single-use gloves follows:

- Gloves reduce the possibility of the dental hygienist coming in contact with blood, saliva, and mucous membranes of the client
- Gloves reduce the likelihood that the dental hygienist will transmit his own endogenous flora to clients
- Gloves reduce the possibility that the dental hygienist will become transiently colonized with microorganisms that can be transmitted to other clients. Single-use of gloves is imperative, since reuse of gloves increases infection risks for other clients[16,61]

See Gloves (OSHA Final Rule for Occupational Exposure to Bloodborne Pathogens) chart for protocol for glove usage.

Risks The specific risks to the ungloved hands of the dental hygienist are HBV, HIV, herpes, and cytomegalovirus (CMV). The numerous small cuts and abrasions on bare hands may provide portals of entry for any of the previously noted pathogens. Ungloved hands are probably the route by which dental hygienists have acquired (1) HBV from clients, (2) herpetic whitlow, and recurring herpetic lesion on the finger (Fig. 7-26), and (3) HIV. As Klein reported, one dentist, without other risk factors other than occupation, was found to be seropositive for HIV antibodies.[17] It was noted that he did not routinely wear gloves when providing dental care and additionally had a history of sustaining needlestick injuries and trauma to his hands. It must be noted that gloves do not prevent needlesticks or instrument punctures; in this case other measures must be taken (see Chapter 8 for local anesthetic administration implementation, and Chapter 9 for instrument handling and recirculation). Gloves do protect the hands when touching blood or other body fluids, mucous membranes, or nonintact skin of all clients and when handling items or surfaces contaminated with blood and saliva. High concentrations of cytomegalovirus (DNA family, herpesvirus group) have been found in saliva and are linked to birth

GLOVES (OSHA Final Rule for Occupational Exposure to Bloodborne Pathogens)

Methods of Compliance—Personal Protective Equipment, Provision, and Use
Gloves must be provided by employer

Accessibility
Gloves must be readily accessible in appropriate sizes whenever there is potential for occupational exposure to bloodborne pathogens. Hypoallergenic gloves, glove liners, powderless gloves, or other similar alternatives must be readily accessible for employees who are allergic to the gloves normally provided

Glove Use
Gloves shall be worn when the employee has potential for direct contact with blood, other potentially infectious material, mucous membranes, nonintact skin, and when handling items or surfaces soiled with blood or other potentially infectious materials

Disposable (Single-Use) Gloves
Disposable (single-use) examination or surgical gloves shall be replaced as soon as feasible when visibly soiled, torn, or punctured, or when their ability to function as a barrier is compromised. *They shall not be washed or disinfected for reuse*

Utility Gloves
Utility gloves may be decontaminated (disinfected) for reuse if the integrity of the glove is not compromised. However, they must be discarded if they are cracked, peeling, discolored, torn, punctured, or exhibit other signs of deterioration

From Department of Labor, Occupational Safety and Health Administration. Occupational exposure to bloodborne pathogens: Final rule. Federal Register 56(235):64004–64182, 1991.

defects, another significant reason for glove use as barriers for the hands.

Clients are protected when the dental hygienist dons disposable single-use gloves because they are at risk for HBV, HIV, and herpesvirus as well. The largest documented outbreak of HBV transmitted from an oral healthcare provider to clients involved an ungloved dentist who infected 55 of his clients;[2] the hepatitis B cross-infection from the dentist resulted in the deaths of two clients. The Florida dentist identified as the probable source of cross-infection of six clients with HIV-1 was reported to have had less than the standard-of-care infection control program in his practice; while the precise mode of disease transmission to the five clients remains uncertain (barrier techniques were reportedly used, but the techniques were not always consistent or in compliance with recommendations), the dentist was not routinely changing gloves for each client. Also herpes simplex virus cross-infection from a dental hygienist in Pennsylvania to 20 clients has been reported.[2,62]

Next to immunization, gloves offer the dental hygienist the most significant barrier to disease transmission, protecting both the dental hygienist and the client from cross-infection.

Types of Gloves There are four types of gloves from which the dental hygienist may select, depending on the specific client care procedure or services to be performed.

Single-Use Nonsterile "Examination" Gloves. The glove type with the greatest volume of use predominantly by the oral healthcare providers during the course of the work day (Fig. 7–27). This glove provides an adequate level of protection for most procedures. "Examination" type gloves are manufactured in either latex or vinyl. Vulcanized or "Straight Dip" latex gloves are preferred over vinyl unless the dental hygienist has a latex allergy (latex allergy should be verified by a dermatologist). The vulcanized latex gloves have minimal manufacturing defects and offer greater elasticity and better fit than does vinyl. A nonvinyl alternative for the dental hygienist with latex sensitivity would be to acquire hypoallergenic gloves (Fig. 7–28)[3,22]

Single-Use Sterile "Surgical" or "Surgeon's" Gloves. Recommended for periodontal and oral surgical procedures because these procedures involve contact with areas of the body that normally are sterile. Sterile surgeon's gloves are available in latex, vinyl, and hypoallergenic materials (Fig. 7–29)

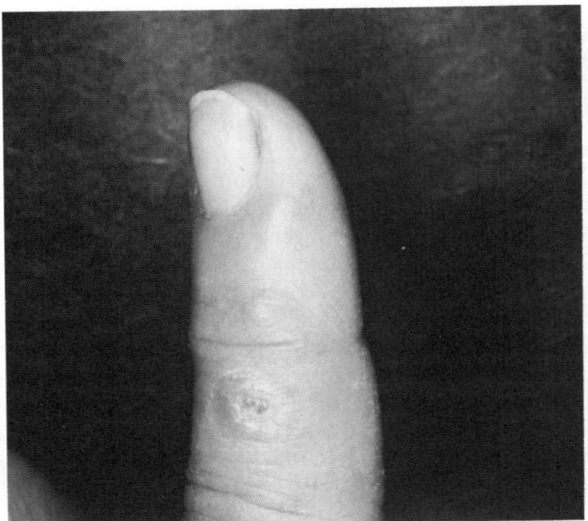

FIGURE 7–26
Herpetic whitlow on index finger.

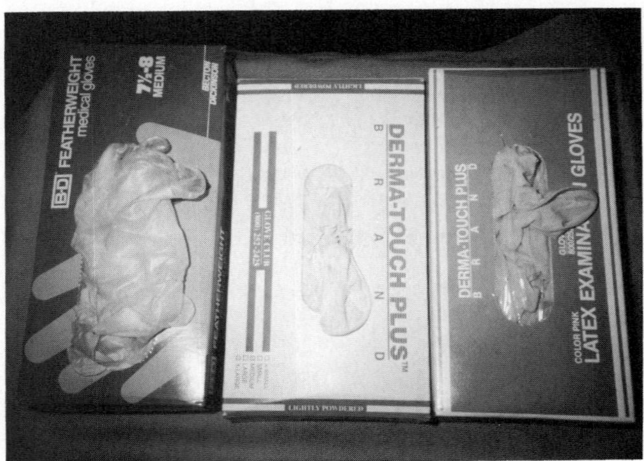

FIGURE 7–27
Single-use nonsterile "examination" gloves.

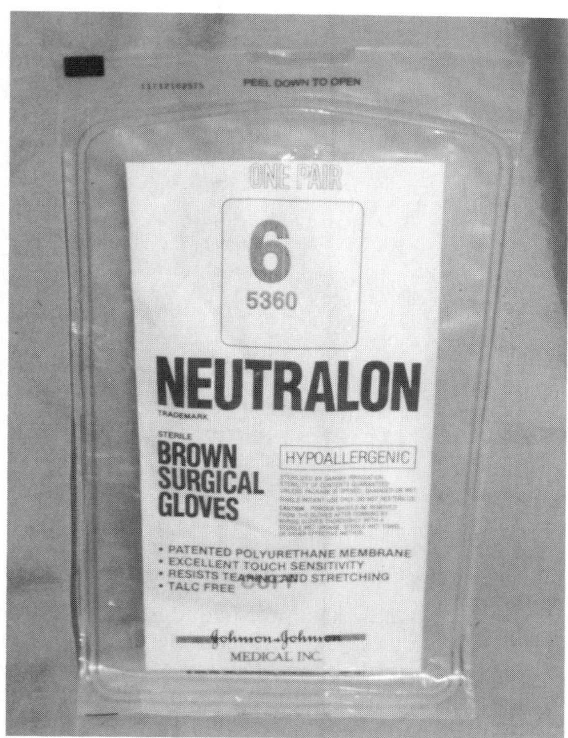

FIGURE 7-28
Hypoallergenic gloves.

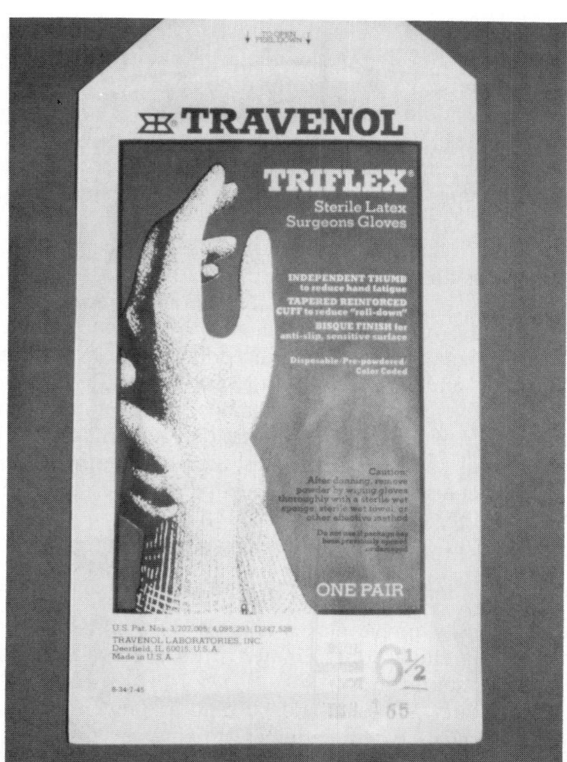

FIGURE 7-29
Sterile "surgical" gloves.

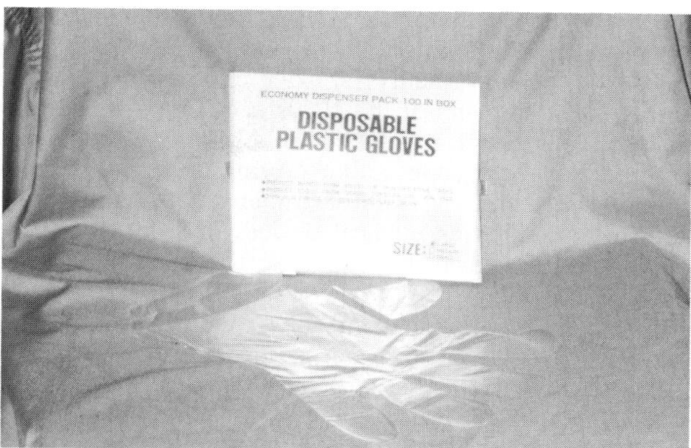

FIGURE 7-30
Nontreatment or food-handler-type gloves.

- **Single-Use Plastic Overgloves (Nontreatment) or "Food-Handler-Type" Gloves.** Slightly larger gloves that may be slipped over the "examination" gloves to prevent cross-contamination when direct client care is interrupted to record data, reference the client chart, or retrieve an equipment item or instrument from a drawer or area that is not easily surface disinfected. Overgloves are manufactured in lightweight plastic (Fig. 7-30)
- **Multiple-Use Utility, "Heavy-Duty," "Heavy Rubber," or Polynitrile Gloves.** Used for nontreatment activities that involve handling of contaminated instruments or exposure to chemicals. The objective is to protect the hands from physical or chemical injury. Heavy-duty, "puncture-resistant" gloves are made of rubber, neoprene, or polynitrile (Fig. 7-31). A significant advantage of polynitrile gloves is that they may be sterilized for reuse on a regular basis. Heavy-duty gloves are not appropriate for handling hot instruments. Heat-resistant gloves (e.g., aluminized, silica fiber, or fiberglass types) are needed for removing hot items from sterilizers[1,63]

Quality Control The quality of gloves is a concern for the dental hygienist, because leakage compromises the ben-

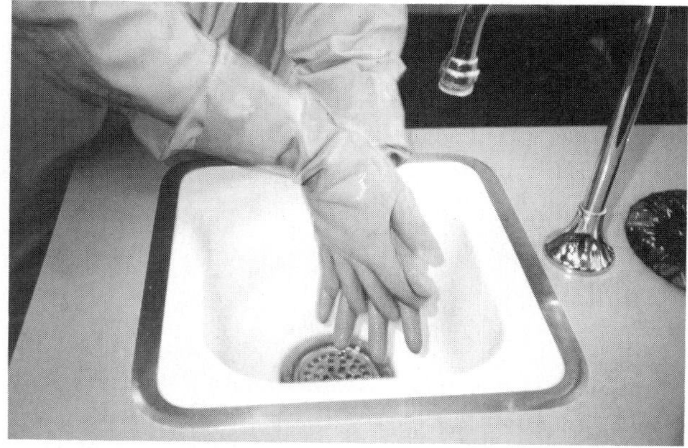

FIGURE 7-31
Polynitrile gloves.

efit of the barrier as a method of prevention of disease transmission. Pinholes exist in 1.5 to 9% of unused gloves.[60] The poor quality of examination gloves on the market in the last half of the 1980s stimulated considerable concern. This concern resulted in regulation of examination and surgeon's glove manufacturing under the auspices of the **Food and Drug Administration** (FDA) after gloves were first classified as medical devices in 1989.[64] In 1990, the FDA published a final rule (effective March 12, 1991) defining acceptable quality, glove sampling plans, and test methods. The test method for glove quality requires filling a glove with 1,000 mL of water, suspending it, and without squeezing the glove, observing it for leaks over a 2-minute period (Fig. 7-32). Rejection occurs for a manufactured lot of surgeon's gloves when 2.5% or more have leaks and for a lot of examination gloves when 4% or more leak. Many gloves manufactured currently exceed the standard of quality.[63,65] The fact that pinholes may be present in both surgeon's and examination gloves reinforces the importance of handwashing as well as the necessity of changing gloves for each client, because microorganisms may enter the pinholes, enter into small cuts or abrasions on the skin and multiply, exit through the same pinhole or tear, and enter into the next client's mouth.[1]

Some dental hygienists wear two pairs of gloves (double gloving) to reduce the chances of body fluids entering through the inherent pinholes in the gloves. Double gloving has not been part of the CDC, ADA, or OSHA guidelines or recommendations and may be considered "overkill." The double thickness of latex reduces dexterity and increases expense. Current standards have increased the quality of gloves manufactured, which should decrease the concerns about defects and protection. If double gloving is preferred by the dental hygienist, it should be done universally and not selectively, based on a client's health history.[65]

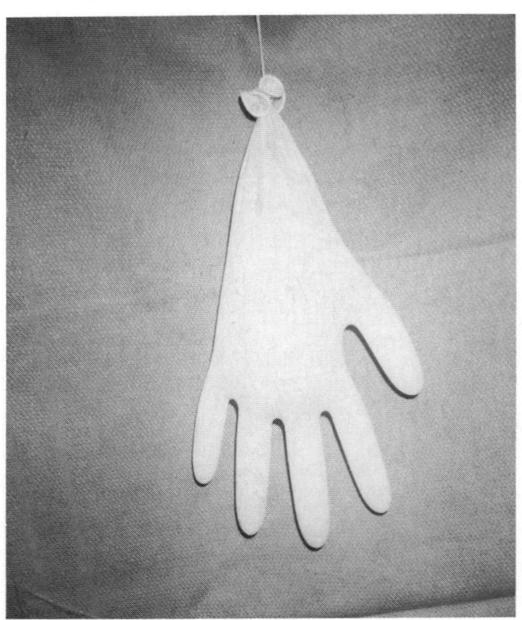

FIGURE 7-32
Glove filled with 1,000 mL of water and suspended for testing and observation of leaks.

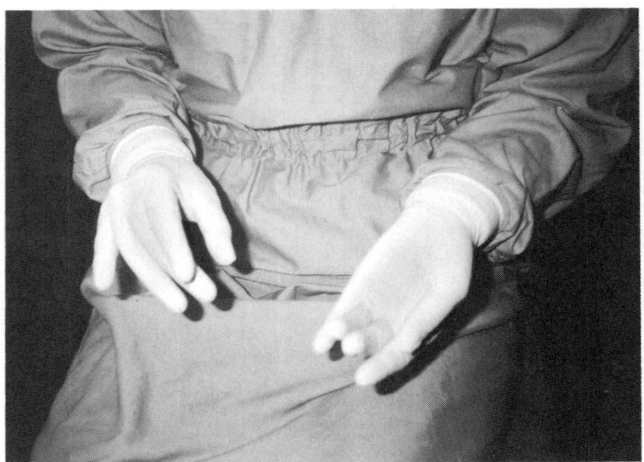

FIGURE 7-33
Latex gloves representing good fit and coverage.

Protocol for Maximizing Effectiveness and Minimizing Cross-Contamination with Gloves

- Use proper handwashing techniques (see previous section for rationale and techniques) prior to donning gloves, an antimicrobial soap and cool to lukewarm water, followed by a thorough drying. Remove rings to prevent puncturing of gloves and harboring of microorganisms
- Gloves must be worn whenever contact with blood, saliva, mucous membranes, or contaminated equipment or surfaces is anticipated
- Use gloves that fit well (Fig. 7-33). Latex gloves are preferred over vinyl because they provide maximum elasticity with less tendency to tear or break
- Gloves should cover the cuffs of the long sleeves of protective clothing of the dental hygienist[66]
- Gloves must be changed for each client[66]
- Gloves should be changed during long appointment procedures. Defects in gloves dramatically increase when they are used beyond 60 minutes. Also, moisture accumulates between the gloves and the skin, causing bacteria and yeast to grow, which is a common source of skin irritation. This dermatitis has been misinterpreted as an allergic response to latex[59]
- Washing of gloves should be avoided, since washing, especially with antimicrobial soap or disinfectants, may cause "wicking," the enhanced penetration of liquids through undetected holes in gloves[67]
- Plastic overgloves must be changed for every client and discarded if torn. It is important to remember that the inside of the overgloves has been contaminated and must be disposed of along with the direct client care gloves after each use
- Discard examination or surgeon's gloves after each use

Protocol for "Heavy-Duty" Nontreatment Gloves

- Heavy-duty nitrile gloves (Fig. 7-34) should be worn when handling contaminated instruments in preparation for sterilization
- Heavy-duty gloves should be used to prevent exposure to chemicals when handling, mixing, or disposing of detergents, cleaners, disinfectants, sterilants, and radiographical and other chemicals[68]

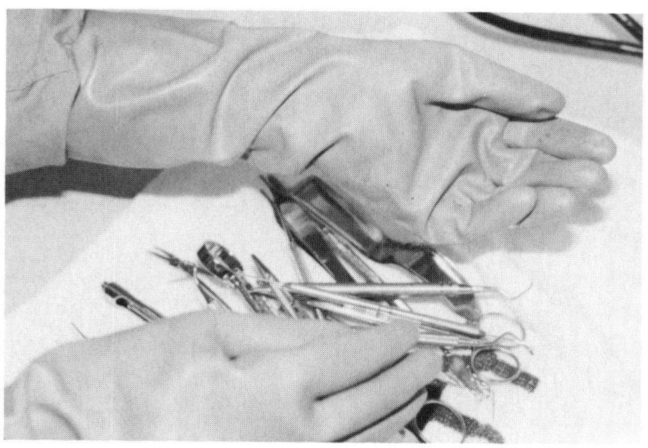

FIGURE 7-34
Polynitrile gloves worn for handling chemicals and preparation of instruments for sterilization.

- Each dental hygienist performing these tasks should have his own pair of gloves, which helps with compliance regarding disinfection, sterilization, and maintenance
- Gloves that are used to handle contaminated items should be viewed as contaminated, and the dental hygienist must take great care to avoid transfer of contamination to other surfaces. Think before you touch
- Polynitrile heavy-duty gloves should be disinfected for reuse and sterilized (autoclaved or chemiclaved) on a regular basis, a minimum of one or two times per week[3]
- Reuse of heavy-duty gloves requires monitoring gloves for tears or cracks, with discarding and replacement as needed

Masks

Objective A mask prevents the transmission of infection by protecting the easily infected mucous membranes of the mouth and nose from direct exposure to droplets (spatter) of blood and saliva (Fig. 7-35). A mask also blocks inhalation of microorganisms from a client's respiratory tract as well as aerosols, artificially generated collections of particles, solid or liquid, suspended in air and capable of airborne infection (see the section on sources of cross-infection while providing dental hygiene care, earlier in this chapter). The mask also protects the client from transmission of pathogens from the dental hygienist's respiratory tract.[1,16,22]

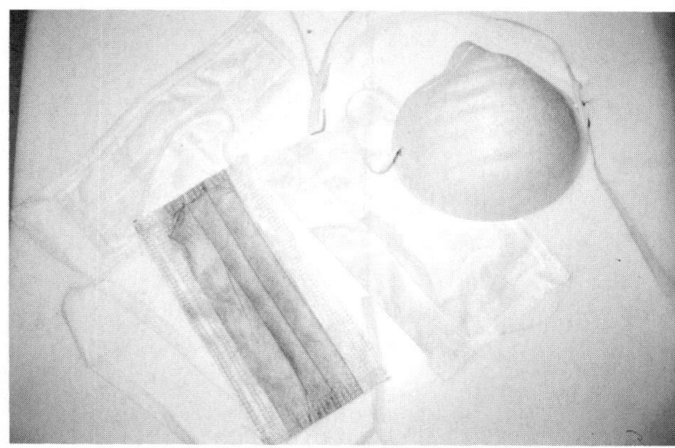

FIGURE 7-35
Assortment of masks.

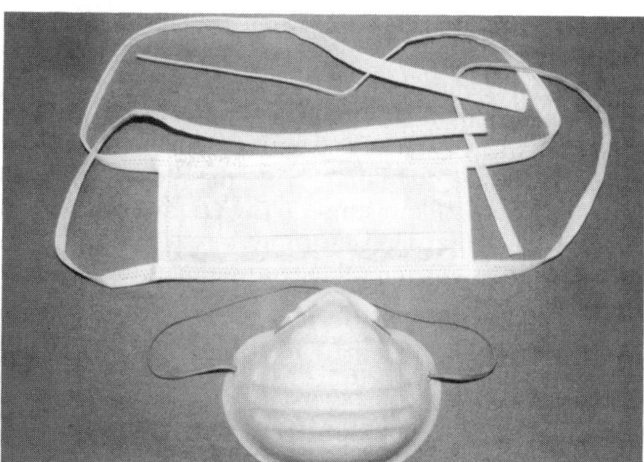

FIGURE 7-36
Two basic types of masks.

Risks to Dental Hygienists Working Without a Mask The risks from airborne microorganisms include tuberculosis and measles (HIV and HBV are not acquired by inhalation). The predominant concern is with the spatter of blood, saliva, and debris and the aerosols associated with the performance of instrumentation procedures, especially polishing, ultrasonic scaling, and use of the air-spray-water (ASW) syringe [see Masks (OSHA Final Rule for Occupational Exposure to Bloodborne Pathogens) chart]. Microorganisms found in aerosols include staphylococci, streptococci, diphtheroids, pneumococci, tubercle bacilli, influenza virus, hepatitis virus, herpesvirus hominis, and neisseria.[1]

Types The two basic types of masks are the dome type and the tie-on mask (Fig. 7-36). Masks should filter at least 95% of droplet particles 3.0 to 3.2 μm in diameter[60] (micron = .001 mm). Variation in filtering efficiencies of

MASKS (OSHA Final Rule for Occupational Exposure to Bloodborne Pathogens)

Personal Protective Equipment—Provision and Use, Accessibility
When there is potential for occupational exposure, the employer shall provide and have readily accessible appropriate personal protective equipment such as masks.

Masks, Eye Protection, and Faceshields
Masks shall be worn whenever splashes, spray, spatter, droplets, or aerosols of blood or other potentially infectious materials may be generated and there is a potential for nose or mouth contamination.

From Department of Labor, Occupational Safety and Health Administration. Occupational exposure to bloodborne pathogens: Final rule. Federal Register 56(235):64004-64182, 1991.

masks ranges from 14 to 99%; when selecting masks, maximize protection by choosing masks made of either glass fibermat or synthetic fibermat, which are the most effective filters.[1] The dome mask with an elastic band for attachment offers the benefit of greater distance between the mask and the face than that with the tie-on mask. This decreases the rate of moistness. When a mask is moist, its effectiveness as a barrier is compromised, since wet fabric serves as a vehicle for microbial transfer.[59]

Protocol for Maximizing Effectiveness and Minimizing Cross-Contamination with Masks

- A new mask should be put on for each client along with protective eyewear prior to handwashing and donning gloves
- A properly applied mask should fit snugly over the mouth and nose so that pathogens cannot enter or escape through the sides. The top edge of the mask should fit below the eyeglasses to minimize fogging of the protective eyewear as the dental hygienist exhales (Fig. 7–37)[16]
- Avoid touching the mask during the appointment, because the surface of the mask becomes a nidus (focus of infection) for spatter and aerosols (Fig. 7–38), and hands can further contaminate the mask, with fingers transmitting moisture and infectious organisms (blood and saliva)[1,3]
- If the mask becomes moist or if the procedure generates a lot of aerosols and moisture, change the mask during the procedure. Cautiously remove the mask overhead, handling it only by the elastic or cloth tie strings (Fig. 7–39). A 1-hour limit of wear for long procedures or a 20-minute limit with high aerosol generation is the time extent of the barrier's effectiveness[1,69]
- At the end of a procedure that generates heavy aerosols, keep the mask on afterwards to prevent direct exposure to airborne organisms[70]
- When appropriate to remove the mask, remove it over the head, avoiding dangling it around the neck (contaminated surface may contaminate the neck). Discard the mask with contaminated waste
- A faceshield may be worn over the mask but does not replace the mask; masks are the barrier of choice for protection from aerosols (Fig. 7–40)

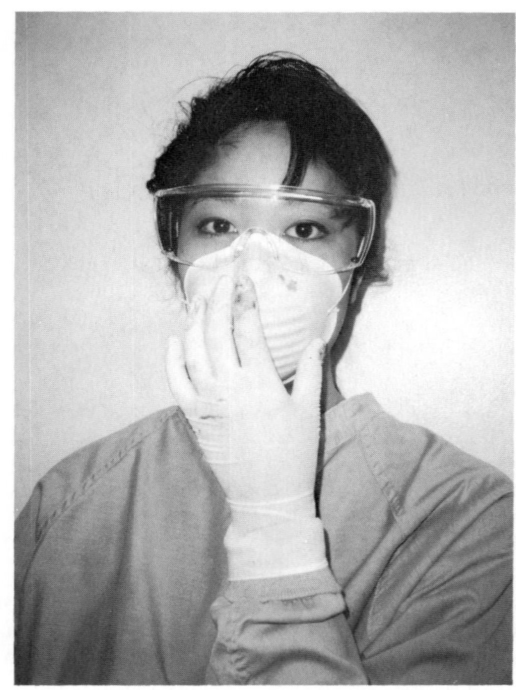

FIGURE 7–38
Visibly spattered mask demonstrating the mask as a nidus for spatter and aerosols.

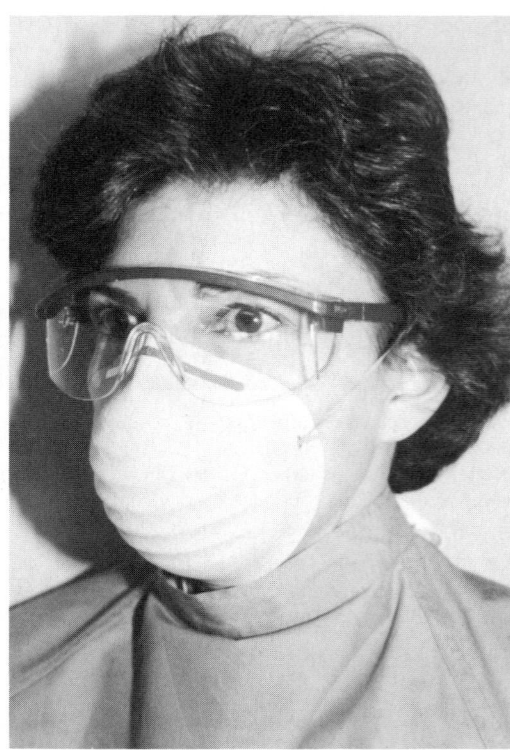

FIGURE 7–37
Close-up of properly applied mask with top edge of mask fitting below protective eyewear.

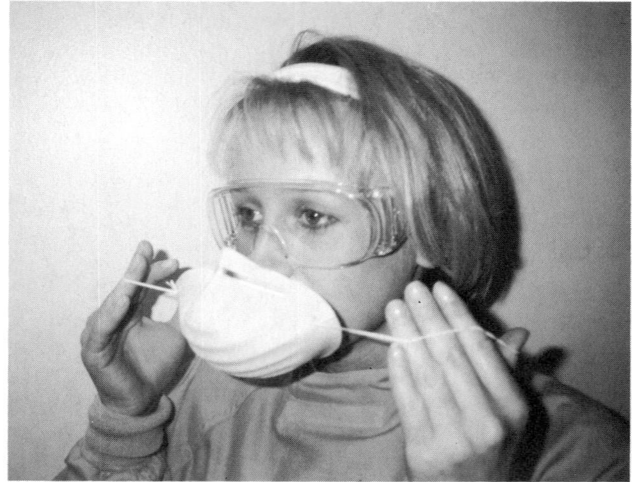

FIGURE 7–39
Remove mask cautiously, handling it only by the elastic or cloth tie strings.

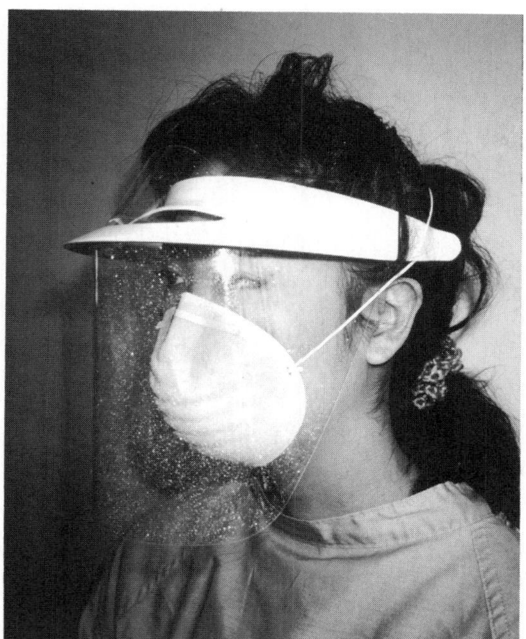

FIGURE 7-40
Faceshield worn over mask.

EYE PROTECTION (OSHA Final Rule for Occupational Exposure to Bloodborne Pathogens)

Personal Protective Equipment—Provision and Use, Accessibility
When there is potential for exposure to blood or other potentially infectious materials, the employer shall provide and have readily accessible appropriate personal protective equipment such as eye protection.

Masks, Eye Protection, and Faceshields
Eye protection devices, such as goggles or glasses with solid side shields, or chin-length faceshields shall be worn whenever splashes, spray, spatter, droplets, or aerosols of blood or other potentially infectious materials may be generated and there is a potential for eye contamination.

From Department of Labor, Occupational Safety and Health Administration. Occupational exposure to bloodborne pathogens: Final rule. Federal Register 56(235):64004–64182, 1991.

Eye Protection

Objective The objective of protective eyewear (Fig. 7–41) is to provide a barrier for the eyes and mucous membranes against microbial injury, physical projectiles, and chemical damage during client care, laboratory procedures, or the handling of chemicals.[22,48]

Risks of Eye Exposure to Debris, Blood, Body Fluids, and Chemicals

- Debris caused by rotary instruments and scaling procedures can cause penetrating injuries that may result in the initial damage of the penetration, infection caused by microorganisms on the projectile, or a secondary injury related to the surgical procedure for removal of the object[48]
- Microorganisms on the debris and within the blood and body fluids may cause conjunctivitis, hepatitis B, or ocular herpes, which is second only to injury as the leading cause of blindness. The dental hygienist should not assume the absence of risk of ocular herpes if no lesion is present, extraorally or intraorally, since the virus is present in saliva prior to the onset of clinical symptoms.[71] Although no HBV infections transmitted through the human eye have been documented, it is feasible, since HBV has been transmitted to a chimpanzee via the eye route in the laboratory[1]
- Many chemicals used in the provision of oral healthcare are incompatible with ocular tissue, such as fluorides, bentonite present in some polishing agents, and solutions associated with disinfection and sterilization. When these substances come in contact with the eye, they may cause necrotized tissue and can result in permanent vision impairment[71]

Types of Protective Eyewear

- Eyeglasses that cover the entire eye orbit, with side extensions for expanded facial coverage (top and side) (Fig. 7–42), offer more protection than do regular eyeglasses, which are open on the top and sides. Occupational eyewear should also be more shatter-resistant than regular eyeglasses. Some protective eyewear may be worn over regular prescription eyeglasses[3]
- Chin-length faceshields (Fig. 7–43) provide a barrier for the entire facial area, ensuring greater coverage to

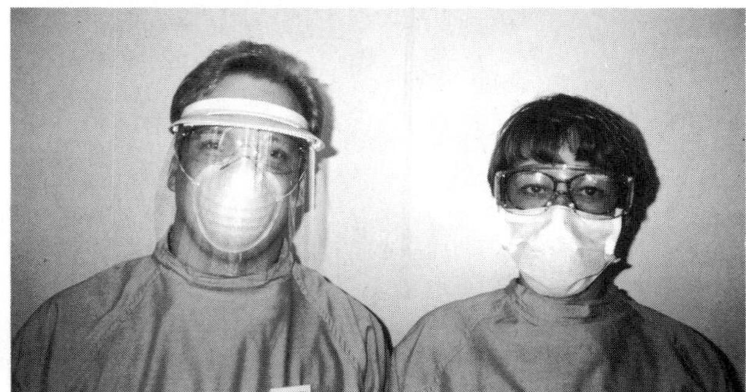

FIGURE 7-41
Protective eyewear as a barrier for eye and mucous membranes.

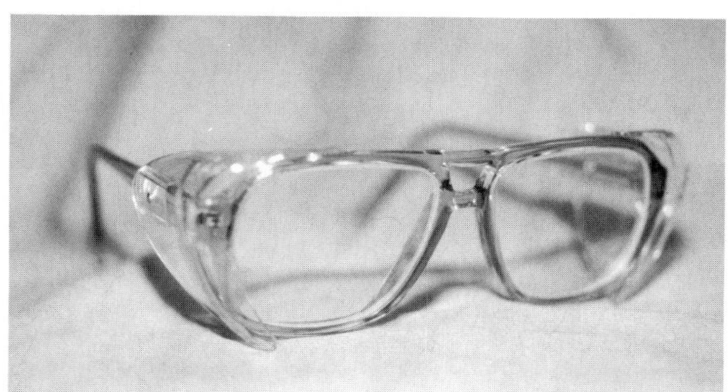

FIGURE 7-42
Protective eyewear worn over regular eyeglasses.

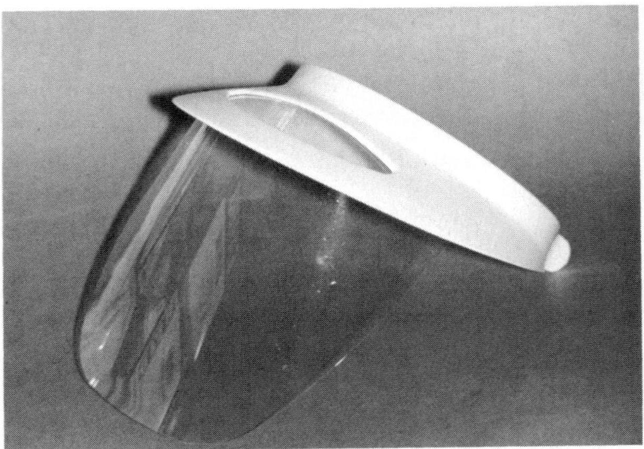

FIGURE 7-43
Chin-length faceshield.

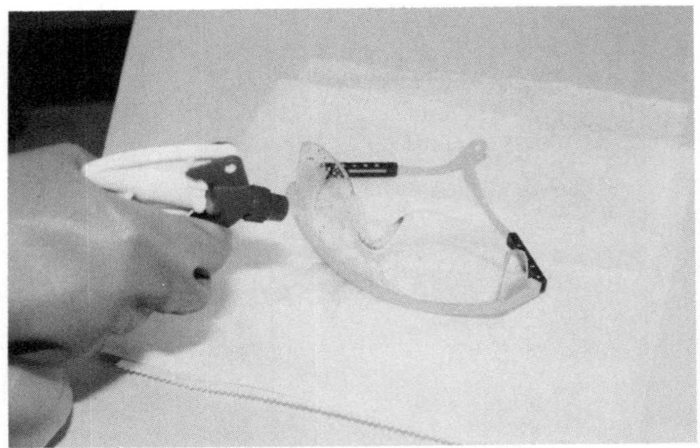

FIGURE 7-45
Protective eyewear being sprayed with EPA-registered surface disinfectant.

protect the face as well as mucous membranes from spatter and aerosols. Faceshields are an alternative to protective eyeglasses or goggles but should not be considered a substitute for a mask.[69] Masks provide maximum protection for the nose and mouth from aerosols and spatter, while faceshields do not.[72] Faceshields may be used as an adjunct to glasses and a mask for high aerosol-generating procedures (e.g., with an ultrasonic scaling instrument). Faceshield quality varies; select one that is shatter-resistant and has minimal visual distortion

Protocol for Maximizing Effectiveness and Minimizing Cross-Contamination with Protective Eyewear

- Disinfected protective eyewear or faceshields should be put on along with a mask prior to handwashing and donning of gloves for client care [see Eye Protection (OSHA Final Rule for Occupational Exposure to Bloodborne Pathogens) chart] (Fig. 7-44)
- Maximize protection by wearing protective eyewear consistently, since selective use could lead to forgetting or misplacing eyewear. Additional nontreatment eye risks in the workplace, such as laboratory procedures, mixing and pouring of chemicals, and use of disinfectants and sterilants, should be recognized[12,70]
- Avoid touching protective eyeglasses or faceshields during client care to minimize contamination of protective equipment with blood and saliva
- Both faceshields and protective eyeglasses must be able to withstand sterilization or disinfection with an ADA- or EPA-approved disinfectant (Fig. 7-45)
- Contaminated protective eyewear should be washed with soap and water, rinsed, and sterilized or disinfected between clients. Multiple eyewear should be available to facilitate decontamination and recirculation of protective equipment[1,3,7]
- Clients should be provided with eye protection (Fig. 7-46) during client care procedures. This eyewear can be tinted to decrease light glare, thus meeting the client's human need for freedom from stress as well as regarding safety

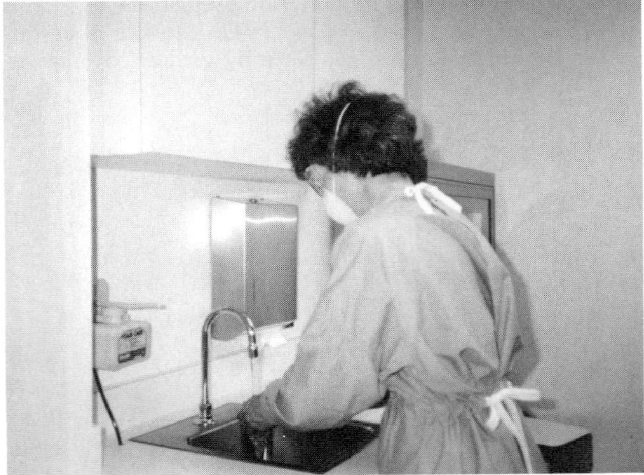

FIGURE 7-44
Dental hygienist wearing protective eyewear and mask prior to handwashing and donning of gloves.

Protective Clothing

Objective Protective clothing (Fig. 7-47) is worn to prevent contamination of skin and underlying clothing from aerosols, spatter, droplets, or sprays of blood or saliva **(bioburden).**

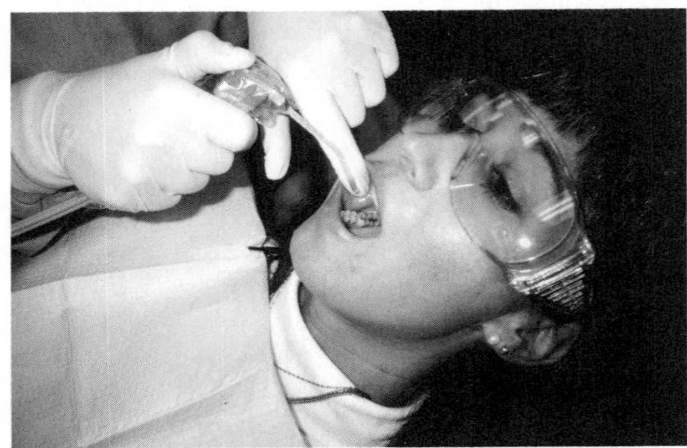

FIGURE 7-46
Client wearing protective eyewear during dental hygiene care.

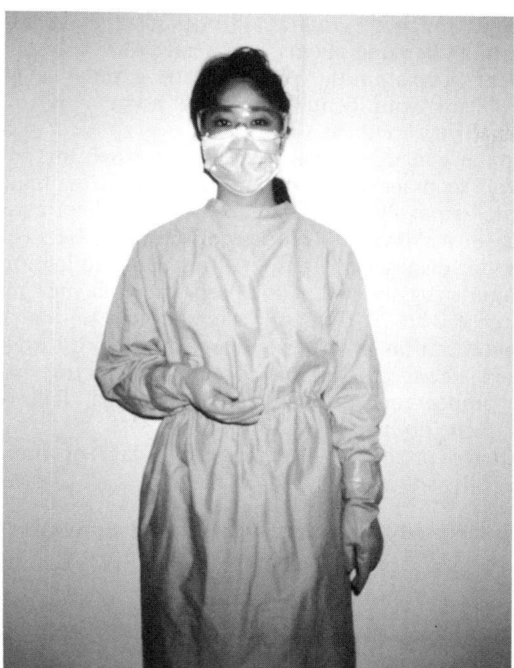

FIGURE 7-47
Clothing protecting the skin and underlying clothing from potentially infectious materials.

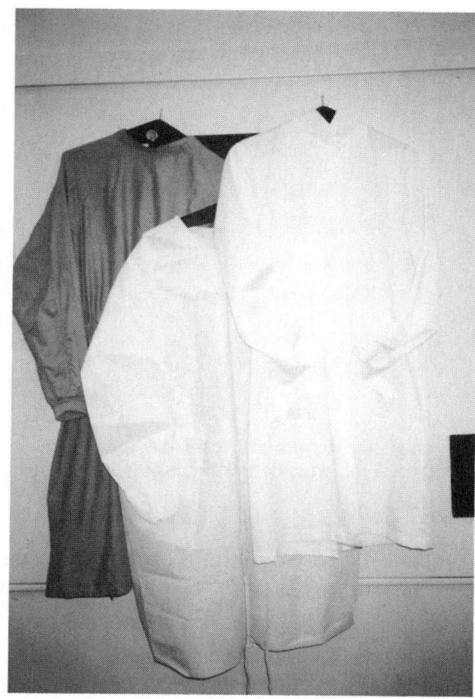

FIGURE 7-48
Assortment of disposable and reusable protective clothing.

Risks in Exposure of Skin and Underlying Clothing to Blood and Other Potentially Infectious Materials In the recent past, it had become fashionable not to provide client care in a clinic gown, but authorities are once again emphasizing the need for this type of clothing. The risks involved in practicing without protective attire are not as clear-cut as those for the absence of gloves, mask, and protective eyewear.

Although large numbers of certain pathogenic microorganisms have been found on soiled linen, the actual risk of disease transmission is negligible.[13] Concerns for the families of dental hygienists have been raised as well when the dental hygienist returns home after providing client care in clothing not protected by gowns, aprons, uniforms, or surgical scrubs. The greatest risk is the exposure of nonintact skin to blood and/or saliva and associated pathogens. The CDC report that clothing exposed to HIV may be safely used after a normal laundry cycle.[13] The primary objective of providing a protective barrier for the skin, together with the recognition that pathogenic organisms are present on attire worn during client care, has influenced the following protocol for the selection and handling of protective clothing, even though no documented case of disease transmission has been reported as a result of contact with contaminated fabric.

Types of Protective Clothing Two broad categories of attire are "disposable" and "reusable" protective clothing (Fig. 7-48). The benefits of reusable clothing are economic and environmental in waste reduction through reuse. The reuse of protective clothing presents unique challenges in the handling and decontamination procedures required for reuse without risk to employees. Although comfort, style, and professionalism are of concern to the dental hygienist, the variety of attire options precludes a comprehensive listing here. The significant criteria for selection of attire should include:

Fabric. Synthetic material is less absorbent and more fluid-resistant. Bleach-safe fabric permits disinfectant use during laundering. Most recently, newer fabrics have been designed to provide antimicrobial apparel (a poly-cotton twill treated with a microbe growth-inhibitor that is durable, safe, and nonallergenic and claims to reduce bacterial growth for the life of the uniform)[73]

Coverage. Regardless of the style or design label attached to the clothing, its fit should be high and close around the neck and permit coverage of street clothing and exposed skin with long sleeves, and it should have reinforced material with fitted cuffs at the wrist to permit gloves to extend over the gown for complete coverage (Fig. 7-49)

Design Extras. Buttons, seams, pockets, and buckles

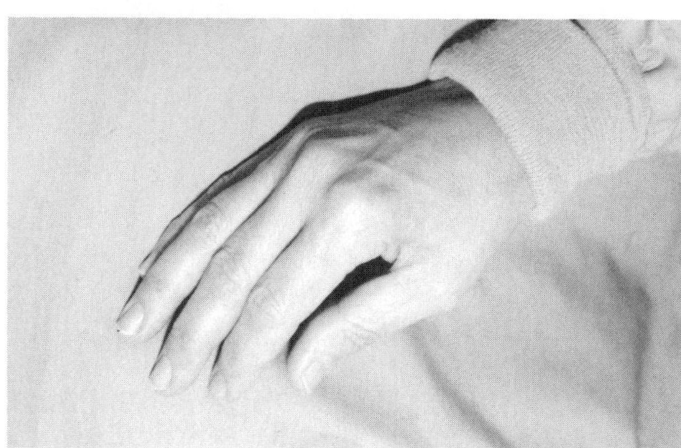

FIGURE 7-49
Complete coverage should include fitted cuffs at the wrist to permit gloves to extend over gown.

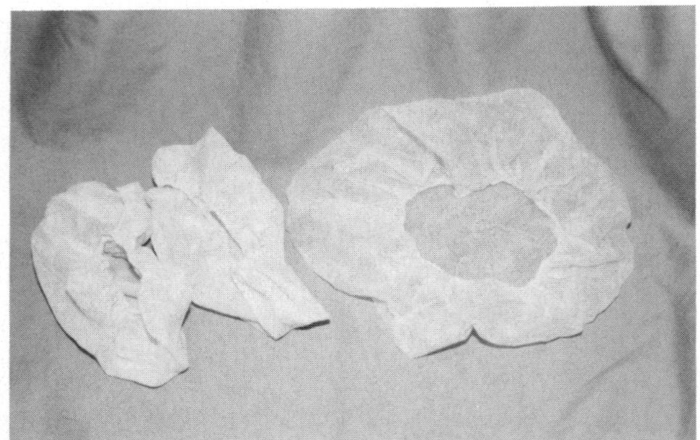

FIGURE 7–50
Head covers and shoe covers are available for use during procedures with potential for gross contamination (splashing of blood).

should be kept to a minimum. Hidden pockets for storage that are protected from most spatters and aerosols are useful features to consider[59,72]

Protocol for Maximizing Effectiveness and Minimizing Cross-Contamination with Protective Clothing

- Put on new or freshly laundered protective clothing first, prior to proceeding with masks, eyewear, and hand preparation (see Protective Clothing Chart)
- Consider additional coverage such as a plastic apron, head cover, and shoe covers (Fig. 7–50) if invasive procedures are likely to result in the splashing of blood and saliva

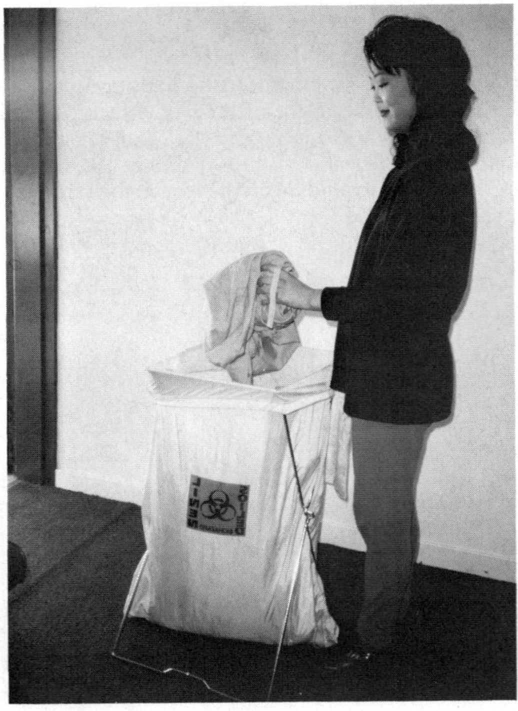

FIGURE 7–51
End-of-day procedure for handling/transport of contaminated protective clothing (placement in leakproof bag).

- Avoid touching clothing throughout the day, inspect clothing between clients, and change if visibly soiled
- Wear gowns in the practice setting only to prevent problems with contaminants at home and in other nonclient care areas
- At the end of the day, carefully remove the gown to avoid contact with contaminated surfaces, handle as little as possible, sort in a separate nonclient care area, bag in leakproof, sealed laundry/disposal bags (Fig. 7–51) for disposal or transport from office to laundry[66]
- Laundering should be done separately, at high temperature (60 to 70°C) in a washcycle with normal bleach concentration. If lower-temperature laundry cycles are used, chemicals suitable for low-temperature washing at proper concentration should be used, followed by machine drying (100°C or higher)[13,22,66]
- Change protective clothing every day, or more frequently if it is visibly soiled

Occupational Exposure, Risks and Protocol

Risk of Occupational Exposure

Dental hygienists may experience occupational exposure to blood and saliva from potentially infected clients via nee-

PROTECTIVE CLOTHING (OSHA Final Rule for Occupational Exposure to Bloodborne Pathogens)

Personal Protective Equipment—Provision and Use, Accessibility

- When there is potential for occupational exposure, the employer shall provide and have readily accessible appropriate personal protective equipment such as gowns, aprons, laboratory coats, clinic jackets or similar outer garments, and head and foot coverings.

Gowns, Aprons, and Other Protective Body Clothing

- Appropriate protective clothing shall be worn when the employee has a potential for occupational exposure. The type and characteristics will depend upon the task and degree of exposure anticipated; however, the clothing selected shall form an effective barrier.
- Gowns, laboratory coats, aprons, or similar clothing shall be worn if there is a potential for soiling of clothes with blood or other potentially infectious materials.
- Fluid-resistant clothing shall be worn if there is a potential for splashing or spraying of blood or other potentially infectious materials.
- Surgical caps or hoods shall be worn if there is a potential for gross contamination such as splashing of blood or other potentially infectious materials on the head.
- Fluid-proof clothing shall be worn if there is a potential for clothing becoming soaked with blood or other potentially infectious materials.
- Fluid-proof shoe covers shall be worn if there is a potential for shoes to become contaminated and/or soaked with blood or other potentially infectious materials.

From Department of Labor, Occupational Safety and Health Administration. Occupational exposure to bloodborne pathogens: Final rule. Federal Register 56(235):64004–64182, 1991.

dlesticks or puncture wounds, cut injuries, and splashes to the mucous membranes of the mouth, nose, and eyes. The list of occupations considered to be at substantial risk for exposure to HIV and/or HBV includes the dental hygienist.[65] The previous section has identified the protective equipment needed as essential components for a universal precautions approach to provide disease transmission protection for both the client and the dental hygienist. Using procedures that limit the spread of blood and saliva, in addition to wearing gloves, masks, protective eyeglasses or faceshields, and protective clothing, reduces the risk of exposure. It is important to keep in mind the fact that there have been no *documented cases* of HIV occupationally transmitted from client to oral healthcare provider.[10] The situation of a known exposure to infected blood and saliva by an HIV-negative dental care provider during dental treatment and a seroconversion of the dental care provider to an HIV-positive status has not occurred at this time.[74] The six dental workers who have become HIV positive from possible, but undocumented, occupational exposures reported inconsistent use of barrier techniques and numerous undocumented needlesticks.[10]

Exposure-Prone Invasive Procedures

There are no routinely used barriers that will prevent the penetration of a needle through a glove. Extreme care must therefore be used when handling blood- or saliva-contaminated "sharps," such as needles, instruments, burs, scalpel blades, broaches, files, and wires (for the protocol on needle use associated with local anesthetic administration see Chapter 8; for sharps handling and waste management see Chapter 9).

The risks increase for both the oral healthcare provider and the client when the care involves performance of invasive procedures. The CDC define invasive procedures as including the following:

> . . . surgical entry into tissues, cavities, or organs, or repair of major traumatic injuries associated with any of the following: . . . the manipulation, cutting, or removal of any oral or perioral tissues, including tooth structure, during which bleeding occurs or the potential for bleeding exists.[13]

Therefore, the majority of the procedures that the dental hygienist performs meet the definition of invasive. The

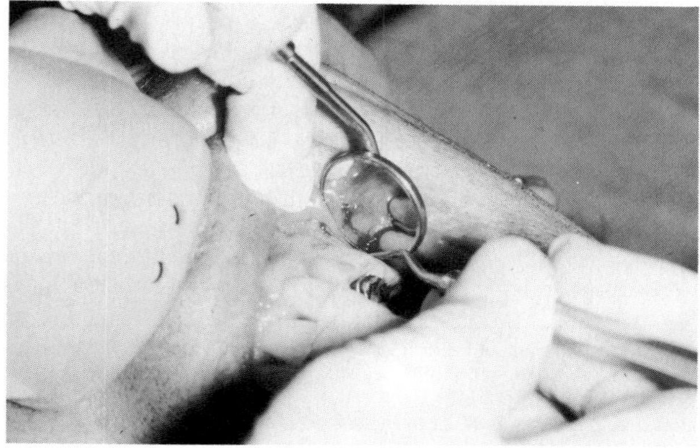

FIGURE 7-52
Scaling and root planing is an invasive procedure, since bleeding or the potential for bleeding is frequent.

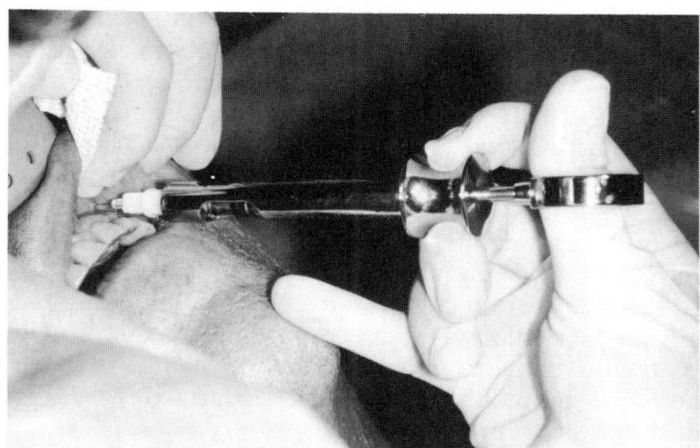

FIGURE 7-53
Administration of local anesthetic involves the simultaneous presence of the dental hygienist's fingers and a needle in a highly confined anatomic site.

most threatening invasive procedures are those considered "exposure-prone." The "characteristics of exposure-prone procedures include . . . the simultaneous presence of the healthcare worker's fingers and a needle or other sharp instrument or object in a poorly visualized or highly confined anatomic site."[20,21] The exposure-prone invasive procedures specific to dentistry have yet to be clearly defined by professional organizations and institutions. Based on the characteristics described by the CDC, periodontal instrumentation associated with scaling and root planing (Fig. 7-52) and administering local anesthetics would seem to fit the exposure-prone invasive procedure category (Fig. 7-53).

Risks for the Dental Hygienist

Performance of exposure-prone procedures presents a recognized risk of percutaneous injury to the dental hygienist. Percutaneous injuries present the greatest potential for transmission of HBV and HIV from client to dental hygienist. Studies indicate that the risk of HBV transmission to healthcare providers after percutaneous exposure to blood that is hepatitis B e antigen (HBeAg) positive is approximately 30%.[76,77] *The presence of HBeAg in the blood serum signifies higher levels of circulating virus and indicates greater infectivity in the individual who is HBsAg positive.*[20,21] In contrast with HBV, the risk of HIV transmission for healthcare providers following percutaneous exposure to HIV-infected blood is 0.3%, which is considerably lower than the 30% for HBV.[78-80] The question of variation in levels of infectivity of HIV is unclear, although it probably differs among individuals and over time for each HIV-infected individual. In contrast with HBV, there is no currently available laboratory test for increased HIV infectivity.[20,21] While it is important to note that dental hygienists, dental assistants, and dental technicians have not had any reported cases of occupationally related HIV infection, percutaneous injury poses the greatest threat of HBV and HIV transmission.[74] Therefore, meticulous care is required when performing exposure-prone invasive procedures.

Exposure-Prone Procedures Significant for Clients

The client may also be at risk if a percutaneous injury occurs during an exposure-prone invasive procedure, such as a local anesthetic needle puncture wound to a finger used to retract the buccal mucosa for access to an injection site, or a wound from a sharp instrument used in a confined area such as the maxillary posterior region. The dental hygienist's blood is likely to contact the client's oral cavity, subcutaneous tissues, and/or mucous membranes, which would put the client at risk for transmission of HIV and HBV as well.[20,21] The risk for HIV transmission is likely to be proportionally lower in comparison to HBV. An accurate assessment of the risk of HIV transmission from an HIV-infected healthcare provider requires studies to carefully evaluate a larger number of clients whose exposure-prone procedures have been performed by HIV-infected healthcare providers.[20,21]

There are many questions to be answered regarding the subject of HIV transmission in the healthcare environment. The public and professional concerns are great, but it should be remembered that despite the testing of hundreds of clients of HIV-infected healthcare workers, the Acer case is still the only known situation in which possible HIV transmission occurred from healthcare provider to clients (there were six clients in this case). Other HIV-infected healthcare providers and incidents of transmission involved clients with identifiable risk factors for HIV. Thus, over the period of 11 years since HIV has been monitored, there has been only one case in which possible provider-to-client HIV transmission occurred.[81]

Percutaneous (Needlestick) Exposure Protocol

All contaminated needlesticks, puncture wounds, or cuts from contaminated sharp dental hygiene instruments should be treated as potentially infectious. The same consideration should be given to contamination of open wounds or mucous membranes by blood and/or saliva. Contact of *intact skin* with blood and/or saliva is not considered as significant an exposure and does not require following the protocol for exposure, yet intact skin exposure should be followed immediately with a thorough washing of the affected site with an antimicrobial soap that has the seal of acceptance of the ADA Council on Dental Therapeutics.

The protocols for wound, nonintact skin, and mucous membrane exposures are as follows:[1,13,57]

- The wound should be bled immediately by squeezing the site, cleansed under running water, and washed thoroughly with an antimicrobial soap
- The client should be consulted, and his consent and cooperation requested in complying with blood testing procedures. The dental hygienist (the exposure recipient) needs to consent to blood testing as well. Pretesting counseling is advised
- Laboratory evaluation of the client's blood, testing for antibodies to HIV (anti-HIV) and hepatitis B surface antigen (HBsAg), should be done on the same day as the exposure
- Protocols for exposure require that the employer provide the dental hygienist with services for counseling, employee and client testing, and follow-up testing and treatment if indicated. The employer should be noti-

POSTEXPOSURE EVALUATION AND FOLLOW-UP (OSHA Final Rule)

Report Exposure to Employer
Following a report of an exposure incident, the employer shall make available a confidential medical evaluation and follow-up to each employee.

Documentation
Documentation must be made of the routes of exposure, HBV and HIV antibody status of the source client(s) (if known), and the circumstances under which the exposure occurred.

Source Client Testing
If the source client can be determined and permission is obtained, collection of and testing of the source client's blood must be made as soon as feasible to determine the presence of HIV or HBV infection.

Exposed Employee Testing
Blood must be collected from the exposed employee as soon as possible after the exposure incident for the determination of HIV and/or HBV status. Actual antibody or antigen testing of the blood or serum sample may be done at that time or at a later date if the employee so requests. Testing requires employee consent: if the employee consents to baseline blood collection but does not give consent for HIV serologic testing, one sample may be held for 90 days in the event that the exposed employee elects to have HIV status determined.

Exposed Employee Follow-Up
Follow-up of the exposed employee shall include antibody or antigen testing, counseling, illness reporting, and safe and effective postexposure prophylaxis according to the U.S. Public Health Service recommendations for medical practice.

Information Provided to Physician
The employer shall provide a copy of OSHA regulations, a description of the employee's duties as they relate to the employee's occupational exposure, documentation of route(s) of exposure and circumstances under which exposure occurred, results of source client's blood testing, if available, and exposed employee's pertinent medical records, including required documentation of vaccination status.

Physician's Written Opinion
The employer shall obtain and provide the employee with the physician's written opinion within 15 days of complete evaluation. The opinion should include the physician's recommended limitations upon the employee's ability to receive the hepatitis B vaccine, documentation if administered, and a statement that the employee has been informed of results of medical evaluation and any medical conditions resulting from exposure which require further evaluation or treatment. Only specific findings or diagnoses which are related to the employee's ability to receive the HBV vaccination may be disclosed in the written opinion. Any other findings or diagnoses shall remain confidential.

From Department of Labor, Occupational Safety and Health Administration. Occupational exposure to bloodborne pathogens: Final rule. Federal Register 56(235):64004–64182, 1991.

fied about the incident and the need to proceed with the established protocol for both the source client and the dental hygienist

- The dental hygienist should also have laboratory assessments for anti-HIV and anti-HBs on the same day. Hepatitis testing is not required if the dental hygienist has received the hepatitis B vaccine and has been post-tested for seroconversion and immunity
- Counseling for the dental hygienist involves a review of the signs and symptoms associated with anti-HIV seroconversion and the entitlement to medical evaluation. The dental hygienist is to be advised to seek medical assessment for any acute febrile illness that may occur within 12 weeks after the exposure, especially any illness with fever, rash, or lymphadenopathy (symptoms associated with recent HIV infection) [see Postexposure Evaluation and Follow-Up (OSHA Final Rule) chart]
- HIV blood test results and treatment recommendations:[58]

Client's Antigen Status	Recipient of Exposure
1. Diagnosed AIDS, anti-HIV positive, refuses testing, or unknown source	1a. Anti-HIV positive: *Post-test counseling and medical evaluation*
	1b. Anti-HIV negative: *Post-test counseling and repeat testing at 6, 12, and 24 weeks*
2. Anti-HIV negative	2a. Anti-HIV positive: *Post-test counseling and medical evaluation*
	2b. Anti-HIV negative: *Post-test counseling and optional follow-up at 12 weeks*

- Hepatitis blood test results and treatment recommendations:[57]

Client's Antigen Status	Recipient of Exposure
1. HBsAg negative	1a. Hepatitis B vaccine, if not already received
2. HBsAg positive	2a. Anti-HBs–positive recipients: *No treatment*
	2b. Hepatitis B vaccine recipient with laboratory-proven seroconversion: *No treatment necessary*
	2c. Hepatitis B vaccine recipient without laboratory-proven seroconversion: *One additional dose of vaccine and one dose of hepatitis B immune globulin (HBIG) if anti-HBs negative on testing*
	2d. Anti-HBs–negative recipient: *HBIG starting within 48 hours after exposure (0.06 mL/kg intramuscularly) and hepatitis B vaccination series started within 7 days*

References

1. Cottone, J. A., Terezhalmy, G. T., and Molinari, J. A. Practical Infection Control in Dentistry. Philadelphia: Lea & Febiger, 1991.
2. Scarlett, M. L., and Furman, L. I. Infection control risk assessment and management for the dental health professional. Journal of Dental Hygiene 61(7):300, 1987.
3. Miyasaki, C., and Maguire, B. (eds.). Teamasepsis, An Infection Control System for the Dental Office, UCSF, American Fund for Dental Health, Center for AIDS Prevention Studies 1989–1990.
4. Department of Labor, Occupational Safety and Health Administration. Proposed rules. Federal Register 52:45438–41, November 27, 1987.
5. Runnells, R. R. Infection Control in the Wet Finger Environment. Salt Lake City: Publishers' Press, 1984.
6. Cottone, J. A. Recent developments in hepatitis: New virus, vaccine, and dosage recommendations. Journal of the American Dental Association 120:501, 1990.
7. Dienstag, J., and Ryan, D. Occupational exposure to hepatitis B virus in hospital personnel: Infection or immunization? American Journal of Epidemiology 115:26, 1982.
8. Sampson, E. Hepatitis B–protection of patient, dentist, and staff. In Proceedings of the 123rd Annual Session of the American Dental Association. Las Vegas: American Dental Association, 1982, pp. 16–20.
9. Schiff, E. R., de Medina, M. D., et al. Veteran's Administration Cooperative Study on Hepatitis and Dentistry. Journal of the American Dental Association 133:390, 1986.
10. Centers for Disease Control. Surveillance for occupationally acquired HIV infection, United States, 1981–1992. Morbidity and Mortality Weekly Report 41, no. 43, October 30, 1992.
11. Crawford, J. J. Clinical Asepsis in Dentistry. 2nd ed. Chapel Hill, NC: University of North Carolina Dental School, 1979.
12. Molinari, J. A., and York, J. Cross contamination visualization. Journal of the California Dental Association 15(9):12, 1987.
13. Centers for Disease Control. Recommendations for prevention of HIV transmission in health care settings. Morbidity and Mortality Weekly Report 36:2-S, August 21, 1987.
14. Miyasaki, C., and Heckman, B. Microbiology and infection control. In Darby, M. L., and Bushee, E. J. (eds.). Mosby's Comprehensive Dental Hygiene Review, 3rd ed. St. Louis: C. V. Mosby, 1994.
15. Crawford, J. J. Cross infection risks and their control in dentistry, an overview. Journal of the California Dental Association 13(2):18, 1985.
16. Potter, P. A., and Perry, A. G. Fundamentals of Nursing, 3rd ed. St. Louis: C. V. Mosby, 1993.
17. Klein, R. S., Phelan, J. A., et al. Low occupation risk of human immunodeficiency virus infection among dental professionals. New England Journal of Medicine 318:86, 1988.
18. Manzella, J. P., McConville, J. H., et al. An outbreak of herpes simplex virus type I gingivostomatitis in a dental hygiene practice. Journal of the American Medical Association 252:2019, 1984.
19. Shaw, F. E., Jr., Barrett, C. L., et al. Lethal outbreak of hepatitis B in a dental practice. Journal of the American Medical Association 255:3260, 1986.
20. Centers for Disease Control. Update: Transmission of HIV infection during an invasive dental procedure—Florida. Morbidity and Mortality Weekly Report 40:2(21–33), January 18, 1991.
21. Centers for Disease Control. Recommendations for preventing transmission of human immunodeficiency virus and hepatitis B virus to patients during exposure-prone invasive procedures. Morbidity and Mortality Weekly Report 40:RR-8, 1991.
22. Department of Veterans Affairs, American Dental Association, Department of Health and Human Services: Infection Control in the Dental Environment. Washington, DC: Learning Resources Service and Eastern Dental Education Center, Veterans Administration Medical Center, 1989.
23. Abel, L. C., Miller, R. L., et al. Studies on dental aerobiology.

IV. Bacterial contamination of water delivered by dental units. Journal of Dental Research 50:1567, 1971.
24. Gross, A., Devine, M. J., and Cutright, D. E. Microbial contamination of dental units and ultrasonic scalers. Journal of Periodontology 47:670, 1976.
25. DeVore, L., and Dean, M. Strategies for oral health promotion, disease prevention and control. In Darby, M. L. (ed.). Mosby's Comprehensive Review of Dental Hygiene, 3rd ed. St. Louis: C. V. Mosby, 1994.
26. American Dental Association Research Institute, Department of Toxicology. Infectious hazards for both dental personnel and patients in the operatory. Journal of the American Dental Association 117(8):374, 1988.
27. Goodwin, A. M. Oral manifestations of AIDS: An overview. Journal of Dental Hygiene 16(7):304, 1987.
28. Wolfsy, C. Clinical features and therapeutics. Paper presented at the annual session of the American Association of Dental Schools, San Francisco, March, 1989.
29. Winkler, J. R., and Robertson, P. B. Periodontal disease associated with HIV infection. Oral Surgery, Oral Medicine, Oral Pathology 73:145, 1992.
30. Keyes, G. G. HIV-positive dental students and faculty: Their right to provide care in light of federal constitutional and anti-discrimination laws. Journal of Law Ethics Dentistry 1:199, 1988.
31. Lyons, S. Risk management or risk taking? A new look at malpractice. Access Newsmagazine of the American Dental Hygienists' Association November 1990, pp. 7–10.
32. DeBiase, C. B. Theory and Practice of Dental Health Education. Philadelphia: Lea & Febiger, 1991.
33. Legalities. Control, The Infectious Disease Newsletter 6(5):1–11, 1991.
34. Dentistry and the media blitz. Control, The Infectious Disease Newsletter 6(5):1, 1991.
35. Zarkowski, P. Legal issues in the practice of dental hygiene. Seminars in Dental Hygiene 2:1, 1990.
36. Weinstein, B. D. Management considerations for an HIV-positive dental student: Ethical and legal commentary. Journal of Dental Education 55(4):238, 1991.
37. American Dental Hygienists' Association Policy on DH Practice Policy No. 43-79. American Dental Hygienists' Association Policy Manual. Chicago: ADHA, 1988.
38. Koelbl, J. J. AIDS at the Medical College of Georgia—a study in institutional ethics. Journal of Dental Education 55(4):235, 1991.
39. American Dental Association. Interim Policy on HIV-infected dentists. Jan. 16, 1991. Chicago: ADA, 1991.
40. American Dental Association. Annual Reports and Resolutions, Report of Council on Ethics, Bylaws, and Judicial Affairs, 1990. Chicago: ADA.
41. Late-breaking item—AADS actions on CDC report on Florida dentist with AIDS. American Association of Dental Schools Bulletin of Dental Education, February 1991, p. 1.
42. Trends (CDC). Control, The Infectious Disease Newsletter 8(1):3, 1993.
43. Kramer, S. Practice management and career development strategies. In Darby, M. L., and Bushee, E. J. (eds.). Mosby's Comprehensive Review of Dental Hygiene, 3rd ed. St. Louis: C. V. Mosby, 1994.
44. Department of Labor, Occupational Safety and Health Administration. Proposed rules. Federal Register 52:45438, November 27, 1987.
45. "A few seconds was all it took." Hepatitis infection changes dentist's life. American Dental Association News, March 7, 1988, pp. 10–11.
46. Slupski, J. Is OSHA becoming a four-letter word? Access 3(6):6, 1989.
47. Miyasaki, C. M., Fowle, M., et al. Demystifying OSHA inspection guidelines. Journal of the California Dental Association 17(12):28, 1989.
48. Macdonald, G. Rationale for protective eyewear. Journal of the California Dental Hygienists, Winter 1987, p. 9.
49. Molinari, J. A., Cottone, J. A., and Gleason, M. J. Hepatitis B and available vaccines. California Dental Association Journal 43–45, October 1992.
50. Choo, Q., Ruo, G., et al. Isolation of a DNA clone derived from a blood-borne non-A, non-B viral hepatitis genome. Science 244:359, 1989.
51. American Dental Hygienists' Association. American Dental Hygienists' Association Position Statement on Prevention of Disease Transmission. June 30, 1992.
52. American Dental Hygienists' Association Council recommends hepatitis vaccine for dentists, students, and auxiliary personnel. ADA News 13:1, August 26, 1982.
53. Macdonald, G. Immunization: The best barrier. California Dental Hygienists' Association Journal February 1991, pp. 2–3.
54. Siew, C., Gruninger, S., et al. Survey of hepatitis B exposure and vaccination in volunteer dentists. Journal of the American Dental Association 114:457, 1987.
55. Perillo, R. Screening of health care workers before hepatitis B vaccination: More questions than answers. Annals of Internal Medicine 103:793, 1985.
56. Centers for Disease Control. Suboptimal response to the hepatitis B vaccine given by injection into the buttock. Morbidity and Mortality Weekly Report 34(8):105, 1985.
57. Centers for Disease Control (ACIP). Protection against viral hepatitis. Morbidity and Mortality Weekly Report 39(RR-2):19, 1990.
58. Molinari, J. A., Cottone, J. A., and Gleason, M. J. Hepatitis B and available vaccines. California Dental Association Journal 43–45, October 1992.
59. Molinari, J. A., Gleason, M. J., et al. Cleaning and disinfectant properties of dental surface disinfectants. Journal of the American Dental Association 117:179, 1988.
60. Otis, L. L., and Cottone, J. A. The use and abuse of gloves in dentistry. Los Angeles, 1989, University of Southern California, School of Dentistry.
61. Williams, W. W. CDC guidelines for infection control in hospital personnel. Infection Control 4(4):325, 1983.
62. Runnells, R. R. Mandatory testing for HIV-1? Acer-Bergalis forces a review. Control, The Infectious Disease Newsletter 6(3):1, 1991.
63. Miller, C. H. Routine gloving common practice. RDH 11:36, 1991.
64. Department of Health and Human Services. Medical devices; patient examination glove: Revocation of exemptions from the pre-market notification procedures and current good manufacturing practice regulations; final rule (FDA, 21 CFR Part 880). Federal Register 54(9):1602, January 13, 1989.
65. Department of Labor, Occupational Safety and Health Administration. Instruction CPL 2-2, 44B Office of Health Compliance Assistance, 27, 90.
66. American Dental Association Council on Dental Materials, Instruments and Equipments; on Dental Practice; and on Dental Therapeutics. Infection control recommendations for the dental office and dental laboratory. Journal of the American Dental Association 116:241, 1988.
67. Centers for Disease Control. Update: Universal precautions for prevention of transmission of human immunodeficiency virus, hepatitis B virus, and other bloodborne pathogens in health care settings. Morbidity and Mortality Weekly Report 37:24(377), June 1988.
68. Miller, C. H. Reduce chance of exposure. RDH 11:4, 32, 1991.
69. Runnells, R. R. Handbook of Dental Infection Control. New York: Johnson & Johnson, 1988.
70. Wilkins, E. M. Clinical Practice of the Dental Hygienist, 6th ed. Philadelphia: Lea & Febiger, 1989.
71. Bond, W. Modes of transmission of infectious diseases. From Proceedings of National Symposium on Infection Control in Dentistry, May 13, 1986. Chicago, Atlanta, U.S. Department of Health and Human Services.
72. Jakush, J. Infection control procedures and products: Cautions and common sense. Journal of the American Dental Association 117:293, 1988.
73. Witherspoon, T. More or less? RDH March 1991.
74. Miller, C. H. Guarding against HIV. RDH August 1991, pp. 38–40.
75. Alter, H. J., Seeff, L. B., et al. Type B hepatitis after needlestick exposure: The infectivity of blood positive for a antigen

and DNA polymerase after accidental needlestick exposure. New England Journal of Medicine 296:909, 1976.

76. Grady, G. F., Lee, V. A., et al. Hepatitis B immune globulin for accidental exposures among medical personnel: Final report of multicenter controlled trial. Journal of Infectious Disease 138:625, 1978.
77. Seef, L. B., Wright, E. C., et al. Type B hepatitis after needlestick exposure: Prevention with hepatitis B immunoglobulin, final report of the Veterans Administration Cooperative Study. Annals of Internal Medicine 88:286, 1978.
78. Gerberding, J. L., Bryant-LeBlanc, C. E., et al. Risk of transmitting the human immunodeficiency virus, cytomegalovirus, and hepatitis B virus to health care workers exposed to patients with AIDS and AIDS-related conditions (ARC). Journal of Infectious Diseases 156:1, 1987.
79. Henderson, D. K., Fahey, B. J., et al. Risks for occupational transmission of human immunodeficiency virus type 1 (HIV-1) associated with clinical exposures: A prospective evaluation. Annals of Internal Medicine 113:740, 1990.
80. Marcus, R. Centers for Disease Control Cooperative Needlestick Study Group. Surveillance of health-care workers exposed to blood from patients infected with the human immunodeficiency virus. New England Journal of Medicine 319:1118, 1988.
81. King, L. J. HIV developments affect healthcare workers. Access 5(7):6, 1991.

Suggested Readings

Ackerman, T. F., Graber, G. C., et al. (eds.). Clinical Medical Ethics: Exploration and Assessment. Lanhan, MD: University Press of America, 1987.

American Dental Association Council on Dental Materials, Instruments, and Equipments; on Dental Practice; and on Dental Therapeutics. Infection control recommendations for the dental office and the dental laboratory. Journal of the American Dental Association 116:241, 1988.

Boyce, J. S. Risk management: An introduction for the dental practice. Dental Hygiene 61:504, 1987.

Callahan, J. C. (ed.). Ethical Issues in Professional Life. New York: Oxford University Press, 1988.

Cottone, J. A., and Molinari, J. A. Hepatitis B vaccines, an update. Journal of the California Dental Association 17(2):11, 1989.

Crawford, J. J. State of the art: Practical infection control in dentistry. Journal of the American Dental Association 110:629, 1985.

Immunization Practice Advisory Committee. Adult immunization. Morbidity and Mortality Weekly Report 33S:1S–685, 1984.

Knoben, J. E., Anderson, P. O., et al. (eds.). Handbook of Clinical Drug Data, 6th ed. Hamilton, IL: Drug Intelligence Publications, 1988.

Lewis, D. L., Arens, M., et al. Cross contamination potential with dental equipment. Lancet 340:1252, 1992.

Molinari, J. A., Merchant, V. A., and Gleason, M. J. Equipment asepsis. Monitor, Newsletter of the University of Detroit School of Dentistry, September 1987, p. 3.

Reis-Schmidt, T. Controlling aerosols, splatter, droplets: Procedures to interrupt mechanisms of disease transmission in the operatory. Infection Control Report March 1988, p. 71.

Reveal, M. ADHA perspective. Journal of Dental Hygiene 6416:18, 1990.

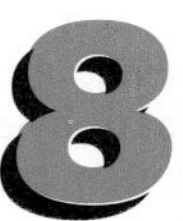

Infection Control Protocols for the Dental Hygiene Process of Care

OBJECTIVES

Mastery of the content in this chapter will enable the reader to:

- Define the terms used
- Identify the design features related to the operatory equipment and environment that reduce the possibilities of cross-contamination
- Describe approaches to operatory organization that facilitate efficient and meticulous preparation prior to receiving the client for dental hygiene care
- Explain the distinctions between cleaning, disinfection, and sterilization, and determine when disinfection is appropriate for reducing sources of microbial cross-contamination
- Discuss Spaulding's classification of instruments and equipment as critical, semicritical, and noncritical (based on use and degree of contamination) as criteria for selection of sterilization or disinfection for the prevention of disease transmission
- Compare surface disinfection and the use of blood- and saliva-impervious disposable surface barriers
- Identify equipment well suited to routine covering with surface barriers
- Identify the qualities of an ideal surface disinfectant, types of disinfectants that are approved by the Environmental Protection Agency (EPA) and the American Dental Association (ADA), and the appropriate techniques for maximizing effective decontamination of surfaces
- Describe the critical steps in surface cleaning and disinfection
- List and briefly explain the steps in the protocol for operatory preparation prior to the dental hygiene appointment
- Develop dental hygiene care protocols with detailed step-by-step procedures customized to meet the requirements of the oral healthcare setting based on current professional and governmental standards or guidelines
- Apply the concept of "defined use areas" within designated contaminated and noncontaminated zones for instruments, items, and material in order to control flow and cross-contamination during procedures (dental hygiene, radiography, and laboratory) in a variety of settings
- Discuss the value of team participation in protocol development and the review process to gain the compliance essential for quality assurance and safe delivery of client care
- Describe the postappointment procedures for operatory decontamination, the initial preparation of instruments for recirculation, and waste handling

THE DENTAL HYGIENE CARE ENVIRONMENT

It is imperative that infection control protocols for each aspect of comprehensive dental hygiene care be developed with attention given to the need for effectiveness and practicality (time and cost requirements). Infection control protocols must be based on an awareness of a working environment's design features and limitations and a scientific understanding of the theory and modes of disease transmission and current research. Establishing procedures that may be efficiently carried out, meticulously followed for every client, and revised as technological advances occur is critical for infection control in the dental hygiene care environment.

Areas to Be Considered Prior to the Dental Hygiene Care Appointment

Aseptic technique, a combination of all efforts made before, during, and after care to prevent entry of microorganisms into the client (e.g., via the sulcular epithelium of the periodontium and the circulatory system), requires lowering the number of microbes present in five areas for the goal of achieving effective asepsis.[1] The five areas that must be considered in controlling pathogenic microorganisms in preparation for dental hygiene care are:

- General clinical environment (operatory design, organization, and cleanliness)
- Client preparation (health history, premedication if indicated for prevention of autogenous infection, and mouth rinse)
- Personal protection (handwashing, gloves, masks, protective eyewear, and clothing)
- Surface decontamination (selection of chemical disinfectant, precleaning for the removal of bioburden [organic debris], and disinfection procedures)
- Instrument recirculation (containment of contaminated instruments, decontamination, sterilization, and storage until reuse)

Aseptic technique, in the strict sense of the term, refers to procedures used in hospital operating rooms, specialized facilities designed and staffed for maximum control of microorganisms, sterile (free of living microorganisms) gowns, gloves, hair covers, shoe covers, air flow controls to collect and filter out microorganisms, and sterile water (no tap water) for use during procedures. This strict aseptic environment (surgical asepsis) required for a hospital operating room is not necessary for the delivery of most dental and dental hygiene care. Exceptions include severely medically compromised clients (e.g., those with active tuberculosis or acute exacerbated leukemia) whose inability to resist infections warrants referral to a hospital dental service equipped to provide care in a strict aseptic environment. Most dental hygiene care, however, can be provided to healthy and medically compromised clients in a dental office environment, depending on the severity of the medically compromised's condition and the potential for posttreatment infection. Although traditional dental environments have a lower level of clinical asepsis than a hospital operating room, they do use a "sterile-clean technique," which provides for use of sterile instruments within a clean, not necessarily sterile, environment. Normally, a totally sterile environment is not necessary for the provision of oral healthcare because the body defense mechanisms of most clients usually are able to control rapidly and eliminate any microorganisms that gain entry into the blood stream (bacteremia). For some clients, however, antibiotic premedication is necessary before the dental hygiene care appointment, and antibiotic prophylaxis after treatment, to prevent bacteremia (see Chapter 10). The approach used in dental hygiene care has as its goal to reduce, as much as possible, the number of microorganisms present in order to minimize the possibility of disease transmission or of inducing autogenous infections. The latter is accomplished by limiting exposure to high numbers of pathogens through the use of effective infection control protocols for the delivery of dental hygiene care.[1]

Operatory and Equipment Design

The increased interest in the prevention of transmission of bloodborne pathogens in the oral healthcare environment has led oral healthcare professionals and dental equipment manufacturers to assess the materials, fixtures, equipment, organization of the workspace, and flow of movement in the clinical environment as they relate to the prevention of disease transmission. This assessment of operatory and equipment design is in response to the demand for an environment that not only enhances the efficient delivery of care but also expedites a practical and thorough program of infection control.

Although the dental hygiene care operatory is not required to be a sterile environment, it is imperative that the general working area and the nondirect client contact equipment be maintained as a disinfected environment.[2] The design of the areas of client care, instrument recirculation, and the laboratory should reflect a functional design philosophy. Initially identifying the services to be rendered in each area, along with the associated infection control requirements, and the projected client activity will provide the list of needs to guide the design process. The equipment, controls for dental units and chairs, cabinetry, countertop surfaces, sinks, faucets, towel dispensers, walls, flooring, evacuation system, and water purity system all have design considerations relevant to infection control (Table 8–1) (see Design Features That Inhibit Efficient Cleaning and Disinfection chart).[1–3]

DESIGN FEATURES THAT INHIBIT EFFICIENT CLEANING AND DISINFECTION

- Numerous crevices
- Uneven surfaces
- Buttons, seams, switches and knurled knobs
- Porous finishes, textured paint
- Surfaces unable to withstand repeated disinfection (wood)
- Fabric-covered, coiled and retractable tubings
- Fabric upholstery
- Carpeting
- Lettering on equipment (air/water), adhesive trims

Data from Cottone, J. A., Terezhalmy, G. T., and Molinari, J. A. Practical Infection Control in Dentistry. Philadelphia: Lea & Febiger, 1991.

TABLE 8–1
EQUIPMENT DESIGN CONSIDERATIONS AND INFECTION CONTROL

Equipment Design Elements	Objective	Rationale	Prevention of Disease Transmission
Chair Form: contoured for body shape	Client comfort	Dental hygiene procedures more time-consuming, technically demanding; longer appointments	Combination of surface covers and surface disinfection
Chair Upholstery: durable, nonorganic materials, seamless (e.g., vinyl covering)	To facilitate surface disinfection, moisture-proof	Majority of chair within 3-foot zone of greatest contamination; potential for cross-contamination significant	Combination of barrier cover and surface disinfection
Chair Operation Control Switches: foot-operated control recommended	To remove potential for cross-contamination	Finger-operated switches contain many crevices, impossible to clean; avoid spraying disinfectant into switch area, which may cause an electrical short-circuit or equipment malfunction.	Disposable surface cover for hand-operated controls; or equipment retrofitted with foot control
Chair Arm- and Handrest: durable covering able to withstand disinfection; avoid seams, crevices	To withstand repeated cleaning and disinfection	"Sling-type" armrest acts as a trap for debris and dirt; frequently touched by dental hygienist and client	Difficult to cover fully, will generally need between-client cleaning/disinfection; include underside of armrests
Chair Headrest and Control: currently lever or strap adjustment for headrest cushion; durable moisture-proof, minimal seams, crevices	To eliminate potential for cross-contamination, ease of surface disinfection	Headrest within the most critical area of contamination (3 feet) and requires adjustment at times during client care	Headrest surface cover needed to protect surface from spatter; currently acts as barrier for adjustment control as well if coverage is adequate
Delivery System: (great variation in design: system includes handpiece, hangers and controls, syringes, hoses, switches, handles, hooks, cart base or arm attachment, surface for tray); suggested features: transparent shield to protect controls or "seamless" membrane control switches minimize crevices and uneven surfaces	To minimize direct contamination and facilitate surface cleaning and disinfection	The delivery system is within the zone of greatest direct microbial transfer (syringe, handpiece, high- and low-volume evacuation have the greatest contamination while hoses are less exposed)	Maximum use of barrier material; analyze each system's design to determine best surface coverage and minimize yet meticulously disinfect parts not covered completely; include underside edges of cart tops; sterilize handpiece, ASW syringe, and/or tip
Suction-tubing and Connectors/ Flow-Control Assemblies: smooth design with crevices minimized	For ease in cleaning and disinfection	Suction/evacuation system becomes readily contaminated, especially finger control valves	Exterior hose ends rinsed, scrubbed, and disinfected; interior of tubing cleaned between clients by flushing with water, and disinfected at end of working day with a commercial cleansing solution
Light: foot-controlled on-off switch, removable handles	To minimize direct contamination	Multiple direct contamination contacts with light handle by dental hygienist's gloved hand occur during care; great potential for direct contamination with hand-operated switch; light shield exposed to spatter, since within 3 feet of oral cavity	Use surface cover on light handle or sterilize if removable; disinfect shield between clients; wipe arm of the light once each day
Dental Hygienist's Chair Design and Upholstery: durable covering; smooth, moisture-proof	To withstand surface disinfection, promote physical comfort with flexibility in adjustment to maximize support (lumbar region), and height position for balance, control, and to promote circulation	Potential for direct contamination if dental hygienist touches the chair-positioning controls or upholstery on chair back; minimizing contact is recommended unless overgloves are worn	Surface cleaning/disinfection or use of barriers placed over chair back and adjustment control

Table continued on following page

TABLE 8–1
EQUIPMENT DESIGN CONSIDERATIONS AND INFECTION CONTROL *Continued*

Equipment Design Elements	Objective	Rationale	Prevention of Disease Transmission
Cabinetry/Countertop: surfaces should be seamless and smooth, constructed of materials such as plastic laminate with 4-inch or full backsplash extending between base cabinetry and upper cabinetry	To create surfaces that are compatible with disinfectants and detergents	Exposed surfaces (vertical and horizontal) that are not practical to cover and that are within 3 feet of the client's mouth must be considered contaminated with spatter	Surfaces that are touched must be cleaned and disinfected or have disposable covers changed between clients; cabinet doors and drawers must be closed during treatment
Sinks: should be located within view of client, deep enough to rinse hands and arms; stainless steel or porcelain	To locate for easy use, near client for observation of handwashing and gloving; constructed of materials to withstand scrubbing with iodophor or sodium hypochlorite solution	Sinks in client care and instrument recirculation areas considered a high contamination risk	Minimize contact with surfaces throughout appointment; disinfect between clients
Faucets: foot- or knee-activated or electric eye–activated water flow	To eliminate potential for cross-contamination	Manual faucets are prone to contamination	Use barrier material if manual faucet; if larger faucet handle use gown-covered forearm to operate; since washing of gloves during procedures is discouraged, sink use is reduced; aerators should not be used because they harbor microorganisms
Soap Dispensers: knee-, foot-, or forearm-controlled	To avoid contamination of dispenser and/or hands or gloves when washing hands before and after client care or rinsing gloves	Manual soap dispensers are considered to be semicritical (high) source of contamination	Manual soap dispensers are to be cleaned/disinfected between clients
Towel Dispensers: paper is material of choice in towels and should be dispensed from holders not contaminated during dispensing	To avoid contamination of the dispenser by touching only the paper-towel hanging down	Crank-type or lever-type dispensers encourage direct contact of dispenser surface by contaminated hands	If towel dispenser is contacted by contaminated gloves, it must be cleaned/disinfected between clients
Walls: vinyl coverings (sheet vinyl) or semigloss paint finish	Wall surfaces that promote ease in cleaning and maintain appearance over time (7–10 years)	Walls in halls, treatment areas, and instrument recirculation areas contribute to the overall cleanliness of the environment	Recommendations regarding housekeeping suggest routine cleaning and removal of soil and cleaning of walls with nontoxic, biodegradable nonabrasive cleaners when visibly soiled
Flooring: seamless vinyl floor covering	Ease in maintenance, ease in confinement and spill clean-up in areas of operatory, laboratory, darkroom, instrument recirculation area, and restroom	Flooring is subject to oral spatter, spills of potentially infective liquids or hazardous chemicals (mercury)	Cleaning and soil removal should be done routinely; maintenance is facilitated by selecting seamless vinyl over carpeting or square tiles
Water-Retraction Valves: (originally designed into older units to prevent water dripping on clients) must be removed from handpiece and syringe	To prevent "suckback" from forming microbial-contaminated bioburden in water lines	Water lines are very susceptible to microbial build-up; fresh water and removal of debris must be ensured	Test for water-retraction valves; install one-way valve in tubing of water line; if needed flush water lines at beginning and end of day and between clients; change water filters frequently

Data from Cottone, J. A., Terezhalmy, G. T., and Molinari, J. A. Practical Infection Control in Dentistry. Philadelphia: Lea & Febiger, 1991; Harfst, S. Accepting the challenge: zone by zone. Control, The Infectious Disease Newsletter 6(3):1–8, 1991; Office Sterilization and Asepsis Procedures (OSAP) Research Foundation. OSAP Office Sterilization and Asepsis Procedures Report 4(2):5, 1991; Pollack, R. Form follows function. California Dental Association Journal 17(2):17, 1989; and Whitacre, R. J., Robins, S. K., et al. Dental Asepsis. Seattle: Stoma Press, 1979.

DESIGNATION OF AREAS ACCORDING TO FUNCTION

Treatment Areas
Care delivery areas where direct intraoral mucosal contact occurs, such as operatories, oral hygiene instruction areas, and radiographic imaging rooms.

Treatment Support Areas
Areas with activities that support the delivery of care where indirect client contact occurs through direct handling of contaminated care support items such as instruments, exposed film, and impressions. Examples of such areas include instrument recirculation centers, radiograph processing rooms, and laboratory areas.

Nontreatment Areas
Areas that require no direct client contact, *no direct mucosal contact, and no contaminated support item contact* are considered to be nontreatment areas, such as reception rooms, business offices, staff lounges, private offices, and lavatory areas.

Data from Cottone, J. A., Terezhalmy, G. T., and Molinari, J. A. Practical Infection Control in Dentistry. Philadelphia: Lea & Febiger, 1991.

Organization of the Clinical Environment

Although the equipment design considerations listed in Table 8–1 most directly affect the quality of an infection control program, the overall office or clinic design plays a role and also should be considered. The designation of areas for specific activities creates efficient workspaces and guides the associated flow of traffic. Proper office design reduces excess cross-contamination by providing direct access to the dental hygiene care space without passage through additional instrument recirculation, treatment, or laboratory areas.[2] Unless the dental hygienist is involved in the design process or employed as an infection control consultant, it may be difficult for her to have any influence on the floor plan and traffic flow. Although the chances of influencing the overall design may be limited, an appreciation of the need to designate specific areas according to function helps reduce excess cross-contamination (see Designation of Areas According to Function chart). For example, since the staff lounge is a nontreatment area, contaminated items should not be taken into this space. Likewise, staff should not eat in the instrument recirculation or laboratory areas, since these treatment support areas involve direct contact with contaminated items, such as instruments or impressions. Strict adherence to the function of each specific area avoids cross-contamination and the potential for cross-infection and ultimately helps ensure the success of the infection control program.

Zones of Contamination and Noncontamination in Client Care Areas

Client care areas have the highest level of microbial-laden spatter and, therefore, require the most careful approach to design and organization. Design should follow function in order to facilitate efficiency and minimize movements away from the oral cavity (zone of contamination). This goal is best accomplished by positioning equipment to promote ease of use and comfort to minimize the zone of contamination. The well-organized operatory space should accommodate only what must be immediately accessible for client care. This minimalist approach is necessary and precludes the display of posters, plants, and other decorative items to avoid their contamination with the numerous pathogens in the immediate area. A simple, uncluttered work area not only presents a clean image for the client but also enhances aseptic technique and infection control efficiency.[2] Preset procedure trays and support armamentarium (instructional models, visual aids, ultrasonic scaling equipment) need to be arranged according to defined areas in the operatory that correlate with degree of contamination. For example, any surfaces (vertical or horizontal) within 3 feet of the client's mouth must be considered contaminated. When the oral healthcare provider is in contact with blood and saliva, she should avoid touching any surface outside this immediate zone of contamination. When items in the armamentarium that are outside the zone of contamination need to be retrieved, methods such as overgloves or sterile pliers should be utilized to prevent contamination (Fig. 8–1). Establishing contaminated and uncontaminated zones (Fig. 8–2) avoids cross-contamination by organizing the location of instruments, support items, and other materials to control their flow during dental hygiene procedures.[4]

Within the scope of the contaminated zone, "use areas" may be designated to further organize the placement, use, and control of the flow of instruments, material, and equipment to minimize occupational exposure and avoid cross-contamination. The "work" or "use areas" within the contaminated zone include the bracket table, the top of the power module or the instrument cabinet, and the area of the countertop closest to the client's oral cavity. The remaining area of the countertop is designated as the noncontaminated area (see Designated Use Areas Within the Dental Hygiene Care Environment chart). The items to be placed in these areas are determined by the specific dental hygiene care procedure being delivered (see dental hygiene standard operating infection control protocols for each component of comprehensive dental hygiene care in the last section of this chapter).[4]

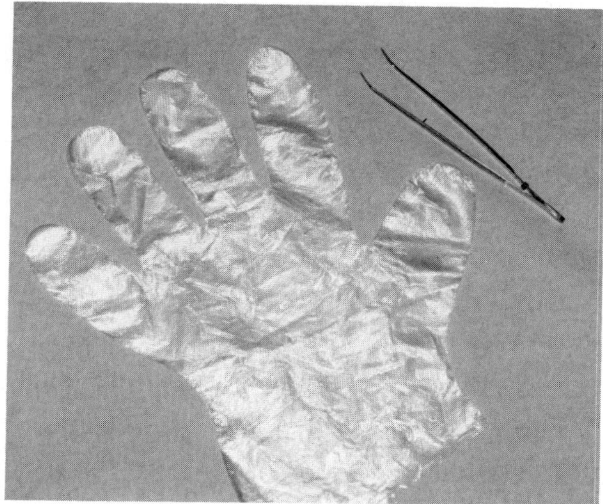

FIGURE 8–1
Overgloves/sterile pliers.

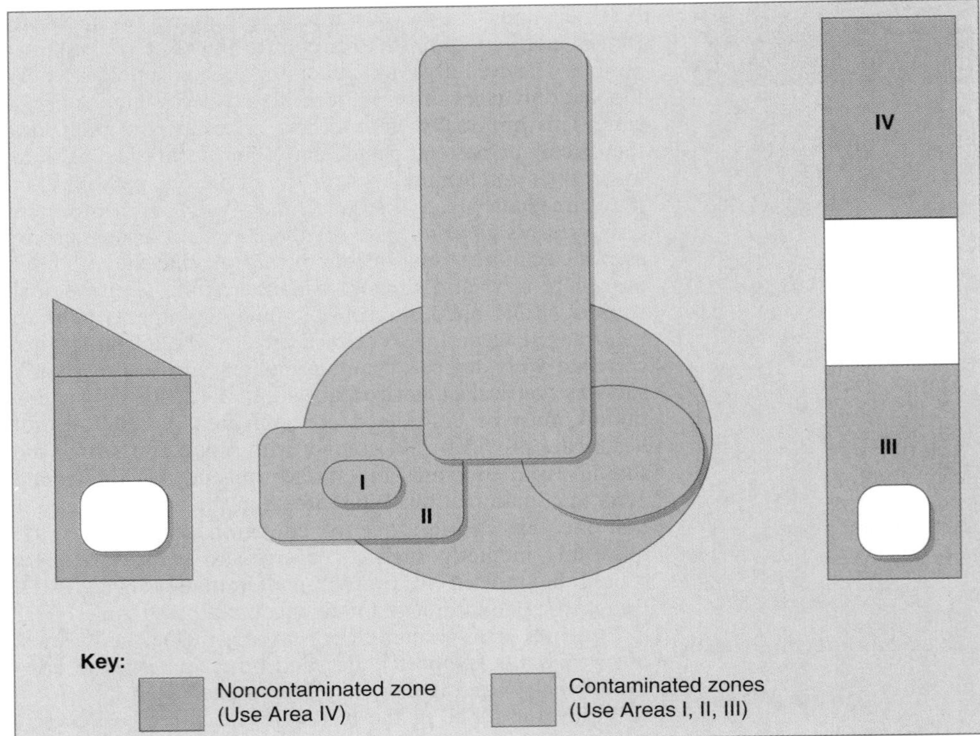

FIGURE 8–2
Operatory zones. I, II, and III indicate contaminated zones. I, bracket table/instrument tray or cassette; II, top of instrument cabinet or power module; III, adjacent countertop area closest to the client's oral cavity. IV indicates noncontaminated zone. IV, remaining area of countertop. (Adapted from Ino, J., and Miyasaki, S. University of California, San Francisco, School of Dentistry Clinic Manual: Infection Control Protocol. San Francisco: UCSF, 1987.)

DESIGNATED USE AREAS WITHIN THE DENTAL HYGIENE CARE ENVIRONMENT

Area I (Contaminated Zone)—The Bracket Table/ Instrument Tray or Cassette
Items within this area are used frequently during dental hygiene care and come into direct contact with mucous membranes and/or body fluids.

Area II (Contaminated Zone)—The Top of the Instrument Cabinet or Power Module
Items within this area are infrequently used during dental hygiene care but will be contaminated (e.g., the suction tips, air/water tip, handpiece, and attachments).

Area III (Contaminated Zone)—The Adjacent Countertop Area Closest to the Client's Oral Cavity
Items placed in this area will eventually become contaminated because of proximity to the source of contamination; apparatus that cannot be cleaned and disinfected properly such as ultrasonic scaling equipment must be protected with a barrier.

Area IV (Noncontaminated Zone)—The Remaining Area of the Countertop
Dental hygiene care items that cannot be sterilized or disinfected and therefore must not be contaminated (e.g., bulk materials such as topical fluoride, plaque control materials, records, forms, and pens) must be covered when not in use and should not be touched without the use of a barrier, such as an overglove.

Adapted from Cottone, J. A., Hars, E., et al. Recommended clinical guidelines for infection control in dental education institution. Journal of Dental Education 55(9):621–630, 1991.

EQUIPMENT AND OPERATORY ENVIRONMENT PROTECTION AND SURFACE DISINFECTION

Classification of Instruments and Equipment

Items that have the greatest potential for transmitting infections are classified as **critical items.** To prevent the transmission of infectious agents in the dental hygiene care environment all critical items must be sterile. Other items with lower potential for transmitting infection are classified as **semicritical items** and should either be sterile or have a high level of disinfection. Although disinfection is a less lethal process than sterilization, high-level **disinfection** refers to the ability to kill some, but not necessarily all, bacterial spores. Less significant items classified as **noncritical items** should receive intermediate-level disinfection, which kills *Mycobacterium tuberculosis* var. *bovis,* hepatitis B virus (HBV), and human immunodeficiency virus (HIV) but does not kill bacterial spores.[5] The classification of instruments and equipment as critical, semicritical, or noncritical was developed by Spaulding for hospital instruments. Therefore, specified use is a major factor in determining whether an item is sterilized, disinfected, or simply cleaned **(sanitization).** Spaulding's classification for instruments and equipment has been adapted for dentistry and directly relates to dental hygiene equipment and instruments (see Spaulding Classification of Instruments and Equipment chart).[5]

Disposable Surface Barriers

While instrument and equipment use and degree of contamination may be useful criteria for determining when to

SPAULDING CLASSIFICATION OF INSTRUMENTS AND EQUIPMENT

Critical: Require Sterilization

Items that penetrate or touch broken skin or mucosa or bone: periodontal probes, explorers, scaling and root planing instruments, needles, and mouth mirrors (Fig. 8–3).

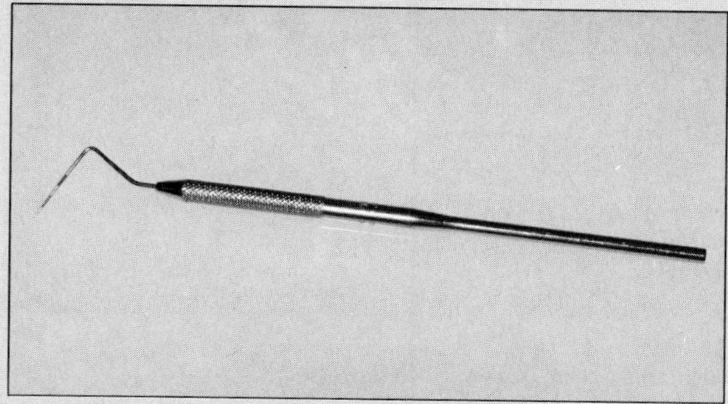

FIGURE 8–3
Example of critical equipment—probe.

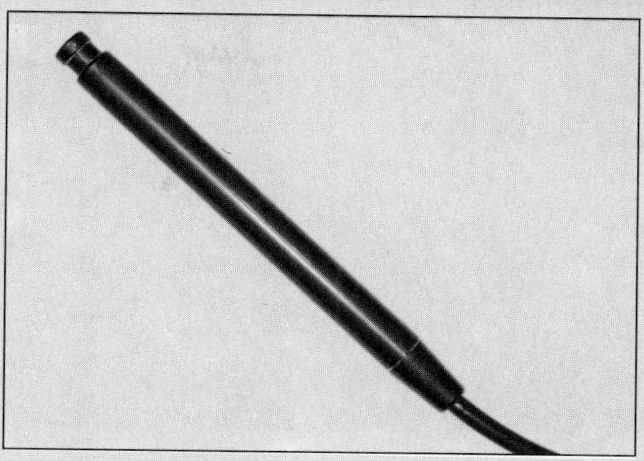

FIGURE 8–4
Example of semicritical equipment—ultrasonic handpiece.

Semicritical: Require Sterilization Whenever Possible, or Subjected to High-Level Disinfection

Items that contact mucous membranes but do not enter sterile body areas such as the blood stream: handpieces, untrasonic scaling handpieces (not tip insert), plastic impression trays, oral photography retractors, and amalgam condensers (Fig. 8–4).

Noncritical Items: Require Intermediate-Level Disinfection (Tuberculocidal)

Items that do not penetrate or contact mucous membranes but are exposed to saliva, blood, and debris by spatter or the touch of contaminated hands: light handles, high- and low-volume evacuators, tubing for handpieces, instrument trays, countertops, and chair surfaces (Fig. 8–5).

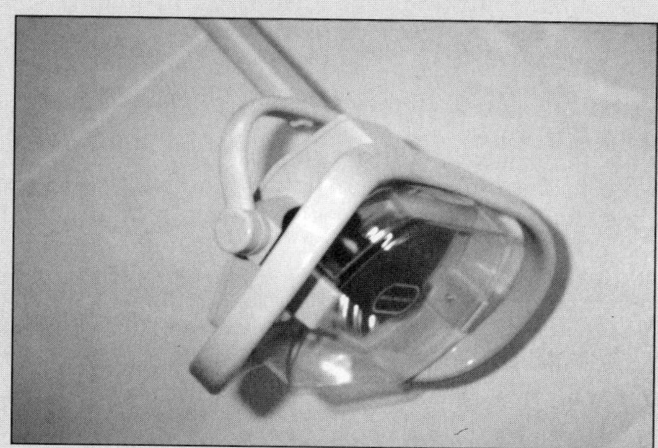

FIGURE 8–5
Example of noncritical equipment—light handle.

Adapted from Spaulding, E. H. Chemical disinfection of medical and surgical materials. In Lawrence, A. S., and Block, S. S. (eds.). Disinfection, Preservation and Sterilization. Philadelphia: Lea & Febiger, 1968, pp. 517–531.

sterilize, disinfect, or clean, the reality of the dental hygiene working environment is such that it is not always possible to sterilize all equipment or surfaces according to Spaulding's criteria (e.g., semicritical—sterilize whenever possible). Instrument and equipment recirculation is addressed in detail in Chapter 9. However, the major task of surface protection, cleaning, and disinfection is presented here as a significant part of the preparation for dental hygiene client care in the healthcare environment.

Use of surface barriers, nonpermeable disposable covers that are discarded after each client, is an alternative to multiple scrupulous cleanings and disinfections. Examples of equipment well suited to routine covering with plastic, aluminum foil, or impervious-backed paper are dental light handles (Fig. 8–6); bracket tables including switches and hose supports (Fig. 8–7); airspray-water (ASW) syringe handles with controls (Fig. 8–8); high- and low-volume evacuation controls; headrests and/or chair backs; counter surfaces in areas of contamination; and x-ray equipment and controls.

Although plastic is the most frequently used barrier material, foil provides good coverage for light handles and switches, while paper is an adequate barrier for counter surfaces and headrest covers. Plastic, foil, or impervious-backed paper are preferred materials because they prevent moisture absorption through the cover to the underlying surface. If moisture is absorbed through the cover to the underlying surface, the purpose of the barrier is negated

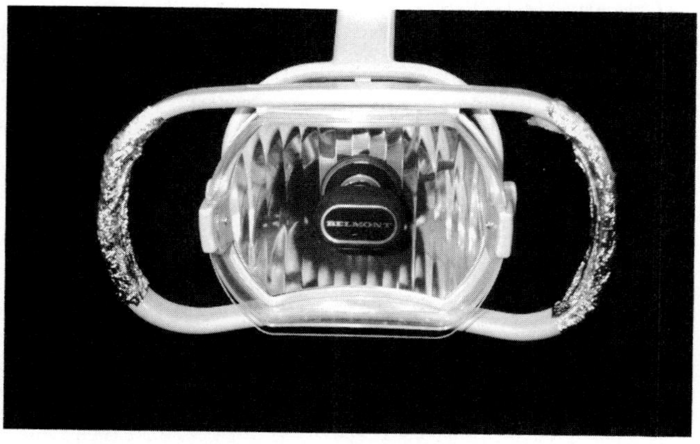

FIGURE 8–6.
Foil on light handle.

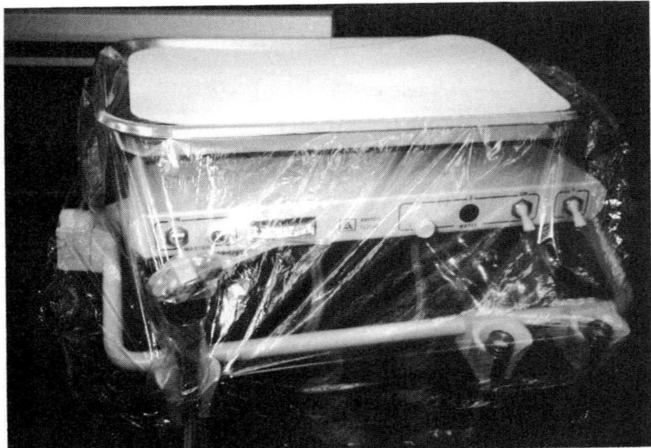

FIGURE 8-7
Plastic barrier on unit controls.

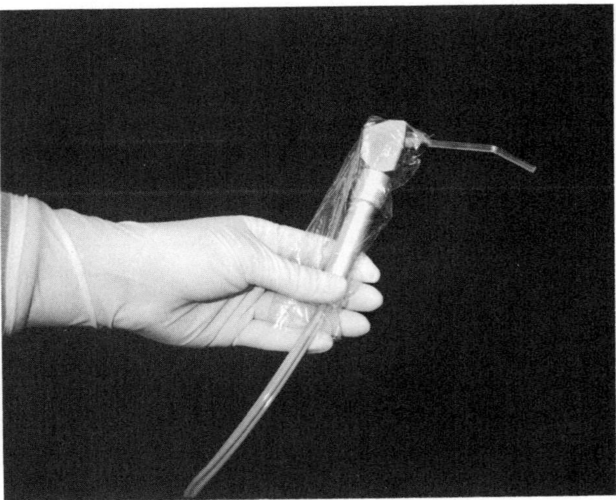

FIGURE 8-8
Plastic barrier or bag on ASW syringes.

and the surface must be disinfected (see Important Factors Related to Disposable Surface Barriers chart).[2]

Surface Cleaning—The Critical Step Prior To Disinfection

The use of disposable surface barriers minimizes the need to clean and disinfect surfaces for items that cannot be sterilized. However, while barriers may reduce the number of times surfaces need to be cleaned and disinfected each day, the necessity of this procedure is not eliminated. When surface barriers provide complete surface protection and are carefully discarded and changed between clients, cleaning and disinfection may be required only at the end of the day.

Cleaning environmental surfaces and contaminated items attached to the dental unit control system (Fig. 8-9) prior to disinfecting them is one of the most overlooked yet critical steps needed to ensure the antimicrobial **(biocidal)** action of the disinfection procedure. Omission of the cleaning step or insufficient cleaning of the surfaces contaminated with blood and saliva and other debris (bioburden) prior to disinfection or sterilization may render those procedures ineffective. *The significance of the initial cleaning step in environmental surface disinfection cannot be overemphasized.* Agencies and organizations, for example, the Centers for Disease Control (CDC) and ADA, responsible for publishing infection control guidelines for healthcare professionals consistently reinforce the importance of **precleaning** as an essential step in ensuring effective disinfection and sterilization.[5-7]

IMPORTANT FACTORS RELATED TO DISPOSABLE SURFACE BARRIERS

Rationale for Use of Nonpermeable Barriers
To protect surfaces and items from contact with hands contaminated by blood and saliva.

Types
Plastic wrap, plastic food bags, aluminum foil, impervious-backed paper, or custom-designed plastic covers/bags.

Targeted Items
All equipment and surfaces prone to contamination that are practical to cover, especially items with crevices, knobs, buttons, uneven surfaces and those made of materials susceptible to damage by chemical disinfectants.

Procedure
Selected barrier must cover the entire surface and edges for adequate protection. Discard and replace after each client; clean and disinfect the surface at the end of the day.

Benefits
Barriers save time since they limit the number of surfaces that must be cleaned and disinfected between clients; with adequate barrier coverage it is only necessary to clean and disinfect the covered surfaces at the end of the day as opposed to between clients.

Alternative Method
Time-consuming, meticulous cleaning and disinfection between clients.

Trends
More custom-designed barrier covers to improve convenience; may increase cost and improve appearance.

Data from Cottone, J. A., Terezhalmy, G. T., and Molinari, J. A. Practical Infection Control in Dentistry. Philadelphia: Lea & Febiger, 1991.

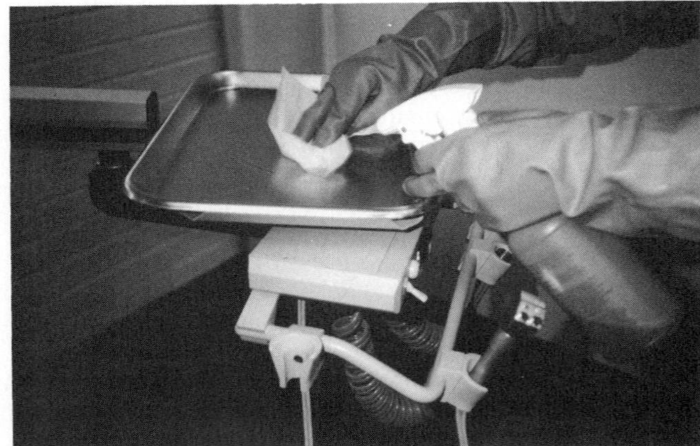

FIGURE 8-9
Heavy-duty nitrile-gloved hands performing initial cleaning step of environmental surface disinfection.

Since there is agreement that the presence of bioburden (organic debris) on uncleaned surfaces reduces or impairs germicidal activity, it is important to select a cleaning agent that effectively penetrates blood, saliva, and other organic debris.[8] Detergents are cleaning agents, or surface-active agents **(surfactants),** that effect a cleansing action by altering the nature of the interface between the surface and the debris by lowering the surface tension. They also contribute an antimicrobial effect by altering the osmotic barrier of the cell membrane, which results in increased cell permeability and loss of cell integrity.[2] Surface-active agents that lower surface tension, possess antimicrobial properties, and penetrate organic debris on inanimate surfaces are anionic soaps and synthetic anionic detergents (see Agents Useful for Cleaning Surfaces chart).[2] Additionally, aqueous (water-based) **disinfectants** that solubilize organic matter or those that contain detergents may serve as both a cleaning agent and a surface disinfectant.[8]

AGENTS USEFUL FOR CLEANING SURFACES (EITHER BY PRECLEANING PRIOR TO DISINFECTION* OR BY CLEANING AND DISINFECTING WITH AGENT CAPABLE OF BOTH FUNCTIONS)

- Anionic soaps*
- Synthetic anionic detergents*
- Aqueous (water-based) disinfectants that contain a detergent (complex phenols and iodophors)**
- Water-based disinfectant solutions that solubilize blood and other organic matter (sodium hypochlorite)**

Data from Cottone, J. A., Terezhalmy, G. T., and Molinari, J. A. Practical Infection Control in Dentistry. Philadelphia: Lea & Febiger, 1991.

Environmental Surface Disinfection

Levels of Surface Disinfection

The selection of chemicals for surface cleaning and disinfection may be confusing because of the number of agents available, manufacturers' biased claims, and misleading assays reported in the scientific literature.[2] The goal of surface disinfection is to maximize microbial inactivation or to kill microorganisms via the most effective and practical alternative mechanism when heat-sterilization is not possible. Disinfectants are classified according to three levels—high, intermediate, and low—based on their efficacy across a wide antimicrobial spectrum (Table 8–2) (see Wide Microbial Spectrum Associated with Levels of Disinfection chart).

It is generally recommended that an intermediate-level disinfectant that is registered by the **Environmental Protection Agency (EPA-registered)** as a tuberculocidal, **hospital-level disinfectant** (Fig. 8–10) with appropriate virucidal activity is appropriate for surface disinfection in the oral healthcare environment.[2,5] Surface disinfectants carrying the ADA Council on Dental Therapeutics seal of acceptance on the product label indicate that the product has documented evidence of bactericidal, tuberculocidal, and virucidal (lipophilic and hydrophilic viruses) activity.[10]

Criteria for an Ideal Disinfectant

Although there are many products with EPA registration and the ADA seal of acceptance, there is no single chemical

TABLE 8–2
LEVELS OF DISINFECTION AND ASSOCIATED GERMICIDAL ACTION

Level	Capability	Essential Criterion	Examples
High	Inactivates resistant bacterial spores and other less resistant microbial forms, such as bacteria (tubercle bacillus, vegetative bacteria), fungi, and viruses (lipid and medium-sized, and nonlipid and small)	Ability to kill bacterial spores required for a high-level classification; with extended exposure times, high-level disinfectants capable of sterilization (6–10 hours); EPA-registered "disinfectant/sterilant" indicated on the product label	2.0–3.2% glutaraldehyde preparations (immersion glutaraldehydes) and ethylene oxide
Intermediate	May not be able to inactivate bacterial endospores; there are differences among intermediate disinfectants in their ability to inactivate small, nonlipid viruses; as a group, will kill other microbial forms, including the second most resistant microorganism, *Mycobacterium tuberculosis*	Ability to kill *M. tuberculosis;* for the dental environment an intermediate-level disinfectant should be EPA-registered as tuberculocidal, hospital-grade (kills three species of basic test bacteria: *Staphylococcus aureus, Salmonella typhimurium,* and *Pseudomonas aeruginosa)* with appropriate virucidal activity	Formaldehyde, chlorine compounds, iodophor, alcohols, complex (synthetic) phenols
Low	Has the narrowest antimicrobial range; may inactivate certain viruses and vegetative bacteria	Will not kill tubercle bacilli, nonlipid viruses, or fungi; unacceptable for disinfection of items and equipment classified as critical or semicritical	Quaternary ammonium compounds, simple phenols and detergents

Adapted from Cottone, J. A., Terezhalmy, G. T., and Molinari, J. A. Practical Infection Control in Dentistry. Philadelphia: Lea & Febiger 1991; and Department of Veterans Affairs, American Dental Association, Department of Health and Human Services. Infection control in the dental environment. Washington, D.C.: Learning Resources Service and Eastern Dental Education Center, VA Medical Center, 1989.

WIDE MICROBIAL SPECTRUM ASSOCIATED WITH LEVELS OF DISINFECTION

Bacterial Endospores
The most resistant microorganisms (having thick-walled bodies with a hard outer shell that protects the living organisms inside; the tough shell is what makes spores so resistant to destruction). The ability to kill bacterial spores requires a **high-level chemical disinfectant/** sterilant (6 to 10 hours exposure). Some intermediate-level disinfectants exhibit sporicidal action.

***Mycobacterium Tuberculosis* (TB)**
The most resistant microorganisms after bacterial endospores, presenting a severe challenge to chemical disinfectants and requiring an **intermediate-level disinfectant.**

Small Nonlipid Viruses
Hydrophilic (nonlipid) viruses do not have a lipid (fat) envelope and are more resistant than lipophilic viruses. Nonlipid viruses such as polioviruses, coxsackie virus, rhinovirus, and rotavirus are more difficult to kill and require an **intermediate-level disinfectant** (alcohol and phenolic compounds (water-based, alcohol-based) may have limited virucidal activity).

Fungi
Simple microscopic plants such as molds and yeasts that are less resistant (e.g., *Candida* and *Aspergillus*). Some **low-level disinfectants** are capable of fungicidal action, and all **intermediate-level disinfectants** produce effective fungicidal action.

Medium-Sized Lipid Viruses
Viruses enclosed in capsids (shells) containing lipids or fat are called lipophilic viruses, such as influenza viruses, HIV, and herpes simplex viruses. They are more easily killed by both **intermediate-** and **low-level disinfectants.**

Vegetative Bacteria
The least resistant to the effects of disinfectants at all levels.

Data from Cottone, J. A., Terezhalmy, G. T., and Molinari, J. A. Practical Infection Control in Dentistry. Philadelphia: Lea & Febiger, 1991.

disinfectant that has all the properties required for an ideal disinfectant (Table 8–3). The ideal disinfectant properties have been identified and are useful criteria for evaluation of available products.

Characteristics of Chemical Agents for Surface Disinfection

Although no one single product meets all the criteria for an ideal environmental surface disinfectant, the categories of EPA- and, formerly, ADA-accepted intermediate-hospital-surface disinfectants include iodophors (e.g., Biocide, Iodo-five), complex (synthetic) phenols (e.g., Omni II, Vitaphene), and chlorine-containing compounds (e.g., Alcide LD, Exspor). The EPA has also given intermediate-hospital-surface disinfectant approval to a class of glutaraldehyde products that contain 0.25 to 0.50% glutaraldehyde (e.g.,

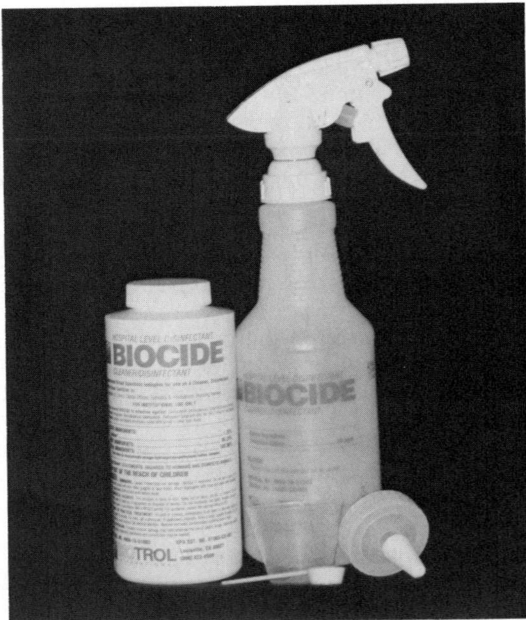

FIGURE 8–10
Bottles of intermediate-level disinfectant, and EPA-registered, tuberculocidal, hospital-grade disinfectant.

Sterall). Other chemicals combined in the glutaraldehyde preparations may enhance the disinfection activity of the products. Glutaraldehydes and other immersion disinfectants and sterilants (sporicidal disinfectants) are discussed in greater detail in Chapter 9 with the subject of instrument and equipment recirculation.

The advantages and disadvantages of using the iodophors, complex (synthetic) phenols, chlorine-containing compounds, and glutaraldehyde products as disinfectants are presented in Table 8–4. Chemical agents, products, and their status for acceptance as environmental surface disinfectants are presented in Table 8–5.

It should be noted that prevention of transmission of bloodborne pathogens (HBV, HIV) in the dental environment requires that the cleaning and/or disinfecting agents used are able to penetrate and remain active in the presence of organic matter such as blood, saliva, and exudate. Two categories of agents that have limited ability to penetrate organic debris on inanimate surfaces or have no ability to penetrate tissue proteins such as those found in blood and saliva are quaternary ammonium compounds and ethyl and isopropyl alcohol preparations.[2] Although alcohols have a broader antimicrobial range than quaternary ammonium compounds, both have been clearly identified as *unacceptable* for surface or instrument disinfection by the ADA Council on Dental Therapeutics and the CDC. Even ADA-approved disinfectants that contain a high percentage of alcohol need to be evaluated carefully, because alcohols are poor cleaning agents in the presence of bioburden. Alcohol denatures proteins, causing them to be insoluble and adherent to most surfaces and leaving a coating of denatured blood and organic debris that can protect the potential pathogens from the biocidal effects of alcohols for prolonged periods.[2,11,12] For effective use of ADA- and EPA-approved disinfectants that are more than 50% ethyl or isopropanol, surfaces must be precleaned with a separate agent that thoroughly removes the bioburden. Meticulous cleaning and disinfection is time-consuming enough with-

TABLE 8–3
CRITERIA FOR AN IDEAL DISINFECTANT

Property	Significance
Broad spectrum	Must have widest antimicrobial spectrum; use of chemicals is a compromise when heat sterilization is not possible; important to maximize the microbial kill and recognize that highly resistant bacterial and mycotic spores may not be affected
Not affected by physical factors	Must be able to penetrate and retain antimicrobial action in the presence of organic matter, such as blood, saliva, exudate, and feces; compatibility with other chemical soaps and detergents used is essential for maximum effectiveness
Fast-acting	Must be rapidly lethal in action on all vegetative forms and spores of bacteria, fungi, protozoa, and viruses; chemicals that require 20 minutes or more to kill *Mycobacterium tuberculosis* would be of little practical value for the oral healthcare provider; contact time must be reasonable to allow use between appointments
Nontoxic	Must be nonirritating to skin and eyes; many disinfectants are irritating and harmful to skin and eyes, and breathing the vapors can cause additional problems
Surface compatibility	Must not be damaging to metal, plastic, cloth, or painted or other surfaces/materials; chemicals may corrode instruments and other metallic surfaces, cause disintegration of plastics, rubber, and cloth, and cause staining from repeated use
Easy to use	Must be easily prepared or mixed for use and readily applied, preferably via a pump-spray bottle for easy delivery, and must serve as both a cleaner and a disinfectant to maximize efficiency; less frequent preparation of chemical product saves time; premixed product or less frequent mixing minimizes chances of not following the directions for preparation requiring strict compliance for maximum microbial control; both cleaning and disinfecting properties combined in one product also provide some protection during the cleaning step by sanitizing any debris spattered during the cleaning step
Residual effect on treated surfaces	Must have prolonged biocidal activity after application; multiple applications of cleaner/disinfectant with residual antimicrobial activity continue biocidal action even after solution has dried
Odorless	Must be odorless; an inoffensive odor, preferably no odor, facilitates continued and routine use of chemical disinfectant
Economical	Cost must not be prohibitively high; reasonable cost is a consideration that influences product selection, utilization, and oral healthcare costs

Adapted from Molinari, J. A., Campbell, M. D., and York, J. Minimizing potential infections in dental practice. Journal of the Michigan Dental Association 64:411, 1982.

TABLE 8–4
CHARACTERISTICS OF CHEMICAL AGENTS FOR ENVIRONMENTAL SURFACE DISINFECTION

Agent	Action	Advantages	Disadvantages
Iodophors	Powerful germicidal action of iodine acts by iodination of proteins and subsequent formation of protein salts	EPA-registered and ADA-accepted Broad spectrum: bactericidal, tuberculocidal, and virucidal against hydrophilic and lipophilic viruses Biocidal activity within 5–10 minutes Economical Effective in dilute solution Few side effect reactions Surfactant carrier maintains surface moistness Residual biocidal action	Not a sterilant Unstable at high temperatures Dilution and contact time are critical Must be prepared daily to ensure tuberculocidal activity May discolor some surfaces Inactivated by hard water; distilled water recommended Inactivated by alcohol[2]
Complex (synthetic) phenols	Phenolic compounds act as cytoplasmic poisons by penetrating and disrupting microbial cell walls, which results in denaturation of intracellular proteins	EPA-registered and ADA-accepted as both an immersion and a surface disinfectant **Synergistic** effect of combining two to three phenols Broad antimicrobial spectrum Tuberculocidal Useful on metal, glass, rubber, and plastic	Not sporicidal Must be prepared fresh daily Can degrade certain plastics and etch glass with prolonged exposure Film accumulation Skin and eye irritation[2]

Table continued on following page

TABLE 8–4

CHARACTERISTICS OF CHEMICAL AGENTS FOR ENVIRONMENTAL SURFACE DISINFECTION

Continued

Agent	Action	Advantages	Disadvantages
		Less toxic and corrosive than glutaraldehyde Economical	
Chlorine compounds	Act primarily by oxidation; elemental chlorine is a potent germicide, killing most bacteria in 15–30 seconds	Some products are EPA-registered and ADA-accepted Rapid antimicrobial action Broad spectrum: bactericidal, tuberculocidal, and virucidal; CDC has recommended sodium hypochlorite (diluted bleach 1:10 to 1:100) as an effective agent in destroying hepatitis B viruses) Economical Effective in dilute solution	Sporicidal only at high concentrations Cannot be reused (no reuselife) Must be prepared fresh daily Activity diminished by organic matter Unpleasant, persistent odor Irritating to skin and eyes Corrodes metals and damages clothing Degrades plastics and rubber[2]
A class of glutaraldehyde surface disinfectants was developed in the mid-1980s, 0.25–0.50% glutaraldehyde, which is a derivation from the 2.0–3.2% glutaraldehyde used as immersion chemical sterilants/disinfectants	Glutaraldehydes have a broad antimicrobial spectrum and, at the lower concentration, have been EPA-approved as intermediate hospital-surface disinfectants		May be sensitizing to the skin Vapor can irritate or injure eyes and nasal passages

TABLE 8–5

CHEMICAL AGENTS FOR CLEANING AND DISINFECTION OF ENVIRONMENTAL SURFACES

Chemical Classification	Product	TB Disinfection Directions and Requirements**	EPA Registration Number	Formerly ADA Accepted*	Hydrophilic Virucide	Cleaning Ability
Chlorine dioxide	• Exspor	4:1:1, 3 min., 20c (AOAC)	(45631-03)	Yes	Yes	Good
Sodium hypochlorite	• Bleach (5.25%)	1:10, 10 min., 20c	—	No	Yes	Good
	• Dispatch	None, 2 min., 20–25c	(56392-7)		Yes	Good
Iodophor	• Biocide, Bi-Arrest	1:213, 10 min., 20c (AOAC)	(4959-16)	Yes	Yes	Good
	Surf-A-Cide	20c (AOAC)		Yes	Yes	Good
	• Iodofive	1:213, 5 min., 20c (AOAC)	(1677-22)	Yes	Yes (10 min.)	Good
	• Asepti-IOC	1:256, 10 min., (AOAC)			Yes	Good
	• Wescodyne	1:213, 25 min., 25c (Quant)			Yes	Good
Phenolic Combinations*** Water-based pump spray *Phenyl* *Amyl* *Chloro*						
9.0% — 1%	• Omni II, ProPhene	1:32, 10 min., 20c (AOAC)	(4685-1)	Yes	Yes	Good
0.28% — 0.03%	Vital Defense-D			Yes	Yes	Good
12.0% 4.0% 10.0%	• Asepti-phene 128	1:128, 10 min., 25c (AOAC)	(303-223)	No	No	Good
Alcohol-Based Aerosol *Phenyl* *Amyl* *Ethanol*						
0.1% — 79%	Lysol IC Disinfectant	None, 10 min., 20c (AOAC)	777-53		Yes	Poor
0.136% — 78.5%	ClinAsept Spray	None, 10 min., 20c (AOAC)	675-25		Yes	Poor
0.12% — 66.6%	Citrace	None, 10 min., 20-25c (AOAC)	56392-2		Yes	Poor
The following products in this group do not demonstrate a hydrophilic virus kill:						
0.176% 0.044% 52.79%	Medicide/ADC Disinfectant Deodorant	None, 10 min. (AOAC)	334-214		No	Poor
0.176% 0.045% 49.95%	Asepti-Steryl	None, 10 min., 25c (AOAC)	206-69		No	Poor

*ADA no longer has a formal acceptance program for surface disinfectants, the formerly accepted products have been subjected to the additional scrutiny required to warrant the seal.

**Test used to TB label claim: Association of Official Analytical Chemists (AOAC).

***Phenyl = ortho phenylphenol; amyl = tertiary amylphenol; chloro = benzyl chlorophenol.

RT = Room Temperature.

Adapted from Office Sterilization and Asepsis Procedures (OSAP) Research Foundation. Guide to chemical agents for disinfection and/or sterilization, May, 1992. Distributed to Foundation members January 1994; and data from Office Sterilization and Asepsis Procedures (OSAP) Research Foundation. Chemical agent for surface cleaning and disinfection, January, 1993. Distributed to Foundation members April 3, 1993.

out having to use a separate product to ensure adequate precleaning prior to use of an ADA- or EPA-approved alcohol-based disinfectant.[2,8,11,12]

SPECIFIC PROTOCOLS FOR PREVENTION OF DISEASE TRANSMISSION DURING THE DENTAL HYGIENE CARE PROCESS

Environmental surface disinfection constitutes a major portion of an effective infection control program, yet it is only one aspect of it. In order to maintain quality assurance and standardization of the many procedures associated with the prevention of transmission of bloodborne pathogens, all techniques or steps for maintaining equipment in the most aseptic condition possible need to be included as part of the infection control program. Each infection control program needs to incorporate into one comprehensive document for aseptic technique accountability a compilation of the following: all infection control protocols and procedures, delineation of responsibilities, a log of infection control activities, a record of requirements established by the Occupational Safety and Health Administration (OSHA) (see Chapter 7), documentation of biological monitors for sterilization equipment, and mechanisms for checking on compliance of dental team members with standard operating procedures. The dental hygienist, a traditional role model in the area of aseptic technique, can make a significant contribution in this endeavor. The expertise of the dental hygienist as clinician, educator, and change agent seems to be a natural match with the role of infection control program planner, consultant, or coordinator.

The following section addresses aseptic technique as it affects all phases of the dental hygiene process. Protocols and standard operating procedures are presented for each aspect of dental hygiene care, including the fundamental

CRITICAL ASPECTS OF SURFACE DISINFECTION

- Product selection—EPA-registered, ADA-accepted disinfectant specified for use as a "surface" disinfectant.
- Aqueous disinfectant with detergent may be used for both cleaning and disinfection.
- Preparation of disinfectant according to manufacturer's directions for **dilution** (if label states to dilute with water, water must be used, not alcohol).
- Specific **use-life** (length of time of effectiveness) must be noted and preparations made accordingly. Some disinfectants must be mixed daily.
- Surfaces must be *cleaned first,* then wiped (Fig. 8–11).
- Paper towels are larger, faster, and less expensive than sponges or gauze.
- Spray delivery is well suited to penetrate crevices:
  Prevent inactivation of germicidal activity or absorption caused by sponges or gauze.
  Spray/wipe (cleaning step), spray (disinfection step).
  Single-use disposable covers best for electrical switches—spray may cause short-circuit of electrical system.
- Disinfectant applied for prescribed time (at least minimum exposure time required for TB kill; if 20 minutes, of limited value, not practical).
- After specified time, any excess disinfectant may be wiped away with a clean paper towel (Fig. 8–12).
- Only items used in zone of contamination (chairside) that are not completely protected by covers need to be cleaned and disinfected between clients.

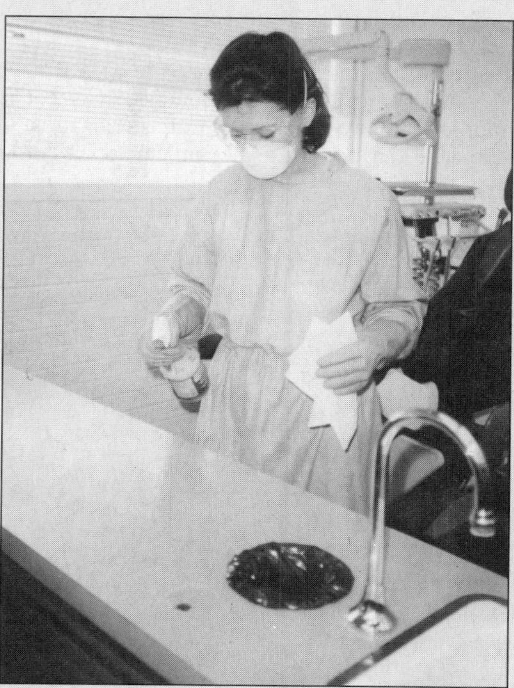

FIGURE 8–11
Spraying surface for initial cleaning step.

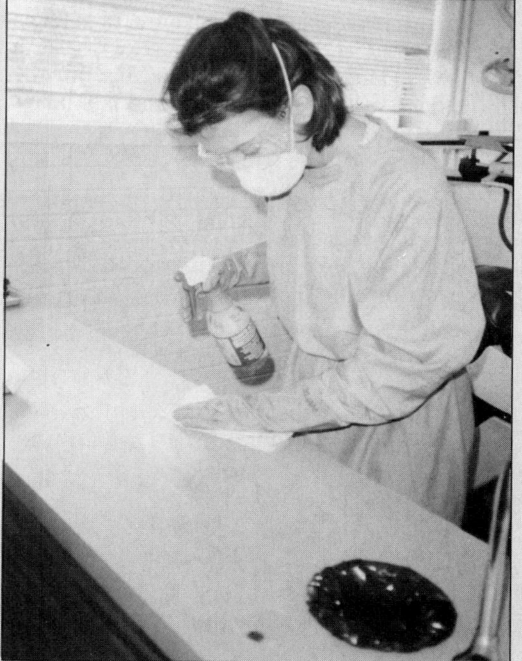

FIGURE 8–12
Wiping sprayed surface—bioburden removal.

preparation of the operatory for the appointment, aseptic technique during dental hygiene care delivery, and postappointment decontamination (see Critical Aspects of Surface Disinfection chart). Chapter 9 addresses instrument and equipment recirculation.

Preparation of the Operatory for the Dental Hygiene Care Appointment

It is critical that the dental team clearly understand the rationale for aseptic techniques and come to a consensus for following prescribed infection control protocols for every aspect of client care. A protocol is an explicit detailed plan, and here the term is used to refer to detailed, step-by-step procedures for prevention of disease transmission during dental hygiene care. Dental hygienists do not provide care in a vacuum, and they may be responsible for the development of the overall infection control program in a practice, clinic, or educational program. Communication and team participation in the protocol development and review process is imperative to gain consensus and to facilitate compliance. Periodic review of protocols to update and ensure that procedures meet or exceed professional and governmental standards also improves communication and compliance. Compliance with the protocols for dental hygiene, oral and maxillofacial radiography, and laboratory procedures is essential for quality assurance and safe delivery of client care (see Standards and/or Guidelines for Infection Control Protocols and Policies chart).

As an example, surface disinfection is a significant part of every protocol and involves every member of the dental team. Consensus should be gained in order to establish the procedure for surfaces to be cleaned and disinfected daily, including surfaces covered by single-use barriers that should be changed between clients and uncovered surfaces that require meticulous cleaning and disinfection between clients.

Operatory preparation involves making sure that *all* surfaces are cleaned and disinfected daily (at the end of the day). In settings in which there is more than one dental hygiene care provider using an operatory, assumptions should not be made regarding surface decontamination.

When previous surface decontamination is unknown, the operatory preparation protocol is the following:

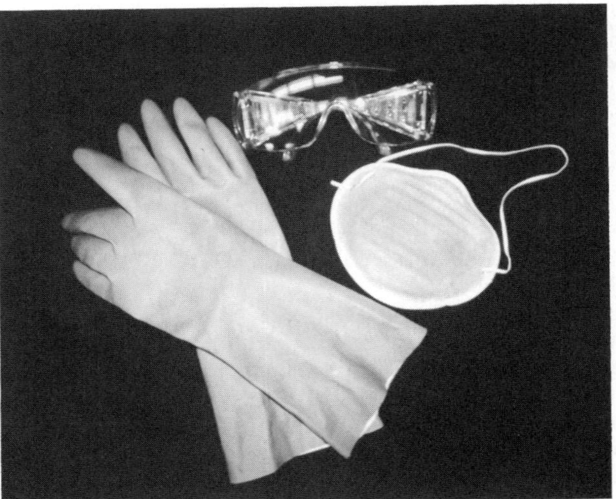

FIGURE 8-13
Protective eyewear, heavy-duty (nitrile) gloves, mask.

Operatory Preparation Protocol

1. Prepare for the operatory preparation infection control procedure by wearing protective eyewear, a mask, and puncture-resistant nitrile gloves (Fig. 8-13).
2. Flush all water lines (e.g., ASW syringes, handpiece water lines, which may be used for sonic scaling device, and/or ultrasonic scaling equipment) (Fig. 8-14) for 3 to 5 minutes at the beginning of the day, for 20 seconds between clients, and for 1 minute after lunch. (Handpieces should be disconnected from hoses during flushing; free running water could damage the bearings.)[2]
3. Suction tubing for low- and high-volume suctions should be flushed with water between client appointments and cleaned and disinfected (Fig. 8-15) at the end of the day with a commercial cleansing solution (see Chapter 9 for procedures to be performed at the end of the day).
4. Clean and disinfect all surfaces (see Critical Aspects of Surface Disinfection chart) (Fig. 8-16).
5. If equipment attached to the unit (e.g., ASW syringes, suction and delivery hoses, and handpieces) is not removable and/or cannot withstand heat sterilization (steam under pressure and unsaturated chemical vapor sterilization

STANDARDS AND/OR GUIDELINES FOR INFECTION CONTROL PROTOCOLS AND POLICIES

Development and revision of infection control protocols and policies should comply with current guidelines and/or standards published by:

- United States Public Health Service Centers for Disease Control (CDC)
- American Dental Association (ADA)
- American Association of Dental Schools (AADS)
- American Dental Hygienists' Association (ADHA)
- United States Occupational Safety and Health Administration (OSHA)
- Environmental Protection Agency (EPA)
- State, local and institutional regulations

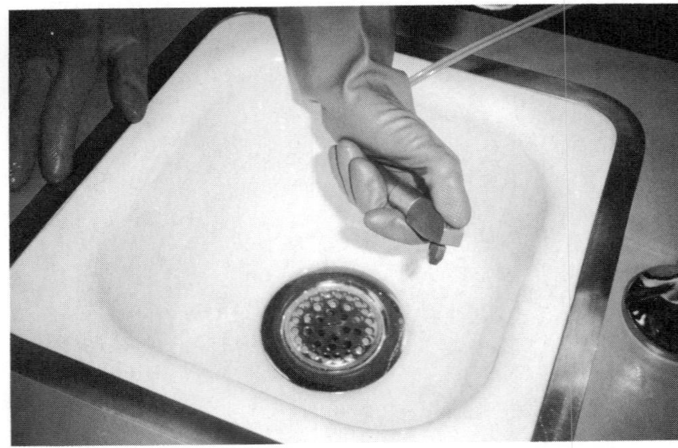

FIGURE 8-14
Air-spray-water syringe being flushed.

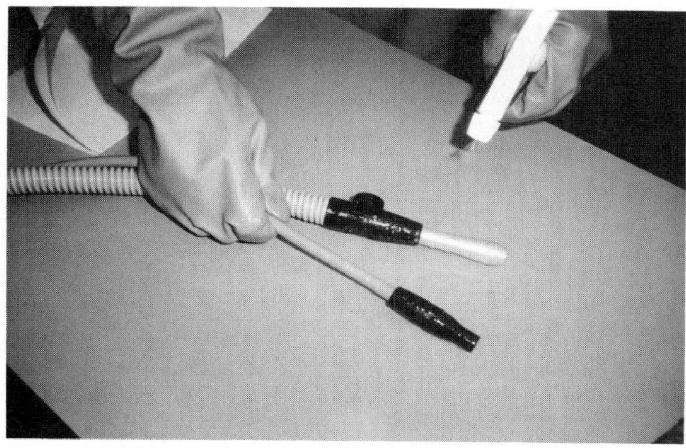

FIGURE 8–15
Suction lines being cleaned and disinfected.

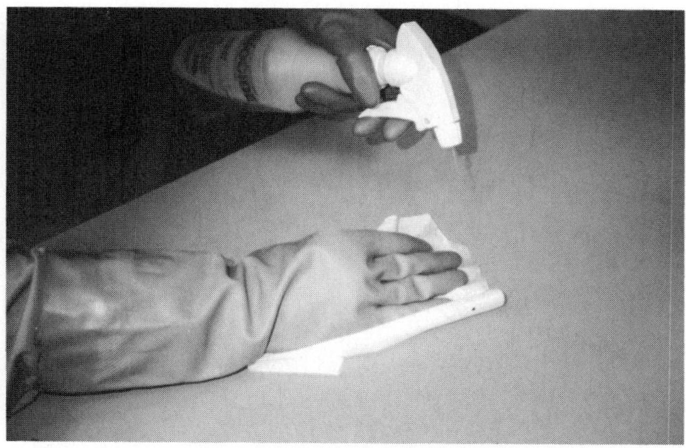

FIGURE 8–16
Spraying surfaces with environmental surface disinfectant.

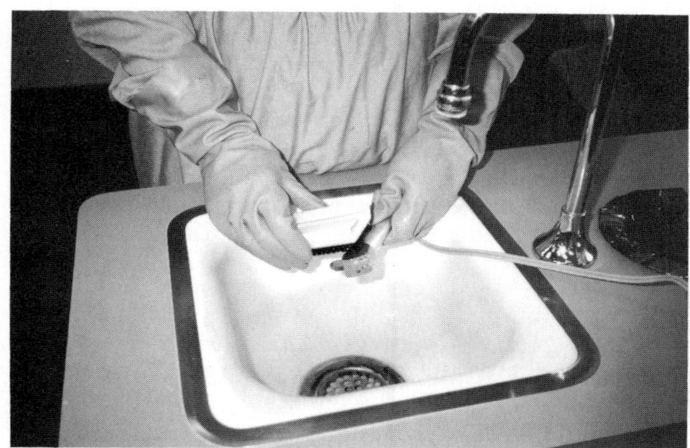

FIGURE 8–17
Brushing air-water syringe.

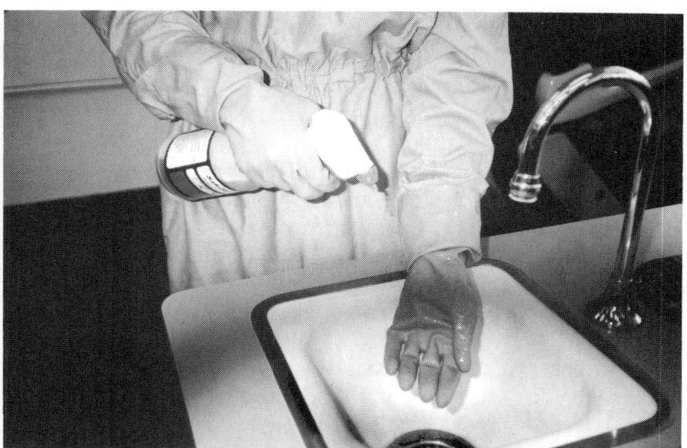

FIGURE 8–18
Spraying nitrile gloves with environmental surface disinfectant.

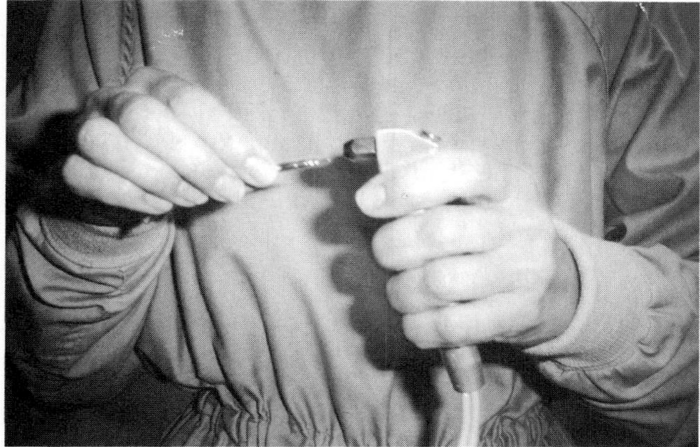

FIGURE 8–19
Clean hands placing air-water syringe tip.

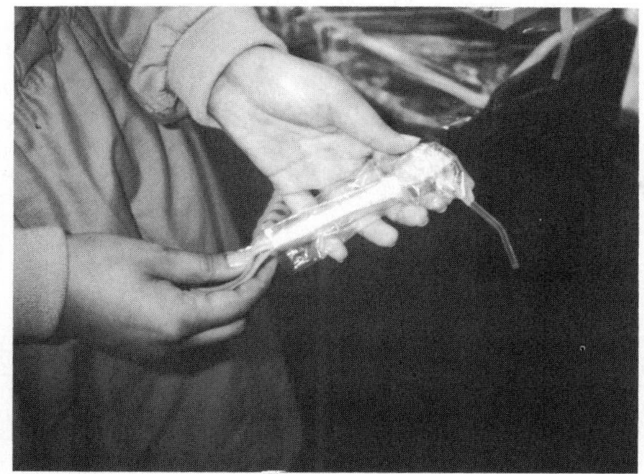

FIGURE 8–20
Placement of barrier over air-water syringe.

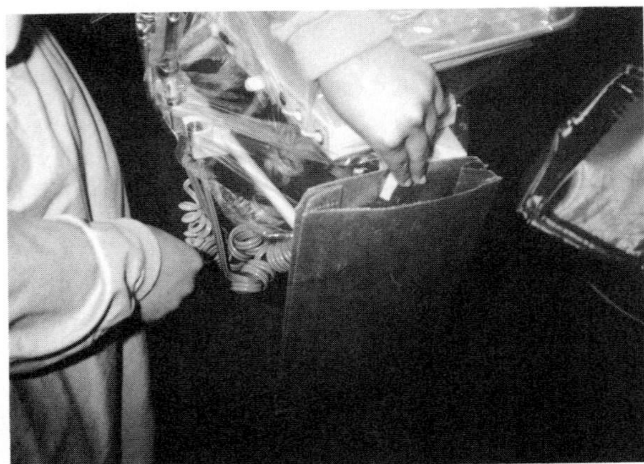

FIGURE 8-21
Attachment of biohazardous-waste bag to unit.

methods), pull it to a nearby sink, clean with disinfectant scrub (using a clean brush) (Fig. 8-17), rinse, dry with a paper towel, wet with an EPA- or ADA-accepted disinfectant for the specified time, and check directions to determine whether air-drying or rinsing is required.[2]

6. Clean and disinfect puncture-resistant nitrile gloves (Fig. 8-18); wash hands.

7. With clean hands, put in place single-use surface barriers; ensure complete coverage of surfaces selected for barrier use in order to prevent cross-contamination. If the ASW syringe is not removable for sterilization, attach sterilized or disposable ASW tips (Fig. 8-19) prior to placement of barrier over handle and control buttons (Fig. 8-20).

8. Attach the biohazardous waste bag (Fig. 8-21) within easy reach for disposal of blood- and saliva-soaked items (see Chapter 9 for waste disposal).

9. Place disposable and sterilized equipment according to use areas within the zone of contamination.

10. Preorganized cassettes or trays and support equipment prepared (Fig. 8-22) according to the schedule for specific dental hygiene care procedures increase efficiency and reduce stress. Sufficient supplies should be included, such as sterile gauze, cotton swabs, and cotton rolls. Frequently needed disposable and protective materials should be readily accessible, which may include low- and high-volume suction tips, client protective eyewear, dental hygienist full-protection eyewear, high-filtration masks, and quality gloves.

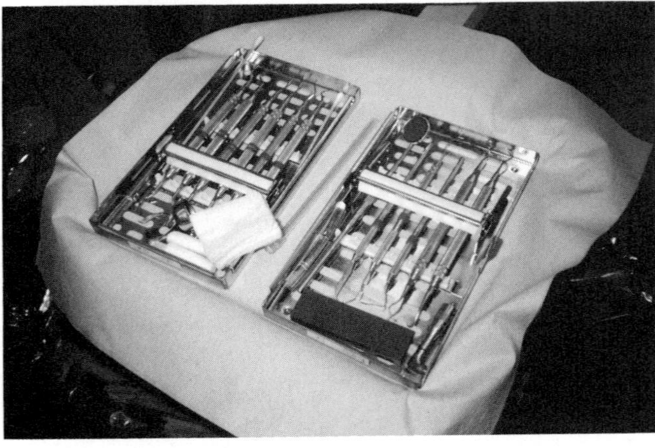

FIGURE 8-22
Cassette with gauze cotton-tips, saliva ejector, and instruments.

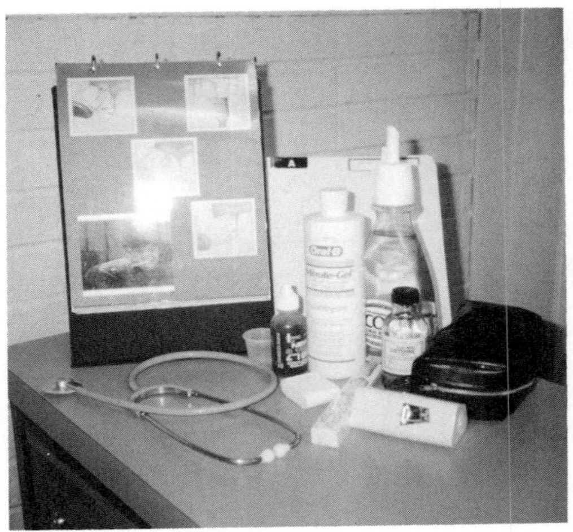

FIGURE 8-23
Client records, visual aids, and supplies in noncontaminated zone.

11. Additional supplies, client education and counseling materials, client records, fresh personal protective barriers, and nontreatment gloves for the appointment should be prepared and placed in the noncontaminated zone (Fig. 8-23). (Items in the noncontaminated area are to be kept to a minimum.)

PROTOCOLS FOR THE DENTAL HYGIENE CARE PROCESS

Protocols for specific procedures that are associated with the different phases of the dental hygiene care process are presented. Each protocol includes infection control considerations particular to the procedure and a table presenting a suggested strategy for organizing the armamentarium according to specific use areas within the contaminated and noncontaminated zones.

The contaminated zone is divided into three use areas (see Fig. 8-2) with use area I (instrument tray/cassette bracket table) representing the use area with the highest concentration of microorganisms; use area II (power module, unit controls) includes additional items that frequently come into contact with the contaminated gloved hand of the operator. The third contaminated zone, use area III (adjacent countertop) is exposed to microorganisms (spat-

TABLE 8-6
PLACEMENT OF EQUIPMENT WITHIN EACH USE AREA DURING CLIENT INTERVIEW

I	II	III	IV
			Forms Pens Pencils Client hand mirror Stethoscope Sphygmomanometer

ter/aerosols only) by virtue of proximity and may hold adjunct items or equipment used during dental hygiene care. The noncontaminated zone is designated as use area IV (section of countertop away from the contaminated zone). Items placed here are to remain noncontaminated and should come into contact only with clean hands, nontreatment gloves (overgloves), or forceps/pliers.

The following protocols are designed to prevent cross-contamination during dental hygiene care.

INFECTION CONTROL PROTOCOLS FOR THE ASSESSMENT PHASE OF THE DENTAL HYGIENE CARE PROCESS

The assessment phase of the dental hygiene care process is presented here with protocols and standard operating procedure examples that emphasize infection control considerations and also the organization of the armamentarium according to use areas during the client interview (Table 8-6), extraoral/intraoral examination, periodontal evaluation, and examination of the teeth.

Client Interview (Histories)

The client interview consists of an assessment of the human needs related to dental hygiene care, the health history, the vital signs (pulse, respiration, and blood pressure), and the dental cultural histories (Fig. 8-24).

- In addition to significant data collection, the time spent during the client interview provides an important opportunity to communicate and establish a rapport with the client prior to donning the personal protection barriers, which may impede direct communication.
- The only pieces of equipment involved in the initial assessments are the stethoscope and sphygmomanometer. The earpieces of the stethoscope should be cleaned and disinfected along with other surfaces cleaned and disinfected at the end of the day.

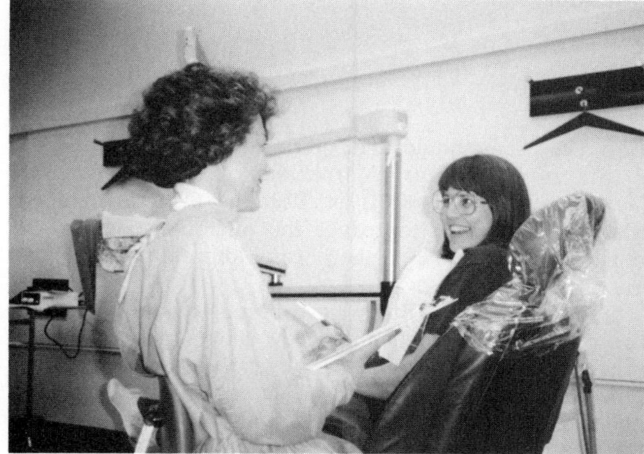

FIGURE 8-24
Client interview.

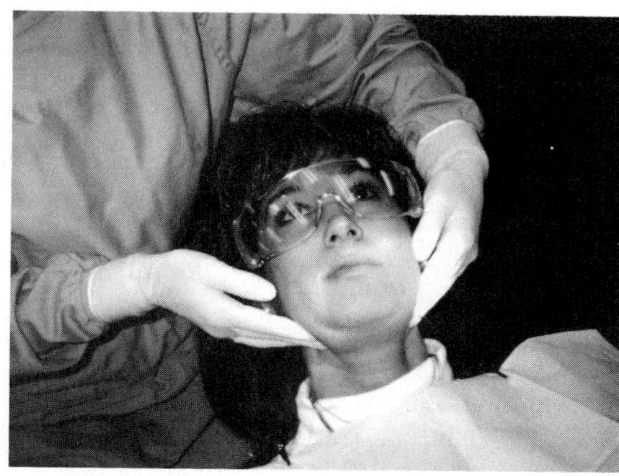

FIGURE 8-25
Extraoral assessment.

Extraoral/Intraoral Assessment

1. The extraoral/intraoral assessment (Fig. 8-25) is the first in a series of assessments that potentially expose the dental hygienist to the blood and saliva of the client. At this time, the dental hygienist should explain the procedure to the client, noting the use of client and dental hygienist protective eyewear, gloves, and mask. Emphasis should be placed on explaining universal precautions and adherence to CDC, ADA, and OSHA guidelines and standards to protect clients and to meet their human needs for safety and conceptualization.

2. Protective attire, disinfected protective eyewear, and a new mask should be put on before handwashing and donning of gloves, as the last step prior to beginning the extraoral portion of the examination.

3. Before proceeding with the extraoral and intraoral assessment, the client should remove any complete or partial prostheses or other removable appliances, such as orthodontic retainers and stay plates. When the dental history indicates use of a night guard (splint) or any other removable preventive or therapeutic intraoral appliance, the client should be requested to present the appliance for assessment if it is available.

- Inspect prostheses, brush to remove soft deposits (either with a new brush to be dispensed to the client or a heat-sterilizable denture brush), and rinse.
- Place in a disposable plastic barrier bag, add mouth rinse (holding solution to prevent drying of contaminants and prostheses) to cover the prosthesis/appliance, and place the bag in a denture cup (Fig. 8-26). The denture cup may be dispensed to the client for home use; if it is not dispensed to the client, reuse of the denture cup by the dental hygienist requires the use of a plastic barrier bag and meticulous cleaning and disinfection.
- The mouth rinse holding solution reduces microorganisms, gives a pleasant taste, and permits nonirritation of tissue on reinsertion of the prostheses or appliance.
- Prior to removing calculus and stain from prostheses, spray or soak the prostheses with disinfectant (Table 8-7 lists biomaterials considerations for selection of disinfectant). (Calculus and stain removal will be presented later in this chapter in the laboratory section under dental hygiene care.)

TABLE 8–7
GUIDE FOR SELECTION OF DISINFECTANT SOLUTIONS

	Iodophors[1]	Chlorine Compound[2]	Glutaraldehydes[3]	Phenolic Glutaraldehydes[4]	Complex Phenolics[3]
Types of Prostheses*/Appliances†					
Removable (acrylic/porcelain)	+	+	–	–	–
Removable (metal/acrylic)	+[5]	+[5]	–	–	–
Appliances (all metal)	–	–	+	?	?
Fixed (metal/porcelain)	–	–	+	?	?
Types of Impression Materials					
Alginate	+	+	–	–	–
Polysulfide rubber base	+	+	+	+	–
Silicone rubber	+	+	+	+	+
Polyether	+[6]	+	+[6]	–	+[6]
ZOE impression paste	+	–	+	+	?
Reversible hydrocolloid	+	+	–	+	?
Compound	+	+	–	+	–

Considerations for selection of product for disinfection of impressions: type of impression material; disinfectants available/used in office; compatibility recommended by manufacturer/ADA; available research data; cost; time required. (CDA, Oct. 1992)

Rinse impression prostheses under running tap water and then immerse‡ for the time recommended for tuberculocidal action with the selected product. Following disinfection, rinse impression prosthesis thoroughly under running tap water to remove any residual disinfectant.

+ = Recommended immersion disinfectant.
– = Not recommended.
? = Data not available or inconclusive.
[1]Prepared at a 1:213 dilution.
[2]1:10 Dilution of commercial bleach or prepared according to manufacturer's instructions for disinfection.
[3]Prepared according to the manufacturer's instructions.
[4]Diluted per the manufacturer's instructions for disinfection.
[5]Use minimal exposure time (10 minutes) to avoid damage to metal.
[6]Use with caution. Check manufacturer's recommendation.
*May also be ethylene oxide–sterilized.
†Prostheses and appliances that have been worn by clients must be thoroughly cleaned prior to disinfection.
‡1991 ADA recommendation, impressions should be immersed for time recommended for TB disinfection (ADA, 1991).

Data from Merchant, V. A. Update on disinfection of impressions, prostheses, and casts. California Dental Association Journal, Oct. 1992, pp. 31–35; Merchant, V. A. A guide for selection of disinfectant solutions. Office Sterilization and Asepsis Procedures Report 6(4):4, 1993.

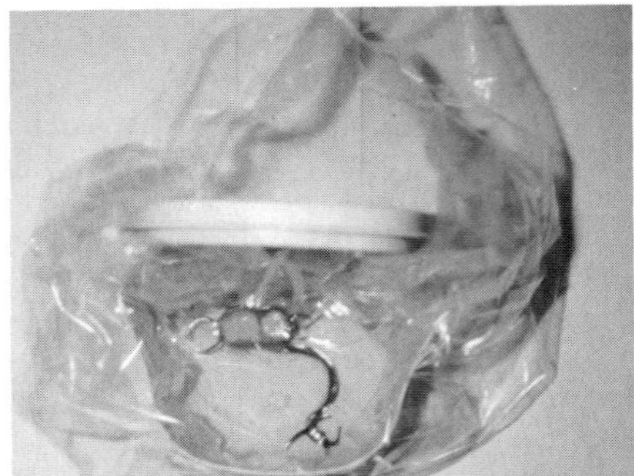

FIGURE 8–26
Prosthesis in holding solution.

4. The client should then prerinse with an antimicrobial mouth rinse, such as chlorhexidine (Peridex; Procter & Gamble, Cincinnati, OH) or Listerine (Warner-Lambert, Morris Plains, NJ), to reduce the microbial count by as much as 98%; even a plain water mouth rinse reduces microbes by 75%.[13]

5. Change gloves if they have become contaminated by the prosthesis or appliances. New gloves may be rinsed briefly and dried to remove the excess powder prior to proceeding with the palpation of the salivary glands, lymph nodes, and temporomandibular joint. A note of caution: washing of gloves should be minimized, and antimicrobial soaps or disinfectants should be avoided because they may cause "wicking," the development of undetected holes that

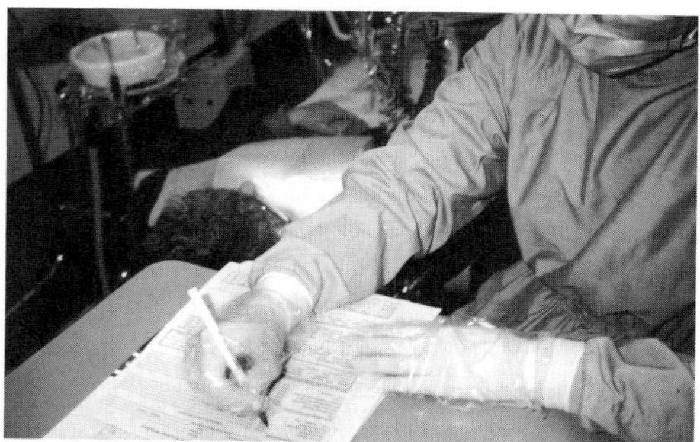

FIGURE 8-27
Overgloved hands recording extraoral and intraoral assessment findings.

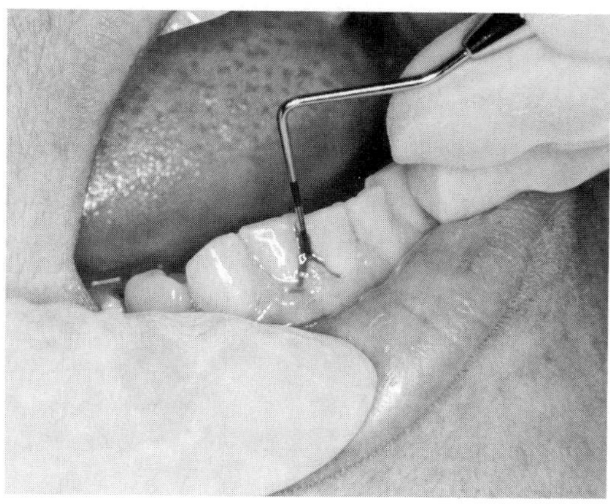

FIGURE 8-28
Probe in contact with blood and saliva.

enhance the penetration of liquids through the gloves.[14] Gloves should be changed whenever a defect is observed or during appointments longer than 60 minutes.

6. Documentation of observations found during the examination creates a great potential for cross-contamination of records unless:

- An assistant is available for recording data gathered
- Voice-activated computers are used for recording data
- The solo dental hygienist uses nontreatment gloves (overgloves) (Fig. 8-27) when documenting findings

7. When plastic overgloves are used for documentation, the dental hygienist should open the gloves before the appointment and place them at the border of the contaminated and the noncontaminated counter areas adjacent to the records. Open gloves facilitate ease in their donning and removal; however, great care should be taken to *avoid contact* between the external surface of the overglove and the contaminated treatment gloves.

8. Overgloves should be clearly recognizable and distinct from treatment gloves. Although the interior of the overglove is contaminated, the exterior must remain clean and uncontaminated.

Table 8-8 shows the placement of equipment within each use area for the extraoral and intraoral assessment.

Periodontal Assessment

1. Probing (Fig. 8-28) increases contact with blood and saliva; therefore, all the previously mentioned barriers and protocols regarding the notation of findings apply here.

2. Manual documentation of periodontal findings by a dental hygienist working alone presents a significant challenge in preventing cross-contamination. Great care is required in donning or removing overgloves in order to enter information into client records. A heat-sterilizable, combination periodontal probe and pen has been developed that may be useful for temporary notation of probe depths, attachment loss, furcation, and mobility classifications on an impervious-backed paper barrier used on the bracket table or tray. Written notations would need to be transcribed from the contaminated barrier later when the dental hygienist has overgloves on or clean ungloved hands in order to avoid contamination of the client's record.

3. The working end of the probe should be wiped with sterile gauze prior to returning it to the instrument tray or cassette in order to prevent blood and saliva from drying on the instrument. Dried bioburden makes the cleaning process difficult, requiring additional time, effort, and risk (if handscrubbing is required to supplement ultrasonic cleaning); if the bioburden is not fully removed it will inhibit the effectiveness of the sterilization process.

4. When the ASW syringe is used to clear the field of visibility, the simultaneous spraying of air and water should be avoided in order to prevent excessive creation of aerosols and spatter.

5. The client's past periodontal records and radiographs, placed on a lighted viewbox, should be accessible for inspection yet positioned just outside the zone of contamination.

Table 8-9 shows the placement of equipment within each use area during the periodontal assessment.

TABLE 8-8
PLACEMENT OF EQUIPMENT WITHIN EACH USE AREA FOR EXTRAORAL AND INTRAORAL ASSESSMENT

I	II	III	IV
Mirror Probe Gauze	Low-volume suction ASW syringe Antimicrobial rinse		Forms Pens Client hand mirror Overgloves

TABLE 8-9
PLACEMENT OF EQUIPMENT WITHIN EACH USE AREA DURING THE PERIODONTAL ASSESSMENT

I	II	III	IV
Mirror Probe Explorer (calculus)	Low-volume suction ASW syringe		Client hand mirror Forms Pens Overgloves Radiographs/viewbox

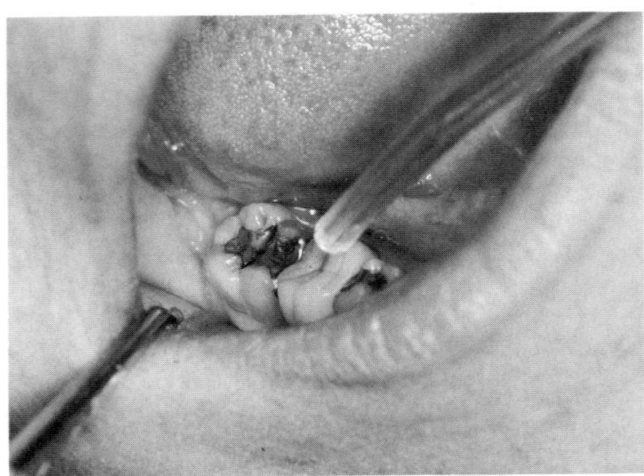

FIGURE 8-29
Air-drying tooth with restoration.

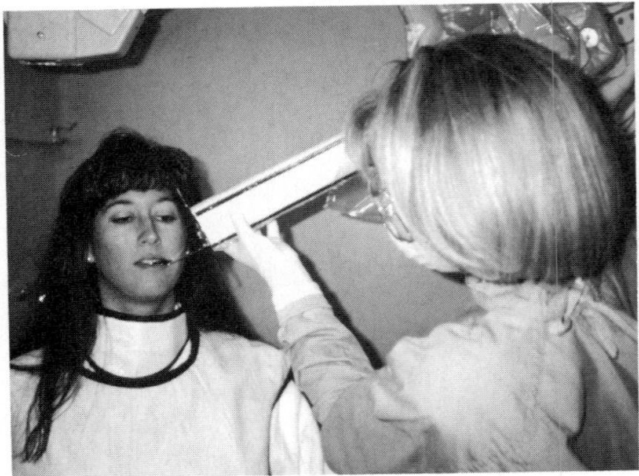

FIGURE 8-30
Barrier-covered position-indicating device (PID) alignment with film holder.

Assessment of the Dentition

1. Assessment of the teeth requires the use of personal barrier precautions mentioned earlier (extraoral/intraoral assessment protocol), since this procedure involves contact with saliva, blood, and other body fluids.

2. Air is frequently used to maximize visibility for inspection of the teeth and restorations (Fig. 8-29). Aerosols are generated, and the potential for spatter exists.

3. Wipe instruments with the 2 in. × 2 in. gauze prior to returning them to the instrument tray or cassette to avoid the presence of dried debris (bioburden) on the working ends of the explorer. Using a moistened gauze to wipe the mirror during the examination not only removes debris but also increases visibility for direct vision.

4. Occasionally, when a tooth is suspected of being nonvital, electrical pulp testing (using the vitalometer) for the assessment of tooth vitality will be necessary. When use of the vitalometer is indicated, clean and disinfect surfaces and protect the unit and controls with a surface barrier. Cover the handpiece and pulp tester tip with an open-ended plastic barrier sheath. The very end of the tip of the pulp tester must be moistened with a small amount of toothpaste or another electrolyte for use as a conductor. A nonconductive plastic barrier over the terminal working end of the pulp tester could cause insufficient conduction, creating a false-negative response.[15] The manufacturer's instructions should be checked to determine whether the entire handpiece or pulp tester tip may be removed and heat-sterilized or, if it is heat-sensitive, submerged in a chemical sterilant. If the handpiece or tip cannot withstand either of these sterilizing methods, the contaminated equipment should be meticulously cleaned and disinfected. When this equipment is not in use, it should be stored in a cabinet yet remain accessible. If such equipment must be left out in the operatory, it should be kept in a noncontaminated area of the operatory and covered to protect it from possible aerosol contamination.

5. Documentation of the findings presents the greatest challenge in the prevention of cross-contamination. The dental hygienist must either use overgloves for recording findings or use an assistant, a voice-activated computer, or a recording device for postappointment transcription of the data collected (Fig. 8-30).

Table 8-10 shows placement of equipment within each use area during examination of teeth.

Oral and Maxillofacial Radiography[17]

The potential for infection control problems associated with dental radiographical procedures was not specifically addressed in infection control literature until recent times.[2] The reason for this may have been the erroneous perception that, since radiographical procedures do not involve the use of sharp instruments or the spatter of blood and saliva, the risk of disease transmission is negligible. The potential for disease transmission does, in fact, exist during radiographical procedures, even though radiographical techniques are predominantly noninvasive except for the use of probes in sialography (radiographical imaging of salivary

TABLE 8-10
PLACEMENT OF EQUIPMENT WITHIN EACH USE AREA DURING ASSESSMENT OF THE DENTITION

I	II	III	IV
Mirror Explorer (for caries detection Sterile 2 in. × 2 in. gauze Dappen dish with small amount of toothpaste (pulp testing) Floss	Low-volume suction ASW syringe	Electrical pulp tester (vitalometer)	Client mirror Forms Pens and/or colored pencils Overgloves Radiographs/viewbox Instructional materials Tube of toothpaste Floss dispenser

TABLE 8–11
PLACEMENT OF EQUIPMENT WITHIN EACH USE AREA DURING ORAL AND MAXILLOFACIAL RADIOGRAPH EXPOSURE

I	II	III	IV
Dental x-ray machine (tube head) (PID) Control panel Exposure switch (area I or II)	Film Film-holding devices Mouth mirror Cotton rolls Extra gloves Exposure switch (area I or II)	Client chair Lead apron Thyroid shield	Radiograph viewing boxes Radiographic film mounts Overgloves Client chart Pens/pencils

glands and ducts). Equipment and supplies associated with intraoral radiographical procedures are contaminated with saliva, and the potential does exist for the presence of blood as well, especially if radiographical exposure is done during or in conjunction with an invasive procedure such as scaling and root planing.[2,16]

Microorganisms have been isolated from surfaces associated with dental radiography in both the exposure area and the processing room. The potential for cross-contamination is extensive, since the procedure involves intraoral film placement; manual alignment of the tube head, extension cone, and/or position-indicating device (PID) (see Fig. 8–30); touching of the control and panel and exposure switch; and removal and temporary storage of each contaminated film. A 20-film intraoral survey requires multiple contacts of saliva-contaminated gloves with equipment.[2] After the required number of radiographical exposures have been made, the contaminated films are transported to the automatic film-processing unit in the darkroom or to the location of the daylight loading box of an automatic processor. The exposure area, the processing room, and the route between exposure and processing areas are susceptible to extensive cross-contamination via saliva-contaminated gloves and film.

The designation of use areas within contaminated and noncontaminated zones in the radiographical exposure area and processing room helps minimize cross-contamination (see Figs. 8–31, 8–36, and 8–39). Delineation of the specified use areas helps organize the placement, use, and flow of equipment and supplies in order to minimize occupational exposure and cross-contamination (Table 8–11).

Preparation for the Intraoral Radiographical Survey Procedure

1. Heavy-duty nitrile gloves, a mask, and protective eyewear should be worn for all cleaning and surface-disinfecting procedures as well as for equipment maintenance procedures in the processing area and for the replenishing of chemicals. Such personal barriers are advised as a precaution because vapors and fine particulates of the chemicals in the x-ray developer and fixer may cause contact dermatitis and irritation of the eyes, nose, throat, and respiratory system.[17]

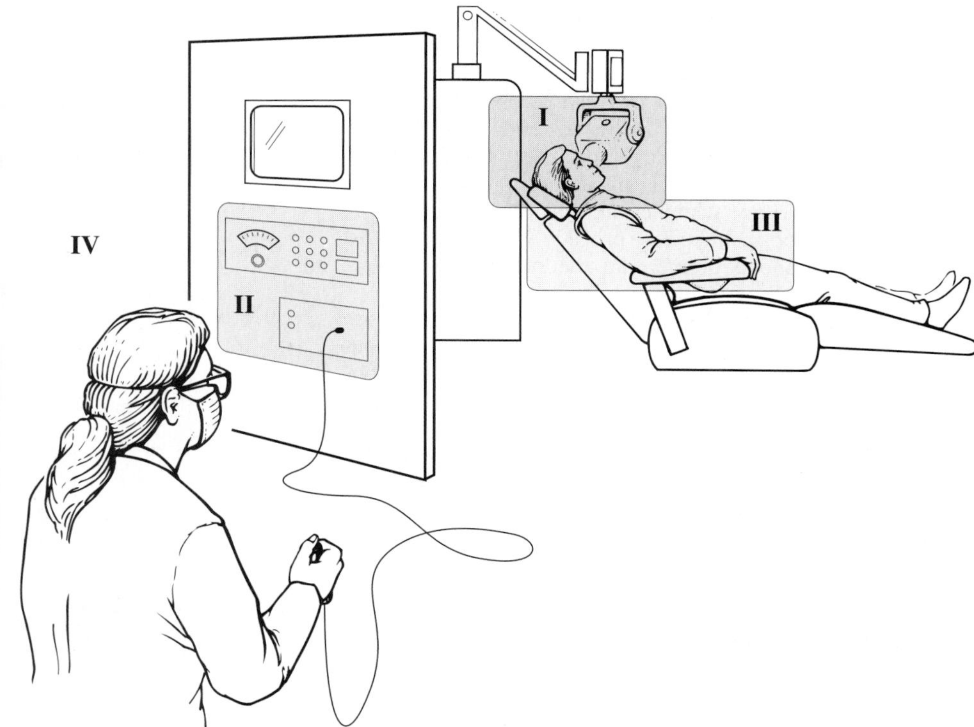

FIGURE 8–31
Graphic of designated use zones within the radiography exposure area. I, II, and III indicate contaminated zones. I, dental x-ray machine (tube head, position-indicating device), control panel (may be located in use area II if mounted on the wall outside dental x-ray room); II, shielded area adjacent to the room housing the dental x-ray machine (the control panel and exposure switch may be located here); the top of the control box, the sill of the observation window, or a wall-mounted shelf or tray may serve as a counter area for placement of the tray set-up with film-holding devices and film. III, client chair, lead apron, thyroid shield, and counter area and/or equipment adjacent to the x-ray machine. IV indicates noncontaminated zone. IV, radiograph mounting and viewing area and/or counter top not immediately adjacent to the dental x-ray machine, control panel, or instrument tray. (Redrawn and adapted from Cottone, J. A., Hars, E., et al. Recommended clinical guidelines for infection control in dental education institutions. Journal of Dental Education 55(9):621, 1991.)

TABLE 8-12
INFECTION CONTROL CONSIDERATIONS FOR ORAL/MAXILLOFACIAL RADIOGRAPHY

Item	Management
Client	Review health and radiological histories
Working surfaces	
Dental radiography chair	Barrier or disinfection
Countertops	Barrier or disinfection
Instruments	
Films	Controlled handling; barrier, disinfection, or sterilization
Film-holding devices	Sterilization *whenever possible;* high-level disinfection is the minimum
Cotton rolls	Dispose with other contaminated waste
Operator's hands	Wash before donning gloves and after removing gloves; use overgloves or have extra gloves to use between exposing and processing procedures
X-ray tube head and position-indicating device	Barrier preferred or disinfection
X-ray control panel	Barrier preferred or disinfection
Lead apron and thyroid shield	Disinfection; as an added precaution, Mylar-backed bib placed over lead apron
Darkroom	
Entrance	Enter with uncontaminated hands
Countertops	Barrier or disinfection
Automatic processor	Feed only uncontaminated films with clean hands
Solutions	Maintain uncontaminated films
Paper waste	Dispose with contaminated waste

Adapted from Manson-Hing, L. R. Fundamentals of Dental Radiography, 3rd ed. Philadelphia: Lea & Febiger, 1990.

2. Proceed with surface disinfection (spray, wipe, spray). Clean and disinfect the following areas of the dental radiography area *if they are touched or not protected by impervious barriers:* operatory chair, tube head, PID, timer switch and control panel, film tray, sill of observation window, sink and faucets, soap dispenser and towel holder, and protective plastic covering of lead apron and thyroid shield (Table 8-12). Remove nitrile utility (heavy-duty) gloves worn for surface disinfection, and prepare gloves for the sterilization or disinfection process. Wash hands and prepare barriers and equipment in the radiography operatory.

3. Dental radiography equipment lends itself well to the use of barrier materials to wrap or cover equipment. Cohesive plastic wrap, aluminum foil, plastic bags, and impervious-backed paper are some of the barrier options. Clinging plastic wrap placed on the machine control panel prior to the procedure is preferred, since electrical connections and irregular surfaces do not lend themselves to thorough saturation with liquid disinfectants (Fig. 8-32).[18] Place plastic barrier bags over the patient chair, PID, tube head, and yoke (Fig. 8-33).

4. Turn on the line switch (on/off button), check controls, and make any necessary adjustments for kVp (kilovolt peak) and exposure settings. The kVp (output) meter needle reading should be selected *before* plastic wrap is placed, since the static charge from the placement of the plastic wrap on some x-ray machines may cause the needle

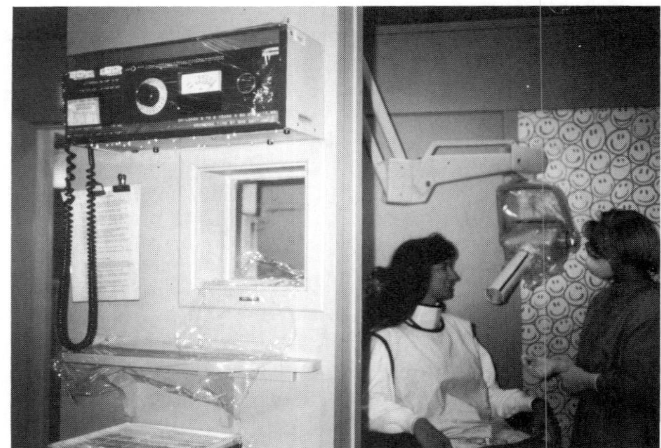

FIGURE 8-32
Plastic wrap placed over control panel of x-ray unit.

to be deflected either low or high on the kVp meter. These false readings must be ignored, and no attempt to adjust the initial kVp setting should be made if the needle is deflected by the presence of the plastic wrap.[19]

5. Cover the timer switch, the control panel, the observation window sill, and the film tray with plastic wrap (secured with masking tape, if necessary, to ensure adherence).

6. Fasten a small contaminated-waste bag to the end of the film tray.

7. Set up the correct number and size of film, sterilized film-holding devices, and mouth mirror; cotton rolls; latex examination gloves (include extra pairs for use in the processing area); overgloves; tissue to wipe saliva from each film; plastic cup to hold exposed film; and sterile napkin chain and plastic-backed napkin or bib (Fig. 8-34). If the client has a removable prosthesis or appliance, set up a denture cup with a plastic bag barrier in which mouth rinse is placed for use as a holding solution for the prosthesis or appliance during radiographical procedures.

8. Review the client chart for health/dental/cultural histories, most recent oral examination, and date or scope of last radiographs. Check the dentist's prescription for radiographs and the client's radiological exposure record.

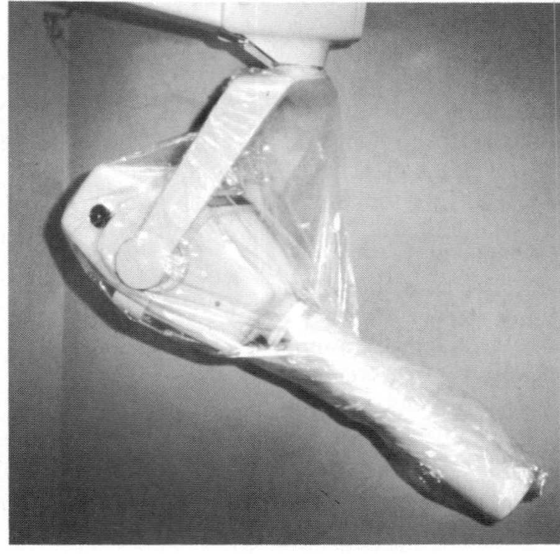

FIGURE 8-33
Plastic barrier bag placed over the PID/tube head of x-ray unit.

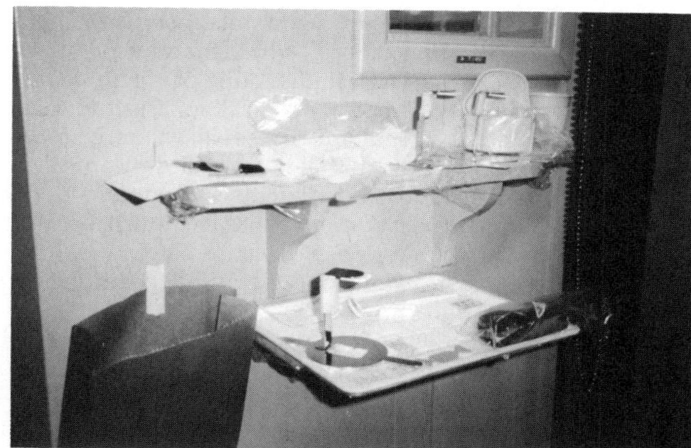

FIGURE 8-34
Armamentarium for radiographic exposure.

Minimizing the Extent of Cross-Contamination in the Radiographical Exposure Area

1. Seat the client, adjust the headrest, and place a lead apron and thyroid shield on the client. Place a plastic-backed bib over the apron as an added precaution or barrier to absorb any saliva that may drip onto the apron area below the client's chin when films are removed after exposure.
2. Complete the health history update, and request the client's signature.
3. Put on protective eyewear, mask, and examination gloves.
4. If the client has a removable prosthesis or appliance, ask the client to remove it and to place it in the small plastic bag containing mouth rinse in the denture cup, and then cover the cup.
5. Using a mirror, inspect the client's mouth for conditions that might alter the usual placement technique; determine the direction of contacts.
6. Prepare the film-holding device, and set the time for the exposure.
7. Place the film in the client's mouth, adjust the PID, and expose the film. Alternatively, there is a two-person technique to eliminate surface contamination during radiographical procedures. With this technique, one person (the dental hygienist) places the film in the client's mouth while the other person adjusts the chair, the PID, and the control panel and makes the exposure. The individual placing the film is the only one capable of cross-contamination. Only the film and holding devices are contaminated. No surfaces are contaminated.
8. Remove the film from the client's mouth; wipe off saliva with a tissue wipe, drop the film into the plastic cup reserved for the exposed contaminated film (Fig. 8-35), and place a new film in the holding device. Repeat this process until all the requested radiographs have been exposed.
9. The client may remain in the operatory or return to the reception room. The dental hygienist then puts on overgloves or removes gloves and washes hands. If the client returns to the reception room, the bib, lead apron, and thyroid shield should be removed.

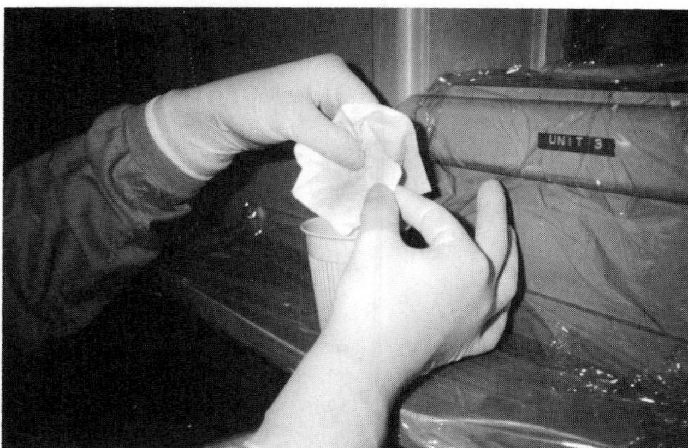

FIGURE 8-35
Film being wiped to remove saliva before placement in cup for transport.

Processing the Radiographs and Minimizing the Potential for Contamination

1. Put on overgloves, or remove examination gloves and wash hands before entering the darkroom. The entrance to the darkroom or the surfaces around the portals to the daylight loading box must remain uncontaminated (Fig. 8-36).
2. After the exposed contaminated film has been carefully placed in a plastic cup to preserve an uncontaminated exterior cup surface, take it to the processing room (Fig. 8-37). Place an impervious-backed paper towel on the designated use area or counter on which films are set, and remove the film packaging material. The film packaging material is to be considered contaminated at this point unless:

The exposed radiographs were sterilized at room tem-

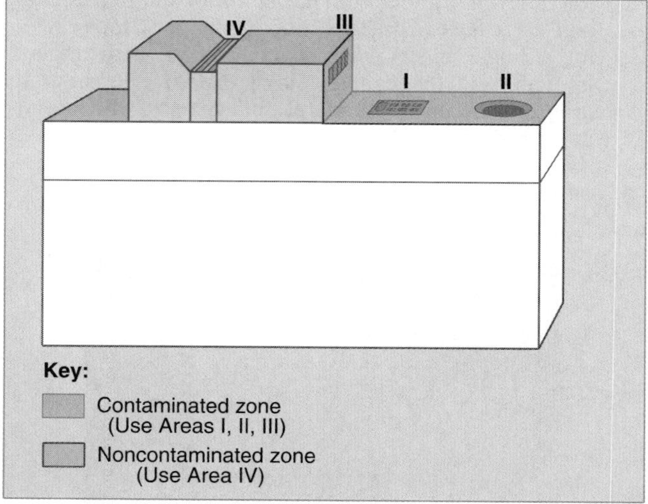

FIGURE 8-36
Designated use zones within the radiographic processing area/darkroom. I, II, and III indicate contaminated zones. I, counter area in the darkroom where film is removed from film packets. II, receptacle for disposing of contaminated waste. III, area adjacent to the section of the automatic processor with slots for accepting the films to begin the development process. IV indicates noncontaminated zone. IV, the automatic processor and the counter top area adjacent to where films exit the processor after the process of developing, fixing, rinsing, and drying.

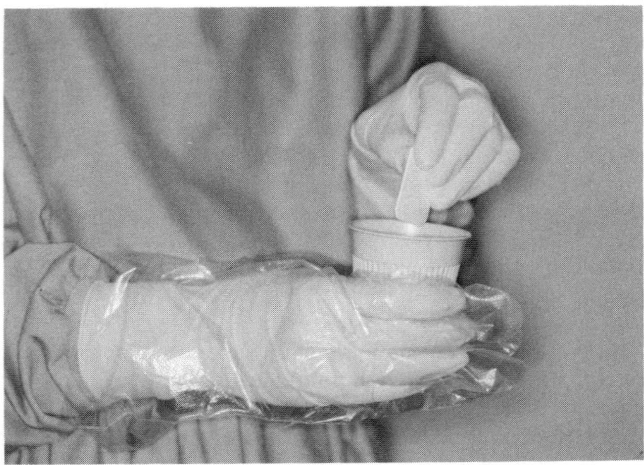

FIGURE 8–37
Cup holding contaminated film (overglove holding noncontaminated exterior with latex glove holding contaminated film packet).

perature with ethylene oxide, an expensive process taking from 24 to 48 hours.

- The exposed radiographs, plastic-covered and tightly sealed, were cleaned and disinfected by immersion in 1:10 sodium hypochlorite (bleach) for 10 minutes.[18] Alternatively, film packets may also be cleaned and disinfected with a spray-wipe technique prior to being opened for processing.[2]
- A barrier was placed on the film prior to intraoral placement and removed after exposure and just prior to processing (Fig. 8–38). Two types of barriers are appropriate here: (1) commercially available polypropylene barrier envelopes for individual film packets, which are to be removed after exposure by tearing away from the film and dropping the film into a cup for removal without contamination of the film packet; and (2) a finger cot (latex barrier designed for protecting a single finger) placed over the film, with the end knotted, and the knot cut after exposure in order to drop out the uncontaminated film onto an uncontaminated surface.

These options for preventing contamination of the film packaging may not be practical when more than a few films need to be exposed. Careful handling of contaminated film packaging may be the only practical approach to take. If the film packaging is contaminated at the time of processing, the best approach to follow is called "controlled handling," in which a conscious effort is required to remember what may and what may not be touched, with attention given to the designated contaminated and noncontaminated use areas within the processing room (Table 8–13).[18]

3. Carefully pour out contaminated films on covered surface area designated as contaminated, remove overgloves, or, if not gloved, put on a new pair of examination gloves to begin removal of contaminated film packaging (Fig. 8–39).

4. Open all film packets while being careful to touch only the packaging and not the film itself. Deposit the film onto an adjacent covered counter surface or into a container designated as noncontaminated.

5. After all film packages have been opened, the gloves may be discarded and hands washed prior to picking up films for placement into the processor; another option is to remain gloved and very carefully handle the films solely by the edge before feeding the film into an automatic processor. Some research has been done that has confirmed that the processing chemicals (developer and fixer) are incapable of sustaining bacterial growth under normal use conditions.[2] If wearing gloves, discard them along with the other contaminated waste, wash hands, and exit the processing area.

Special considerations when using a daylight loading box with an automatic processor:

- Prepare the processor by lining the daylight loading box with plastic wrap as a surface barrier. Place two cups inside the box, one with the exposed film packets and the other for use as a packaging debris receptacle.
- Avoid contamination of the fabric-covered hand portals (light-tight baffles) by entering portals wearing a new pair of examination gloves.
- Handle films solely by the edges and feed them into the processor. Remove gloves and place them in the

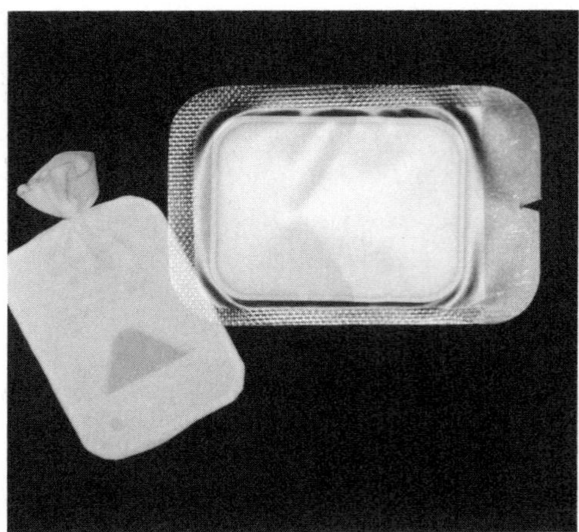

FIGURE 8–38
Barriers designed to prevent contamination of film packaging material (barrier envelope/finger cot with knotted end).

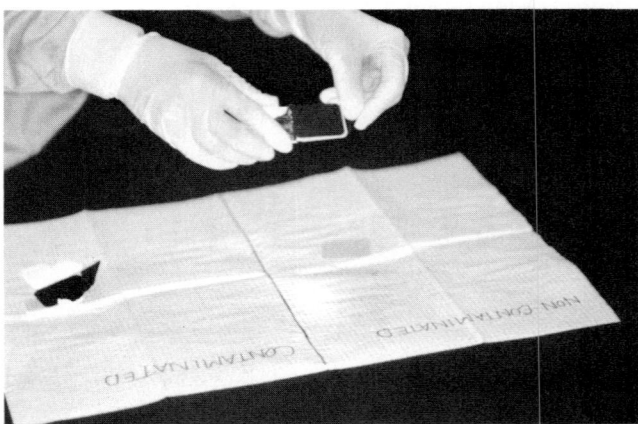

FIGURE 8–39
Paper (e.g., bib) with marks designating contaminated/noncontaminated sections with gloved hands opening packet to drop film on noncontaminated side.

TABLE 8–13
PLACEMENT OF EQUIPMENT WITHIN EACH USE AREA DURING THE PROCESSING OF RADIOGRAPHS

I	II	III	IV
Exposed film packets Examination gloves	Waste receptacle	Packaging separated from film Additional gloves Daylight loading box	Unwrapped exposed film Automatic processor Overgloves

cup holding film packaging debris. Remove hands from the light baffles, and wash hands.

6. Take the processed film to the view box, evaluate the diagnostic quality of the radiographs, and inform the client if any supplemental radiographs or retakes will be required. When additional radiographs are required, repeat the procedures listed previously for the exposure of radiographs. If evaluation of the processed radiographs confirms a completed diagnostic-quality radiographic survey, rinse any prosthesis or appliance (if applicable) thoroughly and return it to the client. Wash hands and discard gloves or overgloves in order to dismiss the client.

Postintraoral Radiographic Survey Procedures

1. Enter the procedures on the client chart.
2. Return to the operatory, put on nitrile gloves, and prepare the film-holding devices for decontamination and instrument recirculation. Film-holding devices and panoramic bite-blocks, according to the Spaulding classification of instruments and equipment, are classified as semicritical because they contact mucous membranes. Semicritical instruments require sterilization whenever possible, and at a minimum, semicritical items should be subjected to high-level disinfection.[20]
3. All disposable materials should be put in a contaminated-waste bag. These include cotton rolls, gloves, overgloves, mask, client napkin, film-drying tissue, the plastic bag liner for the denture cup, and the towel used to return dentures.
4. Remove plastic bags from the client chair and the tube head or the PID; remove all plastic coverings from controls and tray or shelf area. Discard these along with other contaminated waste.
5. Spray-wipe-spray to clean and disinfect surfaces, including the plastic-covered surfaces of the lead apron and thyroid collar and any other surfaces where barriers may have been compromised during the radiographic procedures. In general, all barrier-protected surfaces should be disinfected as part of the protocols for the end of the day. Equipment should be turned off and the manufacturer's recommendations followed regarding maintenance.

Alginate Impressions and Study Models

Impressions[21]

1. Set up the armamentarium (Table 8–14), retrieve the plastic bag with the cleaned and disinfected mixing bowl and the heat-sterilized spatula (the plastic bag used for storage and transport may also serve as a waste bag at the end of the procedure). A prepackaged portion/unit dose packet of alginate should be utilized to prevent cross-contamination of bulk impression materials.
2. Lubricate the client's lips, mix the impression material, prepare the trays (metal is preferred because of its ability to recirculate through heat sterilization; if plastic trays are used they should be disposed of afterwards; Styrofoam adhesive-lined disposable trays are the only other option), and then take the impression.
3. Immediately after the impression is completed, inspect and rinse the impression to remove blood and saliva. Use slowly running water to minimize aerosol and spatter in the sink area.
4. Completely immerse (Fig. 8–40) the impression in disinfectant (iodophor compounds and household bleach or chlorine dioxide may be used with alginate impressions (see Table 8–7).[5,22] Then cover the impression immersed in disinfectant for transport to the laboratory. The impressions should be kept from drying during the disinfection time specified by the impression material manufacturer.
5. Remove excess alginate from the bowl, and dispose of it with the contaminated waste. Clean and disinfect (spray-wipe-spray) the bowl and the spatula, and place them in the plastic bag with the impressions (Fig. 8–41). If an assistant is available to make study models, give the plastic bag with the bowl, spatula, and bagged impressions to the assistant, otherwise the dental hygienist is to don overgloves and transport the bag to the laboratory in order to pour the models.

Laboratory Preparation of Study Models[21]

The dental laboratory presents special problems for infection control because it involves the transfer of contaminated intraoral appliances and other materials (impressions)

TABLE 8–14
PLACEMENT OF EQUIPMENT WITHIN EACH USE AREA WHILE TAKING IMPRESSIONS IN THE OPERATORY

I	II	III	IV
Mirror Dappen dish with lubricant Cotton swabs	Upper and lower rim-lok (metal trays) Low-volume ASW syringe Wax to adjust tray for hard-to-fit client	Bag with mixing bowl, spatula Portion of alginate Graduated cylinder for water	Client chart Overgloves Pens

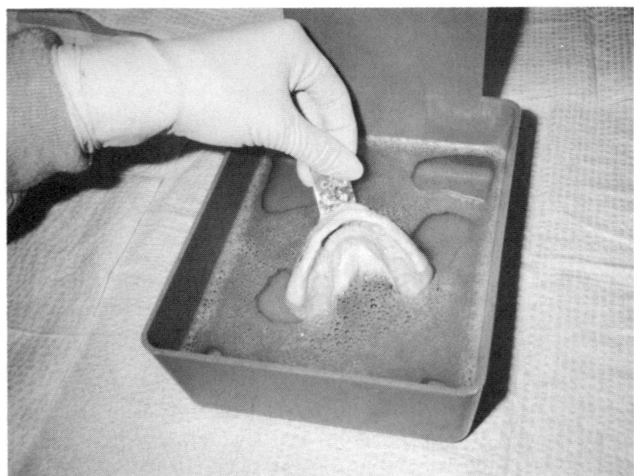

FIGURE 8-40
Alginate impression in metal tray being immersed in disinfectant.

from the operatory to the laboratory and back to the operatory (Fig. 8-42, Table 8-15). Laboratory personnel must recognize that even though the client may not be present, the potential for HBV and other disease transmission exists. Studies have indicated that dental laboratory technicians have the same prevalence of antibodies to HBV as do dental hygienists and dental assistants.[5] The following is a step-by-step infection control protocol for preparing study models in the laboratory (Fig. 8-43).

1. Discard overgloves and previous treatment gloves, and then wash hands.
2. Wrap the vibrator in plastic, and place paper or plastic covers on the well-defined contaminated use area (counter workspace—area III).
3. Place an estimated amount of water in the bowl. Obtain the necessary amount of plaster or stone with a paper cup, and place it in the work area. Prepare identification labels for the impression trays on a contaminated area of the countertop (area III) and a label for the laboratory

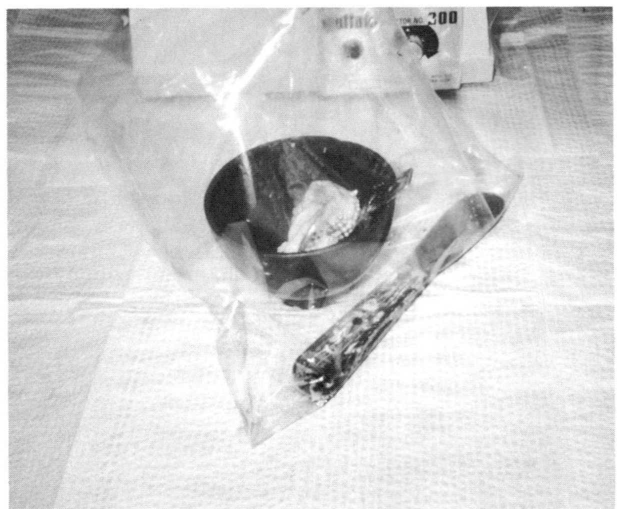

FIGURE 8-41
Plastic bag holding bagged impressions, bowl, and spatula.

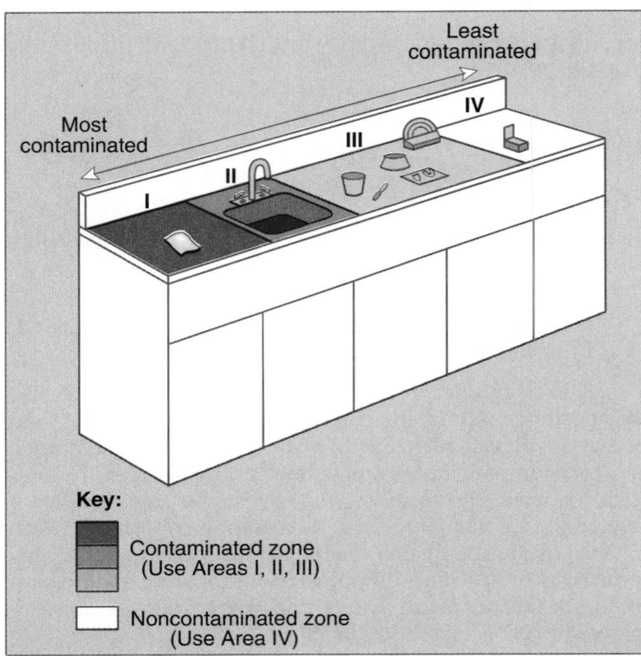

FIGURE 8-42
Laboratory zones for preparation of study models. I, II, and III indicate contaminated zones. I, receiving area; II, sink; III, mixing, vibrating, and setting area. IV indicates noncontaminated zone. IV, packaging for delivery.

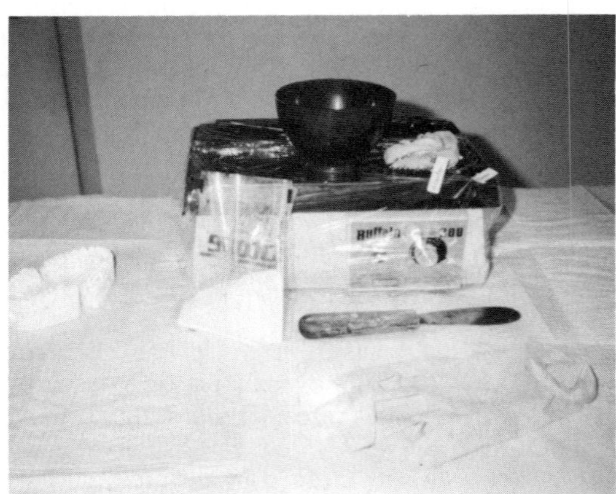

FIGURE 8-43
Laboratory set-up with barrier-covered vibrator, gloves, labels, bowl, and materials.

TABLE 8-15
PLACEMENT OF EQUIPMENT WITHIN EACH USE AREA DURING LABORATORY PREPARATION OF STUDY MODELS

I	II	III	IV
Bag with impressions	Sink	Bowl with spatula Stone/plaster Vibrator Ceramic tile/plastic sheet/glass slab Model trimmer	Labels Lab box

case box on a noncontaminated area of the countertop (area IV).

4. Don new gloves when mixing powder with water to protect the hands from microbes and to serve as a skin protector. (Avoid hand injuries and irritation dermatitis; dental hygienists who have weeping dermatitis or exudative lesions must refrain from direct client contact until the condition has resolved).[25] Remove the disinfected impressions from the disinfectant, and rinse them.

5. Rinse the spatula and any remaining disinfectant from the bowl, add water and then stone or plaster, mix, and pour the impression on the vibrator.

6. Put poured impressions on a sheet of plastic, ceramic tile, or a glass slab, and place them in a designated area for stone or plaster to set (laboratory area III). Wipe impression tray handles to remove gross debris and moisture, place prepared self-adhesive identification labels (client name, date, operator) on the handles. Color-coded identification labels for each operator may be useful.

7. Discard gloves, wash hands, and leave the laboratory.

8. Return to the laboratory after appropriate setting time. Eyewear and a mask must be worn for protection from flying debris. Gloves are required to protect hands and skin from the sharp edges of study models. Separate impression trays from study models.

9. Even though impressions were rinsed and sprayed with disinfectant prior to pouring stone or plaster models, because undercuts of impressions may retain bioburden, the study model should be sprayed before trimming for additional microbial kill. (Caution: spray with iodophor but do not wrap because if unable to dry, the increased moisture and contact with the model will dissolve stone or plaster.)

10. While sprayed models are air-drying, remove and dispose of alginate waste from the tray. If trays are disposable, discard; if they are metal, thoroughly clean and prepare for heat-sterilization (see Chapter 9).

11. Take the air-drying study models to the model trimmer for trimming (all barriers required).

12. Place the trimmed study models to complete air-drying in the plastic laboratory case box or tray (laboratory area IV) prelabeled with the client's name, the date, and the operator. Discard gloves and wash hands. When thoroughly dry, direct labeling of the model is highly recommended (use of marker or identification sticker will suffice).

Oral Photography

1. Prepare the camera and check the batteries. Load the film in advance of the appointment if photographs are anticipated. Retrieve the sterilized mirrors, retractors, and ASW syringe, or use a sterilized syringe tip and cover the disinfected syringe handle and controls with an appropriate barrier.

2. Arrange forms, instruction guides, and/or an oral photography series model for ease in reference during the appointment.

3. Don gloves and place mirrors and retractors in the client's mouth as needed. The potential for contact with blood and saliva, albeit minimal, does exist during this procedure. Cross-contamination of the camera may be eliminated if there is a dental team member to assist with holding the retractors, positioning the mirror, and adjusting the light (Fig. 8–44).

4. When working without assistance, put on overgloves prior to holding the camera to prevent the contamination of the camera body, lens, and flash attachment. Focus and shoot. The use of overgloves eliminates the need for a camera surface barrier. (Use of a barrier for the camera may not be practical, and direct camera surface cleaning and disinfection could prove damaging to the equipment.)

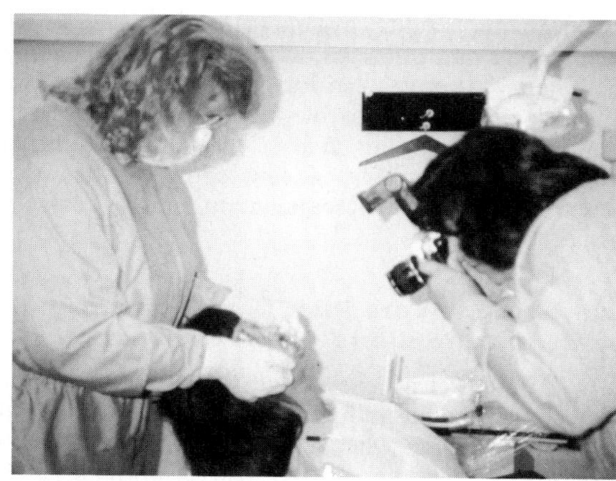

FIGURE 8–44
Ungloved hands holding camera for intraoral photograph with mirrors/retractors being held by gloved assistant.

5. Note of caution: if plastic retractors are used, check the manufacturer's information to determine whether the retractors are able to withstand heat sterilization prior to recirculation. Most plastic retractors are heat sensitive and need chemical sterilization (see Chapter 9 for information on materials and best-suited forms of sterilization). No one method of sterilization works for all items.

Table 8–16 shows the placement of equipment within each use area for taking oral photographs.

INFECTION CONTROL PROTOCOL FOR THE PLANNING PHASE OF THE DENTAL HYGIENE CARE PROCESS

Following completion of the assessment procedures, the dental hygienist reviews the data collected to identify the human need deficits related to dental hygiene care based on specific problems discovered through the client interview, extraoral and intraoral, periodontal, tooth and radiographic assessments. Once the specific dental hygiene diagnoses

TABLE 8–16
PLACEMENT OF EQUIPMENT WITHIN EACH USE AREA FOR TAKING ORAL PHOTOGRAPHS

I	II	III	IV
Mirrors Retractors	ASW syringe		Camera, film, and camera case Client record Instruction guide Model of complete oral photographic series Oral photography consent form Overgloves

have been made, a dental hygiene care plan must be developed with goals and priorities established to meet the needs of the client. Although critical infection control issues such as risk of exposure to bloodborne pathogens are not inherently associated with analysis of problems and dental hygiene care planning, a few considerations should be observed to prevent cross-contamination during this process.

Dental Hygiene Care Plan Development, Plan Presentation, and Client Consent

1. On completion of assessment data collection, prior to review of documented findings for formulation of the dental hygiene care plan, the dental hygienist must remove gloves and wash hands or don overgloves prior to handling the client's records, radiographs, study models, or photographs (Fig. 8–45).
2. Once the plan has been developed, the dental hygienist presents the plan to the client for approval and informed consent. Good communication skills are essential to meet the client's need for conceptualization. Personal barriers used in the prevention of disease transmission such as masks and faceshields may inhibit the communication process. Remove the mask by the elastic or ties and the faceshield by the back of the head band support for the shield in order to avoid contact with the exposed surfaces contaminated by spatter and aerosols generated during the assessment procedures (Fig. 8–46). The mask and faceshield may be temporarily placed on a counter area (area III) designated as contaminated. Masks should not be pulled down and worn around the neck during the presentation of the dental hygiene care plan, since the exposed contaminated surface area would come in contact with the skin on the neck and chin.
3. With the mask removed, communication will be facilitated, since a freer exchange of information may occur with the client's ability to see the face, facial expression, and mouth of the dental hygienist. In addition, the dental hygienist should handle radiographs and other material useful as visual aids with overgloves or clean, ungloved hands. In this way, the dental hygienist will be able to handle and refer to the radiographs and other visual aids for clarification of problems and rationale to support the selected dental hygiene care interventions without contamination of those items kept in the noncontaminated use area.
4. To enhance the client's awareness of periodontal disease, on a personal level, the dental hygienist allows the client to observe some of the problems identified in the client's mouth. The client hand mirror should be removed from the noncontaminated area and given to the client. The dental hygienist should use care in removing overgloves before handling and putting back on the mask and eye protection prior to pointing out areas of bleeding and inflammation for the client to observe.

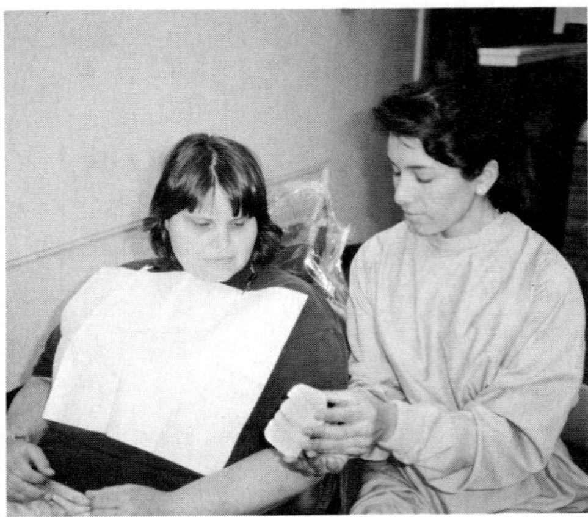

FIGURE 8–45
Dental hygienist presenting case to client using model/radiographs or periodontal assessment data.

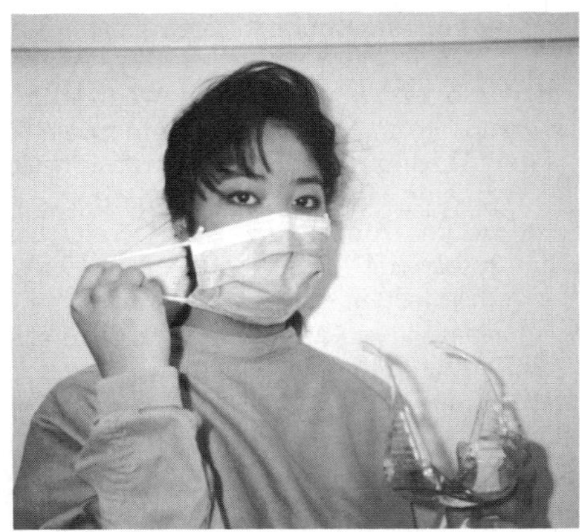

FIGURE 8–46
Mask removal.

Table 8–17 shows the placement of equipment within each use area during the dental hygiene care plan presentation.

INFECTION CONTROL PROTOCOLS FOR THE IMPLEMENTATION PHASE OF THE DENTAL HYGIENE CARE PROCESS

Preventive Care

Personal Mechanical Oral Hygiene Practices

Education of the client throughout the dental hygiene process of care is essential. The client's involvement in each step by use of the hand mirror to observe findings in her

TABLE 8–17
PLACEMENT OF EQUIPMENT WITHIN EACH USE AREA FOR DENTAL HYGIENE CARE PLAN PRESENTATION

I	II	III	IV
Mouth mirror Periodontal probe			Client chart/records Radiographs Study models Intraoral photographs Educational materials Client hand mirror Overgloves or additional gloves

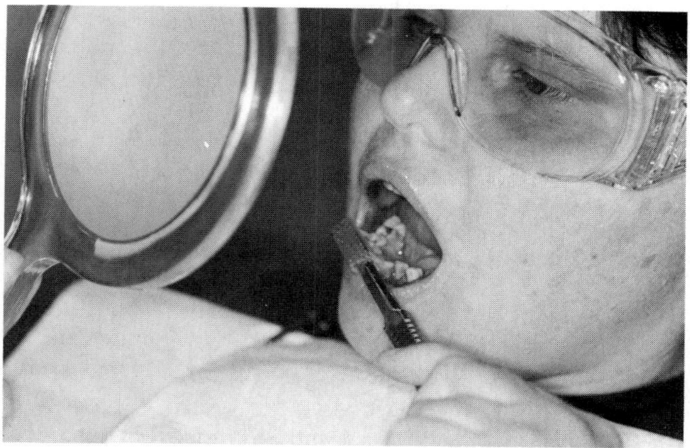

FIGURE 8–47
Close-up of client with disclosed plaque and holding toothbrush against gingival margin. Note protective eyewear.

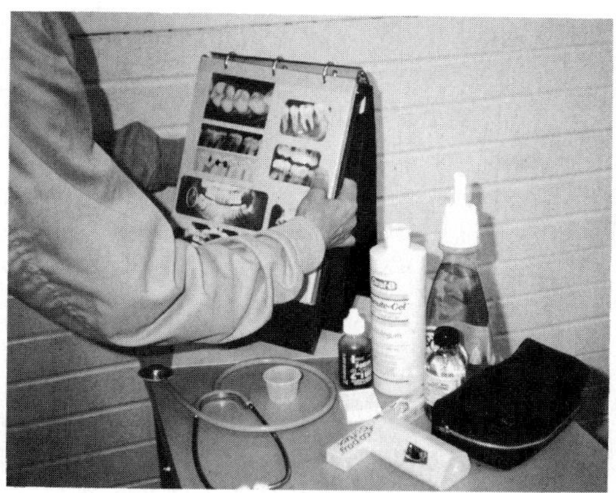

FIGURE 8–48
Dental hygienist without barriers holding visual aid.

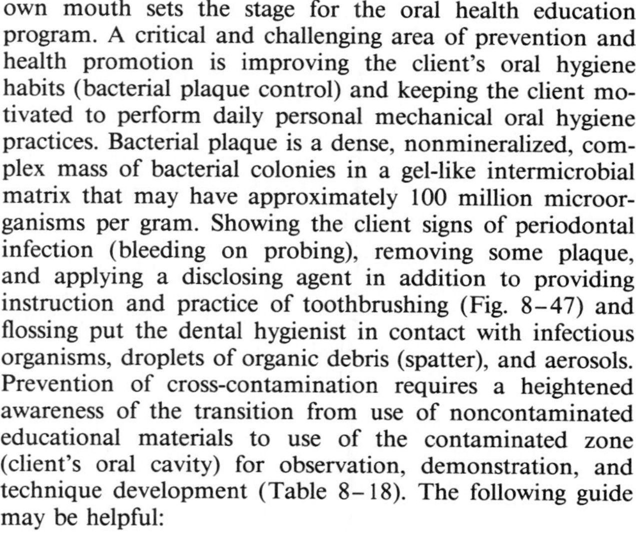

own mouth sets the stage for the oral health education program. A critical and challenging area of prevention and health promotion is improving the client's oral hygiene habits (bacterial plaque control) and keeping the client motivated to perform daily personal mechanical oral hygiene practices. Bacterial plaque is a dense, nonmineralized, complex mass of bacterial colonies in a gel-like intermicrobial matrix that may have approximately 100 million microorganisms per gram. Showing the client signs of periodontal infection (bleeding on probing), removing some plaque, and applying a disclosing agent in addition to providing instruction and practice of toothbrushing (Fig. 8–47) and flossing put the dental hygienist in contact with infectious organisms, droplets of organic debris (spatter), and aerosols. Prevention of cross-contamination requires a heightened awareness of the transition from use of noncontaminated educational materials to use of the contaminated zone (client's oral cavity) for observation, demonstration, and technique development (Table 8–18). The following guide may be helpful:

1. The dental hygiene care plan for client preventive education and assessment data information should be kept in the noncontaminated area. Educational materials, models, and other supporting documentation may be moved for client viewing but should be returned to the noncontaminated area prior to client demonstration of bacterial plaque control techniques and potential exposure to spatter (Fig. 8–48).

2. The dental hygienist must be fully protected with personal barriers (gloves, protective eyewear, mask, and protective clothing) when involved in all intraoral procedures including client demonstration of personal mechanical plaque control techniques (Fig. 8–49). Aerosols and spatter capable of causing airborne infection and direct contamination of skin and mucous membranes are created during all intraoral procedures including toothbrushing, flossing, and use of other supplemental plaque removal devices. Inspection of the client hand mirror after a plaque control technique demonstration frequently reveals the presence of the spatter (particles greater than 50 microns in diameter) sometimes visible yet constantly being produced during such procedures.[2] The protective personal barriers prevent such contamination of skin and mucous membranes.

3. The use of the periodontal probe to point out plaque retention areas, the curet to remove a sample of bacterial plaque, the cotton swab to apply disclosing solution, and the ASW syringe to rinse and dry teeth all require equipment sterilization, flushing of water lines, and an awareness of the continued generation of aerosols and spatter.

4. Toothbrushes, floss, and other items stocked for preventive education should be accessible for dispensing in a noncontaminated area of the operatory. When large floss dispensers are used, avoid contamination of the container either by removing lengths of floss prior to the appointment as part of the tray set-up or by using overgloves for floss retrieval. Toothbrushes and interproximal plaque-removal devices dispensed to the client after intraoral demonstration should be packaged in a bag for transporting home. Covering the toothbrush and interproximal brush prevents contamination of the counter area during the re-

TABLE 8–18
PLACEMENT OF EQUIPMENT WITHIN EACH USE AREA DURING PLAQUE CONTROL INSTRUCTION

I	II	III	IV
Mouth mirror Periodontal probe Curet Dappen dish with disclosing solution Dappen dish with lubricant A single length of floss	ASW	Client hand mirror (after use)	Client chart/records Radiographs Educational materials Client hand mirror (prior to use) Overgloves or additional gloves New toothbrush and any other dispensed plaque-removal devices

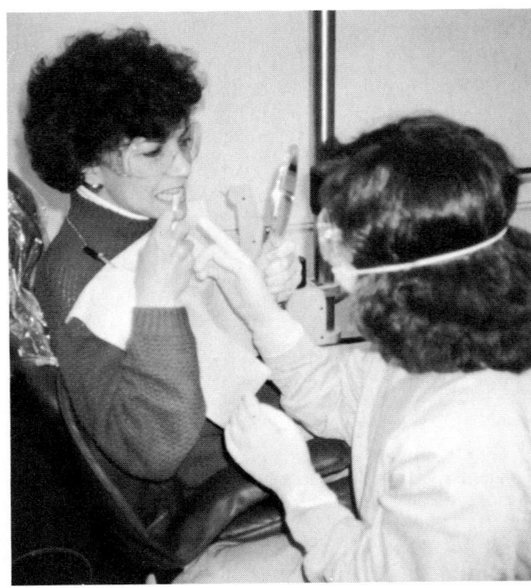

FIGURE 8-49
Dental hygienist is wearing barriers and observing client demonstration of perio aid technique. Client is holding hand mirror.

mainder of the appointment and protects the devices from environmental contamination en route home.

5. Remember to include the client hand mirror among the surfaces and equipment requiring surface disinfection between clients.

Preventive Oral Prophylaxis

Prevention of gingivitis is the objective of the preventive oral prophylaxis, and if that objective is unable to be accomplished the alternative objective is to prevent gingivitis from progressing to periodontitis.[24] The preventive oral prophylaxis procedure includes instruction in personal mechanical oral hygiene practices as well as professional instrumentation to remove supragingival and subgingival tooth and root surface irritants (Fig. 8-50).

Extrinsic stain removal is associated with the oral prophylaxis as well (see protocol on coronal polishing). Aseptic technique considerations for supragingival and subgingival tooth and root surface irritant removal become even more significant with the more technically demanding scaling and root planing associated with nonsurgical therapy for periodontitis-affected clients. Recommendations for preventive oral prophylaxis infection control protocols are presented here; a more extensive protocol is included in therapeutic care section on scaling and root planing.

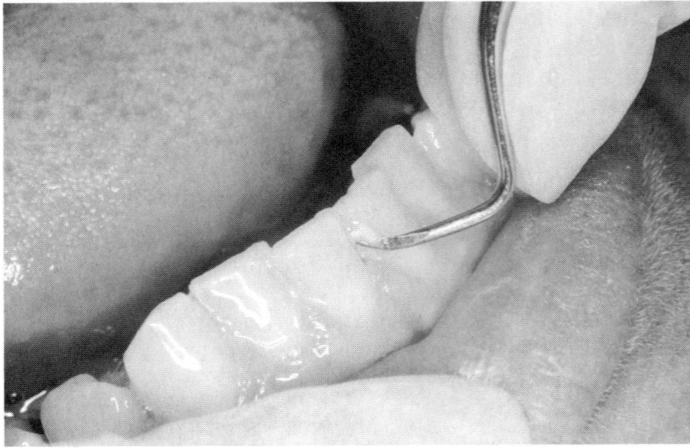

FIGURE 8-50
Intraoral photograph of scaling supragingival calculus (mandibular anteriors facial aspect).

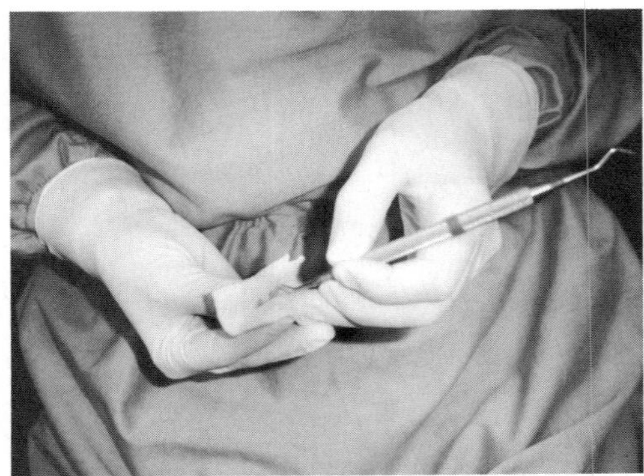

FIGURE 8-51
Wiping curet working end with sterile gauze.

1. During instrumentation to remove supragingival and subgingival tooth and root surface irritants, carefully wipe bioburden from the instrument working ends with sterile gauze. Consistently remove debris from instruments prior to returning them to the instrument tray or cassette to prevent drying of bioburden on curets and the sickle scaler, which would inhibit or prevent effective sterilization (Fig. 8-51).

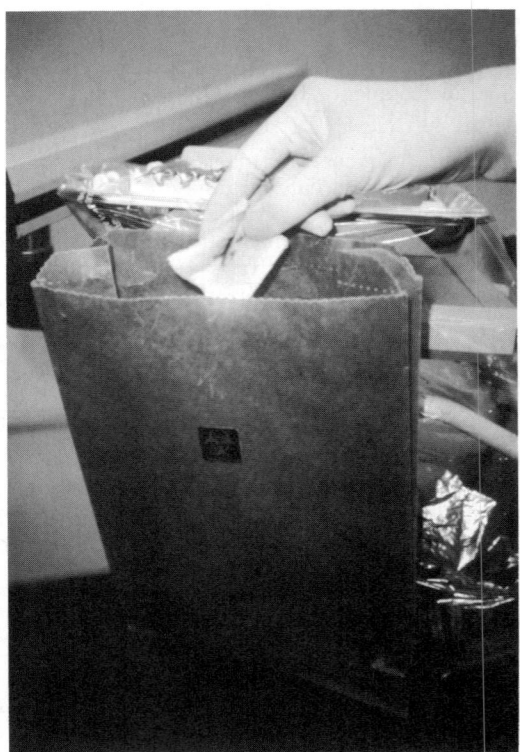

FIGURE 8-52
Used gauze being placed in biohazardous-waste bag.

TABLE 8–19
PLACEMENT OF EQUIPMENT WITHIN EACH USE AREA FOR ORAL PROPHYLAXIS

I	II	III	IV
Mouth mirror Universal curet Sickle scaler Explorer Sterile gauze	ASW syringe Low-volume evacuation		Client chart/ records Radiographs Overgloves or additional gloves

2. Blood-soaked gauze and cotton rolls are classified as medical waste[2] and require disposal in a biohazardous-waste bag. As work is being completed dispose of each gauze immediately in a readily accessible biohazardous-waste bag (Fig. 8–52).

Table 8–19 shows the placement of equipment within each use area for the preventive oral prophylaxis.

Coronal Polishing and Airpolishing Delivery Systems (Extrinsic Stain Removal)

The dental hygiene care plan is developed to meet the needs of the client. An unmet human need related to dental hygiene associated with aesthetics (as part of the need for wholesome body image) may be deficient because of the presence of extrinsic stains that cannot be removed by the client. Selective coronal polishing (Fig. 8–53) or airpolishing may be incorporated into the care plan and requires attention to the following infection control issues:

- All intraoral procedures potentially generate aerosols and spatter.[15] Aerosols increase to tremendous proportions when action-generating equipment is introduced into the intraoral environment (e.g., use of the airspray or combined air-water-spray, the ultrasonic scaling and airpolishing equipment, and use of handpieces). The higher concentration of bacteria-laden aerosols and spatter are found within 2 feet in front of the client, where the dental hygienist is usually positioned.[2] The dental hygienist must use all the standard personal barriers when polishing the teeth. In addition, the dental hygienist should consider the supplemental barrier of a faceshield to be worn along with a mask when working with handpieces and other equipment, such as the airpolisher and ultrasonic or sonic scaling devices, because of the increased concentration of aerosols and volume of spatter generated during care.

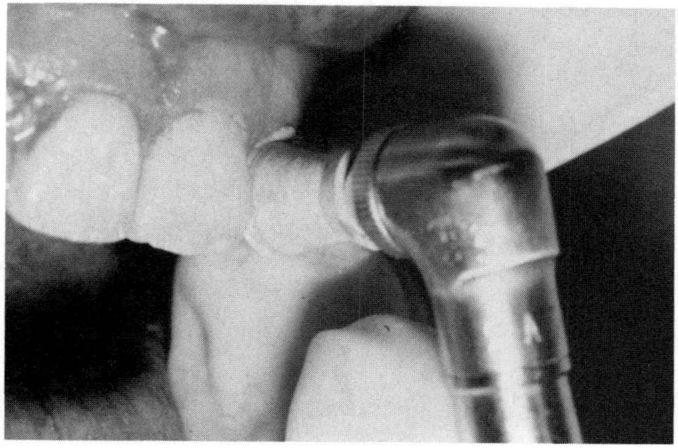

FIGURE 8–53
Rubber cup polishing with heat-sterilizable handpiece.

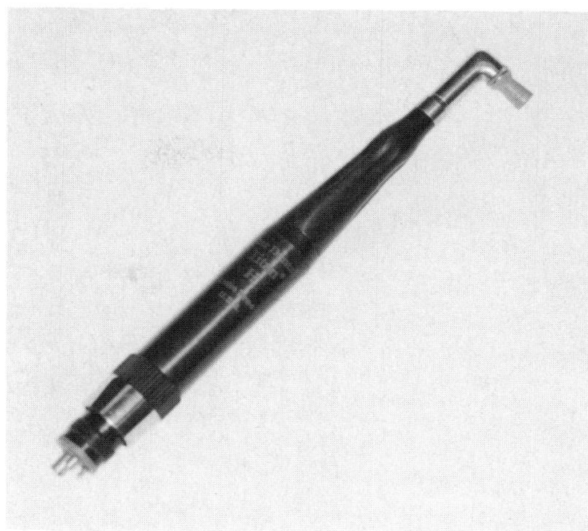

FIGURE 8–54
Low-speed handpiece with prophylaxis angle.

- If a faceshield is added to the personal barriers worn during specific procedures that generate increased amounts of aerosols, it should be consistently worn every time that procedure is performed and not selectively used based on client health history (universal precautions).
- The equipment options for extrinsic stain removal range from the porte polisher (see Fig. 8–58), low-speed handpiece (Fig. 8–54) with prophylaxis angle attachment, to the use of an airpolishing delivery system (see Fig. 8–59). The equipment selected depends on the client's needs and the indications and contraindications of each approach. Aseptic technique requirements associated with polishing include the following:

Handpieces The porte polisher, low-speed handpiece, and handpiece attached to the airpolishing delivery system are classified as semicritical according to the Spaulding classification of inanimate objects because they are items that touch mucous membranes but do not enter sterile body areas.[2] Semicritical objects should be sterilized or disinfected (high-level). The CDC, in the "Recommendations for Prevention of HIV Transmission in Health Care Settings," emphasize handpiece sterilization after each use, since blood, saliva, or gingival fluid may be aspirated into the handpiece or water line.[7] The recommendation statement refers to the high (100,000 to 160,000 revolutions per minute [rpm]) or middle (20,000 to 100,000 rpm) speed handpieces used for the majority of dental procedures and refers to the presence of a water line. A water spray is required to cool the handpiece at the higher revolutions per minute. The low-speed (under 20,000 rpm) handpiece is used for polishing and finishing procedures and does not have a water line, since it does not require the cooling system for heat reduction. It is possible with some high-speed handpieces to adjust the speed from zero to full capacity and therefore, with a lowered speed and proper attachments, use them for tooth polishing, in which case a water line would be involved. Any equipment with a water line requires flushing the water line at the beginning of the

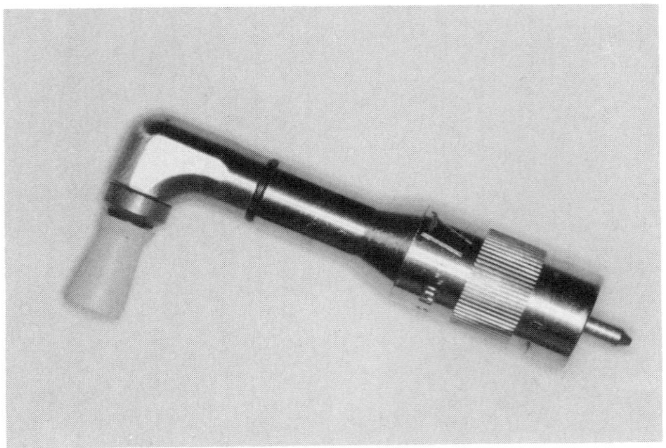

FIGURE 8-55
Prophylaxis angle with rubber cup.

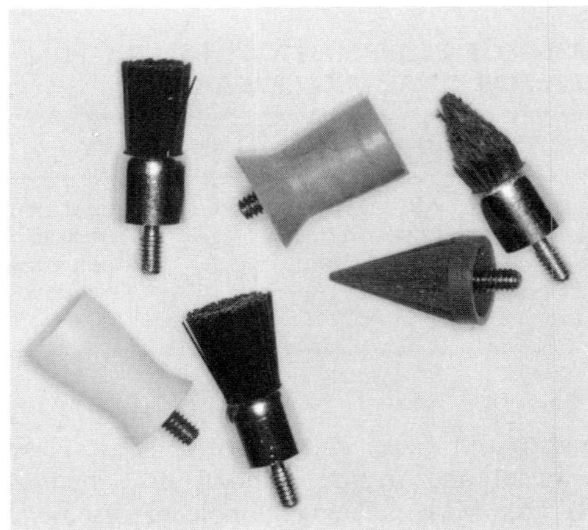

FIGURE 8-57
Rubber cups and bristle brushes.

day and after use with each client to prevent accumulation of microbial-contaminated bioburden in the water lines and to ensure clean water for each client.[2] The handpieces, regardless of speed, should be heat-sterilized not only because microorganisms may be aspirated into the internal mechanism but also because the external surface of handpieces contains a number of grooves and edges that make effective disinfection difficult.[2] Most quality manufacturers of handpieces have produced models that are able to withstand heat sterilization. The CDC have issued a statement calling for "improvements in sterilization and disinfection techniques for certain reusable equipment and devices."[25] Handpiece sterilization probably will be mandated in the near future.[26]

Currently, disinfection of handpieces is considered a compromise *not* a substitute for sterilization. The CDC and ADA have always recommended heat sterilization of handpieces between clients, but not all handpieces can withstand sterilization. Handpieces incapable of withstanding heat sterilization should not be used.[27] Handpieces *cannot* withstand immersion in disinfectant solution, and it should also be noted that use of chemical sterilants such as 2.0 to 3.2% glutaraldehyde is never recommended, since these chemical preparations shorten the life of the handpiece and create the potential for toxic reaction during handling by the dental hygienist.[2]

Contra or Right-Angle Attachments (Prophylaxis Angle) The low-speed handpiece is designed to be used with contra or right-angle attachments to which various polishing and finishing devices are attached (Fig. 8-55). The term "prophylaxis angle" has traditionally been used to refer to the low-speed contra or right-angle attachment for the rubber cup or bristle brushes used for extrinsic stain removal.[15] The prophylaxis angles frequently draw debris, saliva, blood, and other fluids into the internal working mechanisms and require cleaning and heat-sterilization to ensure elimination of all potential pathogens.[2] As with all instruments that come into contact with mucous membranes, only ones that can be heat-sterilized should be selected for use. Almost every type of instrument now is available in sterilizable form, and the ability to withstand heat sterilization should be used as a criterion for purchase. Infection control guidelines must be considered when purchasing equipment. Reusable, heat-sterilizable quality prophylaxis angles provide continued efficacy and efficiency with extrinsic stain removal if manufacturers' care recommendations are consistently followed. The following are aseptic technique recommendations when using the low-speed handpiece and prophylaxis angle attachment.

- Place the handpiece, angle, and rubber cup with pol-

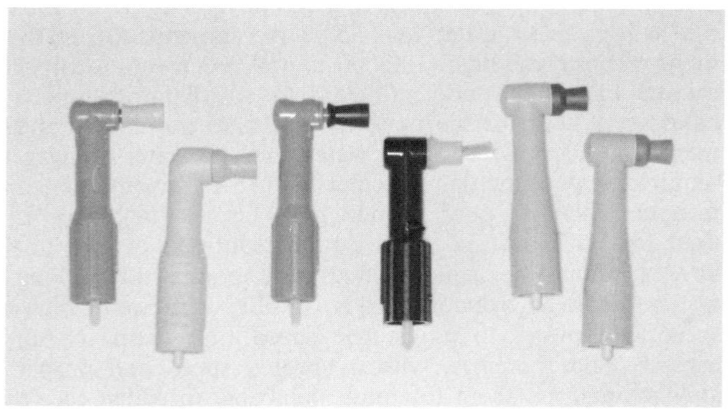

FIGURE 8-56
Disposable prophylaxis angles.

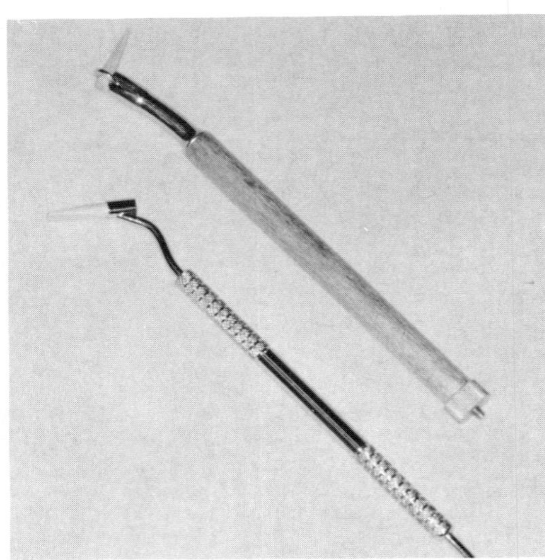

FIGURE 8-58
Porte polishers.

TABLE 8–20
PLACEMENT OF EQUIPMENT WITHIN EACH USE AREA FOR EXTRINSIC STAIN REMOVAL WITH A RUBBER CUP/BRISTLE BRUSH

I	II	III	IV
Mouth mirror Disclosant Cotton swab Lubricant in dappen dish Unit dose of polishing agent Single length of dental floss Single length of dental tape Universal curet Sickle scaler Explorer	Low-speed handpiece Prophylaxis angle Rubber cup/bristle brush Low-volume suction ASW syringe		Client chart/records Client hand mirror Selection of unit dose of polishing agents Radiographs Overgloves or additional gloves Floss dispenser Tape dispenser

ishing agent intraorally prior to starting the rubber cup in motion by pressing on the rheostat (foot control) in order to minimize aerosol generation and spatter.

- Operate the handpiece at the slowest speed possible; this protects the teeth and reduces generation of aerosol and spatter.
- Eliminate or minimize use of the bristle brush attachment to avoid increased generation of aerosol and spatter with occlusal surface stain removal. When use of the rubber cup is inadequate to remove occlusal stain, selectively use a soft bristle brush, angled to adapt to the inclined planes of the cusps, running at the slowest speed possible.[15]
- Use low-volume suction (high-volume suction with four-handed dental hygiene) to evacuate the excess saliva, polishing agent, blood, and debris during the procedure and to contain some of the potential aerosol spray.

Disposable Prophylaxis Angles An alternative gaining wide acceptance and recommendation is the use of disposable prophylaxis angles (Fig. 8–56).[2] Disposable prophylaxis angles (including affixed rubber cups and bristle brushes) are inexpensive and readily available. Criteria for evaluation of disposable prophylaxis angles involve the ability to work throughout the procedure, efficiency in removing stain and bacterial plaque, ability of rubber cup and bristle brushes to conform to tooth surface, ease with which the angle fits into the handpiece, and comfort to the dental hygienist's hand when grasping the angle.[28]

Rubber Cups and Brushes The rubber cup and bristle brush attachments for reusable prophylaxis angles are single-use items to be disposed of after initial use (Fig. 8–57). The cups and brushes retain debris, making sterilization ineffective. After each client, discard the rubber cups and brushes used.[2]

Table 8–20 shows the placement of equipment within each use area for extrinsic stain removal with a rubber cup.

Porte Polisher The porte polisher (Fig. 8–58) is a hand instrument that has an area at the terminal end of the shank into which a wooden point may be inserted for use in rubbing an abrasive agent against the tooth surface for removal of extrinsic stain and plaque. On occasion, this may be the method of choice for coronal polishing. Heat sterilization of the porte polisher is effective and recommended. The wooden points are designed for single use. The use of the porte polisher for coronal polishing produces minimal aerosols.

Table 8–21 shows the placement of equipment within each use area for extrinsic stain removal with a porte polisher.

Airpolishing Delivery System The airpolishing delivery system (also known as airbrasive machine, air-powder abrasive, air-powered slurry, or airabrasive system) involves the use of equipment that delivers air, water, and specially processed sodium bicarbonate particles propelled against the tooth surface under 43 to 58 pounds per square inch (psi) and water pressure of 10 to 50 psi (Fig. 8–59).[29,30] The

TABLE 8–21
PLACEMENT OF EQUIPMENT WITHIN EACH USE AREA FOR EXTRINSIC STAIN REMOVAL WITH A PORTE POLISHER

I	II	III	IV
Porte polisher Wood points Mouth mirror Cotton swab Disclosant in dappen dish Lubricant in dappen dish Unit dose of polishing agent Single length of dental floss Single length of dental tape Universal curet Sickle scaler Explorer	Low-volume suction ASW syringe		Client chart/records Client hand mirror Selection of polishing agent (unit dose) Radiographs Overgloves or additional gloves Floss dispenser Tape dispenser

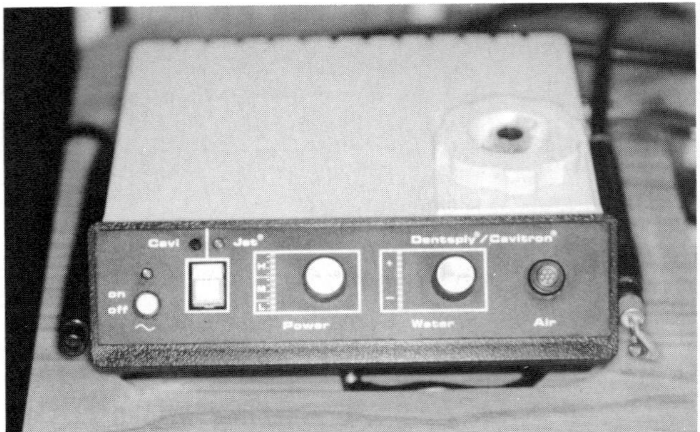

FIGURE 8-59
Airpolishing delivery system.

airpolisher has a power unit with water and air controls, a foot control switch for operation, and a handpiece connected to the unit for delivery of the sodium bicarbonate slurry that exits from the handpiece nozzle. The airpolisher is selectively used for removal of tenacious stains and heavy plaque. Findings from studies also suggest its use prior to bonding procedures, for orthodontically bracketed and banded teeth, for polishing implant prostheses, and for root detoxification. When the unit, controls, and handpiece are in use, they should be protected with surface barriers.[29] Cleaning and disinfection of surfaces not adequately protected with barriers as well as flushing the water line associated with slurry production for 3 to 5 minutes prior to first use during the day are required.[2] Check with manufacturer's recommendation regarding the ability of the equipment to withstand heat sterilization. Companies are continuing to improve products' ability to facilitate optimal standards for heat sterilization. The nozzle working end of the Dentsply/Cavitron PROPHY-JET may be sterilized with any form of heat sterilization, and the adjacent sleeve will withstand autoclave sterilization. Manufacturer research and development are working toward detachable handpieces and cords for improved sterilization of equipment such as the airpolisher.[31] Use of the airpolishing delivery system requires attention to the following infection control issues:

- Clients should use a mouth rinse prior to polishing to reduce the bacterial count in the aerosols generated by polishing. This is especially important if the client did not use an antimicrobial mouth rinse earlier in the appointment.
- Eye protection for the client also is an important safety precaution.

When using the airpolishing delivery system, the following are aseptic technique recommendations:

1. Use recommended precautionary measures for the client, including a preoperative antimicrobial mouth rinse, protective eyewear, complete coverall drape, hair cover, and lubricant to protect the lips from the drying effect of sodium bicarbonate.[15] The dental hygienist should wear the basic personal barriers of gloves, mask, protective eyewear, and protective clothing with the addition of a faceshield for more coverage in the presence of the increased aerosols and spatter. A hair cover for the dental hygienist may be worn for added coverage as well. The action of the sodium bicarbonate slurry being propelled against the tooth surfaces covered with tenacious stain, plaque, and soft deposits creates a copious spray containing oral debris and microorganisms that presents a potential health hazard for both the client and the dental hygienist. When a comparison of the airpolishing delivery system and the slow-speed handpiece was made, it was found that the airpolisher produced more bacterial contamination than the low-speed handpiece and that the airpolisher generated aerosols that contaminated surfaces as far away as 6 feet from the center of operation.[32] An open bay operatory arrangement permits the potential for atmospheric contamination when the airpolisher is used in an open area. Another way of reducing the aerosols once generated and liberated into the environment is the use of a laminar airflow system to lower the number of airborne bacteria.[30,33]

2. Increase the amount of water in the water-powder spray to aid in containing the amount of particles that will be aerosolized. The increase in water reduces the exposure of the client and the dental hygienist to the bacteria-laden particles.[29]

3. Use airpolisher instrumentation technique to minimize generation of aerosols by adhering to the following correct use angulations of the airpolisher handpiece nozzle:

- For adaptation to the facial and lingual surfaces of anterior teeth use a 60-degree angle to the tooth, and hold the handpiece 3 to 4 mm from the tooth surface (Fig. 8-60)
- For adaptation to the facial and lingual surfaces of the posterior teeth use an 80-degree angle to the tooth, and hold the handpiece 3 to 4 mm from the tooth surface
- For adaptation to the occlusal surface use a 90-degree angle to the occlusal plane, and hold the handpiece spray nozzle 3 to 4 mm from the tooth surface
- For prevention of an immediate reflux of the aerosolized spray back onto the operator avoid a 90-degree angle between the facial/lingual tooth surface and the handpiece nozzle[29]

4. Request that an assistant provide high-volume evacuation by holding the plastic suction tip as close to the handpiece nozzle as possible, or parallel to it, in order to significantly reduce exposure of the client and the operator to aerosolized particulates.[29]

5. Position the client to maximize evacuation of the

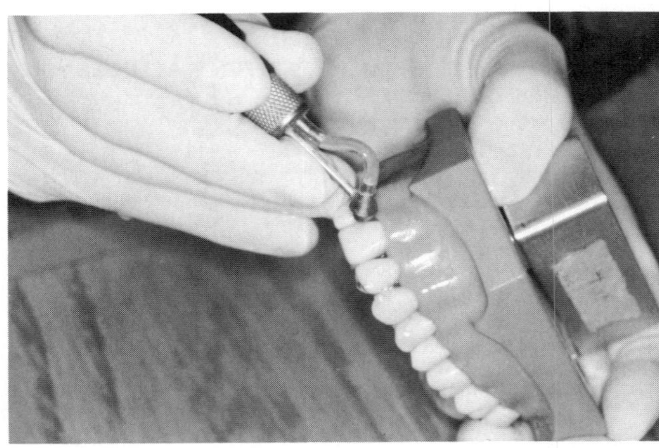

FIGURE 8-60
Nozzle of airpolishing delivery system during activation.

TABLE 8–22
PLACEMENT OF EQUIPMENT WITHIN EACH USE AREA FOR EXTRINSIC STAIN REMOVAL WITH AN AIRPOLISHING DELIVERY SYSTEM

I	II	III	IV
Mouth mirror Cotton swab Disclosant in dappen dish Lubricant in dappen dish Single length of dental floss Single length of dental tape	High-volume suction Airpolisher handpiece with nozzle for slurry delivery	Airpolishing power unit	Client chart/records Client hand mirror Radiographs Overgloves or additional gloves Floss dispenser Tape dispenser

water-powder spray by having the client turn the head as far as possible toward the side that is being airpolished. This adjustment in client position not only permits maximal evacuation but also allows the dental hygienist to retract the buccal mucosa and contain a significant portion of the aerosol spray.[29]

Table 8–22 shows the placement of equipment within each use area for extrinsic stain removal with an airpolishing delivery system.

Professional Application of Topical Fluoride

Fluoride plays an important role in the prevention of dental caries. A program of fluoride therapy may include systemic fluorides, professionally applied fluorides, and client-applied fluorides. Following assessment of the needs of the client and a fluoride history, all aspects of fluoride therapy should be considered when developing an individualized prevention-oriented dental hygiene care plan. Frequently the plan includes the professional application of topical fluoride, especially for clients at high risk for caries. Topical fluoride application also is indicated for adult clients who have caries activity, dentinal hypersensitivity following therapeutic scaling and root planing, orthodontic appliances, and xerostomia due to irradiation or certain medical conditions or in association with specific medications. The specific armamentarium prepared for the procedure depends on the form of topical fluoride (gel or solution) selected for the client. The most widely used form of fluoride for professional fluoride applications is the fluoride gel. The gel form of fluoride lends itself well to the use of trays (Fig. 8–61) because it is more viscous (thick) than the solution and is easier to transfer into the mouth.[30] The professional application of fluoride in a topical form requires attention to the following protocols:

Gel/Tray Method of Topical Fluoride Application

- There are many commercially available disposable trays for use with fluoride gels such as Styrofoam trays, plastic trays with foam insert, and fused plastic and foam trays (Fig. 8–62). Other reusable forms of trays are less desirable because they cannot withstand heat sterilization. If reusable vinyl trays with disposable liners or the air cushion tray system with disposable liners and a tray portal for saliva ejector connection for direct evacuation are used, they must be cleaned and chemically sterilized in 2 to 3.2% glutaraldehyde or ethylene oxide for the manufacturer's recommended time, according to ADA and EPA recommendations.[2]
- Disposable trays (see Fig. 8–62) eliminate the potential for cross-contamination, since they are used once and discarded. Reusable trays present a problem, if chemical sterilization should be inadequate (the time factor involves 6 to 10 hours or more of controlled undisturbed contact), and there is no form of biological monitoring available for quality assurance evaluation of glutaraldehyde chemical sterilants.
- Disposable trays come in a variety of arch sizes to ensure fit. If after try-in, the tray is determined to be either too small or too large, the tray must be discarded and the best-fitting tray selected.

Solution/Paint-On Method of Topical Fluoride Application

- When topical fluoride is in the form of a solution, the method by which it is applied to the teeth requires

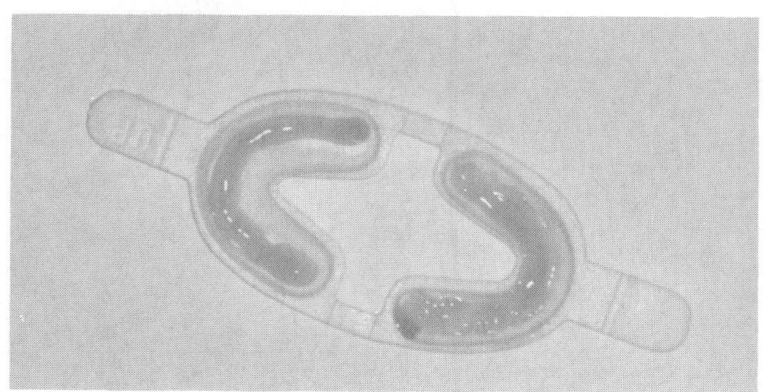

FIGURE 8–61
Gel form of fluoride placement in tray for professional fluoride application.

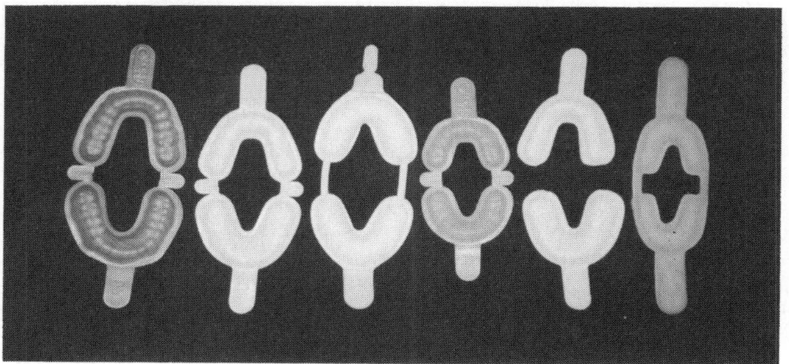

FIGURE 8–62
Variety of commercially available disposable trays for use with fluoride gels.

direct and continuous application with cotton tip applicators and involves the use of two sizes of cotton rolls and cotton roll holders. This method may also be used for gel application if the tray method is inappropriate or contraindicated.

- Isolation of the teeth for drying and the painting on of the fluoride may be accomplished by the use of sterile long and short cotton rolls held in place on the mandible by cotton roll holders called Garmer clamps (Fig. 8–63). The cotton roll holders are made of metal and are able to withstand heat sterilization for reuse.

Additional Factors for Consideration

- Regardless of the form of topical fluoride and the application method selected, evacuation of excess fluoride is critical to prevent inadvertent retention and ingestion of fluoride. The suction system is routinely exposed to large amounts of saliva, blood, excess biomaterials, and medicaments that not only contribute to microbial accumulation but also inhibit the efficiency of the evacuation system (low- and high-volume). The interior of the suction tubing should be flushed with water (Fig. 8–64) between clients and disinfected at the end of the day with a commercial cleansing solution.[2] The outside surfaces (suction tubing and connector/flow control assemblies) must be protected with barriers and/or cleaned and disinfected as well, because of their proximity to the oral cavity and their potential for contamination with blood and saliva. The low- and high-volume suction should be prepared for use during topical fluoride application; the low-volume suction should be set at the maximum level for efficient evacuation of excess fluoride and saliva throughout the timed procedure. The high-volume suction should be set for post–fluoride application removal of excess fluoride.
- The polyethylene bottles used to store the more stable forms of fluoride (acidulated phosphate-fluoride, sodium fluoride) or the polyethylene bottle holding the fluoride (stannous) mixed immediately before the professional fluoride application should be placed in the noncontaminated operatory use area. The bottle containing the bulk supply of fluoride is designated to remain in the noncontaminated area to prevent the external surfaces of the fluoride bottle from being touched with contaminated examination gloves during the course of the appointment. Cross-contamination may be prevented by using overgloves or another barrier for handling the bottle when placing the gel in the tray or solution in a disposable cup for the paint-on technique. If the exterior surface of the bottle is touched, by accident, with contaminated gloves, then cleaning and disinfection of the bottle is imperative.

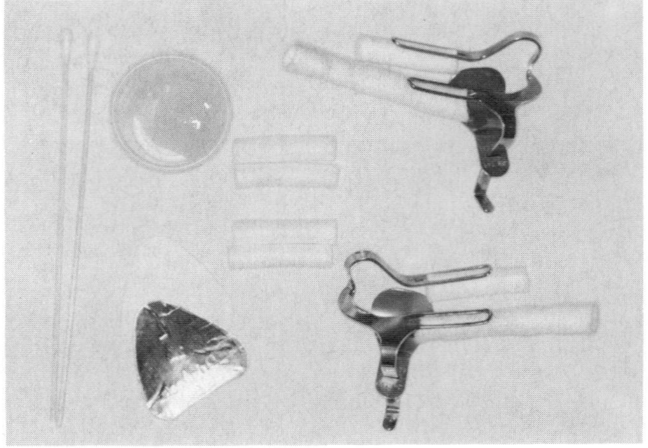

FIGURE 8–63
Armamentarium for paint-on method of topical fluoride application (cotton-tip applicators, cotton rolls, cotton roll holders).

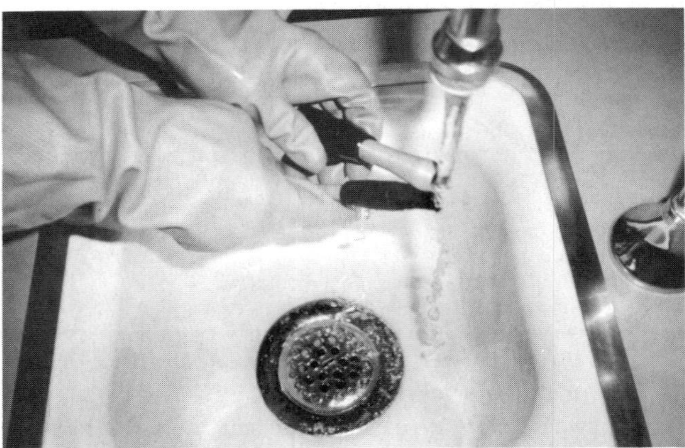

FIGURE 8–64
Flushing high- and low-volume evacuation system (flush with water between clients, vacuum cleaning and disinfection solution at the end of the day) to maximize efficiency.

Specific Infection Control Issues Directly Related to Fluoride Application Procedure

After the client has been educated about the benefits of fluoride, has been advised of the precautions to be taken

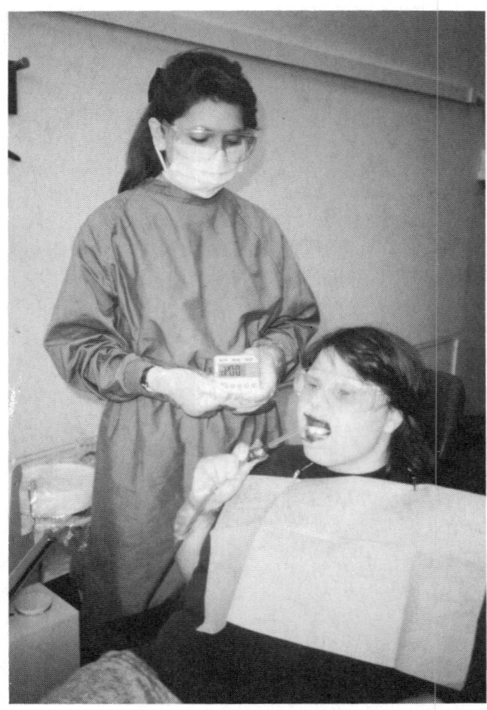

FIGURE 8–65
Dental hygienist setting timer and observing client after inserting fluoride trays into client's mouth.

TABLE 8–23
PLACEMENT OF EQUIPMENT WITHIN EACH USE AREA DURING A PROFESSIONAL APPLICATION OF TOPICAL FLUORIDE FOR TRAY METHOD

I	II	III	IV
Disposable tray (one-third full with fluoride) Cotton rolls Gauze sponges	Low-volume suction High-volume suction Cuspidor		Client chart/records Polyethylene bottle of fluoride Timer Tissues for client Overgloves or additional gloves Client hand mirror

during and following the application, and has given consent, and after the armamentarium has been set up and the fluoride prepared in tray or solution, the initial step of the procedure is to prepare the teeth by drying the field. During this implementation phase the following protocol should be followed:

- Minimize the splashing of saliva by evacuation of excess oral fluids prior to spraying air to dry the surfaces of the teeth.
- All personal barriers must be worn by the dental hygienist and the standard precaution of protective eyewear for the client is also advised.
- Following insertion of trays or with paint-on technique after all surfaces have been covered with fluoride, a timer should be set for 4 minutes (Fig. 8–65). The use of a timer presents another opportunity for cross-contamination unless overgloves are used or a barrier is placed over the timer. Use of a wall clock eliminates the potential for cross-contamination.
- After 4 minutes, remove trays or cotton rolls and Garmer clamps and evacuate excess saliva and fluoride with high-volume suction; wipe excess fluoride from teeth and soft tissues. A combination of evacuation, wiping tissues, and client expectoration provides the most effective clearing of excess agent from the mouth.[34]
- All water and suction lines need to be flushed after professional fluoride application, cleaned, and sterilized or surface disinfected along with the cuspidor. A molded style (seamless construction) dental cuspidor with water flow tubes that are removable and sterilizable has appeared on the market (Pelton & Crane; Charlotte, NC). These modern cuspidor units have improved the ease in cuspidor cleaning and maintenance of an aseptic condition.[35]
- The cotton rolls and/or disposable trays should be disposed of with other contaminated waste but are not considered biohazardous or medical waste because they are not blood-soaked materials.[2]

Tables 8–23 and 8–24 show the placement of equipment within each use area during a professional application of topical fluoride for tray method and paint-on cotton roll technique.

Application of Pit and Fissure Sealants

The dental hygiene care plan may include sealant placement as part of the preventive program for maximizing caries protection (see Chapter 21). Sealants are a safe and highly effective method for reducing or eliminating the caries process occurring in pits and fissures (Fig. 8–66). The clients who can benefit from sealant application include children with newly erupted teeth with pits and fissures, children at high risk for caries (lack of fluoride exposure, lifestyle, behavior patterns, physical or emotional development factors), and other clients who request occlusal sealants as part of a comprehensive preventive program.[34] The application of pit and fissure sealants presents some challenges for the solo operator dental hygienist, such as management of an extensive armamentarium, establishing a dry field to ensure the success of the procedure, and working with materials that may have a limited time for handling prior to setting (autopolymerization). In addition, there appears to be a lack of information, in the literature or from manufacturers, regarding infection control recommendations for the handling of sealant materials and equipment (most applicator handles are multiple use and non–heat-sterilizable). Inferences may be drawn that aseptic technique is not as critical with procedures having less contact with blood and involving predominantly children. Oral healthcare for children should not be accompanied by a lack of concern about the potential for transmission of HBV, HIV, and other microorganisms. Professional re-

TABLE 8–24
PLACEMENT OF EQUIPMENT WITHIN EACH USE AREA DURING PROFESSIONAL APPLICATION OF FLUORIDE WITH PAINT-ON/COTTON ROLL TECHNIQUE

I	II	III	IV
Sterilized Garmer clamps Long cotton rolls (2) Short cotton rolls (4) Saliva absorber for cheek Cotton pliers Disposable cup for fluoride Cotton-tipped applicators (2) Gauze sponges	Low-volume suction High-volume suction Cuspidor		Client chart/records Polyethylene bottle of fluoride Timer Tissues for client Overgloves or additional gloves Client hand mirror

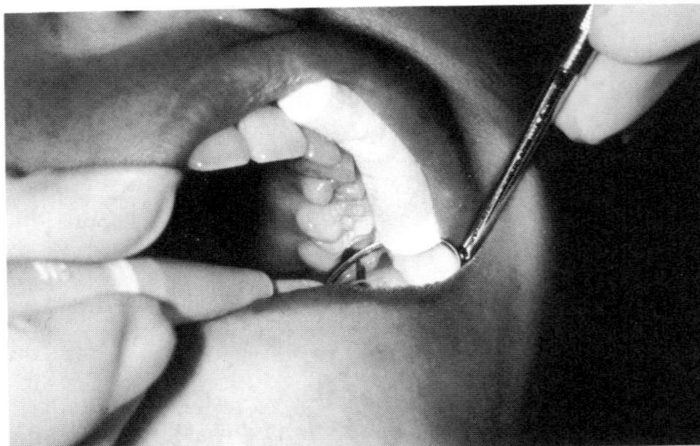

FIGURE 8-66
Pit and fissure sealant placement.

sponsibility and universal precautions require an obligation to protect the client regardless of age as well as the operator and other team and family members.

Prior to the procedure, the dental hygienist should review assessment data, determine the need for sealants, present the care plan to the client or a parent of the client if the client is a child, and gain consent. Aseptic technique considerations and recommendations related to the steps in the application of pit and fissure sealants are as follows:

- Carefully prepare and organize the extensive sealant armamentarium to minimize cross-contamination and to increase efficiency and successful sealant placement (Fig. 8-67). The armamentarium includes sterilized disposable supplies (cotton rolls, cotton pellets [pledgets]); mirror and explorer; equipment for polishing to prepare the occlusal surfaces (see protocol on coronal polishing); rubber dam or Garmer clamps/cotton roll holder(s) for isolation of the teeth; and the sealant kit with a visible light unit (produces an intense blue light) for use with light-activated sealants.

  Equipment surfaces that cannot be sterilized are cleaned and surface disinfected with the spray-wipe-spray technique and protected with surface barriers, if practical. Water and air are critical elements in the technique for pit and fissure sealant placement; they are used for rinsing and drying of the prepared surfaces. Water lines require the usual 3 to 5 minutes of flushing at the beginning of the day and for at least 15 seconds between clients.[2] The air line of the ASW syringe should be flushed prior to use with the sealant procedure as well to ensure that the air spray is free from contaminants. Flushing of the lines should be completed prior to attachment of sterile ASW tip.
- Having an extra pair of hands is always helpful. A dental hygienist working with an assistant not only increases efficiency but also can improve aseptic technique by minimizing cross-contamination and reducing the concentration of aerosols through maximum use of high-volume evacuation. In the cases of sealant placement, an assistant can also affect the quality of the outcome by improving isolation of the field and the handling of biomaterials.
- Both the dental hygienist and the assistant must wear all protective barriers and may choose to use face-shields in addition to a mask, since sealant placement generally involves higher levels of aerosol generation with polishing of the surfaces to be sealed and frequent use of water and air spray. The client's eyes should be protected (protective eyewear) during all dental hygiene care procedures.
- After cleaning the pits and fissures by using either a sharp explorer or the low-speed handpiece and prophylaxis angle with rubber cup/brush and flour of pumice (non-fluoride- and non-oil-containing agent), the field is thoroughly rinsed and evacuated. Isolation and drying of the quadrant may be accomplished with either rubber dam placement or cotton rolls attached to sterilized Garmer clamps. The placement of a rubber dam requires the use of a rubber dam clamp to attach the rubber dam to the tooth at the cementoenamel junction (Fig. 8-68). Generally, this is not tolerated by the client without administration of local anesthetic. A combined restorative (procedure that requires local anesthesia) and sealant appointment provides a situation more conducive to the use of the rubber dam and clamp for sealant isolation.[15]

  The rubber dam provides a means of isolating a specific tooth or area in the dentition, such as a posterior sextant for sealant placement. The role of the rubber dam as a barrier technique for controlling airborne

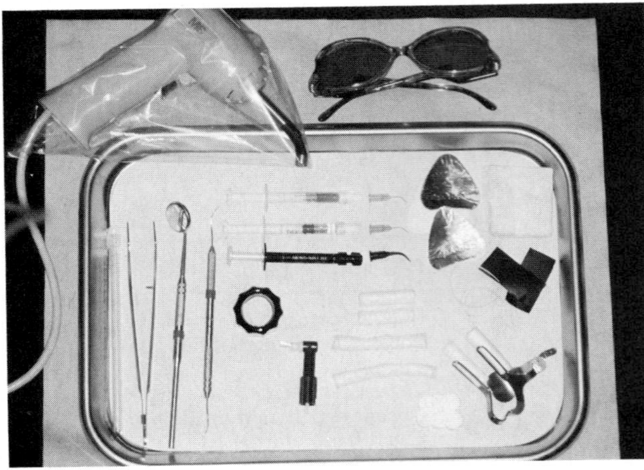

FIGURE 8-67
Armamentarium for sealant placement.

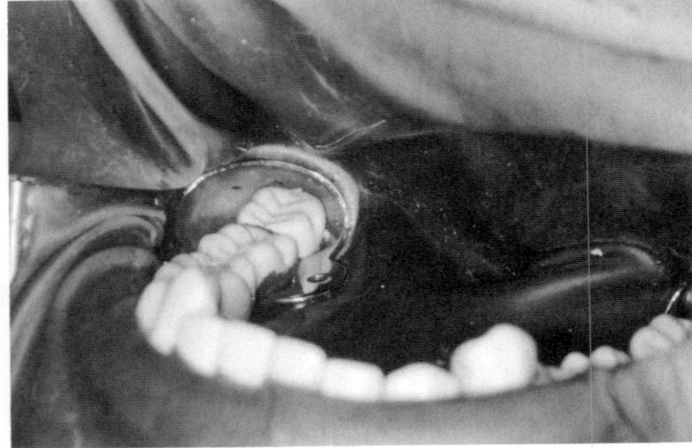

FIGURE 8-68
Rubber dam used for isolation of teeth during sealant placement.

contaminants has emerged in more recent years.[36] A significant reduction in the number of infectious particles in aerosols has been shown with the use of rubber dam isolation.[37] Further reduction in the risk of contamination can be gained with a combination of antimicrobial mouth rinse (CHX) and rubber dam isolation. It should be noted that even with a significant reduction in the number of microorganisms in the mouth subject to aerosolization or spatter, the bloodborne pathogens are not affected by mouth rinsing. Although rubber dam isolation has been shown to reduce infectious particles in aerosols, contaminated aerosols continue to be produced by the ASW syringe and handpiece. All appropriate barriers therefore are constantly required.[38]

- Once isolation has been completed, a dry field must be created. Prior to using the air to dry the tooth surface, the air must be checked to be sure that no contaminants are present in the air line that would compromise the mandatory dry field. Use of a clean mouthmirror surface to evaluate the cleanliness of the air flow from the air syringe may be helpful.
- The cleansed and dried occlusal surface is treated with the etching solution on a single-use cotton pellet/pledget, brush, or plastic sponge held by sterilized cotton pliers. The surface is dabbed with the conditioner according to the manufacturer's directions. The challenge of the aseptic technique is how to handle the small bottles of bulk supply of conditioner without contaminating the bottle, and even more important, the supply of etchant. When preparing for the procedure, place the appropriate amount of etchant needed in a dappen dish, if liquid, or on a single piece of paper pad, if in gel form, and place in use area I. All handling of the bottles should be done with clean hands or while wearing overgloves, and the bottles must remain in the noncontaminated zone (use area IV).
- Rinse and dry the acid-etched surfaces thoroughly. The careful use of a cleaned and disinfected high-volume suction with a sterilized or single-use suction tip increases the effectiveness of the evacuation of water from the etched surface and a combination of water and saliva from the cotton rolls used for isolation. Isolation of the etched surfaces from saliva contamination is critical to the success of sealant application. Drying the surfaces with clean air, free from contaminants, is mandatory prior to sealant application.
- Sealant infection control issues are related primarily to the logistics of dispensing, mixing, delivering the sealant, and light-curing, if indicated. There is considerable variation among dental manufacturers in mechanisms for dispensing sealant material and the accompanying equipment for mixing and delivering the material to the prepared surface. It is incumbent on the dental hygienist to evaluate the range of acceptable products approved by the ADA Council on Dental Materials, Instruments, and Equipment to select the system that will meet the standards for infection control. Acceptable products provide materials that are designed to prevent cross-contamination and equipment that can withstand heat sterilization or has completely disposable items that come in contact with oral fluids during sealant application. Because of the variation among manufacturers, the following addresses infection control issues related to dispensing, mixing, delivering, and light-curing a sealant.

Dispensing

Self-cure sealant—Two liquids of equal amounts are dispensed immediately before mixing, after the surface has been acid-etched, rinsed, and dried. The bottles containing these liquids should be placed within use area IV to avoid indirect contamination by aerosols, spatter, and droplets. Overgloves should be used when touching the bottles to prevent cross-contamination.

Light-cure sealant—The photopolymer type of sealant does not require mixing of two sealant materials just prior to placement but does require an additional piece of equipment, the visible light-curing unit, to solidify the liquid resin after placement on the etched occlusal surface. Since no mixing is required, direct application of the sealant material to the etched occlusal surface is possible. Direct intraoral dispensing to the prepared occlusal surface from the bulk dispenser presents a dilemma with surface contamination of dispenser (bottle/syringe) and the possibility of the tip coming in contact with oral fluids. Some manufacturers provide a disposable cover to shield the tip of the dispenser from microorganisms. The potential exists for the sealant material to become contaminated if any portion of the tip comes in contact with saliva (microorganisms may be drawn into the dispenser). To prevent contamination of the bulk supply of the light-cure sealant, dispense only the required amount of the sealant (unit dose system), immediately prior to the procedure, in a disposable or sterilizable container.

Mixing

A self-cure sealant requires mixing of equal amounts of sealant materials for a specified mixing time, placement time, and setting time (see manufacturer's product information). Potential elements in this step that could compromise aseptic technique are the container in which the two sealant materials are mixed and the stick or stirrer supplied for mixing. Some products provide multiple mixing wells within a single container for use during multiple sealant procedures. To avoid cross-contamination, a unit of mixing wells and stirrer should be used for one client only and then discarded.

Delivery

Equipment supplied with self-cure sealant kits for the purpose of delivering the mixed sealant material to the etched pits and fissures varies in design. Other components of the kit may present handling concerns with regard to cross-contamination, but it is the holder that deposits the sealant on the tooth surface that poses the most significant infection control concern with regard to reuse. When selecting a sealant product, the dental hygienist needs to evaluate the holder/handle and working ends to determine whether they meet the criteria for heat sterilization. A combination with heat-sterilizable holder/handle and single-use disposable tubes, brushes, or ball-shaped applicators is acceptable.

Dispensing

As noted above under "Delivery," with the light-cure sealant material it is possible that the manufacturer intends the bulk dispenser to serve as the mechanism for delivery. Each manufacturer seems to have developed its own system, with variations, including slip-on cannula for direct attachment to and delivery from the bottle; and a separate holder with disposable plastic tips with a ball-type working end, onto which a drop of sealant from the bottle is placed just prior to delivery to the etched surface. Other dental instruments may be suggested for delivery, such as ball-type pluggers, cotton pliers, and a small disposable tube attached to a reusable applicator that draws up a measured amount of sealant for delivery onto the etched surface. All delivery mechanisms, by the nature of their function, come in contact with the tooth structure and associated microorganisms. A system that separates dispensing from delivery prevents any risk of contaminating the bulk supply of sealant material. Use of heat-sterilizable holders/handles for attachment of disposable brush/ball tip/tube for applying the sealant to the occlusal surface facilitates improved aseptic technique.

The light source used to polymerize the light-cure sealant material must be held immediately adjacent (1 to 2 mm) and perpendicular to the sealant. Although the visible light unit does not directly contact the tooth surface, it is subject to coming in contact with oral mucosa, a zone where equipment is exposed to aerosols, spatter, and droplet contamination. Check with the manufacturer regarding recommendations for sterilization or disinfection. Consider the use of barriers if surface disinfection is the only option. Full barrier coverage should not interfere with the functioning of the visible light unit and may greatly simplify meticulous cleaning and surface disinfection.

Visible-light eye protection requires the use of a specific type of lens in protective eyewear or the use of a protective shield, sometimes directly attached to the light-curing unit. This additional piece of equipment requires cleaning and surface disinfection because of the proximity of its use to the oral cavity.

Evaluation

Evaluation of sealant placement involves the use of additional armamentarium items, such as the low-volume suction to maintain a dry field, an explorer, cotton pliers, cotton pellet, ASW syringe for rinsing, a high-volume suction, floss, and articulating paper. Although evaluation is the final step in this procedure, it requires ever-vigilant attention to aseptic technique because it involves multiple pieces of equipment, the potential for generating aerosols, spatter, and droplets, and the ever-present risk of cross-contamination.

Table 8–25 shows the placement of equipment within each use area when applying sealants.

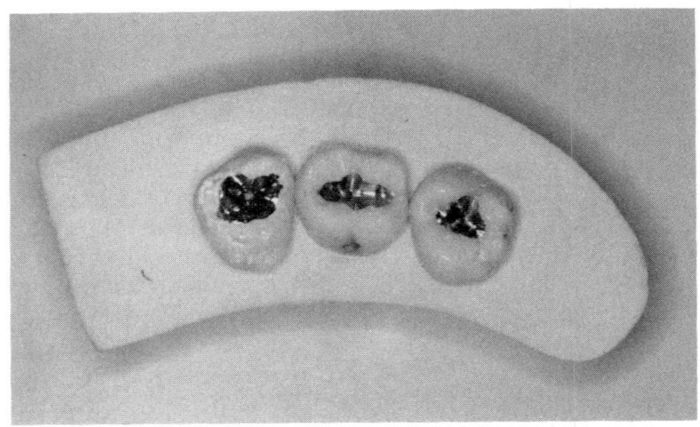

FIGURE 8–69
Amalgam restorations.

Recontouring, Finishing, and Polishing Amalgam Restorations

The dental hygiene care plan may include recontouring and/or finishing and polishing of restorations when the dental hygiene assessments detect amalgam restorations in need of margination (recontouring), finishing, and polishing (Fig. 8–69). In addition, the polishing of newly placed amalgam restorations may be the responsibility of the dental hygienist. The objective of these procedures is to pro-

TABLE 8–25
PLACEMENT OF EQUIPMENT WITHIN EACH USE AREA DURING SEALANT APPLICATION

I	II	III	IV
Mouth mirror Explorer Cotton pliers Cotton pellets Cotton rolls Garmer clamps or rubber dam Triangular saliva absorber (bibulous paper) Flour of pumice in dappen dish Disposable pad or cup with conditioner Mixing well or pad with sealant Applicator with disposable tip, tube or brush or dispenser with predosed amount of sealant to deliver to tooth/teeth Articulating paper Single length of dental floss Gauze sponges Optional: bite block	High-volume suction Low-speed handpiece Angle attachment rubber cup/brush Low-volume suction ASW syringe	Visible light unit* Protective glasses/shield*	Client chart/records Client hand mirror Radiographs Floss dispenser Timer/clock/watch with second hand Sealant kit—bottles of conditioner (acid etchant), universal resin and catalyst, or light-curing sealant material Overgloves or additional gloves

*Required for light polymerized sealant materials (photo-polymerizing material).

TABLE 8-26

PLACEMENT OF EQUIPMENT WITHIN EACH USE AREA DURING RECONTOURING, FINISHING, AND POLISHING AMALGAM RESTORATIONS

I	II	III	IV
Mouth mirror	ASW syringe		Client chart/records
Explorer	Low-speed handpiece		Client hand mirror
Amalgam knife	Contra angle		Radiographs
Gold knife	Low-volume suction		Dental tape dispenser
Cleo-discoid carver	High-volume suction		Dental floss dispenser
Files			Topical fluoride
Curets			Overgloves or additional gloves
Finishing strips			Water-soluble lubricant
Finishing and polishing stones			
Burs			
Mandrel and finishing disks			
Dappen dish with lubricant			
Single length of dental tape			
Dappen dish with flour of pumice			
Rubber cups			
Dappen dish with tin oxide			
Brushes—tapered and wheel			
Single length of floss			
Articulating paper			
Dappen dish with topical fluoride			
Gauze			
Cotton-tipped applicators			

vide the client with a smooth, hard, plaque-resistant surface, a restoration that is lustrous, free from visible and tactile irregularities, and functionally adequate.[15,30,39]

Once the proposed plan that includes finishing procedures has been presented to the client and client consent has been gained, the dental hygienist must determine the armamentarium required to accomplish the objective. Preparation of the items in the armamentarium, arranged in order of use, with a cassette or tray system, improves efficiency and prevents cross-contamination of supplies, cabinets, and other designated noncontaminated areas from exposure to saliva-coated gloves during rushed midappointment equipment retrieval (Fig. 8-70). The specific instruments selected depend on the restoration and the location and extent of the work to be accomplished.

Additionally, recontouring, finishing, and polishing technique methods vary. See Chapter 22 for specific recommendations on technique and armamentarium for these procedures. Table 8-26 shows placement of equipment within each use area during recontouring, finishing, and polishing of amalgam restorations. Aseptic technique considerations/recommendations related to recontouring, finishing, and polishing amalgam restorations are the following:

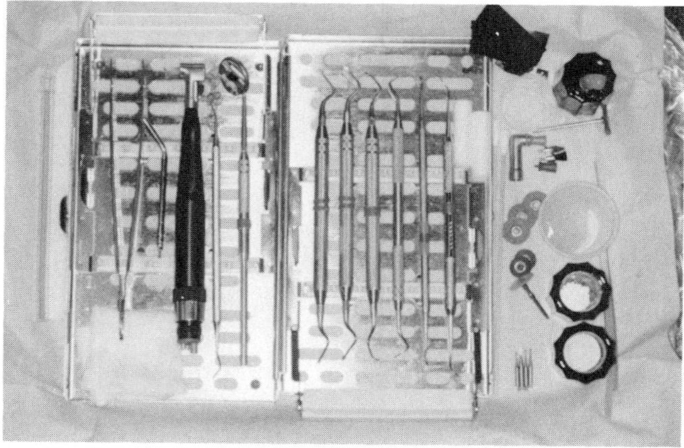

FIGURE 8-70
Armamentarium for amalgam recontouring, finishing, and polishing.

- Personal protective equipment used by the dental hygienist, whenever there is a risk of exposure to bloodborne pathogens, is required for restorative finishing procedures as well. Protective eyewear is advised for the client, especially with the increased level of aerosols, spatter, and droplet formation associated with the use of power/rotary instruments. The protocol for polishing and the use of low-speed handpieces is to be followed as described for extrinsic stain removal (pages 201-203). Chin-length faceshields in addition to masks may be used to supplement coverage during procedures prone to producing higher levels of artificially generated airborne contaminants, including amalgam dust.
- All water and air lines should be flushed, cleaned, and disinfected prior to client care. Cleaning and disinfecting the suction system also is required to protect the client and to increase the efficiency and effectiveness of field evacuation.
- Although control of contaminants in the field of operation is not as critical during recontouring, finishing, and polishing of restorations as it is during the placement of pit and fissure sealants, an area free from saliva contamination is required. The benefits of isolation with a rubber dam have been noted (see sealant protocol—rubber dam), including reduction of airborne contaminants. The use of a rubber dam with finishing procedures also provides a clear field, improves vision and access, protects the client's soft tissues from rotary instruments, and prevents the client

from inhaling particles of amalgam and polishing agents.[15] The client's ability to tolerate the rubber dam clamp without anesthesia must be considered if this optimal approach is selected. Low- or high-volume evacuation of the field either with or without a rubber dam benefits both the client and the operator, since effective evacuation can significantly reduce the aerosolized particulates.[29]

- Recontouring refers to the process of correcting and reshaping older restorations and may include the removal of excess restorative material (margination) to ensure a smooth junction between the tooth and the restoration.[15] When manual instruments (critical items) are used to remove excess amalgam (overhang) at the gingival cavosurface margin in interproximal areas, their insertion generally produces gingival bleeding. This gingival bleeding increases the bioburden on the instruments. Hence the working end of instruments should be carefully wiped before being returned to the tray/cassette to prevent the bioburden from drying on the instrument. Dried blood, debris, and exudate, if not fully removed during the cleaning/decontamination process, can interfere with effective sterilization, requiring more time to sterilize or in some instances preventing sterilization.[2]
- Power-driven instruments used for recontouring, finishing, and polishing include a low-speed handpiece with contra angle attachment and stones (green and white); finishing burs (flame, pear and barrel) and mandrels with different disks (coarse to fine); and rubber cups and mandrel brushes. All items used in the mouth should be heat-sterilized or heat- and pressure-sterilized. Heat-sensitive items that are used intraorally should be phased out from use and replaced with similar products that are not heat-sensitive. Manufacturers are striving to address the needs of the dental community for aseptic technique and are competing for their share of the marketplace. Handpieces and all finishing and polishing instruments and materials are covered by the requirement for heat sterilization. Equipment and devices that touch intact mucous membranes but do not penetrate the client's body surfaces (semicritical) should be sterilized when possible or undergo high-level disinfection if they cannot be sterilized.[25] Heat-sterilizable handpieces and contra angles are available, and the manufacturer's step-by-step instructions for maintenance of handpieces and attachments should be followed. Stones, burs, and mandrels are heat-sterilizable for reuse (see Chapter 9 for specific methods of sterilization that are effective and preferred for all items commonly used in dentistry). Disks (garnet and cuttle) and prophylaxis cups and brushes should be discarded after use, since they do not respond well to heat sterilization or are difficult to effectively sterilize.[2,6]
- To minimize the risk of penetrating the skin with a contaminated instrument, including burs, carefully wipe instrument working ends individually after use, and place the handpiece and contra angle with bur on the handpiece holder with the bur positioned down and away from the operator.
- To reduce heat and pressure when using power-driven instruments use low-speed, light strokes, water and air for cooling, and high-volume evacuation.[15] This careful use of power-driven instruments prevents excessive pressure and heat from producing mercury vapor and amalgam dust.
- As each step of the recontouring, finishing, and polishing procedure is done, a through evacuation with water and suction is advised to flush out amalgam particles and abrasive and polishing agents. Avoid a combination spray (air/water) to reduce aerosols generated. Water spray, in addition to evacuation, provides an effective lavage.

Nonsurgical Periodontal Therapy and Periodontal Maintenance Procedures

The needs of the client frequently require the dental hygienist to implement a plan of care designed to treat periodontitis. Thorough scaling and root planing in conjunction with personal oral hygiene practices are therapeutic measures used to halt the inflammatory process causing destruction of the periodontium and to create a root surface that is biologically acceptable for connective tissue reattachment (Fig. 8–71).[40] The following section presents infection control protocols for therapeutic scaling and root planing and associated procedures (ultrasonic/sonic scaling, local anesthetic agent administration, nitrous oxide–oxygen analgesia, and irrigation with chemotherapeutic agents) that facilitate the therapeutic process.

Therapeutic Scaling and Root Planing

Therapeutic scaling and root planing is a key element in nonsurgical periodontal therapy. The objective of nonsurgical periodontal therapy is to treat disease, arrest periodontal destruction, and increase attachment level. Additional components are the establishment of an effective personal oral hygiene program and recontouring ill-fitting restoration margins (see previous protocol). Ongoing success is dependent on continued effective personal mechanical oral hygiene as well as the commitment of the client to seeking regular and frequent professional care for maintaining health and preventing reestablishment of pathogenic flora.[24]

The thoroughness of root débridement appears to be the most critical element in the promotion of gingival healing and the resultant shrinkage and reduction in pocket depths, and in the provision of an environment that favors the new attachment of epithelial and gingival tissues to the surface of the tooth.[30] Creation of this biologically acceptable root surface is technically demanding, extremely time-consuming (multiple appointments), and often requires local anes-

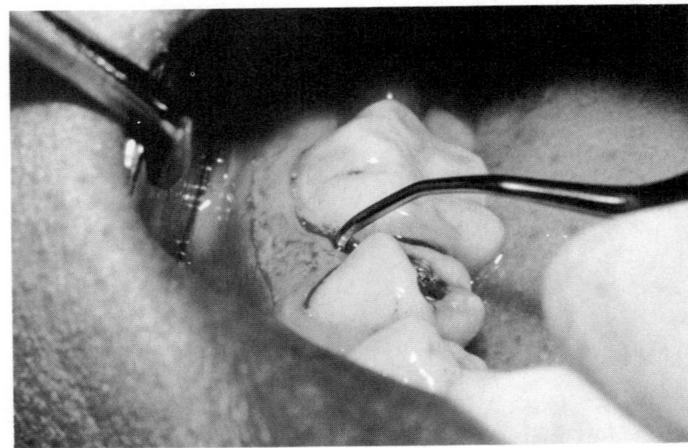

FIGURE 8–71
Instrumentation associated with therapeutic scaling and root planing.

TABLE 8–27
PLACEMENT OF EQUIPMENT WITHIN EACH USE AREA DURING THERAPEUTIC SCALING AND ROOT PLANING

I	II	III	IV
Mouth mirror Subgingival explorer Probe Universal curets Gracey curets Gauze Hoes Files Single length of dental floss (Local anesthetic—see protocol)	ASW syringe Low-volume suction Barrier Protected periodontal charting	Sharpening stone(s) Acrylic testing stick Gauze	Client chart/records Radiographs Additional packets of sterile gauze Petroleum jelly Sterile oil Cassette with supplemental instruments Overgloves or additional gloves Dental floss dispenser

thesia.[24] Scaling and root planing procedures bring the dental hygienist into frequent and direct contact with blood and saliva, generate aerosols and spatter, require handling multiple sharp instruments in a confined area, and generally require the additional risk of needlestick when local anesthetic agent administration is needed to meet the client's need for freedom from pain. The following aseptic technique recommendations for scaling and root planing procedures minimize the potential for cross-infection and cross-contamination. Table 8–27 shows the placement of equipment within each use area for scaling and root planing.

- Because scaling and root planing instruments penetrate the client's vascular system they are classified as critical items that require sterilization.[2,20,25] Sterilized instruments prearranged in instrument cassettes or trays improve efficiency. In addition, a cassette may be wrapped in paper that, when opened, creates a sterile field barrier for the top of the bracket table or instrument tray. The sterile cassette also should include an instrument rack that separates instruments to avoid protruding cutting edges and to decrease the risk of puncture of the skin of the operator. After instrumentation, the cassette is used to transport the contaminated instruments to the instrument recirculation area and is used as the container for immersion of the instruments into the ultrasonic cleaner during the initial decontamination process. This function further reduces the risk of puncture injury incurred with loose instrument placement into the ultrasonic cleaner.
- At the beginning of each appointment in the series of appointments, the dental hygienist should request that the client rinse with an antimicrobial mouth rinse. This rinsing reduces the microbial count in the oral cavity by as much as 98%. This reduction affects the pathogenicity of the aerosols and spatter created during the scaling and root planing procedures.[13] Cleanliness of the water line is critical when spraying into the gingival crevicular areas, providing direct contact between water and a wound-like inflammatory lesion. Standard operatory preparation requires flushing of all water lines for 3 to 5 minutes at the beginning of the day and 20 seconds between clients to prevent such microbial contamination.[2] Exposure to water with high bacterial counts could result in bacteremia.[30]
- Wipe the instrument working ends on sterile gauze prior to returning the instrument to the cassette or tray during the procedure. The gauze wipe helps prevent visible bioburden from drying on instruments. The dried bioburden is difficult to remove and, if it remains on the instrument through the recirculation process, may inhibit effective sterilization.[2]
- Since bleeding may be considerable during scaling and root planing procedures, producing aerosols, spatter, and droplets that carry greater potential for disease transmission and increase the volume of medical waste (blood-soaked materials), a substantial number of sterile gauze sponges should be included as part of the armamentarium, and additional sterile gauze packets in the noncontaminated zone should be available for retrieval if needed. Placement of gauze in the vestibule, adjacent to the teeth being scaled and root planed, increases the ability to isolate and readily blot the area, reducing aerosols and spatter.
- The exacting effort required for complete root planing involves a variety of instruments. Access to instruments and care and efficiency in handling them are concerns for the dental hygienist. A well-organized instrument cassette, in full view of the operator, conveniently placed for good body mechanics (readily accessible) and an approach to instrumentation that minimizes instrument transfer to and from the tray increase efficiency, reduce stress, promote thoroughness, instill client confidence, and decrease the risk of puncture wounds from contaminated sharp instruments.
- Scaling and root planing is time-consuming and exacting and involves instruments that require numerous strokes on each surface. Instrument sharpness must be maintained throughout the procedure to maximize the effectiveness and efficiency of root planing. Therefore the dental hygienist frequently has to resharpen during scaling and root planing and so must use great care with sharpening instruments during procedures to avoid puncturing himself with a contaminated instrument (Fig. 8–72).
- Sterilized sharpening stone(s) and a sterilized acrylic testing stick should be standard components of each cassette or tray set-up for scaling and root planing. Easy access to a sharpening stone facilitates maintenance of instrument sharpness during care and eliminates the need for retrieval of a stone from a noncontaminated area and accompanying use of overgloves. If lubrication of the stone is preferred to facilitate blade movement on the stone and to suspend the metallic particles removed during sharpening, the lubricant should be either a fine sterile oil or a petrolatum and

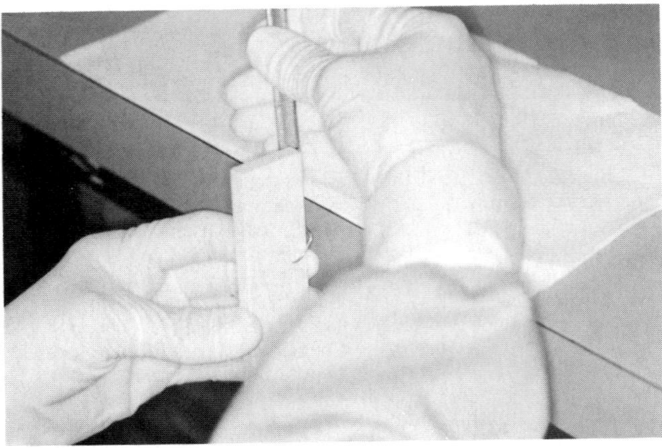

FIGURE 8–72
Instrument with sharpening stone.

should be applied as a thin layer on the stone with a sterile cotton swab. Water also has been used as a lubricant with sharpening stones. The use of a dry stone offers an advantage in eliminating any potential concerns about the sterility of the lubricant, nonsterile instrument sharpening oil, petrolatum, or water and their use during instrumentation.[15]

- Instrument sharpening requires a working surface for the dental hygienist to use to stabilize the instrument or stone, depending on the technique used. A firm, immovable surface within the contaminated area of the operatory should be selected in preparation for instrument sharpening. An example is a section of the countertop in use area III (see Fig. 8–2). Proximity to the dental operating light is important so the light may be directed toward the working surface and instrument during sharpening. A bracket table, cart, or delivery unit suspended above the client are movable surfaces and therefore unsafe and inappropriate for use as a working surface for instrument sharpening. A surface barrier, such as impervious-backed paper, should be placed on the countertop and extended over the edge in order to protect the surfaces from the contaminated gloved hands of the dental hygienist, instrument, stone, plastic or acrylic testing stick, and gauze sponge. Care should be used in moving the instrument from the cassette to the sharpening set-up and while sharpening the contaminated cutting edges of the instruments.
- Care in instrument handling is emphasized to prevent exposure incidents for the oral healthcare team and accidents involving the client as well. Instruments should not be moved or passed across the face of the client. The client should be provided with protective eyewear to serve as a barrier for eyes and mucous membranes against debris, aerosols, and spatter caused by scaling and root planing procedures. If an instrument is dropped during the course of returning instruments to the cassette or transferring an instrument to the instrument-sharpening set-up area, the instrument should be moved off the floor and temporarily placed into the sink or holding solution container to begin the decontamination process. The challenge is to accomplish this efficiently, carefully, and *without* contaminating the instrument cassette, gloves of the operator, and other disinfected surfaces. The use of overgloves is suggested to retrieve the instrument and place the instrument in holding solution or the sink. Discard overgloves with contaminated waste (the interior of the overglove is contaminated with blood and saliva; the glove exterior is contaminated with dust and settled airborne particles from contact with the floor. An additional pair of overgloves needs to be available for use during the remaining portion of the appointment.
- During the process of scaling and root planing, inflamed soft tissues bleed. In addition, the design of the curet, with a continuous cutting edge around both sides of the working end, unavoidably places the trailing edge in contact with the wall of the periodontal pocket during scaling and root planing. This instrumentation causes some unintentional removal of ulcerated sulcular epithelium, junctional epithelium, and superficial layers of the inflamed connective tissue. Removal of retained particles of dislodged calculus, bacteria, debris, diseased root surface, and ulcerated sulcular epithelium and promotion of healing may be enhanced by thoroughly flushing out the crevicular areas with a stream of water.[30] When cleansing the area with irrigation and evacuation, use of the water and air spray combination should be avoided because the forced spray increases the level of blood-contaminated aerosols. Such aerosols are concentrated 2 feet in front of the client, where the dental hygienist is frequently located. The droplet-nuclei type of infectious aerosols may remain suspended in the air for a long time and are spread through the operatory by air currents, contaminating the atmosphere.[2]
- Other methods of minimizing operator exposure to aerosols, spatter, and droplets include optimum client-operator positioning. The client may be in the supine position, with the mouth at the operator's elbow level; the operator's eyes are 14 to 16 inches from the oral cavity. The operator seated behind the client provides for less exposure to aerosols and spatter; retraction of soft tissues adjacent to the intraoral working area reflects liquid aerosols and spatter away from the operator.[15,30]

Soft Tissue Curettage Deliberate soft tissue curettage, the *intentional* removal of the inflamed, ulcerated soft tis-

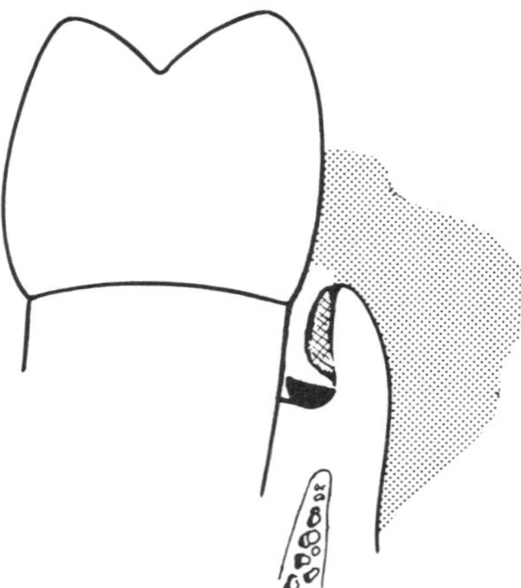

FIGURE 8–73
Cross-sectional diagram of epithelial tissue removed during soft tissue curettage. (From Grant, D. A., Stern, I. B., and Listgarten, M. A. Periodontics in the Tradition of Gottlieb and Orban, 6th ed. St. Louis: C. V. Mosby, 1988, p. 741.)

sue of the periodontal pocket (Fig. 8–73), may be included in the dental hygiene care plan following completion of scaling and root planing. Although the infection control protocol for scaling and root planing is applicable to the soft tissue curettage procedure as well, the following are a few additional suggestions to consider:

- Reserve a separate set of curets specifically for performing soft tissue curettage to ensure sharpness and to facilitate the procedure.
- Irrigate with sterile water or normal saline in a disposable syringe to limit the possibility of bacteremia.[15,30]
- Take great care in using a finger of the nonworking hand to support the outer surface of the facial or lingual gingiva when performing soft tissue curettage to prevent any risk of an exposure wound.
- Use a sterile gauze sponge moistened with normal saline or sterile water to apply pressure for recoaptation of the tissue, to stop bleeding, to help reduce the clot size (thickness), and to promote healing.[15,30]
- Place a periodontal dressing if bleeding does not stop, if papillary tissue is detached, and/or if tissue would benefit from additional protective coverage.

Potential sources of cross-contamination occur during the transition between completion of soft tissue curettage and the preparation of the materials for the periodontal dressing. The container of dressings should be kept in a noncontaminated area and should be handled only with clean hands or overgloves. Once the dressing is placed on the mixing pad and the container returned to the noncontaminated zone, overgloves should be removed because they may be too cumbersome for the mixing procedure. In addition, contaminated gloves should be discarded, hands washed, and new examination gloves donned prior to mixing and rolling the dressing in use area III. Most mixing pads are in tablet form for multiple use, which creates a cross-contamination problem when contaminated gloves are worn during the mixing procedure. The mixing pad must be held around the edges for support during mixing, which would cause cross-contamination of the edges of the additional pages remaining on the pad. An alternative to donning new examination gloves would be to tape a single piece of the mixing pad to the counter area (III) with clean hands prior to initial client contact to avoid contamination of the multiple-use mixing pad.

Table 8–28 shows the placement of the supplemental armamentarium items for soft tissue curettage and periodontal dressing placement.

Ultrasonic and Sonic Scaling The exacting scaling and root planing effort required during nonsurgical periodontal therapy involves an array of instruments selected according to amount, type, and location of calculus and other root surface irritants, and client need. When periodontal assessments reveal large amounts of heavy, tenacious calculus/root surface irritants and/or extrinsic stain, or necrotizing ulcerative gingivitis with the need for initial débridement, the dental hygienist may choose to use an ultrasonic or sonic scaling device as an adjunct to manual scaling and root planing instruments.

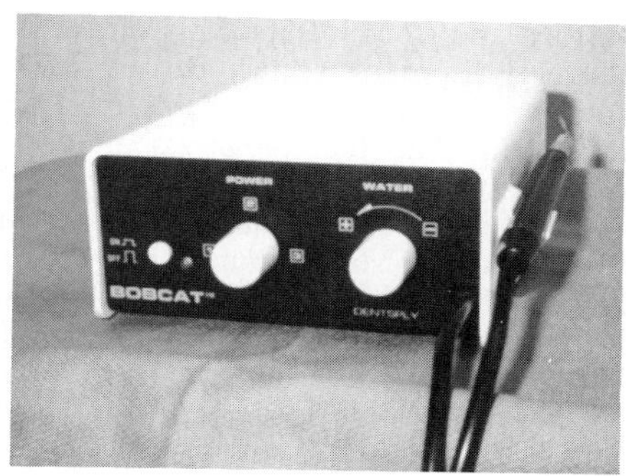

FIGURE 8–74
Ultrasonic scaling unit.

When a review of the completed periodontal assessments leads the dental hygienist to select an ultrasonic or sonic scaling device the following infection control protocol should be considered:

1. Discuss the proposed use of ultrasonic or sonic scaling instrument with the client, explaining advantages and disadvantages. Once client consent is gained, begin equipment preparation.
2. If the ultrasonic scaler (Fig. 8–74) is selected for use:
   - Position the ultrasonic unit within use area III for easy access to electrical controls, handpiece, water connector, and foot control. Connect electrical and water lines, turn on power switch and water control.
   - Flush the water line for 3 to 5 minutes before the first use of the day and for at least 1 minute prior to reuse on the same day. Flushing water through the ultrasonic unit cord and handpiece removes stagnant water and associated microorganisms in the water lines, a potential source of contamination. High concentrations of microorganisms from saliva have been found in the water from ultrasonic scalers and ASW syringes.[41,42] A precedent-setting legal case, McDonald *v.* Beaver State, was settled out of court for an undisclosed amount of money when a client developed bacterial endocarditis following instrumentation with an ultrasonic scaler. Contaminated water from the ultrasonic unit was linked to the bacterial endocarditis.
   - Clean and disinfect (spray-wipe-spray technique) the surfaces of the ultrasonic electrical unit and handpiece assembly. After the surfaces have dried, apply barriers to prevent surface contamination of equipment from aerosols, spatter, and droplets generated during the procedure. The handpiece component receives the most contamination from the gloved hands of the den-

TABLE 8–28
PLACEMENT OF SUPPLEMENTAL ARMAMENTARIUM WITHIN EACH USE AREA FOR SOFT TISSUE CURETTAGE AND PERIODONTAL DRESSING PLACEMENT

I	II	III	IV
Curets (very sharp) Gauze Scissors	Disposable syringe with normal saline	Mixing paper/pad Tongue blades	Periodontal dressing, tube(s)/container Dry foil

tal hygienist and from intraoral placement during scaling. Use of a disposable surface barrier (sleeve), specifically designed for handpieces, helps minimize surface contamination. The handpiece assembly tubing/cord also requires surface cleaning and disinfection and may be protected with a disposable barrier designed for dental unit tubing. Manufacturers are working on developing handpiece assemblies that can withstand heat sterilization; check the manufacturer's recommendations. If the handpiece is not heat-sterilizable, meticulous cleaning and surface disinfection and barrier use is required.

3. If the *sonic* scaling device is selected for use, the following apply:

- At the beginning of the day, flush the handpiece water line for 3 to 5 minutes prior to attachment of the sterilized or disinfected sonic handpiece. The water line should be flushed for 20 seconds between clients, and if an hour or more has passed since sonic scaling was last performed the handpiece water line should be flushed for 1 minute.[2] The sonic scaling device is activated with the same foot control used for low- and high-speed handpieces.
- Sonic scaler handpieces may be fully heat sterilizable; check the manufacturer's recommendations. Replacement of nonsterilizable sonic handpieces should be considered. If the sonic handpiece is not able to withstand heat sterilization, the surfaces of the handpiece require meticulous cleaning and surface disinfection and would benefit from use of a disposable surface barrier sleeve. The handpiece air hose and connector also should be cleaned and disinfected or covered with a barrier during use.

4. Even though most ultrasonic handpiece assemblies and some sonic scalers are not able to withstand heat sterilization, the ultrasonic tip inserts and sonic scaler tips are heat-sterilizable. These working ends contact the blood stream and, because of this, are classified as critical items that require sterilization prior to each use.

5. An adequate spray of water is essential to reduce the frictional heat generated by ultrasonic mechanical vibrations. This water provides a positive irrigation-cleansing effect. Adequate evacuation of the water, however, is necessary to reduce the sprays of oral fluids that contaminate the operator and the surrounding environment. The evacuation system should be cleared by flushing with water between clients and cleaned and disinfected at the end of the day. The ideal evacuation for the ultrasonic or sonic scaler is high-volume suction maintained at the field of operation by an assistant, or a saliva ejector linked to the high-volume suction for the operator working alone.

6. Client preparation for ultrasonic or sonic scaling should include rinsing with antimicrobial mouth rinse, being covered with a plastic drape and absorbent bib, wearing protective eyewear, and being provided with tissues for use.

7. The oral healthcare team working with ultrasonic and sonic scaling devices need the protection of personal barriers, which include the standard gloves, mask, protective eyewear, and protective clothing. The addition of a faceshield (Fig. 8–75) and hair covering should be considered for increased protection from the atomized blood, saliva, and other debris expelled from the mouth when using an ultrasonic or sonic scaling instrument. Measurements of bacterial counts in the air are quantified as viable particles (VPs) per cubic foot of air. For example, the environment of a surgical operating room is considered acceptable at 1 VP per cubic foot of air. When air was sampled 30 minutes after instrumentation with an ultrasonic scaler, a count of 5,000 VPs per cubic foot was measured, which represents a 3,000% increase in bacterial count over background counts. A microbiological analysis of aerosols generated by ultrasonic scalers revealed a predominance (90%) of alpha-hemolytic streptococci, which can remain airborne and viable for as long as 24 hours (see Microorganisms Discovered in Dental Aerosols chart). Currently, no documented airborne infections have been associated with these suspended alpha-hemolytic streptococci.[2]

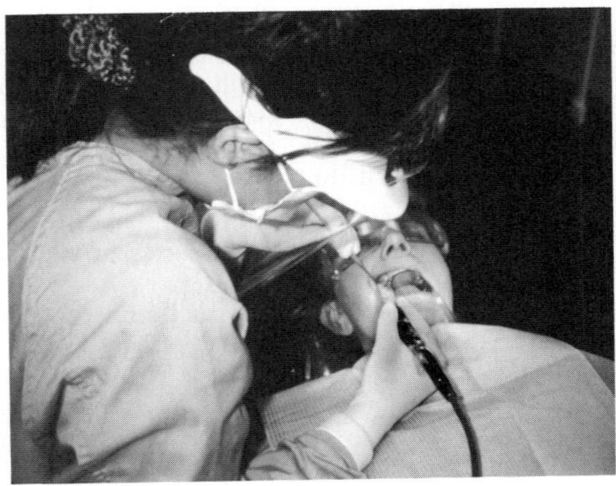

FIGURE 8–75
Water spray (aerosol) generation by ultrasonic scaling device.

The potential for airborne infection combined with the generation of spatter of blood, saliva, and other debris also reinforces the importance of evacuation, proper client positioning (fully supine not only helps with pooling and containment but also prevents gagging, which the semisupine position usually stimulates), and retraction of tissues to deflect the spray of oral fluids.

The air quality of the overall environment can be enhanced with the use of a laminar airflow system, which circulates the air and filters out microorganisms.[30]

MICROORGANISMS DISCOVERED IN DENTAL AEROSOLS

- Staphylococci
- Streptococci
- Diphtheroids
- Pneumococci
- Tubercle bacilli
- Influenza virus
- Hepatitis virus
- Herpesvirus hominis
- Neisseria

Staphylococci are the only organisms on the list usually found in the air.

Data from Cottone, J. A., Terezhalmy, G. T., and Molinari, J. A. Practical Infection Control in Dentistry. Philadelphia: Lea & Febiger, 1991.

TABLE 8–29
PLACEMENT OF EQUIPMENT WITHIN EACH USE AREA FOR ULTRASONIC AND SONIC SCALING

I	II	III	IV
Mouth mirror Subgingival explorer Probe Universal curets Gracey curets Gauze	High-volume suction with wide tip or high-volume suction with adapter for saliva ejector (one operator) Optional: Sonic handpiece and tip Low-volume suction	Ultrasonic unit Electrical generator Ultrasonic scaling handpiece and insert	Client chart/record Radiographs Sterilized supplemental ultrasonic insert(s) Optional: Supplemental sonic tip(s)

8. The tips for the sonic scaler are sharper than the rounded, dull tip of the ultrasonic scaler inserts. Therefore, they have the potential to cut, puncture, or abrade the skin. Care should be used in placing a handpiece with an exposed sonic tip on a port of the unit, since the contaminated tip is capable of causing a skin puncture on the arm of the operator if the tip is placed in the path of arm movement. Insert the handpiece with the tip down into the port, and direct the tip away from the operator and the client. Another option is to place a cotton roll over the tip as a barrier.

Table 8–29 shows the placement of equipment within each use area for ultrasonic and sonic scaling.

Local Anesthetic Agent Administration

Administration of local anesthetic agents is one of the methods of pain control utilized by dental hygienists in jurisdictions where permitted by the dental practice act (Fig. 8–76). Local anesthetic agent administration is frequently incorporated into a dental hygiene care plan for pain control during nonsurgical periodontal therapy to ensure therapeutic scaling and root planing to the full extent of the periodontal pocket and to permit meticulous instrumentation for the removal of tooth and root surface irritants. With the administration of local anesthetics, the oral healthcare provider is put at increased risk for exposure incidents and disease transmission, and critical infection control issues are raised. Once client consent to treatment has been gained, the infection control issues include the following:

1. A room temperature, sterilized *syringe* should be among the instruments included in a nonsurgical periodontal therapy cassette or readily available in single-syringe sterilization bags when unanticipated needs for pain control in conjunction with dental hygiene care arise. The syringe should be inspected to check the harpoon present on the piston (Fig. 8–77) unless the syringe is a self-aspirating type. The harpoon should be sharp and straight; if it is bent it could potentially cause breakage of the anesthetic cartridge glass tube, which may then penetrate the skin.[10,43]

2. Contamination and possible corrosion of the anesthetic solution can be prevented by *avoiding immersion* of cartridges in disinfectant or sterilant solution, or solutions of any kind.[43] The cylindrical glass anesthetic cartridge has a rubber stopper and plunger on one end for harpoon engagement and an aluminum cap on the other end. The aluminum cap holds a thin diaphragm in position to receive the syringe end of the needle, which passes through the diaphragm to allow the flow of the anesthetic solution out of the cartridge and into the needle. The diaphragm is a semipermeable membrane that permits diffusion of solutions through it. When a cartridge is immersed in disinfectant or sterilant solution, the solution diffuses through the semipermeable membrane and contaminates the solution. An extruded rubber plunger may be an indication of such contamination, or contamination may occur without any visible signs. The side effects of administering anesthetic solution that has been contaminated range from a burning sensation on injection to postinjection paresthesia and edema.[45]

If there is concern about the surfaces of a cartridge, spray a piece of gauze with disinfectant and wipe the aluminum cap, diaphragm (Fig. 8–78), and the rest of the cartridge. Opened cans or packets of anesthetics should be stored in a noncontaminated area.

The local anesthetic solution inside the cylindrical glass anesthetic *cartridge* is sterile, and the exterior of the cartridge is considered clean and uncontaminated regardless of packaging—either can or plastic blister packs. Malamed reports that bacterial cultures made from cartridge surface samples taken immediately after opening a container of

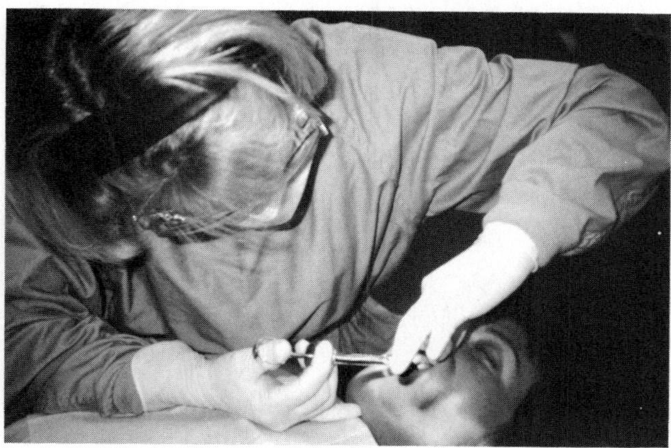

FIGURE 8–76
Local anesthetic agent administration.

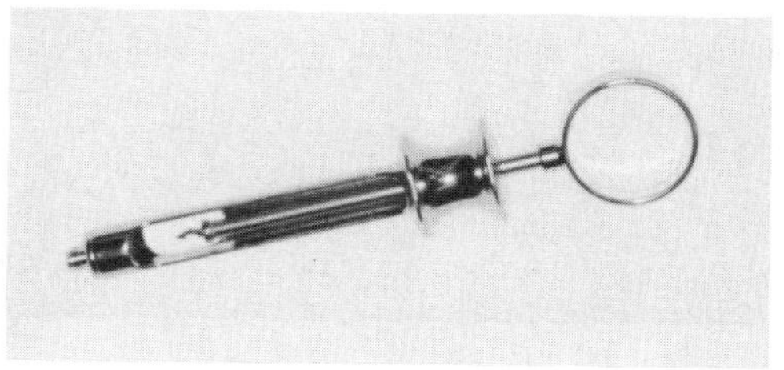

FIGURE 8–77
Unloaded syringe.

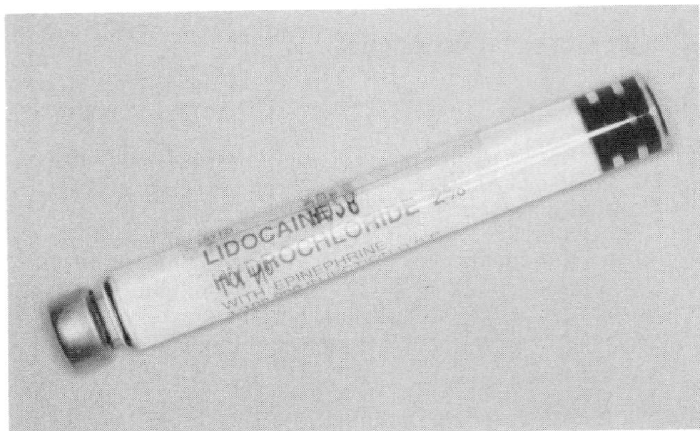

FIGURE 8-78
Local anesthetic agent cartridge.

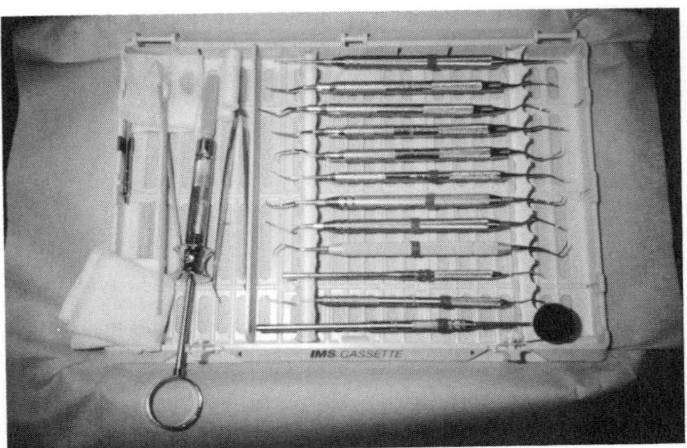

FIGURE 8-80
Instrument cassette with local anesthesia set-up includes unit dose set-up of topical anesthetic.

cartridges usually fail to produce bacterial growth.[43] However, care must be taken to prevent any possible cross-contamination of the opened canister or packet during anesthetic retrieval. The cartridge components cannot withstand heat sterilization.

3. Sharp, stainless steel, sterilized, disposable *needles* are used for the administration of local anesthetic agents. Select the specific needle(s) by gauge (diameter) and length according to the recommended guidelines (see Chapter 23) for the injections to be performed during dental hygiene care. The sterile needle is packaged in a plastic encasement made up of a colored cap over the needle end and a white plastic cap to cover the syringe-penetrating end of the needle (Fig. 8-79). The outer surfaces of the plastic encasement may be considered clean and uncontaminated when removed from the bulk supply as long as they are stored in a noncontaminated area. If for any reason there is a question about the handling of the exterior surfaces of an unopened needle, the plastic encasement may be cleaned and disinfected when preparing the armamentarium.

4. Availability and use of *sterile gauze* are especially important for drying the tissue at the site of the injection because it removes gross debris and reduces the number of microorganisms at the injection site, and dried mucosa permits more rapid uptake of the topical anesthetic agent.

5. A minimal amount of *topical anesthetic agent* to reduce discomfort at the site of the needle penetration should be dispensed and placed on a dappen dish, on a piece of gauze, or on a tongue depressor (Fig. 8-80). The vehicle for holding the topical anesthetic agent should be placed next to the instrument cassette for easy access for application with a sterile cotton-tipped applicator. The bulk container of the topical anesthetic agent must be stored in a noncontaminated area and must not be placed within the zone of contamination. If an additional amount is required during the appointment, a sterile cotton swab should be used in retrieval as well as overgloves or clean hands to prevent contamination of the bulk supply.

6. When loading the syringe, the following method is recommended:

- Remove the sterilized syringe from the cassette or individual syringe sterilization bag. Check the harpoon to be sure that it is straight and sharp unless it is a self-aspirating syringe.
- Insert the cartridge, rubber stopper end first, while the piston is fully pulled back into the syringe.
- Gently press the ring and piston to engage the harpoon in the cartridge rubber stopper (Fig. 8-81). The harpoon must be firmly engaged in the stopper.
- After the cartridge is in place and the harpoon en-

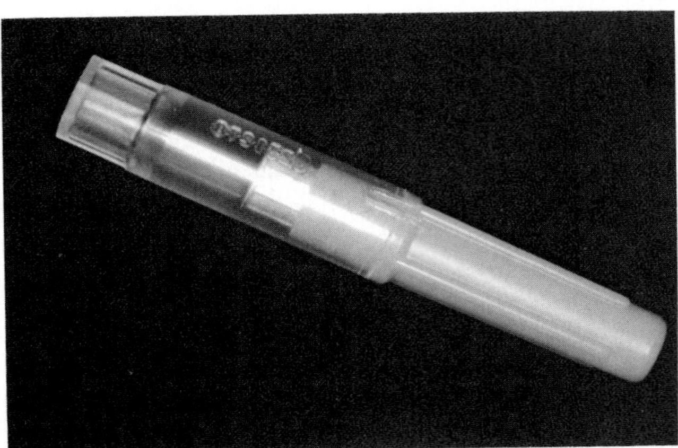

FIGURE 8-79
Sterilized disposable needle, sheathed.

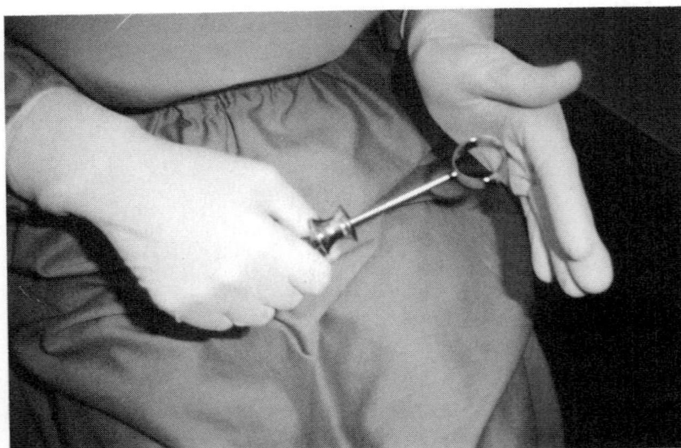

FIGURE 8-81
Syringe with cartridge in place and harpoon being engaged.

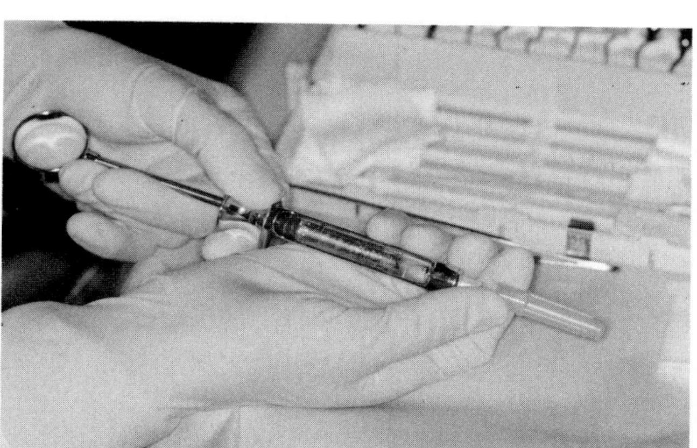

FIGURE 8-82
Needle cap being disengaged from the syringe.

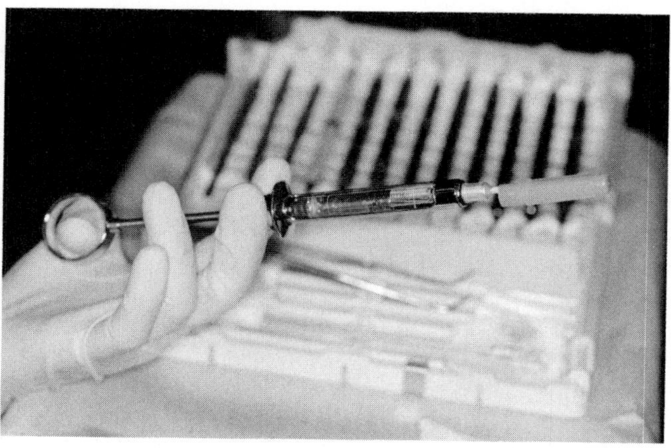

FIGURE 8-84
Needle cap being slipped down toward the hub.

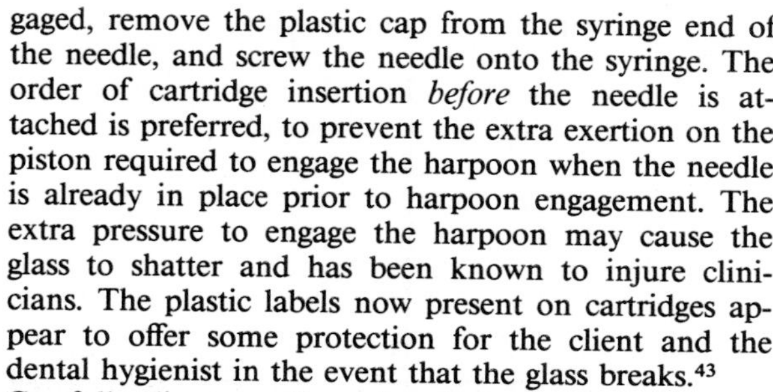

gaged, remove the plastic cap from the syringe end of the needle, and screw the needle onto the syringe. The order of cartridge insertion *before* the needle is attached is preferred, to prevent the extra exertion on the piston required to engage the harpoon when the needle is already in place prior to harpoon engagement. The extra pressure to engage the harpoon may cause the glass to shatter and has been known to injure clinicians. The plastic labels now present on cartridges appear to offer some protection for the client and the dental hygienist in the event that the glass breaks.[43]

- Carefully disengage the colored plastic protective covering or needle cap (Fig. 8-82) at the hub with the hand around the syringe and the needle directed away from the body or the hand. Allow the cap to slide off the needle, and slip it carefully onto the instrument tray. The sheath should always be carefully removed from the needle. Placing one's hand on the end of the cap for removal should be avoided because pulling off the cap may cause the hand to "bounce back," resulting in a needlestick with an exposed needle. After removing the needle cap, inspect the bevel end of the needle to check for a barb or fish-hook type of projection, which increases pain and causes tissue trauma if used for an injection. Expel a few drops of anesthetic solution to check the flow of solution.
- Resheath the needle, using a *one-handed technique* to "scoop up" the cap from the tray onto and over the needle (Fig. 8-83). Tilt the syringe upward (Fig. 8-84), and once the cap has slipped down toward the hub secure the cap to the syringe. The key to preventing needlestick injuries is to use an appropriate one-handed technique for recapping the needle. The greatest risk of a needlestick injury occurs when the needle is moved toward a body part, especially the hand, as in the two-handed technique (Fig. 8-85). Another one-handed technique is the use of a needle-sheath prop device that holds the sheath (cap) at an angle so the needle is resheathed with ease (Fig. 8-86). The sheath holder, or prop, should be heat-sterilizable. Some companies are marketing devices that withstand 400 to 500 autoclave (sterilization) cycles. Check with the manufacturer to be sure that such devices may be sterilized prior to purchasing. Another resheathing alternative is the use of forceps to hold the sheath on the tray while keeping the other hand at a safe distance from the needle, which provides more control over the sheath for recapping the needle (Fig. 8-87). A needle should be promptly resheathed immediately after withdrawal from the tissue and should never be left exposed on the dental hygiene instrument tray.[43-45]

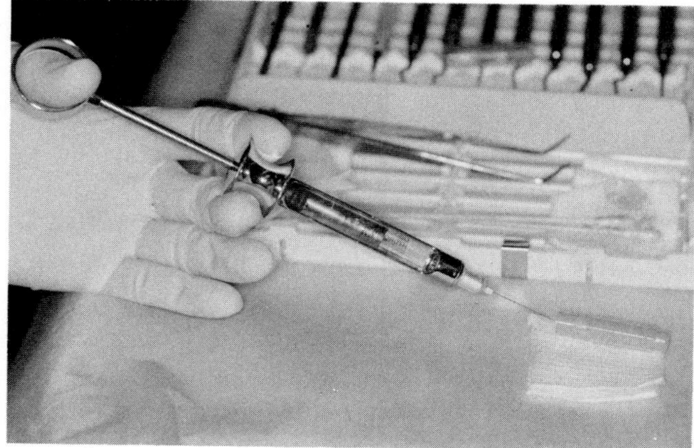

FIGURE 8-83
Needle cap being "scooped up" from the tray onto the needle.

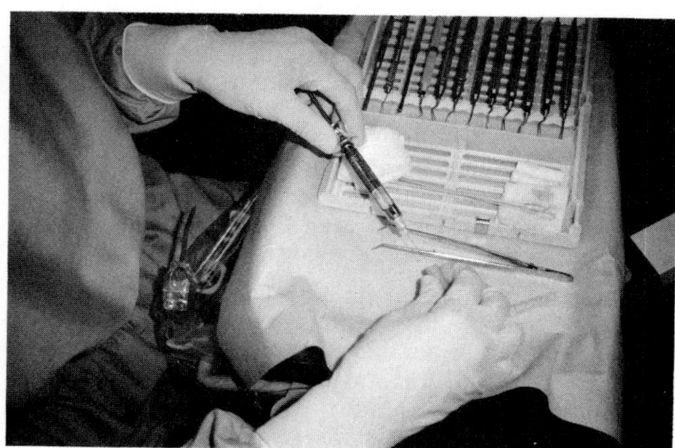

FIGURE 8-85
Two-handed recapping technique showing risk of needlestick injury.

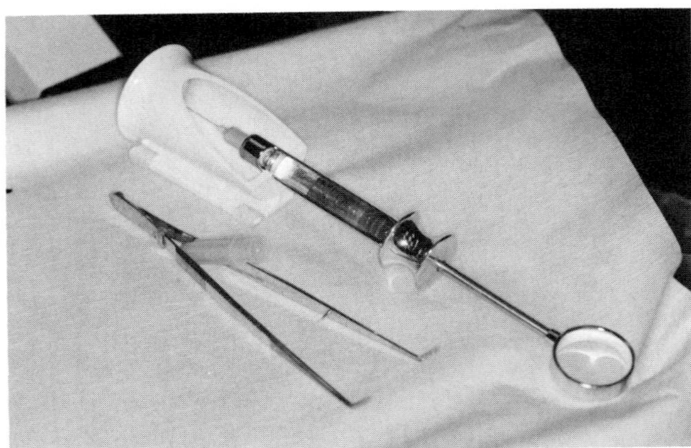

FIGURE 8-86
Needle-sheath propping devices.

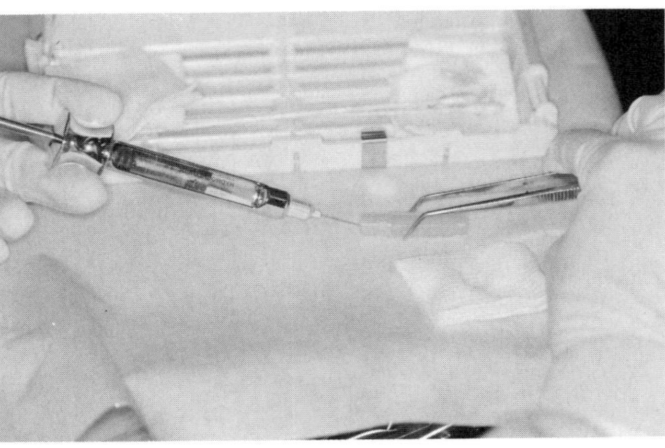

FIGURE 8-87
Forceps used to control sheath (cap) on tray for recapping needle.

7. Administering a local anesthetic agent meets the characteristics of an exposure-prone procedure as described by the CDC: "the simultaneous presence of the healthcare worker's fingers and a needle or other sharp instrument or object in a poorly visualized or highly confined anatomic site."[25] Recommended methods for reducing contaminants and preventing needlestick exposures are as follows:

- Position the client in the supine position to maximize access, ease in rinsing and evacuation, and reduction of aerosols.
- Dry tissue with a sterile gauze, apply topical **antiseptic** (optional), apply topical anesthetic agent, and redry.
- Carefully disengage the needle sheath (see fifth entry in this list).
- Use a new piece of gauze for gentle, yet well-controlled tissue retraction to provide good visibility.
- Using taut tissue retraction, place the finger(s) retracting tissue out of the path of the needle approach to the injection site, and use a firm hand rest to stabilize the syringe.
- Be aware of the position of the uncovered needle tip whether it is inside or outside the client's mouth. The needle should not be touching anything except the client's tissue at the site of the injection. This awareness helps prevent injury or potential exposure of both the client and the operator.[43]

8. The administration of local anesthetic agent in conjunction with dental hygiene care frequently requires multiple injections to provide pain control during therapeutic scaling and root planing of a quadrant or sextant. Multiple injections may necessitate the replacement of empty anesthetic cartridges and the changing of the needle to ensure sharpness and/or appropriate length (long versus short) for a specific injection. When changing a cartridge for additional anesthetic solution the following is recommended:

- Resheath the needle with a one-handed technique.
- Secure the sheath/cap. Recapping needles should include the scoop technique or shields, and holders. Remember when using the "scoop" technique to be sure to tilt the needle upward once the sheath is on the needle. If the sheath starts to slide off the needle, do not attempt to stop the sheath from sliding off, because in the process the sheath may slip off the needle and the exposed contaminated needle and hand may meet to create an exposure incident.
- Carefully place the capped needle on a sterile gauze. The exposed end of the needle inserted in the syringe should be handled with extreme care, since both ends of the used needle are considered contaminated sharps with the potential of causing an exposure incident.
- Malamed[43] recommends removal and reattachment of the needle during a cartridge change to prevent potential breaking of the glass cartridge when additional pressure is required on the harpoon to engage the rubber stopper on the new cartridge. The potential for cartridge breakage is greatest if the needle is not removed. However, the risk of removal and increased handling of a contaminated needle must be weighed against the risk of potential breaking of the glass cartridge. The placement of the plastic label on the glass cartridge has reduced the potential for breaking of glass.
- Retract the piston.
- Remove the cartridge, and dispose of it in a sharps container (Fig. 8-88). A sharps container is a critical element in the overall waste disposal system within the healthcare setting. The majority of exposures that occur among healthcare providers involve sharp instruments; therefore, the handling and disposal of sharps are of utmost importance. The empty glass cartridge is considered infectious, since some body fluids are drawn up into the cartridge during aspiration, and it is

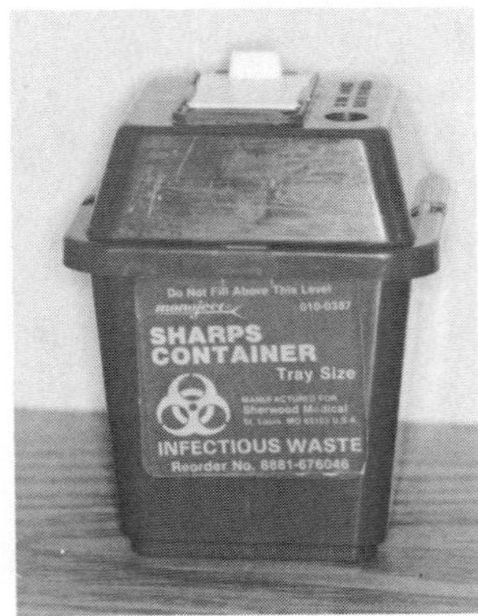

FIGURE 8-88
Sharps container.

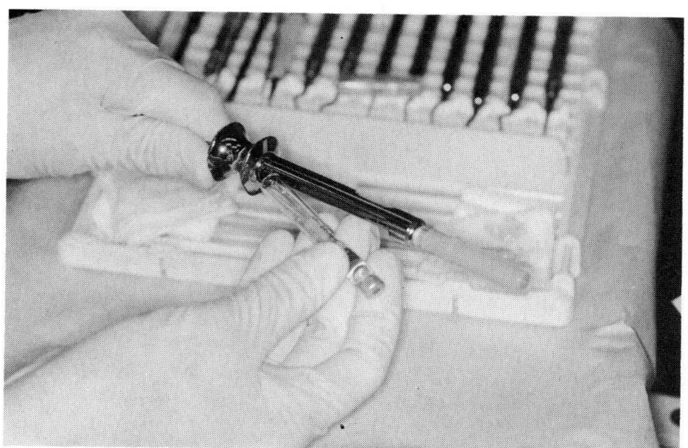

FIGURE 8-89
Cartridge removal from syringe.

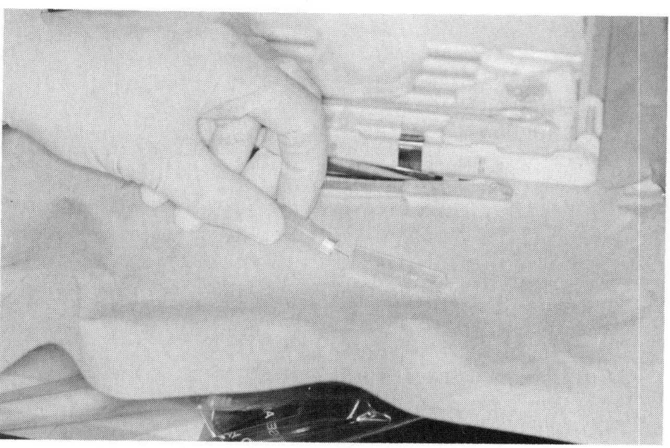

FIGURE 8-90
Exposed syringe-end of needle being recapped by "scooping up" of small cap for disposal.

possible that the glass cartridge could break. The used cartridge is viewed as infectious and potentially a sharp capable of causing a puncture wound. Therefore, cartridges must be disposed of in an impervious container that is rigid, puncture-proof, leak-resistant, and able to be sterilized or incinerated. Sharps containers should be located as close as possible to the area of operation, readily available for immediate disposal of contaminated sharps.[10]

- Replace with a new cartridge.
- Engage the harpoon in the rubber stopper.
- Reattach the needle for multiple use with the same client.
- Discard the needle in the sharps container, and replace it with a new needle after three or four injections to ensure adequate sharpness for comfort and ease of insertion and advancement. Needle replacement also may be required to have the appropriate length needle for a specific injection.

9. After the injection(s) is(are) completed, the procedure for postadministration handling of the armamentarium includes the following:

- Scoop up the sheath with a one-handed technique, and be sure to tilt the syringe up to facilitate the sheath sliding down toward the hub.
- Retract the piston by pulling back on the ring to disengage the cartridge from the needle.
- While the piston is retracted, turn the opening on the side of the syringe downward to enable the cartridge to fall free from the syringe (Fig. 8-89).
- Separate the needle from the syringe with great care. The risk with this step is the chance of accidental exposure with the syringe (inner) end of the needle. Malamed[43] recommends unscrewing and removing the exposed needle from the syringe and scooping up the syringe end into the short cap for protection from exposure during disposal into the sharps container (Fig. 8-90).
- Do not take any other steps before the needle is put into the sharps container (Fig. 8-91). Sharps containers should be readily available within the dental hygiene operatory, located as close as possible to the area of sharps use[10] (see OSHA Rules and Regulations on Work Practice Controls Related to Contaminated Needles and Other Contaminated Sharps chart).
- The rigid, puncture-proof, leak-resistant sharps containers can be sterilized or incinerated. The container should not be overfilled and, when no longer in use, should be closed and disposed of in accordance with federal, state, and local regulations.[10]
- *Note:* Needles or contaminated sharps are considered to be infectious waste and, as such, are in a category with other materials, such as blood components and pathological and microbiological waste materials. Not all medically generated waste is potentially infectious. Epidemiological evidence has shown blood, used sharps, and pathological and microbiological waste to be capable of transmitting communicable disease; therefore, they are subject to federal, state, and local regulations.[46]

Table 8-30 shows the placement of equipment within each use area for the administration of a local anesthetic agent.

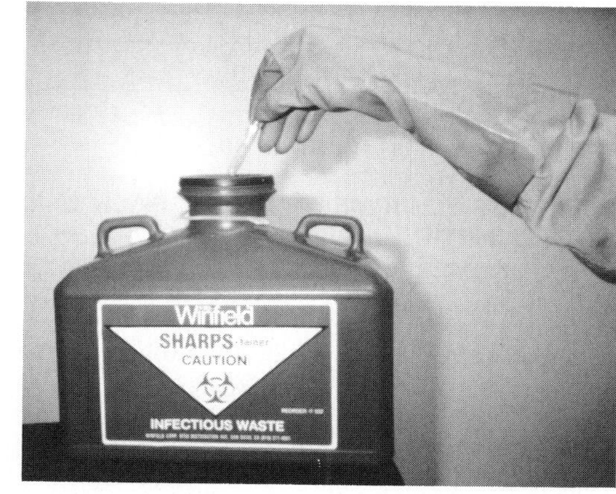

FIGURE 8-91
Covered needle being dropped into sharps container for disposal.

OSHA RULES AND REGULATIONS ON WORK PRACTICE CONTROLS RELATED TO CONTAMINATED NEEDLES AND OTHER CONTAMINATED SHARPS

- Contaminated needles and other contaminated sharps shall not be bent, recapped, or removed . . . unless the employer can demonstrate that no alternative is feasible or that such action is required by a specific medical procedure and such *recapping* or *needle removal* must be accomplished through the use of a mechanical device or a one-handed technique.
- Contaminated sharps (regulated waste) shall be discarded immediately or as soon as feasible in containers that are closable; puncture-resistant; leakproof on the sides and bottom; and labeled with a fluorescent orange or orange-red label with a contrasting BIOHAZARD legend (Fig. 8–92) or color-coded (red containers may be substituted for labels). Containers for contaminated sharps shall be located as close as is feasible to the immediate area where sharps are used.

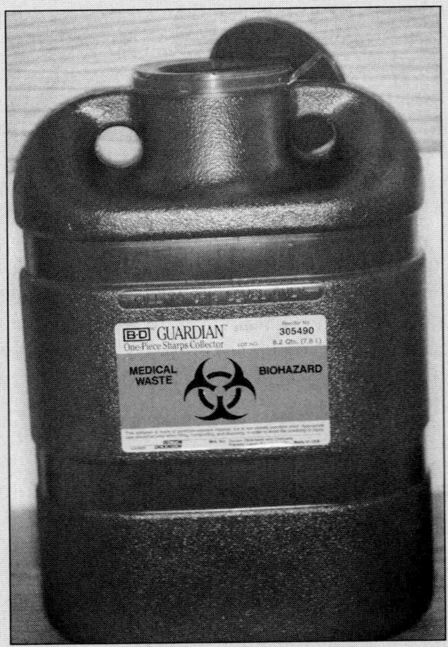

FIGURE 8–92
Sharps container with biohazard label warning.

From Federal Register 56(235):64004–64182, 1991.

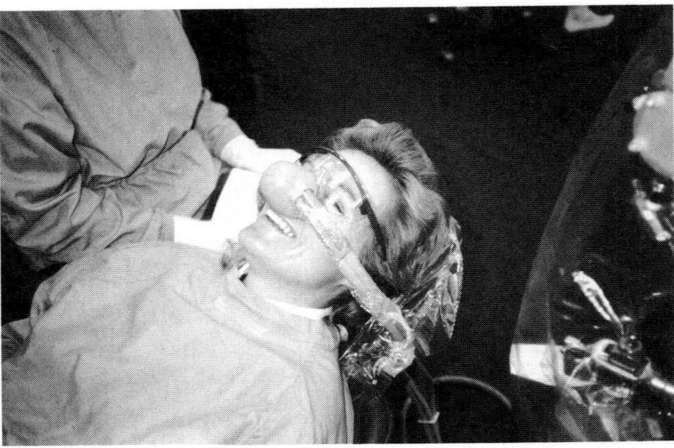

FIGURE 8–93
Client with nitrous oxide–oxygen conscious sedation set-up.

Nitrous Oxide–Oxygen Analgesia

Nitrous oxide–oxygen (N_2O-O_2) analgesia may be a desired method of pain control to help meet the client's need for freedom from pain and stress (Fig. 8–93). N_2O-O_2 analgesia is often part of a dental hygiene care plan to provide therapeutic scaling and root planing and soft tissue curettage and to reduce the anxiety associated with the administration of a local anesthetic agent. Currently 21 states permit the dental hygienist to administer the N_2O-O_2 analgesia for conscious sedation. In other states, the dentist may be required by law to titrate the levels of nitrous oxide and oxygen, with the dental hygienist being responsible for monitoring the client during conscious sedation and oxygenating the client at the completion of dental hygiene care. Once an indication for use and informed consent have been established, the dental hygienist needs to consider the following infection control protocol for the administration of N_2O-O_2 conscious sedation:

1. Before turning on the flow of gases and touching the controls to regulate gas flow for either the portable or the centralized analgesia system, clean and disinfect the surfaces of the equipment to be touched during the administration of conscious inhalation sedation.
2. Cover the control dials/levers, buttons, and liter flow gauges contacted during the procedure with disposable surface barriers (Fig. 8–94). Plastic wrap, foil, and plastic bags as well as custom-designed plastic barriers are effective and increase the efficiency of postprocedure decontamination, since most controls have grooves, crevices, or knurled surfaces that are difficult to clean and thoroughly disinfect

TABLE 8–30
PLACEMENT OF EQUIPMENT WITHIN EACH USE AREA FOR THE ADMINISTRATION OF LOCAL ANESTHETIC

I	II	III	IV
Sterilized disposable needle(s) Sterile syringe Dappen dish with topical antiseptic (optional) Sterile cotton-tipped applicators Topical anesthetic on gauze or dappen dish Sterile gauze	Low-volume ASW syringe	Sharps container	Container of topical antiseptic Container of topical anesthetic agent Container of local anesthetic agent

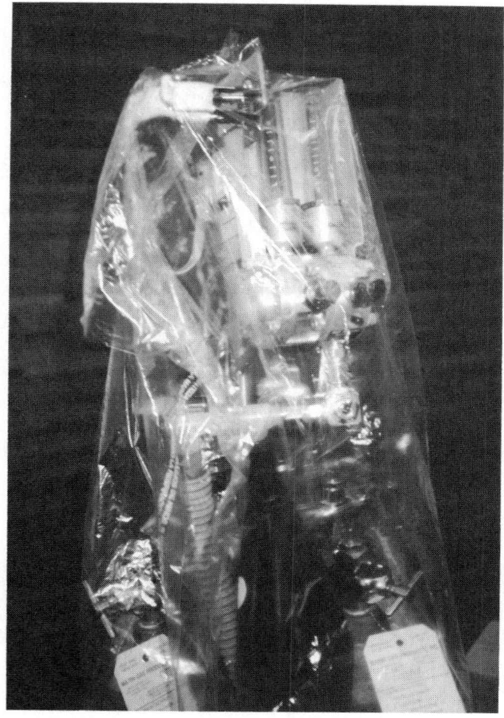

FIGURE 8–94
Use of surface barriers with portable nitrous oxide–oxygen unit.

between clients. Overgloves or other hand barriers can be used to avoid direct contact with the contaminated gloved hand of the dental hygienist. Surface coverage with barriers adds the additional protection of equipment from exposure to aerosols and spatter due to proximity to the working area. A plastic bag large enough to cover the liter flow gauges and the control levers or dials permits clear observation of flow meters and maximizes surface protection. As long as the plastic bag is not broken or compromised in any way during the procedure, cleaning and disinfection of the gas machine may be limited to one time per day.

3. Place the N_2O-O_2 gas machine within the contaminated zone (behind the client) for close monitoring and easy access during the dental hygiene care procedure.

4. Attach the sterilized tubing and nasal mask to the portable gas machine or to the wall hookup for a centralized system. Nasal masks and hoses that can withstand heat sterilization (steam under pressure and unsaturated chemical vapor sterilization methods) should be used. Ethylene oxide sterilization (verifiable method of sterilization) is the more costly and less available method that is recommended for heat-sensitive materials.

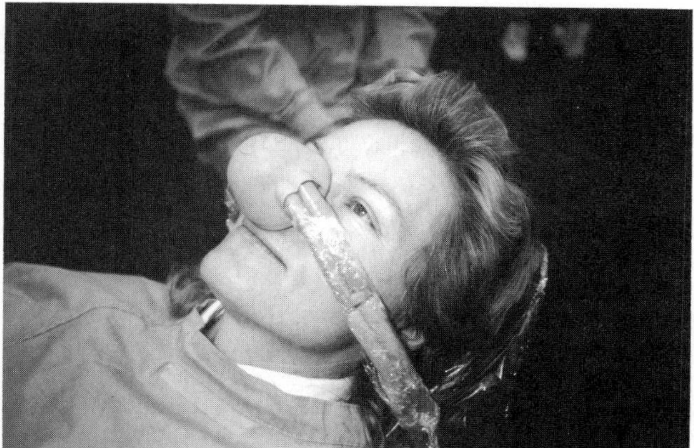

FIGURE 8–96
Nasal mask with barriers on tubing adjacent to oral cavity.

5. Adjust the evacuation system volume setting for maximizing the effectiveness of the scavenging of exhaled gases with a suction-measuring device (Fig. 8–95). The tip of the suction-measuring device is inserted into the attachment mechanism for the high-volume suction. As a result, it becomes contaminated by contact with the interior surface of the evacuation tubing and should be cleaned and disinfected prior to storage for reuse.

6. The tubing on the gas machine that delivers and removes the gases is immediately adjacent to the oral cavity and requires some barriers for minimizing bioburden due to aerosols, spatter, and droplets and to direct contamination by the clinician when adjusting the client's nosepiece during procedures (Fig. 8–96). Foil or plastic wrap on sections of the tubing adjacent to the nosepiece and the oral cavity offers some protection for the surfaces.

7. Once a comfortable conscious sedation level is established, the dental hygienist should document the time this

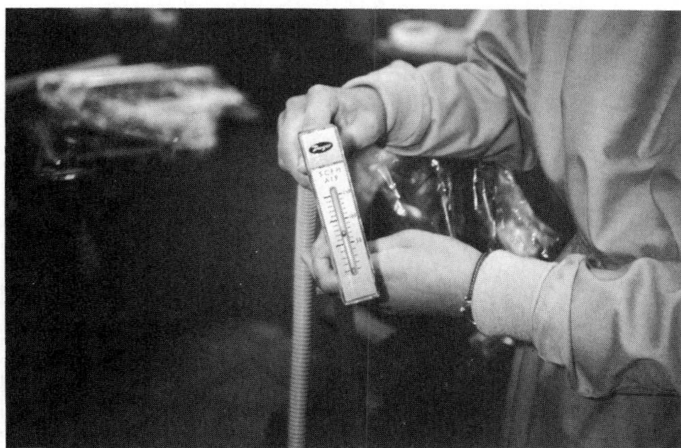

FIGURE 8–95
Flow meter used to establish scavenger flow setting.

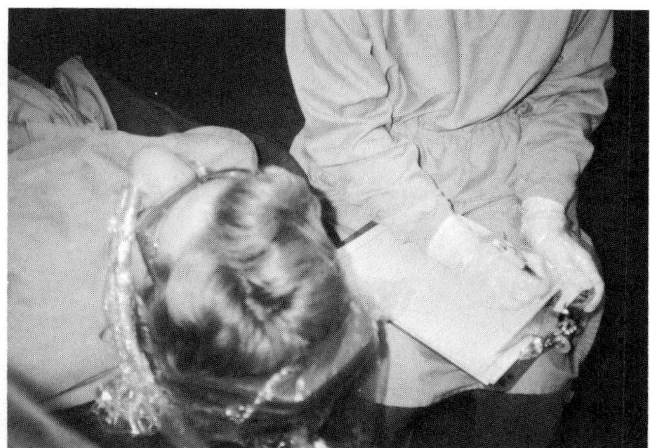

FIGURE 8–97
Overgloved hands documenting baseline nitrous oxide–oxygen levels and time on client record.

TABLE 8–31
PLACEMENT OF EQUIPMENT WITHIN EACH USE AREA FOR THE ADMINISTRATION OF NITROUS OXIDE–OXYGEN CONSCIOUS INHALATION SEDATION

I	II	III	IV
Nasal mask and tubing	Flow meter and controls (behind client)	Flow meter measuring device for scavenger system	Client chart/record

state was reached and the associated levels of nitrous oxide and oxygen. The client record should be in the adjacent noncontaminated area, and overgloves should be used for record entry (Fig. 8–97).

8. Only barrier-protected surfaces on the machine and nasal hood and tubing should be directly contacted by contaminated operator gloves during and after the procedure.

Table 8–31 shows the placement of the equipment within each use area for the administration of N_2O-O_2 conscious inhalation sedation.

Irrigation with Antimicrobial Agents

The professional delivery of antimicrobial agents to subgingival areas to enhance the results of therapeutic scaling and root planing is an area of special interest to the dental hygienist (Fig. 8–98). If professional irrigation with an antimicrobial is incorporated into the dental hygiene care plan to augment thorough scaling and root planing either during initial therapy or during periodontal maintenance care, the following protocol should be considered for asepsis:

1. The mode of antimicrobial delivery must provide access to subgingival areas with safety and ease. A number of effective methods include the use of plastic disposable syringes, powered oral irrigators, ultrasonic units, and air-driven subgingival irrigation handpieces. The working end/tip (cannulas) of the manual, disposable syringe, as well as the air-powered (handpiece) or electrical-powered (oral irrigator) delivery systems must be sterile (see Modes of Professional Delivery of Antimicrobials chart). Such working ends are considered a critical item, according to the Spaulding classification of instruments and equipment. Critical items are those that penetrate or touch broken skin on mucosa or bone.[5,10,20]

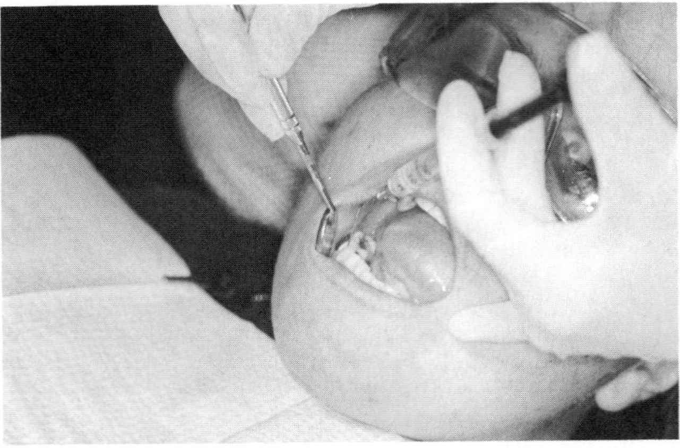

FIGURE 8–98
Subgingival irrigation with antimicrobial agent.

2. Preparation of the armamentarium and placement of equipment in the area of use in the dental hygiene care setting require either attachment of the sterilized handpiece to the dental unit air supply hose (zone II) or convenient placement of the separate oral irrigation device or ultrasonic unit for ease in access during the subgingival irrigation procedure. The oral irrigator or ultrasonic unit surfaces

MODES OF PROFESSIONAL DELIVERY OF ANTIMICROBIALS

- Plastic disposable syringes vary in size and needle gauge. Manual syringes were used in most of the early research on subgingival delivery for antmicrobial agents.[30] They provide the advantage of a single-use disposable product that is sterile until opened. They are lightweight and thus provide good tactile sensation.[43] Following use, the entire disposable syringe should be discarded with the other sharps in the sharps container.[46]
- Powered irrigation devices have been modified for professional subgingival delivery of antimicrobials. The system includes a special heat-sterilizable handpiece(s), disposable cannulas (tips) for subgingival insertion, a variable-length hose (some 6 feet in length) for handpiece connection to the reservoir containing the antimicrobial, foot pedal control, and a covered reservoir for the antimicrobial agent. The cannula attachment is a blunt needle that has either an end-port with the orifice at the end or a side-port with the orifice on the side of the cannula. Selection of the type of cannula is generally considered to be a matter of professional preference.[30]
- Ultrasonic Irrigation Unit: Ultrasonic scaling instruments with a quick-release water connection may be connected to a pressurized container holding the antimicrobial agents. Antimicrobial agents may then be used instead of water as a coolant and irrigant *during instrumentation*. Some ultrasonic instruments have a built-in reservoir for antimicrobial agents (CAVIMED 2000, Dentsply International). Antimicrobial lavage during the use of sonic scaling also is possible if a small fluid reservoir is connected to the lines of a sonic instrument.[47]
- An air-driven subgingival irrigation handpiece may also be used for local delivery of antimicrobial agents. This is accomplished through the use of a heat-sterilizable handpiece designed for subgingival irrigation via attachment to the operatory dental unit air supply and the use of the rheostat as a foot control. The reservoir for the chemotherapeutic agent is built into the handpiece. The disposable cannula is attached to the handpiece for local delivery of the antimicrobial into the subgingival areas.

and controls should be protected with disposable surface barriers, since placement will be in an area of contamination (zone III) in the operatory; the attached foot control also should be conveniently placed for comfort and easy access. Ideally, the use of antimicrobials would be identified as part of the dental hygiene care plan for the appointment so that the equipment could be prepared in advance of the appointment rather than during the appointment. Advance preparation not only increases efficiency but also minimizes the potential for cross-contamination following the completion of therapeutic scaling and root planing. If the dental hygienist decides during the appointment to irrigate subgingivally with an antimicrobial, the use of overgloves or the discarding of gloves and handwashing prior to the preparation of the armamentarium would be required. The amount of antimicrobial agent to be placed in the syringe or reservoir should be enough for only one procedure to avoid waste and to prevent contamination of the reservoir between clients. The transfer of antimicrobial agent from the source container to the disposable syringe, oral irrigator/ultrasonic unit reservoir, or handpiece reservoir requires care to avoid contamination of the source supply and the sterile needle or cannula.

3. Once the armamentarium is prepared and the dental hygienist is appropriately protected for the intraoral procedure, the cannula can be placed into the sulcus or pocket like a periodontal probe (approximately 3 mm), and the syringe plunger slowly pushed or the foot control (if using a handpiece, oral irrigator, or ultrasonic unit) activated for the slow, controlled-pressure delivery of the antimicrobial at a consistent rate and force.[30] The cannula is moved subgingivally around each tooth until all the designated areas have been thoroughly irrigated. The gentle stream of chemotherapeutic agent flushes away calculus, diseased root surface, and plaque fragments as well as provides target delivery of the agent for contact with the subgingival microorganisms.

4. After the subgingival irrigation is completed, any remaining antimicrobial should be discarded. The plastic disposable syringe, the cannula attached to the handpiece, or the oral irrigator must be disposed of in the sharps container. The reservoirs and handpieces should be flushed with water. The handpiece (air-driven ultrasonic unit insert or attachment for oral irrigator) should be prepared for sterilization. Barriers should be removed from the oral irrigator ultrasonic unit. The surfaces of the oral irrigator device or ultrasonic unit should be cleaned and disinfected if the barriers were compromised or at the end of the day if the surfaces were adequately protected.

Table 8–32 shows the placement of equipment within each use area for subgingival irrigation with antimicrobials.

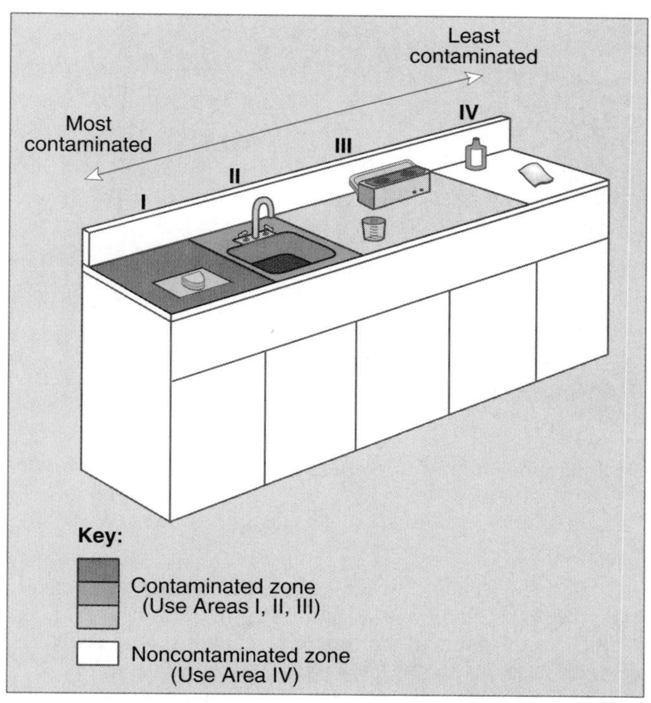

FIGURE 8–99
Laboratory zones for calculus and stain removal from removable dental appliances. I, II, and III indicate contaminated zones. I, receiving area for denture cup with disinfected prosthesis or appliance; II, sink for rinsing appliance; III, location of ultrasonic bath and plastic bag–lined beaker with lid. IV indicates noncontaminated zone. IV, dispensing (storage for solution and supplies)/transport.

Supplemental Dental Hygiene Care

Calculus and Extrinsic Stain Removal from Removable Dental Appliances (Operatory-Laboratory Interface) For the initial care and handling of dental prostheses or appliances, refer to the section on extraoral/intraoral assessment, step 3, earlier in this chapter.

1. The dental hygienist, wearing overgloves, should bring the denture cup with the bagged disinfected prosthesis or appliance to the laboratory (see Figure 8–99 for laboratory use areas and design flow from most to least contaminated use areas).

2. Prepare the equipment. While wearing overgloves, check the ultrasonic bath solution level (ideally, a separate laboratory ultrasonic device should be used exclusively for laboratory procedures and should not be used for cleaning or initial decontamination of instruments for recirculation; see Chapter 9).

TABLE 8–32
PLACEMENT OF EQUIPMENT WITHIN EACH USE AREA FOR SUBGINGIVAL IRRIGATION WITH ANTIMICROBIALS

I	II	III	IV
Mouth mirror Plastic disposable syringe*	Low-volume suction Air-driven subgingival irrigation handpiece*	Oral irrigation unit* Ultrasonic irrigation unit*	Client chart Antimicrobial agent (source container) Client hand mirror Radiographs Overgloves or additional gloves

*Options for antimicrobial delivery system.

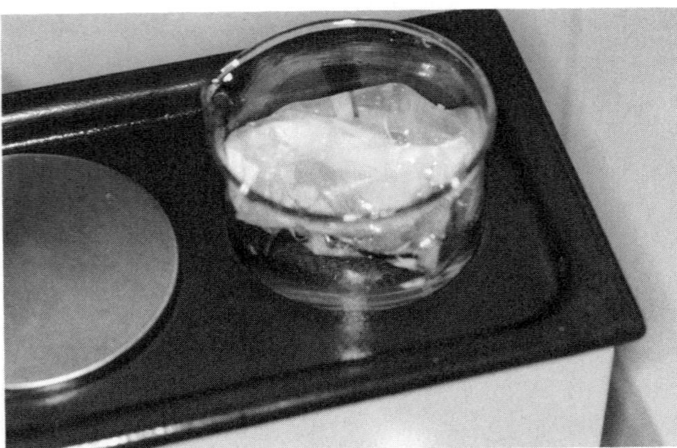

FIGURE 8-100
Small ultrasonic unit with beaker, sealed plastic bag, and prosthesis.

3. Position the ultrasonic cover, the disinfected beaker, and the lid. Place the plastic bag in the beaker (Fig. 8-100), and pour in commercial calculus and stain remover.

4. Open the bag, remove the overgloves, remove the appliance from the bag, discard the paper towel, rinse the appliance, and place it in the solution in a plastic bag-lined beaker.

5. Put on overgloves, seal the bag, set the timer on the ultrasonic cleaner, and follow the manufacturer's recommendation for the length of time in the ultrasonic solution (with heavy stain and calculus, it may take as long as 1 hour). Lids should always be on the bath or beaker whenever the ultrasonic device is in use in order to minimize aerosol generation in the laboratory.

6. The dental hygienist, wearing overgloves, should return to the laboratory after the specified time, remove the lid or lids, remove the bag from the beaker, and transport it back to the operatory.

7. In the operatory, remove overgloves, pour off the solution, rinse the appliance or prosthesis, and inspect and brush it. If calculus remains, minimize hand scaling for the removal of adherent calculus to avoid scratching denture teeth or any acrylic part of the denture.

8. After calculus and stain removal is completed, place the dental appliance in mouth rinse in a bag in the denture cup to ensure a pleasant taste and comfort for the client. Remove it from the mouth rinse, rinse with water, and hand it to the client for reinsertion.

9. If more than one dental team member is involved in procedures, such as calculus and stain removal, which include two areas (operatory and laboratory), the opportunities for cross-contamination are more numerous. Generally, the best protocol is to clean and disinfect objects (contaminated impressions or dental appliances) at every exit and entry point when transferring such items between the operatory and the laboratory. Laboratory contamination and concerns about how appliances may have been handled may be minimized with this procedure if the other dental team member involved brings the "Ziploc-type" bag containing the calculus and stain removal solution to the operatory for the dental hygienist to place the contaminated dental appliance directly into the solution. Either the same person assisting with this procedure could return the bagged and cleaned appliance to the operatory for steps 8 and 9 or the dental hygienist could retrieve the bag containing the appliance after the specified time has passed.

INFECTION CONTROL PROTOCOLS FOR THE EVALUATION PHASE OF THE DENTAL HYGIENE CARE PROCESS

The evaluation phase of the dental hygiene care process (see Chapter 25) involves a review of the initial goals established with the client to determine their level of attainment. The evaluation phase varies in its components, since the goals established for each client may be somewhat different. Infection control considerations during the evaluation phase of the dental hygiene care process therefore depend on the specific outcomes assessment procedures to be done for comparison with initial client data. Once the specific outcomes assessment procedures are identified, utilize the specific infection control protocol for that procedure, as presented earlier in this chapter.

Postappointment Protocol

It is imperative that the oral healthcare team reach a consensus for a prescribed infection control protocol for the prevention of disease transmission *after care* as well as *during client care.* The potential for disease transmission does not leave the operatory along with the client. Blood, saliva, exudate, and organic debris (bioburden) remain on the instruments used, and the surfaces touched or contaminated via spatter or aerosols during delivery of care. Postappointment decontamination presents a number of significant risks, including the required handling of sharps such as the disposal of contaminated local anesthetic needles and the initial preparation and transportation of contaminated *reusable sharps,* such as curets, sickles, and explorers (Fig. 8-101). Compliance with postappointment decontamination protocol is essential to ensure quality infection control.

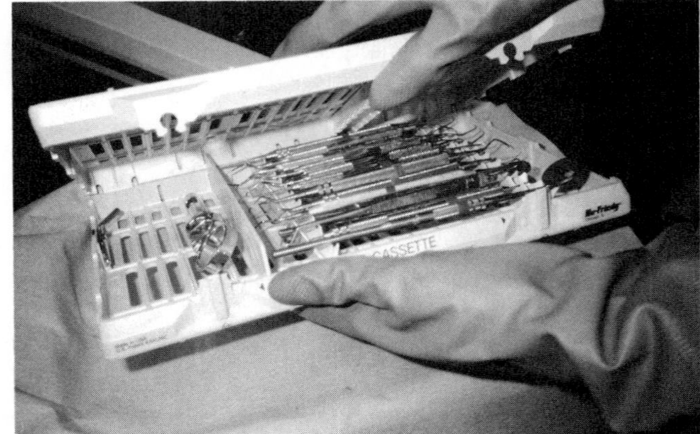

FIGURE 8-101
Closing instrument cassette with nitrile-gloved hands in preparation for transport to recirculation area.

OSHA POST–DENTAL HYGIENE APPOINTMENT HANDLING OF CONTAMINATED INSTRUMENTS (SHARPS)

Immediately or as soon as possible after use, contaminated *reusable sharps* (e.g., curets) shall be placed in an appropriate container until properly reprocessed. These containers shall be puncture-resistant; labeled or color-coded in accordance with this standard; leak-proof on the sides and bottom.

Reusable sharps that are contaminated with blood or other potentially infectious materials shall not be stored or processed in a manner that requires employees to reach by hand into containers where these sharps have been placed.

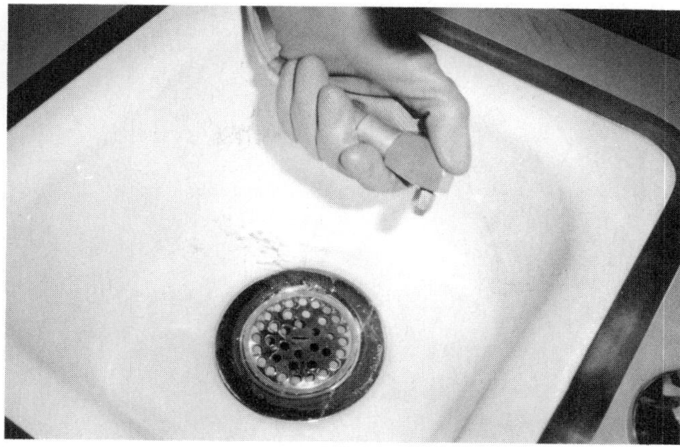

FIGURE 8–103
Water lines being flushed after appointment.

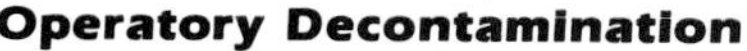

Operatory Decontamination

1. Prepare for the procedure by wearing protective eyewear, a mask, and puncture-resistant nitrile gloves.

2. If a local anesthetic agent was administered, it is necessary to dismantle the syringe according to the protocol for local anesthetic administration. After the recapped needle has been removed from the syringe, re-cover the syringe end of the needle by using a one-handed technique to scoop up the smaller cap prior to disposal. Immediately drop the covered needle into a sharps container (Fig. 8–102), which should be readily accessible within the dental hygiene operatory. Note that needles are *not* to be bent or broken or cut before disposal.[6,7,48] The used glass cartridge is considered infectious, since some body fluids are drawn up into the cartridge when aspiration occurs during local anesthetic administration. The potential for glass breakage in combination with body fluid contamination warrants the cartridge being considered potentially a sharp, and it should be disposed of accordingly.[10]

3. Flush all water lines (e.g., ASW syringes, handpiece water line used with the sonic scaling device, or ultrasonic scaling equipment water line) for 20 seconds as recommended for between client procedures (Fig. 8–103). (A note of caution: when flushing the water line associated with high-speed handpiece use, the handpiece should be disconnected from the hose during flushing; free running water could damage the bearings of the high-speed handpiece.)[2]

4. Remove all disposable surface barriers. Care should be used to avoid touching the clean uncovered surfaces underneath the used disposable surface barrier during removal.[49]

5. Discard blood-soaked gauze immediately during the course of client care in the conveniently placed biohazardous(medical)-waste bag (Fig. 8–104). If contaminated gauze was not previously discarded and remains on the tray/cas-

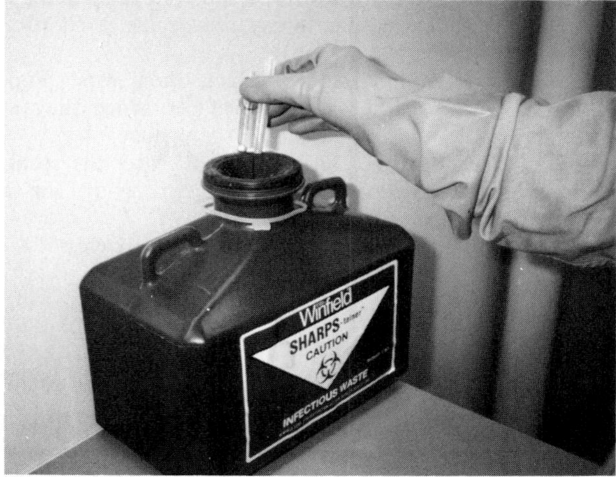

FIGURE 8–102
Nitrile-gloved hand disposing of needle and cartridge in sharps container.

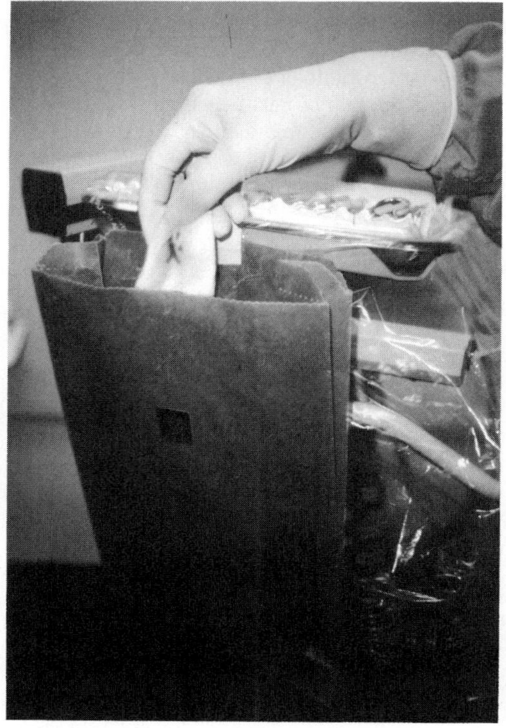

FIGURE 8–104
Disposal of blood-soaked gauze in biohazardous-waste bag.

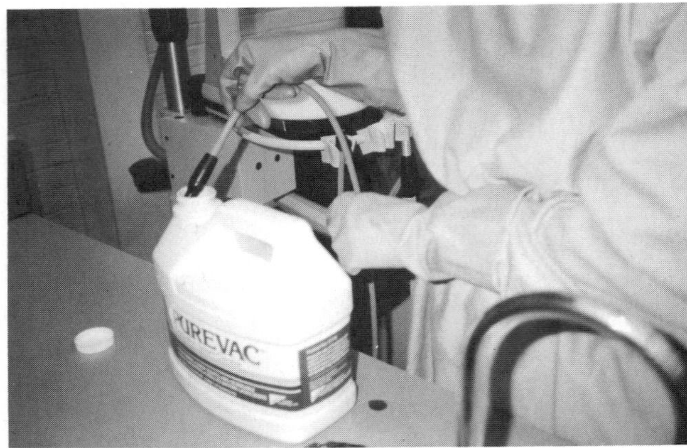

FIGURE 8–105
Cleaning and disinfection of high- and low-volume suction tubing.

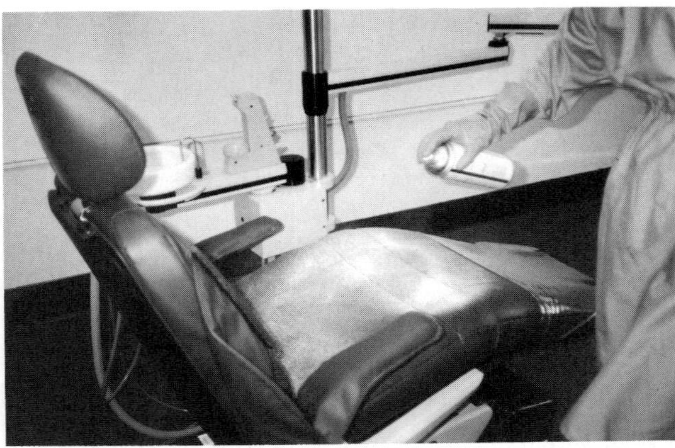

FIGURE 8–107
Spray-wipe-spray technique for surface disinfection.

sette at the end of the appointment, the gauze should be placed in the biohazardous-waste bag as part of the decontamination process.

6. Close the instrument cassette for immediate transport and recirculation (cleaning, packaging, sterilization, cooling or drying, storage, and distribution). If instrument recirculation/processing is not commenced immediately, instruments need to be placed in a presoak solution until time is available for processing instruments.

7. Discard disposable, single-use items, such as low-volume suction tip, high-volume suction tip, and, if applicable, disposable ASW tip, along with the disposable surface barriers with the other contaminated waste (medical solid waste), which by definition is not considered biohazardous or infectious waste[50] (refer to the section on waste handling in this chapter, and to the section on hazardous waste management in Chapter 9). Infectious waste includes the following materials: blood, contaminated sharps, and pathological and microbiological wastes, which have been shown through epidemiological evidence to be capable of transmitting a communicable disease.[46]

8. The suction tubing (interior) should be cleaned between clients by flushing with water and disinfected at the end of the working day with a commercial cleansing solution (Fig. 8–105). The exterior hose ends and flow control assemblies should be rinsed, cleaned and scrubbed, and disinfected.[2]

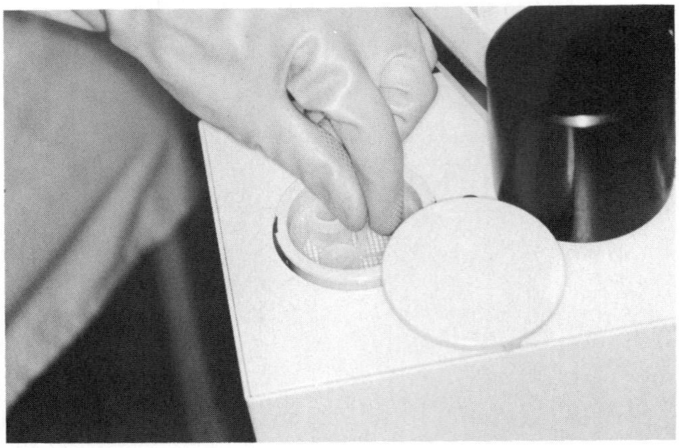

FIGURE 8–106
Disposable sediment trap for the suction-generating system.

9. The sediment trap for the suction-generating system should be cleaned daily, disassembled, and flushed with copious amounts of water[35] (disposable traps may offer convenience in managing the trap-cleaning maintenance procedure) (Fig. 8–106).

10. The extent of environmental surface decontamination depends on the use of surface barriers and their ability to provide complete surface protection. When surface barriers provide thorough surface protection and are carefully discarded and changed between clients, cleaning and disinfection may be required only at the end of the day. The spray-wipe-spray technique (Fig. 8–107) for surface cleaning and disinfection for unprotected surfaces and as an end-of-the-day procedure for all the affected environmental surfaces in the operatory is as follows:

- Select a product and prepare if necessary, preferably an aqueous disinfectant with detergent for both cleaning and disinfection (see section on environmental surface disinfection).
- Deliver product. A spray delivery works well for penetration of crevices (however, avoid direct spraying of electrical switches, since spray may cause a short-circuit of the electrical system).
- Clean surfaces first with product, then wipe. Paper towels work well for wiping surfaces, since they are larger, faster, and less expensive than gauze.
- Spray a second time for disinfection. After the second spray application, permit the surface to air-dry for the prescribed time.
- After the specified time, wipe away any excess disinfectant with a clean paper towel.

References

1. Whitacre, R. J., Robins, S. K., et al. Dental Asepsis. Seattle: Stoma Press, 1979.
2. Cottone, J. A., Terezhalmy, G. T., and Molinari, J. A. Practical Infection Control in Dentistry. Philadelphia: Lea & Febiger, 1991.
3. Pollack, R. Form follows function. California Dental Association Journal 17(2):17, 1989.
4. Cottone, J. A., Hars, E., et al. Recommended clinical guide-

lines for infection control in dental education institutions. Journal of Dental Education 55(9):621, 1991.
5. Department of Veterans Affairs, American Dental Association, Department of Health and Human Services. Infection control in the dental environment. Washington, DC: Learning Resources Service and Eastern Dental Education Center, VA Medical Center, 1989.
6. American Dental Association Council on Dental Materials, Instruments and Equipments; on Dental Practice; and on Dental Therapeutics. Infection control recommendations for the dental office and the dental laboratory. Journal of the American Dental Association 116:241, 1988.
7. Centers for Disease Control. Recommendations for prevention of HIV transmission in health care settings. Morbidity and Mortality Weekly Report 36:2-S, August 21, 1987.
8. Office Sterilization and Asepsis Procedures Research Foundation. Position paper 7-003: Surface disinfection—antimicrobial chemicals for cleaning and disinfecting environmental surfaces and equipment in the dental operatory. Denver: Office Sterilization and Asepsis Procedures Research Foundation, 1988.
9. Cottone, J. A. Recent developments in hepatitis: New virus, vaccine, and dosage recommendations. Journal of the American Dental Association 120:501, 1990.
10. Cottone, J. A., and Molinari, J. A. State of the art infection control in dentistry. Journal of the American Dental Association 122:33, 1991.
11. Molinari, J. A., Gleason, M. J., et al. Comparison of dental surface disinfectants. General Dentistry 35:171, 1987.
12. Molinari, J. A., Gleason, M. J., et al. Cleaning and disinfectant properties of dental surface disinfectants. Journal of the American Dental Association 117:179, 1988.
13. Worrall, S. F., Knibbs, P. J., and Glenwright, H. D. Methods of reducing bacterial contamination of the atmosphere arising from the use of an air polisher. British Dental Journal 163:118, 1987.
14. Centers for Disease Control. Update: Universal precautions for prevention of transmission of human immunodeficiency virus, hepatitis B virus, and other bloodborne pathogens in health care settings. Morbidity and Mortality Weekly Report 37(24):377, June 1988.
15. Wilkins, E. M. Clinical Practice of the Dental Hygienist, 6th ed. Philadelphia: Lea & Febiger, 1991.
16. Brabrandt, B. A. Radiation asepsis. Dental Teamwork 3(1):16, 1990.
17. Miller, C. H., and Palenik, C. J. Infection Control and Management of Hazardous Materials for the Dental Team. St. Louis: C. V. Mosby, 1994, p. 205.
18. Mason-Hing, L. R. Fundamentals of Dental Radiography, 3rd ed. Philadelphia: Lea & Febiger, 1990.
19. Jeffries, D., Morris, J. W., and White, V. P. kVp meter errors induced by plastic wrap. Journal of Dental Hygiene 65:91–93, February 1991.
20. Spaulding, E. H. Chemical disinfection of medical and surgical materials. In Lawrence, A. S., and Block, S. S. (eds.). Disinfection, Preservation and Sterilization. Philadelphia: Lea & Febiger, 1968, pp. 517–531.
21. Tham, M. Personal communication, December 6, 1991.
22. Merchant, V. A. Update on disinfection of impressions, prostheses, and casts. California Dental Association Journal 20:31–35, October 1992.
23. American Dental Association. Handle with care: A hazards communication program for dentistry. ADA News, April 25, 1, 3, 1988.
24. Walsh, M., and Robertson, P. Professional mechanical oral hygiene practices in the prevention and control of periodontal diseases. California Dental Association Journal 13:58–62, December 1985.
25. Centers for Disease Control. Recommendations for preventing transmission of human immunodeficiency virus and hepatitis B virus to patients during exposure-prone invasive procedures. Morbidity and Mortality Weekly Report 40:RR-8, 1991.
26. Current status of handpiece sterilization. Control: The Infectious Disease Newsletter 6(10):1–2, 8, October 1991.
27. Department of Health and Human Services (Public Health Service, Food and Drug Administration). Dental Handpiece Sterilization. Letter, Benson, J. S., Rockville, MD, September 28, 1992.
28. Fleming, L. S., Barnes, C. M., and Russell, C. M. An in vivo comparison of commercially available disposable prophylaxis angles. Dental Hygiene 65(9):441, 1991.
29. Barnes, C. M. The management of aerosols with airpolishing delivery systems. Journal of Dental Hygiene 65:280–282, July–August 1991.
30. Woodall, I. R., Dafoe, B. R., et al. Comprehensive Dental Hygiene Care, 4th ed. St. Louis: C. V. Mosby, 1993.
31. Brinkman, H. Personal communication. Dentsply/Quality Assurance, Long Island City, NY, January 1992.
32. Logothetis, D. D., Gorss, K. B. W., and Eberhart, A. Bacterial airborne contamination with an air-polishing device. General Dentistry 36:496, 1988.
33. White, S. L., and Hoffman, L. A. A practice survey of hygienists using an air-powder abrasive system. Dental Hygiene 65(9):433, 1991.
34. DeVore Rubenstein, L., and Dean, M. Strategies for oral health promotion, disease prevention and control. In Darby, M. L. (ed.). Mosby's Comprehensive Review of Dental Hygiene, 3rd ed. St. Louis: C. V. Mosby, 1994.
35. Young, J. M. Dental equipment asepsis. Dental Clinics of North America 35(2):391, 1991.
36. Forrest, W. R., and Perez, R. S. AIDS and hepatitis prevention: The role of the rubber dam. Operative Dentistry 11:1591, 1986.
37. Cochran, M. A., Miller, C., and Sheldrade, M. The efficacy of the rubber dam as a barrier to the spread of microorganisms during dental treatment. Journal of the American Dental Association 119:141, 1989.
38. Harfst, S. A. Personal barrier protection. Dental Clinics of North America 35(2):3517, 1991.
39. Weed-Fonner, L. Amalgam restoration removing overhangs. RDH 1:32–35, Sept./Oct. 1981.
40. Armitage, G. C. Biological basis of periodontal disease maintenance. Berkeley, CA: Praxis, 1980.
41. Abel, L. C., Miller, R. L., et al. Studies on dental aerobiology. IV, Bacterial contamination of water delivered by dental units. Journal of Dental Research 50:1567, 1971.
42. Gross, A., Devine, J., and Cutright, D. E. Microbial contamination of dental units and ultrasonic scalers. Journal of Periodontology 47:670, 1976.
43. Malamed, S. F. Handbook of Local Anesthesia. St. Louis: C. V. Mosby, 1990.
44. American Dental Association Council on Dental Materials, Instruments and Equipment; on Dental Practice; and on Dental Therapeutics: Infection control recommendations for the dental office and dental laboratory. Journal of the American Dental Association 116:241, 1988.
45. Jakush, J. Infection control procedures and products: Cautions and common sense. Journal of the American Dental Association 117:293, 1988.
46. Miller, C. H. Reduce chance of exposure. RDH 11:4, 32, 1991.
47. Reynolds, M., Lavigne, C., et al. Clinical effects of simultaneous ultrasonic scaling and subgingival irrigation with chlorhexidine. Journal of Clinical Periodontology 19:595, 1992.
48. Department of Labor, Occupational Safety and Health Administration. Occupational exposure to bloodborne pathogens: Final rule. Federal Register 56(235):64004, 1991.
49. Whitacre, R. J. Environmental barriers in dental office infection control. Dental Clinics of North America 35(2):367, 1991.
50. Shaefer, M. E. Hazardous waste management. Dental Clinics of North America 35(2):383, 1991.

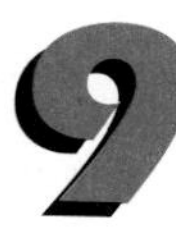

Instrument Recirculation: Containment, Decontamination, Packaging, Renewal (Sterilization), Maintenance, and Dispensing

OBJECTIVES

Mastery of the content in this chapter will enable the reader to:

- Define the terms used
- Discuss the use of universal precautions during instrument processing
- Describe the fundamental principles of prevention of disease transmission as they relate to the design, organization, equipment, materials management, and waste disposal in the instrument recirculation area
- List the protective barriers essential for personal protection when processing contaminated instruments
- Discuss the purposes of instrument holding-solutions (containment) and describe the advantages and disadvantages of various detergents and disinfectants used for this purpose
- Describe the cleaning procedures (decontamination) used in preparation of contaminated instruments as a critical component of the instrument sterilization process
- Describe the methods and materials available for packaging instruments, their appropriateness for various methods of sterilization, and their associated advantages and disadvantages
- Describe the sterilization methods that are rated as acceptable by the appropriate agencies
- Discuss the rationale for heat sterilization of all dental hygiene instruments that are heat stable
- Compare methods of sterilization (instrument renewal), conditions required, mechanisms of microbial destruction, safety precautions, advantages and disadvantages, and indications for use
- Describe liquid chemical germicides registered with the Environmental Protection Agency (EPA) as disinfectants/sterilants, mechanisms of microbial action, conditions required, indications for use, advantages and disadvantages, and safety precautions
- Differentiate between liquid chemical agents approved for instrument immersion and those for environmental surface disinfection
- Evaluate which method of sterilization/disinfection is appropriate for dental hygiene clinical armamentarium, including handpieces
- Describe the procedure to monitor the use and effective functioning of steam, chemical vapor, dry heat, and ethylene oxide gas sterilizers using biological indicators and chemical monitors
- Describe the methods for maintaining sterility (maintenance) of processed instruments prior to recirculation back into dental hygiene care use
- Differentiate among infectious, contaminated, medical, hazardous, and toxic waste
- Describe the appropriate containers for the disposal of sharps and infectious solid wastes along with the regulations regarding waste management

INTRODUCTION

Meeting the client's human need for safety is a professional responsibility of the dental hygienist in the realm of prevention of disease transmission. This responsibility requires that recirculation of instruments used during the delivery of dental hygiene care provide client protection from the spread of infectious disease agents and prevent occupational exposure of the oral healthcare team. The instrument recirculation center must include areas for specific functions arranged in a sequential pattern to facilitate efficient movement of contaminated instruments through the sterilization process with maintenance of sterility until reuse. The design and organization of the instrument recirculation area should promote an efficient yet carefully controlled flow of instruments and include the following:

- A receiving area that promotes *containment* of contaminated instruments by presoaking in an instrument holding solution, and careful handling of biomedical waste
- A *decontamination area* that uses ultrasonic cleaning to remove the bioburden to ensure that the sterilization agent is able to gain access to contaminated instruments
- An area for *instrument packaging* to protect the instruments from recontamination after sterilization until reuse

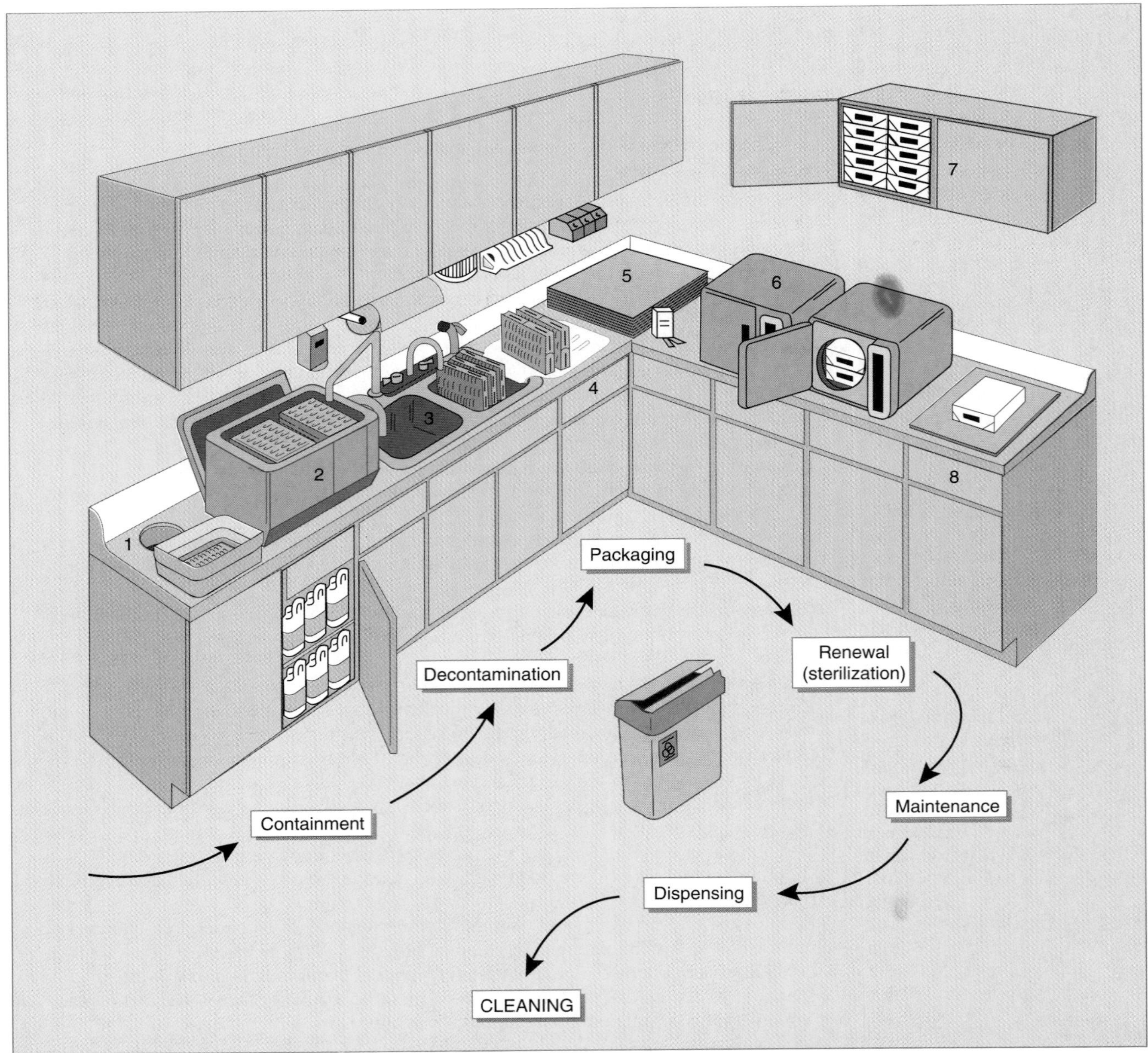

FIGURE 9–1
Overview of floor plan with centralized recirculation area. (Courtesy of Hu-Friedy.)

- A *renewal area,* where the sterilization of all dental hygiene instruments occurs
- *Maintenance* and *dispensing areas*

DESIGN AND ORGANIZATION OF THE INSTRUMENT RECIRCULATION AREA

The instrument recirculation center is also referred to as the central sterilization area or instrument decontamination area. It is the treatment support area within the clinical environment where contaminated instruments are contained and where instrument decontamination, packaging, sterilization, storage and dispensing for reuse occurs (Fig. 9–1). In this and other treatment *support areas,* such as the dental laboratory and the radiograph processing area, *indirect client contact* occurs through direct contact with contaminated instruments or objects.[1] Design and organization of the instrument recirculation area should be carefully considered to facilitate efficiency, to minimize occupational exposure, and to prevent cross-contamination. The philosophy of a universal approach to infection control applies to all contaminated instruments (see Chapter 7).[2] Currently all instruments must be considered contaminated with hepatitis B virus (HBV) and/or other bloodborne pathogens, because of the number of undiagnosed HBV clients and the associated unreliability of the health history.[3] Therefore, contaminated instruments and biohazardous waste are to be handled according to one universal standard protocol. Rigorous adherence to a protocol developed for the handling of instruments and waste after dental hygiene care minimizes the risk of exposure to blood and body fluids of all clients.

While client treatment areas may be sites of the highest level of microbial-laden spatter, the instrument recirculation area is the repository for the instruments and waste contaminated as a result of direct contact with blood and other body fluids. This treatment support area should be limited to use for instrument recirculation and, ideally, should be separate from the laboratory and other treatment support areas. The recirculation area should be centrally located to all the treatment rooms to minimize the distance of transport of contaminated items. In addition, it should have two separate sections of cabinetry, parallel to each other or in an L-shaped design to enhance the flow of the processing procedures.[4] Table 9–1 describes the important design features recommended for the instrument recirculation area.

The recirculation room should be large enough to have clearly defined function areas. Separate function areas facilitate a designated flow, or path, for the instruments. The presence of both contaminated and sterilized instruments in the recirculation center requires organization of the area to consider a flow of instrument processing that goes from areas that deal with contaminated instruments to areas that deal with sterilized instruments. The section of the pathway before sterilization is designated as the contaminated zone of the recirculation center, and the pathway following instrument sterilization of the noncontaminated zone (Fig. 9–2). Clearly identifying the zones of contamination and noncontamination and developing a step-by-step protocol for instrument processing affect exposure control, efficiency, productivity, and quality assurance. The function areas (see Fig. 9–2) located within the contaminated zone are the *containment* or *receiving area* for contaminated instruments, the *decontamination* or *cleaning area,* and the *packaging area* for preparation of instruments prior to renewal. The boundary between the contaminated and the noncontaminated zones is located at the point of processing for sterilization. The noncontaminated zone includes the function areas (see Fig. 9–2) of *renewal* (after sterilization), *maintenance* or storage of instruments until they are needed for use, and in some cases a *dispensing area* for tray preparation and distribution.[1] Because many oral healthcare environments have less than ideal space allocation for the instrument recirculation area, smaller instrument recirculation areas may be encountered. Yet even with space constraints, the dental hygienist may be able to greatly affect the quality of the instrument processing by arranging the instrument recirculation center according to the six functional areas presented in detail.

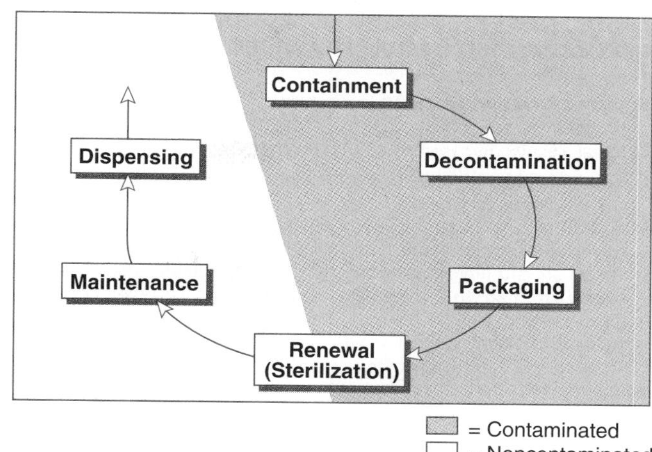

FIGURE 9–2
Recirculation area.

Containment Area

Instrument Transport from the Treatment Area to the Recirculation Center

When the dental hygiene care appointment has concluded, a protocol for postappointment decontamination procedures must be followed. For both postappointment and recirculation infection control protocols the operator must wear all personal barriers as well as heavy-duty (puncture-resistant) nitrile gloves (Fig. 9–3). Heavy-duty gloves are especially important during the implementation of the postappointment and recirculation protocols because of increased risk of a puncture wound with the handling of multiple contaminated instruments. Latex or vinyl examination gloves are inappropriate for instrument processing procedures. The transfer of contaminated instruments and waste must be carefully considered to prevent cross-contamination and potential exposure incidents. Unless the instrument recirculation processing is begun immediately, the contaminated instruments should be put into a **holding solution** container for presoaking to prevent drying of bioburden on instruments, to initiate dissolving of organic debris, and, depending on the agent used, to begin the microbial kill[5] (Fig. 9–4). The interface between the treatment area and containment protocols is the transfer juncture where instruments in a holding solution are transported from the treatment area to the receiving area of the recirculation center for processing. The contaminated utility gloves worn

TABLE 9–1
RECOMMENDED DESIGN FEATURES FOR INSTRUMENT RECIRCULATION AREA

Equipment Design Elements	Objectives
General Recirculation Area	
Cabinetry with two separate parallel sections or L-shaped counter (16–21 linear feet total)	To facilitate a linear flow of instrument processing and designation of defined function areas
Countertop surfaces should be constructed of smooth, nonporous materials of either resin, laminates, processed resin or metal	To create surfaces that are compatible with disinfectants/sterilants and detergents
Cabinets should have melamine interiors, removable shelves, plastic laminate to top and face surfaces and clear glass cabinet doors	To increase ease in surface cleaning and disinfection as well as increased accessibility and visibility
Vinyl wall coverings (sheet vinyl)	To provide ease in care with little or no discoloration from environmental surface disinfection
Seamless vinyl floor covering	To promote ease in maintenance, facilitate confinement and spill clean-up, and provide total wet mopping
Containment Area	
Wall-mounted shelves	To accommodate volume of in-coming trays and cassettes
Sharps container located in containment area	To minimize handling and transport of sharps Disposal into sharps container should occur in operatory (area of use), with supplemental sharps container in recirculation area for overlooked sharps arriving with contaminated trays/ cassettes.
Rectangular countertop trash receptacles, chutes	To deposit disposable items directly from trays without handling
Trash compactor	To minimize bulk of trash and number of times transporting waste to storage, reducing risk of exposure
Decontamination Area	
Large 32-inch-wide stainless steel sink, placed strategically 3–4 feet from counter end	To locate strategically between containment cleaning areas and packaging as well as large enough to accommodate baskets, cassettes, and trays
Foot-controlled, knee-activated or electric-eye faucet activated water flow	To eliminate potential for cross-contamination
Spray attachment for faucet	To accelerate rinsing of instrument baskets and cassettes
Knee-, foot-, or forearm-controlled soap dispensers	To avoid contamination of dispenser and/or hands or heavy-duty nitrile gloves before and after instrument cleaning
Towel dispensers that permit the towel to hang down from the dispenser	To prevent contamination of the dispenser by providing direct access to towel
Large ultrasonic cleaning unit (12 × 13 × 10 inches), recessed in countertop adjacent to sink; reduces noise factor, clutter, and draining of unit	To accommodate size of cassettes and/or volume of instruments for recirculation
Packaging Area	
Sloping sink drains, drainboard	To permit ease in draining cleaned and rinsed cassettes and instruments
Counter space with adjacent shelving	To provide space for packaging instruments for renewal and storage for packaging supplies (wraps, bags, indicator tape, gauze, cotton swabs, and cotton rolls)
Ventilation system	To control the noxious vapors from sterilization procedures and various chemicals
Adjacent counter space area designating pathway flow into noncontaminated zone	To provide space for temporary placement of heat-sterilized instruments (bags/cassettes) for cooling prior to storage
A drawer underneath the sterilizer with ventilation	To accommodate immediate transfer of hot instruments to a "cool-down" drawer as an alternative to using counter space for instrument cooling, where a backlog of instruments may slow down the recirculation process
Maintenance Area (Storage Area)	
Shelving with glass doors	To protect processed instrument bags and cassette wraps from exposure to environmental contaminants (glass doors are preferred to provide ease in instrument inventory and location)
Dispensing Area	
Counter space with adjacent shelving and cabinets/shelves ("slide-out" shelves improve access with base cabinetry storage)	To create an area for preparing customized tray set-ups with access to additional unit-dose supplies, adjunct materials, disposables, restorative materials, and sealants

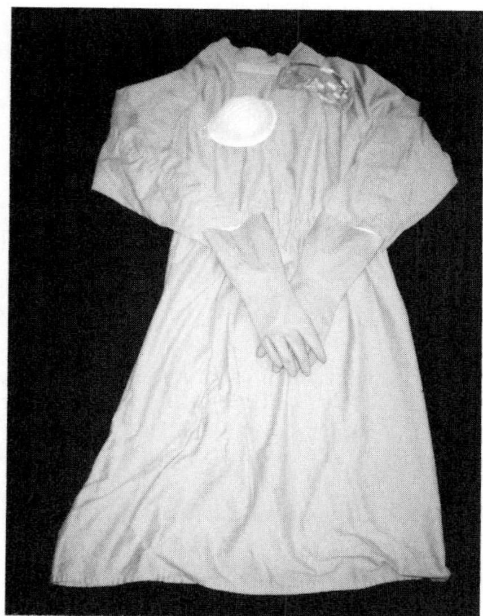

FIGURE 9-3
Protective barriers. Eyewear, clothing, mask, and nitrile gloves.

to decontaminate also are worn to place instruments into the holding solution and to place instruments in the receiving area within the recirculation contaminated zone. During instrument transport, great care must be taken to remember that the nitrile gloves are contaminated. Such gloved hands should be kept above the waist and in front of the body; nothing should be handled or touched. If a surface is contacted, surface disinfection of the newly contaminated areas is necessary.[6]

Instrument Receiving Area

The trays or cassettes of client-contaminated instruments and materials arrive in the receiving area of the recirculation center and are immediately processed, or if a delay is anticipated, the instruments should be placed in a presoaking container (see Instrument Presoaking Protocol [Containment]) (Figs. 9-5 to 9-7). The amount of space adequate for the receiving area depends on the number of oral healthcare providers and their productivity. The number of incoming trays and presoaking containers may require shelves for temporary storage of trays and containers in order to handle the flow.

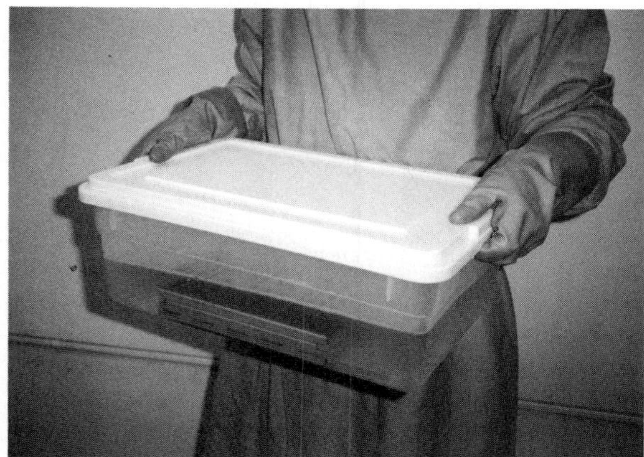

FIGURE 9-4
Holding solution container. Gloved hands holding transportation holding solution.

INSTRUMENT PRESOAKING PROTOCOL (CONTAINMENT)

- Presoaking of instruments is required when processing is not begun immediately after instrument use.
- Wear personal protective attire: heavy-duty nitrile gloves, protective eyewear, mask, and protective clothing.
- Place instruments (reusable sharps) in a container that is puncture-resistant, leak-proof on the sides and bottom, and labeled or color-coded to meet the Occupational Safety and Health Administration (OSHA) standard.[8]
- The solutions used may be plain detergents or detergents containing disinfectants (phenolic compounds) for the benefit of an initial microbial kill and reduction of contamination risks.
- Fill container with enough solution to cover the cassette or to a level above the instruments in the ultrasonic basket.
- If an instrument cassette system is not used, an ultrasonic basket may provide an alternative vehicle for containment of instruments for presoak immersion to reduce the direct handling of contaminated instruments.
- The instrument cassette or ultrasonic basket may be used to retain instruments through the presoaking, ultrasonic cleaning, rinsing, up to and/or through the sterilization process.
- Extended presoaking (2 hours or more) should be avoided to prevent corrosion of some instruments.
- Careful and protected handling is critical even when a disinfectant has been used during the presoaking procedure, since the instruments and the used solution must still be considered contaminated.
- Decant the presoaking liquid into the sink (used solution should be discarded at least once a day), rinse cassette or basket, and proceed with the terminal cleaning step by placing the cassette or basket into the ultrasonic cleaner.
- OSHA cautions against contaminated instruments (reusable sharps) being stored or processed in such a manner that requires the employee to reach by hand into containers where contaminated reusable sharps have been placed.[8]
- The container used for presoaking should be rinsed, cleaned, and disinfected for reuse with the "spray-wipe-spray" technique used for environmental surface disinfection prior to reuse.
- If another member of the team takes responsibility for processing from this point on, the dental hygienist should wash/clean the heavy-duty utility gloves thoroughly, dry/wipe and spray with a disinfectant, and hang up to dry (nitrile gloves may be sterilized by a moist heat method). Wash hands thoroughly with an antimicrobial soap.

Data from Miller,[5] Shaefer,[15] OSAP Report,[29] Cottone et al.[1]

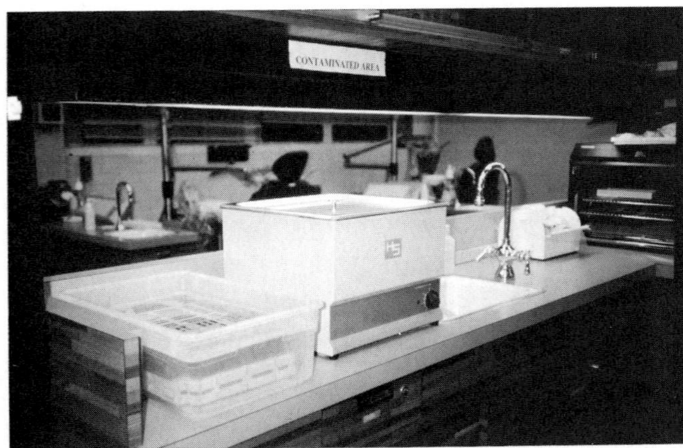

FIGURE 9–5
Receiving area.

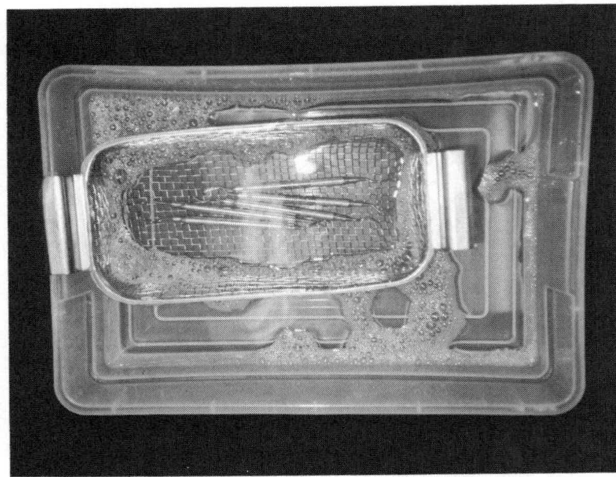

FIGURE 9–7
Basket immersed in holding presoak solution.

Waste Handling

The majority of disposable items such as gloves, surface barriers, masks, and suction tips fall into a broad category of nonbiohazardous **medical** solid **contaminated waste** (Fig. 9–8). Although this waste has been contaminated by contact with blood and saliva, it is not considered **infectious (biohazardous) waste,** since there is no epidemiological evidence that contact with it will result in disease transmission.[1,7] Such disposable items are directed into the appropriate container for the disposal of contaminated waste as required by the local ordinances (see post–dental hygiene appointment waste handling protocol, Chapter 8).

Blood-soaked gauze and body tissues, including extracted teeth and other items, however, are considered to be infectious waste and must be handled according to the guidelines for regulated waste and placed in plastic "biohazard" labeled or color-coded bags for disposal (Fig. 9–9).[1,8,10,11] The small impervious bags used in the treatment area must be transported to the containment area for placement into a larger approved biohazardous waste container (bag or box). A larger biohazardous waste container should be located in the receiving area or containment section within the contaminated zone of the recirculation center for ease in collection of the blood-soaked gauze and other infectious waste (see Classification System for Waste chart) (Fig. 9–10). Sharps, although also considered to be infectious, are handled separately, with disposal into containers made specifically for sharps (Fig. 9–11). Needles and other sharps (e.g., broken curets, burs, anesthetic cartridges, disposable syringes) should be disposed of routinely into a sharps container in the treatment area as close as possible to the point

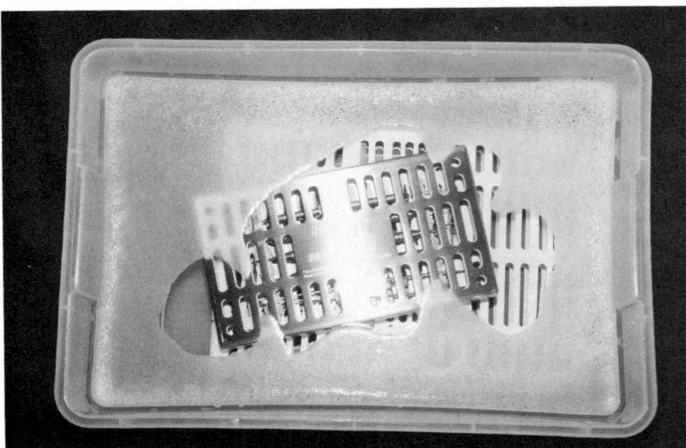

FIGURE 9–6
Container with holding solution covering immersed cassettes.

CLASSIFICATION SYSTEM FOR WASTE

Medical Waste
"Any solid waste which is generated in the diagnosis, treatment or immunization of human beings or animals, in research pertaining thereto, or in the production or testing of biologicals." *

Infectious Waste
Waste that contains a concentration of virulent pathogens sufficient to be considered capable of causing an infectious disease when a susceptible host is exposed to the waste.†

Contaminated Waste
Broadly defined as items having contact with blood and other body fluids; even though all infectious waste is contaminated waste, not all contaminated waste is considered to be infectious (capable of causing an infectious disease). The critical differences in infectivity are the presence of a sufficient quantity of disease-causing organisms harbored in the waste in addition to the provision of a vector (carrier) for the infectious agent to infect a susceptible host.†

Hazardous Waste
Waste posing a risk or peril to humans or the environment.†

Toxic Waste
Waste capable of having a poisonous effect (e.g., the surfacing of chemical wastes in the Love Canal area of New York).†

*EPA, Standards for the tracking and management of medical waste. Federal Register 54:12326–12395, 1989.
†Reis-Schmidt, T. Waste handling and processing standards developing for dentistry: agencies, associations, and legislators respond to waste management issues. Dental Products Report, 46–63, May 1989.

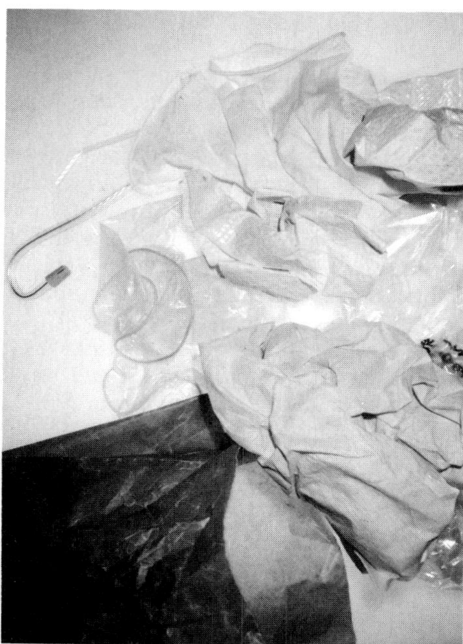

FIGURE 9–8
Disposables: Nonbiohazardous medical waste—gloves, surface barriers, masks, and tips (suction).

of use (Fig. 9–12). An additional sharps container should be located in the receiving area in the event that a needle or other sharp was not disposed of at the point of use in the operatory, or a contaminated reusable sharp breaks in the recirculation area (see Classification System for Waste chart).

Three **classes** of ***regulated waste*** (infectious) in the oral healthcare environment are:[9]

- Blood and blood-soaked items

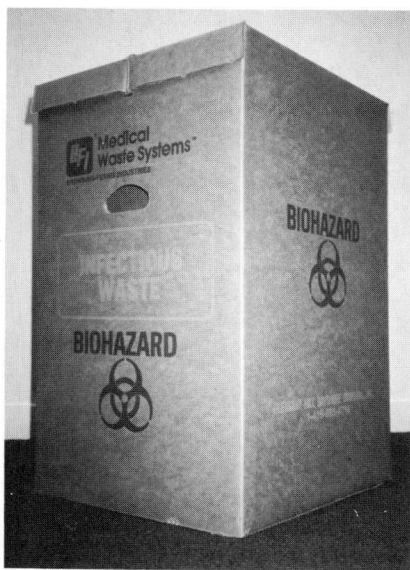

FIGURE 9–9
Small biohazard waste bag.

FIGURE 9–10
Large biohazard waste box.

- Sharps (e.g., needles, disposable syringes, glass cartridges, burs)
- Tissues and extracted teeth

Waste Handling Protocol (Containment)

1. Personal protective barriers should be worn routinely when the dental hygienist is in the instrument recirculation center. Puncture-resistant nitrile gloves are required for the handling of contaminated instruments and disposable sharps. Great care must be used when handling these items, which have the potential for puncturing through even the heavy-duty gloves recommended.

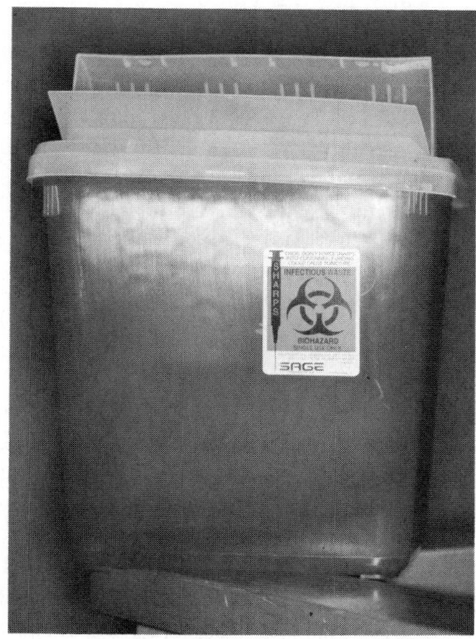

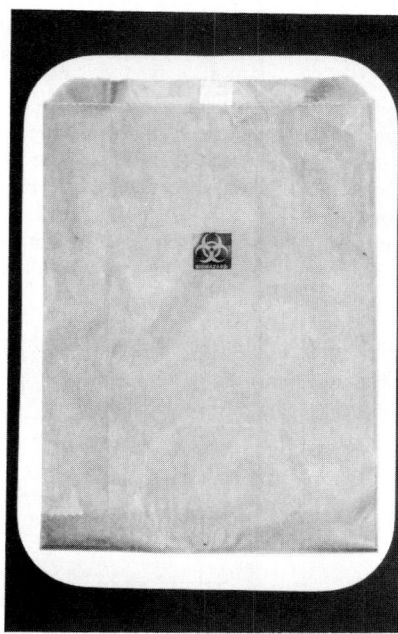

FIGURE 9–11
Sharps container.

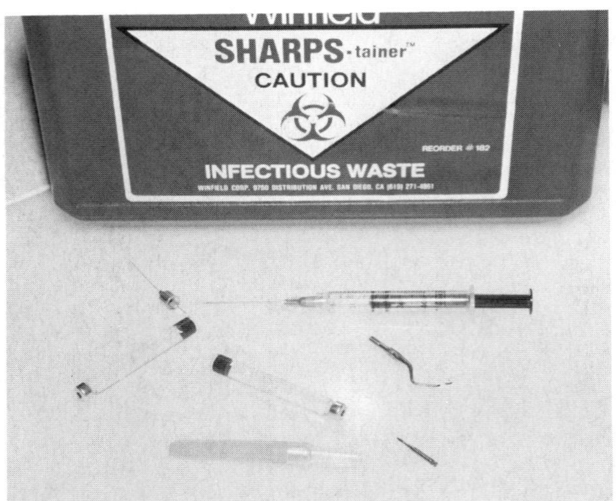

FIGURE 9–12
Assorted sharps: needles, broken curets, burs, cartridges, and disposal syringes.

2. Segregation of waste should be done according to category of waste:

- Sharps
- Saliva- and blood-soaked items (gauze), tissue, extracted teeth
- Other nonsoaked contaminated disposable waste

The concept of "universal precautions" applies to waste materials as well as to clinical infection control procedures. Therefore, the wastes generated during the dental hygiene care of all clients should be handled in a universal manner, according to each specific waste category. Waste generated from a known infectious client should not be accorded any variation in waste handling precautions.[11]

3. Saliva- and blood-soaked items: Small sealed "biohazard" waste bags containing saliva- and blood-soaked gauze should be combined with the other small waste bags in the large, clearly marked (biohazard symbol or red bag) collection container.

4. Nonsoaked contaminated waste: Any other contaminated waste such as client disposable surface barriers, gloves, cotton rolls, *unless* they are soaked with blood and saliva, are not considered biohazardous (infectious) waste. However, some state regulations and proposals include client disposables as regulated waste (e.g., Maryland and Pennsylvania).[11] Check your state and local regulations regarding waste disposal for confirmation (sources: regional EPA, Department of Health, state and local dental societies). The majority of states do not regulate this type of waste, since it is considered to be medical solid waste that may be disposed of along with the rest of the common waste. Generally, such waste is handled carefully and placed in impervious, sealed bags for disposal.

5. Storage: The large biohazard collection receptacle (bag or box) and sharps containers must be safely stored to maintain integrity of containment, prevent odor, and prevent access by unauthorized persons.[11] Check with the regional EPA and state and local waste management authorities to determine whether there is a regulation regarding the length of time that biohazardous waste may be stored at a clinical site. For example, Pennsylvania has storage limit regulations of 3 days for waste if it is stored at room temperature, 5 days if it is refrigerated, and 30 days if it is frozen.[11]

6. Disposal: Requirements for disposal of the three classes (blood and blood-soaked items, sharps, and tissues and extracted teeth) of regulated waste vary greatly according to state and local regulations.[11] The weight of the waste generated determines the classification of "small" versus "large" waste generator. The extent of waste disposal documentation (e.g., waste type, company responsible, licensing, destination) required increases when the provider exceeds the limits for a small generator. The definition of a small waste generator varies geographically as well. San Diego, California, for example, sets the limit at 100 kilograms (kg) (220 pounds) a month, to qualify as a small waste generator. In addition, small waste generators in San Diego are required to have an annual permit to store and dispose of such waste; red bags for solid biohazardous waste and sharps containers for sharps disposal (Title 22 of the California Code of Regulations); and a *biomedical waste management plan document.* The plan must include demographical information about the generator; a 24-hour personnel contact designee; a description of methods and containers for storage, treatment, and disposal of biohazardous wastes; and a statement of assurance that personnel handling biomedical wastes have received appropriate instruction on safe handling of the wastes specified in the plan designed to meet the provisions of the ordinance.[10] By contrast, the jurisdictions (New Jersey, New York, Connecticut, Rhode Island, Louisiana, Washington, D.C., or Puerto Rico) covered by the federal EPA regulations consider a small generator to be less than 50 pounds of regulated medical waste per month. Federally regulated biohazardous wastes must be transported and disposed of in specifically marked containers. Packaging must be rigid, leak-resistant, impervious to moisture, and labeled with a universal biohazard symbol as well as the name and permit number of the generator and transporter. Check state and local regulations before disposing of regulated waste by the US Postal Service or United Parcel Service. In-office methods of decontamination and destroying of regulated waste, such as heat-sterilizing sharps containers, are allowed in some jurisdictions and not others.[11]

7. Records: The extent of waste disposal record keeping required also depends on local regulation. Check with state and federal regulatory agencies to determine the requirements for waste tracking documentation (see Requirements for Compliance with Federal Waste Disposal Laws chart). Small waste generators may be required to keep a log of all medical waste shipments, including the transporter's name,

REQUIREMENTS FOR COMPLIANCE WITH FEDERAL WASTE DISPOSAL LAWS

- Segregate regulated medical waste.
- Package the waste in containers.
- Label the containers.
- Store the waste in a protected/secure area.
- Place the containers in a marked carton for transport.
- Ship to a licensed disposal facility (depending on local laws), or use a licensed waste-hauling firm.

Data from ADA,[11] Molinari and Gleason,[9] and Shaefer.[10]

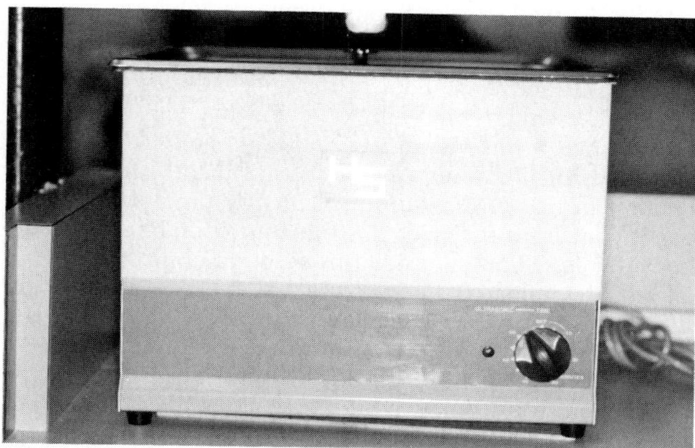

FIGURE 9–13
Ultrasonic cleaning unit.

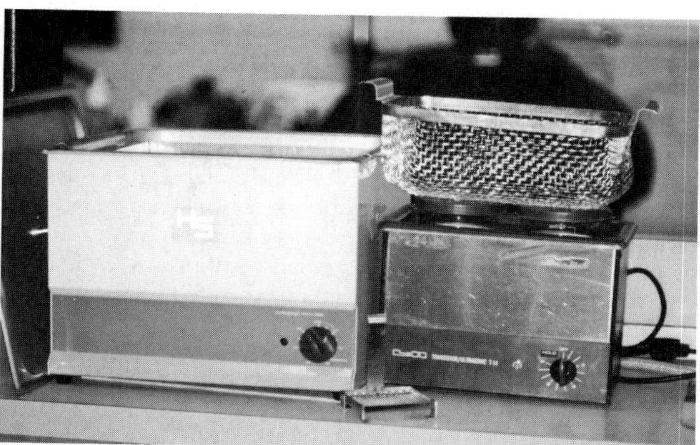

FIGURE 9–14
Different-sized ultrasonic units and basket.

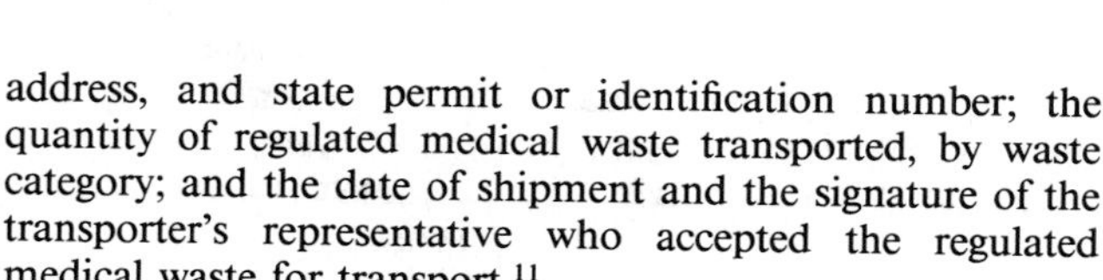

address, and state permit or identification number; the quantity of regulated medical waste transported, by waste category; and the date of shipment and the signature of the transporter's representative who accepted the regulated medical waste for transport.[11]

Decontamination (Cleaning)

Following completion of containment (presoaking and waste disposal), the next step in the recirculation process is decontamination (terminal cleaning) (see Fig. 9–2). Preliminary preparation of the instruments by presoaking prevents the drying of collected bioburden (blood, saliva, and exudate) on the instruments and facilitates the cleaning process yet does not preclude it. The terminal cleaning or decontamination procedure is essential preparation for sterilization. Decontamination involves thorough removal of the softened bioburden, which, if it remains on the surfaces of the instruments, can shelter harmful microorganisms from direct contact with the heat or chemical used for sterilization. The presence of bioburden on instruments inhibits, or lengthens the time required for, effective sterilization.[5] In addition, organic contaminants (bioburden) may inactivate or slow down the action of some chemical **sterilants** and disinfectants.[12]

Ultrasonic Cleaning

The most effective and safest method of terminal cleaning is **ultrasonic cleaning** (Fig. 9–13). Studies have shown ul-

TABLE 9–2
TERMINAL DECONTAMINATION

	Benefits	Concerns
Ultrasonic cleaning	Superior in safety compared with manual cleaning; minimal handling, minimizes risk of puncture wounds Excellent ability to clean all surfaces (grooves and crevices) Hand scrubbing of instruments prior to ultrasonic cleaning is not necessary if instruments have been presoaked and the ultrasonic unit is operating effectively Efficient removal of dried organic contaminants and dental materials Less labor-intensive; other tasks may be done during timed cleaning	Requires frequent changing of solution because of contamination of cleaning solution in tank as instruments are processed Aerosolization of contaminants (never operate without cover) Solution used must be specifically designed for use in an ultrasonic apparatus. (Although an ultrasonic solution could be used as a presoak, not all presoaking solutions are suitable for ultrasonic cleaning, since some may react to heat generated or create hazardous aerosols) Cost of high-quality equipment is expensive, although labor dollars are saved in terms of team members' time
Hand scrubbing	If performed properly, it is possible to clean exposed surfaces thoroughly	Increased potential for exposure to microorganisms with gloved hands immersed in the contaminated cleaning solution as recommended to reduce splattering of debris and microbial contaminants Direct handling of contaminated instruments is dangerous and is not recommended because of increased risk of exposure injury Risk of spatter contamination is increased Time-consuming

Data from Miller,[5,13] Shaefer,[15] and Cottone et al.[1]

trasonic cleaning to be efficient in removal of dried whole blood, saliva, serum, and bacterial plaque as well as dental material cements from instrument surfaces.[13,14] The equipment works by generating high-frequency sound waves that travel through the solution, hitting the instrument surfaces, creating millions of tiny bubbles that collapse in on themselves. The cavitation, or scrubbing action, can reach and clean even the smallest crevice or groove. This ability to reach the tiniest crevice is especially important with difficult to clean items, such as burs and serrated instruments.[15]

Ultrasonic cleaning equipment is available in a variety of sizes to accommodate a range of equipment loads from small to large in volume (Fig. 9–14). Some units are able to process multiple instrument cassettes. Perforated baskets are used to hold the equipment and suspend the items above the bottom of the chamber. The basket acts as a vehicle for transferring instruments from the presoak, into and out of the ultrasonic cleaning tank. Suspending the instruments above the floor of the tank prevents the instruments from interfering with or damaging the energy-producing transducers beneath the tank bottom.[5] A significant advantage of ultrasonic cleaning (see Table 9–2) is the reduction in risk of exposure incidents by minimizing direct hand contact with sharp instruments contaminated with body fluids. The "hands-off" concept minimizes handling of all contaminated instruments whenever possible. This universal precaution is clearly a benefit of ultrasonic cleaning compared with the increased risk of instruments.[1,5,12,15]

Procedure 9–1 presents the steps for effective decontamination of instruments with an ultrasonic cleaner.

Selection of a good cleaning agent enhances the end result for ultrasonic cleaning as well as hand scrubbing,

PROCEDURE 9–1

DECONTAMINATING INSTRUMENTS WITH AN ULTRASONIC CLEANER

Equipment

Nitrile gloves
Ultrasonic cleaning unit
Cleaning solution
Contaminated instruments
Instrument cassette
Face mask and protective eyewear

Steps	Rationale
1. Wear heavy-duty, puncture-resistant nitrile gloves and protective eyewear when processing contaminated equipment. Although wearing a mask to protect the mucous membranes of the nose and oral mucosa is not emphasized as much in the literature on instrument recirculation, such a precaution provides an additional protection in the event of exposure to contaminated aerosols spatter associated with some steps in instrument processing	1. Heavy-duty, puncture-resistant gloves greatly minimize risk of exposure incidents involving contaminated reusable sharps. Protective eyewear and masks prevent exposure of mucous membranes to spatter and aerosols generated in instrument recirculation area
2. Prepare the ultrasonic equipment solution according to the manufacturer's directions to ensure proper dilutions. Maintain the tank solution level at least three-quarters full (1 and a half inches from the top)[1] (Fig. 9–15)	2. Specifically formulated high-quality detergent selection and proper dilution ensure optimal bioburden removal. Maintain solution at the proper level to ensure that all items being decontaminated are completely submerged

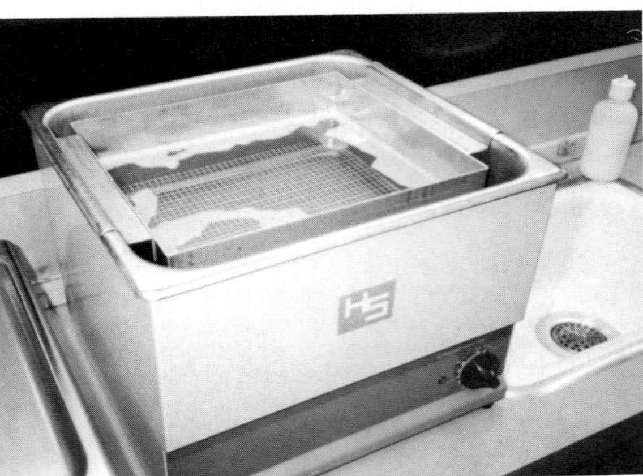

FIGURE 9–15
Ultrasonic cleaning unit.

CONTINUED ON FOLLOWING PAGE

Steps	Rationale
3. Decant the holding solution into the drain of the sink while water is running, before the instrument container is moved from the containment area to the decontamination area (Fig. 9–16). After the presoaking solution is removed, rinse the instruments in the basket or cassette with cool water. Drain off the excess water for additional contaminant reduction prior to immersing the basket or cassette into the ultrasonic solution[15] (Fig. 9–17)	3. The contaminated holding solution is diluted for disposal, since the presoaking solution may be different from the ultrasonic solution. Instruments are rinsed with cool water to remove residual holding solution and some of the softened bioburden. Drain off excess water to prevent dilution of ultrasonic cleaning agent

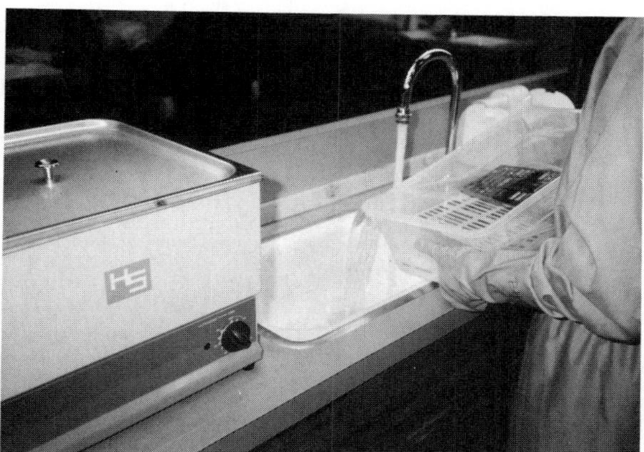

FIGURE 9–16
Decant holding solution into sink.

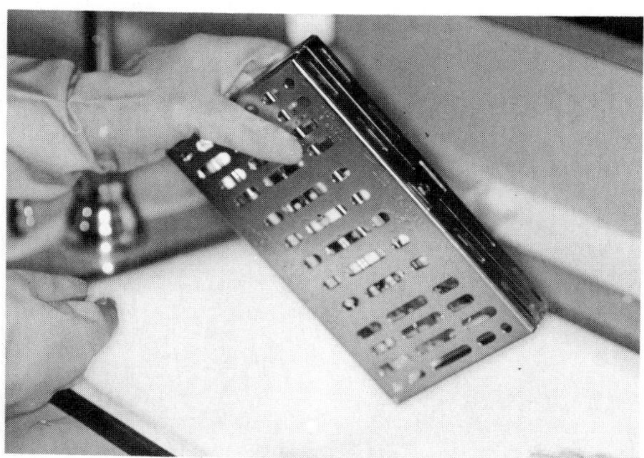

FIGURE 9–17
Drain excess water.

Steps	Rationale
4. After immersion of the instrument container, cover the tank with the lid and set the cleaning time for 6 to 10 minutes or until no visible debris remains (Figs. 9–18 and 9–19). The number of instruments that will fit in the instrument basket depends on the size of the ultrasonic unit, which is usually related to the volume of care and number of dental and dental hygiene care providers. A small ultrasonic cleaner can effectively accommodate 8 to 10 instruments.[1] When cassettes are used for transport from presoaking through ultrasonic cleaning to sterilization, the length of time for cleaning needs to be increased to 15 minutes to ensure effective decontamination.[14]	4. Cover tank with lid whenever it is cleaning to prevent generated aerosols from escaping. Overloading the unit inhibits the ability of the ultrasonic's billions of tiny bubbles to collapse and create the turbulence necessary to effectively clean the surface of all instruments. Time required for effective cleaning may vary, depending on the amount or type of material or instruments and energy of unit

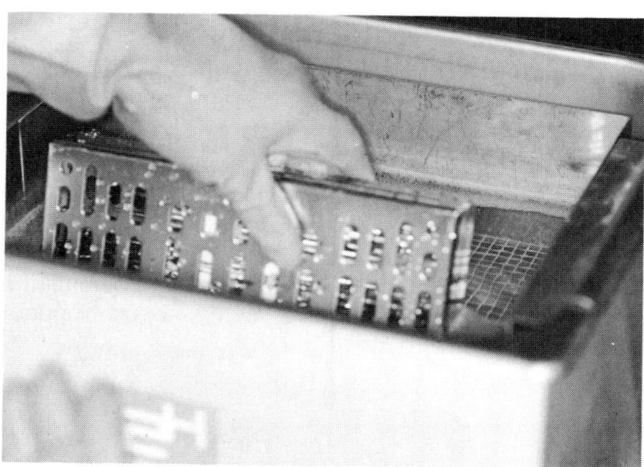

FIGURE 9–18
Immerse instrument cassette into solution.

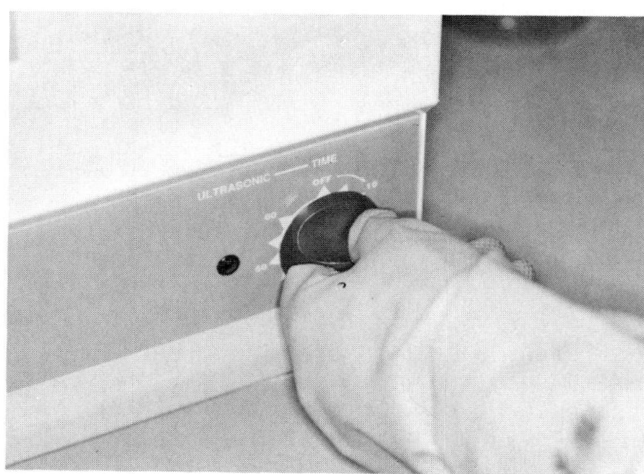

FIGURE 9–19
Set timer.

CONTINUED ON FOLLOWING PAGE

PROCEDURE 9-1

DECONTAMINATING INSTRUMENTS WITH AN ULTRASONIC CLEANER
Continued

Steps	Rationale
5. During the ultrasonic cleaning, a well-fitting cover must remain on the equipment to prevent contaminated aerosols from escaping into the atmosphere of the instrument recirculation center.[1]	5. Cover tank with lid during operation to prevent generated contaminated aerosols from escaping
6. When the timed cleaning cycle has ended, slowly and carefully lift up the basket, allowing excess solution to drain off the instruments into the tank to maintain the level of solution (Fig. 9–20). Transfer the basket to an adjacent sink, and rinse instruments thoroughly under running water (Fig. 9–21). Drain instruments, inspect them, and set them aside for drying and advancement to the packaging area	6. Following ultrasonic cleaning, both instruments and solution are contaminated and, therefore, require careful protected handling

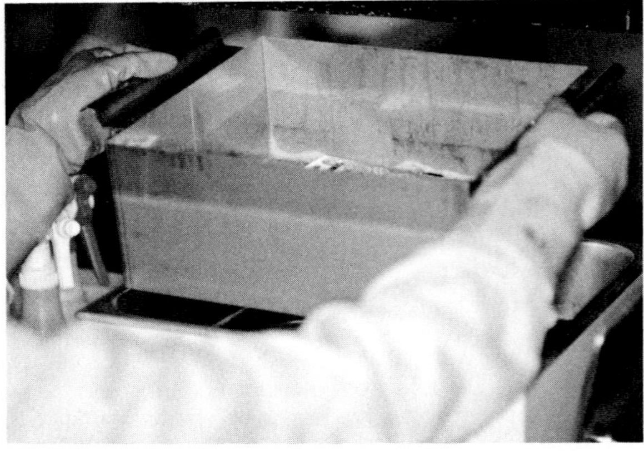

FIGURE 9–20
Lift basket to drain excess solution.

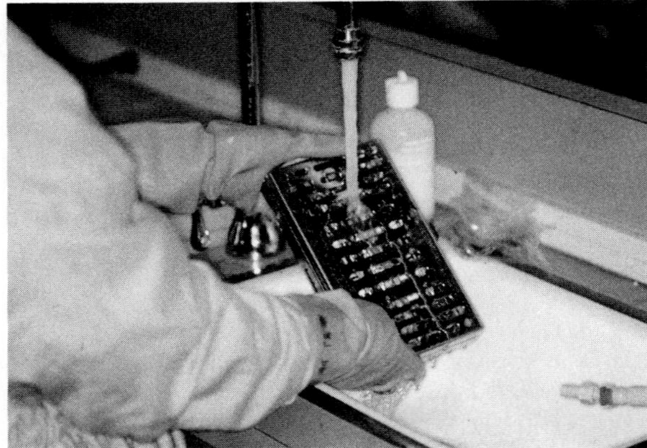

FIGURE 9–21
Rinse instrument cassette.

Steps	Rationale
7. Carefully dry the instruments with a disposable towel to reduce the chance of instrument corrosion. Convection ovens may be used for drying instruments on trays or cassettes as an alternative to hand-drying. Non–stainless steel instruments require the additional protection of a rust inhibitor (sodium nitrite dip or spray) when steam sterilization is the method of renewal[5]	7. Wet carbon steel instruments and burs will rust (sodium nitrite spray will reduce rusting of items)
8. If instrument is accidentally dropped into ultrasonic chamber, retrieve it with tongs or forceps[12]	8. Instruments and solution are contaminated; avoid direct contact, and decrease risk of cuts and punctures
9. Change the solution when it is visibly soiled, but at least once a day[1,5]	9. Maximize effectiveness of solution as a cleaning agent (blood solvent, bioburden penetration, rust inhibition)
10. Drain, rinse, and disinfect (spray-wipe-spray) the ultrasonic cleaning unit at the end of each day[1,5]	10. The tank and solution become contaminated with use
11. Test the ultrasonic unit monthly to evaluate its operation and cleaning efficiency.[1,15] An aluminum foil test may be useful to evaluate the ability of the ultrasonic unit to produce the high-frequency sound waves. The sound waves create the millions of tiny bubbles that collapse and create the cavitation, or scrubbing, action.[16] Place a piece of aluminum foil in the ultrasonic solution, and turn on the unit for the standard time After the cycle is finished, remove foil and inspect for evidence of pitting on the aluminum foil surface. The pitting should be evident if the equipment is generating the high-frequency sound waves necessary to create an effective scrubbing action.	11. Inability of ultrasonic unit to generate high-frequency sound waves prevents effective scrubbing action and therefore may require longer processing, equipment repair or replacement, or increased risk of cuts or punctures due to need for hand scrubbing

Note: Instrument basket/cassette, instruments, and solution are not sterilized or disinfected and must be treated as contaminated *until* they have been sterilized.

should manual cleaning be required. The goal of bioburden removal is enhanced when a cleaning agent is:

- A blood solvent
- Neutral in pH when mixed with water
- Effective against protein soil
- Low in surface tension for soil penetration
- Nondamaging to materials
- Rust inhibiting
- Effective in both hard and soft water
- Easy to rinse[5]

Detergents used with ultrasonic cleaning equipment must be specifically formulated high-quality detergents and mixed according to manufacturer's directions to ensure the optimal ultrasonic cleaning action. Ideally, the same product may be used for both the presoaking process and the ultrasonic cleaning. Detergents containing a rust inhibitor (1% sodium nitrite) are recommended.[1] Initial testing of ultrasonic detergents is showing some indication that these detergents may possess antibacterial activity even though the intent of design was not for use as a disinfectant. It is important to note that once the detergent solution has been used for cleaning instruments, the solution must be treated as contaminated.[12]

Hand scrubbing of instruments is no longer recommended. However, should it become necessary because of ultrasonic malfunction, Procedure 9–2 should be followed to reduce risk and maximize effectiveness.

PROCEDURE 9–2

HAND SCRUBBING METHOD OF INSTRUMENT DECONTAMINATION

Equipment

Heavy-duty (nitrile) gloves
Protective clothing, mask, and eyewear
Long-handled (heat-sterilizable) brush
Very small brush

Steps	Rationale
1. Wear heavy-duty utility (nitrile) gloves in addition to the other personal barriers for protection from direct contact as well as aerosols and spatter (Fig. 9–22)	1. Protection of skin and mucous membranes from direct contact as well as aerosols and spatter
2. Immerse instruments in detergent solution (Fig. 9–23)	2. Minimizes generation of aerosols and spatter; detergent enhances cleaning

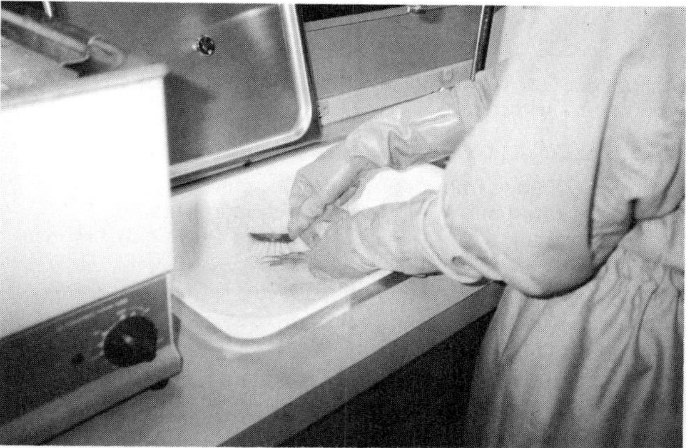

FIGURE 9–22
Handscrubbing with use of heavy-duty (nitrile) gloves and long-handled brush.

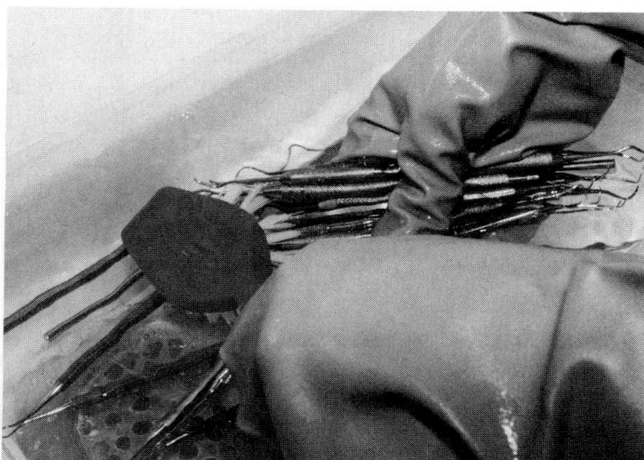

FIGURE 9–23
Handscrubbing with gloved hands under solution.

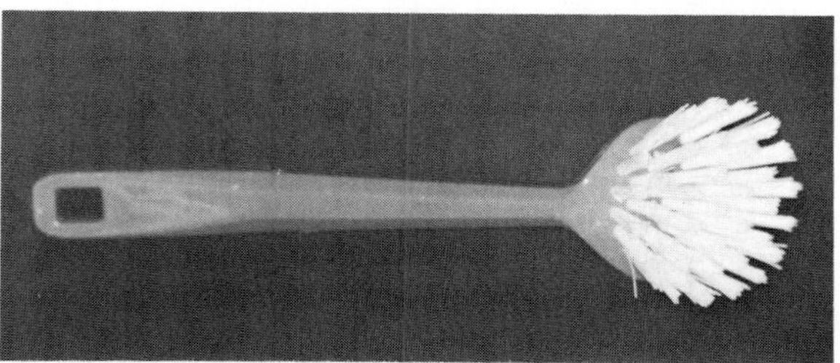

FIGURE 9–24
Long-handled heat-sterilizable brush.

CONTINUED ON FOLLOWING PAGE

PROCEDURE 9–2

HAND SCRUBBING METHOD OF INSTRUMENT DECONTAMINATION
Continued

Steps	Rationale
3. Scrub with a long-handled, heat-sterilizable soft brush (Fig. 9–24)	3. Creates distance between hand and contaminated reusable sharps (reduces exposure risk)
4. Hold brush and instruments under the surface of the detergent solution	4. Minimizes generation of aerosol and spatter
5. Give special attention to grooves, serrations, and hinges. Use a very small brush or pipe cleaner to clean small holes and lumens on equipment	5. Required for effective meticulous cleaning; otherwise bioburden remains, jeopardizing sterilization

Packaging

The next area along the recirculation pathway of processing of instruments is the packaging area. This counter space is located, ideally, on the opposite side of the sink from the receiving (containment) and decontamination (ultrasonic cleaning) areas. The packaging area is within the contaminated zone of the instrument recirculation center. Once the instruments have been cleaned, rinsed, inspected for bioburden removal, and dried, cassettes, functional sets of instruments, and single instruments are packaged (wrapped or bagged) in preparation for the sterilization procedure. The objective of packaging is to provide instruments with poststerilization protection from environmental contamination (see Protocol for Instrument Packaging chart). The instruments remain in the package until they are used; at that time they are unwrapped or opened at chairside to ensure the fullest protection from contamination prior to use. The poststerilization instrument protection and unwrapping/opening in front of clients also helps reassure the clients of instrument sterilization and helps meet their human need for safety.

TABLE 9–3
STERILIZATION METHODS AND COMPATIBLE PACKAGING MATERIALS*

Type of Sterilizer	Single-Use Packaging Material	Conditions Required	Reusable Packaging/ Containers
Steam (autoclave)	Poly film/paper-peel pouches Paper bags Sterilization paper wrap Nylon plastic tubing	Must permit steam penetration and withstand heat	Cloth (muslin) Open glass or metal containers
Unsaturated chemical vapor	Poly film/paper-peel pouches Paper bags Sterilization paper wrap	Must permit chemical vapor penetration and withstand heat	Open containers (glass or metal)
Dry heat	Sterilization paper wrap (some paper may become charred) Aluminum foil Nylon plastic tubing	Must not overly insulate from heat and must withstand heat without melting	Closed containers Solid metal tray with lids Cloth-muslin (cloth may become charred)

* Consult with packaging product manufacturer and sterilizer manufacturer to verify material selection.
Adapted from Miller, C. H. Sterilization: Disciplined microbial control. Dental Clinics of North America 35(2):339–355, 1991.

PROTOCOL FOR INSTRUMENT PACKAGING

- To reduce the chances of corrosion of non–stainless steel instruments it is imperative that instruments be inspected to ensure that they are completely dry prior to processing in a **chemical vapor sterilizer,** a dry heat oven, or a liquid sterilant or by **ethylene oxide gas sterilization.** The drying process may be expedited by the use of a dryer or heat lamp. No specific drying unit has been developed for the dental market at this time.[1] Because of the increased risk of corrosion of the non–stainless steel instruments processed with steam sterilization, a rust inhibitor (dip or spray 1% sodium nitrite) should be applied prior to packaging[5]
- If a lubricant is used on instruments with moving parts, prior to packaging and sterilization, a water-based lubricant product should be used so that it does not interfere with sterilization. Check with the manufacturers to be sure that a lubricant does not leave a film on the instrument that prevents steam penetration. Silicon- or oil-based lubricants pose the greatest chance of leaving a film barrier[5]
- The packaging material selected must be compatible with the particular method of sterilization used (Table 9–3). Some materials may melt in dry heat yet are well suited to the moist heat of steam sterilization. The various types of packaging include sterilization paper bags, paper/poly film "see-through" bags, clear nylon plastic tubing on a roll that is cut and heat-sealed, and cloth wrapping.[5] The packaging selected should also be made of high-quality materials that maintain sterility and promote safe use. Thin paper bags permit sharp instruments to protrude through the wrapping, possibly causing an exposure incident during presterilization handling and/or compromising sterility following processing. Paper sterilization wrapping, materials stamped with an American Dental Association (ADA) acceptance seal or "Made in the United Kingdom"

currently meet the most rigid standards regarding strength of wet paper, air permeability resistance, wet and dry seal strength, tear resistance, and peel characteristics. Packaging materials are designed for *single use;* to use more than once compromises their ability to maintain sterility[1]

- The cassette system provides an excellent mechanism for encasement of a functional set of instruments for the entire instrument recirculation process, from containment of the instruments during presoak to terminal cleaning and drying. In addition, they can be reused to hold instruments for subsequent sterilization.[5] The cassette is perforated to permit instrument access by the presoaking and cleaning solution and by the chemical, steam, or gas during processing (Fig. 9–25). Just prior to

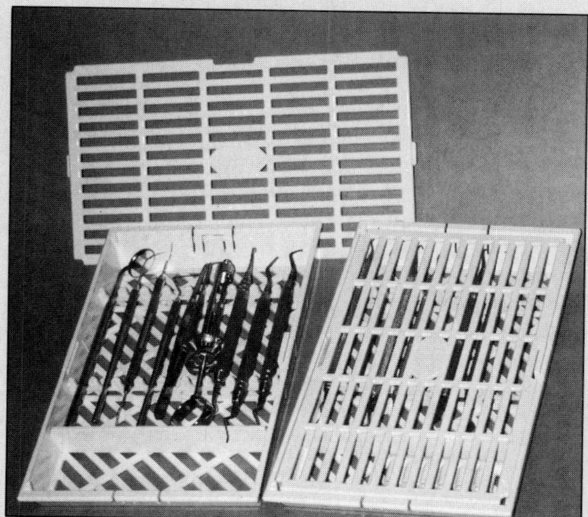

FIGURE 9–25
Instrument cassette.

sterilization the cassette is wrapped to protect the instruments following sterilization. The sterilizers must be of a larger size to adequately accommodate the cassettes for processing. After the cassette is processed, the opened paper wrap may serve as a sterile field barrier on the dental hygiene tray top, while the cassette functions as a sterile instrument tray or rack

- Instrument packaging in bags or pouches such as paper bags, paper/poly see-through bags (facilitates instrument identification), and polyfilm bags made from clear nylon plastic tubing may be used if specified as compatible with the particular method of sterilization. A variety of sizes are available. Select the size of package that is appropriate for the number and size of instruments to be processed. Avoid overloading the package with an excessive number of instruments (Fig. 9–26). Such overloading compromises the packaging as well as the effectiveness of the sterilization process by preventing instrument contact with the chemical, steam, or gas, depending on the process used[1]

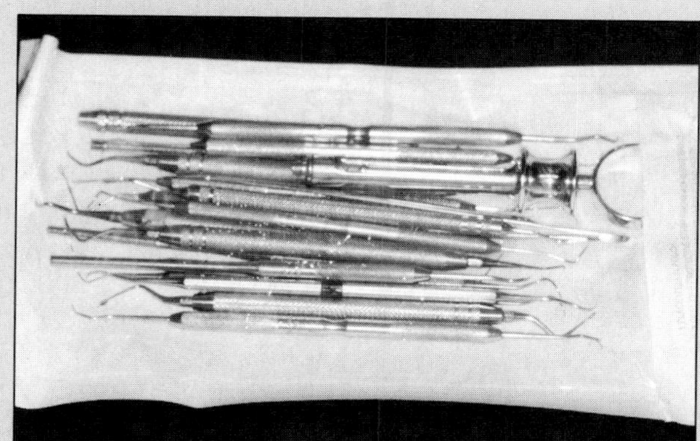

FIGURE 9–26
Packaging. Overloaded packages.

- Before closing the cassette or bag, unit-dose quantities of gauze, cotton rolls, and cotton swabs **(unit-dose system)** should be added to the package. Ease in access, increased efficiency, prevention of cross-contamination from midappointment supply retrieval, and sterilization of disposables that come in contact with critical and semicritical items are the benefits of packaging unit-doses of cotton goods with instruments
- Labeling the packages prior to processing may include such information as the name of the user, identification of contents (unless packaging permits viewing of contents), and date, for less frequently used items (Fig. 9–27). A soft lead pencil is generally recommended for labeling, especially if unsaturated chemical vapor is the method of sterilization used. Chemical vapor dissolves ink-type markings in the chamber, affecting the clarity of the labeling. In addition, the ink settles out on the chamber walls and instruments[15]

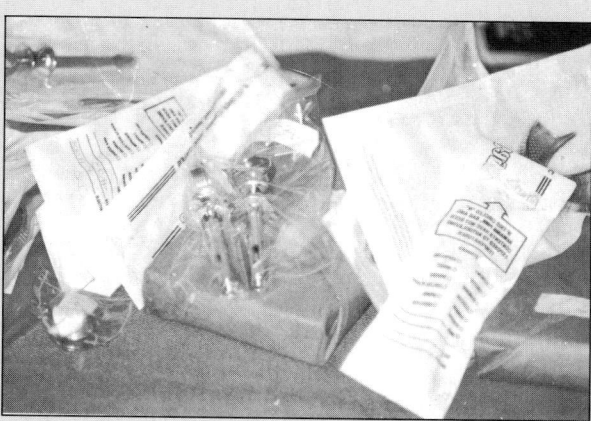

FIGURE 9–27
Labeled packages.

- **Chemical indicators,** sometimes called process indicators, are usually composed of a chemical formulation of indicator ink impregnated on tape, paper, or cardboard. A change in color identifies the items that have been sterilized. The most familiar type of indicators are the chemically treated tapes, labels, and bag markings used as external indicators that change color after brief exposure to high temperatures (Fig. 9–28). Check with the manufacturers to determine which specific sterilization method the process indicators are designed to monitor. External indicator tape is not an accurate temperature indicator, since it generally changes color before adequate sterilization temperatures have been reached.[1,18] It is a good indicator to identify items that have been processed. Therefore, all packages, containers, and bags being processed should have process indicator tape, or marking on the exterior of the

Continued on following page

PROTOCOL FOR INSTRUMENT PACKAGING *Continued*

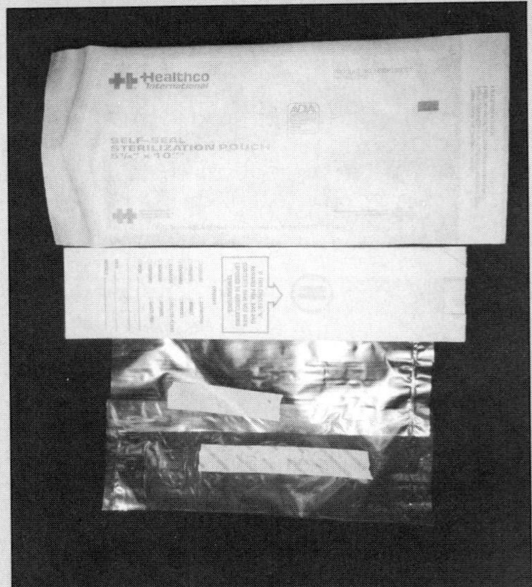

FIGURE 9–28
External process indicator.

packaging, to indicate clearly to all team members which instruments have been processed and which have not[1,19]

- Internal chemical indicators, also referred to as control indicators, "slow-change" indicators, or integrators are more sophisticated than external indicator tape because they test more than one parameter of the sterilizing process. These indicators are paper strips impregnated with a chemical formulation of indicator ink that are designed to be placed *inside* one instrument package per load to ensure that the internal contents have been exposed to the appropriate conditions.[18] Various packaging materials and loading methods can affect the time or temperatures required for sterilization, so these control indicators are designed to test, for example, time as well as temperature. Check with the manufacturer to determine which specific sterilization method the internal chemical indicators are designed to monitor. The routine use of such indicators does not guarantee that the precise conditions for sterilization have been met. Internal chemical indicators are not as effective as **biological monitor indicators** in ensuring that the specific conditions for sterilization have been met, yet they detect gross malfunction or errors in the sterilization procedure. For example, the steam sterilization indicator in Figure 9–29 integrates the processing conditions and records no movement when there is an absence of steam, or an air pocket in the steam sterilizer. An integrator may reveal a partial color change if the parameters for sterilizing have not been satisfied (e.g., inadequate steam pressure, poor packing technique); a uniform and complete color change indicates that processing parameters have been met. Direct contact of the indicator ink with the instrument surfaces inside the package should be avoided to prevent a false-positive internal indicator color change[1]
- All instrument packages should have an external indicator. Internal package monitoring with a "slow-change" chemical indicator should be done at least once a day.[20] Routine monitoring of packages being processed as well as use of internal parameters for processing can alert those responsible for instrument recirculation to sterilization problems. The *only* verifiable method of confirming that sterilization conditions have been met is the use of a calibrated biological monitoring spore test system (see section on quality assurance).

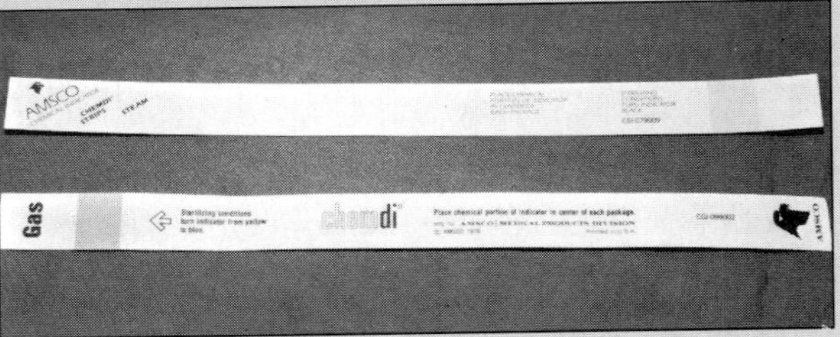

FIGURE 9–29
Examples of chemical indicators (also called "slow-charge" indicators).

- To ensure packaging integrity and to maintain sterility following the renewal procedure, an adequate package seal must be provided. Options include bags that are self-sealed, heat-sealed, or double-folded and sealed with an adequate amount of indicator tape or cassettes and trays sealed with sterilization wrapping paper and tape. Paper clips, staples, or any other devices that do not totally seal the package should not be used under any circumstances[1,5]
- Processing unwrapped instruments (e.g., instruments processed in pans/trays uncovered) is not considered a satisfactory approach to instrument renewal (Fig. 9–30). Sterilization of unwrapped instruments is compromised immediately after processing by contact with contaminated hands or gloves, contaminated surfaces, dental aerosols that tend to remain airborne, and microbe-laden dust particles. A sterilization method that permits constant use of packaging is preferred over the use of a disinfectant or sterilant solution immersion processing, since it is incompatible with instrument packaging[5]

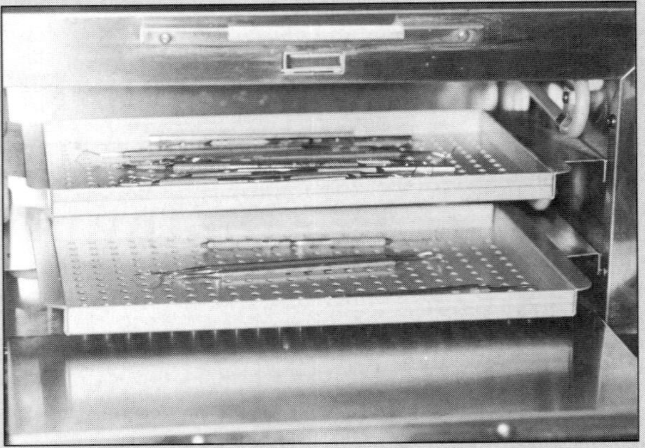

FIGURE 9–30
Trays with unwrapped instruments.

Renewal Process

Once the instruments are packaged and properly sealed and labeled, the renewal process (sterilization) may begin. The sterilizers are located in an area of transition between the contaminated zone and the noncontaminated zone (see Fig. 9–2). The area for renewal must be adequate in size to accommodate more than one method of sterilization, since no one method is suitable for all dental hygiene care items. Most recirculation areas have three methods (steam autoclave, unsaturated chemical vapor, and dry heat) available to accommodate the wide variety of materials requiring sterilization. The contaminated zone adjacent to the sterilizers holds the cleaned, yet contaminated, instruments prior to loading or placement in the chamber for processing. On completion of the sterilization process, the instruments move into the noncontaminated zone for cooling and storage or distribution.

Sterilization or renewal of instruments for reuse on subsequent clients is only one component of the recirculation area activity, yet it is the critical element. Sterilization is the most important component of a comprehensive infection control program, and it is the only component that has the potential for reducing the microbial count to zero.[1,21] Successful and effective sterilization depends on a number of elements, including the selection of the appropriate method of sterilization for the specific material to be processed. The diversity of instruments and items used in comprehensive dental hygiene care requires more than one method of sterilization, since there is no all-purpose sterilizer.[21] A wide selection of items used in dental hygiene and dentistry are presented on Table 9–4, with the recommended/preferred method(s) of sterilization.

Sterilization methods are designed to kill *all* microorganisms. Therefore, the sterilization process, to be effective, must be able to kill the bacterial endospores, commonly known as spores, the microorganism that requires the longest time, hottest temperature, or highest concentration of chemical. When spores are killed, other less resistant microorganisms are killed in the process. Bacterial and mycotic spores are the most heat resistant form of life.[1] The effectiveness of the sterilization process is verified by routine spore testing with the use of biological indicators that contain spores (see quality assurance section).

TABLE 9–4
STERILIZATION AND DISINFECTION OF DENTAL INSTRUMENTS, MATERIALS, AND SOME COMMONLY USED ITEMS*

	Steam Autoclave	Dry Heat Oven	Chemical Vapor	Ethylene Oxide	Chemical Disinfection/ Sterilization	Other Methods/ Commments
Angle attachments*	+	+	+	++	+	
Burs						
Carbon steel	–	++	++	++	–	
Steel	+	++	++	++	+	
Tungsten-carbide	+	++	+	++	+	
Condensers	++	++	++	++	+	
Dappen dishes	++	+	+	++	+	
Endodontic instruments (broaches, files, reamers)						Hot salt/glass bead sterilizer 10 to 15 seconds, 218°C (425°F)
Stainless steel handles	+	++	++	++	+	
Stainless with plastic handles	++	++	–	++	–	
Fluoride gel trays						
Heat-resistant plastic	++	––	–	++	–	
Non–heat-resistant plastic	––	––	–	++	–	Discard (++)
Glass slabs	++	++	++	++	+	
Hand instruments						
Carbon steel	–	++	++	++	–	
		[Steam autoclave with chemical protection (1% sodium nitrite)]				
Stainless steel	++	++	++	++	+	
Handpieces*						
Sterilizable*	(++)*	–	(+)*	++	––	Sterilizable preferably
Contra angles*	–	–	–	++	+	Combination synthetic phenolics or iodophors (–)
Nonsterilizable*	–	–	–	++	+	
Prophylaxis angles*	+	+	+	+	+	Discard (++)
Impression materials						Table 2
Impression trays						
Aluminum metal	++	+	++	++	–	
Chrome-plated	++	++	++	++	+	
Custom acrylic resin	––	––	––	++	+	
Plastic	––	––	––	++	+	Discard (++): preferred
Instruments in packs	++	+ Small packs	++	++ Small packs	––	
Instrument tray set-ups						
Restorative or surgical	+ Size limit	+	+ Size limit	++ Size limit	––	

Table continued on following page

TABLE 9–4
STERILIZATION AND DISINFECTION OF DENTAL INSTRUMENTS, MATERIALS, AND SOME COMMONLY USED ITEMS* *Continued*

	Steam Autoclave	Dry Heat Oven	Chemical Vapor	Ethylene Oxide	Chemical Disinfection/ Sterilization	Other Methods/ Commments
Mirrors	–	++	++	++	+	
Needles						
Disposable	––	––	––	––	––	Discard (++) Do not reuse
Nitrous oxide						
Nosepiece	(++)*	––	(++)*	++	(+)*	
Hoses	(++)*	––	(++)*	++	(+)*	
Orthodontic pliers						
High-quality stainless	++	++	++	++	+	
Low-quality stainless	–	++	++	++	–	
With plastic parts	––	––	––	++	+	
Pluggers	++	++	++	++	+	
Polishing wheels and disks						
Garnet and cuttle	––	–	–	++	––	
Rag	++	–	+	++	––	
Rubber	+	–	–	++	+	
Prostheses, removable	–	–	–	+	+	
Rubber dam equipment						
Carbon steel clamps	–	++	++	++	–	
Metal frames	++	++	++	++	+	
Plastic frames	–	–	–	++	+	
Punches	–	++	++	++	+	
Stainless steel clamps	++	++	++	++	+	
Rubber items						
Prophylaxis cups	–	–	–	++	–	Discard (++)
Saliva evacuators, ejectors						
Low-melting plastic	–	–	–	++	+	Discard (++)
High-melting plastic	++	+	+	++	+	
Stones						
Diamond	+	++	++	++	+	
Polishing	++	+	++	++	–	
Sharpening	++	++	++	–	–	
Surgical instruments						
Stainless steel	++	++	++	++	+	
Ultrasonic scaling tips	+	––	––	++	+	
Water-air syringe tips	++	++	++	++	+	
X-ray equipment						
Plastic film folders	(++)*	––	(+)*	++	+	
Collimating devices	–	––	––	++	+	

* As manufacturers use a variety of alloys and materials in these products, confirmation with the equipment manufacturers is recommended, especially for handpieces and the attachments.
++ Effective and preferred method.
\+ Effective and acceptable method.
– Effective method, but risk of damage to materials.
–– Ineffective method with risk of damage to materials.
Adapted from American Dental Association Council on Dental Materials, Instruments, and Equipments; on Dental Practice; and on Dental Therapeutics. Infection control recommendations for the dental office and the dental laboratory. Journal of the American Dental Association 116:241, 1988.

Disinfection

In contrast to sterilization, **disinfection** is a process intended to kill or remove pathogenic microorganisms, with the exception of bacterial spores.[12] If a microbial killing method yields a lower number of dead microorganisms, it is usually referred to as a disinfection method. There is a range of effectiveness used to categorize disinfectants with the ability to kill tubercle bacillus *(Mycobacterium tuberculosis)* used as the standard for intermediate-grade, EPA-approved disinfectants (see section on disinfectants/surface disinfection in Chapter 7)[5,22] (Fig. 9–31). The Council on Dental Therapeutics acceptance of disinfectants is predicated on tuberculocidal ability.[22]

In the recirculation process, disinfection usually refers to the use of a liquid chemical (disinfectant) at room temperature for immersion renewal of instruments. Dentistry has been deeply entrenched in the use of liquids for instrument treatment over the years and has frequently referred to this process as **"cold sterilization."**[21] This term is a misnomer, since disinfectants do *not* kill all microorganisms including bacterial and mycotic spores. The range of microorganisms killed by disinfectants varies, depending on the chemical itself and how it is used.[12] The immersion disinfectants widely used in dentistry for many years are the quaternary ammonium compounds (e.g., Zephirin, Cetylcide, Mann's solution). Quaternary ammonium compounds are not acceptable for disinfection of instruments or surfaces because they are irregularly virucidal, do not kill tubercle bacilli, and are quickly neutralized by soap and bioburden.[21,23]

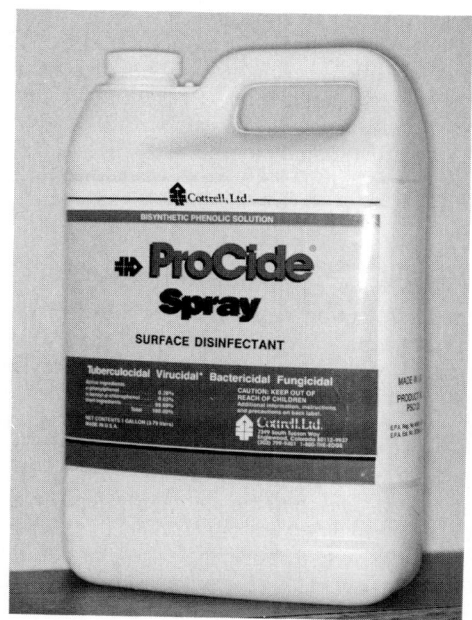

FIGURE 9–31
Bottle of EPA-approved tuberculocidal disinfectant.

Chemical Sterilants/Disinfectants

There are other chemicals, such as glutaraldehydes and chlorine dioxide, that have been shown in laboratory testing to achieve either disinfection or sterilization (kill bacte-

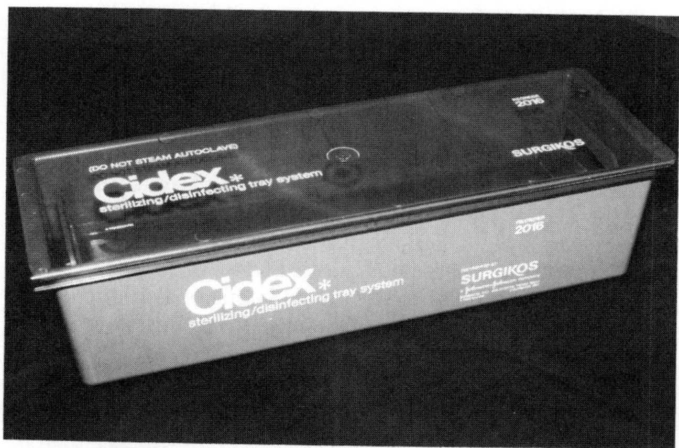

FIGURE 9–32
Container with glutaraldehyde for immersion in sterilant disinfectant.

rial spores), depending on strict adherence to the concentration and the time allowed for contact with the contaminated instruments (Fig. 9–32). Although chlorine dioxide and glutaraldehydes (2.0 to 3.2%), as listed in Table 9–5, have been shown to kill bacterial spores within 6 to 10 hours of contact time, it obviously is not practical to use such a time-consuming process to routinely sterilize a volume of instruments.[13] Any length of contact time shorter than the specified 6 or 10 hours is a disinfection procedure, *not sterilization.* Another significant limitation for the use of an immersion sterilant is the inability to verify sterilization with biological monitors. Spore testing for the routine

TABLE 9–5
STERILANTS: IMMERSION DISINFECTANTS ABLE TO FUNCTION AS STERILANTS UNDER PRESCRIBED CONDITIONS

Immersion Disinfectants/Sterilants		**Sterilant Requirements**				
Chemical Classification	Product(s)	Dilution	Time (hr)	Temp. (°C)	**EPA Reg. No.**	**Formerly ADA Accepted**
Chlorine dioxide	Exspore	4:1:1	6	20	45631-03	Yes
Glutaraldehydes						
2% Glutaraldehyde acidic	Banicide Sterall Wavicide 01	FS	10	21	15136-1	Yes
3.2% Glutaraldehyde alkaline	Cidex Plus	FS	10	20	7078-14	Yes
	Coe Cide *XL* Plus Aristocrat Plus 30 Maxicide Plus 30 Metricide Plus 30	FS	10	20	46781-4	Yes
2% Glutaraldehyde alkaline	Cidex 7	FS	10	20	7078-1	Yes
	Germ-X	FS	10	20	10352-29	Yes
	Baxter/Omnicide Glutall K-Cide Omnicide Procide	FS	10	20	46851-2	Yes
	Coe Cide XL Maxicide Metricide Protec-top Vital Defense-S	FS	6	20	46781-2	Yes

FS, Full strength. 20°C = 68°F.
Data from JADA,[38] Balanyk,[22] Office Sterilization and Asepsis Procedures Research Foundation,[29] and Cottone and Molinari.[24]

verification of microorganisms killed during sterilant immersion is not possible in the clinical setting. The only type of monitoring available for glutaraldehydes is a dipstick, which is used to estimate chemical concentration (free aldehyde remaining), not to determine microbial kill.[13,22] Additional disadvantages associated with the sporicidal glutaraldehydes are possible toxicity, skin and mucosal irritation for client and operator, offensive vapor, corrosion of some metals, the instability of the active solution, and relatively high cost. Although chlorine dioxide requires fresh solution for use and corrodes most metals, it is nontoxic.[22]

If a contaminated item can be immersed, immersion in a liquid sterilant is an appropriate alternative sterilization method only if the item would be destroyed by heat sterilization and no other verifiable method of sterilization is available (e.g., gas sterilization) (see Protocol for Use of Immersion Disinfectants/Sterilants for Sterilization chart). Chemical sterilants should not be used as a substitute for heat sterilization when items are able to withstand repeated heat sterilization processing.[24]

PROTOCOL FOR USE OF IMMERSION DISINFECTANTS/STERILANTS* FOR STERILIZATION

- Select a chemical/product that has an EPA registration number and ADA acceptance
- Nitrile gloves, protective eyewear, and masks should be worn when preparing (diluting/pouring), using, and discarding immersion disinfectants/sterilants
- Special care must be used to follow the manufacturer's directions for use (specific dilution or full-strength, temperature and time)
- Items to be immersed must be precleaned and *dried* (water affects dilution and effectiveness of the sterilant)
- Carefully submerge items/instruments for the length of time specified by the manufacturer and maintain temperature required (see Table 9–5 for products and variation in times and temperatures)
- If more than one team member is responsible for instrument recirculation, label or note that the liquid sterilant is in use, and specify time the renewal process† will be completed
- Lift items out of solution, permit excess sterilant to drain off items into sterilant bath
- Rinse with sterile water and immediately protect from contamination. Dry and at once cover with a sterile towel. Since items renewed by liquid sterilants have no "shelf life," packaging for processing is not feasible. Contamination by the environment occurs immediately after items are removed from the solution. Noncritical items may be rinsed with tap water unless the water is known or suspected to be contaminated
- Evaluate product's ability to be reused; check manufacturer's directions, date prepared, and time limit for use; monitor with chemical indicator† tap water unless the water is known or suspected to be contaminated
- Evaluate product's ability to be reused; check manufacturer's directions, date prepared, and time limit for use; monitor with chemical indicator to evaluate effectiveness level of glutaraldehyde concentration
- Recognize limitations with use of immersion sterilants. Whenever possible, select the methods of sterilization preferred by the Centers for Disease Control (CDC) and the ADA

*Liquid sterilants should be used only on clean plastics or other items that do not physically withstand heat sterilization and cannot be sterilized by ethylene oxide.

†Renewal by liquid sterilants cannot be monitored by biological indicators, and therefore sterilization is not verifiable.

Universal Sterilization

Instrument recirculation requires sterilization of everything that can be sterilized, and disinfection in place of sterilization is a compromise.[21] A guiding tenet of every infection control program should be the determination not to disinfect when you can sterilize.[1] The methods of sterilization that can be verified by spore testing are the preferred methods. Heat, heat/pressure, or gas methods are verifiable and recommended for *all* reusable dental hygiene instruments contaminated with blood or saliva. Selectively disinfecting some instruments, while sterilizing others is not a safe approach to preventing disease transmission to clients from instruments. Some states (Indiana and Ohio) have adopted laws requiring sterilization rather than disinfection of reusable instruments. Other states are considering similar legislation as well. Sterilizing all reusable instruments (universal sterilization) through the use of the preferred methods, accompanied by routine biological monitoring, helps ensure high-quality client care and prevent the spread of disease[25] (Fig. 9–33).

The concept of universal sterilization is based on the concept of universal precautions for the prevention of transmission of bloodborne pathogens established to protect the client, oral healthcare team members, and their families. Treating all clients as if they are known carriers of the human immunodeficiency virus (HIV) or HBV, and applying the highest standards of infection control based on scientific rationale, are fundamental concepts for infection control, since it is impossible to determine which clients are carriers.[5] The concept of universal precautions should be transferred to the recirculation area, where each contaminated instrument should be viewed as having the potential for carrying HBV or HIV. The guideline that emerges from this concept is to sterilize every item contaminated with blood and saliva—not only those items used in direct

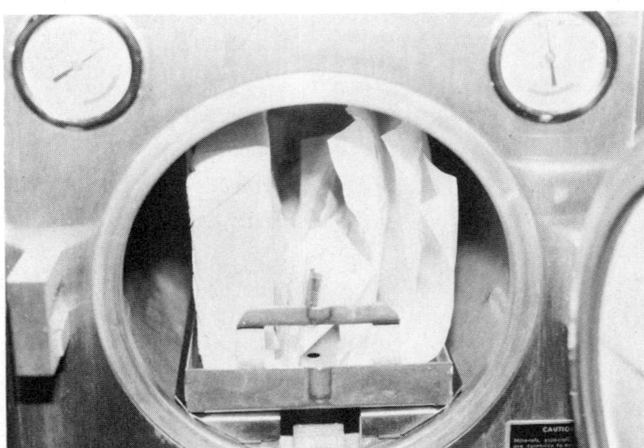

FIGURE 9–33
Open sterilizer with a variety of packages and spore vial.

client contact but also items indirectly contacted by the blood- and saliva-coated gloved fingers of the dental hygienist. Even though an instrument is not going to be used for a procedure that penetrates soft tissue (critical item according to Spaulding classification, see Chapter 8), it may accidentally penetrate the tissues or may be a source of microorganisms transferred to a subsequent client. Even the smallest amount of contamination may be significant; for example, the tip of an explorer that has been dipped into whole saliva may contain approximately 50,000 microorganisms, which are not even visible to the naked eye.[5] The procedures and protocols related to recirculation, presented previously, and those that follow are designed to lead to practical and effective sterilization for the killing of all forms of microorganisms. Therefore, all instruments, even those used for dental hygiene care on clients with known HIV infection or a HBV carrier state, should be handled in the same manner, treated with the same disciplined microbial control. A universal protocol for instrument recirculation is part of the universal precautions for prevention of transmission of bloodborne pathogens and requires one standard of infection control for all clients.

TABLE 9–6
COMPARISON OF VERIFIABLE METHODS OF STERILIZATION

Method	Standard Sterilizing Conditions*	Advantages	Precautions	Spore Testing
Steam autoclave	20 min at 121°C (250°F) (15 psi)	Time efficient Good penetration Sterilize water-based liquid	Do not use closed containers May damage plastic and rubber items Non–stainless steel metal items corrode Use of hard water may leave deposits	*Bacillus stearothermophilus* strips, vials, or ampules
Unsaturated chemical vapor	20 min at 132°C (270°F) (20–40 psi)	Time efficient No corrosion Items dry quickly after cycle	Do not use closed containers May damage plastic and rubber items Must use special solution Predry instruments, or dip them in special solution Provide adequate ventilation Cannot sterilize liquids	*Bacillus stearothermophilus* strips
Dry heat				
Dry heat oven	60–120 min at 160°C (320°F)	No corrosion Can use closed containers Large capacity per cost Items are dry after cycles	Longer sterilization time Cannot sterilize liquids May damage plastic and rubber items Do not open door before end of cycle Predry instruments	*Bacillus subtilis* strips
Rapid heat transfer	12 min at 191°C (375°F) (for wrapped items) 6 min at 191°C (375°F) (for unwrapped items)	No corrosion Short cycle Items are dry after cycle	Cannot sterilize liquids May damage plastic and rubber items Do not open door before end of cycle Small capacity per cost Predry instruments Unwrapped items quickly contaminated after cycle	*Bacillus subtilis* strips
Ethylene oxide	10–16 hr at 61°C (110°F)	No corrosion Ideal for items damaged by heat and/or moisture	Long turn-around time Requires poststerilization aeration Insufficient aeration can cause tissue irritation Requires spark shield to prevent potential for explosion Requires adequate ventilation because of gas toxicity	*Bacillus subtilis* strips or vials

* These conditions do not include warm-up time, and they may vary, depending on the nature and volume of the load. Sterilizing conditions in sterilizers should be defined by results of routine spore testing.

Adapted from Miller, C. H. Take the safe approach to prevent disease transmission. RDH 9(5):35, 1989; with permission.

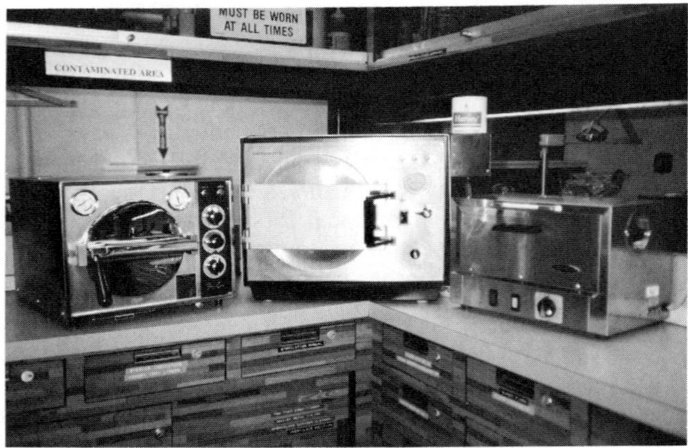

FIGURE 9–34
Autoclave, chemiclave, and dry-heat sterilizers.

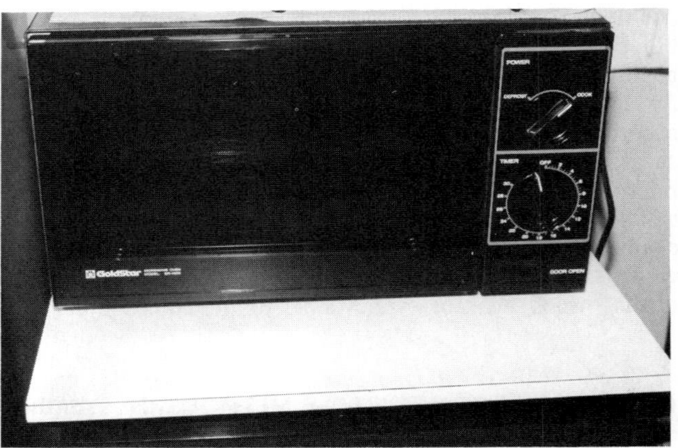

FIGURE 9–35
Microwave.

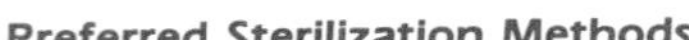

Preferred Sterilization Methods

The three preferred methods for sterilization of instruments able to withstand repeated exposure to high temperatures are steam under pressure (autoclave), unsaturated chemical vapor (chemiclave), and dry heat sterilization (Fig. 9–34). These three processes all have the element of heat in common.[1,7,26] The heat sterilization methods are more efficient and reliable than the chemical sterilant/disinfectant immersion process. Reliability is related to the fact that sterilization with these methods may be verified by spore testing. The only chemical method included with the preferred methods of sterilization is ethylene oxide gas, which is a verifiable low-temperature process with excellent penetration power used in hospitals and large clinics (Table 9–6). Gas sterilization, however, is used in only a few dental offices.[5]

Other methods of sterilization have been or are currently being investigated. Hydrogen peroxide vaporization appears to hold the most promise as a low-temperature method with practical application for future use in oral healthcare settings. Additional research and development have gone into evaluation of the use of ionizing radiation, ultraviolet (UV) light, and microwaves for killing microorganisms. Ionizing radiation is a low-temperature method of sterilization used on a large scale in industry without practical application for the oral healthcare environment. Ultraviolet light appears to have significant limitations unless the UV light has access to all surface areas; at most, it is currently considered to be a form of disinfection rather than sterilization. The use of standard microwave ovens and gas-plasma microwave has also been investigated, with limited useful application (Fig. 9–35). Incompatibility with metal instruments is a major limitation.[5]

The verifiable methods of sterilization are presented in the following section with information on specific sterilizing conditions, action on microorganisms, advantages and precautions, and spore testing included in Table 9–7. Successful instrument sterilization depends on the selection of the preferred method to ensure microbial kill with minimal instrument deterioration and on a disciplined approach to operation, maintenance, and routine biological monitoring of the sterilization equipment.[5,27] The recommended times, temperatures, and pressure conditions associated with methods of sterilization may vary, depending on the model and use. The operating conditions must be monitored

TABLE 9–7
SPORE TESTING IN STERILIZATION MONITORING USE OF BIOLOGIC INDICATORS

Situation	Rationale
Weekly monitoring of routine use and function	To detect sterilization failure from improper use or malfunction; will alert recirculation personnel to check and correct packaging procedures and sterilizer loading, operating, and functioning
When a new type of tray, cassette, and/or packaging material is used	To ensure that the sterilizing agent (steam, gas, etc.) is getting inside to the surfaces of the instruments
During and after initial training of new recirculation area operators	To verify proper operation of the sterilizer
During the first use of a new sterilizer	To make sure that the sterilizer is functioning and that unfamiliar operating instructions are being followed
During the first cycle of use after any sterilization equipment repair	To verify that the sterilizer is functioning properly
After any change in sterilizer loading procedure	To make sure that the sterilizing agent has access to each item
With sterilization of every implantable device allowing enough lead time for sterilization to be verified	To ensure sterilization of items to be implanted into tissues

Adapted from Miller, C. H. Sterilization: Disciplined microbial control. Dental Clinics of North America 35(2):339–355, 1991.

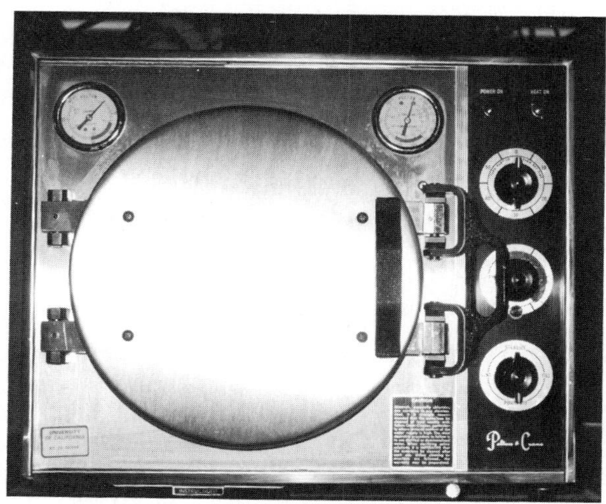

FIGURE 9–36
Autoclave.

weekly with biological indicators to confirm that the values established for operation are effective.[27]

Steam Sterilization (Steam Under Pressure or Steam Autoclave)

The use of saturated steam under pressure is the oldest, best known, and most widely used physical method of sterilization in oral healthcare.[1,5,21] Sterilization by steam autoclave with moist heat under pressure can be accomplished in 15 to 20 min at 121°C (250°F) with steam pressure of 15 lb per in.^{2} (psi). Effective use of the autoclave depends on the ability of the steam to penetrate the packaging material in order for sterilization of the items to occur (Fig. 9–36; see Procedure 9–3 for assuring effective performance of the steam autoclave). Thus, use of solid, nonporous packaging or closed containers (e.g., items wrapped/sealed in aluminum foil, vials, or tubes with solid lids/caps) is not recommended because they prevent the passage of steam to the package contents.[1,5]

PROCEDURE 9–3

ASSURING EFFECTIVE PERFORMANCE OF THE STEAM AUTOCLAVE

Equipment

Autoclave	Indicator tape	Biological monitor
Packaging material	Slow-change chemical indicator	

Steps	Rationale
1. Check operating conditions (cycle time, temperature and pressure gauges) daily (Fig. 9–37)	1. Suboptimal operating conditions cause sterilization failures (insufficient time or temperature to kill)

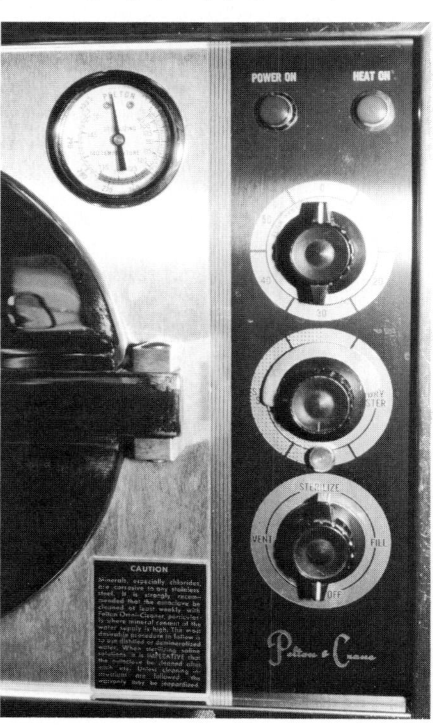

FIGURE 9–37
Close-up of autoclave showing gauges.

CONTINUED ON FOLLOWING PAGE

PROCEDURE 9–3

ASSURING EFFECTIVE PERFORMANCE OF THE STEAM AUTOCLAVE

Continued

Steps	Rationale
2. Keep operations manual in an accessible location within the noncontaminated zone of the recirculation center for ease of reference (Fig. 9–38). Review manual periodically	2. Operation of sterilizing equipment varies, and most sterilization failures are due to errors in following operation instructions

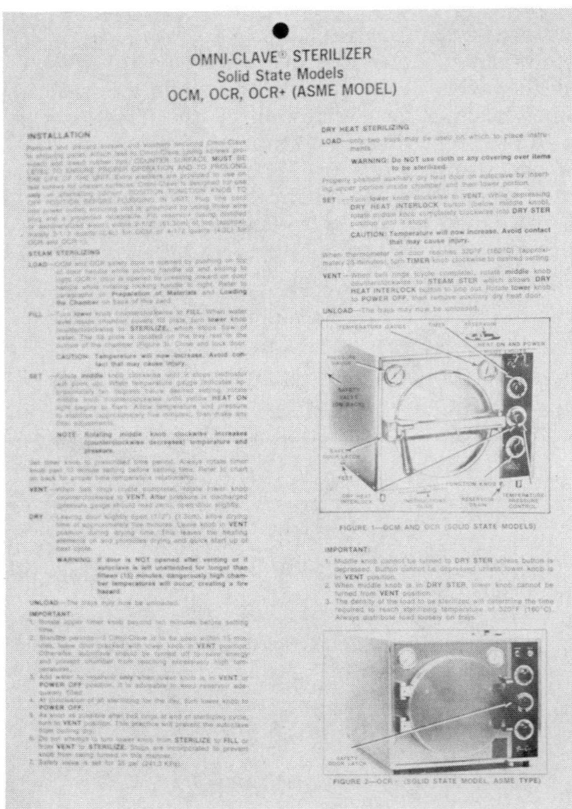

OMNI-CLAVE® STERILIZER
Solid State Models
OCM, OCR, OCR+ (ASME MODEL)

FIGURE 9–38
Operations manual.

Steps	Rationale
3. Use distilled or deionized water instead of water from community supply	3. Use of hard water may leave deposits on instruments
4. Select packaging materials designed for use in a steam autoclave (plastic tubing, poly film paper pouches, *open metal* or *glass containers* (Fig. 9–39)	4. Use of packaging not designed for steam autoclave prevents sterilizing agent (steam) from penetrating to instruments inside

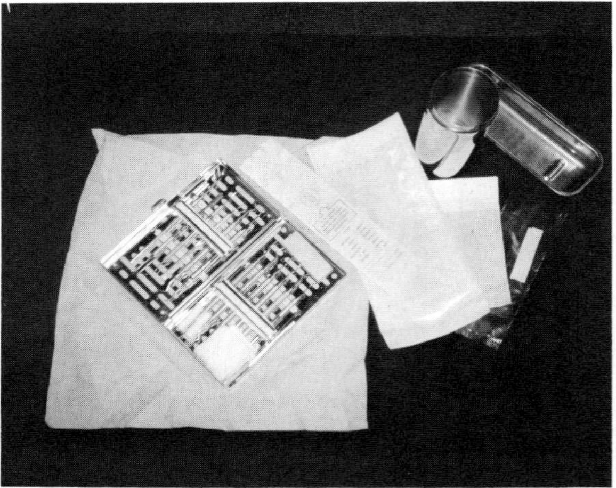

FIGURE 9–39
Various packaging materials.

Steps	Rationale
5. Avoid use of sealed or closed containers or aluminum foil for packaging materials	5. Closed containers and impervious packaging does not permit direct contact of steam with contacts
6. Prevent the formation of interior air pockets by packaging instruments securely without wrapping them so tightly that steam penetration is precluded	6. Interior air pockets (inside packaging) may not permit penetration of sterilizing agent (steam)
7. Enhance steam access to packages by placing wrapped packages on edge, with no more than two layers of packs on each shelf. The upper layer should be placed perpendicular and cross-wise to the one below; avoid packaging contact with the chamber walls (Fig. 9–40). If opened containers are used they should be placed on their sides	7. Allows for thorough contact of steam with all chamber contents

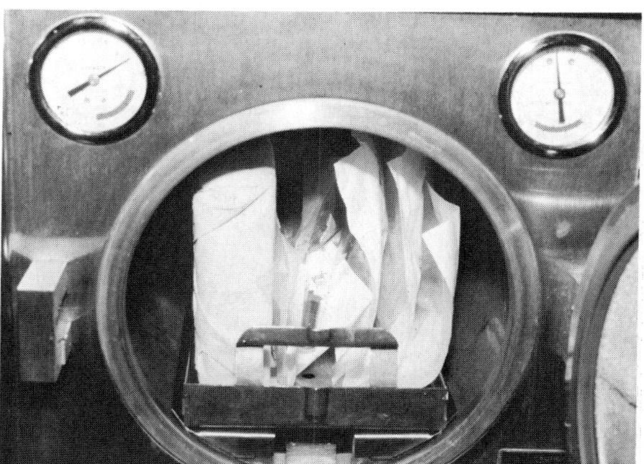

FIGURE 9–40
Packages loaded into autoclave.

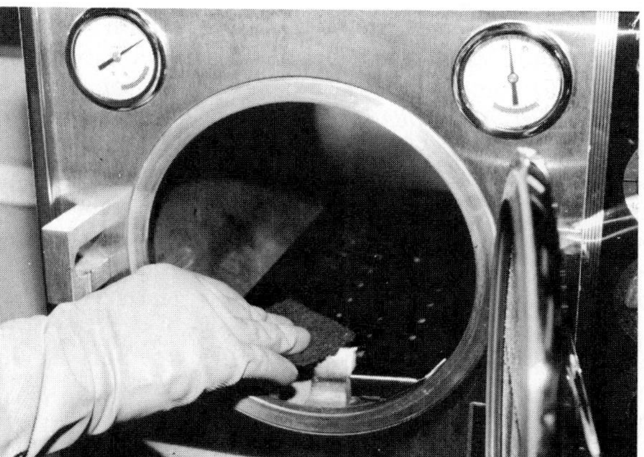

FIGURE 9–41
Nitrile-gloved hand washing interior for maintenance.

Steps	Rationale
8. Inspect all fittings and seals regularly, especially the door gasket (see operations manuals for guidelines)	8. Ill-fitting seals and gaskets may inhibit achieving proper sterilizing conditions (pressure and temperature)
9 Maintain equipment by washing all internal surfaces weekly with a mild detergent, and rinse well (Fig. 9–41). Locate the discharge line and remove the plug at the opening. Using a funnel, flush the line with 3 to 4 quarts of hot water to clean the screen/strainer	9. Poor equipment maintenance may result in sterilization failure
10. Use indicator tape or markings on all packages processed for clear identification of items processed (not an accurate predictor of sterilization) (Fig. 9–42). Place a slow-change chemical indicator into one item once a day, and use a biological monitor (spore test) once a week	10. External indicator (rapid-change) tape on packages prevents confusion by identifying packages that have been processed; slow-change indicators (internal packaging) assess instrument exposure to temperature and steam, time and temperature, or time; biological monitoring verifies that the renewal process kills highly resistant bacterial spores (main guarantee of sterilization)

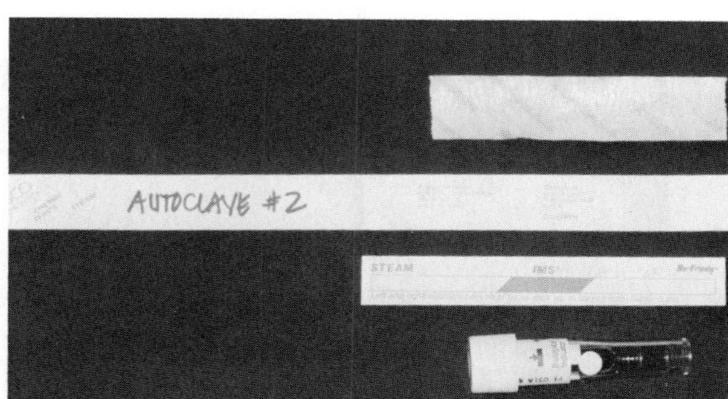

FIGURE 9–42
(Top to bottom) Postrenewal indicator tape, integrator, spore test vial.

Adapted from Miller, C. H., and Palenik, C. J. Improving the performance of the office sterilizer. Dental Asepsis Review 11(1):1–2, 1990.

The fact that the autoclave is quick (relatively short renewal cycle time), easy to use, and reliable (based on biological monitoring) and penetrates packaging materials well has contributed to the widespread use of the steam autoclave. Steam heat processing is dependent on 100% water vapor and heat to kill microorganisms by a process of denaturation (coagulation of protein). Water saturation, so critical to the quick killing of spores, causes the disadvantages of rusting, corroding, and dulling of instrument cutting edges (primarily carbon steel) and requires additional recirculation time to permit drying prior to reuse or storage. The combination of moisture and elevated temperatures negatively affects certain plastics, rubber, and other materials, which makes the steam autoclave an inappropriate method of sterilization for these items.[21]

Steam sterilizers have been used for "flash sterilization," a term used to describe the use of higher than normal temperature and shorter than normal time. By elevating the temperature to a minimum of 132°C (270°F) for 3 minutes, *unwrapped instruments* and other nonporous items may be sterilized for a minimal turn-around time (Fig. 9–43). Porous items or anything with a lumen, such as reusable air-water syringe tips, rubber or plastic items, and towels, requires 10 minutes at or above 132°C (270°F). The American Association of Medical Instrumentation, the standards-setting organization related to sterilizers and other medical devices, states regarding "flash sterilization" that "steam sterilization by the unwrapped method is not recommended if time permits the use of the preferred, wrapped methods."[17] A situation appropriate for flash sterilization would be if an instrument(s) was dropped or some other unplanned urgent need came along (see Flash Sterilization Guidelines chart). The shorter cycle time requires an even more disciplined approach to procedures to avoid any processing error and to permit steam under pressure immediate and complete access to all external and exposed surfaces and internal surfaces. Any barrier (e.g., bioburden, packaging, contact with other instruments) preventing immediate access of steam to contact all surfaces of the items delays the killing process. The major drawback with the flash method of sterilization is the lack of packaging to maintain the sterility of the processed instruments once the steam autoclave door is opened.

FLASH STERILIZATION GUIDELINES

Conditions: 132°C (270°F), 3 minutes for metal hand instruments (nonporous); 10 minutes for rubber or plastic or items with lumens (porous)

- Restrict use for unplanned urgent need and emergency situations
- Ensure proper preparation (decontamination, inspection, arrangement of separate items on tray for maximum steam exposure)
- Enhance steam access to all surfaces of items by using perforated trays, disassembling items with removable parts, opening hinged instruments, and placing items with concave surfaces open side down
- Ensure direct delivery of unwrapped sterilized instruments (sterilizer in treatment area) for immediate use.

Adapted from Miller, C. H. Flash method not for routine use. RDH 12:14, 1991.

Unsaturated Chemical Vapor

Another preferred method of sterilization that has been widely used over the past 40 years is chemical vapor sterilization (see Guidelines for Assuring Performance of the Unsaturated Chemical Vapor Sterilizer chart). Like the steam autoclave, chemical vapor sterilization uses heat (131°C [270°F]) and pressure (20 psi). Instead of using steam (100% water saturation), however, the chemical vapor system uses a solution of specific amounts of alcohol, acetone, ketone, and formaldehyde and water (8 to 12%)[21] (Fig. 9–44). The ratio of each of the chemicals must be so precise that premixed chemical solution, for use in the reservoir of the chemical vapor sterilization system, must be purchased from the manufacturer.[1] Heat, water, and chemical synergism is the critical factor contributing to the efficacy of the chemical vapor system of sterilization. To be effective, the chemical vapor must permeate the packaging material and condense on all the surfaces of the instruments in order for the gas to destroy the microbes and viruses.[28] The chemical vapor penetrates packaging at a

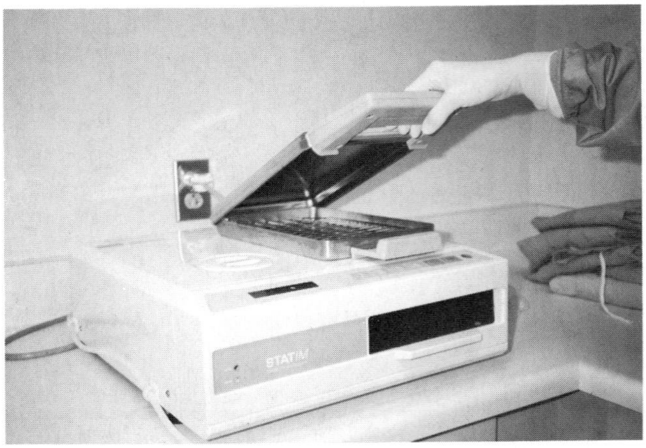

FIGURE 9–43
Autoclave with capability of rapid or flash sterilization.

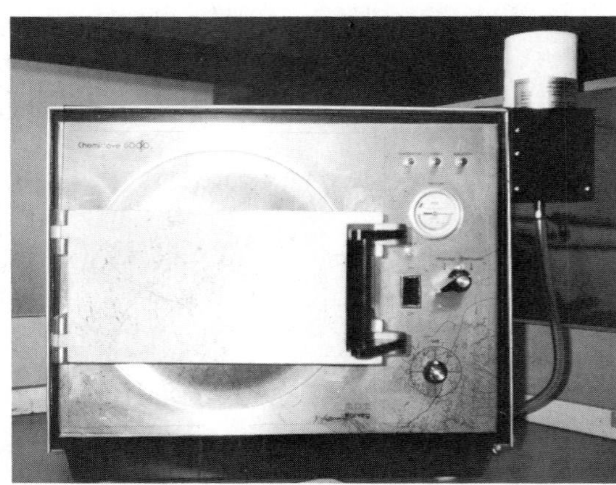

FIGURE 9–44
Unsaturated chemical vapor sterilizer.

GUIDELINES FOR ASSURING PERFORMANCE OF UNSATURATED CHEMICAL VAPOR STERILIZERS

- Check cycle time, temperature and pressure gauges daily (Fig. 9–45)

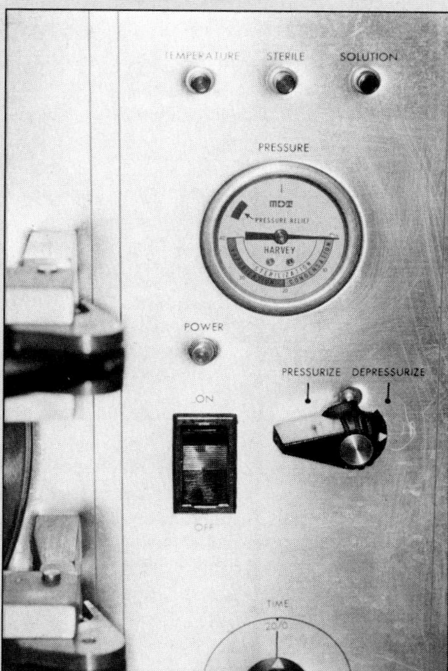

FIGURE 9–45
Close-up of chemiclave showing gauges.

- Keep the operations manual in an accessible location within the noncontaminated zone of the recirculation center for reference. Review manual periodically
- Use chemical solution prepared by the manufacturer, and maintain an adequate level of solution for operation (Fig. 9–46)

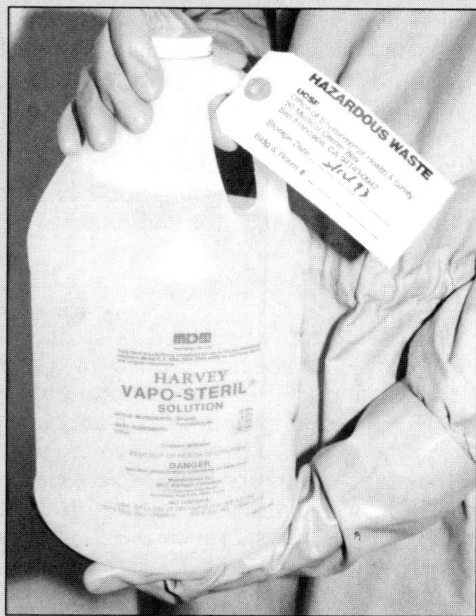

FIGURE 9–46
Chemical solution bottle.

- Select packaging materials designed for use in the chemical vapor sterilizer (paper, paper-plastic tubing, plastic—heat-sealed is best (Fig. 9–47). Perforated metal or plastic cassettes are to be wrapped in paper for processing and storage after sterilization. If glass or metal containers are used, their lids must be kept ajar

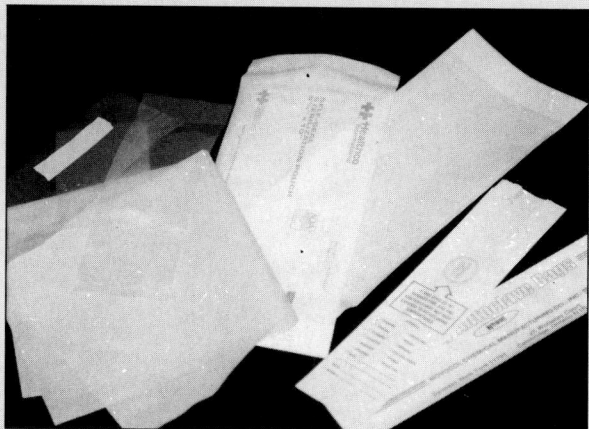

FIGURE 9–47
Assorted packaging materials.

- Avoid use of sealed containers or aluminum foil for packaging materials
- Prevent the formation of interior air pockets by packaging instruments securely without wrapping so tightly that gas penetration is precluded
- Enhance gas access and penetration to instruments by dispersing packs and cassettes throughout the chamber to allow adequate space between items. Items should not touch. *Avoid overloading* (Fig. 9–48)

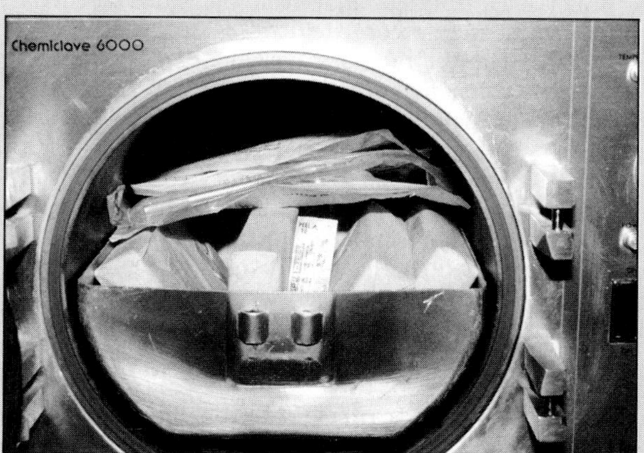

FIGURE 9–48
Chemiclave chamber with packaged items.

- Inspect all fittings and seals, especially the door gasket; refer to operations manual for adjustment or replacement procedures
- Maintain equipment by cleaning the unit weekly according to the manufacturer's recommendations
- Place indicator tape on all packages processed for clear identification of items processed (not an accurate

Continued on following page

GUIDELINES FOR ASSURING PERFORMANCE OF UNSATURATED CHEMICAL VAPOR STERILIZERS *Continued*

predictor of sterilization) (Fig. 9–49). Place a slow-change chemical indicator into one item once a day, and use a biological monitor (spore test) once a week

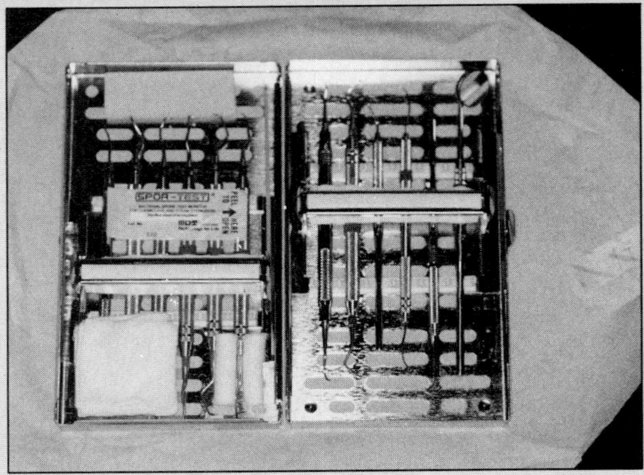

FIGURE 9–49
Package with postrenewal indicator tape. Biological monitor strip.

Data from Miller, C. H., and Palenik, C. J. Improving the performance of the office sterilizer. Dental Asepsis Review 11(1):1–2, 1990.

slower rate than saturated steam under pressure. Therefore, 30 minutes is required for the chemical vapor sterilizer's cycle[1] (20 minutes plus the 10 minutes required for the temperature and pressure to rise to the appropriate level).[21]

For both steam sterilization and chemical vapor sterilization, the two heat and pressure methods, the two cycle times are similar, and they have the advantage of automatic, preset cycle timing.[1] However, the slower penetration of chemical vapor compared with steam does pose some limitations on the type of packaging that can be used with unsaturated chemical vapor. For example, muslin (cloth), absorbent materials, or heavy textile wrappings preclude effective penetration of the chemical vapor to the instruments.[21] Packaging materials should be checked to be sure they are compatible with unsaturated chemical vapor sterilization. Other important considerations for successful vapor penetration and sterilization involve operation, loading, monitoring, and maintenance.

An important advantage of the chemical vapor sterilization method is the reduction in water content and the resultant prevention of rusting, corrosion, and dulling of metals because of the lack of moisture on the instruments prior to and during processing.[1,5,21] Because metal instruments rust if the water content in a sterilizer solution is 15% or greater, the chemical vapor sterilization method is designed not to exceed the 15% water vapor threshold. The solution for the vapor method contains 8 to 12% water. Additional moisture brought in on instruments, however, could raise the water content above the threshold and cause rusting or spotting of non–stainless steel instruments.[1,15,21] Therefore, instruments must be thoroughly dried before packaging to consistently realize the benefit of corrosion and dullness prevention.[1,15]

The short cycle time, prevention of rust and corrosion, and the fact that instruments are dry at the end of the sterilization cycle are advantages of the unsaturated chemical vapor method of instrument recirculation when compared to the autoclave method.[1] A drawback, however, is the special chemical solution required by this form of sterilization. The chemical solution increases the cost and creates a need for adequate ventilation to deal with the chemical vapors released when the door of the chamber is opened at the end of the cycle. The odor from the heated chemical solution in the surrounding area is unpleasant and may cause some operator discomfort if the air circulation is inadequate for removal of the fumes. Many toxicity studies have been conducted by the manufacturer to determine irritation and other side effects from working around the residual vapor, particularly the presence of formaldehyde. The vapors are not considered harmful. Yet, discomfort may occur if the air circulation is poor unless the model is equipped with a special filtration device to reduce the fumes from the chamber at the end of the cycle.[1,21]

Dry Heat Sterilization

Dry heat is another preferred method of sterilization (Fig. 9–50). The absence of moisture created by water (steam autoclave) or chemical solutions (unsaturated chemical vapor) as part of the sterilization process affects the conditions that must be met in order for all microorganisms to be killed through the use of dry heat. Moist heat coagulates proteins within microorganisms. Because with dry heat microbial proteins are more resistant to the denaturation process, the length of time and the level of temperature required for sterilization are increased. The lack of efficiency with the standard dry heat sterilizing oven is reflected in the recommended operating conditions of 320°F (160°C) for 2 hours or 340°F (170°C) for 1 hour.[1,21] The standard dry heat sterilizing oven may not be practical for routine

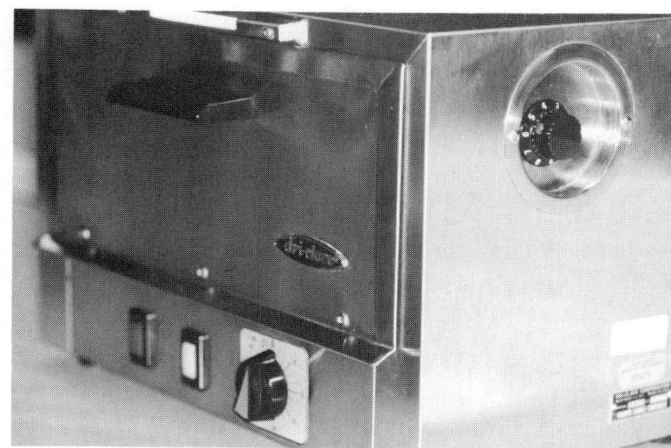

FIGURE 9-50
Dry heat oven sterilizer showing gauges.

use in busy healthcare settings because of the long turnaround or may be used only on occasion as an alternative approach to sterilization.[21]

Even though the use of hot air to kill microorganisms in a standard dry heat sterilization oven is less efficient, the significant advantage with the absence of water vapor is the prevention of rust or dulling of susceptible instruments and cutting edges.[1] For precautions note that higher temperatures preclude dry heat sterilization from being used on many rubber and plastic-based materials. The melting of some plastics or adhesive tapes could release toxic gases.[20] Additionally, the high temperatures will melt the solder of most impression trays, weaken some fabrics, and char or scorch other fabrics and paper materials.[1]

Dry heat sterilization ovens use either conduction (direct contact with a heat source) or convection (heated air) *with* or *without* forced air circulation units. The heat distribution of convection ovens may be irregular, resulting in substantial temperature variation within the chamber[21] (Fig. 9-51). Large versions of the smaller countertop convection oven are available from scientific supply companies. Large forced air circulation ovens have an internal circulation fan that gives a more even heat distribution in the chamber.[5,30] Dry heat oven sterilization in the oral healthcare environment is best accomplished by commercial equipment that has been tested and approved by the U.S. Food and Drug Administration (FDA).[1]

The effectiveness of a sterilization method is dependent on the ability of element(s) used to kill microorganisms to penetrate through the packaging and to have access to all surfaces of the item being renewed. Dry heat sterilization requires that all the instruments reach the optimal temperature (warm-up time) and that the temperature be sustained for the prescribed time.[5] Verifying the oven temperature alone may be misleading, as it represents the temperature of the oven and not that of the instruments. The instrument load temperature can be determined with a thermocouple and pyrometer.[31]

Once the load temperature has been reached, the sterilization time must be sufficient and sustained without opening the oven to put in additional items; otherwise the complete cycle must be started over. The two most frequent misuses of dry heat sterilization are insufficient exposure time and interruption of the cycle to add items without starting the time interval over again.[1,5]

Advances in dry heat sterilization technology are evolving and include *rapid heat transfer.* This type of oven utilizes a controlled internal air flow system that causes the instruments to warm faster as the hot (elevated temperature of 375°F) air is rapidly circulated within the chamber (Fig. 9-52). The increased temperature and air circulation may result in sterilization in 6 to 12 minutes—6 minutes for unwrapped instruments for immediate reuse and 12 minutes for wrapped instruments.[5] The rapid heat transfer sterilizer has been authorized by the FDA for commercial distribution as a medical device in the United States since 1987. It is approved by the Underwriters Laboratory under the product category "Medical and Dental Equipment, Professional" and has been professionally recognized with a seal from the ADA.[16]

Packaging materials for dry heat sterilization are more limited than for the steam autoclave and chemical vapor sterilization methods. Plastic and poly film wrapping materials melt in dry heat sterilizers. Although a few packaging materials survive all three types of sterilization, it is important to check with the packaging manufacturer to confirm appropriateness for dry heat sterilization.[5,21] Thick instrument wraps and oversized packages can also have an effect on the length of time required to ensure sterility.[1]

The arrangement of the instruments for loading in the oven for sterilization is very important in order for the hot

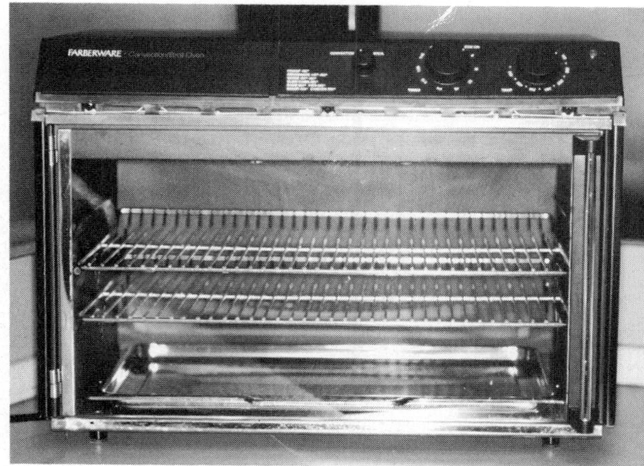

FIGURE 9-51
Convection oven.

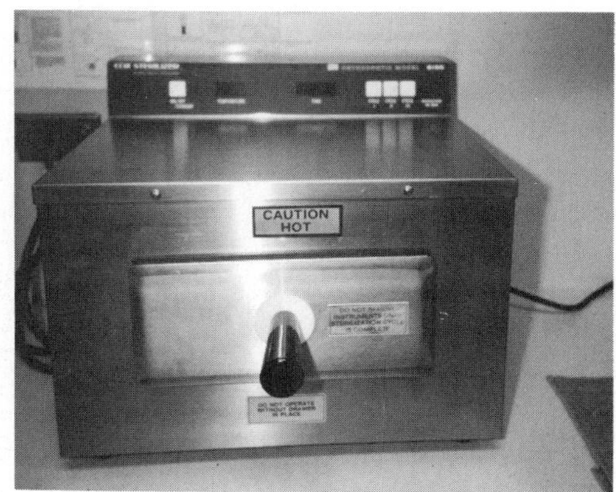

FIGURE 9-52
Rapid heat transfer oven sterilizer.

GUIDELINES FOR ASSURING PERFORMANCE OF DRY HEAT STERILIZERS

- Check operating conditions (cycle timing and operating temperature) daily
- Keep the operations manual in an accessible location within the recirculation center noncontaminated zone for ease of reference. Review manual periodically
- Use packaging materials specifically designed for dry heat sterilization (some plastic pouches or tubing, aluminum foil, closed or open glass/metal containers or trays (Fig. 9–53)

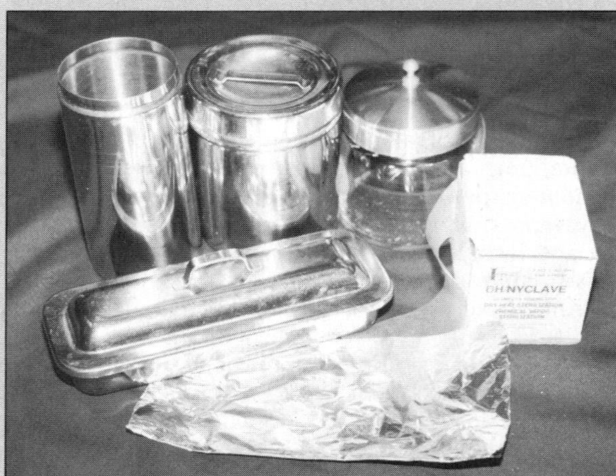

FIGURE 9–53
Assorted packaging materials most suited for dry heat sterilization.

- Do *not* sterilize plastic items or adhesive tapes; there is potential for release of toxic gases
- Avoid overloading. Separate items on *all levels* by at least 0.5 inch. Cassettes or packages should be no more than two layers deep, with the top layer at a right angle to the bottom layer. Air circulation is essential (Fig. 9–54)

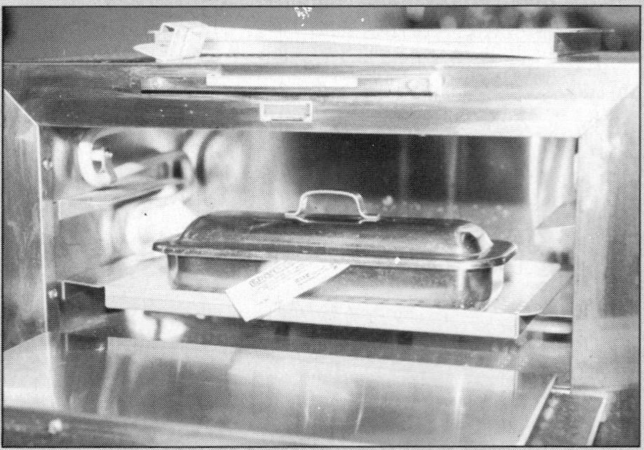

FIGURE 9–54
Packages in dry heat oven.

- Select an oven with an air circulation fan to provide more even heat distribution within the chamber
- Allow time for a warm-up period after the chamber has been loaded, prior to starting the sterilization cycle. Some ovens do this automatically; however, even these should be routinely monitored
- Do not interrupt the cycle by opening the door. The entire cycle *must be restarted* if such an interruption in sustaining the temperature occurs
- Maintain equipment by cleaning the unit with a mild detergent once a week (Fig. 9–55). The unit should be rinsed well and allowed to air-dry. Check the chamber and door insulation at this time

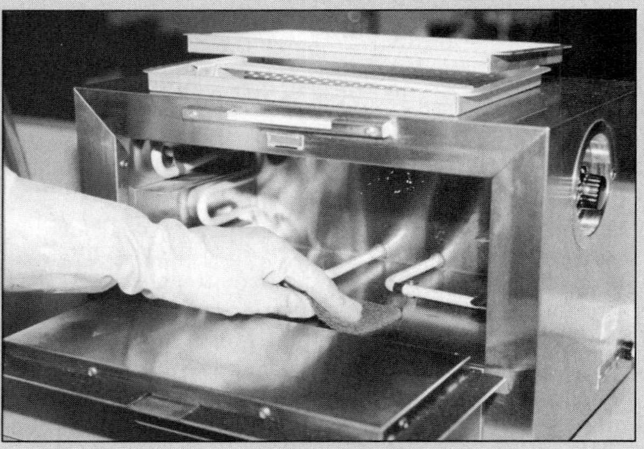

FIGURE 9–55
Nitrile-gloved hand with detergent cleaning oven.

- Place a slow-change chemical indicator into one package or cassette once a day, and use a biological monitor (spore test) once a week (Fig. 9–56)

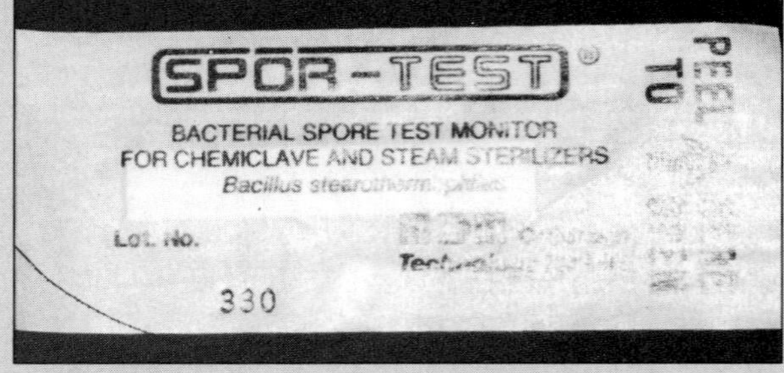

FIGURE 9–56
Spore test monitor.

Data from Miller, C. H., and Palenik, C. J. Improving the performance of the office sterilizer. Dental Asepsis Review 11(1):1–2, 1990.

air to have access to all instruments. Packages and cassettes should be placed on their edges rather than stacked flat. A second layer should be placed perpendicular to the bottom layer.[5] There should be a space (approximately 0.5 inch) between instrument packages and cassettes to ensure uniform hot air distribution during the cycle. Overloading the oven should be avoided if the space for hot air access is limited. Otherwise some instruments may be sterilized while others in the same batch are not because of stratification and the creation of air pockets (see Guidelines for Assuring Performance of Dry Heat Sterilizers chart).

Ethylene Oxide

Ethylene oxide gas is a method of sterilization, frequently used in the hospital environment or in a manufacturing arena for sterilizing commercial products[32] (see Table 9–6). This colorless gas (sporicidal/virucidal) penetrates at room temperature and is among the preferred sterilization methods because it is verifiable with biological monitors. Sterilization is accomplished by the ethylene oxide acting as an alkylating agent that irreversibly inactivates cellular nucleic acids and proteins. The fact that sterilization may be accomplished at room temperature makes ethylene oxide ideal for items damaged by heat and/or moisture. The ADA and CDC recognize ethylene oxide as an acceptable method of sterilization[1] (see Guidelines for Assuring Performance of Ethylene Oxide Sterilizers chart).

Ethylene oxide sterilization units are expensive however, and the cycle times range from 1 and a half hours to 12 hours, depending on the type of unit (Fig. 9–58). The unit that has a heating element is more expensive but takes less time than the unheated portable model that sterilizes at room temperature in 12 hours. The more affordable portable models are impractical for most oral healthcare settings because of the long turn-around time for instrument sterilization.[30] In addition, these portable models require post-sterilization aeration (10 to 16 hours for nonporous items; 24 to 48 hours for porous materials) to dissipate the residual ethylene oxide gas (Fig. 9–59). Insufficient aeration of items can cause tissue irritation (painful burns) when the residual gas on item surfaces contacts epithelial tissues.

GUIDELINES FOR ASSURING PERFORMANCE OF ETHYLENE OXIDE STERILIZERS

- Check operating conditions (cycle time and temperature) daily (Fig. 9–57)

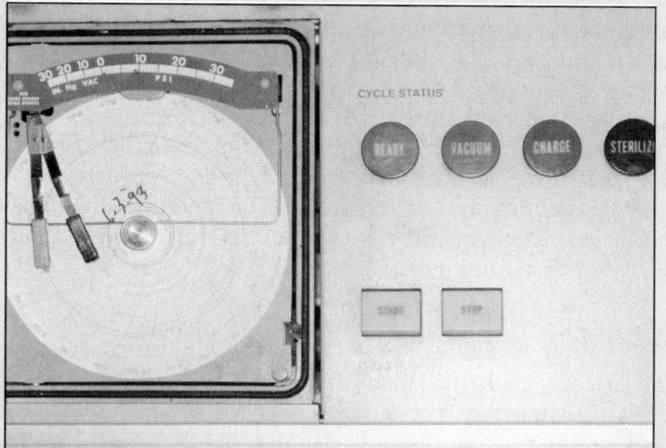

FIGURE 9–57
Close-up of gauges.

- Keep the operations manual in an accessible location within the noncontaminated zone of the recirculation area for ease of access and review of procedures for the gas sterilizer and for the aeration equipment
- Verify gas supply
- Select packaging materials designed for use with ethylene oxide sterilization, such as gas-permeable paper and plastic bags, perforated metal/plastic trays, or cassettes wrapped with paper. (Sealed metal or glass containers and aluminum foil are unacceptable, since gas must be allowed to penetrate wrap or container.)
- Avoid overloading the chamber with bags/cassettes in order to permit gas access to all item surfaces during the sterilization process. Large quantities of wrapped goods or towels are more reliably sterilized by steam autoclave
- Check the seal, fittings, and door gasket of the unit as well as the ventilation system
- Maintenance
- Each package of instruments to be sterilized should be sealed with indicator tape specifically designed for ethylene oxide use. At least once a day a Biologic Company's slow change chemical indicator should be placed inside a bag or cassette; a biological indicator should be used once a week

Adapted with permission from Cottone, J. A., Terezhalmy, G. T., and Molinari, J. A. Practical Infection Control in Dentistry. Philadelphia: Lea & Febiger, 1991; and American Dental Association Council on Dental Materials, Instruments, and Equipment; on Dental Practices; and on Dental Therapeutics. Infection control recommendations for the dental office and the dental laboratory. Journal of the American Dental Association 116:241–248, 1988.

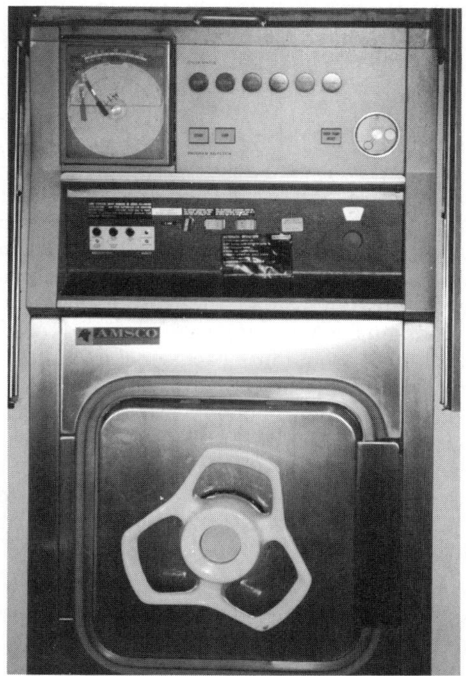

FIGURE 9–58
Ethylene oxide gas sterilizer.

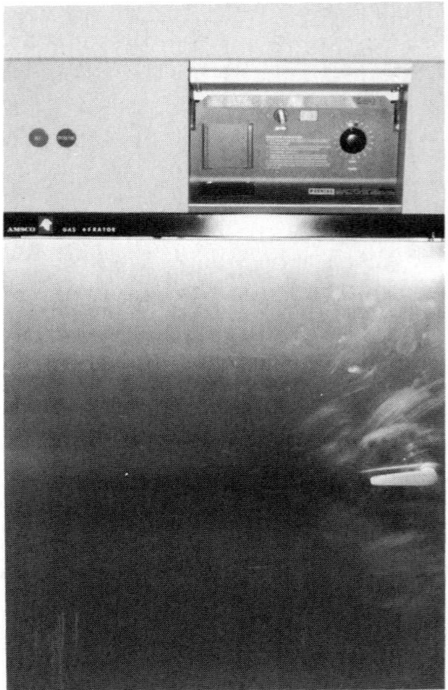

FIGURE 9-59
Aerator for poststerilization aeration.

When aeration is adequate for the porous materials, tissue irritation is prevented, since the vapor evaporates without leaving a residue.[1]

It should be noted that the nature of pure ethylene oxide is rather toxic, allergenic, and slow in action and forms explosive mixtures with air. For professional or commercial use, ethylene oxide is prepared to contain carbon dioxide or an inert gas to form a more stable active combination. The potential for explosion still exists, however, during the sterilization cycle in the presence of a flame or spark. Therefore, items must be processed in a special container with a spark shield. The fact that ethylene oxide causes irritation to eyes and nose, is toxic to skin, and has mutagenic or carcinogenic effects requires safe handing procedures and adequate ventilation in the recirculation area.[1,32]

QUALITY ASSURANCE

Factors affecting *quality assurance* aspects of instrument recirculation relate to time limitations, supplies, equipment regular maintenance, weekly biological monitoring, and meticulous record keeping.[33] Time constraints may affect compliance with protocols in the instrument recirculation process. Additional compromises of quality would be incurred if supplies (solutions, packaging materials, process indicators, and biological monitors) were inadequate for instrument recirculation, maintenance of renewal equipment, and monitoring of processing effectiveness. It is critical that equipment selected for instrument renewal be sterilized with one of the preferred and verifiable methods. Some of the variables that affect the efficiency of the sterilizer include:[34]

- Instrument cleaning
- Wrapping of instruments
- Proper loading
- Operating temperature
- Exposure time
- Maintenance

ELEMENTS ESSENTIAL TO ENSURING INSTRUMENT STERILIZATION

- Quality sterilization equipment and maintenance
- Comprehensive operator training
- Correct operation of sterilization equipment
- Use of biological indicators to monitor the effectiveness of sterilization procedures

The oral healthcare team members' compliance with regard to recirculation protocols is the critical element for ensuring the quality of prevention of disease transmission. It is essential to provide written protocols for each area of the instrument recirculation center and a training program for all members of the oral healthcare team along with written protocols. The team member responsible for coordinating the instrument recirculation center also assists with protocol training, equipment purchase and maintenance, and monitoring of the sterilization performance, including maintenance of records of the biological indicator testing results[35] (see Elements Essential to Ensuring Instrument Sterilization chart).

Biological Indicators

The use of biological indicators (spore tests) is the only mechanism currently available to verify the effectiveness of sterilization procedures and equipment operation. Biological indicators (BIs) contain highly resistant, nonpathogenic, bacterial spores that are more difficult to kill than any other microbes. Currently, there is no mechanism, technique, or product available to prove sterility of the instruments processed. As a result, a risk exists that a nonsterile item may be present in a load of renewed instruments. Through the implementation of the essential elements of sterilization quality assurance, however, it is possible to achieve a 99.9999% or better probability of success. Such a probability means that the possibility of the presence of a nonsterile item is 1 in 1,000,000.[5,36]

The Food and Drug Administration developed an index of probable sterility called "sterility assurance level" (SAL) or microbial safety index. The probability of one surviving microorganism in 1,000,000 is equal to an SAL of 6. An SAL of 4 would have a probability of one survivor in 10,000; and an SAL of 3 would have a probability of one survivor in 1,000. Sterilization validation with the use of biological indicators has been accepted by the FDA with the standard SAL of 6 required to indicate that the sterilization process is effective.[37] The specific spore species selected for the biological indicators is based on the sterilization method being monitored (see Table 9-7). The reliability of the biological indicators in identifying sterilization failures is dependent on the specific type and variable number of microorganisms present on the indicator.[34] *Bacillus stearothermophilus* is a standard organism considered to be the spore most resistant to steam and chemical vapor sterilization. *Bacillus subtilis* is the spore most resistant to dry heat and ethylene oxide sterilization.[5,28] The biological indicator selected should be suited for the specific method of sterilization to be monitored. For monitoring a combination of methods of sterilization, dual species biological indicators (containing both types of spores) would be an appropriate choice.[5] Biological indicators used to test

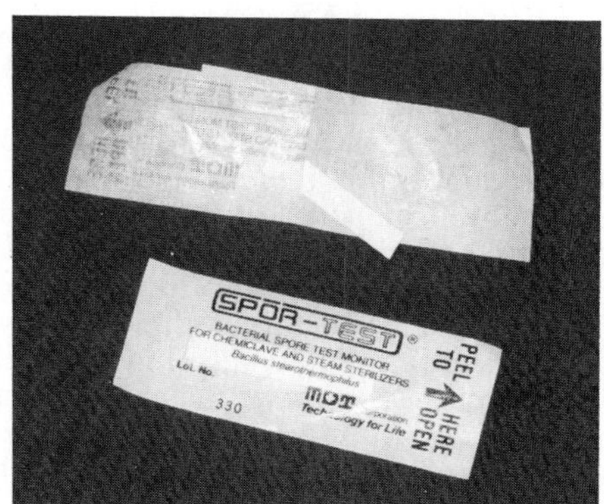

FIGURE 9–60
Spore strips.

sterilizers should contain approximately 10,000 (10^4) to 1,000,000 (10^6) spores.[34]

The packaging of the spores for biomonitoring varies. *Spore strips,* filter paper strips impregnated with the microorganisms, are encased in an envelope through which the sterilizing agent must be able to penetrate (Fig. 9–60). Spore strips may be used for verifying steam, chemical vapor, dry heat, or ethylene oxide gas sterilization. *Spore vials* are self-contained vials that have *vents* to permit access of the sterilizing agents (Fig. 9–61). They contain a small paper disc or strip of spores plus a small ampule of culture medium that is crushed and mixed with the spores *after* the renewal processing. Spore vials are better suited for use with steam and ethylene oxide sterilizers. The *spore ampule* biological indicator is a *sealed glass ampule* containing *B. stearothermophilus* spores encased with a vial of culture medium. It is effective only for monitoring steam sterilization. There are no biological monitoring tests for any liquid chemical sterilants (e.g., glutaraldehydes, chlorine dioxide).[5]

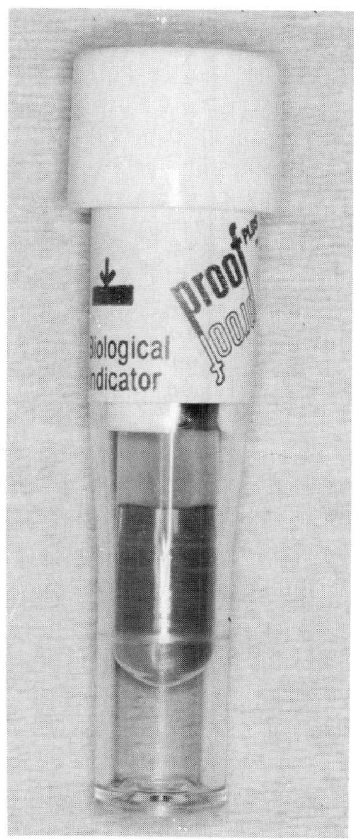

FIGURE 9–61
Spore vial.

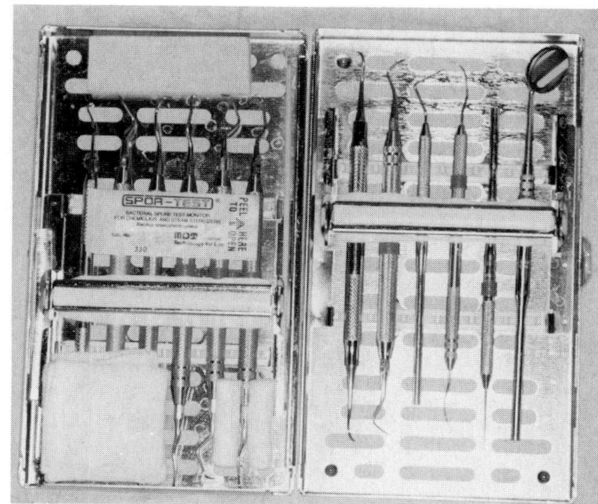

FIGURE 9–62
Open cassette with strip placed inside.

Both the CDC and the ADA recommended that biological indicators be used at least weekly to ensure the quality of sterilization procedures.[7,38] The states of Indiana and Ohio have laws that mandate spore-testing (weekly and monthly, respectively) of dental office sterilizers, and it is likely that other states will follow.[5,39,40] There are other quality assurance indications for use of biological indicators in addition to routine verification of proper use and functioning of the sterilizing equipment[5] (see Table 9–7).

The steps for routine biomonitoring include the following:

1. Placement of the strip, vial, or ampule inside an instrument cassette or package (Fig. 9–62)
2. Processing of the package along with other items in the usual size load
3. Retrieval of the biological indicator after sterilization
4. Incubation of the test indicator along with a control biological indicator from the same lot number of the test (Fig. 9–63). The processing conditions such as time, tem-

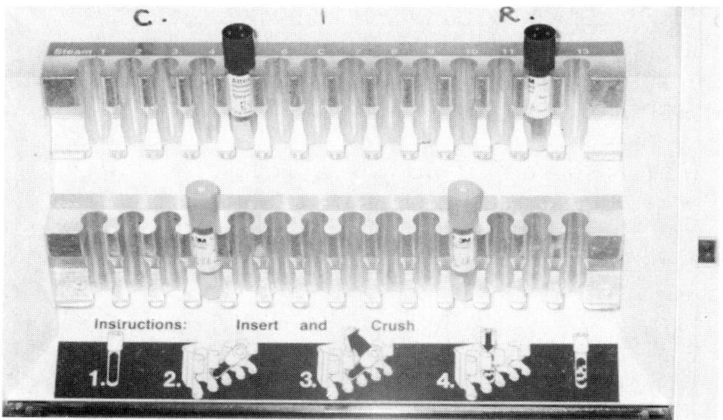

FIGURE 9–63
Incubator with test indicator and control biological indicator.

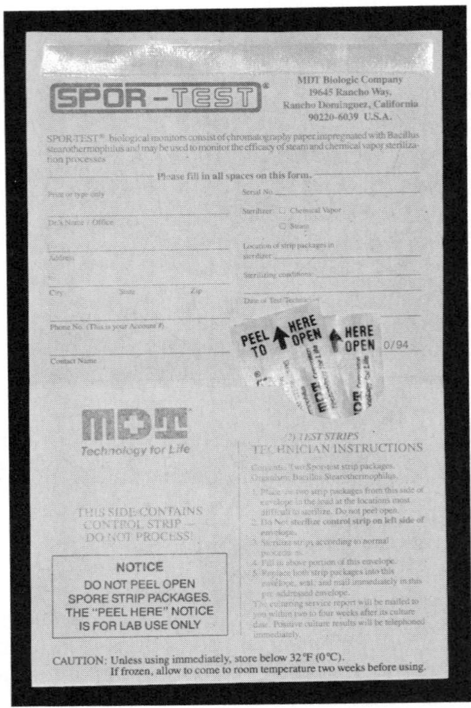

FIGURE 9-64
Mailer for spore testing service (envelope and strips).

perature, and pressure as well as biomonitoring test results should be recorded.

An alternative to in-office incubation is subscribing to the convenience of spore testing through a mail-in sterilization monitoring service available commercially or through some dental schools (Fig. 9-64). If on-site incubation is preferred, both test and control biological indicators should be assessed for growth of any remaining live spores after the prescribed incubation period. A control, biological indicator test must be done with every test to ensure that microbial growth will occur when the biological indicator is processed in conditions inadequate for sterilization. *The control must always show growth in order for the test to be valid.* The results of the spore testing must be recorded and kept on file (Fig. 9-65).

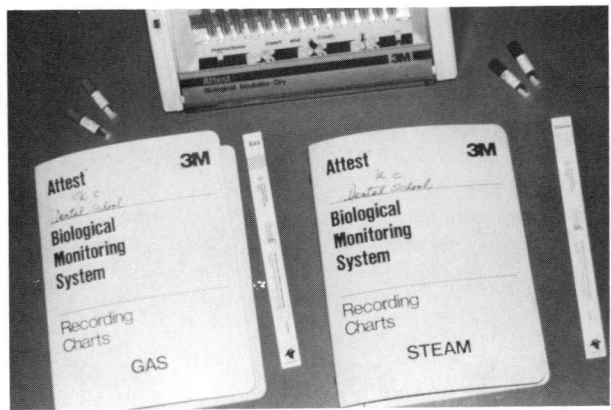

FIGURE 9-65
Record-keeping books of spore testing for the evaluation of sterilizing equipment for documentation.

When a test biological indicator shows microbial growth, sterilization failure is evident and that biological indicator should be analyzed to ascertain that the growing organisms are the same as the challenge organisms. If evidence supports a sterilization failure, it is necessary to pin-point and correct the cause of the sterilization failure. A number of studies done on sterilization performance show variations in failure rates when comparing performance of specific types of sterilizers (autoclave, dry heat, chemical vapor); yet all found high rates of sterilization failure for overall (total) sterilizer performance.[35] In two Minnesota studies that spanned a 10-year period, operator error was determined to be a major cause of sterilization failure.[35,41] Therefore, the importance of comprehensive operator training is key to maintaining high-quality instrument recirculation procedures.

Although the use of biological indicators is not a magical solution for problems with instrument sterilization, spore tests are the only definitive verification mechanisms available for evaluation of the sterilization process. Chemical indicators (heat- and steam-sensitive indicators) and chemically treated tapes are useful external indicators of processing and gross malfunction. The ultimate approach to minimizing risk of infectious disease transmission for clients and the dental team requires implementing and maintaining high-quality instrument sterilization procedures.[1,5,35]

Poststerilization Procedures

Maintenance (Storage)

The goal of aseptic technique during poststerilization procedures is to protect sterilized instruments from recontamination between renewal and reuse. The recirculation area designed to receive the renewed instruments after sterilization must be clearly identified as a noncontaminated zone to prevent mingling of sterile packages with nonsterile packages (see Fig. 9-2). The noncontaminated zone includes areas for cooling, storage, and dispensing. Any drying required prior to cooling should be accomplished at the conclusion of the sterilization cycle within the steam autoclave chamber. Wet packaging materials may indicate removal of packages too soon after the sterilization cycle, overloading of the chamber, improper arrangement of the packs in the chamber, use of inappropriate packaging material, or sterilizer malfunction. Wet poststerilization packaging compromises sterility, since microorganisms may penetrate through the material and the integrity of packaging may be broken. In addition, compressed or torn pack-

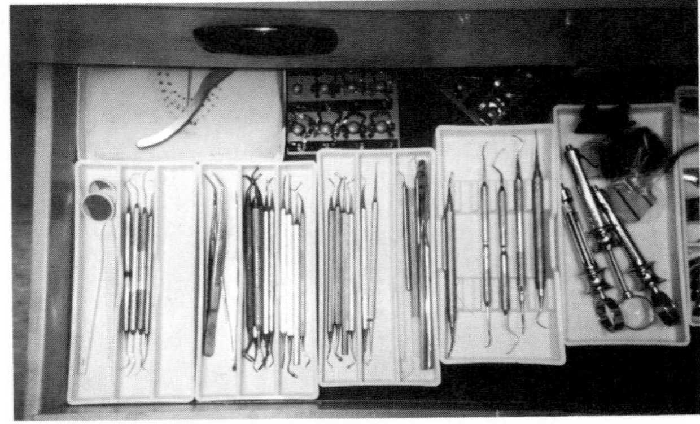

FIGURE 9-66
Trays with unwrapped instruments.

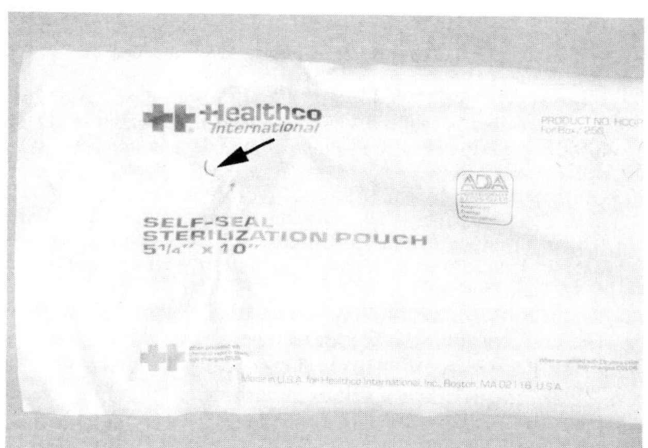

FIGURE 9-67
Torn paper packaging with instrument protruding.

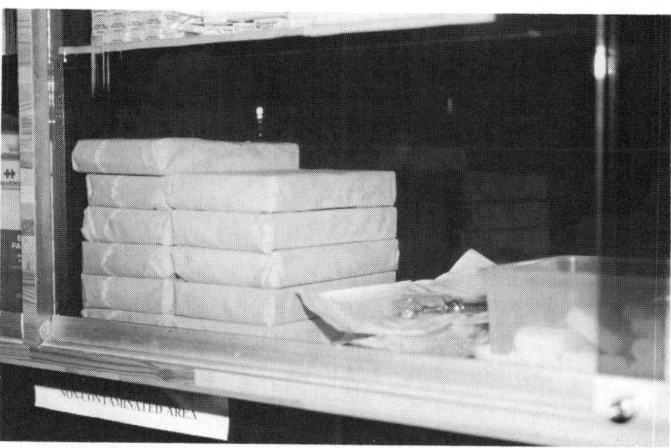

FIGURE 9-69
Cassettes or packages of sterile instruments stored behind glass doors.

ages, packages that drop on the floor, or packages touched with contaminated heavy-duty gloves are considered contaminated. The sterility of *unwrapped instruments* is compromised immediately after sterilization of instruments[5] (Figs. 9-66 and 9-67).

The noncontaminated zone should include counter space adjacent to the sterilizers for cooling of instrument cassettes, trays, and packages after removal from heat sterilizers (Fig. 9-68). Cooling of instruments permits ease in handling for storage. The cooling area should be designated to permit packages to remain untouched and protected from contaminants in the environment.[5,15]

Once instruments have cooled, packages are stored until they are needed in the treatment area. Instrument storage requires continued protection from recontamination. Ideally, the noncontaminated storage area is on shelving protected by glass doors to provide dry, low-dust storage; located in low-traffic areas, away from floors, outside walls, and ceilings; and protected from moisture and heat sources that would affect packaging integrity.[5,15]

A guiding rule for minimizing time between sterilization and reuse is to date packages and rotate on a "first in, first out" basis (Fig. 9-69). The shelf life of minimally handled, well-protected and sealed sterile packages is considered to be 1 month (Fig. 9-70).

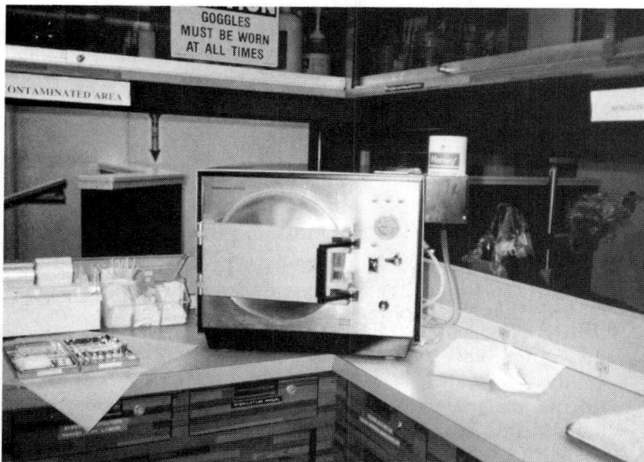

FIGURE 9-68
Noncontaminated area adjacent to sterilizers.

The shelf life of sterile packages depends on the following:[1,5]

- Maintenance of packaging material integrity
- Storage protected from environmental factors of dust, moisture, and heat
- Reduced handling to prevent contamination
- Maximum storage time limit of 30 days

Dispensing

The last area in the flow of procedures in the recirculation center is the dispensing area (see Fig. 9-2). The noncontaminated dispensing area is the area where sterilized instruments and disposable items (e.g., sterile gauze packets, disposable saliva ejectors) are assembled. The selected instrument cassette or tray is combined with the unit dose disposable supply items required for the dental hygiene care procedure planned (Fig. 9-71). All materials and equipments kept in the dispensing area are sterile or disinfected and noncontaminated. Contamination must be meticulously avoided. The dispensing area is the preferred location for disposable supplies such as cotton swabs, cotton rolls, and client napkins rather than the treatment areas. Avoiding dispensing of supplies within each treatment area minimizes the risk of contamination due to potential aerosols and spatter of oral fluids so prevalent in the operatory.[15] The use of drawers in treatment areas for

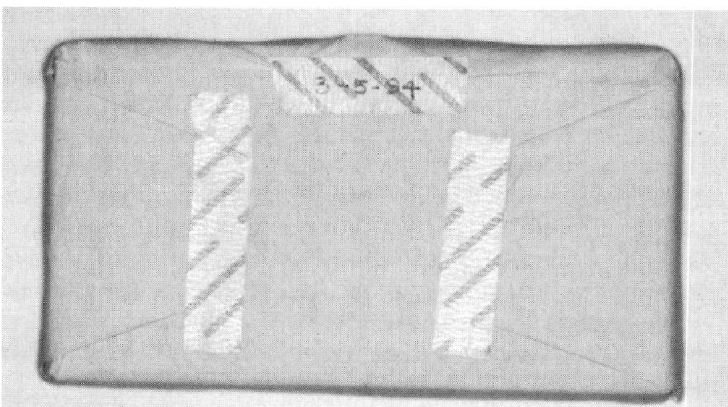

FIGURE 9-70
Dated label on sterilized package/cassette.

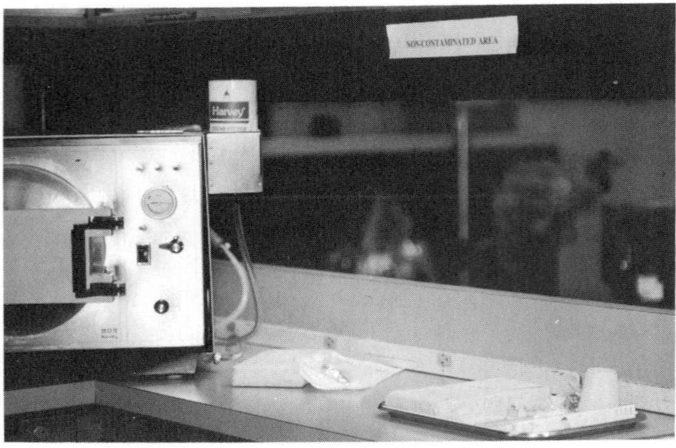

FIGURE 9-71
Dispensing section. Recirculation area with cassette, packages, and unit dose items prepared for transport to treatment area.

unwrapped or wrapped instrument distribution and supply item dispensing is plagued with great potential for cross-contamination.[5] Sterilized instrument cassettes, trays, and packages can be unwrapped and opened at chairside for use.[5] Opening sterile packages at chairside in front of the client preserves sterility up to the time of the dental hygiene care and helps meet the client's human need for safety, reassuring them of the high standard of infection control.

References

1. Cottone, J. A., Terezhalmy, G. T., and Molinari, J. A. Practical Infection Control in Dentistry. Philadelphia: Lea & Febiger, 1991.
2. Centers for Disease Control. Recommendations for prevention of HIV transmission in health care settings. Morbidity and Mortality Weekly Report 36:2-S, August 21, 1987.
3. Cottone, J. A. Recent developments in hepatitis: New virus, vaccine, and dosage recommendations. Journal of the American Dental Association 120:501, 1990.
4. Pollack, R. Form follows function. California Dental Association Journal 17(2):17, 1989.
5. Miller, C. H. Sterilization: Disciplined microbial control. Dental Clinics of North America 35(2):339, 1991.
6. Rosenbaum, W. Gloving—can it be a time bomb? Control, The Infectious Disease Newsletter 6(9):4, September 1991.
7. Centers for Disease Control. Recommended infection control practices for dentistry. Morbidity and Mortality Weekly Report 35:237, 1986.
8. Department of Labor, Occupational Safety and Health Administration. Occupational exposure to bloodborne pathogens: Final rule. Federal Register 56(235):64004, 1991.
9. Molinari, J. A., and Gleason, M. J. Medical waste controversies. California Dental Association Journal 18(4):37, 1990.
10. Shaefer, M. E. Hazardous waste management. Dental Clinics of North America 35(2):383, 1991.
11. American Dental Association. Infectious waste disposal in the dental office, Q & A. Journal of the American Dental Association (Suppl.) S211:1, August 1989.
12. Miller, C. H. Infection alert—instrument sterilization. Dental Assistant 4-5:43, March-April 1990.
13. Miller, C. H. Instrument cleaning involves multiple steps. American Dental Association News, May 1990, pp. 23-24.
14. Miller, C. H., and Hardwick, L. M. Ultrasonic cleaning of dental instruments in cassettes. General Dentistry 36:31, 1988.
15. Shaefer, M. E. Central sterilization area. Office Sterilization and Asepsis Procedures Research Foundation Report 4(3):1, 4, 1991.
16. Ask the experts. Control, The Infectious Disease Newsletter. 3(5):6, 1988.
17. Miller, C. H. Flash method not for routine use. RDH 12:14, 1991.
18. Whitacre, R. J., Robins, S. K. et al. Dental Asepsis. Seattle: Stoma Press, 1979.
19. Miller, C. H., and Palenik, C. J. Sterilization, disinfection, and asepsis in dentistry. In Block, S. S. (ed.). Sterilization, Disinfection, and Preservation. Philadelphia: Lea & Febiger, 1991, pp. 676-695.
20. Office Sterilization and Asepsis Procedures Research Foundation. Position paper 4-002, Instrument sterilization: Improving the performance of the office sterilizer. Office Sterilization and Asepsis Procedures Research Foundation Report, Issn 1041-4142, Summer 1991.
21. Runnells, R. R. Heat and heat/pressure sterilization. California Dental Association 13:46-49, October 1985.
22. Balanyk, T. E. Chemical sterilizing/disinfecting solutions: Which ones are best for what? Oral Health 77:42, May 1987.
23. American Dental Association Council on Dental Therapeutics. Quaternary ammonium compounds not acceptable for disinfection of instruments and environmental surfaces in dentistry. Journal of the American Dental Association 97:855, 1978.
24. Cottone, J. A., and Molinari, J. A. State of the art infection control in dentistry. Journal of the American Dental Association 122:33, 1991.
25. Miller, C. H. Sterilization and disinfection: What every dentist needs to know. Journal of the American Dental Association 123(3):46, 1992.
26. American Dental Association Council on Dental Materials. Instruments and equipment: Sterilizers and sterilization devices. In Dentists' Desk Reference: Materials, Instruments, and Equipment, 2nd ed. Chicago: The American Dental Association, 1983.
27. Miller, C. H., and Palenik, C. J. Indiana dental infection control laws, part II. Dental Asepsis Review 11(4):1, 1990.
28. Crawford, J. J. Clinical Asepsis in Dentistry, 2nd ed. Mesquite, Texas: R. A. Kostad, 1978.
29. Office Sterilization and Asepsis Procedures Research Foundation. Glutaraldehyde for Instrument Sterilization. January 1993. Distributed to Foundation members, April 3, 1993.
30. Department of Veterans' Affairs, American Dental Association, Department of Health and Human Services. Infection control in the dental environment. Washington, DC: Learning Resources Service and Eastern Dental Education Center, VA Medical Center, 1989.
31. Crawford, J. J., and Jackson, R. J. Principles of sterilization and disinfection. In McGhee, J. R., Michalek, S. M., and Cassell, G. H. (eds.). Dental Microbiology. New York: Harper & Row, 1982.
32. American Dental Association Council on Dental Therapeutics. Sterilization or disinfection of dental instruments. In Accepted Dental Therapeutics, 40th ed. Chicago: The American Dental Association, 1984.
33. Reveal, M. ADHA perspective. Journal of Dental Hygiene 6416:18, 1990.
34. Nickerson, A., Bhuta, R., et al. Monitoring dental sterilizers' effectiveness using biological indicators. Journal of Dental Hygiene 64:69, 1990.
35. Hastreiter, R. J., Molinari, J. A., et al. Effectiveness of dental office instrument sterilization procedures. Journal of the American Dental Association 122(10):51, 1991.
36. Association for the Advancement of Medical Instrumentation (AAMI). Selection and use of chemical indicators for steam sterilization monitoring in health care facilities. Arlington, VA: AAMI, 1988.
37. Keller, J. J. Sterilization monitoring. Control, The Infectious Disease Newsletter 6(6-7):4, 1991.
38. American Dental Association Council on Dental Materials, Instruments, and Equipments; on Dental Practice; and on Dental Therapeutics. Infection control recommendations for the dental office and the dental laboratory. Journal of the American Dental Association 116:241, 1988.
39. Indiana State Board of Health, Dental Health Division. Indiana public law 123-1988, dental on-site compliance review check list. Indianapolis, IN: February 1, 1990.
40. Ohio State Dental Board of Examiners. Infection Control Rules. Columbus, OH: November 1, 1987.
41. Simonsen, R. J., Schachtele, C. F., and Joos, R. W. An evaluation of sterilization by autoclave in dental offices (abstr. 1236). Journal of Dental Research 58A:400, 1979.

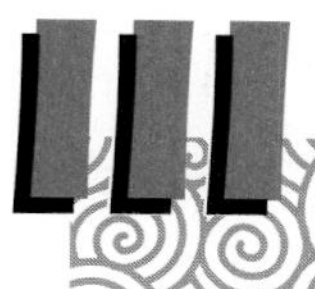

III DENTAL HYGIENE ASSESSMENTS

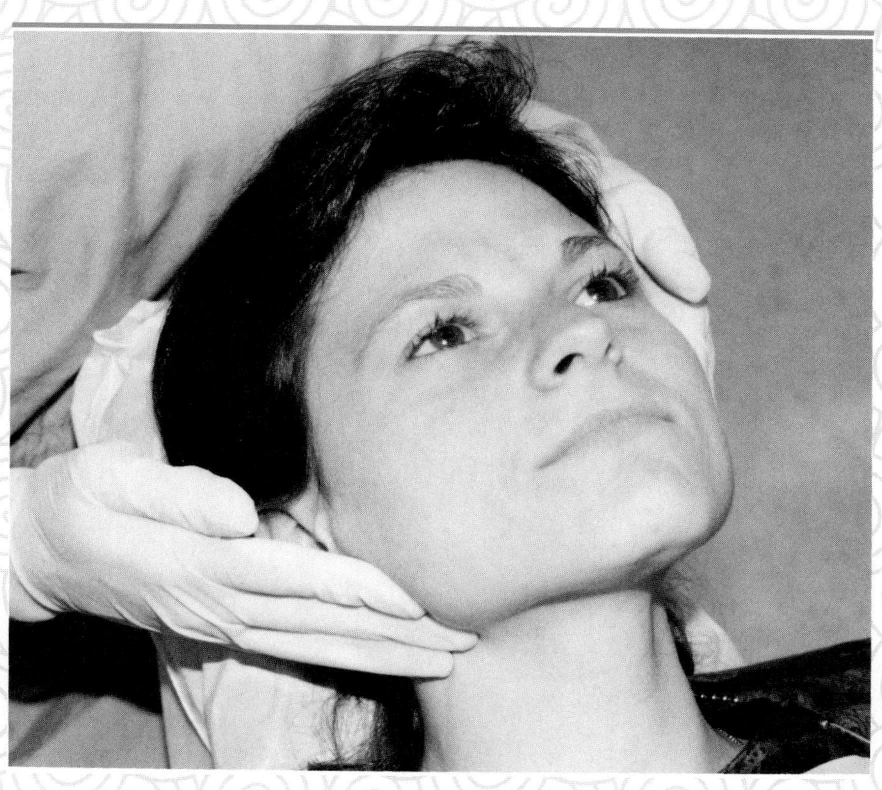

10 Assessment of Client Health History Data and Vital Signs

OBJECTIVES

Mastery of the content in this chapter will enable the reader to:

- Identify and describe the vital signs
- Describe when it is appropriate to take the vital signs
- List and describe the advantages and disadvantages of the three types of thermometers
- Obtain a client's temperature using a mercury-in-glass thermometer
- Obtain a client's radial pulse
- Describe the technique to measure a client's respiration
- Obtain a client's respiration rate
- List and describe the advantages and disadvantages of the three types of manometers
- Describe the technique to measure a client's blood pressure using an aneroid or mercury manometer and stethoscope
- List the normal ranges for the vital signs
- Identify the appropriate equipment utilized for taking vital signs
- List the uses of the ***Merck Manual***
- Identify and describe factors that can influence the vital signs
- Describe the purposes of the client's health history
- Describe how a health history and knowledge of vital signs are related to meeting the client's human need for safety
- List the four indices of the *Physicians' Desk Reference (PDR)*
- Obtain information about prescription drugs that the client is taking by utilizing the *PDR*
- Recognize disease conditions for which dental hygiene care is contraindicated
- Recognize medications or allergies that may alter the dental hygiene care plan
- Recognize signs of undiagnosed disease conditions from reports by the client in the health history
- Avoid emergency situations in the oral healthcare environment by careful evaluation of the client's health history
- Identify and describe the conditions that warrant prophylactic premedication
- Describe the protocol for prophylactic premedication
- Discuss indications for seeking medical consultation regarding the client's health status

HEALTH HISTORY

Throughout the dental hygiene process of care, the dental hygienist collects accurate information about the client's health status to meet the client's human need for safety. Initially, information about the client's health status is obtained during the client's health history interview prior to dental hygiene care. The health history enables the dental hygienist to:

- Identify client human needs related to oral health and disease and provide comprehensive dental hygiene care
- Assess overall physical and emotional health and nutritional status
- Identify conditions that necessitate precautions to ensure that oral healthcare meets the client's need for safety and that medical emergencies are prevented
- Assist in the medical and dental diagnosis of various conditions

- Identify conditions for which the client should be referred for evaluation
- Establish baseline information about the client's health status
- Maintain legal documentation as a mechanism for managing risks

The health history form is completed by the client and verified by the dental hygienist at the first visit and then reviewed at each appointment to verify and document changes. A complete and thorough health history provides information concerning the client's health and well-being, including current measurements of blood pressure, pulse, and respiration. In addition, a health history should contain information about the client's past and present medical and dental conditions, risk factors for disease, medications being taken, undiagnosed conditions, and allergies or unusual reactions. The health history also should include a section on personal and social history that elicits information about the client's lifestyle, cultural practices related to health and disease, past and present emotional problems, and general state of mind (see also Appendix I, Tobacco Use Assessment Form, at the end of this chapter). The major rationale for taking the client's health history is to identify any of the following:

- Diseases or medications that contraindicate dental or dental hygiene care
- Diseases or conditions that require special precautionary measures for the client prior to care
- Reactions to drugs
- Infectious diseases that endanger others
- Special physiological states such as pregnancy

Assessment of the Client's Health Status

Table 10–1 provides a comprehensive list of items that can be included on the written health history form with additional follow-up questions that should be verbally asked by the dental hygienist during client assessment. Prior to the oral health history interview, the dental hygienist should mentally evaluate the client for the following:

- How is the overall appearance of the client?
  - Emotions: happy, depressed, fearful?
  - Physical gait: injuries, diseases, functional status?
  - Color/pallor?
  - Eyes: alert, bright, glassy, focused?
  - Dress and personal hygiene?
- Does the client respond well to questions? Are the responses correct, applicable, coherent?
- Is the client using any type of assistive device (e.g., cane, walker)?
  - How dependent is the client on the device?
  - Does the client prefer that you assist him? (Client independent or reliant on others?)
- Does the client have any obvious impairments in function that the dental hygienist may need to know more about?
- Could the client be under the effects of a medication? Alcohol? Illegal drug? (Client is sleepy, incoherent, distracted, depressed, moody, uninterested? Slurred speech?)
- Does the client seem emotionally stable? Is the client eager to talk and to share, or disoriented, depressed and gloomy, irritable, angry, scared/anxious?
- If the client does not seem emotionally stable, could the emotional state be related to medications, stroke, other systemic problems, or psychiatric problems?
- Is the client potentially dangerous to self? To the dental hygienist?
- Is the client at risk for a medical emergency?
- Is there a potential language or cultural barrier that needs to be overcome?

There are standard forms for the written health history (Fig. 10–1). However, workers in each oral healthcare setting should determine their needs for a health history form, and review and update the form on a periodic basis.

The health history form constitutes a legal document that provides past and present information about the client's health. Therefore, the health history form should be completed by the client in nonerasable ink (pencil is not acceptable), and comprehensive information should be recorded. The client should sign the written health history form at each appointment to indicate its accuracy. If the client is a minor (younger than 18 years of age), a parent or legal guardian should sign and date the health history form. The signature also grants permission for services to be rendered during the appointment.

To meet the client's ongoing human need for safety, the health history should be updated at each appointment by documenting changes in the client's health since the last visit. After reviewing the health history with the client, the dental hygienist should date (month, day, and year) and sign the chart entries in nonerasable pen. Entries should be carefully written and legible; mistakes should be neatly lined out and initialed. Since the client's chart is a legal record, mistakes should never be covered with correction fluid or lined out until the entry is illegible. Positive answers to the health history questionnaire can be marked in red or highlighted for easy visibility at the initial appointment. Any YES or positive responses on the health history should be explained in full. The client's health history is confidential information that cannot be shared with others without the permission of the client. Confidentiality is essential for meeting the client's human need for territoriality.

Use of the *PDR* and *Merck Manual* in the Dental Hygiene Process of Care

Before dental hygiene care, medications currently taken by the client should be investigated and documented. Some medications taken by the client can alter treatment outcomes, may be contraindicated with medications used for dental and dental hygiene treatment, or indicate the need for a medical consultation prior to initiating dental or dental hygiene care. The ***Physicians' Desk Reference (PDR),*** an essential guide for dental hygiene practice, provides valuable information about prescription drug products. For example, as shown in Figure 10–2, a drug's action, usage, contraindications, adverse reactions, warnings, and precautions are available and readily accessible via the *PDR*. The *PDR* also displays colored pictures of the dispensed form of medications, so a visual identification can be made when the client cannot verbally identify his medication. Sections of importance to the dental hygienist found in the *PDR* are described in Table 10–2. These sections are color-coded in the *PDR* for easy access by the practitioner.

Product information can be retrieved if the medication can be identified in sections 2 to 4 of the *PDR*. The sections most commonly used are the Product Category Index and Product Name Index. Once the medication is identi-

Text continues on page 280

TABLE 10–1
HEALTH HISTORY ITEMS EXPLAINED

Item	Purpose	Additional Questions	May Indicate a Deficit in the Human Need For:
Date	To indicate when the form was last completed		
Date of birth	To indicate the client's age accurately (asking "How old are you?" will not reflect the client's current age if a new health history is not completed every year) To indicate if the client is a minor, and the need for a consenting adult to sign the health history To alert the dental hygienist that young children need morning appointments To assist in identifying some oral conditions that are age related To be considered in the development of educational strategies To identify older people who are prone to orthostatic hypotension		Safety
Name, telephone, home address, employer information	Necessary to conduct the business aspect of the practice		Safety
Height and weight	Necessary to calculate drug dosages A marked change in weight may indicate an undiagnosed disease process		Safety Nutrition
Occupation	To determine if a factor in disease etiology via exposure to occupational hazards, stains, nutrition, occlusal wear To determine, in part, educational level of the client To determine the potential for financial barriers to care		Safety Conceptualization and problem solving
Previous dentist's name, address, and phone	To determine where to send for previous radiographs To call for consultation on a preexisting condition		Safety
Physician's name, address, and phone	To consult on disease conditions, problems, or suspected undiagnosed conditions To contact in an emergency		Safety
What is your estimate of your general health?	To reveal a significant medical problem or disability To reveal client's determination of own health To identify client who is a hypochondriac or emotionally disturbed	How important is the client's health to her?	Value system
Why are you now seeking dental hygiene or dental care?	To reveal chief complaint in the client's own words To reveal a need for immediate treatment or referral to a specialist	Type of problem? Date of onset of symptoms? How important is the client's oral health to her?	Value system

Table continued on following page

TABLE 10–1
HEALTH HISTORY ITEMS EXPLAINED *Continued*

Item	Purpose	Additional Questions	May Indicate a Deficit in the Human Need For:
When was your last physical examination?	To reveal a significant medical problem To identify clients who do not obtain regular healthcare	What was it for? Any problems found? Was it with the same physician noted above or was it with a specialist?	Value system Safety
Is the client currently under the care of a physician? If so, what for?	To indicate any surgery or anticipated surgery To determine if the client is seeking care from other physicians To determine if the person is at risk for a medical emergency	What is the nature of the condition? What type of treatment has the client had or is the client having?	Safety
Is the client taking any medications? List them.	To identify: Current medications the client is taking Medications contraindicated for dental and dental hygiene treatment Medications contraindicated with dental medications Potential drug interactions The cause of **xerostomia**	What is the type of medication, dosage, and reason for its use?	Safety
Has the client taken any medications within the past year?	To reveal a prior condition or problem	What was the type of medication, dosage, and reason for its use?	Safety
Is the client allergic to any medication?	To indicate any medication that should not be prescribed for the client in the course of dental or dental hygiene treatment	When was the allergy determined? What is the type of medication? What type of reaction occurred?	Safety
Has the client experienced an unusual reaction to penicillin, aspirin, iodine, sulfa drugs, or other medications?	To identify medications that should not be given to the client (iodine may be an ingredient in disclosing solution, the use of which should be avoided with clients reporting an allergy to iodine)	What were the circumstances? What type of reaction did the client have (e.g., allergic reaction or a stress reaction)?	Safety
Have there been any changes in the client's health within the past year?	To identify an illness that may reflect on the client's oral care A recent change may indicate an alteration in local anesthetic solution	What type of illness did the client have? What treatment was involved? Were there any relapses or problems involved?	Safety
Has the client ever been hospitalized?	To alert for recurrence in oral cavity if hospitalized for cancer To identify factors that may influence the client's oral care To identify local anesthesia precautions that may be needed if prior history of problems To determine if the client has a compromised health condition	What was the reason for hospitalization? Did any problems occur? Were there any complications?	Safety

TABLE 10–1
HEALTH HISTORY ITEMS EXPLAINED *Continued*

Item	Purpose	Additional Questions	May Indicate a Deficit in the Human Need For:
Has the client lost or gained more than 10 pounds in the last year?	To determine if the client has an undiagnosed condition, such as uncontrolled diabetes, acquired immunodeficiency syndrome (AIDS), tuberculosis, anxiety, stress, carcinoma, heart failure, eating disorder, thyroid problems	When did this occur? What was the cause? Did the client change or start new medication?	Nutrition Freedom from pain/stress
Does the client have or has she ever had any of the following conditions: Heart disease	To alert the dental hygienist that prophylactic premedication may be required To identify clients that may need minimal stress and shorter appointments To identify clients who may have increased bleeding if they are taking **anticoagulants**	What type of heart disease? Any medication? Type? Has the client taken prophylactic antibiotic premedication for previous dental or dental hygiene care?	Safety
Heart failure	To identify clients who may need a medical consultation for surgical procedures To identify clients who may need minimal stress and shorter appointments	When did it occur? Any medication? Type?	Safety Freedom from pain/stress
Heart attack	To identify clients who may be taking nitroglycerin, which will need to be available and readily accessible during treatment To identify clients who have had a heart attack within the last 6 months and for whom dental or dental hygiene treatment is contraindicated	When did it occur? If hospitalized, how long? Any complications? Any medication? Type? Any recurrences?	Safety Freedom from pain/stress
Rheumatic fever	To identify clients who may need prophylactic antibiotic premedication for heart valve damage	When did it occur? Any complications? Has the client taken prophylactic antibiotic premedication for previous dental or dental hygiene care?	Safety
Rheumatic heart disease	To identify clients who may need prophylactic antibiotic premedication	When did it occur? If hospitalized, how long? Any complications? Has the client taken prophylactic antibiotic premedication for previous dental or dental hygiene care?	Safety
Pacemaker	To identify clients for whom ultrasonic vibrations from the ultrasonic scaler or the ultrasonic cleaner are contraindicated To recognize that a medical consultation may be needed prior to dental or dental hygiene care	When did the client receive it? Any complications?	Safety

Table continued on following page

TABLE 10–1
HEALTH HISTORY ITEMS EXPLAINED *Continued*

Item	Purpose	Additional Questions	May Indicate a Deficit in the Human Need For:
Heart murmur	To identify clients with organic heart murmurs, which may indicate the need for prophylactic antibiotic premedication The cardiologist or physician of record should be contacted if the client is unsure about premedication	When was the condition diagnosed? Was the heart murmur functional or organic? Has the client taken prophylactic antibiotic premedication for previous dental or dental hygiene care?	Safety
Mitral valve prolapse	To identify clients who may need prophylactic antibiotic premedication	When was the condition diagnosed? Has the client taken prophylactic antibiotic premedication for previous dental or dental hygiene care?	Safety
Chest pain	To identify the need to minimize stress, and shorter appointments may be indicated	When was the onset of the condition? What causes the condition to occur? Was the client under the care of a physician? Any medications? Type?	Safety Freedom from pain/stress
Swollen ankles	To identify clients with conditions such as kidney disease, heart disease, an obstruction in the leg, anemia, and pregnancy (standing for long periods can cause this condition)	Does the client know the cause of the condition? Was the client under the care of a physician for the condition? Any medications? Type?	Safety
Artificial heart valves	To identify the need for prophylactic premedication To identify clients taking anticoagulants, which may cause gingival bleeding	When were the valves placed? Any complications? Any medications? Type?	Safety
Angina pectoris	To alert the dental hygienist about the need for shorter appointments To decrease stress To identify the need for good pain control To identify clients taking nifedipine, which can cause gingival enlargement	When did the condition occur? If hospitalized, how long? Any complications? Recurrences? Any medications? Type?	Safety Freedom from pain/stress
Lung disease	To identify clients who may not be able to recline fully in the dental chair because of compromised breathing	When was the condition diagnosed? What type of lung disease? Any medications? Type?	Safety
High blood pressure	To identify the need to take the client's blood pressure on a regular basis prior to dental and dental hygiene care To identify the cause of xerostomia To reveal if the condition is a symptom of other disease states To identify clients who may experience dizziness when the dental chair is returned to the upright position	When was the condition diagnosed? Was the condition controlled? Is the client currently seeking care from a physician for the condition? Any medications? Type?	Safety

TABLE 10–1
HEALTH HISTORY ITEMS EXPLAINED *Continued*

Item	Purpose	Additional Questions	May Indicate a Deficit in the Human Need For:
High blood pressure *Continued*	To alert the dental hygienist that alternative choices of local anesthetic may be indicated		
Stroke	To identify clients: Who may have physical impairments that may limit their oral hygiene behaviors or require modified oral hygiene aids Taking anticoagulants, which is a consideration prior to dental surgery Who have had a stroke within the last 6 months and for whom dental treatment and dental hygiene treatment is contraindicated	When did the condition occur? If hospitalized, how long? Any complications? Any recurrences? Any medications? Type? Any physical/mental impairments? Communication disorders? Any difficulty with oral hygiene? Does the client measure his blood pressure? Does the client use special devices to carry out daily self-care behaviors?	Safety Self-determination, responsibility
Anemia	To identify clients with a decreased ability to carry oxygen in the blood	When was the condition diagnosed? Any medications? Type?	Safety
Bruise easily	To reveal a possible blood disorder To indicate a need for a medical consultation	When was the condition noticed? Is the client seeking care from a physician for the condition?	Safety
Prolonged bleeding	To reveal a blood disorder To reveal the use of anticoagulants or aspirin To reveal a condition that should be a consideration for dental surgery and for scaling and root planing	When did this condition occur? How long was the bleeding? What were the circumstances? Is the client seeking care from a physician for the condition?	Safety
Hemophilia	To indicate the need for a medical consultation prior to surgery or any invasive procedure To identify clients at risk for increased bleeding To indicate that block injections should be avoided if possible	Any medication? Type? Any complications or problems?	Safety
Drug addiction	To avoid the client going into relapse by administering or giving narcotic medications or alcohol-containing products	When did the condition occur? What type of drug was involved? Is this currently a problem?	Safety Freedom from pain/stress
Blood transfusion	To identify client who may have been exposed to hepatitis or human immunodeficiency virus (HIV)	When did the transfusion occur? What were the circumstances? Any problems or complications?	Safety
Blood disorder	To indicate that the client's physician may need to be consulted about prophylactic antibiotic premedication	When was the condition diagnosed? Any medications? Type? Is the client in remission?	Safety

Table continued on following page

TABLE 10–1
HEALTH HISTORY ITEMS EXPLAINED *Continued*

Item	Purpose	Additional Questions	May Indicate a Deficit in the Human Need For:
Blood disorder *Continued*	or problems with immunosuppression To indicate potential changes in the care plan		
Fainting **(syncope)**	To identify clients predisposed to fainting in the oral care environment To reveal conditions such as transient ischemic attacks (prestroke), postural hypotension **(orthostatic hypotension)** and anemia To indicate the need for humanistic behaviors during care	When did the condition occur? What was the cause? Any problems associated with it? How often has it occurred?	Safety
Convulsions	To identify clients with undiagnosed epilepsy	When did the condition occur? What was the cause? Any problems associated with it? Did the client seek care from a physician for the condition?	Safety
Epilepsy	To alert the dental hygienist that the client may have an epileptic seizure in the oral healthcare environment To identify clients taking an anticonvulsant To identify clients who may be taking valproic acid, which may cause increased bleeding, or phenytoin sodium, which may contribute to gingival hyperplasia	What type of seizures are they? How often do they occur? When was the last one? What are the signs that signal the onset of a seizure? How long does it last? If hospitalized, how long?	Safety Skin and mucous membrane integrity of head and neck
Frequent headaches	To indicate chronic tension or other disease states	When does the condition occur? What type of headache is it? Any medications? Type?	Safety Freedom from pain/stress
Frequently exhausted	To indicate conditions that may be drug related or emotionally related, or indicate chronic fatigue syndrome or anemia To indicate inability to maintain daily oral health behaviors	When does the condition occur? What was the cause? Is the client seeking care from a physician for the condition? Any medications? Type?	Freedom from pain/stress Skin and mucous membrane integrity of head and neck Self-determination, responsibility
Depressed/anxious	To indicate: Conditions that may be drug related or indicate an emotional problem The need to limit stress Inability to maintain oral health behaviors	Is the client seeking care from a physician? Any medications? Type?	Freedom from pain/stress Self-determination, responsibility
Psychiatric treatment	To indicate that changes may be needed in the care plan To indicate that the client may be taking various kinds of medications	What type of condition is it? Is the client seeking care from a physician? Any medications? Type?	Freedom from pain/stress Self-determination, responsibility

TABLE 10–1
HEALTH HISTORY ITEMS EXPLAINED *Continued*

Item	Purpose	Additional Questions	May Indicate a Deficit in the Human Need For:
Immunosuppression	To indicate a systemic disease, such as lupus or AIDS To reveal clients with compromised healing To reveal clients who have greater susceptibility to disease To identify need for possible prophylactic antibiotic premedication	What is the cause of the condition? When was the condition diagnosed? Any medications? Type?	Safety Skin and mucous membrane integrity of head and neck
Herpes	To identify clients for whom dental and dental hygiene treatment is contraindicated if active oral lesions are present	How long has the client had the condition? Is it an oral condition? Does it recur and what causes the recurrence? When did it last recur?	Safety Skin and mucous membrane integrity of head and neck
Venereal disease	To identify clients for whom dental and dental hygiene treatment is contraindicated if open weeping oral sores are present	When was the condition diagnosed? What type of condition was it? Any medications? Type? Any recurrences?	Safety Skin and mucous membrane integrity of head and neck
Jaundice	To reveal conditions such as hepatitis infection	When did the condition occur? What was the cause?	Safety
Hepatitis A	To identify clients who may have liver damage and bleeding problems To alert the dental hygienist that the client may be prone to drug toxicity reactions	When did the condition occur? Any complications?	Safety
Hepatitis B	To reveal that the client may have liver damage and may be unable to metabolize drugs such as local anesthetics at a normal rate To reveal clients who are chronic carriers of the virus (antigen positive)	When did the condition occur? Any complications? Was the client tested following infection to rule out a carrier state (presence of antibodies)?	Safety
Liver disease	To reveal clients with a history of hepatitis or jaundice To reveal a condition such as liver cirrhosis To alert the dental hygienist that the client is prone to drug toxicity reactions in the event of local anesthetic administration	What type of liver disease? When was the condition diagnosed? Any medications? Type?	Safety
Thyroid disease	Clinically hypothyroid clients are unusually sensitive to central nervous system depressants (e.g., sedatives), sensitive to cold, and tend to gain weight Clinically hyperthyroid clients are unusually sensitive to heat, tend to lose weight without dieting, and have an increased appetite	What type of thyroid disease? When was the condition diagnosed? Any medications? Type?	Safety

Table continued on following page

TABLE 10–1
HEALTH HISTORY ITEMS EXPLAINED *Continued*

Item	Purpose	Additional Questions	May Indicate a Deficit in the Human Need For:
Thyroid disease *Continued*	Untreated thyroid disease may lead to life-threatening situations		
Kidney disease	To reveal clients who may have damaged kidneys and cannot excrete drugs at a normal level To indicate that the client may need antibiotic premedication	What type of kidney disease? When was the condition diagnosed? Any medications? Type? Is the client unusually sensitive to heat or cold? Is the client unusually sensitive to drugs or medications?	Safety
Frequent urination	To indicate disease states such as diabetes To indicate the use of medications such as diuretics or substances in the diet	When did this condition occur? Is the client aware of the cause of the condition? Has the client sought care from a physician for the condition?	Safety
Often thirsty	To indicate unsuspected conditions such as diabetes if the client responds to questions concerning increased weight loss and increase in appetite To indicate an underlying systemic or drug reason for xerostomia	When did this condition occur? Is the client aware of the cause of the condition? Has the client sought care from a physician for the condition?	Safety Skin and mucous membrane integrity of head and neck
Diabetes	To indicate that the dental hygiene appointment should be made soon after the client takes her **insulin** and eats To alert the dental hygienist that the client may have a tendency to heal more slowly and to need regular maintenance To alert the dental hygienist to be prepared for diabetes-related emergencies	When was the condition diagnosed? What type of diabetes is it? Any medications? Type? Is the diabetes controlled? How often is blood or urine glucose monitored? Does the client have hypoglycemic episodes? How often?	Safety Skin and mucous membrane integrity of head and neck
Persistent cough	To indicate conditions such as a respiratory problem or infection due to smoking, carcinoma, bronchitis, tuberculosis To alert the dental hygienist that the client may have compromised respiration	When did the condition start? Is the client aware of the cause of the condition? Has the client sought care from a physician for the condition? Any medications? Type?	Safety
Emphysema	To alert the dental hygienist that nitrous oxide–oxygen analgesia is contraindicated for dental treatment	When was the condition diagnosed? Any medications? Type?	Safety
Bronchitis	To alert the dental hygienist that the client may have compromised respiration	When did the condition occur? Any medications? Type? Any recurrences?	Safety
Tuberculosis	To indicate that dental and dental hygiene treatment should be deferred if the	When was the condition diagnosed? Any medications? Type?	Safety

TABLE 10–1
HEALTH HISTORY ITEMS EXPLAINED *Continued*

Item	Purpose	Additional Questions	May Indicate a Deficit in the Human Need For:
Tuberculosis *Continued*	disease recently diagnosed; the client should be on medication (usually isoniazid) for at least 2 weeks and not actively coughing, sneezing, or wheezing		
Asthma	To alert the dental hygienist that stress may precipitate an attack, and therefore steps should be taken to make the appointment as unstressful as possible	When did the condition last occur? How often does it occur? If hospitalized, how long? When was the condition diagnosed? What causes the condition? Any medications? Type?	Safety Freedom from pain/stress
Sinus problem	To identify clients who are prone to headaches or pain in the maxilla To identify clients who may have an allergy To alert the dental hygienist that the client may have problems breathing with a rubber dam	When does the condition occur? Any medications? Type? Is the client prone to headaches or pain in the maxilla?	Safety
Hay fever/hives/skin rash	To alert the dental hygienist to an unsuspected or undiagnosed drug allergy To alert the dental hygienist that dental or dental hygiene care should be deferred during periods when the client may experience an acute condition	When does the condition occur? What causes the condition? Any medications? Type?	Safety
Swollen joints/arthritis	To identify the client who: May have increased bleeding time from medications, such as aspirin and nonsteroidal antiinflammatory medication May have difficulty moving, especially in the morning May have joint replacements and may need prophylactic antibiotic premedication May need modified dental hygiene aids May need shorter appointments May have difficulty opening her mouth	What joints are swollen? Temporomandibular joint affected? What causes the condition? Any medications? Type?	Self-determination, responsibility
Glaucoma	To identify clients who may have visual impairments	When was the condition diagnosed? Any surgery performed? Any medications? Type?	Skin and mucous membrane integrity of head and neck
Measles/chickenpox/scarlet fever	To facilitate the diagnosis of enamel hypoplasia or pigmentation if high fevers were experienced	When did the condition occur? Any complications?	Biologically sound dentition
Mumps	To rule out mumps in the diagnosis if the client had a previous infection	When did the condition occur? Any complications?	

Table continued on following page

TABLE 10–1
HEALTH HISTORY ITEMS EXPLAINED *Continued*

Item	Purpose	Additional Questions	May Indicate a Deficit in the Human Need For:
Cancer treatment	To alert the dental hygienist: To watch for recurrence in the oral cavity If the client received radiation treatment to the head and neck region, there will be decreased healing and decreased secretion by the salivary glands To clients with compromised healing, in whom invasive surgery should be avoided To identify clients who may need fluoride supplements, home fluoride therapy, or salivary replacement therapy To identify clients who may be receiving long-term therapy with medications	What type of cancer was diagnosed? When did the treatments occur? Is the cancer in remission? Any medications? Type?	Safety Skin and mucous membrane integrity of head and neck Wholesome body image
Ulcers	To identify clients who may be apprehensive about dental and dental hygiene care To alert the dental hygienist that the client may have acute or chronic anxiety To identify clients who may be taking tranquilizers and antacids	When was the condition diagnosed? Any medications? Type? Is the client on a restricted diet?	Freedom from pain/stress
Cortisone treatment	To alert the hygienist that the client may be immunosuppressed	What was the treatment for? When did the treatment occur? Any complications?	Safety Freedom from pain/stress
Shortness of breath	To indicate conditions such as heart disease, obesity, emphysema, anemia, and asthma	When did the condition occur? What was the cause? Did the client see a physician? Any medications? Type?	Safety Freedom from pain/stress
Does the client use more than two pillows to sleep?	To indicate cardiovascular disease conditions (e.g., congestive heart failure)	Is there a reason for using two pillows?	Safety Freedom from pain/stress
Is the client pregnant?	To alert the dental hygienist that elective treatment is usually avoided in the first trimester To identify clients who may have difficulty in the supine position, especially in later stages of pregnancy, and who are prone to orthostatic hypotension	How many months? Any complications?	Safety Skin and mucous membrane integrity of the head and neck
Is the client taking birth control pills?	To alert the dental hygienist to gingival bleeding problems that might be partially related to the woman's hormonal balance To alert the dental hygienist to the fact that some antibiotics may alter the effectiveness of birth control medication	Name and type of medication	Safety Skin and mucous membrane integrity of the head and neck

TABLE 10–1
HEALTH HISTORY ITEMS EXPLAINED *Continued*

Item	Purpose	Additional Questions	May Indicate a Deficit in the Human Need For:
When was the client's last dental visit? X rays?	To indicate: If the client seeks regular dental treatment If recent oral radiographs should be requested To alert the dental hygienist that oral radiographic exposure should be limited if radiographs taken recently	What treatment was performed? Any problems? What type of radiographs were taken?	Safety Value system
Complications during dental treatment?	To avoid the same complication or similar complications	What type of complication occurred? What was the treatment for the complication?	Safety
Unusual reaction to dental treatment?	To identify clients prone to allergic reactions and to syncope or "fainting" To alert the dental hygienist that report of this condition should be followed up with a medical consultation if cause of reaction is unknown	What type of reaction occurred? What treatment was performed? What caused the reaction?	Safety Freedom from pain/stress
Nervous about dental treatment?	To recognize need for sympathy, patience, short appointments, and possibly antianxiety agent, e.g., valium or nitrous oxide–oxygen analgesia	What causes the nervousness? What has been done to alleviate this nervousness?	Freedom from pain/stress
Do the client's teeth affect her general health?	To assess the client's biological understanding of dentistry	In what way?	Value system
Are the client's teeth sensitive?	To indicate conditions such as recession, bruxism, sinus problems, periapical problems, eating disorders, improper self-care techniques	What causes the sensitivity? If cause is not known, ask the client about bruxing, sinus problems, home care technique	Freedom from pain/stress Biologically sound dentition
Is the client dissatisfied with the appearance of her teeth?	To alert the dental hygienist that the client may need referral to an orthodontist or prosthodontist To indicate that porcelain restorations should be used instead of gold	What causes the dissatisfaction? Any treatment performed prior?	Wholesome body image
Injury to face and jaw?	To identify clients: With temporomandibular joint disorders Who may have difficulty opening or have problems with long appointments Who may have malocclusion, devitalized or ankylosed teeth	What type of injury? Any treatment? Any complications?	Skin and mucous membrane integrity of head and neck Nutrition
Difficulty chewing food?	To indicate conditions such as ill-fitting dental appliances, missing teeth, dental caries	What causes this difficulty?	Biologically sound dentition Nutrition

Table continued on following page

TABLE 10-1
HEALTH HISTORY ITEMS EXPLAINED *Continued*

Item	Purpose	Additional Questions	May Indicate a Deficit in the Human Need For:
Bleeding gums?	To indicate conditions such as periodontal disease, blood disorder, trauma, neoplasm, nutritional deficiency, immunosuppression	What causes the gums to bleed? How often does it occur?	Skin and mucous membrane integrity of head and neck Self-determination, responsibility Nutrition
Sores in mouth?	To indicate condition such as herpes, recurrent aphthous ulcers, nutritional deficiency, trauma, immunosuppression	When did the sores occur? How long did they last? Is the cause known?	Freedom from pain/stress Nutrition Skin and mucous membrane integrity of head and neck
Sores slow to heal?	To indicate a premalignant or malignant lesion and also uncontrolled diabetes	When did the sores occur? How long did the sores last? What is the cause?	Safety Skin and mucous membrane integrity of head and neck
Personal/Social/Cultural History Items			
Substance use/abuse (e.g., tobacco, alcohol consumption)	To alert the dental hygienist: That tissue changes may be present with tobacco use That the client may have poor nutritional status That the client may be uncooperative To avoid alcohol-containing products such as mouthrinses for clients who are recovering alcoholics To possible cocaine use To identify clients with stained teeth To alert the hygienist to past or present problems with alcohol	What type of tobacco is used? How often and how much? How long has the tobacco been used? How often is alcohol ingested? How much is ingested?	Safety Freedom from pain/stress Nutrition
Tea/coffee consumption	To identify clients with stained teeth To alert the dental hygienist that the client may be prone to dental caries if taking tea or coffee with honey, sugar, or creamer substitute	How often is it consumed? How much is consumed?	Biologically sound dentition
Oral habits	To alert the hygienist to oral habits that may be deleterious to a client's oral health (e.g., holding things in mouth like pins, needles, paper clips may cause abrasion; pushing gums with fingernail may cause recession; thumbsucking, which may contribute to malocclusion)	What type of habit? Frequency, duration, and intensity of habit?	Freedom from pain/stress

fied in a particular color-coded section, the reader is referred to the Product Information Section to obtain extensive information about the particular medication. Boldfaced numbers in the *PDR* access either color photographs of the dispensed form of the drug or information concerning the medication.

The *PDR,* published yearly, reports new or revised information about prescription drug products. Other related publications include the ***PDR Drug Interactions and Side Effects Index*** and the ***PDR for Nonprescription Drugs.***

The *Merck Manual* is a standard reference handbook on diseases, including their etiology, signs and symptoms,

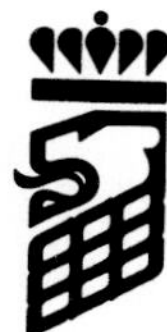

G.W. HIRSCHFELD
SCHOOL OF DENTAL HYGIENE AND DENTAL ASSISTING

DENTAL HYGIENE SERVICES CLINIC

For safe, personalized dental hygiene care, a complete and accurate health history is necessary. Dental procedures may complicate or be complicated by existing conditions elsewhere in the body; general health factors influence response to care. Please give each question careful consideration. If your answer is YES to the question, put a circle around YES. If your answer is NO to the question, put a circle around NO. To specify condition, circle the appropriate condition. Answer all questions and fill in blank spaces when indicated. Answers to the following questions are for our records only and will be considered CONFIDENTIAL.

HEALTH HISTORY

Date of Birth ____________

Social Security Number ____________

Marital Status ____________

Sex: M or F

Address ____________
____

Phone ____________

Physician ____________

Address ____________
____

Phone ____________

Address ____________
____

Phone ____________

Emerg. Contact ____________ (relationship)

Address ____________
____

Phone ____________

Address ____________
____

Phone ____________

Dentist ____________

Address ____________
____

Phone ____________

1. How would you rate your present health?
   Good Fair Poor
   a. Has there been any change in your general health within the past year? Yes No
      If yes, explain ____________
2. My last physical examination was on ____________
   a. Lab tests: ____________ Results of Exam and tests: ____________
3. Are you now under the care of a physician? Yes No
4. Who? ____________
5. Have you been hospitalized or had a serious illness within the past five (5) years? Yes No
   a. If so, what was the problem? ____________
6. Do you have or have you had any of the following diseases or problems?
   a. Rheumatic fever or rheumatic heart disease Yes No
   b. Congenital heart disease Yes No
   c. Heart trouble of any kind (heart murmur, heart attack, coronary insufficiency, coronary occlusion, angina, arteriosclerosis, stroke, pacemaker) Yes No
      1) Do you have chest pain when you exercise? Yes No
      2) Are you ever short of breath after mild exercise? Yes No
      3) Do your ankles swell? Yes No
      4) Do you get short of breath when you lie down? Yes No
      5) Do you use an extra pillow when you sleep? Yes No
   d. Cancer Yes No
   e. Allergy or hay fever Yes No
   f. Asthma or bronchitis Yes No
   g. Hives or a skin rash Yes No
   h. Fainting spells, seizures or epilepsy, headaches Yes No
   i. Diabetes Yes No
      1) Do you have to urinate (pass water) more than six times a day? Yes No
      2) Are you thirsty much of the time? Yes No
      3) Does your mouth frequently become dry? Yes No
      4) Weight gain or loss of more than 10 lbs? Yes No
      5) Slow healing? Yes No
   j. Hepatitis, jaundice or liver disease Yes No
   k. Arthritis Yes No
   l. Inflammatory rheumatism (painful, swollen joints) Yes No
   m. Stomach ulcers Yes No
   n. Kidney trouble Yes No
   o. Tuberculosis—Positive TB or PPD Test?, Chest X-ray? ____________ Yes No
   p. Do you cough a lot or cough up blood? Yes No
   q. High blood pressure or low blood pressure Yes No
   r. Venereal disease—syphilis, gonorrhea, chlamydia Yes No
   s. Oral herpes/cold sores/fever blisters Yes No
   t. Mononucleosis Yes No
   u. Joint replacement/implants Yes No

FIGURE 10–1
Sample health history form. (Adapted from G. W. Hirschfeld School of Dental Hygiene and Dental Assisting, Old Dominion University, Norfolk, VA.)

Illustration continued on following page

v. HIV positive Yes No
w. Nervous system disorders—cerebral palsy, etc. Yes No
x. Emotional or mental system disorders Yes No
y. Other ______

7. Have you had abnormal or severe bleeding after tooth extractions, surgery, or injury? Yes No
a. Do you bruise easily? Yes No
b. Have you ever required a blood transfusion? Yes No
If so, explain the circumstances ______

8. Do you have any blood disorder? (bleeder, leukemia) Yes No
9. Do you have anemia? Yes No
10. Have you had surgery or x-ray treatment for a cancer, tumor, growth, or any other condition? Yes No
11. Have you had medical x-rays in the last five years? Yes No
12. Are you taking any of the following?
a. Antibiotics or sulfa drugs Yes No
b. Anticoagulants (blood thinners) Yes No
c. Medicine for high blood pressure Yes No
d. Cortisone (steroids) Yes No
e. Tranquilizers Yes No
f. Aspirin Yes No
g. Insulin, tolbutamide (Orinase) or similar drugs Yes No
h. Digitalis or drugs for heart trouble Yes No
i. Nitroglycerin Yes No
j. Antihistamines Yes No
k. Other ______

13. Are you taking any other drug or medicine? Yes No
If so, what? ______
Condition for which taken ______
14. Have you taken any of the above in the past six months? Yes No
If so, why ______
15. Are you allergic or have you reacted adversely to:
a. Local anesthetics Yes No
b. Penicillin or other antibiotics Yes No
c. Sulfa drugs Yes No
d. Barbiturates, sedatives, or sleeping pills Yes No
e. Aspirin Yes No
f. Iodine Yes No
g. Codeine/narcotic Yes No
h. Other ______
16. Are you employed in any situation which exposes you regularly to x-rays or other ionizing radiation? Yes No
17. Are you wearing contact lenses? Yes No
18. Do you have any disease, condition, or problem not listed above that you think I should know about? Yes No
If so, please explain ______

WOMEN SHOULD ANSWER THE FOLLOWING:

19. Are you pregnant? Yes No
If yes, Trimester: ______

Comments on Positive Responses:	Contraindication for Treatment: (PDR Information)

DENTAL HISTORY

1. Reason for visit ______
2. Who referred you to our clinic? ______
3. Are you under the care of a dentist? Yes No
4. What was the approximate date of your last dental appointment? ______ Treatment received: ______
5. How would you rate the dentistry performed in your mouth in the past? Good Fair Poor
6. When was your last professional dental hygiene care appointment? ______
7. When did you last have x-rays taken? ______
a. What kind of x-rays? ______
8. How would you rate your present oral health? Good Fair Poor
9. Do you have or have you ever had any lumps or sores in your mouth or on your lips? Yes No
10 How often do you brush your teeth? ______
11. Do you avoid any area of your mouth when brushing? ______
12. What type of toothbrush do you use? ______
13. What other aids do you use (floss, irrigation, rubber tips)? ______
14. Do you use any of the following at home:
a. Fluoridated water Yes No
b. Fluoride toothpaste Yes No
c. Fluoride rinse/gel Yes No
d. Other Yes No
15. Do your gums bleed? Yes No
a. When ______
16. Have you ever been treated for trenchmouth or other gum diseases? Yes No
17. Do your teeth ever feel sore when you bite on them? Yes No
18. Do you ever:
a. clench or grind your teeth? Yes No
b. chew on one side? Yes No
c. breathe through your mouth? Yes No
d. have difficulty swallowing? Yes No
e. smoke? What, and how much? Yes No
f. other oral habits (thumbsucking, nail biting, foreign objects)? Yes No
19. Do hot, cold, or sweet beverages cause discomfort or pain in your mouth? Yes No
20. Have you ever received nutritional counseling? Yes No
21. What do you eat between meals? ______
22. Have you ever had:
a. orthodontic treatment? Yes No
b. endodontic treatment? Yes No
c. extractions? Yes No
d. jaw surgery? Yes No
e. dental implants? Yes No
23. Have you had any serious trouble associated with any previous dental care? Yes No
If so, explain ______
24. Are you nervous about dental care? Yes No
25. Have you ever had severe pains of the face or head? Yes No
26. Do you have sinus problems? Yes No

FIGURE 10–1 *Continued*

To my knowledge, the preceding information is correct and I consent to having dental hygiene care at Old Dominion University.

INITIAL APPOINTMENT

Date	Blood Pressure	Pulse + Resp.
Signature of Client	Signature of Student Hygienist	Instructor

CONTINUED CARE APPOINTMENTS

CHANGES ____________________

Date	Blood Pressure	Pulse + Resp.
Signature of Client	Signature of Student Hygienist	Instructor

CHANGES ____________________

Date	Blood Pressure	Pulse + Resp.
Signature of Client	Signature of Student Hygienist	Instructor

CHANGES ____________________

Date	Blood Pressure	Pulse + Resp.
Signature of Client	Signature of Student Hygienist	Instructor

CHANGES ____________________

Date	Blood Pressure	Pulse + Resp.
Signature of Client	Signature of Student Hygienist	Instructor

CHANGES ____________________

Date	Blood Pressure	Pulse + Resp.
Signature of Client	Signature of Student Hygienist	Instructor

CHANGES ____________________

Date	Blood Pressure	Pulse + Resp.
Signature of Client	Signature of Student Hygienist	Instructor

CHANGES ____________________

Date	Blood Pressure	Pulse + Resp.
Signature of Client	Signature of Student Hygienist	Instructor

FIGURE 10–1 *Continued*

PAVABID® Plateau CAPS® ℞
[*pav'uh-bid*]
(papaverine hydrochloride) 150 mg

COMPOSITION
Each capsule contains:
Papaverine hydrochloride .... 150 mg
in a specially prepared base to provide prolonged activity.
Also contains: calcium stearate, starch, stearic acid, sucrose, talc, and other ingredients.

ACTION AND USES
The main actions of papaverine are exerted on cardiac and smooth muscle. Like quinidine, papaverine acts directly on the heart muscle to depress conduction and prolong the refractory period. Papaverine relaxes various smooth muscles. This relaxation may be prominent if spasm exists. The muscle cell is not paralyzed by papaverine, and still responds to drugs and other stimuli causing contraction. The antispasmodic effect is a direct one, and unrelated to muscle innervation. Papaverine is practically devoid of effects on the central nervous system.
Papaverine relaxes the smooth musculature of the larger blood vessels, especially coronary, systemic peripheral, and pulmonary arteries. Perhaps by its direct vasodilating action on cerebral blood vessels, papaverine increases cerebral blood flow and decreases cerebral vascular resistance in normal subjects; oxygen consumption is unaltered. These effects may explain the benefit reported from the drug in cerebral vascular encephalopathy.
The direct actions of papaverine on the heart to depress conduction and irritability and to prolong the refractory period of the myocardium provide the basis for its clinical trial in abrogating atrial and ventricular premature systoles and ominous ventricular arrhythmias. The coronary vasodilator action could be an additional factor of therapeutic value when such rhythms are secondary to insufficiency or occlusion of the coronary arteries.
In patients with acute coronary thrombosis, the occurrence of ventricular rhythms is serious and requires measures designed to decrease myocardial irritability. Papaverine may have advantages over quinidine, used for a similar purpose, in that it may be given in an emergency by the intravenous route, does not depress myocardial contraction or cause cinchonism, and produces coronary vasodilation.

INDICATIONS
For the relief of cerebral and peripheral ischemia associated with arterial spasm and myocardial ischemia complicated by arrhythmias.

PRECAUTIONS
Use with caution in patients with glaucoma. Hepatic hypersensitivity has been reported with gastrointestinal symptoms, jaundice, eosinophilia, and altered liver function tests. Discontinue medication if these occur.

ADVERSE REACTIONS
Although occurring rarely, the reported side effects of papaverine include nausea, abdominal distress, anorexia, constipation, malaise, drowsiness, vertigo, sweating, headache, diarrhea, and skin rash.

DOSAGE AND ADMINISTRATION
One capsule every 12 hours. In difficult cases administration may be increased to one capsule every 8 hours or two capsules every 12 hours.

HOW SUPPLIED
PAVABID® (papaverine hydrochloride) Capsules are available in bottles of 100 (NDC 0088-1555-47). Capsules are imprinted with MARION/1555.

CAUTION
Federal law prohibits dispensing without prescription.
Shown in Product Identification Section, page 417
Issued 2/89

FIGURE 10–2
Sample of information available in the *Physicians' Desk Reference.* (Redrawn from Physicians' Desk Reference, 47th ed. Montvale, NJ: Medical Economics Data, a division of Medical Economics Company, Inc., 1993, pp. 1392–1393. Copyright *Physicians' Desk Reference®* 1993, 47th Edition, published by Medical Economics Data, Montvale, NJ 07645. Reprinted by permission. All rights reserved.)

diagnostic indicators, and treatment. Essential facts about medical conditions identified on the health history can be found in the latest edition of the *Merck Manual.* Dental hygienists who are confronted with medical conditions with which they are unfamiliar will find readily available, concise descriptions of most diseases in this reference book.

Prophylactic Antibiotic Premedication

Manipulation of mucosal tissues that results in bleeding during dental or dental hygiene procedures may cause a transient bacteremia. Although bacteremias rarely persist for more than 15 minutes, infectious microorganisms in the blood stream may lodge on damaged or abnormal areas of the heart valves, lining of the heart, and also the underlying connective tissue and cause **bacterial endocarditis** or **endarteritis** (see Chapter 29, section on types of diseases). These conditions can be life-threatening.

Prophylactic antibiotic premedication should be given to clients who are susceptible to bacterial endocarditis (an infection of the lining of the heart and also the underlying connective tissue) before initiating any dental hygiene care that could induce gingival or mucosal bleeding. Prophylactic antibiotic premedication also should be given to clients who may have difficulty resisting infections, that is, clients with unstable diabetes, persons undergoing anticancer chemotherapy, or persons taking immunosuppressive medications. Prophylactic antibiotic premedication is recommended by the American Heart Association[1] for, but not limited to, clients with:

- Prosthetic joint replacement
- Past history of rheumatic fever that results in valvular heart damage
- Recent history of acute rheumatic fever
- Prosthetic cardiac valves, including **bioprosthetic cardiac valves** (made from biological tissue) and **homograft** (human tissue graft) **cardiac valves**
- Previous bacterial endocarditis, even in the absence of heart disease
- Most congenital cardiac malformations
- Acquired valvular dysfunction, even after valvular surgery
- Hypertrophic cardiomyopathy in which the heart muscle increases in weight especially along the septum, which affects the blood flow from the atria to the ventricles
- **Mitral valve prolapse with valvular regurgitation** (the mitral valve is pushed back too far during ventricular contraction, and blood regurgitates back through the mitral valve, back into the left atrium)
- Organic heart murmur
- Ventriculoatrial shunts to relieve hydrocephalus and arteriovenous shunts
- Reduced capacity to resist infection (e.g., anticancer chemotherapy, immunosuppressive medications, acute leukemia, renal transplantation, and dialysis)

The standard prophylactic regimen recommended by the American Heart Association is presented in Table 10–3.[1] Cardiologists generally believe that premedication is not necessary for indwelling transvenous cardiac pacemakers and implanted defibrillators. Cardiac surgery, in and of itself, is not an indication for premedication.

Lifetime coverage of premedication has been suggested for all total joint replacements (TJRs). The opinion of an orthopedic physician is essential before dental hygiene care is initiated. The suggested premedication for orthopedic replacements is presented in Table 10–4.

Indications for Medical Consultation

The client's physician should be consulted if the client reveals a condition that may threaten the client's safety during dental hygiene care. Immediate medical consultation, via telephone, with the client's physician and referral to the physician are indicated if the client reveals a condition that precludes dental hygiene care or needs immediate medical

TABLE 10–2
SECTION DESCRIPTIONS FOR THE *PHYSICIANS' DESK REFERENCE*

Section Name	Color of Index	Purpose
1. Manufacturer's index (e.g., Parke-Davis, Lederle, Procter & Gamble)	White	Provides the name, addresses, and emergency phone numbers of the manufacturers whose products are listed in the *PDR*
2. Product Name index (e.g., Motrin)	Pink	Lists the name given to the product by the manufacturer, also referred to as the brand name. These are in alphabetical order If the client knows the product name refer to this section
3. Product Category index (e.g., antiinflammatory agents)	Blue	Lists products in the appropriate category for type of medication; represents the product's action in the body If the condition for prescription is known refer to this section
4. Generic and Chemical Name index (e.g., ibuprofen)	Yellow	Lists products and their generic and chemical names If only the generic or chemical name is known refer to this section
5. Product Identification Section	Full color	Provides color pictures of the products listed in sections 2 to 4
6. Product Information Section	White	Drug descriptions divided into clinical pharmacology, indications and contraindications, warnings and precautions, and adverse reactions

attention. Medical consultation should be documented in writing from the client's physician. A sample medical consultation form is shown in Figure 10–3. Telephone consultation with the client's physician should be documented in the client's dental record and followed up with a written consultation form. When the written consultation form is received from the physician, it should be placed in the client's chart.

Medical consultations are recommended for the following conditions:

- A condition that may need prophylactic antibiotic premedication
- Suspicion of an undiagnosed condition
- Abnormal vital signs
- The client is receiving radiation therapy

When the dental hygienist requests information in writing from the client's physician, the request should be duplicated and placed in the client's dental chart. For convenience, the medical consultation can be placed on three pages, NCR-type paper, which defers the duplication process.

VITAL SIGNS

The vital signs are measurements of a person's temperature, pulse, respiration, and blood pressure. Properly taken, the vital signs are indicators of a person's present health status. The list that follows explains when it is appropriate for the dental hygienist to measure and record the client's vital signs.

- During the client's initial visit to obtain baseline readings
- At least once a year for a client who is within normal limits
- If there is a significant change in the client's health history
- At each appointment for a client with readings that exceed the normal limits but are being currently monitored by a physician
- Before the administration of a local anesthetic of nitrous oxide–oxygen analgesia
- Before and after surgical procedures
- If the client reports symptoms that indicate a potential emergency situation

Preceding list adapted from Potter, P. A., and Perry, A. G. Fundamentals of Nursing, 3rd ed. St. Louis: C. V. Mosby, 1993, p. 564.

Abnormal vital signs may indicate health problems, undiagnosed conditions, or the need for referral to a physician. Abnormal readings also may be attributed to a variety of environmental factors, such as extreme temperature changes, physical exertion, diet, stress, improperly used equipment, and unreliable equipment. To obtain readings that are true indicators of the client's present condition, the dental hygienist should:

- Be knowledgeable about the normal range for vital signs
- Be familiar with the client's health history, past or present treatment(s), and medications
- Be knowledgeable about and skillful with the equipment used for measuring vital signs
- Take the vital signs in an organized and systematic manner
- Verify significant changes in the client's vital signs and communicate them to the client, dentist, and physician of record

If abnormal readings are obtained, the client should be questioned about possible environmental causes of the abnormal readings, and measuring of the vital signs should be repeated when the conditions are altered or removed. If no environmental factors can be determined, readings that exceed normal limits suggest a potential medical problem, and the client should be referred to a physician.

TABLE 10–3
RECOMMENDED STANDARD PROPHYLACTIC REGIMEN FOR ADULTS AND CHILDREN TO PREVENT BACTERIAL ENDOCARDITIS

Medication	Child or Adult	Initial Dose	Follow-Up Dose
Amoxicillin V* (oral)	Adult	3.0 g 1 hour before procedure	1.5 g 6 hours after initial dose
	Child	50 mg/kg of body weight 1 hour before procedure	½ of initial dose 6 hours after initial dose
Erythromycin stearate (oral)	Adult	1.0 g 2 hours before the procedure	500 mg 6 hours after initial dose
	Child	20 mg/kg of body weight 1 hour before procedure	½ of initial dose 6 hours after initial dose
Clindamycin (oral)	Adult	300 mg 1 hour before procedure	150 mg 6 hours after initial dose
	Child	10 mg/kg of body weight 1 hour before procedure	½ of initial dose 6 hours after initial dose

**Note:* Amoxicillin is now recommended because it is better absorbed and provides higher sustained serum levels. However, the use of penicillin rather than amoxicillin is rational and acceptable.

Adapted with permission from Dajani, A. S., Bisno, A. L., et al. Prevention of bacterial endocarditis. JAMA 264(22):2919–2922, 1990. Copyright 1990, American Medical Association.

Body Temperature

Body temperature is regulated by the hypothalamus, which acts as the body's thermostat. The hypothalamus senses changes in temperature and sends impulses out to the body to correct temperature changes. For example, on a hot day the hypothalamus detects a rise in body temperature and sends signals to the skin to perspire and lower its temperature. In cold weather, the hypothalamus detects a lowering of the body's temperature and signals the body to shiver to produce an increase in the body's temperature. Normally, the hypothalamus regulates the body's temperature at a certain set-point (37°C or 98.6°F for the average adult). When a person experiences the flu, the infectious agent (e.g., virus) secretes substances that affect the hypothalamus by raising its set-point for temperature past the normal temperature. The hypothalamus is deceived and perceives that the body's current temperature of 37°C is too low. The body is directed to conserve and produce heat. This produces a body temperature higher than normal, referred to as a fever. Until the higher set-point is reached, a person may feel chills and shiver. The body experiences an increased need for oxygen as the body's metabolism increases, and adequate nourishment is needed. A person who is feeling feverish should be kept comfortably warm until her temperature reaches the higher set-point. Once that point is reached and the person feels neither hot nor cold, excess clothing and wrapping should be removed. If the person's temperature is elevated for a prolonged time, fluids are needed to prevent dehydration.

No single temperature is normal for all people. As the body produces heat, it is also losing heat. Therefore, for the body temperature to be maintained at a stable level, there must be a balance between heat loss and heat production. As a client ages, the normal temperature range gradually drops because the mechanisms that control thermoregulation start to deteriorate. In cold weather, the body temperature may drop as low as 35°C (95°F) in an elderly client. In the event that a client's body temperature falls below the normal level, steps should be taken to control the body heat lost to the environment (e.g., covering the client with clothing, exposing the client to warmer air or water, and reducing wind drafts). Table 10–5 lists factors that may affect body temperature.

Body Temperature Measurement Sites

Table 10–6 indicates possible body sites for temperature measurement. The oral cavity is the most common site

TABLE 10–4
RECOMMENDED ANTIBIOTIC REGIMEN FOR ADULTS AND CHILDREN WITH TOTAL JOINT REPLACEMENTS

Medication	Initial Dose	Follow-Up Dose
Cephalexin (Keflex)	2 g orally 1 hour before procedure	1 g 6 hours after initial dose
Clindamycin (Cleocin) For persons allergic to cephalexin	600 mg orally 1 hour before procedure	600 mg 6 hours after initial dose

Adapted from Cioffi, G. A., Terezhalmy, G. T., and Taybos, G. M. Total joint replacement: A consideration for antimicrobial prophylaxis. Oral Surgery, Oral Medicine, Oral Pathology 66(1):124–129, July 1988.

NAME

Use this space for the client's name, address, date of birth, and social security number

REQUEST FOR CONSULTATION

TO: ______

FROM: ______

REQUEST:

Sample Request:

(___client's name___) is being seen in the UCSF School of Dentistry for dental hygiene treatment. It is anticipated that the care may extend over several months with a series of appointments of 3 hours duration. The treatment we are recommending involves scaling and root planing, the smoothing of the unattached surfaces of the tooth by removing calculus and/or cementum. I expect to use lidocaine 2% with 1/1:00,000 epinephrine, the maximum dose of which would be 8 cc per 3-hour appointment. Your client's blood pressure reading on date was ______ right arm seated. (Specific areas in the health history that are of concern are discussed in this space, for example, heart murmur, rheumatic fever, hepatitis, gonorrhea, and high blood pressure, i.e.:) The client's health record revealed a history of heart murmur. Since scaling and root planing procedures do contact the blood stream, causing a transitory bacteremia that could result in subacute bacterial endocarditis, we are requesting this medical consultation. Would you recommend prophylactic antibiotic coverage to prevent such an infection? Please evaluate ___client's name___ and report your findings, including contraindications for dental hygiene treatment. Thank you for your attention to this matter.

Signature of Requesting Dentist

RECOMMENDATION:

THIS SPACE IS FOR THE MEDICAL CONSULTANT'S REPLY.

Signature of Consultant | Date

DENTAL RECORD COPY

FIGURE 10–3
Sample medical consultation form. (Adapted from University of California, San Francisco, School of Dentistry, San Francisco, CA.)

TABLE 10–5
FACTORS THAT AFFECT BODY TEMPERATURE

Factors	Effects
Exercise	Increases body temperature
Hormonal influences	
Before ovulation	Decreases body temperature
During ovulation	Increases body temperature to baseline or higher
Menopause	Periodically increases body temperature
Time variations	
Early morning	Temperature at minimum level
Daytime	Body temperature rises
Evening	Body temperature peaks
Stress (physical and emotional)	Increases body temperature
Warm environment	Increases body temperature
Cold environment	Decreases body temperature
Infection	Increases body temperature

used for measuring body temperature in the oral healthcare setting. Caution should be taken to prevent inaccurate readings if hot or cold food or liquids have been ingested or if the client has been smoking. Alternative sites should be used when there is potential for inaccurate readings or when the client's safety is a consideration. For example, an unconscious client, infants, small children, or a mentally challenged client may have difficulty with the placement of the oral thermometer or may bite on the thermometer and break it.

Thermometers

There are three types of **thermometers** available for measuring body temperature. Table 10–7 describes the three types of thermometers. The mercury-in-glass thermometer is probably the most common type for use at home and in professional practice. The electronic (digital) thermometer consists of a probe attached to a digital readout. Disposable

TABLE 10–6
SITES FOR BODY TEMPERATURE MEASUREMENT

Site	Advantages	Limitations
Oral cavity	Most accessible site; comfortable for client	Should not be used for clients who: Could be injured by the thermometer (e.g., clients with very dry mouth) Are unable to hold the thermometer properly Have had oral surgery, or trauma to face or mouth Are experiencing oral pain Breathe only with mouth open Have a history of convulsions Are experiencing a shaking chill Are unconscious
Rectum	Most reliable measure of body temperature	Should not be used for clients who: Have recently had rectal surgery Have a rectal disorder, such as a tumor or hemorrhoids Cannot be positioned for proper thermometer placement, such as those in traction
Axilla	Safest method because it does not involve invasion of a body cavity	Least accurate method of obtaining body temperature

TABLE 10–7
TYPES OF THERMOMETERS FOR MEASURING BASAL BODY TEMPERATURE

Name	Types Available	Disadvantages	Advantages
Mercury-in-glass	Oral Stubby Rectal	Longer reading time May break	Low price Availability Reliability, accuracy Can be used with a disposable cover or sheath
Electronic (digital)	Oral Rectal	Potential for inaccuracies due to shorter reading time (must control environmental variabilities, such as recent intake of hot or cold fluid, smoking)	Disposable sheaths available for maintaining infection control Short reading time Decreased client discomfort Efficient for healthcare professional Easy to read
Disposable	Oral	Cost	Short reading time Disposable Good for maintaining infection control

PROCEDURE 10–1

TAKING AN ORAL TEMPERATURE MEASUREMENT WITH A MERCURY-IN-GLASS THERMOMETER

Equipment

Mercury-in-glass thermometer Disposable sheath	Protective barriers for the clinician

Steps	Rationale
1. Wash hands with antimicrobial soap; don barriers	Reduces chances of transmitting microorganisms
2. Ask the client if hot or cold substances were recently ingested	This can alter the client's true temperature
3. Hold the end of the thermometer opposite the mercury end with your fingertips	This prevents contamination of the bulb to be inserted into the client's mouth
4. Place disposable cover or sheath on thermometer	This prevents cross-contamination
5. Before inserting the thermometer in the client's oral cavity read the mercury level	Mercury is to be below 35°C (96°F). The thermometer reading must be below the client's actual temperature before use
6. If the mercury is above the desired level shake the thermometer so that the mercury moves toward the bulb. Grasp the tip of the thermometer securely and stand away from any solid objects. Sharply flick the wrist downward as though you were cracking a whip. Continue until the reading is at the appropriate level	Brisk shaking lowers the mercury level in the glass tube. Standing in an open spot prevents breakage of the thermometer
7. Ask the client to open his mouth and gently place the thermometer under the tongue lateral to the lower jaw	Heat from superficial blood vessels under the tongue produces the temperature readings
8. Ask the client to hold the thermometer with the lips closed	The lips hold the thermometer in the proper position during recording
9. Leave the thermometer in place for 3 full minutes	The thermometer should remain in place for a minimum of 3 minutes and no longer than 6 minutes
10. Carefully remove the thermometer	
11. Remove and discard the disposable cover	The cover should be removed to allow maximum visibility and should be discarded in the appropriate manner to prevent cross-contamination
12. Read the thermometer	
13. Wash the thermometer in soap and water. Disinfect the thermometer with a hospital-approved and tuberculocidal disinfectant	Prevents cross-contamination in the event that the disposable cover breaks or tears
14. Store the thermometer in its sterilized container after shaking down the mercury again	Proper storage prevents breakage and contamination. The container for the thermometer should be sterile
15. Record the client's temperature, the date, and the time of day on the chart	Vital signs should be recorded immediately, before they are forgotten
16. Inform the dentist of readings above 38°C (99.6°F)	A client's experiencing fluctuations in temperature should be referred to her physician for immediate consultation

plastic sheaths can be used over the probe end as a protective barrier for infection control. The mercury-in-glass thermometer should be handled carefully to avoid breakage and inadvertent spillage of the contents. If a mercury-in-glass thermometer is broken, it should be cleaned up immediately to prevent mercury contamination or poisoning. A mercury clean-up kit for such use can be purchased for the oral healthcare setting from dental supply companies.

Pulse

The **pulse,** the intermittent beat of the heart that is felt through the walls of an artery, is an indicator of the integrity of the cardiovascular system. The most common site for assessing the pulse is located on the thumb side of the inner wrist **(radial pulse)** (Fig. 10–4). The fingertips of the first three fingers are used to feel for the pulse (a throbbing sensation). Never use the thumb to feel for the pulse, since it has a pulse of its own that can be mistaken for the client's. If the radial pulse cannot be felt, the carotid pulse, located on the side of the neck, is an alternative. The pulse is recorded in beats per minute (BPM).

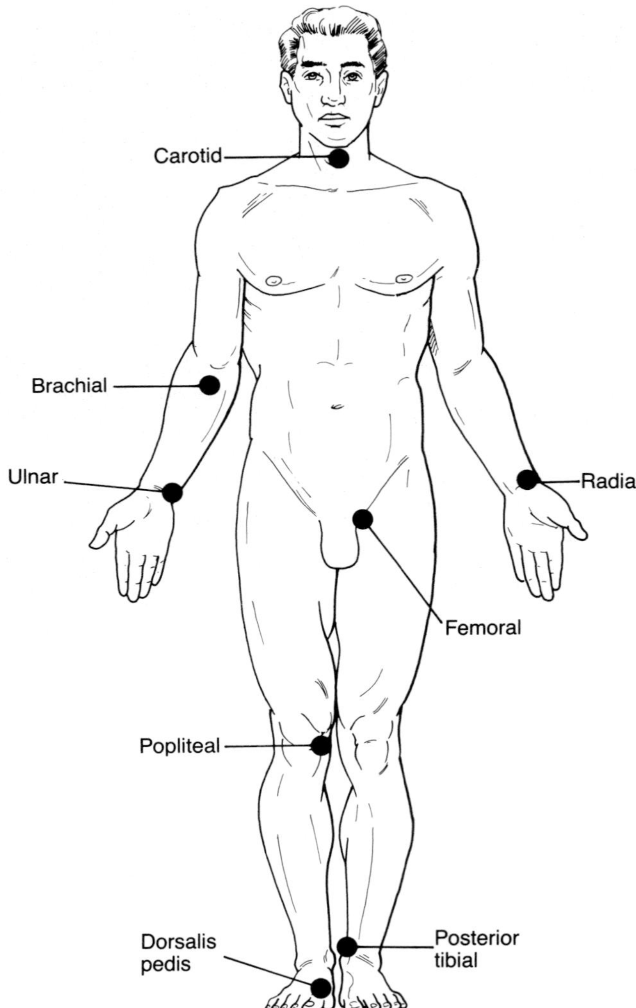

FIGURE 10–4
Sites for pulse assessment. (Redrawn from Miller-Keane Encyclopedia and Dictionary of Medicine, Nursing, and Allied Health, 5th ed. Philadelphia: W. B. Saunders, 1992, p. 1245.)

TABLE 10–8
NORMAL VALUES FOR VITAL SIGNS IN CHILDREN AND ADULTS

Vital Sign	Normal Range
Body temperature (oral)	*Child:* 4 years: 37.3°C (99.2°F) 12 years: 36.7°C (98.0°F) *Adult:* 36°C–36.7°C 97°F–99.6°F Normal average: 37°C (98.6°F)
Pulse rate	*Infant:* 100–160 BPM *Age 4 years:* 80–120 BPM *Adolescent to adult:* 60–100 BPM
Respiration rate	*Infant:* 30–60 breaths/minute *Age 2 years:* 20–30 breaths/minute *Age 6 years:* 18–26 breaths/minute *Adult:* 12–20 breaths/minute
Blood pressure	*Age 4 years:* <85 mm Hg systolic <60 mm Hg diastolic *Adult:* <140 mm Hg systolic (when diastolic is <90 mm Hg) and <85 mm Hg diastolic *Age more than 60 years:* 140–170 mm Hg systolic <90 mm Hg diastolic

The normal heart rate for an adult at rest can range from 60 to 100 BPM. However, there are factors that can affect the heart rate. Fever, acute pain, anxiety, atropine, hemorrhage, and exercise prior to taking the pulse can increase the pulse rate. Digitalis and long-term exercise are factors that can decrease the pulse rate. Postural changes also can influence the pulse rate. A person who lies down will have a decreased rate; standing or sitting results in an increased rate. Children usually have a more rapid heart rate than that of adults (Table 10–8).

If on initial evaluation the client's heart rate falls under 60 BPM or rises above 110 BPM, the client should be evaluated for causative factors or conditions. If no cause can be determined, a medical consultation should be obtained from the client's physician. If the client is experiencing five or more premature ventricular contractions (PVCs) per minute, a medical consultation should be considered. A PVC is a break, or skip, in the normal rhythm, and the dental hygienist will detect an interruption in successive pulse waves. A medical consultation is also recommended for a client who presents with alternating strong and weak heart beats, which may indicate ventricular failure, high blood pressure, and/or coronary heart disease. A full, bounding pulse may indicate high blood pressure. A weak, thready pulse usually is found in clients with hypotension and also is a sign of shock.

PROCEDURE 10–2

MEASURING THE RADIAL PULSE

Equipment

Wristwatch with a second hand

Steps	Rationale
1. Use a wristwatch with a second hand	Allows the clinician to make an accurate assessment
2. Wash hands with antimicrobial soap	Washing reduces the chances of transmitting infectious microorganisms
3. Explain the purpose and method of procedure to the client	Explanations relieve the client's anxiety and facilitate cooperation during the procedure
4. Have the client assume a sitting position, bend the client's elbow 90 degrees, and support his lower arm on the armrest of the chair. Extend the wrist with the palm down	Proper positioning fully exposes the radial artery for palpation
5. Place the first three fingers of your hand along the radial artery and lightly compress them against it	The fingertips are most sensitive to vibration
6. Obliterate the pulse initially, and then relax pressure so that the pulse is easily palpable	The pulse is more accurately assessed with moderate finger pressure. Too much pressure occludes the pulse, and too little prevents the examiner from feeling the pulse with regularity
7. When the pulse can be felt regularly use the watch's second hand and begin to count the rate, starting with zero and then 1, and so on	The rate is determined accurately only after the examiner is certain that the pulse can be palpated. Timing should begin with zero. The count of 1 is the first beat felt after timing begins
8. If the pulse is regular, count for 15 seconds and multiply the total by four	A regular rate is accurately assessed in 15 seconds
9. If the pulse is irregular, count for a full minute	The longer time ensures an accurate count
10. Assist the client to a comfortable position	
11. Record heart rate, rhythm of the heart (regular or irregular), the quality of the pulse (thready, weak, bounding), and the date in the chart	Vital signs should be recorded immediately on the client's record

Respiration

The **respiration** rate is assessed by counting the rise and fall (inspiration and expiration) of the client's chest. This vital sign can be altered by the client if the client is aware that it is being measured. The dental hygienist should attempt to make this assessment without making the client aware of the hygienist's intention. To do this, the respiration rate can be measured before or after taking the client's pulse rate. The dental hygienist's hand remains on the client's radial pulse while the hygienist inconspicuously counts respiratory rate.

The normal adult range for respiration rate is 12 to 20 breaths per minute. Children have a more rapid respiratory rate (20–30 breaths per minute for a 6-year-old child) than that of adults. Young children also tend to have a less regular breathing cycle. Advancing age produces an increase in the respiration rate.

Narcotic administration produces an abnormally slow and shallow respiratory rate. Exercise, pain, anxiety, long-term smoking, fever, and alkalosis all produce an abnormally rapid respiratory rate. Abnormally deep but regular respiratory cycles may indicate diabetic ketoacidosis. Disorders of the brainstem, which contains the respiratory control center, may impair respiration. If an abnormal respiratory rate is detected, the client should be referred to her physician for a medical consultation and evaluation.

PROCEDURE 10–3

MEASURING RESPIRATIONS

Equipment

Wristwatch with second hand

Steps	Rationale
1. Use a wristwatch with a second hand	Allows the dental hygienist to make an accurate assessment
2. Place your hand along the client's radial artery and inconspicuously observe the client's chest	Allows the dental hygienist to make the assessment without the client's awareness of the process
3. Observe the rise and fall of the client's chest. Count complete respiratory cycles (one inspiration and one expiration)	
4. For an adult count the number of respirations in 30 seconds and multiply that number by two. For a young child count respirations for a full minute	The respiratory rate is equivalent to the number of respirations per minute. Young infants and children breathe in an irregular rhythm
5. If an adult has respirations with an irregular rhythm, or respirations are abnormally slow or fast, count for a full minute	Accurate interpretation requires assessment for at least a minute
6. While counting, note whether depth is shallow, normal, or deep and whether rhythm is normal or one of the altered patterns	The character of ventilatory movements may reveal specific alterations or disease states
7. Record the date and the client's respirations per minute in the chart	Vital signs should be recorded immediately

Blood Pressure

Blood pressure is the force exerted by the blood against the arterial walls when the heart contracts. Blood pressure is an important indicator of present cardiovascular function. The blood pressure also indicates the risk of future cardiovascular morbidity and mortality. Chronic hypertension causes thickening and loss of elasticity in the arterial walls, which can lead to serious disorders, such as heart failure, stroke, and kidney failure. There are no adverse effects from "low blood pressure" unless the client is in a state of shock or is affected by a condition that may lower the blood pressure. In fact, the lower the blood pressure the better the long-term prognosis for cardiovascular health. An acute change in blood pressure can indicate an emergency situation, such as shock or rapid hemorrhaging.

Blood pressure is measured in millimeters of mercury (mm Hg). The two measurements taken for blood pressure are the systolic blood pressure and the diastolic blood pressure. The systolic blood pressure measures the maximum pressure occurring in the blood vessels during cardiac ventricular contraction **(systole),** and the diastolic measures the minimum pressure occurring against the arterial walls as a result of cardiac ventricular relaxation **(diastole).** The normal systolic and diastolic measurements for adults 18 years and older are less than or equal to 140/85 mm Hg. The top number of a given blood pressure is always the systolic measurement, and the bottom number is the diastolic measurement. In children in the United States, fewer than 3% have arterial hypertension. Table 10–9 lists the classifications of hypertension in the young.

TABLE 10–9
CLASSIFICATION OF HYPERTENSION IN THE YOUNG BY AGE GROUP

	Significant Hypertension	Severe Hypertension
≤2 years	Systolic ≥112 Diastolic ≥74	≥118 ≥82
3–5 years	≥116 ≥76	≥124 ≥84
6–9 years	≥122 ≥78	≥130 ≥86
10–12 years	≥126 ≥82	≥134 ≥90
13–15 years	≥136 ≥86	≥144 ≥92
16–18 years	≥142 ≥92	≥150 ≥98

Adapted from Report of the Second Task Force on Blood Pressure Control in Children—1987. Pediatrics 79(1):1–25, January 1987, p. 38. Reproduced by permission of Pediatrics, copyright 1987.

Factors Influencing Blood Pressure

Several factors can influence blood pressure. Increasing age, anxiety, fear, pain, emotional stress, chronic renal failure, smoking, and diets high in fat content are some conditions that can raise blood pressure. At menopause, a woman tends to have a higher blood pressure compared with a man of the same age. Medications, hemorrhage, fasting, rest, fainting, and shock can lower blood pressure. Blood pressure also can vary according to the time of day it is

TABLE 10–10
BLOOD PRESSURE GUIDELINES USED IN THE DENTAL HYGIENE PROCESS OF CARE

Blood Pressure (mm Hg)	Dental and Dental Hygiene Therapy Considerations
<140 systolic and <90 diastolic	No unusual precautions related to client management based on blood pressure readings. Recheck in 6 months
140 to 159 systolic and/or 90 to 94 diastolic	Recheck blood pressure prior to dental or dental hygiene therapy for three consecutive appointments; if all exceed these guidelines, seek medical consultation. No unusual precautions related to client management based on blood pressure readings are needed. Stress-reduction protocol if indicated, such as administration of nitrous oxide–oxygen analgesia, should be considered
160 to 199 systolic and/or 95 to 114 diastolic	Recheck blood pressure in 5 minutes. If still elevated, seek medical consultation prior to dental or dental hygiene therapy. No unusual precautions related to client management based on blood pressure readings. Stress reduction protocol if indicated, such as administration of nitrous oxide–oxygen analgesia
>200 systolic and/or >115 diastolic	Recheck blood pressure in 5 minutes. Immediate medical consultation if still elevated. Dental or dental hygiene therapy, routine or emergency treatment may be performed if the blood pressure is only slightly above 200 systolic or 115 diastolic, and nitrous oxide–oxygen analgesia lowers the blood pressure below 200 systolic or 115 diastolic. If blood pressure is not reduced using nitrous oxide–oxygen analgesia, only (noninvasive) emergency therapy with drugs (analgesics, antibiotics) is allowable to treat pain and infection. Refer to hospital if immediate dental therapy is indicated

Adapted from Malamed, S. F. Handbook of Medical Emergencies in the Dental Office, 4th ed. St. Louis: C. V. Mosby, 1993, p. 33.

taken. For example, it is normally lowest in the morning and gradually rises during the morning and afternoon.

A medical consultation is indicated for clients with abnormal blood pressure readings (Table 10–10).

Blood Pressure Equipment

Although electronic equipment is available for blood pressure measurement, it is not generally used by healthcare providers. The following is a description of equipment used to assess blood pressure in the healthcare environment.

Sphygmomanometer There are different types of manometers (Table 10–11). The parts of a manometer are similar, however, regardless of the type available (Fig. 10–5). The parts include an occlusive cloth cuff, a pressure bulb, and a release valve on the pressure bulb. Large adult cuffs (Fig. 10–6) and thigh cuffs also are available.

Stethoscope The **stethoscope** is used to amplify sound. The stethoscope consists of two earpieces, plastic or rubber tubing, and a chestpiece. The chestpiece consists of two sides, the bell and the diaphragm (Fig. 10–7). Either end of the chestpiece can be used; however, the bell end is recommended because it is designed to transmit low-pitched sounds if it is held lightly against the skin.

The proper cuff size of the sphygmomanometer is necessary for an accurate blood pressure reading. The bladder width should encircle 40 to 50% of the upper arm. The bladder width multiplied by 2.5 defines the ideal arm circumference; for example, the ideal arm circumference for a sphygmomanometer with a bladder width of 15 cm is $15 \times 2.5 = 37.5$ cm. Therefore, a bladder width of 15 cm has the more accurate reading for a person with an arm circumference of 37.5 cm. Table 10–12 provides information about systolic and diastolic adjustments for bladder width that do not fit accurately.

When the bladder within the occluding cuff is deflated, the blood begins to flow intermittently through the brachial artery, producing rhythmic, knocking sounds. These sounds

TABLE 10–11
TYPES OF MANOMETERS

Name	Advantages	Disadvantages
Mercury	Most accurate	Bulky
Aneroid	Lightweight Portable Compact	Needs to be recalibrated to mercury manometer
Electronic	Less chance of operator error	Difficult to check accuracy

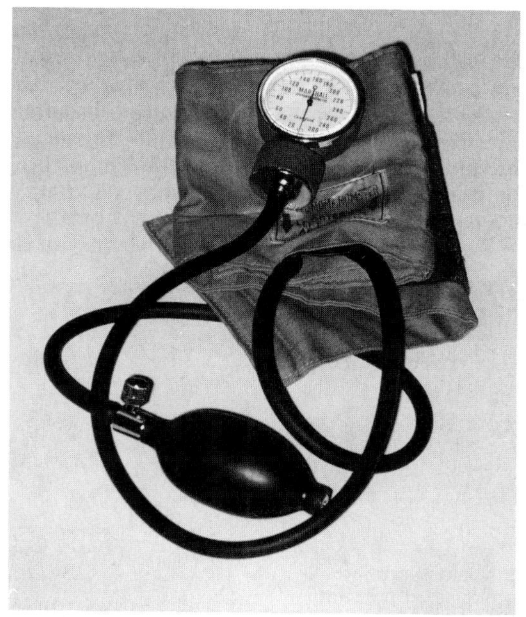

FIGURE 10–5
Manometer.

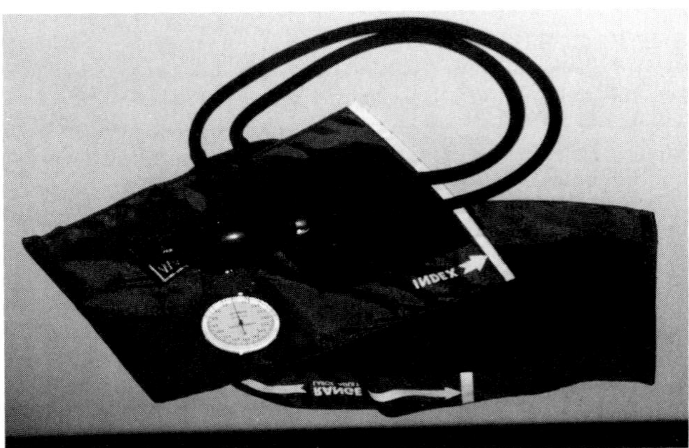

FIGURE 10-6
Large adult cuff.

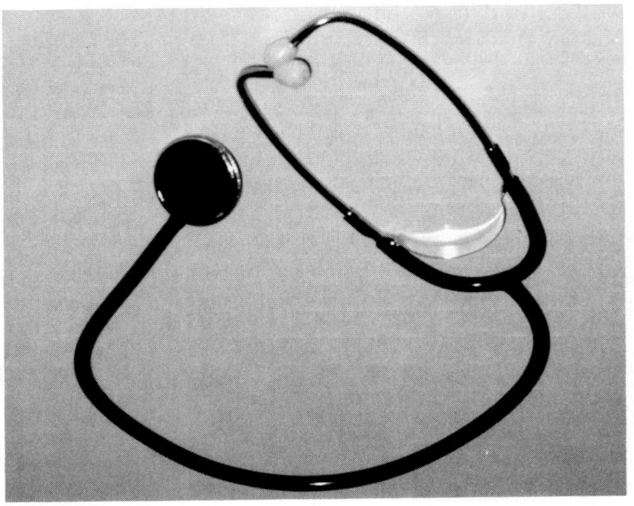

FIGURE 10-7
Stethoscope.

are referred to as Korotkoff sounds. As the cuff is deflated further, the Korotkoff sounds become less audible, and the pulse sound eventually disappears. There are five Korotkoff sounds that are described in phases (see Description of Korotkoff Sounds chart, on opposite page).

Technical Hints for Taking and Interpreting Blood Pressure Measurements

- The systolic blood pressure is the number on the sphygmomanometer when the first sound is heard. The diastolic blood pressure is the number on the sphygmomanometer when the last sound is heard.
- Falsely low readings can occur if too wide a cuff is used
- Falsely high readings can occur under the following conditions: unsupported arm, cold hands of operator, cold equipment
- Deflating the cuff too slowly results in a high diastolic reading
- Inaccurate inflation of the cuff results in a low systolic reading
- Deflating the cuff too quickly, improper use of the stethoscope, or a poor-fitting stethoscope results in falsely low systolic and falsely high diastolic readings (e.g., on a small child or an obese person). This error

TABLE 10-12
RECOMMENDED IDEAL ARM CIRCUMFERENCE, ARM CIRCUMFERENCE RANGES, AND CORRECTION OF SYSTOLIC AND DIASTOLIC READINGS FOR ADULT BLOOD PRESSURE CUFFS OF DIFFERENT BLADDER WIDTHS AT VARIOUS ARM CIRCUMFERENCES

Bladder width (cm)	12		15		18	
Ideal arm circumference (cm)	30.0		37.5		45.0	
Arm circumference range (cm)	26–33		33–41		41	
Arm circumference (cm)	***SBP**	**†DBP**	**SBP**	**DBP**	**SBP**	**DBP**
26	+5	+3	+7	+5	+9	+5
28	+3	+2	+5	+4	+8	+5
30	0	0	+4	+3	+7	+4
32	−2	−1	+3	+2	+6	+4
34	−4	−3	+2	+1	+5	+3
36	−6	−4	0	+1	+5	+3
38	−8	−6	−1	0	+4	+2
40	−10	−7	−2	−1	+3	+1
42	−12	−9	−4	−2	+2	+1
44	−14	−10	−5	−3	1	0
46	−16	−11	−6	−3	0	0
48	−18	−13	−7	−4	−1	−1
50	−21	−14	−9	−5	−1	−1

*Systolic blood pressure.
†Diastolic blood pressure.
Reproduced with permission from Recommendations for Human Blood Pressure Determination by Sphygmomanometers. Report of a special task force appointed by the steering committee, American Heart Association. American Heart Association, 1987, p 10. Copyright American Heart Association.

DESCRIPTION OF KOROTKOFF SOUNDS

Phase I: first pulse sound—starts faintly and becomes clear tapping sound
Phase II: second pulse sound—murmur or swishing sound
Phase III: third pulse sound—sound is crisp and increases in intensity
Phase IV: fourth pulse sound—muffled sound
Phase V: when the last sound is heard

Reproduced and adapted with permission from Recommendations for human blood pressure determination by sphygmomanometers. Report of a special task force appointed by the steering committee, American Heart Association. American Heart Association, 1987, p. 4. Copyright American Heart Association.

can be prevented by using the proper cuff size and accurate technique

- The Special Task Force appointed by the Steering Committee, American Heart Association, recommends recording three readings of blood pressure for children. The first reading is taken when the first sound appears; the second reading is taken before the pulse disappears and can be distinguished when the pulse becomes muffled (phase IV); and the third reading is the last sound heard (phase V). In adolescents and adults, phase V sounds best represent diastolic pressure
- There may be difficulty hearing the pulse if the bell-shaped end is pressed too tightly against the skin
- An auscultatory gap is often present in clients with hypertension. This gap appears between the first and

PROCEDURE 10–4

ASSESSING BLOOD PRESSURE BY AUSCULTATION

Equipment

Blood pressure cuff or sphygmomanometer
Stethoscope

Steps	Rationale
1. Determine the proper cuff size	The proper cuff size is necessary so that the correct amount of pressure is applied over the artery. The bladder width should be 40 to 50% of the upper arm circumference. Bladder width multiplied by 2.5 defines the ideal arm circumference (e.g., the ideal arm circumference for a bladder width of 15 cm is 15 × 2.5 = 37.5 cm). Cuffs that are too small for a client's arm produce artificially high blood pressure readings; cuffs that are too large produce artificially low readings
2. Wash hands with antimicrobial soap	Washing reduces the chances of transmitting infectious microorganisms
3. Explain the purpose of the procedure	Explanations reassure the client. Ideally, the client should not have eaten or smoked 30 minutes prior to the procedure. The dental hygienist must attempt to obtain a blood pressure reading that is representative of the client's blood pressure under "ordinary" circumstances. The blood pressure should be taken in a quiet area after 5 minutes of rest by the client. Screen the client for other environmental or biological factors, such as anxiety, distention of the urinary bladder, exertion, pain, changes in climate temperatures, and prescribed drugs or other medications that also may influence blood pressure measurements
4. Assist the client to a comfortable sitting position, with arm slightly flexed, forearm supported, and palm turned up	This position facilitates cuff application. Having the arm above heart level would produce a falsely low reading
5. Expose the upper arm fully	Exposing the upper arm ensures proper cuff application
6. Palpate the brachial artery. Position the cuff approximately 1 inch above the brachial artery	Proper positioning of the cuff facilitates an accurate reading
7. Center the arrows marked on the cuff over the brachial artery	Inflating the bladder directly over the brachial artery ensures that proper pressure is applied during inflation
8. Be sure the cuff is fully deflated. Wrap the cuff evenly and snugly around the upper arm	This ensures that proper pressure will be applied over the artery
9. Be sure the manometer is positioned at eye level	Eye level placement ensures accurate reading of mercury level

CONTINUED ON FOLLOWING PAGE

PROCEDURE 10–4

ASSESSING BLOOD PRESSURE BY AUSCULTATION *Continued*

Steps	Rationale
10. If the client's normal systolic pressure is not known, palpate the radial artery and inflate the cuff to a pressure 30 mm Hg above the point at which radial pulsation disappears. Deflate the cuff and wait 30 seconds	This determines the maximal inflation point and prevents auscultatory gap. The 30-second delay prevents venous congestion and falsely high readings
11. Place the stethoscope earpieces in the ears and be sure sounds are clear, not muffled	Each earpiece should follow the angle of the examiner's ear canal to facilitate hearing
12. Place the diaphragm (or the bell) of the stethoscope over the brachial artery	Proper stethoscope placement ensures optimal sound reception. The American Heart Association recommends use of the bell for hearing low-pitched Korotkoff sounds clearly
13. Close the valve of the pressure bulb clockwise until tight	Tightening the valve prevents air leak during inflation
14. Inflate the cuff to 30 mm Hg above the client's normal systolic level	Proper cuff inflation ensures accurate pressure measurement
15. Slowly release the valve, allowing the mercury to fall at a rate of 2 to 3 mm Hg per second	Too rapid or slow a decline in the mercury level may lead to an inaccurate reading
16. Note the point on the manometer at which the first two consecutive beats are heard	The first **Korotkoff sound** indicates the systolic pressure. Blood pressure levels should be recorded in even numbers
17. Continue cuff deflation, noting the point on the manometer at which sound muffles (phase IV) for children or when the sound disappears (phase V) for adults	The American Heart Association recommends recording the fifth Korotkoff sound as the diastolic pressure in adults. In certain clients, such as children, the Korotkoff sounds do not disappear and may be heard until the pressure in the cuff falls near to 0 mm Hg. Therefore, phase IV, which is a muffled pulse sound heard before the last pulse sound, is a more reliable index for children
18. Deflate the cuff rapidly. To determine an average blood pressure and to ensure a correct reading, wait 30 seconds and then repeat the procedure for the same arm	Continuous cuff inflation causes arterial occlusion, resulting in numbness and tingling in the client's arm. The delay prevents venous congestion and falsely high readings and provides an accurate assessment of the client's blood pressure. The blood pressure reading is repeated on the same arm because there may be as much as 10 mm Hg difference in readings between arms
19. Remove the cuff from the client's arm. Assist the client to a comfortable position and cover upper arm	This maintains the client's comfort
20. Fold the cuff and store it properly in a cool, dry place	Proper maintenance of supplies contributes to instrument accuracy. Sunlight and heat may compromise rubber tubing
21. Calculate the average of the two blood pressure readings. Record on the client's chart the average blood pressure, the date, cuff size, and which arm was used for measurement	Vital signs should be recorded immediately. When phase IV is recorded, phase V (which is when the last sound is heard) is also recorded (e.g., 110/68/52)

Adapted from Potter, P.A., and Perry, A.G. Fundamentals of Nursing, 3rd ed. St. Louis: C.V. Mosby, 1993, pp. 588–589.

second systolic sounds. Therefore, it is important that the dental hygienist assess the point at which the pulse is obliterated while increasing the pressure in the bladder prior to taking the blood pressure by ascultation. It is also important that the dental hygienist increase the bladder pressure 30 mm Hg higher than the point at which the pulse is obliterated when measuring blood pressure

Obesity Falsely high blood pressure measurements may be obtained if a standard-size blood pressure cuff and accurate technique are used to measure blood pressure of an obese person. Following are alternative techniques for measuring the blood pressure of obese persons.

Moderately obese—use large adult cuff
Morbidly obese—use thigh cuff (18-cm wide) (arm circumference >41 cm)

Children and Adolescents Cuffs used for children and adolescents may be labeled newborn, infant, child, small adult, and large adult. The dental hygienist should not rely on the age of the client, however, for the basis of cuff selection. The bladder width should be 40% of the arm circumference.

Special Populations Several special population groups are prone to hypertension:

- Forty-five percent of the elderly population, 65 years or older, have a blood pressure greater than 160

Adapted from Recommendations for human blood pressure determination by sphygmomanometers. Report of a special task force appointed by the steering committee, Copyright American Heart Association. American Heart Association, 1987, p. 22.

Name____ Date____________

1. Do you **use** tobacco in any form? yes_____ no_____

1a. If no, have you **ever used** tobacco in the past? yes_____ no_____

How long did you use tobacco? years_____ months_____

How long ago did you stop? years_____ months_____

If you are **not currently** a tobacco user, no other questions should be answered. Thank you for completing this form.

Questions 2 to 10 are for ***current*** *tobacco users only.*

2. **If you smoke,** what type? (check) How many? (number)

Cigarettes	_____	cigarettes per day	_____
Cigars	_____	cigars per day	_____
Pipe	_____	bowls per day	_____

3. **If you chew/use snuff,** what type? How much?

Snuff	_____	days a can lasts	_____
Chewing	_____	pouches per week	_____

Other (describe) ______________________ amount_____ per_____

3a. **How long** do you keep a chew in your mouth? minutes_____

4. **How many days** of the week do you use tobacco? 7 6 5 4 3 2 1

5. **How soon** after you wake up do you first use tobacco? within 30 minutes_____ more than 30 minutes_____

6. Does the person **closest to you** use tobacco? yes_____ no_____

7. **How interested are you** in stopping your use of tobacco? not at all_____, a little_____, somewhat_____, yes_____, very much_____

8. Have you **tried to stop** using tobacco before? yes_____ no_____

8a. How long ago was your **last try** to stop? years_____ months_____

9. Have you **discussed stopping** with your physician? yes_____ no_____

10. If you decided to stop using tobacco completely during the next two weeks, **how confident are you** that you would succeed?

not at all_____, a little_____, somewhat_____, very confident_____

Thank you for completing this form.

From: Mecklenburg, R. E., Christen, A. G. et al. How to Help Your Patients Stop Using Tobacco. US Dept of Health and Human Services, Public Health Service, National Institutes of Health NIH Publ 91-3191, September, 1991, p 45.

mm Hg systolic or greater than 96 mm Hg diastolic. Two-thirds have greater than 140 mm Hg systolic or greater than 90 mm Hg diastolic. Medical intervention may be introduced when the diastolic pressure is greater than 90 mm Hg. Systolic pressure may be treated nonpharmacologically or with antihypertensive therapy to reduce the pressure to 140 to 160 mm Hg

- The prevalence rate of hypertension in African Americans is considerably higher than in the white population, and hypertension tends to appear earlier in life in this group. Deaths related to hypertension are disproportionately higher among African Americans, especially in the younger population
- Hypertension experienced during pregnancy is termed "preeclampsia" or chronic (essential) hypertension. Medical intervention is beneficial in reducing maternal and fetal mortality
- Clients who have had an acute stroke may experience an increase in blood pressure

The technique for obtaining blood pressure measurements in children is identical to that described for adults; however, in children, the fourth Korotkoff sound best represents the diastolic pressure. In adolescents and adults, the fifth Korotkoff sound is the best indicator of diastolic pressure.

Reference

1. Dajani, A. S., Bisno, A. L., et al. Prevention of bacterial endocarditis. JAMA 264(22):2919, 1990.

Suggested Readings

Malamed, S. F. Handbook of Medical Emergencies in the Dental Office, 4th ed. St. Louis: C. V. Mosby, 1992.

NIH Publication No. 93-1088, The Fifth Report of the Joint Committee on Detection, Evaluation, and Treatment of High Blood Pressure, January 1993.

O'Toole, M. (ed.). Miller-Keane Encyclopedia and Dictionary of Medicine, Nursing, and Allied Health, 5th ed. Philadelphia: W. B. Saunders, 1992.

Potter, P. A., and Perry, A. G. Fundamentals of Nursing, 3rd ed. St. Louis: C. V. Mosby, 1993.

Wilkins, E. M. Clinical Practice of the Dental Hygienist, 6th ed. Philadelphia: Lea & Febiger, 1989.

11 Extraoral and Intraoral Clinical Assessment

OBJECTIVES

Mastery of the content in this chapter will enable the reader to:

- Define the key terms used
- Recognize the normal anatomy of the head and neck area
- Recognize and describe signs of common oral disease and deviation from normal
- Follow proper methods and sequence in performing extra- and intraoral examinations
- Apply appropriate follow-up and referral protocol when abnormal or atypical tissue changes warrant further evaluation
- Review common normal but atypical findings of skin and oral mucosa as well as some abnormal and pathological oral mucosal lesions
- Explain self-examination techniques for the oral cavity to the client
- Discuss the procedures for preparing exfoliation cytology slides and sending them to the pathology laboratory with appropriate documentation
- Discuss the procedure for applying toluidine blue staining to a suspended dysplastic or malignant lesion
- Identify categories of oral lesions and terms used to describe their location, distribution, size, color, surface texture, attachment, and consistency
- Explain classifications of cytology specimens
- Describe and document significant findings in the client's record using precise, descriptive terms

INTRODUCTION

The oral tissues are sensitive indicators of general health. Changes in these structures may be the first indication of subclinical disease processes in other parts of the body. For example, some systemic diseases that first manifest themselves in the oral cavity include diabetes, human immunodeficiency virus (HIV) infection, nutritional deficiencies, and leukemia. A variety of skin and oral mucosal lesions observed may or may not be symptomatic. Recognition, treatment, and follow-up evaluation of specific lesions may be of great significance to the general and oral health of the client. Taking the appropriate action with an individual following the recognition of an abnormal extraoral or intraoral condition is imperative for promoting optimal client wellness, controlling morbidity, and, in the case of cancer, possibly preventing premature death. Educating clients through instruction in self-examination techniques to identify signs outside of normal in their own mouth engages them in "co-therapy," allowing them to assume some responsibility for the care and control of their own oral health.

For professional dental hygienists practicing within a human needs framework, information obtained from the extra- and intraoral assessments can facilitate the identification of human need deficits related to the integrity of the skin and mucous membranes of the head and neck area; a biologically sound dentition; freedom from pain and stress; nutrition; self-determination and responsibility, and values. For example, assessment of the need for integrity of the skin and mucous membranes of the head and neck area and for freedom from pain and stress occurs through observation of the head and neck area and an overall appraisal of the client upon reception and seating. Once the client is seated and the health/dental/cultural histories and vital signs have been obtained, careful examination of the oral cavity and adjacent structures allows the hygienist to assess soft tissue and periodontal health status which may indicate deficits in the needs for nutrition and for integrity of the skin and mucous membranes of the head and neck area. In addition, abnormalities of teeth and restorations and ill-fitting dentures relate to the need for a biologically sound dentition; and the presence of bacterial plaque and other soft and hard deposits on the teeth relate to the need for self-determination and responsibility and may indicate that oral hygiene care has a low priority in the client's value system.

This chapter focuses on assessing extraoral and intraoral deviations from normal other than those related to the periodontium, oral hygiene, and tooth structure. (Tooth, periodontal, and oral hygiene assessments are covered in detail in Chapters 12 and 13.)

THE ORAL CAVITY

Normal Anatomy and Surrounding Structures

Knowledge of the general histology and categories of oral mucosa is necessary to understanding their appearance and function. The **oral mucosa,** or the lining of the oral cavity, is a mucous membrane composed of connective tissue covered with stratified squamous epithelium. There are three categories of oral mucosa:

- Masticatory mucosa
- Specialized mucosa
- Lining mucosa

The **masticatory mucosa** covers the hard palate and gingiva and is attached firmly to the tissue underneath. Because these areas are directly exposed to masticatory forces, they are keratinized. **Specialized mucosa** is limited to the upper surface or dorsum of the tongue. Keratinized and used for mastication, it also serves the special function of taste sensation. The remainder of the oral mucous membrane, **lining mucosa,** is unkeratinized. Lining mucosa covers the

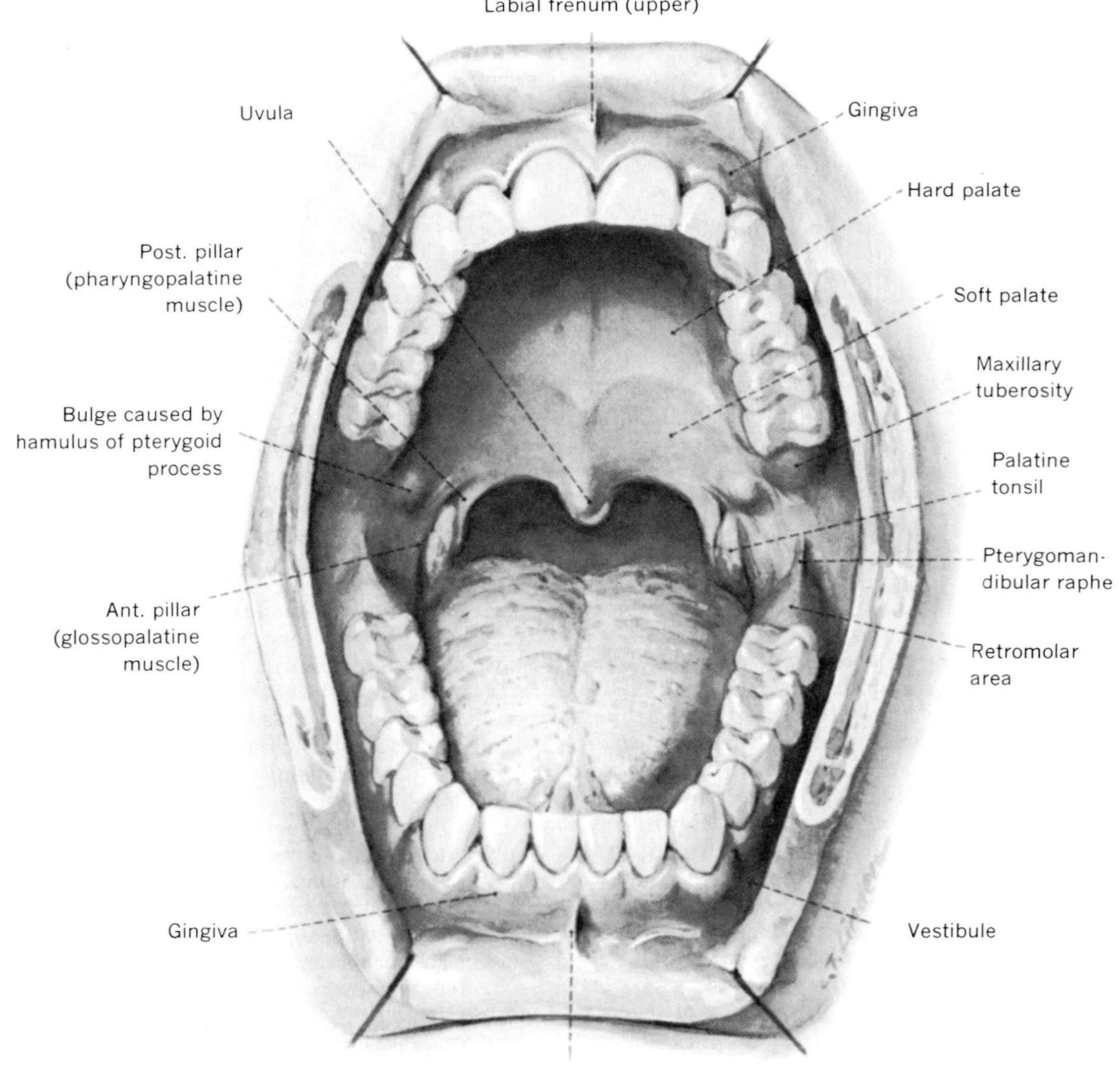

FIGURE 11–1
Anatomical landmarks in the oral cavity. (From Massler, M., and Schour, I. Atlas of the Mouth, 2nd ed. Chicago: American Dental Association, 1958, Plate 1. Copyright © 1958. Reprinted by permission of ADA Publishing Co., Inc.)

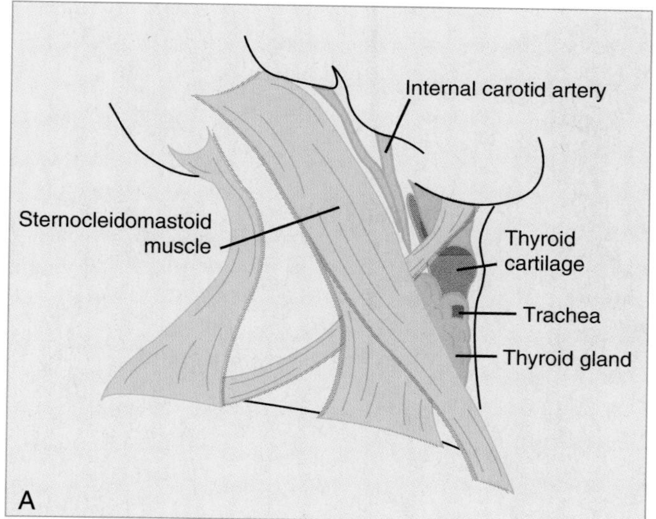

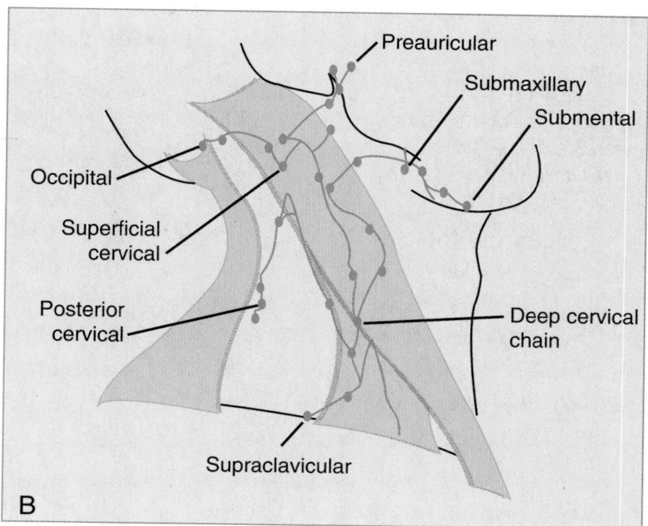

FIGURE 11–2
A, Location of the thyroid gland and major muscle groups of the neck. *B*, Lymph nodes of the head and neck. (Redrawn from Potter, P. A., and Perry, A. G. Fundamentals of Nursing: Concepts Process, and Practice, 3rd ed. St. Louis: C. V. Mosby, 1993, pp. 546–547.)

inner surfaces of the cheeks and lips, the floor of the mouth, the ventral surface (under surface) of the tongue, and the soft palate.

It is necessary for the dental hygienist to understand and identify normal physical characteristics of the head and neck area in order to be able to distinguish abnormal variation among clients.

The anatomical landmarks in the oral cavity, as shown in Figure 11–1, are used as a general point of reference during an intraoral examination. The tongue is an important potential lesion site and must be examined carefully. Figure 11–2 shows the location of the thyroid gland and the major muscle groups and lymph nodes of the neck. Figure 11–3 identifies the sublingual and submandibular salivary glands and associated structures. Figure 11–3 also shows the normal anatomy of the ventral surface of the

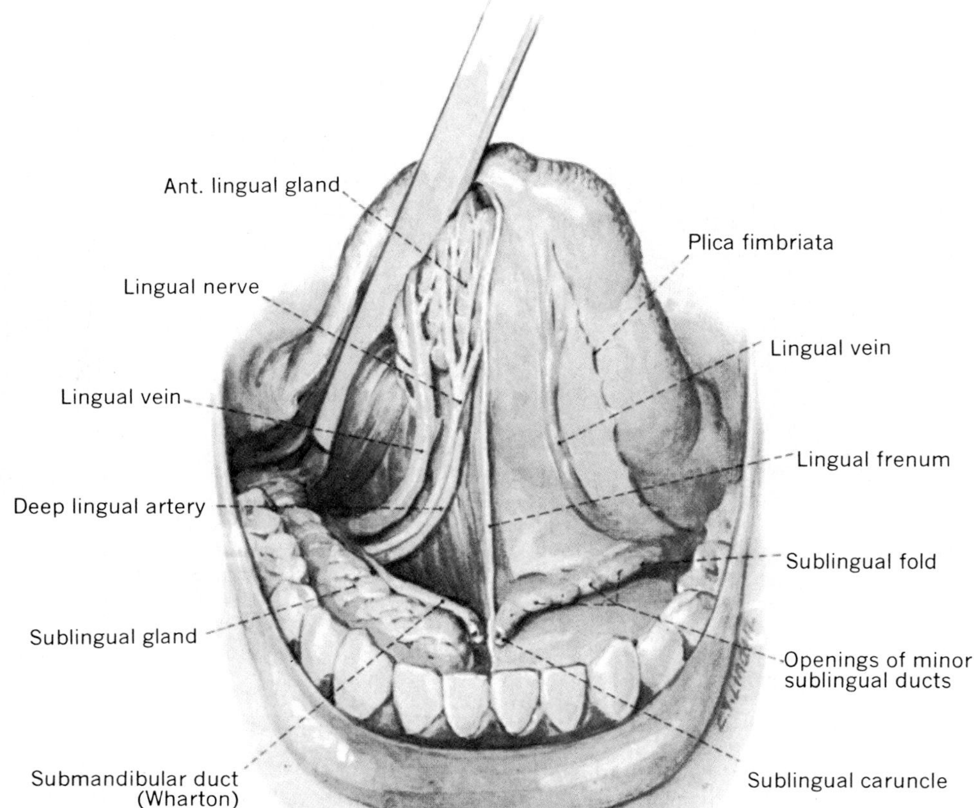

FIGURE 11–3
Normal anatomy of the ventral surface of the tongue and associated structures. (From Massler, M., and Schour, I. Atlas of the Mouth, 2nd ed. Chicago: American Dental Association, 1958, Plate 2. Copyright © 1958. Reprinted by permission of ADA Publishing Co., Inc.)

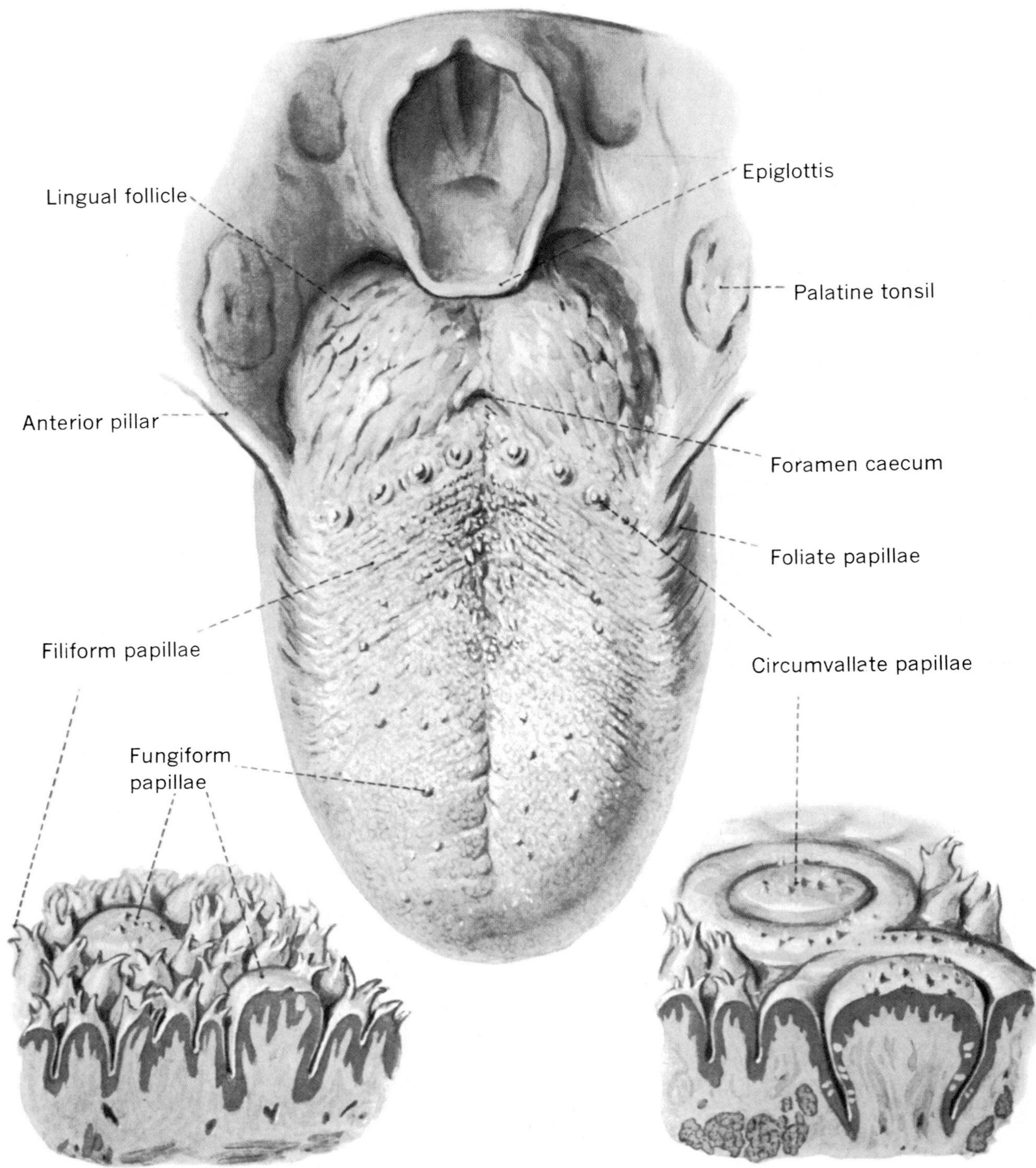

FIGURE 11–4
Normal anatomy of the dorsal surface of the tongue and relationship of papillae. (From Massler, M., and Schour, I. Atlas of the Mouth, 2nd ed. Chicago: American Dental Association, 1958, Plate 42. Copyright © 1958. Reprinted by permission of ADA Publishing Co., Inc.)

tongue and associated structures. Figure 11–4 illustrates the normal anatomy of the dorsal surface of the tongue and shows a magnification of its papillae. These structures must be visually and manually examined at each initial oral healthcare appointment for the control and prevention of oral disease.

Skills Used in the Extraoral and Intraoral Assessment Sequence

Extraoral Examination

The skills of direct **observation, palpation, auscultation,** and **olfaction** are basic to client assessment. These skills and examples of their application are described in Table 11–1. Table 11–2 describes the types of palpation techniques used. The dental hygienist must establish an examination sequence and follow it systematically during client assessment. The recommended sequence for a thorough extra- and intraoral examination is outlined and illustrated in Table 11–3. The client is observed during reception and seating to note physical characteristics and abnormalities and to make an overall appraisal. The client should be seated in an upright position with the clinician facing him. Good lighting and exposure of the area being assessed are essential (e.g., collar and tie loosened, glasses removed). The client's head, face, eyes, and neck are observed and the skin of the face and neck is evaluated.

If lesions are observed, clients should be asked how long they have had the lesions, if the lesions have changed, and whether they are painful. The clinician then extraorally palpates the following structures in the head and neck area, using firm but gentle bilateral circular compressions with the fingertips to identify enlargements, pain, and hard lymph nodes:

- **Anterior border of the mandible**—this structure is palpated bilaterally from a position behind the client to examine the soft tissue and underlying bone; the bimanual palpation starts at the midline and moves posteriorly to the angles of the mandible
- **Occipital nodes**—these nodes are bilaterally palpated at the base of the skull while the client's head is tilted forward (see Fig. 11–2*B*)
- **Auricular lymph nodes**—bilateral palpation occurs around the ear (i.e., above, behind, and in front of the ear) (see Fig. 11–2*B*)
- **Superficial and deep cervical lymph nodes** along the sternocleidomastoid muscle—the client is asked to turn his head to the right and lower his chin to increase visibility of and accessibility to the muscle. Supporting the chin with one hand, the dental hygienist grasps the muscle behind the ear and palpates bidigitally its entire length to check for deep cervical lymph nodes. After the client moves his head to an upright and forward position, circular compressions are applied with fingertips anterior and posterior to the muscle to check the superficial cervical nodes. Note all enlarged nodes for firmness, mobility, and tenderness. Repeat the process for the opposite side of the neck (see Fig. 11–2*B*).
- **Temporomandibular joint**—fingers are placed bilaterally just anterior to the ear while the client opens and closes his jaw slowly several times. Auscultation also is used to detect popping or clicking of the joint. If clicking is present, the client should be asked about associated pain.
- **Parotid gland**—fingers are placed bilaterally in front of the tragus of the ear; using gentle circular compressions with the fingertips, the dental hygienist palpates to the border of the mandible
- **Submental and submandibular glands**—the client is asked to bend the head slightly forward to gain access to the deep tissues of the submandibular area. Starting at the midline of the mandible, the dental hygienist palpates posteriorly to the angle of the mandible noting any lumps, tenderness, mobility, or firmness of lymph nodes.
- **Thyroid gland**—the thyroid gland lies in the anterior lower neck in front of and to the side of the trachea (see Fig. 11–2*A*). Standing in front of the client the dental hygienist observes the lower part of the neck while the client extends the neck and swallows. The action of swallowing should cause a bulge in the gland. To palpate the gland, the dental hygienist stands either in front of or behind the client. The client lowers the chin. The dental hygienist palpates the lower trachea (the isthmus) bilaterally with the fingertips while the client swallows. To examine each lobe, the dental hy-

Text continued on page 313

TABLE 11–1
SKILLS USED IN CONDUCTING THE EXTRAORAL AND INTRAORAL ASSESSMENT

Skill	Definition	What Is Being Assessed
Direct observation (inspection)	The act of viewing and watching the client to collect data	Client movement; body structure and symmetry; skin and mucous membrane color, texture, consistency, contour and form; and client knowledge, attitude and behavior
Palpation	The act of using the sense of touch to collect client data	Tenderness, texture, masses/tumors, variations in structure, and temperature
Auscultation	The act of listening to and detecting body sounds in order to determine variations from normal	Sounds made by the temporomandibular joint, e.g., clicking; hoarseness and general quality of speech which may be indicative of problems with the vocal cords
Olfaction	The act of sensing body odors to detect variations from normal and potential disease entities	Alcohol breath caused by alcohol abuse; halitosis associated with dental caries, periodontitis, acute necrotizing ulcerative gingivitis; sweet fruity ketosis associated with diabetic acidosis; and fetid sweet odor caused by a respiratory infection (Pseudomonas bacteria)

TABLE 11–2
PALPATION METHODS FOR ASSESSING THE ORAL CAVITY

Type	Definition	Technique
Digital palpation	Use a single finger to move or press against tissue	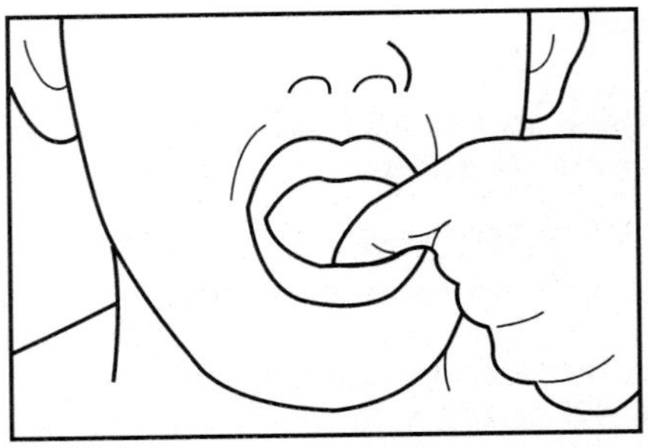 Use index finger to detect the presence of exostosis on the border of the mandible
Bidigital palpation	Use one or more fingers and a thumb to move or compress tissue	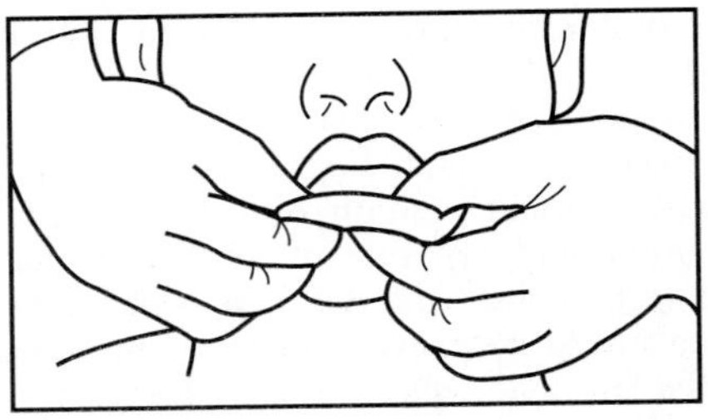 Palpate the lip.
Bimanual palpation	Use index finger of one hand and fingers and thumb of other hand simultaneously to move or compress tissue	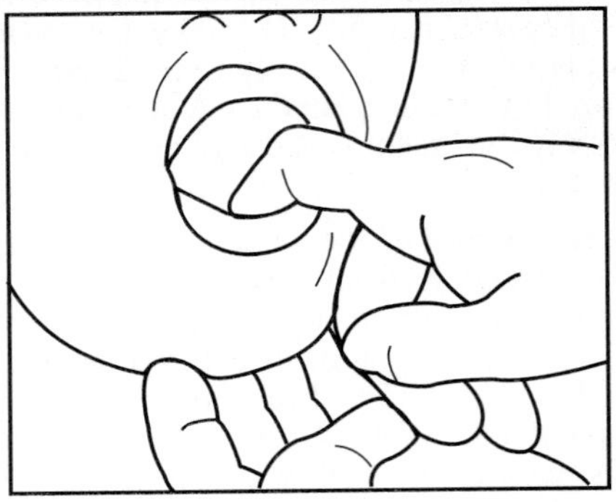 Palpate floor of the mouth with the index finger of one hand while pressing the same area extraorally with finger of the opposite hand under the chin
Manual palpation	Use all fingers of one hand to simultaneously move or compress tissues	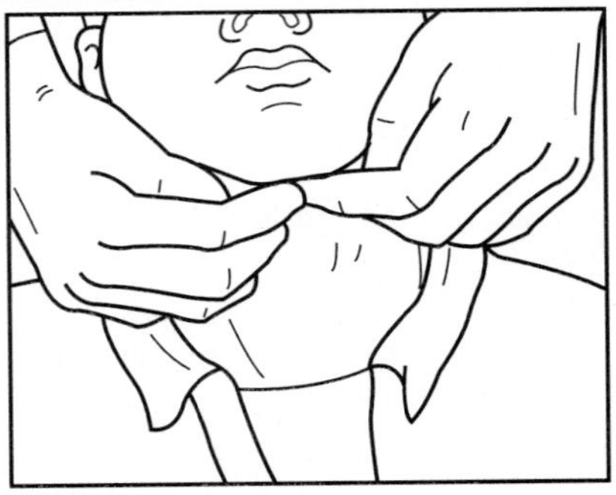
Bilateral palpation	Use a finger of both hands simultaneously to move or press tissue on contralateral sides of the head/body	Use both hands to examine the subauricular nodes
Circular compression	Move finger tips in a deliberate, rotating fashion over tissues to be examined and at the same time exert pressure	

TABLE 11–3
CONDUCTING EXTRAORAL AND INTRAORAL EXAMINATIONS

Equipment

Protective barriers, mouth mirror, 2 × 2 gauze, explorer, periodontal probe, tongue blade, hand mirror, cup of water to facilitate swallowing

Extraoral	Steps	Rationale	Normal Findings	Atypical Findings	Abnormal Findings
Face, head, and neck	With client sitting upright and relaxed, visually observe the symmetry, head and neck, including the skin, eyes, nose, mouth, ears, and areas of unusual pigmentation. Ask client to remove glasses	This step allows the clinician to check for signs of nutritional deficiency and/or signs of systemic disease, possible asymmetry from tumor or abnormal growth and development	Face and head should be symmetrical; skin should be continuous, firm and pigmented in relation to the normal variations associated with race and ethnicity. Eyes should be clear and exhibit normal responses to light stimulus	Moles, freckles, scars; facial grimacing during swallowing	Skin cancer, melanoma, alveolar/soft tissue abscesses, paralysis of facial nerve (Bell's palsy), tumors of jaw and parotid gland; jaundiced appearance of skin and eyes, pinpoint pupils; strained breathing (flared nostrils or roped breathing)

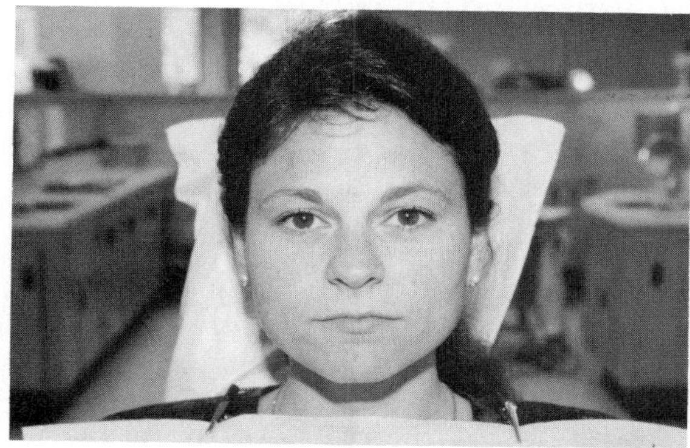

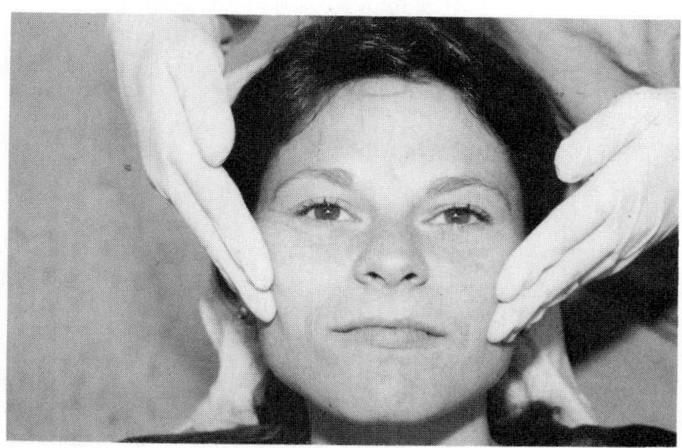

Extraoral	Steps	Rationale	Normal Findings	Atypical Findings	Abnormal Findings
Parotid gland, masseter muscle, and temporalis muscle	Visually observe and bilaterally palpate the parotid glands and parotid nodes located superior to the angles of the mandible. Test the functioning of each gland by wiping it with gauze and compressing it with a gloved finger to observe salivary flow. Place the fingers of each hand over the masseter muscle and ask client to clench the teeth together several times. Repeat on temporalis muscle	This step allows the clinician to check for signs of gland dysfunction: enlargement, tumors, calcified areas, tender enlarged nodes (lymphadenitis), and form and function of the masseter and temporalis muscles	Gland should be the color of the buccal mucosa and easily milked to express saliva	Prominent Stensen's duct, blocked duct of parotid gland	Sialolithiasis (salivary stone), parotitis (inflammation of parotid gland), excessive or inadequate salivary flow; tenderness and pain in the masseter and/or temporalis muscle; enlarged nodes (adenopathy) or masses; lymphadenitis. Tender, soft, enlarged and freely movable nodes may suggest acute infection

Table continued on following page

TABLE 11–3
CONDUCTING EXTRAORAL AND INTRAORAL EXAMINATIONS *Continued*

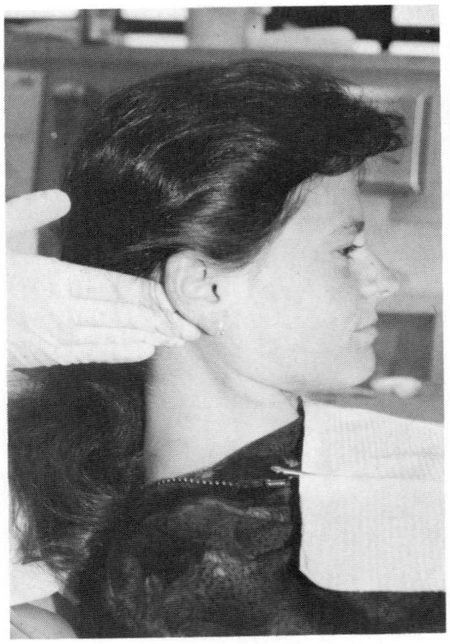

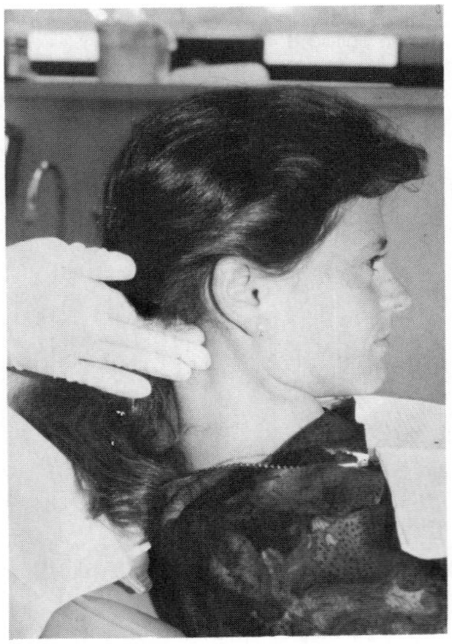

Extraoral	Steps	Rationale	Normal Findings	Atypical Findings	Abnormal Findings
Auricular lymph nodes (anterior, posterior, superior, inferior)	Bilaterally palpate the auricular lymph nodes, including the anterior, the posterior, the superior, and the inferior nodes	This step allows the clinician to check for tender, enlarged nodes (lymphadenitis) or masses indicating local or systemic infection; these nodes drain the ear areas and may indicate infection in that area	Nodes should not be clinically palpable or visible	Palpable, nontender node may be the result of scar tissue from a past chronic infection	Hard, nontender, and fixed nodes may suggest a chronic infection or even malignancy
Occipital lymph nodes	Have client tilt head toward the chest to bimanually palpate the occipital region located at base of the head	This step allows the clinician to check for tender, enlarged nodes or masses indicating local or systemic infection; these nodes drain the area and may indicate infection in that area	Nodes should not be clinically palpable or visible	Palpable, nontender node may be the result of scar tissue from a past chronic infection	Enlarged nodes (adenopathy) or masses; lymphadentitis. Tender, soft, enlarged and freely movable nodes may suggest acute infection. Hard, nontender and fixed nodes may suggest a chronic infection or even malignancy

TABLE 11–3
CONDUCTING EXTRAORAL AND INTRAORAL EXAMINATIONS *Continued*

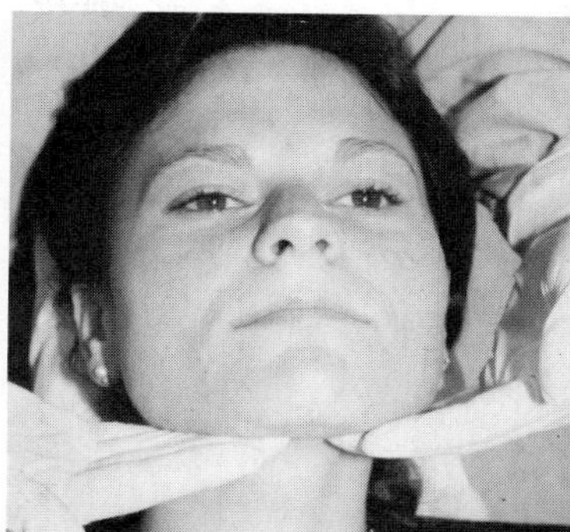

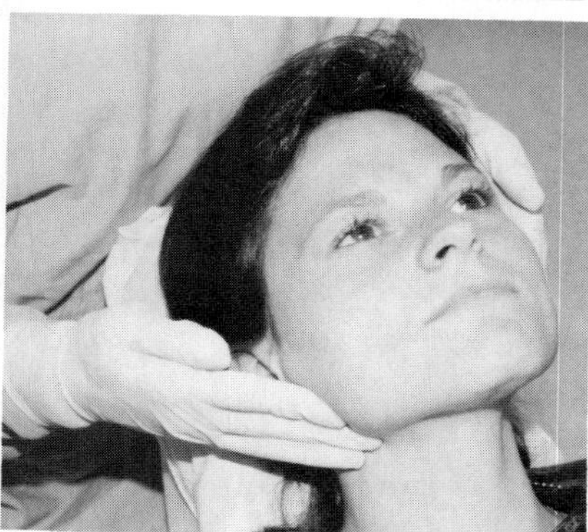

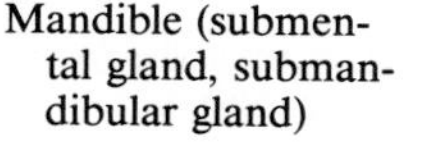

Extraoral	Steps	Rationale	Normal Findings	Atypical Findings	Abnormal Findings
Mandible (submental gland, submandibular gland)	"Cupping" the mandible with the thumb and fingers, palpate bilaterally and draw the tissue against lateral border of mandible. Palpate the mentalis muscle using digital compression; observe the function of the mentalis muscle during swallowing. From behind the client, use bidigital and circular compression to palpate from the symphysis to the posterior borders of the mandible, the submental region, and the submandibular region	This step allows the clinician to assess the submental, sublingual, and submandibular glands and lymph nodes	Mandible should be symmetrical, with continuous borders. Nodes should not be clinically palpable or visible	Exostosis of bone; facial grimacing during swallowing; crepitus	Tumors, bony or soft tissue masses; deviations in symmetry; tenderness; enlarged nodes (adenopathy) or masses; lymphadenitis. Tender, soft, enlarged and freely movable nodes may suggest acute infection. Hard, nontender and fixed nodes may suggest a chronic infection or even malignancy
Thyroid gland and larynx	In anterior lower neck, locate area just below "Adam's apple" to bidigitally palpate the gland. Place fingers on one side of trachea and gently push the thyroid gland towards the other side of the neck. With other hand, exert circular digital compression on the gland tissue. Ask client to swallow—gland should rise up and then down. Assess larynx with bilateral palpation	This step allows the clinician to check for masses; enlargement may be a manifestation of thyroid dysfunction	Thyroid gland should not be clinically visible; thyroid should rise up and down during swallowing; larynx should be freely movable when palpated and deliberatly moved	Prominent "Adam's apple"	Enlargement, soft tissue masses, immobility, evidence of thyroid surgery; lack of movement during swallowing 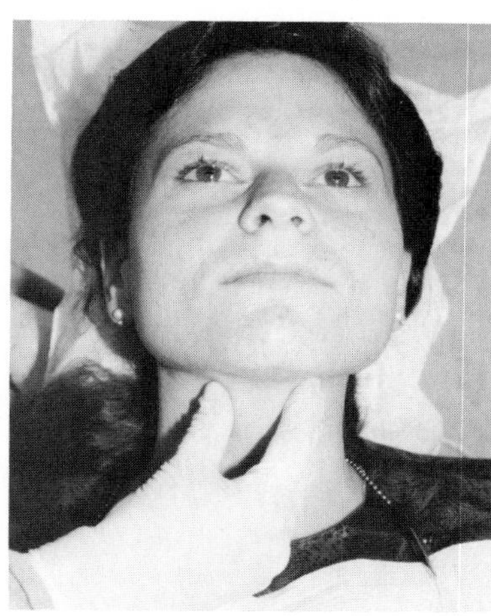

Table continued on following page

TABLE 11–3
CONDUCTING EXTRAORAL AND INTRAORAL EXAMINATIONS *Continued*

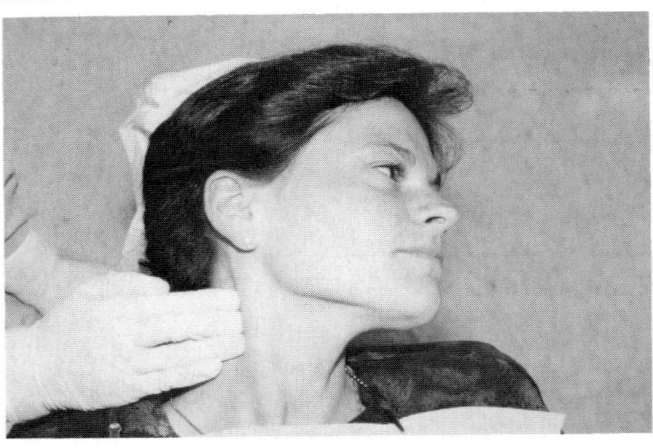

Extraoral	Steps	Rationale	Normal Findings	Atypical Findings	Abnormal Findings
Superficial cervical lymph nodes	Have client turn his head to one side. Next, alongside the exposed part of the neck, place fingers of both hands next to the sternocleidomastoid muscle. Palpate in a continuous manner from underneath the mandibular to the shoulder. Repeat for other side of the neck	This step allows the clinician to check for enlarged nodes or masses indicating local or systemic disease	Nodes should not be clinically palpable or visible	Enlarged neck muscles; palpable, nontender node may be the result of scar tissue from a past chronic infection	Enlarged nodes (adenopathy) or masses; lymphadenitis. Tender, soft, enlarged and freely movable nodes may suggest acute infection. Hard, nontender and fixed nodes may suggest a chronic infection or even malignancy
Deep cervical lymph nodes	Have client look straight ahead. Next, place your hand along the sternocleidomastoid muscle. Ask him to turn toward your hand and to look downward. Push your fingers into the deep tissues alongside the muscle. Palpate with thumb and index finger	This step allows the clinician to check for enlarged nodes or masses indicating local or systemic disease	Nodes should not be clinically palpable or visible	Enlarged neck muscles; palpable, nontender node may be the result of scar tissue from a past chronic infection	Enlarged nodes (adenopathy) or masses; lymphadenitis. Tender, soft, enlarged and freely movable nodes may suggest acute infection. Hard, nontender and fixed nodes may suggest a chronic infection or even malignancy

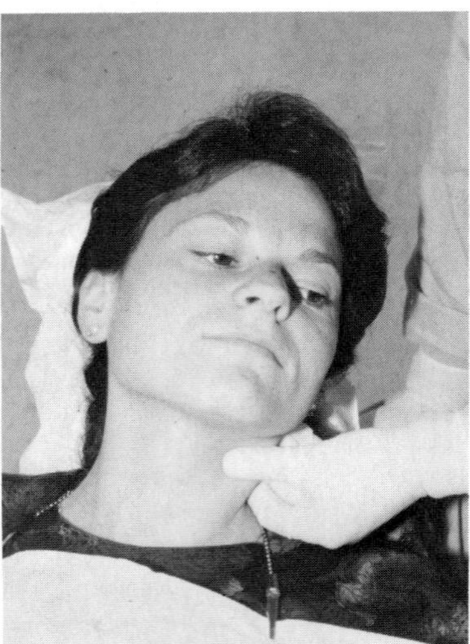

TABLE 11–3
CONDUCTING EXTRAORAL AND INTRAORAL EXAMINATIONS *Continued*

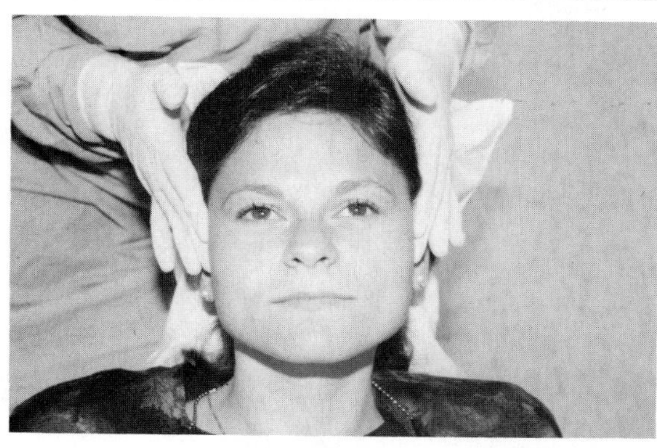

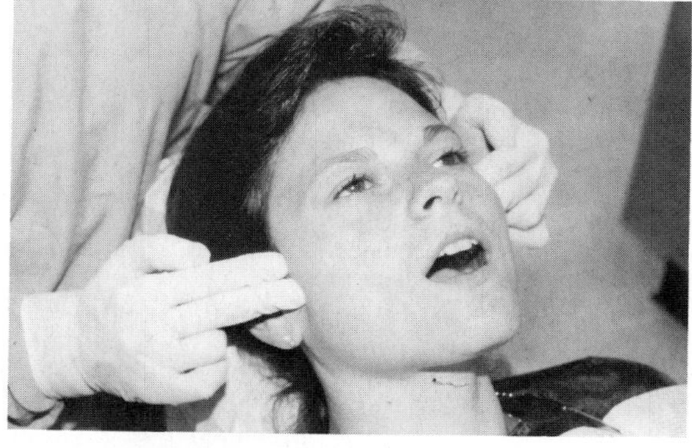

Extraoral	Steps	Rationale	Normal Findings	Atypical Findings	Abnormal Findings
TMJ (temporomandibular joint)	Bilaterally place fingers of hand just anterior to the outer meatus (tragus) of ears. Ask client to open and close mouth several times. Use auscultation to identify abnormal sounds from the joint. Ask client to move the opened jaw left, then right, and then forward	This step allows the clinician to assess for TMJ dysfunction	Movement should be smooth, continuous and sound-free; both sides of the joint should function similarly; both joint and associated musculature should be free of pain	Limitations of movement, discomfort during appointment	Clicking, popping, crepitus (a crackling sound), deviation, dysfunction, subluxation (an incomplete or partial dislocation); pain on movement
Lips	Ask client if he is experiencing any areas of discomfort in the mouth. Seat the client in a supine position and sit beside his head. Use one or several fingers to retract the corners of the mouth. Retract the lower lip down and out and	This step allows the clinician to assess skin of lips and vermilion border for changes in color, form, texture, signs of nutritional deficiency, or fungal infection	The lips should be a continuous pinkish-red color, or pigmented in relation to the normal coloration of the client's skin, firm in texture, free of lesions, semimoist, and an apparent border between the lips and the skin of the face.	Dryness, cracks, irritation from lip biting, herpetic lesions	Signs of vesiculoerosive disease (skin disease with bullous erosive oral mucous membranes), oral cancer, masses, lesions, mouth breathing, angular cheilosis, candidiasis, cheilitis

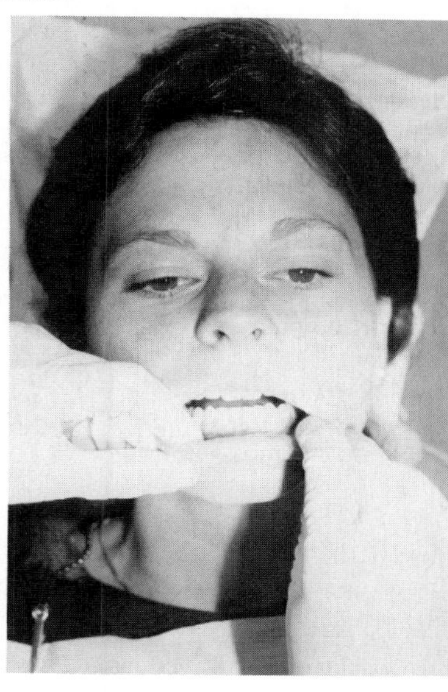

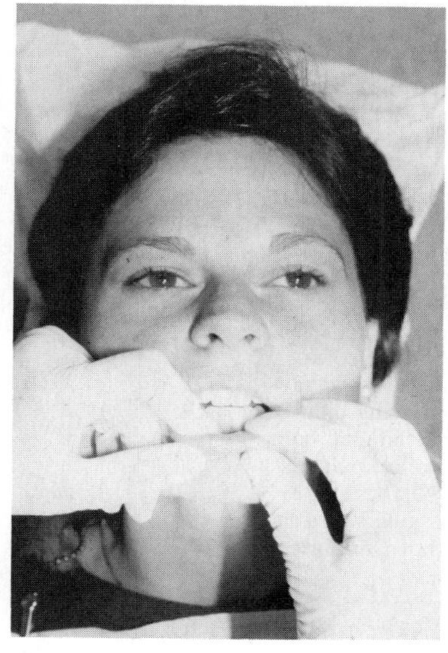

Table continued on following page

TABLE 11–3
CONDUCTING EXTRAORAL AND INTRAORAL EXAMINATIONS *Continued*

Extraoral	Steps	Rationale	Normal Findings	Atypical Findings	Abnormal Findings
	look at the inside of the lower lip. Palpate by using your thumb and forefinger in a systematic manner from one corner of the mouth to the other. Use same technique for the upper lip		Commissures should be continuous and intact		
	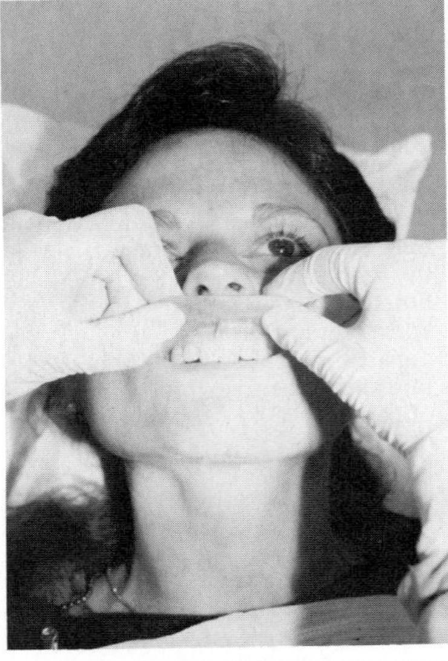		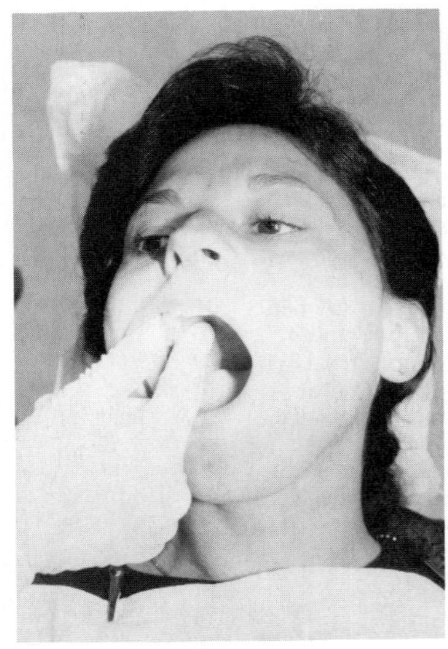		
Labial and alveolar mucosa and gingiva	Invert and inspect upper labial mucosa. Check labial frena for tightness, tissue tags, or scarring; inspect general state of free and attached gingiva, mucogingival junction, and alveolar mucosa. Palpate labial mucosa using bilateral, bidigital compression; palpate alveolar mucosa and gingiva using digital compression	This step allows the clinician to assess mucous membranes for signs of disease, and to locate gross signs of periodontal disease	Mucosa should be a continuous pinkish-red color, or pigmented in relation to the normal coloration of the client's skin, firm in texture, free of lesions, and moist	Traumatic lesions, abrasions, signs of smokeless tobacco use, tight frenum attachment, mucocele, lip biting, Fordyce's granules (ectopic sebaceous glands), amalgam tattoo	Signs of vesiculoerosive disease, recurrent aphthous ulcers, masses, lesions, oral cancer, gingival recession and inflammation, mouth breathing
Buccal mucosa (see left-hand and center figures on next page)	Have client turn to one side. Use one or several fingers of one hand to retract the cheek. Use mouth mirror to reflect light and inspect the buccal mucosa. Palpate buccal mucosa with your thumb and first fingers and bimanually. Repeat for other side	This step allows the clinician to evaluate mucous membranes for signs of disease, enlargements or masses within the parotid gland/Stensen's duct	Mucosa should be a continuous pinkish-red color, or pigmented in relation to the normal coloration of the client's skin, firm in texture, free of lesions, and moist. The parotid papilla and Stensen's duct should be visible anatomical landmarks opposite the area of the maxillary molars	Traumatic lesions, linea alba (white line on buccal mucosa adjacent to where teeth occlude), Fordyce's granules (ectopic sebaceous glands), cheek biting	Lichen planus, leukedema, oral cancer, blocked Stensen's duct

TABLE 11–3
CONDUCTING EXTRAORAL AND INTRAORAL EXAMINATIONS *Continued*

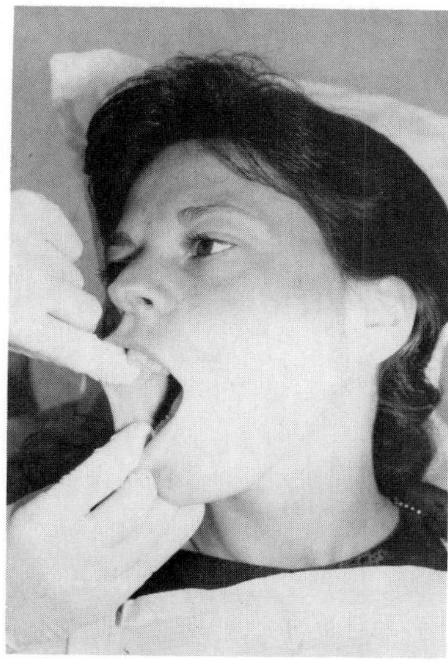
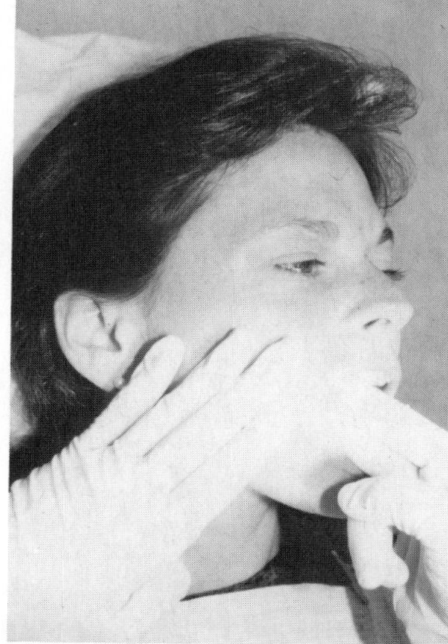
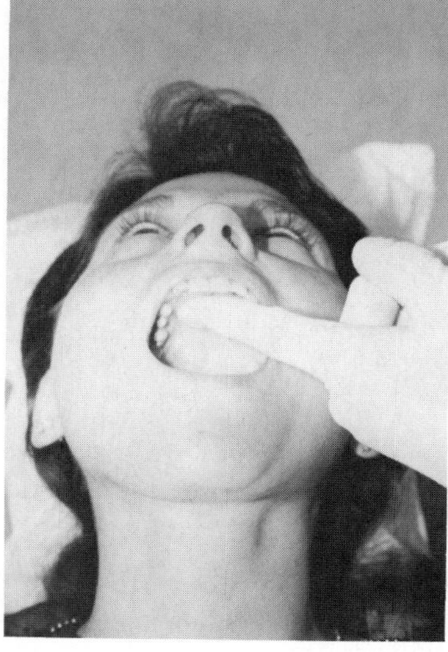

Extraoral	Steps	Rationale	Normal Findings	Atypical Findings	Abnormal Findings
Hard and soft palate and alveolar ridges	Have client tilt his head back slightly. Use mouth mirror to intensify light source and view the hard and soft palate including maxillary tuberosities and retromolar areas. Compress hard and soft palate with first or second finger of one hand. Avoid digital compression on this soft palate to prevent initiating the gag reflex. Palpate and visually examine the alveolar ridges	This step allows the clinician to check hard palate, palatine raphe, incisive papilla, rugae for changes in color, form, and texture. Furthermore, the clinician can assess soft palate for changes in form and texture. To assess for signs of abscesses, swellings, exostoses, or tenderness	Pink in color or pigmented in relation to the normal coloration of the client's skin. Anatomical structures to observe are incisive papilla, medial palatal raphe, palatal rugae, palatine fovea, demarcation between hard and soft palate, anterior and posterior palatine pillars, and uvula	Hard palate: petechiae (pinpoint discoloration of mucous membrane from hemorrhage), torus palatinus, food burns, scarring from third molar extractions, opercula, impacted third molars Soft palate: petechiae, bifid uvula Alveolar ridges: exostoses	Denture stomatitis, denture-related candidiasis (fungal infection), nicotine stomatitis, oral cancer Any lesions or ulcers Abscesses, fistulas, swellings
Oropharynx	Visually assess by asking client to say "ah" 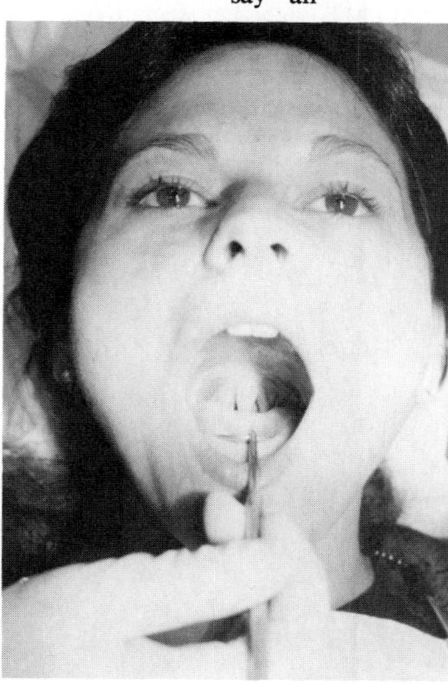	This step allows the clinician a wide view of the palatine and pharyngeal tonsils, posterior pharyngeal wall, uvula, anterior and posterior pillars for signs of infection or disease	Pinkish-red in color or pigmented in relation to the normal coloration of the client's skin	Prominent tonsillar tissues in children, sore throat, postnasal drip	Tonsilitis, oral cancer, lesions, masses

Table continued on following page

TABLE 11–3
CONDUCTING EXTRAORAL AND INTRAORAL EXAMINATIONS *Continued*

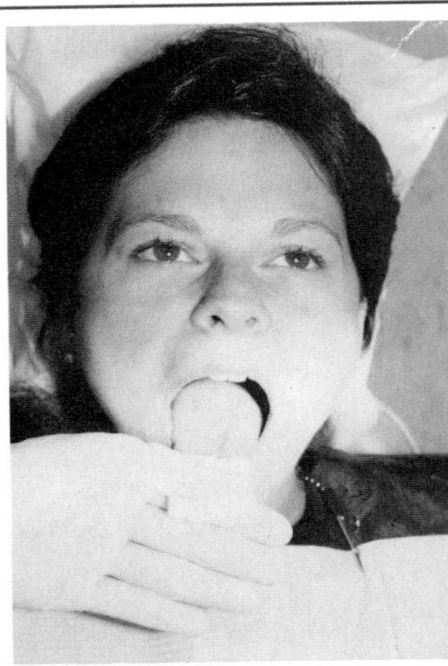
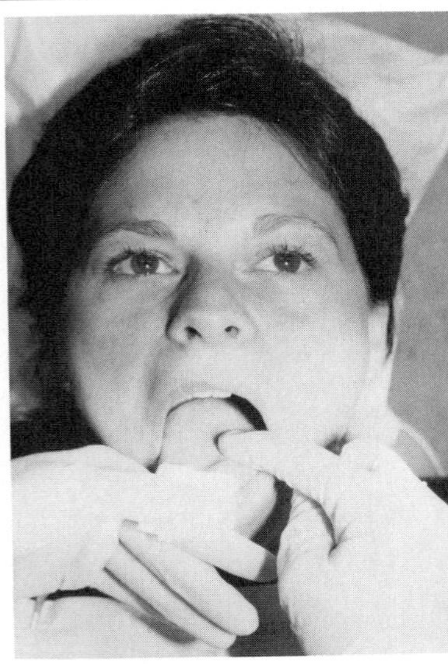
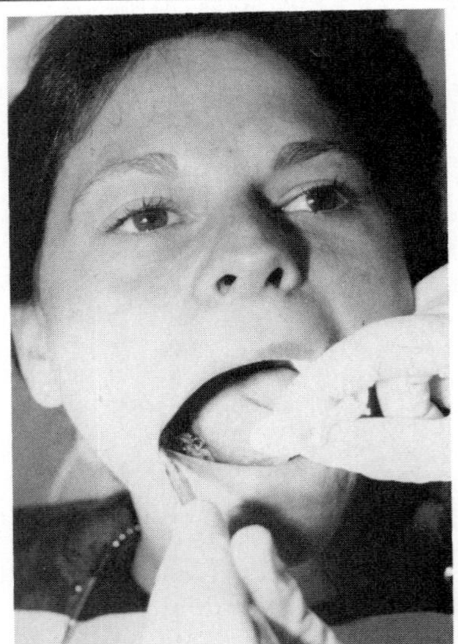

Extraoral	Steps	Rationale	Normal Findings	Atypical Findings	Abnormal Findings
Tongue	Visually inspect dorsal surface; ask client to extend tongue onto piece of gauze. With one hand, firmly grasp tongue and turn it slightly on its side to view lateral borders by digital palpation with the other hand. Ask client to touch the roof of mouth with the tip of the tongue to assess ventral surface. Ask client to touch facial surface of the maxillary molars with	This step allows the clinician to check filiform, fungiform, circumvallate, and foliate papilla as well as foramen cecum and lingual tonsils; to check ventral surface of tongue for signs of oral cancer; to evaluate oral cleansing capabilities of the tongue; to evaluate swallowing pattern	Bilateral symmetry, extremely vascular, reddish-pink in color and moist; may be pigmented in relation to the normal coloration of the client's skin	Fissured or geographic tongue, median rhomboid glossitis (smooth rhomboidal elevation without papillae on posterior ⅓ of tongue), lingual varicosities (enlarged lingual veins), plica fimbriata (feathery folds of tissue on the ventral surface of the tongue), coated tongue, macroglossia (enlarged tongue), tongue thrusting behavior during swallowing	Hairy leukoplakia (hair-like extensions of keratin on lateral border of tongue indicating HIV infection), other signs of oral cancer

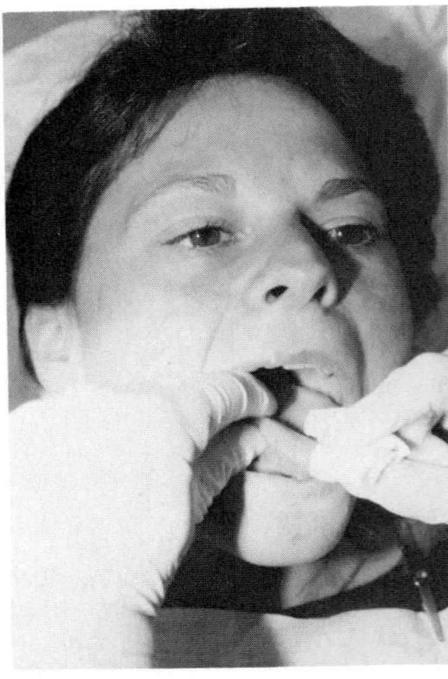
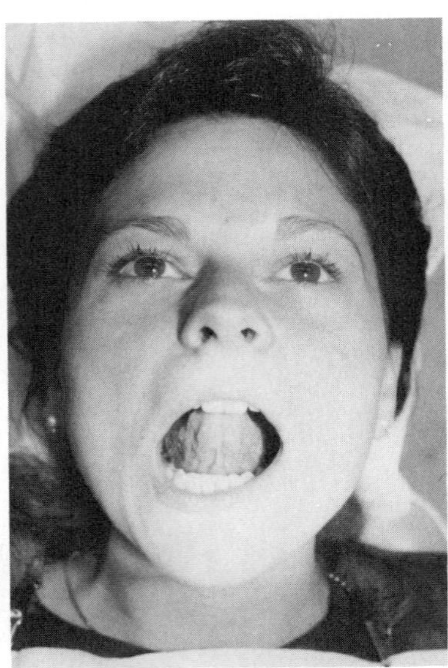
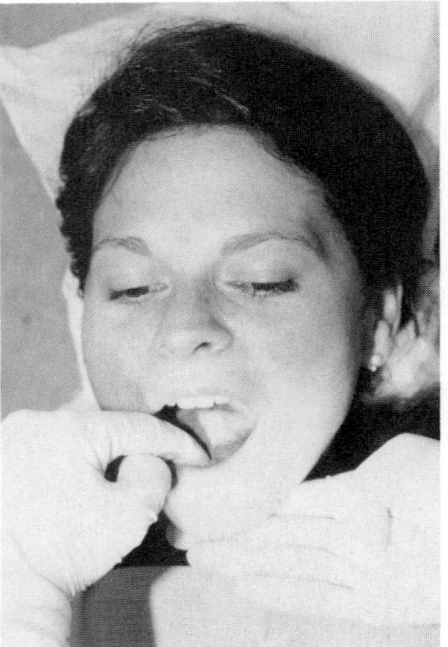

TABLE 11–3
CONDUCTING EXTRAORAL AND INTRAORAL EXAMINATIONS *Continued*

Extraoral	Steps	Rationale	Normal Findings	Atypical Findings	Abnormal Findings
	the tip of the tongue. While holding lips apart, ask client to swallow and observe swallowing pattern				
Floor of mouth	Along with visual observation, bimanually palpate the entire floor of mouth; use a finger of one hand, and finger and thumb of another under the chin to palpate. Test functioning of the submandibular gland by wiping each Wharton's duct with gauze and compressing it with a gloved finger to observe salivary flow	This step allows the clinician to detect enlargement or masses, Wharton's duct, sublingual caruncle, lingual frenum	Bilateral symmetry, extremely vascular, reddish-pink in color and moist. Anatomical structures to observe are lingual vein, plica fimbriatic, lingual frenum, sublingual caruncle, Wharton's duct, sublingual folds, and plica fimbrata	Varicosities, limitations of movement of tongue, tight frenum attachment, blocked salivary duct	Tenderness, color changes, ankyloglossia, any enlargement or induration, or signs of oral cancer

gienist has the client turn the head slightly toward the side being examined. For example, during examination of the right lobe the client lowers the chin and turns his head slightly to the right. The hygienist's left hand gently moves the gland to the right while the right hand gently palpates the lobe. The process is repeated for the left lobe. Enlargement of the isthmus as the client swallows or lack of movement should be noted because they may be signs of thyroid dysfunction. Masses and nodules also should be noted.

Intraoral Examination

After the extraoral examination is complete, document abnormal or atypical findings in the client record. Proceed to the *intraoral assessment*. For clients who wear dentures, provide them with a tissue and denture cup and ask them to remove their dentures. After making an initial inspection intraorally with a mouth mirror, the dental hygienist should observe and palpate the following structures:

- **Lips**—normally lips are pink in light-skinned individuals or pigmented with melanin in dark-skinned individuals, uniform in color, slightly moistened, symmetrical, and smooth. Inspect them for color, texture, hydration, contour, and the presence of lesions. Also check for cracks at the corner of the mouth (called "angular cheilitis"). Apply lubricant to cracked and dry areas to meet the client's need for freedom from pain.
- **Oral mucosa**—normal oral mucosa is glistening pink or pigmented with melanin and uniform in color. Normal hyperpigmentation of the oral mucosa is seen in 10% of whites after the age of 50 and in up to 90% of African-Americans by the same age. Small, whitish bumps just below the mucosal lining are ectopic sebaceous glands (called **Fordyce's granules**). Have the client open his mouth slightly and gently pull the lower lip away from the teeth to observe the labial mucosa for color, hydration, and lesions. Bidigitally palpate it for hard masses and tenderness. Repeat the process for the upper lip. Then gently pull the buccal mucosa slightly away from the teeth to observe for swellings, lesions, and color changes (white or red patches); palpate bidigitally for hard masses or tenderness. Note that opposite the second molar is a soft tissue flap, the **parotid papilla,** that marks the opening of **Stenson's duct** to the parotid gland. Dry the area and observe the flow of saliva from each duct. Retract mucosa enough to inspect the vestibular area.
- **Tongue**—normally, the tongue appears medium red in color with smooth lateral margins and free mobility. Melanin pigmentation may be observed in dark-skinned individuals. The dorsal surface should not be exceptionally smooth. It is covered with whitish hair-like **filiform papillae** which may become stained with tobacco or coated as a result of poor oral hygiene. Less numerous **fungiform papillae,** mushroom-shaped and red in color, are scattered among the filiform papillae and contain taste buds for sweet, sour, and salt stimuli. In addition, the **circumvallate papillae** are larger and broader and located in a V formation on the posterior section of the dorsal surface of the tongue and contain taste buds responsible for sensing bitter taste. The **foliate papillae** contain taste buds responsible for sour and acidic stimuli and are found along a series of vertical ridges on the posterior lateral borders of the tongue. A gauze square is wrapped around the anterior one-third of the tongue to obtain a firm grasp while the client extends it. If the client is forced to extend the tongue too far the gag reflex is triggered. The dor-

sal surface is palpated digitally. The tongue is turned slightly on its side to inspect its base and lateral borders (common sites for oral cancer) for abnormal color, swellings, masses, or lesions. Bidigitally palpate the lateral surfaces of the tongue. Have the client lift his tongue to inspect and digitally palpate the ventral surface. Note the **lingual vein** and the **plica fimbriata** (feathery folds of tissue next to the lingual vein).

Atypical variations of the tongue include the geographic tongue, the fissured tongue, and the coated tongue. The **geographic tongue** is a condition in which there is a sporadic and uneven distribution of papillae, or de-papillation lending an unusual "topographic" appearance. A **fissured tongue** is a condition in which fissures or grooves are observed on the tongue, most frequently down the midline. A **coated tongue** displays a yellow or whitish covering on all or a portion of the tongue's dorsal surface.

- **Soft palate and oral pharynx**—while the tongue is extended, observe the soft palate for color change and lesions. Gently place the mouth mirror or tongue blade on the middle of the tongue and ask the client to say "ah." As he does this, observe the uvula and the pharynx for deviations in color and signs of lesions. Normally, pharyngeal structures are pink, well-hydrated, and devoid of lesions.
- **Hard palate**—have the client point his chin to the ceiling. Observe the surface of the hard palate. Digitally palpate the hard palate for lesions, swellings, hard masses, and color change. In approximately 15 to 20% of the population the hard palate has a **torus palatinus** (a projection of bone) in the midline.
- **Floor of the mouth**—while the client lifts the tongue to the roof of the mouth, observe the mucosa of the floor of the mouth for lesions, swelling, or color change. Observe the **sublingual caruncle,** a small round area at the base of the lingual frenum which is the opening of **Wharton's duct** of the submandibular salivary gland. Wipe the caruncle with gauze and observe the saliva flow from the duct. Bimanually palpate the sublingual area by placing the right index finger intraorally and the fingertips of the left hand extraorally under the chin to feel the tissue between the two hands. Note any tenderness or swelling.
- **Gingiva**—the gingiva is that part of the oral mucous membrane attached to the teeth and the alveolar processes of the jaws. The color of normal gingiva is pale pink but may vary according to degree of vascularity, epithelial keratinization (thickness), and pigmentation. The papillae of anterior teeth that are in contact fill the interproximal spaces to the contact point. The papillae of posterior teeth are normally flatter and "saddle-like." When there are spaces between the teeth, the papillae tend to be flatter. With increasing age the papillae may atrophy slightly (together with the underlying alveolar crest); therefore, a more blunt contour may be considered normal for older clients, even in between anterior teeth in contact. The texture (surface) of the gingiva is generally stippled, and stippling is usually present in varying degrees on facial surfaces of the attached gingiva. A stippled surface is often described as "orange peel" in appearance. The consistency of the gingiva upon bidigital palpation should be firm and the attached part tightly anchored to the teeth and underlying alveolar bone. (See Chapter 13 for a detailed discussion of gingiva.)

Palpate the maxillary tuberosity and the retromolar area using digital compression. Use the mouth mirror to facilitate lighting and direct observation. Note any abnormal growth of tissue, **exostoses,** abnormal bony growths from the surfaces of bone, lesions, and tenderness. The general extra- and intraoral examinations are now complete. After documenting all pertinent findings in the client record, the dental hygienist initiates specific periodontal, oral hygiene, and tooth assessments (see Chapters 12 and 13).

Table 11–3 provides a detailed rationale for examining recommended structures and lists common and abnormal findings that may be observed during an extra- and intraoral assessment.

TABLE 11–4
CATEGORIES OF ORAL LESIONS

Lesion	Lesion Category	Size (cm)	Description	Example
	Macule	< 1	Flat, nonpalpable	Freckle, petechiae
	Papule	< 0.5	Palpable, circumscribed, solid elevation in skin	Elevated freckle
	Nodule	0.5–2	Elevated solid mass; deeper and firmer than papule	Wart

TABLE 11-4
CATEGORIES OF ORAL LESIONS *Continued*

Lesion	Lesion Category	Size (cm)	Description	Example
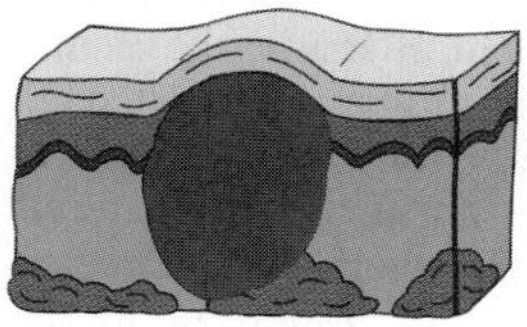	Tumor	> 1–2	Solid mass; may extend deep through subcutaneous tissue	Epithelioma
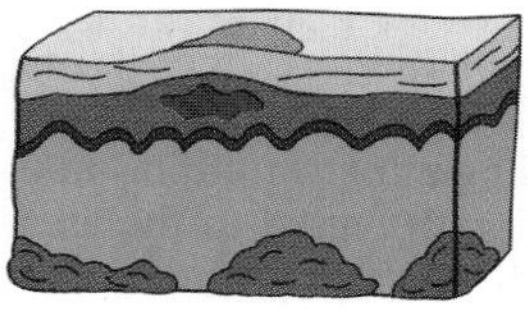	Wheal	Varies	Elevated area of superficial localized edema; irregularly shaped	Hive
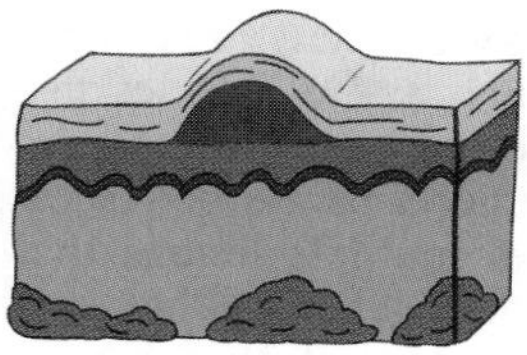	Vesicle	< 0.5	Circumscribed elevation of skin filled with serous fluid	Herpes labialis
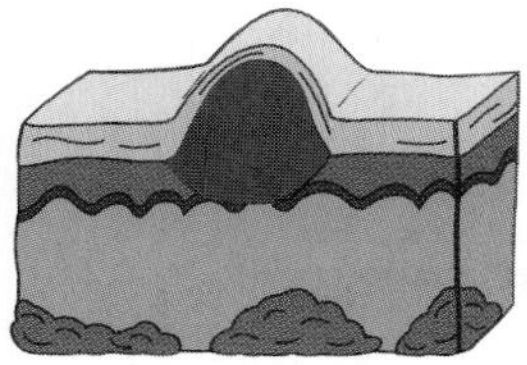	Pustule	Varies	Similar to vesicle; lesion filled with pus	Acne
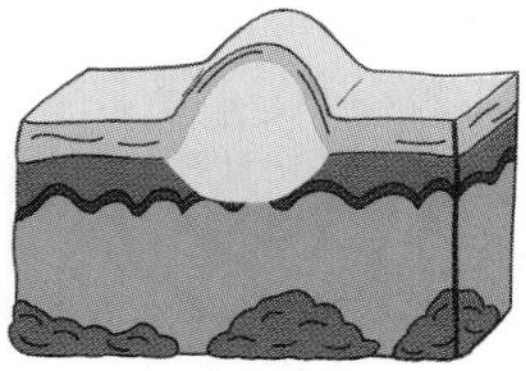	Bulla	> 0.5	Circumscribed bleb containing clear, watery fluid or blood	Blister
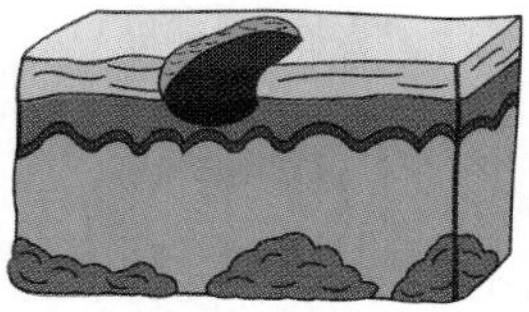	Ulcer	Varies	Deep loss of epidermis, may extend to dermis	Recurrent aphthous ulcer
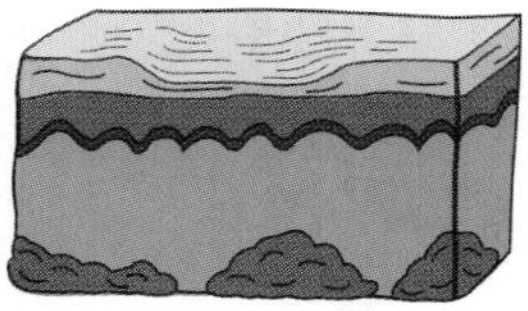	Atrophy	Varies	Thinning of skin with loss of normal skin furrow; shiny and translucent skin	Oral mucosa often found in the elderly
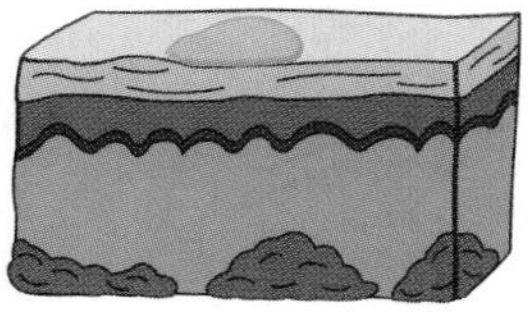	Plaque	> 0.5	A discrete, slightly elevated area of altered texture or coloration	Candidiasis

Redrawn and modified from Potter, P. A., and Perry, A. G. Fundamentals of Nursing: Concepts, Process, and Practice, 3rd ed. St. Louis: C. V. Mosby, 1993, p. 526.

Describing and Documenting Significant Findings

Following the observation of atypical or abnormal findings, the dental hygienist must describe and record them accurately in the client's permanent record. The ability to describe an oral lesion is critical to the assessment process because precise descriptive terms enable the dental hygienist to communicate with the dentist and other healthcare professionals, to identify the lesion and facilitate its accurate dental diagnosis. The terms listed in Table 11–4 provide the terminology used to categorize and describe oral lesions.

A complete description of each abnormal finding includes a written statement in the client's record about the location, distribution, size, color, surface texture, and attachment of the lesion. On palpation, consistency, mobility, symptomatology, and associated **lymphadenopathy** (hardening and enlargement of the lymph nodes) also should be evaluated and recorded. A sample form used for collecting data during an extraoral and intraoral assessment is shown in Figure 11–5.

Location and Distribution

The precise **location** of a finding should be recorded in the client's record along with its description. The location is important because some lesions characteristically occur in specific areas and this information can help the dentist formulate a differential dental diagnosis. For example, herpes labialis characteristically recurs in the same location on the upper and lower lip; in HIV-positive clients, hairy leukoplakia occurs on the lateral borders of the tongue. When describing the location of an oral lesion the dental hygienist should identify the specific anatomical part (e.g., upper lip, labial mucosa, tongue); specify its anatomical relationship (e.g., anterior/posterior, dorsal/ventral, lateral/medial, inferior/superior), and specify whether it is located on the right side of the mouth, on the left side, or in the midline.

In addition to its location, **distribution** of the lesion should be stated when describing it. Distribution of a lesion refers to whether the lesion is single or multiple and whether it is localized or generalized with regard to the area affected. A mucocele (a distended epithelial-lined space filled with mucinous secretions) is an example of a single lesion that is well-demarcated. Herpes simplex virus manifesting on the gingiva often presents as multiple lesions, referring to several lesions of a specific type. Multiple lesions may be described as being either separate or coalescing. The term **"separate"** describes multiple lesions that are discrete and do not run together, whereas the term **"coalescing"** describes lesions with margins that merge.

ORAL/ FACIAL SOFT TISSUE EXAMINATION RECORD

PATIENT'S NAME: ____________________

PATIENT'S I.D. #: ____________________

N = Normal O = Other use "Notes" section

Date:	N	O	N	O	N	O	N	O
EXTRAORAL								
Skin – Face								
– Neck								
* Vermilion Borders								
Parotid Glands								
Lymph Nodes								
Anterior Cervical								
Posterior Cervical								
Submental								
Submandibular								
Supraclavicular								
INTRAORAL								
Labial Mucosa								
Labial Vestibules								
Anterior Gingivae								
Buccal Vestibules								
Buccal Gingivae								
Tongue – Dorsal								
* – Ventral								
* – Lateral								
* Lingual Tonsils								
* Floor of Mouth								
Lingual Gingivae								
* Tonsillar Pillars								
* Pharyngeal Wall								
* Soft Palate								
Uvula								
Hard Palate								
Palatal Gingivae								
Submandibular Glands								

RIGHT LEFT

* *High risk sites for squamous carcinoma*

FIGURE 11–5
Extraoral and intraoral assessment form. (Courtesy of the American Cancer Society. Developed by the Dental Professional Education Subcommittee. American Cancer Society, California Division, Inc.)

RECOMMENDATIONS:

1. Establish an examination sequence and follow it routinely.
2. Tell the patient you are performing a complete Soft Tissue Examination.
3. Examine **ALL** areas each time.
4. Use visual inspection **AND** palpation.
5. Record **ALL** findings — Normal or Abnormal.
6. Remove dental appliances before the examination.
7. Suggested descriptive terms: hard, soft, well-circumscribed, ill-defined, indurated, sessile, pedunculated, hemorrhagic, ulcerated, edematous, normal in color, red, white, speckled, color other than normal.

NOTES

FOLLOW-UP TAKEN

Biopsy ______

Results ______

Referral to Dr. ______

Other ______

This chart is a general guideline. Neither the American Cancer Society nor the California Dental Association assume liability for individual evaluation or recommendations.

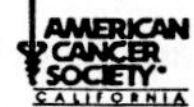

Developed by the Dental Education Subcommittee
American Cancer Society, California Division, Inc.

FIGURE 11–5 *Continued*

"Localized lesions" refers to lesions that are limited to a single area, whereas **"generalized lesions"** describes lesions involving more than one area in the oral cavity.

The majority of oral lesions occur singly. Examples of single lesions are the *mucocele,* and *amalgam tattoo* or *argyrosis* (a localized gray-blue discoloration from inadvertent disposition of silver amalgam fragments). Multiple lesions may be localized or generalized, and may indicate a systemic disease of a dermatological nature. Examples of dermatological diseases include *erythema multiforme* (a disease of unknown cause with bullous erosive involvement of the oral mucous membranes), and *lichen planus* (a skin disease with oral manifestations that vary from flat or slightly elevated lesions with striae to extensive areas of ulceration or erosion).

Size

The size of oral lesions varies, but generally a lesion is not tolerated by the client when it is larger than 1 to 2 cm. Size can be measured with a periodontal probe, in addition to using the teeth that border the lesion as markers. For example, an appropriate statement documenting lesion size in a client's chart may be entered as follows: lesion measures 4 × 5 mm and covers the attached gingiva extending from the apices of tooth number 24 to number 25.

Color

Oral lesions may display a variety of colors depending on the type of tissue or combination of tissues of which they are composed. Lesion colors that can be observed normally are red **(erythroplakia)** and white **(leukoplakia)**. Other less common colors may include blue, purple, yellow, black, or gray. Lesions of normal color exhibit the same color as the adjacent tissue. Lesions of a red color may be the result of increased vascularity, thinning, or loss of the surface mucosa. White lesions may be the result of hyperkeratosis of the surface epithelium or decreased vascularity. Blue lesions may be the result of increased melanin or blood or to the presence of amalgam particles. Yellow lesions usually contain lipid material.

Surface Texture

Texture refers to the surface appearance or characteristics of the tissue. The surface characteristics of a lesion are important to note during clinical assessment because they are taken into account when establishing a list of possible dental diagnoses (differential diagnosis). Lesions of surface epithelial tissues frequently have a rough surface, whereas those of deeper tissues may have a smooth surface (Table 11–5).

TABLE 11-5
TERMS USED TO DESCRIBE SURFACE TEXTURE OF A LESION

Term	Description
Smooth	Deep lesions that push up and stretch surface tissue
Papillary	Rough surface resembling small nodulations or elevated projections
Verrucous	Rough, wart-like surface with multiple irregular folds
Crust	A hard outer layer or covering composed of dried serum, pus, blood, or a combination
Cratered	Centrally depressed like a bowl or saucer
Indurated	Hardness primarily as a result of an increase in the number of epithelial cells
Pseudomembrane	A loose membranous layer of exudate containing organisms formed during an inflammatory reaction of the surface tissue

Modified from Wilkins, E. M. The Clinical Practice of the Dental Hygienist. Philadelphia: Lea & Febiger, 1989. Used with permission.

Attachment

If a lesion has a broad base of attachment as wide as the lesion itself, its attachment is described as **sessile. Pedunculated** lesions have a narrow pedicle, or stalk-like base of attachment (Fig. 11-6).

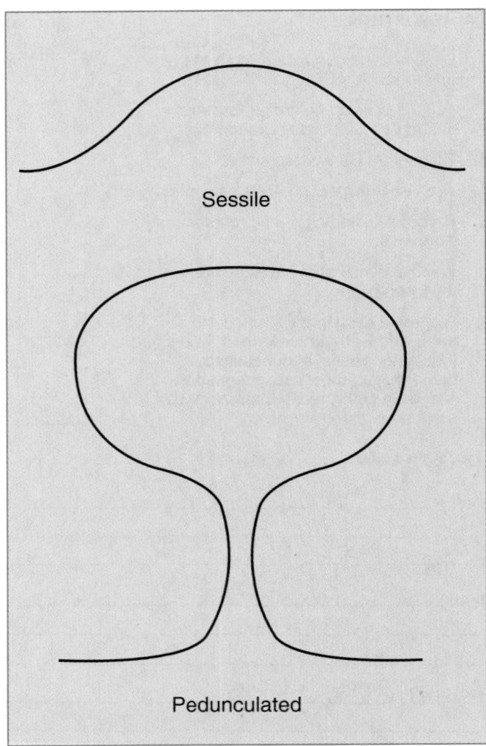

FIGURE 11-6
Types of base or attachment of a lesion.

Consistency

Consistency refers to the degree of firmness or density or degree of movement of the tissue. Therefore, consistency cannot be evaluated by visual examination alone. Palpation (feeling by touching) is required to categorize the consistency of a lesion (Table 11-6).

Symptomatology

By directing questions to the client, the dental hygienist can elicit symptoms related to the finding. A **symptom** is a subjective condition reported by the individual. A **sign** is an objective condition that can be directly observed. Specifically, the dental hygienist can determine and record in the client's permanent record:

- Whether the lesion is known or unknown to the client
- If the lesion is known to the client, how long it has been present, and if there have been any changes in its size and appearance (signs)
- Whether the client has related symptoms: pain, tingling, burning, or numbness, etc.

TABLE 11-6
TERMS TO INDICATE CONSISTENCY OF AN ORAL LESION

Term	Description
Fluctuant	A lesion that conveys a wave-like motion usually owing to a liquid content
Soft	A lesion composed chiefly of cells without much intervening fibrous connective tissue
Firm	A lesion that is harder than the adjacent mucosa indicating a high content of fibrous connective tissue
Indurated	Hardness primarily as a result of an increase in the number of epithelial cells
Hard	A lesion that contains bone or other calcified material
Mobile	A lesion which can freely move upon palpation

Modified from Wilkins, E. M. The Clinical Practice of the Dental Hygienist. Philadelphia: Lea & Febiger, 1989. Used with permission.

Associated Swelling and Enlargement of Lymph Nodes

To determine whether the oral lesion has systemic involvement or has invaded nearby tissues, it is important to identify swollen or enlarged lymph nodes near the area of the lesion. This identification is made possible by palpation of lymph nodes during the extra- and intraoral assessment procedure. Oral cancer spreads primarily by local direct extension and lymphatic permeation.[2] Involved lymph nodes are freely movable at first, but as they gradually become replaced by tumor tissue, they increase in size and may attain considerable proportions. The tumor then breaks and ulcerates into the surrounding tissue and becomes fixed to vital structures such as the carotid artery.[2] Therefore, swollen, soft, mobile lymph nodes are of less concern than those that are hard and immobile. Figure 11-7 depicts descriptions of lesions for entry into a client's record.

Examine and palpate the tongue, including the dorsal and ventral surfaces, lateral border, and base. Wrap the tongue with a piece of gauze and retract it to observe the posterior one-third: first to one side, then to the other. Observe the mucosa of the floor of the mouth. Palpate the floor of the mouth. Examine the hard and soft palates,

Example No. 1:

Chart Entry:
Positive finding on intraoral examination: lower right labial mucosa, single white sessile nodule 2 × 2 mm with a slightly rough surface; nonmobile on palpation. Client is asymptomatic with no associated lymphadenopathy. Client has been informed and will return for follow-up visit in 2 weeks—possible biopsy or referral to oral surgeon if the lesion changes in nature or does not resolve.

Date the entry; have the entry initialed by DDS and RDH.

Example No. 2:

Chart entry:
Positive finding on extraoral examination: upper left vermilion border, multiple coalescing vesicles 5 × 7 mm in total area; slightly red in color with a crust. Lesions have been known to the client for 5 days and began with associated tingling and itching in the area prior to appearance of the lesions. Client reports a history of similar "cold sores" in the area.

Date the entry; have the entry initialed by DDS and RDH.

FIGURE 11–7
Sample descriptions of lesions for entry into the client's dental record.

oropharyngeal and tonsillar areas, back of the throat, and uvula.

ORAL CANCER

Oral cancer accounts for 3% to 4% of all cancers each year (see Chapter 34). Oral cancer is more common than cancers of the brain, liver, bone, stomach, cervix, and ovaries; it is more common than leukemia. If oral cancer is detected early, the cure rate is over 90%. Unfortunately, by the time of dental or medical diagnosis, about two-thirds of oral cancers are advanced lesions leading to high morbidity and mortality. Annually, oral cancer kills more people than cervical cancer and costs society more than $2 billion in treatment and lost wages. Many of these malignant conditions could be arrested if detected earlier. Dental hygienists have a unique opportunity during client assessment to detect oral cancer while it is still asymptomatic, innocuous, and unsuspected.

Although tumors may arise at any site in the oral cavity, the most common sites are:

- The lateral border of the tongue
- The oropharynx, the soft and hard palate
- The lower lip
- The floor of the mouth

The client often complains of a "sore" or "irritation" in the mouth. Sometimes, a client seeks consultation because of a "lump in the neck" that represents a metastasis (the spread of cancerous cells to other parts of the body via the blood and lymph systems) from an oral cancer lesion of which the person may be completely unaware.[2] Common signs of oral cancer are described in the Common Signs of Oral Cancer chart.

COMMON SIGNS OF ORAL CANCER

Ulceration
Loss of skin surface with a gray to yellow center surrounded by a red halo resulting from destruction of epithelial integrity owing to discrepancy in cell maturation, loss of intercellular attachments, and disruption of the basement membrane

Erythema
A red area of variable shape and size reflecting inflammation, thinness, and irregularity of epithelium, and lack of keratinization

Induration
Hardness primarily as a result of an increase in number of epithelial cells from an inflammatory infiltrate

Fixation
A nonmobile lesion occurring as a result of abnormally dividing cells invading to deeper areas and onto muscle and bone

Chronicity
Failure to heal

Lymphadenopathy
Disease process affecting the lymph nodes resulting in hardening and enlargement of the nodes

Adenopathy
Any disease of the glands, especially of the lymphatic glands

Leukoplakia
A white patch on the mucosal surface

Leukoplakia, reflecting excess keratin production, is often related to localized conditions (irritation from badly fitting dentures, broken teeth, tobacco use, or combustion and heat contact). A variety of other factors also may be involved including heavy alcohol consumption and vitamin A or B complex deficiency. Although most oral leukoplakias are benign and represent a callus type of formation, all lesions should be biopsied to rule out malignancy. Leukoplakia is considered precancerous, with malignant transformation rates between 3% and 5%.[3]

Tobacco users experience a significantly higher risk of developing cancer of the mouth, larynx, pharynx, and esophagus than those who do not use tobacco. Body sites that are most consistently exposed to cancer-producing tobacco byproducts (especially tars) include the lips, oral cavity, larynx, pharynx, and esophagus. Pipe smoking seems to have a significant causal relationship to lip cancer. Any form of smoking that is combined with habitual drinking is associated with high rates of head and neck cancer. Cancer can produce a thickening anywhere on the oral mucosa, causing a crater-like defect, with or without an ulcer and bleeding, or an outward raised growth of tissue. Usually painless in the early stages, these lesions, bright red or red in color, may be very innocent looking. Often, the first symptoms are noticed when body function is affected.

The Self-Examination Technique for Observing the Oral Cavity

Dental hygienists are often the oral health professionals consulted by clients for general oral complaints and therefore have the responsibility of referring all clients with oral lesions to the dentist for dental diagnosis. This client-dental hygienist interaction is an opportunity to teach the client simple self-examination techniques, empowering them with the skills to note any changes in an extra- or intraoral condition. For example, if a lesion is noted on the lower right labial mucosa, the client can simply be handed a mirror and shown where the lesion is and what it looks like. The client also should be instructed to check this area daily to observe change in lesion size, color, shape, texture, or symptoms. Together with the client, the dental hygienist can influence the potential outcome of a life-threatening disease.

General self-examination of the oral mucosa, tongue, gingiva, and palate to promote prevention and early identification of lesions can be demonstrated during the assessment phase of dental hygiene care. It involves educating the client in basic normal oral anatomy and structures. Routine self-examination also should be encouraged. The major concepts for prevention of oral cancer useful in educating clients are early detection through the routine extraoral and intraoral assessment and self-examination techniques to identify possible cancerous lesions, and eliminating high-risk behaviors that predispose one to oral cancer such as alcohol and tobacco use. For more information on oral cancer and dental hygiene care for persons with cancer, see Chapter 34.

PROCEDURE 11–1

TEACHING ORAL CANCER SELF-EXAMINATION

Equipment

Large mirror
Gauze
Good lighting
Protective barriers for the dental hygienist

Steps	Rationale
1. Have client sit in front of a large mirror under good lighting	Client must have a clear view of the face, neck, and mouth
2. Explain to the client that he is looking for: ■ Any sores on the face, neck, or mouth that do not heal within 2 weeks ■ Any red, white, or dark patches in the mouth ■ Any swellings, lumps, thickenings, bumps, or growths ■ Repeated bleeding for no apparent reason ■ Pain or loss of feeling in any area of the face, neck, or mouth ■ Hoarseness that does not go away within 2 weeks	Client must have a good idea of the early signs of cancer
3. Ask client to look at her facial symmetry in the mirror. Client should report any unilateral lumps, bumps, swellings, or growths	Both sides of the face should be similar, but not necessarily identical

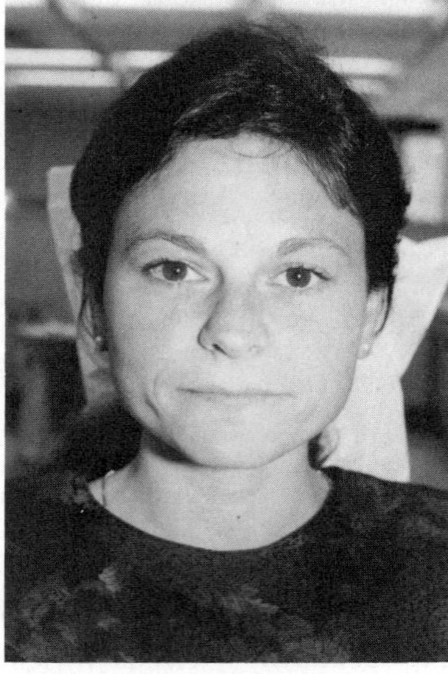

Steps	Rationale
4. Ask client to observe the skin for lumps, changes in skin color, changes in color or size of a mole (remove eyeglasses for this step)	Changes in the color of the skin or the size and color of a mole may be an early cancer warning sign
Ask client to use both hands to palpate simultaneously both sides of the entire face and neck	Palpating both sides at the same time will allow for the identification of unilateral growths or swellings

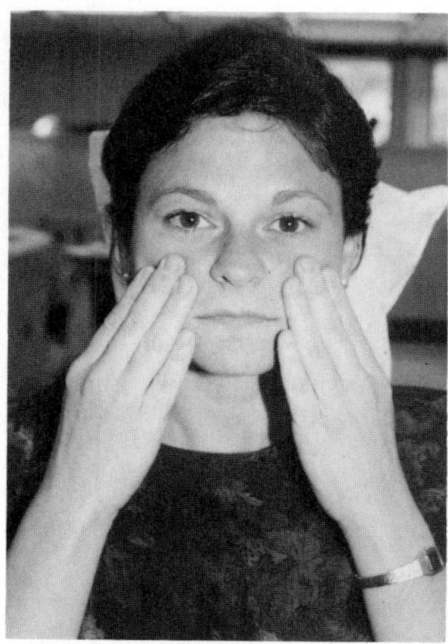
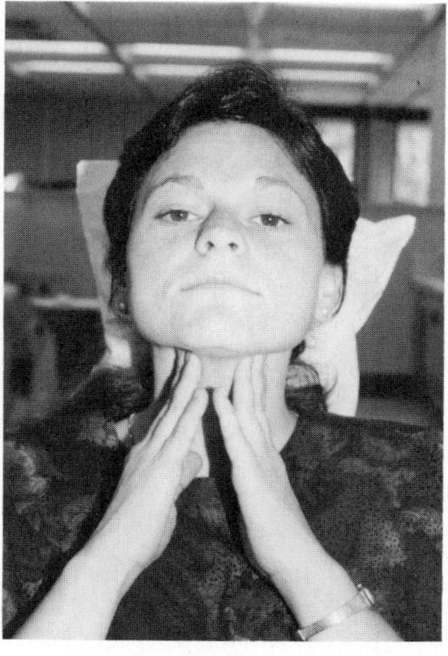

Steps	Rationale
5. Ask client to place her fingers on the "Adam's apple" and swallow	Adam's apple should move freely during a swallow
Ask client to grasp the "Adam's apple" and move it from side to side	Adam's apple should be freely movable

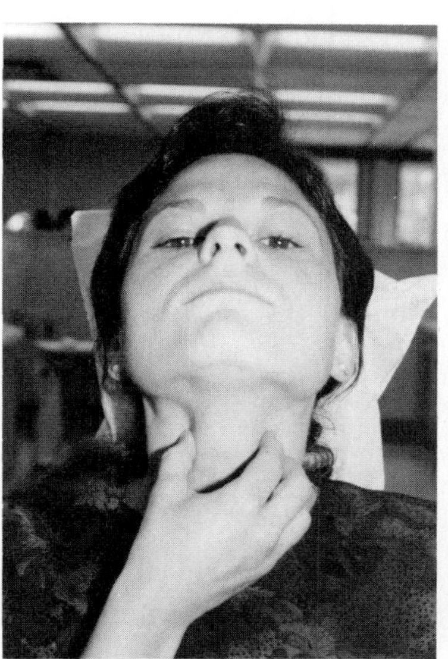
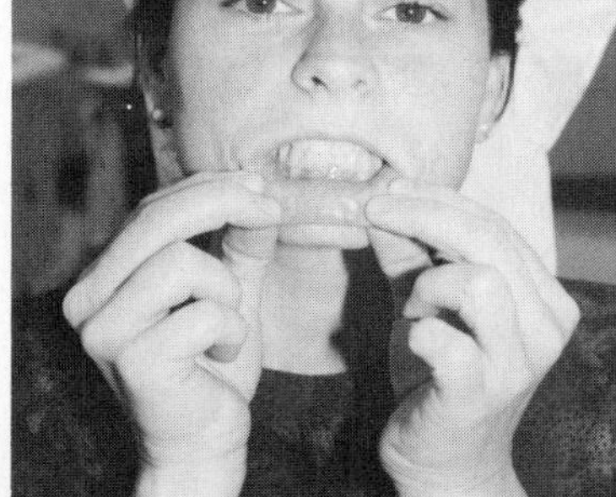
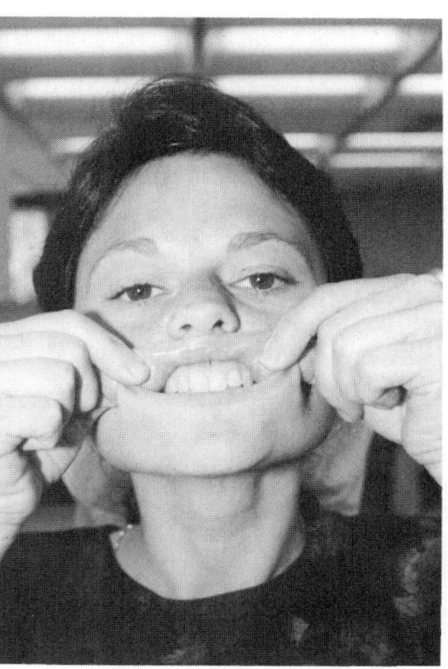

Steps	Rationale
6. Ask client to grasp the lower lip with index finger and thumb of both hands and palpate. Invert lower lip to view the mouth side. Repeat the procedure on the upper lip.	Early cancer warning signs may be apparent either visually or through bilateral palpation

CONTINUED ON FOLLOWING PAGE

PROCEDURE 11–1

TEACHING ORAL CANCER SELF-EXAMINATION *Continued*

Steps	Rationale
7. Ask client to retract cheek with fingers to view the inside of the cheek. Put thumb inside the cheek and the index and middle fingers on outside of cheek to palpate the entire cheek tissue. Repeat on each side of face.	Cheek should be firm and continuous, free of any lumps or lesion, and appear continuous in color

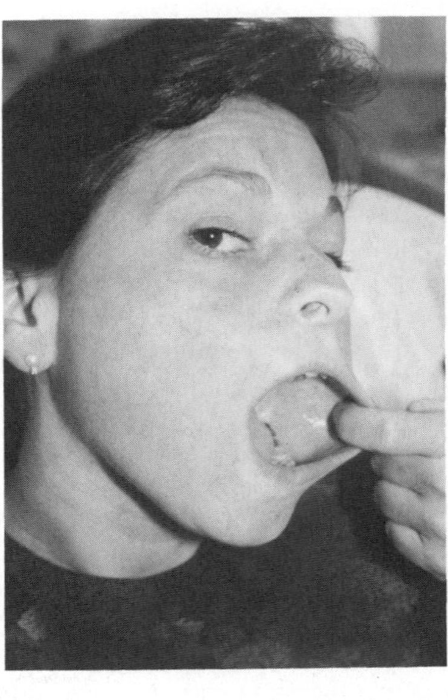

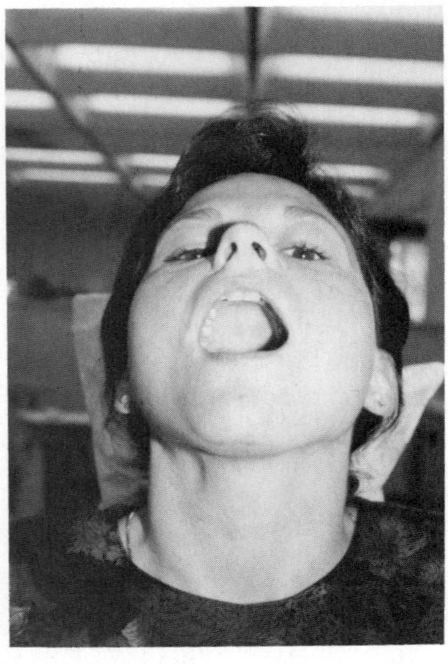

Steps	Rationale
8. Ask client to tilt head back to view the hard palate and soft palate for changes in color. Instruct client to use his thumb or index finger to compress the tissue against the roof of the mouth. Client should be taught that a palatine torus is normal.	Area should be firm and continuous, free of lumps or lesions (except for tori) and appear continuous in color
9. Client should be instructed to retract lips to view the gingivae for variations in color, bleeding, ulceration, lumps, swellings, or areas of pus drainage	Client must have a clear idea of signs that are outside of the range of normal
10. Teach client to touch the roof of his mouth with the tip of his tongue and then view the underside of the tongue and floor of the mouth. Show client how to use the index finger of one hand and fingertips of the opposite hand to bimanually palpate the floor of the mouth.	Client should know that the floor of the mouth is a primary site for oral cancer

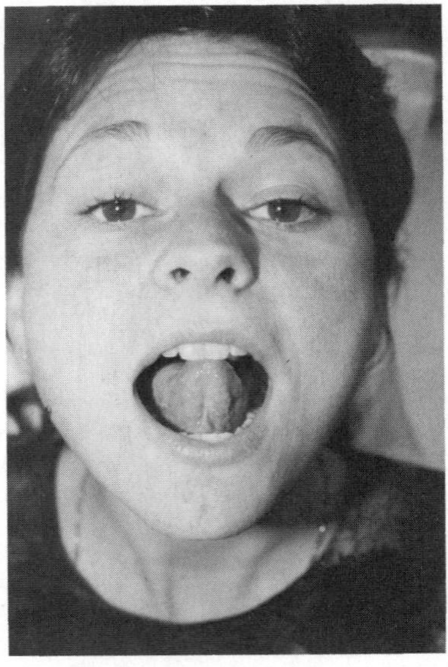

Steps	Rationale
11. Ask client to extend the tongue to view it for variations in color, ulceration, lumps, or swellings. Then instruct the client to use a gauze square to grasp the tongue. Teach client to gently pull the tongue to one side, and then the other, to view the posterior sides of the tongue. Ask client to extend the tongue forward and bidigitally palpate the entire body of the tongue.	Client should know that the lateral borders of the tongue are primary sites for oral cancer

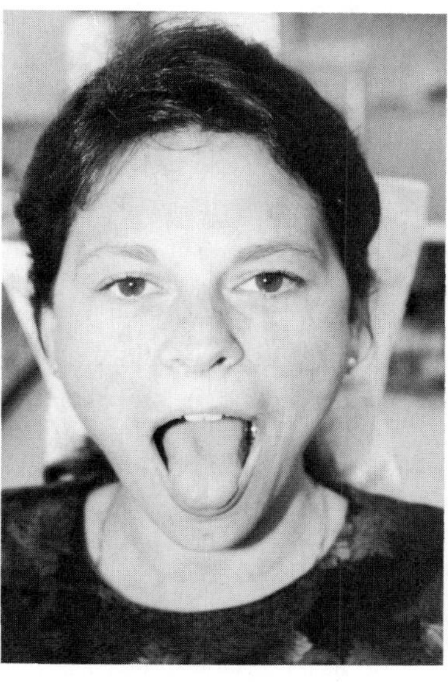

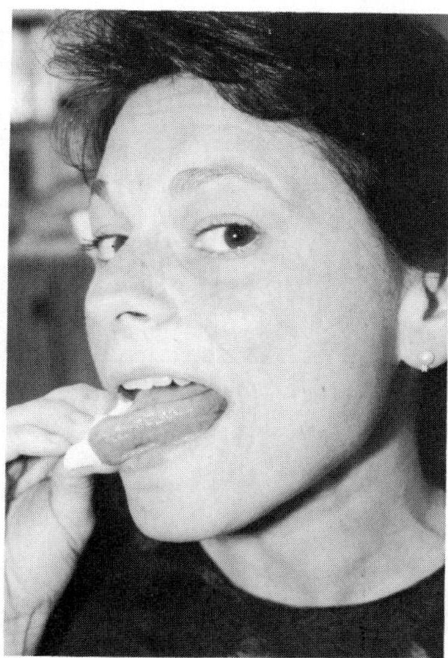

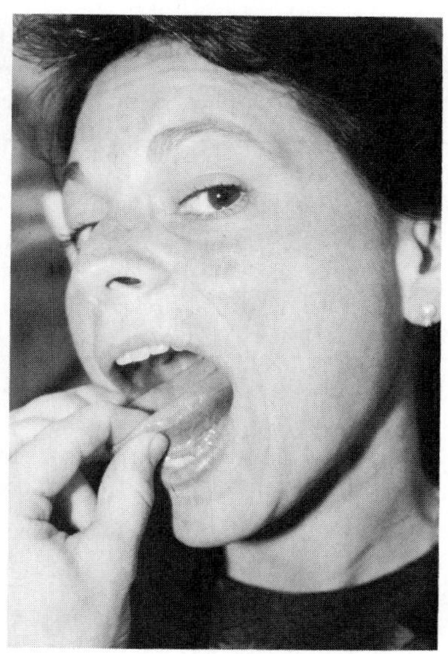

Steps	Rationale
12. Instruct client on risk factors for oral cancer, e.g., use of tobacco products, alcohol use	Clients who abuse tobacco products and alcohol should be informed about cessation programs and resources in the community

CARE FOR THE CLIENT WITH A SUSPICIOUS LESION

On identification of a lesion, the client must be informed of its existence. The clinician should use appropriate verbal skills, and pertinent information must be provided in writing if the client is referred to a specialist for further treatment. The dental hygienist collaborates with the dentist who determines the course of action to take to protect the client's well-being. Specialists who may collaborate in developing a differential diagnosis and providing treatment are oral pathologists, oral surgeons, and oral medicine specialists. Procedures following identification of a lesion during an extra- and intraoral examination may include exfoliative cytology, biopsy, staining tissue with toluidine blue dye for pathology examination, and continued careful evaluation of the client.

Biopsy is the only method of definitively diagnosing a cancer. Obviously, immediate biopsy of every oral lesion is impractical and contraindicated when other simple, reliable, and acceptable techniques are available to support the need for a biopsy. Exfoliative cytology and toluidine blue staining are such techniques.[2]

Exfoliative Cytology

Exfoliative cytology is a technique used for observing the microscopic morphology of individual cells after they have been obtained from a tissue, spread on a slide, fixed, and

CLASSIFICATIONS OF CYTOLOGY SPECIMENS

Unsatisfactory
Specimen is inadequate for diagnosis

Class I
Normal

Class II
Atypical cells, but not cancer

Class III
Possible for cancer

Class IV
Probable for cancer

Class V
Positive for cancer

stained (see Procedure 11–2). Surface scrapings (cytologic smear) of a lesion may be a reliable indicator of precancerous (dysplastic) or cancerous (neoplastic) changes.[2] However, a thorough examination of cellular scrapings must be made by a competent pathologist to make a proper assessment and correctly report the histological findings of the cytological smear. The pathologist may classify the cytology specimen according to one of the categories listed in the Classification of Cytology Specimens chart. Exfoliative cytology is performed infrequently or selectively, based on the sound clinical judgments of the dentist and dental hygienist and accessibility to a reputable laboratory. Exfoliative cytology is intended as an adjunct to—not a substitute for—biopsy.[2]

PROCEDURE 11–2

PREPARING EXFOLIATION CYTOLOGY SLIDES

Equipment

Pencil	Tongue blade or small metal spatula
Protective barriers	Laboratory mailing container
Glass slides	Basic information forms
Gauze	Fixative

Steps	Rationale
1. Put on gloves and other protective barriers before handling slides	Prevents contamination of the slide and maintains infection control.
2. Using a pencil, label two glass slides with the client's name, date, and area from which the specimens will be obtained	Two specimens give the pathologist a more complete picture of the histological components of the lesion
3. Wipe the site to be sampled with a wet gauze square; do not dry	This step removes the debris from the site to be sampled; cells that are dried become distorted
4. Scrape the lesion with a wet tongue blade or a small metal spatula; use slight rolling and scraping motions	This picks up the sample of cells; a wet tongue blade prevents the cells from being absorbed into the wood
5. Spread the sampled material on the center of the slide over a 20 mm area	This ensures a thin sample for microscopic evaluation
6. Immediately fix the cells by spraying the slide with a commercial fixative, 70% alcohol, or a commercial hairspray; do not allow the smear to dry before fixation	This ensures that the cells do not dry out and become distorted
7. Obtain a second sample by repeating steps 3 to 6	A second specimen gives the pathologist a more complete picture of the histological components of the lesion
8. Allow both slides to dry completely in an area free from possible contamination	Prevents contamination of the slide and maintains infection control
9. Complete the basic information form that will be forwarded	Including information such as the dentist's name and address, client's name and address, and a complete clinical description of the lesion is necessary for documentation
10. Package slides and basic information form in the mailing container provided by the pathology laboratory	Using mailing containers provided by the pathology laboratory increases the likelihood that the slides will arrive intact and ready for analysis. The specimen is stained in a laboratory by a modified Papanicolaou-Traut technique using Moyer's hematoxylin, orange B, eosin, and light green.
11. Record procedure in the client's record	This is done for legal purposes and to facilitate continuity of care
12. Note on calendar when the pathology report is due back; the slide can be made ready by the laboratory in less than 1 hour	This ensures that the report is not overlooked or ignored
13. Read the pathology report from the laboratory and make sure that findings are shared with the client	This ensures that client is informed and that appropriate follow-up care is obtained
14. Guide the client to receive the appropriate follow-up care, as recommended by the dentist	Increases the likelihood that client will adhere to recommendations

Toluidine Blue

Toluidine blue is a **metachromatic** dye (stains certain tissue a different color) that has been effectively used as a nuclear stain to confirm clinical impressions of abnormal cellular changes.[2] This technique, done in collaboration with the dentist, can accelerate the dentist's or physician's decision to biopsy and precedes diagnosis and treatment of cancerous and precancerous tissue (see Procedure 11–3).

PROCEDURE 11–3

TOLUIDINE BLUE STAINING OF A SUSPECTED DYSPLASTIC OR MALIGNANT LESION

Equipment

Toluidine blue dye	1% acetic acid solution
Cotton-tipped applicator	Other protective barriers

Steps	Rationale
1. Wear appropriate protective barriers	Maintains infection control
2. Apply dye liberally to the suspected area in the oral cavity with a cotton-tipped applicator	Dye is taken up by the oral tissue
3. Apply a 1% acetic acid solution to the suspected area	The acid removes the dye from healthy tissues; the dye is retained in the precancerous and malignant sites
4. Share findings with the client	This ensures that client is informed
5. Guide the client to receive the appropriate follow-up care as recommended by the dentist	Increases the likelihood that client will adhere to recommendations

Because toluidine blue is regarded as a nuclear stain, selective dye uptake by dysplastic (abnormal) and malignant cells, which contain quantitatively more nucleic acids than normal tissue, is the premise for its use. However, the most probable explanation to toluidine blue binding to precancerous and cancerous tissue is the immediate binding by mucopolysaccharides (sugars) which are found in higher quantities in tissues that are actively growing, such as tumors and tissues that are healing.[2]

Toluidine blue staining is a useful adjunct to careful examination, clinical judgment, and biopsy.[2]

Biopsy

The decision to perform a biopsy, after any unusual oral lesion is identified, is made by the dentist. Biopsy is the surgical removal and microscopic examination of a section of tissue or other material from the living body for the purpose of diagnosis, to estimate prognosis, and to monitor the cause of disease.[4] **Excisional biopsy** indicates that the entire lesion is removed for assessment. **Incisional biopsy** indicates that only a representative section is taken. The steps in taking a biopsy are as follows.

1. Identification of the suspected lesion.
2. Preparation of the lesion site for biopsy by anesthetizing it with a local anesthetic.
3. Incision is made (using a scalpel or "punch" biopsy instrument).
4. Hemostasis of the incision site is achieved by applying pressure with sterile gauze.
5. Specimen is placed in 10% normal buffered formalin for histological processing.[2]
6. Specimen is sent to a qualified laboratory for evaluation.

After the specimen is obtained and properly packaged for transport to a laboratory, it is analyzed by a pathologist. A report of the findings is then issued by the pathologist after assessing the histological appearance of the suspected lesion in conjunction with the clinical diagnosis. This report is then sent to the dentist to determine any further action. The report should be discussed with the client.

References

1. Potter, P. A., and Perry, A. G. Fundamentals of Nursing: Concepts, Process, and Practice, 3rd ed. St. Louis: C. V. Mosby, 1993, p. 526.
2. Silverman S., Jr. Oral Cancer. New York: American Cancer Society, 1990.
3. Christen, A. G., McDonald, J. L., et al. A Smoking Cessation Program for the Dental Office (Monograph). Kansas City, MO: Indiana University School of Dentistry. 1990.
4. Wilkins, E. M. The Clinical Practice of the Dental Hygienist. Philadelphia: Lea & Febiger, 1989, pp. 111–112.

12 Assessment of the Dentition

OBJECTIVES

Mastery of the content in this chapter will enable the reader to:

- Discuss the components of tooth assessment
- Explain the purposes, characteristics, and procedures of dental charting
- Describe the classification of quadrants, sextants, and tooth surfaces
- Describe the classification of permanent and primary teeth
- Explain the major tooth numbering systems
- Describe the classification of ideal occlusion and malocclusion
- Describe normal and abnormal anterior teeth relationships
- Describe some common tooth anomalies that may be observed during assessment

INTRODUCTION

Tooth assessment is used to determine whether the client's need for a biologically sound dentition is in deficit and is related to the client's human need for freedom from pain/stress, for nutrition, for safety, and for wholesome body image. Complete and accurate records and charting of the existing conditions of the teeth provide the initial and ongoing documentation used in providing optimal client care and managing risks associated with litigation.

Dentition charting is the graphic representation of the condition of the client's teeth observed on a specific date. The data recorded are based on clinical and radiographical assessment and the client's report of symptoms. The exact location and condition of all teeth, restorations, and dental caries noting normal and abnormal findings are documented carefully on a detailed dentition chart as a permanent part of the client's record. The data collected are used collaboratively with the dentist in planning, implementing, and evaluating dental and dental hygiene care for the client. The purpose of this chapter is to provide the fundamental concepts related to tooth assessment and documentation. Dental charts, quadrants, sextants, types of teeth, tooth surfaces, classification of dental caries and restorations, tooth numbering systems, charting methods, dental anomalies, and identification of malocclusion are discussed.

PURPOSES AND CHARACTERISTICS OF TOOTH ASSESSMENT AND DOCUMENTATION

Tooth assessment and its documentation on the client's chart initially occurs during the assessment phase of the dental hygiene process, and this information is updated regularly during the implementation and evaluation phases of dental hygiene care. Documentation of tooth assessments on a client's dentition chart serves numerous purposes: care planning, enhancement of professional communication, legal documentation, forensic applications, and financial audits.[1]

Care Planning—Documentation of tooth assessment findings on the client's dentition chart provides the visual description of the client's current dental status. After the collection of these and other data, the clinician is able to formulate an accurate and comprehensive dental hygiene care plan

Communication—Accurate documentation of tooth assessment findings enhances communication with the client, and about the client to other members of the oral health team. It also assists communication with third-party payors, such as insurance companies and health maintenance organizations

Legal Documentation—The client's record is a legal document and admissible evidence in a court of law. Comprehensive charting of tooth assessment findings documents the level of care provided

Forensic Uses—During forensic investigations the record of the client's dentition is often the only means of identifying a deceased person; therefore, accuracy and completeness of these records are essential

Financial Audits—The client's dentition chart assists in the verification of oral healthcare provided and may be the key record in a financial audit

An ideal chart for tooth assessment incorporates key characteristics. The chart should be *comprehensive* in that it contains sufficient space for initial recording of data as well as for successive findings. The chart format should be *un-*

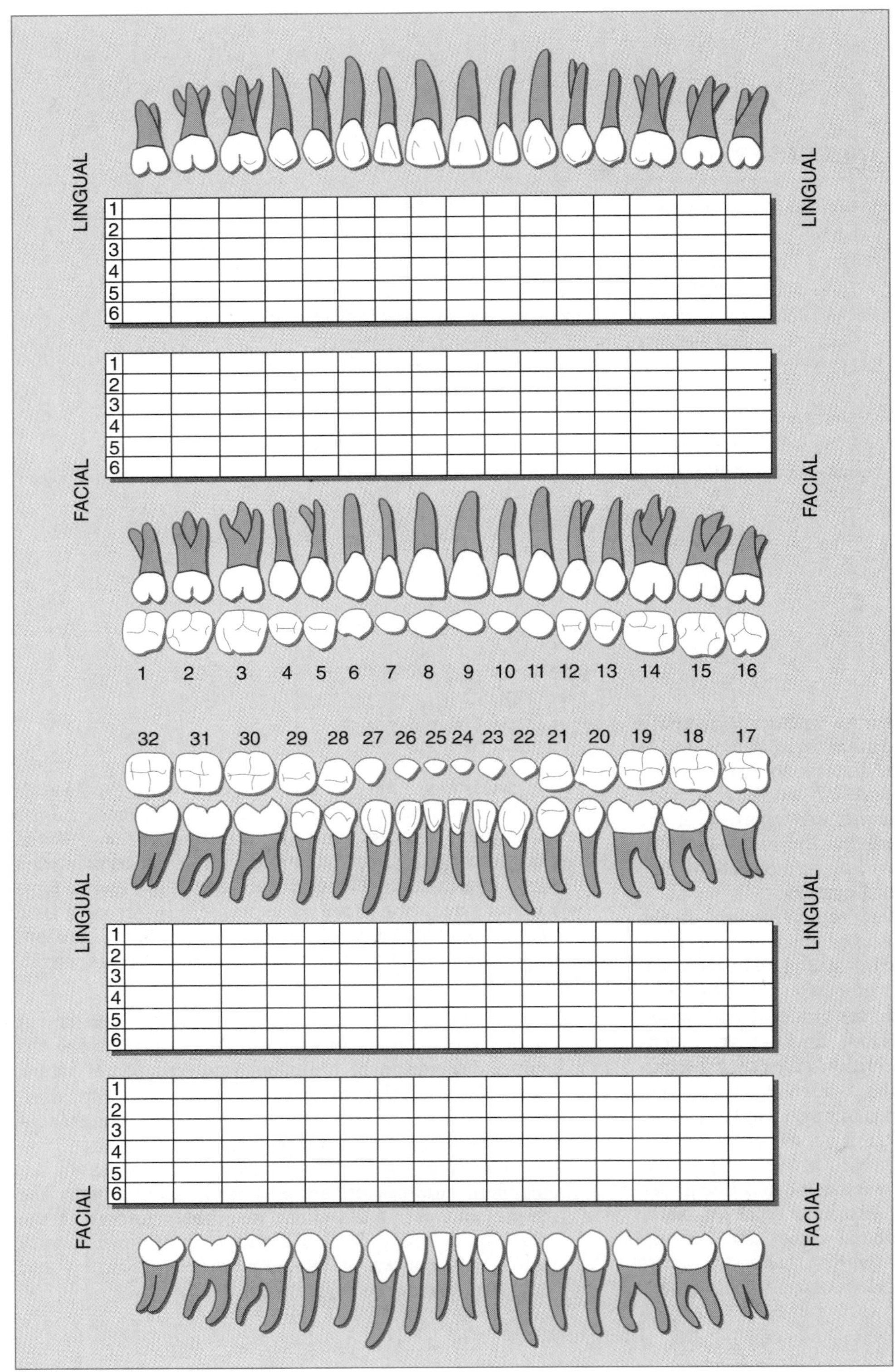

FIGURE 12–1
Example of an anatomical chart.

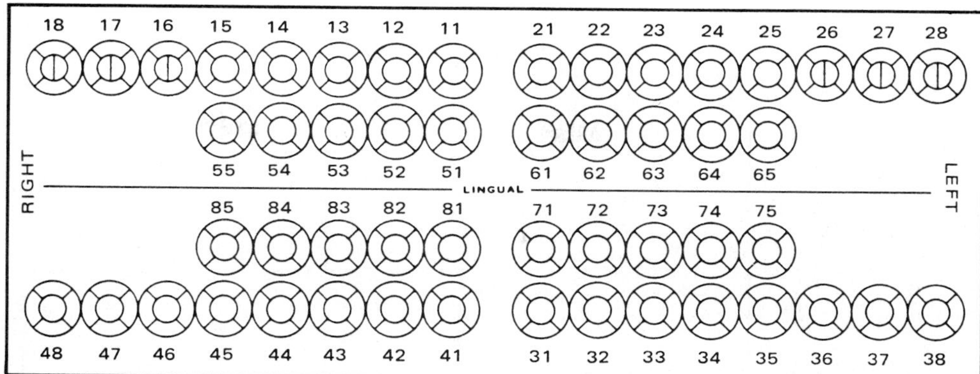

FIGURE 12–2
Example of a geometrical chart. (Courtesy of Colwell Systems, Inc., Champaign, IL.)

complicated so that all oral health professionals can use and interpret it with ease. The chart should be a part of the permanent client record and be *accessible* for reference during all appointments, thus facilitating continuity, sequencing, and ongoing documentation of care.[1]

TYPES OF CHARTS FOR TOOTH ASSESSMENT

Charts for tooth assessment are available in several formats; the most commonly used present anatomical or geometrical representations of the teeth (Fig. 12–1). Anatomical charts give the most realistic graphic descriptions, with the anatomy of the crown and root(s) of each tooth usually provided with facial, occlusal, and lingual views (Fig. 12–2). Geometrical charting uses geometrical drawings that represent "stylized anatomy." The occlusal surfaces are usually the only surfaces shown on geometrical charts. As a result, these charts may be easier to interpret, yet their comprehensiveness is limited because of the lack of surface views provided.

Quadrant and Sextant Classification

To facilitate communication about specific areas of the dentition and individual teeth, the dentition is divided into quadrants and sextants, and each tooth is divided into specific surfaces and zones.

Quadrants

If one were to draw an imaginary line dividing the client's face into two equal halves longitudinally, then the maxillary and mandibular arches of the mouth would be divided into two mirror images or halves. This imaginary longitudinal line that bisects the client's face is referred to as the midline. Then if one were to draw horizontally a second imaginary line that divided the maxillary arch from the mandibular arch, the combination of the imaginary horizontal and vertical midlines would divide the client's mouth into four equal sections termed **quadrants (Q)** (Fig. 12–3). Each quadrant of the mouth contains either five or eight teeth, depending on whether the client has primary or permanent dentition. Quadrants of the permanent dentition are numbered 1 through 4, and those of the primary dentition 5 through 8. The maxillary right is referred to as quadrant 1 in the permanent dentition or quadrant 5 in the primary dentition. Continuing in a clockwise pattern around the dentition, the maxillary left is designated as quadrant 2 (permanent) or quadrant 6 (primary). The mandibular left is referred to as quadrant 3 (permanent) or quadrant 7 (primary), and the mandibular right is designated as quadrant 4 (permanent) or quadrant 8 (primary).

Sextants

Another means of dividing the primary and permanent dentition into sections is created by drawing additional imaginary lines between the canine and the first premolar teeth, thereby creating divisions between the anterior and the posterior teeth. Dividing the dentition in this manner creates six areas called **sextants (S).** Each anterior sextant contains incisors and canines, while premolars and/or molars are found in the posterior sextants. Like quadrants, sextants are numbered clockwise beginning at the client's maxillary right (Fig. 12–4).

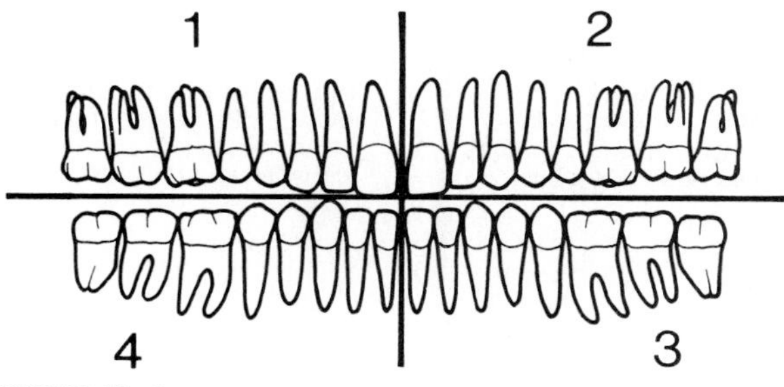

FIGURE 12–3
Quadrant classification in the permanent dentition. (Adapted from Nield, J. S., and Houseman, G. A. Fundamentals of Dental Hygiene Instrumentation, 2nd ed. Philadelphia: Lea & Febiger, 1988. Used with permission.)

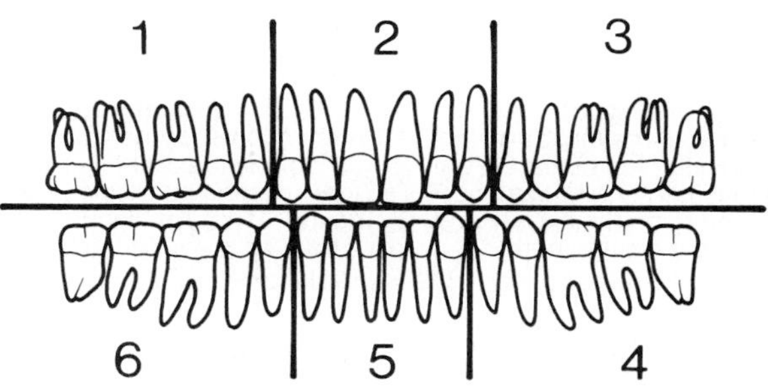

FIGURE 12–4
Sextant classification in the permanent dentition. (Adapted from Nield, J. S., and Houseman, G. A. Fundamentals of Dental Hygiene Instrumentation, 2nd ed. Philadelphia: Lea & Febiger, 1988. Used with permission.)

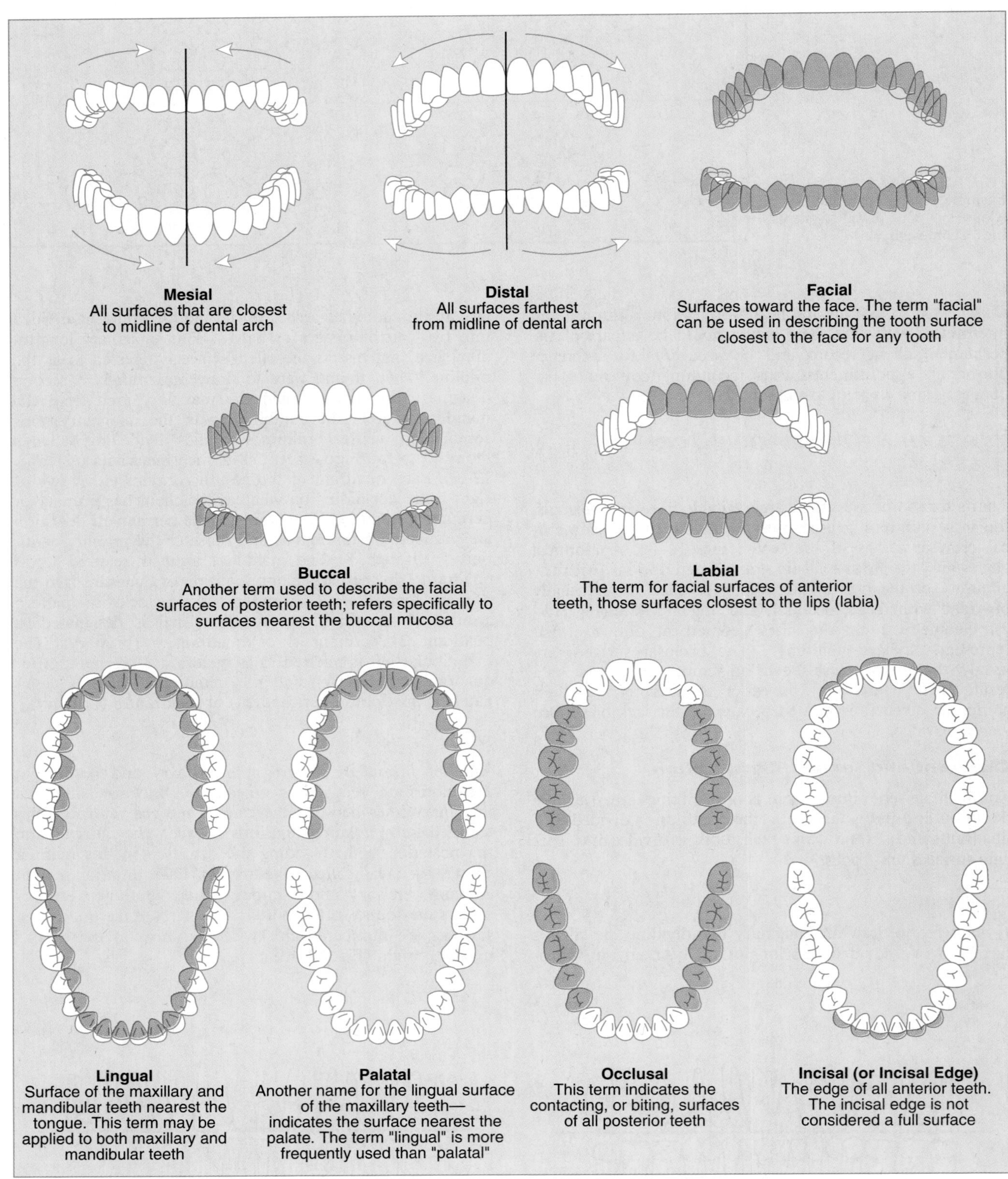

Mesial
All surfaces that are closest to midline of dental arch
Distal
All surfaces farthest from midline of dental arch
Facial
Surfaces toward the face. The term "facial" can be used in describing the tooth surface closest to the face for any tooth
Buccal
Another term used to describe the facial surfaces of posterior teeth; refers specifically to surfaces nearest the buccal mucosa
Labial
The term for facial surfaces of anterior teeth, those surfaces closest to the lips (labia)
Lingual
Surface of the maxillary and mandibular teeth nearest the tongue. This term may be applied to both maxillary and mandibular teeth
Palatal
Another name for the lingual surface of the maxillary teeth—indicates the surface nearest the palate. The term "lingual" is more frequently used than "palatal"
Occlusal
This term indicates the contacting, or biting, surfaces of all posterior teeth
Incisal (or Incisal Edge)
The edge of all anterior teeth. The incisal edge is not considered a full surface

FIGURE 12–5
Classification of tooth surfaces. (Adapted from Wootton, D. The Art of Dental Scaling. Burlington, VT: University of Vermont, 1991.)

TOOTH SURFACES AND ZONES

Teeth have several surfaces and zones. The differentiation of **tooth surfaces** and **zones** provides a means of pinpointing specific areas of the tooth for accurate assessment, charting, treatment, and evaluation. In addition to an incisal edge, each anterior tooth has four surfaces: mesial, distal, facial (or labial), and lingual. Each posterior tooth has five surfaces (Fig. 12–5):

- Mesial
- Distal
- Facial (buccal)
- Lingual
- Occlusal

Tooth Zones

Another arbitrary means of dividing teeth is the division into zones of imaginary thirds. These tooth zones are named according to the areas in which they are found. The root of the tooth is divided into the apical, middle, and cervical thirds (Fig. 12–6).

The crown of the tooth can be divided into the following three directions:[10]

Cervicoocclusal Division—Dividing the crown of the tooth horizontally, from cervical to occlusal areas, creates divisions defined as the occlusal (incisal), middle, and gingival thirds (see Fig. 12–6*A*)

Mesiodistal Division—Lines drawn vertically on the facial or lingual surface of the crown, from the mesial to distal, create the mesial, middle, and distal thirds (see Fig. 12–6*B*)

Faciolingual (or Buccolingual) Division from the Proximal View—Lines drawn vertically on the mesial or distal view of the crown create thirds called facial (labial or buccal), middle, and lingual (see Fig. 12–6*C* and *D*)

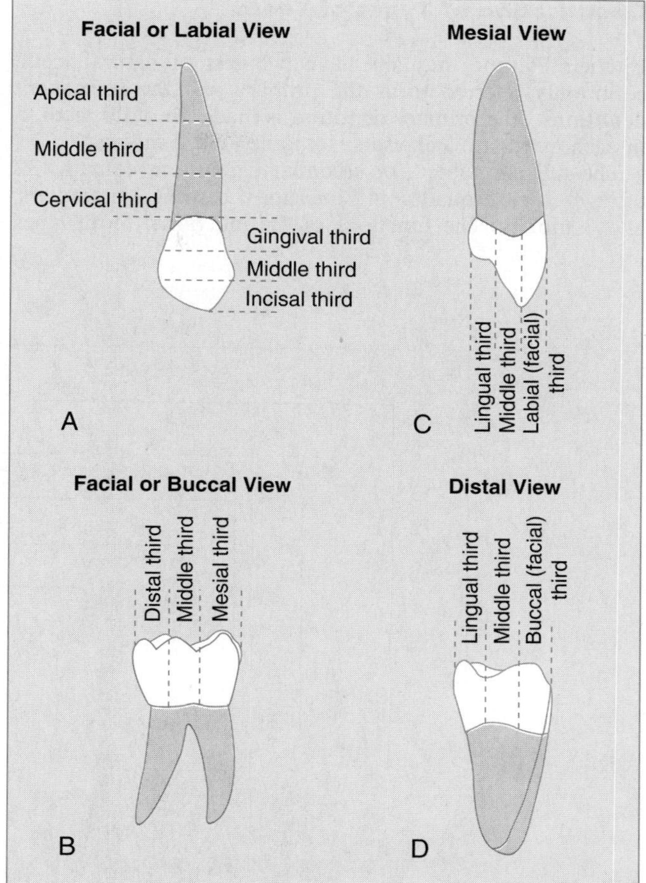

FIGURE 12–6
Diagram of a maxillary canine and a mandibular first molar to show the manner in which the parts of a tooth may be divided.

TABLE 12–1
CLASSIFICATION OF PRIMARY AND PERMANENT TEETH

Type	Primary Dentition	Total Number	Permanent Dentition	Total Number	Function
Incisor*	Central incisor Lateral incisor	1 per quadrant 1 per quadrant Total = 8	Central incisor Lateral incisor	1 per quadrant 1 per quadrant Total = 8	Cutting Incising
Canine†	Primary canine	1 per quadrant Total = 4	Permanent canine	1 per quadrant Total = 4	Cutting Tearing
Premolars‡	No premolars found in the primary dentition	0	First premolar Second premolar	1 per quadrant 1 per quadrant Total = 8	Tearing Holding Grinding
Molar§	First primary molar Second primary molar	1 per quadrant 1 per quadrant Total dentition = 8	First permanent molar (6-year molar) Second permanent molar (12-year molar) Third permanent molar (wisdom tooth) Total of 12 permanent molars	1 per quadrant 1 per quadrant 1 per quadrant Total = 12	Grinding

* The central and lateral incisors in both the primary and the permanent dentition are in the first and second tooth positions from the midline in each quadrant.

† The canines in both the primary and the permanent dentition are in the third tooth position from the midline in each quadrant.

‡ The first and second premolars are in the fourth and fifth tooth positions from the midline in each permanent quadrant.

§ The molars are in the fourth and fifth tooth positions from the midline in each primary quadrant and in the sixth, seventh, and eighth tooth positions from the midline in each permanent quadrant.

Classification of Types of Teeth

In their lifetime, humans have two sets of natural teeth, commonly referred to as the primary and the permanent dentitions. The primary dentition is made up of 20 teeth, 5 in each quadrant: 2 incisors, 1 canine, and 2 molars.

The full permanent, or secondary, dentition contains 32 teeth, 8 in each quadrant: 2 incisors, 1 canine, 2 premolars, and 3 molars. The functions of the individual tooth types are similar in the primary and the permanent dentition. The classification of primary and permanent teeth is provided in Table 12–1 and Figures 12–7 and 12–8.

TOOTH NUMBERING SYSTEMS

Tooth numbering systems were developed to simplify the task of identifying individual teeth without using their full

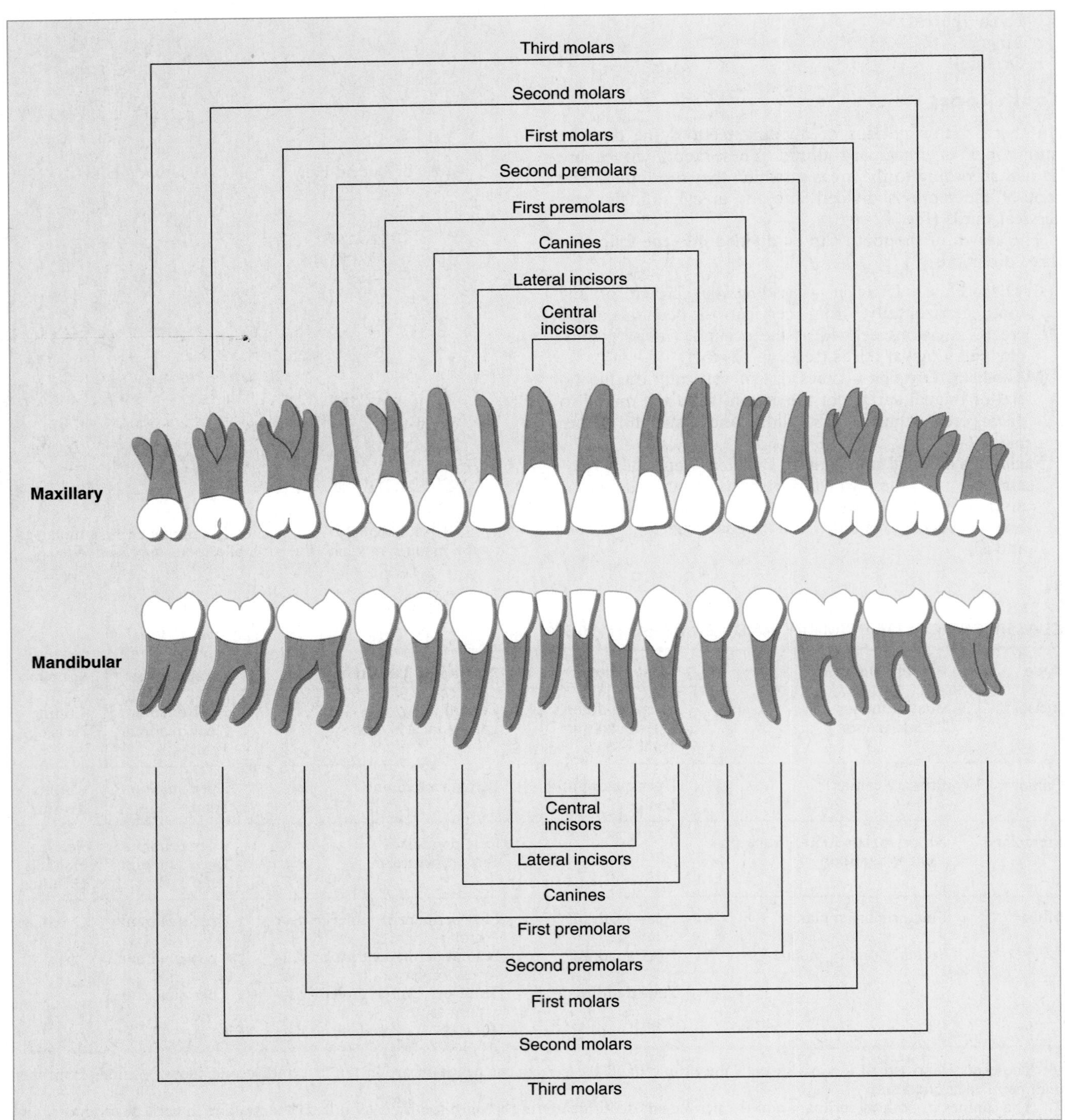

FIGURE 12–7
Classification of permanent teeth.

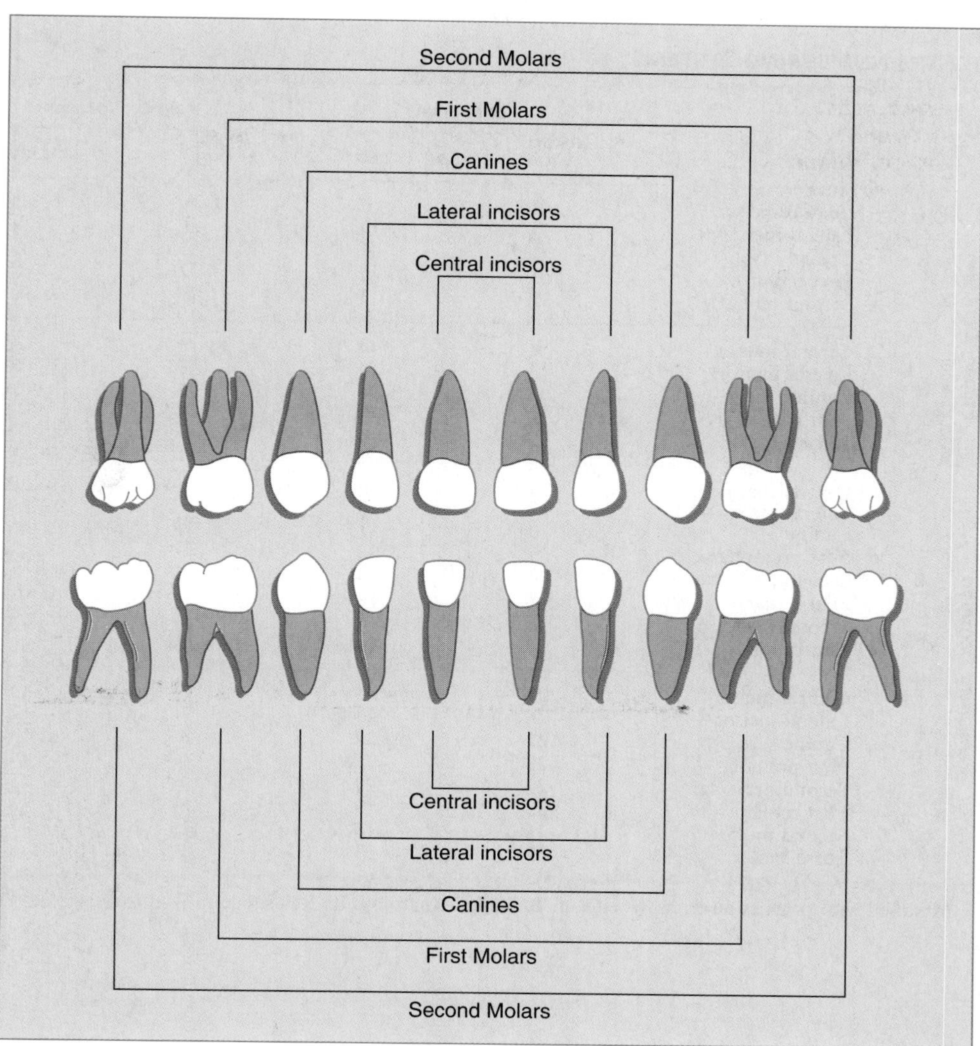

FIGURE 12-8
Classification of primary teeth.

name designations. Such systems are essential for charting and recording procedures. The three most commonly used are the Universal Numbering System, the International Numbering System, and the Palmer Numbering System. Table 12-2 summarizes these systems.

Universal Numbering System

The **Universal Numbering System,** officially adopted by the American Dental Association in 1975, is the most widely used. This system provides a standard sequential numbering system for all permanent teeth. The permanent teeth are numbered 1 through 32, beginning with the maxillary right permanent third molar designated tooth no. 1, and following a clockwise pattern around the maxillary arch the left maxillary third molar is designated tooth no. 16. The mandibular numbering begins with no. 17, which identifies the left mandibular third molar, and following clockwise around the mandibular arch the right mandibular third molar is no. 32 (Fig. 12-9). The primary dentition is identified in the same order; however, alphabetical letters, capitals "A" to "T," identify the individual teeth. Letter "A" designates the maxillary right second molar, and following clockwise around the maxillary and mandibular arches the mandibular right second molar is designated by the letter "T" (see Fig. 12-9).

International Numbering System (Federation Dentaire International [F.D.I.])

The **International Numbering System** uses a two-digit system to identify each tooth. The first digit indicates the quadrant in which the tooth is located, while the second digit identifies the specific tooth. For quadrant designations, numbers 1 to 4 are used to specify permanent quadrants, and numbers 5 to 8 to designate primary quadrants. The second digit identifies the specific tooth in the quadrant: the numbers 1 through 8 are used for permanent teeth, and the numbers 1 through 5 for primary teeth. In each dentition, tooth no. 1 is the central incisor. In primary dentition, tooth no. 5 is the second primary molar, and in secondary dentition tooth no. 8 is the third permanent molar (Fig. 12-10). The pronunciation of the International system is emphasized by the hyphenated notation; for example, "1-6" is pronounced "one six," rather than "sixteen."

TABLE 12–2
TOOTH NUMBERING SYSTEMS

	Tooth	Universal		Palmer Notation		International (F.D.I.)	
		Right	Left	Right	Left	Right	Left
Primary Dentition, Maxillary Teeth	Central incisor	E	F	A⌋	⌊A	51	61
	Lateral incisor	D	G	B⌋	⌊B	52	62
	Canine	C	H	C⌋	⌊C	53	63
	First molar	B	I	D⌋	⌊D	54	64
	Second molar	A	J	E⌋	⌊E	55	65
Primary Dentition, Mandibular Teeth	Central incisor	P	O	A⌉	⌈A	81	71
	Lateral incisor	Q	N	B⌉	⌈B	82	72
	Canine	R	M	C⌉	⌈C	83	73
	First molar	S	L	D⌉	⌈D	84	74
	Second molar	T	K	E⌉	⌈E	85	75
Permanent Dentition, Maxillary Teeth	Central incisor	8	9	1⌋	⌊1	11	21
	Lateral incisor	7	10	2⌋	⌊2	12	22
	Canine	6	11	3⌋	⌊3	13	23
	First premolar	5	12	4⌋	⌊4	14	24
	Second premolar	4	13	5⌋	⌊5	15	25
	First molar	3	14	6⌋	⌊6	16	26
	Second molar	2	15	7⌋	⌊7	17	27
	Third molar	1	16	8⌋	⌊8	18	28
Permanent Dentition, Mandibular Teeth	Central incisor	25	24	1⌉	⌈1	41	31
	Lateral incisor	26	23	2⌉	⌈2	42	32
	Canine	27	22	3⌉	⌈3	43	33
	First premolar	28	21	4⌉	⌈4	44	34
	Second premolar	29	20	5⌉	⌈5	45	35
	First molar	30	19	6⌉	⌈6	46	36
	Second molar	31	18	7⌉	⌈7	47	37
	Third molar	32	17	8⌉	⌈8	48	38

Modified with permission from Woelfel, J. B. Dental Anatomy: Its Relevance to Dentistry, 4th ed. Philadelphia: Lea & Febiger, 1990.

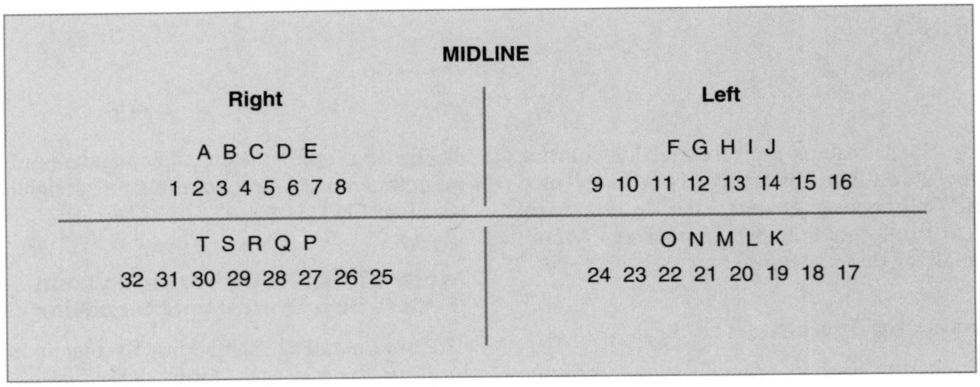

MIDLINE

Right	Left
A B C D E	F G H I J
1 2 3 4 5 6 7 8	9 10 11 12 13 14 15 16
T S R Q P	O N M L K
32 31 30 29 28 27 26 25	24 23 22 21 20 19 18 17

FIGURE 12–9
Universal Numbering System.

PERMANENT DENTITION	
Q_1	Q_2
1-8 1-7 1-6 1-5 1-4 1-3 1-2 1-1	2-1 2-2 2-3 2-4 2-5 2-6 2-7 2-8
4-8 4-7 4-6 4-5 4-4 4-3 4-2 4-1	3-1 3-2 3-3 3-4 3-5 3-6 3-7 3-8

PRIMARY DENTITION	
Q_1	Q_2
5-5 5-4 5-3 5-2 5-1	6-1 6-2 6-3 6-4 6-5
8-5 8-4 8-3 8-2 8-1	7-1 7-2 7-3 7-4 7-5

FIGURE 12-10
The International Numbering System.

Palmer Numbering System

A grid that identifies the quadrants is the basis of the **Palmer Numbering System.** The client's mouth is represented by a grid as the operator views it: ┘, maxillary right; └, maxillary left; ┐, mandibular right; ┌, mandibular left. The tooth numbers are similar to those in the International Numbering System in the permanent dentition, from tooth no. 1 designating the central incisor to tooth no. 8 denoting the third molar. The number is placed within the grid symbol; two examples are:

8┘ Maxillary right third permanent molar
┌6 Mandibular left first permanent molar

In the primary dentition, the same quadrant grid symbols are used; however, instead of digits, capital alphabetical letters "A" (central incisor) through "E" (second primary molar) indicate the tooth. For example:

┌D Mandibular left primary lateral incisor
D┘ Maxillary right primary first molar

TOOTH DAMAGE AND DEVELOPMENTAL ANOMALIES

Acquired tooth damage and developmental anomalies recognized by the dental hygienist during the assessment phase of care must be called to the attention of the dentist.

Tooth Damage*

Tooth damage can be caused by any process that results in a loss of the integrity of the tooth surface. Dental caries is a bacteria-caused form of tooth damage. The other common forms of tooth damage (attrition, abrasion, erosion, and fracture) are the result of mechanical or chemical assault to the tooth structure.

Dental Caries

Dental caries is an infectious, bacteria-caused disease characterized by the acid dissolution of enamel and the eventual breakdown of the more organic, inner dental tissues.[2] *Streptococcus mutans* is the microorganism identified as the primary causative agent in this process, which leads to cavitation and possible tooth loss. Through a complex process, a sticky dextran matrix is produced and colonized by these acidogenic bacteria. This inhabited mucogelatinous coating, termed "bacterial plaque," is harbored in the recesses in and around the dentition. It is nourished by elements within the diet. Refined sugars (sucrose in particular) are efficiently assimilated by the bacteria and result in the production of acid and a rapid drop in pH. The release of acid over an extended period of time demineralizes the tooth structure adjacent to the bacterial plaque and eventually results in cavitation. Within this cavitation, the demineralization continues, promoted by episodes of acid release as the bacteria act on new substrate. Tooth cavitation is best referred to as a **"carious lesion."** However, it is more commonly termed a "cavity," and the affected tooth is said to be "carious" or "decayed."

Attrition

Dental **attrition** is the tooth-to-tooth wear of the dentition. All teeth wear from opposing tooth contact. Excessive wear is pathological and may be caused by bruxism, grinding, or clenching (Fig. 12-11). The restoration of teeth presenting excessive attrition may include the complete tooth coverage offered by a crown.

Abrasion

Dental **abrasion,** pathological tooth wear due to a foreign substance, is commonly seen as a result of traumatic tooth-

*This section was contributed by Cheryl Cameron, RDH, PhD, and Glen E. Gordon, DDS.

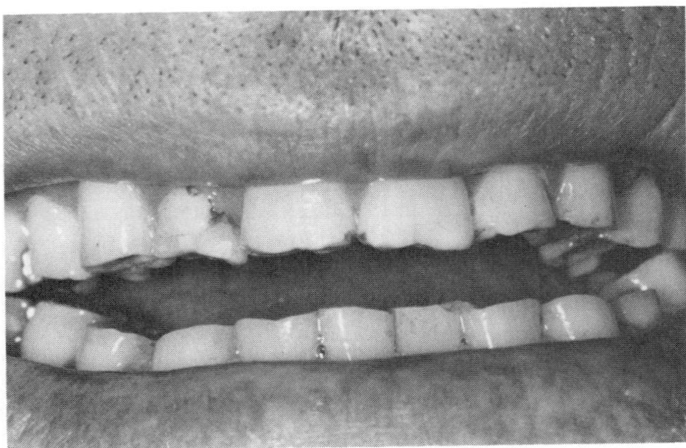

FIGURE 12–11
Attrition. (Courtesy of Cheryl Cameron, RDH, PhD, and Glen E. Gordon, DDS.)

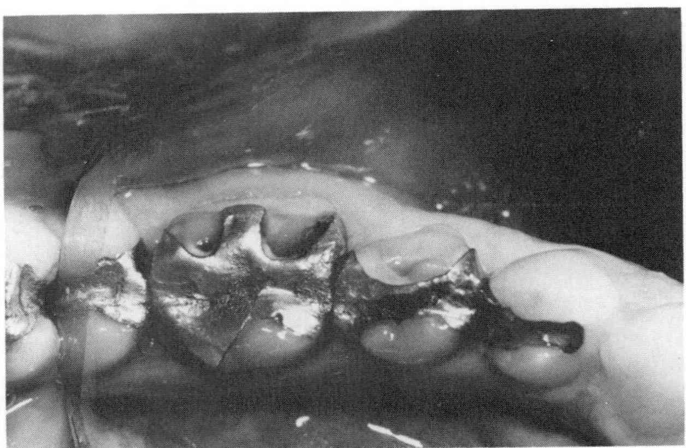

FIGURE 12–13
Erosive action causes local destruction of tooth enamel. (Courtesy of Cheryl Cameron, RDH, PhD, and Glen E. Gordon, DDS.)

brushing and appears as notches worn into the teeth near the gumline (Fig. 12–12). Occlusal abrasion often is seen on teeth that oppose porcelain crowns. Very coarse diets, uncleaned foods, and dusty environments also can contribute to the loss of occlusal enamel. It is not uncommon for pipe smokers and seamstresses to exhibit incisal abrasion as a result of clenching foreign objects between the anterior teeth.

Erosion

Dental **erosion,** the loss of tooth surface as a result of chemical agents, has recently received considerable attention because of the prevalence of anorexia and bulimia.[3] Excessive vomiting can be associated with these disorders as an individual strives for the ultimate thinness. The repeated regurgitation of stomach acids through the oral cavity results in the dissolution of the dental tissues on the lingual and incisal/occlusal surfaces of the maxillary teeth. Tooth erosion also results from habits such as holding mouth fresheners, cough drops, or candies in the mucobuccal fold. The erosive action of these lozenges causes local destruction of tooth enamel (Fig. 12–13).

Tooth Fracture

Tooth fractures may range from small chips of the enamel to breaks that penetrate deeply into the tooth (Fig. 12–14). Minor enamel fractures often require nothing more than polishing of the rough surfaces. More severe fractures require various levels of restoration. Some fractured teeth may not be restorable and, as a result, require removal.

Types of Dental Caries*

The classification of dental caries is intended to describe the rate, direction, and/or type of disease progression. The terms of classification include acute, or rampant, caries; chronic caries; arrested caries; recurrent caries; and backward caries. These terms permit the oral healthcare practitioner to communicate the urgency with which restorative therapy should be delivered. As these terms are not specific regarding tooth and surface, they must be combined with other cavity classification terminology to permit location-specific communication.

*This section was contributed by Cheryl Cameron, RDH, PhD, and Glen E. Gordon, DDS.

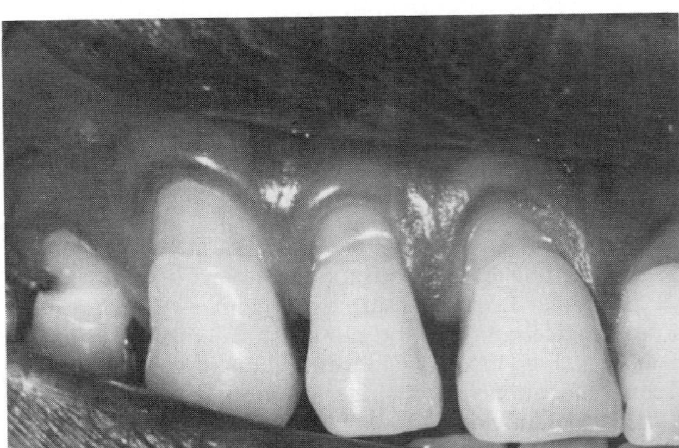

FIGURE 12–12
Abrasion. (Courtesy of Cheryl Cameron, RDH, PhD, and Glen E. Gordon, DDS.)

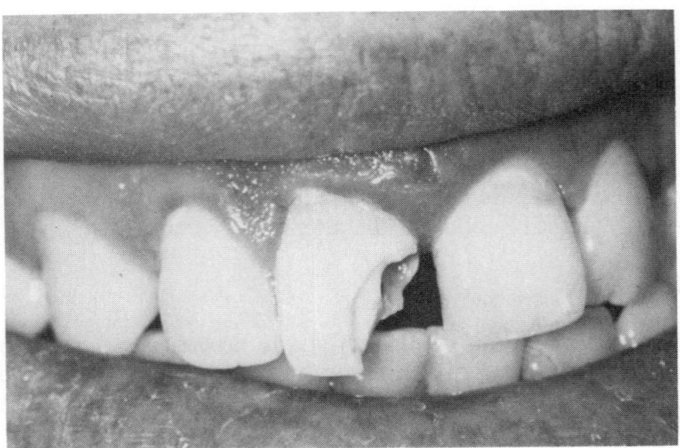

FIGURE 12–14
Tooth fracture. (Courtesy of Cheryl Cameron, RDH, PhD, and Glen E. Gordon, DDS.)

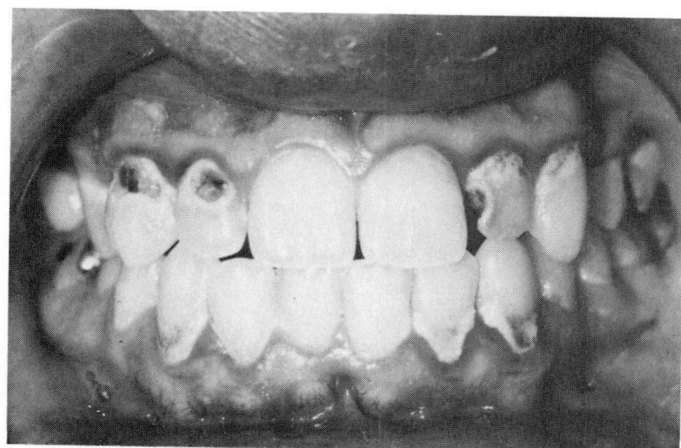

FIGURE 12–15
Rampant caries. (Courtesy of Cheryl Cameron, RDH, PhD, and Glen E. Gordon, DDS.)

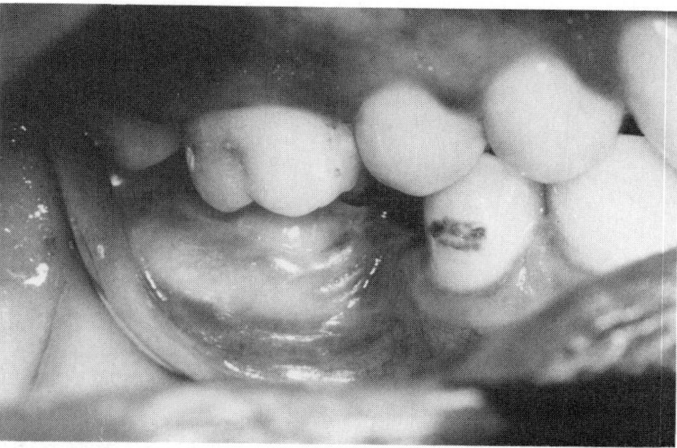

FIGURE 12–17
Arrested caries. (Courtesy of Cheryl Cameron, RDH, PhD, and Glen E. Gordon, DDS.)

Acute or Rampant Caries

Acute, or **rampant, caries** describes a rapidly progressive decay process that requires urgent intervention to gain control. The lesions are usually numerous and may be large. The decayed dentin is very soft and moist and is often light in color (Fig. 12–15). Rampant caries is often associated with the effects of nursing bottle syndrome in infants.[4]

Chronic Caries

Chronic caries describes a slowly progressive decay process that requires routine intervention. The carious dentin is firm and often brown to black. In large open cavities the decayed dentin can be scooped out in large segments and has the consistency of firm leather (Fig. 12–16).

Arrested Caries

Dental decay is not a continuous demineralization process. Evidence supports a continuous demineralization-**remineralization** process that can be tipped out of balance by changes in diet and oral environment. Since the saliva provides the constituents that enable enamel to remineralize after an acid attack, a reduction in salivary flow or salivary buffering capacity may cause rapid demineralization. Conversely, demineralized lesions may recalcify as a result of an improved oral environment. **Arrested caries** describes such a demineralization-remineralization process. Arrested lesions may be noticed because of their light or brown color, but they feel firm and glass-like when explored (Fig. 12–17).

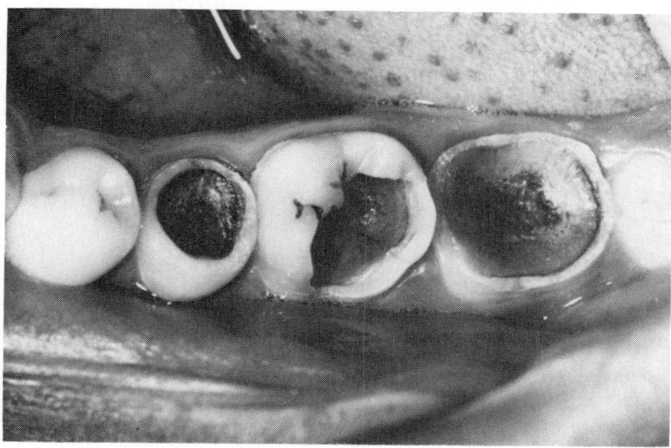

FIGURE 12–16
Chronic caries. (Courtesy of Cheryl Cameron, RDH, PhD, and Glen E. Gordon, DDS.)

Recurrent Caries

Recurrent caries describes new decay that occurs at the margin(s) of existing restorations. These lesions pose a special threat because they may go undetected and invade the tissue beneath the restoration (Fig. 12–18).

Backward Caries

Backward caries describes the lateral spread of decay at the dentinoenamel junction. This undermining process frequently results in a carious lesion with a small opening at the surface and extensive breakdown and cavitation within the tooth. The significance of this progression of caries

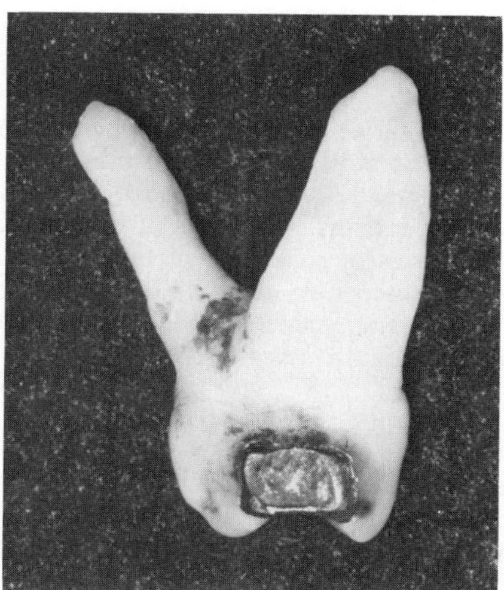

FIGURE 12–18
Recurrent caries. (Courtesy of Cheryl Cameron, RDH, PhD, and Glen E. Gordon, DDS.)

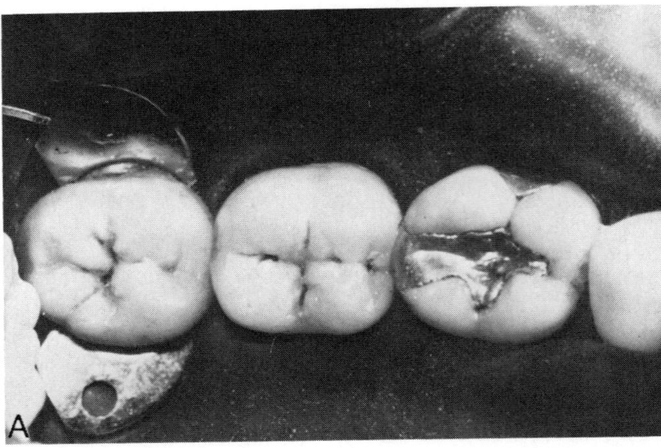

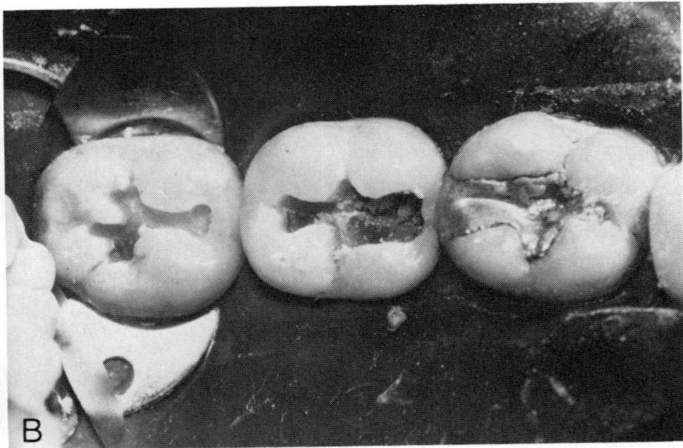

FIGURE 12-19
A, Mandibular molars with small carious openings in the occlusal pits and fissures. These lesions present a sticky (tug-back) texture when explored. *B*, Initial opening in cavities (shown on left) reveals extensive lateral spread of caries at the dentinoenamel junction. (Courtesy of Cheryl Cameron, RDH, PhD, and Glen E. Gordon, DDS.)

relates primarily to cavity preparation and treatment. On clinical examination, a carious lesion may appear to require a simple restoration, but during dental treatment require a complex restoration (Fig. 12-19).

Location of Carious Lesions*

Carious lesions are often referred to by their specific location on a tooth. This mechanism of description may be best suited for describing the dental problem to the client. The description of the location may include anatomical representations such as pit and fissure caries, smooth surface caries, and root caries. Another method of describing the location of a carious lesion is to identify the specific surface(s) on a tooth with a lesion. It is not uncommon for noncarious tooth surfaces to become involved in the restoration process because of the need for access or cavity design. For example, a tooth with a carious lesion on the distal surface may require the involvement of the occlusal surface or a distoocclusal cavity preparation for restoration. Thus, another form of classification is by the number or identification of involved surfaces rather than carious surfaces.

Pit and Fissure Caries

Pit and fissure caries is most frequently found in the grooves and crevices of the occlusal surfaces of premolars and molars (see Fig. 12-19). It is also found in the lingual pits of maxillary incisors, facial pits of mandibular molars, and lingual grooves of maxillary molars. Pits and fissures are particularly susceptible to a carious attack because of the protected bacterial niche provided by the inadequately coalesced developmental lobes of enamel.

Smooth Surface Caries

Smooth surface caries is found on the facial, lingual, mesial, and distal surfaces of the dentition (Fig. 12-20). The proximal smooth surfaces are the most susceptible to dental caries because of the shelter that is provided for the bacterial plaque colonies. The gingival one-third of the facial and lingual surfaces also are more susceptible to caries because of the increased difficulty associated with cleaning this less bulbous portion of the crown.

Root Caries

Root caries is found on the root surfaces of teeth. Also referred to as "senile caries," root caries is most frequently found in the elderly population, in whom root exposure is common because of gingival recession. Root caries presents a unique set of considerations for restorative therapy be-

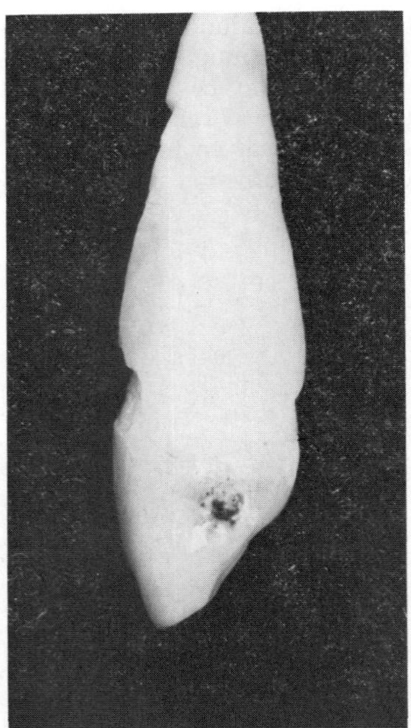

FIGURE 12-20
Smooth surface caries. (Courtesy of Cheryl Cameron, RDH, PhD, and Glen E. Gordon, DDS.)

*This section was contributed by Cheryl Cameron, RDH, PhD, and Glen E. Gordon, DDS.

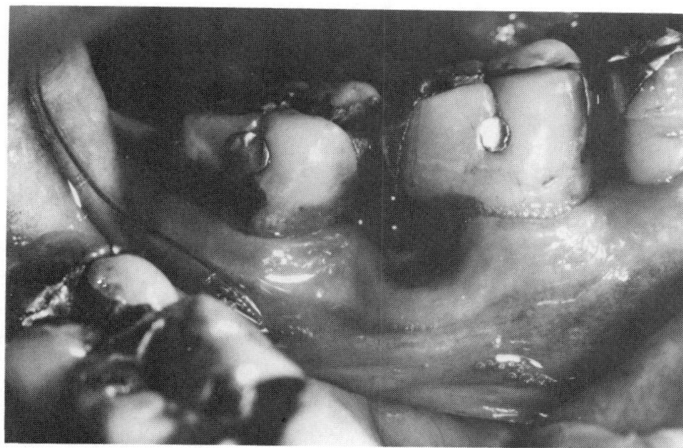

FIGURE 12–21
Root caries are found on the root surfaces of teeth. (Courtesy of Cheryl Cameron, RDH, PhD, and Glen E. Gordon, DDS.)

cause of the location of the lesions, the difficulty of adequate plaque control, and the chemical composition of the root surface.[5] As the lesion progresses, it may encircle the tooth at the gumline, making it very difficult to isolate and restore (Fig. 12–21).

DEVELOPMENTAL ANOMALIES

During tooth formation, dental anomalies may arise from a disruption in the stages of tooth development (odontogenesis), causing one or more of the tissues of the tooth bud to be disrupted. These disturbances may be the result of local, systemic, or hereditary factors. The extent of the manifestation of the disturbance is dependent on the stage of dental development and the duration and nature of the assault.

Dental anomalies include anomalies of the number of teeth and anomalies of dental tissues. The following discussion briefly describes the more frequently noted dental anomalies. (Tooth anomalies with variation in root form are presented in Chapter 19.)

Anomalies of Number of Teeth

Hyperdontia is the presence of extra teeth beyond the normal complement. Hyperdontia is commonly referred to as supernumerary or supplemental teeth. Supernumerary teeth are extra teeth of abnormal shape, whereas supplemental teeth are extra teeth of normal shape. When an extra tooth occurs in the midline between the maxillary anterior incisors, it is referred to as a "mesiodens" (Fig. 12–22). These supernumerary teeth are usually misshaped, small, and peglike. A natal tooth is a supernumerary tooth that erupts prior to birth, while a neonatal tooth is a supernumerary tooth that erupts shortly after birth.[6]

Hypodontia is the absence of one or more teeth and also may be called **anodontia.** The failure of all teeth to develop is termed **complete anodontia,** while the absence of one or several teeth is called **partial anodontia.** Anodontia is usually associated with defects of ectodermal structures, such as is found with the disorder ectodermal dysplasia.

While complete anodontia is extremely rare, partial anodontia is more common. The teeth most frequently observed as congenitally missing are third molars, followed sequentially by maxillary lateral incisors and mandibular premolars. The teeth least frequently absent are first permanent molars.

Anomalies of the Dental Tissues

Anomalies of the teeth can be subdivided into several categories: those affecting the total tooth and those affecting the individual dental tissues, including enamel, dentin, cementum, and pulp.

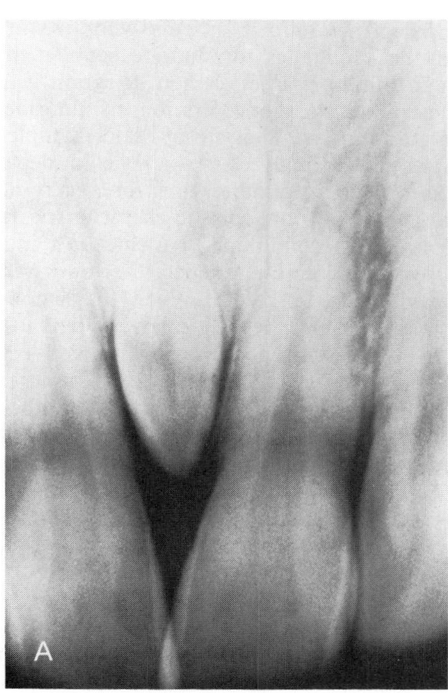

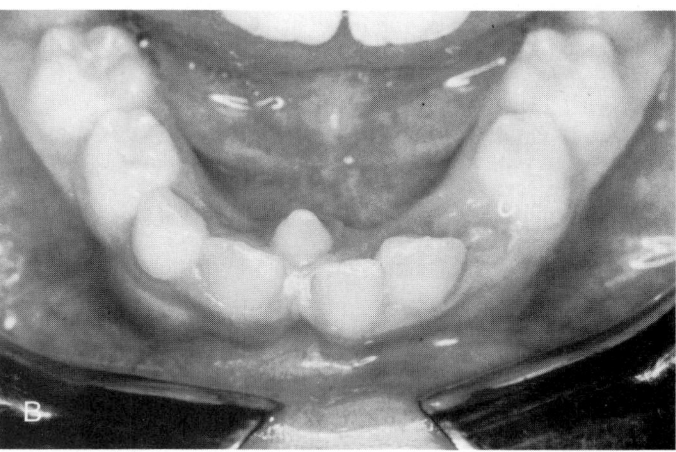

FIGURE 12–22
Mesiodens. (With permission from Regezi, J. A., and Sciubba, J. J. Oral Pathology: Clinical-Pathologic Correlations, 2nd ed. Philadelphia: W. B. Saunders, 1993, p. 505.)

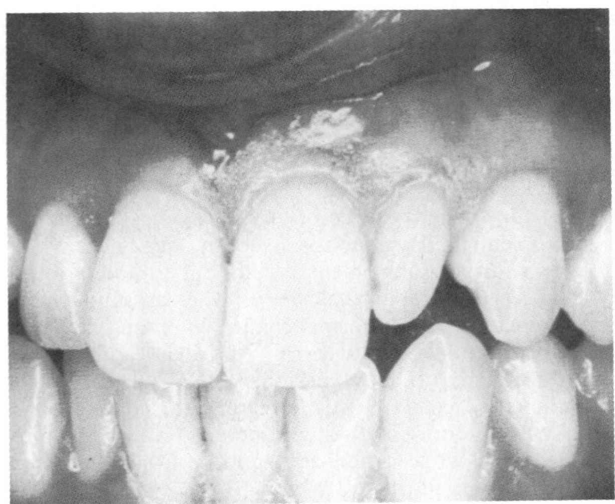

FIGURE 12–23
Microdontia. (Courtesy of Dr. George Blozis.)

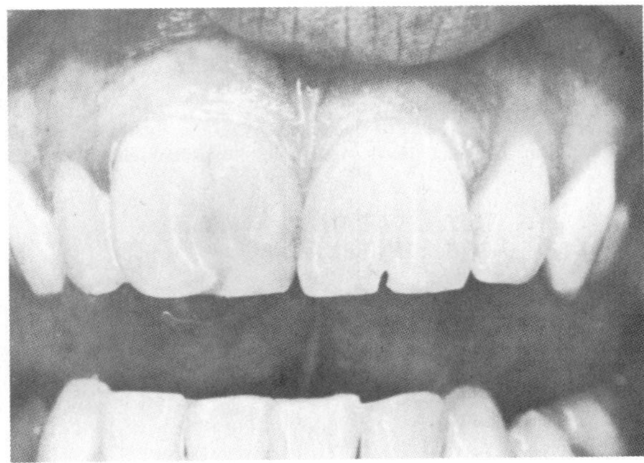

FIGURE 12–24
Gemination. (Courtesy of Dr. George Blozis.)

Anomalies of the Whole Tooth

Macrodontia refers to larger than normal teeth. These teeth may be larger in width, length, or height.[6]

Microdontia is a developmental anomaly in which the teeth are smaller than normal. This condition may affect one tooth, several teeth, or all teeth within the dentition. Many supernumerary teeth are small and can be classified as microdonts (Fig. 12–23).

In **gemination,** a large tooth results from the splitting of a single tooth germ that attempts to form two teeth (Fig. 12–24). This twinning usually results in a partially or completely divided crown attached to a single root with one canal.[6]

Dens in dente (also called *dens invaginatus*) is defined as a tooth within a tooth. It is caused by invagination of the enamel organ during development and is most frequently observed on the lingual aspect of the maxillary lateral incisors. A deep crevice usually runs between the oral mucosa and the inner surface of the tooth where the anomaly is found.[6] This crevice increases the likelihood of early dental caries; consequently a preventive restoration may be considered in order to prevent internal decay.

Dilaceration is the severe distortion of a crown or root caused by trauma during tooth formation. It is usually manifested as a severely angulated root. Extraction of a tooth with a dilacerated root often creates a treatment problem for the dentist because of the root angulation.[7]

Intrinsic staining of dental tissues may occur when the antibiotic tetracycline is administered during tooth formation. The tetracycline is deposited in the forming enamel and dentin, resulting in permanent staining ranging from mild yellow to yellow-brown or gray coloration. The dental hygienist may play a role in the prevention of intrinsic staining by educating pregnant women and mothers about the side effects of tetracycline consumption during pregnancy and early childhood.

Anomalies of Enamel Formation

An insult to ameloblasts during tooth formation may result in abnormal enamel development, referred to generally as **enamel dysplasia.** Enamel dysplasia encompasses two types of abnormal enamel development, enamel hypoplasia and enamel hypocalcification.

Enamel hypoplasia is the result of a disturbance of the ameloblasts during matrix formation (Fig. 12–25). **Enamel hypocalcification** is a defect occurring to the enamel as the result of a disturbance during mineralization (Fig. 12–26). The clinical differentiation of these lesions is such that enamel hypoplasia produces a pitted or rough striated enamel surface, whereas enamel hypocalcification produces a white spotted appearance of the enamel surface; however, the enamel surface is generally smooth in texture.

Many factors—local (e.g., trauma), systemic (e.g., diseases, nutritional deficiencies, excess systemic fluoride), hereditary, and idiopathic (unknown)—may cause anomalies of enamel formation.

When excessive amounts of systemic fluoride are responsible for enamel hypoplasia or enamel hypocalcification, this condition is classified as *dental fluorosis.* This condition may range from mild fluorosis, associated with white flecking, to severe situations in which the teeth are deeply pitted and/or brown-stained. Clients who live in a rural setting may be candidates for fluoride supplements; however, prior to initiating a supplement program it is important to determine the concentration of fluoride in the drinking water through analysis of water samples. These water samples can be analyzed by local health departments.

Congenital syphilis is another, now rare, cause of enamel hypoplasia, and several hypoplastic characteristics are often associated with this condition. "Hutchinson's incisors" is the term used to denote the notched or screwdriver appearance of syphilitic incisor teeth. When the lateral incisors display a conical shape, they are often referred to as "peg-laterals." It is important to note that not all peg-laterals occur as the result of syphilis. A peg-lateral is, in essence, a microdont and can stem from a variety of other causes. The term "mulberry molars" is used to describe the mottled mulberry-shaped molars also associated with congenital syphilis[6] (Fig. 12–27).

Amelogenesis imperfecta is a form of enamel dysplasia resulting from hereditary factors. For example, many patterns of inheritance are associated with this disorder, such as autosomal dominant, recessive, or X-linked. Amelogenesis imperfecta is the partial or total malformation of enamel. The dentin and pulp of these teeth develop normally, whereas the enamel is easily chipped or worn away.

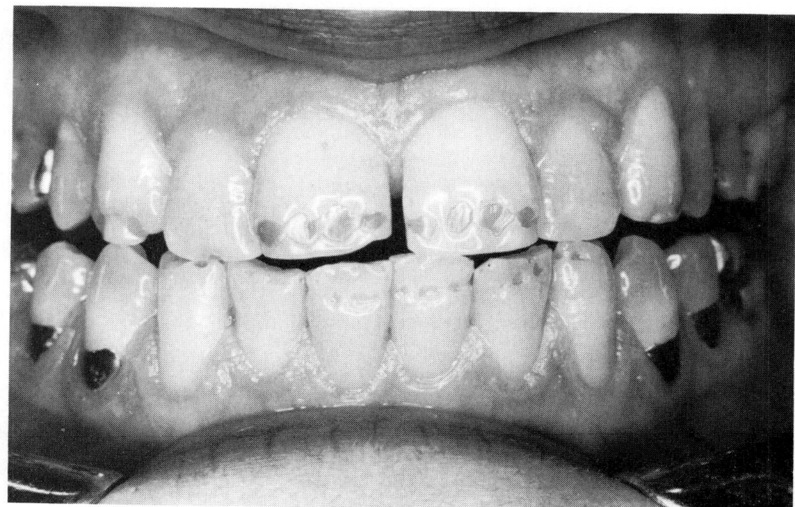

FIGURE 12-25
Enamel hypoplasia. (With permission from Regezi, J. A., and Sciubba, J. J. Oral Pathology: Clinical-Pathologic Correlations, 2nd ed. Philadelphia: W. B. Saunders, 1993, p. 507.)

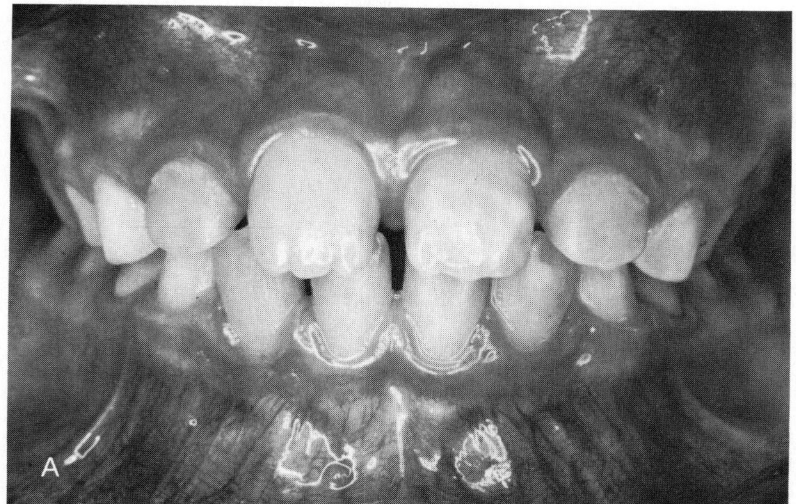

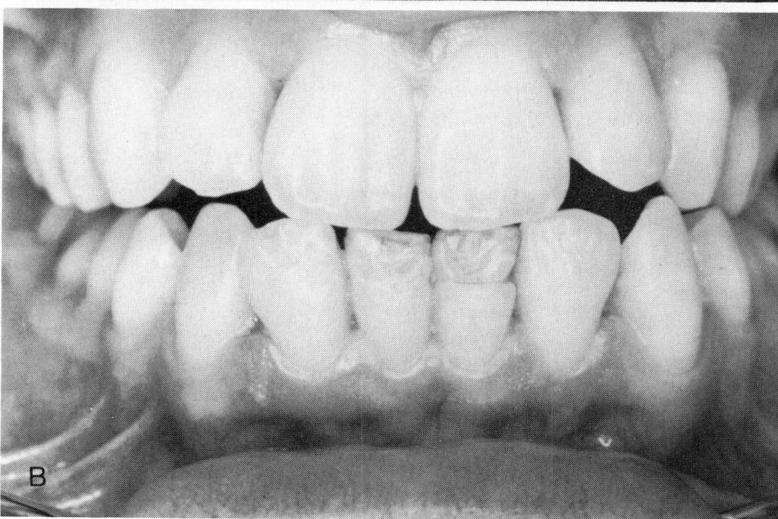

FIGURE 12-26
Enamel hypocalcification. (With permission from Regezi, J. A., and Sciubba, J. J. Oral Pathology: Clinical-Pathologic Correlations, 2nd ed. Philadelphia: W. B. Saunders, 1993, p. 507.)

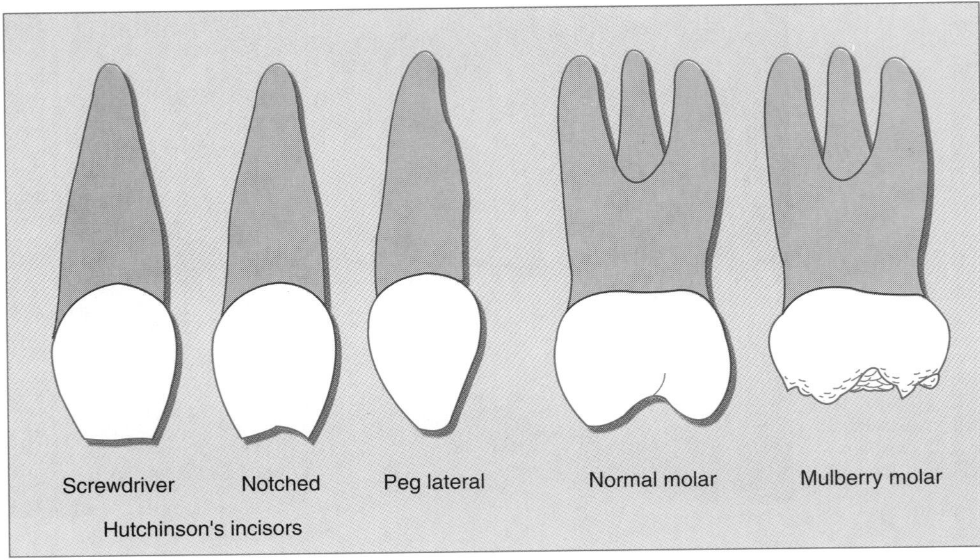

FIGURE 12–27
Syphilitic enamel hypoplasia. (Redrawn from Giunta, J. L. Oral Pathology. St. Louis: CV Mosby, 1989, pp. 55 and 58.)

Several anomalies involving enamel are not classified as enamel dysplasia, two of which are **enamel pearls** (see Chapter 19) and dens evaginatus.

Dens evaginatus, also referred to as *tuberculated cusp,* is a small mass of enamel or accessory cusp projecting on the occlusal surface of molars and premolars (Fig. 12–28). It is believed to form from an outpouching of the enamel epithelium during the early stages of odontogenesis. The mass of tissue contains normal pulp and is subject to occlusal wear, risking exposure from the evaginated pulp chamber.[7]

Anomalies of Dentin Formation

Dentinogenesis imperfecta is the irregular formation or absence of dentinal development. Dentinogenesis imperfecta is associated with a dominant inherited disorder that is characterized by faulty formation of connective tissues. The dentin displays a softer consistency as a result of increased water and organic content. Enamel formation occurs normally. The enamel easily breaks away from the dentin, however, and the teeth are prone to rapid wear[7] and dentinal hypersensitivity. Dental treatment usually includes placement of crowns to preserve existing crown structure.

Dentin dysplasia is a mesenchymal dysplasia and differs from dentinogenesis imperfecta in that the enamel does not readily chip away. The teeth exhibit normal color and little evidence of attrition. However, teeth with dentin dysplasia show retarded root formation and a lack of supporting bone. The lack of periodontal support may likely have serious periodontal implications; therefore, referral to a periodontist is recommended.

Anomalies of Pulp Formation

Taurodontism, meaning "bull-like" teeth, is an inherited phenomenon and thus is genetically determined (Fig. 12–29). The crowns of these teeth develop normally; however, the pulp chambers are much enlarged at the expense of the dentinal walls.[8]

CLASSIFICATION OF DENTAL CARIES AND RESTORATIONS

There are several formats used to classify and describe both dental caries and dental restorations. Caries are commonly classified either by Black's classification or by the Simple/Complex/Compound system.

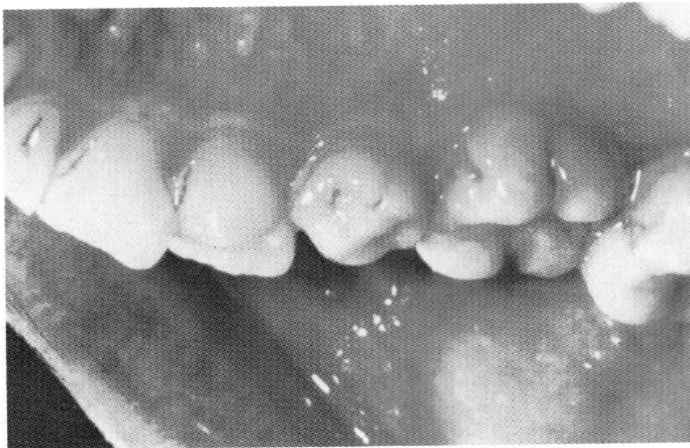

FIGURE 12–28
Dens evaginatus. (Courtesy of Dr. Margot Van Dis.)

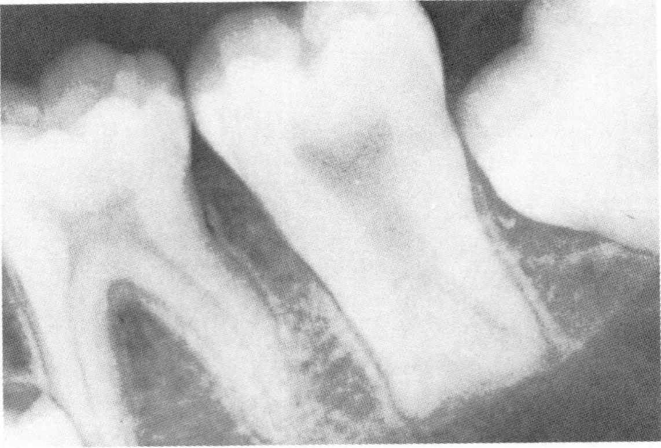

FIGURE 12–29
Taurodontism. (Courtesy of Dr. George Blozis.)

Black's Classification of Dental Caries and Restorations

The most commonly used system to classify both dental caries and restorations was established by G. V. Black in the early 1900s and provides a precise description of the types and location of the dental caries and restorations. This descriptive system consists of six classifications, as follows.

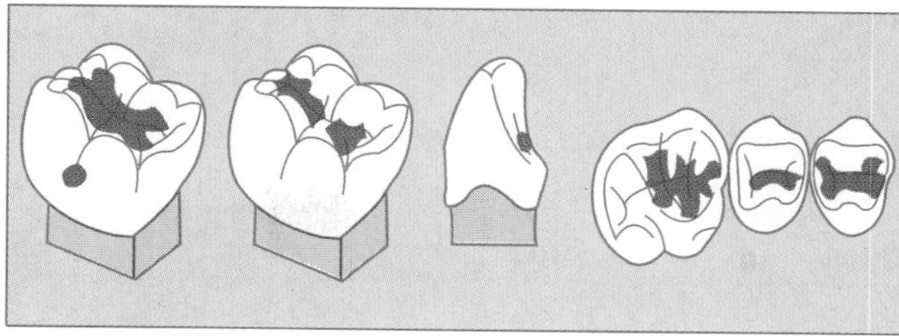

FIGURE 12–30
Class 1, Black's classification of dental caries and restorations. (Redrawn from Northern Alberta Institute of Technology: Instructional Resource #1399, 1993.)

Class 1 (Fig. 12–30)

Class 1 dental caries or restorations occur in the following:

- Occlusal surfaces (pits and fissures) in premolars and molars
- Occlusal two-thirds of the facial or lingual surfaces of molars
- Lingual surfaces of maxillary incisors

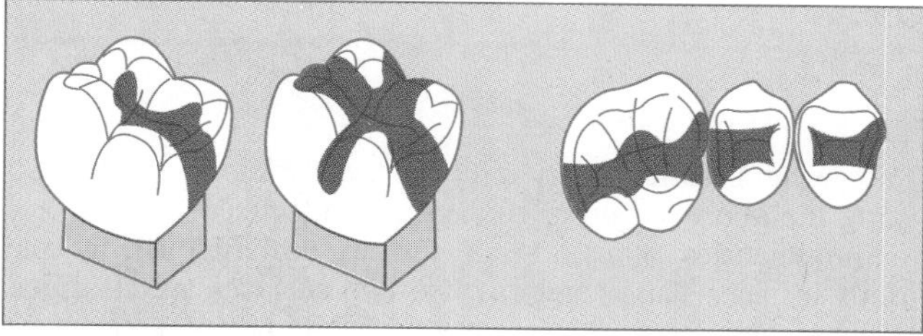

FIGURE 12–31
Class 2, Black's classification of dental caries and restorations. (Redrawn from Northern Alberta Institute of Technology: Instructional Resource #1399, 1993.)

Class 2 (Fig. 12–31)

Class 2 dental caries or restorations occur in the following:

- Proximal surfaces of posterior teeth
- Occlusal surfaces—usually involved

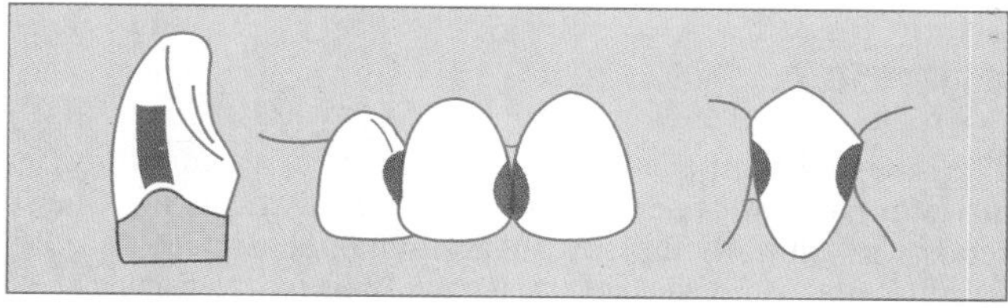

FIGURE 12–32
Class 3, Black's classification of dental caries and restorations. (Redrawn from Northern Alberta Institute of Technology: Instructional Resource #1399, 1993.)

Class 3 (Fig. 12–32)

Class 3 dental caries or restorations occur in the following:

- Proximal surfaces of incisors and canines. Incisal angle —*not* involved

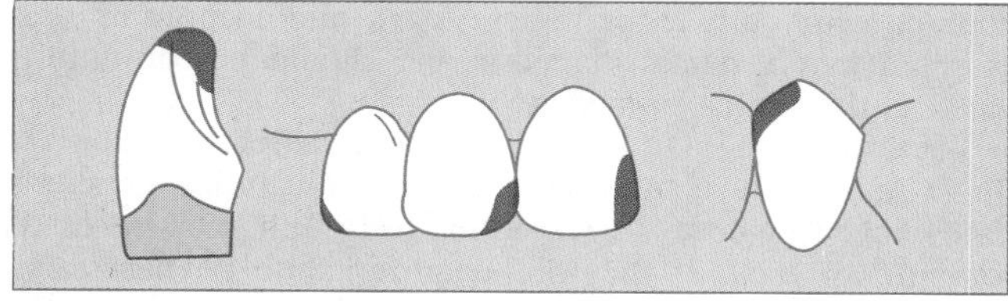

FIGURE 12–33
Class 4, Black's classification of dental caries and restorations. (Redrawn from Northern Alberta Institute of Technology: Instructional Resource #1399, 1993.)

Class 4 (Fig. 12–33)

Class 4 dental caries or restorations occur in the following:

- The proximal surfaces of incisors and canines, including the incisal angle

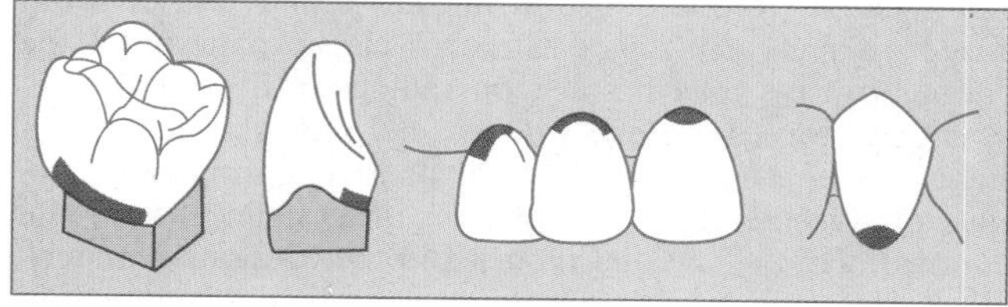

FIGURE 12–34
Class 5, Black's classification of dental caries and restorations. (Redrawn from Northern Alberta Institute of Technology: Instructional Resource #1399, 1993.)

Class 5 (Fig. 12–34)

Class 5 dental caries or restorations occur in the following:

- Gingival third of facial or lingual surfaces of any tooth

Class 6 (Fig. 12–35)

Class 6 dental caries or restorations involve the following:

- Incisal edge of anterior teeth and the cusp tips of posterior teeth

Classification by Complexity

This system of classification identifies dental caries and restorations by the names of the surfaces that they involve.

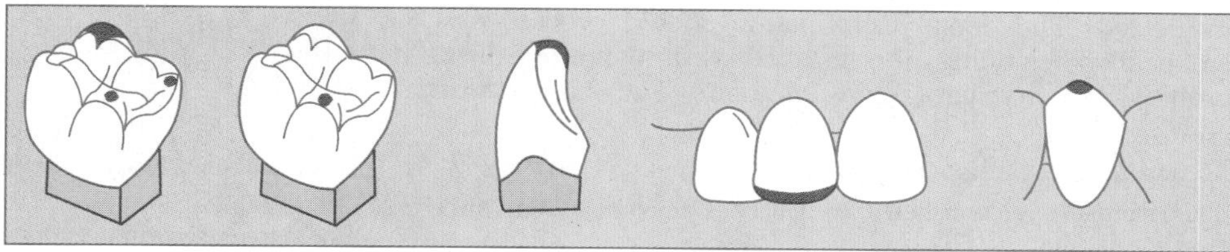

FIGURE 12–35
Class 6, Black's classification of dental caries and restorations. (Redrawn from Northern Alberta Institute of Technology: Instructional Resource #1399, 1993.)

TABLE 12–3
SIMPLE, COMPOUND, AND COMPLEX DESIGNATIONS FOR DENTAL CARIES AND RESTORATIONS

Simple	Abbreviation	Compound	Abbreviation	Complex	Abbreviation
Buccal	B	Mesioocclusal	MO	Mesioincisodistal	MID
Facial	F	Distoocclusal	DO	Mesiolinguodistal	MLD
Gingival	G	Occlusobuccal	OB	Mesioocclusobuccal	MOB
Incisal	I	Distolingual	DL	Mesioocclusodistal	MOD
Lingual	Li	Distoocclusal	DO	Mesioocclusodistobuccolingual	MODBL
Labial	La				
Occlusal	O				

The usual practice is to refer to the caries or restoration using the abbreviation of the surfaces affected.

Simple caries or restorations are those involving only one tooth surface. Those that involve two surfaces are classified as **compound caries** or restorations, while **complex caries** or restorations involves more than two surfaces.

Table 12–3 outlines examples of simple, compound, and complex designations for dental caries or restorations.

TOOTH ASSESSMENT*

The assessment of the biological integrity of the dentition is an essential component of overall client assessment. Client reports of pain elicited by sugar intake, sensitivity to cold stimuli, and objectionable taste are frequently due to advanced carious lesions or leaking/defective restorations. Tooth abrasions and erosions may be sensitive to toothbrushing, acidic foods, and cold stimuli. Incomplete fractures of teeth may elicit sharp pain during chewing and contact with cold foods. These signs and symptoms are essential to the dental diagnosis and should be communicated to the dentist immediately.

Tooth assessment must include both radiographical and direct (clinical) evaluations. Bite-wing radiographs are standard diagnostic tools for posterior teeth and may be used for anterior teeth if they are determined to be necessary during the clinical examination. The bite-wing radiograph produces the best image of the tooth crowns—the main area of concern for tooth restoration. Carious lesions appear as radiolucent images on radiographs because dental caries causes localized demineralization and loss of tooth tissue. In the early stages of decay, classic patterns of the carious process may be seen on radiographs, since the destruction proceeds in line with enamel rods and along dentinal tubules. Depending on their density, restorative materials produce relatively radiopaque images. Because of the contrast between the oral tissues and the restorative materials, radiographs readily illustrate the fit and contours of restorations (Fig. 12–36).

Direct examination can be done well only if the teeth are clean and dry and visualized in good light. When bacterial plaque and saliva coat the teeth, lesions and defects may go undetected. The dental examination should proceed systematically, beginning, for instance, with the most distal tooth in the maxillary right quadrant. The examination should be continued around the arch, through the last tooth in the maxillary left quadrant. Then the mandibular arch should be examined in reverse order, beginning with the most distal tooth in the mandibular left quadrant and ending with the last tooth in the mandibular right quadrant. Cotton roll isolation can be helpful in maintaining a dry environment, and forced air-drying is essential for the individual examination of each tooth. A sharp explorer is used to check grooves and pits in enamel, discolored root surfaces along the gingival margin, and suspicious margins of restorations. Moderate pressure is applied with the explorer, and control of the force using a proper fulcrum is important. Care should be exercised to avoid gouging of restorations and causing pain from undue exploring of known sensitive areas. An area may be considered carious, regardless of color, if it feels soft when explored. The withdrawal of the explorer tip from the true lesion produces the feeling of "tug-back," as though the explorer were stuck into a piece of leather. Color is not a foolproof indicator of caries, since carious dentin can range in color from nearly white to shades of black. If a dark area on a tooth is hard, regardless of the color, it is rarely an active carious lesion. The caries process often undermines otherwise intact enamel (backward caries), producing a "pearly" appearance. In this case, color may be an indicator of the extent of the carious lesion. Marginal ridges, especially in anterior teeth, should be examined under a well-directed light. The careful use of a nonmagnifying, front-surface mirror for transillumination may show undermining decay, which can then be substantiated by exploring the lesion. Early recurrent caries at the proximal margins of a restoration may go

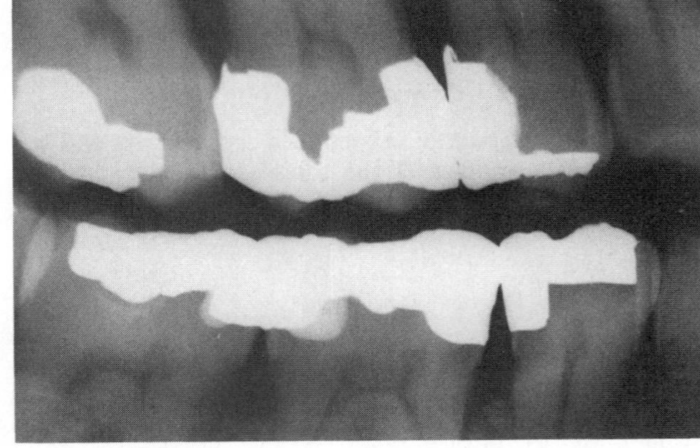

FIGURE 12–36
Radiograph showing restorations.

*This section was contributed by Cheryl Cameron, RDH, PhD, and Glen E. Gordon, DDS.

clinically undetected because of the difficulty in exploring these areas. Thus, radiographical diagnosis can be essential for supplementing tactile findings.

The clinical examination is also used to assess tooth damage and defective restorations unrelated to dental caries. Abraded areas, erosions, and fractures should be noted; however, careful exploration is required, since these are often sensitive areas. The tactile examination of overhangs, open margins, short margins, poor contours, and other restorative defects observed in the radiographical survey is important for verification. Suspected open proximal contacts should be visually corroborated by viewing through the contact against a white background, such as the rubber glove surface. If light passes through the contact, it is judged to be open. The use of floss only in assessing the status of an open contact may result in an inaccurate diagnosis. A slightly open contact may resist the passing of dental floss and, yet, result in food impaction and gingival inflammation.

Charting Tooth Assessment Data

To facilitate planning, the tooth assessment charting procedure is conducted at the client's assessment appointment(s). Charts are subsequently updated at each reappointment. Although no set sequences are required for charting, clinicians are advised to devise a routine to avoid deleting important information. The systematic approach most often advocated is as follows:

1. Chart all missing or unerupted teeth first, to prevent the wrongful identification of existing teeth
2. Chart in blue ink existing amalgam or tooth-colored restorations
3. Chart in blue ink gold restoration, crowns, and bridges, and follow by notating the presence of partial and/or complete dentures
4. Complete the tooth charting by recording signs of dental caries, and watch areas in red ink and other miscellaneous chartable items (e.g., hypoplasia, appliances) in blue ink
5. The use of abbreviations to explain the symbols is optional for recording on the chart (Table 12–4). Figure 12–37 illustrates an example of a completed chart along with a descriptive key of the charted symbols
6. Periodontal charting of gingival and mucogingival lines, probing depth, attachment loss, recession, furcation involvement, mucogingival problems, abnormal frenum attachments, and mobility of teeth is described in Chapter 13
7. Protocol for updating the chart should be established in each oral healthcare setting to avoid a cluttered and unreadable chart. One suggestion is to photocopy the original chart and to highlight the changes in a different color of ink on the chart copy. This avoids recharting the original findings, and the process can be repeated many times[9]

Text continued on page 354

TABLE 12–4
CHARTING SYMBOLS FOR TOOTH ASSESSMENT

Chartable Item	Description	Charting Procedure	Charting Symbol	Abbreviations
Missing teeth	Teeth that are not present because of extraction or are congenitally missing	Place vertical line through facial, occlusal, and lingual surfaces Chart in blue ink	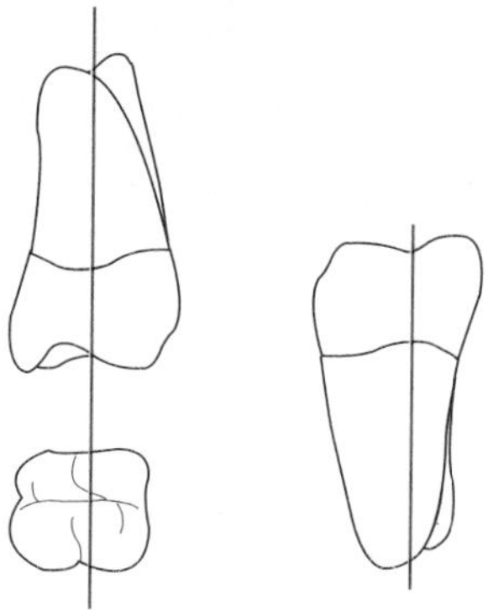	M
Unerupted teeth	Teeth that have not yet erupted Term may also be used for impacted teeth	Circle facial, occlusal, and lingual surfaces of tooth Chart in red ink	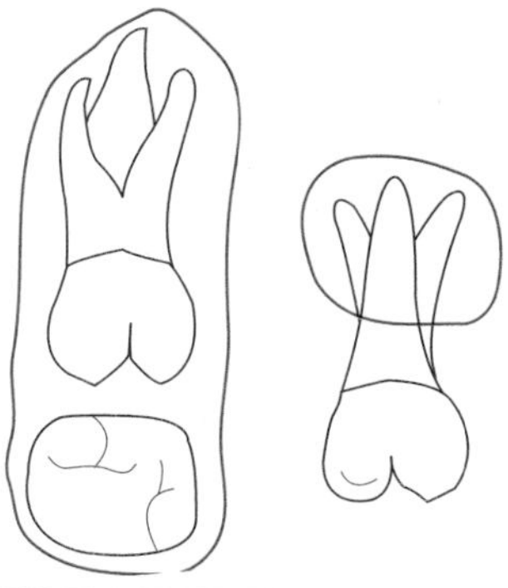	U

Table continued on following page

TABLE 12–4
CHARTING SYMBOLS FOR TOOTH ASSESSMENT *Continued*

Chartable Item	Description	Charting Procedure	Charting Symbol	Abbreviations
Teeth to be extracted	Teeth to be extracted because of pathological or orthodontic reasons	Place X over facial, occlusal, and lingual surfaces Chart in red ink	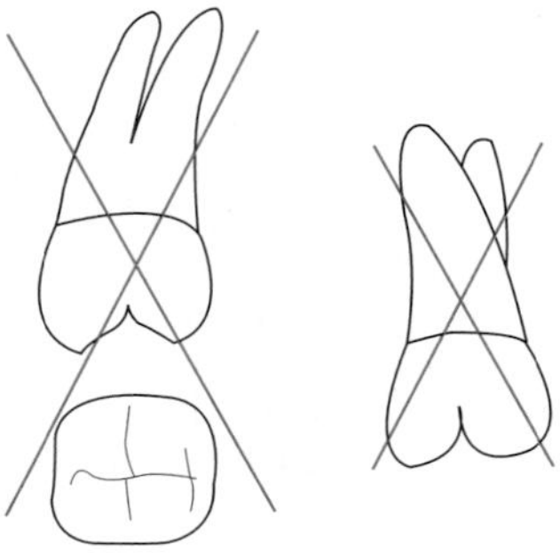	Ex
Amalgam restorations	Alloy of silver and mercury; silver or dark gray in color; widely used as a restorative material	Chart surfaces where the restorations appear Outline and shade in blue the shape of restoration For precise notation Black's classification can be used	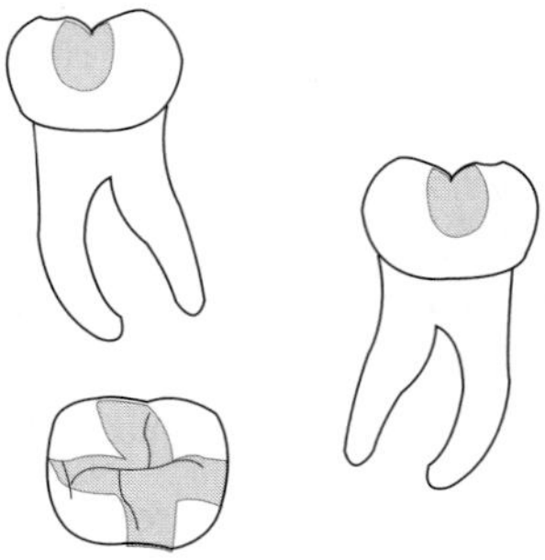	A
Tooth-colored restorations	Composite resin is a tooth-colored restorative material. Usually placed in anterior teeth, for restoring facial and/or proximal surfaces where aesthetics are a major concern, but found in posterior areas for the same reason	Outline exact size and shape of restoration Shade with blue ink Chart surfaces involved Can be further identified using Black's classification	TC(4) 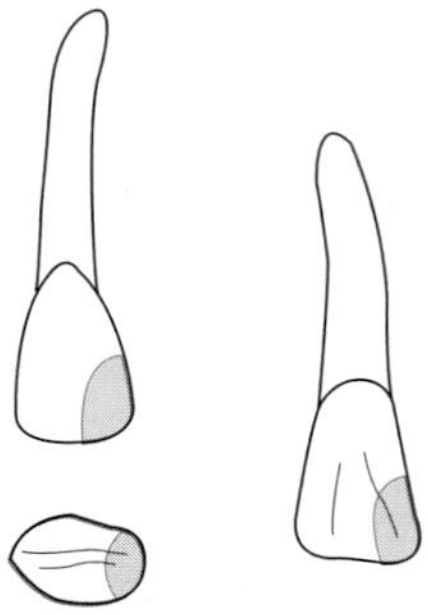	TC, tooth-colored S, silicate R, resin CR, composite resin
Temporary restorations	Temporary filling cements (i.e., a zinc oxide–eugenol cement) may be placed as an interim measure for a displaced restoration or between phases of treatment while observing pulpal reaction. Distinguishable by its creamy, yellow color	Chart temporary restorations the same as amalgam or tooth-colored restorations in blue ink, but distinguish from amalgams with the abbreviation	TR 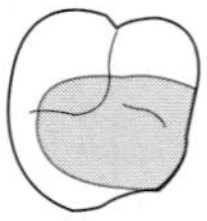	Temp

TABLE 12–4
CHARTING SYMBOLS FOR TOOTH ASSESSMENT *Continued*

Chartable Item	Description	Charting Procedure	Charting Symbol	Abbreviations
Veneer	An aesthetic veneer or layer of tooth-colored material that is used to cover the unsightly area of a tooth Typical indications for veneers include teeth with facial surfaces that are malformed, discolored, or abraded. Technique for replacing labial surface is used	Outline and shade in surface of tooth where veneer is found Chart in blue ink	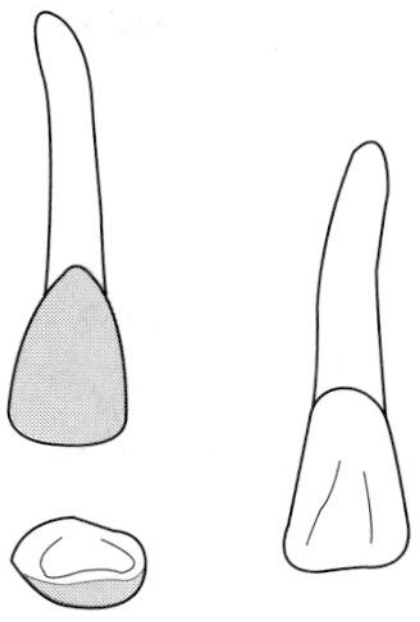	Ven
Gold restorations	Gold restorations are noted by the yellow gold luster. Several types of gold restorations are found, including cast gold restorations (onlays, inlays, crowns)	See below		
Full gold crown	A cast yellow-gold crown covering the entire surface and all of the crown surfaces	Outline and fill in with diagonal lines covering all surfaces of the crown Chart in blue ink	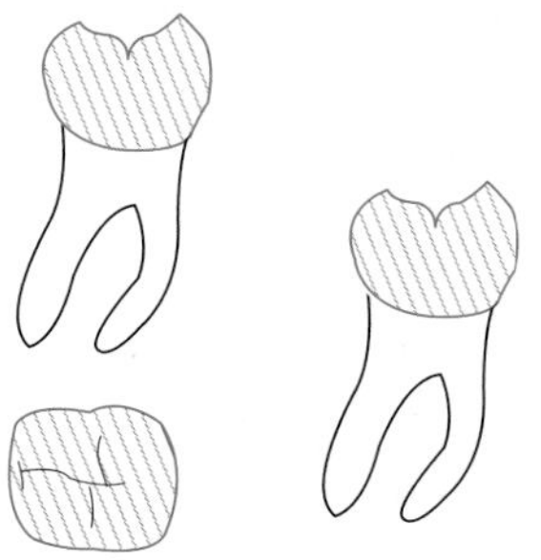	FGC
3/4 gold crown	Covers less than 3/4 of tooth surfaces	Outline and fill in with diagonal lines placed on all surfaces or portion of surfaces covered by crown Chart in blue ink	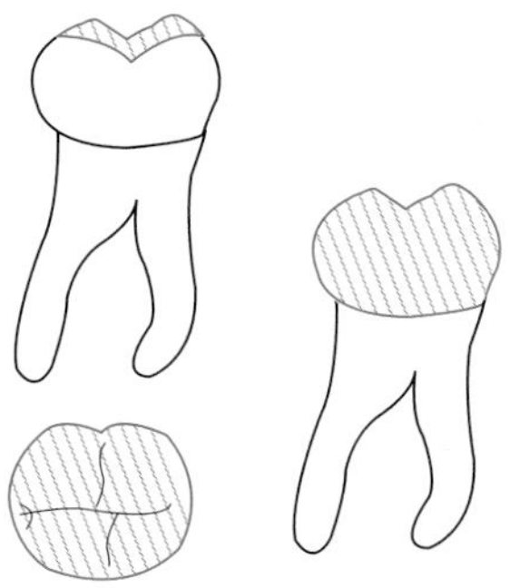	3/4 GC
Ceramic-metal crowns	White-gold alloy crown with bonded acrylic or porcelain facing. Provides a tooth-colored appearance	Chart similarly to gold crowns Abbreviation can be used to distinguish it from full gold or 3/4 gold crowns Chart in blue ink	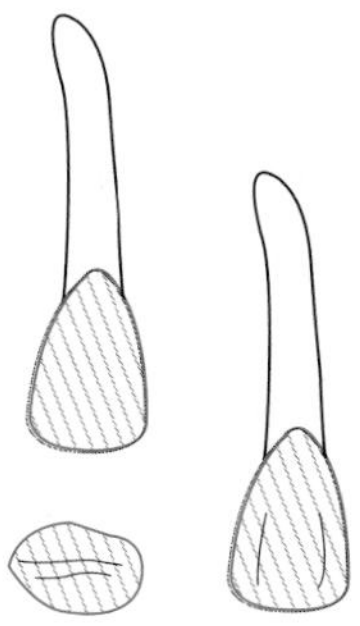	GCPF (gold crown porcelain face) GCAF (gold crown acrylic face)

Table continued on following page

TABLE 12–4
CHARTING SYMBOLS FOR TOOTH ASSESSMENT *Continued*

Chartable Item	Description	Charting Procedure	Charting Symbol	Abbreviations
Gold inlay	A cast gold restoration that is placed within the prepared tooth cavity and does not cover the cusps	Outline the shape of the restoration on the surfaces where it appears Chart in blue ink	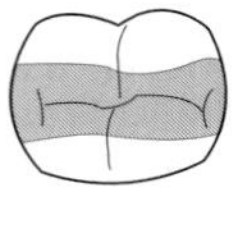	GI
Gold onlay	A cast gold restoration with the cusp tips covered in gold for added strength	Outline and color the shape of the restoration on the surfaces where it appears Chart in blue ink	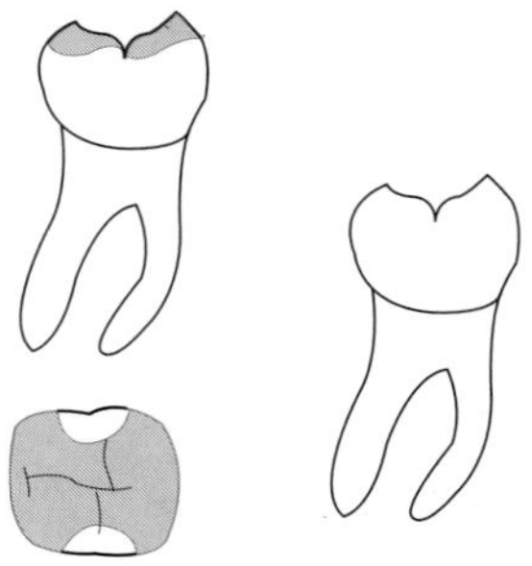	GO
Gold foil	A noncasted gold restoration that is currently not widely used in dental practice. Thin particles of gold are manually placed in the cavity preparation	Outline and color the shape of the restoration Chart in blue ink	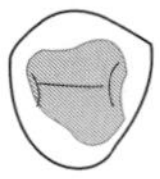	GF
Fixed bridges	A bridge unit serves to restore a functional unit by replacing one or more missing teeth. A fixed bridge consists of abutment and pontic teeth splinted together	Outline abutment and pontic teeth in blue ink and fill in with diagonal lines on occlusal, facial, and lingual surfaces Chart the pontic teeth as extracted and draw a vertical line through their roots. The type of crowns may be identified with abbreviations (e.g., FGC, GCPF) Place two horizontal lines between the occlusal surfaces of the teeth to represent the splinted unit	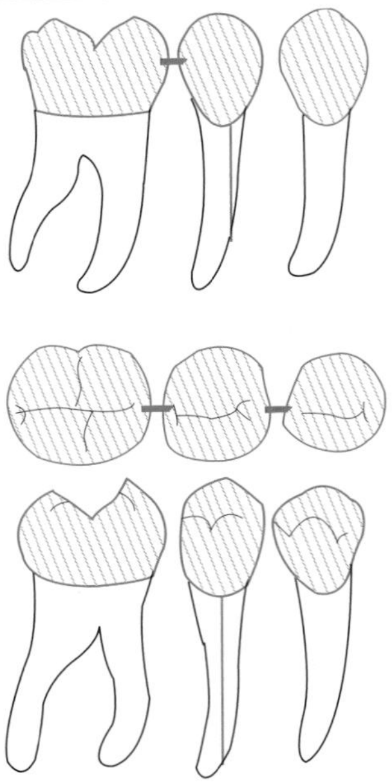	Each tooth may be labeled with the appropriate abbreviations FGC GCPF 3/4 GC
Dental implants	A stable functional replacement for one or more missing teeth that consists of an osseointegrated anchor, an abutment, and a prosthetic tooth or appliance	Place a dental implant stamp over the teeth involved. If no stamp is available, make a written comment under the teeth involved	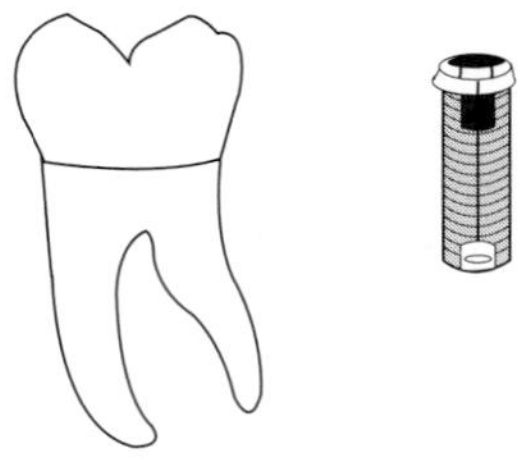	IMPL

TABLE 12–4
CHARTING SYMBOLS FOR TOOTH ASSESSMENT *Continued*

Chartable Item	Description	Charting Procedure	Charting Symbol	Abbreviations
Dental caries (see pp. 335–339 and 342–344 for further discussion)	Technically known as a carious lesion, commonly referred to as a cavity	Outline the carious area(s) in red on the surfaces where the caries appear. Suspect carious surfaces can be labeled for observation On completion of the restorations fill in the red areas with blue ink	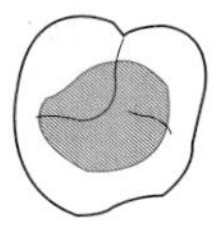	C
Recurrent decay	Recurring caries around the margin of an existing restoration	Outline the area of recurrent decay in red	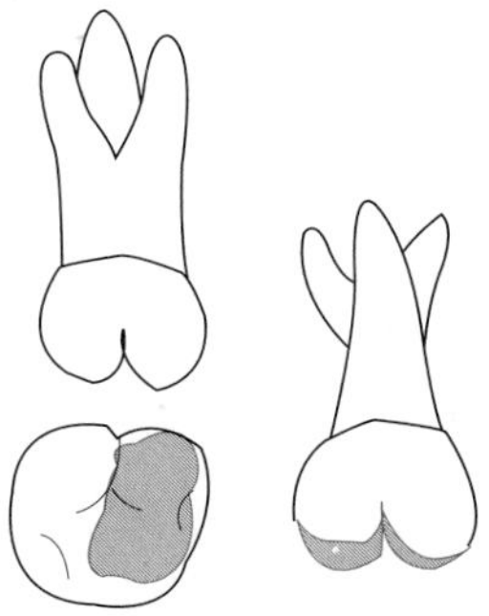	RD
Defective restorations	Defective restoration may be due to, for example, marginal ditching, voids, fracture lines, or improper anatomical contours	Chart the defective restoration similarly to recurrent decay Outline the restoration in red, and label it with an abbreviation Differentiate between recurrent decay and defective restoration with suitable abbreviation	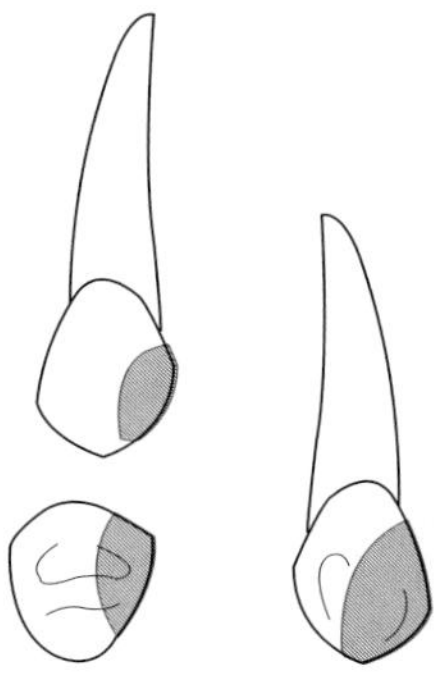	DR
Appliances				
Partial or complete dentures	Removable dentures for partial or full replacement of the dentition	Chart the missing teeth with vertical lines through all surfaces. Join vertical lines with a horizontal line at the root apex, and label appropriately to indicate upper or lower, and partial or complete denture	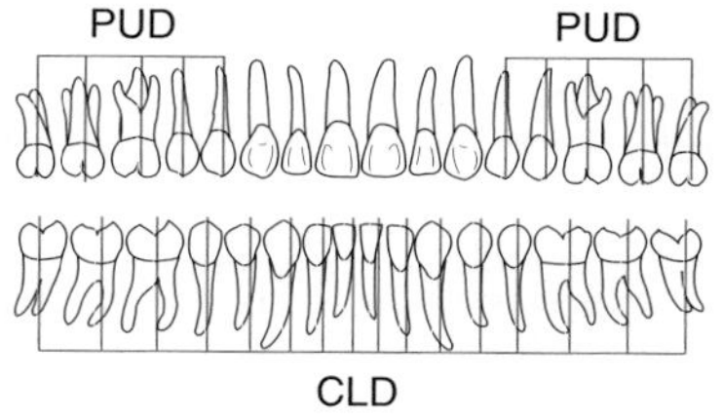 PUD PUD CLD	PUD, partial upper denture PLD, partial lower denture CUD, complete upper denture CLD, complete lower denture
Orthodontic/temporomandibular (TMJ) appliance	Placed for the shifting or stabilization of teeth (i.e., bands, night guards, retainers, space maintainers)	These appliances need not be charted on the tooth surfaces but should be identified as present in the record section of the chart		

Table continued on following page

TABLE 12–4
CHARTING SYMBOLS FOR TOOTH ASSESSMENT *Continued*

Chartable Item	Description	Charting Procedure	Charting Symbol	Abbreviations
Miscellaneous				
Overhanging Restorations	Projections of restorative material that extend beyond the curvature of tooth	Chart with triangular symbols in the interproximal area Chart in blue ink	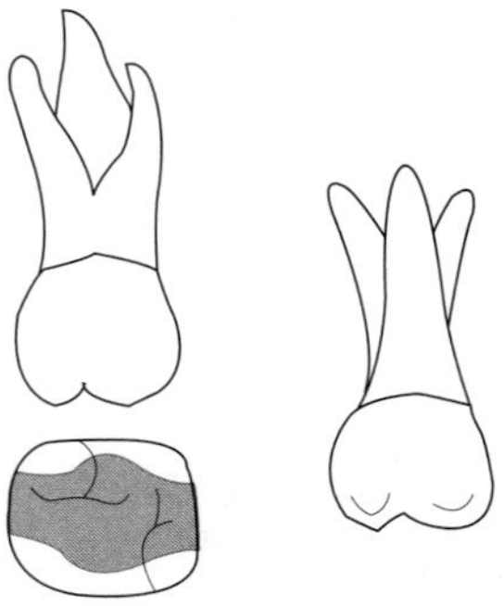	OH
Dental sealants	A plastic resin coating placed on occlusal surface to seal pits and fissures against caries	Encircle and color in with abbreviation Chart on occlusal surface in yellow or green pencil	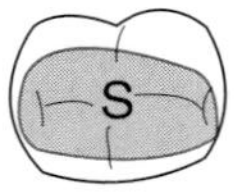 S	S
Root tip	A remaining root tip, likely from surgical extraction of tooth	Chart tooth as missing, and place abbreviation symbol near root apex Chart in blue ink	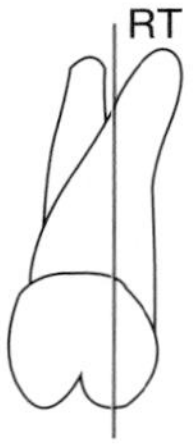 RT	RT
Root canal	Removal of pulp tissue and replacement with endodontic filling material	Place vertical line through pulpal area of root Label with abbreviation Chart in blue ink	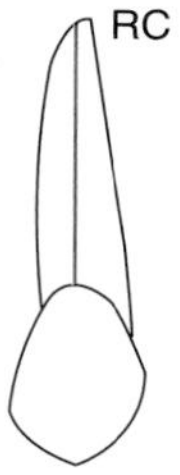 RC	RC
Acquired Dental Defects				
(see pp. 335–336 for further discussion) Decalcification or hypocalcification	Appears chalky white in color, possibly an incipient carious lesion. Usually softer than adjacent enamel	Outline the area, and label with abbreviation Chart in blue ink	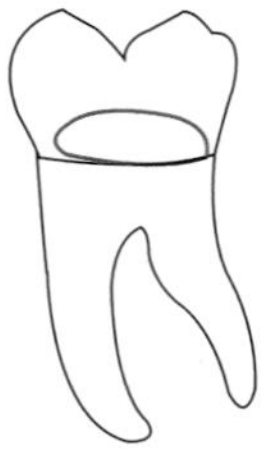 Decal	Decal

TABLE 12–4
CHARTING SYMBOLS FOR TOOTH ASSESSMENT *Continued*

Chartable Item	Description	Charting Procedure	Charting Symbol	Abbreviations
Attrition	Mechanical wear from the forces of mastication of the incisal or occlusal surfaces	Place a horizontal line over the affected surfaces Chart in blue ink	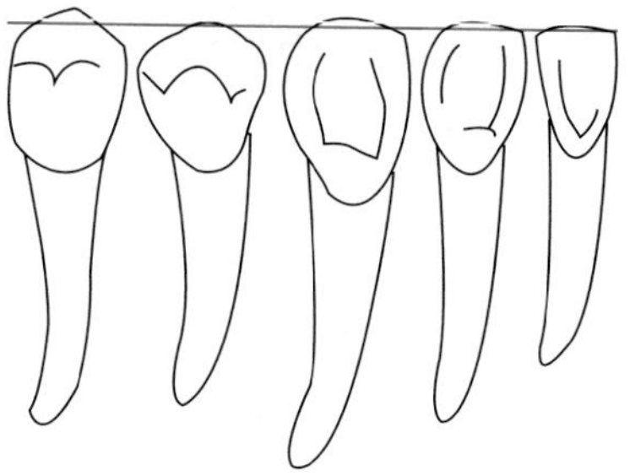	ATT
Abrasion	Mechanical wear caused by improper toothbrushing or other habits (i.e., chewing on pencils, pipe smoking)	Chart two horizontal lines in blue ink	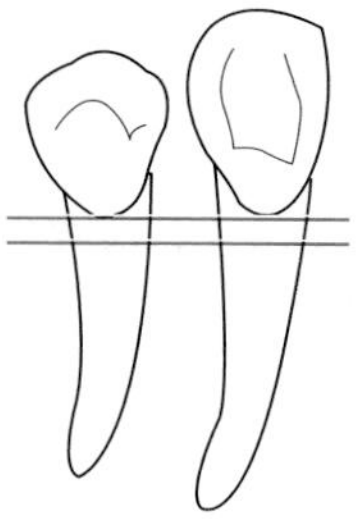	Abr
Dental Anomalies				
(see pp. 339–342 for further discussion) Enamel hypoplasia or enamel hypocalcification	Enamel defect resulting from a variety of systemic or traumatic influences. The surface is pitted and rough with enamel hypoplasia, while white flecking appears with enamel hypocalcification	Chart using wavy lines to denote the irregularity of enamel with symbol Indicate with abbreviation	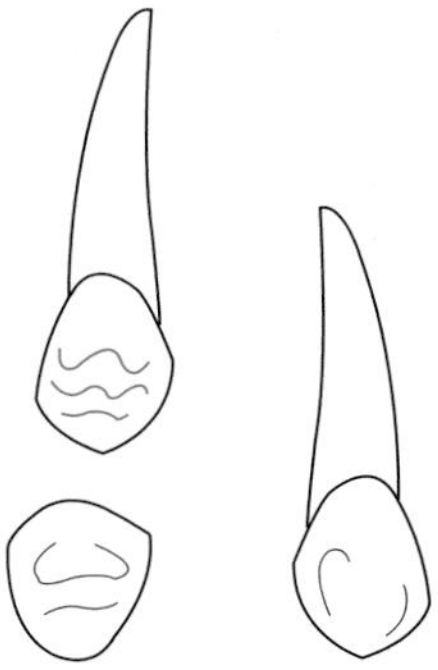	Hypoplas
Supernumerary teeth	Extra teeth	Draw additional tooth in location found Chart in blue ink Label with abbreviation	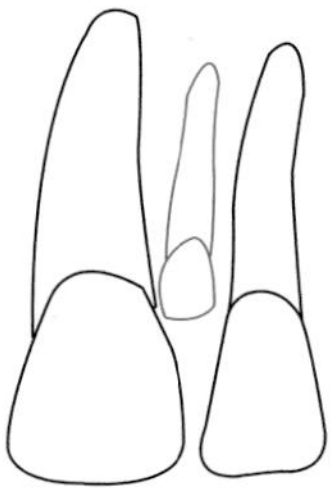	Su
Other Dental Anomalies				
	Other anatomical variations, such as dens in dente, should be clearly indicated in the record section of the dental chart			

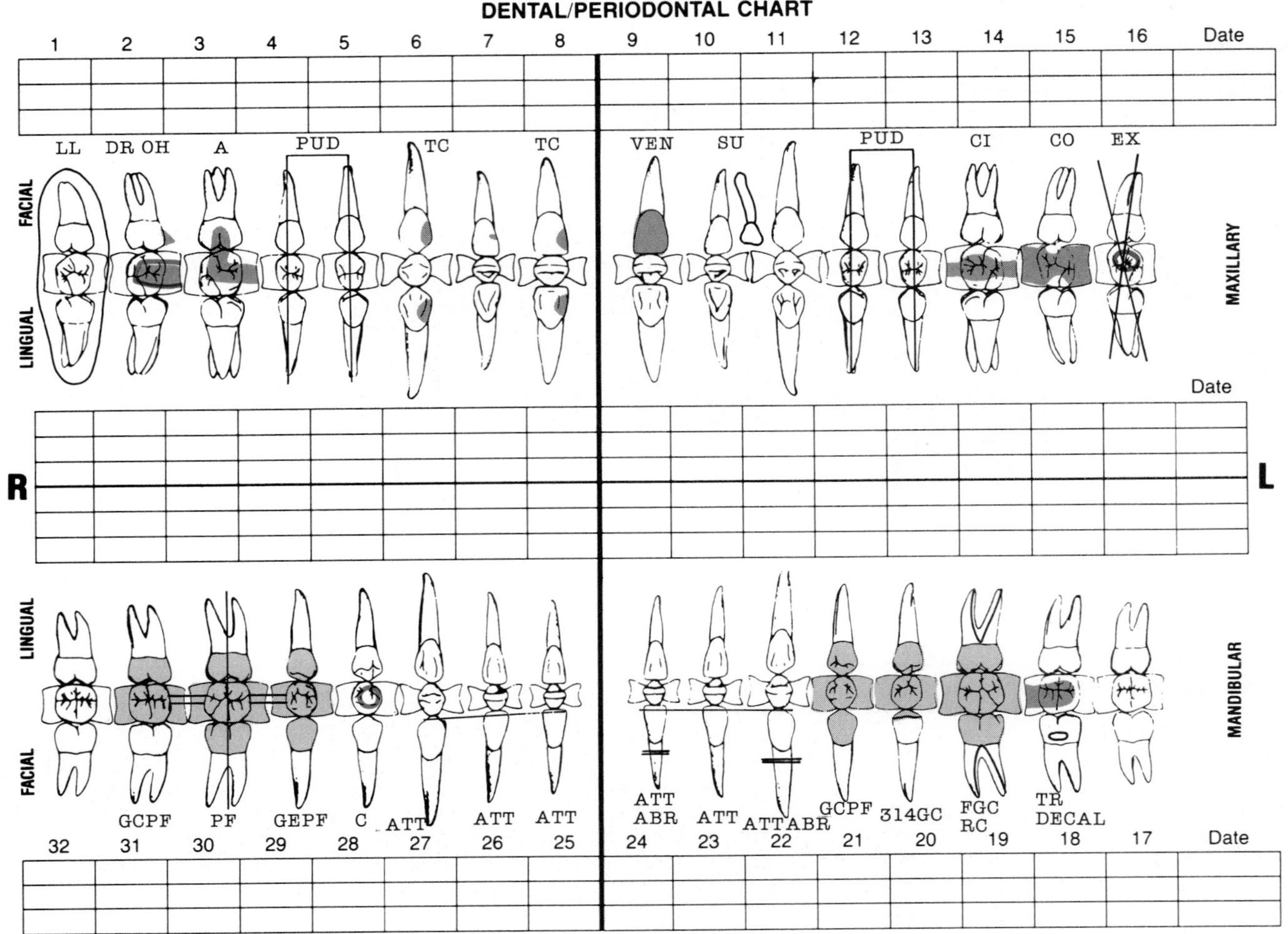

PEDO

A	B	C	D	E	F	G	H	I	J

R | | | | | | | | | | | L

T	S	R	Q	P	O	N	M	L	K

COMMENTS

FIGURE 12–37
Charting symbols.

Tooth Number	Description of Charting Symbols
#1	Unerupted
#2	Defective restoration, overhang
#3	Amalgam, class 2
#4	Extracted, partial upper denture
#5	Extracted, partial upper denture
#6	Dental implant
#7	Tooth-colored restoration with recurrent decay
#8	Tooth-colored restoration, class 4
#9	Veneer
#10	Supernumerary #10
#12	Extracted, partial upper denture
#13	Extracted, partial lower denture
#14	Gold inlay
#15	Gold onlay
#16	Extracted, with root tip remaining
#18	Temporary restoration, decalcification
#19	Full gold crown, root canal
#20	3/4 gold crown
#21	Gold crown acrylic face
#22	Attrition, abrasion
#23	Attrition
#24	Attrition, abrasion
#25	Attrition
#26	Attrition
#27	Attrition
#28	Gold foil
#29	Fixed bridge, gold crown porcelain face
#30	Fixed bridge, pontic gold crown porcelain face
#31	Fixed bridge, full gold crown
#32	Caries, class 1

FIGURE 12–37 *Continued*

OCCLUSION

Thorough assessment of the dentition includes classifying occlusion and documenting any malrelationship of teeth that is present. The dental hygienist's role is to assess and document these situations.

Occlusion is defined as the contact relationship between maxillary and mandibular teeth when the jaws are in a fully closed position. **Centric occlusion** is the relationship between maxillary and mandibular occlusal surfaces that provides the maximum contact and/or intercuspation.

Malocclusion is the malportioned relationship or deviation in the relationship of maxillary and mandibular teeth when they are in centric occlusion. Malocclusion may arise

Occlusal Relationships in Centric Occlusion	Molar Relationships	Canine Relationships	Anterior Relationships	Face Profile
Normal occlusion 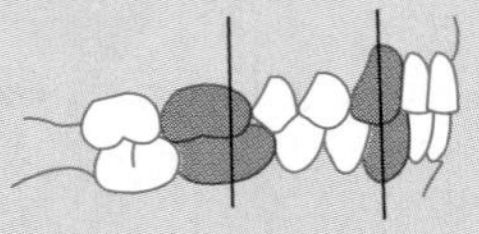	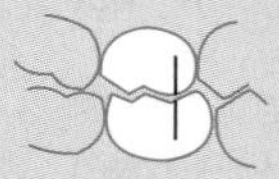	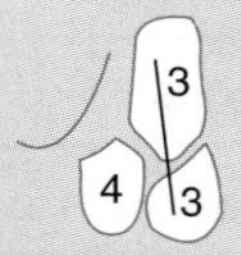 3 4 3	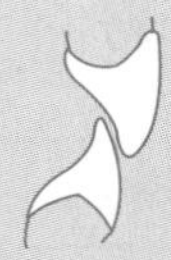	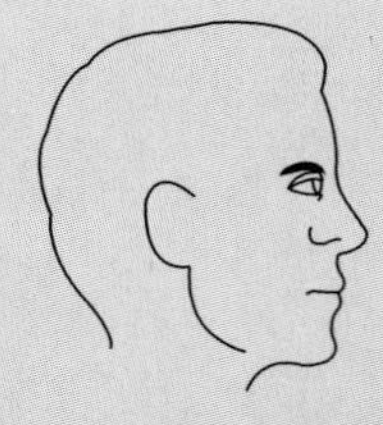 Orthognathic profile
Class I Malocclusion	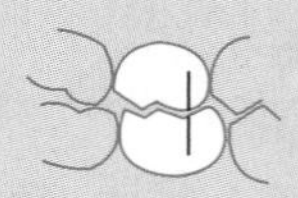	Malpositions of individual or groups of teeth may occur	Malpositions of individual or groups of teeth may occur	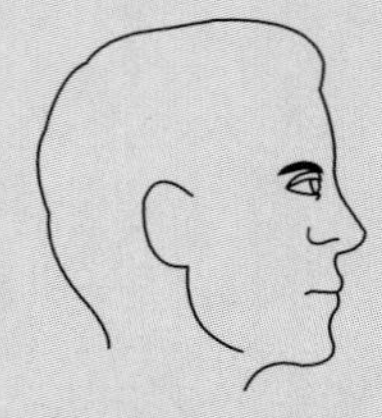 Orthognathic profile
Class II Class II Division 1 Distal occlusion 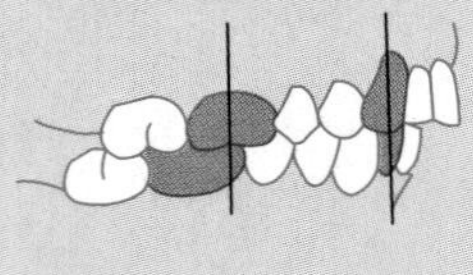	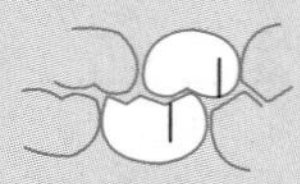	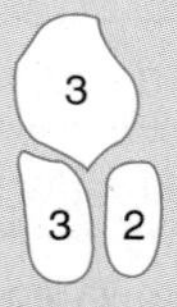 3 3 2	Division 1 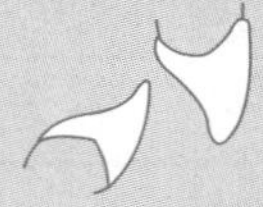 Division 2 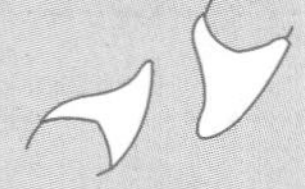	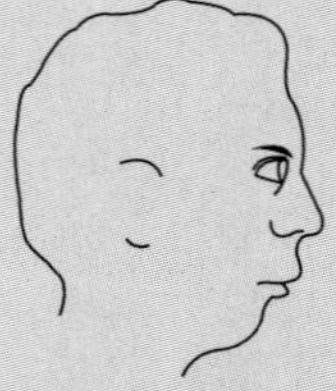 Retrognathic profile
Class II Division 2 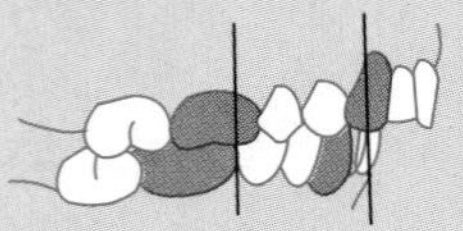	Same as class II division 1	Same as class II division 1	Same as class II division 1	Same as class II division 1
Class III Mesial occlusion 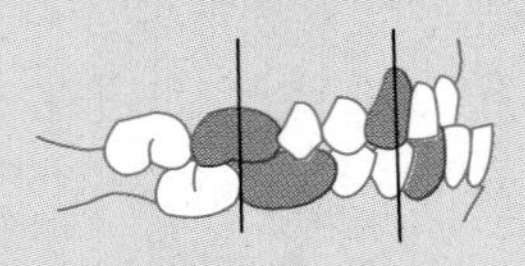	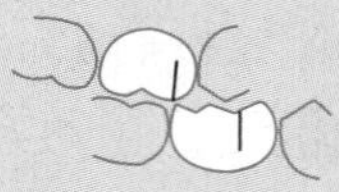	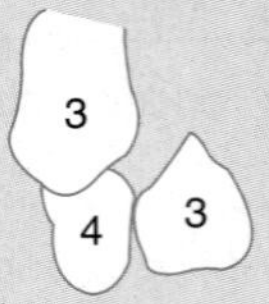 3 4 3	Anterior crossbite 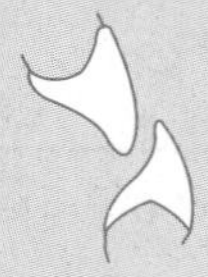	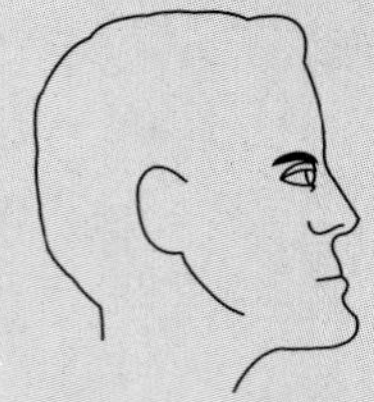 Prognathic profile

FIGURE 12–38
Classification of malocclusion. (Adapted and redrawn from Woelfel, J. B. Dental Anatomy: Its Relevance to Dentistry, 4th ed. Philadelphia: Lea & Febiger, 1990.)

from numerous factors, including abnormalities in the size or arrangement of teeth, arch or occlusal relationships. Malocclusion may be detrimental to an individual's well-being, oral health, and interpersonal relations and may adversely affect the function of the teeth and an individual's overall appearance. It may also affect bodily function because of temporomandibular joint (TMJ) pain and inadequate nutrition associated with malocclusion.

As part of the dental hygiene assessment, occlusion is classified on both the right and the left sides of the dentition. Malocclusal conditions and TMJ dysfunctions are referred to the dentist for further evaluation.

In 1887, Dr. Edward H. Angle established a system of classification of malocclusion. Although many classification systems for occlusion have been considered, Angle's is the most widely implemented.

Because of their stability within the dental arch, the first permanent molars were selected by Angle as the indicator teeth to assess the relationship between the maxilla and the mandible. Currently, the relationship of the canines and the relationship of the anterior teeth, specifically the overjet and overbite measurements, are also evaluated and incorporated with the occlusal assessment. There are three types of malocclusion as defined by Angle, class I, class II, and class III. Class II is subclassified into divisions 1 and 2.

Normal Occlusion

In **normal occlusion,** the molar relationship is such that the mandibular permanent molar is situated mesially to the maxillary permanent first molar. Specifically, the mesiobuccal cusp of the maxillary permanent first molar occludes with the buccal groove of the mandibular permanent first molar. In the canine relationship, the maxillary permanent canine occludes with the distal half of the mandibular permanent canine and the mesial half of the mandibular first premolar.

Class I Malocclusion

In **class I malocclusion** the molar and canine relationships are similar to normal occlusion. The difference between normal occlusion and class I malocclusion is that one or more of the following aspects may be present: the anterior teeth may have crowded alignment; abnormal buccolingual tooth position (e.g., crossbite) may be present; or the presence of premature occlusal contacts. The facial profile associated with class I malocclusion is classified as straight or orthognathic[10] (Fig. 12–38).

Class II Malocclusion

Class II and III malocclusions are referred to as skeletal malocclusions because of the differences in the size or the abnormal relationship of the maxilla and the mandible. **Class II malocclusion,** also referred to as distal occlusion, is characterized by the buccal groove of the mandibular first permanent molar being distal to the mesiobuccal cusp of the maxillary first permanent molar by at least the width of a premolar. The canine relationship is such that the distal surface of the mandibular permanent canine is distal to the mesial surface of the maxillary permanent canine by at least the width of a premolar. If the distance is less than the width of a premolar, it is classified as "tendency toward class II." An individual with a class II malocclusion usually has a retrognathic facial profile, that is, a small receded chin due to the apparently small mandible in relationship to the maxilla.

Two subdivisions of the class II malocclusion are used to indicate the relationship of the anterior teeth.

In class II division 1, the anterior incisors are facially inclined. In class II division 2, one or more of the maxillary incisors are lingually inclined or retruded (see Fig. 12–38).

Class III Malocclusion

In **class III malocclusion** the mandible is relatively large compared with the maxilla; thus, a prognathic profile results. The molar relationship is such that the buccal groove of the mandibular first permanent molar is situated mesial to the mesiobuccal cusp of the maxillary first permanent molar by at least the width of a premolar, while the distal surface of the mandibular permanent canine is mesial to the mesial surface of the maxillary permanent canine by at least the width of a premolar (see Fig. 12–38). Similar to the case with the class II, if the distance of movement in the molars or canine is less than the width of a premolar, the classification of occlusion is labeled "tendency toward class III."

Anterior Teeth Relationships

Overjet

Overjet is the horizontal overlap, or distance, between the lingual surface of the maxillary incisors and the labial surface of the mandibular incisors (Fig. 12–39).

Overjet is measured when the client's teeth are closed in centric occlusion and the tip of the periodontal probe is placed at a right angle to the labial surface of the mandibular incisor at the base of the incisal edge of the maxillary incisor. The measurement is taken from the labial surface of the mandibular incisor to the lingual surface of the maxillary incisor. The labiolingual width of the maxillary incisor is not included in the recorded measurement. The dental hygienist is then able to measure and record the overlap in millimeters.

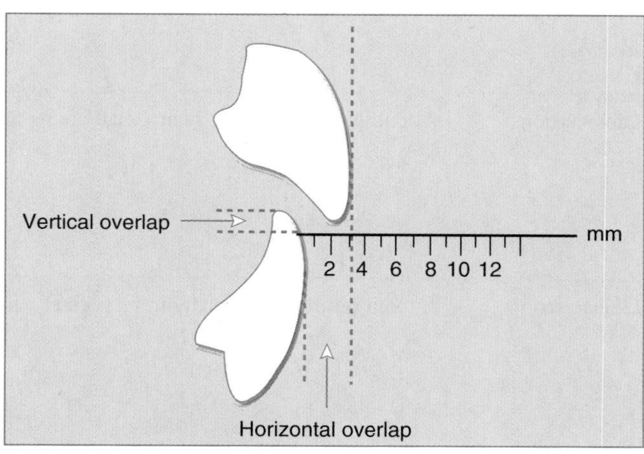

FIGURE 12–39
Vertical overlap (overbite) and horizontal overlap (overjet).

TABLE 12–5
MALRELATIONSHIPS OF INDIVIDUAL OR GROUPS OF TEETH

Malrelationship	Description
Openbite	Abnormal vertical spaces between mandibular and maxillary teeth most frequently observed in the anterior teeth; however, may occur in posterior areas 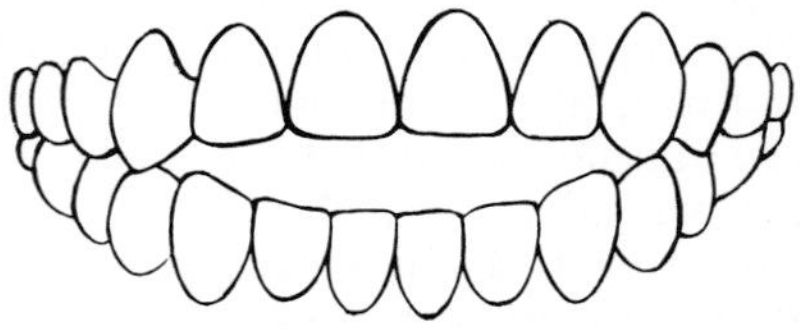
Underjet	Maxillary incisors are lingual to mandibular incisors; this could also be referred to as an anterior crossbite 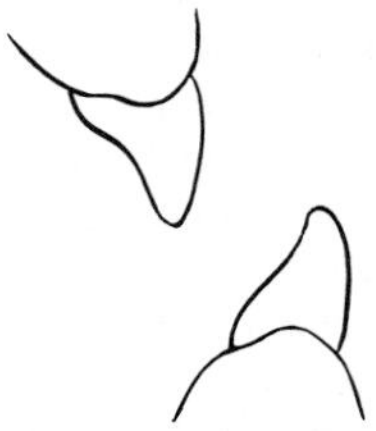
Edge-to-edge bite	The incisal edges of the anterior teeth occlude together. No overlap of the incisal teeth 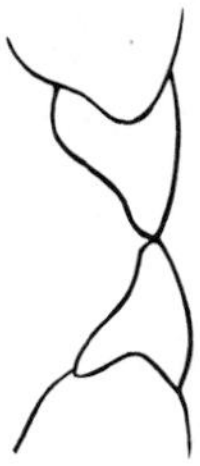
End-to-end	The cusp tips of the molars occlude cusp to cusp 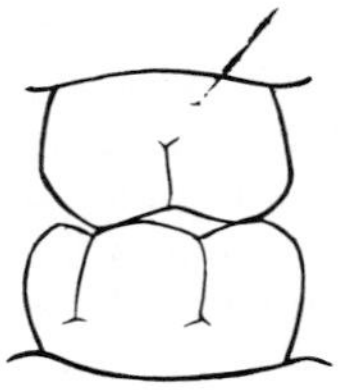
Crossbite	The normal maxillary teeth are positioned lingual to the mandibular teeth. May occur unilaterally or bilaterally Anterior crossbite; Posterior crossbite (Facial, Lingual) 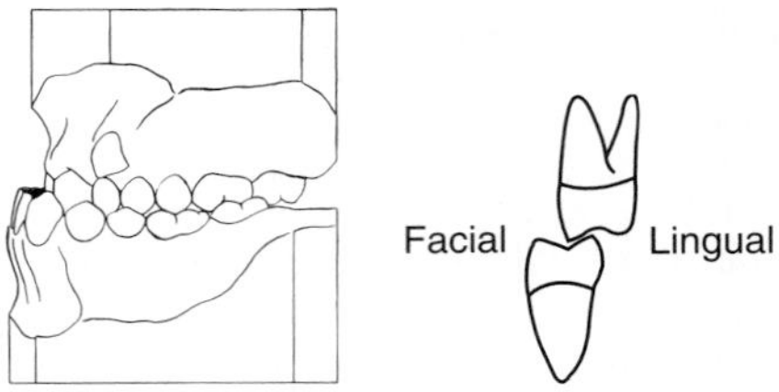
Labioversion	A tooth positioned labially or facially to its normal position 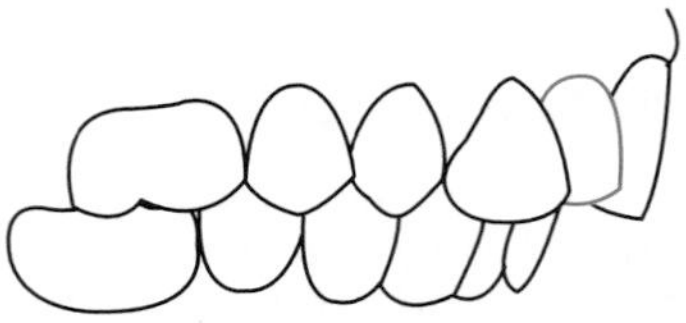
Linguoversion	A tooth positioned lingually to its normal position 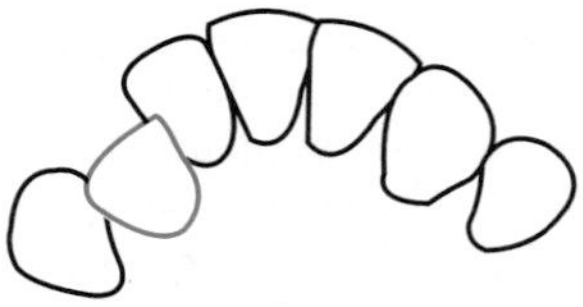

Art for the first four figures redrawn from Wilkins, E. M. Clinical Practice of the Dental Hygienist, 6th ed. Philadelphia: Lea & Febiger, 1989, p. 228; art for "crossbite" figure redrawn from Begg, P. R., and Kesling, P. C. Begg Orthodontic Theory and Technique, 3rd ed. Philadelphia: W. B. Saunders, 1977.

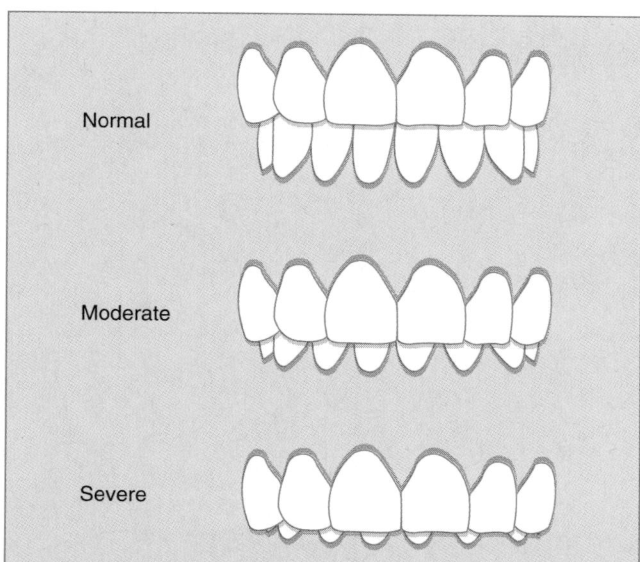

FIGURE 12–40
Classification of overbite.

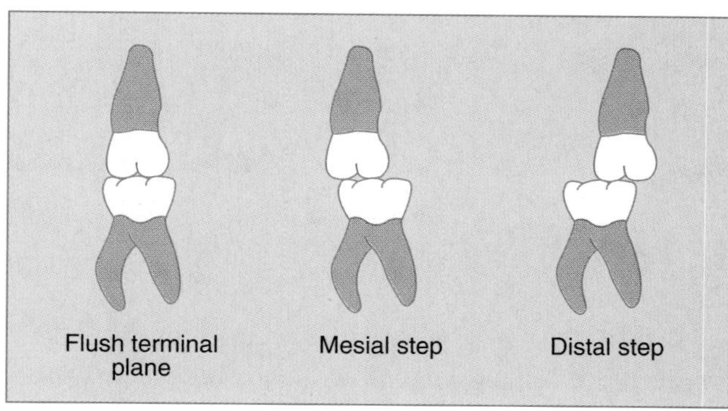

FIGURE 12–41
Occlusal relationship of primary molars.

Overbite

Overbite is the vertical overlap of the maxillary and mandibular incisor teeth (see Fig. 12–28). Overbite is classified as normal, moderate, or severe based on the depth of the overlap. Overbite is considered normal if the maxillary incisors develop within the incisal third of the mandibular incisors. Moderate overbite occurs when the maxillary incisors overlap into the middle third of the mandibular incisors, and severe overlap when the incisal edges of the maxillary teeth reach to the gingival third of the mandibular incisors (Fig. 12–40).

Overbite is measured when the client's maxillary and mandibular teeth are closed in centric occlusion: the tip of the periodontal probe is placed at the incisal edge of the maxillary incisor at right angles to the mandibular incisor. As the client opens his jaws the probe is placed vertically against the mandibular incisor to measure the distance to the incisal edge of the mandibular incisor.[9]

It is customary to measure the overbite in millimeters and to include a classification of normal, moderate, or severe with the recorded measurement (Table 12–5). These variations should be documented in writing on the client's chart.

Primary Occlusion

Similar to permanent occlusion, ideal primary occlusion is referred to as normal occlusion. In normal occlusion the primary canine relationship is in a position similar to that noted with normal permanent occlusion. This normal molar relationship of the primary molar teeth is referred to as a flush terminal plane.

A **flush terminal plane** occurs when the primary molars erupt in an end-to-end position. If spacing between the primary mandibular teeth exists (primary space), following the eruption of the first permanent molar, the permanent molar will put pressure on the first and second primary molars, causing forward movement of the mandibular primary canine and mandibular primary first molar. This movement then facilitates the development of a normal permanent molar relationship. Corresponding to Angle's class I malocclusion is a primary tooth relationship called a **mesial step.** In this case the distal surface of the mandibular second primary molar is mesial to the distal surface of the second primary maxillary molar. The equivalent of Angle's class II malocclusion in the primary dentition is called a **distal step** relationship. This occurs when the distal surface of the mandibular second primary molar is distal to the distal surface of the second primary maxillary molar. An equivalent of class III malocclusion is almost never seen in the primary dentition because of the normal pattern of craniofacial growth in which the mandible lags behind the maxilla[11] (Fig. 12–41).

References

1. Sturdevant, C. M., Barton, R. E., Sockwell, C. L., and Strickland, W. D. (eds.). The Art and Science of Operative Dentistry, 2nd ed. St. Louis: C. V. Mosby, 1985.
2. Menaker, L. The Biologic Basis of Dental Caries. New York: Harper & Row, 1980.
3. Roberts, M. W., and Tylenda, C. A. Dental aspects of anorexia and bulimia nervosa. Pediatrician 16(3–4):178, 1989.
4. Ripa, L. W. Nursing caries: A comprehensive review. Pediatric Dentistry 10(4):268, 1988.
5. Billings, R. J. Restoration of carious lesions of the root. Gerodontology 5(1):43, 1986.
6. Giunta, J. L. Oral Pathology. Baltimore: Williams & Wilkins, 1989.
7. Robinson, H. B. G., and Miller, A. S. Color Atlas of Oral Pathology. Philadelphia: J. B. Lippincott, 1990.
8. Ibsen, O. A. C., and Phelan, J. A. Oral Pathology for the Dental Hygienist. Philadelphia: W. B. Saunders, 1992.
9. Woodall, I. R., Dafoe, B. R., et al. Comprehensive Dental Hygiene Care, 4th ed. St. Louis: C. V. Mosby, 1993.
10. Woelfel, J. B. Dental Anatomy: Its Relevance to Dentistry, 4th ed. Philadelphia: Lea & Febiger, 1990.
11. Proffit, W. R. Contemporary Orthodontics. St. Louis: C. V. Mosby, 1986.

Suggested Reading

Grant, A., Stern, I. S., and Listgarten, M. A. Periodontics, 6th ed. St. Louis: C. V. Mosby, 1988.

13 Periodontal and Oral Hygiene Assessment

OBJECTIVES

Mastery of the content in this chapter will enable the reader to:

- Define the key terms used
- Describe healthy periodontium related to clinical signs, histological characteristics, and radiographic findings
- Identify the four objective parameters of the periodontal assessment
- Evaluate radiographs for three periodontal parameters
- State limitations of the radiographic survey
- Distinguish between gingivitis and periodontitis
- Identify five categories of periodontitis as defined by the American Academy of Periodontology
- Identify three methods of microbiological identification of periodontitis
- Differentiate between pocket depth and attachment loss
- Determine which assessment methods are realistic for clinical, epidemiological, or motivational use
- Assess the client's need for periodontal treatment modalities
- Utilize a standard notation system for periodontal record-keeping
- Describe at least two indices for measuring bacterial plaque and gingival bleeding

INTRODUCTION

The **periodontium** is the supporting structure of tissues that surrounds the teeth. A major objective of dental hygiene care is to promote the health of the periodontium and to collaborate with the dentist to bring diseased periodontal tissues to a state of health that can be maintained by the client.

The purpose of this chapter is to focus on the specific components of periodontal and oral hygiene assessments and their application to dental hygiene care.

ASSESSMENT TOOLS

Performing conscientious and thorough periodontal and oral hygiene assessments is a key role of the dental hygienist. Basic tools include a good source of light, compressed air to dry the tissues, a mouth mirror, an explorer, and a periodontal probe.

There are many kinds of periodontal probes available. All are calibrated in millimeters for use by the dental hygienist in assessing the health of the periodontium (see Chapter 18). Figure 13–1 shows the marquis probe with its colored bands to indicate different measurement levels and the Williams probe, which is calibrated with the 4- and 6-mm calibrations missing to facilitate reading the probe. When a probe is inserted into the space between the tooth and the gingiva, the calibrations show the depth of the space in millimeters (Fig. 13–2). Probing depths are used to monitor periodontal health and disease.

HEALTHY PERIODONTIUM

Recognizing the basic characteristics of the healthy periodontium is essential for accurate periodontal data collection. The healthy periodontium consists of four physical units:

- Gingiva
- Cementum
- Periodontal ligament
- Alveolar process or supporting bone

Gingiva

Gingiva is masticatory oral mucosa that surrounds the teeth. It covers the alveolar process and the cementoenamel

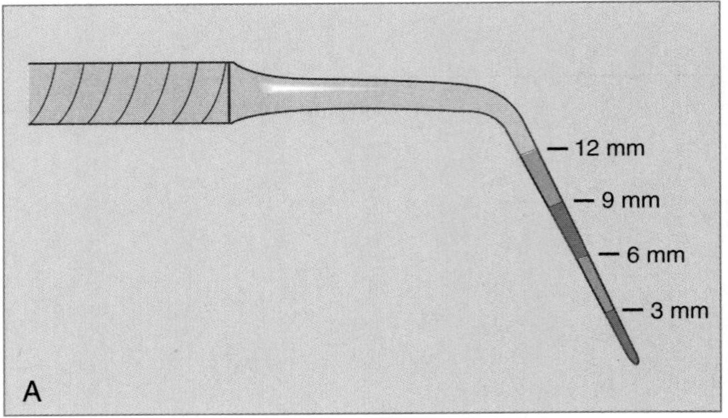

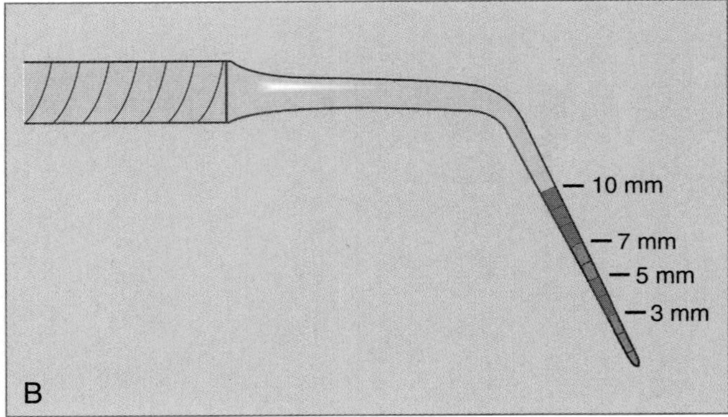

A, Marquis probe calibrated with colored bands to indicate 3, 6, 9, and 12 mm levels of penetration.
B, Williams probe calibrated in 3, 5, 7, and 10 mm increments.

junction (CEJ) of the tooth. Histologically, the gingiva has a protective layer of stratified squamous epithelium, covering a dense, fibrous connective tissue. The gingiva can be divided into marginal gingiva (or free gingiva), alveolar gingiva (or attached gingiva), and the interdental gingiva (or interdental papilla) (Fig. 13–3).

The gingival tissue closest to the crown is called the **marginal** or **free gingiva.** Marginal gingiva is not directly attached to the alveolar bone. In healthy adult dentitions, the marginal gingiva is located on the tooth enamel 0.5 to 2 mm coronal to the CEJ and fits tightly around each tooth. The edge of the marginal gingiva that is nearest to the incisal or occlusal area of the tooth is called the **gingival margin** or the **crest of the gingiva.** The gingival margin marks the opening of the gingival sulcus (Fig. 13–4).

Gingival Sulcus

The space between the marginal gingiva and the tooth is called the **gingival sulcus** or **gingival crevice.** The healthy gingival sulcus measures 0.5 to 3 mm from the gingival margin to the base of the sulcus. Most authorities refer to 3 mm or less as acceptable measurements for the depth of the sulcus in periodontal health. The boundaries of the gingival sulcus are the sulcular epithelium and the tooth. **Sulcular epithelium** is a thin layer of nonkeratinized stratified squamous epithelium. It is the nonkeratinized continuation of the keratinized epithelium covering the marginal gingiva. The sulcular epithelium is clinically significant in that it is a semipermeable membrane which, in the presence of mature plaque, may allow bacterial endotoxins to penetrate into the underlying tissue.

Inside the gingival sulcus the sulcular epithelium attaches to the tooth at the coronal portion of the **junctional epithelium** (JE). The junctional epithelium is a cuff-like band of squamous epithelium that completely encircles the tooth. Histologically the apex, or base of the sulcus, is formed by the junctional epithelium (see Fig. 13–4). This thin layer of epithelium covers the gingival connective tissue layer. The junctional epithelium is 15 to 20 cells thick where it joins sulcular epithelium and tapers down to one or two cells thick at the apical end. The **epithelial attachment** is the inner part of the junctional epithelium attached to the tooth by hemidesmosomes and the basement lamina.

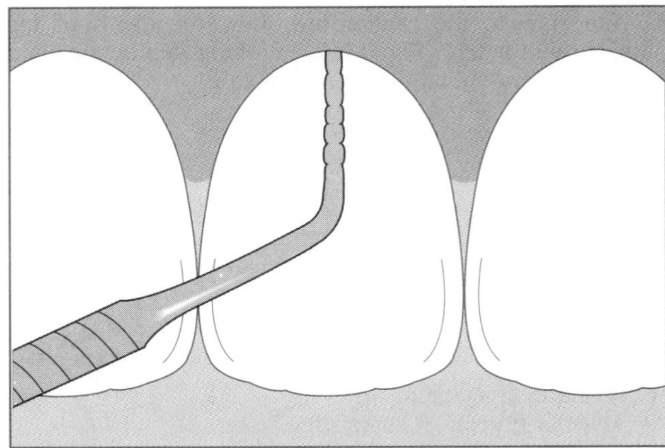

FIGURE 13–2
Williams probe inserted into a gingival sulcus. The calibrations show a depth of 4 mm. (Probe readings are rounded up to the next highest millimeter. Here, the 3-mm mark is covered up so the measurement is read "4 mm.")

Gingival Crevicular Fluid

Gingival crevicular fluid (GCF), sometimes called sulcular fluid, is a serum-like fluid secreted from the underlying connective tissue into the sulcular space. Little or no fluid is found in the healthy gingival sulcus, but gingival crevicular fluid has been found to flow after one day without bacterial plaque control and to increase with the presence of gingival inflammation.[1] The GCF is part of the body's defense mechanism and is able to transport antibodies and certain systemically administered drugs.

Gingival Groove

From the facial aspect, the **gingival groove** corresponds to the base of the gingival sulcus (see Fig. 13–3). Research indicates that the gingival groove is clinically visible in only one-half of the population. The marginal gingiva connects with the alveolar gingiva at the gingival groove. The **alveolar** or **attached gingiva** is continuous with the marginal gingiva and is covered with stratified squamous epithelium. The alveolar gingiva covers the crestal portion of the alveolar bone and the roof of the mouth. It is firmly attached to

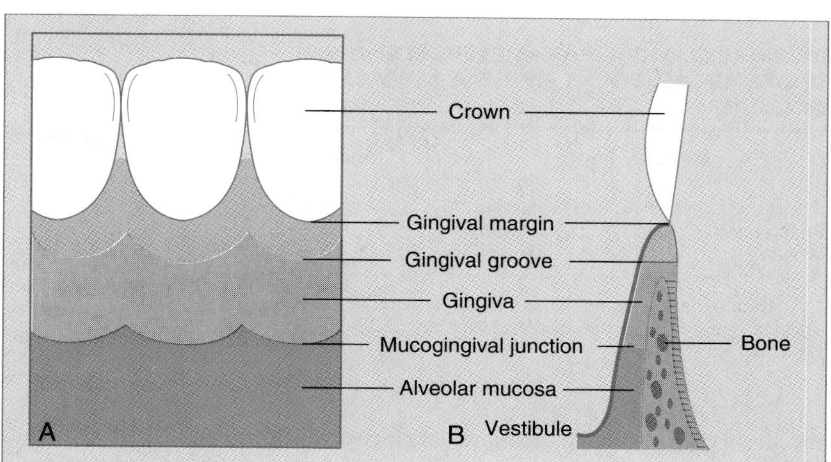

FIGURE 13-3
Anatomical relationship of normal gingiva in facial view (*A*) and in cross-section (*B*).

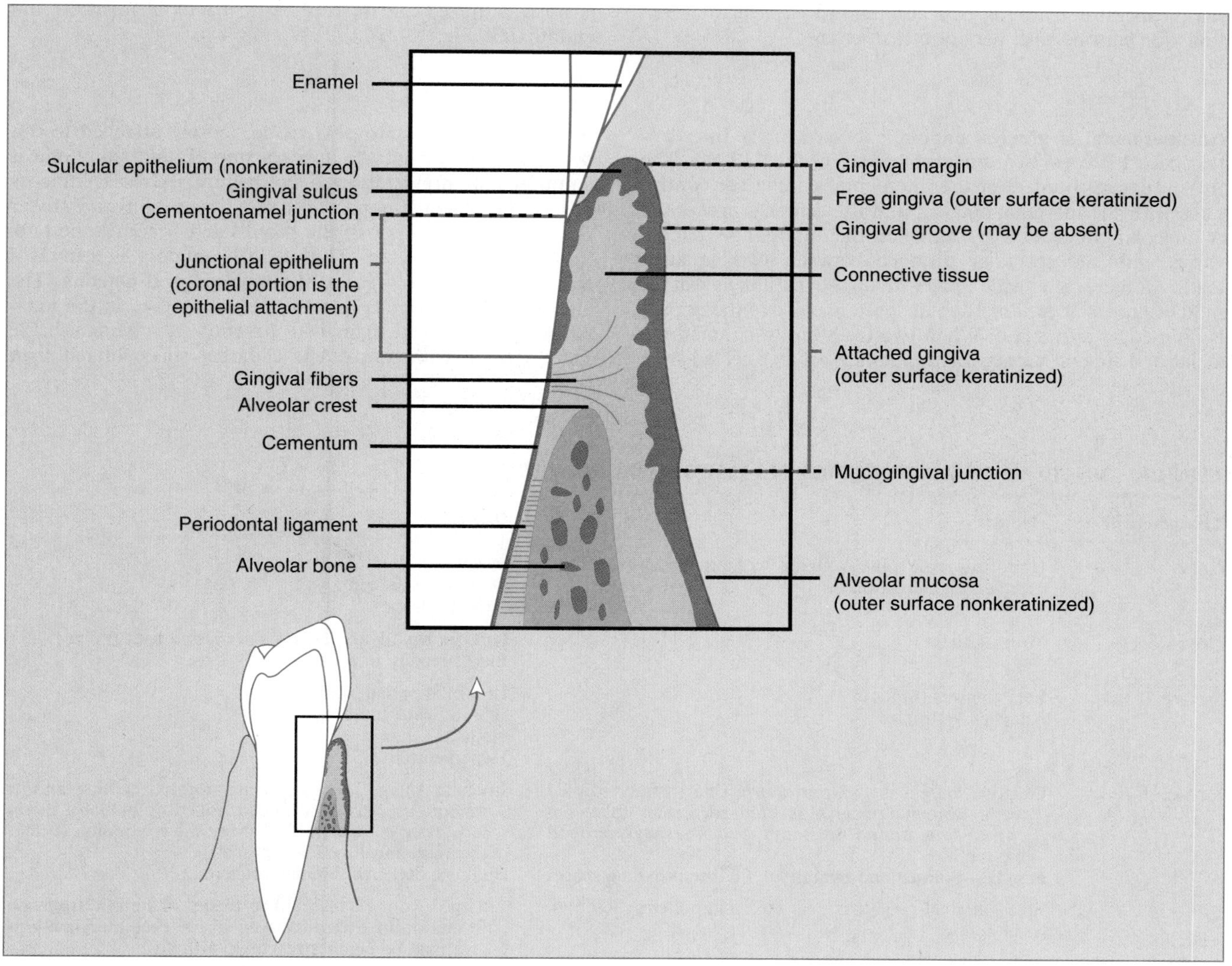

FIGURE 13-4
The gingiva and other periodontal tissues in cross-section.

TABLE 13–1
NORMAL CLINICAL PARAMETERS FOR THE WIDTH OF ALVEOLAR GINGIVA (ATTACHED GINGIVA)

Maxillary (mm)		Mandibular (mm)	
Incisors	3.5–4.5	Incisors	2.9–3.9
Premolars	1.9–2.4	Premolars	1.7–2.1
Molars	2.1–3.0	Molars (lingual)	1.9–4.0

Adapted from Ainamo, J., and Loe, H. Anatomical characteristics of gingiva. Journal of Peridontology 37:5–13, Jan.–Feb. 1966.

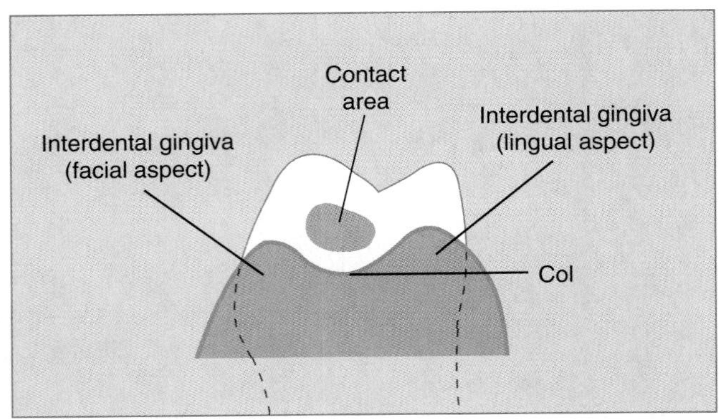

FIGURE 13–5
The col.

the alveolar bone, unlike the marginal gingiva which has no attachment fibers. The mandibular facial and lingual alveolar gingiva and the maxillary facial alveolar gingiva are demarcated from the alveolar mucosa by the mucogingival junction; the width of alveolar gingiva varies throughout the mouth (Table 13–1). The facial aspect of the maxillary anterior teeth has the widest alveolar gingiva. In general, at least 1 mm of alveolar gingiva is sufficient for gingival health.[1] This minimum width measurement has significance for planning educational and clinical interventions for persons with periodontal disease.

Gingival Papilla

An **interdental** or **gingival papilla** is located in the interdental space between two adjacent teeth (see Fig. 13–3). The tip and lateral borders of the interdental papilla are continuous with the marginal gingiva, and the center is composed of alveolar gingiva. The shape of the interdental papilla varies with the space or distance between two adjacent teeth. If there is a wide space, then the papilla is flat or saddle-shaped. If the interdental space is narrow, the papilla is pointed or pyramidal. When two teeth are in contact, the facial and lingual aspects of the papilla are connected by a **col.** A col is a saddle of interdental gingiva that connects the facial and lingual aspects of the papilla. The interdental papilla may appear as two papillae, with this smooth saddle shape or depression between the papillae. The center of the col is not keratinized, which makes it susceptible to disease. Most periodontal infections begin in the col area because it is nonkeratinized and susceptible to bacterial invasion and endotoxins (Fig. 13–5).

Alveolar Mucosa

Alveolar mucosa is movable tissue, loosely attached to underlying bone. Its surface appears smooth and shiny and is composed of nonkeratinized epithelium. Alveolar mucosa covers the alveolar bone. This same type of tissue covers the vestibule and floor of the mouth and becomes the buccal and labial mucosa. The alveolar mucosa is separated from the alveolar gingiva at the **mucogingival junction.** The alveolar mucosa blends into the palatal gingiva in the maxilla so that no mucogingival junction is distinguishable there. The alveolar mucosa is a darker shade of red than

TABLE 13–2
CLINICAL GINGIVAL CHARACTERISTICS IN HEALTH AND DISEASE

Characteristic	Health	Disease
Color	Uniformly pale pink with or without generalized dark brown pigmentation	Bright red Dark red, blue-red Pink if fibrotic
Consistency	Firm, resilient	Soft, spongy, dents easily when pressed with probe Bleeds readily to probing
Surface Texture	Free gingiva—smooth Attached—stippled	Loss of stippling, shiny Fibrotic with stippling Nodular Hyperkeratotic
Contour	Gingival margin is 1–2 mm above CEJ in fully erupted teeth. Marginal gingiva is knife-edge, flat; follows a curved line around the tooth, and fits snugly around the tooth Papilla—pointed and pyramidal; fill interproximal spaces	Irregular margins from edema, fibrosis, clefting and/or festooning. May be rounded, rolled or bulbous; therefore more coronal to CEJ. May show recession so that the anatomical root is exposed Bulbous, flattened, blunted, cratered
Size	Free marginal gingiva is near CEJ and adheres closely to the tooth	Enlarged from excess fluid in tissues or fibrotic from the formation of excess collagen fibers. Free marginal gingiva may be highly retractable with air
Probing Depth	0–4 mm; no apical migration of JE	>4 mm with or without apical migration of JE

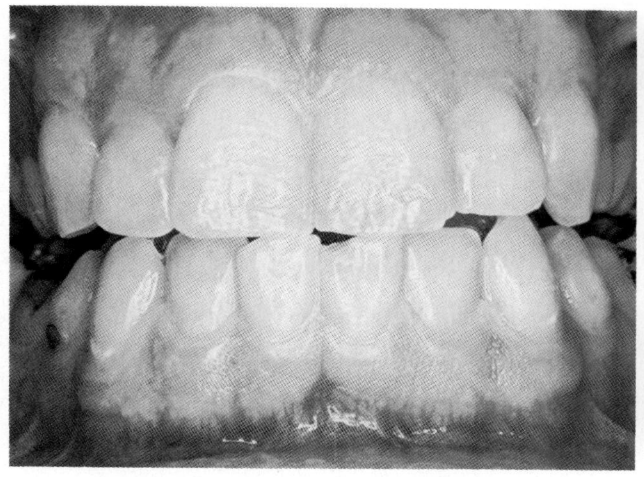

A

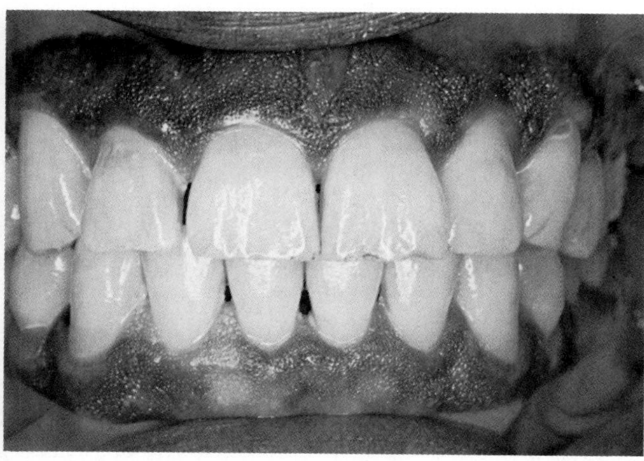

B

FIGURE 13–6
A, Clinically normal gingiva in light-skinned individuals. *B*, Clinically normal pigmented gingiva in dark-skinned individuals. (With permission from Glickman, I., and Smulow, J. B. Periodontal Disease: Clinical, Radiographic, and Histopathologic Features. Philadelphia: W. B. Saunders, 1974, p. 3.)

gingiva because of its richer blood supply and the thin, nonkeratinized epithelial layer that covers it. The difference between firm alveolar gingiva and the loose alveolar mucosa can be easily demonstrated to the client.

Appearance of Gingiva

Clinically, gingiva has distinctive *color, consistency, surface texture, contour,* and *size* in health and disease (Table 13–2). Gingiva is considered healthy when the color is uniform and consistent. Gingival color varies according to the degree of vascularity, amount of melanin pigmentation present, the degree of epithelial keratinization present, and the thickness of the epithelium. In light-skinned individuals, pale pink or salmon pink describes the color of healthy gingiva when compared with the red alveolar mucosa. Pigment-containing cells in the basal layer of epithelium are commonly present in persons of dark complexion (Fig. 13–6). Therefore, some individuals normally have brown melanin pigmentation distributed throughout the gingiva. The healthy alveolar gingiva is resilient and of firm consistency. It is firmly bound by gingival fibers running between connective tissue and the alveolar periosteum, which may give it a stippled appearance or texture.

The healthy gingiva, when visually examined, air-dried, and probed, does not bleed or exude fluids. It may or may not have an overall stippled texture. The presence of stippling varies with individuals and areas of the mouth. In addition, the contour, size, and shape of the gingiva are dependent on location, tooth size, and tooth alignment. Healthy gingiva does not feel hypersensitive to air or touch. Educating clients about the clinical appearance of healthy gingiva prepares them to participate knowledgeably in decision-making about their health and is fundamental for teaching self-examination techniques.

Cementum

Cementum is a mineralized bone-like substance that covers the roots of teeth and also provides attachment and anchorage for the periodontal fibers. Cementum is usually a very thin cellular layer, not as hard as dentin, and it lacks blood vessels and nerves. In health the cementum is not exposed to the oral environment but is protected by the periodontal ligament.

Periodontal Ligament

The fibrous attachment of the teeth to the bone is called the **periodontal ligament.** The width of the periodontal ligament, seen in radiographs only as a black (radiolucent) space, depends upon age, stage of eruption, and the function of the tooth. Collagen fibers of the ligament are inserted into the cementum, and they prevent tooth mobility by securing the tooth into its socket in the alveolar bone. The ligament also functions in the formation of periodontal tissues by housing cementoclasts, fibroclasts, and osteoblasts; in the resorption of periodontal tissues by housing cementoclasts, fibroclasts, and osteoclasts; in carrying nutrients through blood vessels to the cementum, bone, and gingiva; and in proprioception. The periodontal ligament is connected to cementum and bone by collagen fibers called **Sharpey's fibers.** The hemidesmosome, an attachment structure on some epithelial cells, aids the attachment of the periodontal fibers to cementum or tooth. In health, the periodontal ligament is attached to the root, thereby protecting it from visual or tactile exposure.

Alveolar Bone

The alveolar bone is composed of compact or cortical bone and of spongy bone that is marked by trabecular spaces when seen on radiographs. The compact bone is the outside wall of the alveolar bone, where the periodontal ligament fibers are anchored and the rich vascular supply penetrates. The spongy bone is the interior of the alveolar bone, and it is plastic. It can increase and decrease in response to physical pressure, function, and bacterial infection and inflammation. The alveolar crest, the portion of the alveolar bone located between the teeth, varies in size

TABLE 13–3
CLINICAL PERIODONTAL CHARACTERISTICS IN GINGIVITIS AND PERIODONTITIS

Characteristic	Gingivitis	Periodontitis
Gingival inflammation	Acute	Acute or chronic
Position of junctional epithelium	At the CEJ	Below the CEJ (attachment loss)
Position of gingival margin	Greater than 1–2 mm above the CEJ (gingival pocket)	Variable
Bleeding upon probing	Present	May be present
Exudate	May be present	May be present
Furcation involvement	Absent	May be present
Tooth mobility	Absent	May be present
Bone loss	Absent	May be present

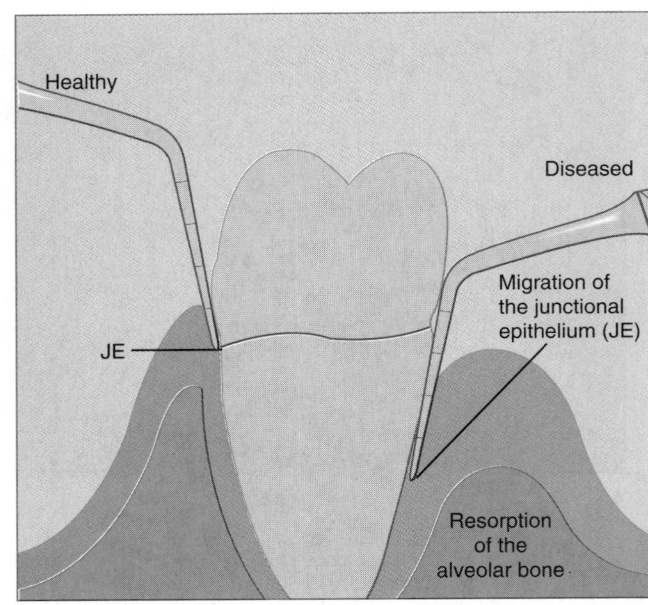

FIGURE 13–7
Some clinical parameters in health and in periodontitis.

and shape, depending upon tooth position. (See the section on clinical use of radiographs, page 376, for radiographic signs of periodontal health related to the alveolar bone.)

DISEASED PERIODONTIUM

Understanding the characteristics of the healthy periodontium provides a foundation upon which to recognize signs of disease. The term "periodontal disease" includes both gingivitis and periodontitis. "Gingivitis" means inflammation of the gingival tissue. In gingivitis, the marginal gingiva shows signs of inflammation, but there is no apical migration of the junctional epithelium beyond the CEJ. Also, in gingivitis there is no bone loss (Table 13–3). Although most forms of gingivitis are plaque-induced, secondary factors apparently modify the clinical characteristics of the disease and have resulted in the subclassifications (see Classification of Gingivitis chart).

"Periodontitis" means inflammation of the supporting tissues of the teeth. In periodontitis there is apical migration of the junctional epithelium from the CEJ and there may be bone loss. Periodontitis, therefore, is the extension of the inflammatory process into the connective tissue and alveolar bone that supports the teeth (see Table 13–3). The progression of periodontitis involves the destruction of connective tissue attachment at the most apical portion of a periodontal pocket. Associated with this attachment loss is the apical downgrowth of the subgingival flora, apical migration of the junction epithelium, and resorption of alveolar bone (Fig. 13–7).

Traditionally, periodontitis was considered a bacterial plaque-induced, nonspecific inflammatory lesion that progressed slowly and at a constant rate. In addition, all individuals were viewed as being equally susceptible to periodontitis. These concepts have been found to be overly simplistic and partially inaccurate. The current view of periodontitis maintains that there are several forms of periodontitis, all of which are infections caused by groups of microorganisms indigenous to the oral cavity.[2] (See Classification of Periodontal Disease chart).[3] In general, adult periodontitis has attachment loss of about 0.25 mm per year. It thus progresses much more slowly than the other forms of periodontitis, which may average 1 to 2 mm of attachment loss per year. The current view of progression

CLASSIFICATION OF GINGIVITIS

Acute necrotizing ulcerative gingivitis
A gingival infection of complex etiology (e.g., plaque, stress, poor diet) characterized by necrosis of the tips of the gingival papillae (punched out papilla with overlying gray pseudomembrane), spontaneous bleeding, pain and fetor ovis

Steroid hormone-influenced gingivitis
Includes puberty gingivitis, pregnancy gingivitis, and gingivitis associated with birth control medication and steroid therapy from increased growth of *Bacteroides* when steroid hormones are elevated; characterized by an exaggerated response to plaque, reflected by intense inflammation, redness, edema, and enlargement; may progress to a pyogenic granuloma (pregnancy tumor)

Medication-influenced gingival overgrowth
Occurs as a result of phenytoin use, to control seizure disorders; cyclosporin, used for immunosuppressive therapy in transplant patients; and nifedipine

Desquamative gingivitis
Characterized by sloughing of the gingival epithelium leaving an intensely red surface; represents oral manifestations of erosive lichen planus, benign mucous membrane pemphigoid, bullous pemphigoid, pemphigus vulgaris, and allergic reactions

HIV-associated gingival diseases
Characterized by extreme redness in the gingiva, linear gingival erythema; or a fiery red edematous gingivitis not limited to the attached gingiva, now called necrotizing (ulcerative) gingivitis

Based on American Academy of Periodontology. Proceedings of the World Workshop in Clinical Periodontics. July 23–27, 1989, Princeton, NJ.

TABLE 13–4
MICROBIAL SPECIES ASSOCIATED WITH PERIODONTAL DISEASES

Organism	GI*	AP	LJP	HIV	I
Actinobacillus actinomycetemcomitans	−	++	+++	+	+
Porphyromonas gingivalis†	−	+++	−	+	−
Prevotella intermedia	++	+	++	++	
Bacteroides forsythus	−	+++	−	?	?
Fusobacterium species	+++	++	−	+	+
Peptostreptococcus micros	−	+++	−	++	++
Wolinella recta	+	++	+	+++	+
Treponema denticola	++	++	−	++	+
Enteric rods/ pseudomonads	+	+	−	++	+
Streptococcus species	+++	−	−	−	−
Actinomyces species	+++	−	−	−	−

* GI, Gingivitis; AP, adult periodontitis; LIP, localized juvenile periodontitis; HIV, HIV-periodontitis; I, periimplantitis

† Formerly *Bacteroides gingivalis.*

+++ = strong association, ++ = moderate association, + = weak association, − = no association.

From Slots, J., and Taubman, M. Contemporary Oral Microbiology and Immunology. St. Louis; Mosby–Year Book, 1992, p. 429.

of periodontitis is that some affected sites lose connective tissue attachment in short-lived bursts and other sites lose attachment in small increments at a more or less continuous rate. All forms of periodontal disease, however, appear to be related to qualitative changes in the bacteria composing the subgingival flora. Susceptibility to periodontitis appears to be associated with host responses to periodontal pathogens.[2] Although it is not known which specific microorganisms or groups of microorganisms cause the progression of periodontitis, microbial species associated with some periodontal diseases are identified. These are listed in Table 13–4.

Recognition of periodontal changes by the dental hygienist is important in identifying signs of disease, and in bringing these signs to the attention of the dentist and client.

Signs of Inflammation (Gingivitis)

The epithelium of the col and of the marginal gingiva is the site where inflammation begins as a result of bacterial invasion or endotoxin irritation. Bacterial endotoxins and enzymes released from gram-negative bacteria cause a breakdown of epithelial intercellular substances that produce ulceration of the sulcular epithelium. This ulceration permits enzymes and toxins to penetrate further into the underlying connective tissue. Inflammation in the connective tissue results in dilation and increased permeability of cap-

CLASSIFICATION OF PERIODONTITIS

I Adult Periodontitis

May begin in adolescence, but is not clinically significant until after age 35. The following levels of periodontal case classification have been identified:

- Early periodontitis: Progression of gingival inflammation into the alveolar bone crest and early bone loss resulting in attachment loss (pocket formation) of 2–4 mm
- Moderate periodontitis: A more advanced state of the previous condition, with increased destruction of periodontal structures associated with moderate-to-deep pockets (5–7 mm), moderate to severe bone loss and tooth mobility. There may be furcation involvement in multirooted teeth
- Advanced periodontitis: Further progression of periodontitis with severe destruction of the periodontal structures with increased pocket depth, usually 8 mm or greater with increased tooth mobility and furcation involvement

II Early Onset*

Occurs prior to age 35 and is associated with rapid rate of progression of tissue destruction; host defense defects and composition of subgingival flora. The following subclassifications have been identified:

- Prepubertal periodontitis: onset occurs between eruption of the primary teeth and puberty; occurs in localized and generalized forms
- Juvenile periodontitis: onset during the circumpubertal period. Characteristic features include familial distribution, relative paucity of microbial plaque; preponderance of *Actinobacillus actinomycetemcomitans.* (Aa) in the associated flora; and less acute clinical signs of inflammation than would be expected based on the severity of destruction. The localized form is confined mostly to permanent first molars and/or incisors. In the generalized form these teeth may be the most affected but other teeth, if not all, are involved
- Rapidly progressive periodontitis: Similar to generalized juvenile periodontitis in that inflammation may be less than expected but the age of onset is usually in the 20s or later; severity is not greater around first molar and incisors compared to other teeth; familial distribution is not as related; and pigmented bacteroides rather than Aa may be predominant in the flora

III Periodontitis associated with systemic disease

Several systemic diseases such as diabetes mellitus Type I, Down syndrome, Papillon-Lefevre syndrome, HIV infection and AIDS predispose the individuals who have them to periodontitis which may be the early-onset type

IV Necrotizing ulcerative periodontitis (NUP)

Acute inflammation that involves the supporting structures of the periodontium, not just the marginal gingiva, and is known for recurrent episodes of the disease

V Refractory periodontitis

Represents periodontal conditions that are unresponsive to thorough treatment or with recurrent disease at a few or many sites

*Overlap exists among categories and cases exist that do not clearly fit into any single category

Based on American Academy of Periodontology. Proceedings of the World Workshop in Clinical Periodontics. July 23–27, 1989, Princeton, NJ. 1989.

TABLE 13–5
TERMINOLOGY USED TO DESCRIBE OBSERVATIONS ASSOCIATED WITH THE CLINICAL ASSESSMENT OF THE GINGIVA

Characteristic	Terminology	Description	Example
Gingival Color	Location: Distribution: Severity: Quality:	Generalized or localized Diffuse, marginal, or papillary Slight, moderate, severe Red, bright red, pink, cyanotic	Localized slight marginal redness linguals of numbers 18, 19, 30, 31, all other areas coral pink, uniform in color
Gingival Contour	Location: Distribution: Severity: Quality:	Generalized or localized Diffuse, marginal, or papillary Slight, moderate, severe Bulbous, flattened, punched out, cratered	Localized moderately cratered papilla #6–11, #22–27, all other areas within normal limits
Consistency of Gingiva	Location: Distribution: Severity: Quality:	Generalized or localized Diffuse, marginal, or papillary Slight, moderate, severe Firm (fibrotic), spongy (edematous)	Generalized moderate marginal sponginess more severe on facial #8, #9, all other areas coral pink with moderate, generalized melanin pigmentation
Surface Texture of Gingiva	Location: Distribution: Quality:	Generalized or localized Diffuse, marginal, or papillary Smooth, shiny, eroded, stippling	Localized smooth gingiva on facial #7, #8, all other areas with generalized stippling

illaries, resulting in redness of tissue, edema, bleeding, and an exudate. Thus, the four characteristic signs of gingival or periodontal inflammation are:

- Changes in color
- Bleeding on probing
- Swelling or edema
- Presence of exudate from the gingival sulcus[3]

Color Change

When performing an assessment of the gingiva, the first thing to note is the color of the gingival tissue. Erythema, or reddened gingiva, is common in the process of inflammation. This reddened color of the gingiva indicates an increase in the vascular supply as a result of the body's effort to defend itself against bacterial plaque or foreign objects (i.e., a popcorn shell). A bright red color indicates acute inflammation of the gingiva.

A magenta or purple coloration of the gingival tissue also may be detected. This coloration may indicate venous congestion (cyanosis) in the connective tissue as a result of a chronic inflammatory condition. Thus, magenta-colored or cyanotic gingival tissue signals a longer duration of the inflammation. It is important to monitor and record the slightest change of color in the gingiva, as well as changes in its contour, consistency, and texture. Documentation should indicate the location, distribution, severity, and quality of such changes. Table 13–5 summarizes this terminology and provides examples for describing gingival color, contour, consistency, and texture. Clients should be informed of these findings and taught to monitor their own gingival health. Using the hand mirror, the dental hygienist should point out gingival color to the client and compare an inflamed periodontal area of the client's mouth to one that is healthy. This instruction assists the client in developing a concept of periodontal health.

Bleeding on Probing

Use of a periodontal probe to measure the depth of a healthy sulcus (one with an intact layer of sulcar epithelium) does not produce bleeding. Therefore, bleeding on probing is one of the earliest signs of the presence of inflammation. It has been reported, however, that bleeding on probing (BOP) predicts attachment loss only 30% of the time. Furthermore, fibrotic tissue that results from chronic inflammation may bleed very little or not at all. Nevertheless, BOP always signals the presence of inflammation and has value in identifying clients at risk for periodontal disease progression.

BOP always should be recorded in the client record and monitored. The dental hygienist should explain to the client that BOP is caused by soft tissue inflammation and is a significant sign of gingival infection. Moreover, the hygienist should point out that bleeding, or its absence, upon brushing or flossing gives the individual a self-test for monitoring personal gingival health status at home. Cessation of bleeding correlates with reduced inflammation, repair of gingival connective tissue, pocket reduction, and gain of attachment levels.[6] Absence of bleeding usually signifies periodontal health. The wooden toothpick or triangular interdental Stimudent, as well as other common oral hygiene devices used by clients, also can be used to detect gingival bleeding.

Swelling or Edema

Microorganisms in plaque produce harmful toxins and enzymes that result in increased permeability of the blood vessels in the connective tissue underlying the gingival epithelium. This increased permeability of blood vessels allows lymphocytes, plasma cells, and extracellular fluid to accumulate in gingival connective tissue. This accumulation results in enlarged, edematous tissue. When there is no apical

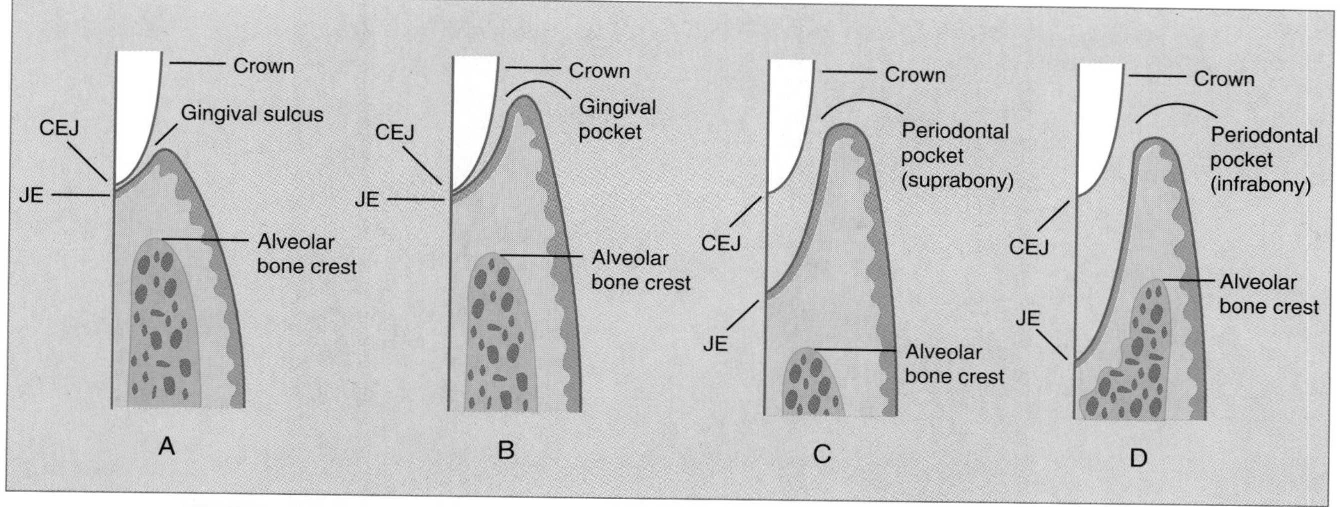

FIGURE 13–8
Comparison of the relationship of the junctional epithelium (JE) to the cementoenamel junction (CEJ) and alveolar bone in health (*A*), gingival pocket (gingivitis) (*B*), suprabony periodontal pocket (periodontitis) (*C*), and infrabony periodontal pocket (periodontitis) (*D*).

migration of the junctional epithelium, the sulcus becomes deepened from this edematous enlargement of the gingival tissue, producing a **gingival pocket.** This gingival pocket is also called an artificially deepened sulcus or a **pseudopocket** because the marginal gingiva has moved coronally, not apically. Deeper periodontal structures are not involved and there is no migration of the junctional epithelium.

A gingival pocket can be reversed to a healthy gingival sulcus by the client's daily plaque control regimen supplemented by professional mechanical oral hygiene care. When bacterial plaque is controlled and calculus is removed, the inflammation subsides and the gingival enlargement decreases, with a resultant decrease in the depth of the gingival pocket. Gingival pockets are always suprabony, because the base of the pocket is coronal to the crest of the alveolar bone (Fig. 13–8).

It is important for dental hygienists to be aware that gingival enlargement also may be the result of ingestion of certain drugs. For example, phenytoin (a drug used to control seizures), cyclosporin (an immunosuppressant drug used for persons with organ transplants to prevent rejection), and nifedipine (a drug used in the treatment of angina and ventricular arrhythmia) all cause enlargement of the gingival tissue.

Changes in Texture and Contour

Swelling or edema produces texture and contour changes in the gingiva (Fig. 13–9). In gingivitis, the texture of the gingiva becomes shiny smooth as a result of loss of stippling and edema. Contour changes occur as a result of gingival enlargement such that the position of the gingiva is high on the enamel, partly or nearly covering the anatomical crown. The marginal gingiva becomes rounded or rolled rather than knife-edged or slightly rounded and closely adapted to the tooth. In chronic inflammation the gingival surface may even become nodular or fibrotic (Fig. 13–10).

Interdental Papillae Changes

While examining the color, texture, size, and shape of the gingiva, the clinician gives careful attention to the gingival papilla. When the col area is inflamed, degeneration of the epithelial and connective tissue layer can result in either a blunted papilla, a split interdental papilla, or a cratered papilla (Fig. 13–11). Such degradation usually indicates a loss of the alveolar bone. In addition, self-induced trauma, for example, from improper use of dental floss, may cause laceration of the gingival papillae.

Exudate

Gingival crevicular fluid (GCF) may be found in healthy gingiva, but significantly increases in the presence of inflammation. GCF is measured by isolating a site, drying it with air, and inserting a small paper strip into the pocket or sulcus for 3 to 5 seconds. Electronic devices can measure the gingival crevicular fluid volume of the paper strip.

In mild inflammation, GCF contains plasma proteins, proteolytic enzymes like those in saliva, and both living and dead white blood cells such as polymorphonuclear leukocytes (PMNs) and lymphocytes and may be referred to as "inflammatory exudate." The inflammatory components cleanse and defend the sulcus against bacterial invasion by engulfing bacteria and by developing antibodies against plaque. Other inflammatory components of GCF in the presence of gingival disease include bacterial products such as endotoxins (fragments of bacterial cell walls) and byproducts of connective tissue cell breakdown.

The GCF is called **suppuration** when it is a clear serous liquid, and **purulent exudate** when it contains living and dead PMNs, bacteria, necrotic tissue, and enzymes. When a purulent exudate is present in the pocket, pus can be noticed during probing and expressed clinically by applying pressure to the base of a pocket with one's finger and moving it coronally. Although this purulent exudate is a dramatic sign of inflammation, it is not indicative of the severity of inflammation or pocket depth. Some shallow and some deep pockets have pus formation, and some do not. The presence of pus is, however, a good indicator of

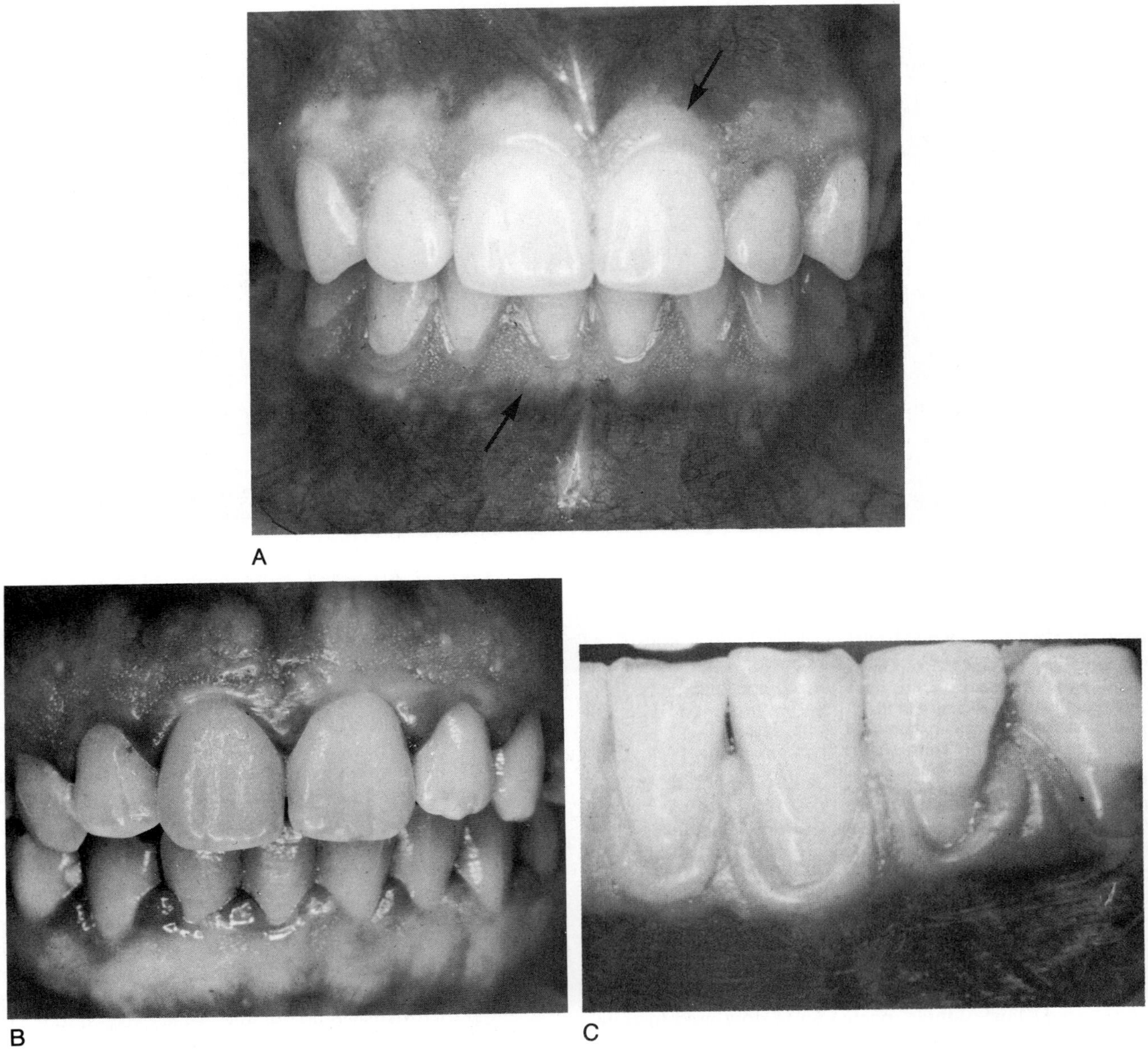

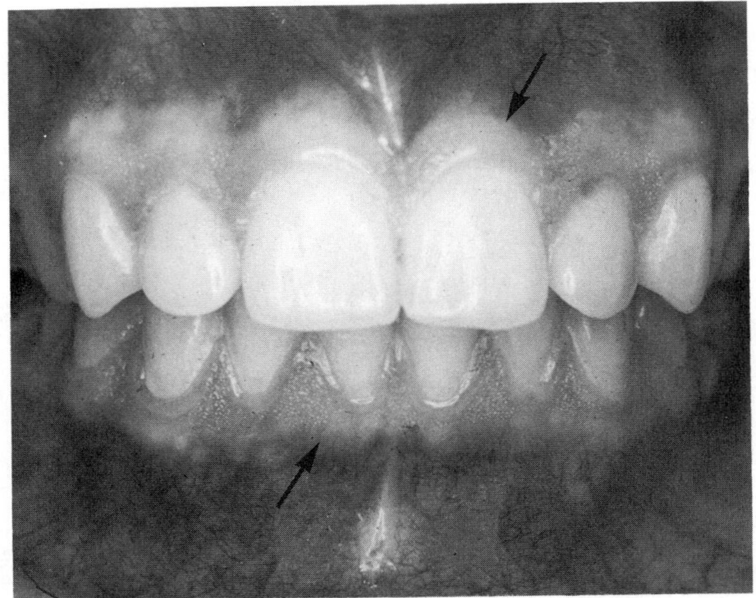

A

B

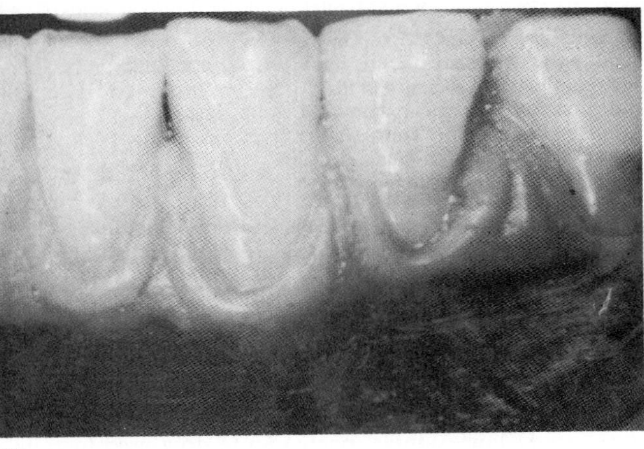

C

FIGURE 13–9
A, Normal gingiva. Note the demarcation (mucogingival line) (*arrows*) between the attached gingiva and the darker alveolar mucosa. Interdental gingiva is closely adapted to the tooth and is pointed or slightly rounded. *B*, Edema associated with papillary gingivitis. *C*, Life-saver-like enlargement of the gingival margin characteristic of McCall's festoons. (With permission from Carranza, F. Glickman's Clinical Periodontology, 7th ed. Philadelphia: W. B. Saunders, 1990, pp. 15, 112, and 124.)

active periodontal destruction. Suppuration correlates with specific attachment loss only 2% to 30% of the time, so it is not a reliable predictor of disease progress.[4] Suppuration is not always clinically evident. When suppuration or purulent exudate is observed, it should be recorded for each area found.

Documentation of the Clinical Evaluation of the Gingiva

When performing a clinical examination of the gingiva changes in gingival color, consistency, surface texture, contour, and size should be described with regard to *location* (generalized throughout or localized to a specific area); *distribution* (diffuse, marginal, or papillary); *severity* (slight, moderate, severe); and *quality*. Table 13–2 compares gingival characteristics associated with health and disease. Consensus from the 1989 World Workshop in clinical periodontics emphasized that "the term 'healthy periodontium' is appropriate for sites that are disease-free but have extensive attachment loss and recession [described below] resulting from previous episodes of periodontitis. For example, sites that have been successfully treated fall into this category."

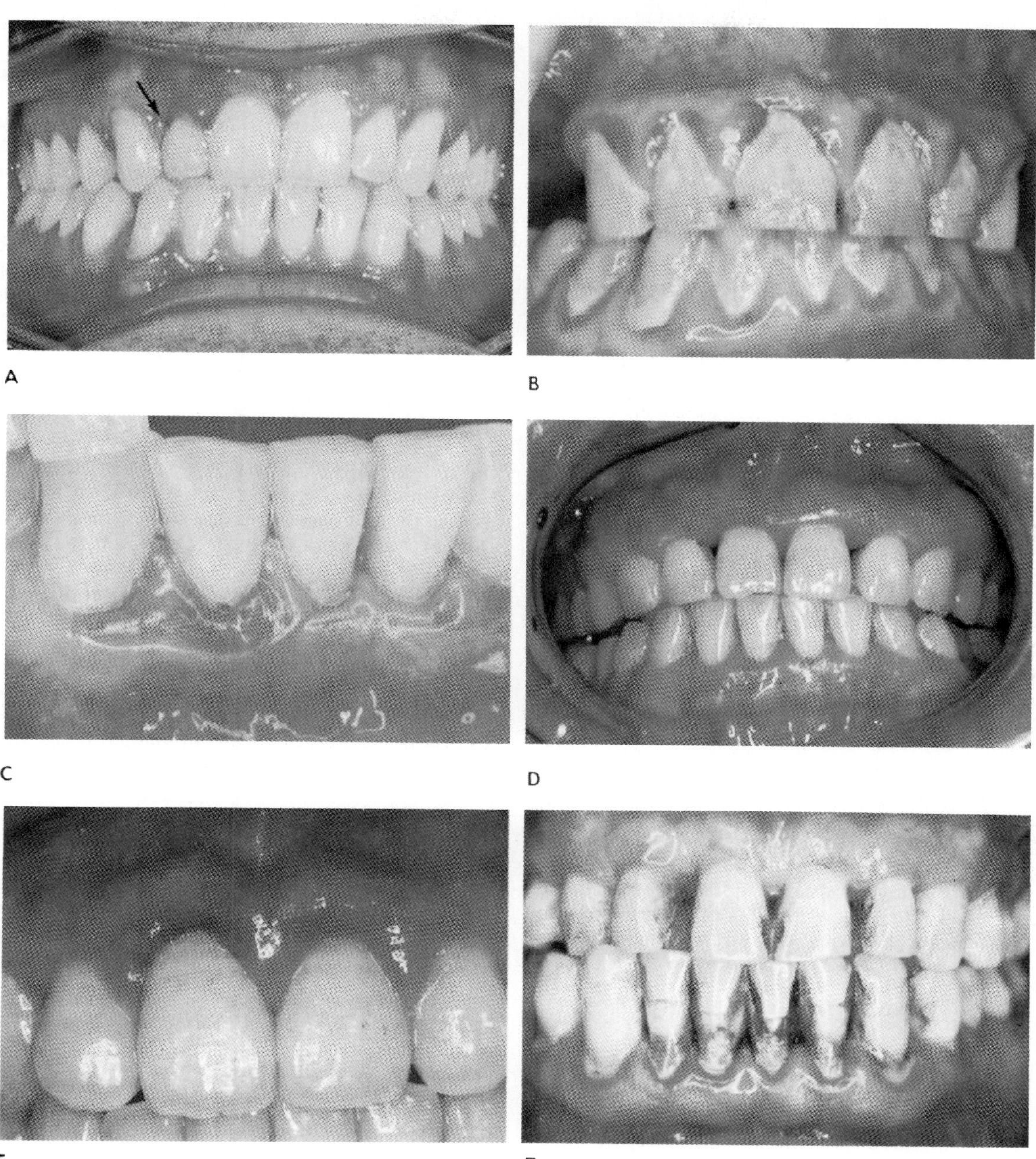

FIGURE 13–10
A, Incipient marginal gingivitis. Note slight puffiness and bleeding (*arrow*) around upper right lateral incisor. *B*, Edematous type of gingival inflammation. Note loss of stippling, increase in size, abundant plaque and materia alba, and change in color. *C*, Close-up view of edematous type of gingival inflammation. Note the red, shiny, smooth gingiva. *D*, Fibrotic type of gingival inflammation. Pockets of moderate depth are present, but the gingiva retains its stippling in some areas. *E*, Severe generalized gingival inflammation and inflammatory gingival enlargement. *F*, Fibrotic gingival inflammation. Note the abundant calculus and the gingival recession. The patient has pockets of moderate to severe depth in the mandibular anterior teeth and shallower pockets in the maxillary teeth. (With permission from Carranza, F. Glickman's Clinical Periodontology, 7th ed. Philadelphia: W. B. Saunders, 1990, p. 492.)

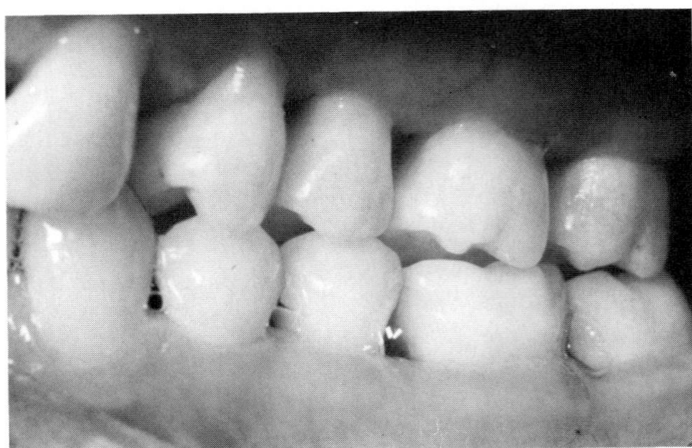

FIGURE 13–11
Cratered and missing interdental papilla.

Signs of Disease Progression (Periodontitis)

Periodontal Pocket

Probing depth is the distance from the gingival margin to the base of the sulcus or pocket as measured by the periodontal probe (Fig. 13–12). Unlike a gingival pocket, a periodontal pocket is a pathologically deepened sulcus caused by plaque. When the coronal end of the junctional epithelium (the surface that forms the actual sulcus/pocket bottom) comes in contact with bacterial plaque, it detaches from the tooth. At the same time, the apical end of the junctional epithelium migrates apically, thus deepening the sulcus into a periodontal pocket. As inflammation causes apical migration of the junctional epithelium it also causes gradual alveolar bone resorption, which reduces the level of bone support for the tooth (see Fig. 13–7).[7]

Periodontal pockets may be **suprabony** or **infrabony** pockets. In a suprabony periodontal pocket the junctional epithelium has migrated below the CEJ but remains above the crest of the alveolar bone. In infrabony pockets the junctional epithelium has migrated below the crest of the alveolar bone (see Fig. 13–8).

Periodontal pockets may be present in the absence of clinical signs of gingival inflammation or recession. Therefore, clinical probing is the only accurate way to assess the gingiva for the presence of periodontal pockets. Because periodontal pockets can develop at any point around a tooth, the probe must be inserted around the entire circumference of the tooth. The deepest reading at each of the six tooth surfaces (Fig. 13–13) is the one that should be recorded on the client's peridontal charting form. The probe is moved or "walked" along the pocket bottom and angled to keep the tip in contact with the tooth (Fig. 13–14). If calculus is encountered, the probe should be teased over the calculus (Fig. 13–15) or the calculus should be removed to allow insertion of the probe to the bottom of the pocket.

The interproximal area is the hardest area for the client to clean and therefore is where periodontal pockets tend to form. To probe the interproximal area just apical to the contact, *place the probe up against the interdental contact and tilt the probe mesially or distally as appropriate to keep the tip touching the tooth* (Fig. 13–16). Failure to tilt the probe enough to keep its tip in contact with the tooth surface is a common error and causes inaccurate interproximal probing depth readings (Fig. 13–17). The interproximal tooth surfaces should be probed from both the facial and lingual sides of each tooth so that all of the epithelial attachment of the junctional epithelium is explored (Fig. 13–18).

Because pockets with shallow probing depths have been found to exhibit more rapid disease progression than pockets with deep probing depths, it is very important to observe and record signs of inflammation along with shallow depths when assessing periodontal probing depths.[8]

Attachment Loss

Attachment loss is the best indicator of damage to the periodontium. It is determined by comparing the distance from the CEJ to the base of the sulcus or pocket over time

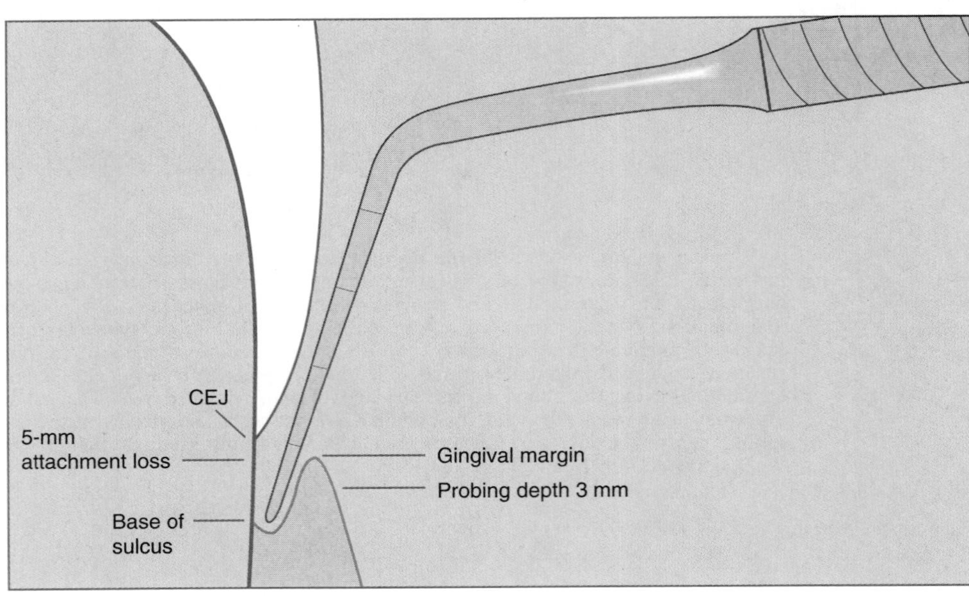

FIGURE 13–12
Probing depth and attachment loss measurement on same tooth using the Williams probe.

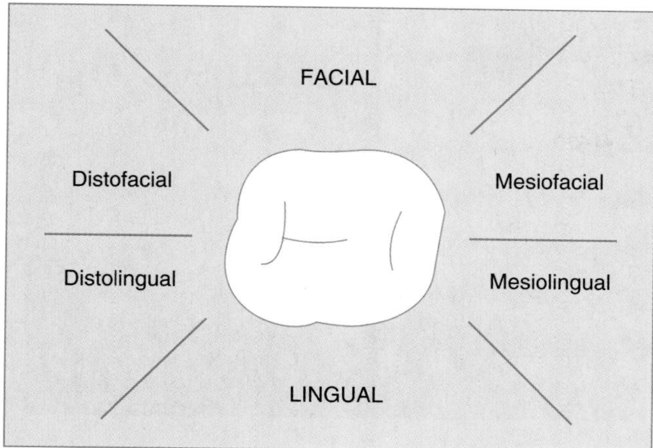

FIGURE 13–13
Occlusal view of the six tooth surfaces.

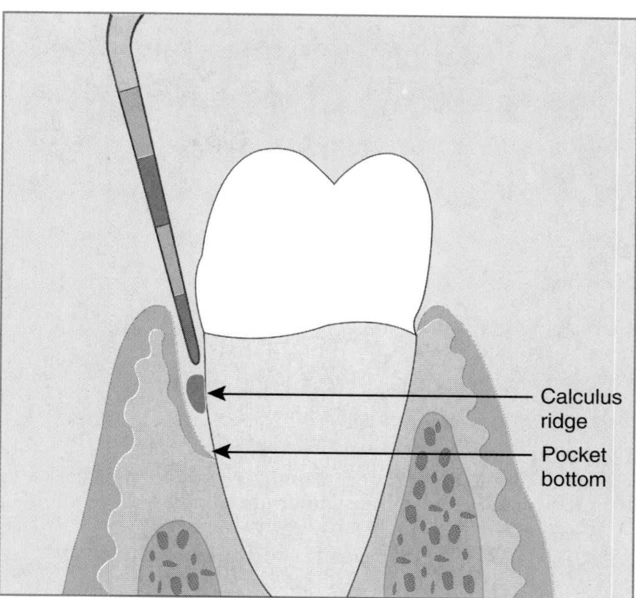

FIGURE 13–15
Probe blocked by calculus. (With permission from Praxis Publishing. Taken from Section of Instructional System Design, Department of Periodontology, UCSF School of Dentistry, 1978.)

as measured by the periodontal probe. Consequently, attachment loss includes both periodontal pocket depth and recession measurements (see Fig. 13–12). Increase in attachment loss over time indicates actual progression of periodontal disease. Consequently, regular documentation of attachment loss in the client record is important to allow tracking of periodontal disease activity.

Recession

Gingival recession is the reduction of the height of the marginal gingiva to a location apical to the CEJ (Fig. 13–19). It has importance in the periodontal assessment because it signifies attachment loss and can produce significant discomfort for the client. Causes of gingival recession are numerous. Chronic exposure to bacterial plaque, toothbrush abrasion, floss cuts, occlusal trauma, root instrumentation, and polishing with an abrasive prophylaxis paste or air polisher have all been known to result in migration of the junctional epithelium and cause recession. Once the root surface is exposed to the oral environment by gingival recession, the connective tissue rarely reattaches because collagen breaks down when exposed to the oral environment, and cementoblasts grow only on root surface adjacent to the periodontal ligament.

Areas of recession may be sensitive, because the exposed cementum may be lost, exposing dentin. As a result, exposed nerve endings in the dentin may be stimulated mechanically (e.g., by toothbrushing), chemically (e.g., by acidic foods), or thermally (e.g., by cold air or food at extreme temperature), producing sensitive teeth. Noting areas of dentinal hypersensitivity on the client record provides information for planning care, because clients with

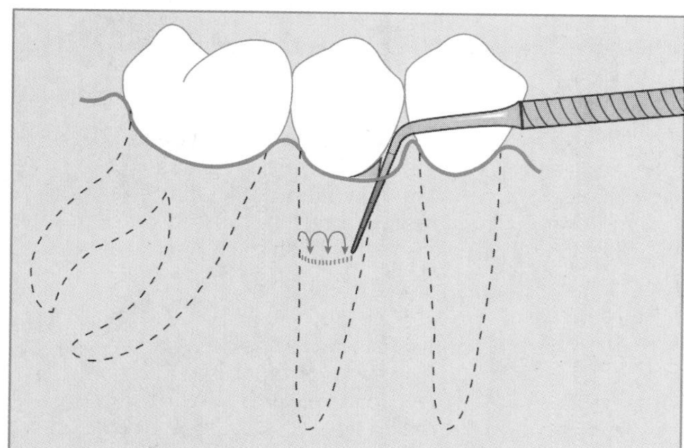

FIGURE 13–14
Facial view showing how the probe is moved around the tooth in short steps, reestablishing contact with the pocket bottom at each step.

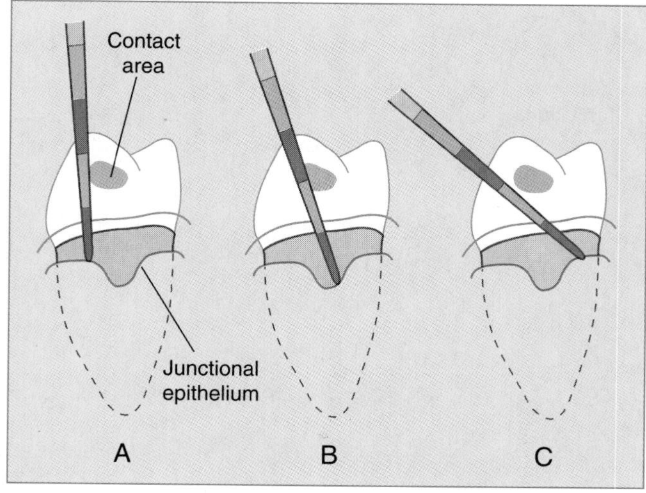

FIGURE 13–16
A, Incorrect technique for probing the interproximal area. *B*, Correct technique. *C*, Incorrect technique. (Redrawn with permission from Perry, D., Beemsterboer, P., and Carranza, F. Techniques and Theory of Periodontal Instrumentation. Philadelphia: W. B. Saunders, 1990, p. 34.)

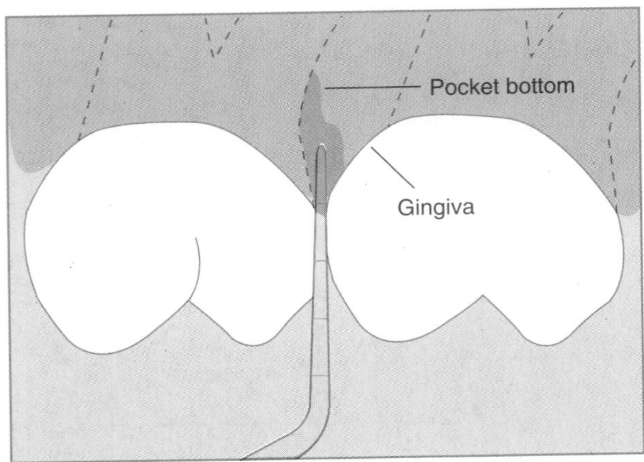

FIGURE 13-17
Failure to tilt the probe far enough to keep its end in contact with the tooth surface. Probe is resting on the pocket wall, resulting in an inaccurate probing depth measurement.

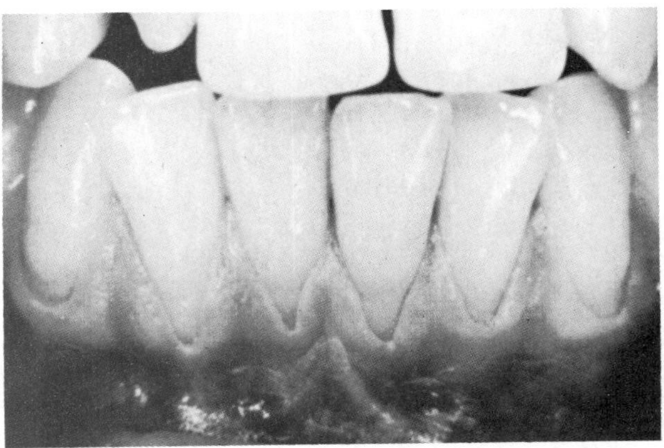

FIGURE 13-19
Gingival recession. Note excellent condition of the gingiva. (With permission from Carranza, F. Glickman's Clinical Periodontology, 7th ed. Philadelphia: W. B. Saunders, 1990, p. 121.)

hypersensitivity may require more time and possibly local anesthetic for effective tooth instrumentation.

Probing depths, recession, and sensitive teeth, along with all gingival changes, must be accurately recorded and monitored to provide a reference for the client's disease activity over time.

Furcation Involvement

Furcation involvement, or loss of attachment between the roots of posterior teeth, needs to be identified, classified, and monitored (see Classification of Furcations chart; Fig. 13-20). The client must be informed about areas of furcation involvement and taught home care techniques to manage these areas. The Nabors furcation probe (Fig. 13-21) is often used to detect and measure furcation involvement. Radiographs confirm, but do not always show, this condition.

Tooth Mobility

Tooth mobility is the degree to which a tooth is able to move in a horizontal or apical direction. Although tooth mobility is caused by loss of bone and periodontal ligament support associated with periodontitis, it has been found to vary during the day according to diet and stress.[9] Children, young adults, and some women exhibit more movement than other groups.[10] Tooth mobility is not a cause of periodontal disease but may contribute to it, and thus it is

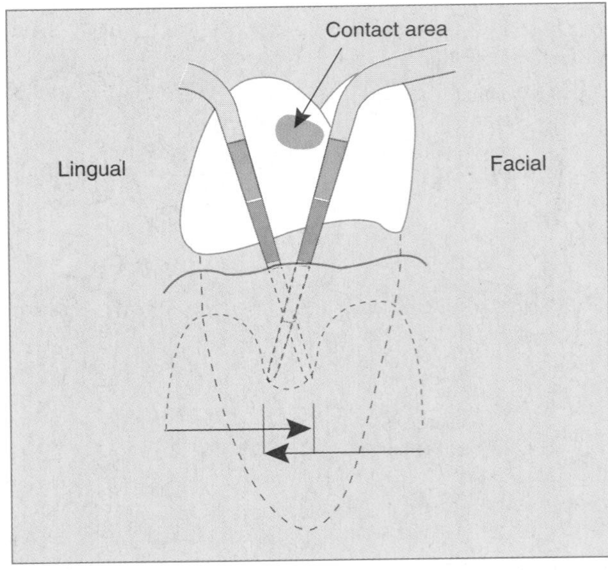

FIGURE 13-18
Proximal view of tooth being probed from both facial and lingual sides so that all of the junctional epithelium is explored. (Redrawn with permission from Carranza, F. Glickman's Clinical Periodontology, 7th ed. Philadelphia: W.B. Saunders, 1990, p. 494.)

CLASSIFICATION OF FURCATIONS

Class I
Beginning involvement. The clinician can detect the concavity of the furcation with an explorer or probe but cannot enter it. This type of defect cannot be detected radiographically. Charted as /\ directly on the furcation of the tooth involved.

Class II
Cul-de-sac involvement. The clinician can enter the furcation area with an explorer or probe, but cannot penetrate through to the opposite side. A slight radiolucency in the furcation area may be seen on the radiograph. Charted as △ directly on the furcation of the tooth involved.

Class III
Through and through involvement. The clinician can pass an explorer or probe all the way through the furcation to the opposite side. A definite radiolucency in the furcation area is visible on the radiograph. Charted as ▲ directly on the furcation of the tooth involved.

Adapted from Ramfjord, S. P., and Ash, M. M. Periodontology and Periodontics. Philadelphia: W. B. Saunders, 1979.

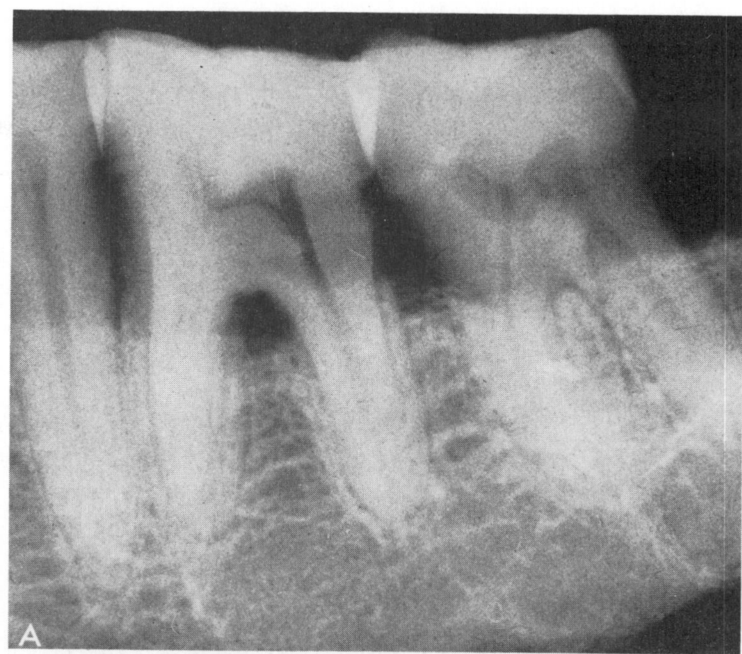

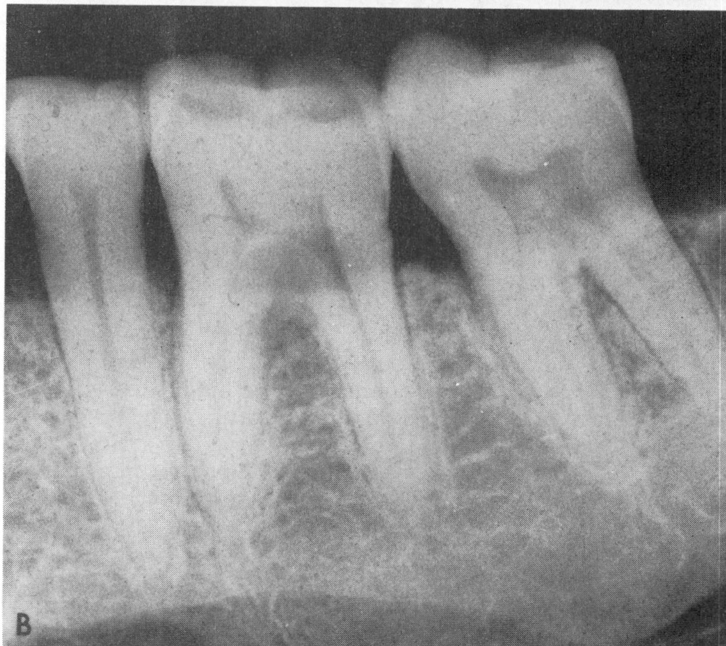

FIGURE 13–20
Furcation involvement. *A*, Triangular radiolucency in bifurcation area of mandibular first molar indicates furcation involvement. *B*, Same area, different angulation. The triangular radiolucency in the bifurcation of the first molar is obliterated, and involvement of the second bifurcation is apparent. (With permission from Carranza, F. Glickman's Clinical Periodontology, 7th ed. Philadelphia: W. B. Saunders, 1990, p. 510.)

assessed along with attachment levels. To test for mobility, place an instrument handle on the lingual surface of the tooth and gently push on the facial surface with another instrument (e.g., a periodontal probe or mouth mirror). The feeling of movement is most acute at the contact points between two teeth. The classification of mobility should be recorded directly on the charting form to allow comparative readings at successive appointments (see Classification of Mobility chart).

Occlusal Traumatism

Occlusal traumatism is a degenerative, noninflammatory periodontal condition that results in the destruction of the

CLASSIFICATION OF MOBILITY

Class I°
Tooth can be moved up to 1 mm in any direction

Class II°
Tooth can be moved more than 1 mm in any direction but is not depressible in the socket

Class III°
Tooth can be moved in a buccolingual direction and is depressible in the socket

Adapted from Parr, R. W., Pipe, P., and Watt, S. Recognizing Periodontal Disease. San Francisco: Praxis Publishing, 1978.

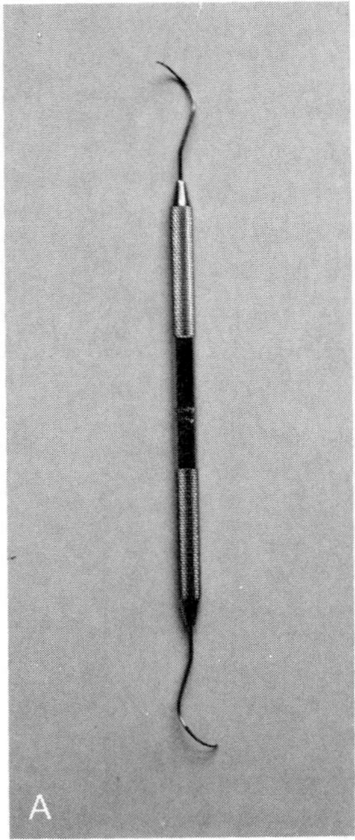

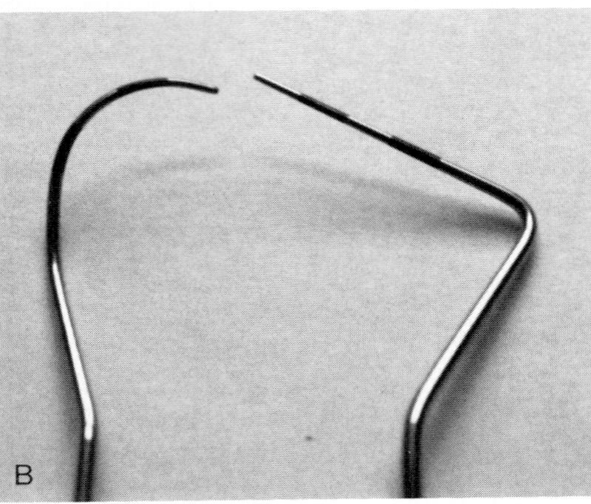

FIGURE 13–21
A, Nabor's furcation probe. *B*, Comparison of the working ends of the Nabor's furcation probe and the Marquis probe.

supporting structures of the teeth because they cannot withstand the forces acting upon them. Clinical and radiographic signs of occlusal traumatism include discomfort in a localized area, loss of supporting bone, widening of the periodontal ligament space, loss of lamina dura, wear facets, tooth mobility, and root fracture. Histologically, there is also a breakdown of the fibers of the periodontal ligament.

Occlusal trauma may be primary or secondary in nature. *Primary occlusal traumatism* occurs when destruction of the supporting structures is caused by excessive occlusal forces acting on an otherwise normal periodontium. Excess occlusal forces in primary occlusal traumatism may be caused by bruxism, clenching, malocclusion, or iatrogenic factors such as a poorly made dental restoration or appliance. *Secondary occlusal traumatism* is caused by occlusal forces acting on an already diseased periodontium.

Occlusal trauma exacerbates periodontal disease because the supporting structures are already weakened or damaged. Elimination of the etiological factors of gingivitis and periodontitis comes first, with occlusal adjustment a secondary treatment by the dentist.

Inadequate Alveolar Gingiva

Areas with a limited zone of alveolar gingiva (also called "attached gingiva") should be noted, shown to the client, and explained during the periodontal assessment. Inadequate alveolar gingiva is defined as less than 1 mm of keratinized alveolar gingiva. These areas are often sensitive, can be difficult to maintain, and can develop into a mucogingival problem because the thin zone of attachment usually reflects a reduced blood supply and a potential for quick loss of supporting bone and connective tissue. Recession and high frena or muscle attachments may add to the reduction of alveolar mucosa. These are chronic conditions that must be recorded and monitored. It is critical to consider these conditions when planning root planing and periodontal surgery. Although good oral hygiene can maintain periodontal health with almost no alveolar gingiva, high frenum attachments or the use of the tooth as a crown and bridge abutment may indicate surgical intervention to widen the zone of alveolar gingiva.[1]

Mucogingival Problems

Mucogingival problems are those conditions wherein the junctional epithelium or attachment level is apical to the mucogingival junction and there is no alveolar gingiva (Fig. 13–22). When pockets extend up to or beyond this point, the area must be monitored very closely for the potential of tooth loss because of reduced periodontium and vascular supply to this defect. Conscientious home care and precise root planing are indicated. In the absence of pocket formation, gingival grafts may be performed by the dentist to cover root surfaces with a transplanted piece of gingival tissue from a donor site in a neighboring area, such as the palate. However, in many cases, the condition can be maintained nonsurgically.[1] Frenectomy is a surgical technique to correct a high frenum attachment associated with pocket formation and mucogingival problems. It is usually performed in conjunction with pocket elimination methods.

RADIOGRAPHIC ASPECTS OF PERIODONTAL ASSESSMENT

A radiograph is a projection of a three-dimensional object onto a two-dimensional film. Consequently, not all periodontal defects are visualized on radiographs. Therefore, radiographs are to be used only as an adjunct to clinical periodontal assessment. The clinician must interpret the radiographic image and relate it to what is seen in the client's mouth.

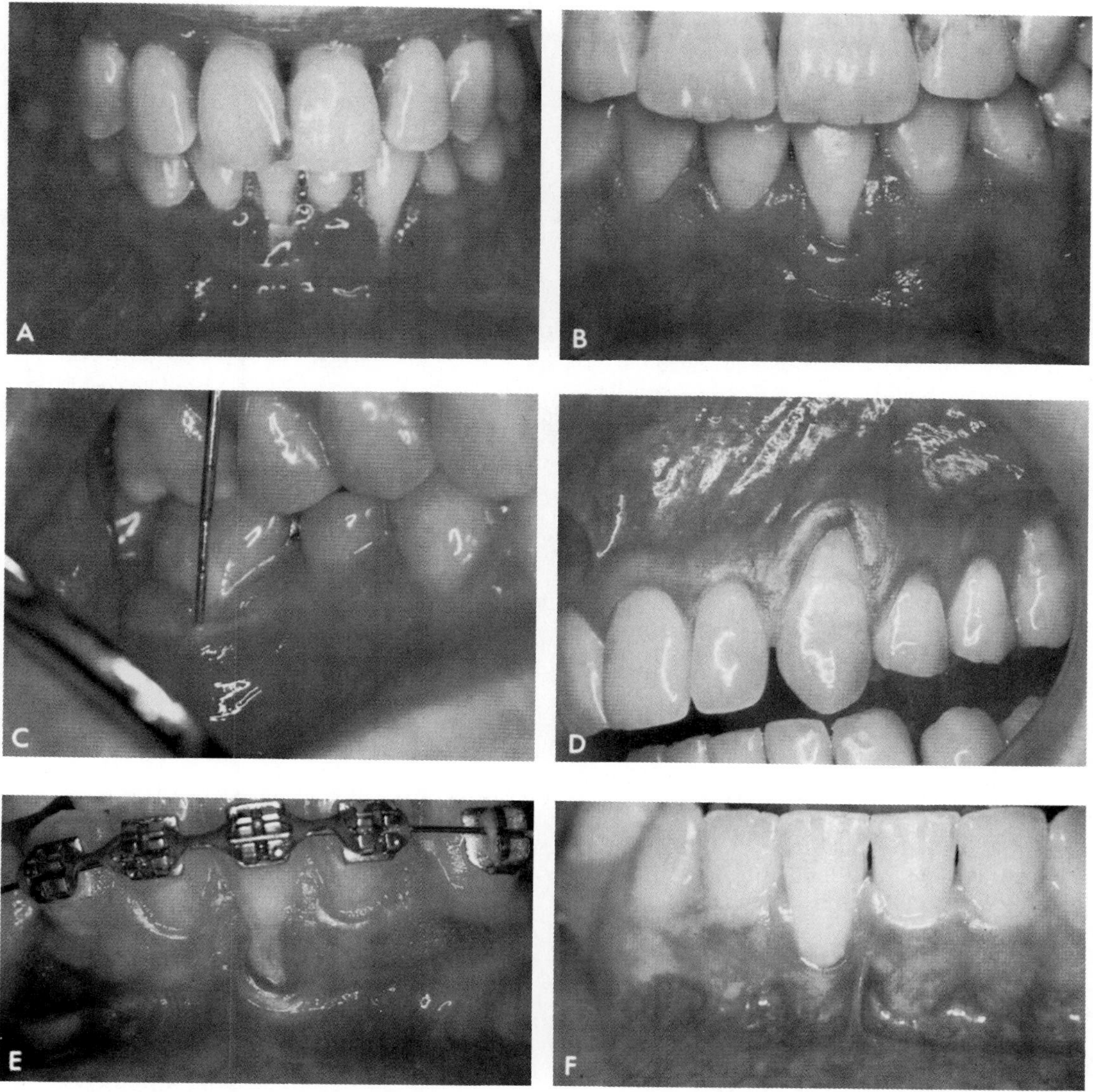

FIGURE 13-22
Mucogingival defects. *A*, Irregular gingival contours, pocket furcations, and recession with severe gingival inflammation. *B*, Gingival recession and inflammation. Bottom of pocket is beyond mucogingival junction. *C*, Recession on mesiobuccal root of lower first molar. Probe indicates presence of shallow pocket with absence of attached gingiva. *D*, Gingival recession and cleft on upper cuspid. *E*, Advanced gingival recession and inflammation. *F*, After scaling and root planing and adequate plaque control, gingival condition has improved markedly. (With permission from Carranza, F. Glickman's Clinical Periodontology, 7th ed. Philadelphia: W. B. Saunders, 1990, p. 905.)

Types of Radiographs, Recommended Technique, and Exposure

The complete dental survey consists of a combination of 14 or more periapical films that show each tooth in its entirety and its existing periodontium. The bite-wing survey consists of two to four films that show the interdental area and bone crest of the posterior teeth in a clenched position. Vertical bite-wings (Fig. 13-23) allow the best view of the alveolar crest with bone loss, and are recommended. A panograph is a single film of the whole dentition. It is not used for periodontal assessment because the complete dental survey allows more periodontal abnormalities to be visualized. Interproximal areas are better viewed when the x-ray passes between the teeth in question. This targeting of the x-ray beam can be achieved in the bite-wing survey and in periapical radiographs.

The paralleling technique of exposing radiographs produces standardized films that are the most anatomically correct and easily read by the clinician. By placing the film parallel to the long axis of the tooth and passing the central x-ray beam through interproximal areas of one or several teeth, the hygienist can obtain an accurate radiographic projection of one or several teeth. Good clinical presentation of these films requires proper placement, exposure, and processing. A current set of radiographs is important for periodontal assessment. Recommendations from the American Dental Association as to frequency of exposure defer to dentists' professional judgment on a case-by-case

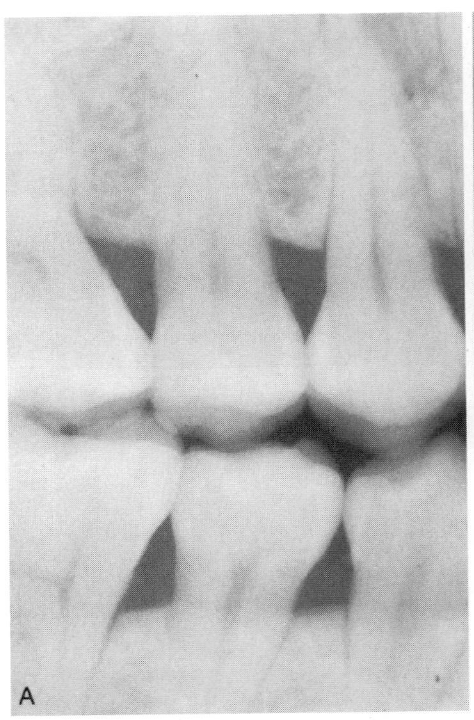

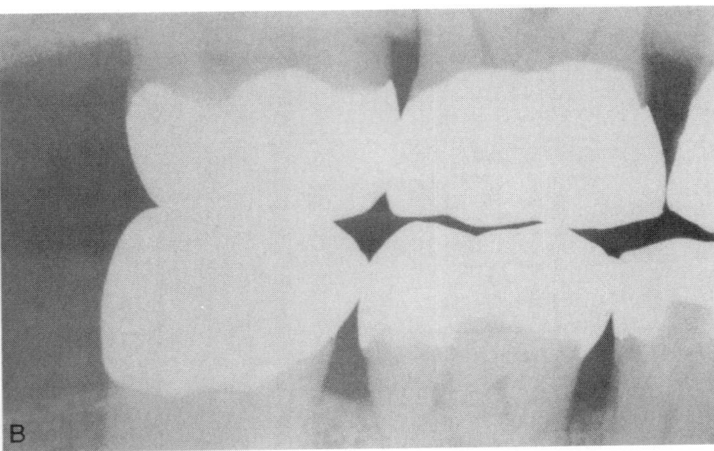

FIGURE 13-23
A, Vertical bitewing radiograph. *B*, Horizontal bite-wing radiograph.

basis after they perform a thorough oral examination and take a thorough health history.[11] Findings from a study that analyzed serial bite-wing radiographs from more than 700 individuals are summarized in the criteria listed in Table 13-6 for exposure schedules for radiographs.[12,13,14] Care must be taken to consider clients' health, safety concerns, and radiologic history when exposing them to further radiation.

Clinical Use of Radiographs

Clinical signs of the health status of the periodontium should be confirmed by examining a complete dental series and bite-wing survey of radiographs. Radiographs are examined as a set and individually. Initially, the complete dental series is scanned for missing, impacted, or primary teeth; restorations; endodontic repair; implants; anomalies; and periapical pathosis. Radiographs are then examined for periodontal assessment factors: alveolar crest location, intact lamina dura, furcation involvement of posterior teeth, and bone loss.

In health, the alveolar crest is 1 mm apical to the CEJ of adjacent teeth. If a line were drawn to connect the CEJs of adjacent teeth, it should be parallel to the alveolar crest (Fig. 13-24). In addition, in health the lamina dura (the radiographic image of the cortical bone that surrounds the root of the tooth) should be dense, radiopaque (white), and continuous. The trabecular pattern of the spongy aspect of the alveolar bone is regular and less opaque than the lamina dura, although there is no relationship between trabecular bone patterns and health, disease, or age. The width of the periodontal ligament space is not necessarily indicative of periodontal health or disease, but it should be noted as baseline information to be used in subsequent radiographic examinations. Cortical bone, enamel, and metal are all radiopaque on the film, because the x-ray beam is halted by their density.

The dental hygienist should view the lamina dura and trabeculation between the posterior roots in the furcation of the tooth. The degree of furcal health is hard to determine with great accuracy from radiographs, but radiopacity (light or white areas) in the furcation may mean intact alveolar

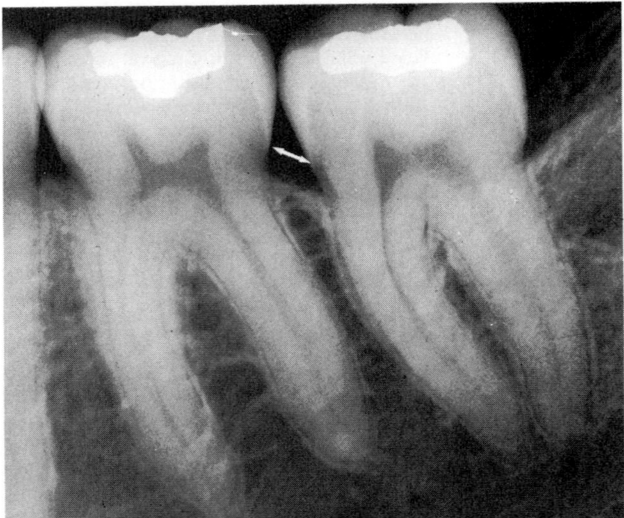

FIGURE 13-24
Crest of interdental septum normally parallel to a line drawn between the CEJ of adjacent teeth (*arrow*). (With permission from Carranza, F. Glickman's Clinical Periodontology, 7th ed. Philadelphia: W. B. Saunders, 1990, p. 502.)

TABLE 13–6
RECOMMENDATIONS FROM THE DENTAL PATIENT SELECTION CRITERIA PANEL FOR PRESCRIBING DENTAL RADIOGRAPHS

	Children			
	Primary Dentition (Before Eruption of First Permanent Tooth)	Transitional Dentition (After Eruption of First Permanent Tooth)	**Adolescents (All Permanent Teeth Present Except Third Molars)**	**Adults**
I. Radiographic examination of new patient without previous radiographs*	Posterior bite-wing examination if proximal surfaces of primary teeth cannot be visualized and probed and child can be expected to cooperate for exposure	Full-mouth examination posterior bite-wings or panoramic examination with posterior bite-wings†	Full-mouth examination w/posterior bite-wings	Full-mouth examination and posterior bite-wings‡
II. Radiographic examination of recall patient				
A. Caries or other high-risk factors§	Posterior bite-wing examinations at 6-month intervals or until no caries are evident		Posterior bite-wing examination at 6 to 12 month intervals or until no caries are evident	Posterior bite-wing examination at 12 to 18 month intervals
B. No caries and no other high-risk factors	Posterior bite-wing examination if proximal surfaces of primary teeth can be visualized and probed and child can be expected to cooperate for exposure; posterior bite-wing examination repeated every 12 to 24 months	Posterior bite-wing examination every 12 to 24 months	Posterior bite-wing examination every 18 to 36 months	Posterior bite-wing examination every 24 to 36 months
C. Periodontal diseases or history of periodontal treatment	Selected periapical or bite-wing should be made for those areas where periodontal diseases (except gingivitis) can be demonstrated clinically			
D. To assess growth and development		Full-mouth or panoramic examination	Periapical or panoramic radiographs to view third molars	
E. With signs or conditions other than caries or periodontal disease*	Radiographs as indicated by history, signs or symptoms			

These guidelines are to be used by the dentist only after a review of the health history and a clinical examination have been completed. The recommendations used in the chart are subject to clinical judgment and may not apply to every patient, given individual susceptibility, health care practice, and experience.

* Clinical situations for which radiographs may be indicated include the following: previous pulpal therapy; deep carious lesions, large or deep restorations; history of pain; evidence of swelling; positive neurologic findings in face and jaws; trauma to teeth, jaws, or lips; mobility of teeth; unexplained bleeding; unexplained sensitivity of teeth; evaluation of sinus condition; unusual spacing or migration of teeth; unusual tooth structure, calcification, or color; evaluation of growth abnormalities or eruption; altered occlusal relationships; aid in diagnosis of systemic disease; familial history of dental anomalies; postoperative evaluation for diagnostic purposes; missing teeth because of unknown history of unexplained absence; localization of foreign bodies within jaws; evaluation of temporomandibular joint.

† Clinical evidence of periodontal disease (except gingivitis) indicates periapical and bite-wing views rather than panoramic.

‡ Full-mouth examination with bite-wings is preferred, but panoramics and bite-wings may be substituted in the clinical absence of periodontal diseases (except gingivitis).

§ High-risk group includes patients demonstrating any of the following: high level of caries experience, history of recurrent caries, existing poor-quality restorations.

With permission from U.S. Food and Drug Administration: The selection of patients for x-ray examinations: Dental radiographic exposures. HHS Publication 88-3273. Washington, DC, November 1987.

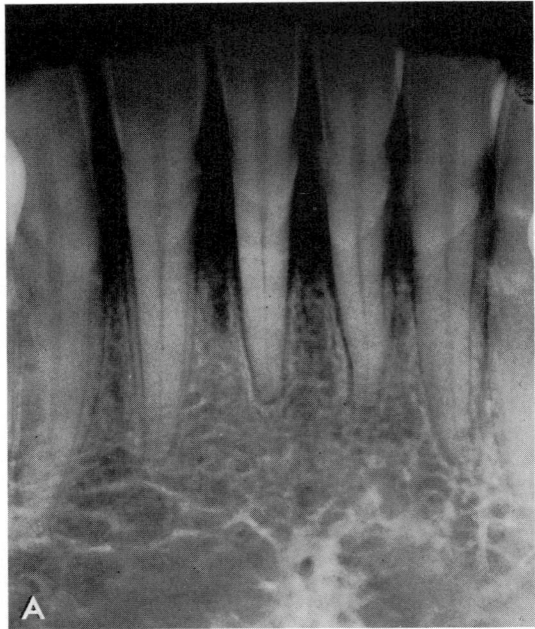

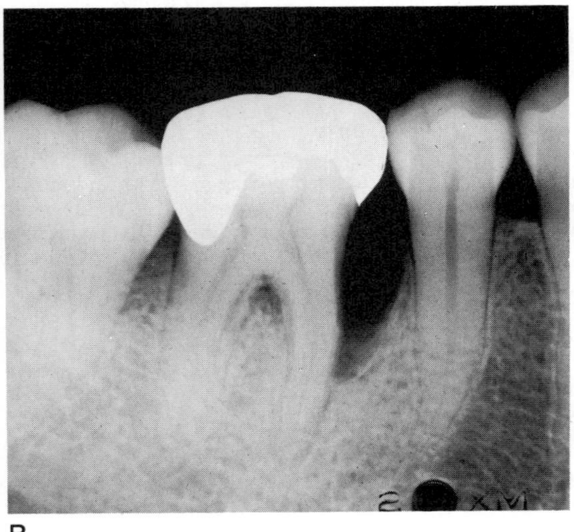

FIGURE 13-25
A, Horizontal bone loss around mandibular anterior teeth. *B*, Vertical bone loss on the mesial surface of the first molar. Note also the furcation involvement. (With permission from Carranza, F. Glickman's Clinical Periodontology, 7th ed. Philadelphia: W. B. Saunders, 1990, p. 57 and 253.)

bone. The horizontal angle of the x-ray beam, if not perpendicular to the long axis and furcation of the tooth, disguises bone loss there. Radiographs also show the crown-to-root ratios. The proportionate ratio of root length to crown size is usually uniform for the whole dentition, and this fact is verified by radiographs.

The first radiographic evidence of bone loss may be loss of height in the alveolar crest. In disease, radiographs show horizontal and vertical patterns of bone loss (Fig. 13-25). Horizontal bone loss is observed when the loss of alveolar bone is spread over an area at the same rate from tooth to tooth. Vertical, or angular, bone loss is found when a tooth has lost more bone than the one next to it.

Radiographs confirm oral findings. For example, if the dental hygienist obtains probing depth readings of 2 to 3 mm but observes bone loss on the radiograph, probing depth measurements should be rechecked. In this case the radiographs provide a check of clinical findings for periodontal probing.

Standardized radiographs exposed using the paralleling technique provide a guide to the root surface and can be a roadmap for scaling and root planing. For example, Figure 13-26 shows root position, bone destruction, dental caries, and large calculus deposits in the premolar area.

Radiographs also provide a serial record of the client's periodontal status, giving the dental hygienist a basis for comparison with new findings. Radiographs show the history of disease progression, allowing the dental hygienist to follow bone levels over time. Standardized radiographs are most helpful in making longitudinal comparisons and in providing objective documentation of clinical findings. Periodontal probing and other clinical findings are subjective assessments, but radiographs present objective data that two or more clinicians can observe at the exact same time.

Limitations

Radiographs are to be used as an adjunct to clinical periodontal assessment. They are not to be used alone to assess periodontal status because of the following limitations:

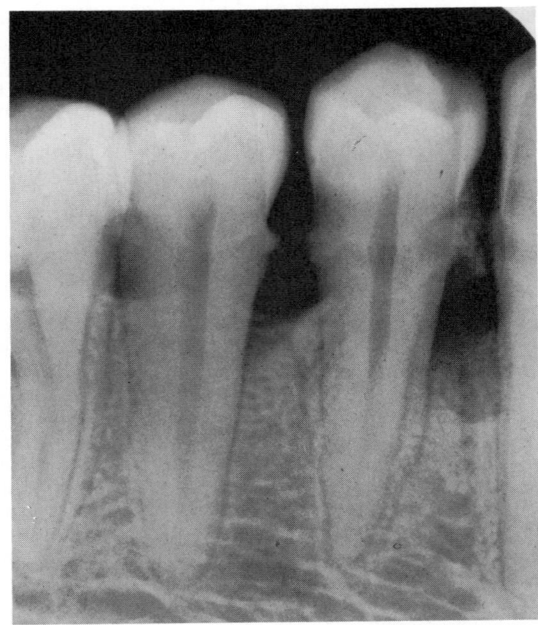

FIGURE 13-26
Radiograph showing bone destruction and dental caries in the mandibular premolar area. Note the heavy calculus deposits. (With permission from Carranza, F. Glickman's Clinical Periodontology, 7th ed. Philadelphia: W. B. Saunders, 1990, p. 248.)

- Projection factors such as cone-to-film distance, angulation, technique, and film positioning can distort or obscure radiographic images. For example, healthy alveolar bone is evenly located 1 mm apical to the tooth's CEJ, and the alveolar crest should parallel an imaginary line drawn from the CEJ of one tooth to the CEJ of the adjacent tooth. In the radiographic view, this bone position may be distorted by x-ray angulation, suggesting vertical bone loss.
- Exposure errors such as cone cuts and imbalance of kVp and mA disguise anatomy and pathosis. Proper exposure of the complete dental and bite-wing series utilizes the widest range of contrast (grays) so that minute changes in bone density and mineralized calculus are visualized. Increased kVp and lower mA produce this broad contrast range and reduce exposure time for the client, but this combination also lengthens processing time. Shortened processing time decreases contrast and reduces information for the clinician.
- Facial and lingual supporting bone are not visualized because they are obscured by the more radiodense tooth. Therefore, facial and lingual bone loss cannot be detected from radiographs.
- Early interdental bone loss is not detectable on radiographs because horizontal alveolar bone loss may not be seen until 20% of the original bone height and density is lost.[15] By the time one sees it radiographically, the bone loss is so far advanced that it is easily detected clinically by probing.
- Bony interdental craters, resulting from vertical bone loss, are not well imaged because facial and lingual ridges of the teeth may be superimposed, and because the dense facial and lingual walls of bone obscure the crater. Interdental craters, therefore, are detected only with the periodontal probe.
- Radiographs do not show soft tissues or connective tissue attachment and consequently cannot show soft tissue changes. Pockets cannot be measured from radiographs except by using radiopaque markers, such as a periodontal probe or silver point placed at the depth of the sulcus before exposure.
- Although such radiographic images as a "moth-eaten" alveolar crest, a discontinuous lamina dura, increased trabeculation, and a thickened periodontal ligament space are suggestive of periodontal abnormality, they are not pathognomonic for periodontitis.[16]
- Normal anatomy can be mistaken for abnormalities on radiographs. Darkened or radiolucent areas, such as the mental and incisive foramina located in apical regions, may masquerade as lesions.
- Although all teeth are radiographically examined for the presence of calculus, films are not the best indicators of calculus. Only highly mineralized deposits may be seen as radiopacities on the radiograph.

Because of these limitations, radiographs must be used only in conjunction with clinical findings to determine a client's periodontal and oral hygiene status. In general, however, the radiographic examination is helpful in observing normal anatomy and the tooth crown-to-root ratio; noting distinctions between vertical and horizontal bone loss; confirming clinical findings and topography of root surfaces, the CEJ, caries, margins of restorations; and viewing the presence of a variable periodontal ligament space.

ASSESSMENT OF PERIODONTAL DISEASE ACTIVITY

The progression of periodontal disease is the "pathogenic process in which connective tissue attachment at the most apical portion of a periodontal pocket is destroyed."[2] Related to this attachment loss is the apical migration of the junctional epithelium and resorption of alveolar bone. Progression of most forms of periodontitis appears to be associated with qualitative changes in the subgingival flora.

At the current time there are no diagnostic tests that have been proven to identify progressing or "active" periodontitis lesions other than longitudinal assessments of radiographs and probing attachment levels. However, in the near future many tests designed for this purpose will be marketed. Some tests are likely to have considerable clinical value, others will be useless. Before purchasing these tests, it is important to make sure that data from well-controlled studies justify their use.[2]

Assessment of periodontal disease activity is an attempt to determine how rapidly periodontitis is progressing and how susceptible the client is to periodontal infections. Statistical concepts commonly used to explain the reliability of diagnostic tests for measuring progression of periodontitis are **sensitivity** and **specificity**. Sensitivity refers to the degree of the test's ability to provide a positive result when clinical signs of disease are also positive. Specificity refers to the test's ability to provide a negative result when there are no clinical signs of disease. A diagnostic test that could detect all progressing sites without registering a false negative (100% sensitivity) and could identify all nonprogressing sites without registering a false positive (100% specificity) would be an ideal test. Such a test would have sensitivity and specificity values of 1.00. Table 13–7 lists clinical indicators of periodontal disease progression and evaluates them for sensitivity and specificity. For example, according to data in Table 13–7, gingival redness correlates with the presence of periodontitis only 27% of the time, and lack of gingival redness correlates with lack of disease 67% of the time.

Tests for Disease Activity

Measure of Attachment Loss

An increase in the distance measured from the CEJ to the base of the sulcus or pocket currently is the best measure for disease progression. Flaws in this measure, however, are related to the fact that the probe's penetration can vary with its thickness, the insertion force, and the degree of inflammation in the tissues.[17] In addition, it is difficult to position the periodontal probe in exactly the same position from one appointment to another. The dental hygienist must be aware of these limitations and try to compensate for them by using standardized equipment and techniques as much as possible.

Clinical Signs of Inflammation

Redness, swelling, bleeding on probing, and suppuration have been reported to have relatively good diagnostic specificity (in Table 13–7 values range from 0.67 to 0.99), but they have poor sensitivity (in Table 13–7 values range from 0.02 to 0.32). Two long-term studies of persons on

TABLE 13–7
EVALUATION OF CLINICAL PARAMETERS FOR MEASURING PROGRESSION OF PERIODONTITIS

	Sensitivity	Specificity	False Positive Ratio	Sensitivity False Positive Ratio	Predictability P_{F+}	P_{F-}
Gingival redness	0.27	0.67	0.34	0.8	0.98	0.03
Plaque	0.47	0.65	0.36	1.3	0.96	0.03
BOP	0.32	0.82	0.18	1.8	0.95	0.03
Supporation	0.02	0.99	0.01	2.0	0.95	0.03
Pocket depth < 4 mm	0.34	0.25	0.75	0.5	0.99	0.07
Pocket depth 4–6 mm	0.41	0.83	0.17	2.4	0.93	0.02
Pocket Depth > 6 mm	0.25	0.92	0.08	3.1	0.91	0.03
Attachment level < 4 mm	0.09	0.30	0.70	0.1	0.99	0.09
Attachment level 4–6 mm	0.61	0.81	0.19	3.2	0.91	0.02
Attachment level > 6 mm	0.30	0.89	0.11	2.7	0.92	0.02

Adapted from Haffajee, A. D., Socransky, S. S., and Goodson, J. M. Clinical parameters as predictors of destructive periodontal disease activity. Journal of Clinical Periodontology 10:257, 1983. ©1983 Munksgaard International Publishers Ltd., Copenhagen, Denmark.

periodontal maintenance programs found that sites that did not bleed on probing were almost certain not to show further loss of attachment.[5] Of sites that did bleed on probing at four consecutive visits, 30% lost 2 mm or more of probing attachment. These findings suggest that whereas bleeding on probing may have some clinical value as an indicator of increased risk of progression, the continuous absence of bleeding on probing is a reliable indicator that periodontal health will be maintained.[2]

Monitoring of Periodontal Pocket Temperatures

Although measuring small changes in pocket temperatures over time has been suggested as a way of objectively measuring inflammation,[18,19] the value of such an approach in detecting disease progression has not been established.

Microscopic Assessment of Subgingival Plaque

A sample of subgingival plaque is placed on a slide and immediately viewed under a darkfield or phase contrast microscope to identify motile and nonmotile bacteria and to categorize bacteria into general morphotypes (e.g., cocci, rods, spirochetes). With this method there is a good correlation (0.80) between increased percentages of subgingival spirochetes and disease progression in untreated persons. Unfortunately, the pathogenic potential and the number of microorganisms required to cause disease cannot be determined by this method.

Microbiological Assessment of Subgingival Plaque

A number of bacteria, found in untreated persons with periodontitis, have been suggested as possible periodontopathogens:

- Spirochetes
- *Porphyromonas (Bacteroides intermedius) gingivalis*
- *Bacteroides forsythus*
- *Prevotella (Bacteroides) intermedia*
- *Campylobacter rectus (Wollinella recta)*
- *Eikenella corrodens*
- *Capnocytophaga sputigena*
- *Actinobacillus actinomycetemcomitans*
- *Fusobacterium nucleatum*
- *Peptostreptococcus micros*
- *Selenomonas sputigena*
- *Eubacterium alactolyticum*
- *Haemophilus aphrophilus*
- *Treponema denticola*

Which of these organisms, singly or in groups, is responsible for the progression of periodontitis is not known. Nevertheless, sufficient research exists to implicate these microorganisms as potential periodontopathogens, so that methods have been devised to detect their presence in subgingival flora as a measure of disease activity. Methods to do this include the following:

Microbiological Cultural Analysis A sample of subgingival plaque is collected and cultured in the laboratory to determine the presence of specific microorganisms—marker bacteria—associated with the progression of periodontitis (e.g., *Actinobacillus actinomycetemcomitans, Prevotella intermedia,* and *Porphyromonas*). However, this method is time-consuming and relies on bacterial samples that must be specially handled so they can survive several days in transport to the laboratory. Consequently it is not a test that is readily used by the clinician.

Immunologic Methods Antibodies specific for particular bacterial species are applied to plaque samples and antibody-antigen reactions are detected by a variety of methods such as direct and indirect immunofluorescence, rapid enzyme immunoassay, and latex agglutination tests. Although direct and indirect immunofluorescence is a test that is valuable as a research tool, it requires considerable expertise and expense to perform in evaluating plaque samples. Other assays are only moderately sensitive, but their results can be read in the oral healthcare setting within minutes.

DNA Probes Fragments of bacterial deoxyribonucleic acid (DNA) are used in hybridization reactions to probe for complementary DNA in subgingival plaque samples. Tests for *Porphyromonas gingivalis, Prevotella intermedia,* and *Actinobacillus actinomycetemcomitans* are commercially available.

Bacterial Enzymatic Activity Chemicals that indicate the presence of enzymes produced by periodontopathogens are applied to plaque samples. Such tests may have value in detecting relative levels of certain periodontopathogens.

Assessments of Cell Death or Tissue Breakdown Products Aspartate aminotransferase (AST) is an enzyme released upon death of cells. In preliminary research, marked elevations in AST levels were reported in GCF samples obtained from sites with severe gingival inflammation[20] or with recent attachment loss.[20,21,22] In addition, enzyme-linked immunoadsorbent assays (ELISA) to detect collagen breakdown products in gingival crevicular fluid are being pursued as possible diagnostic tests. Finally, preliminary research suggests that the content of sulfated glycosamino glycans in gingival crevicular fluids is elevated in persons with periodontitis.

Assessment of Inflammatory Mediators Offenbacher and colleagues have shown that the mean levels of prostaglandin E_2 (PGE_2) in samples of GCF collected from the entire mouth had a high degree of sensitivity (0.76), specificity (0.96), and predictability (0.92–0.95) when used as a test to determine whether persons with periodontitis were in remission or about to undergo an episode of attachment loss.[23]

Subtraction Radiography

Subtraction radiographic methods, though not widely available, can detect very small changes in the density of alveolar bone when digitized images of two standardized radiographs taken at different times are subtracted from one another.[24,25] In a recent study,[26] the progression of periodontitis was monitored in 21 persons over 9 months by use of a manual periodontal probe and computer-assisted densitometric image analysis of standardized radiographs. Whereas the periodontal probe detected clinical attachment loss in a mean of 6% of the sites per person, the radiographic analysis detected loss of radiographic density in alveolar bone in a mean of 38% of sites per person—a higher prevalence of disease progression than previously reported in the literature. These findings suggest that the current view that gingivitis progresses to periodontitis in only a small percentage of sites and in short bursts of disease activity may need to be reexamined.

ORAL HYGIENE ASSESSMENT

The recognition of bacterial plaque is of significant importance in client education. Self-care is the client's responsibility for and contribution toward his own health. Self-care has pattern and sequence and, when effectively performed, contributes greatly to the quality of oral health. Since the classic studies on periodontal disease report that 50 to 90% of the population has periodontal disease, there is evidence to suggest that the oral hygiene self-care techniques of many individuals need improvement. Assessment data collected on oral hygiene status assists the dental hygienist in recognizing human need deficits (e.g., self-determination and responsibility, conceptualization and problem-solving), communicating these deficits to clients, and instructing them in effective techniques for bacterial plaque control.

Oral hygiene assessment includes evaluating the presence and amount of hard and soft deposits on the teeth as well as evaluating the client's knowledge, skill, and motivation related to using personal oral hygiene cleaning devices. Table 13–8 and Figures 13–27 and 13–28 show soft and hard deposits that accumulate on teeth. Bacterial plaque is the most important of these deposits because it is the cause of dental caries and periodontal diseases. Stain and calculus serve to trap bacteria plaque, and they have cosmetic implications for the client. Therefore, the amount and extent of plaque, stain, and calculus are important oral hygiene variables for the dental hygienist to evaluate during the assessment phase of the dental hygiene process of care.

TABLE 13–8
HARD AND SOFT ACQUIRED DEPOSITS

Term	Classification	Definition
Acquired pellicle and exogenous dental cuticle	Acellular, nonmineralized layer	An unstructured, homogenous film adhering to tooth surfaces, firm surfaces in the oral cavity, and old calculus. May be stained by tar products and tannin
Plaque	Cellular, nonmineralized layer	A soft, dense, transparent matrix of microorganisms that adheres to the acquired pellicle
Materia alba	Cellular, nonmineralized layer	Loose deposit of microorganisms, desquamated epithelial cells and broken down food debris; white to yellowish white in color; has cottage cheese-like appearance. Can be removed with rinsing and water irrigation
Food debris	Cellular, nonmineralized layer	Unstructured particles that remain in the mouth after eating and that are removed with irrigation unless impacted between the teeth
Extrinsic stain	Cellular may be mineralized or nonmineralized	Discolorations that accumulate on the external surface of the tooth via pellicle, plaque, or calculus that can be removed by toothbrushing, scaling, and/or polishing
Supragingival calculus	Cellular, mineralized layer	Mineralized bacterial plaque permeated with moderately hard calcium phosphate crystals; superficially covered with bacterial plaque; usually white or yellowish-white in color but may be stained darker
Subgingival calculus	Cellular, mineralized layer	Mineralized bacterial plaque; adheres to tooth structure in the gingival sulcus; organic matrix of bacteria permeated with hard calcium phosphate crystals. May be stained dark green to green-black; superficially covered with bacterial plaque

Adapted from Schroeder, H. E., and Hirzel, H. C. A method of studying dental plaque morphology. Helvetica Odontologica Acta 13(1):22, 1969.

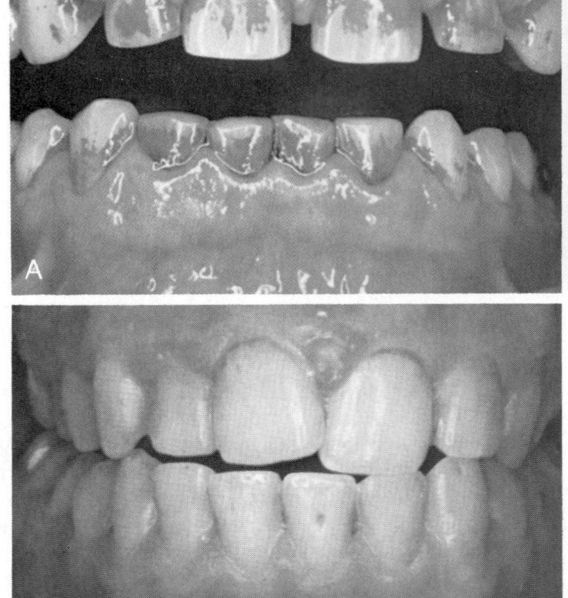

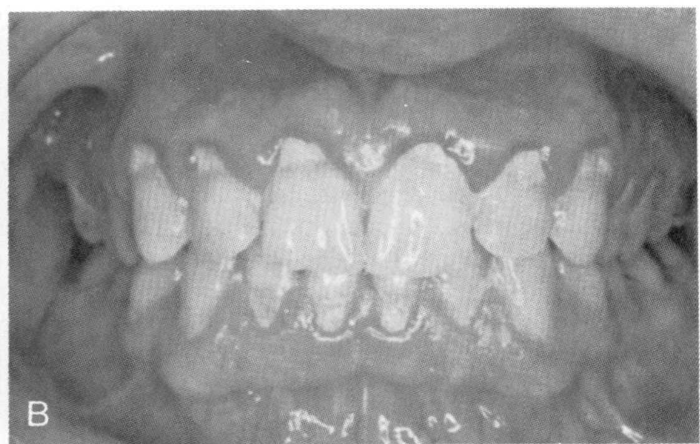

FIGURE 13–27
Deposits on tooth surfaces. *A*, Disclosed supragingival plaque covering one-half to two-thirds of the clinical crowns. (Courtesy of Dr. S. Socransky.) *B*, Material alba generalized throughout the mouth, with heaviest accumulation near the gingiva. Note the gingivitis present. *C*, Green stain on anterior teeth. Note the inflamed, enlarged interdental papilla between the maxillary central incisors. (*B* and *C* from Carranza, F. Glickman's Clinical Periodontology, 7th ed. Philadelphia: W. B. Saunders, 1990, p. 347.)

Bacterial Plaque

Bacterial plaque is a dense, nonmineralized, highly organized mass of bacterial colonies in a gel-like intermicrobial matrix. In the periodontally healthy person, bacterial plaque initially is composed of a preponderance of gram-positive rods and coccal forms with few spirochetes and motile forms. Examples of some of the predominant microorganisms present in this health-associated plaque are *Streptococcus mitis, Actinomyces* species, and *Streptococcus oralis* (*sanguis II*). In bacterial plaque associated with gingivitis, there is an increase in thickness and mass of plaque with an increase of gram-negative motile rods and spirochetes. Examples of some of the predominant organisms are *Fusobacterium nucleatum*, various species of *Prevotella* and *Treponema,* and *Campylobacter rectus* (*Wolinella recta*). In advancing periodontitis the plaque is characterized by a zone of gram-positive organisms that attach to the tooth surface and a loosely adherent zone of gram-negative organisms and spirochetes adjacent to the pocket wall. Important periodontitis-associated organisms include *Porphyromonas gingivalis* (*Bacteroides gingivalis*), *Prevotella intermedia* (*Bacteroides intermedius*), *Bacteroides forsythus, Treponema denticola, Peptostreptococcus micros* and other microorganisms.

Clinically, plaque is a transparent film of bacteria that accumulates on teeth every 12 to 24 hours. To help reveal plaque in the mouth, a variety of disclosing agents are on

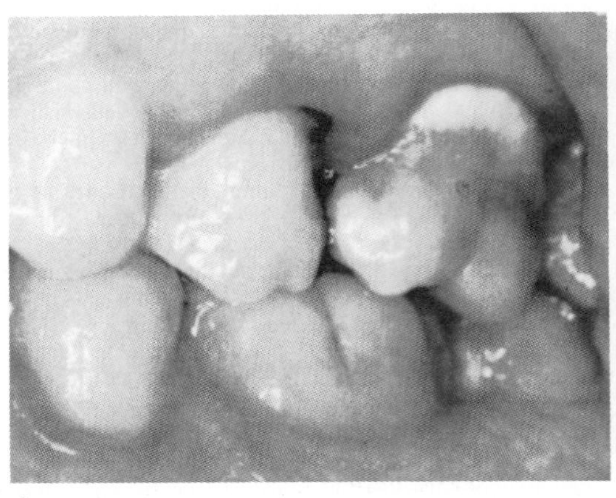

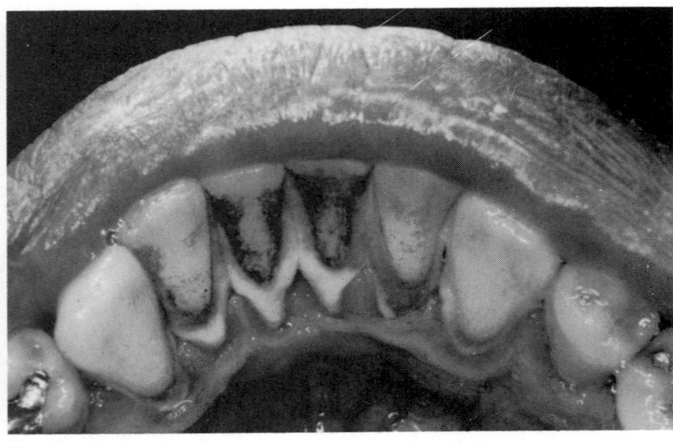

FIGURE 13–28
A, Calculus on molar opposite Stensen's duct. *B*, Calculus and stain on lingual surface in relation to orifice of submaxillary and sublingual glands. (From Carranza, F. Glickman's Clinical Periodontology, 7th ed. Philadelphia: W. B. Saunders, 1990, p. 391.)

STAGE 1	Proteins in the saliva attach to the tooth enamel to form PELLICLE PROTEIN + TOOTH = PELLICLE
STAGE 2	Microorganisms in the saliva colonize the pellicle to form EARLY PLAQUE (gram + aerobic cocci and rods predominate) PELLICLE + MICROORGANISMS = PLAQUE
STAGE 3	Plaque microorganisms multiply and change as plaque ages (IN MATURE PLAQUE gram-facultative and anaerobic filamentous forms and fusobacteria predominate, followed by the appearance of spirochetes. Mature plaque has a greater proportion of pathogenic types of microorganisms and is more associated with disease than early plaque) PLAQUE + TIME = MATURE PLAQUE

FIGURE 13–29
The three stages of bacterial plaque formation. (Based on Katz, S., McDonald, J. L., and Stookey, G. K. Preventive Dentistry. Upper Montclair, NJ: DCP Publishing, 1976, p. 74.)

the market, in either liquid or tablet form, that contain dye or other coloring agents. When applied to the teeth the agent imparts its color to the plaque, but it can be rinsed readily from clean tooth surfaces.

Plaque is classified by its location: *supragingival plaque* is on the clinical crown of the tooth above the margin of the gingiva; *subgingival plaque* is on the part of the tooth beneath the margin of the gingiva.

Generally, there are three stages to plaque formation (Fig. 13–29). First, an **acquired pellicle** forms on the tooth surface. The acquired pellicle is an acellular (contains no bacteria or other cell forms) organic tenacious film that is composed of glycoproteins from the saliva. Within minutes after a tooth surface is thoroughly cleaned and polished the acquired pellicle begins to form on the exposed tooth surface. Second, bacteria from indigenous oral microflora attach to the pellicle and form microbial colonies in layers as the bacteria grow and multiply. An intermicrobial substance is formed mainly from saliva and from polysaccharides produced by certain bacteria from sucrose in the diet. The polysaccharides are sticky and facilitate the adhesion of plaque to the tooth surface. Unlike food debris, plaque is not removed by oral irrigation. Third, as plaque ages, a change in the types of microorganisms occurs within plaque (Fig. 13–30). Plaque that is 1 to 2 days old consists primarily of cocci. By days 2 to 4 the filamentous forms grow and replace the cocci. By days 4 to 7, filamentous forms increase, and rods and fusobacteria appear. By days 7 to 14, vibrios and spirochetes appear, and more gram-negative and anerobic microorganisms appear. Bacterial plaque, if not mechanically disturbed, produces a greater proportion of those microorganisms associated with periodontal disease.

The plaque that forms on the tooth adjacent to and under the margin of the gingiva is of particular concern with regard to periodontal disease. The longer the plaque remains undisturbed, the older it becomes and the greater is its pathogenic potential. In periodontal disease there is a shift in the plaque bacteria to higher proportions of gram-negative and anerobic bacteria.

Stain

There are two basic types of stain that can be observed on client's teeth: intrinsic and extrinsic. **Intrinsic stain** results from alterations during the development of the tooth (embryonic to 6 years of age), related to events such as antibiotic use, fevers, accidental trauma, infection, and exposure to a high amount of systemic fluoride. Intrinsic stains cannot be removed by scaling and polishing because they are incorporated into the enamel. Examples of intrinsic stains include dental fluorosis—a mottled, opaque or brownish discoloration caused by ingesting excessive quantities of fluoride during enamel formation—and tetracycline stain—a yellow, brown or orange discoloration within the substance of the tooth from ingestion of the antibiotic when the tooth is developing.

Extrinsic stains are removable and result from the presence of certain bacteria or from the use of such substances as tobacco, coffee, tea, certain drugs, wine, and food.[27] Brown, black, green, metallic, and tobacco extrinsic stains have been studied to identify how and why they attach to the teeth (see Fig. 13–27*C*). Results of these studies indicate that a smooth enamel surface does not stain. Formation of acquired pellicle or plaque is required for extrinsic stains to attach to the tooth. Chromogenic bacteria (*Actinomyces,* and occasionally *Bacteroides melaninogenicus*), foods (with tannin, such as coffee, tea, and red wine), and chemicals (like metals, chlorhexidine, alexidine) usually stain the pellicle or accumulated plaque. The root surface is more porous than enamel, and thus cementum and dentin surfaces may stain permanently.

Green and black line stains are thought to result from gram-positive microorganisms embedded in the pellicle along the gingival margin. Both are found more commonly in childhood but may occur despite good oral hygiene in middle-aged women. Extrinsic stain usually can be scaled or polished away. However, green stain may become embedded in demineralized enamel under the chromogenic plaque. As a result, this stain becomes intrinsic, and attempts to remove it by scaling may result in removal of decalcified enamel. Personal oral hygiene practices such as toothbrushing help to prevent stain from reforming, and fluoride rinses act to harden the underlying tooth structure. The exact nature of stains can be determined microscopically, but usually the same information is determined by questioning the client about causes. Diet, oral hygiene, tobacco products, coffee, tea, red wine, and industrial exposure all may contribute to extrinsic stains (Table 13–9).

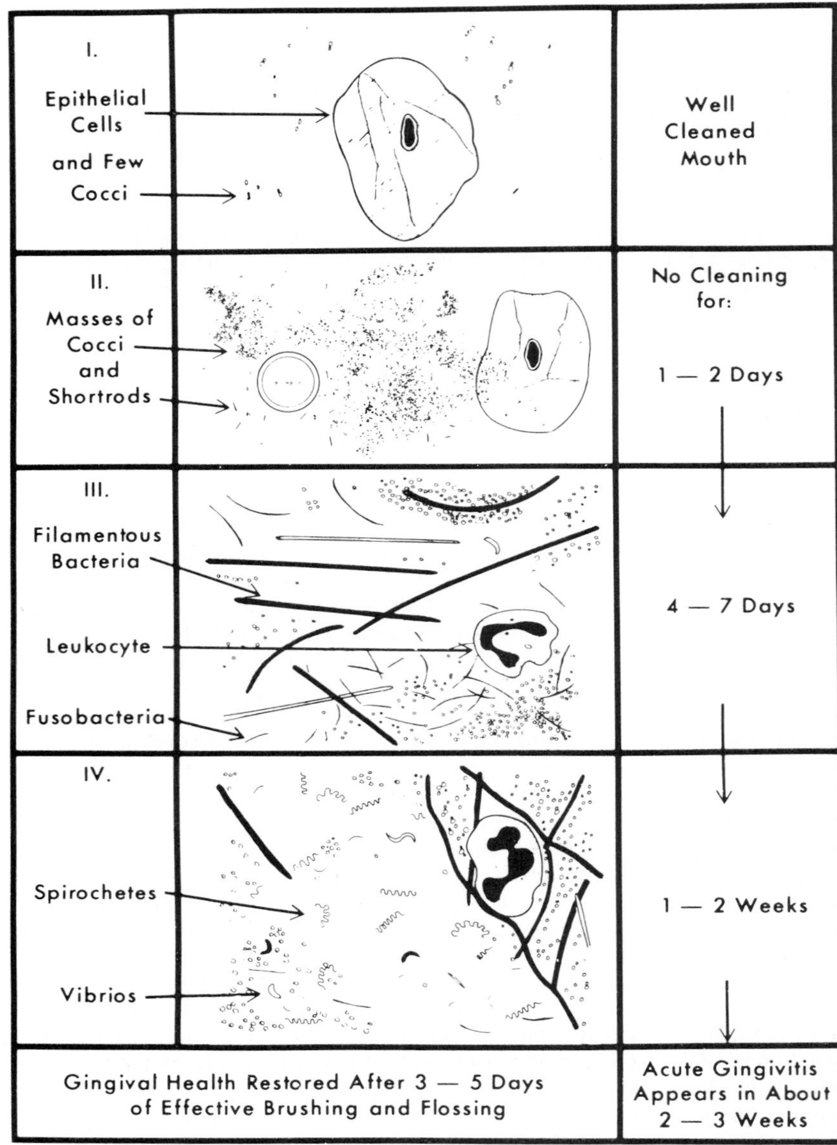

FIGURE 13–30
Plaque microorganisms. On the right are the time intervals from 1 day to 3 weeks. On the left are the changes in the plaque content that take place as plaque ages. As the numbers of microorganisms increase, the numbers of defense cells (leukocytes) also increase. (With permission from Crawford, J. J. Microbiology. In Barton, R. E., Matteson, S. R., and Richardson, R. E. The Dental Assistant, 6th ed. Philadelphia: Lea & Febiger, 1988, p. 74.)

Calculus

Calculus, also known by the lay term "tartar," is calcified plaque (see Figs. 13–27*C* and 13–28*A* and *B*). Calculus is discovered on visual examination, probing or exploring, and on radiographic survey. Characteristics and classifications of calculus are described in Table 13–8 and in greater detail in Chapter 18. The rough surface of calculus retains bacterial plaque and keeps it in contact with gingival tissue, promoting inflammation. Therefore, calculus is associated with the progression of periodontal disease and should be removed from the tooth surface.

Skill, Motivation, and Compliance

Assessment of the individual client's oral hygiene skill and motivation is critical for establishing an effective plaque control program. In clinical practice, disclosants have been successfully used to evaluate a client's ability to remove plaque as well as to evaluate the efficacy of specific oral hygiene devices in removing plaque. McConaughy and colleagues found that clients' acceptance of oral hygiene recommendations improves when they are taught oral hygiene skills in small steps to match their individual needs and when they receive supervised practice sessions with immediate feedback from the dental hygienist.[28]

Periodontal and Oral Hygiene Indices

There are many ways of quantifying periodontal health and oral hygiene status. However, the specific method selected is influenced by whether the purpose is to document research findings related to a large group or to evaluate the status of a single individual, the results of which are used to identify professional care needs and to communicate to the client an assessment of his self-care behaviors. For example,

TABLE 13–9
TYPES OF STAINS

Type	Source	Clinical Approach
Extrinsic Stain		
Green	Chromogenic bacteria from poor oral hygiene; most often seen in children with enamel irregularities	Should not be scaled because of underlying demineralized enamel. Have client remove during toothbrush instruction and reinforcement
Black-line stain	Iron in saliva; often seen in females with good oral hygiene	Firmly scale because of calculus-like nature as well as polish for complete removal
Orange	Chromogenic bacteria from poor oral hygiene	Lightly scale and then polish
Tobacco	Tars from smoking and chewing and dipping spitting tobacco	Lightly scale and then polish
Food	Food and beverage pigment	Lightly scale and then polish
Drug	Chlorhexidine, stannous fluoride, extended antibiotic use	Scale and then polish
Intrinsic Stain		
Fluorosis (white-spotted to brown-pitted enamel)	Excessive fluoride ingestion during enamel development	Cannot be removed by scaling and polishing
Hypocalcification (white spots on enamel)	High fever during enamel formation; endocrine and other metabolic causes	Cannot be removed by scaling or polishing
Decalcification (white to brown enamel —may be smooth or rough)	Acid erosion of enamel caused by bacterial plaque	Cannot be removed by scaling and polishing—recommend daily 0.05% sodium fluoride rinses for remineralization
Tetracycline (grayish brown discoloration)	Ingestion of tetracycline during tooth development	Cannot be removed by scaling or polishing

if the dental hygienist is to survey the prevalence of periodontal disease and plaque in a particular population (epidemiological research), it is important to use indices used by other researchers so that the results can be compared. However, if the dental hygienist intends to assess a single individual's periodontal and oral hygiene status for the purpose of developing a care plan for that person, it is important to select an assessment method that is simple, cost-effective, and easily understood to motivate the client to adopt recommended oral hygiene behaviors. The following section presents periodontal and oral hygiene indices commonly used in research and client care.

Indices Used in Research

Periodontal and oral hygiene are used in epidemiology to quantify the prevalence and incidence of disease and oral debris in specific populations. *Prevalence* refers to the number of cases existing at a specific point in time per specified number of persons. For example, the statement "52% of 1,328 college baseball athletes reported using dental floss daily" is a statement of floss use prevalence. *Incidence* refers to the number of new cases per specified number of persons occurring in a specified period of time, typically 1 year. For example, the statement "40,000 new cases of periodontitis were diagnosed in the United States from 1992 to 1993" is a statement of incidence. *Severity* refers to how much destruction is present at one time. For instance, 5 mm of attachment loss is a standard often used to indicate the need for periodontal treatment. Periodontal and oral hygiene indices are used in research to describe prevalence, incidence, and severity of disease in populations and to serve as outcome measures when testing the efficacy of approaches to care, such as when fluoride toothpaste is tested to determine its effectiveness in preventing periodontal disease.

Popular periodontal and oral hygiene indices often used in research are listed and compared in Table 13–10. Usually a subset of teeth described by Ramfjord is used in evaluating groups of people. Based on large-scale studies, Ramfjord determined that measurement of six teeth (#3, #9, #12, #19, #25, #28) were representative of those for the entire dentition. These six teeth are called the Ramfjord teeth.[29] When data collection is limited to a few representative teeth, the index is called "simplified." Methods of substitution are always calibrated in the simplified index. In some studies missing teeth are not counted, and in others the clinician is required to substitute missing teeth with the next most distal tooth. Other indices require substitution by going mesially or across the arch to the contralateral tooth.

A limitation of indices is that each index usually measures only one variable, and thus more than one index frequently is needed. For example, the Gingival Index of Silness and Loe provides information about the presence and severity of gingival inflammation in a population at a given time, but it provides no information about the cause of the inflammation. In contrast, the Plaque Index of Podshadley does provide information on the location and thickness of plaque (the cause of the inflammation), but does not provide information about inflammation. Moreover, indices that measure the same variable often do not have the same focus. For example, the thickness of plaque is important in the Silness and Loe Plaque Index, but not in the Turesky modification of the Quigley-Hein Index (see Table 13–10).

In choosing a good index for measuring periodontal

Text continued on page 390

TABLE 13–10
PERIODONTAL AND ORAL INDICES

Index	Author	Measures	Procedure for Use	Rating Score
Oral Hygiene Indices				
Simplified Oral Hygiene Index	Greene and Vermillion (1964)	Oral debris and calculus	Divide the dentition into sextants. Using the side of the tip of the periodontal probe or explorer estimate oral debris and supragingival and subgingival calculus on the facial and lingual surfaces of the teeth. Select one tooth from each quadrant with the greatest amount of debris or calculus and score the facial and lingual surfaces using the following criteria: Oral Debris Index 0 = No debris or stain present 1 = Soft debris covering not more than one-third of the tooth surface being examined, or the presence of extrinsic stains without debris, regardless of surface area covered 2 = Soft debris covering more than one-third but not more than two-thirds of the exposed tooth surface 3 = Soft debris covering more than two-thirds of the exposed tooth surface Calculus Index 0 = No calculus present 1 = Supragingival calculus covering not more than one-third of the exposed tooth surface being examined 2 = Supragingival calculus covering more than one-third but not more than two-thirds of the exposed tooth surface, or the presence of individual flecks of subgingival calculus around the cervical portion of the tooth 3 = Supragingival calculus covering more than two-thirds of the exposed tooth surface or a continuous heavy band of subgingival calculus around the cervical portion of the tooth Separately determine the Debris Index (DI) and Calculus Index (CI) by totaling the scores and dividing the total by the number of sextants. Add the DI and CI to determine the OHI-S.	OHI-S 0.0–1.2: Good oral hygiene 1.3–3.0: Fair oral hygiene 3.1–6.0: Poor oral hygiene DI-S or CI-S: 0.0–0.6: Good oral hygiene 0.7–1.8: Fair oral hygiene 1.9–3.0: Poor oral hygiene
Plaque Index (PI)	Silness and Loe (1967)	Plaque accumulation	Four gingival scoring units, mesial, distal, buccal, and lingual, are examined on the following teeth: #3, #9, #12, #19, #25, and #28. A mouth mirror, dental explorer, and air are used to score the tooth surfaces for plaque using the following criteria: 0 = No plaque 1 = A film of plaque adhering to the free gingival margin and adjacent area of the tooth. The plaque may be recognized only after application of disclosing agent or by running the explorer across the tooth surface 2 = Moderate accumulation of soft deposits within the gingival pocket that can be seen with the naked eye or on the tooth and gingival margin 3 = Abundance of soft matter within the gingival crevice and/or the tooth and gingival margin PI for area is obtained by totaling 4 plaque scores per tooth. If sum of PI scores per tooth is divided by 4, PI	Excellent: 0 Good: 0.1–0.9 Fair: 1.0–1.9 Poor: 2.0–3.0

TABLE 13–10
PERIODONTAL AND ORAL INDICES *Continued*

Index	Author	Measures	Procedure for Use	Rating Score
			score for tooth is obtained. PI score per person is obtained by adding PI scores per tooth and dividing by number of teeth examined. May be obtained for a segment or group of teeth	
Plaque Index	Turesky Modification of Quigley and Hein (1970)	Plaque accumulation	0 = Absence of plaque 1 = Discontinuous band of plaque at the gingival margin 2 = >1 mm continuous band of plaque at gingival margin 3 = <1 mm band of plaque but > the gingival 1/3 of the tooth surface 4 = Plaque covering < 1/3 but > 2/3 of the tooth surface 5 = Plaque covering 2/3 or more of the tooth surface	
Patient Hygiene Performance (PHP)	Podshadely and Haley (1968)	Plaque accumulation	Teeth disclosed: The following six teeth are evaluated: #3, #8, #14, #19, #24, and #30. Each tooth is divided into 5 areas: 3 longitudinal thirds, distal, middle, and mesial; the middle third is subdivided horizontally into incisal, middle, and gingival thirds. Score per person is obtained by totaling 5 subdivision scores per tooth surface and dividing by number of tooth surfaces examined	
Plaque Index	Ramfjord (1967)	Plaque	Apply disclosing agent, request client to rinse with water. For teeth #3, #9, #12, #19, #25, and #28, 4 surfaces (facial, lingual, mesial, and distal) are scored using the following criteria: 0 = No plaque 1 = Plaque present on some but not all interproximal, facial, and lingual surfaces of the tooth 2 = Plaque presents on all interproximal, facial, and lingual surfaces, but covering less than one-half of these surfaces 3 = Plaque extending over all interproximal, facial, and lingual surfaces, and covering more than one-half of these surfaces Add the plaque scores for each tooth and divide by the number of teeth examined.	
Calculus Index	Ramfjord (1967)	Calculus	An explorer or probe may be used to locate subgingival calculus and determine its extent. For teeth #3, #9, #12, #19, #25, and #28, 4 surfaces (facial, lingual, mesial, and distal) are scored using the following criteria: 0 = No calculus 1 = Supragingival calculus extending only slightly below the free gingival margin (not more than 1 mm) 2 = Moderate amount of supra- and subgingival calculus, or subgingival calculus only 3 = Abundance of supra- and subgingival calculus Add scores for each surface and divide by the number of surfaces (4) for tooth score. Add the scores for the individual teeth and divide by the number of teeth to determine the calculus score for an individual.	

Table continued on following page

TABLE 13–10
PERIODONTAL AND ORAL INDICES *Continued*

Index	Author	Measures	Procedure for Use	Rating Score
Periodontal Disease Indices				
Community Periodontal Index of Treatment Needs (CIPTN)	Ainamo (1982)	Periodontal status and treatment needs	For adults (20 years and older), divide the dentition into sextants. Evaluate all teeth except third molars. For children and adolescents (7–19 years of age) divide the dentition into sextants but evaluate only the first molars in posterior; right central incisor in maxilla; and the left central incisor in mandibular anterior. Use the WHO periodontal probe marked at 3.5-, 2.0-, 3.0-, and 3.0-mm intervals from the tip with color-coding between 3.5 and 5.5 mm and a ball 0.5 mm in diameter at the working tip. Score according to the following criteria: Code 0 = Healthy periodontal tissues Code 1 = Bleeding after gentle probing Code 2 = Supra- or subgingival calculus or defective margin of filling or crown Code 3 = 4- or 5-mm pocket Code 4 = 6-mm or deeper pathological pocket Mark one score to represent each sextant. Record only the highest code that corresponds with the most severe condition. Patients are classified (0, I, II, III) into treatment needs according to the highest coded score recorded during the examination. Criteria for classification are: 0 = No need for treatment (Code 0) I = Oral hygiene instruction (Code 1) II = Oral hygiene instruction plus scaling and root planing, including elimination of plaque retentive margins of fillings and crowns (Codes 2 and 3) III = I + II + complex periodontal therapy that may include surgical intervention and/or deep scaling and root planing with local anesthesia (Code 4)	To identify high and low priorities for treatment in a community, calculations of the number and percentage of individuals with the following can be made: a. No sextant scoring each code b. 1 to 2 sextants scoring Code 1, 2, 3, or 4 c. 3 to 4 sextants scoring Code 1, 2, 3, or 4 d. 5 to 6 sextants scoring Code 1, 2, 3, or 4
Gingival Index (GI)	Loe and Silness (1963)	Gingival Inflammation	A score of 0 to 3 is assigned to mesial, distal, buccal, and lingual surfaces of teeth #3, #9, #12, #19, #25, and #28. A blunt instrument, such as a periodontal probe, is used to assess bleeding potential based on the following criteria: 0 = Normal gingiva 1 = Mild inflammation—slight change in color, slight edema. *No bleeding on probing* 2 = Moderate inflammation—redness, edema, and glazing. *Bleeding on probing* 3 = Severe inflammation—marked redness and edema. Ulceration. *Tendency to spontaneous bleeding* Totaling scores around each tooth yields GI score for area; divide by 4, score for tooth is determined. Totaling all scores and dividing by number of teeth examined provides GI score per person. Can be used on selected or all erupted teeth	0.1–1.0: Mild gingivitis 1.1–2.0: Moderate gingivitis 2.1–3.0: Severe gingivitis

TABLE 13–10
PERIODONTAL AND ORAL INDICES *Continued*

Index	Author	Measures	Procedure for Use	Rating Score
Periodontal Index (PI)	Russell (1967)	Gingival inflammation pocket presence and mobility	A score for each individual is obtained by arriving at a score for mesial, distal, facial and lingual surfaces of all teeth in the mouth, adding the scores, and dividing by the total number of teeth. The following scoring system is used: 0 = Negative: neither overt inflammation in the investing tissues nor loss of function due to destruction of supporting tissues 1 = Mild gingivitis: an overt area of inflammation in the free gingivae, but this area does not circumscribe the tooth 2 = Gingivitis: inflammation completely circumscribes tooth, but there is no apparent break in epithelial attachment 4 = Not used in the field study 6 = Gingivitis with pocket formation: epithelial attachment has been broken and there is a pocket (not merely a deepened gingival crevice due to swelling in the free gingivae). No interference with normal masticatory function; the tooth is firm in its socket and has not drifted 8 = Advanced destruction with loss of masticatory function: tooth may be loose; may have drifted; may sound dull on percussion with a metallic instrument; may be depressable in its socket	0.0–0.2: Clinically normal 0.3–0.9: Gingivitis 0.7–1.9: Incipient destructive disease 1.5–5.0: Established destructive disease 3.8–8.0: Terminal states of disease
Periodontal Disease Index	Ramfjord (1967)	Extent of periodontal disease	Six teeth are examined: #3, #9, #12, #19, #25, and #28. PDI assesses gingivitis, gingival sulcus depth, calculus, plaque, occlusal and incisal attrition mobility, and lack of contact. Criteria used for evaluation are: 0 = Absence of inflammation 1 = Mild to moderate inflammatory gingival changes not extending all around tooth 2 = Mild to moderately severe gingivitis extending all around tooth 3 = Severe gingivitis, characterized by marked redness, tendency to bleed, and ulceration 4 = Gingival crevice in any of 4 measured areas (mesial, distal, buccal, lingual), extending apically to cementoenamel junction but not more than 3 mm 5 = Gingival crevice in any of 4 measured areas extending apically to cementoenamel junction (3–6 mm) 6 = Gingival crevice in any of 4 measured areas extending apically more than 6 mm from cementoenamel junction PDI score is obtained by totaling scores of the teeth and dividing by number of teeth examined	Group score of 3.5 = severe gingivitis for epidemiologic purposes. Care must be taken when interpreting the PDI on an individual basis.
Sulcular Bleeding Index (SBI)	Muhlemann and Son (1971)	Gingival inflammation and bleeding on probing	Four gingival units are scored each tooth: the marginal gingiva, labial and lingual (M units), and the papillary gingiva, mesial and distal (P units). Probe each of the four areas. Hold the	

Table continued on following page

TABLE 13–10
PERIODONTAL AND ORAL INDICES *Continued*

Index	Author	Measures	Procedure for Use	Rating Score
			probe parallel with the long axis of the tooth for M units, and direct the probe toward the col area for P units. Wait 30 seconds after probing before scoring, using the following criteria: 0 = Healthy appearance of P and M, no bleeding on sulcus probing 1 = Apparently healthy P and M showing no change in color and no swelling, but bleeding from sulcus on probing 2 = Bleeding on probing *and* change of color caused by inflammation. No swelling or macroscopic edema 3 = Bleeding on probing *and* change in color and slight edematous swelling 4 = (1) Bleeding on probing *and* change in color *and* obvious swelling (2) Bleeding on probing and obvious swelling 5 = Bleeding on probing and spontaneous bleeding *and* change in color, marked swelling with or without ulceration Scores for the 4 units are totalled and divided by 4. By totaling scores for individual teeth and dividing by the number of teeth, the SBI is determined	
Eastman Interdental Bleeding Index	Caton and Polson (1985)	Interdental gingival bleeding	0 = Absence of bleeding when a triangular toothpick is depressed 2 mm inserted interproximally 4 times, and checked 15 seconds later 1 = Bleeding after above procedure	

health or oral health status, it is important to choose an instrument that:

- Is simple to use
- Is painless to the client
- Takes a minimal amount of time to execute
- Is cost-effective in terms of time, money, and armamentarium
- Has clear criteria for standardization and reproducibility
- Uses numerical values on a smooth, graduated scale
- Is statistically valid and reliable

It is essential to calibrate examiners before using any oral index for research purposes. With regard to measuring probing depths, examiners are considered to be calibrated if each one's measurements are within 1 mm, plus or minus, of the others. Some plaque indices require that disclosing solutions be applied and rinsed away after application, whereas others require no rinsing, or the use of no disclosant. However, whether in research or practice, the dental hygienist should standardize all aspects of data gathering.

Procedures for use may vary with different standard indices (see Table 13–10). The Community Periodontal Index of Treatment Needs (CPITN) is of special interest because it provides information on determining periodontal status as well as treatment needs. A special periodontal probe with color-coded gradations was designed for this index. It has a 0.5-mm ball tip to prevent severing of junctional epithelium and to allow some tactile sensation as the clinician probes the tooth surface in the pocket. Shallow pockets are represented by reporting a sulcus less than a color-coded gradation from 3.5 to 5.5 mm, a finding that indicates no special treatment is needed. Deeper pockets measuring within the color gradation require professional scaling. The deepest pockets, where the color-coded gradation cannot be seen (more than 5.5 mm), require complex treatment, described as scaling and root planing under local anesthesia, with or without surgical exposure for access.

Sextants of the mouth or the full mouth can be assessed by the CPITN, but in epidemiological studies only 10 teeth are examined. Only the worst score per sextant is recorded. This may underestimate the number of deep pockets in older adult populations that generally have many areas of attachment loss, and overestimate shallow pockets in younger age groups that have many healthy sulci. Other indices are shown in Table 13–10.

Indices Commonly Used for Individual Client Care

Indices that assess an individual client's periodontal and oral hygiene status or demonstrate personal progress also are used in dental hygiene. Indices performed on an individual to promote personal awareness are best evaluated over the entire dentition or mouth, rather than simplified

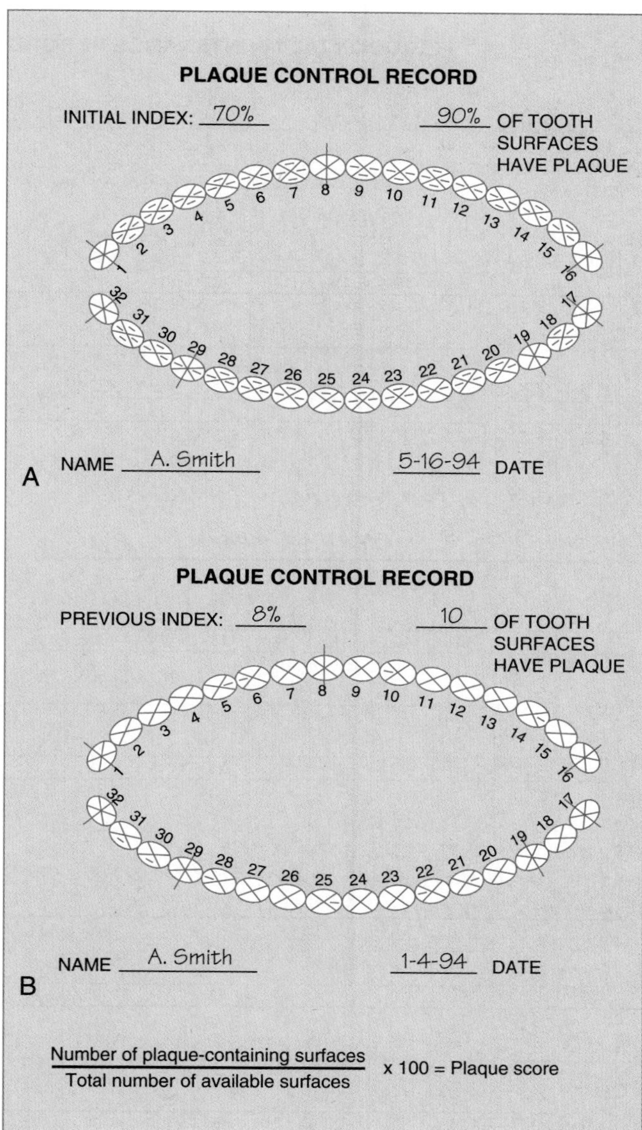

FIGURE 13–31
Plaque control record form. *A*, 70% of tooth surfaces have plaque at initial appointment. *B*, 8% of the tooth surfaces have plaque at a follow-up visit. (Redrawn with permission from O'Leary, T. J., Drake, R. B., and Naylor, J. E. The plaque control record. Journal of Periodontology 48:38, 1972.)

to a narrow field. The absence of inflammation, as measured by lack of bleeding on probing while monitoring attachment level, is the most valid test for gingival health. The Eastman Interdental Bleeding Index (EIBI), shown in Table 13–10, is an example of an index used to quantify gingival and oral hygiene status for individual clients and to motivate desired behavioral change.

One of the most straightforward plaque indices appropriate for use in client care is O'Leary's Plaque Control Record, designed for use with a disclosing solution, and described in Table 13–10. In addition, the Plaque Control Record provides a simple method of identifying and recording the presence of plaque on the mesial, distal, facial, and lingual surfaces at the gingival margin (Fig. 13–31). Plaque observed is recorded by striking a dash through the appropriate surface or surfaces. After all teeth are examined and scored for plaque, the index is computed by dividing the number of plaque-containing surfaces by the total number of available surfaces. The score that results is the percentage of tooth surfaces in the mouth with plaque. Use of the form over time also allows the client to visualize and monitor his own plaque control progress and therefore facilitates client motivation and behavioral change.

Stain can be quantified by a score similar to the plaque score described above, wherein a minimum percentage of stained areas is acceptable. Stain removal is not only an aesthetic concern to clients, it is also important to the health of the periodontium because stain is associated with the presence of plaque.

DOCUMENTATION AND RECORD KEEPING

The dental hygienist evaluates the information collected throughout the assessment phase of care and records all pertinent findings at each appointment. Such records allow the hygienist to monitor the effects of the client's personal oral hygiene efforts, the progress of healing after professional care, and the status of periodontal health over time. In addition, the data collected on periodontal and oral hygiene status facilitate assessment of the client's human needs for skin and mucous membrane integrity of the head and neck, a biologically sound dentition, self-determination and responsibility, and conceptualization and problem-solving.

A properly planned and organized record-keeping system provides easy recording of and ready access to important information. The format should be brief, complete, comprehensible and permanent. Legal and insurance requirements have changed the simple data collection system of the past into a more complex system that requires ongoing and thorough documentation of the client's oral hygiene and periodontal status at each visit. Documentation protocols should be based on current information related to plaque accumulation and to the following anatomical changes; inflammation, attachment levels (probing depth and gingival recession), furcation involvement, tooth mobility, the width of alveolar gingiva, mucogingival problems, and bone loss determined from radiographs. Today, records of observations must demonstrate the dental hygienist's awareness of the client's periodontal status to legal authorities, as well as to the client.

The dental hygiene record must provide a form for documentation of the baseline or initial data collected about the client. This form should be carefully organized before the client is seen, so that all required data are included and there is one standard location for the information. A well-thought-out record form eliminates having to search for more details or for critical information, thus signalling inadequate record keeping to the client or to the healthcare professionals with whom the dental hygienist collaborates. At subsequent client visits, changes in the baseline conditions are further documented and these data are compared with this baseline information. Diligent record keeping is the key to tracking frequency of care, disease episodes, and the success rate of interventions. Analysis of trends is based upon comparing findings with the baseline data and is as critical to the dental hygiene practitioner as it is to the dental hygiene researcher.

PERIODONTAL MAINTENANCE RECORD

CASE TYPE (I) II III IV V

Watch Status: ~~1~~ (2) (3) 4 5 6 (7) (8) 9 10 11 12 13 14 15 ~~16~~
~~32~~ (31) (30) 29 28 27 26 25 24 23 22 21 (20) (19) 18 ~~17~~

Special Instructions: *needs antibiotic pre-med* For: *Jane Doe*

A = (ACUTE) erythema, swelling, stippling loss, poor tone
C = (CHRONIC) fibrous enlargement, reverse architecture
B = bleeding
S = suppuration
M = minimum attached gingiva
P = mucogingival pocket
Mobility: slt = I° mod = II° adv = III°
Furcations: slt = V mod = ∇ adv = ▼

1/5/94 DDS ✓ $ *68.00*

	ur	ua	ul		lr	la	ll
buc	2	1	2		1	1	2
I.P.	2	2	2		2	2	2
ling	2	2	2		2	2	2

33

OH Routine: *TB 1x/day*
Demonstrated: *BASS Tech & Floss*
Dispensed: *P39 TB & Floss*
DH: (RP) (polish) Fl2
QRP: UR UL LR LL

UPPER	1	2	3	4	5	6	7	8	9	10	11	12	13	14	15	16
		✓	✓											✓	✓	
buccal	X	423	525	323	323	313	315	413	212	333	313	434	333	333	434	X
palatal		325	524	323	323	323	323	324	313	212	333	434	333	333	434	

LOWER	32	31	30	29	28	27	26	25	24	23	22	21	20	19	18	17
lingual	X	325	423	333	333	333	333	333	333	333	333	434	334	434	334	X
buccal		325	524	333	333	333	323	323	323	323	333	434	325	534	334	

BP WNL, Took premed, A, B thru/out; mod supra & subgingival calculus used microultrasonic & scaled & polished + recall 3 mos. P.W.

4/7/94 DDS ✓ $ *68.00*

	ur	ua	ul		lr	la	ll
buc	1	1	1		1	1	1
I.P.	2	2	2		2	2	2
ling	0	1	0		2	1	2

24

OH Routine: *TB 2x/day*
Demonstrated: *Floss, TPK in furca*
Dispensed: *P39 TB & Floss*
DH: (RP) (polish) Fl2
QRP: UR UL LR LL

UPPER	1	2	3	4	5	6	7	8	9	10	11	12	13	14	15	16
		✓	✓											✓	✓	
buccal	X		5 5				4	5 5								X
palatal		5	4 4													

LOWER	32	31	30	29	28	27	26	25	24	23	22	21	20	19	18	17
lingual	X	5	4										4	4		X
buccal		5	4										5	5		

took premed. B b/t #2 & #3 and b/t #31, #30, #20 & #19 discussed relationship of plaque to perio disease & importance of using TPK & of flossing to improve perio health. recall 3 mos. P.W.

7/6/94 DDS ✓ $ *68.00*

	ur	ua	ul		lr	la	ll
buc	1	0	1		1	0	0
I.P.	1	0	1		1	0	1
ling	1	0	1		1	1	1

12

OH Routine: *TB 2x/day Flosses 3x/wk*
Demonstrated: *TPK & Floss on post teeth*
Dispensed: *P39 TB & Floss, TPKs*
DH: (RP polish) Fl2
QRP: UR UL LR LL

UPPER	1	2	3	4	5	6	7	8	9	10	11	12	13	14	15	16
		✓	✓											✓	✓	
buccal	X		4 4				3	4 3								X
palatal		3	4 3													

LOWER	32	31	30	29	28	27	26	25	24	23	22	21	20	19	18	17
lingual	X	4	4										4	4		X
buccal		4	3										4	4		

took premed; OH much improved — tissue looks healthy! B only b/t #31 & #30 & b/t #20 & #19; recall 3 mos. needs to use TPK more often to clean furcations P.W.

10/5/94 DDS ✓ $ *68.00*

	ur	ua	ul		lr	la	ll
buc	1	0	0		1	0	0
I.P.	0	0	0		0	0	0
ling	1	0	0		1	0	0

4

OH Routine: *TB 2x/day Floss & TPK 1x/day*
Demonstrated: *TB on post teeth*
Dispensed: *P39 TB & Floss*
DH: (RP) (polish) Fl2
QRP: UR UL LR LL

UPPER	1	2	3	4	5	6	7	8	9	10	11	12	13	14	15	16
		✓	✓											✓	✓	
buccal	X		4					3	3							X
palatal																

LOWER	32	31	30	29	28	27	26	25	24	23	22	21	20	19	18	17
lingual	X		4													X
buccal																

took premed, BP WNL, tissue looks healthy — no bleeding recall 6 mos. P.W. (dexterity very good — Jane is motivated)

PROFESSIONAL PRESS
P.O. Box 7638
Berkeley, California 94707-9991
(415) 525-5998

GP/PMR-1

FIGURE 13–32
Kramer-Rhodes periodontal data collection form for comparisons at successive visits. (Courtesy of S. Kramer and P. Rhodes)

Noting conditions that are beyond normal limits, or variations from previous conditions, allows for the analysis of trends. This longitudinal evaluation not only is critical for providing optimal dental hygiene care, but also is important for meeting third-party requirements for periodontal data on client needs and treatment outcomes. Moreover, notations on records of client perceptions, needs, and desires alert other personnel of special client considerations, and facilitate oral health education and continuity of care for the client.

As new assessment techniques and technologies become available, their results should be integrated into the periodontal and oral hygiene record-keeping system. Figure 13–32 and Table 13–11 provide an example of a record-keeping system developed by Kramer and Rhodes that reflects the elements of satisfactory record keeping for documenting periodontal maintenance care. This system provides divisions for data collection for several appointments on the same page. Each appointment segment allows oral hygiene assessment, periodontal observations, dental hygiene care provided, and adjunctive data to be recorded. By eliminating drawings of the teeth and substituting boxes with tooth numbers, improvement or deterioration in the client's periodontal condition or oral hygiene skills quickly can be observed over a series of appointments. Key points related to the documentation of oral hygiene and periodontal status are discussed separately below, using the Kramer-Rhodes form as a sample record-keeping format.

Sample Record-Keeping Format

Oral Hygiene Assessment

Maintaining a record of the oral hygiene behavior and status of the client is part of overall dental hygiene assessment. Such records provide the client and the clinician with data to use as a baseline reference for subsequent visits. Clinician awareness of oral hygiene products and instruction that previously have been given to the client provides for continuity of care and assures that educational interventions are appropriately designed to build on past knowledge.

In the portion of the Kramer-Rhodes form used to record bacterial plaque scores, client oral hygiene routine, demonstrated oral hygiene techniques, and products dispensed to the client, the mouth is divided into upper and lower arches with corresponding scoring boxes for the upper right (UR), upper anterior (UA), upper left (UL), lower right (LR), lower anterior (LA), and lower left (LL) sextants of the dentition. With the aid of a disclosing agent, the hygienist scores plaque for buccal (facial), interproximal, and lingual surfaces of all teeth using a scale of 0 to 3 as described in the Simple Scoring System for Oral Hygiene chart. The dental hygienist then determines the mean plaque scores for buccal (bucc), interproximal (ip), and lingual (ling) surfaces in each sextant and records each in the corresponding box. The scores in the boxes are totaled and the sum for the entire dentition is recorded in the largest square. A score of 10 or less is recommended as an indication of client success with bacterial plaque control.[30]

Documenting the client's plaque index score at each visit serves to monitor plaque accumulation over time and to motivate clients to initiate or continue positive home care behavior. Also the hygienist is provided with valuable information about the efficacy of client oral hygiene efforts in each sextant of the mouth. This information can be used to refine oral hygiene techniques, to recommend appropriate oral hygiene devices, and to demonstrate the relationship between bacterial plaque and inflammation. Comparing plaque scores at subsequent appointments facilitates evaluation of client skill development and acceptance of oral hygiene recommendations. In addition, the listing of techniques demonstrated and products dispensed alerts the clinician to the home care recommendations presented at earlier sessions. This documentation allows the clinician to reinforce instructions and encourage the client in the effective use of techniques and products. Clients expect a continuing conversation about their success with recently recommended products and devices, and a form that documents this information facilitates such interaction.

At the top of the Kramer-Rhodes periodontal maintenance form is an area for the date and fee to be entered. The term "DDS" is circled and initialed when the dentist examines the client after the dental hygienist has completed the assessment and the dental hygiene care procedure.

At the bottom of the portion of the Kramer-Rhodes form shown in Figure 13–32 the dental hygienist circles the specific dental hygiene care provided (scaling/root planing [RP], polishing [polish] and/or topical fluoride application [F]) and records his initials. Quadrants receiving quadrant root planing (QRP) on that date are identified by circling UR, UL, LR, or LL, on the QRP line, allowing records to

TABLE 13–11

CODE INDEX FOR THE PERIODONTAL MAINTENANCE RECORD (PMR)

A	Acute inflammatory signs: edema, redness
B	Bleeding on probing
C	Chronic inflammatory signs: magenta coloration, connective tissue alteration: hyperplastic or fibrotic tissue, reverse architecture
S	Suppuration
M	Mucogingival concerns such as minimal gingival mucosa, or a frenum pull
P	Mucogingival pocket where the junctional epithelium is located apical to the mucogingival junction (no gingival mucosa)
R	Recession noted in millimeters
→	Inclusive area
#	Attachment loss in millimeters. Probing depth (lower, clear boxes) or Recession (blue boxes)
	Large Box is used for cumulative plaque score (or stain, calculus) or letter grade
	Small Boxes indicate areas where plaque has accumulated
QRP	Quadrant root planing
F	Fluoride application or rinse

Adapted from Kramer, S. M. The Periodontal Maintenance Record (unpublished). 1991.

SIMPLE SCORING SYSTEM FOR ORAL HYGIENE

0 = No plaque present
1 = Light plaque (at gingival margin)
2 = Moderate plaque (covering half the tooth surface)
3 = Heavy plaque (up to the incisal/occlusal edges)

Courtesy of S. Kramer and P. Rhodes.

UNIVERSITY OF CALIFORNIA – SCHOOL OF DENTISTRY
SPECIALIZED PERIODONTAL EXAMINATION RECORD

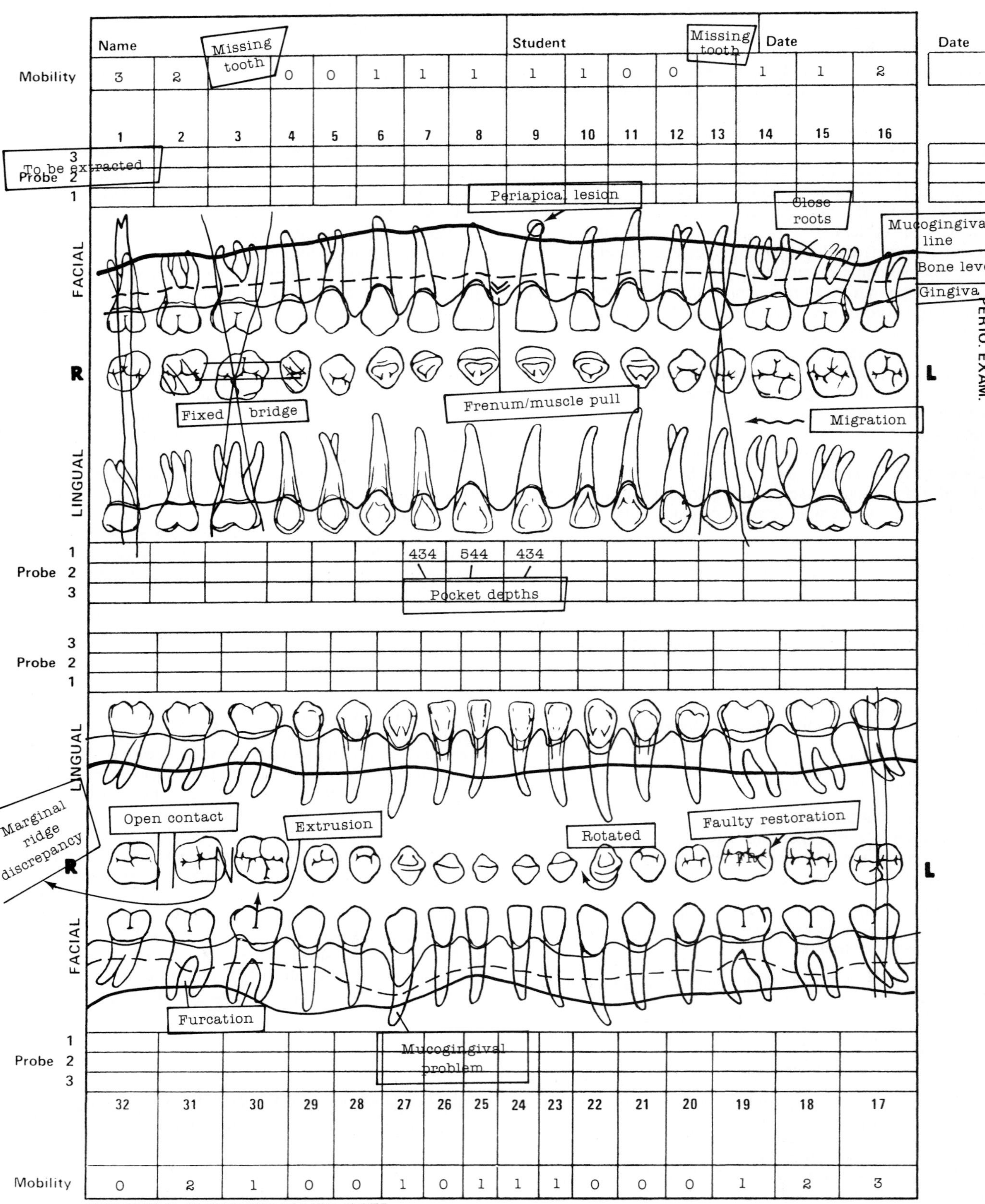

UCSF DENTAL CLINIC FORM 61-5 (Front) 8/77

FIGURE 13–33
Periodontal examination record. (Courtesy of University of California, San Francisco, School of Dentistry.)

reflect when treatment concentration is rotated by quadrant or arch from one appointment to the next.

Periodontal Assessment

In addition to documenting oral hygiene status, it is necessary to monitor periodontal status from appointment to appointment. The Kramer-Rhodes form allows one to record six-point probing depths in the white boxes adjacent to specific tooth numbers. In addition, findings of inflammation, aberrant tissue form, bleeding, suppuration, minimum attached gingiva, tooth mobility, and furcation involvement are recorded in the gray boxes using the codes given at the top of the chart and in Table 13–11.

Initially, complete six-point probing measurements are recorded for each tooth; however, only changes are recorded at subsequent visits. The practitioner is able to identify an improvement or decline in periodontal status by vertically scanning the form for any particular tooth or area. Comparison of notations from appointment to appointment facilitates periodontal diagnosis, treatment planning and monitoring by the dentist-dental hygienist team.

Additional notes are made in the blank space below the charting notes. These notes should include such information as significant health history updates, personal data, and pain control used according to type, amount, and duration (as with nitrous oxide/oxygen analgesia) or according to area (as with local anesthetic agent administration).

The documentation form should list factors that may negatively affect the outcome of care. For example, the dental hygienist should note when the client's plaque score is consistently high; and when gingival inflammation and healing are affected by stress, nutrition, medications, and systemic conditions. Client noncompliance, tardiness, cancellations, and missed appointments also should be recorded to demonstrate that the client may be responsible for a less than satisfactory result. The example of a Kramer-Rhodes form shown in Figure 13–32 over a 1-year period demonstrates how a system like this clearly and easily organizes data.

The top left corner of the Kramer-Rhodes form notes the periodontal case type (I through V as defined in Classification of Periodontal Disease chart) and those teeth that are to be watched most carefully. Also noted are special instructions regarding medical concerns, pain control, or client positioning.

Other Documentation Formats

Other methods of recording findings provide a more graphic display of the client's periodontal health status. Figure 13–33 is an example of a charted dentition with the bone level drawn from radiographic and probing measurements. Recession levels are quickly visualized by another line (the dotted or color-coded line) to show marginal gingiva. Other codes, such as for mobility, are added to the form, using the criteria described in the Classification of Mobility chart, and bleeding is specified. This form, however, does not show chronological changes in plaque location, periodontal condition, mobility, or home care, nor does it record the history of care, instruction, oral hygiene routine, or products/devices dispensed and demonstrated. Another charting form must be used to record changes in the dentition and periodontium.

Accurate and thorough recording of the assessment information is critical to the formulation of proper dental and dental hygiene diagnoses. Whether the client is an individual in a private office or a subject in an epidemiological study, assessment information needs to be documented to reflect client status, continuity of care, and communication with other healthcare providers. Furthermore, when oral health status is consistently monitored and clients are routinely informed about assessment findings, they can be full participants in their health and dental hygiene care.

THE DECISION-MAKING MATRIX

The participation of clients in the decision-making about their health is an important aspect of dental hygiene care. Assessment data are shared with the individual client to gain feedback during the course of information gathering. The client's values regarding periodontal health may differ from those of the dental hygienist and need to be evaluated during the assessment phase of care. Satisfaction with the explanations and priorities proposed by the dental hygienist is vital to the client's acceptance of recommended care.

The Periodontal Decision-Making Matrix

Figure 13–34 illustrates a decision-making matrix used by the dental hygienist in providing dental hygiene care. Decisions are the result of objective clinical and radiographic information collected and recorded during the assessment phase of dental hygiene care and collaboration with the dentist and the client. Objective assessment data can be further evaluated in follow-up assessments.

The health and personal history information can influence the choice of treatment modalities.[31] For example, the host defense mechanisms and presence of disease may compromise care results, as can nutritional status, the effects of tobacco, alcohol, medications, stress, oral habits, and emotional factors. The client's level of motivation and degree of assumption of responsibility also affect oral hygiene care instruction and outcome of care. Such factors must be considered in the decision-making process.

Dental factors such as occlusal trauma and oral appliances also influence the outcome of care. Occlusal trauma may exacerbate, but does not cause, periodontal disease. Orthodontic treatment often entails trauma to gingival tissue and compromises oral hygiene. In addition, each situation needs to be assessed to identify the client's perception of her needs, level of dexterity in plaque control, and the degree of anatomical access for professional and self-maintenance.

There are three main nonsurgical mechanical oral hygiene procedures that the dental hygienist provides:

- The preventive oral prophylaxis
- Therapeutic scaling and root planing
- Periodontal maintenance (see Chapter 17).[32]

If elimination of inflammation and arresting disease progression can be achieved by root planing, then no further treatment is necessary. If scaling and root planing fail to achieve these objectives, then surgical access may be necessary. Surgery by the dentist, based solely on probing depths, is not necessarily warranted.[3]

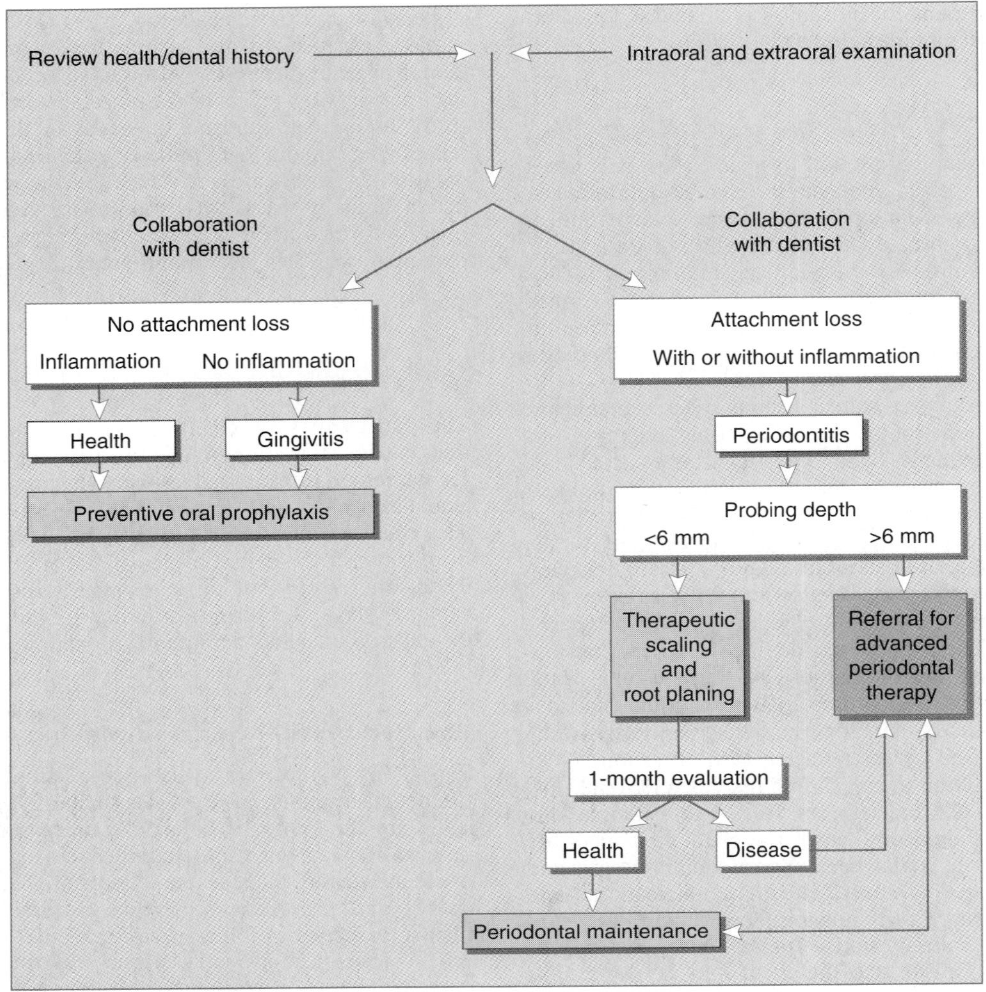

FIGURE 13–34
Decision tree for periodontal assessment and treatment of the adult client.

References

1. Carranza, F. A. Glickman's Clinical Periodontology, 7th ed. Philadelphia: W. B. Saunders, 1990.
2. Armitage, G. C. Biologic Basis of Periodontal Maintenance Therapy. Berkeley, CA: Praxis, 1980.
3. The American Academy of Periodontology. Proceedings of the World Workshop on Periodontics, Princeton, NJ, July 23-27, 1989.
4. Haffajee, A. D., Socransky, S. S., and Goodson, J. M. Clinical parameters as predictors of destructive periodontal disease activity. Journal of Clinical Periodontology 10:257, 1983.
5. Lang, N. P., Joss, A., et al. Bleeding on probing—a predictor for the progression of periodontal disease? Journal of Clinical Periodontology 13:590, 1986.
6. Canton, J., Proye, M., and Polson, A. Maintenance of healed periodontal pockets after a single episode of root planing. Journal of Periodontology 53:420, 1982.
7. Department of Periodontology, University of California School of Dentistry. Recognizing Periodontal Disease. Berkeley, CA: Praxis, 1978.
8. Greenwell, H., Bissada, N. F., and Wittwer, J. W. Periodontics in general practice: Perspectives on periodontal diagnosis. Journal of the American Dental Association 199:537, 1989.
9. Fedi, P. F. The Periodontic Syllabus, 2nd ed. Philadelphia: Lea & Febiger, 1989.
10. Grant, D. A., Stern, I. B., and Listgarden, M. A. Periodontics in the Tradition of Gottlieb and Orban, 6th ed. St. Louis: C. V. Mosby, 1988.
11. American Dental Association Council on Dental Materials, Instruments, and Equipment. Recommendations in radiographic practices. Journal of the American Dental Association 109:764, 1984.
12. Shwartz, M., Pliskin, J. S., et al. Benefits of Alternative Schedules for Bitewing Radiographs, NCHSR Research Summary Series, DHHS Publication No. (PHS) 87-3407, Grant HS 04858. US Department of Health and Human Services, Public Health Service, National Center for Health Services Research and Health Care Technology Assessment, February 1987.
13. Kogon, S. L., and Stephens, R. G. Selective radiography instead of screening partonography—a risk/benefit evaluation. Canadian Dental Association Journal 48:271, 1982.
14. Brooks, S. L. A study of selection criteria for intraoral dental radiography. Oral Surgery 62:234, 1986.
15. Lang, N. P., and Hill, R. W. Radiographs in periodontics. Journal of Clinical Periodontology 4:16, 1977.
16. Greenstein, G., Polson, A. M., Iker, H., and Meitner, S. Associations between crestal lamina dura and periodontal status. Journal of Periodontology 52:362, 1981.
17. Armitage, G. C., Svanberg, G. K., and Loe, H. Microscopic evaluation of clinical measurements of connective tissue attachment levels. Journal of Clinical Periodontology 4:173, 1977.
18. Kung, R. T., Ochs, B., and Goodson, J. M. Temperature as a

periodontal diagnostic. Journal of Clinical Periodontology 17:557, 1990.

19. Meyerov, R. H., Lenmer, J., et al. Temperature gradients in periodontal pockets. Journal of Periodontology 62:95, 1991.
20. Persson, G. R., and Page, R. C. Effect of sampling time and repetition on gingival crevicular fluid and aspartate aminotransferase activity. Journal of Periodontal Research 25:236, 1990.
21. Chambers, D. A., Imrey, P. B., et al. A longitudinal study of aspartate aminotransferase in human gingival crevicular fluid. Journal of Periodontal Research 26:65, 1991.
22. Imrey, P. B., Crawford, J. M., et al. A cross-sectional analysis of aspartate aminotransferase in human gingival crevicular fluid. Journal of Periodontal Research 26:75, 1991.
23. Offenbacher, S., Odle, B. M., and Van Dyke, T. E. The use of crevicular fluid prostaglandin E2 levels as a predictor of periodontal attachment loss. Journal of Periodontal Research 21:101, 1986.
24. Jeffcoat, M. K., and Reddy, M. S. A comparison of probing and radiographic methods for detection of periodontal disease progression. Current Opinions in Dentistry 1(1):45, 1991.
25. Jeffcoat, M. K. Diagnosing periodontal disease: New tools to solve an old problem. Journal of the American Dental Association 122(1):54, 1991.
26. Deas, D. E., Pasquali, L. A., et al. The relationship between probing attachment loss and computerized radiographic analysis in monitoring progression of periodontitis. Journal of Periodontology 62(2):135, 1991.
27. Allen, D. L., McFall, W. T., and Jenzano, J. W. Periodontics for the Dental Hygienist. Philadelphia: Lea & Febiger, 1987.
28. McConaughy, F. L., Lukken, K. M., and Toevs, S. E. Health promotion behaviors of private practice hygienist. Journal of Dental Hygiene 65:222, 1991.
29. Ramfjord, S. P. The periodontal disease index. Journal of Periodontology 38:602, 1967.
30. Kramer, S. M. The Periodontal Maintenance Record (PMR). Unpublished manuscript, 1991. Available from the author at: 1870 San Pedro Ave., Berkeley, CA 94707.
31. Hall, W. B. (ed.). Decision Making in Periodontology. St. Louis: C. V. Mosby, 1988.
32. Walsh, M. M., and Robertson, P. B. Professional mechanical oral hygiene practices. Journal of the American Dental Hygienists' Association 63:242, 1989.

Suggested Readings

Ainamo, J., Barnes, D., et al. Development of the World Health Organization (WHO) Community Periodontal Index of Treatment Needs (CPITN). International Dental Journal 32:281, 1982.

Ainamo, J., and Loe, H. Anatomical characteristics of gingiva. Journal of Periodontology 37:5, 1966.

Ainamo, J., and Talari, A. The increase with age of the width of attached gingiva. Journal of Periodontal Research 1:182, 1976.

Amato, R., Caton, J. G., Polson, A. M., and Espeland, M. A. Interproximal gingival inflammation related to the conversion of a bleeding to a non-bleeding state. Journal of Periodontology 57:63, 1986.

Armitage, G. C., Dickinson, W. R. et al. Relationship between the percentage of subgingival spirochetes and the severity of periodontal disease. Journal of Periodontology, 53:550, 1982.

Armitage, G. C. Assessment of periodontal disease "activity." Unpublished manuscript, University of California, San Francisco, 1990.

Axelsson, P. and Lindhe, J. Effect of controlled oral hygiene procedures on caries and periodontal disease in adults. Journal of Clinical Periodontology, 5:133, 1978.

Badersten, A., Nilveus, R., and Egelberg, J. Effect of non-surgical periodontal therapy. VIII. Probing attachment changes related to clinical characteristics. Journal of Clinical Periodontology 14:425, 1987.

Barnett, M. L. Inhibition of oral contraceptive effectiveness by concurrent antibiotic administration: A review. Journal of Periodontology 56:18, 1985.

Barnett, M. L., Gilman, R. M., Charles, C. H., and Bartels, L. L. Computer-based thermal imaging of human gingiva. Journal of Periodontology, 60:628, 1989.

Bragger, D., Pasquali, L., et al. Computer-assisted densitometric image analysis in periodontal radiography. A methodology study. Journal of Clinical Periodontology 15:27, 1988.

Bragger, U., Nyman, S., et al. The significance of alveolar bone in periodontal disease. Journal of Clinical Periodontology 17:379, 1990.

Caffesse, R. G., Nasjleti, C. J., Kowalski, C. J., and Castelli, W. A. The effect of mechanical stimulation on the keratinization of sulcular epithelium. Journal of Periodontology, 53:89, 1982.

Canton, J., and Polson, A. The interdental bleeding index: a simplified procedure for monitoring gingival health. Compendium of Continuing Education in Dentistry 6:88, 1985.

Canton, J., Proye, M., and Polson, A. Maintenance of healed periodontal pockets after a single episode of root planing. Journal of Periodontology 53:420, 1982.

Canton, J. G. Periodontal diagnosis and diagnostic aids. In The American Academy of Periodontology. Proceedings of the World Workshop on Periodontics, Princeton NJ, July 23–27, 1989, pp. I-1 to I-22.

Carranza, F. A., and Perry, D. A. Clinical Periodontology for the Dental Hygienist. Philadelphia: W. B. Saunders, 1986.

Caton, J., Eaton, K. A., et al. Removal of root surface deposits. Journal of Clinical Periodontology 12:141, 1985.

Darby, M. L. Mosby's Comprehensive Review of Dental Hygiene, 3rd ed. St. Louis: C. V. Mosby, 1994.

Delta Dental Plans. Dentist's Handbook, Los Angeles, 1989.

DeVore, C. H., Hicks, M. J., and Claman, L. A. A system for insuring success of long-term supportive periodontal therapy. Journal of the American Dental Hygienists' Association 63:214, 1989.

Duckworth, J. E., Judy, P. F., Goodson, J. M., and Socransky, S. S. A method for the geometric and densitometric standardization of intraoral radiographs. Journal of Periodontology 54:435, 1983.

Engelberger, T., Hefti, A., Kallenbeger, A., and Rateitschak, K. H. Correlations among Papillary Bleeding Index, other clinical bleeding indices and histologically determined inflammation of gingival papilla. Journal of Clinical Periodontology 10:579, 1983.

Flischman, S. L. Clinical index systems used to assess the efficacy of mouth-rinses on plaque and gingivitis. Journal of Clinical Periodontology 15:506, 1988.

Flynn, T. R. Odontogenic Infections. Oral and Maxillofacial Surgery of North America 3:311, 1991.

Genco, R. J. (ed.). Contemporary Periodontics. St. Louis: C. V. Mosby, 1990.

Glossary of Periodontic Terms. Journal of Periodontology 57 [Suppl], 1986.

Golub, L. M., Goodson, J. M., et al. Tetracyclines inhibit tissue collagenases. Effect of ingested low-dose and local delivery systems. Journal of Periodontology 56[Special Issue]:93, 1985.

Greene, J. C., and Vermillion, J. R. The oral hygiene index: A method for classifying oral hygiene status. Journal of the American Dental Association 61:172, 1960.

Greene, J. C., and Vermillion, J. R. The simplified oral hygiene index. Journal of the American Dental Association 68:7, 1964.

Grondahl, H. G., Grondahl, K., and Webber, R. L. A digital subtraction technique for dental radiography. Oral Surgery, Oral Medicine, Oral Pathology 55:96, 1983.

Haffajee. A. D., Socransky, S. S., and Ebersole, J. L. Survival analysis of periodontal sites before and after periodontal therapy. Journal of Clinical Periodontology 12:553, 1985.

Kalkwarf, K. L. Effect of oral contraceptive therapy on gingival inflammation in humans. Journal of Periodontology 49:560, 1978.

Kay, H. M., and Wilson, M. The *in vitro* effects of amine fluoride on plaque bacteria. Journal of Periodontology 59:266, 1988.

Kornman, K. S. Nature of periodontal diseases: Assessment and diagnosis. Journal of Periodontal Research 22:192, 1987.

Lindhe, J., Westfelt, E., et al. Healing following surgical/non-surgical treatment of periodontal disease. Journal of Clinical Periodontology 9:115, 1982.

Lindhe, J., and Nyman, S. Scaling and granulation tissue removal in periodontal therapy. Journal of Clinical Periodontology 12:374, 1985.

Lindhe, J. (ed.). Textbook of Clinical Periodontology, 2nd ed. Copenhagen: Munksgaard, 1989.
Listgarten, M. A., Lindhe, J., and Helden, L. Effect of tetracycline and/or scaling on human periodontal disease. Journal of Clinical Periodontology 5:246, 1978.
Listgarten, M. A., and Rosenberg, M. M. Histological study of repair following new attachment procedures in human periodontal lesions. Journal of Periodontology 53:333, 1979.
Listgarten, M. A., Schifter, C. C., et al. Failure of a microbial assay to reliably predict disease recurrence in a treated periodontitis population receiving regularly scheduled prophylaxes. Journal of Clinical Periodontology, 13:768, 1986.
Lobene, R. R., Mankodi, S. M., et al. Correlations among gingival indices: A methodology study. Journal of Periodontology 3:159, 1989.
Loe, H. The gingival index, the plaque index and the retention index systems. Journal of Periodontology 38:610, 1967.
Lucas, R. M., Howell, L. P., and Wall, B. A. Nifedipine-induced gingival hyperplasia. Journal of Periodontology 56:211, 1985.
Magnusson, I., and Listgarten, M. A. Histological evaluation of probing depth following periodontal treatment. Journal of Clinical Periodontology 7:26, 1980.
Muhlemann, H. R., and Son, S. Gingival sulcus bleeding–a leading symptom in initial gingivitis. Helvetica Odonotologica Acta 15:107, 1971.
O'Leary, T. J., Drake, R. B., and Naylor, J. E. The plaque control record. Journal of Periodontology 43:38, 1972.
O'Leary, T. J., The impact of research on scaling and root planing. Journal of Periodontology 57:69, 1986.
Oliver, R. C., Holm-Pedersen, P., and Loe, H. The correlation between clinical scoring, exudate measurements and microscopic evaluation of inflammation in the gingiva. Journal of Periodontology 40:201, 1969.
Page, R. C. Gingivitis. Journal of Clinical Periodontology 13:345, 1986.
Parr, R. W., Pipe, P., and Watt, S. Recognizing Periodontal Disease. San Francisco: Praxis Publishing, 1978.
Passo, S. A., Reinhardt, R. A., DuBois, L. M., and Cohen, D. M. Histological characteristics associated with suppurating periodontal pockets. Journal of Periodontology 59:731, 1988.
Periodontal Maintenance Record (PMR). Professional Press, P. O. Box 10520, Oakland, CA 94610, 1991.
Perry, D. A., and Newman, M. E. Occurrence of periodontitis in an urban adolescent population. Journal of Periodontology 61:185, 1990.
Perry, D. A., Beemsterboer, P., and Carranza, F. A. Techniques and Theory of Periodontal Instrumentation, Philadelphia: W. B. Saunders, 1990.
Persson, R., Swedsen, J., and Daubert, K. A. Longitudinal evaluation of periodontal therapy using the CPITN index. Journal of Clinical Periodontology 16:569, 1989.
Podshadley, A. G., and Haley, J. V. A method for evaluating oral hygiene performance. Public Health Report 83:259, 1968.
Polson, A. M., and Caton, J. G. Current status of bleeding in the diagnosis of periodontal diseases. Journal of Periodontology 56[Special Issue]:1, 1985.
Quigley, G. A., and Hein, J. W. Comparative cleansing efficiency of manual and power brushing. Journal of the American Dental Association 65:26, 1962.
Ramfjord, S. P., and Ash, M. M. Periodontology and Periodontics. Philadelphia: W. B. Saunders, 1979.
Rateitschak-Pluss, E. M., Hefti, A., Lortscher, R., and Thiel, G. Initial observation that cyclosporin-A induces gingival enlargement in man. Journal of Clinical Periodontology 10:237, 1983.
Research words. Perio Reports 1:25, 1989.
Renvert, S., Widstrom, M., et al. On the inability of root debridement and periodontal surgery to eliminate *Aa* from periodontal pockets. Journal of Clinical Periodontology 17:351, 1990.
Reinhart, T., Killoy, W., et al. The effectiveness of a patient applied tooth desensitizing gel. Journal of Clinical Periodontology 17:123, 1990.
Rethman, M., Ruttiman, U., et al. Diagnosis of bone lesions by subtraction radiography. Journal of Periodontology 56:324, 1985.
Robertson, P. B., Walsh, M. M., et al. Periodontal effects associated with the use of smokeless tobacco. Journal of Periodontology 61:438, 1990.
Russell, A. L. The periodontal index. Journal of Periodontology 38:585, 1967.
Saglie, F. R., Newman, M. G., Carranza, F. A., and Pattison, G. L. Bacterial invasion of gingiva in advanced periodontitis in humans. Journal of Periodontology 53:217, 1982.
Schluger, S., Yuodelis, R. A., and Page, R. C. Periodontal Disease, 2nd ed., Philadelphia: Lea & Febiger, 1990.
Silverman, S., Migliorti, C. A., et al. Oral findings in people with high risk for AIDS: A study of 375 homosexual males. Journal of the American Dental Association 112:187, 1986.
Suzuki, J. B. Diagnosis and classification of periodontal diseases. Dental Clinics of North America 32:195, 1988.
Taggert, J. E. Lecture on Epidemiology of Periodontal Disease. University of California, San Francisco, 1990.
Tal, H., and Rosenberg, M. Estimation of dental plaque levels and gingival inflammation using a simple oral rinse technique. Journal of Periodontology 61:339, 1990.
Tanner, A., and Bouldin, H. The microbiota of early periodontitis lesions in adults. Journal of Clinical Periodontology 16:467, 1989.
Turesky, A., Gilmore, N., and Glickman, I. Reduced plaque formation by the chloromethyl analogue of vitamin C. Journal of Periodontology 41:41, 1970.
Walsh, M. M., Heckman, B., et al. Comparison of manual and power toothbrushing with and without adjunctive oral irrigation, for controlling plaque and gingivitis. Journal of Clinical Periodontology 16:419, 1989.
Walsh, M. M., and Robertson, P. B. Professional mechanical oral hygiene practices. Journal of the American Dental Hygienists' Association 63:242, 1989.
Wilkins, E. M. Clinical Practice of the Dental Hygienist, 6th ed. Philadelphia: Lea & Febiger, 1989.
Winkel, E. G., Abbas, F., et al. Experimental gingivitis in relation to age in individuals not susceptible to periodontal destruction. Journal of Clinical Periodontology 14:499, 1987.
Woodall, I. R., Dafoe, B., et al. Comprehensive Dental Hygiene Care, 3rd ed. St. Louis: C. V. Mosby, 1989.
Yankell, S. L., Moreno, O. M., et al. Effects of chlorhexidine and four microbial compounds on plaque, gingivitis and staining in beagle dogs. Journal of Dental Research 61:1089, 1982.

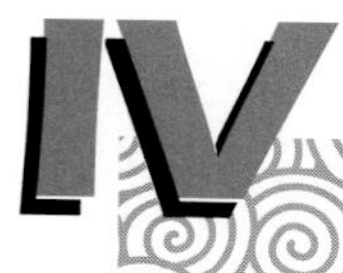

IV DENTAL HYGIENE DIAGNOSIS AND CARE PLAN

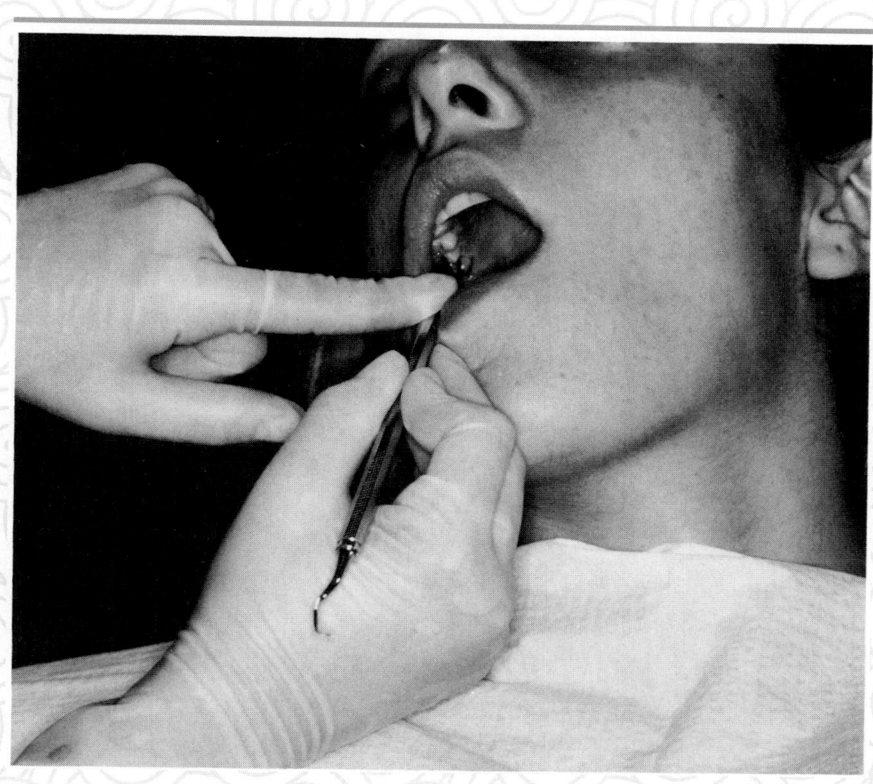

14 Dental Hygiene Diagnosis

OBJECTIVES

Mastery of the content in this chapter will enable the reader to:

- Define the key terms used
- Discuss the steps of the dental hygiene diagnostic process
- Differentiate between a dental hygiene diagnosis and a dental diagnosis
- Explain the advantages of using the dental hygiene diagnosis for the client, other health professionals, and the profession of dental hygiene
- Discuss the limitations of the dental hygiene diagnosis
- Identify appropriate dental hygiene diagnoses supported by clinical assessment data
- Use the guidelines for writing dental hygiene diagnoses when developing diagnostic statements
- Identify needed dental hygiene interventions as related to the dental hygiene diagnosis
- Apply human need theory to support decision making throughout the dental hygiene diagnostic process

INTRODUCTION

Diagnosis Defined

According to the dictionary, **diagnosis** is "an analysis of the cause and nature of a problem or situation, or a statement of its solution."[1] The process is generic but can be applied to specific disciplines. A diagnosis becomes discipline-specific when it is derived from the phenomena central to that discipline.

Miller introduced the concept of the dental hygiene diagnosis and advanced it as "an appropriate term to describe the expression of dental hygiene judgment and decision making ability."[2] The American Dental Hygienists' Association has included dental hygiene diagnosis as integral to its Standards of Applied Dental Hygiene Practice. Identification of dental hygiene diagnoses as a step in the dental hygiene process of care has no doubt stimulated the dental hygiene diagnosis movement. Although the dental hygiene profession has accepted diagnosis as part of the dental hygienist's role, there is no fully acceptable definition of what a dental hygiene diagnosis is. Therefore, the Standards of Applied Dental Hygiene Practice cannot be fully implemented until a definition of the dental hygiene diagnosis is universally accepted by the dental hygiene profession and is developed and integrated into practice.

When dental hygiene practitioners use a process of care, and the theory and behaviors that reflect a conceptual model, it is logical to identify the client's problem related to dental hygiene care (diagnosing) based upon assessment findings. Diagnosis is a critical thinking process by which clinical data about the client are analyzed and assigned a diagnostic label. Therefore, after completing the assessment phase of the dental hygiene process, the work of diagnosing begins (Fig. 14–1).

The dental hygiene diagnostic process presented here uses human need theory as its basis with emphasis on the client's 11 human needs related to dental hygiene care. This chapter introduces the concept of the dental hygiene diagnosis, distinguishes it from that of a dental diagnosis, addresses the problems that dental hygienists diagnose, and discusses a method of formulating dental hygiene diagnostic statements.

Dental Hygiene Diagnosis Defined

Using human need theory as a conceptual framework, dental hygiene diagnosis is the identification of a client's human need deficit related to dental hygiene care. A **dental hygiene diagnosis** is a clinical diagnosis made by a professional dental hygienist that identifies an actual or potential human need deficit related to oral health or disease that the dental hygienist is educated and licensed to treat. The dental hygiene diagnosis focuses on problems or potential problems that are related to oral health and disease, rather than on the disease itself. It is derived from the dental hygiene assessment and requires interventions within the scope of dental hygiene practice. The dental hygiene diagnosis:

- Is derived from pertinent client data
- Identifies human need deficits related to oral health that can be fulfilled through dental hygiene care

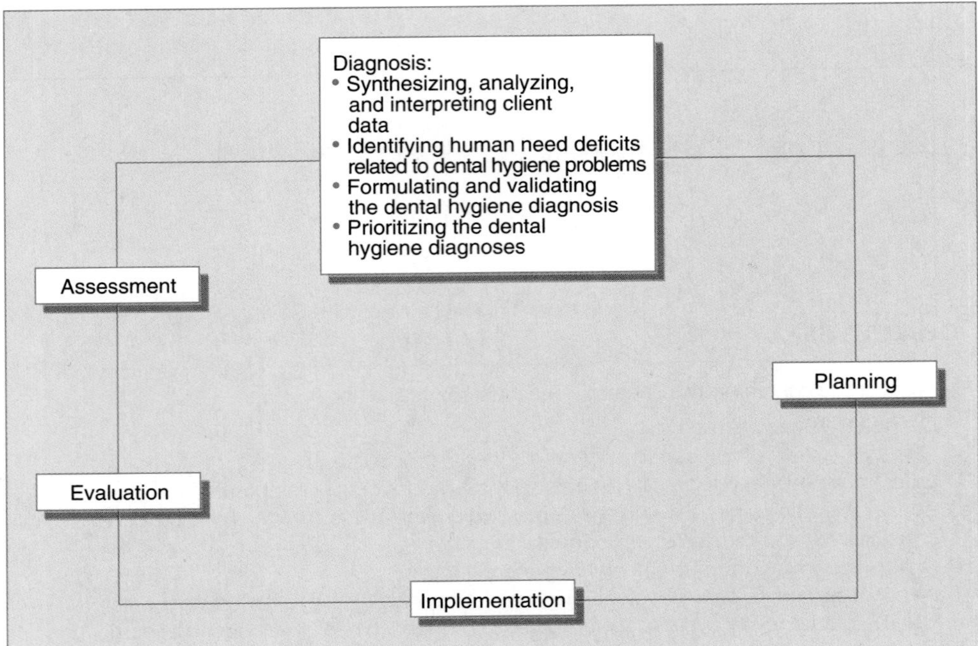

FIGURE 14–1
The concept of diagnosis within the dental hygiene process. The term *dental hygiene diagnosis* is used to describe actual or potential oral health problems that can be prevented or resolved by dental hygiene interventions.

- Is a necessary behavior for planning and implementing effective dental hygiene care and evaluating its outcomes

Making a dental hygiene diagnosis includes identifying the following:

- Human need deficits that relate to the client's oral health or disease
- Factors contributing to or causing the human need deficits (etiologies)
- Evidence to support the dental hygiene diagnosis
- Strengths the client can draw on to prevent or resolve the problem
- A focus for prioritizing subsequent care

In making a dental hygiene diagnosis, the dental hygienist must discriminate problems that are within the scope of dental hygiene practice from those that are not. Hence, the dental hygiene diagnostic process requires that the dental hygienist have a concrete understanding of the domain of dental hygiene and that collaboration between the dental hygienist and dentist occurs.[3]

In the past, dental hygiene students were cautioned to "not diagnose." Instead, they were encouraged to identify dental problems and then communicate their findings using phrases such as:

> Mr. Jones has *suspicious* areas on teeth numbers 14, 19, and 32.
>
> Ms. Smith has *signs* of periodontal disease around teeth numbers 22 to 26.
>
> There *appears* to be a radiolucent area at the apex of tooth number 8.

Such observations are neither dental diagnoses nor dental hygiene diagnoses. Dental hygiene professionals frequently lament the obscurity that such phraseology creates for the client and the feelings of embarrassment for the dental hygienist. Applying the human needs conceptual model, the dental hygiene diagnosis might be that "the client has a deficit in the human need for a sound dentition due to inadequate oral health behaviors as evidenced by the specific clinical and radiographic signs of dental caries." The appropriate dental hygiene intervention is to refer to a dentist for dental diagnosis and treatment. Another dental hygiene diagnosis might be that "the client has a deficit in the human need for self-determination and responsibility due to inadequate oral health behaviors as evidenced by the specific clinical and radiographic signs of dental caries." The appropriate dental hygiene intervention is to initiate bacterial plaque control strategies and both in-office and at-home fluoride therapy.

If the state law permits preliminary diagnostic services provided by the dental hygienist, the dental hygienist could say:

> Mr. Jones, my preliminary diagnosis suggests dental caries on teeth numbers 14, 19, and 32; however, the final dental diagnosis must be made by the dentist.
>
> Ms. Smith, the periodontal probing depths of 5 to 7 mm, mobility of 2, and bleeding all around teeth numbers 22 to 26 suggest moderate periodontitis; however, the final diagnosis must be confirmed by the dentist.
>
> Mrs. Carson, your son has a radiolucent area on the apex of tooth number 8 suggesting a pathological condition; however, a dental diagnosis must be made by the dentist.

All of these aforementioned scenarios suggest a dental hygiene diagnosis of "a deficit in the human need for a sound dentition" or a "deficit in the human need for skin and mucous membrane integrity of the head and neck" with the dental hygiene intervention calling for a referral to a dentist. For example, when a dental hygienist identifies oral disease during the assessment phase of the dental hygiene process, such as gingivitis or early periodontitis, this is called a preliminary diagnosis that must be referred to a dentist for a definitive diagnosis and treatment, or for possible delegation by the dentist back to the dental hygienist for care.

When the client manifests signs and symptoms of states that require dental treatment by a licensed dentist, a dental referral is indicated for the best treatment of the client and for the protection of both the dental hygienist and client.

Dental Hygiene Diagnosis Versus Dental Diagnosis

Legal, professional, and social responsibilities require that clear distinctions be made between a dental hygiene and a dental diagnosis. "For consumer protection, there are legal and professional boundaries in diagnosis and treatment."[4] **Dental diagnoses,** like **medical diagnoses,** identify disease, whereas dental hygiene diagnoses focus on identifying human need deficits as they relate to oral health, wellness, and disease prevention. Dental diagnoses identify problems for which the dentist directs or provides the primary treatment; dental hygiene diagnoses identify human need deficits related to oral health that can be met by dental hygienists within the scope of dental hygiene practice. A dental diagnosis remains the same until the oral disease is eliminated; a dental hygiene diagnosis may change as the client's human need deficits, behavior, and responses change (Table 14–1). The dental hygiene diagnosis is no more a usurpation of the dentist's role than is the dental diagnosis a usurpation of the physician's role in medical diagnosis. All are different and serve different purposes.

Dental diagnoses are derived from data in the dental domain that are used to assess biological problems related to dental treatment of oral disease. In the context of the human needs conceptual model, dental hygiene diagnoses are derived from data in the dental hygiene domain that are used to assess 11 human needs related to dental hygiene care, the prevention of oral disease, and the promotion of wellness. Examples of the diagnostic process used in other domains include the competent automotive mechanic's diagnosis of a car's problem before servicing its parts; the physician's diagnosis of a disease before initiating medical care; and the teacher's diagnosis of Johnny's learning problem before designing an intervention to improve learning.[2] Even certain salespersons diagnose personal skin care needs at the department store cosmetic counter prior to selecting facial products. So, too, the dental hygienist diagnoses client problems within the domain of dental hygiene to prevent oral disease and promote wellness.

TABLE 14–1
DENTAL HYGIENE DIAGNOSIS VERSUS DENTAL DIAGNOSIS

Dental Hygiene Diagnosis	Dental Diagnosis
Identifies a human need deficit related to dental hygiene care	Identifies oral diseases
Identifies problems (human need deficits or disturbances) treated by dental hygienists within the scope of dental hygiene practice	Identifies problems for which the dentist directs the primary treatment
Often deals with the client's perceptions, beliefs, attitudes, motivations regarding his own oral health and wellness	Often deals with the actual pathophysiological changes in the body
May apply to alterations in individuals or groups	Applies to disease in individuals only
May change as the client's responses and behaviors change	Remains the same for as long as the disease is present

Taxonomy of Dental Hygiene Diagnoses

The use of the dental hygiene diagnosis creates a need for an acceptable system of classification that facilitates its use. A taxonomy or classification system fulfills this need by identifying the client problems that can be resolved by professional dental hygiene care.

A taxonomy creates a standardized language for communicating about client dental hygiene problems and clarifies oral health problems (and strengths) amenable to dental hygiene interventions. Therefore, a classification or taxonomy of dental hygiene diagnoses is valuable for the enhanced communication it provides. The dental hygiene diagnostic taxonomy allows dental hygienists to identify more precisely than ever before what it is that dental hygienists do and to communicate this to other dental hygienists, clients, and health professionals.

The Taxonomy of Dental Hygiene Diagnoses and Their Definitions Based on Human Needs Theory chart provides a focus for building clinical knowledge about the phenomena of concern in dental hygiene and allows dental hygienists to articulate and assess dental hygiene problems they prevent and sometimes treat from a human needs perspective. It should be clear from reviewing the taxonomy of dental hygiene diagnoses that the system is based upon human need deficits of the client rather than on pathological conditions as are found in a taxonomy of dental diagnoses. The dental hygiene diagnostic taxonomy uses descriptors that focus on the client's human needs related to oral health and disease and to his interaction pattern, thus emphasizing the client as an integrated human being rather than as a disease entity. The Taxonomy of Dental Hygiene Diagnoses and Their Definitions Based on Human Needs Theory chart shows how this series of diagnoses fits into a human needs theoretical framework. As dental hygienists begin to use this diagnostic taxonomy, modifications are made and new diagnostic categories substituted. The clinical validity of this taxonomy should be tested to ensure intra- and interdiagnostician reliability. Such research should be given high priority in dental hygiene.

DENTAL HYGIENE DIAGNOSTIC PROCESS

The dental hygiene diagnostic process is a problem-solving approach to the delivery of dental hygiene care. It outlines the intellectual activity of the dental hygienist (Fig. 14–2). The process relates *what* a dental hygienist does in practice with *why* he does it.

The dental hygiene diagnosis, an essential step in the dental hygiene process, helps dental hygienists focus knowledge on the phenomena central to dental hygiene care for the benefit of the client and collaborating dentist. The dental hygiene diagnosis further enhances the focus of the den-

TAXONOMY OF DENTAL HYGIENE DIAGNOSES AND THEIR DEFINITIONS BASED ON HUMAN NEEDS THEORY

Wholesome Body Image
The need to have a positive mental representation of one's own body boundary and how it looks to others.

Freedom From Pain/Stress
The need to be exempt from physical and emotional discomforts

Skin and Mucous Membrane Integrity of Head and Neck
The need to have an intact and functioning covering of the person's head and neck area, including the oral mucous membranes and gingiva, which defend against harmful microbes; provide sensory information; and resist injurious substances, and trauma

Nutrition
The need to ingest and assimilate sufficient amounts of carbohydrates, proteins, fats, vitamins, minerals, trace elements, and fiber required for growth, repair, and maintenance of structurally and functionally competent bodily parts

Safety
The need to experience freedom from harm or danger involving the integrity of the body's structure and environment around the person

Conceptualization and Problem Solving
The need to grasp ideas and abstractions, to reason, to make sound judgments about one's life and circumstances

Territoriality
The need to possess a prescribed area of space or knowledge that a person denotes as one's own, maintains control over, and defends if necessary, and is acknowledged by others as owning

Biologically Sound Dentition
The need to have intact teeth, and restorations that defend against harmful microbes and provide for adequate function and aesthetics

Appreciation and Respect
The need to be acknowledged for achievement, worth, service, or merit and to be regarded favorably, with admiration and approval by others

Self-determination and Responsibility
The need to exercise accountability for one's behavior and actions

Value System
The need to have an internalized designation of the importance of people, institutions, things, activities, and experiences in one's life

Adapted from Yura, H., and Walsh, M. B. (eds.). The Nursing Process. Norwalk: Appleton & Lange, 1988.

tal hygienist in practice because the diagnosis reflects the domain of dental hygiene.

Goals are developed in conjunction with the client and are derived from the data base established from the assessment and diagnosis. Goals specify how a client can move toward promotion, maintenance, or restoration of oral wellness. Planning, dental hygiene interventions, and client outcomes are guided by the dental hygiene diagnosis. "Diagnoses contain the links between the client's problem and etiology that guide the identification of (dental hygiene) interventions and facilitate the definition of expected outcomes to evaluate the efficacy of (care)." [5,6]

Synthesis, Analysis, and Interpretation of Assessment Data

Dental hygienists identify problems (formulate dental hygiene diagnoses) that are of concern to dental hygiene and that dental hygienists may treat in collaboration with the dentist. Experienced dental hygienists begin to synthesize, analyze, and interpret data while they are still collecting it during the assessment phase. The dental hygienist looks for significant data or clusters of data that signal the presence of an actual or potential human need deficit related to an oral health deficit, and then develops a dental hygiene care plan that facilitates the human need fulfillment.

Using Standards

To identify oral health deficits that are integrated into a human needs framework, the dental hygienist can compare observed data (objective and subjective) with an accepted standard. Appropriate standards include normative values for the client's age, race, and illness category. For example, a child's gingival architecture may be normal given the child's developmental level, but abnormal at another age. Similarly, a blood pressure of 150/90 might be within the expected range for an individual with hypertension under the control of a physician. Gordon's criteria for how standards may be used to recognize significant data follow:[7]

- Changes in a client's usual health patterns that are unexplained by expected norms for growth and development
- Deviation from an appropriate population norm
- Behavior that is nonproductive in the whole person context
- Behavior indicating a developmental lag or evolving dysfunctional pattern

Recognizing Patterns

Dental hygiene diagnoses should always be based on a number of significant pieces of information rather than on a single sign or symptom. The danger of arriving at a dental hygiene diagnosis from a single cue is evident from this example. The dental hygienist may diagnose a woman as a client with a deficit in the human need for nutrition, related to noncompliance as evidenced by too much sugar in the diet, but may have misinterpreted the observed data. The dental hygienist erroneously identified the etiology as noncompliance when really the etiology is rooted in the belief system of the client's culture. Gathering complete data to support a recognizable pattern prevents the dental hygienist from formulating an erroneous diagnosis.

Identifying Human Need Deficits

The next step in the diagnostic process is to determine the client's human need deficits related to the oral health problem. It is here that the dental hygienist must distinguish between oral health problems that only a dentist is quali-

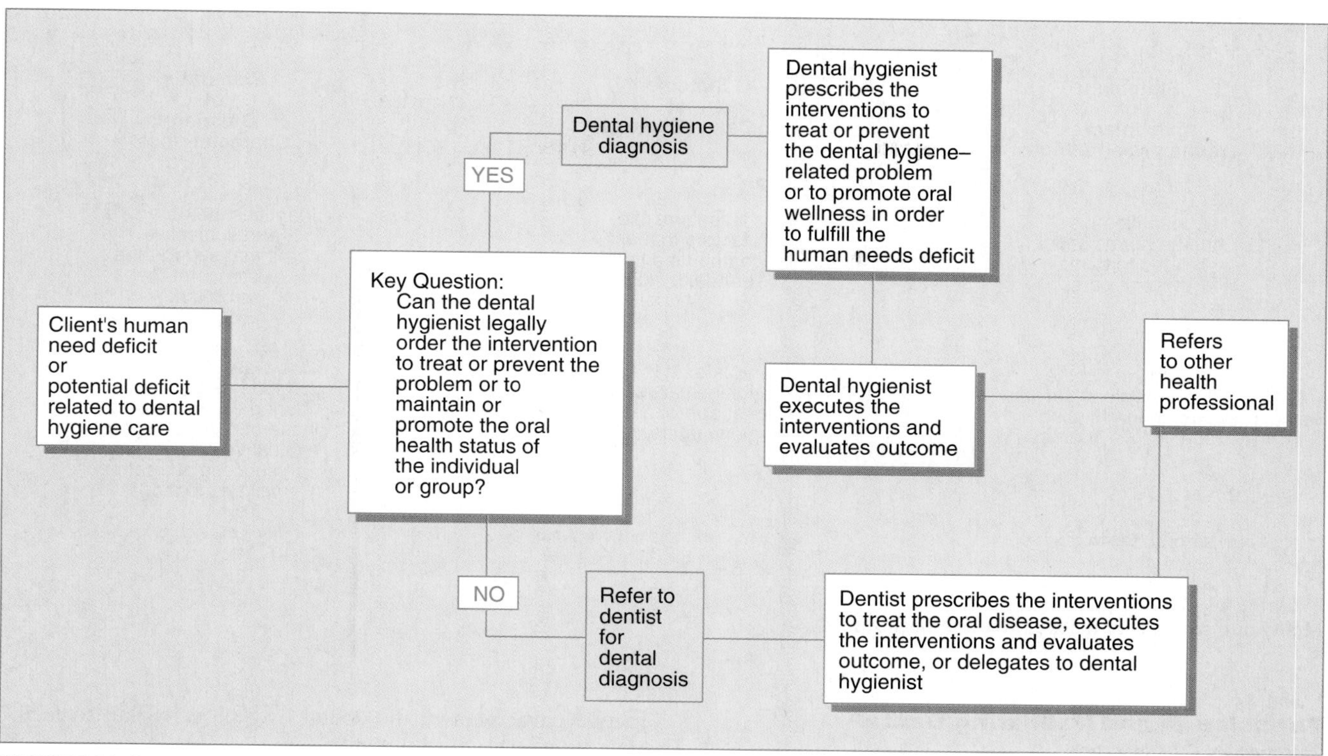

FIGURE 14–2
Flow chart of the dental hygiene diagnostic process.

fied to treat (dental diagnosis), therefore requiring a dental referral, and oral health problems that generate a need for dental hygiene care (dental hygiene diagnosis). Such analysis determines whether the data require a dental diagnosis, a dental hygiene diagnosis, or a medical diagnosis.

The client also may present information identified during the assessment indicating that the client is at risk for developing a potential human need deficit from a health problem. For example, the dental hygienist records that a client has signs of possible uncontrolled diabetes mellitus, but the results were not confirmed at the last physical examination. The dental hygienist then predicts the deficits or problems this client is likely to experience as a result of scaling and root planing, such as longer healing period than normal and a potential for infection. These deficits are related to the human needs for safety and for skin and mucous membrane integrity. These dental hygiene diagnoses have implications for dental hygiene interventions, such as collaboration with and referral to the dentist and the physician of record, analysis of the client's diet and nutrition, review of the client's medication schedule, reduction of the length of the dental hygiene care appointment, need for premedication, use of antibacterial rinses for postoperative care, and the establishment of a personal oral hygiene program, just to mention a few.

Identifying Strengths

At times, a client may present with no human need deficits related to oral health or disease. These individuals may take their oral health for granted and not know how to build on this strength for greater levels of oral wellness. This situation is an opportunity for the dental hygienist to discuss observed strengths with the client and to plan oral health promotion interventions to maintain and expand wellness.

After interpreting and analyzing the client's data, the dental hygienist reaches one of four basic conclusions, all of which require different actions. These conclusions and actions are shown in Table 14–2.

TABLE 14–2
POSSIBLE CONCLUSIONS AND ACTIONS TAKEN BY THE DENTAL HYGIENIST AFTER ANALYZING CLIENT ASSESSMENT DATA

Conclusion	Dental Hygiene Actions
No human need deficits related to dental hygiene care	Initiate oral health promotion strategies to achieve higher levels of oral wellness Reinforce client's oral health beliefs and behaviors
Possible human need deficit related to an oral health problem	Collect more assessment data to validate suspected problem that may require a dental hygiene diagnosis, a dental diagnosis, or a medical diagnosis
Actual or potential human need deficit related to dental hygiene care that requires a dental hygiene diagnosis	Plan, implement, and evaluate dental hygiene care
Actual or potential human need deficit requiring a diagnosis by another healthcare professional	Consult with and refer to appropriate healthcare professional and work collaboratively to solve the problem

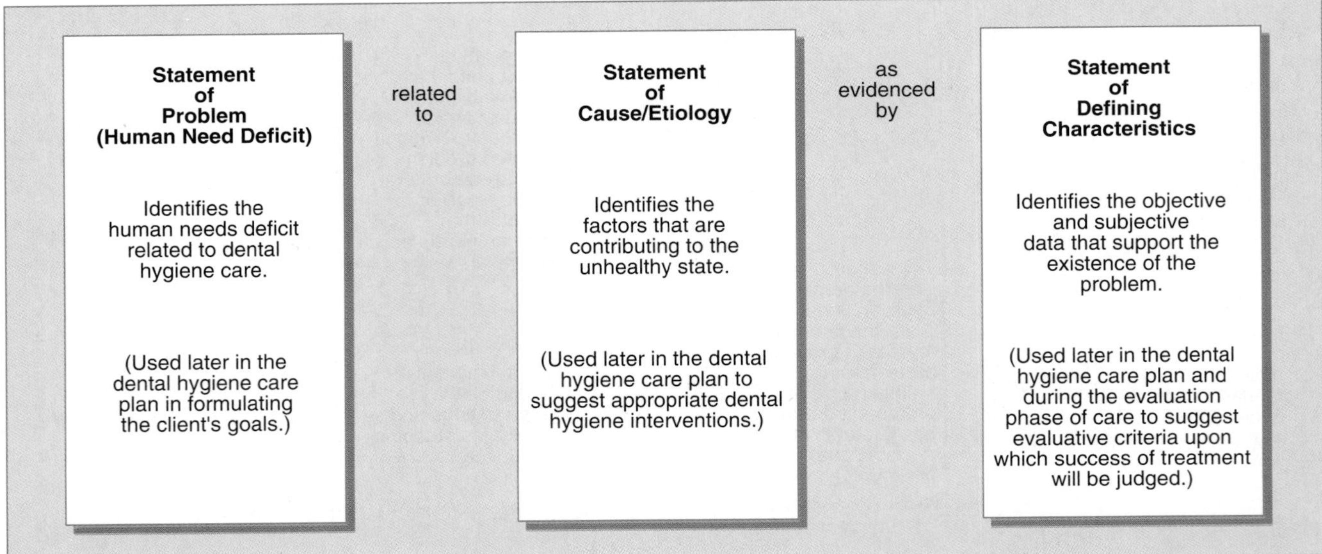

FIGURE 14–3
Model of three parts of a dental hygiene diagnosis.

Formulating and Validating Dental Hygiene Diagnoses

Writing Dental Hygiene Diagnoses

More than one human need may be found in deficit, and multiple dental hygiene diagnoses may be identified. The dental hygienist therefore formulates and validates dental hygiene diagnoses and prioritizes them prior to planning care.

Formulation of the dental hygiene diagnosis is based on the identification of the client's human need deficits as supported by the clinical assessment data. Because people are self-motivated to satisfy human needs, dental hygiene care is predicated on the assumption that the client is an active participant in the dental hygiene care plan to facilitate human need fulfillment.

According to Gordon's structural format, there are three components that must be included in a diagnosis statement:[8]

- The **oral health problem** or potential health problem amenable to dental hygiene intervention
- The probable cause or etiological factor(s)
- The defining signs and symptoms (Fig. 14–3)

Table 14–3 presents some examples of accurate dental hygiene diagnostic statements. Potential health problems do not require etiological specification. In these situations, the observed risk factors (or signs and symptoms) are also the

TABLE 14–3
FORMULATION OF DENTAL HYGIENE DIAGNOSTIC STATEMENTS

	Problem (Dental Hygiene Diagnosis)	Etiology	Defining Characteristics
Defined	Client's human need deficit related to dental hygiene care for which the dental hygienist is educated and licensed to treat	Factors causing or maintaining the unhealthy oral state or response	The subjective and objective data collected in the dental hygiene assessment that suggest the existence of a problem or potential problem
Examples	Skin and mucous membrane integrity of the head and neck deficit	Related to lack of skill and motor ability	As manifested by gingival bleeding, periodontal probing depths of 5 to 7 mm, and arthritis in the hands
	Safety deficit (potential for oral infection)	Related to knowledge and skill deficit, stressful lifestyle, inadequate nutrition	*Note:* Potential problems may not have defining characteristics in the diagnostic statement
	Safety deficit (potential for oral injury)	Related to early age of client and regular participation in contact sports	Client does not wear a mouth protector
	Self-determination and responsibility deficit	Related to inadequate parental supervision of home care	As manifested by gingival bleeding, signs of active caries, and parent indicating that "John brushes his own teeth"
	Wholesome body image deficit	Related to a class II, division I malocclusion	As manifested by client's consistent derogatory remarks about her teeth

cause. For example, the 11 diagnostic categories presented in the Taxonomy of Dental Hygiene Diagnoses and Their Definitions Based on Human Needs Theory chart comprise possible dental hygiene diagnoses. The **dental hygiene diagnostic categories** identify human need deficits related to dental hygiene care and the client's responses. Each diagnostic category has a cluster of critical defining characteristics that must be observed in the client during the assessment. The critical defining characteristics are the conditions that must be evident for the diagnostic label to be used correctly (Table 14–4).[4]

The diagnostic categories enable the dental hygienist to summarize the dental hygiene process data collected during client assessment. In the human needs conceptual model, the organizing principle that directs the dental hygiene diagnostic categories is human needs theory. The critical defining characteristics are the best predictors for judging the presence of a human need deficit related to an oral health problem or a potential problem. It is the critical defining characteristics that enable the dental hygienist to focus on the true problem and to eliminate others (differential diagnoses). More importantly, they provide a mechanism so that the traditional "shotgun" approach characteristic of "routine" dental hygiene care (45-minute appointment for an oral prophylaxis, bite-wing radiographs, fluoride application, and 6-month recall) is no longer an appropriate standard of care.

To classify and standardize dental hygiene diagnoses and interventions, a diagnostic statement should be accompanied by a noting of the objective signs observed by the dental hygienist, subjective symptoms reported by the client, and etiological factors that led to the making of the diagnosis. Thus, a dental hygiene diagnosis is written as a three-part statement. One part of the statement describes the presenting problem, one part states the etiology,[4,9–14] and a third part describes the defining characteristics (i.e., signs and symptoms). An example is "a deficit in the human need for skin and mucous membrane integrity of

TABLE 14–4
TAXONOMY OF DENTAL HYGIENE DIAGNOSIS BASED ON THE HUMAN NEEDS CONCEPTUAL MODEL OF DENTAL HYGIENE WITH *POSSIBLE* ETIOLOGY, DEFINING CHARACTERISTICS, AND CLIENT GOALS

Human Need Related to Oral Health	Dental Hygiene Diagnosis Based on Human Needs	Related to (Cause/Etiology)	As Evidenced by (Defining Characteristics)	Goal/Expected Behavior
Freedom from pain/ stress	Deficit in the need for freedom from pain/ stress	Immunosuppression Inadequate self-monitoring Anesthesia, paresthesia Oral surgery, dental procedure, dental hygiene procedure Untreated dental disease Lack of resources	Client-specific indicators: e.g., too much anxiety, fear, inability to experience pain relief, lack of appropriate pain signals, overresponse to painful stimuli	Client-specific
Self-determination and responsibility	Deficit in the need for self-determination and responsibility	Need for parental supervision of oral hygiene Partial self-care deficit Total self-care deficit Educational deficit Skill deficit Lack of motivation Impaired physical, mental ability Role conflicts	Client-specific indicators: e.g., various physical indicators of oral disease, client's health-seeking behavior	Client-specific
Nutrition	Deficit in the need for nutrition	Recent acquisition of implants, appliances Sugar in diet Fluoride deficit Knowledge deficit Lack of resources (time, money) Recent oral or maxillofacial surgery	Client-specific indicators: e.g., physical indicators of oral status; socioethnocultural indicators; lack of knowledge about diet and nutrition	Client-specific
Wholesome body image	Deficit in the need for a wholesome body image	Acquisition of oral prosthesis Visible dental disease or disorder Halitosis Malocclusion Acquisition of orthodontic appliances	Client-specific indicators: e.g., physical indicators of oral disease; client's subjective responses of dissatisfaction with his oral condition	Client-specific

Table continued on following page

TABLE 14–4
TAXONOMY OF DENTAL HYGIENE DIAGNOSIS BASED ON THE HUMAN NEEDS CONCEPTUAL MODEL OF DENTAL HYGIENE WITH *POSSIBLE* ETIOLOGY, DEFINING CHARACTERISTICS, AND CLIENT GOALS *Continued*

Human Need Related to Oral Health	Dental Hygiene Diagnosis Based on Human Needs	Related to (Cause/Etiology)	As Evidenced by (Defining Characteristics)	Goal/Expected Behavior
Safety	Deficit in the need for safety	Participation in sports Improper use of oral healthcare product Educational deficit Paresthesia, anesthesia Oral habit Potential for oral infection Potential for oral injury Concern about infection control, radiation safety, fluoride safety, previous negative experience	Client-specific indicators: e.g., physical indications of oral injury, or potential for oral injury, vital signs, client's subjective expectations that reveal threats to safety	Client-specific
Skin and mucous membrane integrity of the head and neck	Deficit in the need for skin and mucous membrane integrity of the head and neck	Inadequate oral health behaviors	Client-specific indicators: e.g., various physical indicators of oral disease	Client-specific
Conceptualization and problem solving	Deficit in the need for conceptualization, problem solving	Educational deficit, lack of knowledge	Client-specific indicators: e.g., client inability to verbalize information about various oral disease processes	Client-specific
Territoriality	Deficit in the need for territoriality	Physical proximity of the healthcare provider as determined by psychosociocultural factors	Client-specific indicators: e.g., client's verbal and nonverbal indicators of discomfort with proximity, position, body mechanisms	Client-specific
Biologically sound dentition	Deficit in the need for a biologically sound dentition	Nutrition and diet Educational deficit Nonadherence Inadequate self-monitoring	Client-specific indicators: e.g., physical indicators of oral disease, defect, or disability; poorly fitting appliances; presence of calculus, plaque, stain, abrasion, attrition	Client-specific
Appreciation and respect	Deficit in the need for appreciation and respect	Lack of acceptance	Client-specific indicators: e.g., client's subjective expressions of dissatisfaction	Client-specific
Value system	Deficit in the need for a value system regarding oral health	Client's belief system Client's culture Client's life pattern Nonadherence Lack of knowledge or educational deficit Inadequate self-monitoring Health-seeking behaviors of client	Client-specific indicators: e.g., client's verbalization about the importance of oral health, client's lifestyle, client's oral health behaviors	Client-specific

CASE STUDY. DENTAL HYGIENE CARE PLAN: YOUNG WOMAN WHO RECENTLY OBTAINED ORTHODONTIC APPLIANCES

Brenda Smith, age 16 and a junior in high school, received full orthodontic appliances 1 month ago. Although she wanted the orthodontic appliances to correct the severe crowding of her anterior teeth, she now is experiencing an adjustment problem. She decided to visit her dental office of record for a 3-month checkup because she was treated last for gingivitis prior to placement of the orthodontic appliances. Upon assessment, the dental hygienist found loss of weight, slight gingivitis, and fair bacterial plaque control. All other findings were within normal limits. Ms. Smith verbalized that not very many 16-year-olds at her school wear braces, that she couldn't wait to get them off, and that she can't stand to look at herself in the mirror. One of her high school friends said that she looked weird. She obviously is experiencing high anxiety since the orthodontic appliances were placed. She said that she has a difficult time eating because food sticks to the appliances and she feels embarrassed if the appliances are retaining food. She no longer likes to eat with her friends in the school cafeteria or when she is out on weekends.

Dental Hygiene Diagnosis	Due To or Related To	As Evidenced By	Goal/Expected Behavior
Deficit in the human need for a wholesome body image	• Acquisition of orthodontic appliance	• Unwillingness to smile • Constant negative referral to the appliances and the way they look • Anxiety about wearing the appliances	• Increase in smiling behavior after 1 month • Verbalizes acceptance of appliance after 2 months • Client states that she is interested in pursuing her social life
Deficit in the human need for nutrition	• Inability to eat • Lack of desire to eat	• Loss of weight • Anxiety about wearing the orthodontic appliances	• Client experiences adequate nutrition after 1 month • Client's weight becomes stabilized after 2 months

DENTAL HYGIENE INTERVENTIONS

1. Assess Ms. Smith's perception of her oral condition and appearance prior to wearing orthodontic appliances.
2. Listen to client's comments.
3. Compliment client on appearance.
4. Assist Ms. Smith in visualizing her altered body image and the temporary status of the orthodontic appliances. Emphasize that the altered body image is a normal part of wearing orthodontic appliances.
5. Assist Ms. Smith in concentrating on the positive aspects of her oral health (e.g., no decay, no periodontal disease).
6. Actively reinforce accomplishments such as bacterial plaque control, no gingival bleeding.
7. Encourage Ms. Smith to talk with others who wear orthodontic appliances in order to share concerns and feelings.
8. Conduct nutritional counseling with Ms. Smith to encourage nutritional foods that can be eaten with orthodontic appliances.
9. Describe dietary needs of adolescents.
   - Explain using basic food pyramid.
   - Review a basic food plan.
10. Instruct Ms. Smith in how to record a food diary.
11. After about 1 week, review food diary and lead Ms. Smith to identify areas of concern that might be contributing to undernutrition.
    - Discuss alternative food choices (e.g., foods that are less retentive).
    - Explain how good nutrition will enable her to cope better with the appliances.
12. Review oral hygiene care for orthodontic appliances with specific emphasis on what can be done to keep appliances looking clean while away from home.
13. Continually monitor her anxiety level, emotional status, and attitude toward orthodontic appliances.
14. After 1 month, check with client about eating habits and body weight.
15. After 2 months, check with client about eating habits and body weight.

CASE STUDY. DENTAL HYGIENE CARE PLAN: CHILD WITH LOCALIZED JUVENILE PERIODONTITIS

Devan Sacks, age 12, is a new client in the dental practice and has been scheduled for dental hygiene care. Devan is in the seventh grade and is one of the star players on the girls' soccer team. She is accompanied by her mother Margaret (age 32) and her sister (Bridget), age 10. After completing health and dental histories, the dental hygienist initiates the assessment phase of the dental hygiene process of care including a baseline assessment of human needs related to dental hygiene care, a complete tooth and periodontal assessment, and dental hygiene education and skill level assessment. Significant findings include 6-mm probing depths around tooth numbers 19 and 30 and 4- to 5-mm pockets around tooth numbers 22 to 27. Oral hygiene was generally poor and tooth mobility of periodontally involved teeth ranged from 2 to 3. Client has a knowledge deficit regarding bacterial plaque, periodontal disease process, and status of the oral cavity.

Dental Hygiene Diagnosis	Due To or Related To	As Evidenced By	Goal/Expected Behavior
Deficit in the human need for safety	• Plays on soccer team	• Does not use a mouth protector • Plays soccer three times each week	• Verbalizes belief in the value of a mouth protector • Wears mouth protector at all soccer games and practice sessions • Parent verbalizes emergency care for an avulsed tooth
Deficit in the human need for skin and mucous membrane integrity of the head and neck and in the human need for conceptualization and problem solving	• Knowledge deficit about the periodontal disease process, bacterial plaque, and state of oral cavity	• Probing depth of 4 to 5 mm • Poor oral hygiene • Tooth mobility of 2 and 3	• Decrease bacterial plaque score from 3 to 0 within 1 month • Verbalize the periodontal disease process • Describe the unhealthy signs in her mouth; describe the healthy signs

DENTAL HYGIENE INTERVENTIONS

1. Assess client's present level of knowledge of reasons for a mouth protector.
2. Teach client about the value of a mouth protector for children who play in sports.
3. Teach parent and client emergency care for an avulsed tooth.
4. Construct a mouth protector and discuss use and care with the client; fit mouth protector.
5. After 1 week, evaluate fit and client response to the mouth protector.
6. Teach both child and parent about the periodontal disease process.
   - Explain the disease process of localized juvenile periodontitis
   - Use signs and symptoms of health and disease found in the client's own mouth as a teaching aid
7. Work collaboratively with the dentist and periodontist to carry out successful root planing and antimicrobial therapy.
8. Teach child and parent about bacterial plaque.
9. Teach child and parent personal skills (e.g., toothbrushing and flossing).
10. Evaluate knowledge and skill acquisition after 1 month.
11. Modify plan as needed.
12. Refer back to dentist or periodontist.

CASE STUDY. DENTAL HYGIENE PLAN: YOUNG CHILD WITH RAMPANT CARIES

Blake Olds, age 4, was brought to the dental hygiene clinic by his mother Caren, age 28. Caren is unemployed and on public assistance; therefore, finances are always a major concern. Blake has been in pain associated with his teeth. His mother reported that "he has been crying on and off for about four days, saying that his mouth hurt." The dental hygienist conducted a complete health, dental, and cultural history and initiated the assessment phase of the dental hygiene process of care with a baseline assessment of human needs related to dental hygiene care. Because of the immediacy of the need for relieving the child from pain, she collaborated with the attending dentist who extracted J, K, and L at that visit and who prescribed an antibiotic to control the infection. After the oral surgery, the client was dismissed and the dental hygienist analyzed the findings. Blake's significant findings included rampant caries and

CASE STUDY. DENTAL HYGIENE PLAN: YOUNG CHILD WITH RAMPANT CARIES *Continued*

periapical abscesses on J, K, and L, with caries also on A, B, E, F, I, M, O, P, S, and T. Because of extraction and interproximal caries, the maintenance of space for the permanent teeth is a major concern. Although there were no significant periodontal probe depths, there is green and orange extrinsic stain, heavy materia alba, and bacterial plaque throughout the mouth.

Dental Hygiene Diagnosis	Due To or Related To	As Evidenced By	Goal/Expected Behavior
Deficit in the human need for freedom from pain	• Rampant caries	• Patient's expression of pain and mother's report	• Refer to dentist for emergency care
Deficit in the human need for a biologically sound dentition	• Lack of financial resources	• Signs of caries and rampant caries • Presence of periapical abscesses • Space loss that could create a future malocclusion	• Assist parent in identifying dental care resources for low-income individuals • Refer client to dentist for care
Deficit in the human need for self-determination and responsibility	• Lack of parental supervision of daily oral hygiene • Too much autonomy for self care on the part of the child • Skill deficit of parent and client	• Heavy materia alba and bacterial plaque • Green/orange extrinsic stain present • Lack of a systematic and efficient method of toothbrushing	• Client shows improved oral hygiene within 1 month • Client cleans oral cavity once a day by himself; mother cleans client's oral cavity once a day • Parent demonstrates appropriate skill in cleaning client's mouth
Deficit in the human need for conceptualization and problem solving	• Knowledge deficit of parent and client	• Inability to explain the disease process and etiology • Lack of understanding about concepts of oral disease prevention	• Parent can explain the disease process and etiology; client can explain in age-appropriate terms • Parent verbalizes cost of preventing oral diseases vs. cost of treating them • Parent verbalizes the value of preventing further tooth or space loss for Blake • Parent verbalizes that she sees a visible change in Blake's teeth and gums

DENTAL HYGIENE INTERVENTIONS

1. Assess oral hygiene knowledge, attitude, and skill level of the client and the parent.
2. Instruct client and parent on basic oral hygiene:
   - Knowledge of etiology
   - Use of a toothbrush and positioning of client
   - Frequency of toothbrushing
3. Conduct nutritional counseling for caries control with the parent.
4. Discuss value of daily fluoride treatment until caries are controlled.
5. Discuss reasons for restoring the primary teeth:
   - Maintenance of space
   - Prevention of malocclusion
   - Prevention of need for costly orthodontics
6. Compliment client on the good job he is doing.
7. Refer parent to community facility where oral healthcare can be obtained on a sliding scale payment basis.
8. Complete scaling, selective polishing, and fluoride therapy; obtain prescription for daily fluoride therapy.
9. One month after, evaluate effectiveness of interventions.
10. Modify as necessary; maintain collaboration with treating dentist.

GUIDELINES FOR WRITING DENTAL HYGIENE DIAGNOSES

- Phrase the dental hygiene diagnosis as a client oral health problem or alteration in oral health state
- Indicate what the problem is related to; the problem and etiology should be linked by the phrase "related to"
- Indicate the evidence for the problem and etiology by stating the defining characteristics as observed in the client; the defining characteristics should be linked to the diagnostic statement by the phrase "as manifested by"
- Use language that avoids emotionalism or value judgment
- Be sure that the dental hygiene diagnosis is not a medical or dental diagnosis

the head and neck related to skill deficiency in removing bacterial plaque as evidenced by plaque and gingival bleeding scores of 5 and 3, respectively."

A dental hygiene diagnosis regarding a potential dental hygiene-related problem is written as a "potential problem with its presenting risk factors as the defining characteristics."[15] For example, a potential for human need deficits related to the needs for safety and for freedom from stress exists as a result of the use of "spit" tobacco. Such dental hygiene diagnoses should be documented as a permanent entry on the client's record. Some additional guidelines for writing dental hygiene diagnoses are presented in the Guidelines for Writing Dental Hygiene Diagnoses chart.

As dental hygienists begin to formulate dental hygiene diagnoses, it is expected that misunderstanding of the concept will translate into error. The most frequent errors found in dental hygiene diagnostic statements include: the presence of emotional terms, a dental diagnosis, etiology presented as the diagnosis, signs and symptoms presented as the diagnosis, and writing the diagnosis in terms of the client's needs rather than in terms of the client's response. These common errors are listed in Table 14–5 with guidelines on how these errors can be corrected.

As dental hygienists begin to work with the diagnostic process, dental hygiene diagnoses are expanded and refined. This classification needs to be further developed and research is needed on the diagnostic process, the validation of dental hygiene diagnoses, and the identification of interventions that work for each diagnosis.

To practice the process of arriving at a dental hygiene diagnosis, use the format shown in Figure 14–4. The dental hygienist can begin by reviewing the three case studies shown with their respective dental hygiene diagnoses, client goals, and dental hygiene interventions. These cases exemplify the dental hygiene diagnostic process, which can then be applied in the clinical setting.

TABLE 14–5
COMMON ERRORS IN WRITING DENTAL HYGIENE DIAGNOSES

Type of Error	Example of Poor Dental Hygiene Diagnosis	Correction Required	Example of Corrected Dental Hygiene Diagnosis
Emotionalism expressed in the diagnosis	Poor self-care related to laziness	Eliminate words that express emotionalism	Value deficit related to low priority ascribed to oral cleanliness as evidenced by heavy plaque accumulation
Dental diagnosis instead of a dental hygiene diagnosis	Moderate gingivitis and localized juvenile periodontitis	Avoid using dental diagnostic terms	Deficit in skin and mucous membrane integrity: Need for preliminary dental diagnosis, and refer to dentist for dental diagnosis
Citing etiology as the diagnosis	Knowledge deficit related to nonadherence	Use human need framework	Deficit in self-determination and responsibility related to a lack of manual dexterity and motivation as evidenced by poor oral hygiene
Identifying signs and symptoms as the client problem	Generalized gingival bleeding and attachment levels of 5–8 mm	Use signs and symptoms to focus on and validate the actual problem	Deficit in skin and mucous membrane integrity related to a lack of skill and motor ability as manifested by gingival bleeding and attachment loss of 5–8 mm
Writing the diagnosis in terms of client needs and not deficit	Needs education about the disease process and oral health products	Write the diagnosis in terms of client problem or responses rather than need	Deficit in conceptualization: Potential for oral disease related to a lack of knowledge about disease process and oral health products

Adapted from Taylor, C., Lillis, C., and LeMone, P. Fundamentals of Nursing, 2nd ed. Philadelphia: J. B. Lippincott, 1993, pp. 258–259.

Dental Hygiene Diagnosis	Due To	Evidenced By	Goal / Behavior

FIGURE 14-4
Worksheet for making a dental hygiene diagnosis.

Validation of the Dental Hygiene Diagnosis

Once the diagnosis is formulated, it must be validated. An affirmative response to each of the statements in Figure 14-5 validates the dental hygiene diagnosis.[16] The importance of validation is discussed also in Chapters 15 and 25.

What is Not a Dental Hygiene Diagnosis?

A dental hygiene diagnostic statement is written in terms of a client problem for which the dental hygienist provides the primary therapy. In writing dental hygiene diagnostic statements for the client record, the dental hygienist avoids dental diagnoses, medical diagnoses, medical pathology, and dental pathology because these are outside of the scope of dental hygiene practice. Table 14-6 provides examples of conditions that are *not* dental hygiene diagnoses.

OUTCOMES OF THE DENTAL HYGIENE DIAGNOSES

Collaboration and independent decision making is an important dimension of professionalism. Dental hygiene diagnoses require critical thinking and facilitate the development of dental hygienist autonomy and accountability by focusing on the phenomena that are uniquely dental hygiene and by providing a language for communication of the phenomena.[5,17-19] Autonomy is the "right to self-determination and governance without external control in which its membership defines and delineates the services that constitute practice."[20] Accountability is the "responsibility incurred by individuals and members to be morally obligated and answerable to a higher authority for services rendered."[20] The dental hygiene diagnosis, by identifying the client's human needs that can be fulfilled through dental

1. The database is complete, accurate, and based on a concept of dental hygiene. Yes ____ No ____
2. Data reflect the existence of a pattern. Yes ____ No ____
3. Both subjective and objective data support the existence of the human need deficit related to dental hygiene care identified in the dental hygiene diagnosis. Yes ____ No ____
4. The dental hygiene diagnosis is based on scientific knowledge. Yes ____ No ____
5. The dental hygiene diagnosis can be prevented, controlled, or resolved by dental hygiene interventions. Yes ____ No ____
6. Given the same data, other qualified dental hygiene practitioners would formulate the same dental hygiene diagnosis. Yes ____ No ____

FIGURE 14-5
"Yes" answers to all of these statements validate the dental hygiene diagnosis.

TABLE 14–6
WHAT A DENTAL HYGIENE DIAGNOSIS IS NOT

It Is Not A	Example	Rationale
Dental diagnosis	Myofascial pain disorder Class III malocclusion Advanced periodontal disease Oral carcinoma	Although there is dental hygiene care associated with dental diagnoses, the disease or disorder is not primarily amenable to dental hygiene intervention Dental hygiene's concern is for the person and the oral health behaviors in which they engage
Dental pathology	Leukoplakia	Dental hygienists need to understand the pathology underlying disease states to plan appropriate dental hygiene care; however, the focus is on the person's response and not the pathology The person's response to leukoplakia is the domain of dental hygiene
Diagnostic test, treatment, appliance	Pulp tester Antibiotic therapy Antimicrobial therapy Oral prosthetic appliances	Dental hygiene's concern is the individual's oral health behavior and response to the diagnostic test, treatment, or equipment If the need for antimicrobial therapy reveals a conceptualization or self-determination deficit, this is the dental hygiene diagnosis
Therapeutic need of the client	Client's need to learn the relationships among bacterial plaque, diet, and periodontal disease	The dental hygiene diagnosis should be written as a client oral health problem rather than as a client need Example: Conceptualization deficit related to a lack of knowledge of the relationships among bacterial plaque, diet, and periodontal disease
Dental hygiene treatment goal	To develop self-care behaviors to control bacterial plaque interproximally	The dental hygiene diagnosis should be written from the client's perspective, not the dental hygienist's perspective Example: Self-determination deficit related to lack of financial resources
Single sign or symptom	Bacterial plaque on lingual surfaces of all teeth	A dental hygiene diagnosis is not developed until a pattern or cluster of significant cues is identified The clustering of signs and symptoms leads to the dental hygiene diagnosis but in itself is not the diagnosis In this situation, no dental hygiene diagnosis is indicated until more data are collected, synthesized, analyzed, and interpreted
Unvalidated dental hygiene diagnosis	Previous example leads dental hygienist to the dental hygiene diagnosis: Deficit in conceptualization and problem solving	Unvalidated, this is a premature dental hygiene diagnosis that may not focus on the client's true problem More defining characteristics need to be identified before the dental hygiene diagnosis can be validated

Adapted from Taylor, C., Lillis, C., and LeMone, P. Fundamentals of Nursing, 2nd ed. Philadelphia: J. B. Lippincott, 1993, p. 260.

hygiene care, has the potential to alleviate ambiguity about the role of the dental hygienist and allows for a clearer definition of the scope, domain, and focus of dental hygiene practice. "Diagnosis by dental hygienists is not, and should not be, an attempt to move into the domain of the dentist; it is a vehicle for distinguishing roles professionally and legally."[2]

Dental hygiene diagnosis facilitates the delivery of quality dental hygiene care and quality assurance, and it provides a mechanism for charging for dental hygiene services. Because dental hygiene diagnoses are based on a logical classification system, the taxonomy of dental hygiene diagnoses, communication and collaboration among oral health professionals are facilitated as is the application of computerized information systems for operation and research. For example, the future use of the human needs conceptual model of dental hygiene and dental hygiene diagnoses appears promising for the development of a computerized system of diagnosis and care planning, with expansion to a system of cost accounting for dental hygiene. Diagnosis fosters clinical practice that is directed and capable of outcomes evaluation, which has implications for education, research, regulatory mechanisms, and direct access to care.

The dental hygiene diagnosis is a valued and essential

step in the dental hygiene process. Through the dental hygiene diagnosis, the domain of dental hygiene practice is reality. Used correctly, it is a significant tool for individualizing client care and ensuring that the dental hygienist focuses professional attention on the true oral health problem and its cause within the context of the total person. Only then can appropriate interventions be applied and outcomes evaluated to meet client needs.

References

1. Stein, J. (ed.). The Random House College Dictionary (rev. ed.). New York: Random House, 1982.
2. Miller, S. Dental hygiene diagnoses. RDH, July/August 1982, pp. 46–54.
3. Darby, M. L. Collaborative model of practice—the future of dental hygiene. Journal of Dental Education 47:9:589, 1983.
4. Gordon, M. Conceptual issues in nursing diagnosis. In Chaska, N. L. (ed.). The Nursing Profession: A Time to Speak. New York: McGraw-Hill, 1983.
5. Maas, L. Nursing diagnoses in a professional model of nursing: Keystone for effective nursing administration. Journal of Nursing Administration 16:39, 1986.
6. Bulechek, G., and McCloskey, J. Nursing diagnosis and interventions. In Bulechek, G, and McCloskey, J. (eds.). Nursing Interventions: Treatments for Nursing Diagnosis. Philadelphia: W. B. Saunders, 1985, pp. 1–18.
7. Gordon, M. Nursing Diagnosis: Process and Application, 2nd ed. New York: McGraw-Hill, 1987.
8. Gordon, M. Nursing diagnosis and the diagnostic process. American Journal of Nursing 76:1298, 1976.
9. Yura, H., and Walsh, M. B. The Nursing Process, 5th ed. New York: Appleton & Lange, 1988, p. 129.
10. Carpenito, L. J. Nursing Diagnoses: Application to Clinical Practice, 4th ed. Philadelphia: J. B. Lippincott, 1992.
11. Little, D. E., and Carnevali, D. I. Nursing Care Planning, 2nd ed. Philadelphia: J. B. Lippincott, 1976.
12. Marrines, A. The Nursing Process: A Scientific Approach to Nursing Care, 3rd ed. St. Louis: C. V. Mosby, 1983.
13. Mundinger, M. O., and Jauron, G. D. Developing a nursing diagnosis. Nursing Outlook 23:94, 1975.
14. Soares, C. Nursing and medical diagnosis: A comparison of essential and variant features. In Chaska, N. L. (ed.). The Nursing Profession: Views through the Mist. New York: McGraw-Hill, 1978.
15. O'Hearn, C. A. S. Nursing diagnosis: a phenomenological structural description and multidimensional taxonomy or typological redefinition. In Chaska, N. L. The Nursing Profession Turning Points. St. Louis: C. V. Mosby, 1990.
16. Price, M. R. Nursing diagnosis: making a concept come alive. American Journal of Nursing 80(4):668, 1980.
17. Peplaw, H. Further explanatory notes on nursing: a social policy statement. Paper presented at Nurses' Day, Des Moines, IA: Iowa Nurses Association, 1983.
18. King, I. Analysis of views on issues and trends related to nursing diagnosis and national conference. In Kim, M. J., McFarland, G. K., and McLane, A. M. (eds.). Classification of Nursing Diagnosis: Proceedings of the Fifth National Conference. St. Louis: C. V. Mosby Company, 1984, p. 567.
19. McCloskey, J. Analysis of views on issues and trends related to nursing diagnosis and national conference. In Kim, M. J., McFarland, G. K., and McLane, A. M. (eds.). Classification of Nursing Diagnoses: Proceedings of the Fifth National Conference. St. Louis: C. V. Mosby, 1984, p. 567.
20. Baer, C. L. Nursing diagnosis: a futuristic process for nursing practice. Topics in Clinical Nursing 5:89, 1984.

Suggested Readings

Alfaro, R. Application of Nursing Process: A Step-by-Step Guide. Philadelphia: J. B. Lippincott, 1986.

American Dental Hygienists' Association. Standards of Applied Dental Hygiene Practice. Chicago: American Dental Hygienists' Association, 1985.

Gurenlian, J. R. The politics of diagnosis. Access 8(2):11, 1994.

Heidgerken, L. Nursing research—its role in research activities in nursing. Nursing Research 11:140, 1962.

Korchen, S. Modern Clinical Psychology. New York: Basic Books, 1976.

Taylor, C., Lillis, C., and LeMone, P. Fundamentals of Nursing, 2nd ed. Philadelphia: J. B. Lippincott, 1993.

15 Dental Hygiene Care Plan

OBJECTIVES

Mastery of the content in this chapter will enable the reader to:

- Define the key terms
- Discuss the purposes of developing a dental hygiene care plan
- Discuss the role of the client in developing the dental hygiene care plan
- Identify phrases that can be used to increase client participation in dental hygiene care planning
- Write client-centered goals that contain a subject, a verb, a criterion for measurement, and a time dimension
- Discuss the concept of informed consent as it relates to the dental hygiene process of care
- Develop a dental hygiene care plan derived from a dental hygiene diagnosis
- Discuss the importance of collaborating with other healthcare professionals during the planning phase of the dental hygiene process
- Integrate the dental hygiene care plan with the appointment plan

INTRODUCTION

Planning is that phase of the dental hygiene process in which priorities are set, client goals are established, and interventions and outcome measures are determined (Fig. 15-1). The primary purpose of the planning phase of the dental hygiene process is to develop the plan of care, which, once implemented, will result in the resolution of an oral health problem amenable to dental hygiene care, the prevention of a problem, or the promotion of oral health. Therefore, **care plan,** rather than treatment plan, is consciously used to denote the broad range of preventive, educational, therapeutic, and support services within the scope of dental hygiene practice. In recognition of clients' human need for self-determination, the dental hygienist actively involves clients, according to their ability and motivation, in all aspects of the dental hygiene process and obtains the informed consent of the client (or client's guardian) prior to the initiation of professional care. This philosophy is particularly relevant during the planning phase of care. The tangible outcome of the planning phase is the dental hygiene care plan.

To formulate a care plan, the professional dental hygienist must:

- Possess a sound background in dental hygiene theory
- Be thoroughly familiar with the standards for professional dental hygiene care
- Possess the ability to collect, analyze, and interpret client data
- Develop dental hygiene diagnoses
- Formulate client goals
- Select appropriate dental hygiene interventions
- Be able to synthesize this aforementioned information into a written plan
- Be able to view the dental hygiene care plan within the context of the total treatment plan developed by the dentist

The intent of this chapter is to apply the principles of dental hygiene care planning that enable the dental hygienist to write comprehensive dental hygiene care plans that meet the human needs of clients and that support the dental treatment plan developed by the dentist.

Total Dental Treatment Plan

The general dentist, or dental specialist, develops a total dental treatment plan for the client. This usually includes the dental diagnosis, the essential services that need to be carried out by the dentist, dental hygienist, and client to eliminate or control disease, and the prognosis. The total dental treatment plan includes:

- Emergency treatment
    - Relief of pain
    - Laboratory tests for suspected pathology
- Preventive care
- Educational services
- Initial preparation
- Treatment
    - Endodontic

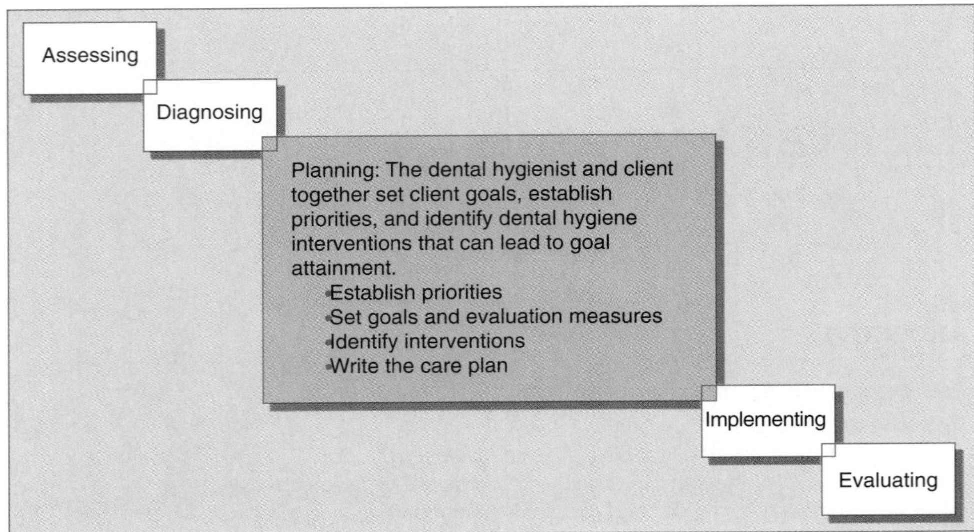

FIGURE 15–1
Planning phase of the dental hygiene process.

Periodontal
Restorative
Prosthetic
Orthodontic

- Maintenance

To best meet the needs of the client, the dental hygiene care plan must support the total dental treatment plan. This requires communication and collaboration between the dental hygienist and the dentist.

Client Involvement in the Dental Hygiene Process

Too often, individuals receiving care in the oral healthcare setting are referred to as the "class II cavity preparation in treatment room two" or "the perio case at 4:00 P.M." These apparently harmless phrases communicate an insensitivity to the individual who is the focus of the dental hygiene care. The dental hygienist who is practicing within a human needs framework would more aptly refer to these persons as "Mrs. Smith who has a human need for a biologically sound dentition as evidenced by a class II cavity on tooth number 19" or "Mr. Jones who has a deficit in skin and mucous membrane integrity of the head and neck as indicated by his class IV periodontal disease."

The oral healthcare professional who views the person as the focus of attention is more likely to establish a collaborative, co-therapeutic relationship with the client. This philosophy of care sets the stage for active client participation in identifying needs, priorities, goals, and interventions. Clients who are encouraged to participate in the process of care are more likely to communicate their wants, needs, and expectations than to relinquish all decision-making about their oral care to the dentist or dental hygienist. Individuals are more likely to express commitment to a care plan if they shared in the development of goals, priorities, interventions, and even appointment planning. Furthermore, when persons have been a part of the planning process and have a key role in the overall success of the plan, the likelihood of compliance is augmented.

Involving the client in the dental hygiene process is a difficult concept for most dental hygienists to implement. The following scenario is presented to analyze some strategies that may be used by the dental hygienist to involve the client in the dental hygiene care planning process.

> Mrs. Riner, one of the key points you conveyed to me earlier today was that you are experiencing bleeding when you brush and that you can't seem to eliminate the odor in your mouth. Is that still your primary concern? (Allow client to respond.) Let us together examine your mouth and see if we can identify the factors that might be contributing to the bleeding and odor (dental hygienist gives client a large mirror; dental hygienist also uses mouth mirror and probe). (Client begins to point out gingival bleeding as hygienist shows client pocket depths and attachment loss.) The areas of bleeding seem to correlate with the areas of bacterial plaque and calculus accumulations. Would you agree that you need a better way of removing bacterial plaque on a daily basis? (Allow client to respond.) If you agree, I would like to explain the disease process that we are seeing in your mouth and what you can do at home to prevent further disease. After you have mastered the home care, I would like to schedule you for two, 1-hour appointments that would be devoted to the removal of calculus and bacterial toxins from your teeth, polishing your teeth, and then fluoride therapy for root desensitization and dental caries prevention. Is this set of priorities and the appointment scheduling acceptable to you? (Allow client to respond. Observe both verbal and nonverbal communication.) When this has been completed, we should have you return after 1 month to evaluate your home care and gingival healing. (Do you have any suggestions for how we can best work together?) (Are you interested in having this done?) (Are you interested in achieving this goal?)

Although the scenario is short, some of the verbal statements made by the dental hygienist operationalize the philosophy of a client-oriented dental hygiene process of care. Phrases that can be used by the dental hygienist who is interested in making the client the central focus of care are listed in the box below.

Certainly there are times when specific goals are valued more highly by the dental hygienist than by the client. When this occurs, the dental hygienist should provide an explanation for his professional judgment, with a clear message that the client's wants and needs are equally important to the overall care plan. While these points are important for obtaining client commitment and compliance with the final dental hygiene care plan, dental hygienists must also keep in mind that respecting the client's role as a co-therapist and as a partner in decision-making is an effective risk management strategy for avoiding malpractice.

There are also times when the client disagrees with the dental hygienist's recommended care plan. The client may not want certain procedures or may choose to delay care despite the dental hygienist's careful explanations and rationales. Such disagreements between dental hygienist and client may manifest themselves in the client's:

- Refusal of fluoride therapy, radiographs, or antimicrobial agents
- Noncompliance with a referral to a dental specialist or physician
- Nonadherence to a specific oral home care technique
- Decision to terminate care prior to goal attainment
- Refusal to give up a behavior, such as her use of tobacco, that increases the risk of oral disease

Although disappointing to the dental hygienist, such client responses must be carefully analyzed to determine how or why the client arrived at that decision. In such situations, further discussion with and education of the client is warranted. Of course, if the client continues to refuse professional advice, this occurrence should be documented in the client's permanent record. Documenting *informed refusal* is a risk management strategy for the potential threat of malpractice (see Chapter 39).

In some situations, the client may request care that, in the opinion of the dentist or dental hygienist, is unwarranted, inappropriate, or dangerous. If the dental hygienist is faced with this dilemma, she should refuse to provide the care and encourage the client to seek a second professional opinion.

Establishing Priorities

To establish priorities in care, the dental hygienist considers the dental and dental hygiene diagnoses and, in **collaboration** with the dentist, determines their urgency. Although many criteria can be used to determine priorities, the following considerations prove helpful:

The degree to which the dental hygiene diagnosis relates to a human need deficit that:

- threatens the client's well-being (it is importtant to distinguish deficits that pose the greatest threat to the client's comfort, health, and safety from those that are non–life-threatening and/or not related to a current oral disease)
- can be addressed simultaneously with other diagnoses
- is viewed as a priority by the client (client preferences)

Once these criteria are applied to the dental hygiene diagnoses, the dental hygienist rank-orders the human need deficits in the priority that they will be addressed.

Other than meeting the client's human need for freedom from pain, which in most instances constitutes emergency care, most dentists and dental hygienists would probably identify the client's ability to assume responsibility for the control of his own oral disease (human need for self-determination and responsibility) as a top priority. The establishment of priorities is always influenced by factors such as:

- The attitudes of the client
- The philosophy of the healthcare provider
- Goals of the collaborating dentist
- Health status of the client
- Whether or not the client is experiencing any discomfort

After the list of dental hygiene diagnoses are prioritized, the process of goal setting can begin.

Basing care plans on dental hygiene diagnoses, rather than on oral symptoms alone, ensures that care will be comprehensive, individualized, and focused on the human needs of the client. It also directs the dental hygienist's attention to the causes of the signs and symptoms and, hence, to what dental hygiene interventions can be used to control or eliminate the etiology, as opposed to providing the same routine care to all clients. Since signs and symptoms related to dental hygiene problems may have numer-

COMMON PHRASES USED BY THE DENTAL HYGIENIST TO MAXIMIZE CLIENT INVOLVEMENT IN THE DENTAL HYGIENE PROCESS

- Here is a hand mirror. Let's examine your mouth together.
- What was your primary reason for seeking dental hygiene care?
- Is this set of priorities acceptable to you?
- Is this care plan acceptable to you?
- What would you like to achieve as a result of dental hygiene care?
- How will you feel if this goal is attained?
- Are you satisfied with the plan of care we just discussed?
- How important is your oral health?
- Where would you like me (the dental hygienist) to start first?
- When and where is it easiest for you to clean your mouth (or your dependent's mouth)?
- Can you think of a better way that we can accomplish this goal?
- Let's compare how your gingiva looks today with how it looked 2 weeks ago.
- What are you willing to do to keep your mouth healthy?

ous etiologies, it holds that interventions must be carefully selected to ensure that the fundamental cause is being addressed in dental hygiene care. For example, a dental hygiene diagnosis of a human need deficit in the area of wholesome body image may be due to:

- Client dissatisfaction with the color of his teeth
- Client embarrassment because of a disfiguring malocclusion
- A teenage boy's distress about having to wear an orthodontic appliance that he views as unattractive
- A teenage girl's embarrassment over the monthly herpetic lesion that she develops in association with her menstrual cycle
- A middle-aged man's loss of self-esteem associated with mobile teeth and halitosis from adult-onset periodontal disease
- A resident of a nursing home who has misplaced her denture and who no longer wants to interact with friends and family

All these problems require the establishment of unique client goals and varying dental hygiene interventions to resolve them. Figure 15–2 uses the aforementioned examples as the basis for establishing goals and planning dental hygiene interventions that focus on the unique needs of the client who is dissatisfied with the color of his teeth. Another example of a dental hygiene care plan is shown in Figure 15–3.

Writing Client-Centered Goals

A **client-centered goal** is defined as the desired end result that the client is to achieve through specific dental hygiene interventions. Client-centered goals must be directly related to the dental hygiene diagnosis. The direct link between the dental hygiene diagnosis and the client-centered goal increases the likelihood of dental hygiene care that meets the needs of the client. It also underscores the importance of the client as the main focus of dental hygiene care.

At least one goal and one intervention should be established for each dental hygiene diagnosis. Examples of client-centered goals related to the dental hygiene diagnosis are presented in Table 15–1.

As discussed in Chapter 3, goals may be cognitive, affective, or psychomotor in nature. Cognitive goals target increases in the client's knowledge. Human needs related to dental hygiene care that provide the basis for cognitive goals are wholesome body image; nutrition; safety; and conceptualization, rationality, and problem solving. Psychomotor goals reflect the client's skill development and skill mastery. The human need related to dental hygiene care that provides the basis for psychomotor goals is the human need for self-determination and responsibility. Affective goals address the desired changes in client values, beliefs, and attitudes. Human needs that provide the basis for affective goals are the needs for a wholesome body image; freedom from pain/stress; safety; territoriality; and appreciation and respect.

Client's Name: ______________________________

OBJECTIVE DATA

1. Health history reveals no significant findings
2. Class II extrinsic stain
3. Class II calculus
4. Class III intrinsic tetracycline stain

SUBJECTIVE DATA

1. Client verbalized "I wish that my teeth were a whiter color," and "My teeth seem to be darkening with my age."

Dental Hygiene Diagnosis	Due To or Related To	As Evidenced By	Goals/Expected Behavior
Human need deficit in wholesome body image	• Client's dissatisfaction with the color of his teeth	• Client verbalizes that he doesn't like the color of his teeth • Client asked if there is anything that can be done to make his teeth whiter	• Increase the whiteness of the client's tooth color by 6/28

DENTAL HYGIENE INTERVENTIONS

1. Measure color of client's teeth using a color scale.
2. Refer client to dentist for consultation of cosmetic bleaching options.
3. Recommend that client uses tooth-whitening toothpastes with fluoride available on the market.
4. Educate client about the normal color of teeth.
5. Remove all calculus deposits and extrinsic stains from the client's teeth.

EVALUATIVE STATEMENTS

1. The color of client's teeth will lighten by at least two values on the color scale.
2. The client will verbalize his satisfaction with the color appearance of his teeth.

FIGURE 15–2
Dental hygiene care plan for a client who wants whiter teeth.

Client's Name: ____________________

OBJECTIVE DATA

1. Health history reveals no human immunodeficiency virus (HIV) infection and no risk factors associated with HIV infection.

SUBJECTIVE DATA

1. Client verbalized "I am frightened about the cases of people getting AIDS from their dentist," and "I had a friend who died from AIDS within the past year."

Dental Hygiene Diagnosis	Due To or Related To	As Evidenced By	Goals/Expected Behavior
Human need deficit in safety	• Fear about acquiring AIDS as a result of dental hygiene care	• Client's continual discussion of the case of the Florida dentist who infected six of his clients with HIV	• By 9/9, client will state the three modes of HIV transmission • By 9/9, client will verbalize confidence in her ability to find and obtain quality dental/dental hygiene care • By 12/2, client will verbalize decreased anxiety about acquiring AIDS from a dental practice

DENTAL HYGIENE INTERVENTIONS

1. Assess client's knowledge of HIV transmission; reinforce known modes of transmission.
2. Provide client with information about the universal precautions used in the practice.
3. Answer client's questions and address concerns.
4. Provide client with accurate reading material about AIDS transmission.

EVALUATIVE STATEMENTS

1. Client will verbalize the three basic modes by which HIV infection is acquired.
2. Client will indicate that she is impressed by the infection control procedures used in the dental practice.
3. Client will verbalize that she would recommend the practice to her friends and that she looks forward to her next appointment in 1 year.

FIGURE 15–3
Dental hygiene care plan for a client who is afraid of contracting AIDS at the dental office.

TABLE 15–1
EXAMPLES OF CLIENT-CENTERED GOALS AS RELATED TO THE DENTAL HYGIENE DIAGNOSIS

Dental Hygiene Diagnosis	Goals
Human need deficit in freedom from stress (related to parent's divorce as evidenced by a thumb-sucking habit)	By 1/14, parent will report decreased thumb-sucking behavior in the client during television watching By 2/15, parent will report no thumb-sucking behavior in the client during television watching By 2/30, parent will report no thumb-sucking behavior during bedtime
Human need deficit in nutrition (related to a lack of knowledge about nutrition, a history of periodontal problems, as evidenced by junk food eating and the beginning of periimplantitis)	By 3/12, client will exhibit the ability to make informed food choices required for healing, repair, and maintenance of the periodontium
Human need deficit in skin and mucous membrane integrity of the head and neck (due to subgingival plaque accumulation in 4-mm pockets as evidenced by visible plaque and gingival bleeding)	By 5/11, the client will verbalize the benefits of daily subgingival irrigation with an antimicrobial to control plaque and gingivitis By 5/11, the client will demonstrate the proper use of an oral irrigator for the at-home target delivery of an antimicrobial to the subgingival areas of the mouth By 6/15, the client will exhibit a gingival bleeding score of no more than 2
Human need deficit in freedom from stress (due to abuse of spit tobacco as evidenced by a 6-mm, white lesion in the oral vestibule adjacent to teeth nos. 22, 23, and 24)	By 10/4, the client will verbalize the risks associated with the daily use of spit tobacco and describe a plan for discontinuing its use By 11/15, the client will reduce the frequency of use of spit tobacco By 12/20, the client will complete a program for spit tobacco cessation By 1/15, client reports that he no longer uses tobacco

These goals, if achieved, resolve client deficits in knowledge, values, and skills, respectively. For example, a client may intellectually grasp the importance of daily bacterial plaque control in a class III furcation (cognitive) but still need instruction from the dental hygienist in using an interdental brush and antimicrobial agent to control disease in the area (psychomotor). Both cognitive and psychomotor goals would need to be established in the dental hygiene care plan of this client.

Adopting a format for each client-centered goal simplifies the act of goal writing (see Guidelines for Writing Client-Centered Goals). Each client-centered goal should have a *subject,* a *verb,* a *criterion for measurement,* and a *time dimension.* The subject is the client (or client's caregiver); the verb is the action desired of the client; the criterion is the observable behavior or tangible outcome expected; and the time dimension denotes when the subject is to have achieved the goal. Methods used for the evaluation of client-centered goals are discussed in Chapter 25.

Developing an Evaluative Strategy

Chapter 25, Evaluation of Dental Hygiene Care, specifically addresses the evaluation phase of the dental hygiene process. However, during the planning phase, an evaluation strategy is identified and reflected in the written plan of care.

Most dental hygiene care plans contain an **expected outcome** that reflects the evidence that will be used to determine if the client's goal was *met, partially met,* or *not met at all.* Each goal must correspondingly have an expected outcome. The expected outcome becomes an **evaluative statement,** when on evaluation of care, the dental hygienist makes one of the following decisions—goal met, goal partially met, or goal not met—and indicates this in writing. If the goal was partially met or not met, the dental hygienist reassesses the client, discusses the findings with the dentist, and, perhaps, modifies the dental hygiene diagnosis and care plan. Hence, the cyclical nature of the process of care is again in motion. Without an evaluative statement, the value of dental hygiene care is too easily overlooked.

GUIDELINES FOR WRITING CLIENT-CENTERED GOALS

- Prepare each goal, or set of goals, from only one dental hygiene diagnosis.
- Make sure that the goals, if met, will resolve the problem reflected in the dental hygiene diagnosis.
- Collaborate with the dentist to ensure that the dental hygiene and dental care plans are mutually supportive.
- Involve the client in goal setting.
- Make sure that the client values the goals set.
- Write goals that are observable and measurable.
- Use active verbs to denote the critical client behavior expected in the goal, such as the following:

define	plan	exhibit
describe	demonstrate	increase
discuss	perform	decrease
explain	use	affirm
verbalize	choose	detect
purchase	report	communicate
replace	eliminate	stop
complete	guide	finish
remove		

Selected Dental Hygiene Interventions

Dental hygiene interventions, like client goals, are derived from the dental hygiene diagnosis, including the cause and the evidence that supports the diagnosis. If dental hygiene care is to be effective, the dental hygienist must select interventions that specifically address the underlying factors contributing to the client's human need deficit related to dental hygiene care.

For example, many factors may contribute to a client's deficit in the need for a biologically sound dentition (dental caries): deficit in knowledge about caries prevention, high intake of sugars, skill deficit in toothbrushing and flossing, deficit in the nutrient of fluoride, inability to value good oral hygiene, low self-esteem, and inadequate financial resources as a barrier to oral healthcare, just to mention a few. Thus, not every client with a high caries rate is cared for in the same way. Professional dental hygiene care involves the careful tailoring of dental hygiene interventions to meet the unique needs of the client, as directed by the dental hygiene diagnosis.

The Dental Hygiene Care Plan

The **dental hygiene care plan** is the written blueprint that directs the dental hygienist and client as they work together to meet the client's goals for oral health. Primarily, the plan increases the likelihood that the oral healthcare team will work collaboratively to deliver client-focused, goal-oriented, individualized care to clients. The care plan facilitates the monitoring of client progress, ensures continuity of care, serves as a vehicle for communication among healthcare professionals, and increases the likelihood of quality care (see Rationale for Developing a Formal Dental Hygiene Care Plan chart).

The dental hygiene care plan is prepared on the day that the dental hygienist completes the assessment and diagnosis phases of the dental hygiene process and in conjunction with the overall dental treatment plan prepared by the dentist. The plan must clearly specify the dental hygiene diagnoses, client goals, dental hygiene interventions, and evaluative strategies. To save space, the plan uses standardized

RATIONALE FOR DEVELOPING A FORMAL DENTAL HYGIENE CARE PLAN

- To individualize dental hygiene care
- To focus care on priorities
- To facilitate communication and collaboration among healthcare professionals
- To establish client-centered goals
- To have a foundation on which evaluation of dental hygiene interventions can be based
- To evaluate the client's response to dental hygiene care (outcomes)
- To promote professional dental hygiene practice

CHARACTERISTICS OF A WELL-WRITTEN DENTAL HYGIENE CARE PLAN

- Reflects the purposes of dental hygiene, which are to:
  - Develop and maintain the individual's capacity to perform the behaviors essential to oral health and the mastery of self-care and the environment.
  - Prevent oral disease whenever possible using primary, secondary, and tertiary preventive interventions.
  - Promote oral wellness.
- Is consistent with the needs of the client.
- Identifies the dental hygiene diagnosis, related client goals, and dental hygiene interventions.
- Is compatible with the dental treatment plan prepared by the dentist.
- Identifies the dental hygienist's responsibilities, if any, for fulfilling components of the dental treatment plan.
- Is based on current standards of professional dental hygiene care.
- Meets the psychosociocultural needs, as well as the physical needs, of the client.
- Reflects the dental hygienist's role as clinician, educator/health promoter, manager, researcher, change agent, client advocate.
- Establishes the priorities of care.

abbreviations, and key phrases as specified in the policy manual of the healthcare institution with which the dental hygienist is affiliated (see Characteristics of a Well-Written Dental Hygiene Care Plan chart).

Once written and shared with the client, the care plan becomes a legal contract between the dental hygienist and the client. When one begins to write the dental hygiene care plan, each assessment finding should be scrutinized to determine its relationship to a potential human need deficit. Human need deficits, supported by assessment findings, become the dental hygiene diagnoses in the care plan. Once the diagnosis is made, the dental hygienist establishes, in conjunction with the client, client-centered goals. From the established client goals, interventions and expected outcomes can be drafted. With client input, priorities for each goal are established, and then appointment planning can begin.

Once priorities are established, the dental hygienist must estimate the time necessary to complete each intervention (see Time Estimates for Some Dental Hygiene Procedures chart). Of course, the speed and experience of each dental hygienist and the oral conditions of the client affect the ultimate time required for quality, comprehensive client care.

Many suggestions for dental hygiene care plans appear in the dental hygiene literature.[1,2] Each dental hygiene care facility may have its own format. The care plan format should provide the dental hygienist with an opportunity to document assessment findings, dental hygiene diagnoses, client-centered goals, dental hygiene interventions, evaluative outcomes anticipated from care, and the expected date of goal attainment. Although formats may differ, the critical point is that these factors are documented in the client's permanent record and are followed rigorously to ensure quality dental hygiene care.

The dental hygienist can assess the comprehensiveness of the care plan by answering the following questions:

- Does the care plan address the client's human need deficits related to oral health that are amenable to or affect the outcomes of dental hygiene care?
- Has the cultural diversity of the client been considered?

TIME ESTIMATES (IN MINUTES) FOR SOME DENTAL HYGIENE PROCEDURES

	Dental Hygiene Student	Dental Hygiene Practitioner
Assessment/Diagnosis		
Health/dental/cultural history	10	10
Dental charting	15	10–15
Periodontal assessment	30	10–15
Intraoral photographs	15	5
Reassessment	15	5
Planning		
Care planning	15	10
Implementation		
Oral health instruction	30	15–30
Scaling and root planing	1–12 hr	1–4 hr
Extrinsic stain removal	20	10
Fluoride therapy	5	5
Desensitization therapy	5	2
Antimicrobial irrigation therapy	10	5
Impressions	15	5
Athletic mouth protector	30	15
Study models	30	10
Ultrasonic scaling	15–60	10–40
Tobacco cessation therapy	30–60	15–45
Dietary counseling therapy	30–60	15–45
Evaluation	1 hr	30 min

- What might be the client's response to the care plan? For example, will the client express interest, worry, fear, discontent, or lack of enthusiasm?
- How can the dental hygienist best present the care plan to elicit client cooperation?
- How can client involvement be maximized in the care plan?
- What alternative care plans should be offered to the client?
- What is the dental hygienist's response if the client refuses care?

Informed Consent and the Dental Hygiene Care Plan

Most consumers no longer view healthcare professionals as infallible. Clients expect to participate in their dental hygiene care and have a right to accept or refuse care. To enable the client to participate in care, the dental hygiene care plan must be presented to the client. Failure to present the care plan to the client can result in services performed without the client's knowledge or permission. This scenario can result in a violation of tort law known as **technical assault.**

Informed consent is a legal term that means that the client must be knowledgeable about what the healthcare provider plans to do and must give permission for the plans to be carried out. A key element in informed consent is that the client must have enough information to make a rational choice. To meet the requirements of informed consent, the client must receive, in understandable language, the following information from the healthcare provider:

- the nature of the condition
- the proposed care plan
- the risks involved (if any)
- the potential for failure
- the expected outcomes if the problem goes untreated
- the alternative procedures that might be used

In addition to the requirements of informed consent, the client giving consent must:

- be legally competent
- be informed
- give consent to a specific treatment
- give consent to a procedure that is legal
- give consent under truthful conditions, for example, the consent cannot be obtained through fraud, deceit, or trickery

Although informed consent is given when a client voluntarily comes to the oral healthcare setting and sits in the dental chair, his implied consent applies only to the assessment, diagnosis, and planning components of the dental hygiene process of care. The dental hygienist cannot assume that the client consents to any further care (see Chapter 39, Ethical and Legal Decision Making in Dental Hygiene). The dental hygienist must keep in mind that the client must provide **expressed consent,** orally or in writing, for specific procedures to be performed.

APPOINTMENT PLANNING

Once the dental hygiene care plan has been formulated, it must be operationalized into specific appointments. In most oral healthcare settings, the dental hygiene care can be provided to meet the expressed preference of clients. Keep the following points in mind when planning appointments:

- Estimated time needed for each procedure
- The logic of grouping procedures that are interrelated
- Client's tolerance for long sessions
- Client's scheduling requirements, for example, early morning only, time limitations
- Client's preferences

Figures 15–4 through 15–9 are sample dental hygiene care plans and appointment sequences for clients with various dental hygiene diagnoses. In each example, the CDT-1 Procedure Code from the American Dental Association Council on Dental Care Programs is given to show how these various procedures can be billed for third-party reimbursement.[3]

A. DENTAL HYGIENE CARE PLAN

Dental Hygiene Diagnosis	Goals	Evaluative Statements or Expected Outcomes	Dental Hygiene Interventions
Deficit in skin and mucous membrane integrity of the head and neck	• By 8/4, client will have healthy gingiva with no bleeding, swelling, or tenderness	• No evidence of gingival inflammation or periodontal attachment levels greater than 3 mm present in oral cavity. Client complies with recommended treatment to reverse gingivitis	• Perform therapeutic procedures as outlined in appointment plan
		• No evidence of bleeding on probing gingival tissues	• Provide appropriate ''continuous care'' every 4 to 6 months
	• By 9/4, client will demonstrate proper oral self-care skills	• Client reports successful use of oral self-care aids	• Demonstrate proper angulation of toothbrush and wrap method for floss/dentotape
	• By 9/4, client will disrupt/remove bacterial plaque every 24 hours	• Client achieves a score of no more than 1.7 on the Patient Hygiene Performance Index	• Involve client in the design of an oral self-care skills/regimen • Recommend daily use of brush and floss and an effective antimicrobial mouth rinse (Listerine)
	• By 9/10, client will describe the disease process and how it is related to gingivitis	• Client verbalizes the etiology and control of gingivitis	• Explain disease process and its role in gingivitis

B. SAMPLE APPOINTMENT PLAN

(Dental Hygiene Diagnosis: Deficit in the human need for skin and mucous membrane integrity of the head and neck)

Description: Edematous and erythematous gingiva; bleeding; loss of stippling; no attachment loss; shallow pockets 0 to 3 mm and pseudopockets 4 mm in depth.

Four Appointments (or as needed):

FIRST APPOINTMENT (1 HOUR)	CDT-1 PROCEDURE CODE
• Initial intra- and extraoral examination (includes health/dental cultural history, head and neck examination, oral cancer examination, dental/periodontal charting)	00110
• Complete intraoral series of radiographs, including bitewings	00210
• Document and present findings to client	N/A
SECOND APPOINTMENT (1 HOUR)	
• Inform client of diagnosis and recommended care plan, and obtain informed consent	N/A
• Periodontal scaling performed in the presence of gingival inflammation (ultrasonic scaling and hand-scaling entire mouth)	04345
• Oral hygiene instructions	01330
• Postoperation instructions	N/A
THIRD APPOINTMENT, 1 WEEK LATER (45 MINUTES)	
• Prophylaxis (hand-scale and polish)	01110
• Oral hygiene instruction	01330

FIGURE 15–4
A, Dental hygiene care plan. *B*, Appointment plan.

SAMPLE APPOINTMENT PLAN *Continued*

FOURTH APPOINTMENT, 2 WEEKS LATER (30 MINUTES)

• Periodic oral examination (reevaluation of tissue, probe, charting, and client attitude)	00120
• Oral hygiene instruction	01330
• Client scheduled for oral health continued care (recall) appointment:	
continuing care (cc)—45 minutes at 2, 3, 4, or 6 months	1110
periodontal maintenance (PM)—1 hour procedures at 2, 3, 4, or 6 months (or as needed)	4910

TOTAL TIME: approx. 3 hr, 15 min

FIGURE 15–4 *Continued*

Dental Hygiene Diagnosis	Goals	Evaluative Statements or Expected Outcomes	Dental Hygiene Interventions
Deficit in skin and mucous membrane integrity of head and neck.	• By 1/10, client will maintain periodontal tissues in a healthy state with no further destruction	• No evidence of bleeding on probing the periodontal tissues • No evidence of further loss of periodontal attachment • No evidence of active disease in pockets, such as exudate or further bone loss • No evidence of further destruction of alveolar bone or connective tissue attachment	• Teach client to use bleeding as an indicator of active disease progression • Involve client in determining when plaque removal can best fit into his lifestyle and schedule • Perform therapeutic procedures as outlined in appointment plans based on type of disease
Deficit in self-determination and responsibility	• By 6/3, client will demonstrate effective oral self-care skills	• Client reports successful use of oral self-care aids	• Assess client's psychomotor skill level • Demonstrate plaque control measures • Recommend use of antimicrobial rinse at home
	• Client will describe the disease process and how it relates to periodontitis • By 6/3, client disrupts/removes bacterial plaque every 24 hours	• Client explains the relationship between bacterial plaque and periodontal disease progression • Client achieves a score of no more than 1.5 on the Patient Hygiene Performance Index	• Teach client about the progression of periodontal disease • Teach client about plaque formation and pathogenicity
	• By 2/15, client assumes responsibility for the management of periodontal conditions by practicing daily oral self-care skills	• Client demonstrates successful use of self-care skills	• Involve client as co-therapist in the design of self-care skills program • Periodically contact client by telephone to monitor motivational level
	• By 2/15, client verbally communicates openly with the dental hygienist and participates in decision making about his dental hygiene care	• Client will verbalize his role in preventing the occurrence of oral diseases in his own mouth	• Explain important role of the client in preventing oral disease over the lifespan
	• By 6/15, client participates in treatment of periodontitis by attending all dental hygiene care and continued care appointments	• Client complies with treatment and maintenance visits and referrals to specialist • Client actively seeks dental	• Schedule peridontal maintenance appointments in advance • Provide appropriate follow-up care (dental hygiene evaluation)

FIGURE 15–5
Dental hygiene care plan for a client with periodontal disease. (Data from American Academy of Periodontology, Current Procedural Terminology for Periodontics, 5th ed. Washington, DC: The Association, 1987; and Code on Dental Procedures and Nomenclature: Report from the Council on Dental Care Programs. Journal of the American Dental Association 122:91, 1991.)

Figure continued on following page

Dental Hygiene Diagnosis	Goals	Evaluative Statements or Expected Outcomes	Dental Hygiene Interventions
		hygiene services and periodontal maintenance procedures	
Deficit in wholesome body image	• Client will have normal breath with no halitosis	• No evidence of halitosis associated with periodontal disease	• Perform therapeutic procedures as outlined in appointment plans based on type of disease
	• Client accepts dental hygiene/periodontal interventions as a coordinated effort toward comprehensive care	• Client has realistic expectations for alterations in appearance of periodontal conditions	• Liaison with other dentists to coordinate various treatment interventions (e.g., aesthetics, implants)
	• Client accepts dental hygiene/periodontal interventions as a coordinated effort toward comprehensive care	• Client has realistic expectations for alterations in appearance of periodontal conditions	• Liaison with other dentists to coordinate various treatment interventions (e.g., aesthetics, implants)
		• Client expresses greater acceptance of periodontal conditions	• Provide client with verbal and nonverbal reinforcement demonstrating acceptance of client's disease state
		• No evidence of bacterial plaque and calculus deposits	• Provide education regarding client's expressed dissatisfaction with periodontal condition
		• No evidence of bleeding and inflamed gingival tissues	• Provide periodontal maintenance procedures every 2 to 4 months
Deficit in value system	• By 9/4, client will regularly attend recommended appointments	• Client actively seeks regular dental hygiene services and periodontal maintenance procedures	• Explain periodontal disease in terms of the need for long-term control over the lifespan, rather than as a disease that is curable • Provide appropriate periodontal maintenance procedures every 2 or 4 months or as needed • Refer to periodontist for periodontal therapy and pocket elimination

FIGURE 15–5 *Continued*

SAMPLE APPOINTMENT PLAN

(Dental Hygiene Diagnosis: Deficit in the human need for skin and mucous membrane integrity of the head and neck and freedom from pain and stress.)

Description: Inflammation has progressed past the gingiva into the periodontal structures and the alveolar bone crest with slight bone loss evident. Pocket depths are 4 to 5 mm, with loss of connective tissue attachment in the range of 2 to 4 mm.

Five Appointments (or as needed):

FIRST APPOINTMENT (1 OR 1½ HOURS)	CDT-1 PROCEDURE CODE
• Initial intra- and extraoral examination (includes health/dental/cultural history, head and neck examination, oral cancer examination, dental/periodontal charting)	00110
• Complete intraoral series of radiographs, including bitewings	00210
• Document and present findings to client	N/A
• Periodontal (therapeutic) scaling performed in the presence of gingival inflammation (if applicable*)	4345
SECOND APPOINTMENT (1 HOUR)	
• Inform client of diagnosis and recommended care plan, and obtain informed consent	N/A
• Periodontal (therapeutic) scaling and root planing, half of mouth, maxillary right quadrant and mandibular right quadrant	04341
• Local anesthesia: list type and number of carpules (if applicable)	9215
• Nitrous oxide–oxygen analgesia (if applicable)	9230
• Oral hygiene instruction	01330
• Subgingival irrigation with antimicrobial agent	09630
• Postoperative instructions	N/A
THIRD APPOINTMENT, 1 WEEK LATER (1 HOUR)	
• Periodontal (therapeutic) scaling and root planing, half of mouth, maxillary left quadrant and mandibular left quadrant	04341
• Local anesthesia: list type and number of carpules (if applicable)	9215
• Nitrous oxide–oxygen analgesia (if applicable)	9230
• Oral hygiene instruction	01330
• Subgingival irrigation with antimicrobial agent	09630
• Postoperative instructions	N/A
FOURTH APPOINTMENT, 1 WEEK LATER (45 MINUTES)	
• Prophylaxis (hand-scale and polish)	01110
• Oral hygiene instruction	01330
• Application of desensitizing medicants (if applicable)	09910
FIFTH APPOINTMENT, 2 WEEKS LATER (30 MINUTES)	
• Periodic oral examination (reevaluation of tissue, probe, charting, and client attitude)	00120
• Oral hygiene instruction	01330
• Client scheduled for continued care (recall) appointment: periodontal maintenance (PM)—1 hour procedure at 2, 3, 4, or 6 months (or as needed)	

TOTAL TIME: approx. 4 hr, 15 min–4 hr, 45 min

* Procedure should be completed initially if heavy, tenacious calculus is present supragingivally or acute necrotizing ulcerative gingivitis (ANUG) is present throughout the dentition.

FIGURE 15–6
Sample appointment plan for a client with signs of early periodontitis. (Data from American Academy of Periodontology, Current Procedural Terminology for Periodontics, 5th ed. Washington, DC: The Association, 1987; and Code on Dental Procedures and Nomenclature: Report from the Council on Dental Care Programs. Journal of the American Dental Association 122:91, 1991.)

SAMPLE APPOINTMENT PLAN

(Dental Hygiene Diagnosis: Deficit in the human need for skin and mucous membrane integrity of the head and neck and freedom from pain and stress.)

Description: Inflammation has progressed to an advanced stage with exudate, recession, tooth mobility, and some furcation involvement. Pocket depths are 6 to 7 mm, with loss of connective tissue attachment of 5 to 6 mm. Offensive mouth odor unique to periodontal disease.

Seven Appointments (or as needed)

FIRST APPOINTMENT (1 OR 1½ HOURS)	CDT-1 PROCEDURE CODE
• Initial intra- and extraoral examination (includes health/dental/cultural history, head and neck examination, oral cancer examination, dental/periodontal charting)	00110
• Complete intraoral series of radiographs, including bitewings	00210
• Document and present findings to client	N/A
• Periodontal (therapeutic) scaling performed in the presence of gingival inflammation (if applicable*)	4345
SECOND APPOINTMENT (1 HOUR)	
• Inform client of diagnosis and recommended care plan, and obtain informed consent	N/A
• Periodontal (therapeutic) scaling and root planing, maxillary right quadrant	04341
• Local anesthesia: list type and number of carpules (if applicable)	9215
• Nitrous oxide–oxygen analgesia (if applicable)	9230
• Oral hygiene instruction	01330
• Subgingival irrigation with antimicrobial agent	09630
• Postoperative instructions	N/A
THIRD APPOINTMENT, 1 WEEK LATER (1 HOUR)	
• Periodontal (therapeutic) scaling and root planing, mandibular right quadrant	04341
• Local anesthesia: list type and number of carpules (if applicable)	9215
• Nitrous oxide–oxygen analgesia (if applicable)	9230
• Oral hygiene instruction	01330
• Subgingival irrigation with antimicrobial agent	09630
• Postoperative instructions	N/A
FOURTH APPOINTMENT, 1 WEEK LATER (1 HOUR)	
• Periodontal (therapeutic) scaling and root planing, maxillary left quadrant	04341
• Local anesthesia: list type and number of carpules (if applicable)	9215
• Nitrous oxide–oxygen analgesia (if applicable)	9230
• Oral hygiene instruction	01330
• Subgingival irrigation with antimicrobial agent	09630
• Postoperative instructions	N/A
FIFTH APPOINTMENT, 1 WEEK LATER (1 HOUR)	
• Periodontal (therapeutic) scaling and root planing, mandibular left quadrant	04341
• Local anesthesia: list type and number of carpules (if applicable)	9215
• Nitrous oxide–oxygen analgesia (if applicable)	9230
• Oral hygiene instruction	01330
• Subgingival irrigation with antimicrobial agent	09630
• Postoperative instructions	N/A
SIXTH APPOINTMENT, 1 WEEK LATER (30 MINUTES)	
• Prophylaxis (hand-scale and polish)	01110
• Oral hygiene instruction	01330
• Application of desensitizing medicants (if applicable)	09910

FIGURE 15–7
Sample appointment plan for a client with signs of moderate periodontitis. (Data from American Academy of Periodontology, Current Procedural Terminology for Periodontics, 5th ed. Washington, DC: The Association, 1987; and Code on Dental Procedures and Nomenclature: Report from the Council on Dental Care Programs. Journal of the American Dental Association 122:91, 1991.)

Figure continued on following page

SAMPLE APPOINTMENT PLAN

SEVENTH APPOINTMENT, 2 WEEKS LATER (30 MINUTES)

• Periodic oral examination (reevaluation of tissue, probe, charting, and client attitude)	00120
• Oral hygiene instruction	01330
• Bacteriological studies for determination of pathological agents (applicable if no response to current therapy occurs)	00415
• Referral to periodontist (if indicated)	N/A
• Client scheduled for oral health continued care (recall) appointment: periodontal maintenance (PM)—1 hour procedure at 2, 3, or 4 months (or as needed)	4910

TOTAL TIME: approx. 6 hr, 15 min

---

* Procedure should be completed initially if heavy, tenacious calculus is present supragingivally or ANUG is present throughout the dentition.

FIGURE 15–7 *Continued*

SAMPLE APPOINTMENT PLAN

(Dental Hygiene Diagnosis: Deficit in the human need for skin and mucous membrane integrity of the head and neck and freedom from pain and stress.)

Description: Further progression reveals major alveolar bone loss, bleeding, extensive tooth mobility, recession, exudate, and definite furcation involvement. Pocket depths are 8 mm and more, with extensive loss of connective tissue attachment of 7 mm or more. Offensive mouth odor unique to periodontal disease.

Nine Appointments (or as needed)

FIRST APPOINTMENT (1 OR 1½ HOURS)	CDT-1 PROCEDURE CODE
• Initial intra- and extraoral examination (includes health/dental/cultural history, head and neck examination, oral cancer examination, dental/periodontal charting)	00110
• Complete intraoral series of radiographs, including bitewings	00210
• Document and present findings to client	N/A
• Periodontal (therapeutic) scaling performed in the presence of gingival inflammation (if applicable*)	4345

SECOND APPOINTMENT (1 HOUR)

• Inform client of diagnosis and recommended care plan, and obtain informed consent	N/A
• Periodontal (therapeutic) scaling and root planing, maxillary right posterior sextant	04999
• Local anesthesia: list type and number of carpules (if applicable)	9215
• Nitrous oxide–oxygen analgesia (if applicable)	9230
• Oral hygiene instruction	01330
• Subgingival irrigation with antimicrobial agent	09630
• Postoperative instructions	N/A

THIRD THROUGH SEVENTH APPOINTMENTS, EACH 1 WEEK LATER (1 HOUR EACH VISIT)

Same procedures and codes as indicated in appointment 2 except location:
3rd appointment—mandibular right posterior sextant
4th appointment—maxillary left posterior sextant
5th appointment—mandibular left posterior sextant
6th appointment—maxillary anterior sextant
7th appointment—mandibular anterior sextant

FIGURE 15–8
Sample appointment plan for a client with signs of severe periodontitis. (Data from American Academy of Periodontology, Current Procedural Terminology for Periodontics, 5th ed. Washington, DC: The Association, 1987; and Code on Dental Procedures and Nomenclature: Report from the Council on Dental Care Programs. Journal of the American Dental Association 122:91, 1991.)

Figure continued on following page

SAMPLE APPOINTMENT PLAN

EIGHTH APPOINTMENT, 1 WEEK LATER (45 MINUTES)

• Prophylaxis (hand-scale and polish)	01110
• Oral hygiene instruction	01330
• Application of desensitizing medicants (if applicable)	09910

NINTH APPOINTMENT, 2 WEEKS LATER (30 MINUTES)

• Periodic oral examination (reevaluation of tissue, probe, charting, and client attitude)	00120
• Oral hygiene instruction	01330
• Bacteriological studies for determination of pathological agents	00415
• Referral to periodontist (if indicated)	N/A
• Client scheduled for continued care (recall) appointment: periodontal maintenance (PM)—1 hour procedure at 2, 3, or 4 months (or as needed)	04910

TOTAL TIME: approx. 8 hr, 15 min

Note: If a full complement of teeth are not present in the oral cavity, the care can be completed by quadrants rather than sextants. The time per appointment could be increased, and the number of appointments could be decreased.
* Procedure should be completed initially if heavy, tenacious calculus is present supragingivally or ANUG is present throughout the dentition.

FIGURE 15–8 *Continued*

SAMPLE APPOINTMENT PLAN

(Dental Hygiene Diagnosis: Deficit in the human need for skin and mucous membrane integrity of the head and neck and freedom from pain and stress.)

Description: Rapid destruction of the periodontium with serious progression and no response to normal therapy.

FIRST APPOINTMENT (1 HOUR)	CDT-1 PROCEDURE CODE
• Initial intra- and extraoral examination (includes health/dental/cultural history, head and neck examination, oral cancer examination, dental/periodontal charting)	00110
• Complete intraoral series of radiographs, including bitewings	00210
• Bacteriological studies for determination of pathological agents	00415
• Document and present findings to client	N/A
• Inform client of diagnosis	
• Provide immediate referral to periodontist	N/A

FIGURE 15–9
Sample appointment plan for a client with signs of periodontitis who is not responding to normal therapy. (Data from American Academy of Periodontology, Current Procedural Terminology for Periodontics, 5th ed. Washington, DC: The Association, 1987; and Code on Dental Procedures and Nomenclature: Report from the Council on Dental Care Programs. Journal of the American Dental Association 122:91, 1991.)

References

1. Wilkins, E. M. Clinical Practice of the Dental Hygienist, 6th ed. Philadelphia, Lea & Febiger, 1989, pp. 291–296.
2. Woodall, I. Comprehensive Dental Hygiene Care, 4th ed. St. Louis: Mosby–Year Book, 1993.
3. American Dental Association. Code on Dental Procedures and Nomenclature: Report from the Council on Dental Care Programs. Journal of the American Dental Association 122:91, 1991.

V IMPLEMENTATION AND EVALUATION

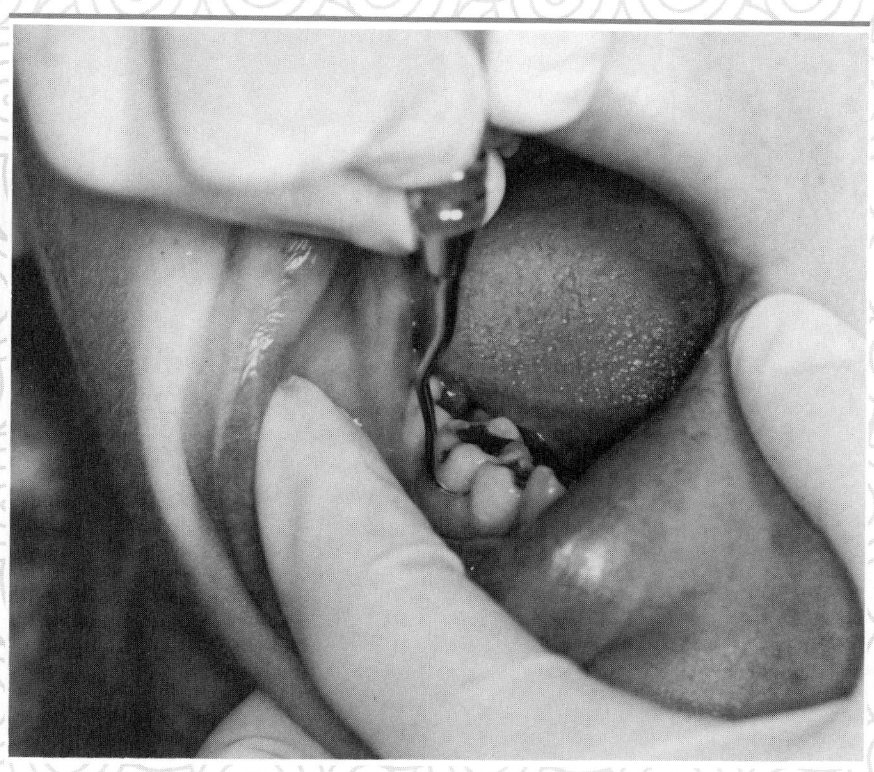

16 Personal Mechanical Oral Hygiene Care and Chemotherapeutic Plaque Control

OBJECTIVES

Mastery of the content in this chapter will enable the reader to:

- Define the key terms used
- Relate human need theory to personal mechanical oral hygiene care
- Discuss how the dental hygiene practitioner can assist clients with disease prevention and oral health promotion at various stages of the life cycle
- Describe the role of bacterial plaque and the susceptible host in dental caries and inflammatory periodontal diseases
- Describe the process by which a plaque control product receives the Seal of Acceptance of the American Dental Association
- List the characteristics of an acceptable manual toothbrush
- Describe the advantages of various powered toothbrushes and indications for their use
- Explain the technique, advantages, and disadvantages of each of the following toothbrushing methods: Bass, Stillman's, and Charters'
- Describe the methods for evaluation of toothbrushing and interdental care
- Discuss appropriate use and indications for the following interdental plaque control devices: waxed dental floss, unwaxed dental floss, dental tape, interproximal brushes and swabs, wooden toothpicks and wedges, knitting yarn, gauze strips, and pipe cleaners
- Discuss the purpose of various ingredients commonly found in dentifrices and mouth rinses
- Discuss indications for use of oral irrigation as an adjunct to mechanical plaque control
- Relate the ADA Guidelines for Acceptance of Chemotherapeutic Agents for the Control of Supragingival Plaque and Gingivitis to the evaluation of related literature
- Discuss appropriate use and indications for chemotherapeutic agents including chlorhexidine, stannous fluoride, phenolic compounds, sanguinarine, quarternary ammonium compounds, prebrushing rinses, and oxygenating agents
- Discuss the following dental caries activity tests: Snyder test, modified Snyder test, methyl red sugar test, and *Streptococcus mutans* count
- Explain the advantages and limitations of using phase contrast microscopy in dental hygiene care
- Discuss legal and ethical considerations related to the client in an effective plaque control program for personal oral hygiene care

INTRODUCTION

The dental hygiene process of care focuses on oral health promotion and disease prevention. Clients are integrally involved in the process of care because their active participation is critical to their maintenance of health and wellness.

Dental caries and periodontal diseases are the most prevalent bacterial infections in humans.[1] These diseases are caused by specific microorganisms found in the oral cavity. A review of the microbiology of **bacterial plaque** and of the oral diseases in which it plays a major etiological role is essential prior to any discussion of plaque control. The clinical rationale for oral hygiene care is based on the clear, essential role of bacterial plaque in the initiation and progression of dental caries and periodontal diseases.

Bacterial Plaque

Initiation and progression of oral diseases are related to the interaction of host, agent, and environmental factors. Prevention and control of caries and inflammatory periodontal diseases depend, in part, on the control of bacterial plaque (the agent) because it is considered to be the primary etiological factor for these diseases. Thus, prevention of bacterial colonization or disruption of plaque deposits is the basis of mechanical plaque control regimens.

Streptococcus mutans, S. mitis, S. sanguis, Lactobacillus species, and *Actinomyces viscosus* have been found to be initial colonizers on tooth enamel. *Streptococcus* and *Lactobacillus* consume large quantities of oxygen and produce potentially harmful products. These species have been associated with dental caries. If supragingival plaque is allowed to grow and mature, it causes gingivitis, which changes the environment because of alteration of the relationship of the gingival margin to the tooth surface as the gingival tissue becomes inflamed.

This altered environment allows subgingival plaque to colonize and adhere to other bacteria, the tooth, or the epithelial tissue lining the sulcus or pocket. Gram-negative anaerobic bacteria, which are believed to be the primary pathogens in periodontitis, become well established. Subgingival plaque may be attached or loosely adherent.

Attached subgingival plaque is similar in structure to supragingival plaque. The inner layers are dominated by gram-positive rods and cocci. Some gram-negative rods and cocci also are found. The apical borders of subgingival bacteria near the junctional epithelium are dominated by gram-negative bacteria, with some filaments present. Attached plaque has been associated with calculus formation, root caries, and slowly progressive adult periodontitis.

Loosely adherent subgingival plaque (unattached plaque) is found adjacent to the gingival epithelium or pocket lumen. It consists primarily of gram-negative rods and cocci, as well as motile organisms and spirochetes that are not highly organized. Loosely adherent plaque microflora have been associated with rapid periodontal destruction (Fig. 16–1).

Total elimination of all bacterial plaque is an unrealistic goal. A more reasonable approach would be to prevent disease by methods that can reduce bacterial plaque below the individual's threshold for disease.[2] Interactions between the host and the oral microorganisms are dynamic. In health, there is a balance between the two. If the balance shifts in favor of the microflora, disease results. Diet, stress, systemic disease, inadequate professional oral care, and environmental risk factors can affect the balance. The disease threshold undergoes changes, and the host is unable to defend himself against the microbial challenge. Thus, continual monitoring of plaque control effectiveness and revision of methods when necessary are essential components of a disease prevention program.

Another approach to controlling bacterial plaque is to alter its composition. Current research on mechanical plaque removal and chemotherapeutic agents is directed toward this goal. At the present time, however, there is no device or agent that can prevent plaque formation or render plaque nonpathological. As a result, it seems reasonable to conclude that regular, efficient mechanical plaque removal is requisite to disease prevention. Increasing host resistance also is an important component of the formula for maintaining a favorable balance between the oral microflora and the host.

Dental Caries

Dental caries results when the host (the tooth) becomes susceptible to the cariogenic microorganisms found in the oral cavity. Diet appears to be the major environmental factor affecting the development of cariogenic bacterial plaque. An appropriate interaction of microbes, dietary

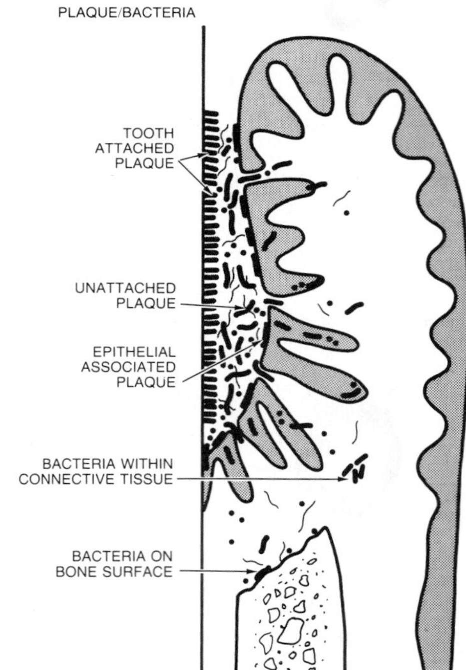

FIGURE 16–1
Diagrammatic representation of subgingival plaque organization. Tooth-associated or attached plaque contains primarily gram-positive organisms. The attached plaque is always covered with a layer of loosely adherent unattached plaque of predominantly gram-negative motile bacteria. This unorganized layer is attached to the pocket epithelial surface. Bacteria associated with the pocket surface may invade the epithelium and connective tissue and alveolar bone (not drawn to scale). (With permission from Newman, M. G., and Saglie, R. S. The role of microorganisms in periodontal disease. In Carranza, F. A. [ed.]. Glickman's Clinical Periodontology, 6th ed. Philadelphia: W. B. Saunders, 1984, p. 351.)

components, host factors, and time results in caries development. Attention to each of these factors is necessary for the prevention of dental caries.

Control of bacterial plaque is important because cariogenic microorganisms, such as *S. mutans* and *Lactobacillus,* are capable of producing lactic acid. These acids cause demineralization of the tooth surface and also aid in retention of bacteria in the plaque. Cariogenic bacteria also synthesize extracellular polysaccharides (e.g., dextran and levan) when exposed to carbohydrates in the diet. These polysaccharides serve as substrates that facilitate acid production and form the majority of the extracellular plaque matrix.[1] Thus, consideration of carbohydrate intake is another component of dental caries control.

The susceptibility of the host is another factor in the dental caries process. Chemotherapeutic agents such as fluoride serve to strengthen the host by processes of remineralization, which render the enamel less vulnerable to plaque acids. Physical barriers such as pit and fissure sealants also provide assistance in areas that cannot be effectively managed by mechanical plaque control and fluoride therapy (see Chapter 12, section on types of dental caries).

Inflammatory Periodontal Diseases

Although bacterial plaque is believed to cause gingivitis and various forms of periodontitis **(inflammatory periodontal disease)**, it is now known that the host response to periodontal pathogens also has a major influence on the role of various microorganisms in the initiation and progression of periodontal diseases. When there is a balance between the host and its parasites, health results and there is minimal tissue destruction. Local or systemic factors that decrease host resistance can alter the balance. Clinical responses to plaque microbes, such as inflammation, bleeding, or loss of attachment, are modulated by host factors that result in disease progression during periods of disease activity.

Documented differences exist between supragingival and subgingival plaque. Although supragingival plaque composition does not differ dramatically from that in gingivitis and periodontitis, subgingival plaques do vary with various forms of periodontal disease.

Bacteria also have been found within diseased periodontal tissues in gingivitis and periodontitis. Widened intercellular spaces in the gingival epithelium or pocket lining allow for penetration of organisms from subgingival plaque. It is unclear whether bacteria actually invade the tissue or whether their presence there results from displacement or manipulation.

Periodontal diseases are no longer regarded as infections to which everyone is equally susceptible. We currently believe that some people are "at risk" more than others, and much progress is being made toward identifying those individuals or groups.

Host immunological responses are important to any infection. In periodontal disease, they can provide protection against infecting agents by modulating the effects of the microorganisms, but they also can contribute to tissue destruction and disease pathogenesis through cytotoxic, anaphylactic, or cell-mediated reactions. An impaired immunological response (e.g., when antibody levels are not adequate in response to certain pathogens) can result in the most severe types of periodontitis, such as the early-onset forms (see Chapter 13).

PLAQUE CONTROL

"Plaque control" refers to the daily removal of bacterial plaque from the teeth and adjacent oral tissues, or to the prevention of its accumulation. It is essential that dental hygiene clinicians engage their clients in proper techniques for the control of bacterial plaque because successful dental hygiene care is dependent on long-term, personal plaque control. The client is an integral co-therapist in the dental hygiene process of care.

Mechanical removal of bacterial plaque, through the use of toothbrushes and other oral physiotherapy aids, is the most widely accepted mechanism for plaque control. These cleansing devices are indispensable because there are, to date, no chemotherapeutic agents that totally prevent the formation of bacterial plaque in the oral cavity.

Product Selection and Evaluation

Dental hygienists are responsible for advising the public about oral hygiene devices (oral physiotherapy aids) and their proper use. In the recent past, there has been a virtual explosion of technology and information on oral hygiene products and their role in oral disease prevention and plaque control. Conflicting information in both lay and professional literature means that dental hygienists must be familiar with research methodologies, current research findings, and available products and their uses in order to make appropriate recommendations to clients.

The American Dental Association (ADA) Council on Dental Therapeutics gathers and disseminates information to assist professionals in selection and use of therapeutic agents. The Council evaluates new products for safety and effectiveness. Its purview includes:

- Dental therapeutic agents that are offered to the public or the profession
- Adjuncts to dental therapeutic agents
- Dental cosmetic agents that are offered to the public or the profession

Evaluation of dental materials and devices is carried out by another body, the ADA Council on Dental Materials, Instruments and Equipment. When dental materials and devices claim some therapeutic value, they are considered cooperatively by both councils.[3]

Commercial products are examined by the ADA Council on Dental Therapeutics at the request of the manufacturer or distributor or at the initiation of the Council. Generally, the manufacturer submits research to substantiate the effectiveness of the product. Products that do not claim therapeutic value (e.g., cosmetic mouthwashes and dentifrices, denture cleansers, etc.) are not considered by the council. Decisions of the council are based upon available scientific data. Product approval is granted for a 3-year period and is renewable. After consideration of a product, the Council on Dental Therapeutics classifies it as "accepted," "provisionally accepted," or "unacceptable." *Accepted* products have adequate evidence of safety and effectiveness and may use the **ADA Seal of Acceptance** or an authorized statement provided by the council. *Provisionally accepted* products have reasonable evidence of usefulness and safety but lack sufficient documentation for acceptance. Further investigation is indicated. *Unaccepted* products have no substantial evidence of usefulness or have questionable safety.[3]

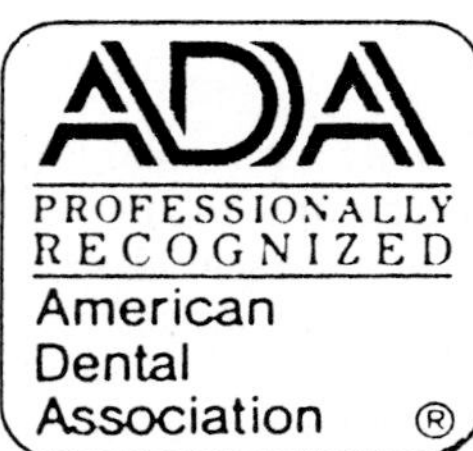

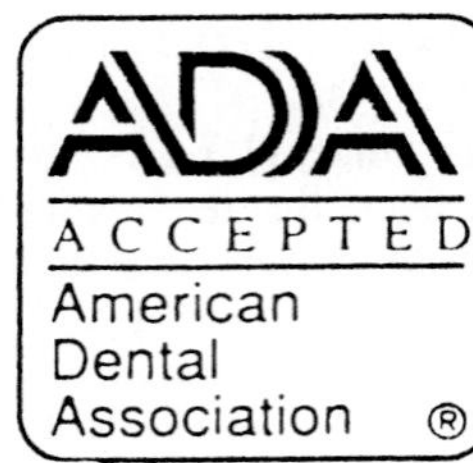

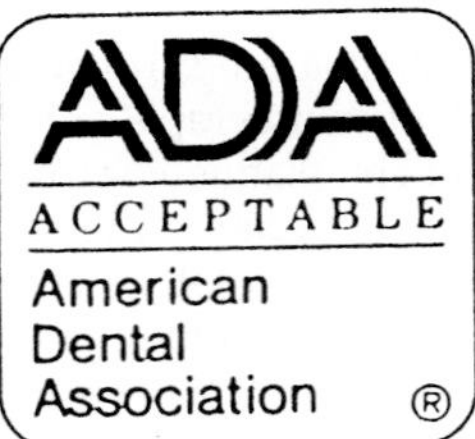

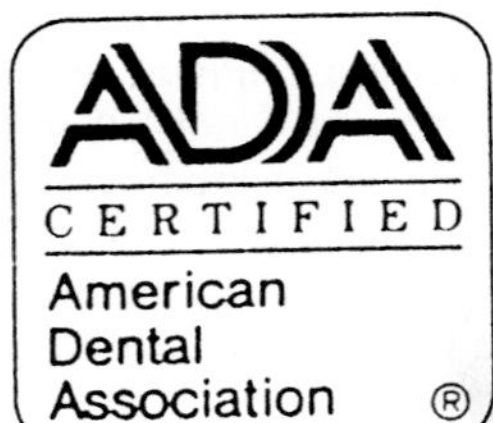

Clinical products that carry these seals have been evaluated by the ADH Council on Dental Therapeutics or the Council on Dental Materials, Instruments, and Equipment and have been found to be safe and effective for specific purposes. The Council on Dental Therapeutics periodically prepares and publishes guidelines for acceptance of certain types of products. For example, guidelines are available for acceptance of fluoride dentifrices[4] and chemotherapeutic products for the control of bacterial plaque and gingivitis.[5] Below are guidelines for acceptance of chemotherapeutic products for the control of supragingival bacterial plaque and gingivitis.[5]

- Characteristics of the study population should represent typical product users
- The active product should be used in a normal regimen and compared with a placebo control or, where applicable, an active control
- Crossover or parallel study designs are acceptable
- Studies should be a minimum of 6 months in duration
- Two studies conducted by independent investigators are required
- Microbiological sampling should estimate plaque qualitatively to complement indices that measure plaque quantitatively
- Plaque and gingivitis scoring and microbiological sampling should be conducted at baseline, at 6 months, and at an intermediate period
- The microbiological profile should demonstrate that pathogenic or opportunistic microorganisms do not develop over the course of the study
- The toxicological profile of products should include carcinogenicity and mutagenicity assays in addition to generally recognized tests for drug safety

A product may not be accepted if:

- It does not fall within the purview of the Council on Dental Therapeutics
- There is insufficient scientific evidence of its safety or effectiveness
- It has not been submitted for consideration[3]

Bacterial Plaque Control on Facial, Lingual, and Occlusal Tooth Surfaces

Manual Toothbrushes

The manual toothbrush is the most commonly used device for the removal of bacterial plaque from the facial, lingual, and occlusal surfaces. The Chinese are given credit for developing the first bristle toothbrush, which was introduced into the Western world in the sixteenth century.[6] Since that time, many improvements have been made and many varieties of toothbrushes have been developed. Currently there is no evidence that one type of toothbrush is superior, as long as individuals are properly motivated and instructed in its use.

Parts of the Toothbrush

Manual toothbrushes have several parts (Fig. 16–2). The *head,* or working end, contains the tufts of bristles. The head of an adult toothbrush should be approximately 1 to $1\frac{1}{4}$ inches (25.4 to 31.8 mm) long and $\frac{5}{16}$ to $\frac{3}{8}$ inches (7.9 to 9.5 mm) wide. The size of the head should be selected based upon the size of the client's mouth. It should be large enough to remove plaque efficiently, yet small enough to facilitate access to all areas of the mouth. There are various toothbrush sizes on the market (Fig. 16–3). Smaller sizes are available for children. The *handle* is the portion of the toothbrush that is grasped by the hand during use. Most handles are aligned in a straight plane with the head of the toothbrush, although some designs have modified the handle. Handles may be angled like a dental mirror, curved, or offset. Consumers can select the handle shape of their preference, with only a few considerations. The toothbrush handle should be easy to grasp, free from sharp projections, durable, and lightweight, regardless of its design. The *shank* of the toothbrush is the segment that connects the head and the handle. It is frequently constricted so that it is narrower than the rest.

The head of the toothbrush contains tufts made of nylon filaments or natural bristles made of boar's hair. *Tufted* toothbrushes are five or six tufts long and two or three tufts across; *multitufted* toothbrushes have 10 or 12 tufts in three or four rows (Fig. 16–4). Multitufted filaments or bristles are in closer proximity, allowing the user to generate greater force while brushing and, thus, better cleansing action.[7] The multitufted design also allows for improved delivery of dentifrice to the tooth surfaces. The filaments or bristles do take longer to dry between uses, so many professionals recommend that their clients rotate use of more than one toothbrush per day. Toothbrush filaments or bristles should be allowed to air dry between uses. One advan-

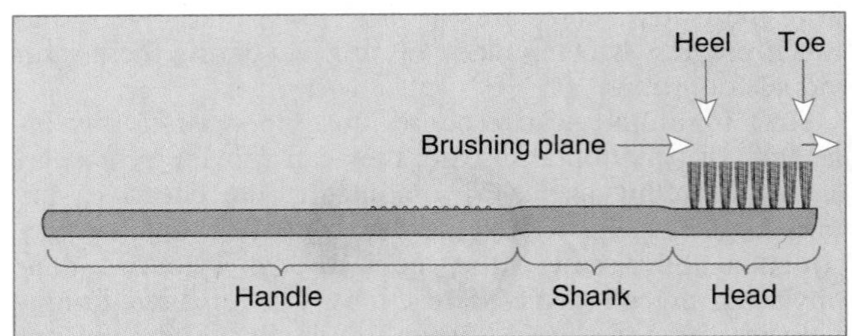

FIGURE 16–2
Parts of a manual toothbrush.

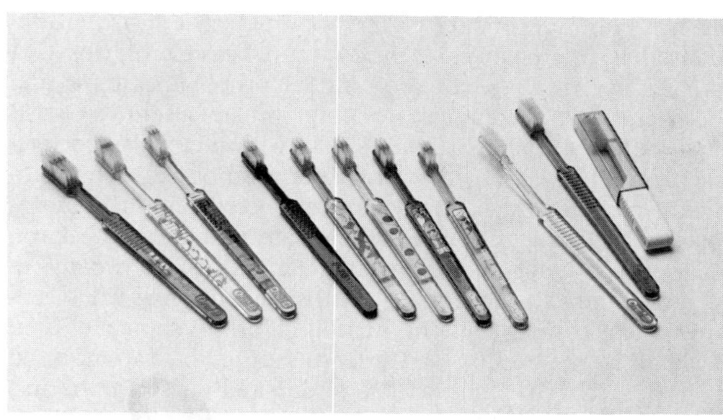

FIGURE 16–3
Various sizes of toothbrushes available for clients of different age groups or for various sizes of the mouth. (Courtesy of Oral-B Laboratories.)

tage of synthetic nylon filaments is that they dry faster than natural filaments.

The *brushing plane* is the surface of the brush used for cleaning the teeth and tissues (see Fig. 16–2). In some toothbrushes, it is flat with all filaments or bristles of the same length. Other toothbrushes have uneven planes. None of these designs has proven to be more effective than another. Some authors state that the straight-trimmed brushing plane is preferred for optimal cleaning, adaptability, and safety.[8,9] Uneven planes may injure the gingiva, because the longer filaments may be pressed too hard in the attempt to use the shorter bristles. Some toothbrushes, however, have been specifically designed with an uneven brushing plane for cleaning around orthodontic fixed appliances. There is no consensus to support clinically significant differences in various toothbrush designs. The ADA's Council on Dental Materials and Devices states that the proper type of toothbrush is dependent largely on the toothbrushing method employed, the positioning of the teeth, and the manipulative skills of the user. The brush must, however, "conform to individual requirements in size, shape, and texture, and be easily and efficiently manipulated, readily cleaned and aerated, impervious to moisture, durable and inexpensive."[10]

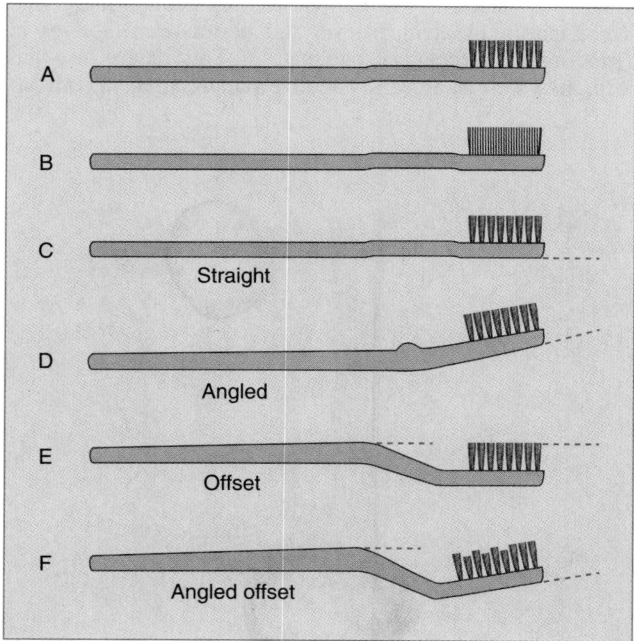

FIGURE 16–4
Toothbrush bristle and handle design. *A,* Tufted toothbrush. *B,* Multitufted toothbrush. *C,* Straight handle. *D,* Angled handle. *E,* Offset handle. *F,* Angled offset handle.

It is clear, however, that nylon filaments are superior to natural bristles made of hog or boar hair. Nylon filaments flex up to 10 times more before breaking; rinse clean and dry more readily; do not split or abrade; and are more resistant to accumulation of bacteria and fungi.[6,9,11] Stiffness of natural bristles also cannot be standardized. Soft nylon filaments are less traumatic to gingival tissues when used for sulcular brushing. For all of these reasons, dental hygienists should recommend toothbrushes with nylon filaments to consumers.

Nylon toothbrush filaments have a uniform shape with a range of diameters from 0.15 mm to 0.4 mm. The stiffness or firmness of the bristle varies with its diameter. Bristle hardness is primarily related to the diameter of the filament because most bristles are 10 to 12 mm long. Toothbrushes are marketed for consumers as extra soft, soft, medium, and hard. Generally, those from 0.007 to 0.009 mm are considered soft, 0.010 to 0.012 mm are considered medium, and 0.013 to 0.015 mm are classified as hard. Soft bristles are recommended for sulcular cleaning and have been shown to be more flexible and to clean proximal surfaces more effectively.[12] Some people prefer medium-hard brushes because they feel that their teeth are cleaner after brushing with a stiffer brush. The concern about use of harder toothbrush filaments or bristles relates primarily to the potential for hard and soft tissue abrasion. Soft filaments are universally considered preferable for sulcular brushing.

The end of the toothbrush filament can be cut bluntly or rounded. Originally, all brush ends were cut; however, end-rounding has become increasingly more common in modern-day manufacturing processes to reduce gingival abrasion.

A scanning electron microscope study examined end-rounding acceptability in eight types of toothbrushes introduced in recent years by quality manufacturers.[13] The results showed significant differences in end-rounding acceptability, from 22% to 88%. The authors concluded that some toothbrushes have unacceptable end-rounding, which may more likely produce gingival abrasion. Further studies are needed to determine the clinical significance of these variations in end-rounding of toothbrush bristles.

Several other factors, besides quality of bristle end-rounding, may affect toothbrushing-induced trauma. Hardness of the bristle, worn bristles, pressure applied by the client during brushing, improper brushing techniques, and abrasiveness of dentifrices used can all influence degree of trauma. Controlled studies of various toothbrush designs are difficult to complete because of the many variables that influence effectiveness and potential damage. Detrimental effects of toothbrushing are discussed in more detail later in this chapter.

It is generally recommended that toothbrushes be replaced at the first sign of the bristles becoming worn, splayed, or frayed.[6,9] The average life of a toothbrush has been estimated at approximately 3 months.[6,14] The ADA recommends toothbrush replacement every 3 to 4 months.[15]

A recent study of dentists' and dental hygienists' attitudes toward toothbrush replacement indicates that practitioners recommend that their clients replace their toothbrushes usually at 3 months when filaments are bent or splayed.[16] Another consideration affecting frequency of toothbrush replacement relates to toothbrush contamination. One author recommends that individuals with oral infections change toothbrushes as often as every 2 weeks.[17] A subsequent study found that toothbrushes were a source of pathogens after approximately 1 month of use.[18] In a related investigation, the herpes simplex virus was introduced into toothbrush bristles. If the brushes were kept in a moist environment, the virus could be recovered 1 week later.[19] It is unknown whether these organisms have any relevance to oral disease in clients who use toothbrushes harboring pathogens. Clients can be instructed to soak their toothbrushes in a solution of household bleach and water (1 : 10) to control toothbrush contamination and crossinfection. Further study on replacement may be indicated. Some commercially available toothbrushes (Oral-B Laboratories) have bristles with a patented dye that fades as the bristles become worn, thus alerting the consumer that replacement is indicated.

Dental hygiene clinicians, as educators and consumer advocates, are influential in helping consumers select toothbrushes. For most clients, a soft multitufted toothbrush with soft, end-rounded nylon filaments, a small enough head to adapt to all areas of the mouth, and a wide and long handle to secure a good grasp is desirable. If a client perceives some benefit from a specific design feature and no detrimental effects are noted, the dental hygienist should not change the type of toothbrush. Components of thorough toothbrushing instruction follow:

- Toothbrush selection and replacement
- Sequence of toothbrushing
- Duration of toothbrushing
- Frequency of toothbrushing
- Toothbrushing method(s)
- Evaluation of toothbrushing effectiveness
- Detrimental effects of improper toothbrushing (safety evaluation)
- Tongue brushing

Powered Toothbrushes

Many studies have been conducted to compare the effectiveness of manual versus powered toothbrushes. Traditionally, powered toothbrushes were designed with a variety of brushing motions including:

- A reciprocating (back-and-forth) motion
- An arcuate (up-and-down) motion
- A combination of these two motions

Studies of these conventional electric toothbrushes have shown that there is no difference in plaque removal when compared with a manual toothbrush.[20–22] However, when assessing effects on gingivitis, results are mixed.

Recently, electrically powered toothbrushes have been redesigned to have counter rotational, rotary, or reciprocal rotating tufts of bristles (Fig. 16–5). The counter-rotational brush (Interplak) has 10 tufts of two different lengths that each rotate independently. The rotary electric brush (Rotadent) has interchangeable hollow-cup brushes or tips that are similar in shape to professional prophylaxis cups and brushes. The reciprocal rotating brush (Braun Oral-B Plaque Remover) has a round head with a cup-shaped bristle design. These devices have been compared to conventional plaque control methods for effectiveness in reducing plaque and gingivitis. Studies indicate that these mechanical oral hygiene devices have shown improvement in plaque removal, subgingival cleansing, and gingival bleeding when compared with manual toothbrushing.[23] When evaluating the results of these studies, it is important to consider that the novelty of a new powered toothbrush might initially influence the motivation of the user. Initially, consumers use new powered toothbrushes frequently, but after 3 months use decreases significantly. The same variations in frequency of use of manual toothbrushes are not evident.[24] Because of this motivational factor, studies of the effectiveness of powered toothbrushes should be conducted for a long term.

Published studies of counter-rotational electric toothbrushes (Interplak) have been based on short-term trials. All of these studies, however, did show reductions in quantity of plaque when compared to manual toothbrushes.[12,25,26] Only one study[12] measured effects of this toothbrush on gingivitis. Although gingivitis was reduced at 4 months in the group that used the counter-rotational, power-assisted toothbrush, a 6-month follow-up telephone survey showed that subjects were not using the device twice daily as they had during the study. The Interplak cannot be used with conventional forms of toothpaste; however, the manufacturer markets its own brand of dentifrice.

Recently, long-term studies of rotary electric toothbrushes (Rotadent) have been published. These studies showed that the rotary-powered toothbrush alone was equally as effective as manual toothbrushing, floss, and toothpicks in reducing plaque and periodontal diseases in periodontal maintenance patients.[24,27] This device also has been shown to significantly reduce plaque, gingival inflam-

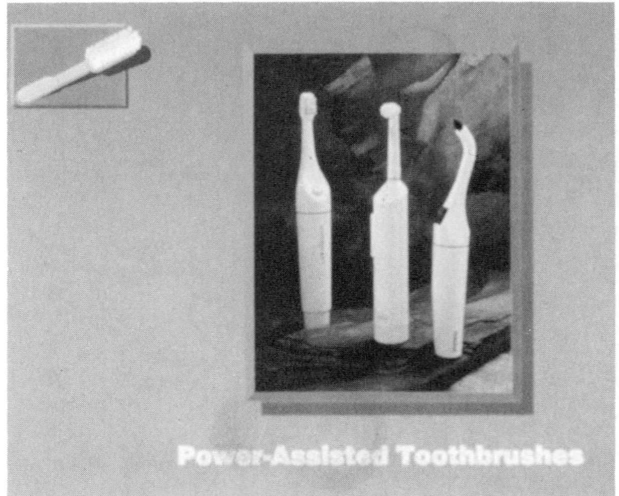

FIGURE 16–5
Examples of electrically powered mechanical plaque control devices: Interplaque, Braun/Oral-B, Rotadent (*left* to *right*). (Compliments of Oral-B Laboratories.)

mation, and bleeding when used by orthodontic clients, as compared to a control group.[27] The rotary electric toothbrush should not be used with dentifrice. Dental hygienists can recommend alternating use with a manual brush for application of a fluoride dentifrice once daily, or use of a fluoride mouth rinse for the benefit of taste and caries prevention.

Short-term studies of the reciprocal rotating toothbrush (Braun Oral-B Plaque Remover) have shown that it is equal to or more effective than manual toothbrushes in bacterial plaque removal. Gingival bleeding also was reduced by 35%.[28,29] The Braun Oral-B Plaque Remover has the advantage of compatibility with commercial toothpaste.

For most clients, the choice between a manual toothbrush and a powered toothbrush is largely a matter of personal preference. Powered toothbrushes have some advantages for people with special needs. Clients who brush less diligently can benefit from a powered toothbrush.[30] Individuals with less fine motor control, physically challenged individuals, and older adults also might find a powered toothbrush to be beneficial. Caregivers often prefer using a powered toothbrush without dentifrice for bedridden or comatose clients, or for people who cannot control swallowing reflexes. As stated earlier, rotary electric toothbrushes also can be useful for clients with orthodontic appliances or for those undergoing dental hygiene care for periodontal maintenance.

A new electronic toothbrush (Sonicare) employs low-frequency acoustic energy to help prevent and control periodontal diseases by altering bacterial adherence. Laboratory studies show that the adherence of *Actinomyces viscosus* is altered. Further study in humans is indicated to determine clinical effectiveness.

Toothbrushing Methods

Many different methods of toothbrushing have been developed (Table 16–1). The best methods will dislodge bacterial plaque and debris, stimulate the gingiva, and deliver fluoridated dentifrice to the tooth surface.

Regardless of the specific toothbrushing method employed, the client must be taught to brush thoroughly. Many clients spend too little time brushing or they brush haphazardly. Dental hygiene practitioners need to stress the importance of thorough plaque removal when teaching others about proper toothbrushing. Clients should be encouraged to develop a standardized sequence of toothbrushing. For example, the practitioner may suggest that the client begin brushing on the facial surface of the most posterior tooth in the maxillary arch. The brushing sequence may follow around the arch from the right molar region, to the right premolars, to the anteriors, to the left premolars, and finally to the left molar regions. The client then begins on the maxillary lingual surfaces of the left posterior segment, brushing each surface until reaching the right posteriors. The same sequence is then repeated on the mandible. After brushing all maxillary and mandibular facial and lingual surfaces, the occlusal surfaces in each quadrant are brushed. There are many possibilities for sequencing, but the individual should be encouraged to select a logical sequence and use it consistently to avoid omission of any area. Also, each brush placement must overlap the previous one for thorough coverage.

TABLE 16–1
TOOTHBRUSHING METHODS AND INDICATIONS FOR THEIR USE

Method	Technique	Indications
Bass (sulcular)	Bristles are directed apically at a 45-degree angle to the long axis of the tooth Gentle force is applied to insert bristles into sulcus Gentle but firm vibratory strokes without removing bristle ends from sulcus	Sulcular cleansing Periodontal health Periodontal disease Periodontal maintenance
Stillman's	Bristles are directed apically and angled similar to Bass Bristles are placed partly on cervical portion of teeth and partly on adjacent gingiva Short back-and-forth strokes are employed and the brush head is moved occlusally with light pressure	Progressive gingival recession Gingival stimulation
Charters'	Bristles are directed toward the crown of the tooth Bristles are placed at the gingival margin and angled 45 degrees to the long axis of the tooth Short back-and-forth strokes are used for activation	Orthodontics Temporary cleaning of surgical wounds Fixed prosthetic appliances Gingival stimulation
Modified Bass, Stillman's, and Charters'	Add a roll stroke Roll tufts occlusally after cervical area is cleaned by prescribed method	Cleaning of entire facial and lingual surfaces
Horizontal scrub	Bristles are activated in a gentle, horizontal scrubbing motion	Not recommended because transition to another technique may be difficult
Fone's (circular)	Bristles are activated in a circular motion	Young children with primary teeth; otherwise not recommended
Leonard	Vertical strokes are used with teeth in an edge-to-edge position	Not recommended
Roll stroke	Bristles are pointed apically and rolled occlusally	Used in conjunction with Bass, Stillman's, or Charters'

Duration of toothbrushing also should be stressed during toothbrushing instructions. It has been shown that the average brushing time varies from approximately 45 to 90 seconds. Dental professionals frequently recommend that clients brush their teeth for 3 minutes. However, it has been shown that thorough toothbrushing actually requires 5 minutes to consistently yield adequate reductions in bacterial plaque.[31] Even with 5 minutes of toothbrushing, interproximal cleansing aids are needed to achieve effective plaque control.

Several teaching strategies can be used with clients to increase their brushing time. The client can be instructed to count 10 brushing strokes in each area before proceeding to the next area of the mouth. Another strategy involves timing toothbrushing with the use of an egg timer or a clock.

In addition to thoroughness of toothbrushing, frequency must be considered. There is no standard recommendation for how many times per day all clients should brush because of variable plaque retention factors, variations in client dexterity, and various plaque formation rates. It could be hypothesized that, for the average person, thoroughly cleaning the teeth once every 24 hours should prevent gingival disease because bacterial plaque is colonized in that amount of time. Unfortunately, most people cannot attain the goal of 100% bacterial plaque removal in a single oral hygiene session. For this reason, it is generally recommended that clients brush *at least* twice daily in order to control bacterial plaque and halitosis. Brushing before bedtime and after a period of sleep should be encouraged, and thus clinicians often suggest cleaning the teeth in the morning and at night. The frequency of toothbrushing should be increased in people with more rapid plaque and calculus formation.

There are several toothbrushing methods that vary in their efficiency in controlling plaque (see Table 16–1).

The Bass Method

The **Bass,** or sulcular, **toothbrushing method** is universally accepted as the most effective; therefore, it is the most commonly recommended. This technique is designed to clean the cervical one-third of the crown of the tooth as well as the area beneath the gingival margin. It has been demonstrated to be more effective than other methods in cleaning the gingival zones of the teeth.[32] Thus, it can be recommended for clients who are periodontally healthy, for clients with periodontal disease, or for periodontal maintenance clients.

The toothbrush can be grasped with a palm grasp or a pen grasp.[33] The toothbrush bristles are directed apically and angled 45 degrees to the long axis of the teeth (Fig. 16–6). Gentle force is then applied to insert the bristles into the gingival sulcus and interproximal embrasures until the gingiva blanches. The stroke is activated with a gentle, but firm, vibratory motion. This vibratory motion consists of short back-and-forth strokes. Approximately 10 strokes should be completed without removing the bristle ends from the sulcus before proceeding to the next area. The brush head is moved to the next tooth or group of teeth by overlapping with the completed area. It must be repositioned at the proper 45-degree angle with the bristles directed apically into the sulcus.

On the facial and lingual surfaces of the posterior teeth, the toothbrush head is positioned parallel with the arch. The rows of bristles closest to the tooth surface are angled into the sulcus. On the anterior teeth, the toothbrush head also can be placed parallel to the arch (or horizontally) when brushing the labial surfaces, but it should be placed parallel with the long axis of the teeth (or vertically) when brushing the lingual surfaces (see Fig. 16–6). Thus, on the lingual surfaces of the anterior teeth, the heel of the tooth-

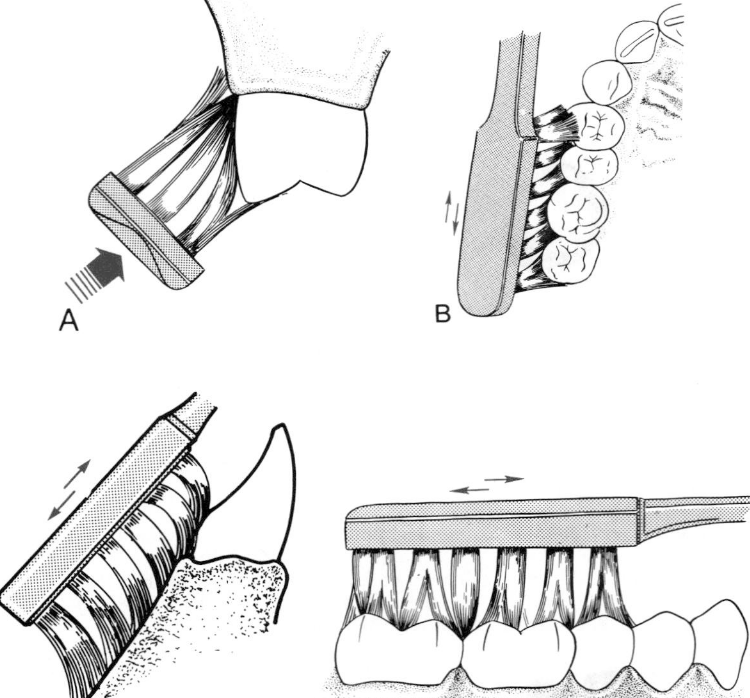

FIGURE 16–6
The Bass toothbrushing method. *A,* Intrasulcular position. *B,* Correct position on facial surface of posterior teeth. *C,* Correct position of lingual surfaces of anterior teeth. *D,* Correct position on occlusal surfaces. (With permission from Carranza, F. A. Glickman's Clinical Periodontology, 7th ed. Philadelphia: W. B. Saunders, 1990, pp. 693, 689, 696, and 697.)

brush is used and the vibratory motion is changed to a short up-and-down stroke. After brushing all facial and lingual surfaces in a sequence, the occlusal surfaces should be cleaned. The bristles are pressed firmly into the occlusal surface so that the ends can penetrate into the pits and fissures and a back-and-forth brushing stroke is activated. The brush is advanced section by section until all occlusal surfaces have been cleaned.

Use of a soft, nylon-bristled brush is indicated when the Bass method is employed.[34] Otherwise, potential for gingival trauma exists. Dental hygiene clinicians also should be aware of common technique problems encountered by individuals who have been taught to use the Bass technique. Some clients exert too much pressure, or use too long a stroke, when attempting the vibratory motion. These errors can result in tissue laceration or gingival sensitivity. Obtaining the proper angle of the bristles also is difficult to achieve and the toothbrush bristles may not be angled into the sulcus. This error results in inefficient strokes, and plaque is allowed to remain at the gingival margin. Sometimes, clients place the bristles on the attached gingiva rather than at the gingival margin, thereby neglecting the tooth surface and traumatizing the attached gingiva. The lingual surfaces of the anterior teeth can be problematic for the client because of the need to position the brush vertically in those areas. If the arm is not raised high enough to direct the bristles toward the gingival margin, only the incisal one-third of these surfaces are cleaned. It is critical for the dental hygienist to observe and evaluate each client's toothbrushing skills so that problems or errors can be corrected. Oral hygiene skill assessment must be repeated periodically to help clients achieve optimal efficiency while toothbrushing.

The Stillman's Method

The **Stillman's toothbrushing method** was developed originally to provide gingival stimulation.[35] The toothbrush is positioned and angled (toward the apex) similarly to the Bass method, but the bristles are placed partly on the cervical portion of the tooth and partly on the adjacent gingiva (Fig. 16–7). The strokes are activated in a short back-and-forth motion while the brush head is moved simultaneously in an occlusal direction. Approximately five to 10 strokes are completed in each region and the brush is moved to the next area. This process is repeated in a sequence until all regions are thoroughly cleaned. Once again, brush placement is vertical on the anterior lingual surfaces and the heel of the brush is used. The occlusal surfaces are brushed with the bristles perpendicular to the occlusal plane.

In the Stillman's method, the toothbrush bristle ends are not directed into the sulcus; therefore, it can be recommended for clients with progressing gingival recession. It is considered less traumatic to the gingival tissue than scrub or sulcular brushing. Of course, a soft brush and light pressure should be recommended in these cases. The added advantage of gingival stimulation has been questioned because, although it has been found to increase circulation and keratinization, no definite clinical benefits have been demonstrated.

The Charters' Method

The Charters' method was developed originally to increase cleansing effectiveness and gingival stimulation in the interproximal areas.[36] It is now known that interproximal surfaces are not cleaned adequately by any toothbrushing method, but the Charters' technique has its advantages. In this technique, the bristles are pointed toward the crown of the tooth rather than apically (Fig. 16–8). Like the Bass and Stillman's methods, the toothbrush is positioned horizontally and parallel with the arch in all areas except the lingual area of the anterior teeth and the occlusal surfaces. The bristles are placed at the gingival margin and directed toward the occlusal surface at a 45-degree angle to the long axis of the tooth. A short back-and-forth motion is used for activation. The process is repeated in a sequence around the mouth until all areas are cleaned. The Charters' method can be recommended for orthodontic clients or for clients with fixed prosthetic appliances to clean the area between the appliance and the gingival margin. It also is useful for clients immediately following periodontal surgery during healing of surgical wounds. It also can provide gingival stimulation if the bristles are placed partly on the gingiva.

Modified Bass, Modified Stillman's, and Modified Charters' Methods

The Bass, Stillman's, and Charters' methods of toothbrushing were designed to concentrate on the cervical portion of

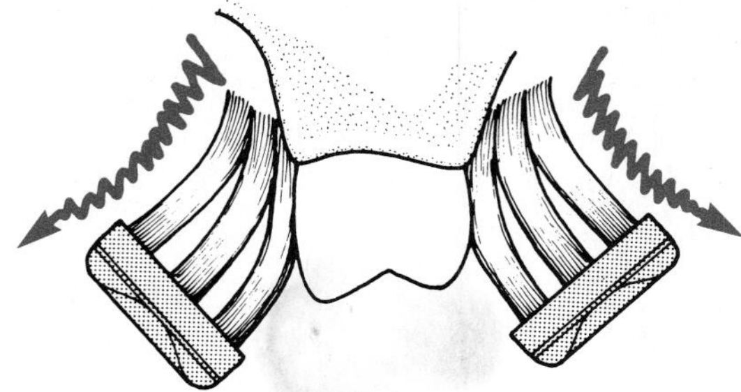

FIGURE 16–7
Stillman's toothbrushing technique—position and placement of bristles. (With permission from Carranza, F. A. Glickman's Clinical Periodontology, 7th ed. Philadelphia: W. B. Saunders, 1990, p. 698.)

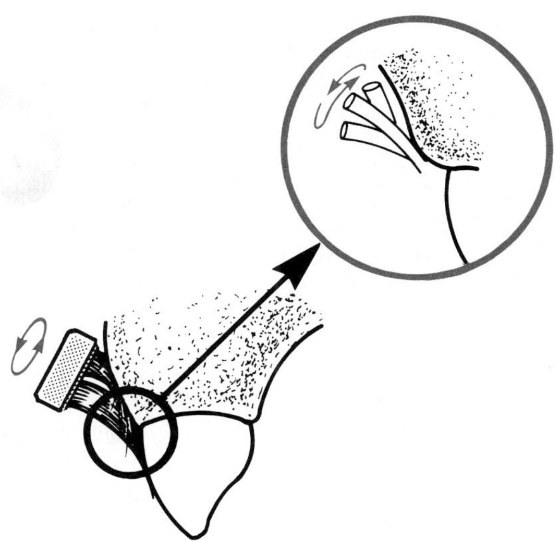

FIGURE 16–8
Charters' toothbrushing method—position and placement of bristles. (With permission from Carranza, F. A. Glickman's Clinical Periodontology, 7th ed. Philadelphia: W. B. Saunders, 1990, p. 699.)

the teeth and the adjacent gingival tissues. Each of these methods can be modified to add a roll stroke. The toothbrush bristles are rolled occlusally to clean the entire facial and lingual surfaces after the cervical area is cleaned. Clinicians need to stress the importance of thoroughly completing the original stroke before rolling the toothbrush bristles occlusally. If the client rolls too prematurely, the vibratory or back-and-forth strokes are ineffective for plaque removal.

Horizontal Scrub

The horizontal scrub technique is probably the most commonly used toothbrushing method. It is considered detrimental because the unlimited scrubbing motion exerts pressure on the facial tooth prominence, resulting in gingival recession and gingival and tooth abrasion.

Circular Method

The method may be recommended as an easy-to-learn first technique for young children. With the teeth closed, the upper and lower facial surfaces of the teeth are brushed simultaneously with large, circular strokes. For lingual surfaces, small, circular strokes are used on each arch separately.

Evaluation of Toothbrushing

Prior to presentation of oral hygiene instruction, the clinician begins by questioning the client about the type of toothbrush used, frequency of toothbrushing, duration of toothbrushing, and toothbrush replacement practices. Next, the client is asked to demonstrate the toothbrushing method routinely used at home. Observation of the client's technique and skill is important in determining the need for modification and reinforcement. The information gained through the client interview and the observation of toothbrushing is then correlated with gingival conditions found during the periodontal assessment and with presence of bacterial plaque and calculus. If the client is using an acceptable toothbrushing technique, the teeth are relatively plaque-free, the gingival tissues are healthy with no bleeding, and no detrimental effects are noted, there is no need to modify the current methods used by the client. Positive recognition and reinforcement should be given to the client at that time. In contrast, clients who exhibit signs of active disease (e.g., signs of gingival inflammation or signs of dental caries, plaque deposits, or signs of trauma) need toothbrushing instruction to assist them with improving their oral health. Instruction and practice are indicated at that time, as well as at subsequent appointments, to evaluate client progress. A discussion of methods used to assess toothbrushing follows.

Disclosing Agents and Their Applications

Disclosing agents are materials used to make the presence of bacterial plaque visible. Available in liquid or tablet form, they contain an ingredient that stains plaque present on the teeth so that it can be seen. Erythrosin dye is the most commonly employed agent; it stains bacterial plaque red. Fluorescein is a dye that can be applied to the teeth without obvious staining. A special ultraviolet light is used to make this agent visible to the client and clinician. Two-tone disclosing agents that stain thicker plaque blue and thinner plaque red also are available. Disclosing agents ideally should provide a distinct staining of deposits that does not rinse off immediately, should have a pleasant taste, and should be nonirritating to the oral soft tissues.

Because staining of the oral soft tissue inhibits the clinician's assessment of signs of disease, disclosing agents should not be applied to the teeth until after completing the oral and periodontal assessment, and findings are shown to the client. Theory regarding plaque and gingival inflammation also should be presented prior to disclosing deposits, so that the client understands the correlation between oral hygiene and periodontal status. After performing the gingival assessment and providing the client with needed theoretical background about the composition and effects of bacterial plaque, a nonpetroleum-based jelly can be applied to the lips to prevent them from staining. Petroleum-based jellies are not recommended because they can break down latex and contribute to weakening of the protective barrier of the clinician's gloves.

Technique for disclosing depends upon the type of product used. Solutions can be applied as a concentrate with a cotton swab, or diluted with water in a cup for the client to use as an oral rinse. Tablets are chewed and swished around the mouth by the client. Excess disclosing agent is expectorated or suction and evacuation devices are used to remove it from the mouth after staining. Clean tooth surfaces do not absorb the dye unless roughness is present (e.g., decalcification, hypocalcification, restorations, cementum). Pellicle, bacterial plaque, debris, and calculus absorb the disclosing agent. This discriminate staining characteristic makes the disclosing agent an excellent oral hygiene aid because the client is able to use it at home for self-evaluation and motivation. Being able to see the plaque deposits helps individuals improve the effectiveness of their home care (Fig. 16–9).

After application of the disclosing agent, the client is given a hand mirror to observe the location of stained deposits. The dental hygiene practitioner assists the client in identifying deposits and correlates findings with signs of gingival inflammation identified prior to staining. Toothbrushing techniques are then modified to improve efficacy in areas of concern. Instruction and demonstration by the clinician are followed by observation of the client's technique during practice. Each area of concern should be practiced because the client may have difficulty adapting the toothbrushing method in a particular region.

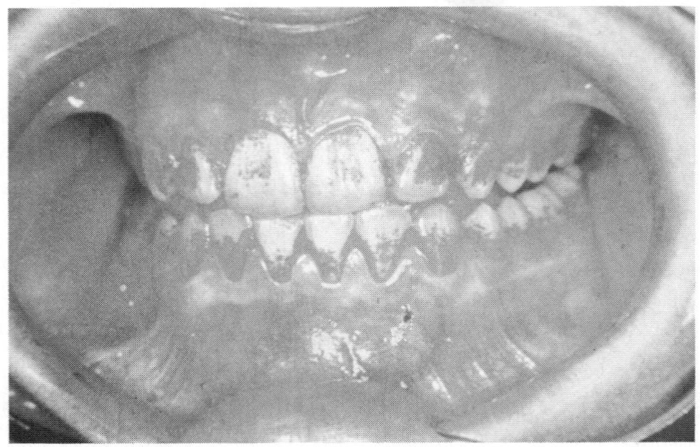

FIGURE 16–9
Bacterial plaque that has been stained using a disclosing agent.

Gingival Evaluation

The color, size, shape, and consistency of the gingiva are examined for signs of inflammation. Periodontal probing also is completed to detect bleeding upon probing and pocket formation. These findings are then reviewed with the client and correlated with the presence of bacterial plaque. The person also should be commended for areas of improvement. Quadrants that have been treated with nonsurgical periodontal therapy can be compared and contrasted with untreated quadrants. Some dental hygiene practitioners also use gingival or bleeding indices to calculate a numerical score for the client (see Chapter 13).

Detrimental Effects of Improper Toothbrushing

The dental hygiene practitioner needs to evaluate damage resulting from toothbrushing in addition to toothbrushing effectiveness. The individual may be removing plaque deposits but also causing trauma from improper toothbrushing, horizontal scrubbing, excessive pressure, use of medium to hard bristles or worn bristles, use of an abrasive dentifrice, or adaptation difficulties around prominent root surfaces. Changes can be detected anywhere in the mouth, although they are most frequently seen on the facial tooth surfaces. Canines are particularly susceptible because of their position in the mouth and the prominence of their roots. Location of trauma is often inversely related to left- or right-handedness.

Initially, toothbrush trauma results in gingival abrasion, which can appear as redness, scuffing, brushing, or punctate lesions. Long-term detrimental effects include gingival recession, gingival clefts, or festooning of the gingiva (Fig. 16–10). In addition, tooth abrasion, the wearing away of the tooth surface, usually cementum and dentin, in the cervical areas, can be caused by toothbrush trauma. Tooth abrasion can result in cervical notches apical to the cementoenamel junction and dentinal hypersensitivity.

If detrimental effects from toothbrushing are noted, the dental hygienist should question the client in an attempt to discover the causative factors. Observation of the client's toothbrushing also is indicated. To meet the client's human need for safety, corrective measures are then discussed and correlated with the clinical findings indicating toothbrush trauma. Recommendations may include use of a soft toothbrush with end-rounded bristles, replacement of a worn toothbrush, use of a less abrasive toothpaste, or modifications in toothbrushing technique.

Long-term Evaluation

Long-term evaluation of the effectiveness of oral hygiene practices is based upon the client's periodontal health status, rather than on the presence of bacterial plaque deposits. Plaque may be present because the person was unable to brush prior to the dental hygiene appointment. Absence of plaque may be the result of thorough brushing immediately prior to the appointment rather than to daily plaque removal. Evaluation of the gingival tissues for signs of inflammation yields more valid findings. Comparisons of previous and current probing depths and periodontal attachment levels at a 1-month and a 3-month interval after active treatment also provides valuable information regarding long-term effectiveness.

Special Toothbrushing Considerations

At times, clients avoid toothbrushing because it is uncomfortable for them. This avoidance syndrome usually compounds problems because of the effects of accumulated bacterial plaque. Special toothbrushing instructions are needed for individuals who may want to avoid toothbrushing. Clients who are in pain have a basic need to free themselves from pain. For example, persons with acute necrotizing ulcerative gingivitis or acute injuries to the soft tissue may be sensitive to toothbrushing. Recommending supragingival brushing and an extra soft brush and explaining the importance of oral cleanliness help these clients. Clients who are undergoing periodontal or oral surgeries need similar instructions. Some people also want to avoid toothbrushing around new dental appliances. Teaching them specific methods for toothbrushing and interdental care in the restored areas is important for maintenance of oral health.

Tongue Brushing

To cleanse the mouth thoroughly, tongue brushing should be incorporated with toothbrushing. The dorsum of the tongue is a primary source of oral microorganisms. Tongue brushing can reduce the number of these organisms, improve the client's taste perception, and contribute to overall cleanliness. After extending the tongue, the toothbrush head is placed horizontally across the tongue and the bristles are directed posteriorly. The bristles are then drawn forward with light pressure to cleanse the tongue. This brushing motion is repeated until the tongue is free of a coating or debris. Care should be taken not to scrub the tongue with the toothbrush.

Interdental Care

Toothbrushing is an effective means of cleaning the facial, lingual, and occlusal surfaces of the teeth. It is ineffective,

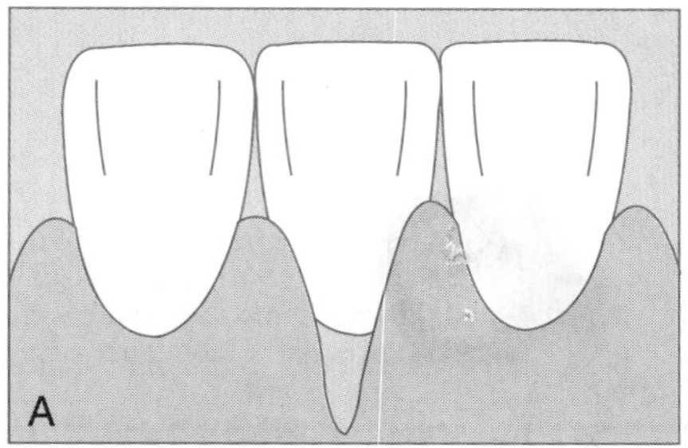

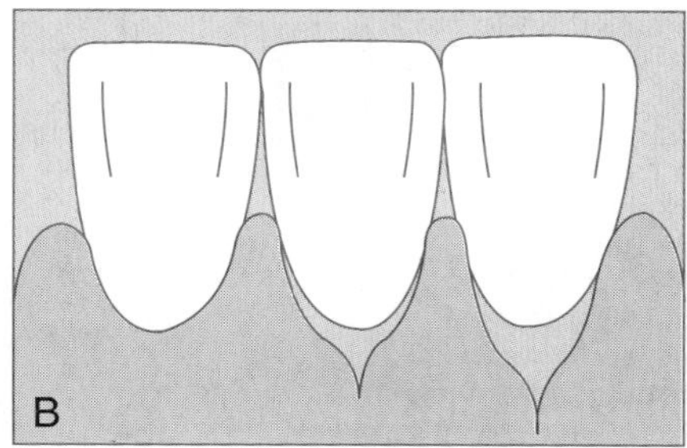

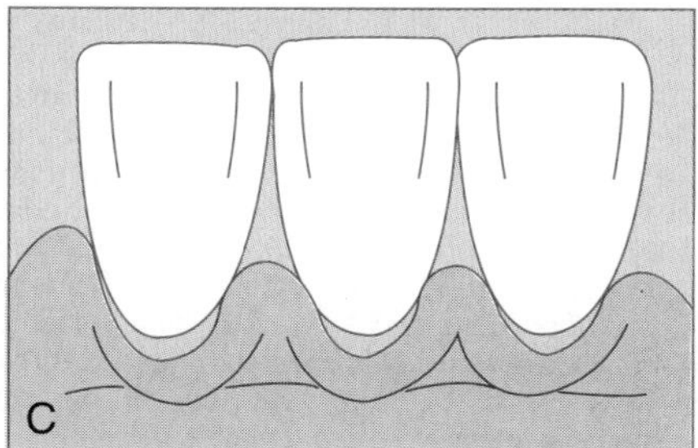

FIGURE 16–10
A, B, C, Gingival festooning.

TABLE 16–2
EXAMPLES OF VARIOUS MECHANICAL ORAL HYGIENE PRODUCTS

Products	Indications for Use	Contraindications/Limitations	Teaching Tips
Power-Assisted Toothbrushes Braun Oral-B Plaque Remover Interplak, Bausch & Lomb Rotadent, Pro-Dentec	Individuals who prefer power-assisted toothbrushes Clients who brush less diligently Individuals with less fine motor control Physically-challenged clients Older adults Caregivers of bedridden or comatose clients Orthodontic or periodontal maintenance therapy	Cost may be a limiting factor for lower socioeconomic groups If fluoridated toothpaste cannot be used with the device, another form of fluoride delivery should be recommended	Recommend careful review of manufacturer's instructions to client Stress importance of fluoridated toothpaste or alternative delivery of fluoride when toothpaste is contraindicated Caregivers can be instructed to use without toothpaste
Interdental Brushes Interdental brushes and handle, Oral-B Laboratories Proxabrush handle and brushes, John O. Butler End-tufted or uni-tufted brush (Oral-B, Butler) Interproximal brush with handle, Lactona Perio Pak, Crescent Dental Manufacturing	Type II or III embrasures Exposed furcation areas Difficult access areas Post-periodontal surgery Fixed dental appliances	Normal gingival contour Type I embrasures	Select size of brush slightly larger than area to be cleaned Clients can be taught to use interdental brushes to deliver chemotherapeutic agent(s) to specific sites
Toothpicks, Toothpick Holders, and Wooden Wedges Interdental handle, Oral-B Laboratories Perio-aid, Marquis Dental Manufacturing Stim-u-dent Wedge Stimulators, Johnson & Johnson Orapik and Dental Pik, Dental Concepts Inc.	Type II embrasures Clients who refuse floss Accessible furcation areas Shallow pockets or normal sulcus depths Clients who already use toothpicks for removal of food debris	Do not clean area of tooth contact Can force bacteria or debris into gingival attachment if used improperly Difficult to adapt on lingual surfaces	Client can be given a choice of hand-held method or holder Caution client not to direct tip of toothpick or wedge apically to avoid trauma and periodontal abcess formation Suggest gentle use tangential with gingival papillae
Oral Irrigation Devices (Self-Applied) Water Pik, Teledyne Oral Irrigator, Braun Via Jet, Viadent	Delivery of antimicrobial chemotherapeutic agents Gingival bleeding and inflammation Orthodontics or fixed prosthetic appliances Removal of oral debris	Cost may be a limiting factor Used only as an adjunct to other mechanical oral hygiene aids Effectiveness in treatment of moderate to advanced periodontitis requires further study	Can have dentist prescribe antimicrobials Client should be instructed how to use tip properly and cautioned about power setting Encourage client to carefully read manufacturer's instructions Stress importance of continued need for toothbrushing and interdental plaque removal
Dental Floss and Tape John O. Butler Johnson & Johnson Gore Oral-B Laboratories	Type I embrasures	Type II and III embrasures	Recommend careful movement of floss between contact areas and beneath gingival margin Stress the importance of hearing a "squeaky clean" sound
Floss Holders	Type I embrasures Clients with large hands Clients who lack manual dexterity or who are physically challenged Clients who prefer not to put hands into mouth Caregivers	Type II and III embrasures	Recommend that floss be kept taut on the holder Same as for dental floss and tape
Floss Threaders John O. Butler Johnson & Johnson	Type I embrasures Clients with fixed orthodontic or dental appliances	Type II and III embrasures	Same as for dental floss and tape
Variable Diameter Dental Floss, Knitting Yarn, Gauze Strips, and Pipe Cleaners Oral-B Laboratories for Superfloss	Type II embrasures Clients with proximal tooth surfaces adjacent to wide interproximal spaces or exposed furcation areas	Type I embrasures	Recommend careful movement of product against soft tissue Avoid scratching soft and hard tissues with pipe cleaner wire

however, for thorough plaque control in the interdental areas.[37,38] Because periodontal diseases most commonly begin in the col area, removal of bacterial plaque from the interproximal tooth surfaces is essential for its prevention and control. Prevention of proximal caries also requires routine removal of plaque deposits coupled with fluoride therapy. Thus, toothbrushing must be supplemented with effective interdental care.

A wide variety of oral physiotherapy aids are available for supplemental plaque control. The dental hygienist needs to evaluate information from the periodontal and oral hygiene assessments coupled with client dexterity and preference in order to select the most appropriate interdental oral hygiene aids for a client. Information should be considered, such as

- Contour and consistency of the gingival tissues
- Probing depths
- Attachment levels
- Size of the interproximal embrasures
- Tooth position and alignment
- Condition and types of restorative work present
- The human needs of the client

The dental hygienist must evaluate oral conditions, client priorities, and planned care goals to determine which oral hygiene aid will most effectively clean the interdental areas to improve or maintain periodontal health status. A general rule to follow is that the simplest, least time-consuming procedures that will effectively control bacterial plaque and maintain oral health should be recommended. The client must have the dexterity and ability to perform the suggested techniques. Also, if one device works, the dental hygienist should choose it over two devices that would accomplish the same goal. Recommended oral care regimens must be practical for the client. Studies have shown that both client acceptance and effectiveness of oral hygiene recommendations improve when the number of aids is limited.[39,40]

If the client's current oral hygiene regimen is effective in maintaining oral health, the dental hygienist should reinforce it rather than changing it to a "more ideal" method. Even the ideal interdental aid is not effective if the client does not use it. Thus, if a client prefers a specific interdental aid or technique, the clinician can assist him by evaluating its use, modifying the technique to maximize efficacy, and discussing potential detrimental effects that can result from incorrect use. Each of these factors is considered when selecting the most appropriate interdental aid for a particular client. Table 16–2 summarizes a variety of mechanical oral hygiene devices available with teaching and selection tips for the dental hygienist. A discussion of various aids available for interdental care follows.

Dental Floss and Tape

Dental floss is the most frequently recommended aid for cleaning proximal tooth surfaces of clients with normal gingival contour and embrasures. Carranza defines three types of interproximal embrasures.[6] Figure 16–11 provides an illustration of these various embrasure types and their recommended interdental care. Dental floss should be recommended only for individuals with type I embrasures.

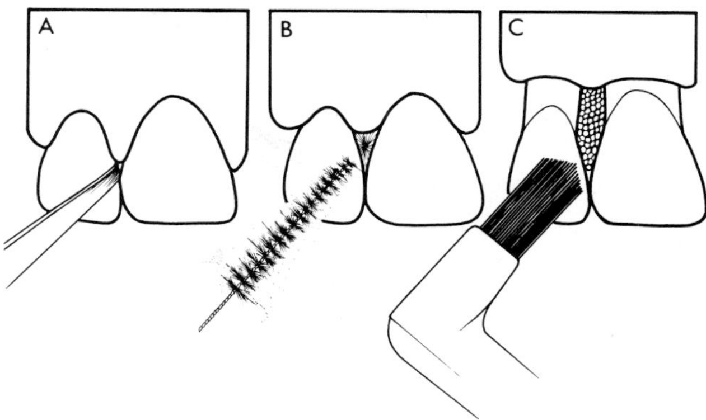

FIGURE 16–11
Types of embrasure spaces and interdental care. *A,* Type I embrasures are totally occupied by the interdental papillae; floss and wooden wedge is recommended. *B,* Type II embrasures are characterized by a slight to moderate recession of the interdental papillae; interproximal brush is recommended. *C,* Type III embrasures are characterized by extensive recession or complete loss of interdental papillae; unitufted brush is recommended. (With permission from Carranza, F. A., and Perry, D. A. Clinical Periodontology for the Dental Hygienist. Philadelphia: W. B. Saunders, 1986, p. 204.)

There is consensus that floss is more effective when interdental spaces are covered by the papillae and that, as recession becomes more pronounced, floss becomes progressively less effective, as shown in Figure 16–12.[41]

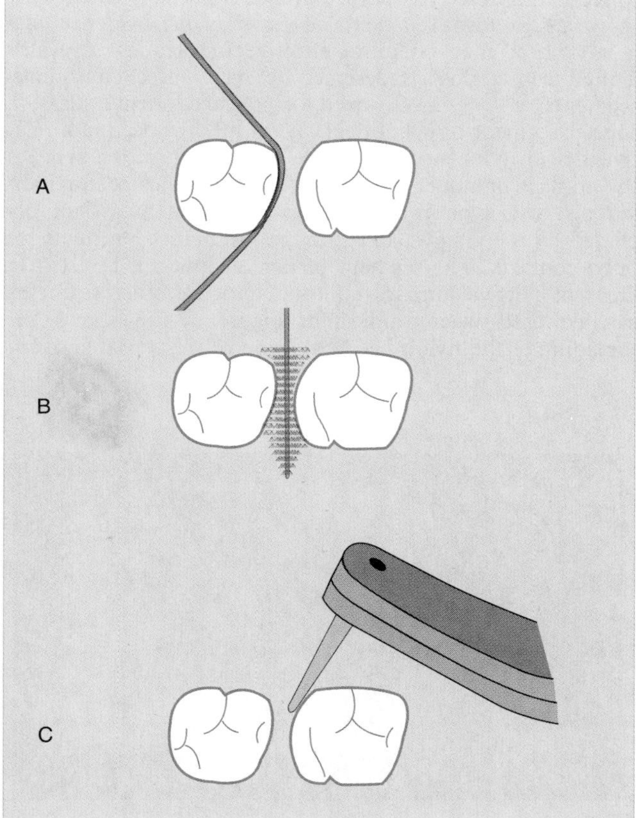

FIGURE 16–12
Use of interdental plaque control devices. *A,* Dental floss. *B,* Interdental brush. *C,* Toothpick in holder.

Several types of dental floss are available commercially:

- Unwaxed
- Waxed
- Variable diameter
- Braided
- Polytetrafluoroethylene

Most floss products are made of nylon and some are impregnated with flavorings.

Studies have shown that there is no difference in the effectiveness of unwaxed versus waxed dental floss.[42–44] *Unwaxed dental floss* is generally recommended for clients with normal tooth contacts because it slides through the contact area easily. It is the thinnest type of floss available. Concern that waxed floss may be inappropriate to use because it leaves a waxy film on tooth surfaces has been dispelled. Wax residue is not left on teeth that are coated by saliva.[44] *Waxed dental floss* is recommended for clients with tight proximal tooth contacts, moderate to heavy calculus deposits prior to scaling and root planing, or defective and overhanging restorations. In these cases, unwaxed floss may shred or tear more easily, resulting in frustration and discomfort for the client. Waxed floss and *polytetrafluoroethylene floss* (e.g., Gore, Glide) are preferred by some clients because of their ability to slide through tight contacts and resist fraying.

Dental tape or ribbon is a waxed floss product that is wider and flatter than conventional dental floss. This flat-sided surface is preferred by some, particularly when the surface area to be flossed is large.

Variable diameter dental floss (e.g., Super Floss), or tufted dental floss, has been found to be equally as effective as waxed or unwaxed dental floss;[44,45] some evidence suggests that it may be more effective in plaque removal.[46] Tufted dental floss is designed to have three continuous segments: a length of waxed or unwaxed dental floss; a shorter segment of cylindrical, nylon meshwork; and a relatively rigid nylon needle capable of being threaded beneath the contact or under fixed bridges. It is indicated for individuals with type II embrasures, furcation areas not occluded by the gingiva, fixed bridges, implant abutments, or open contacts. The segment of dental floss can be used in areas of normal gingival contour, and the other segments can be used where indicated. Figure 16–13 shows the threading of the nylon needle portion of this variable diameter dental floss; Figure 16–14 shows use of the tufted portion.

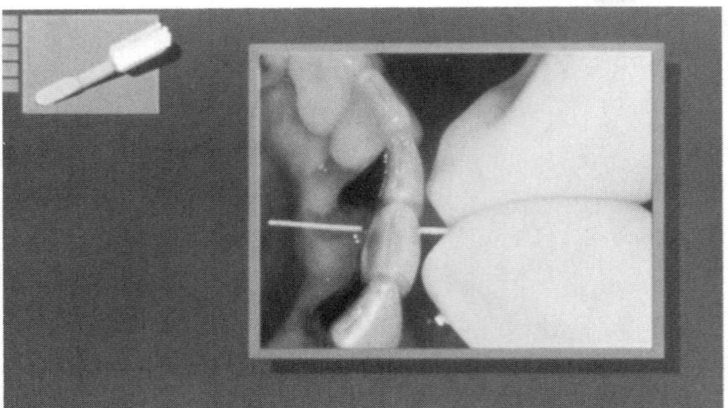

FIGURE 16–13
Use of the nylon tip on variable-diameter dental floss for threading floss subgingivally to a fixed bridge. (Compliments of Oral-B Laboratories.)

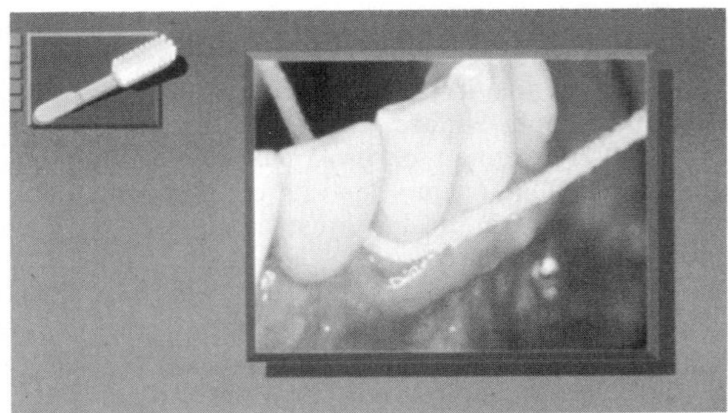

FIGURE 16–14
Use of tufted dental floss in type II embrasure. (Compliments of Oral-B Laboratories.)

Braided nylon floss (e.g., Postcare) is intended for cleaning dental implant posts. It is sold on a spool or with a stiff nylon end for threading. The braided nylon resembles a cord, can be washed after use, and is reused after drying.

Flossing Methods and Flossing Devices

Several flossing methods can be used. The client should be instructed to start with a piece of floss that is long enough to clean all proximal tooth surfaces (approximately 18 inches).

Wrapping Floss Around Fingers The floss can be wound around the fingers or tied in a loop. If winding the floss around the fingers, either the forefingers or middle fingers of each hand can be used. This method may require more dexterity, so children or those who have less manipulative ability with their hands may prefer to tie the floss in a circle by securing both ends together in a knot. The floss is grasped between the forefingers and thumbs on each hand and a small section ($\frac{1}{2}$ inch) is pulled taut between the fingertips. This section of floss is eased past the contact area in a gentle sawing motion. The client is instructed to be careful not to snap or force the floss through the contacts because injury to the gingiva can result. Once the floss is beneath the contact in the interdental space, the adjacent interproximal surfaces are cleaned separately. The floss is wrapped in a C-shape around one tooth and moved up and down the tooth surface from the base of the gingival sulcus to the contact approximately six times. Care must be taken when moving the floss to clean the adjacent tooth surface. Floss should be transferred supragingivally to the papillae to avoid cutting the gingiva. When the tooth surface is clean, a "squeaky clean" sound can be heard by the person during flossing. The floss is then removed from the area cleaned and inserted into the next contact area for bacterial plaque removal. A sequence is followed until all interproximal surfaces have been flossed, including the distal surfaces of the most posterior tooth in each quadrant. A new, unused portion of floss can be used for each interdental space, or when the used portion of floss becomes soiled or frayed.

Using a Floss Holder Another method of flossing, which is considered easier for some clients, involves the use of a *floss holder.* These devices are generally Y-shaped or C-shaped yokes with a handle. The floss is tightly secured between the two prongs and the client manipulates the floss by holding the handle. The technique of flossing used to cleanse interdentally is identical to the other flossing methods described. Floss handles are recommended for clients with large hands, people who are physically challenged or lack normal dexterity, caregivers who assist others with flossing, or clients who prefer not to put their hands in their mouths. Research has shown that reductions in bacterial plaque and gingivitis are equivalent with use of hand flossing and floss holders.[47,48]

Using a Floss Threader Another device designed to assist clients with flossing is the *floss threader.* It is a blunt-ended needle-like device made of stiff yet flexible plastic. The floss is threaded through the floss threader and the blunt end, or nylon tip, is inserted under the tooth contact or pontic to thread the floss from the facial through the interdental space to the lingual surface (see Fig. 16–11). Once the floss is threaded through the contact, it can be used in the usual manner to cleanse the adjacent tooth surfaces. The floss threader is useful when floss cannot be passed through the contact because an appliance is present that occludes the contact area. Thus, it is recommended for clients with fixed bridges, orthodontic appliances, or fixed orthodontic retainers such as a "lingual bar."

Evaluation of Flossing

Evaluation of flossing is similar to the evaluation of toothbrushing. The clinician observes the client's flossing technique for *efficiency, effectiveness,* and *safety* at various intervals throughout the process of care. Disclosing solution and plaque, bleeding, and periodontal indices can be used to assess plaque removal effectiveness. Evaluation of gingival and periodontal conditions also is necessary for long-term evaluation. Oral signs of gingival trauma (e.g., floss cuts, gingival clefts, gingival abrasion) should be used for the safety evaluation.

When bacterial plaque remains interproximally despite regular use of floss, the dental hygienist needs to observe the client's technique, reassess the type of embrasure involved, and suggest modifications. A common error is failure to wrap the floss in a C-shape around the proximal surface of the tooth or failure to recommend the appropriate interdental aid. If the floss is not wrapped tightly to create friction, but used in a straight line, it does not disrupt the deposits of bacterial plaque. Another common error is using too long a piece of floss between the fingers. This error leads to reduced control friction, and insertion difficulties between the teeth. Specific technique errors can be identified by observing the client's flossing. *Frequent reinstruction is necessary because flossing is a difficult skill to master.*

Bleeding during flossing can be a result of trauma or an indication of gingival inflammation. When clients with inflamed gingiva initiate flossing, the gingiva bleeds because of the ulcerations in the sulcular lining that occur during the active disease process. *Clients must be aware that bleeding is not a sign that flossing should be avoided in those areas, but rather an indicator of inflammation and active disease that needs to be controlled.* Bleeding from inflammation subsides with regular bacterial plaque removal and professional oral hygiene care. Focusing on gingival bleeding as an immediate, tangible indicator of periodontal infection may be a more effective means of motivating clients to comply with oral hygiene recommendations than emphasizing oral cleanliness and future oral health.[49,50]

Detrimental effects of flossing also should be noted. Clients who use floss incorrectly or who use excessive pressure can cause damage to the gingival tissues. Floss cuts or clefts occur on the facial or lingual surfaces adjacent to the papillae or across the papillae themselves.[51] They are most frequently caused by snapping the floss through the contacts or by cutting across the papillae when cleaning adjacent tooth surfaces.

Individuals who report that they do not floss should be questioned to determine the reason(s). If they simply do not like or value the procedure (human need deficient in value system), the clinician can find out why and perhaps recommend an alternative interdental aid or a floss holder. If they have difficulty with the technique or with developing the habit (human need deficient in self-determination and responsibility), suggestions can be made to assist them. If they are unaware of the importance of flossing (human need deficient in conceptualization and problem solving), they must be taught about the disease process and the unique susceptibility of the interdental area. If they understand the importance of flossing, but just do not because they are too busy (human need deficient in value system), the dental hygienist might determine with the client his values and priorities and then show how interdental oral hygiene practices can help achieve that priority or fit into that value system. Studies have shown that only 10 to 20% of Americans floss daily.[37,47] When the dental hygienist's approach is based upon the unique human needs of the client, instruction is truly individualized and client acceptance is more likely.

Irregular flossing also might be a concern for some medically compromised persons. During vigorous flossing, bacteremia may result. The occurrence of bleeding and resultant bacteremia increases when gingival inflammation is present. People with congenital heart disease, rheumatic heart disease, heart or vascular prostheses, joint replacements, or other conditions that require antibiotic premedication prior to dental hygiene care should be cautioned about the potential hazards of occasional (rather than routine) flossing.[52] Regular flossing presents no problem for clients with these medical conditions.

Interdental Brushes and Swabs

Interdental brushes are available in various sizes and shapes (see Table 16–2). The most common brushes are conical-shaped or tapered (like an evergreen tree) and are designed to be inserted into a plastic, reusable handle that is angled to facilitate interproximal adaptation. Attendees of the 1989 World Workshop in Clinical Periodontics concluded that interproximal brushes are the superior interproximal cleaning device when space exists for their use.[41] Studies have shown that interproximal brushes are equal to or more effective than floss for bacterial plaque removal and for reducing gingival inflammation in type II embrasures, type III embrasures, and exposed furcation areas.[53–55] Concave proximal root surfaces can be reliably reached and cleansed by interdental brushes (Fig. 16–15). The size of the brush selected is related to the size of the gingival embrasure or furcation area to be cleaned (see Fig. 16–11). The interdental brush should be slightly larger than the embrasure space so that it can effectively clean exposed, irregular, or concave root surfaces. It is inserted interproxi-

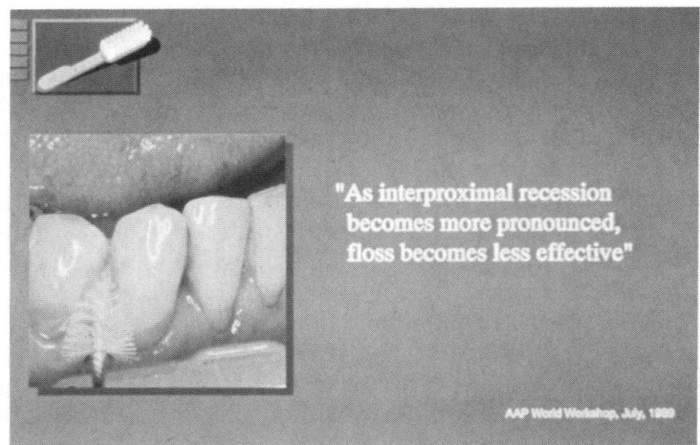

FIGURE 16–15
Proper insertion of interdental brush. (Compliments of Oral-B Laboratories.)

mally and activated with a back-and-forth motion in a facial-lingual direction (see Fig. 16–15). Interdental brushes also can be used for target delivery of chemotherapeutic agents to localized areas. For example, such brushes can be dipped into a solution of 0.12% chlorhexidine gluconate and then used in a furcation defect.

Uni-tufted or *end-tufted toothbrushes* are indicated for type III embrasures, difficult to reach areas, or around fixed dental appliances. They are designed with a smaller brush head that has a single tuft or a small group of tufts (see Fig. 16–11). The bristles are directed into the area to be cleaned and activated with a rotating motion.

Swab tips also are available in various sizes for bacterial plaque removal in type II and III embrasures, furcations, or around fixed dental appliances and orthodontic bands. They also can be used for application of antimicrobial or desensitizing chemotherapeutic agents.

Wooden Toothpicks and Wedges

Many people prefer to use **toothpicks** for interdental bacterial plaque control because of their availability and because of peer acceptance.[11] Attendees of the 1989 World Workshop in Clinical Periodontics concluded that mounted toothpicks are effective in specific sites when space exists for their use.[41] Studies have shown that the toothpick is equally as effective as dental floss in reducing interproximal plaque and bleeding.[50,56] With careful angulation, the toothpick can negotiate smaller root concavities and therefore is indicated for clients with fixed prosthetic appliances, orthodontic bands, type II embrasures, accessible furcations that are small in size, or shallow periodontal pockets. It is unlikely that any mechanical oral hygiene device can remove bacterial plaque from pockets greater than or equal to 5 mm. As pockets become deeper, oral hygiene care becomes increasingly difficult for the client. Thus, the goal of periodontal therapy is pocket reduction and elimination. The toothpick can, however, be useful for cleaning around the gingival margin or in shallow periodontal pockets.

Clients should be taught proper use of the toothpick to effectively remove bacterial plaque without causing damage to the gingiva. The toothpick can be used supragingivally or can be inserted subgingivally at a 45-degree angle to the tooth surface. The tip should maintain contact with the tooth surface and be angled into root concavities or around the margins of dental appliances. It should not be pointed directly into the epithelial attachment. The end of the toothpick can be moistened with saliva to soften it prior to use. If it becomes too frayed, it should be replaced to prevent particles of wood from breaking off in the sulcus or pocket.

A *toothpick holder* (e.g., Perio Aid) can be used to facilitate interproximal adaptation of the toothpick, especially on the lingual surfaces and in the posterior teeth. A round toothpick is secured into the end of an angled plastic handle. The longer end of the toothpick is then broken off cleanly and the end remaining in the toothpick holder is used to cleanse the tooth surface (see Fig. 16–12). Its use would be indicated for the same oral conditions as wooden wedges and toothpicks; however, some clients prefer a holder. Both techniques can be introduced during oral hygiene instruction and each individual can determine his own preference.

Soft triangular toothpicks (e.g., Stim-u-dent) or **wedge stimulators,** are wooden or plastic oral hygiene devices designed for interdental cleansing and stimulation. They are inserted interproximally with the base of the triangle resting on the gingival papilla, the tip pointing occlusally or incisally, and the sides of the toothpick against the adjacent tooth surfaces (Fig. 16–16). The toothpick is activated with a back-and-forth motion tangential with the gingiva. Bacterial plaque is disrupted and removed by using either side of the triangular toothpick or the end. Triangular toothpicks are indicated for clients who need gingival stimulation, for type II embrasure spaces, or for the client who refuses dental floss. They are not recommended for periodontal pockets because they are effective only in supragingival plaque removal and reducing gingival inflammation in the coronal regions of the sulcus rather than in apical regions.[57,58]

The wooden triangular toothpick also can be used during the periodontal assessment for detection of gingival bleeding points.[59] Interdental bleeding following this method of stimulation forms the basis of the Eastman interdental bleeding index.[58,60]

Miscellaneous Interdental Oral Hygiene Aids

When large embrasure spaces or areas of missing teeth are present, household items can be used for bacterial plaque control. *Knitting yarn* or *gauze strips* can be used to clean proximal tooth surfaces adjacent to wide interproximal spaces. *Pipe cleaners* also can be used for type II embrasures or exposed furcation areas. These items may be less expensive or more accessible for some people.

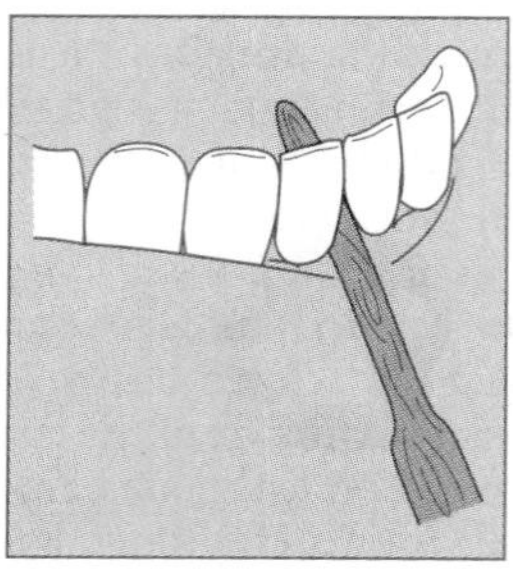

FIGURE 16–16
Use of wooden wedge.

Auxiliary Oral Hygiene Care

Gingival Stimulation

Massaging the gingiva with a toothbrush or an interdental oral physiotherapy device can lead to improved circulation, increased keratinization, and epithelial thickening. Whether these changes in the gingiva provide any clinical benefits is questionable.[11,23] It appears that improved gingival health resulting from oral hygiene practices is more directly related to bacterial plaque removal than to gingival stimulation.

The *interdental tip stimulator,* or rubber tip stimulator, attached to the end of a toothbrush or a plastic handle, has been suggested for use to stimulate the gingiva and to recontour gingival papillae following periodontal therapy. With regard to plaque removal, the literature regarding this device provides conflicting findings, with some studies indicating that the rubber tip is effective in removing plaque and others showing that it does not remove plaque effectively.[54,61] Its use may increase tissue tone.[62] The interdental tip stimulator is contraindicated for areas in which the gingival contour is normal or where the tissue is healthy. It can cause injury to the gingiva if used improperly. The tip should be used only supragingivally, angled coronally, and inserted interproximally tangential with the papillae. Gentle pressure is exerted on the gingiva in a rotary motion. In general, gingival stimulation receives a low priority in a disease control program. Its value in oral health promotion is in need of research.

Dentifrices

Dentifrices, sold as toothpastes, gels, or tooth powders, can be cosmetic or therapeutic.[11] Cosmetic dentifrices assist in cleaning and polishing the teeth; therapeutic dentifrices also contain an active ingredient to reduce dental disease. For example, fluoride dentifrices reduce the occurrence of dental caries, and desensitizing toothpastes reduce dentinal hypersensitivity. Several antimicrobial toothpastes have been sold to reduce bacterial plaque, and antitartar products are available to reduce calculus formation.

Toothpastes contain water, abrasive agents, polishing agents, humectants, binders, preservatives, foaming agents, flavorings, and colorings. The ADA does not consider acceptance for ordinary cleansing dentifrices, but it does consider dentifrices that are marketed for therapeutic or prophylactic effects.[63]

The ADA Council on Dental Therapeutics periodically publishes information on the relative abrasiveness of dentifrices. Laboratory studies that control for type of toothbrush bristle used, pressure applied, number of strokes, and other related variables are conducted periodically to assess the abrasiveness of various products. The ability of a toothpaste to remove stains is related to its level of abrasiveness. Clients who rapidly form dental stains may want to use a dentifrice with a higher abrasiveness. They should be cautioned, however, because abrasives can dull the tooth luster and cause tooth abrasion over time. Also, use of excessive toothbrushing force coupled with an abrasive dentifrice can cause cervical notches on teeth and gingival recession. Some commonly used abrasives are silicon oxide, aluminum oxide, and polyvinyl chloride. These agents do not react with fluoride.

Humectants, such as mannitol or sorbitol, are added to maintain moisture and consistency of the dentifrice. Binding agents, or gums, are used to thicken the paste or gel. Preservatives prevent microbial growth from occurring. The foaming or sudsing action of the dentifrice is created by adding detergents to the formula. Sodium lauryl sulfate and sodium n-lauryl sarcosinate are the most commonly used detergents. As mentioned earlier in this chapter, some powered toothbrushes cannot be used with dentifrices that foam. Flavorings, sweeteners, and colorings are added to make the product more pleasing to the consumer.

The dental hygiene practitioner makes recommendations to clients regarding selection of a dentifrice. Therapeutic dentifrices are available to aid in the control of dental caries, calculus formation, and dentinal hypersensitivity.

The regular use of a fluoride dentifrice is important for clients of all ages. It has been shown to reduce the incidence of dental caries. Sodium fluoride, sodium monofluorophosphate, and stannous fluoride are considered safe and effective agents for use in dentifrices. The ADA Seal of Acceptance is earned by products that are proven to have an anticariogenic effect.

Research is being conducted on dentifrices containing various microbial agents to evaluate their effectiveness in reducing bacterial plaque and gingivitis. Examples of active ingredients currently under study include sanguinaria, zinc citrate, triclosan, and copper citrate. Although many antimicrobial agents have been investigated in the past, their incorporation into dentifrices presents problems of compatibility with other dentifrice components. For example, chlorhexidine is the most widely accepted antiplaque agent; however, it is inactivated when incorporated into a dentifrice. Because the most commonly used oral hygiene device is a toothbrush, it is logical to consider dentifrice as a delivery system for antimicrobials. The American Academy of Periodontology Research Science and Therapy Committee has outlined problems associated with this delivery system.[23] The primary concern is the fact that a manual toothbrush reaches an average of less than 1 mm subgingivally, and only occasionally 2 to 3 mm. Any antimicrobial agent delivered in this manner fails to reach the deeper subgingival sites associated with periodontitis. At the present time, no dentifrice has received the ADA Seal of Acceptance for antiplaque and gingivitis effectiveness.

Anticalculus, or tartar control, dentifrices (e.g., Crest and Colgate) have demonstrated effectiveness in reducing the formation of calculus when compared with conventional dentifrices. They contain soluble pyrophosphates as the anticalculus agent as well as fluoride for anticariogenic benefits. The ADA Seal of Acceptance, however, is granted only for anticariogenic properties despite their proven effectiveness in reducing calculus deposits, because the ADA considers this property to be cosmetic rather than therapeutic.

Some dentifrices, however, have been accepted by the ADA Council on Dental Therapeutics for their effectiveness in reducing dentinal hypersensitivity. These products can be recommended to clients who experience hypersensitivity. Like home fluoride therapy, their use can be coupled with professional application of a desensitizing agent. The most common active ingredients are potassium nitrate, strontium chloride, and sodium citrate. These ingredients are in over-the-counter dentifrices (e.g., Denquel, Sensodyne, Protect, Promise) available to consumers. Some dentifrices also contain fluoride and have received the ADA Seal of Acceptance for both anticariogenic and antihypersensitivity effectiveness. These products are preferred for individuals with dentinal hypersensitivity because of their dual benefits.

Mouth Rinses

Like dentifrices, **mouth rinses** can be cosmetic, therapeutic, or both. Mouth rinses (mouthwashes) are a popular and simple delivery system, and thus they present a logical mode for delivery of therapeutic agents. They also provide a mechanism for rinsing oral debris and bacterial deposits dislodged during mechanical oral hygiene practices. Cosmetic benefits include a reduction in number of oral microorganisms, short-term halitosis control, and a pleasant taste and sensation in the mouth. Mouth rinses that claim no therapeutic value are not included in the ADA acceptance program.

Commercial mouth rinses generally contain an active ingredient to reduce the number of oral microorganisms, a flavoring agent, an astringent, ethyl alcohol, and water. The active ingredient may or may not have therapeutic qualities, but usually it provides a temporary benefit through mechanical reduction of oral microorganisms. The astringent (e.g., citric acid, zinc chloride) provides an invigorating sensation in the mouth, and the flavoring agent provides the pleasant taste. The ethyl alcohol acts as a solvent and a taste enhancer. Many products contain between 11% and 27% alcohol, although a few products are available that contain no alcohol (Table 16–3). Consumers should be advised to read the labels on commercial products to determine alcohol content. Alcohol-containing mouth rinses can be dangerous if ingested by small children, resulting in intoxication, illness, or fatalities depending upon dosage and body weight.[11] The American Academy of Pediatrics has recommended that alcohol content be limited to less than 5%, that package volume be minimal to prevent lethal dosages, and that safety caps be employed.[64] Adult clients who object to alcohol, recovering alcoholics or substance abusers, or clients taking medications that react adversely with alcohol (e.g., metronidazole) should be informed of alcohol content in commercial mouth rinses and guided in the selection of alcohol-free mouth rinses.

Dental hygiene clinicians also need to consider the pH of the mouth rinse when making recommendations to clients (see Table 16–3). A pH below 5 may have a demineralizing effect on exposed cementum. Clients with gingival recession, postperiodontal surgical cases, and those in periodontal maintenance therapy may benefit from a less acidic mouth rinse.

Some mouth rinses also contain sodium, which can result in sodium intake during rinsing.[65] Table 16–3 provides information on sodium content in various products. People on sodium-restricted diets (those with hypertension, congestive heart disease, fluid retention disorders, etc.) should be aware that some brands of mouthwash may be a significant source of sodium.

Therapeutic mouthwashes are available for control of dental caries, bacterial plaque, and gingivitis. Several products have received the ADA Seal of Acceptance. Mouth rinses that have a beneficial effect on supragingival plaque and gingivitis are discussed later in this chapter within the section on chemotherapeutic agents. Fluoride-containing mouth rinses are discussed in Chapter 21. Mouthwashes do not have a therapeutic effect on subgingival periodontopathic microorganisms because they do not significantly penetrate subgingivally.[38] Thus, at the present time, there is currently no mouth rinse accepted by the ADA Council on Dental Therapeutics for use in treatment of periodontitis. Studies are being conducted to determine whether home subgingival irrigation systems may improve the effectiveness of chemotherapeutic agents in the treatment of periodontitis.

Some clients prepare their own mouthwashes at home. Ingredients frequently used include sodium chloride (salt), sodium bicarbonate (baking soda), and hydrogen peroxide. Approximately ½ teaspoon of salt or baking soda per 8 ounces of water is used for preparation. Hydrogen peroxide is diluted with water in equal parts. Extensive short-term and long-term studies evaluating the use of baking soda and peroxide as adjuncts to home care have demonstrated no added value over mechanical oral hygiene alone. Further, chronic use of hydrogen peroxide may have numerous adverse effects (see Oxygenating Agents).[66,67] The routine unsupervised use of medicated mouthwashes is not recommended.[63]

Antibacterial mouth rinses are recommended for use prior to and during professional oral hygiene care. Pretreatment rinsing can reduce the number of microorganisms in the oral cavity and thereby reduce the aerosol contamination occurring during dental hygiene care procedures. Clients also appreciate the provision of a pleasant-tasting rinse after completion of professional oral hygiene care.

Oral Irrigation

Powered **oral irrigation** devices (e.g., Water Pik, Braun), first introduced in 1966,[68] were designed to produce a single jet stream of water that was forced through an irrigation tip with adjustable pressure. These commercial water jet devices became quite popular with the general public. They also were recommended to clients by oral healthcare pro-

TABLE 16–3
EXAMPLES OF MOUTH RINSES: pH, ALCOHOL, AND SODIUM CONTENT

Product	pH	Alcohol Content (%)	Sodium Content (mg/L)	Sodium Retention (mg/15 mL)
Cepacol	6.0	14.0	144	1.9
Regular Listerine	5.0	26.9	*	*
Peridex	5.5	11.6	*	*
Plax	*	7.0	5320	28.3
Scope	5.5	18.0	*	*
Viadent	3.0 (paste 4.0)	11.5	144	0.7

*Data not available.

Data adapted from Ciancio, S. G. Pharmacology of oral antimicrobials. In The Academy of Periodontology's Perspectives on Oral Antimicrobial Therapeutics. Littleton, MA: PSG Publishing Co., Inc., 1987, p. 33; and Wagner, M. J., et al. Sodium retention in mouthwashes. Journal of Clinical Preventive Dentistry 11:21, 1989.

fessionals, especially for those with orthodontic appliances or fixed prostheses, for the removal of food debris. To prevent the possibility of periodontal abscess formation, clients were instructed to direct the irrigator tip at a 90-degree angle to the long axis of the tooth surface, avoid excessive pressure, and never direct the tip subgingivally. Research conducted at that time, however, indicated that oral irrigation failed to remove attached plaque stained with a disclosing agent, which led to skepticism about the therapeutic value of oral irrigation.

In the 1970s, the significance of unattached or loosely attached plaque was related to the specific plaque hypothesis. Suspected pathogens found in unattached plaque were associated with various forms of periodontal diseases. In the 1980s, oral irrigation was given renewed attention when it was suggested that supragingival irrigation may disrupt subgingival areas of unattached bacterial plaque.[23]

With the advent of chemical plaque control (i.e., the use of antimicrobial agents to reduce or eliminate pathogenic organisms from the bacterial composition of plaque), oral irrigating devices have been evaluated as possible systems for local or target delivery of antimicrobials directly into the pocket. In this regard, fractionated multijet irrigators (with many streams) or pulsating irrigators have been developed to dissipate the force with which antimicrobials are delivered to the pocket. In addition, irrigators with specially adapted low-pressure subgingival delivery tips have been developed to increase periodontal pocket access.

Supragingival irrigation with **chemotherapeutic agents,** in conjunction with mechanical oral hygiene measures, has some benefit in controlling gingivitis.[41] Recently, however, the use of supragingival irrigation with antimicrobials has been suggested for controlling subgingival bacterial plaque and periodontitis.[68–70] The latter concept raises the issue of how far into the sulcus or pocket the antimicrobial agent is able to penetrate with supragingival irrigation or with shallow subgingival placement of the tip. Studies have shown that irrigators used according to manufacturer's instructions can penetrate subgingivally from 3 to 6 mm.[68,71–73] Use of a cannula, or needle-like tip, can provide 100% penetration to the depth of a pocket; however, safety is a concern with client use. A tapered plastic tip (e.g., Sulcus Tip) can deliver to an average depth of 42%, and a soft rubber tip (e.g., Pik Pocket) has 80% penetration of the solution.[71] Attendees of the 1989 World Workshop in Clinical Periodontics[38,41] concluded the following:

- Calculus deposits must be removed prior to oral irrigation to maximize penetration
- The irrigator tip must be placed in the gingival crevice for maximal penetration, but this task may limit client performance
- Supragingival irrigation with a jet irrigator may frequently provide secondary subgingival penetration of 3 mm

Attendees of the workshop also concluded that supragingival irrigation, as an adjunct to conventional oral hygiene, may be of value in the treatment of gingivitis.

Subgingival irrigation with various antimicrobials such as chlorhexidine, tetracycline, stannous fluoride, oxygenating agents, and others is another area of current interest. Devices have been developed for in-office use by professionals as well as for home use by clients. When performed professionally by the dental hygienist, subgingival irrigation takes valuable chair time, is performed only infrequently, and has produced questionable results.[23] Most studies have shown that professional oral irrigation performed in conjunction with root planing has no demonstrated advantage over root planing alone.[41] Results of studies evaluating self-applied, daily supragingival irrigation with antimicrobials for the control of bacterial plaque and gingivitis show much more promise at this time.

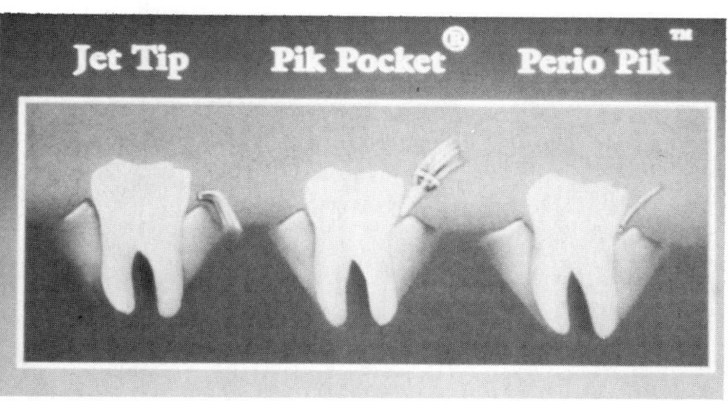

FIGURE 16–17
Oral irrigation tip replacement. (Compliments of Teledyne Water Pik.)

Using an Irrigating Device Clients who use oral irrigating devices need professional instruction for proper use. After turning on the unit and adjusting the water stream, the client should place the irrigation tip intraorally. The tip is placed into the gingival crevice interproximally and directed at a 90-degree angle to the long axis of the tooth, unless using the subgingival tip, which is directed subgingivally (Fig. 16–17). The tip is moved around the mouth in a sequence until all areas needing irrigation are treated. Caution should be taken to avoid excessive pressure, to limit duration of use in each area, and to follow manufacturer's instructions. Particles and bacteria from the crevice can be forced into the soft tissues and periodontal abscesses may develop if excessive water pressure is used and if the supragingival tip is pointed apically.

Oral irrigators with supragingival tips also can be recommended for debris removal. Clients with orthodontic appliances, fixed bridges, implants, splints, or other areas of debris accumulation may find oral irrigation useful. Also, irrigators with various supragingival and subgingival tips provide an effective delivery system for antimicrobial chemotherapeutic agents. It should be emphasized, however, that oral irrigation is an adjunct to mechanical plaque control, not a substitute for it.

Chemotherapeutic Agents for the Control of Bacterial Plaque

There is no convincing evidence of a linear relationship between the quantity of bacterial plaque and the extent of periodontal disease. Rather, the relationship between the amount of plaque and the threshold for disease is most likely dependent on the specific bacterial composition of the plaque and the resistance of the host. A supplemental method for plaque control is to alter the bacterial composition of plaque in such a way that health cannot convert to disease.[2] Use of antimicrobial agents as adjuncts to mechanical oral hygiene is promising for the prevention and

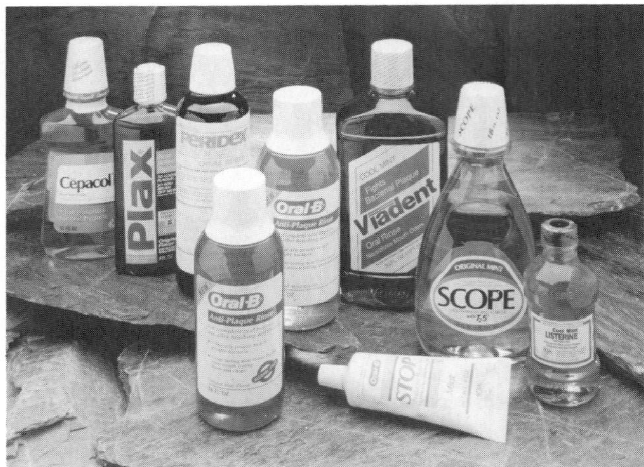

FIGURE 16–18
Various chemotherapeutic products available to consumers. (Compliments of Oral-B Laboratories.)

control of periodontal disease. Figure 16–18 shows a variety of chemotherapeutic products available on the market.

Current periodontal literature is full of articles and studies that describe the effectiveness of various antimicrobial agents. It is important for dental hygiene practitioners to be able to evaluate this literature to determine which findings are valid. In 1986, the ADA established guidelines for acceptance of chemotherapeutic products for the control of bacterial plaque and gingivitis.[5] Any product claiming therapeutic effect that has not been accepted by the ADA Council on Dental Therapeutics either has not been submitted for consideration or has been found to be lacking in scientific evidence of therapeutic effectiveness, safety, or both.[74] Consumers should be advised to look for the ADA Seal of Acceptance when purchasing products containing chemotherapeutic agents for the control of bacterial plaque and gingivitis.

Evaluating Chemotherapeutic Agents

The ADA guidelines for acceptance of chemotherapeutic agents for the control of bacterial plaque and gingivitis specify criteria used by the Council on Dental Therapeutics to evaluate product research. The guidelines do not pertain to evaluating the management of periodontitis or other periodontal diseases.

A term that dental hygienists should understand when evaluating chemotherapeutic oral rinses is **substantivity.** Substantivity is the ability of an active agent to be retained in the oral cavity and to continue to be released over an extended period of time without losing its potency. Oral antimicrobial rinses are divided into first-generation agents and second-generation agents. First-generation agents have been available for some time, as over-the-counter antibacterial rinses. They are antibacterial, but they have less substantivity (or ability to remain in the mouth and work effectively) than second-generation agents. This means that first-generation agents probably need to be used more frequently to obtain the same results.

Second-generation agents have antibacterial activity plus proven substantivity. According to Ciancio,[75] chlorhexidine has high substantivity and stannous fluoride has moderate substantivity. Both of these agents require prescriptions for client use. All of the other agents currently available have lower substantivity and are available over the counter. For these reasons, chlorhexidine and stannous fluoride are classified as second-generation agents, and all of the others as first-generation agents.

Chlorhexidine

Chlorhexidine is a bisbiguanide that was first synthesized and used as a disinfectant for skin and mucous membranes. Clinical trials have clearly documented that chlorhexidine is currently the most effective antiplaque and antigingivitis agent. It has been shown to reduce plaque by 55% and gingivitis by 45%.[38,75] A mouth rinse containing 0.12% chlorhexidine (Peridex) is approved by the ADA on a prescription basis for treatment of gingivitis; as shown in Table 16–3, the product has 11.6% alcohol and a pH of 5.5.[38,75] It is recommended that the client rinse for 30 seconds with $\frac{1}{2}$ ounce of Peridex after brushing and flossing twice a day.

The mode of action of chlorhexidine is to bind to hydroxyapatite and glycoprotein to prevent pellicle formation. It also absorbs to the bacterial cell surface and may interfere with cell attachment. Chlorhexidine has great substantivity in that it is available in an active form for prolonged periods of time (8 to 12 hours) in the mouth. Staining of teeth, tongue, and anterior restorations, a bitter taste, soft tissue ulcerations, and transient loss of taste are reported side effects. Because chlorhexidine may temporarily affect the sensation of taste, it should be used after meals to minimize taste alteration. Clients should not rinse with water immediately after it is used to decrease the medicinal aftertaste. Rinsing may increase the undesirable taste because it removes the flavor-masking agents from the oral cavity. In addition, practitioners should be cautious about recommending a chlorhexidine mouth rinse for clients with anterior facial restorations with rough or pitted areas because it may stain them permanently.

Stannous Fluoride

There is growing evidence that stannous fluoride (SnF_2) has more antiplaque properties than sodium fluoride (NaF). Interestingly enough, it is the stannous ion, not the fluoride, that has the greatest antimicrobial effect. Tin from the stannous ion enters the cell, clogs the metabolism, and affects the growth and adherence properties of the bacteria. Numerous animal and clinical studies have demonstrated that stannous fluoride reduces dental plaque, and some have also indicated a decrease in gingivitis.[76–78]

Several 0.4% stannous fluoride gels carry the ADA Seal of Acceptance (e.g., STOP and Gel Kam). ADA acceptance is for anticaries activity and safety; they have not been accepted for reductions in plaque and gingivitis.

Phenolic Compounds (Essential Oils)

The only product in the **phenolic compounds** category that has been adequately studied is Listerine (see Table 16–3). It has received the ADA Seal of Acceptance as an effective agent for reduction of bacterial plaque and gingivitis. Listerine is a mixture of three phenolic-derived essential oils —thymol, menthol, and eucalyptol, which are combined with methylsalicylate. The mechanism of action appears to be related to alteration of the bacterial cell wall. This product has a low substantivity and is safe. Adverse effects reported have been a burning sensation, bitter taste, and a possible staining of teeth. Twice daily usage without concern for dentifrice interactions favors compliance. Long-term studies evaluating the clinical effects of Listerine indicate that bacterial plaque can be reduced by 25 to 28% and gingivitis can be reduced by an average of 30% compared to baseline levels.[38,74]

Sanguinarine

Sanguinarine, a benzophenathridine alkaloid, is an alcohol extract from the root of the plant *Sanguinaria canadensis.* This antiplaque substance is currently available in over-the-counter mouth rinse and dentifrice products (see Table 16–3). It is marketed as a mouth rinse and a dentifrice (Viadent). The activity of sanguinarine is attributed to its ability to interfere with bacterial glycolysis and bind to plaque to prevent adherence of microorganisms. Sanguinarine is retained for about 2 to 4 hours in the mouth. Research indicates that sanguinarine is less effective than chlorhexidine, and no side effects are observed.[79–81] Short-term clinical studies employing various experimental conditions have evaluated sanguinarine. The agent appears to reduce bacterial plaque and gingivitis somewhat; however, a consistent degree of efficacy has not been documented. Effectiveness is enhanced when both the mouth rinse and the dentifrice are used.[74,82–84]

Quaternary Ammonium Compounds

Quaternary ammonium compounds have been evaluated in a number of short-term studies relative to their effect on plaque and gingivitis. In these studies, an average plaque reduction of 35% less than baseline scores has been reported with mixed effect on gingival health.[38] Cepacol and Scope are two well-known representatives of this group with concentrations of 0.05 and 0.045% cetylpyridinium chloride (CPC), respectively (see Table 16–3). The mechanism of action is related to increased bacterial cell wall permeability that favors lysis, decreased cell metabolism, and a decreased ability for bacteria to attach to tooth surfaces. These agents are categorized as cationic, which favors their attraction to tooth surfaces and bacterial plaque. They alter surface tension and have a low substantivity and a high safety factor.[75]

Prebrushing Rinses

Plax is a **prebrushing mouth rinse** containing sodium benzoate and other nontoxic surfactants (see Table 16–3). It contains 7.5% alcohol. Short-term studies have shown some reductions in bacterial plaque; however, a number of investigations not supported by the manufacturer have shown no effect on plaque reduction when compared to a placebo.[74] Reductions in gingivitis have not been documented. Proof of the clinical efficacy of this product awaits long-term studies that include comparisons with normal toothbrushing and measures of periodontal disease. Safety is not a concern. Sodium content contraindicates use for clients on sodium-restricted diets (see Table 16–3).

Oxygenating Agents

Several products containing **oxygenating agents** are available on the market (e.g., Amosan, Orthoflur, Oxyfresh). The American Academy of Periodontology[67] has published a review of oxygenating agents. Long-term studies have shown no beneficial effects on reductions in bacterial plaque and gingivitis when compared to controls. Safety is an issue with hydrogen peroxide. Chronic use of hydrogen peroxide has been shown to cause serious side effects including carcinogenesis, tissue damage, hyperkeratosis, oral ulcerations, hyperplasia, and black hairy tongue syndrome.[67] Short-term use of oxygenating oral rinses is intended for oral wound cleansing. A soothing effect has been reported.

Client Selection for Chemotherapeutic Adjuncts

Antimicrobials are not indicated for use with all clients. They are recommended for clients who have problems with plaque control; clients with extensive fixed prostheses, splinting, orthodontics, implants, or overdentures; and clients in the immediate postperiodontal surgery period during the healing phase. Use of chlorhexidine has been suggested for clients with compromised immune systems. The first attempt to control bacterial plaque and gingivitis should be made by personal and professional mechanical plaque control methods. When these attempts are unsuccessful, or when problems are anticipated, chemical agents can be introduced and used until health is attained. Reevaluation of clinical parameters is indicated after 3 to 12 weeks of use. If the gingiva is healthy, chemotherapeutic therapy should be discontinued until it is needed again. The unsupervised use of antimicrobials over extended periods of time is not recommended. Cost factors also should be considered. Products with effective chemotherapeutic agents are costly. If mechanical plaque control adequately removes soft deposits, the expense cannot be justified. Clients who may benefit from chemotherapeutic products should be encouraged to purchase them for use in conjunction with mechanical oral hygiene care.

Specific Educational Supplements

At times, dental hygienists use specific educational supplements for teaching clients about effective plaque control. Of course, the client's own mouth is always the most suitable model for demonstration of technique and description of oral conditions. Sometimes, however, audiovisual aids and other educational resources are useful for clarifying theoretical background information. Dental caries activity tests and phase contrast microscopy are two adjuncts that may be used as instructional and motivational tools in a bacterial plaque control program. They can provide a clear, visual picture of theories related to oral hygiene care.

Dental Caries Activity Tests

Caries activity tests provide information about acid-forming microorganisms or their activity in the mouth. They do not test specific sites of bacterial plaque accumulation, but rather sample oral microorganisms from the saliva. As such, results are often inconsistent and are not reliable predictors of dental caries incidence. Rather, caries activity tests provide a means of demonstrating pH changes in the mouth that can be related to the concept of acid production while discussing the caries process with a client. Caries activity tests illustrate that sugar and other cariogenic foods result in acid production by the bacteria in the mouth. Several different caries activity tests are available for use by the dental hygiene clinician or for caries-related programs presented by the oral health educator.

The *Snyder test*[85] is an agar test that contains bromcresol green. This medium turns yellow when exposed to substances with a pH below 5.0. The lower the pH, the more rapidly this color change occurs. A saliva sample is obtained from the client's mouth by having the person chew paraffin for 3 minutes and expectorate the pooled saliva into a sterile bottle. The Snyder medium is then prepared in a test tube. After shaking the saliva sample for mixing, it is added to the agar with a pipette. The sample is then incubated at 32°C for 3 days, and changes in color are compared with a control agar and recorded each day. The rate of color change from green to yellow is related to the degree of caries activity. A marked change within 24 hours indicates significant acid production. The less expensive and more convenient *modified Snyder test* is similar except that less agar is used and it is inoculated with saliva by use of a wire loop.[86] Another modification of the Snyder test is the *swab test.*[87] In this method, saliva is collected by wiping a sterile cotton swab on the buccal gingiva of each quadrant. The swab tip is then inserted into the test tube of bromcresol green medium and allowed to remain there throughout a 48-hour incubation period at 32°C. This method eliminates the need for the client to chew paraffin in order to obtain the sample of saliva and saves incubation time.

The *methyl red sugar test,*[88] or spot plate colormetric test, shows a change in color from red to yellow when pH is lowered from 6.3 to 4.2. A bacterial plaque sample is taken from the distal surfaces of the most posterior maxillary tooth using a curet. The plaque sample is placed on a white porcelain tile and covered with a few drops of methyl red indicator. Sugar is then sprinkled on the sample and a color change is observed over a 10- to 30-minute time period. The more red that is present around the plaque sample, the greater the acid production. This test is perhaps the most practical for the clinical setting because it can be completed during a single appointment and does not require incubation.

The *Streptococcus mutans count* estimates the quantity of *S. mutans* colonies found in a sample of saliva.[89] Because dental caries has been associated with *S. mutans,* this test can be used to count colonies present in the mouth and correlate that information with the possibility of dental caries development. A saliva sample is obtained by moistening a tongue depressor with saliva in the mouth. The tongue depressor is used to inoculate the specialized agar, and the agar is incubated anaerobically for 48 hours at 32°C. Caries activity is correlated with the density of colonies formed.

Phase Contrast Microscopy

The *phase contrast microscope* is used to examine living cells and microbes in a fluid medium. A film of bacterial plaque is placed on a slide and immersed in water. The morphology and activity of the live organisms are maintained and the viewer can determine size, shape, and motility of bacteria present in the plaque sample.

Phase contrast microscopy is employed in the dental hygiene process of care primarily as an adjunct to oral hygiene instruction and motivation. It was formerly used as an assessment tool; however, the advent of current technology for more specific microbial assessment (e.g., nucleic acid and antibody probes) has rendered phase contrast microscopy outmoded and inaccurate as a diagnostic test. Extensive data have been accumulated indicating that specific bacterial species and genotypes are associated with various periodontal diseases. Phase contrast microscopy does not identify species, but rather depicts only morphotypes (shapes) such as cocci, rods, and spirochetes. It also shows motility of live bacteria, a feature that is impressive to clients. Because no single morphotype is solely pathogenic, however, it cannot be used for diagnostic purposes.[66]

Phase contrast microscopy has several advantages as an educational supplement. It can be used to show clients colonies of plaque bacteria taken from their own teeth. The importance of bacteria in the etiology of periodontal disease can be emphasized and plaque can be visualized as a mass of various types of bacteria. Thus, it may be a useful motivational strategy. Microscopic demonstrations also can be used to show plaque maturation because complexes of plaque are more likely to occur with the aging of the plaque mass. As such, repeated phase contrast microscopy demonstrations throughout dental hygiene care can emphasize the value of additional therapeutic endpoints beyond clinical parameters.[66] Although the technology does not assess specific pathogens, it can show an absence of colonized bacteria in a state of health. The progress of a client's bacterial plaque control, therefore, can be documented through dramatic visual presentation.

The phase contrast microscope can be linked to a television screen so that clients are able to view the microorganisms in a plaque sample taken from their own mouths. Highly motile bacteria provide a visual representation of the significance of plaque in the initiation and progression of periodontal disease. This graphic demonstration can be impressive to clients and, hypothetically, enhances motivation.

The technique is very sensitive to the quality of the equipment and the expertise of the user. The slide is prepared with a drop of water at each site to be inoculated with a plaque sample. The sampling sites are selected by the clinician based upon the state of health or disease and the goals of the demonstration. A curet is used to obtain the plaque samples from the gingival crevice, placed into the water droplet, and gently dispersed. The cover slip is then placed over the prepared sample and the slide is mounted in the microscope for viewing. The clinician then focuses on the specimen while viewing it through the eyepieces of the microscope. It can then be viewed on the television screen or through the eyepieces.[90]

The evaluation of the sample can be discussed with the client emphasizing previously discussed theories related to plaque and periodontal disease. For example, in health, the phase contrast microscope reveals an absence of motile organisms and bacterial complexes that are loosely organized. More mature plaque complexes show a variety of motile forms and appear as highly organized masses. Areas of health and disease can be compared and correlated with presence of mature bacterial plaque.

Ethical and Legal Considerations

According to the Principles of Ethics of the American Dental Hygienists' Association, it is the dental hygiene practitioner's ethical responsibility to "provide oral health care using the highest level of professional knowledge, judgment and ability" and to "use every opportunity to increase public understanding of oral health practices."[91] The success of professional oral hygiene care is dependent upon the involvement of the client as a co-therapist. Thus, the dental hygienist must use current information to select appropriate plaque control devices and methods for each client and employ effective instructional and motivational techniques to teach the client to use them properly. This ethical obligation can be fulfilled only by making a life-long commitment to reviewing scientific literature related to preventive interventions and applying the knowledge gained to client care. It requires allocation of time for instruction, repetition, reinforcement, and continual assessment of each client's oral health practices. The public looks to the dental hygienist for sound advice concerning the prevention and control of oral diseases. As clinicians, consumer advocates and oral health educators, dental hygienists continually are involved in assisting people to achieve their oral health goals for a lifetime.

The legal standard of care also requires that dental hygienists educate clients about oral self-care. The American Academy of Periodontology outlines standards of care in the 1991 Guidelines for Periodontal Therapy.[92] Care plans should include evaluation of the presence and distribution of bacterial plaque and calculus, plans for educating the client in daily personal oral hygiene, consideration of adjunctive chemotherapeutic agents, assessment of the client's bacterial plaque control effectiveness, and reinstruction where needed. Upon completion of dental hygiene care the legal records of the client should reveal that the client has been counseled on why and how to perform an effective daily personal oral hygiene program. Monitoring the client's progress also should be recorded. Malpractice cases for failure to recognize and treat periodontal disease can be related to failure to teach adequate plaque control measures to clients.

PREVENTION OF ORAL DISEASE THROUGHOUT THE LIFE CYCLE

Prevention and control of oral diseases are enhanced when appropriate interventions are introduced throughout the life cycle.

In-utero and Infant Care

The dental hygienist teaches expectant mothers about prenatal care and nutrition. A well-balanced diet promotes the oral health of the mother and provides the developing fetus with essential nutrients. Vitamins, proteins, and minerals (especially calcium and phosphorus) for tissue construction and mineralization of the teeth and bones are needed. No direct evidence shows that prenatal fluoride reduces the incidence of dental caries in the child, and this message must be transferred to the pregnant woman.

The dental hygienist explains that fluoride must be present in the infant's daily diet because it benefits both teeth and bones during the mineralization process. The dental hygienist analyzes the baby's fluoride intake from the drinking water, if any, and determines the appropriate daily fluoride supplement.

Nursing bottle syndrome also should be explained to the mother. *Nursing bottle syndrome* is a form of rampant caries that is attributed to prolonged or habitual use of a nursing bottle containing milk, fruit juice, or other sweetened liquids, usually as an aid to sleeping. The dental hygienist should advise avoidance of milk or sweet juices at naptime or bedtime, and recommend use of plain water. Mothers can also be taught to clean the infant's newly erupted teeth, gingiva, and tongue at bathtime. This is best accomplished by use of gauze or a washcloth.

Preschool and Elementary School Children

Children develop manual dexterity at various rates. Oral hygiene practices require fine motor skills and dexterity for effective performance. Dental hygienists counsel parents about slowly shaping their child's toothcleaning habits while accepting low levels of fine motor skills in this age group. Preschool children can be encouraged to accept some responsibility for their oral health. The initial goal is to familiarize the child with oral hygiene aids; however, parents need not be concerned about their child's plaque removal effectiveness at first. The parent should be taught to perform thorough oral hygiene procedures for the child, at least once a day.[93] For example, the parent could clean the child's mouth each evening at bedtime, while the child is encouraged to use the toothbrush independently after breakfast. The experience should be fun.

There will be a time when the child prefers self-care. Even then, the parent should assist the child in thorough plaque removal, supervise his oral hygiene practices, and periodically evaluate effectiveness. School-age children can receive lessons on toothcleaning and, as dexterity permits, can be encouraged to perform oral hygiene procedures themselves while being observed by a parent. It is important for the dental hygienist to teach parents how to help the child through demonstrations and positive reinforcement.

Intrinsic incentives are more effective than extrinsic incentives for motivating children to perform regular, physical activities.[94] For example, having a "prettier smile," "fresh breath," and a "good taste in your mouth" may be better long-term motivational factors than prizes or rewards. Positive social reinforcement, and a minimum of criticism and negative reinforcement, also are important when motivating children to perform oral self-care behaviors.[93] Assisting the parent in selecting appropriate oral physiotherapy aids and identifying a good time and environment for daily oral hygiene care can help to make it a positive experience.

Adolescents

Adolescents generally prefer to be treated as adults and want to make their own decisions. Although it may not be outwardly apparent, adolescents are usually concerned with their body image and their health. Developing rapport with adolescents and actively listening to them are critical to effective oral hygiene instruction and client motivation. Dental caries and chronic gingivitis are frequent oral problems in adolescence. Oral effects of tobacco use, eating disorders, athletic injuries, and oral contraceptives also can be detected. The dental hygienist needs to provide a clear explanation of the etiology and pathogenicity of oral diseases and conditions present. Dietary counseling and oral hygiene instruction are important components of adolescent educational sessions. Evaluation of the need for topical fluoride, in combination with systemic fluoride, also is indicated.

Juvenile periodontitis can affect young individuals who are otherwise healthy. Destruction of the periodontium is usually disproportionate to local factors. If the disease is detected early it may respond well to local periodontal therapy supplemented with systemic antibiotics such as tetracycline.[95]

Adults

Adults are affected by dental caries and various periodontal diseases such as chronic gingivitis, adult periodontitis, and occlusal trauma. Mechanical and chemotherapeutic plaque control measures for this age group have been discussed throughout this chapter.

Older Adults

Preventive measures for the aging population become increasingly important as people live longer and maintain their natural dentition throughout life. Tooth loss increases with age from increased severity and incidence of untreated dental caries and periodontal diseases. The presence of root caries also is a concern in this age group because cementum is often exposed as a result of gingival recession. Fluoride therapy and periodontal maintenance therapy are important aspects of dental hygiene care for older adults.

Xerostomia, frequently reported by these clients, can be drug-induced or may result from radiation therapy or systemic illness. Suggesting mouth rinses or saliva substitutes can be helpful. Stressing the critical importance of daily bacterial plaque removal and self-applied high concentration fluoride and reviewing dietary habits is indicated for clients with xerostomia.

Sensitivity to the needs and concerns of older adults may assist the dental hygiene practitioner in working with them. At times, their self-esteem is low because of changes in social status, work habits, economic stability, or family life. Depression and loneliness and chronic degenerative diseases such as osteoporosis or Alzheimer's disease also may affect their physical well-being and quality of life. A detailed health history provides the dental hygienist with needed background information.

Successful involvement of these older clients lies in allowing enough time to treat them humanistically. Their voluntary reactions may be slowed and physical or sensory impairments may require modifications of conventional oral hygiene devices and techniques (see Chapters 26 and 30.) Assisting the client with improving current methods, rather than attempting to change life-long habits, also may be considered. Expression of personal concern for the client is a key strategy for building rapport and motivating behavioral change.

References

1. Newman, M. G., and Sanz, M. Oral microbiology with emphasis on etiology. In The American Academy of Periodontology's Perspectives on Oral Antimicrobial Therapeutics. Littleton, MA: PSG Publishing Co., Inc., 1989, p. 1.
2. Kornman, K. S. The role of supragingival plaque in the prevention and treatment of periodontal diseases. Journal of Periodontal Research. Suppl 5, 1979.
3. American Dental Association. Accepted Dental Therapeutics, 39th ed. Section on provisions for acceptance of products by the Council on Dental Therapeutics. 1981, pp. xvii–xxi.
4. American Dental Association. Council on Dental Therapeutics guidelines for acceptance of fluoride-containing dentifrices. Journal of the American Dental Association, 110:545, 1985.
5. American Dental Association. Council on Dental Therapeutics guidelines for acceptance of chemotherapeutic products for the control of supragingival plaque and gingivitis. Journal of the American Dental Association 112:529, 1986.
6. Carranza, F. A. Glickman's Clinical Periodontology, 7th ed. Philadelphia, W. B. Saunders, 1990, pp. 684–711.
7. Burgett, F. G., and Ash, M. M. Comparative study of the pressure of brushing with three types of toothbrushes. Journal of Periodontology 45:410, 1974.
8. Frandsen, A. Mechanical oral hygiene practices, In Loe, H., and Klienman, D. (eds). Dental Plaque Control Measures and Oral Hygiene Practices Workshop. Oxford: IRL Press, Ltd., 1986.
9. Wilkins, E. Clinical Practice of the Dental Hygienist, 6th ed. Philadelphia: Lea & Febiger, 1989, pp. 301–336.
10. American Dental Association. Accepted Dental Therapeutics, Section on Homecare in the Control of Dental Plaque: Toothbrushing, 40th ed. Chicago, American Dental Association, 1984, pp. 386–387.
11. Harris, N. O., and Christen, N. O. Primary Preventive Dentistry, 3rd ed. Norwalk, CT: Appleton & Lange, 1991, pp. 79–162.
12. Baab, D. A., and Johnson, R. H. The effect of a new electric toothbrush on supragingival plaque and gingivitis. Journal of Periodontology 60:336, 1989.
13. Silverstone, L. M., and Featherstone, M. J. A scanning electron microscope study of the end rounding of bristles in eight toothbrush types. Quintessence International 19:87, 1988.
14. Silverstone, L. M. Periodontal Dentistry. London: Update Books, 1978, p. 153.
15. American Dental Association. Basic Brushing Pamphlet. Chicago, 1984.
16. Abraham, N. J., et al. Dentists' and dental hygienists' attitudes toward toothbrush replacement and maintenance. Journal of Clinical Preventive Dentistry 12:28, 1990.
17. Vittel, P. Particles of advice on when to change toothbrushes. Chicago Tribune, Aug. 24, 1986; Tempo, Sec. 2.
18. Glass, R. T., and Lare, M. M. Toothbrush contamination. A potential health risk? Quintessence International 17:39, 1986.
19. Glass, R. T., and Jensen, H. G. More on the contaminated toothbrush: The viral story. Quintessence International 19:713, 1988.
20. Kendrick, A. J., et al. A two-year comparison of hand and electric toothbrushes. Journal of Periodontal Research 3:224, 1968.
21. Niemi, M. L., et al. Gingival abrasion and plaque removal with manual versus electric toothbrushes. Journal of Clinical Periodontology 13:709, 1986.
22. Walsh, M. M., et al. Comparison of manual and power toothbrushing, with or without adjunctive oral irrigation, for controlling plaque and gingivitis. Journal of Clinical Periodontology 16:419, 1989.
23. American Academy of Periodontology, Research, Science, and Therapy Committee. Local delivery of antimicrobials: Adjuncts of periodontal therapy. Chicago, American Academy of Periodontology, 1991.
24. Boyd, R. L., et al. Effect on periodontal status of rotary electric toothbrushes versus manual toothbrushes during periodontal maintenance. II. Microbiological results. Journal of Periodontology 60:396, 1989.
25. Coontz, E. J. The effectiveness of a new oral hygiene device on plaque removal. Quintessence International 14:1, 1983.
26. Lungarten, W. P., et al. The effectiveness of a powered toothbrush on plaque removal in periodontal patients. Compendium of Continuing Education, Dentistry 9:658, 1988.
27. Boyd, R. L., et al. Effect on periodontal status of rotary electric toothbrushes versus manual toothbrushes during periodontal maintenance. I. Clinical results. Journal of Periodontology 60:390, 1989.
28. Ainamo, J., et al. Effect of Manual versus Powered Toothbrushes. Helsinki: University of Helsinki (in press).
29. Van der Weijden, G. A., et al. The Plaque Removal Efficacy of a Reciproque Rotating Toothbrush. Amsterdam: Academic Centre for Dentistry (in press).
30. Glass, R. L. A clinical study of hand and electric toothbrushing. Journal of Periodontology 36:332, 1965.

31. Hawkins, B. F., and Lainson, P. A. Duration of toothbrushing for effective plaque control. Quintessence International 17:361, 1986.
32. Gibson, J. A., and Wade, A. B. Plaque removal by the Bass and Roll brushing techniques. Journal of Periodontology 48:456, 1989.
33. Niemi, M. L., et al. The effect of toothbrush grip on gingival abrasion and plaque removal during toothbrushing. Journal of Clinical Periodontology 14:19, 1987.
34. Bass, C. C. The optimum characteristics of toothbrushes for personal oral hygiene. Dental Items International 70:697, 1948.
35. Stillman, P. R. A philosophy of treatment of periodontal disease. Dental Digest 38:315, 1932.
36. Charters, W. J. Immunizing both hard and soft mouth tissues to infection by correct stimulation with a toothbrush. Journal of the American Dental Association 15:87, 1928.
37. Chen, M. S., and Rubinson, L. Preventive dental behavior in families: A national survey. Journal of the American Dental Association 105:43, 1982.
38. Ciancio, S. G. Nonsurgical periodontal treatment. Proceedings of the World Workshop in Clinical Periodontics, American Academy of Periodontology, Section II:1, 1988.
39. Heasman, P. A., et al. An evaluation of the effectiveness and patient compliance with plaque control methods in the prevention of periodontal disease. Clinical Preventive Dentistry 11:24, 1989.
40. Johansson, L. A., et al. Evaluation of cause-related periodontal therapy and compliance with maintenance care recommendations. Journal of Clinical Periodontology 11:689, 1984.
41. Consensus Report: Discussion, Section II. Proceedings of the World Workshop on Clinical Periodontics. Chicago, American Academy of Periodontology, 1989, pp. II13–17.
42. Hill, H. C., et al. The effects of waxed and unwaxed dental floss on interdental plaque accumulation and interdental gingival health. Journal of Periodontology 44:411, 1973.
43. Wunderlich, R. C., et al. The effect of waxed and unwaxed dental floss on gingival health. Journal of Periodontology 53:397, 1982.
44. Ong, G. The effectiveness of 3 types of dental floss for interdental plaque removal. Journal of Clinical Periodontology 17:463, 1990.
45. Stevens, A. W. A comparison of the effectiveness of variable diameter vs. unwaxed dental floss. Journal of Periodontology 51:666, 1980.
46. Spindel, L., and Person, P. Floss design and effectiveness of interproximal plaque removal. Journal of Clinical Preventive Dentistry 9:3, 1987.
47. Kleber, C. J., and Putt, M. S. Evaluation of a floss-holding device compared to hand-held floss for interproximal plaque, gingivitis, and patient acceptance. Journal of Clinical Preventive Dentistry 10:6, 1988.
48. Kresh, C. H. Finger-manipulated and floss-holder flossing: A comparison of the habit formation. General Dentistry 24:35, 1976.
49. Muhlemann, H. R. Psychological and chemical mediators of gingival health. Journal of Preventive Dentistry 4:6, 1977.
50. Walsh, M. M., et al. Use of gingival bleeding for reinforcement of oral home care behavior. Community Dental Oral Epidemiology 13:133, 1985.
51. Hallmon, W. W., et al. Flossing clefts: Clinical and histologic observations. Journal of Periodontology 57:501, 1986.
52. Carroll, G. C., and Sebor, R. J. Dental flossing and its relationship to transient bacteremia. Journal of Periodontology 59:691, 1980.
53. Mauriello, S. M., et al. Effectiveness of three interproximal cleaning devices. Clinical Preventive Dentistry 9:18, 1987.
54. Smith, B. A., et al: Effectiveness of four interproximal cleaning devices in plaque removal and gingival health. American Journal of Dentistry 1:57, 1988.
55. Smukler, H., et al. Interproximal tooth morphology and its effect on plaque removal. Quintessence International 20:249, 1989.
56. Wolffe, G. N. An evaluation of proximal cleansing agents. Journal of Clinical Periodontology 3:148, 1976.
57. Bouwsma, O., et al. Effect of personal oral hygiene on bleeding interdental gingiva: Histologic changes. Journal of Periodontology 59:80, 1980.
58. Caton, J., et al. Effects of personal oral hygiene and subgingival scaling on bleeding interdental gingiva. Journal of Periodontology 60:84, 1989.
59. Haffajee, A. D., et al. Clinical parameters as predictors of destructive periodontal disease activity. Journal of Clinical Periodontology 10:257, 1983.
60. Caton, J. Periodontal Diagnosis and Diagnostic Aids. Proceedings of the World Workshop in Clinical Periodontics 1:1, 1989.
61. Cantor, M. T., and Stahl, S. S. The effect of various interdental stimulators upon the keratinization of the interdental col. Periodontics 3:243, 1965.
62. Grant, D. A., et al. Periodontics, 6th ed. St. Louis: C. V. Mosby, 1988.
63. American Dental Association. Accepted Dental Therapeutics, Section on Dentifrices and Mouthwashes, 1982, Chicago, American Dental Association, pp. 369–378.
64. American Academy of Pediatrics, Committee on Drugs. Ethanol in liquid preparations intended for children. Pediatrics 73:405, 1984.
65. Wagner, M. J., et al. Sodium retention in mouthwashes. Journal of Clinical Preventive Dentistry 11:21, 1989.
66. American Academy of Periodontology, Research, Science, and Therapy Committee. Current Understanding of the Role of Microscopic Monitoring, Baking Soda, and Hydrogen Peroxide in the Treatment of Periodontal Disease. Chicago, American Academy of Periodontology, 1991.
67. American Academy of Periodontology, Research, Science, and Therapy Committee. Hydrogen Peroxide—Use or Abuse? Chicago, American Academy of Periodontology, 1991.
68. Ciancio, S. G. (ed.) Oral irrigation—a current perspective. Biological Therapies in Dentistry 3:33, 1988.
69. Ciancio, S. G. Effect of a chemotherapeutic agent delivered by an oral irrigation device on plaque, gingivitis, and subgingival microflora. Journal of Periodontology 60:310, 1989.
70. Flemming, T. F., et al. Chlorhexidine and irrigation in gingivitis. I. Six months of clinical observations. Journal of Periodontology 61:112, 1990.
71. Ciancio, S. G. (ed.). Powered oral irrigation and control of gingivitis. Biological Therapies in Dentistry 5:21, 1990
72. Cobb, C., et al. Ultrastructural examination of human periodontal pockets following the use of an oral irrigation device in vivo. Journal of Periodontology 59:155, 1988.
73. Eakle, W., et al. Depth of penetration in periodontal pockets with oral irrigation. Journal of Clinical Periodontology 13:39, 1986.
74. American Academy of Periodontology, Research, Science, and Therapy Committee. Chemical Agents for the Control of Plaque. Chicago, American Academy of Periodontology, 1991.
75. Ciancio, S. G. Pharmacology of oral antimicrobials. In The American Academy of Periodontology's Perspectives on Oral Antimicrobial Therapeutics. Littleton, MA: PSG Publishing Co., Inc., 1987, pp. 25–35.
76. Boyd, R. L., et al. Effects on gingivitis of two different 0.4% Sn F2 gels. Journal of Dental Research 67:2, 1987.
77. Tinanoff, N., et al. Clinical and microbiological effects of daily brushing with either NaF or SnF2 gels in subjects with fixed or removable dental prostheses. Journal of Clinical Periodontology 16:284, 1989.
78. Tinanoff, N., et al. Daily use of stannous fluoride gels reduces plaque and gingivitis in adults. Journal of Dental Research Vol. 67, Abstract No. 770, 1988.
79. Grossman, E., et al. A clinical comparison of antibacterial mouthrinses: Effects of chlorhexidine, phenolics, and sanguinarine on dental plaque and gingivitis. Journal of Periodontology 60:435, 1989.
80. Moran, J., et al. A clinical trial to assess the efficacy of sanguinarine-zinc mouthrinse (Viadent) compared with chlorhexidine mouthrinse (Corsodyl). Journal of Clinical Periodontology 15:612, 1988.
81. Quirynen, M., et al. Comparative antiplaque activity of sanguinarine and chlorhexidine in man. Journal of Periodontology 17:223, 1990.
82. Hannah, J. J., et al. Long-term clinical evaluation of toothpaste and oral rinse containing sanguinaria extract in control-

ling plaque, gingival inflammation, and sulcular bleeding during orthodontic treatment. American Journal of Orthodontic Dentofacial Orthopedics 96:199, 1989.
83. Harper, D. S., et al. Clinical efficacy of a dentifrice and oral rinse containing sanguinaria extract and zinc chloride during six months of use. Journal of Periodontology 61:352, 1990.
84. Harper, D. S., et al. Effect of six months use of a dentifrice and oral rinse containing sanguinaria extract and zinc chloride upon the microflora of the dental plaque and oral soft tissues. Journal of Periodontology 612:359, 1990.
85. Snyder, M. L. A simple colorimetric method for the estimation of relative numbers of lactobacilli in the saliva. Journal of Dental Research 19:349, 1940.
86. Sims, W. A modified Snyder test for caries activity in humans. Archives of Oral Biology 13:853, 1968.
87. Grainger, R. M., et al. Swab test for dental caries activity: An epidemiological study. Canadian Dental Association Journal 31:515, 1965.
88. Arnim, S. S., and Sweet, A. P. Acid production by mouth organisms: Use of methyl red for patient education. Dental Radiography and Photography 29:1, 1956.
89. Kohler, B., and Bratthall, D. Practical method to facilitate estimation of *Streptococcus mutans* levels in saliva. Journal of Clinical Microbiology 9:584, 1979.
90. Devore, L. R., and Dean, M. C. Strategies for oral health promotion, disease prevention and control. In Darby, M. L. (ed.). Mosby's Comprehensive Review of Dental Hygiene, 3rd ed. St. Louis: C. V. Mosby, 1994, pp. 478–517.
91. American Dental Hygienists' Association. Principles of Ethics, Association Policy Manual. Chicago: American Hygienists' Association, 1989.
92. American Academy of Periodontology, Research, Science, and Therapy Committee. Guidelines for Periodontal Therapy. Chicago: American Academy of Periodontology, 1992.
93. Weinstein, P., et al. Oral Self Care: Strategies for Preventive Dentistry. Seattle: University of Washington, 1991, pp. 121–145.
94. Fox, K. Motivating children for physical activity: Towards a healthier future. Journal of Physical Education, Recreation and Dance, Sept., 1991, p. 34.
95. American Academy of Periodontology, Research, Science, and Therapy Committee. Periodontal Diseases of Children and Adolescents. Chicago: American Academy of Periodontology, 1991.

17 Professional Mechanical Oral Hygiene Care for the Prevention and Control of Periodontal Diseases

OBJECTIVES

Mastery of the content in this chapter will enable the reader to:

- Define three categories of professional mechanical oral hygiene care and the objectives of, indicators for, and components of each category
- Define the key terms
- Explain the periodontal benefit associated with tooth polishing with a rubber cup
- Explain the periodontal benefit associated with therapeutic scaling and root planing
- Explain the role of the dental hygienist in the prevention and treatment of periodontal disease within the dental hygiene process of care

INTRODUCTION

Although clear microbial patterns for adult periodontitis have not been firmly established, shifts in the subgingival microflora to higher proportions of gram-negative facultative and anaerobic bacteria have been consistently associated with the disease.[1–5] As illustrated in Figure 17–1, gram-positive cocci and rods (aerobic bacteria) predominate in the subgingival microflora, or plaque, in periodontal health; but, in disease, motile rods and spirochetes (facultative and anaerobic bacteria) predominate. A major approach to the prevention and treatment of periodontal disease is to reverse this microbial shift and maintain a microflora consistent with periodontal health. Currently, frequent and thorough plaque removal performed personally and professionally is the only available method for maintaining a subgingival microflora associated with periodontal health,[6–9] and in the dental office it is the dental hygienist who plays the major role in providing such care.[10–12] In fact, the 1981 position paper prepared for the American Association of Public Health Dentistry by its Subcommittee on Preventive Periodontics reported that although "in the global scheme of preventive periodontics, the general dentist . . . is the *pivotal* element . . . it is the dental hygienist, of all those in the dental professional hierarchy, who is the *critical* element . . ."[13]

The dental hygienist's goals are to prevent the initiation of periodontal disease in healthy clients and to arrest the disease in clients who are already affected. Because dental hygiene care directly involves the periodontium, the dental hygienist is in an ideal position to collect data for the assessment of the periodontal tissues, recognize periodontal disease, collaborate with the dentist in planning care, present findings and recommended treatment options to the client, and participate in the provision of therapy for all levels of periodontal disease.

PROFESSIONAL MECHANICAL ORAL HYGIENE CARE

Professional mechanical oral hygiene care refers to the mechanical plaque control procedures that can be performed by the dental hygienist to prevent and control periodontal diseases. These procedures are often generally referred to as "a prophy," "having your teeth cleaned," or "scaling and root planing." The broad and interchangeable use of these general terms to refer to more than one type of professional mechanical oral hygiene procedure often causes ambiguity and confusion among clients and oral health professionals as to exactly what level of care is being referred to. To clarify the relative merits of the mechanical aspects of dental hygiene care devoted to the prevention and control of

HEALTH
Gram-positive (gr+) aerobes
(cocci, rods)
DISEASE
Gram-negative (gr−) facultative bacteria & anaerobes
(motile rods & spirochetes)

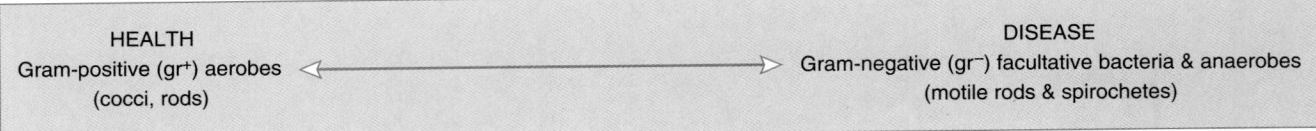

FIGURE 17–1
Bacterial composition of subgingival plaque in health and disease.

periodontal disease, the following three separate categories of professional care are delineated:

- The preventive oral prophylaxis
- Therapeutic periodontal scaling and root planing (also known as nonsurgical periodontal therapy)
- Professional periodontal maintenance care

These three categories of professional care share a number of features, particularly instrumentation of a tooth surface and establishment of an effective personal and professional oral hygiene program. However, the objective, rationale, and skill level required *differ* for each category of professional care (Table 17–1). Recognizing these differences is important for providing appropriate care to a client and for scheduling an appropriate amount of time for delivering the care.[14]

Preventive Oral Prophylaxis

As pointed out in Chapter 13, in gingivitis there is no apical migration of the junctional epithelium. But even though the junctional epithelium remains at the cementoenamel junction (CEJ), the gingival tissue becomes inflamed and edematous from the presence of bacterial plaque and its by-products. The enlarged gingival tissue forms gingival pseudopockets that are 4 to 5 mm deep (see Chapter 13, Figure 13–8).

Although calculus is not the cause of periodontal disease, it originates as persisting deposits of bacterial plaque that eventually mineralize. The rough, porous surface of the calculus retains plaque and can make even the most diligent and skillful personal oral hygiene effort ineffective. Consequently, the dental hygienist must scale calculus deposits from teeth because they interfere with plaque control. "Scaling is the instrumentation of the crown and root surfaces of the teeth to remove bacterial plaque, calculus, and (extrinsic) stain from these surfaces."[15]

The objective of the preventive oral prophylaxis, commonly thought of as a professional tooth cleaning, is to prevent the initiation of gingivitis or, failing that, the conversion of gingivitis to periodontitis. In addition, the preventive oral prophylaxis is performed for cosmetic reasons in clients who accumulate extrinsic stains on the surfaces of their teeth. The preventive oral prophylaxis consists of

- Periodontal and oral hygiene assessment
- Client instruction in personal oral hygiene procedures
- Supragingival and subgingival scaling, often followed by coronal or selective polishing, to remove acquired deposits from all tooth surfaces

Because the root surface is not exposed in a gingival pocket, root instrumentation is not performed. The scaling procedure, however, usually involves some inadvertent removal of the soft tissue lining of the sulcus and gingival pocket, but this should be minimal in a healthy periodontium. The scaling may be followed by a coronal polish to remove extrinsic stain and plaque; by an application of topical fluoride and sealants to prevent dental caries; and by margination and polishing of restorations to promote tissue health and longevity of restorations. In addition, an ultrasonic scaler to remove calculus, plaque and extrinsic stain, or an air-powder polishing unit to remove stain and plaque, also may be used.

TABLE 17–1
PROFESSIONAL MECHANICAL DENTAL HYGIENE CARE MODALITIES

	Preventive Oral Prophylaxis	**Therapeutic Scaling and Root Planing**	**Professional Periodontal Maintenance Care**
Objective	To prevent/control gingivitis	To treat periodontitis; to achieve connective tissue reattachment	To maintain attachment level and periodontal health in individuals who have been treated for periodontitis
Continued Care Interval	3–6 months or as needed	1 month evaluation; repeat as needed	3–4 months or as needed
Dental Hygiene Action*	Scaling to remove calculus, extrinsic stain, and bacterial plaque to promote a healthy oral environment	Scaling and root planing to eliminate microorganisms, endotoxins, rough cementum, and calculus to reduce inflammation, promote connective tissue regeneration, and make the root surface biologically acceptable to the gingival tissues	Closely monitors periodontal status, scaling, and root planing to prevent return of pathogenic subgingival microflora
Required Time	Usually one appointment	Several appointments (up to 8 hours) with use of a local anesthetic	One appointment

* Includes assessment of oral health behaviors and client education.

During the preventive oral prophylaxis, a topical anesthetic for pain control may be administered for clients with sensitive gingiva; however, administration of a local anesthetic is rarely indicated. The preventive oral prophylaxis procedure usually takes 45 to 60 minutes and a standard continued care (recall) interval is 3, 4, or 6 months, depending on the amount of calculus and extrinsic stain the client tends to form.

The preventive oral prophylaxis differs from the periodontal maintenance procedure (described later) in that it is *not* a formal phase of periodontal treatment and usually does not involve root planing. Rather, the preventive oral prophylaxis is the procedure used for maintaining an already healthy periodontium or for controlling gingivitis. Periodontal therapy (either surgical or nonsurgical) does not precede a preventive oral prophylaxis. The selection of this category of care is based upon the periodontal assessment data collected by the dental hygienist at the beginning of the appointment.

Findings from studies of clients with periodontitis who received an oral prophylaxis on a regular basis, but who had *not* been treated periodontally, either surgically or nonsurgically, indicate that such care had no significant effect on the gain of attachment despite the performance of some subgingival instrumentation.[16-19] Thus, the preventive oral prophylaxis is inappropriate periodontal care for clients with periodontitis. Rather, the preventive oral prophylaxis is strictly a preventive procedure, mainly involving supra- and subgingival instrumentation and the establishment of a personal oral hygiene program for the client. The preventive oral prophylaxis is indicated for clients who are periodontally healthy or who at most have gingivitis (see Indications for and Components of the Preventive Oral Prophylaxis chart).

Tooth Polishing

The Rubber Cup Polish

Periodontal Benefit. Tooth polishing is the mechanical removal of bacterial plaque and extrinsic stain from tooth surfaces and restorations. Tooth polishing is a finishing procedure designed to make a tooth free of plaque and stain. Historically, this was accomplished by the use of a motor-driven rotary rubber cup and prophylaxis paste.[15] The therapeutic periodontal benefit of rubber cup polishing performed after scaling has not been well defined. Although several studies have evaluated the contribution of tooth polishing to periodontal health, in most of them the procedure as studied was performed every 2 weeks for periods ranging from 6 months to 3 years, as part of an intensive oral hygiene program. In these studies the oral hygiene program also included reinforced instruction in oral hygiene, toothbrushing, interdental cleaning, and, usually, application of topical fluoride.[20-25] These additional oral hygiene measures make it difficult to distinguish the actual effect of rubber cup polishing on periodontal health.

In clients with gingivitis, Walsh and colleagues studied the periodontal benefit of a single rubber cup polishing procedure performed immediately after the scaling associated with the traditional professional preventive oral prophylaxis performed at 3-, 4-, or 6-month intervals.[26] A split-mouth design was used in that study in which teeth on one side of the mouth were polished and teeth on the other side were not. Immediately after a baseline examination in which clinical and microscopic parameters of periodontal health were assessed, all teeth were scaled without the use of a local anesthetic, and one side of the mouth was randomly selected for polishing. Six weeks later the subjects returned and the clinical and microscopic assessments were repeated. The selection of a 6-week interval as the time period for this study was based on the research of Mousques and colleagues, who demonstrated that a pathogenic microflora was reestablished in subgingival plaque 42 days after a single episode of scaling.[27]

Findings from this study indicated a statistically significant improvement in the clinical and microscopic assessments of periodontal status in subjects who received scaling; they did not indicate further significant improvement from addition of a rubber cup polish to the scaling procedure. Further investigation, however, is needed to determine with more certainty the periodontal benefit of tooth polishing with a rubber cup.

Client Preference. Little is known about the attitudes of clients toward rubber cup polishing as a component of a preventive oral prophylaxis. Schifter and colleagues surveyed dental school clients and determined that 48% of the sample objected to the idea of not having their teeth polished as part of their cleaning.[28] Cross and Carr surveyed private practice and dental school clients and found that most persons in both groups accepted **selective polishing** (i.e., polishing only teeth with extrinsic stain and visible plaque) when they were given a thorough explanation of its rationale before the procedures.[29] Walsh and colleagues surveyed 30 subjects after they had had all their teeth scaled, but only the teeth on one side of their mouths polished, to gain insight into their expectations about the procedures that should be included in a preventive oral prophylaxis.[30] Findings revealed that 83% of the respondents expected polishing as part of the procedure, and 17% did not. Fifty-three percent stated that they would feel dissatisfied or cheated if they paid for an oral prophylaxis and it did not include polishing. Fifty-seven percent of all subjects noticed some desirable difference on the polished side. These findings differ from those of Shifter and colleagues, who reported that less than one-half of surveyed dental school clients objected to the idea of not having their teeth polished in a professional dental cleaning.[28] The findings of

INDICATIONS FOR AND COMPONENTS OF THE PREVENTIVE ORAL PROPHYLAXIS

Indications

- Client has healthy periodontal tissues or gingivitis
- Client has no periodontal probing depths greater than 4 mm

Components

- Client education
- Supra- and subgingival scaling
- Tooth polishing (optional)
- Supportive therapy for comprehensive care (e.g., placement of pit and fissure sealants, athletic mouth protector construction, fluoride therapy)

Continued Care Interval

- 3, 4, or 6 months, depending on formation of calculus and bacterial plaque, or as needed

Walsh and colleagues also differ from those of Cross and Carr, who reported that only 20% of dental school clients and 4% of private practice clients objected to not having their teeth polished.[29] In the latter study, however, clients received either a traditional or a selective polishing procedure and were thoroughly instructed beforehand on the rationale for whichever treatment was given. On the other hand, in the study by Walsh and colleagues, subjects received traditional polishing on one side of their mouth and no polishing on the other.[30] No attempt was made to educate them about treatment benefit; subjects were merely informed that the researchers were evaluating whether polishing had any periodontal benefits. This leads to the conclusion that unless clients are educated as to why their teeth should not be polished, most may object to a deviation from the traditional rubber cup polishing procedure.

Air-Powder Abrasive Systems

See Chapter 18 and the section on air-powder abrasive systems in extrinsic stain removal.

Plaque Control Instruction

Educating clients on the significance of bacterial plaque and its relationship to the periodontal disease process is important during the preventive oral prophylaxis. Only if the client understands the link between plaque and disease and removes the bacteria routinely can periodontal health be maintained. Therefore, plaque control instruction must be included in the preventive oral prophylaxis to educate the client about the periodontal disease process, to identify areas of plaque accumulation and related signs of inflammation visible at that appointment, to demonstrate techniques for the removal of plaque, and to dispense special oral hygiene devices required for plaque removal. (See Chapter 16, Personal Mechanical Oral Hygiene Care.) When a client presents completely free from signs of inflammation, the dental hygienist and the client have achieved their potential for periodontal health maintenance.

Therapeutic Periodontal Scaling and Root Planing

In periodontitis, unlike gingivitis, the junctional epithelium migrates apically from the CEJ, resulting in connective tissue attachment loss, forming a periodontal pocket, and exposing the root surface to the oral environment (see Chapter 13, Figure 13–8). The purpose of therapeutic periodontal scaling and root planing is to treat periodontitis by establishing conditions conducive to reattachment of connective tissue and healing of the periodontal tissues. The objective for this category of professional mechanical oral hygiene care is to eliminate microorganisms, calculus, and other irritants on and within the tooth surface to reduce inflammation, promote connective tissue regeneration, and make the root surface biologically acceptable to the gingival tissues.[31] The fact that the objective is to achieve connective tissue reattachment makes this procedure therapeutic rather than preventive, and thus the procedure is also referred to as nonsurgical periodontal therapy.

A dental diagnosis of early-to-moderate periodontitis (see Chapter 13, Table 13–5) signals the need for treatment with therapeutic periodontal scaling and root planing. In these cases, the dental hygiene therapy may be considered a definitive nonsurgical periodontal therapeutic procedure if connective tissue reattachment to the root surface is achieved. Periodontal scaling and root planing also may be the treatment of choice for some clients with a dental diagnosis of moderate-to-advanced periodontitis for whom surgery is contraindicated (see Indications for and Components of Therapeutic Periodontal Scaling and Root Planing chart). In these cases the dental hygiene therapy is considered a nondefinitive, nonsurgical periodontal therapeutic procedure, with the expectation of some connective tissue reattachment. Finally, periodontal scaling and root planing may be used as a presurgical procedure to improve the health of the tissues in preparation for periodontal surgery. In this situation, the expectation is that after therapeutic scaling and root planing the tissues will be less acutely inflamed and thus more easily manipulated, less likely to bleed during the surgery, and more likely to heal rapidly afterward. Depending on the success of the presurgical dental hygiene therapy and the improved plaque control of the client, the surgery itself may be less complex.

Therapeutic periodontal scaling and root planing are performed after periodontal assessment, diagnosis, care planning, and case presentation in collaboration with the dentist and include plaque control instruction as well as scaling and root planing to remove plaque, calculus, and other irritants on and within the tooth surfaces. This nonsurgical therapeutic procedure generally involves subgingival instrumentation by quadrant with a local anesthetic for pain control. (Some complex cases require instrumentation by sextant and, hence, six appointments.) The procedure is technically demanding and extremely time-consuming,[32]

INDICATIONS FOR AND COMPONENTS OF THERAPEUTIC PERIODONTAL SCALING AND ROOT PLANING

Indications

- Client who has periodontitis-affected sites with 4- to 6-mm pockets
- Client who has pockets 6 mm or more and is scheduled for periodontal surgery (presurgical procedure)
- Client who declines surgery or who cannot undergo surgery for medical or psychological reasons

Components

- Client education
- Local anesthetic agent administration
- Supra- and subgingival scaling
- Root planing
- Soft tissue curettage (optional procedure to be performed **after** scaling and root planing)
- Subgingival irrigation with antimicrobial agent (optional)
- Interventions to control dentinal hypersensitivity (Table 17–3)

Continued Care Interval

- One-month evaluation (scaling and root planing repeated depending on the periodontal status of the client)
- Periodontal maintenance care every 3–4 months if health achieved at 1-month evaluation

usually requiring an experienced clinician 1 hour per quadrant to complete. Therefore, unlike the preventive oral prophylaxis previously described or the periodontal maintenance procedure (described later), nonsurgical periodontal therapy requires several appointments. Typically it is performed in four 1-hour appointments, when one quadrant at a time is treated, or in two 2-hour appointments, when one upper and one lower quadrant are treated in each visit. Often the clinician irrigates inflamed pockets with an antimicrobial agent to decrease pathogens and promote healing of the tissues following periodontal scaling and root planing. The dentist also may consider drug therapy for treating specific periodontal infections (Table 17–2).

The following postoperative instructions for therapeutic periodontal scaling and root planing should be discussed with the client and documented in the client's record:

- There may be some discomfort for a few days
- Prescribed medication for discomfort should be taken as directed on the container. If *not* given a prescription for pain control, take two Tylenol tablets every 4 hours as needed. If discomfort continues, call dentist.
- Expect some tooth sensitivity especially to cold temperatures
- Within 24 hours begin to remove plaque daily by brushing and interdental cleaning
- For the first 1 to 2 days avoid hot and spicy foods (aggravates "raw" tissues) and nuts and tiny seeds (pieces wedge into tissues), then pursue nutritional eating habits

Therapeutic periodontal scaling and root planing is followed by a 1-month evaluation of tissue response and plaque control effectiveness. Research findings indicate that surgical therapy and nonsurgical periodontal therapy (therapeutic periodontal scaling and root planing) are equally effective in treating certain types of adult periodontitis.[20]

Root Instrumentation

Root instrumentation is divided into two separate procedures: *scaling* and *root planing.* The objective of scaling is simply to remove acquired deposits. Root planing is an extension of scaling in which the objective, as the name suggests, is to create a clean, smooth, hard root surface. "Root planing is a definitive procedure designed to remove cementum or surface dentin that is rough, impregnated with calculus, or contaminated with toxins or micro-organisms." Also known as root detoxification, root planing is the critical component of nonsurgical periodontal therapy.[15]

The purposes of root planing are to:

- Ensure complete removal of all acquired deposits on the root surface (e.g., bacterial plaque, residual calculus)
- Create a smooth surface that will retard bacterial plaque formation because rough root surfaces serve as reservoirs for subgingival plaque
- Detoxify the root surface by removing altered or necrotic cementum and surface dentin that may harbor microorganisms and their toxins, which act as an irritant to the periodontal tissues
- Reduce gingival inflammation and promote connective tissue reattachment and healing of the periodontal tissues

Studies have indicated that after careful root planing the root surface can consist of either cementum or dentin. It has been reported that, in general, after root planing the root surface is dentin about 60% of the time, cementum

TABLE 17–2
DRUGS CONSIDERED FOR TREATING VARIOUS PERIODONTAL INFECTIONS

Bacterial Diagnosis	Dental Diagnosis	Drugs Used
Specific		
Anaerobic infection		
Spirochetes	Necrotizing ulcerative periodontitis	Tetracycline
* *Bacteroides gingivalis*	Juvenile periodontitis	Metronidazole
Bacteroides forsythus	Adult periodontitis	Clindamycin
* *Bacteroides intermedius*		Tetracycline
Fusobacterium nucleatum		Spiramycin
Eubacterium species		Penicillin
Microaerophilic infection		
* *Actinobacillus actinomycetemcomitans*	Localized juvenile periodontitis	Tetracycline
Eikenella corrodens	Juvenile periodontitis	
Wolinella recta	Adult periodontitis	Erythromycin
Facultative or aerobic infections		
Pseudomonas species	Refractory periodontitis	Use antibiotic sensitivity pattern to make choice
Proteus species	Periodontal abscess	Use antibiotic sensitivity pattern to make choice
Streptococcus faecalis		Nystatin
Candida		Amphotericin B
Nonspecific		
Plaque overgrowth	Gingivitis	Chlorhexidine

* Also commonly found in gingivitis.

Adapted from Loesche, W. J. Future directions in antiinfective therapy. In Genco, R. J., Goldman, H. M., and Cohen, D. W. (eds.). Contemporary Periodontics. St. Louis: C. V. Mosby, 1990, p. 671.

and dentin about 25% of the time, and cementum only about 15% of the time.[33] Cementum exposed to periodontal pockets contains endotoxins—substances that promote bone resorption and prevent gingival fibroblast attachment.[34-37] There is good scientific justification for removing toxic cementum in order to promote healing of soft tissue adjacent to the root surface. Because loss of cementum may uncover dentin and expose dentinal tubules and may stimulate nerve endings, interventions to control dentinal hypersensitivity are frequently indicated (Table 17–3).

Because nonsurgical periodontal therapy is performed in a closed environment, the clinician cannot directly view the roots while instrumenting them. Studies on extracted teeth have documented that thorough "blind" root planing is extremely difficult to perform.[32,36,38,39] In order to perform therapeutic scaling and root planing successfully in a closed environment, clinicians must rely on their tactile sensitivity and their knowledge of root morphology. Therefore, it is critical for the dental hygienist to develop a three-dimensional mental picture of the root morphology of the different types of teeth. Such mental visualization provides a road map for the clinician that contributes to successful root planing. Besides studying the roots of extracted teeth, an effective way of developing three-dimensional mental pictures of different types of roots is to observe periodontal surgery being performed on roots one personally has scaled and root planed.

Nonsurgical periodontal therapy is considered much more difficult to perform than scaling and root planing at the surgical site when the gingiva is reflected back and one can observe the root directly. In 1981, a panel report of a workshop under the auspices of the National Institute for Dental Research said, "Not only are scaling and root planing fundamental procedures in the treatment of periodontics, but they are among the most difficult techniques in all of clinical dentistry in which to develop a minimum level of proficiency."

Studies on Clinical Effects. Studies have shown that therapeutic scaling and root planing combined with an intensive maintenance program both decreases gingival inflammation and pocket depths and increases probing attachment level in moderate or deep pockets for a prolonged period.[20,25,40-47] Although some studies have indicated that plaque and calculus cannot be completely removed from deep periodontal pockets by subgingival scaling,[48,49] many more studies have documented that thorough scaling and root planing, with or without periodontal surgery, followed by frequent professional periodontal maintenance care with

TABLE 17–3
DESENSITIZING AGENTS

Self-Applied Desensitizing Agents	Active Ingredient	Method of Action	Method of Application
Denquel Sensitive Teeth Toothpaste*	Potassium nitrate	Exact mechanism of action unknown. Partial occlusion of dentinal tubules/desensitizing action on fine nerve fibers at dentinal pulp junction	Toothbrush
Mint Sensodyne Toothpaste*	Potassium nitrate	Same as Denquel toothpaste	Toothbrush
Sensodyne SC Toothpaste*	Strontium chloride	Calcium is displaced by strontium and strontium apatite complex is formed	Toothpaste
Protect Toothpaste*	Dibasic sodium citrate	Precipitation of dentinal or salivary proteins by polyglycoid	Toothbrush
Gel Kam*	0.4% Stannous fluoride	Occlusion of dentinal tubules with tin and fluoride particles	Toothbrush/custom tray/paint on
Professionally Applied Desensitizing Agents	**Active Ingredient**	**Method of Action**	**Method of Application**
Sodium fluoride paste*	33% NaF, 33% kaolin, 33% glycerin	Deposition of insoluble salts into dentinal tubules	Burnish into tooth surface for 1–5 minutes
Stannous fluoride solution or gel (e.g., Dentin Bloc)	0.717% Fluoride solution, NaF, SnF_2, hydrogen fluoride	Occlusion of dentinal tubules with tin and fluoride particles	Apply with cotton pellet for 1 minute, do not burnish
Protect Dentin Desensitizer	Potassium oxalate	Occlusion of dentinal tubules due to formation of calcium oxalate crystals	Isolate area, apply with cotton pellet, keep area wet for 2 minutes
Sensodyne Sealant Kit	6% Ferric oxalate	Occlusion of dentinal tubules due to formation of calcium oxalate crystals	Apply with brush tip applicator
Iontophoresis	2% NaF ion	Penetration of fluoride ion into dentinal tubules	Isolate area with cotton rolls/rubber dam, low voltage battery supplies (+) current to tooth. 2% NaF applied with brush applicator to complete the circuit

TABLE 17–3
DESENSITIZING AGENTS *Continued*

Professionally Applied Desensitizing Agents Seldom Used	Active Ingredient	Method of Action	Method of Application
Dibasic calcium phosphate	Dibasic calcium phosphate	Deposition of minerals into dentinal tubules	Burnish with porte polisher
Sodium silicofluoride	Sodium silicofluoride	Formation of calcium gel which provides an insulating barrier for the tooth/root surface	Saturated solution of 0.6% rubbed into area for 5 minutes
Formalin	Formalin 40%	Partial occlusion of dentinal tubules due to formation of a smear layer	Cotton-tip application followed by burnishing
Calcium hydroxide	Calcium hydroxide	Exact mechanism of action unknown. Blocks dentinal tubules/promotes formation of peritubular dentin	Burnish with porte polisher
Sodium silicofluoride/calcium hydroxide	Sodium silicofluoride/5% calcium hydroxide	Reduction in openings of dentinal tubules	2-step process: sodium silicofluoride is painted on and allowed to react for 2 minutes; 5% calcium hydroxide is painted on and allowed to stand for 1 minute.
Zinc chloride/potassium ferrocyanide	40% Zinc chloride/20% potassium ferrocyanide	Formation of smear layer as a result of burnishing action	2-step process: 40% zinc chloride rubbed into surface of teeth and allowed to remain for 1 minute, followed by application of 20% aqueous solution of potassium ferrocyanide vigorously rubbed into surface until an orange precipitate is formed.
Corticosteroids	N/A	Decrease of pulpal inflammation	Rub into sensitive area
Fluoride varnish	N/A	Surface sealing agent	Painted on during restorative procedure
Unfilled resins	N/A	Surface sealing agent	Restorative procedure
Acid etching and bonding	N/A	Surface sealing agent	Restorative procedure
Glass ionomer cement followed by bonding	N/A	Surface sealing agent	Restorative procedure
Lasers	N/A	Surface alteration	Restorative procedure

* ADA approved.
Prepared by Maureen E. Fannon, RDH, MS, Clinic Coordinator, Foothill Community College.

plaque control reinstruction and subgingival instrumentation arrest periodontal destruction for years.[20,25,40–46,50] These studies also indicated, however, that instrumentation of subgingival areas measuring less than 3 mm deep produced a permanent loss of attachment. Based on this finding, it is recommended that therapeutic periodontal scaling and root planing be directed only at areas with clinical signs of disease.[14]

In addition to supporting the clinical effectiveness of therapeutic scaling and root planing for the treatment of adult periodontitis, several studies have shown that these procedures produce a significantly higher proportion of coccoid cells and a lower proportion of motile rods and spirochetes in the subgingival flora, thus producing a microbial shift toward organisms associated with periodontal health. However, repopulation with organisms associated with periodontal disease has been reported to occur within as little as 1 month to as much as 6 months after thorough subgingival instrumentation.[50–53]

A study by Walsh and colleagues showed that therapeutic periodontal scaling and root planing significantly improved clinical signs of periodontal health and significantly altered the subgingival flora in periodontitis-affected persons.[53] These effects persisted throughout the 3-month study period. Figure 17–2 shows the clinical results of that study. At the baseline examination before treatment, the two groups showed no statistically significant differences in clinical variables. One month after treatment, however, the group treated with scaling and root planing showed significant reductions in all clinical indices. Plaque, bleeding tendency, probing depth, and attachment loss were all significantly less than in the untreated control group and significantly lower than they had been before treatment.

Microscopic results are shown in Figure 17–3. The control group showed no major changes in microscopic pattern throughout the study. However, in the scaling and root planing group, 1 month after treatment there was a significant increase in the proportion of cocci and nonmotile rods and a significant decrease in the proportion of motile rods and spirochetes. These changes were still evident at 3 months. Analysis of differences between groups at 3 months showed that values for the scaling and root planing

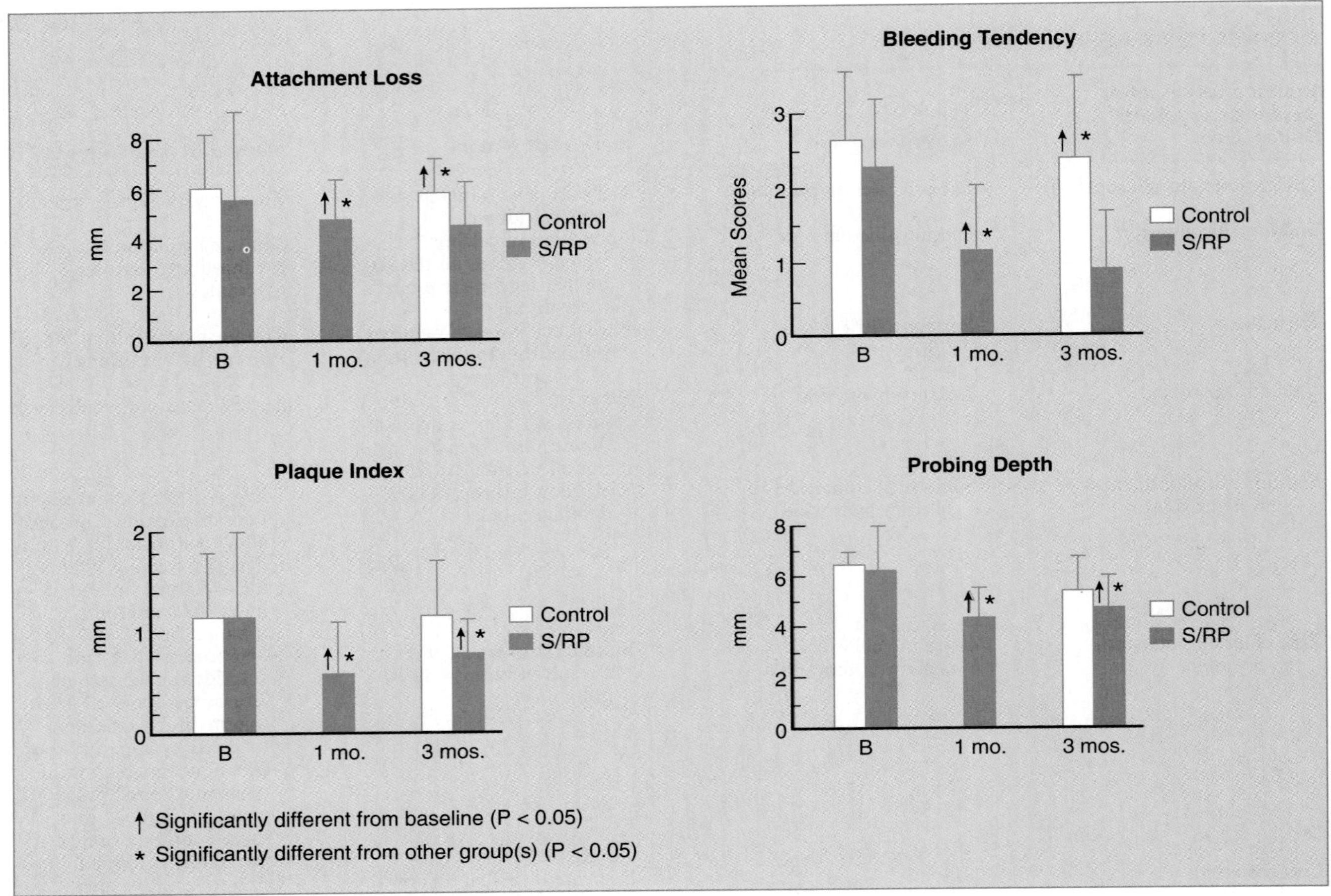

FIGURE 17–2
Clinical assessments of bacterial plaque, gingival bleeding, probing depths, and attachment loss at 1 and 3 months after scaling and root planing compared with a no-treatment control group. (Adapted from Walsh, M., Buchanan, S. A., Hoover, C. I., Newbrun, E., Taggart, E. J., Armitage, G. C., and Robertson, P. B. Clinical and microbiologic effects of single-dose metronidazole or scaling and root planing in treatment of adult periodontitis. Journal of Clinical Periodontology 13:151, 1986. © 1986 Munksgaard International Publishers Ltd., Copenhagen, Denmark.)

group for cocci, motile rods, and spirochetes (microflora associated with health) were significantly different from values for the control group.

For the bacteriological culture analysis shown in Figure 17–4, no significant changes in obligate anaerobes or black-pigmented *Bacteroides* (now classified in the genus *Porphyromonas*) occurred in the control group; however, in the scaling and root planing group 1 month after treatment the percentage of these organisms, which are associated with periodontal disease, was significantly lower than baseline values, and remained significantly lower at 3 months.

Thus, in addition to improving clinical signs of periodontal health, therapeutic scaling and root planing also alter the subgingival microflora in such a way as to cause a shift to the microorganisms associated with health. The inevitability of repopulation, however, requires regular and frequent subgingival instrumentation of teeth of susceptible persons. It is interesting that subgingival instrumentation does not appear to reduce the levels of *Actinobacillus actinomycetemcomitans,*[54–56] the pathogen associated with juvenile periodontitis. The reason for this is unclear but may be the result of the ability of the organism to invade gingival tissue.

Plaque Control Instruction

A bacterial plaque control program must be established and reinforced as an integral part of the therapeutic scaling and root planing procedure. Because bacterial plaque must be controlled daily to prevent gingivitis and periodontitis, the client must understand the cause-and-effect relationship between the retention of plaque and the presence of disease in the periodontium and his responsibility in long-term periodontal maintenance care. At each appointment, the plaque control instruction is based on the presence and location of disease, as well as on the amount and location of plaque and calcified deposits. At the beginning of therapy, the tissues may demonstrate a variety of architectural abnormalities, including edema, recession and pocketing, each requiring special oral hygiene devices that can reach the accumulated plaque. As therapeutic periodontal scaling and root planing progress and the tissues begin to respond, the gingival architecture changes to a healthier contour, and the periodontal pockets and attachment loss are reduced. This result then requires another change in the oral hygiene devices and techniques used by the client. Hence, plaque control is constantly being reeval-

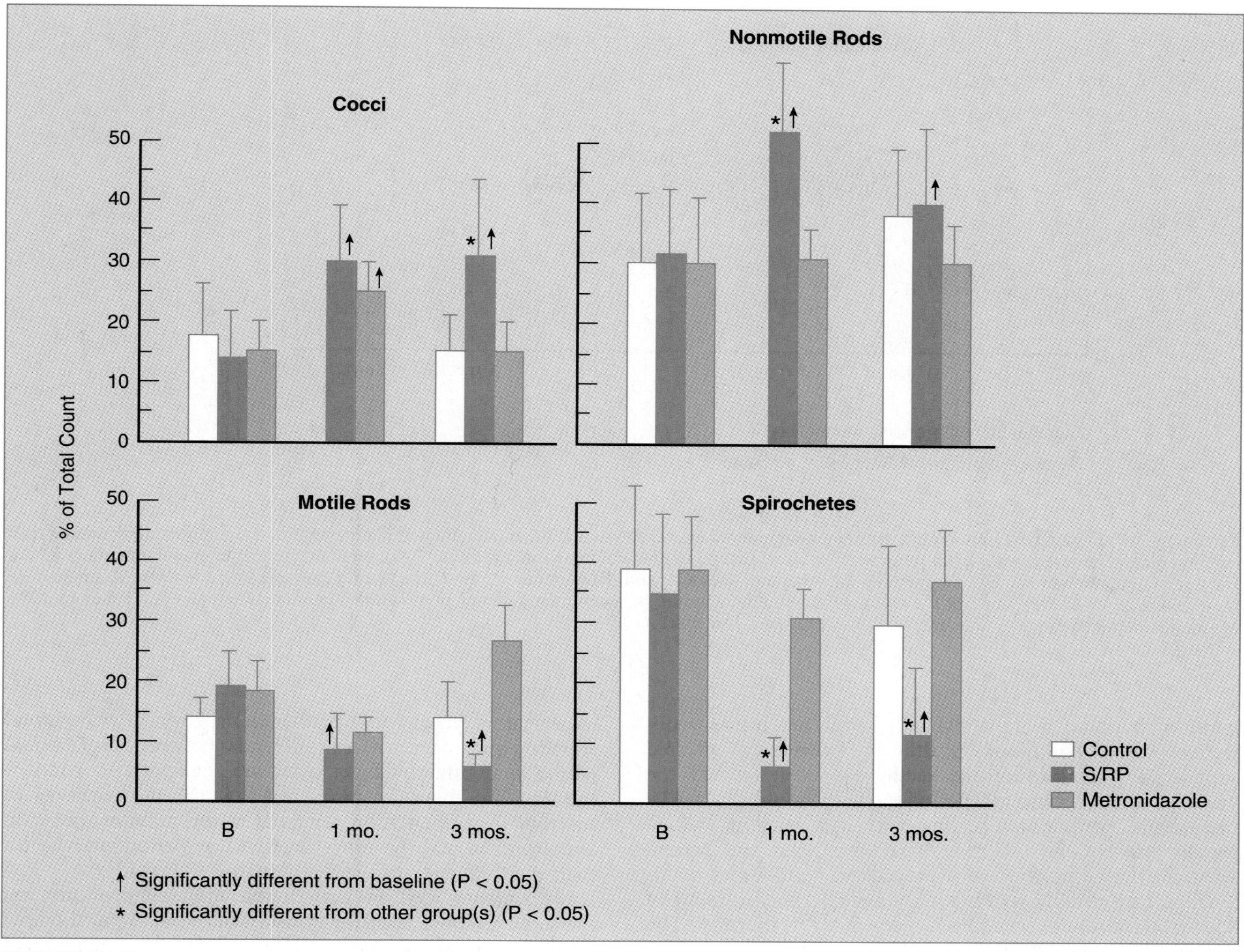

FIGURE 17–3
Microscopic patterns of subgingival plaque at 1 and 3 months after scaling and root planing compared with a no-treatment control group. (Adapted from Walsh, M., Buchanan, S. A., Hoover, C. I., Newbrun, E., Taggart, E. J., Armitage, G. C., and Robertson, P. B. Clinical and microbiologic effects of single-dose metronidazole or scaling and root planing in treatment of adult periodontitis. Journal of Clinical Periodontology 13:151, 1986. © 1986 Munksgaard International Publishers Ltd., Copenhagen, Denmark.)

uated and instructions revised based on the current assessed needs of the client.

The 1-Month Evaluation

The results of therapeutic periodontal scaling and root planing are evaluated approximately 1 month after the completion of therapy. At this appointment, a thorough periodontal examination is performed, with the results recorded as a benchmark to be used as a basis for comparison in later periodontal evaluations. The extent of tissue response determines whether the nonsurgical periodontal therapy has succeeded to the point where the client can enter the maintenance phase of care, or whether the client requires referral to a periodontist for surgical intervention. If the 1-month evaluation demonstrates a sufficient improvement, with a reduction in acute gingival inflammation, pocket depths, and attachment loss, an interval should be established for the client's first maintenance visit, usually 8 to 10 weeks after the 1-month evaluation. If the client presents at the 1-month evaluation with sites of acute gingival inflammation, it may indicate the presence of residual bits of calculus or root roughness, requiring immediate additional therapeutic scaling and root planing or further sessions of oral hygiene instruction to improve bacterial plaque control.

In the event that the findings at the 1-month evaluation visit indicate the need for referral to a specialist for surgical treatment and the client declines the recommendation, this refusal is to be documented in the client record and an informed refusal form signed by the client indicating that the consequences of nondefinitive treatment are understood. In an attempt to prevent further deterioration, a 2-month interval for professional periodontal maintenance care is recommended.

Professional Periodontal Maintenance Care

Once therapy—surgical or nonsurgical—is completed and a state of periodontal health has been established, the principal concern is to maintain periodontal health. This pro-

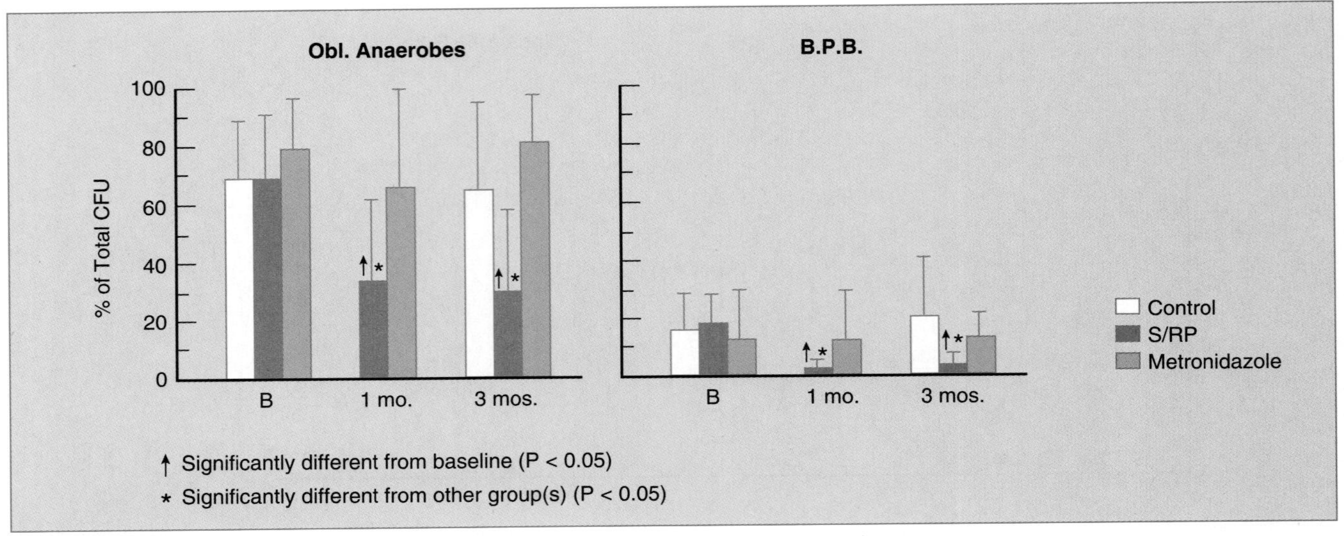

FIGURE 17–4
Percentage of obligate (obl.) anaerobes and black-pigmented bacteroides (B.P.B.) in subgingival plaque at 1 and 3 months after scaling and root planing compared with a no-treatment control group. (CFU, colony-forming units.) (Adapted from Walsh, M., Buchanan, S. A., Hoover, C. I., Newbrun, E., Taggart, E. J., Armitage, G. C., and Robertson, P. B. Clinical and microbiologic effects of single-dose metronidazole or scaling and root planing in treatment of adult periodontitis. Journal of Clinical Periodontology 13:151, 1986. © 1986 Munksgaard International Publishers Ltd., Copenhagen, Denmark.)

gram of periodic professional care, with the primary objective being continued health of previously affected supportive structures of the teeth, has been termed the "maintenance" phase of periodontal therapy.[57,58] Unlike therapeutic periodontal scaling and root planing, which usually involve the use of a local anesthetic and several visits for the completion of a procedure, periodontal maintenance care usually requires only a single appointment of 45 to 60 minutes, scheduled every 3 to 4 months. The periodontal maintenance appointment consists of periodontal assessment and documentation; evaluation of bacterial plaque control effectiveness and demonstration of techniques and devices to achieve improvement, if needed; supragingival and subgingival scaling; and possibly, selective tooth polishing with a rubber cup and interventions to manage dentinal hypersensitivity. The frequently repeated subgingival instrumentation serves to prevent reestablishment of the pathogenic subgingival flora initially responsible for the disease process. Within 1 to 3 years after the therapeutic scaling and root planing, periodic site-specific root planing may be required in locations showing acute inflammation or increasing pocket depth accompanied by root roughness. Sometimes the complete process of therapeutic scaling and root planing is repeated every 3 to 5 years, depending on the periodontal status of the client.

It has been demonstrated that periodontal therapy (surgical or nonsurgical) without periodontal maintenance is of little value for restoring periodontal health.[59] On the other hand, many studies indicate that the state of periodontal health resulting from thorough therapeutic scaling and root planing in the initial phase of periodontal treatment, with or without periodontal surgery, can be maintained provided that professional periodontal maintenance care is carried out every 3 months.[6,21,50,60–65] In addition, studies indicate that when periodontal maintenance was carried out every 3 months, client oral hygiene practices appeared to be a less critical factor in preventing loss of attachment.[60,62,65] Some investigators suggest that further destruction of periodontal support may occur if the intervals between professional periodontal maintenance care are extended beyond 4 months, but they also point out that the thoroughness of the root instrumentation rendered at the maintenance care appointment may be more decisive for periodontal health than the frequency of the maintenance interval.[33,66]

Instruments used in periodontal maintenance care are the same as those used for nonsurgical periodontal therapy. Topical or local anesthetic and agents for the treatment of dentinal hypersensitivity may or may not be used, depending upon the need for pain control.

The procedures used in periodontal maintenance care are:

- Scaling, to remove supra- and subgingival calculus and extrinsic stains
- Root planing, to prevent reestablishment of the pathogenic subgingival flora
- Selective tooth polishing, to remove extrinsic stain and bacterial plaque from the tooth surface
- Selective subgingival irrigation with antimicrobial agents

In addition, ultrasonic scalers to remove calculus and extrinsic stains also may be employed.

THE DENTAL HYGIENE PROCESS OF CARE IN THE PREVENTION AND TREATMENT OF PERIODONTAL DISEASE

Assessment

Chronic inflammatory periodontal disease often goes unrecognized by clients because the disease is slow and painless and without dramatic symptoms. Nevertheless, the disease often produces changes in gingival color, consistency, surface texture, contour, and size, and a bleeding response when the gingiva is disturbed by dental hygiene instrumentation, probing, flossing, brushing, or even eating. These visible signs of disease, which clients may ignore, are obvious to the educated eye and are easily assessed and documented by the dental hygienist on an ongoing basis. As part of this periodontal assessment, the dental hygienist routinely uses a periodontal probe to measure probing depth (the distance from the gingival margin to the base of the sulcus or pocket) and attachment loss (the distance from the CEJ to the base of the sulcus or pocket) (Fig. 17–5). The band of alveolar gingiva also is measured to determine adequacy of its width or the presence of a mucogingival concern. In addition, the dental hygienist tests for the presence of furcations and tooth mobilities and classifies and records all positive findings suggestive of past and current periodontal disease activity. (See Chapter 13: Periodontal and Oral Hygiene Assessment). When no signs of disease are evident, "WNL," indicating "within normal limits," should be recorded to document that an assessment was done and findings were within a healthy range.

Baseline data are collected and documented at the client's initial visit, allowing the dental hygienist to identify signs of the presence and extent of periodontal disease and to establish a basis for comparison with new findings at subsequent opportunities. Gingival inflammation, bleeding upon probing, and the presence of periodontal pockets and attachment loss are the most predictive signs of chronic inflammatory periodontal disease. Such data are factored into the dental hygienist's assessment of deficit in the client's need for integrity of the skin and mucous membranes of the head and neck.

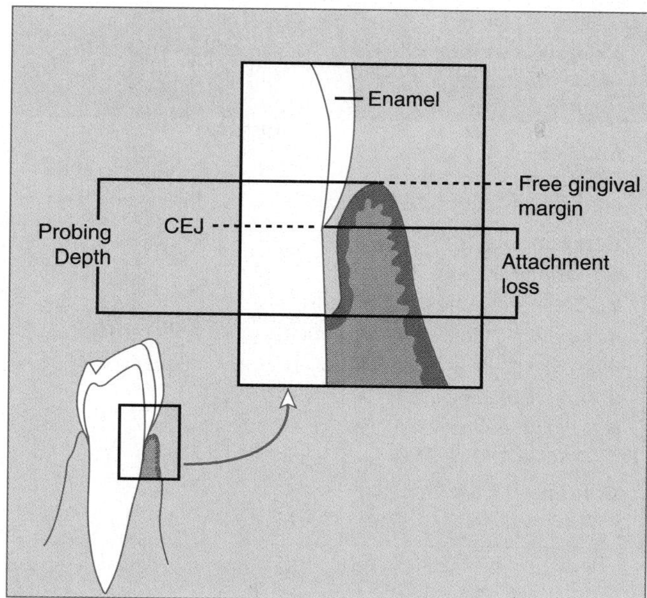

FIGURE 17–5
Shows attachment loss as the distance between the cementoenamel junction (CEJ) and the base of the pocket, and probing depth as the distance between the free gingival margin and the base of the pocket.

Dental Hygiene Diagnosis and Care Planning

After the assessment phase of care, the dental hygienist reviews the findings and collaborates with the dentist to establish a dental hygiene diagnosis and care plan. These phases of care are followed by the case presentation.

The case presentation is the first step in client education, and it is often the responsibility of the dental hygienist to assure that the client comprehends the findings and the recommendations as well as alternatives for care. The case presentation consists of:

- Presenting the findings of the examination
- Discussing the significance and consequences of these findings
- Offering options for care in the form of an initial care plan, as well as explaining other possible therapies
- Initiating an open discussion with the client to assure accurate perception of the client's needs, to affirm the client's understanding of and desire for treatment, and to establish agreement on the care plan between the client and the professional

During the case presentation it is imperative to stress that the client must assume responsibility for adhering to the recommended behaviors, cooperating in care, and obtaining lifelong periodontal maintenance care.

Implementing Care

Scaling, root planing, and tooth polishing are initiated when indicated to help meet the client's needs for oral mucous membrane integrity, a biologically sound dentition, and a wholesome body image. During the early stages of periodontal disease, treatment is simple and is within the scope of dental hygiene care. Even with a dental diagnosis of moderate periodontitis, the dental hygienist has a key role in therapy, either in preparing a tooth for surgery or perhaps in providing the total instrumentation to arrest the disease process. For example, for clients with early-to-moderate periodontal disease, the dental hygienist may be the primary therapist who educates the client and performs all the root instrumentation necessary to arrest and reverse the disease process. For clients with advanced periodontal conditions, the dental hygienist may provide the oral health education and all initial therapy in preparation for surgical reconstruction by the dentist or periodontist. In addition, all long-term follow-up periodontal care may be done under the direction of the dental hygienist, including periodic assessment, ongoing plaque control education, and frequent professional periodontal maintenance care.

Because bacterial plaque control is essential to the successful prevention and treatment of chronic inflammatory periodontal disease, periodontal care for virtually all clients coming to the oral health care setting includes plaque control education and some form of professional mechanical oral hygiene care; it is the dental hygienist who has the primary responsibility for providing that care[67] (see Indications for and Components of Professional Periodontal Maintenance Care chart).

Evaluation

Because periodontal disease may be both sporadic and site-specific, dental hygienists must continually monitor the periodontal status of their clients. Periodically, a complete periodontal examination and charting should be performed, and at each successive appointment changes from previous

INDICATIONS FOR AND COMPONENTS OF PROFESSIONAL PERIODONTAL MAINTENANCE CARE

Indications
Client has previously been treated for periodontitis and an acceptable state of periodontal health has been achieved

Components
- Client education
- Supra- and subgingival scaling
- Subgingival irrigation with antimicrobial agent (optional)
- Topical or local anesthetic agent may be needed
- Tooth polishing (optional)
- Supportive therapy for comprehensive care (e.g., fluoride therapy)

Continued Care Interval
Every 3 to 4 months or as needed

measurements should be recorded and communicated to the client.

Legal and Ethical Issues

It is essential that dental hygienists continuously and scrupulously monitor each client's periodontal status to identify changes in the health condition and to determine the appropriate level of care needed, whether it be preventive oral prophylaxis, therapeutic scaling and root planing, periodontal maintenance care, or referral to a periodontist. Such decisions should be made in collaboration with the dentist and should be based upon the current periodontal assessment findings, as compared with the previous records. In assessing whether a client has active periodontal disease, currently the most reliable standard to use is a change in attachment level. Additional signs used to assess periodontal disease activity are the presence of bleeding and acute gingival inflammation and an increase in probing depth. Complete and accurate documentation of the proceedings of each appointment and evidence to support less-than-adequate client cooperation are to be entered in the client record by the dental hygienist.

It is also the responsibility of the dental hygienist to inform the client of clinical findings at each visit. The client needs to understand the consequences of active and chronic periodontal disease and the expectations, goals, and limitations of all types of professional mechanical oral hygiene procedures. Furthermore, during initial and ongoing periodontal maintenance, the dental hygienist teaches the oral hygiene techniques necessary to remove plaque and motivates the client to assume responsibility for a successful oral hygiene regimen. Such clinician and client discussions and client level of understanding should be documented in the client record.

The dental hygienist has a valuable role in providing care for the prevention and control of periodontal diseases. For the client new to the practice, the dental hygienist introduces the concepts of periodontal health and disease; informs and educates the client as to his level of periodontal health and the location of disease; and, via dental hygiene instrumentation, treats active periodontal disease by performing all the initial procedures necessary to eliminate the etiological factors. For the client in ongoing care, the dental hygienist establishes a relationship of professional care in which all aspects of periodontal health are continually monitored. By making vigilant observations, keeping accurate and thorough records, communicating through an open dialogue with the client, and applying skill to the technically demanding procedures of scaling and root planing, the dental hygienist can successfully help the client to achieve and maintain the best periodontal health possible.

References

1. Socransky, S. S. Microbiology of periodontal disease—present status and future considerations. Journal of Periodontology 48:497, 1977.
2. Slots, J., Mashimo, P., Levine, M. J., and Genco, R. J. Periodontal therapy in humans. I. Microbiological and clinical effects of a single course of periodontal scaling and root planing, and of adjunctive tetracycline therapy and root planing. Journal of Periodontology 50:496, 1979.
3. Page, R. C., and Schroeder, H. E. Periodontitis in man and other animals: A comparative review. Basel: Karger, 1982 p. 330.
4. Savitt, E. D., and Socransky, S. S. Distribution of certain subgingival microbial species in selected periodontal conditions. Journal of Periodontal Research 19:111, 1984.
5. Slots, J., and Genco, R. J. Black-pigmented Bacteroides species, Capnocytophaga species, and Actinobacillus-actinomycetemcomitans in human periodontal disease: Virulence factors in colonization, survival, and tissue destruction. Journal of Dental Research 63:412, 1984.
6. Lindhe, J., and Nyman, S. Long-term maintenance of patients treated for advanced periodontal disease in adults. Journal of Clinical Periodontology 11:504, 1984.
7. Axelsson, P., and Lindhe, J. The effect of a plaque control program on gingivitis and dental caries and periodontal disease in adults. Journal of Clinical Periodontology 5:133, 1977.
8. Axelsson, P., and Lindhe, J. Effect of controlled oral hygiene procedures on caries and periodontal disease in adults. Journal of Clinical Periodontology 5:133, 1978.
9. Listgarten, M. A. Prevention of periodontal disease in the future. Journal of Clinical Periodontology 6:61, 1979.
10. Zaki, H., and Stallard, R. The role of the dental hygienist in preventive periodontics. Journal of Periodontology 42:233, 1971.
11. Friedman, L., and French, C. Survey of preventive practice by dental hygienists. Journal of Preventive Dentistry 2:10, 1974.
12. Reap, C. The hygienists' broad role in examination and counseling. Dental Survey Dec:10, 1976.
13. Periodontal disease in America: A personal and national tragedy. Position paper prepared for the American Association of Public Health Dentists by the AAPHD Subcommittee on Preventive Periodontics. Journal of Public Health Dentistry 43:106, 1983.
14. Walsh, M. M., and Robertson, P. B. Professional mechanical oral hygiene practices in the prevention and control of periodontal diseases. California Dental Association Journal 12:58, 1985.
15. American Academy of Periodontology. Consensus Report of the Committee on Periodontal Diagnosis and Diagnostic Aids, 1989.
16. Suomi, J. D., Greene, J. C., et al. The effect of controlled oral hygiene procedures on the progression of periodontal disease in adults: Results after third and final year. Journal of Periodontology 42:152, 1971.
17. Zamet, J. S. A comparative clinical study of three periodontal surgical techniques. Journal of Clinical Periodontology 2:87, 1975.
18. Waite, I. M. A comparison between conventional gingivectomy and non-surgical regime in the treatment of periodontitis. Journal of Clinical Periodontology 3:173, 1976.
19. Ciancio, S. G., Slots, J., et al. The effect of short-term admin-

istration of minocycline HCL on gingival inflammation and subgingival microflora. Journal of Periodontology 53:557, 1982.

20. Lindhe, J., Westfelt, E., Nymans, S., Socransky, S. S., Heijl, L., and Bratthall, G. Healing following surgical/nonsurgical treatment of periodontal disease. A clinical study. Journal of Clinical Periodontology 9:115, 1982.
21. Nyman, S., Rosling, B., and Lindhe, J. Effect of professional tooth cleaning after periodontal surgery. Journal of Clinical Periodontology 2:80, 1975.
22. Axelsson, P., and Lindhe, J. (1974) The effect of a preventive program on dental plaque, gingivitis and caries in school children. Results after one and two years. Journal of Clinical Periodontology 3:126, 1974.
23. Rosling, B., Nyman, S., and Lindhe, J. The effect of systematic plaque control on bone regeneration in infrabony pockets. Journal of Clinical Periodontology 3:38, 1976a.
24. Rosling, B., Nyman, S., Lindhe, J., and Jern, B. The healing potential of the periodontal tissues following different techniques of periodontal surgery in plaque-free dentitions. A 2-year clinical study. Journal of Clinical Periodontology 3:233, 1976b.
25. Morrison, E. C., Ramfjord, S. P., and Hill, R. W. Short-term effects of initial, non-surgical periodontal treatment (hygienic phase). Journal of Clinical Periodontology 7:199, 1980.
26. Walsh, M. M., Heckman, B. H., Moreau-Dittinger, R., and Buchanan, S. A. Effects of a rubber cup polish after scaling. Journal of Dental Hygiene November:494, 1985a.
27. Mousques, T., Listgarten, M. A., and Stoller, N. H. Effect of sampling on the composition of the human subgingival microbial flora. Journal of Periodontal Research 15:137, 1980.
28. Schifter, C. C., Hangorsky, C. A., and Emling, R. C. A philosophy of selective polishing. RDH, March/April 1:34, 1981.
29. Cross, G. N., and Carr, E. H. Patients' acceptance of selective polishing. Dental Hygiene 57(12):20, 1983.
30. Walsh, M. M., Heckman, B. H., and Moreau-Dittinger, R. Polished and unpolished teeth. Patient response after an oral prophylaxis. Journal of Dental Hygiene July:306, 1985b.
31. Ramfjord, S. P. Root planing and curettage. International Dental Journal 30:23, 1980.
32. Frandsen, A. Mechanical oral hygiene practices. In the state-of-the-science papers of the Dental Plaque Control Measures and Oral Hygiene Practices workshop. Bethesda, MD, February, 1985, pp. 26–28, 109–149.
33. Armitage, G. C. Biologic Basis of Periodontal Disease. Berkeley, California: Praxis Publishing Company, 1980.
34. Jones, W. A., and O'Leary, T. J. The effectiveness of *in vitro* root planing in removing bacterial endotoxin from the roots of periodontally involved teeth. Journal of Periodontology, 49:337, 1978.
35. Patters, M. R., Landesberg, R. L., et al. Bacteroides gingivalis antigens and bone resorbing activity in root surface fractions of periodontally involved teeth. Journal of Periodontal Research 17:122, 1982.
36. O'Leary, T. J., and Kafrawy, A. H. Total cementum removal: A realistic objective? Journal of Periodontology 54:221, 1983.
37. Cogen, R. B., Garrison, D. C., and Weatherford, T. W. Effect of various root surface treatments on the attachment and growth of human gingival fibroblasts: Histologic and scanning electron microscopic evaluation. Journal of Clinical Periodontology 11:531, 1984.
38. Van Volkinburg, J. S., Green, E., and Armitage, G. C. The nature of root surfaces after curette, and cavitron and alphasonic instrumentation. Journal of Periodontal Research 11:374, 1976.
39. Eaton, E. A., Kieser, J. B., and Davies, R. M. The removal of root surfaces deposits. Journal of Clinical Periodontology 12:141, 1985.
40. Hughes, T. P., and Caffesse, R. G. Gingival changes following scaling, root planing and oral hygiene. A biometric evaluation. J Periodontology 49:245, 1978.
41. Proye, M., Caton, J., and Polson, A. Initial healing of periodontal pockets after a single episode of root planing monitored by controlled probing forces. Journal of Periodontology 53:296, 1982.
42. Hill, R. W., Ramfjord, S. P., et al. Four types of periodontal treatment compared over the two years. Journal of Periodontology 52:655, 1981.
43. Cercek, J. F., Kiger, R. D., et al. Relative effects of plaque control and instrumentation on the clinical parameters of human periodontal disease. Journal of Clinical Periodontology 10:46, 1983.
44. Pihlstrom, B. L., McHugh, R. B., Oliphant, T. H., and Ortiz-Campos, C. Comparison of surgical and non-surgical treatment of periodontal disease. A review of current studies and additional results after 6–1/2 years. Journal of Clinical Periodontology 10:524, 1983.
45. Knowles, J., Burgett, F., et al. Comparison of results following three modalities of periodontal therapy related to tooth type and initial pocket depth. Journal of Clinical Periodontology 7:32, 1980.
46. Badersten, A., Nilveus, R., and Egelberg, J. Effect of non-surgical periodontal therapy. I: Moderately advanced periodontitis. Journal of Clinical Periodontology 8:57, 1981.
47. Waerhaug, J. Healing of the dentoepithelial junction following subgingival plaque control. I. As observed in human biopsy material. Journal of Periodontology 49:1, 1978.
48. Rabbani, G. M., Ash, M. M., and Caffesse, R. G. The effectiveness of subgingival scaling and root planing in calculus removal. Journal of Periodontology 52:119, 1981.
49. Badersten, A., Nilveus, R., and Egelberg, J. Effect of non-surgical periodontal therapy. II. Severely advanced periodontitis. Journal of Clinical Periodontology 11:504, 1984.
50. Axelsson, P., Lindhe, J. Effect of controlled oral hygiene procedures on caries and periodontal disease in adults. Results after 7 years. Journal of Clinical Periodontology 8:239, 1981.
51. Listgarten, M. A., and Hellden, L. Relative distribution of bacteria at clinically healthy and periodontally diseased sites in humans. Journal of Clinical Periodontology 5:115, 1978a.
52. Listgarten, M. A., Lindhe, J., and Hellden, L. Effect of tetracycline and/or scaling on human periodontal disease. Clinical microbiological and histological observations. Journal of Clinical Periodontology 5:246, 1978b.
53. Walsh, M., Buchanan, S. A., et al. Clinical and microbiologic effects of single-dose metronidazole or scaling and root planing in treatment of adult periodontitis. Journal of Clinical Periodontology 13:151, 1986.
54. Kornman, K. S., and Robertson, P. B. Clinical and microbiological evaluation of therapy for juvenile periodontitis. Journal of Periodontology 56:(8)443, 1985.
55. Renvert, S., Wikstrom, M., Dahlen, G., Slots, J., and Egelberg, J. Effect of root débridement on the elimination of *Actinobacillus actinomycetemcomitans* and *Bacteroides gingivalis* from periodontal pockets. Journal of Clinical Periodontology 17(6):345, 1990.
56. Renvert, S., Wikstrom, M., Dahlen, G., Slots, J., and Egelberg, J. On the inability of root débridement and periodontal surgery to eliminate *Actinobacillus actinomycetemcomitans* from periodontal pockets. Journal of Clinical Periodontology 17(6):351, 1990.
57. Parr, R., Pipe, P., and Watts, T. Periodontal Maintenance Therapy. Berkeley, CA: Praxis, 1982.
58. Shick, R. A. Maintenance phase of periodontal therapy. Journal of Periodontology 52:576, 1981.
59. Becker, W., Berg, L., and Becker, B. E. Untreated periodontal disease: A longitudinal study. Journal of Periodontology 50:234, 1979.
60. Pihlstrom, B. L., Ortiz-Campos, C., and McHugh, R. B. A randomized four-year study of periodontal therapy. Journal of Periodontology 52:227, 1981.
61. Yukna, R. A., and Williams, J. E. Five year evaluation of the excisional new attachment procedure. Journal of Periodontology 51:382, 1980.
62. Knowles, J. W., Burgett, F. G., et al. Results of periodontal treatment related to pocket depth and attachment level. Journal of Periodontology 50:225, 1979.
63. Ramfjord, S. P. Morrison, E. C., et al. Oral hygiene and maintenance of periodontal support. Journal of Periodontology 53:26, 1982.
64. Garrett, J. S. Effects of non-surgical periodontal therapy on

periodontitis in humans. Journal of Clinical Periodontology 10:515, 1983.

65. Westfelt, E., Nyman, S., Socransky, S., and Lindhe, J. Significance of frequency of professional tooth cleaning for healing following periodontal surgery. Journal of Clinical Periodontology 10:448, 1983.
66. Lindhe, J., Westfelt, E., et al. Healing following surgical/non-surgical treatment of periodontal disease. A clinical study. Journal of Clinical Periodontology 9:115, 1984.
67. Parr, R. W., Watts, T., et al. Subgingival Scaling and Root Planing. University of California at San Francisco, 1976.

Suggested Readings

Haffajee, A. D., Socransky, S. S., and Goodson, M. M. Comparison of different data analyses for detecting changes in attachment level. Journal of Clinical Periodontology 10:298, 1983.

Kornman, K. The microbiologic etiology of periodontal disease. Compendium of Continuing Education in Dentistry 7[Suppl.]: 173, 1986.

Listgarten, M. A. Structure of the microbial flora associated with periodontal health and disease in man. Journal of Periodontology 47:1, 1976.

Loe, H., and Silness, J. Periodontology disease in pregnancy. I. Prevalence and severity. Acta Odontologica Scandinavica 21:533, 1963.

Loe, H., Theilade, E., and Jensen, S. B. Experimental gingivitis in man. Journal of Periodontology 36:177, 1965.

Loesche, W. J. Clinical and microbiological aspects of chemotherapeutic agents used according to the specific plaque hypothesis. Journal of Dental Research 58:2404, 1979.

Loesche, W. J., Syed, S. A., et al. Treatment of periodontal infections due to anaerobic bacteria with short-term treatment with metronidazole. Journal of Clinical Periodontology 8:29, 1981.

Morrison, E. C., Lang, N., Loe, H., and Ramfjord, S. Effects of repeated scaling and root planing and/or controlled oral hygiene on the periodontal attachment level and pocket depth in beagle dogs. I. Clinical findings. Journal of Periodontal Research 14:428, 1979.

Parr, R., Pipe, P., and Watts, T. Periodontal Maintenance Therapy. Berkeley, CA: Praxis, 1982.

Silness, J., and Loe, H. Periodontal disease in pregnancy. II. Correlation between oral hygiene and periodontal condition. Acta Odontologica Scandinavica 22:121, 1964.

University of California School of Dentistry, San Francisco (UCSF) Department of Periodontology. Recognizing Periodontal Disease. Berkeley, CA: Praxis, 1978.

18 Instrumentation Theory for Professional Mechanical Oral Hygiene Care

OBJECTIVES

Mastery of the content in this chapter will enable the reader to:

- Define the key terms used
- Differentiate between food debris, materia alba, bacterial plaque, supra- and subgingival calculus
- Describe the formation of supragingival and subgingival calculus
- List and describe the essential components of the dental unit
- List and describe the essential components of the dental chair
- Describe ways to reduce aerosol contamination when using the three-way syringe
- List and describe the assessment instruments used by the dental hygienist during periodontal instrumentation
- List and describe the working instruments used by the dental hygienist during periodontal instrumentation
- Discuss variations found in instrument handles regarding size, shape, and pattern
- Discuss variations found in instrument shank length, curvature, and flexibility
- Describe a proper grasp for working instrumentation
- Discuss the importance of proper instrument blade adaptation and angulation
- Discuss the major criticisms of using extraoral fulcrums
- List the steps in customizing fulcrum placement for a tooth surface
- Describe indications for using finger flexing movements during scaling procedures
- Discuss the advantages and disadvantages of sharp instruments
- List the four basic functions of the dental mouth mirror
- Explain the advantages and disadvantages of the front-surface, concave-surface, and flat-surface mouth mirror
- List and describe the uses of the periodontal probe
- Describe the technique for reading a periodontal probe
- List and describe the uses of the dental explorer
- Describe how the design of the sickle scaler impedes its use in subgingival instrumentation
- Illustrate the difference between the universal curet and the Gracey curet design in terms of blade-to-shank angulation
- Describe the limitations of the hoe, file, and chisel scalers
- Discuss the primary use and limitations of ultrasonic scalers
- Compare different extrinsic stain removal techniques in terms of efficiency, client comfort, and operator safety
- Discuss the theory about cumulative trauma disorders and periodontal instrumentation
- Discuss symptoms of carpal tunnel syndrome, its causes and treatment
- Demonstrate flexion and hyperextension of the wrist
- Discuss operator positioning that could be incorporated into "protective" scaling strategies for the dental hygienist
- List the various intraoral and extraoral fulcrums used during periodontal instrumentation
- Explain the concept of reinforcement scaling and its relationship to instrument control, fulcrum placement, and "protective" scaling
- List the various reinforcement scaling techniques used during periodontal instrumentation

A prerequisite for successful assessment and treatment of periodontal disease is the dental hygienist's understanding and application of professional mechanical oral hygiene instrumentation. Such instrumentation is the cornerstone of clinical dental hygiene care and comprises a large and complex set of skills that require exquisite manual dexterity, patience, fortitude, and a keen understanding of the potential and limitations of all the various dental hygiene instruments available today. This chapter presents instrumentation theory associated with clinical dental hygiene care. It begins by discussing the various acquired deposits found in the oral cavity. It then focuses on principles of optimal instrumentation, including (1) the use of the dental unit, chair, and operator stool; (2) the use of **assessment instruments** such as the periodontal probe to measure pocket depth and attachment loss or the explorer to detect tooth irregularities and acquired deposits; (3) the use of **treatment instruments,** such as scalers and curets, to remove acquired deposits from the tooth and to smooth and detoxify the root surface; and (4) the use of polishing instruments to remove bacterial plaque and extrinsic stain.

Practice and experimentation with a variety of instruments applied to mannequins and to persons exhibiting variable amounts and types of calculus and disease states are requisite to mastering instrumentation skills. In addition to the importance of mastery of hand skills, operator safety also is a significant issue. In this chapter, the common uses of dental hygiene equipment and instruments are evaluated for their possible secondary effects on operator safety and injury. When indicated, instrumentation techniques with protective mechanisms for the prevention of operator injury are presented.

Integration of the technical aspects of dental hygiene instrumentation, with knowledge of oral biology, tooth morphology, periodontics, and dental hygiene is crucial for the provision of optimal oral healthcare. With this integration, the ability to provide clinical dental hygiene care associated with the management of hard and soft tissues is comprehensive enough to meet the challenge of contemporary professional dental hygiene practice (Fig. 18-1).

ACQUIRED DEPOSITS AND METHODS FOR REMOVAL

Food Debris

Food debris is readily visible in interproximal areas and may be impacted into tissue or sulcular areas where there are open contacts. Food debris identification and removal with periodontal instruments is a relatively easy task performed simply by lifting the food out and wiping or rinsing it away.

Materia Alba

Materia alba is a soft, loose layer of cellular and broken down food debris (Fig. 18-2). Characteristically, it is white to yellowish-white in color, thicker interproximally and at the gingival margin than on the middle and incisal thirds of

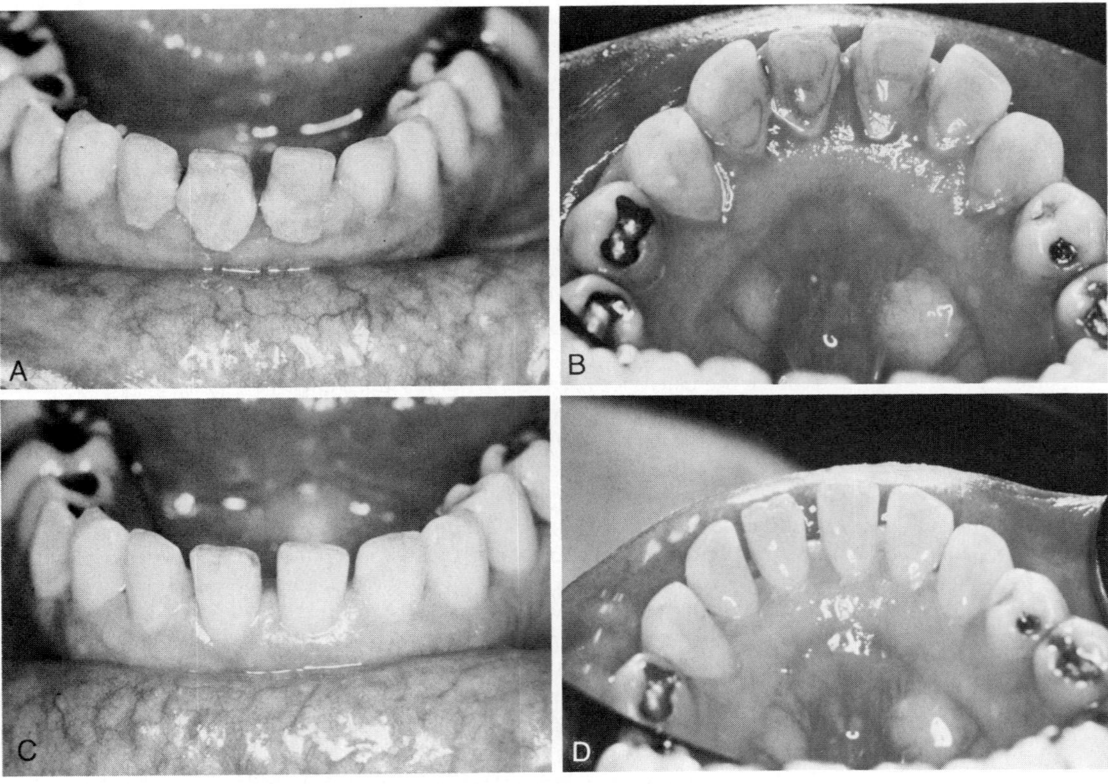

FIGURE 18-1
A and *B*, Severe inflammation. *C* and *D*, Significant reduction of inflammation following therapeutic scaling and root planing.

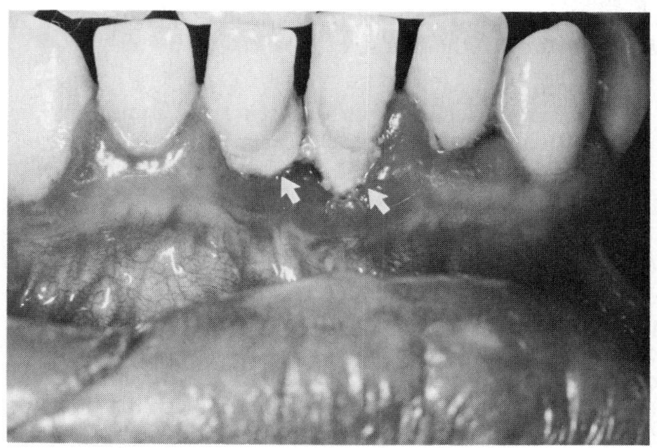

FIGURE 18–2
Materia alba on supragingival calculus.

the crown and, when longstanding, appears bubbly in texture. Others have described its cottage cheese–like appearance.[1] Materia alba is removed with various professional and self-polishing techniques. Where the rubber cup or porte polisher is inaccessible, scaling instruments or even well-adapted dental floss and toothbrushing can remove materia alba.

Acquired Pellicle

The **acquired pellicle** is a thin, clear, unstructured organic membrane that forms over exposed tooth surfaces and restorations within minutes after removal by professional and self-polishing techniques. It is composed from glycoproteins from saliva and gingival sulcus fluid and can become stained with disclosing solution or other extrinsic stain. In coating dental structures, it possibly provides a barrier against acid attack; however, it does provide a nidus for the formation of bacterial plaque and later calculus formation.

Bacterial Plaque

Bacterial plaque is a dense, organized matrix of microorganisms and the cause of dental caries and periodontal diseases (Fig. 18–3). Plaque forms on the surface of the acquired pellicle and on hard and soft surfaces in the oral cavity. The microbial composition of dental plaque differs greatly depending on the age of the plaque, its location on supragingival and subgingival surfaces, and its association with health or disease. Mature plaque is easily recognized during assessment procedures with a periodontal probe or an explorer. Materia alba is material loosely adherent to the tooth surface and should not be mistaken for the firmly adherent bacterial plaque. Materia alba can be removed by vigorous rinsing (water irrigation methods), scaling, and polishing. Bacterial plaque is removed by thorough home care procedures, scaling, and polishing. See Chapters 13 and 16 for a detailed discussion of bacterial plaque.

Calculus

Dental calculus is mineralized bacterial plaque. Classified by its location, supragingival calculus is located above the gingival margin and subgingival calculus is located below the gingival margin (Fig. 18–4). The presence of calculus provides a nidus for new pellicle, bacterial plaque, and additional calculus to form. Thus begins a cycle of supragingival and subgingival deposit accumulation, eventual periodontal soft tissue inflammation, cemental alteration, and progressive periodontal disease. It is important for the dental hygienist to understand the basic differences in formation and attachment of supragingival and subgingival calculus to interpret the significant clinical differences observed during periodontal instrumentation.

Supragingival Calculus

Supragingival bacterial plaque finds its mineral source for calculus formation in the saliva. Most often the sites closest to the salivary gland ducts accumulate the heaviest supragingival calculus deposits. The facial surfaces of maxillary posterior teeth and the mandibular anterior lingual surfaces are therefore commonly affected by supragingival calculus accumulation. **Supragingival calculus** can attach to any hard surface including enamel, restorative materials, prosthetic appliances, or exposed cementum. However, supragingival calculus attaches differently to enamel and restorative surfaces than it does to cementum. Attachment to supragingival enamel and restorative surfaces is by means of the acquired pellicle, which is a very weak mode of

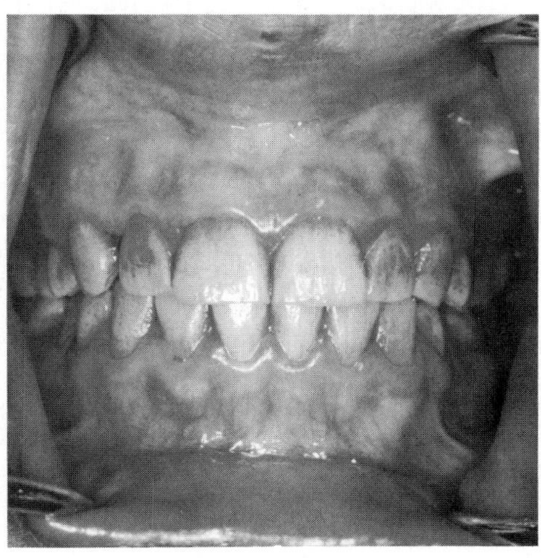

FIGURE 18–3
Bacterial plaque.

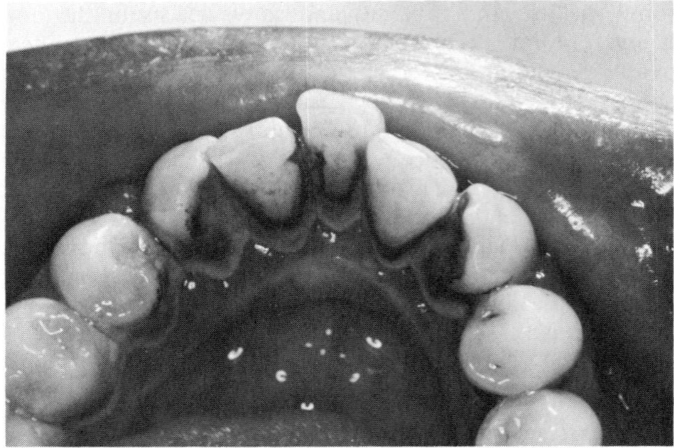

FIGURE 18-4
Supragingival and subgingival calculus and stain.

attachment. There is no actual penetration of the calculus into enamel surfaces. Calculus attached to the exposed roots of teeth in areas of recession, however, actually penetrates the root surfaces. Because of the different modes of attachment between calculus on enamal and cemental surfaces, the dental hygienist usually finds that supragingival calculus on enamel is easier to remove than supragingival calculus on root surfaces.

When supragingival calculus on enamel is difficult to remove, it is usually the result of crown anatomy in which the calculus has formed in narrow fissures or depressions making it less accessible to the curet, sickle scaler, or other scaling instrument. Malalignment of the teeth also makes access difficult for supragingival interproximal areas.

When supragingival calculus formation is light, it is not readily visible because the wetting action of saliva causes it to blend into the color of the tooth surface. Drying the tooth surface with air from the air-water syringe turns calculus a chalky white and enhances its visibility. Another method used to help identify the presence of supragingival calculus is *transillumination.* Transillumination, a method in which light is shined through the teeth, also may reveal dark, opaque areas of calculus. The presence of calculus may be confirmed by tactile sensation derived from using an explorer to detect rough tooth surfaces. If the rough surface does not change even after scaling instrumentation, the presence of hypocalcification, fluorosis, or decalcification of the tooth surface should be considered.

The appearance of heavy supragingival calculus may range from a smooth flat surface to a very rough, irregular surface depending on the client's oral hygiene behaviors, alignment of the dentition, and action of tongue, buccal mucosa, and lips. Heavy calculus may resemble the tooth in color or may be stained by food or tobacco products. This type of calculus is fairly easy to detect.

Subgingival Calculus

Subgingival bacterial plaque finds its mineral source for calculus formation from the gingival sulcus fluid and inflammatory exudate. Therefore, subgingival calculus may be found in almost any area of the mouth especially where gingival inflammation or periodontal disease already exists. Most often these are areas such as the interproximal and lingual tooth surfaces that are difficult to reach by the client. **Subgingival calculus** may attach to cementum or dentin by any of the following means:

- An acquired pellicle
- Mechanical locking into undercuts and minute irregularities in the tooth surface
- Direct contact between calcified intercellular matrix and the tooth surface[2]

Subgingival calculus removal becomes more difficult when it is attached by means other than the acquired pellicle. It requires technical ability, knowledge of root morphology, and analytical skills to differentiate subgingival calculus from tooth structure. As the gingival tissue becomes more inflamed, decreased visibility from bleeding may make subgingival exploration and scaling difficult. Continuous use of a saliva ejector and cotton gauze squares for blotting the gingival tissue in the immediate area is helpful. If bleeding is profuse, infiltration of a local anesthetic with epinephrine may be necessary for additional hemostasis.

The shape of calculus adds to the difficulty of calculus removal. As one might expect, calculus can be found to occur in any possible shape and size. Large, rough, irregular calculus deposits are easily distinguishable from root anatomy and therefore are fairly easy to detect. Detection problems occur when calculus is difficult to distinguish from tooth surface. For example, small, smooth, flat calculus deposits, indistinguishable from root anatomy, are very difficult to assess and remove. This type of calculus may form in subgingival areas where the client employs less-than-adequate oral hygiene. It also may result from inadequate instrumentation on the part of the dentist or dental hygienist. When only superficial layers of calculus are removed, or the instrument is not manuevered into depressions in root anatomy, the deeper layers remain attached to cementum but with a smoothed outer surface. This remaining calculus is described as **burnished calculus.** Any one of a host of problems ranging from difficult detection to inadequate instrumentation technique (e.g., fulcrum, pressure, adaptation, angulation) and inadequate instrument sharpening may account for burnished calculus.

The more tenacious the calculus, the more problems there are with inadequate scaling resulting in burnished calculus. When calculus is tenacious, it does not always break off in one piece cleanly to the cemental surface. Often, the calculus fractures off in smaller pieces or needs to be shaved off in layers before the cemental surface is reached. The deepest underlying layers of calculus may actually be embedded into the root surface, thereby necessitating the removal of both calculus and some cementum to achieve a calculus-free surface. Prior to reaching a completely smooth surface, the layers of calculus may become so smooth that they are difficult to distinguish from root anatomy.

Subgingival calculus often is naturally darker than supragingival calculus because it is stained by blood pigments. Its color may range from light to dark shades of brown, green, and black; this is often helpful in identifying subgingival calculus. However, direct vision of residual calculus is sometimes difficult because of the gingival inflammation and subsequent hemorrhage that often accompany therapeutic scaling and root planing of periodontally involved teeth. It may be best to reexamine the area on subsequent appointments. After a period of healing (approximately 10 to 14 days), some remaining deposit originally subgingival in location may become supragingival as a result of gingival tissue shrinkage from healing and reduced inflammation. Moreover, at that time, gingival bleeding may be diminished or controlled, allowing the dental hygienist to gently retract the marginal tissue with compressed air or an explorer to detect residual, possibly burnished calculus.

When assessing the difficulty of removing subgingival calculus, it is useful to think in terms of its *quantity, shape,* and *tenacity.* A large tenacious flat sheet of calculus requires more strength, skill, and effort to remove than smaller more bulbous, nontenacious pieces of calculus. Correct instrument selection and use, blade sharpness, and well-supported fulcrums with the possible addition of reinforced support from the nondominant working hand are useful in removing these types of subgingival calculus deposits.

Stain

Stain is categorized by its location and source. It may be *extrinsic* (i.e., located on hard tooth structure, on calculus, on restorations, or on removable appliances). Foods, tobacco, antimicrobial plaque agents, chromogenic bacteria, metallic dust, and other drugs are usually responsible for extrinsic stains (see Fig. 18–4). Stain is indicative of areas in which the client needs to improve oral hygiene behaviors. In areas where stain becomes thick and rough, its surface becomes another nidus for plaque formation and subsequent gingival inflammation. Stain should be removed for this reason and for the aesthetic value afforded the client.

Stain also may be *intrinsic* (i.e., located within the tooth structure). Intrinsic stains are caused by defects during tooth development and by administration of tetracycline and/or excessive fluoride during mineralization of tooth structures. Other reasons for intrinsic tooth discoloration may relate to techniques used in endodontic therapy, to restorative materials, and to stannous fluoride topical application. Intrinsic stain is impossible for the dental hygienist to remove. Correct identification, however, aids in providing the client with accurate information on the etiology of the stain and possible options to remedy it if the individual desires further dental treatment, such as professional and at home bleaching procedures or cosmetic restorative procedures (see the section on extrinsic stain removal).

THE DENTAL TREATMENT AREA

The Dental Unit, Chair, and Operator Stool

The basic **dental treatment area** consists of the dental unit, the dental chair, the operating light, and the operator's stool. The dental unit services or contains the ports for essential items such as the handpiece lines, three-way syringe (i.e., for air, water, and air with water), evacuation system, light post, and moveable instrument tray(s). Other optional items that may be included are a timed cuspidor and cup filler (Table 18–1 and Fig. 18–5).

The dental chair is a contoured chair that offers an articulating headrest and foot or side controls. It comes with many helpful options that make provision of care easier for the provider (Table 18–2).

The dental light may mount into the dental unit or ceiling (tract light fixture), although there is slightly more ver-

TABLE 18–1
THE DENTAL UNIT

Item	Description
Handpiece lines	The electrical and air compression lines that attach to the slow-speed handpiece used for polishing
Air-water-spray or three-way syringe	Provides air, water, or a combination of air and water; attaches to a disposable or autoclavable tip
Evacuation system	Contains a high-speed and a low-speed suction attachment. The slow speed is usually on a smaller diameter hose than the high speed. The dental hygienist usually attaches a disposable, bendable suction tip that fits on the end of the slow-speed suction device. A larger disposable plastic or stainless steel autoclavable tube obliquely cut on one end fits on the high-speed suction line
Light post	Attaches to a unit mount dental light
Instrument trays	Moveable stainless steel tray(s) for instruments
Cuspidor	A moveable cup or bowl for clients to expectorate into; it may have a timed water flush mechanism. The cup may be lined with a disposable paper cup
Cup filler	Usually an automatic water cup filler that is sensitive to the weight of the water in the cup

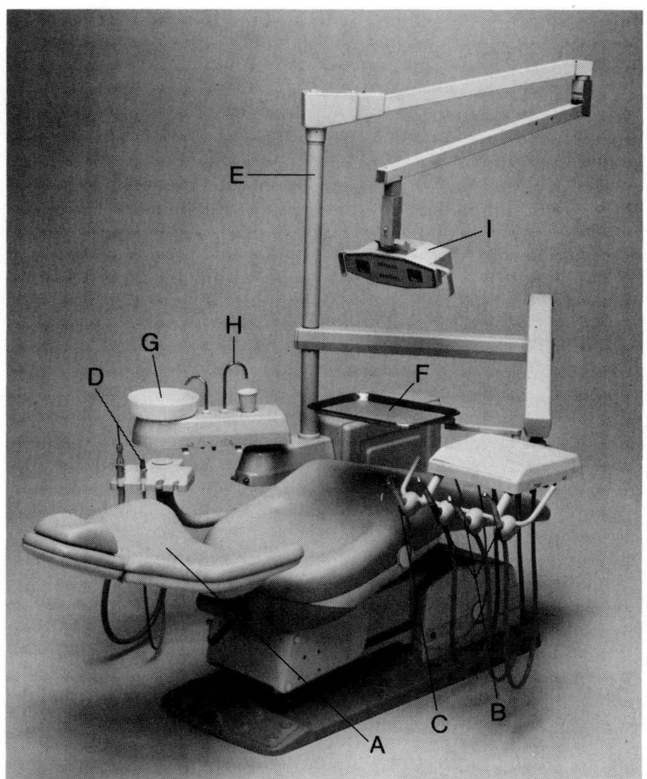

FIGURE 18–5
Proma dental unit and client chair. Contoured dental chair (A), handpiece lines (B), three-way syringe (C), evacuation system (D), light post (E), movable instrument tray (F), cuspidor (G), cup filler (H), light (I).

TABLE 18–2
DENTAL CHAIR

Item	Description
Contoured seat with lumbar support and arm slings	Provides comfortable support for long appointments. Beneficial for apprehensive, insecure, or elderly clients
Articulating thin headrest	A moveable headrest that may be set in a wide range of positions usually with the push of a button. Allows the operator to position the client's head in a preset position as needed. The thin, narrow version allows the operator to work in closer around the client's mouth
Foot or side controls	Controls to lift the back of the chair or the entire chair from a fully supine to the upright position. Provides operator with numerous options for access to different areas of the mouth. Side of chair control buttons requires a disposable barrier or surface disinfectant after each client. Foot controls allow the operator extra versatility and efficiency of motion
360-degree rotation	A lever usually located at the base of the dental chair (and manipulated with the foot) allows the chair to be rotated 360 degrees around. Although this range of motion is usually not indicated, it does allow the operator to move the chair. This is particularly beneficial for left-handed operators when the chair is positioned next to the wall or for times when it is necessary to sit or stand on the opposite side of the client for better access
Low base	Allows the dental chair to be placed in a very low position, close to the floor. Beneficial for times when the operator would like to extend arms in order to use more upper arm and body strength while scaling
Pivoting armrest	Allows the client more room to sit up, rise, and stand when entering or leaving the dental chair

satility with the unit-mounted design. Key aspects of lighting include intensity, pattern, and color. Less eye strain results when the light is sufficient, portrays no significant pattern, and renders natural coloring to hard and soft tissues.

The operator's stool should be a stable seat that does not easily tip if the operator chooses to sit a little forward. A stool with a five-caster base is much more stable than a four-caster base. It should also provide adjustable lumbar back support. A lever to adjust chair height, which is usually located under the seat, is essential. The chair with a lever is more efficient and versatile than a chair that requires turning the stool to raise or lower the seat. A foot control near the base of the chair to adjust height is probably best in that it eliminates the need for a hand adjustment as well as the necessity to clean the area between clients. Lastly, the seat is more comfortable when it is flat rather than contoured because repositioning is easier for the operator.

Light, Water, and Air

Although the air-water spray (AWS) or three-way syringe and dental light are technically part of the dental hygiene unit, they are essential assessment and evaluation tools to be used throughout the examination. The light must be beamed directly to the area being examined or instrumented. If the operator's head, hand, or arm interferes, the light should be readjusted or the operator should move to properly illuminate the working area. The dental light is a strong light. Directing it away from the client's oral cavity does not lessen its effect. Because most lamps emit some heat, it is wise to avoid placing it too close to the client or operator's face. The dental light may be positioned from any angle to illuminate an extraoral or intraoral structure (Fig. 18–6).

Water is necessary for flushing loose calculus, bacterial plaque, materia alba, food debris, blood, suppuration, and polishing agents, and simply to keep the client's tissues and throat moist if opening or suction causes dryness. When using the water spray, the stream should be directed in a horizontal or oblique direction along the lingual, facial, or occlusal surfaces. Scaling instruments such as curets may be used to clean out residual loose calculus and tissue debris from subgingival areas.

Because of the need to reduce aerosol contamination in the oral healthcare setting, use of the air-water combination is not recommended. To reduce the amount of spraying necessary, the dental hygienist should systematically work from the posterior to the anterior regions. Thus, the products of scaling and polishing do not interfere with new areas of instrumentation. The suction generally satisfies the client's need for removal of excess saliva until scaling of segments of the dentition has been completed. To spray, the syringe tip should be directed so that the spray of water flows over the face of the mouth mirror or the facial or lingual tooth surfaces. If the syringe tip is positioned so that the water is delivered at a 90-degree angle, the water and debris splatter back to the operator. To guard against further contamination, the dental hygienist should cover the mouth opening as much as possible with a gloved hand. The client's cheek may be pulled over to cover and protect the practitioner from splatter.

During the final or evaluation stage of scaling, the air spray alone is a valuable tool in assessment. The tooth and tissues to be evaluated should be dried with a 2 × 2 gauze square, suctioned, or both to reduce splatter and prevent recontamination of the dried surfaces with saliva. Air should be directed onto the tooth or into the sulcus if the subgingival area is to be examined. The area should be sprayed until it is thoroughly dry. Supragingival and subgingival calculus appears chalky white, yellow, brown, gray, or black.

Clients who have dental caries, sensitive cementoenamel junctions, or dentinal hypersensitivity object to the cold temperatures generated by the air or water. For these clients, the use of a tactile method of evaluation with the explorer is a more suitable mode of assessment.

ASSESSMENT AND TREATMENT INSTRUMENTS

All instruments used by the dental hygienist in caring for clients with healthy or diseased periodontium may be divided into two catagories:

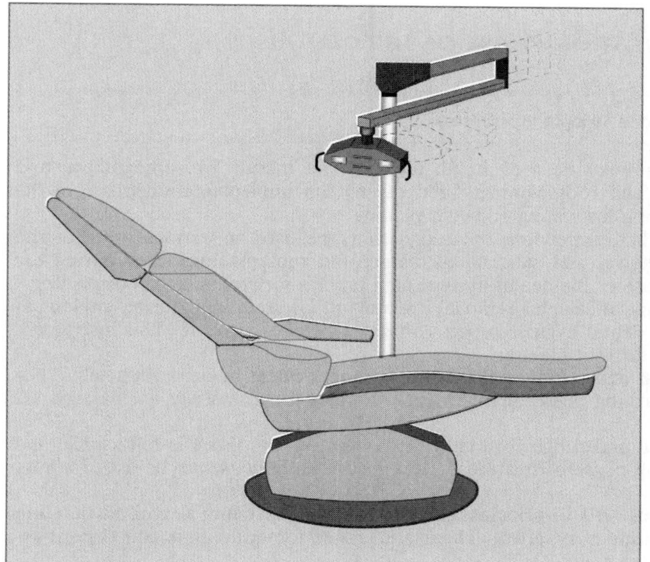

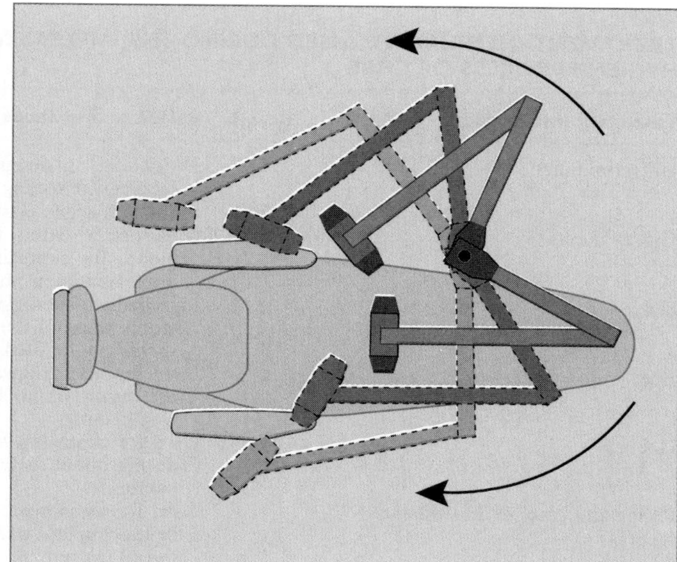

FIGURE 18-6
Dental operatory light positions.

- Assessment instruments that provide the operator with information
- Treatment instruments with which the provider performs scaling, root planing, and extrinsic stain removal

Within each category, various subdivisions may be made with some very specific uses for each instrument. Differences in manufacturing design and metallurgy further subdivide categories. These specific design differences are addressed later in this chapter. Tables 18-3 and 18-4 list the basic assessment and treatment instruments and describe their general usage. Some examples of assessment and treatment instruments are seen in Figure 18-7.

With the exception of the slow-speed handpiece and the air polishing device, all of these instruments consist of three basic parts:

- Handle
- Shank
- Working end

Variations in these fundamental design characteristics of all periodontal instruments are important because they determine the purpose, effectiveness, efficiency, and comfort of use for the operator. A good instrument should support all of these functions. The following discussion of the handle, shank, and the working end apply to all assessment and treatment instruments with the exception of the ultrasonic scaling handpiece, the slow-speed handpiece, and the air polishing device.

Handle

When selecting an instrument, handle specifications are primarily of benefit to the operator. Nevertheless, they *should not* be considered secondary or less important than any other part of the instrument. If the operator is not comfortable, the quality of work eventually suffers.

The most comfortable handles are of medium diameter. Large handles lead to an uncomfortable grasp and tend to be very bulky and cumbersome, making rotation of the instrument difficult. The diameter of large-handled instruments also makes it difficult to reach posterior areas as the extra circumference causes the instrument handle to rub on the teeth of the opposing arch. Slender handles lead to cramping of the hands after prolonged use.

Handle shape or circumference may be round or hexagonal. Both are quite comfortable when a suitable surface

TABLE 18-3
ASSESSMENT INSTRUMENTS USED BY THE DENTAL HYGIENIST

Assessment Instruments	Basic Use and Sequence Within Appointment
Mouth mirror	Indirect vision, indirect illumination, transillumination, and retraction of buccal mucosa and tongue; for use throughout appointment
Periodontal probe	Measurement of probing depth, clinical attachment level, relative attachment level, amount of attached gingiva, gingival recession, furcation invasion, bacterial plaque, gingival inflammation, assessment of bleeding points, and pathological lesions. Used during assessment and again during the evaluation phase of the process of care
Nabor's probe	A furcation classification instrument to be used during assessment and again during the evaluation phase of the process of care
Explorer	Detection of calculus, irregular cementum, junctional epithelium, dental caries, irregular root anatomy, margins or restorations, external resorption and osseous exposures. For use during assessment, implementation, and evaluation phases of the process of care

TABLE 18–4
TREATMENT INSTRUMENTS USED DURING THE IMPLEMENTATION PHASE OF THE DENTAL HYGIENE PROCESS OF CARE

Treatment Instruments	Basic Use and Sequence Within Appointment
Universal curet	Depending on design, may be used in all areas of the mouth for supragingival and subgingival scaling and root planing. Used during the implementation phase of the dental hygiene process for scaling and root planing
Gracey curets	Area-specific curets that, depending on design, may be used in various areas of the mouth for supragingival and subgingival scaling and root planing. Used during the implementation phase of the dental hygiene care process for scaling and root planing
Sickle	Principally a supragingival calculus removal instrument. Used initially during implementation phase of the dental hygiene process for gross calculus removal. This instrument *should not* be used for root planing
File	Used for supragingival and subgingival calculus removal where tissue is retractable. For use during initial scaling phase of treatment. This instrument *should not* be used for root planing
Hoe	Used for supragingival and subgingival calculus removal where tissue is retractable, and during initial scaling phase of treatment. This instrument *should not* be used for root planing
Plastic and graphite instruments	Used for assessment as well as calculus and bacterial plaque removal around titanium dental implant abutment cylinders. There are probes for evaluation and deposit removal instruments for scaling
Ultrasonic scaling devices	Used for supragingival and subgingival calculus removal, and during initial scaling phase of treatment. Not recommended for titanium dental implant abutment cylinders
Slow-speed handpiece	Used for bacterial plaque and extrinsic stain removal after scaling and root planing are complete. Recommended for use with a fine abrasive agent for polishing titanium dental implant abutment cylinders. The prophylaxis angle, rubber cup, point or brush, and polishing agent are part of the armamentarium
Porte polisher	Used as an alternative to the slow-speed handpiece for extrinsic stain and bacterial plaque removal in difficult-to-reach areas. Ideal for clients who do not tolerate handpiece vibration and heat, or for high-risk individuals when an aerosol could be a problem. A good instrument to use on nonambulatory clients who must be treated in an area other than the oral healthcare setting where there is no access to the dental handpiece. May be used for calculus and bacterial plaque removal around titanium dental implant abutment cylinders
Air polishing abrasive system	Used for bacterial plaque and stain removal after scaling and root planing are complete. Contraindicated for use around titanium dental implant abutment cylinders

pattern is used. Many different patterns, pattern sizes, and depths are cut into the handle of the instrument. The depth of the pattern cut into the handle can determine the comfort level to the practitioner. Some patterns are cut so deep that they feel as if they are biting into the skin when pressure is placed on the instrument, even with the benefit of the glove.

Handle weight is the final consideration in handle selection. There are solid- and hollow-handled instruments. Most clinicians find that hollow handles are lighter and less

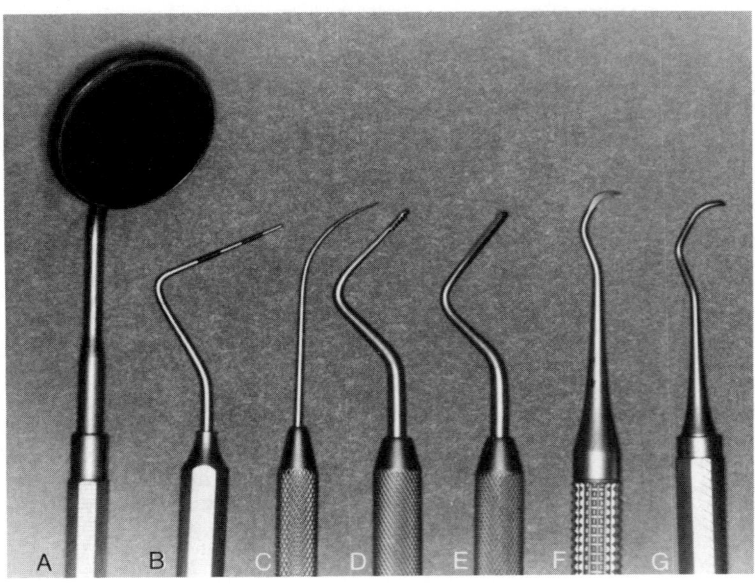

FIGURE 18–7
Assessment instruments: mirror (A), periodontal probe (B), explorer (C). Working instruments: file (D), hoe (E), sickle (F), curet (G).

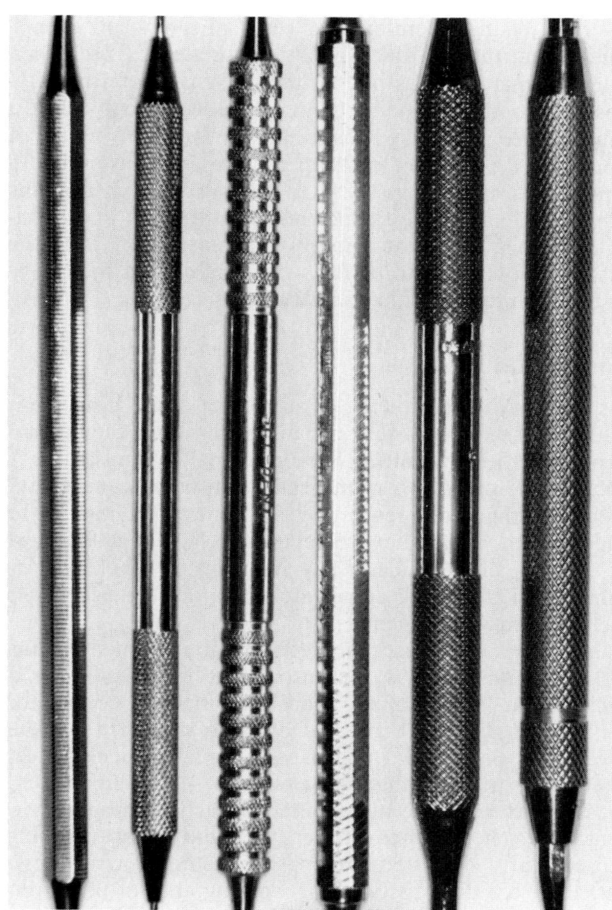

FIGURE 18-8
Observe handle variations of size, shape, and pattern.

strenuous to use and improve tactile sensitivity more than solid-handled instruments (Fig. 18-8).

Shank

The shank of an instrument connects the working end (which is the end that determines the purpose of the instrument such as an explorer or a periodontal probe) to the handle and is the major factor determining the use of each particular instrument. Differences among instruments in shank design relate to:

- Length
- Angle
- Strength

Length

Depending on the particular instrument, shank length ranges from short to long (Fig. 18-9). Generally, instruments with longer shanks are used for individuals with deep periodontal pockets because of the need to insert the working end of the instrument into the bottom of a pocket. This pocket depth or distance can be 10 mm or more in some individuals. The longer shank also is indicated when fulcruming away from the area being instrumented such as on the opposite arch or on an extraoral area. The **fulcrum** is the source of stability for the working hand. It may rest intraorally near the tooth being instrumented, on teeth across from the same arch being instrumented, on teeth on the opposite arch from the area being instrumented, or extraorally on the client's face or chin. (The concept of the fulcrum is discussed further later in the chapter.) Thus, an instrument with a long shank is preferable for instrumenting anterior or posterior teeth with deep periodontal pocket depths, or recession, or when the operator needs to fulcrum a great distance from the area being instrumented. The shorter shank is best suited for instruments used on anterior teeth, when fulcruming close to the area being instrumented is possible and when there are shallow pocket depths.

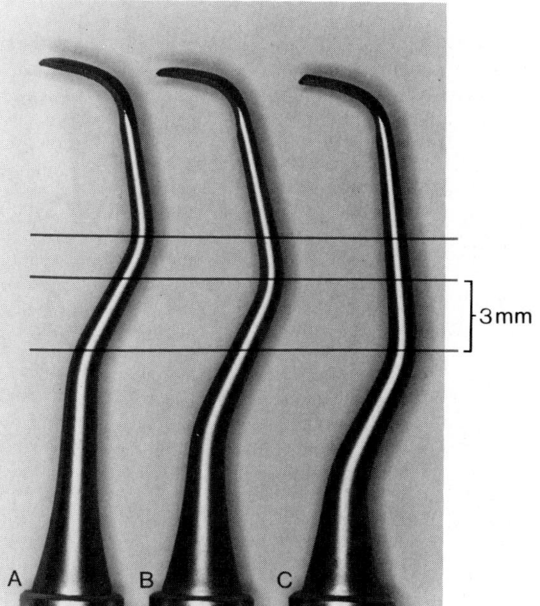

FIGURE 18-9
Comparison of shank lengths. Gracey 1-2 (A), Gracey 5-6 (B), Gracey After-Five 5-6 (C).

Angle

Most periodontal instruments, ultrasonic scaler tips, motor-driven prophylaxis angles, and air polishers have shanks that are curved or bent in at least one and usually two places (Fig. 18-10). The degree and angle of this curvature or bend also determines the area(s) in which this instrument is effective. Generally, the smaller the angle and number of bends an instrument's shank has, the more suitable the instrument is for use on anterior teeth. The more acute the angle and number of bends, the more suitable the instrument is for use on posterior teeth.

The fulcrum, however, also plays a major role in directing the use of the instrument despite the angle of the shank. Although generally, the straighter-shanked instruments are used in anterior areas and the more curved-shanked instruments are used in posterior areas, this does not always have to be the case. For example, clinicians who use a variety of fulcrums ranging from intraoral to extraoral to allow the working end access to deep periodontal areas find that shank angle does not limit the usefulness of the instrument. In other words, fulcrum versatility allows greater flexibility in use of instruments in nontraditional

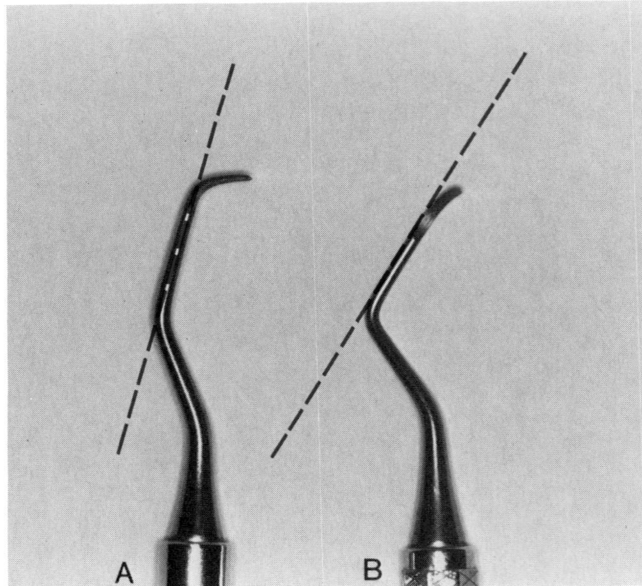

FIGURE 18–10
Comparison of shank bends or curvatures. Gracey curet 5–6 (A), Universal curet (Columbia 4R–4L) (B).

areas. Thus, in some cases straighter shanked instruments may be used for scaling of posterior teeth and considerably more curved instruments may be used in anterior areas.

The portion of the shank from the last bend or curve to the working end is termed the terminal shank. Its position as it relates to the working end is important in determining the correct positioning of the angulation of the curet blade and usually is kept parallel to the long axis of the tooth.

Strength

All shanks taper in diameter from the handle as they approach the working end. Shank strength is a function of the thickness and type of metal used. Some manufacturers actually designate the flexibility of their instruments' shanks. There are definite benefits in using instruments with less flexible shanks. The most important advantage is strength. When scaling teeth with heavy calculus, much less operator effort is needed if the instrument does not bend or flex away from the tooth when pressure is exerted. The practitioner must work harder to direct equivalent lateral pressure against the tooth when the instrument shank flexes. In addition, if the instrument shank is long or if fulcruming away from the working area is required, it results in further dissipation of pressure exerted by the operator. Consequently, in these cases use of an instrument with a strong shank is important. In scaling teeth of individuals with light calculus or in fulcruming close to the working area, there is a savings in operator effort, although it is less noticeable when using an instrument with a strong shank. However, if the operator's saved effort is multiplied by 8 to 10 clients treated per day, the savings become more meaningful.

Nevertheless, arguments against stronger-shanked or rigid-shanked instruments claim a decreased tactile sensitivity with rigid-shanked instruments compared to flexible-shanked instruments. Perhaps it is more a matter of experience, just as the use of gloves thought to interfere with tactile sensitivity was later ruled out. Many clinicians find the rigid shanks comfortable with all types of clients. Others find that flexible shanks are better to use when scaling clients' teeth as part of the preventive oral prophylaxis or periodontal maintenance. The decision to select a rigid- or flexible-shanked instrument is largely a matter of habit and the type of instrument one is accustomed to using. However, it is prudent to learn to use instruments with rigid shanks. The savings in operator effort and possible avoidance of operator injury such as tendonitis of the wrist are most likely to be felt when scaling and root planing teeth with rigid-shanked instruments.

Working End

It is the working end or the terminal end of the instrument attached to the shank that actually determines the general purpose of the instrument. For the dental hygienist, this is probably the most important detail in instrument selection. There are slight differences between manufacturers as to shape, length, width, bend or curvature, and metallurgy of the working ends of identically named and numbered instruments. These small details are important considerations when selecting instruments.

Aside from differences between instrument manufacturers, the working end of an instrument is designed for a specific task. For example, if an instrument is needed for assessing the distance between the marginal gingiva and the base of the periodontal pocket, the dental hygienist must select an instrument that has a working end calibrated to measure distance. The periodontal probe is such an instrument. The general shape and length of the probe's working end are fairly consistent among all manufacturers. However, there are differences in the working ends of periodontal probes with respect to their intervals of millimeter markings and the presence or absence of color-coded probe markings for easier reading. Some working ends of probes are slender whereas others are heavy or even flat-surfaced. The decision about type of periodontal probe to use is based on personal preference for millimeter markings at selected intervals (e.g., 3 mm, 6 mm, 9 mm, 12 mm color coded or some other interval variation the manufacturer has chosen to produce). The decision also may rest on how the dental hygienist feels about using a very thin, pointed probe tip versus a heavier tip that may not pass through the junctional epithelium as easily.

The design of the working ends among scaling instruments varies considerably. Therefore when deciding on which instrument to use for scaling purposes, the criteria for instrument selection are more complex. The dental hygienist's decision is based on experience with using different scaling and root planing instruments, periodontal probing depths present, the gingival tissue tone, and the quantity and type of calculus to be scaled. If there is heavy subgingival calculus, one of the types of treatment instruments the dental hygienist uses is the curet. Within this category of treatment instrument, there is a range in variation among manufacturers of the same instrument (e.g., differences in blade size, length, shape, and metallurgy). Curet selection should be dependent on the amount and tenacity of calculus, pocket depth, alignment of teeth, root proximity, use of intraoral or extraoral fulcrums, and tissue tone. For example, a wide, heavy blade is needed for removal of heavy subgingival calculus; a long blade is necessary for removal of deep subgingival and interproximal calculus; and the shape or curvature of the blade is important for specific area(s) being scaled.

Moreover, curets are further subdivided based on whether their blades are made of stainless steel or carbon steel. Stainless steel instruments maintain adequate sharpness for scaling and root planing and do not rust or discolor when sterilized with saturated steam, or with formalin-alcohol vapor. On the other hand, carbon steel blades tend to feel sharper clinically and hold their sharpened edges longer after prolonged use compared to stainless steel blades.[3,4] However, carbon steel is more brittle and tends to break more easily than stainless steel blades. Carbon steel instruments also are more likely to corrode or rust when sterilized. Carbon steel has a tendency to oxidize (rust) after saturated steam sterilization,[5] or when moisture content of a formalin-alcohol vapor sterilizer reaches 15% or greater. Because of this tendency for oxidation of the carbon steel metal, commercially available corrosion inhibitors are recommended for use with the autoclave to reduce oxidation of carbon steel instruments. Manufacturer instructions concerning dilution of ultrasonic cleaners and chemical disinfection solutions and length of time instruments should remain in solution should be carefully monitored. Dry heat sterilization, however, does not present a problem for carbon steel instruments.

The final selection of a treatment instrument for scaling purposes usually is personal preference relative to which instrument works best with a given instrumentation technique (grasp, fulcrum, wrist, and finger action), scaling and root planing objectives, and desired efficiency in terms of time management. If, for example, a practitioner's scaling technique involves using extraoral fulcrums, area-specific curets are ideal instruments to use. If the client presents with no significant periodontal disease, universal curets may easily accomplish the task of scaling with more efficiency in terms of time management than area-specific curets that require different instruments for different areas of the tooth.

Depending on the manufacturer, the working end of instruments may be double-ended or single-ended. The double-ended instrument has exact, mirror images on the opposite ends. This is necessary because the same curvature of blade does not adapt to each side of the same tooth. For example, the distal surface from the facial aspect of the tooth requires the mirror image of the same instrument to scale the distal surface from the lingual aspect. These same double-ended instruments may be manufactured as single-ended instruments (i.e., only one end has a working blade, requiring the practitioner to have twice as many instruments). Single-ended instruments are inefficient because of the necessity of picking up and replacing instruments to and from the work area every time one chooses to work from the opposite aspect of the same tooth. Instrument cleaning, packaging, sterilization, and storage efforts also are doubled.

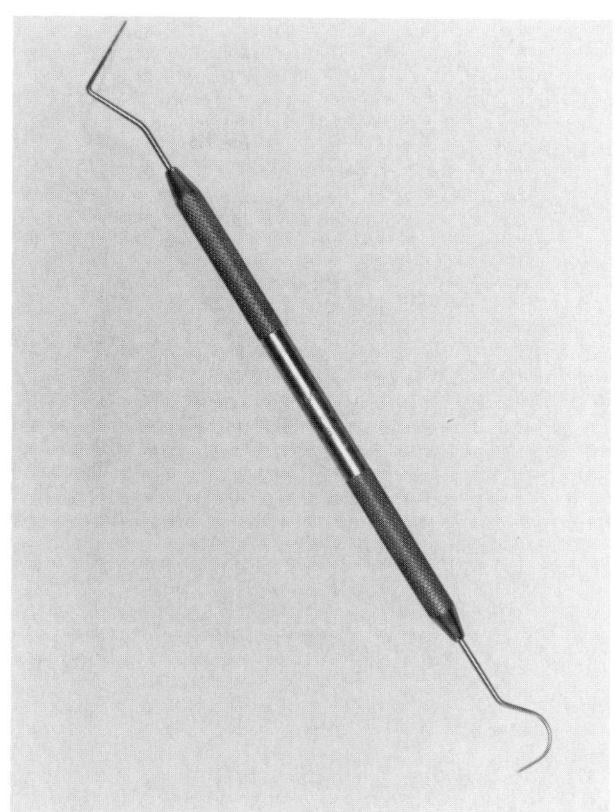

FIGURE 18–11
Double-ended instrument with a periodontal probe on one end and an explorer on the opposite end.

Some assessment instruments do not have mirror-image working ends such as the periodontal probe and the straight explorer. Such instruments may be manufactured so that one side is a periodontal probe and the other side is an explorer. They are double-ended but actually have two different instruments on the same handle (Fig. 18–11).

Whether the instrument is double-ended or single-ended, it should be balanced. This means that the working end is in alignment or centered over the long axis of the instrument handle.[1] When the instrument is balanced, the pressure exerted by the hand and fingers against the handle and shank is directed to the working end (Fig. 18–12).

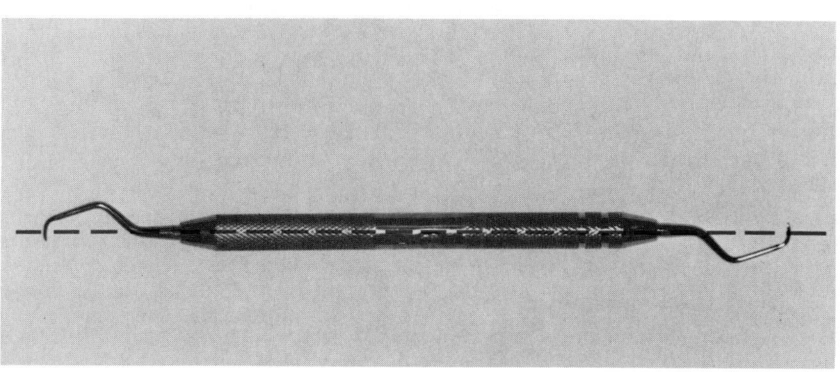

FIGURE 18–12
Balanced instrument. When the working end is centered over the long axis of the handle, the instrument is balanced.

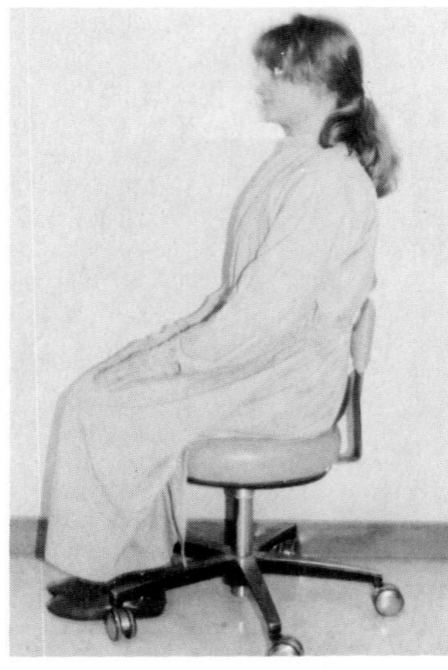

A

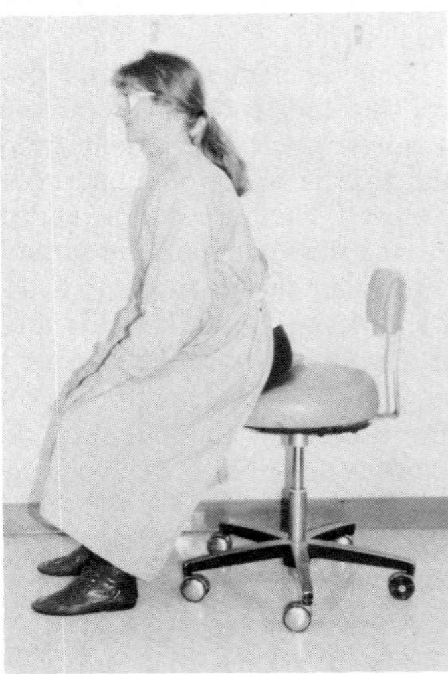

B

- Adjust operator stool so that the dental hygienist's feet are flat on the floor with thighs also parallel to the floor.
- Body weight should be centered on the seat of the chair.
- Back is straight with the maintenance of the lumbar curve. A chair with a lumbar roll positioned in the small of the back may be helpful.
- Shoulders are relaxed and parallel to the floor and are not raised.
- Attempt to sit tall and elevate the chest bone. This step helps keep the head in alignment with the back.
- Eyes, rather than the head, are directed downward to the field of operation. Sit close enough to the client's oral cavity to avoid slumping.
- The distance from the client's oral cavity to the eyes of the operator should be approximately 14 to 16 inches.
- Client's mouth and instrument tray should be at, or slightly lower than, the dental hygienist's elbows.
- The dental hygienist's upper arms should be relaxed, with elbows close to the body.
- The dental hygienist should try to recapture this balanced position at least four times during a one-hour appointment. Balanced sitting contributes to muscle relaxation and thereby decreases midback, upper shoulder, and neck pain.
- For variations on the basic ergonomic approach, see section on protective scaling.

FIGURE 18–13
Basic ergonomic approach to balanced operator seating during the dental hygiene process of care. *A*, Dental hygienist is seated correctly in a balanced position. *B*, Incorrect position. Back and neck are forward, and thighs are not parallel to the floor.

FUNDAMENTAL TECHNIQUES OF INSTRUMENTATION

Operator and Client Positions

Operator and client positioning facilitates proper instrumentation technique. In learning and practicing **operator positioning,** the dental hygienist attempts to achieve a state of musculoskeletal balance that protects the body from strain and cumulative injury. Figure 18–13 outlines the principles for achieving a balanced seating position.

Operator positioning in relation to the client is described in accordance with the face of a clock. The client's head is the center of the clock, and the operator may move in any position from about 8:00 to 4:00 around the client (Fig. 18–14).

The predominant positions used by the right-handed clinician are from 8:00 to 2:00; however, it is not out of the question for this operator to be positioned at 4:00 when irregular tooth positions or access require extreme cross-arch fulcruming. The predominant positions for the left-handed practitioner are from 10:00 to 4:00 with variations required at times at the 8:00 mark. Tables 18–5 and 18–6 list the accessible areas of a client's mouth from various clock positions for both right-handed and left-handed operators.

Operator position may need modification to meet deficits in the client's human need for territoriality. A client's verbal and nonverbal expressions of discomfort related to the proximity of the operator during dental hygiene care are indicators of deficits in this human need. The comfort of the client is a primary concern throughout the process of care and is important for achieving both a good quality of care and client satisfaction. A variety of client positions are used throughout the dental hygiene process. These client positions are demonstrated and described in Figure 18–15.

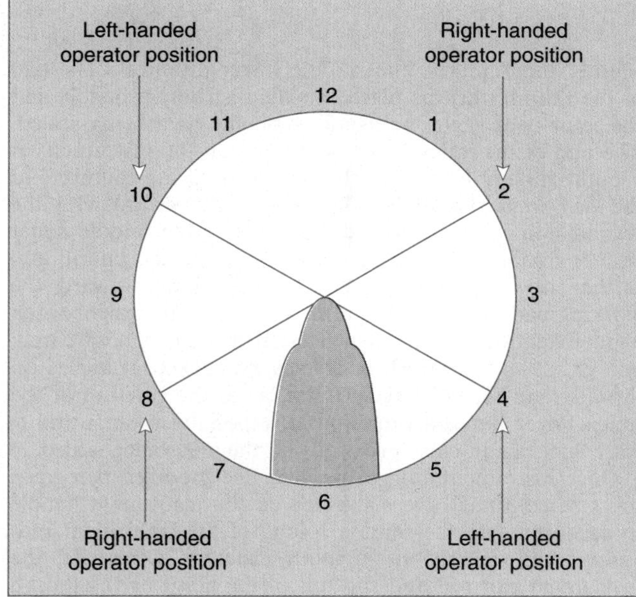

FIGURE 18–14
Possible operator positions around the client. Right-handed operator: 8:00–2:00. Left-handed operator: 4:00–10:00.

TABLE 18–5
GENERAL POSITIONS FOR RIGHT-HANDED PRACTITIONERS

Clock Position	Accessible Areas of the Mouth for the Right-handed Dental Hygienist
8:00–9:00	All surfaces of: Mandibular right quadrant Maxillary right quadrant Mandibular left quadrant Maxillary left quadrant (Exception: labial and lingual of maxillary and mandibular anteriors)
10:00–12:00	Mandibular right mesials Mandibular anteriors (all surfaces) Mandibular left posterior mesials
12:00–2:00	Mandibular left posterior mesials (facial approach) Maxillary right posterior (distal and lingual surfaces)
2:00–4:00	Mandibular right distal, last tooth only

Instrument Blade Selection

After the appropriate instrument has been selected, the next step is to determine the correct working end of the instrument to use for the tooth surface to be evaluated or scaled. For some instruments such as the periodontal probe and the 3-A explorer, the working end is universal and works on all surfaces. The practitioner may find some instruments, however, that work well on all mesial and distal surfaces but only on the anterior teeth. An example of such an instrument is the straight sickle scaler. The majority of treatment instruments are site-specific with a definite side of the blade that should be used against the tooth. The criteria for selecting the correct working end to use is discussed under sections on specific instruments.

After establishing a comfortable operator position and selecting the appropriate instrument and working end, the dental hygienist begins the procedure for scaling and/or root planing. For discussion purposes, this procedure is broken down into its component parts of grasp, fulcrum, insertion, adaptation, angulation, lateral pressure, stroke di-

TABLE 18–6
GENERAL POSITIONS FOR LEFT-HANDED PRACTITIONERS

Clock Position	Accessible Areas of the Mouth for the Left-handed Dental Hygienist
3:00–4:00	All surfaces of: Mandibular left quadrant Maxillary left quadrant Mandibular right quadrant Maxillary right quadrant (Exception: labial and lingual of maxillary and mandibular anteriors)
12:00–2:00	Mandibular left mesials Mandibular anteriors (all surfaces) Mandibular right posterior mesials
10:00–12:00	Mandibular right posterior mesials (facial approach) Maxillary left posterior (distal and lingual surfaces)
8:00–10:00	Mandibular left distal, last tooth only

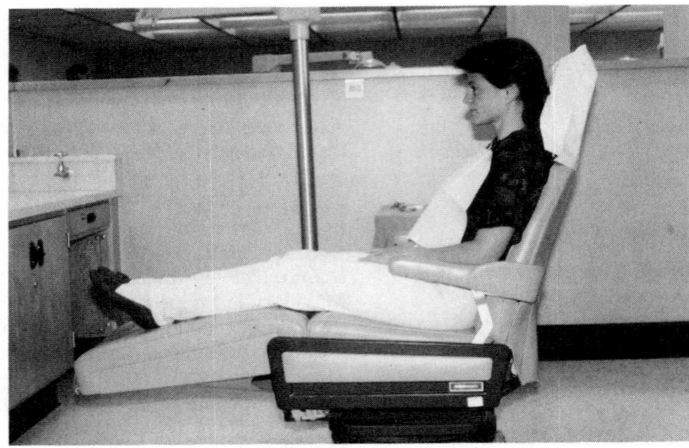

A

USES
- Assessment of health and dental history, vital signs, and extraoral signs of health and disease
- Exposing radiographs
- Educating client
- Administering professional fluoride therapy

DENTAL LIGHT POSITION
- Dental light is not usually used with the services provided in this position

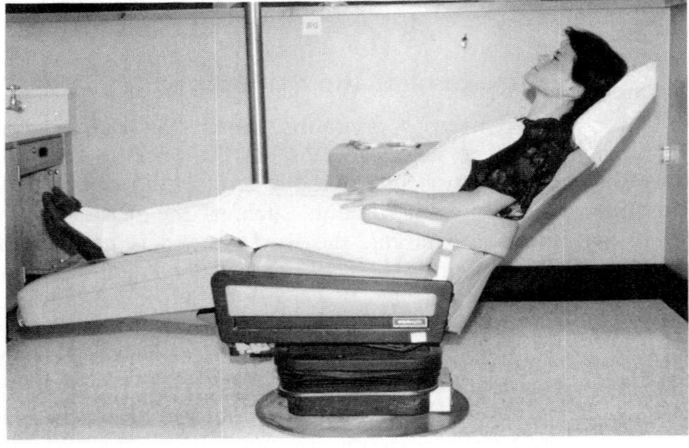

B

USES
- Dental hygiene instrumentation on clients who have difficulty in breathing (e.g., persons with a history of cardiovascular disease or respiratory disease)

DENTAL LIGHT POSITION
- Beam of light is directed into the mouth at about a 45-degree angle

FIGURE 18–15
Basic client body positions used during the dental hygiene process of care. *A*, Basic upright position. Client is seated in an 80-degree to 90-degree angle. *B*, Semi-upright position. Client is seated in a 45-degree angle.

rection, stroke length, and reinforcement. A discussion of modification of these fundamental aspects of periodontal instrumentation also is provided for enhanced instrument versatility.

Grasp

The **pen grasp** is an instrument hold used when the exacting or directive type of pressure used in scaling and root planing is *not* required. As shown in Figure 18–16, the thumb and index finger pads are well situated on the instrument handle, but the middle finger slips down and the instrument rests on the side of the finger near the first knuckle. The pen grasp may be used when light, easy probing or exploring into nonperiodontally involved areas is performed. Much heavier pressure also may be used with this grasp on the mouth mirror for retraction of the buccal mucosa, tongue, or other soft tissues.

Comparison of the pen grasp to the modified pen grasp is illustrated in Figure 18–16. The **modified pen grasp** is the standard grasp used for periodontal instrumentation. When correctly applied, it is a sensitive, stable, and strong grasp because of the tripod effect that the position of the thumb, index finger, and middle finger produces. The pad of the thumb must be placed on the instrument handle and the joint bent slightly depending on the area being scaled. The pad of the index finger should be on the instrument at a point slightly higher on the handle than the thumb, and the first joint should be slightly bent downward with the second joint cocked upward. The side of the middle finger near the nailbed should be placed opposing the thumb and further down the instrument on the shank toward the working end. The middle finger may remain straight when using extended fulcrums (such as cross arch, opposite arch, and extraoral fulcrums); or it may be cocked at angles on the first and second knuckles similar to the position of the index finger but less pronounced, especially when working with fulcrums in close proximity to the area being scaled.

Once instrumentation is initiated, the modified pen grasp must be continually reestablished on the instrument handle to accommodate the minute rolling of the instrument into and around depressions of tooth structure. Otherwise, the instrument can roll and slip out of the grasp or the thumb and fingers end up in an undesirable position on the instrument handle, which may not allow for optimal pressure to be placed against the instrument for adequate assessment

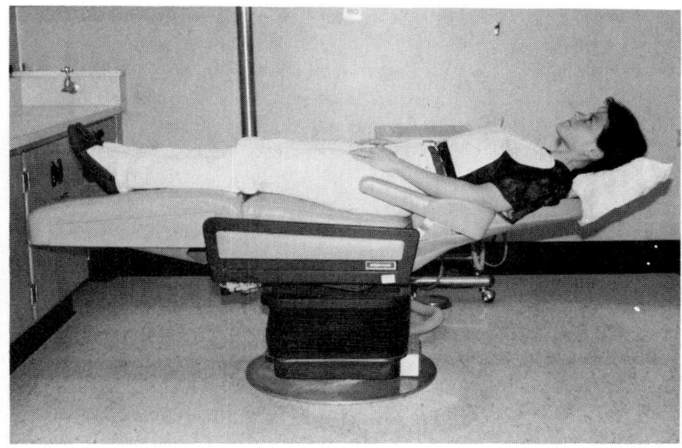

USES

- For mandibular instrumentation, the client's back and head may be readjusted so that the mandible is parallel with the floor when the mouth is open.
- For maxillary instrumentation, the client's back and head may be readjusted so that the maxilla is perpendicular to the floor when the mouth is open.

C

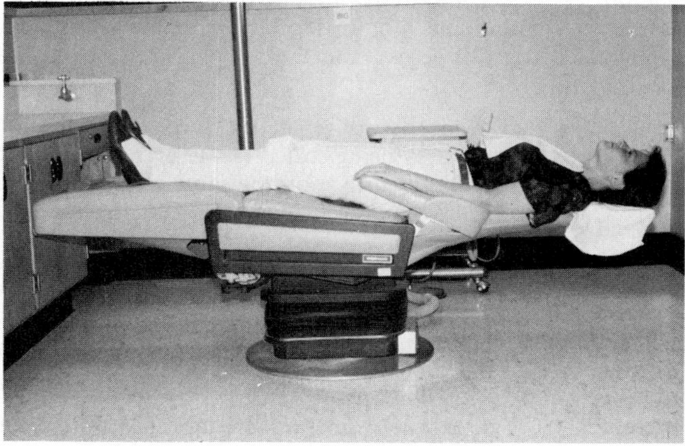

DENTAL LIGHT POSITION

- Mandibular: Direct the beam of light into the oral cavity perpendicular to the horizontal plane of the mandible.
- Maxillary: Direct the beam of light into the oral cavity at about a 45-degree angle to the floor.

D

FIGURE 18–15 *Continued*
C, Supine position that has been modified for mandibular instrumentation. *D*, Supine position that has been modified for maxillary insertion.

or instrumentation. The thumb, index, and middle fingers also are flexed to allow the instrument to be manipulated in various directions around the tooth surface, and to allow equal pressure to be applied against root structure during the course of the stroke. Although, historically, dental hygienists were taught to avoid digital movement during instrumentation, it now appears that such digital movement, when combined with the movement of the wrist, facilitates accurate, even scaling and root planing strokes in deep periodontal pockets during nonsurgical periodontal therapy. Moreover, the most protective situation for the dental hygienist when scaling in deep pockets occurs when both finger movement and wrist (or arm) movement can be used, minimizing stress to one particular area such as the hand or wrist. The degree to which finger flexing is required for successful instrumentation (versus wrist movement and even arm movement) varies, according to the fulcrum used, the area being scaled, the instrument used, and the depth of the periodontal pocket. In certain areas, either finger flexing or wrist movement is used.

Another grasp that is sometimes used is the **palm-thumb grasp** (Fig. 18–17). With this grasp, the instrument is held with all four fingers wrapped tightly around the handle and the thumb placed on the shank in a direction pointing towards the tip of the instrument. This is a very awkward, uncontrolled grasp because the thumb provides the only source of pressure and the opposing fingers clumsily wrap around the handle and do not provide a means of turning the instrument or modifying the effect of the thumb. The palm-thumb grasp provides little in the way of tactile sensitivity during scaling procedures and is not recommended for periodontal instrumentation either supragingivally or subgingivally. It is quite suitable, however, when used for holding the instrument during sharpening procedures. Because the palm-thumb grasp is a very stable grasp that does not allow the instrument to move on its own as the stone passes over the blade, it is ideal for use during instrument sharpening. Table 18–7 categorizes grasp by instrument selection.

Fulcrum

The action of applying lateral pressure against the tooth surface with a sharp blade or pointed instrument necessitates a stable fulcrum. The **fulcrum** is the source of stability or leverage on which the finger rests and pushes against to

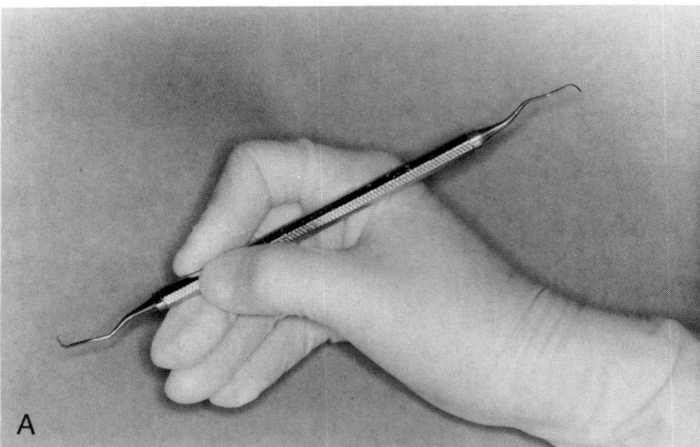

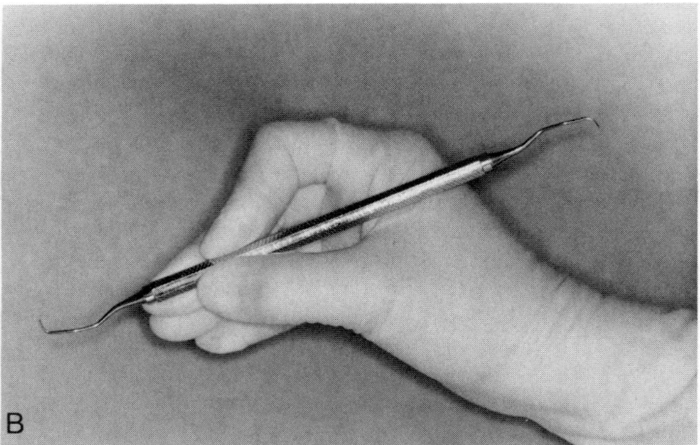

FIGURE 18–16
Comparison of the pen grasp and the modified pen grasp. *A*, Pen grasp. *B*, Modified pen grasp.

hold the instrument with control during stroke activation. When there is no fulcrum, the instrument uncontrollably slips off of the tooth surface when even a slight amount of lateral pressure is exerted.

There are two basic classifications of fulcrums:

- Intraoral fulcrums
- Extraoral fulcrums

The **intraoral fulcrum** is a traditional fulcrum established inside the mouth against tooth surface. The pad of the ring finger usually is positioned on the occlusal, incisal, or facial surface of a tooth close to the one being instrumented. The middle finger should remain in contact with the ring finger even when it is bent during finger flexing or when making digital movements. If the middle finger splits away from the ring finger, control and/or strength diminish from the stroke. With the added support of the middle finger, a built-up stable fulcrum is accomplished.

The intraoral fulcrum also may rest on the operator's finger. Because such a fulcrum is inside the oral cavity, it is still classified as an intraoral fulcrum (Fig. 18–18).

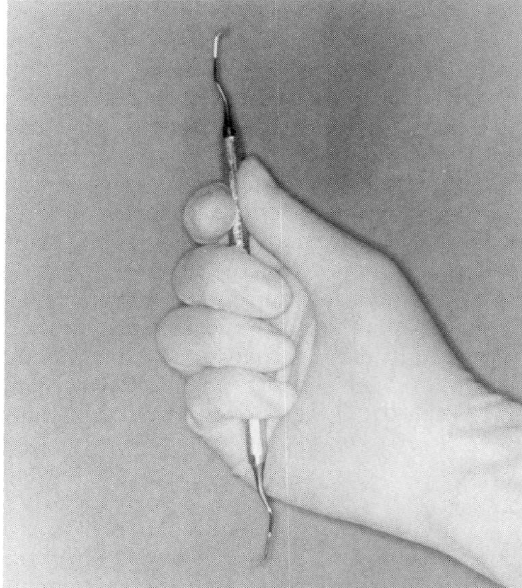

FIGURE 18–17
Palm-thumb grasp is used for instrument-sharpening procedures.

The intraoral fulcrum may be located in different areas within the mouth depending on the area to be scaled, the angle of access, and the pocket depth. It may be positioned on:

- A tooth surface on the same arch positioned near to the area being scaled **(same arch fulcrum)** (Fig. 18–19)
- A tooth surface on the same arch but positioned across from the area being scaled (i.e., on the opposite quadrant or cross arch)—**(cross arch fulcrum)** (Fig. 18–20)
- A tooth surface on the opposing arch from the arch being scaled **(opposite arch fulcrum)** (Fig. 18–21)
- The operator's own finger (e.g., fulcrum on index or thumb) that is located within the oral cavity (see Fig. 18–18).

The **extraoral fulcrum** is established outside of the mouth and predominantly is used when instrumenting teeth with deep periodontal pockets. The extraoral fulcrum is placed against the person's jaw or on a broad surface such as the side of the face. The extraoral fulcrum does not use a small finger point source as does the intraoral fulcrum. Rather, the extraoral fulcrum is accomplished by placing the broad side of the palm or back of the hand against the chin or outer cheek. The extraoral fulcrum does not use light pres-

TABLE 18–7
GRASP AND INSTRUMENT SELECTION

Grasp	Instrument
Pen grasp	Mouth mirror Periodontal probe Explorer
Modified pen grasp	Mouth mirror Periodontal probe Explorer Curets Sickles Hoes Files Plastic instruments Ultrasonic and sonic instruments Porte polisher Slow-speed handpiece
Palm-thumb grasp	Holding instrument during sharpening procedures

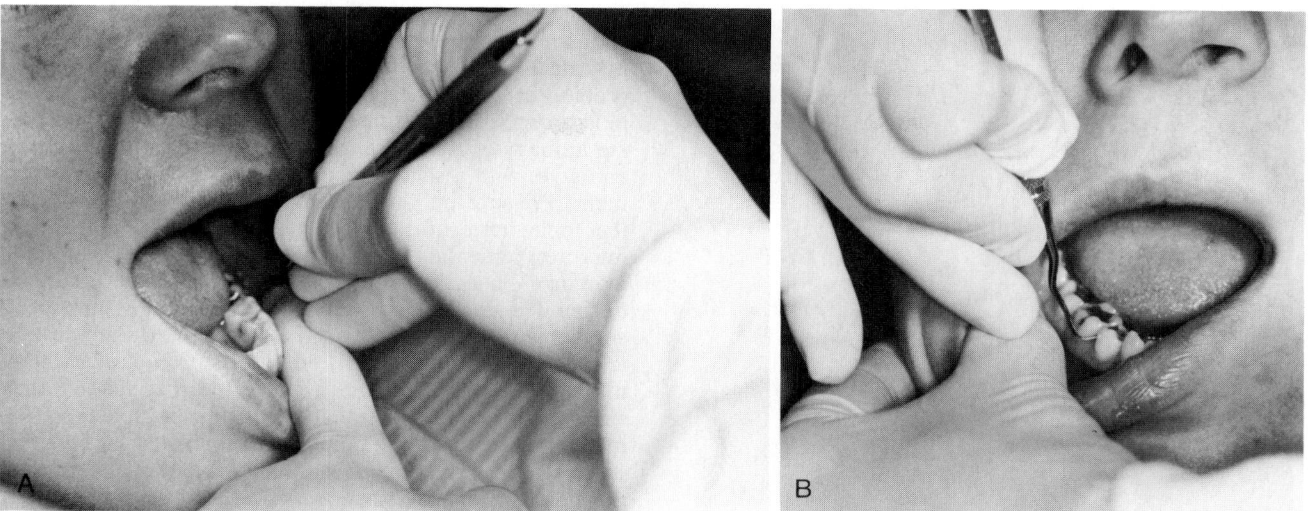

FIGURE 18–18
Intraoral fulcrums. *A*, Fulcrum on operator's index finger. *B*, Fulcrum on operator's thumb.

sure against the skin of the client's face. Rather, the palm or back side of the hand rests with moderate pressure against the bony structures of the face and/or mandible. This extraoral fulcrum has been described as a palm-up or a palm-down position.[6] The extraoral fulcrum provides an excellent means of control and stability for access into periodontally involved areas that may be cumbersome or physiologically strenuous for the dental hygienist to instrument using intraoral fulcrums. Often, the extraoral fulcrum allows a direct "line of draw" in which the instrument may be pulled straight down, as opposed to twisting with the wrist, for effective scaling in areas such as the maxillary posterior regions.

Criticism of extraoral techniques stems from fear of loss of fulcrum stability, when fulcruming farther away from the working area, when grasping the instrument farther

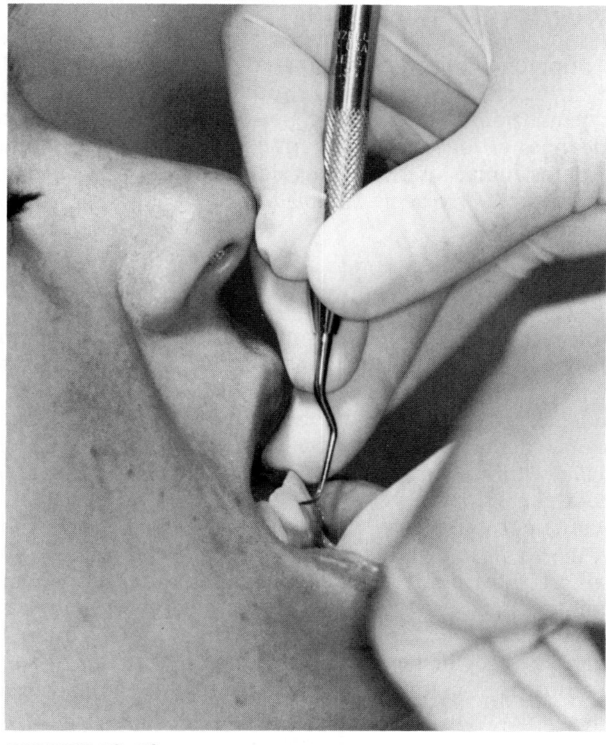

FIGURE 18–19
Same arch fulcrum positioned near area being scaled.

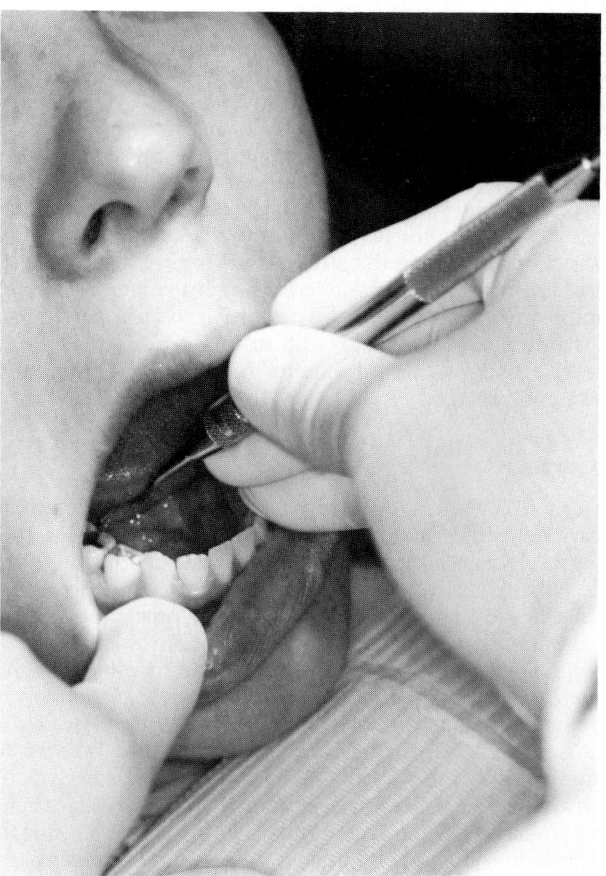

FIGURE 18–20
Cross arch fulcrum is positioned on the same arch but across from area being scaled; fulcrum on opposite quadrant.

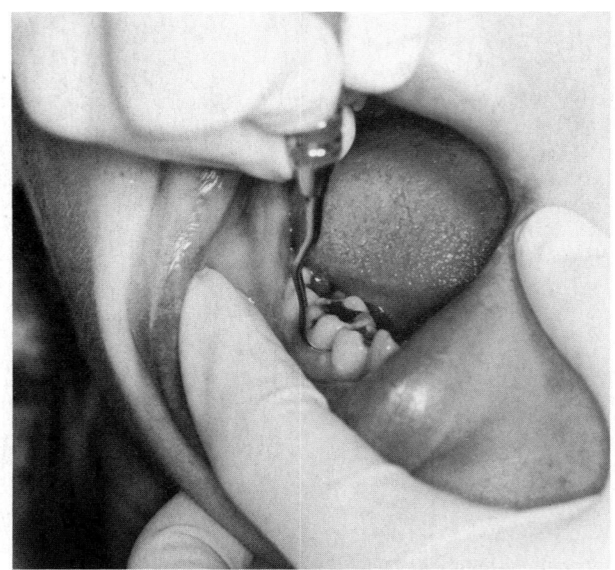

FIGURE 18-21
Opposite arch fulcrum from the arch being scaled.

away from the working end, and/or when stabilizing the instrument against a slightly mobile surface such as the skin rather than on a solid tooth. In reality, fulcruming away from the immediate working area does not necessarily diminish the stability of the fulcrum. Rather, when instrumenting a tooth surface in a deep periodontal pocket, the leverage and, therefore, lateral pressure may be increased and extended throughout the length of a long *working stroke* (scaling or root planing stroke). The loss of control from extending the grasp away from the working end of the instrument can be easily overcome by using reinforcement from the nonworking index finger or thumb to the shank or handle close to the working end of the instrument. Lastly, the extraoral fulcrum allows the operator to change the action of pulling the stroke from the wrist to the lower arm, upper arm, and shoulder. Using instrumentation techniques such as these may be protective to the operator and of significance in avoiding future injury and stress to the nerves, tendons, and ligaments of the dental hygienist's wrist and elbow.

Insertion

Insertion is the act of placing an assessment or treatment instrument into subgingival areas. The purpose of insertion may be to measure the sulcus or pocket depth, to explore the subgingival areas, or to scale and/or root plane subgingival areas. Whatever the purpose is, the procedure must be as atraumatic and accurate as possible. Knowledge of root morphology combined with careful assessment of gingival soft tissues, radiographic interpretation, and appropriate instrument selection is most helpful in achieving these goals.

Assessment instruments are usually thin and pointed for better access into subgingival areas and increased tactile sensitivity. As with all sharp-pointed instruments, extreme care must be taken when the point is inserted directly towards the junctional epithelium. Too much pressure and lack of proper grasp, fulcrum, and contact points with the instrument as it glides down subgingivally may cause perforation through the attachment apparatus. Straight instruments such as the periodontal probe are easily manipulated as long as the side of the tip and the rest of the working end stays close to the root when inserting it. A gentle, delicate touch using fairly light pressure is required when probing or initially exploring subgingivally. With such exploratory strokes, the junctional epithelium offers a moderate amount of resistance, feels slightly elastic to the touch, and gives with a slight amount of pressure from the instrument. Pressure on the instrument may be increased after the topography of the pocket is understood in order to interpret cemental irregularities, calculus, and restorative margins. When inserting a curved explorer, the tip should be pointed apically and the side of the tip should be in contact with the tooth surface being explored. Care must be taken to avoid tissue distension with the rounded bend and to avoid directing the point right at the root surface. Inaccurate deposit assessment and possibly scratching of the root surface result if the pointed tip is directed into the root surface. The only time this is done intentionally is when the dental hygienist suspects root caries or furcation involvement.

Careful insertion of a bladed treatment instrument into subgingival areas essentially involves closing the angle of the cutting edge of the blade relative to the tooth surface to avoid tissue trauma with the opposite side of the blade and to reach the base of the pocket on the downstroke of insertion. With the curet, the closed blade angulation is from 0 to 10 degrees. With sickle scalers that have a sharp-pointed back because of their triangular design, the angulation of insertion is slightly more than 10 degrees, but much less than the more open "working" angulation (which is the angle of the cutting edge of the blade against the tooth that produces a grip or bite to the tooth surface).

Reinsertion is the act of returning the instrument down into the subgingival areas after an assessment or working stroke has been accomplished. The reinsertion stroke angulation is slightly closed compared to that of a working stroke. The working end of the instrument should remain in contact with the tooth until instrumentation is complete. A common error with the reinsertion stroke is the lifting off of the instrument from the tooth surface during the act of reinsertion. The dental hygienist should use the same guidelines of following tooth structure down on reinsertion as in the initial insertion to avoid tissue trauma as well as for accurately replacing the blade for continuous, overlapping strokes.

Adaptation

With regard to pointed assessment instruments, **instrument adaptation** refers to the alignment or placement of the side of the first few millimeters of the periodontal probe or straight explorer against the tooth. With assessment instruments, adaptation is important because it provides the clinician with an accurate measurement or with information about the smoothness of the tooth surface. If the instrument is not well aligned against the tooth surface, it will be off the tooth and into soft tissue. This leads to client discomfort as well as to misinterpretations regarding probing depths and the presence of calculus deposits or cemental irregularities. Only in instances when a tooth surface is being assessed for dental caries is the point or tip of such an instrument used with pressure against the tooth. Assessment instruments such as the periodontal probe and the explorer are always thin, pointed instruments by design to reach deep, sometimes tight subgingival pockets and to facilitate tactile sensitivity. Because they have to reach under

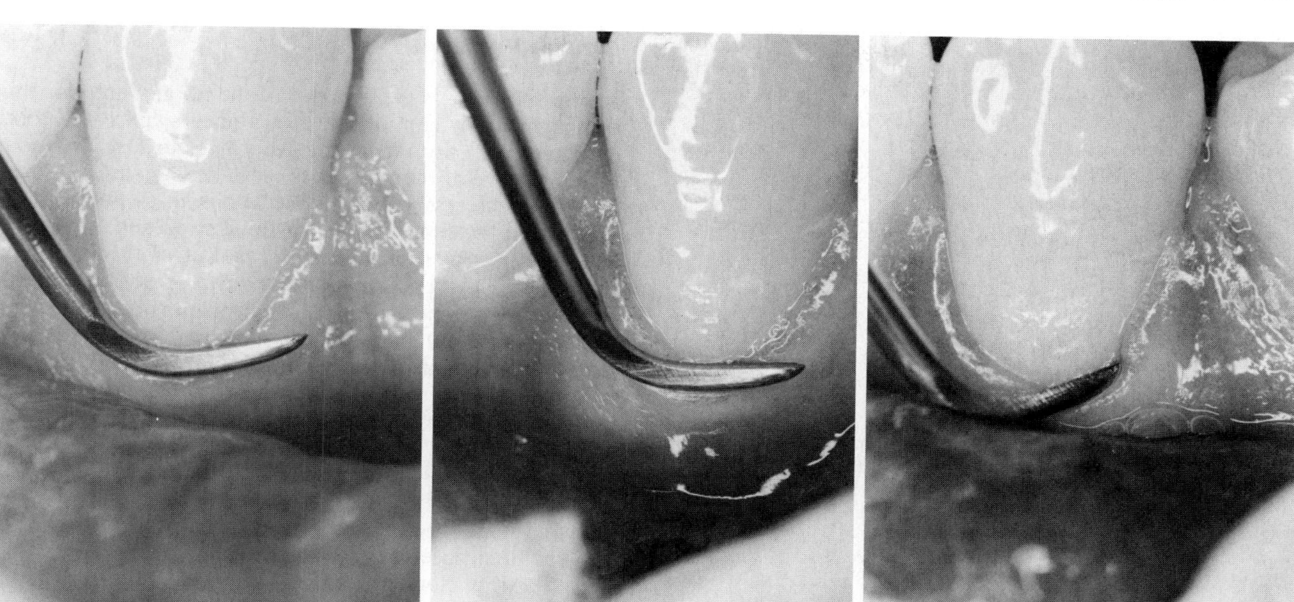

FIGURE 18–22
Comparison of various adaptations of bladed instrument. *A*, Upper third of blade. *B*, Middle third of blade. *C*, Lower third of blade.

tight tooth contacts to detect calculus and into minute pits and fissures to detect dental caries, explorers have fine, delicate working ends. As indicated earlier, the point or tip of an explorer may be used for caries detection. However, the side of the tip must always be in contact with tooth structure to accurately assess the presence of cemental irregularities and acquired deposits and to avoid tissue trauma. The remainder of the explorer's working end should be as closely adapted to the subgingival tooth surface as possible to avoid excessive distension of tissues, excessive pressure against the instrument from the pocket wall, and the possible use of the point for detection instead of the side of the tip of the instrument. There is only one working end with the straight periodontal probe and explorer. Although the correct working end is automatically determined, proper adaptation to the tooth surface must be maintained.

With a bent explorer such as the double-ended pigtail explorer, there is a correct and incorrect working end for different tooth surfaces. The first 2 to 3 mm of the side of the toe (or side of the tip of the instrument) must adapt to an area between the base of the pocket and the contact of the next tooth. The rest of the working end should not excessively distend the sulcular tissues.

With treatment instruments used for scaling and root planing, adaptation is the close relationship of the working blade to the tooth surface. It is a critical component of an effective working stroke. When the working blade is well adapted to the tooth surface, it instruments more root surface than a poorly adapted blade. It also causes less damage to the root surface and/or soft tissues. If only the toe or tip is in contact with the tooth, there is a chance that the tooth surface may become gouged or overinstrumented. If the middle or upper third of the blade is in contact with tooth surface and the lower third is off the tooth, the toe is in an open position and may cause tissue trauma to sulcular epithelium. The adaptation position most effective and causing the least amount of hard or soft tissue damage occurs when the lower third of the working blade remains in contact with the tooth surface during scaling and root planing procedures (Fig. 18–22).

For treatment instruments that have sharp, pointed tips such as sickle scalers, the dental hygienist uses adaptation guidelines similar to those presented for assessment instruments. If the instrument is a simple straight sickle scaler, for example, there is only one end to use. Proper adaptation with the side of the toe to avoid tissue trauma is as important with the sickle scaler as it is with the periodontal probe and the explorer. Proper adaptation is important for meeting the client's need for freedom from pain.

If the sickle scaler has a bent shank and is double-ended, there is definitely one bladed side that is preferable. The correct end produces the closest adaptation of the blade to the tooth surface and maintains a shank position parallel to the plane of the tooth surface being scaled. The angulation (relationship of the cutting edge to the tooth surface) should be between 45 and 90 degrees to the tooth surface (Fig. 18–23).

Adaptation of the curet follows many of the same principles previously discussed. In general, the most desirable portion of the curet blade to contact the tooth surface is the lower third of the blade. However, when broad, flat areas of tooth surface are scaled, the middle third of the blade can be used in addition to the lower third of the blade. Most instrumentation difficulties lie in conforming instruments to the varying convexities and concavities found on tooth structures (see Chapter 19). Especially when instrumenting periodontitis-affected teeth, proper adaptation of the curet blade is a continuing process because of root morphology. Instrumentation is further complicated when there is close root proximity on multiple rooted teeth or from the adjacent tooth. Tooth alignment also complicates procedures, particularly for the novice. In situations such as these, the dental hygienist finds the most successful adaptation is use of the lower third of the blade.

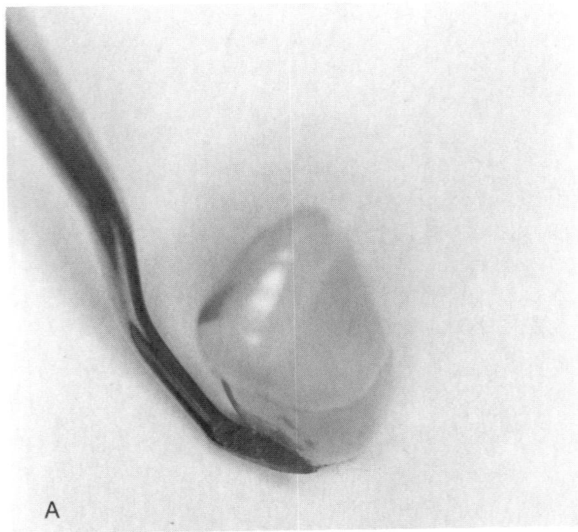

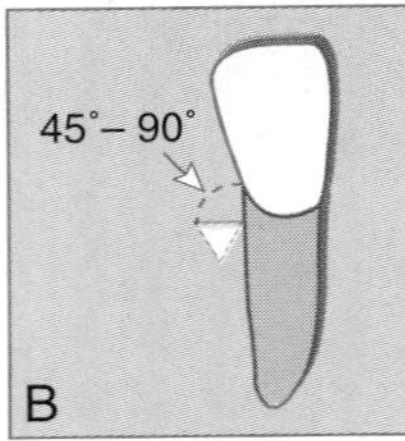

FIGURE 18–23
A and *B*, The correct working angulation of the blade to the tooth should be between 45 and 90 degrees for the sickle scaler.

Angulation

Angulation of a bladed instrument refers to the relationship of the cutting edge to the tooth surface (see Fig. 18–23). Specifically, this is the measurement from the face of the blade to the tooth surface being scaled. An angulation of between 45 and 90 degrees is ideal for removing calculus and planing roots. This standard allows a range of 45 degrees in which to modify the angulation. The closer the angulation is to 45 degrees, the more the instrument cuts or bites into the tooth surface. The closer to 90 degrees, the more the instrument slides over the tooth surface. Therefore, a closer angulation near 45 degrees is recommended when there is heavy deposit to remove and it is necessary to grab the root surface effectively. A more open angulation closer to 90 degrees is recommended when a smoothing, shaving root planing stroke is desired. Just as in performing proper adaptation, it often is necessary to modulate angulation of the blade. An example of such a situation is when there is heavy calculus only at the base of a 6-mm pocket with smooth cementum directly above. Angulation of the blade is closer and the pressure applied is heavier at the base of the pocket to remove the calculus. The angulation is more open and the pressure applied is lighter towards the mouth of the pocket for root planing. The procedure is followed by several more rather open strokes of less than 90 degrees for overall root planing from the junctional epithelium to the cementoenamel junction. Later in this chapter, design of different working instruments and correct angulation interface between the face of the blade and the tooth surface are discussed.

Lateral Pressure

Lateral pressure is the pressure of the tip and anterior third of the working end of the instrument against the tooth. This pressure may range from very light to firm depending on the nature of the roughness on the tooth surface. Therefore, it is necessary to use gradations of pressure during exploratory, scaling, and root planing strokes.

The grasp, fulcrum, and basic control of the instrument must be strengthened as pressure is increased. This is the reason why the beginning dental hygiene student may experience difficulty in physically applying firm lateral pressure. Knowing the correct amount of lateral pressure to apply is a challenging aspect of instrumentation that requires experience, patience, and tactile sensitivity to acquire.

The **exploratory stroke** is used for detection and is usually performed with an explorer or periodontal probe. The curet also may perform an exploratory function to assess the tooth surface during actual scaling or root planing strokes. An exploratory stroke may use light-to-firm lateral pressure. Light lateral pressure during exploration is recommended for detecting light spicules of subgingival calculus. In this case, heavier lateral pressure is insensitive for fine deposit exploration. Situations that require the use of moderate-to-firm pressure during exploration include the detection of flat, burnished calculus or in distinguishing restorative margins from tooth anatomy.

The **scaling stroke** is used for removing calculus from supragingival and subgingival areas. All treatment instruments may be used for gross scaling, but the curet is the instrument of choice for definitive scaling and root planing. As in the exploratory stroke, the lateral pressure used with the scaling stroke ranges from light to firm. The difference, however, is that with the scaling stroke, the magnitude of what is considered firm is far greater during scaling than exploring. During scaling, the action of the instrument may quickly change from a scaling stroke to an exploratory stroke. This change in lateral pressure is done specifically to break off calculus but not to overinstrument a clean area above or below that calculus. It is performed also to assess areas previously scaled without having to stop and pick up an explorer. It is very efficient to be able to work in this manner, and to reserve the actual exploration procedure with an explorer until major areas have been scaled.

The practitioner uses assessment data on pocket depth, tissue tone, bleeding index, and bone loss to determine the degree of periodontal involvement and the probable amount of lateral pressure needed for calculus detection and scaling. Generally, the more periodontally involved the client's teeth are, the more suspicious the dental hygienist should be of local contributing factors such as subgingival calculus. If the calculus occurs in the form of ledges, then any amount of pressure is likely to detect it. If, however, the calculus formation is flat and smooth, medium or even firm exploratory strokes may be necessary to detect the deposit.

The density of the calculus may be determined by radiographs and most accurately by "hardness" when felt with the explorer. Dense calculus appears more radiopaque than lighter, easier-to-remove calculus. Dense calculus feels hard, like tooth structure, as opposed to the porous feel of lighter calculus. In situations where there is dense calculus and naturally grainy or rough root surfaces, the calculus is likely to be embedded into the root surface. Calculus deposits that are both dense and tenacious make scaling significantly more difficult than when calculus deposits are light.

The older and more dense the calculus, usually the more tenacious it is. The practitioner should increase the lateral pressure of the scaling stroke as the tenacity and density of the calculus increases. Too little lateral pressure on instrumentation may cause burnishing of tenacious calculus on cementum. To avoid indiscriminately applying too heavy lateral pressure on instrumentation causing unnecessary gouging and overinstrumentation of root surfaces, the dental hygienist should evaluate the changes occurring on the root surface during instrumentation with the curet using exploratory strokes or by using a dental explorer. Lighter lateral pressure during scaling strokes is indicated for light and easy-to-remove calculus.

The **root planing stroke** is used for shaving embedded calculus from cemental surfaces and smoothing roots. The rationale for root planing lies in the fact that clean, smooth roots are more biologically acceptable for connective tissue reattachment than rough roots. In addition, the client's ability to maintain soft tissue health is improved because bacterial plaque control is made easier when the roots are smooth. Root planing requires extremely good control and dedication to smoothing subgingival surfaces evenly from the junctional epithelium to the cementoenamel junction. Knowledge of root morphology, a sense of the dimensions of this subgingival space, and the area the curet has covered are important to successful root planing. The root planing stroke is a longer stroke than the scaling stroke and may begin with firm lateral pressure if there is significant root roughness to smooth. The change to lighter lateral pressure should occur rather quickly as the curet moves to even out the surface of the cementum.

The thickness of cementum varies but is thinnest at the cervical third of the tooth (0.02 to 0.05 mm). In scaling and root planing tooth structure with such a thin covering of cementum it is easy to visualize how removal of cementum often occurs during indiscriminate root planing, leading to exposure of dentin and dentinal hypersensitivity. To avoid hypersensitive reactions, the dental hygienist should explore the area carefully and discriminately use lateral pressure during scaling and root planing with the purpose of removing only subgingival calculus and altered cementum, smoothing the root surface, and removing as little healthy cementum as possible to achieve good results.

Often the practitioner can visualize subgingival areas by rinsing, removing tissue tags, and retracting gingival tissues with the explorer or curet. If it is not possible to determine how complete the root planing is, the practitioner should compare the smoothness of other areas of the client's mouth with that of the root-planed teeth to assess need for further root planing. If probing depth is minimal and the area is accessible to good oral hygiene techniques, additional scaling may be unnecessary. Where pocket depth is a problem and bacterial plaque control difficult, more root planing may be indicated.

The dental hygienist must analyze the clinical manifestations of the periodontal pathology and decide whether further instrumentation will make a significant difference in light of the client's treatment goals and plan of care. If the area in question is scheduled to receive periodontal surgery, overscaling the area may prove costly in terms of conserving the cementum. If in doubt about whether more instrumentation will make a positive difference, the dental hygienist should refrain from further root planing and reevaluate the area in 2 weeks or at the next maintenance care appointment to determine the client's soft tissue reaction to root roughness.

Stroke Direction

Three basic **stroke directions** are useful for both assessment and treatment instruments:

- The vertical stroke
- The horizontal stoke
- The oblique stroke

It is useful to employ all three or combinations of the three directions for accurate identification of deposit in subgingival areas. Using combinations of different stroke directions is referred to as using a "basketweave of strokes" (Fig. 18–24). This variety is especially useful when using the explorer in assessing deposit or tooth structure. When stroke direction is varied there is a greater possibility that a piece of burnished or smooth calculus may be detected because the instrument may catch one side of the calculus when all other sides may be smooth. Both the explorer and probe are activated beginning with a gentle insertion or downward stroke into the pocket. This exploratory stroke is used as part of the detection process as long as the side of the tip is well adapted to the tooth surface.

The working stroke of the curet, sickle, file, and hoe is performed with a pull stroke. The direction of the pull stroke may be vertical, horizontal, or oblique and it is not directed towards the junctional epithelium. The push or insertion stroke with working pressure is not recommended with treatment instruments because it could potentially violate the integrity of the client's intact junctional epithelium by forcing dental calculus and bacterial plaque through the membrane, potentially causing periodontal abscess formation.

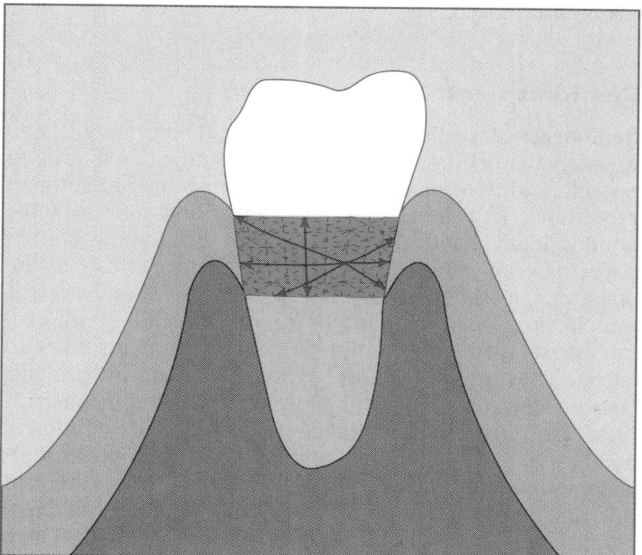

FIGURE 18–24
This diagram illustrates vertical, horizontal, and oblique stroke directions. (Redrawn from Pattison, A., and Pattison, G. Periodontal Instrumentation, 2nd ed. Norwalk, CT: Appleton & Lange, 1992, p. 349.)

Once an efficient stroke direction has been established, it is best to keep moving forward in the direction of the toe of the instrument. Short, overlapping strokes for calculus removal and longer, overlapping strokes for root planing maximize root coverage.

Stroke Length

The **stroke length** is limited by the tissue tone, the morphology of the tooth structure, and client's periodontal probing depth measurements. Loose and inflamed tissue accommodates the movement of long, sweeping, overlapping strokes. However, if the tissue is healthy or fibrotic in tone and positioned tight against the tooth, short, overlapping, well-adapted strokes are indicated to prevent trauma to the tissue.

Short, overlapping strokes and a firmly planted fulcrum provide for good operator-controlled strokes. When managing the curvatures common to most root surfaces, shorter strokes do not pass over deposits in root depressions as easily as longer strokes and therefore are more reliable. On relatively flat areas such as the palatal roots of maxillary molars, however, one may use long stroke lengths and still maintain a controlled, effective movement.

Deep periodontal pockets allow for greater flexibility in stroke length than shallow pockets because of greater root surface area from apical migration of the connective tissue attachment apparatus. When there is recession that has occurred over the lifespan or as a result of surgery there also may be significant root surface. Therefore, with greater pocket depth or more exposed root surface area, it is easier to vary stroke length than when pocket depth is very shallow with little recession.

The scaling stroke to remove calculus is a short pull stroke. The short stroke is best for calculus removal because the increased pressure needed to remove a calculus deposit reduces stroke control. A short stroke facilitates a controlled stroke. For root planing, the stroke length should be increased and the pressure lightened once the calculus has been removed.

Reinforcement

Reinforcement scaling is the use of the nondominant hand to support the instrument or the working hand and to provide additional lateral pressure during instrumentation procedures. In general, the index finger and thumb of the nondominant hand do the work of reinforcing. Either finger or both may be applied to the instrument or to the operator's working hand, usually near the thumb or the muscle area near the thumb **(thenar muscle).** Reinforcements are used only with treatment instruments such as curets. They are not necessary with assessment instruments because control and lateral pressure are not difficult with these instruments. The dental hygienist finds reinforcements useful for additional support and lateral pressure in deep periodontal pockets, particularly when using extended fulcrums (cross arch, opposite arch, and extraoral fulcrums) placed away from the immediate area being scaled. There are several reinforcements that the dental hygienist may use to make scaling easier and more controlled and accurate. Each of these reinforcements is discussed later in this chapter.

Customizing Instrumentation for Periodontitis-affected Teeth

When instrumenting periodontally involved teeth, the method of scaling and root planing varies from one individual to the next because of individual facial anatomy, alignment of teeth, and extent of periodontitis. Some individuals have large dental arches, and others have very small ones; some present with nearly perfect alignment of dentition, and others may have severely overlapping, crowded teeth; and others have limited ability to open their mouth for access into posterior regions. Clients may have normal, healthy periodontium or moderate-to-severe periodontal problems even within the same arch. Each of these general variations requires customization of basic instrumentation technique to treat successfully a particular individual. This procedure for customizing instrumentation in periodontitis-affected individuals allows the dental hygienist to reach almost any area of the mouth, to reach both sulcus areas with minimal probing depth and deep periodontal pockets, and to manage difficult root anatomy with the control and strength needed for effective care. To customize adaptation, angulation, grasp, fulcrum, reinforcement, and operator position for each tooth surface in the mouth, the dental hygiene practitioner should:

1. **Grasp the instrument with a modified pen grasp.** Remember that this is the best grasp when applying a treatment instrument against a tooth surface.
2. **Find the general operator position for the area to be scaled.** Refer to the general operator positions in Tables 18–5 and 18–6).
3. **Find the general fulcrum position for the area to be scaled.** This may be intraoral (same quadrant, cross arch, or opposite arch) or extraoral.
4. **Close angulation and insert the instrument to reach the base of the sulcus or pocket.** This is to avoid trauma and most importantly to reach the bottom of the pocket.
5. **Adapt the instrument to the tooth surface.** Initially adapt at least the first 2 to 3 mm of the blade to the tooth surface.
6. **Angulate the instrument to the tooth surface.** Adjust the angulation of the blade between 45 and 90 degrees for scaling and root planing. The dental hygienist should feel the instrument bite the tooth surface.
7. **Stabilize or firm up the grasp to the instrument handle.** During the manipulations that occur while adapting and angulating the instrument to the tooth surface, the grasp may have changed. Because the handle is positioned for the tooth surface, it changes the angulation if the handle is moved back to the original grasp; therefore, the position of the grasp must be adjusted to the new position of the instrument handle.
8. **Establish a firm fulcrum.** The hand may now be in a slightly different position than it began when the general fulcrum position was found. Within the space of this new-found position that the grasp has moved into, a stable fulcrum position may be established. This fulcrum may be moved to the opposite arch or to an extraoral position because many times the fulcrum close to the area being scaled does not allow correct adaptation and angulation.
9. **Establish a stable and comfortable operator position to facilitate unit movement.** The practitioner moves his body position so that the hand, arm, and possibly the shoulder are in line with the direction of the stroke and can move as

one unit. This helps distribute the workload and mitigates the stress on the hands and wrist. The body position may range from 8:00 to 4:00 for both the right- and left-handed clinician, depending on the area to be scaled.

10. **Apply reinforcement with the nondominant hand as needed.** The further the fulcrum is from the area being scaled, the more useful reinforcement with the nondominant hand becomes. The reinforcement hand can provide stabilization, additional pressure, additional pulling strength, support for the client in opening his mouth, and retraction of lips and buccal mucosa.

11. **Initiate the working stroke.** This action should be the final step of the sequence after all previous actions have been satisfied.

Much of the clinician's success with this customizing procedure depends on finding the correct fulcrum. To accomplish this, the dental hygienist must be able to fulcrum intraorally near the tooth being scaled, cross arch, opposite arch, or on the index finger or thumb of the nondominant hand, or find a comfortable position using extraoral fulcrums. Moreover, the dental hygienist must feel free to use reinforcement techniques during scaling procedures. If the shape of the tooth surface changes to the degree that this position no longer works, the process must be repeated from that point and possibly the fulcrum altered to accommodate the change. With experience, the entire process becomes second nature and adjustments may be made within seconds.

Table 18–8 illustrates the steps in accomplishing an effective stroke that is adjusted to work with the plane of the tooth surface being scaled versus a more traditional method of instrumentation that is based on setting the fulcrum first. The latter method of setting the fulcrum first does not allow for variations in probing depths or alterations in root anatomy, which affect the amount and direction of lateral pressure that can be applied to the root surface. For instance, as probing depth increases on the distal aspect of a mandibular molar from 3 mm to 10 mm, the dental hygienist may find a change in the plane of the root surface from a vertical to a slightly more oblique or horizontal inclination. In subgingival instrumentation of periodontitis-affected teeth, such slight changes in the plane of a tooth surface alter stroke effectiveness. By setting the fulcrum first and not readjusting the fulcrum as the instrument maneuvers into pocket depth, the practitioner is limited in producing effective lateral pressure.

TABLE 18–8
CUSTOMIZING INSTRUMENTATION TO THE ROOT SURFACE OF PERIODONTITIS-AFFECTED TEETH

Noncustomized Basic Instrumentation Technique	Customized Instrumentation Technique
Grasp instrument	Grasp instrument
Establish fulcrum	Establish "general" operator position
Close angulation and insert instrument into pocket	Establish "general" fulcrum position
Adapt instrument to tooth surface	Close angulation and insert instrument into pocket
Angulate instrument to tooth surface	Adapt instrument to tooth surface
Apply reinforcement as needed	Angulate instrument to tooth surface
Initiate working stroke	Position grasp to instrument handle
	Reestablish fulcrum
	Reestablish operator position
	Apply reinforcement as needed
	Initiate working stroke

Instrument Sharpening

Rationale

The major objective of **instrument sharpening** is to restore blade sharpness while preserving the original contours and angles of the instrument. In theory, the objective and procedure appear straightforward; in reality, consistent excellent instrument sharpening is a difficult skill requiring intimate knowledge of blade design, accuracy, and practice. Sharpening techniques are further complicated by differences in types of instrument.

Prior to learning sharpening techniques, it is often valuable to examine the design of each new instrument before using it. Attention to the angle of the lateral surface of the blade to the flat face as well as the possible curvature of the blade is important. Absence of a bevel along the cutting edge and a consequent inability to reflect light if shined upon it—signs of a sharp cutting edge—also should be observed. Testing for sharpness by feeling the way the new instrument blade grips a testing stick at working angulation also is a good method of establishing a reference point for future testing for sharpness of the cutting edge and understanding the sharpening objective.

The basic clinical outcome of using sharp versus dull instruments is delineated in Table 18–9. By using sharp instruments, the practitioner improves the comfort level of the client and decreases operator fatigue by working to remove dental deposits effectively. Effective instrumentation meets the human needs for freedom from pain and stress and for safety. Moreover, sharp instruments are easier to control than are dull instruments because, unlike dull instruments, they do not slip easily over tooth surfaces.

To maintain effectiveness and quality of care for the client, at the first sign of instrument dullness, the dental hygienist should sharpen the instrument. Methods for sharpening individual instruments are discussed under each instrument subheading.

TABLE 18–9
CLINICAL OUTCOMES USING SHARP VERSUS DULL INSTRUMENTS

Outcome	Sharp Instrument	Dull Instrument
Tactile sensitivity	Increased	Decreased
Working efficiency	Increased	Decreased
Lateral pressure	Decreased	Increased
Probability of burnished calculus	Decreased	Increased

Sharpening Stones

Various natural and synthetic stones are available for sharpening dental instruments (Fig. 18–25). The sharpening stone is composed of abrasive crystals that are harder than the metal of the instrument. The Arkansas stone is an example of a natural stone with a fine texture that is manufactured in a variety of shapes for sharpening instruments. Conical and cylindrical Arkansas stones are available for sharpening the face of curets, a practice that tends to weaken the blade. The India stone also is a natural stone that comes in a medium texture. Natural stones such as the Arkansas and India are usually lubricated with clear, fine oil to facilitate the movement across the stone, reduce friction, and reduce the problem of metallic particles embedding into the surface of the stone. Petrolatum may be used in place of oil and is water-soluble, which makes clean-up prior to sterilization easier than with an oiled stone.

Synthetic stones used for instrument sharpening are the ruby and carborundum stones. The ruby stone is a mounted rotary stone and the carborundum stone is manufactured as a hand-held rectangular stone with rounded edges that may be adapted to the face of a curet. Both of these stones are coarse and are lubricated with water.

Sharpening stone selection is primarily determined by the amount of sharpening required to reestablish a cutting edge. Fine stones such as the Arkansas or medium-textured India stones are preferable for the novice or for sharpening during client treatment when little sharpening is required for reestablishment of a cutting edge. Coarsely surfaced stones remove metal at a faster rate than finely surfaced stones and should be used on instruments requiring significant recontouring. Less pressure, fewer strokes, and greater accuracy are needed with coarsely textured stones. Rotary-mounted stones, such as the ruby stone, are considerably more abrasive than coarse hand-held stones because the stone is mounted on a metal mandrel and used in a motor-driven handpiece. For this reason, the mounted rotary stone should be used only when major recontouring of dental instruments is required. Lack of good control, friction, and rapid wearing of the instrument are disadvantages of the rotary-mounted stone.

Instrument Sharpening Technique

To begin sharpening procedures, the proper stone must be selected for the amount of sharpening to be done. The stone must first be properly sterilized (if the instruments are to be used directly on a client) and lubricated. The technique for using hand-held sharpening stones is performed by:

- Moving the instrument over the stone, or
- Moving the stone over the instrument

Using either method, the movement is initiated by the operator's dominant hand. The first technique is recommended for sharpening flat surfaces as found on the hoe or sickle scaler. The second technique is recommended for sharpening curets. To guard against accidental injury during sharpening when moving the stone against the instrument, care must be observed in length of stroke, grasp of stone, and grasp of instrument. Short, even, continuous strokes tend to keep the instrument on the stone. The hand holding the instrument should assume a palm-thumb grasp and be supported against a firm object such as a cabinet top, or the operator's own elbow may be pulled close to the body to support the wrist and hand holding the instrument. The fingers holding the stone should not be wrapped around the stone on the long side exposed to the cutting surface, but positioned behind the cutting surface or at the short ends of the stone (Fig. 18–26).

Prior to initiating the sharpening stroke, proper angulation of the stone to the surface of the instrument is assumed and continuous sharpening motions at this constant angle are made across the length of the cutting edge. (Correct angulation of stone to cutting surface will be discussed under each individual instrument.) The amount of pressure applied should be determined by the amount of recontouring necessary to produce a sharp blade. The

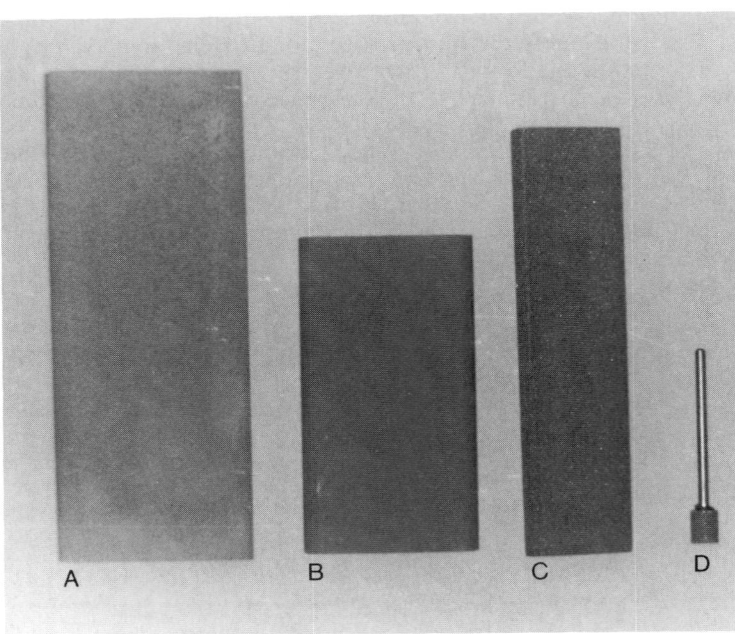

FIGURE 18–25
Arkansas stone (A), India stone (B), Carborundum stone (C), mounted rotary ruby stone (D).

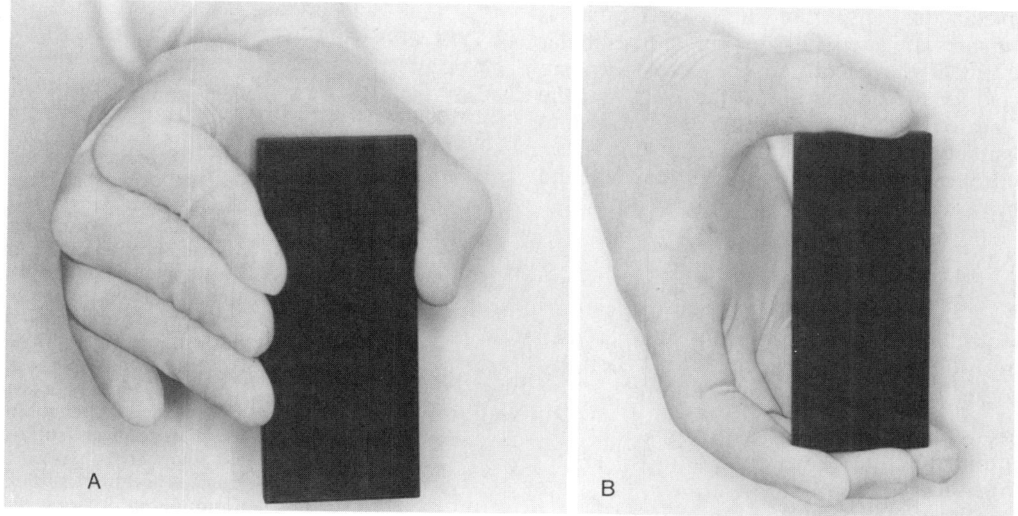

FIGURE 18–26
A, Incorrect finger position on stone; fingertips are exposed to possible injury if stone slips. *B*, Correct finger position on stone.

greater the pressure exerted against the blade with the stone, the more metal is removed. Prudent advice for instrument conservation is to limit sharpening procedures to only what is necessary. The last sharpening stroke(s) should be away from the face of the instrument in a downward motion to remove small metal particles or flash that adhere to the edges of the instrument. The practitioner should wipe the blade with a 2 × 2 gauze square to aid in removing oil and metal shavings floating on the surface of the instrument.

Testing for sharpness may be done by visual inspection or by comparing the sharpness before and after the procedure using a plastic testing stick. When using visual inspection, it is important to have a strong light such as the dental light for viewing. With this test the sharp instrument does not reflect light at the junction between the face and the lateral side of the instrument. In contrast, the dull instrument is beveled on the cutting edge and reflects light back to the observer. The tactile test requires the use of a hard plastic stick that engages the blade of the instrument at proper working angulation. It is important when using this method to test the instrument fully across the length of the blade and to resharpen any area that allows the instrument to slip over the stick.

When testing for sharpness, the dental hygienist also should examine the shape of the sharpened blade. To protect the client against unnecessary instrument breakage, all instruments that have lost their original strength or are too fine to remove heavy deposit or reach deep pockets should no longer be used in such areas. Instruments that have been sharpened down and are of moderate or fine dimensions may be used for the healthier individual with little calculus formation and shallower probing depths. The instrument is retipped or finally discarded when it is no longer functional or is of danger to the client from possible breakage.

Managing Instrument Tip Breakage

When an instrument breaks subgingivally, only the tip breaks off, leaving it for the dental hygienist to locate. To retrieve the small metal fragment, it is essential that the dental hygienist stop instrumentation as soon as the instrument tip has broken and inform the client. Slow-speed or high-speed aspiration (suction) should be discontinued and the client should use a cup to expectorate into (in case the tip is floating in saliva) until the tip is found. Techniques for locating the broken piece include reinstrumentation with another instrument, use of magnetic-tip Periotrievers shaped like thick explorers or probes (Fig. 18–27), and open flap periodontal surgery. Radiographic examination is helpful during these exploration processes for more accurate identification of the metal tip. It should be noted that even new instruments, especially curets, break if they are lodged in a tight area such as under a contact and are twisted or pulled in a direction in which the toe may not be released. If the broken tip cannot be clinically located or if it is not visible on a radiograph of the area, the dental hygienist should suspect that the tip may be outside of the

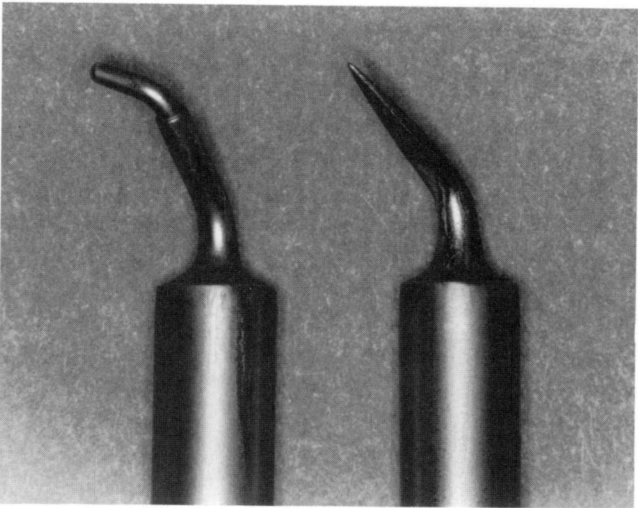

FIGURE 18–27
Magnetic broken tip retrievers (Schwartz periotrievers).

sulcus. A complete visual inspection of the oral cavity is begun. Gauze squares are used to wipe out the vestibular areas and areas under the client's tongue. They then are carefully inspected for the broken tip. In the event that the tip cannot be located, a chest radiograph is indicated to rule out the possibility that the client has aspirated it.

Infection control methods used with instruments and sharpening stones are presented in Chapter 9.

MOUTH MIRROR

The dental mouth mirror is an important adjunct used during all phases of the dental hygiene process. Basically, the mirror performs four functions (Table 18-10):

- Indirect vision
- Indirect illumination
- Transillumination
- Retraction of tissues and tongue

Moistening the face of the mouth mirror by gently rubbing it against the buccal mucosa or dipping it in a commercial mouthwash prevents the mirror from fogging up.

TABLE 18-11
TYPES OF MOUTH MIRROR SURFACES

Type	Advantages and Disadvantages
Front surface	The mirror surface is on the front of the glass, therefore, the image produced is simply the mirror image of the area reflected. This mirror is the most commonly used because there is no distortion or magnification of the image
Concave surface	Causes magnification of the image. Because each movement of the instrument visualized with this mirror is magnified, the operator needs to learn to relate the scale of movement and the image differently from the way it actually appears. This is much more difficult and confusing to learn to use than the front-surface mirror. It does not allow the operator to see as wide a range as the front surface and causes distortion, even dizziness for some clinicians. Not recommended unless eye strain or vision is a significant problem
Flat surface	The image appears doubled or shadowed. Not recommended for periodontal procedures

TABLE 18-10
FUNCTIONS OF DENTAL MOUTH MIRROR

Function	Reason for Use
Indirect vision	The most difficult function of the four to master and work with. Reflection in mirror provides indirect vision of area. Use when it is too difficult to view the tooth or area directly such as the distal surfaces of last molars or when a direct vision approach requires an awkward or strenuous operator position
Indirect illumination	Use to catch more of the light and direct increased illumination to intraoral areas. Additional light is reflected onto working area. When the mirror is being used in this capacity, it cannot be used for indirect vision at the same time. Therefore, operator and client position must be adjusted for direct-vision scaling
Transillumination	Use to reflect light back onto anterior tooth surfaces, which are thin enough to allow light to pass through. Essentially a shadowing technique for visualization of anterior teeth. In doing so, areas of various density or darkness such as dental caries and calculus will contrast and be readily visible
Retraction	A pulling away of soft tissue for illumination, visualization, and protection of client's tissue. Use with the face of the mirror towards the buccal mucosa, lips, or tongue to retract tissues for light to illuminate the working area and or protect the soft tissues during instrumentation. The face of the mirror should be turned towards the working area to provide indirect vision while at the same time retracting soft tissue

The traditional mouth mirror is composed of two parts: (1) handle, and (2) mirror, each with a threaded design or cone socket attachment. The handle and mirror components should be separated, washed, and autoclaved after each appointment. Unlike the mirror heads which eventually become clouded or scratched, handles rarely need to be replaced. Wrapping the mirror heads separately during sterilization minimizes some of the scratching.

Mirror heads come in a variety of sizes from 5/8- to 2-inch diameters. Mirror size selection should be made by the size of the client's mouth, the operator's ability to place the mirror and instrument within a confined space, and the operator's comfort in holding and using a certain size mirror head. In addition to mirror size, there are three types of mirror faces to choose from (Table 18-11):

- Front surface
- Concave surface
- Flat surface

The mouth mirror generally is held with a modified pen grasp; however, other grasps also may be used. The pads of the thumb, index, and middle fingers all rest on the shank and handle of the instrument with the modified pen grasp. It is the most stable grasp because the pads of the thumb and fingers are controlling the instrument. Because of its stability, the modified pen grasp should be used when there is resistance to the mirror head such as during the retraction of buccal mucosa or the tongue (Fig. 18-28).

When there is no resistance, and indirect vision, indirect illumination, or transillumination are the goals, the standard pen grasp is adequate and perhaps desirable. The standard pen grasp yields a very loose grasp that generally allows easy, fluid movement of the mirror head around the mouth. This range of movement is beneficial when examining or comparing large oral areas (Fig. 18-29).

To hold the mouth mirror for indirect vision or illumination as well as reinforce with the nondominant hand, the mirror must be held between the middle and ring fingers.

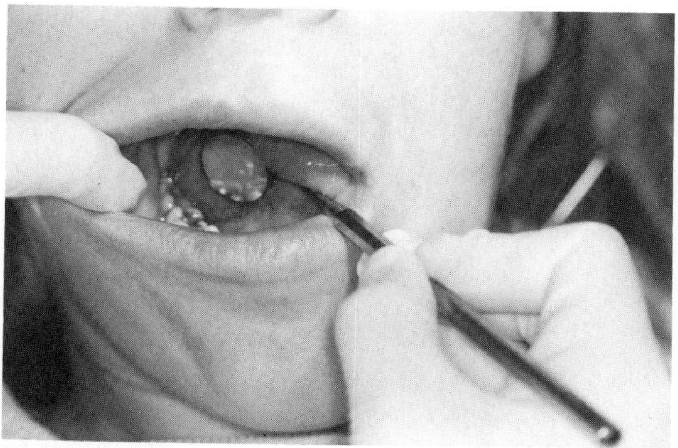

FIGURE 18–28
The modified pen grasp is used for stability when there is resistance (e.g., the tongue) against the mirror head.

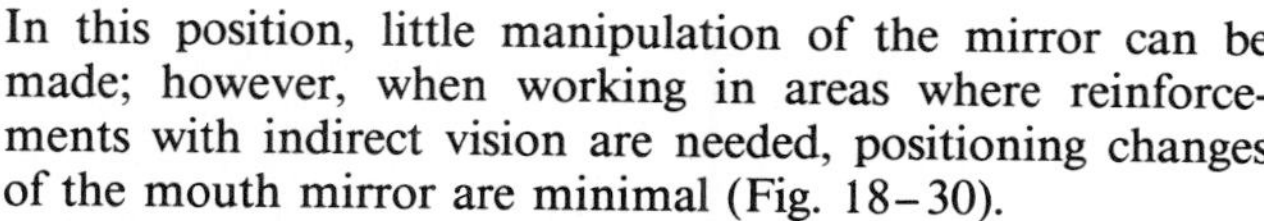

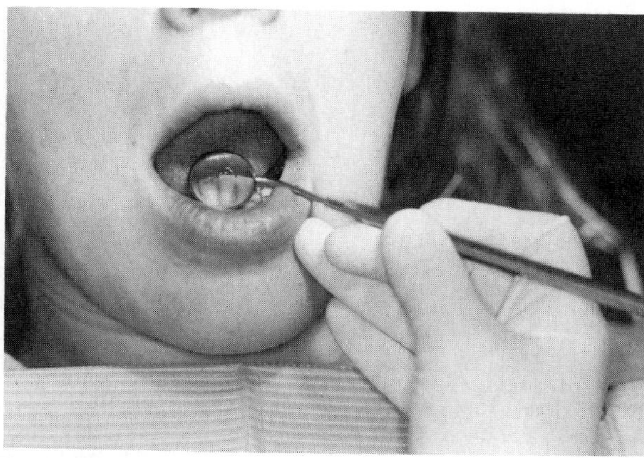

FIGURE 18–29
A looser standard pen grasp is adequate for visualization of illuminated areas.

In this position, little manipulation of the mirror can be made; however, when working in areas where reinforcements with indirect vision are needed, positioning changes of the mouth mirror are minimal (Fig. 18–30).

Because the mouth mirror is the instrument routinely used for retraction, care must be taken to avoid tissue trauma with the handle or shank of the instrument, particularly at the corners of the mouth. This injury may be as slight as soreness to initiation of herpetic lesions on the client's lips and commissures. Trauma can be avoided by maintaining less pressure on stretched lips. In addition, the mouth mirror should never be allowed to rest on sublingual tissue because doing so causes discomfort to the client. Figure 18–31 illustrates a less traumatic method of mouth mirror use. The index finger also may be an excellent alternative for retraction when the operator wishes to avoid using the mouth mirror.

PERIODONTAL PROBE (see Chapter 13)

Design and Use

The periodontal probe is a slender, tapered, blunt instrument with millimeter markings used to determine:

- Probing depth
- Clinical attachment level
- Relative attachment level
- Amount of attached gingiva
- Gingival recession
- Furcation invasion
- Bleeding on probing
- Size of atypical or pathological lesions
- Distance between teeth

In each of these cases, the calibrated markings or tissue response (bleeding) are noted and recorded in the client's record (Table 18–12).

Variations in millimeter markings, as well as other design differences, are found among manufacturers. For example, the Marquis probe is marked at the 3-, 6-, 9-, and 12-mm intervals, the Williams probe is marked at the 1-, 2-, 3-, 5-, 7-, 8-, and 9-mm intervals. Differences in markings and shapes among probes are shown in Figure 18–32. Some probes are color-coded for ease in reading. Personal operator preference determines selection of interval and color-coded markings of the periodontal probe. In the case of dental implants, which require the use of plastic probes, safety against potential injury and scratching the titanium implants determines instrument selection (see Chapter 28).

Shape (round and tapered to flat and tapered) and thickness of the periodontal probe also may differ among manufacturers. When the probe design is flat and too thick or wide, it is difficult to manipulate the instrument into and around narrow, tight areas for accurate measurement. Conversely, if the probe is too fine and sharp, there is danger of trauma and perforation through the nonkeratinizing junctional epithelium resulting in inaccurate readings. If too fine a probe is selected, client comfort and safety become important factors to consider. Thin instruments are also subject to bending and damage during sterilization procedures.

Variations in shank design of the periodontal probe are shown in Figure 18–33. This periodontal probe (Hu-Friedy Novatech) design features a right-angle tip that is color-coded. It offers ease of access in posterior distal surfaces.

Probing depth is the measurement of the distance between the gingival margin and the base of the sulcus or

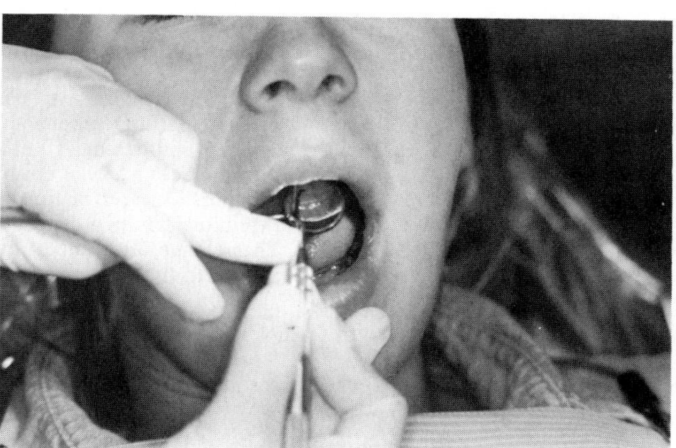

FIGURE 18–30
Use of the mirror hand for mirror placement and reinforcement of scaling instrument.

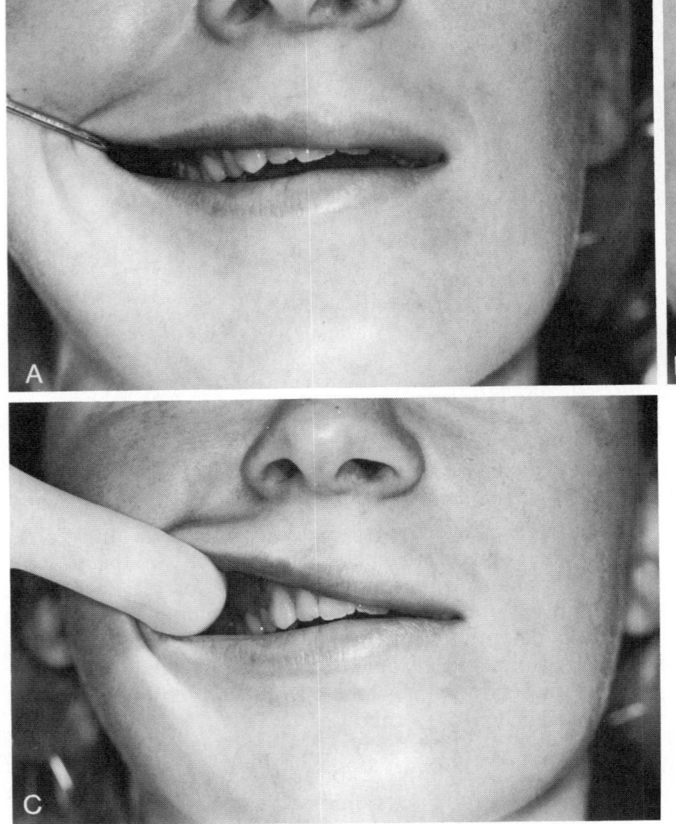

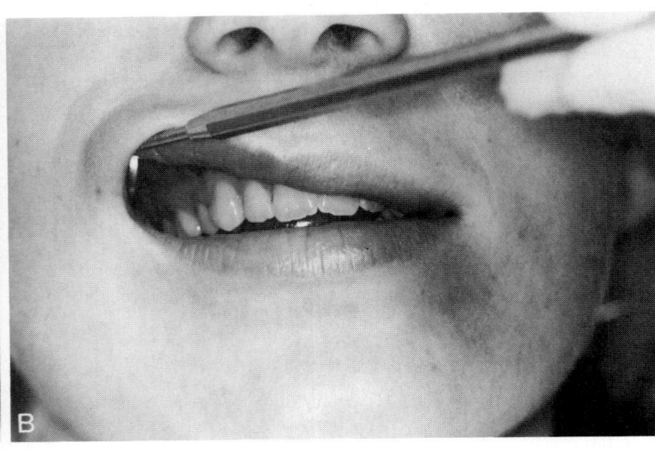

FIGURE 18–31
A, Mouth mirror is traumatic to corners of the mouth. *B*, Mouth mirror is positioned with less trauma to the corner of the mouth. *C*, Index finger is used in place of the mouth mirror for retraction.

TABLE 18–12
PERIODONTAL PROBE: USE, TECHNIQUE, AND SIGNIFICANCE OF RESULTS

Used for Measurement of	Technique and Significance of Results
Probing depth	Measures probing depth from marginal gingiva to junctional epithelium. The instrument is held with a modified pen grasp and a fulcrum is established. Because the technique does not involve significant control or pressure, the fulcrum may be extended crossarch or even extraorally for better access into posterior areas. The technique involves "walking" the tip, keeping the side of the tip and as much of the length of the instrument against the tooth and as parallel as possible. The tip is tilted into the center of the interproximal regions with the side close to the contact region. Six measurements are taken around each tooth (distofacial, facial, mesiofacial, distolingual, lingual, and mesiolingual). The deepest measurements are recorded for each surface. Within any sextant, it is easier to record all facial surfaces, then all lingual surfaces. Probing depth is an important indicator of past disease activity
Clinical attachment level	The clinical attachment level is the measurement from the cementoenamel junction to the junctional epithelium. The technique is similar to probing depth, except that the depth is measured from the junctional epithelium to a fixed reference point. When measuring from a fixed reference point, a clearer picture of bone loss can be determined, especially when there is recession and minimal probing depths
Relative attachment level	The relative attachment level is the measurement from a fixed reference point on the tooth or a stent to the junctional epithelium. The technique is similar to assessing probing depth and offers a record of a past disease activity
Amount of attached gingiva	The attached gingiva is the keratinized stratified squamous epithelium firmly attached to the cementum and alveolar bone. To measure the amount of attached gingiva, the base of facial or lingual probing depth (on the mandible) is measured, recorded, and visualized as it might appear on top of the attached gingiva. From this topographical line of the junctional epithelium, the surface of the attached gingiva is measured down to the line of the mucogingival junction. This is the amount of attached gingiva. Adequate attached gingiva is an important safeguard against future mucogingival defects and recession when there is bone loss
Gingival recession	Gingival recession is the measurement from the gingival margin to the cementoenamel junction. This measurement is another indicator of apical migration of the attachment apparatus

TABLE 18–12
PERIODONTAL PROBE: USE, TECHNIQUE, AND SIGNIFICANCE OF RESULTS *Continued*

Used for Measurement of	Technique and Significance of Results
Furcation invasion	Furcation invasion is classified in the following manner: Class I: The probe detects the curvature of the roots and furcation but cannot extend more than 1 mm under the furcation Class II: The probe extends more than 1 mm under the furcation, but does not pass through the furcation Class III: The probe passes through between the roots under the furcation because there is no bone or tissue attached under the furcation. In the case of mandibular molars, the tip of the instrument passes clear through from facial to lingual or vice versa. In maxillary facial molar furcations, the palatal root is felt The periodontal probe may be used to detect, measure, and classify the degree of furcation invasion. The No. 2 Nabor's probe is a specialized probe used for furcation detection and classification. Its curved shank and blunted end make it ideal for detection of furcations interproximally. Detection of furcation invasion is critical to the therapy and long-term prognosis of the tooth and adjacent bone
Bleeding on probing	Observation of bleeding on light probing should be noted because it is a primary clinical indicator of gingival inflammation
Pathological lesions	An important aspect of oral pathology is an accurate description of the size and shape of the lesion. The periodontal probe is an excellent and readily available instrument for measurement of pathological lesions
Distance between teeth	The periodontal probe may be used to measure the distance between teeth (diastema), overjet, and migration of teeth with severe periodontal disease

pocket. Three models have been used to describe the episodic nature of periodontal destruction:

- Continuous paradigm
- Random burst theory
- Asynchronous multiple burst hypothesis

These have challenged the concept of the validity of using probing depth as a measurement of disease activity. More accurately, this form of measurement represents a record of past disease activity and is used for monitoring the client's response to care.

Degree of probe tip inaccuracy is related to probe design, pressure applied, contour of the tooth, contour of the periodontal defect, degree of inflammation, and accompanying loss of collagen fibers. Various pressure-controlled measuring devices have been developed and are used to standardize research methodologies but are cumbersome and inconvenient for the practicing dental hygienist.

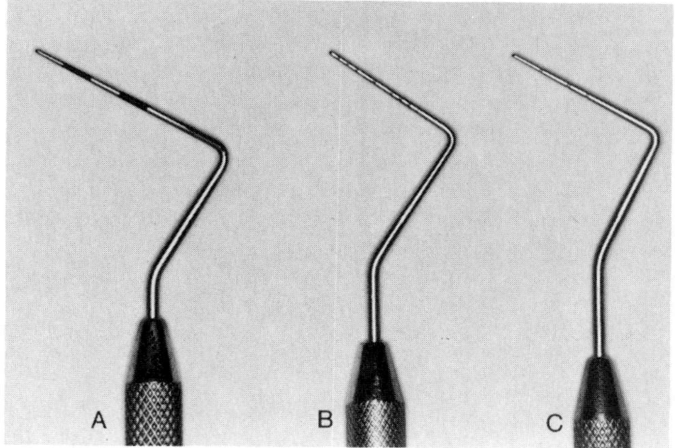

FIGURE 18–32
Examples of periodontal probes. Note the differences in markings. *A*, Marquis color-coded probe with markings at intervals of 3, 6, 9, and 12 mm. *B*, Williams probe with marking at intervals of 1, 2, 3, 5, 7, 8, 9, and 10 mm. *C*, Michigan "O" probe with markings at intervals of 3, 6, and 8 mm.

The readings are recorded for the deepest areas of the distolingual, lingual, mesiolingual, distofacial, facial, and mesiofacial surfaces of each tooth. Thus, each tooth should have six probe depth recordings. Probing depths of 4 mm or more represent periodontal pockets.[8] When probing the full mouth, the practitioner should begin the probing sequence from the distal surface. The periodontal probe may be held with a pen grasp or a modified pen grasp because control and sensitivity may be accomplished with either grasp. The dental hygienist should select any intraoral or extraoral fulcrum that allows access into the area being assessed. The instrument is advanced by moving up and down and forward in 1- to 2-mm increments, gently inserting to the junctional epithelium on each downstroke. The least amount of trauma to the client occurs when the side of the probe maintains contact with the tooth during stroke activation. When using a flat-shaped periodontal probe, it is important for the operator to keep the flat side of the instrument against the tooth. For accuracy of interproximal readings, the probe should be slightly angled to examine the site under the col area and at the same time positioned vertically to touch the contact between the adjacent teeth (Fig. 18–34). Measurement of the probing depth is made by reading the marking on the probe where the gingival margin lies or by adding the increments above the gingival margin and subtracting from the total number of markings on the probe.

Measurement of the *clinical attachment level* is "the relative probing depth corresponding to the distance from the cemento-enamel junction (CEJ) to the location of a periodontal probe tip."[9] Like the measurement of probing depth, clinical attachment level is a measurement of the consequences of periodontitis and not a measurement of current disease activity. Longitudinal monitoring of probing attachment level is a reliable method for determining the stability of the periodontal supporting structures.

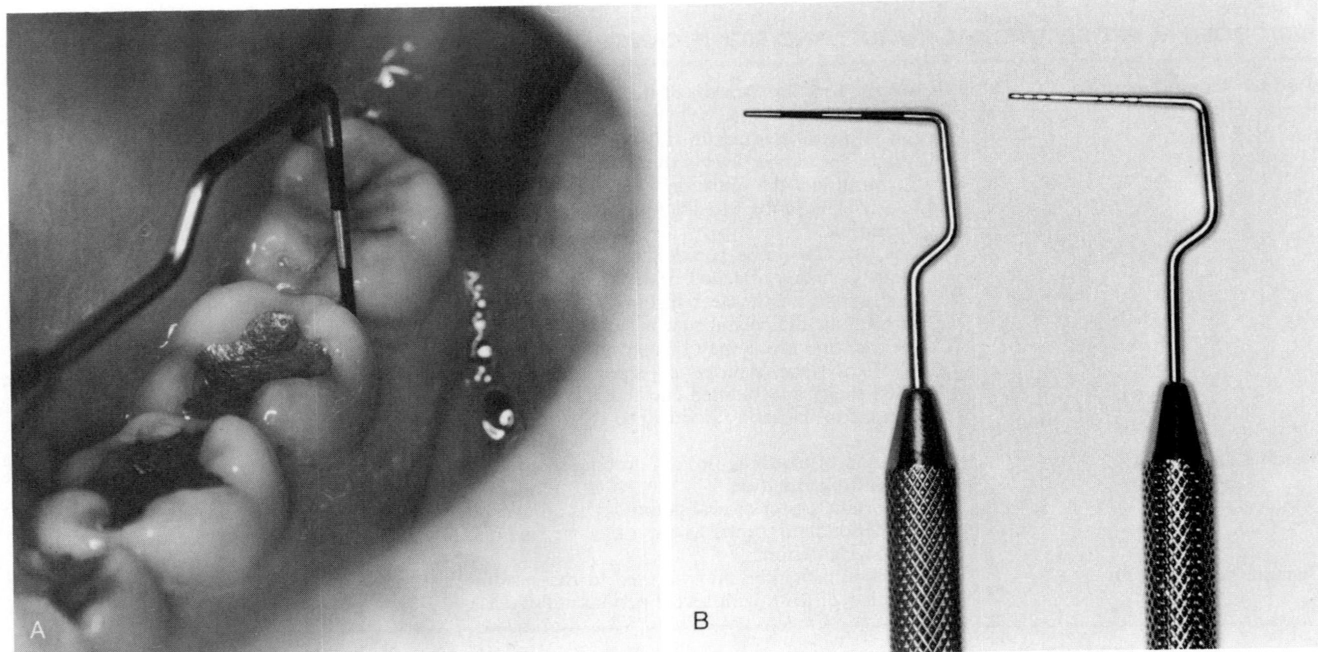

FIGURE 18–33
A, The Hu-Friedy Novatech periodontal probe with its upward bend is designed for access in posterior areas. *B*, The type of probe tip may differ, as illustrated in this photograph.

The *relative attachment level* is "the distance from a fixed reference point on the tooth surface (such as the CEJ) or a stent to the location of a periodontal probe tip."[9] Like measurement of probing depth and clinical attachment level, it offers a historical measurement of disease activity.

Adequacy of attached gingiva is determined with the periodontal probe by observing the mucogingival junction, measuring the distance from the mucogingival junction to the gingival margin, measuring pocket depth, and calculating the difference between the two. *Gingival recession* is simply the distance measured from the cementoenamel junction to the gingival margin.

The No. 2 Nabor's probe is a specialized probe used for the detection and classification of furcations. Because classification of furcation involvement (Classes I, II, III) is based on the degree of penetration of a probe between the roots of multirooted teeth, the Nabor probe, with its curved shank and blunted tip, is well suited for subgingival

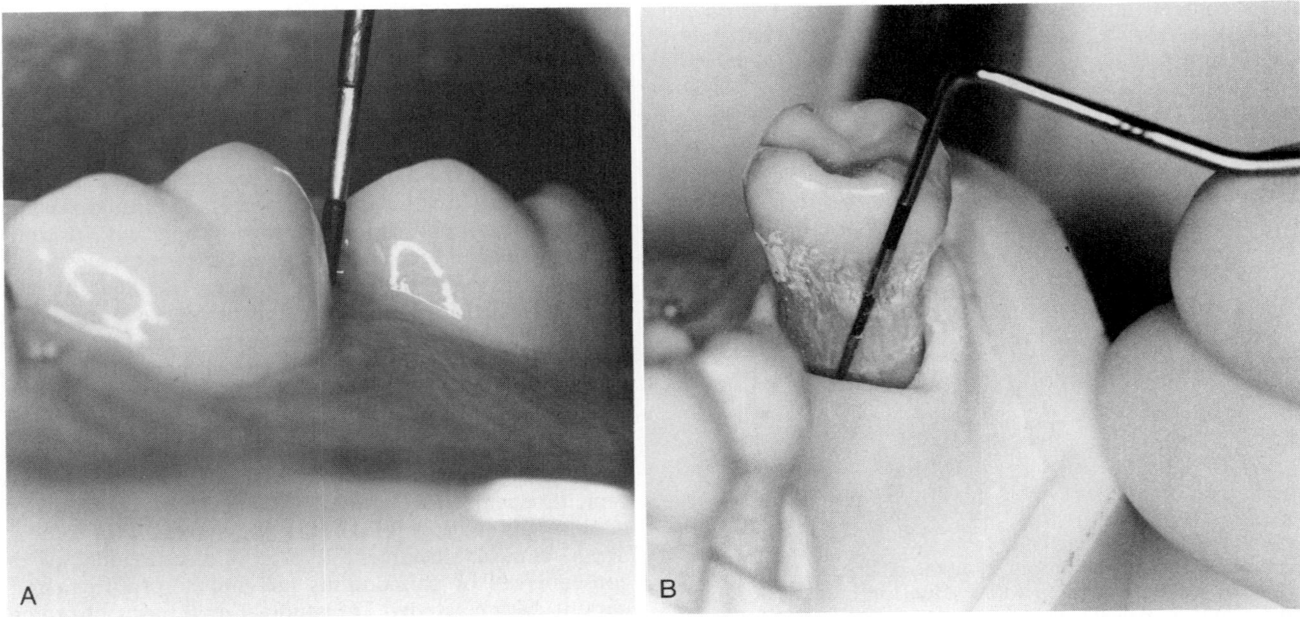

FIGURE 18–34
A and *B*, For proximal readings, the periodontal probe is slightly angled under the col and positioned vertically to touch the contact area between the adjacent teeth.

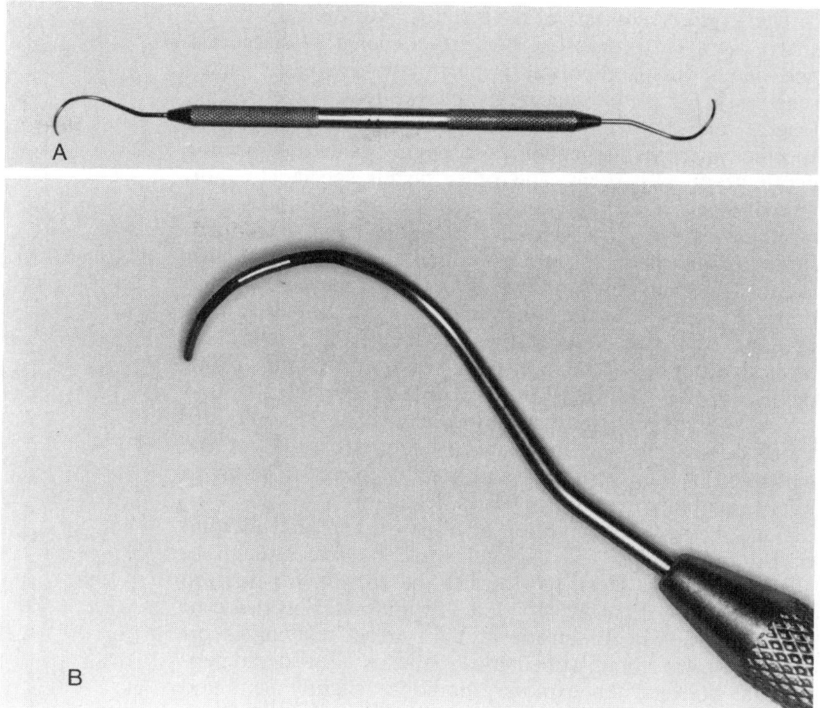

FIGURE 18–35
A and *B*, Nabor's probe is plain or color-coded (as shown) and is used for furcation classification.

insertion and furcation classification. The color-coded Nabor probe allows the clinician to more accurately classify furcations and is shown as a color-coded Nabor probe in Figure 18–35.

The blunted tip of the periodontal probe makes it ideal to determine (but not measure) bleeding tendencies on probing. If gentle probing elicits bleeding, this observation should be noted on the client's record as a clinical indication of inflammation. Gingival bleeding is associated with significant increases in spirochetes, motile bacterial forms, and increased flow of gingival crevicular fluid.[10–12] However, evidence of bleeding has been shown to have only a 30% predictive value in determining future clinical attachment loss. Cessation of bleeding has been related to a significant reduction in gingival inflammation and is used to monitor the effects of periodontal treatment.[13,14]

By compressing the side of the probe tip against the attached gingiva, the dental hygienist may atraumatically evaluate tissue tone, collecting additional information on the overall periodontal health of the individual. More information may be obtained by performing a standard dental index such as the Silness and Loe plaque index or Muhlemann sulcus bleeding index, both of which use the periodontal probe in their assessment (see Chapter 13). Some practitioners use the periodontal probe to identify subgingival calculus; however, most dental hygienists find the dental explorer more reliable for deposit assessment because of its curvature and finer tip.

Measurement of suspected pathological lesions is important for complete recording of size, in addition to a diagram of the shape and verbal description of intraoral and extraoral lesions, whether or not the lesion is biopsied. The periodontal probe is used to measure the dimensions of small lesions and the side and tip of the instrument is used to palpate, lift, or rub over the lesion to examine other characteristics that may be helpful to the dentist making a differential diagnosis. If the lesion is determined to be innocuous and therefore is not excisionally biopsied, it should be monitored by evaluating the size (with a periodontal probe), shape, and visual description on subsequent appointments (see Chapter 11).

The periodontal probe also is used to measure the distance between teeth (diastema) as well as the amount of overjet a person may exhibit. In individuals with severe periodontal disease, tooth migration is an indicator of further loss of support structures, and the stability or degree of movement over time may be monitored with the periodontal probe.

EXPLORER

Design and Use

The astute clinician uses many diagnostic indicators such as tissue response, bleeding, and radiographic surveys to determine the presence of subgingival deposits. However, tissue response to calculus varies by individual, and radiographs are two-dimensional, making it difficult to visualize flat, burnished calculus deposits obscured by restorations or located on facial or lingual surfaces of teeth. The explorer is designed to be manipulated into and around the tooth at various angles and may be used to detect or assess many of the following problems even before they become obvious by other clinical or radiographic parameters:

- Supragingival calculus
- Subgingival calculus
- Cemental irregularities
- Dental caries
- Decalcification
- Irregularities in margins of restorations
- Secondary caries around restorations
- Morphological crown and root anomalies
- External root resorption

The explorer consists of a very fine, wire-like tip with a sharp point that comes in a variety of lengths, diameters, and bends. Shank diameter is narrow for increased tactile sensitivity. The differences in curvature of the shank, length, and diameter make different explorers useful for specific purposes dependent on tissue, calculus, probing depth, tooth alignment, and other details specific to individual clients.

When reviewing the various explorers, general categorizations may be made about the use of this assessment instrument. The explorer should be selected by the task it is to perform. Heavier, wider, or even medium-diameter explorers are best suited for caries detection or exploration around restorations. Such explorers are sturdy and do not deform or bend as they are manipulated under and around caries and metallic margins. Fine, elongated explorers are more difficult to use for caries detection because of the deflection of the instrument and inability of the operator to apply adequate pressure for caries detection.

For subgingival exploration of root structure and identification of calculus, the explorer must be fine enough to allow for tactile sensitivity but at the same time not too thin. Explorers that are too thin flex and catch in tissue or on root structure in fibrotic or tight areas, relaying incorrect messages about subgingival deposits. For deep periodontal pockets, the explorer should be slightly bent and long enough (such as the Hu-Friedy 3-A extra long explorer or the ODU 11–12) to reach to the apical regions (i.e., 12 to 13 mm deep). For shallow sulcus areas, examining cementoenamel junctions and under contact areas, a short explorer (such as a pigtail explorer) is easily adapted because it is short and acutely bent. These short, curved explorers are usually double-ended and area-specific, that is, each end works best on specific surfaces of the tooth. Comparisons of these and other explorers are seen in Figure 18–36.

The modified pen grasp is used with the dental explorer. When exploring shallow, light, or obvious calculus, the dental hygienist uses a grasp with light to moderate strength. The grasp should become firmer when more pressure needs to be exerted against the tooth or when the dental hygienist needs to distinguish between tooth structure and burnished calculus.

The most important rule governing fulcrum placement when exploring is that the fulcrum be flexible enough to allow the explorer to move from the cementoenamel junction to the apex of the pocket with correct insertion and adaptation. Almost any scaling fulcrum could be used as an exploring fulcrum; however, the reverse may not always be true because a scaling fulcrum needs more stability. The exploratory fulcrum could be located close to the area being explored, cross arch, or extraoral. As the fulcrum moves further from the area being explored, the dental hygienist's grasp on the handle of the instrument also moves further away from the working end. This distance does not diminish the hygienist's ability to explore the area, nor does it lessen the dental hygienist's ability to control this particular instrument. Rather, it enhances the important factor of access into interproximal regions and deep periodontal pockets.

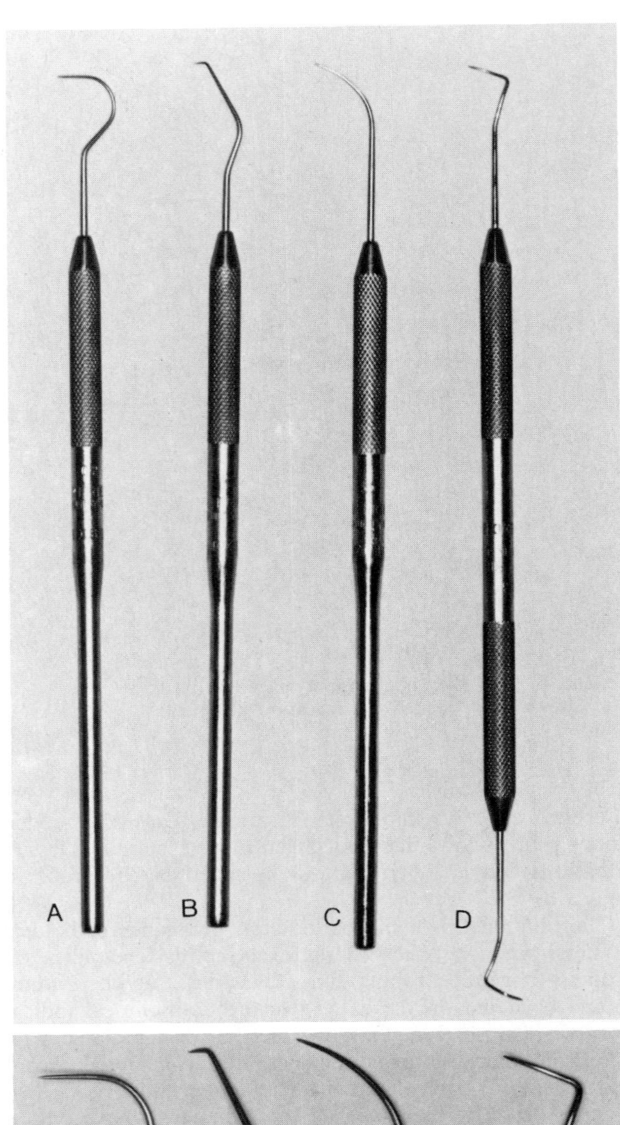

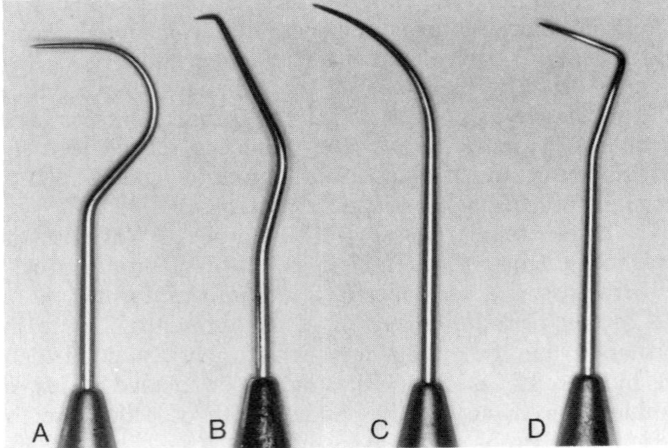

FIGURE 18–36
Top and *Bottom,* No. 23 Shepherds hook explorer (A). No. 17 Orban explorer (B). Hu-Friedy No. 3-A extralong explorer (C). Pig-tail explorer (double-ended) (D).

Concept of Tactile Sensitivity

Tactile sensitivity is the ability to distinguish relative degrees of roughness and smoothness on the tooth surface. Experience in detecting light calculus when it is almost completely scaled and in feeling heavy calculus when it has been burnished is a prerequisite for developing good tactile sensitivity. The skill may be improved by attention to stroke direction, pressure, type of calculus, and type of root surface being explored.

For calculus detection with an explorer, the dental hygiene practitioner uses a variety of stroke directions (vertical, horizontal, and oblique) to form a "basketweave" of strokes, as described earlier. This is particularly helpful when problems of differentiation between calculus and root structure occur. The dental hygienist should practice different strokes when instrumentation has been particularly difficult in a certain area or when it is necessary to be particularly thorough in calculus detection (such as in a very deep pocket or in an area where there is a periodontal abscess).

In periodontal instrumentation, tactile sensitivity also is important in distinguishing between the sulcular soft tissue wall, the junctional epithelium, and possible osseous exposures. The explorer tip should not stop on the sulcular wall if the instrument is inserted properly and the tip remains well adapted to the tooth surface to the base of the pocket. If the explorer contacts soft tissue, it bounces and snags along the wall until the instrument is properly adapted. As one follows the root of the tooth down to the base of the pocket, the nonkeratinizing junctional epithelium is the base of the pocket. The junctional epithelium feels different depending on the state of health of the periodontium. In healthy sulci, the junctional epithelium is firm and elastic in nature. In the inflamed state, the junctional epithelium is soft and easily penetrable with a sharp-pointed instrument. If osseous exposure occurs because of heavy instrumentation and exceptionally friable soft tissue, the sensation at the base of the pocket is much like that of heavy, porous calculus. To differentiate calculus from an osseous exposure, the dental hygienist should attempt to move around and under the area. If it is calculus, the junctional epithelium is felt under the deposit. If the roughness is an osseous exposure, the dental hygienist will find it impossible to move the explorer down and under the area.

The practitioner uses light pressure when faced with light calculus, little pocket depth, and friable tissue. Increased pressure is required when trying to distinguish burnished calculus or when overinstrumentation may have caused irregular changes in root structure. Pressure should be decreased, however, after thorough root planing to get an overview of the final product.

The practitioner determines the potential for smoothing the roots of periodontitis-affected teeth. If it is possible to attain smooth roots, this should be one of the goals throughout care. If there remains a certain level of roughness after a good attempt at root planing, the practitioner may have to accept this and adjust the maintenance interval, educate the person on optimal methods of bacterial plaque control for problem areas, and collaborate with the dentist or periodontist for other periodontal treatment options.

Sharpening Techniques

Occasionally the dental explorer needs sharpening. Fine explorers become dull through general use and frequently are made dull when used for caries detection in pits and fissures and around restorations. Decreased tactile sensitivity is evident when fine changes in root texture are not evident or when the explorer glides over the plastic testing stick instead of catching on irregularities. To sharpen the tips of explorers, the instrument is held with a modified pen grasp, dragged and rotated along the stone at an angle that keeps the tip and 2 to 3 mm of the terminal end in contact with the stone. Two to three rotations around the tip on the stone sufficiently sharpens the dental explorer (Fig. 18–37).

SICKLE SCALER

Design and Use

The sickle scaler is designed with either a straight or bent shank. The straight-shanked sickle scalers are anterior scaling instruments and are often single-ended because the same end may be used mesially and distally. The bent-shanked sickle scalers may be used for anterior as well as posterior areas of the mouth and are usually double-ended with one end designed for scaling mesial tooth surfaces and the other end for scaling distal tooth surfaces.

The working end of the sickle scaler is a two-sided blade with the face and two sides forming the two cutting edges.

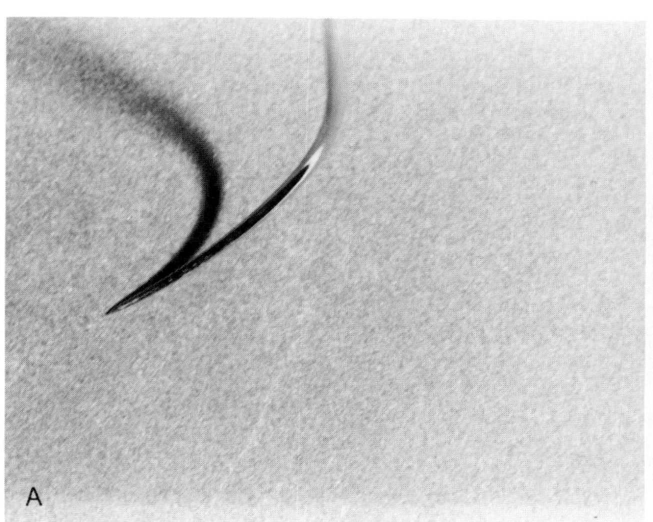

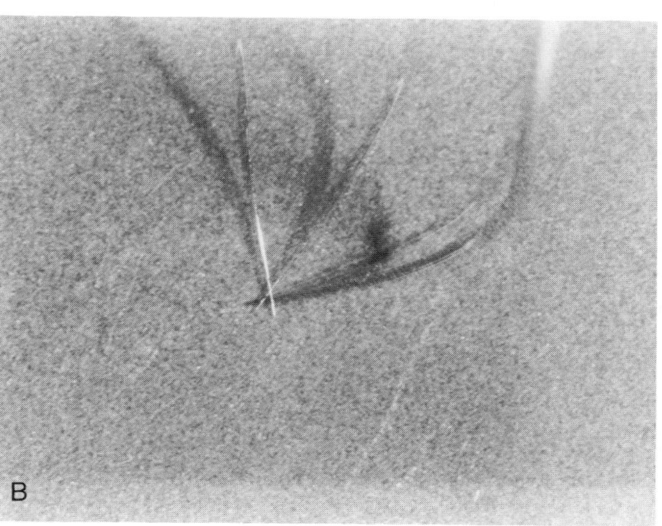

FIGURE 18–37
A and *B*, The dental explorer is sharpened by lightly dragging and rotating the first 2 to 3 mm along the sharpening stone.

The two sides join together in a V shape to form the back of the instrument. Because the sides form a V shape, this instrument is very sturdy in terms of strength even after it has been sharpened many times. Therefore, it is valuable for removal of heavy calculus. However, the extra width from the face to the back of this working end makes it difficult to close the angulation of most sickles without traumatizing the sulcular epithelium with the V-shaped back during subgingival instrumentation. This problem is accentuated with large sickle scalers. Small sickle scalers such as the Morris scaler (Fig. 18–38) cause less trauma and may be easier to use for subgingival scaling. The Morris sickle scaler is a straight-shanked instrument particularly well suited for tight anterior areas.

The tip of the sickle scaler always ends in a sharp point. The advantage of this design feature is the ability to reach between very tight contacts. The disadvantage is that with a sharp tip and a straight cutting edge, the instrument does not adapt well to rounded tooth surfaces. Some part of the instrument is always off the tooth. This problem of adaptation and a V-shaped back imposing on the sulcular wall makes the sickle scaler largely a supragingival scaling instrument. Only in situations of heavy subgingival calculus and very loose tissue may the sickle scaler be used subgingivally. Instrumentation techniques for sickle scalers require a stable modified pen grasp and fulcrum relatively close to the area being scaled because of the need to control adaptation of the toe and cutting edge of this instrument. A pull stroke action in a vertical or oblique direction is made against the tooth surface.

Sharpening Techniques

The sharpening method for the sickle scaler requires the stone to remain stationary and the instrument to move over the stone. The stone is secured with the nondominant hand, the instrument held with a modified pen grasp, and the lateral surface positioned at an angle of 100 to 110 degrees to the stone. The practitioner notes that the entire lateral surface on a flat-surfaced sickle scaler lies against the stone. For curved sickle scalers, small portions of the lateral surfaces are sharpened at a time beginning from the portion nearest the shank. The working hand is stabilized with a fulcrum on the stone and short, firm strokes are applied for sharpening. Because the sickle scaler has two cutting edges, the instrument is turned over and the procedure is repeated for the other lateral surface of the blade. Occasionally the face of the sickle scaler is sharpened. For this surface, the stone either must be positioned near the edge of the table or held up so that the entire face may be sharpened against the surface of the stone. The practitioner tests for sharpness using visual or tactile methods described earlier.

UNIVERSAL CURET

Design and Use

The universal curet is used for supragingival and subgingival scaling and root planing in all areas of the mouth. It is designed with paired mirror-image working ends placed on a single-handle instrument. These working ends are identified by the name of the manufacturer, inventor, or school that developed the particular design. On double-ended instruments, this name is followed by two numbers (e.g., Columbia 13–14) that designate each working end. Universal curets are available also as single-ended instruments that must be purchased in pairs because both ends are necessary in instrumenting a tooth.

The universal curet blade has two lateral surfaces that form two parallel cutting edges on both sides of the flat face (inner surface) of the blade. The two cutting edges form a rounded tip (or toe) at the terminal end of the blade. The lateral surfaces converge to form the rounded back of the blade. This design reduces the chances of subgingival trauma to both sulcular tissues and tooth structure. Both cutting edges of a universal curet blade are parallel and curved upward toward the toe of the blade (Fig. 18–39). The curvature of the blades defines the area(s) in which the instrument is most useful.

The face of the universal curet blade is positioned 90 degrees to the lower shank. There is a bend above the lower shank so that the handle is not parallel with the lower shank (Fig. 18–40). Therefore, to close angulation for scaling to an angle between 45 and 90 degrees, the handle

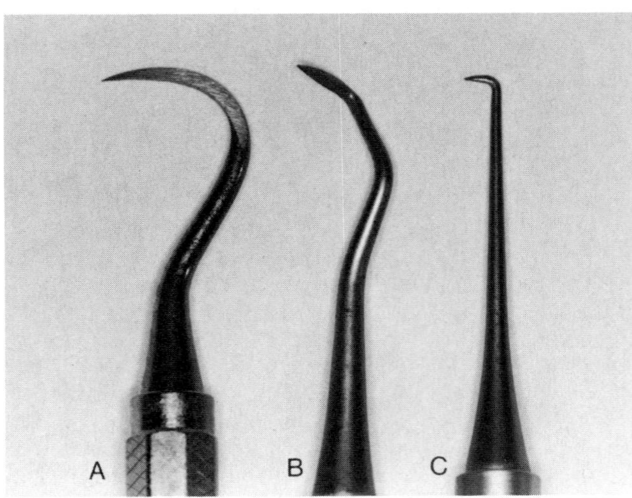

FIGURE 18–38
Comparison of various sickle scalers. Curved sickle (A); posterior (double-ended) sickle (B); and Morris sickle (C).

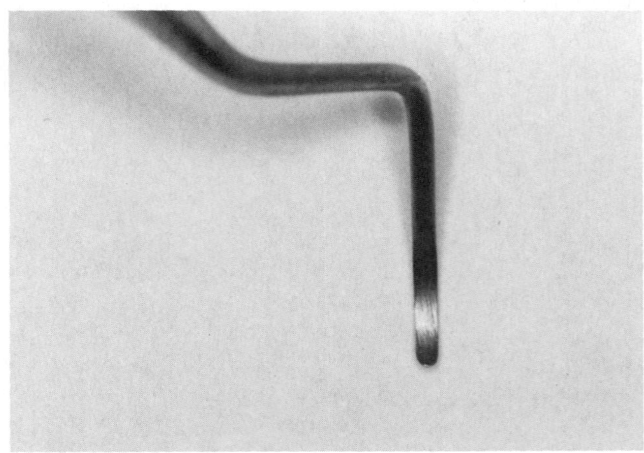

FIGURE 18–39
Both cutting edges of a universal curet blade are parallel and curved upward toward the toe of the blade.

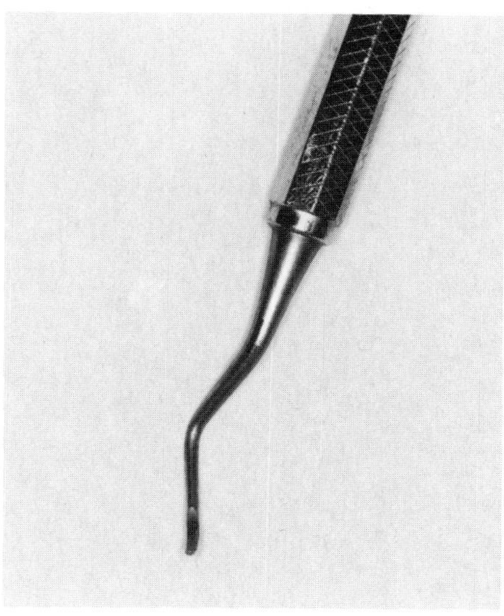

FIGURE 18-40
The handle of the universal curet is not parallel with the lower shank.

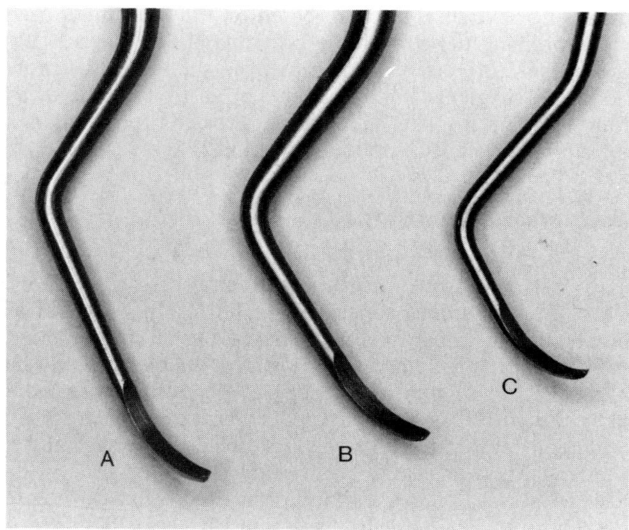

FIGURE 18-42
Universal curets: Columbia 2R-2L (A). Columbia 4R-4L (B). Columbia 13-14 (C).

and lower shank of the universal curet must be tilted slightly toward the tooth (Fig. 18-41).

One double-ended or a pair of single-ended universal curets can be used to scale all areas of the dentition of a periodontally healthy mouth. Scaling with a universal curet is more difficult when there is increased pocket depth. In these cases, combinations of universal curets may be necessary to reach all areas. The Columbia 13-14, for instance, is a short acutely curved universal curet. This instrument works well in anterior areas or in areas with slight-to-moderate probing depths and is often paired with the Columbia 4R-4L for use in deeper, more posterior areas. The Columbia 2R-2L is even longer than the Columbia 4R-4L and is ideal for use in areas of deep facial or lingual pocket depth (Fig. 18-42).

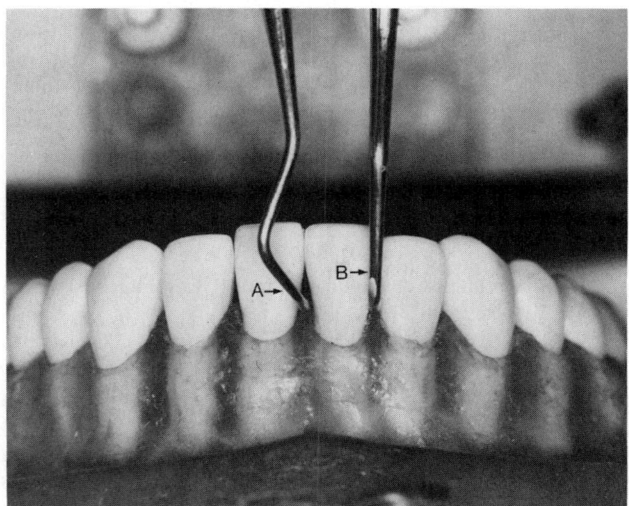

FIGURE 18-41
To close angulation with the universal curet (A), the handle is tilted toward the tooth surface more than the Gracey curet (B). This angulation is due to the differences in the relationships of the faces of the blades and the lower shanks of the two instruments.

Because the ends of a double-ended universal curet or paired universal curets are mirror images, they are used in the same manner but for mirror-image surfaces. This application is especially true in posterior regions. If, for example, one end is used for the distal interproximal surface from the facial surface, then the opposite end is used for the mesial interproximal surface from the lingual aspect. The end that works best for the straight facial aspect is the same end used for the mesial surface. The end that works best for the straight lingual aspect is the same end used again for the mesial aspect from the lingual surface. Therefore, the working ends of the universal curet are not the same for the facial and lingual surfaces in posterior areas.

In anterior areas, the correct side of the instrument is not so critical. Both cutting edges of the universal curet blade may be used for scaling and root planing in anterior areas. Only the angulation or the degree to which the blade is open is different from one end to the other when the ends of the instrument are exchanged. The cutting edge that offers a more open angulation is better for traction and reduces calculus burnishing. However, the type of tissue is a major consideration in selecting the cutting edge for anterior scaling. If the tissue is tight and fibrotic and the pocket depth very shallow, the dental hygienist should choose the cutting edge that offers a closer blade angulation to the tooth surface. If the tissue is loose, the cutting edge that offers a more open angulation, better traction, and less burnishing action is a better choice because the soft tissue is loose and there is less chance of inadvertent soft tissue curettage against the wall of the pocket with the opposite cutting edge.

Because the curets are critically important instruments in scaling and root planing, the dental hygienist needs to select the best instruments made from many different manufacturers. The universal curets are made in several varieties of metals, each with specific strengths and weaknesses (see the section on the "working end" in this chapter). The shank strength and thickness of the blade when new are also factors to consider in instrument selection.

The practitioner uses a modified pen grasp and selects an

intraoral or extraoral fulcrum based on the techniques used in customizing the stroke to a particular tooth surface. Basically, the more periodontally involved the tooth, the more the dental hygienist will find the need to fulcrum away from the working site. A working stroke is initiated in a vertical, horizontal, or oblique direction.

Sharpening Techniques

Curets become dull through general use but are dull particularly after vigorous instrumentation of heavy calculus. When the instrument appears to be burnishing calculus or the practitioner must increase pressure and close angulation for the instrument to grip tooth surface, the curet should be sharpened. The dental hygienist notices that the more accurately the curet has been sharpened (i.e., the angulation of the lateral surface to the face of the blade is correct and a definite cutting edge has been established), the longer the curet feels sharp. Thus, it is important to perform accurate sharpening to lengthen the time interval between sharpenings and to preserve as much metal as possible by not having to sharpen as often. Because the cutting edge of the universal curet is two-sided and includes the rounded toe as well, the method for sharpening this curet includes all of these areas. It is recommended, however, that the toe of the universal curet be preserved as long as possible because the toe itself is not usually used in instrumentation except occasionally under the floor of furcations or under tooth contacts. When the toe is sharpened each time the lateral surfaces are sharpened, there is unnecessary reduction of the length of the blade, eventually making the instrument inaccessible to interproximal areas.

The universal curet may be sharpened either by moving the instrument over the stone or the stone over the blade. The former method requires the stone to be placed on a stable surface such as a tabletop, the curet held in a modified pen grasp, angulation of the face to the surface of the stone positioned between 100 to 110 degrees, and the curet blade moved at this angulation from the lower third of the blade to the midline of the toe. Each side of the universal curet blade is sharpened as needed. The latter method requires the stone to be held in the dominant hand and the instrument held with a palm-thumb grasp secured against a firm surface (tabletop) or the elbow drawn close to the body for support. The instrument is held with the face of the blade parallel to the floor and the stone positioned on the lateral surface at a 100- to 110-degree angle. The stone is moved with short, light-to-firm vertical strokes, depending on the amount of sharpening needed, and slowly passed across the entire cutting edge at consistent angulation. It is important to maintain consistent angulation for an evenly sharpened blade. To do this, the stone should not be lifted from the blade; both the upward and downward stroke are used for sharpening. Even pressure should be used along the cutting edge to prevent changing the normal shape of a curet blade. Figure 18–43 illustrates the cross-sectional views of curet blades resulting from common sharpening errors. The most common error is to place more pressure as the stroke nears the toe producing a blade with converging lateral sides connected by a point instead of parallel lateral sides connected by a rounded toe (Fig. 18–44). The method of moving the stone over the instrument is slightly easier than moving the instrument because as the stone is moved, the practitioner notices a light film of lubricant and/or sharpening byproducts (sludge) accumulating on the surface of the face, and angulation of lateral surface to stone is easier to visualize. Both sides of the blade should be sharpened if dull. The last stroke(s) should be in a downward motion towards the back of the instrument to reduce the possibility of a wire edge on the face of the blade. Figure 18–45 compares both methods of sharpening the universal curet.

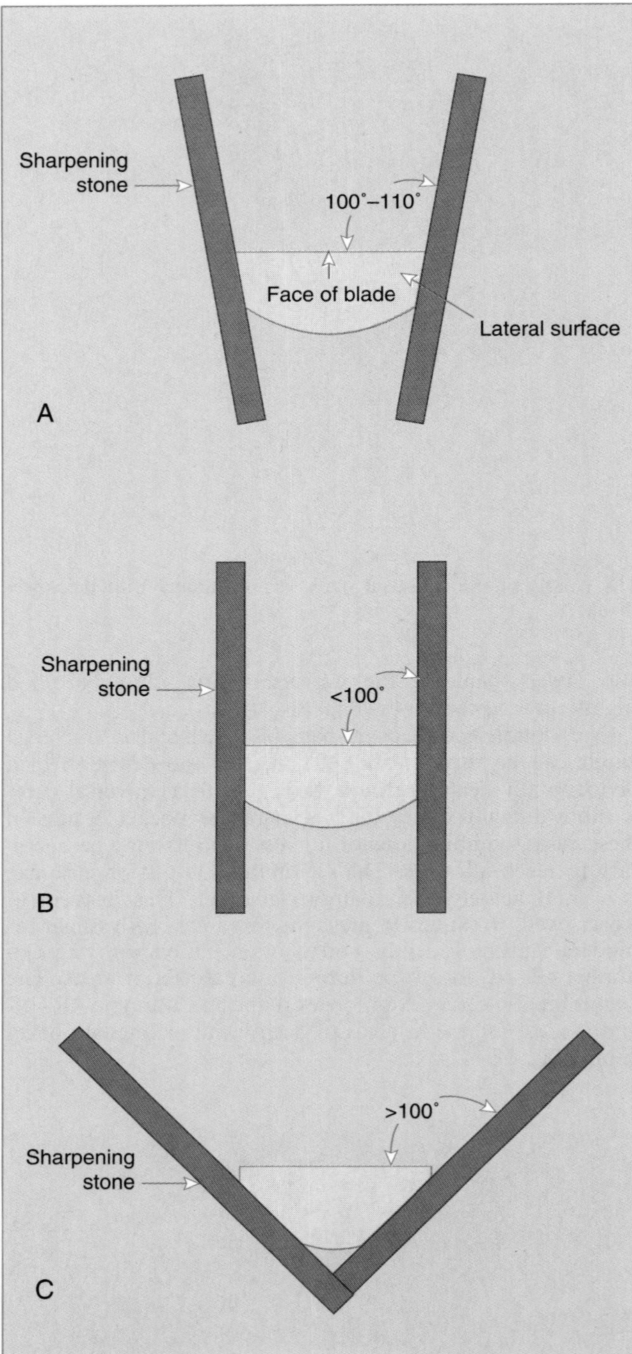

FIGURE 18–43
A, Correct instrument sharpening. *B* and *C*, Common sharpening errors.

The face of the curet blade may be sharpened with a cone-shaped sharpening stone, the rounded side of a sharp-

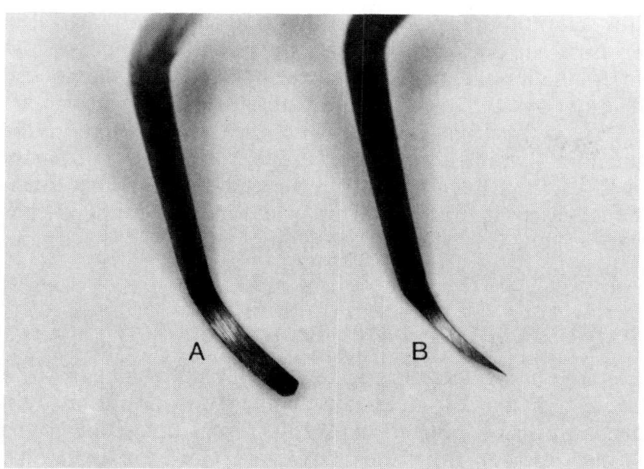

FIGURE 18–44
Parallel lateral cutting edge of a Gracey curet 5–6 (A). Converging lateral cutting edge due to too heavy pressure of the sharpening stone near the toe of the blade of a Gracey curet 5–6 (B).

ening stone, or a mounted rotary stone. Often these methods produce unreliable results because it is difficult to maintain even pressure across the face. If too much metal is reduced (as with the rotary stone) the strength of the blade from face to back is weakened. This dimension from face to back is significant because it is an important factor in providing strength to an instrument that uses a pulling action such as the curet. When all sharpening has been completed, the instrument is wiped with a 2 × 2 gauze square and tested for sharpness.

A curet has lost its sharpness if tactile sensitivity decreases during light root planing strokes, if it does not grasp tooth structure unless the practitioner uses inordinate amounts of pressure, or if its angulation must be further closed for the instrument to maintain a working relationship with the tooth surface. Figure 18–43 illustrates the cross-sectional views of curet blades resulting from common sharpening errors.

GRACEY CURET (AREA-SPECIFIC CURETS)

Design and Use

Gracey curets were developed by Dr. Clayton H. Gracey of Michigan in the late 1930s. The designation of "area-specific" curets means that each of the instruments in this collection was designed to scale specific areas of the mouth (e.g., anterior versus posterior) as well as specific tooth surfaces (e.g., mesial versus distal). Although they were originally designed to be used with a push stroke, Gracey curets were later modified to be pull instruments. Because these instruments were designed with specific areas in mind, the dental hygienist will find them particularly effective for instrumenting teeth with slight to severe periodontitis in individuals who require therapeutic scaling and root planing by quadrant or sextant.

The complete collection of Gracey curets consists of seven mirror-image pairs of instruments. Table 18–13 lists each Gracey curet by number and areas of use. Although Gracey curets were designed to be used in specific areas of the mouth (area-specific), it is possible to use Gracey curets in other areas of the mouth than those originally intended by Dr. Gracey. Because of this, dental hygiene educators often provide instruction for full-mouth periodontal instrumentation using a select few of the entire collection. The instruments selected usually represent basic anterior- and posterior- as well as mesial- and distal-specific instruments. An example of such a selection is the Gracey 5–6, 7–8, 11–12, and 13–14 (Fig. 18–46). Table 18–14 outlines the far-reaching potentials of this combination of Gracey curets.

The basic reason why Gracey instruments are ideal for instrumenting periodontitis-affected teeth lies with the relationship of the face of the blade to the lower shank. The Gracey curet is honed so that the face is "offset" or at an angle to the lower shank. (The lower shank is the last bend of the shank closest to the working end.) Whereas the universal curet's face is at 90 degrees, the Gracey curet is at a 60- to 70-degree angle to the lower shank. With this angle

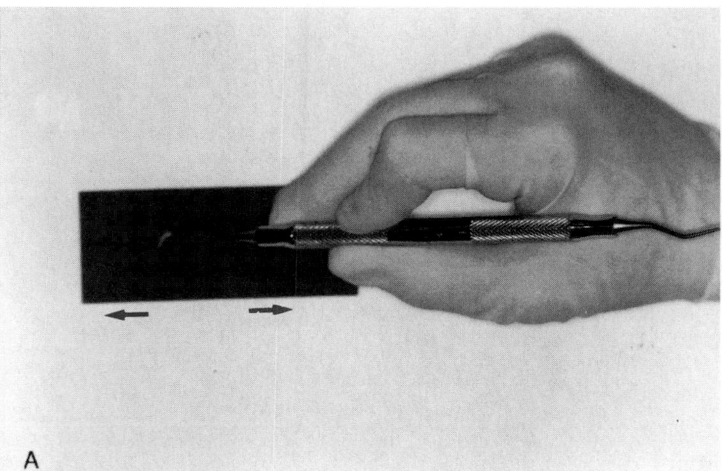

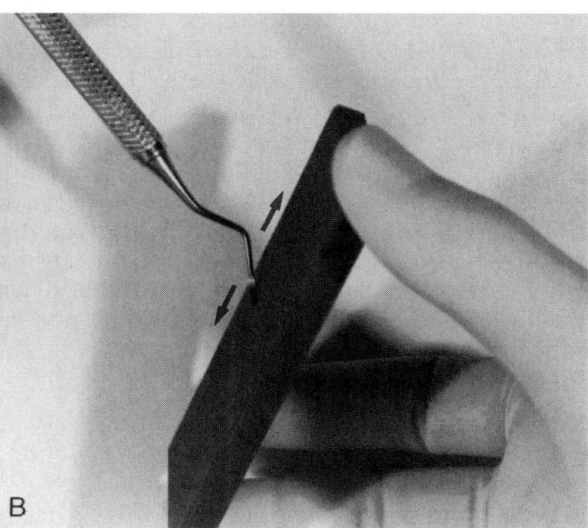

FIGURE 18–45
A, Sharpening by moving instrument over the sharpening stone. *B*, Sharpening by moving sharpening stone over instrument.

TABLE 18–13
GRACEY CURETS (AREA-SPECIFIC CURETS)

Gracey Curet	Area of Use
Gracey 1–2	Anterior teeth
Gracey 3–4	Anterior teeth
Gracey 5–6	Anterior and premolar teeth
Gracey 7–8	Posterior teeth (facial and lingual)
Gracey 9–10	Posterior teeth (facial and lingual)
Gracey 11–12	Posterior teeth (mesial)
Gracey 13–14	Posterior teeth (distal)

of the face to the lower shank, when proper angulation of the cutting edge to the tooth surface is achieved, the lower shank is parallel to the tooth surface being scaled. This automatically places the blade against the tooth at a 40-degree angle. Therefore, when using Gracey curets, it is important to observe the relationship of the lower shank to the surface being scaled to help determine if correct angulation is achieved.

Like the universal curet, the Gracey curet has two bladed sides that come together to form a rounded toe. But unlike the universal curet, which has two useful cutting edges because both blades run parallel to each other, the Gracey curet has only one designated cutting edge. The correct cutting edge is determined by examining the curvatures of the blade. The blade of the Gracey curet is not only bent in a curve, but also it is bent so that one cutting edge is elongated. This longer curved side of the Gracey curet as shown in Figure 18–47 is the correct cutting edge. When the lower shank is held perpendicular to the floor with the face of the blade up, this cutting edge is slightly lower than the shorter edge. Together with the basic bend of the blade, this elongation makes Gracey instruments particularly efficient in adapting to root morphology.

Gracey After-Five Series

Design and Use

In response to the continued challenge of periodontal instrumentation and new knowledge about the value of nonsurgical periodontal therapy, two variations of Gracey curets have been introduced as the Gracey "After-Five" series and the "Mini-Five" series of instruments. The Gracey After-Five series is a modified set of Gracey curets that are exactly like the traditional Gracey curets except that the lower shank of the instruments are an additional 3 mm longer (Fig. 18–48). Gracey After-Five curets are particularly useful in areas with significant pocket depth or recession. Because the shanks are longer than those of the traditional Gracey curets, they often require an extended fulcrum such as an opposite arch, cross arch, or extraoral fulcrum. Often a reinforcement with the nondominant hand is helpful for additional control.

Gracey Mini-Five Series

Design and Use

The second variation of the basic curet is the Gracey Mini-Five series of curets with a terminal shank that is 3 mm longer than and a working blade that is half the length of the traditional Gracey curet (Fig. 18–49). The advantage of this series of Gracey curets is that it is particularly useful in areas of narrow deep pocketing in which it is impossible to insert the long, regular blade straight down into the pocket. The options for the dental hygienist in these situations are to use a horizontal stroke with the toe directed to the junctional epithelium or to use a shortened instrument such as the Mini Five with a vertical stroke. Other situations where this instrument is of use include rounded convexities or concavities found going into and out of root depressions and around line angles.

Shank Design and Metallurgy

Certain manufacturers make the Gracey curet with a "rigid" shank that does not dissipate the power used in generating a working stroke. This design differentiates the "rigid" Gracey from the "finishing" Gracey curet which has a more flexible shank. The rigid shank is essential when performing heavy scaling and root planing. It is also quite effective when less lateral pressure is required. The rigid shank does not diminish tactile sensitivity. Rather, it en-

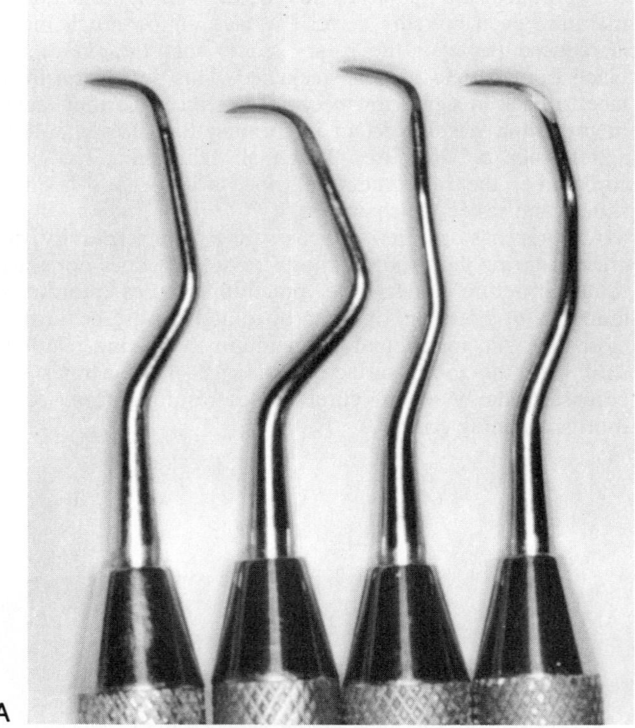

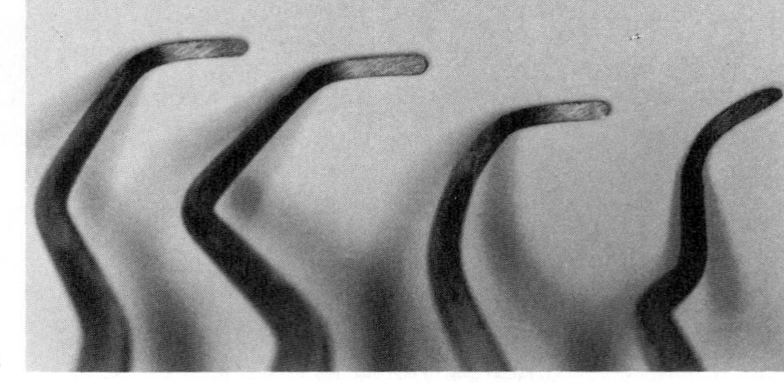

FIGURE 18–46
A and *B*, Hartzell Gracey curets 5–6, 7–8, 11–12, and 13–14.

TABLE 18–14
EXTENDED AREAS OF USE FOR A SELECT COMBINATION OF GRACEY CURETS

Gracey Curet	Area of Use	Stroke Direction		
		Vertical /	Horizontal /	Oblique
5–6	Anterior			
	Mesial	**X**	x	x
	Distal	**X**	x	x
	Facial	x	**X**	**X**
	Lingual	x	**X**	**X**
	Posterior (premolars)			
	Mesial	**X**	x	**X**
	Distal	**X**		**X**
	Facial	x	**X**	**X**
	Lingual		**X**	**X**
	Posterior (molars)			
	Mesial	**X**		x
	Distal (limited access)	**X**		x
	Facial		**X**	**X**
	Lingual	x	**X**	**X**
7–8	Anterior			
	Mesial	**X**	x	x
	Distal	**X**	x	x
	Facial	x	**X**	**X**
	Lingual	x	**X**	**X**
	Posterior (premolars)			
	Mesial	**X**	x	x
	Distal	**X**	x	x
	Facial	x	**X**	**X**
	Lingual	x	**X**	**X**
	Posterior (molars)			
	Mesial	**X**		x
	Distal (limited access)	**X**		x
	Facial	x	**X**	**X**
	Lingual	x	**X**	**X**
11–12	Anterior			
	Mesial	**X**	x	x
	Distal	**X**	x	x
	Posterior (premolars)			
	Mesial	**X**	x	x
	Posterior (molars)			
	Mesial	**X**	x	x
13–14	Anterior			
	Mesial	**X**	x	x
	Distal	**X**	x	x
	Facial	x	**X**	x
	Lingual	x	**X**	x
	Posterior (premolars)			
	Distal	**X**	x	x
	Lingual		**X**	**X**
	Posterior (molars)			
	Distal	**X**	x	x
	Lingual	x	**X**	**X**

Capital and boldface = most commonly used stroke direction.

hances control and energy needed to make any direction of stroke under any degree of pressure.

Because the finishing Gracey has a more flexible shank, it bends under pressure. A significant amount of lateral pressure is lost in the flexion that occurs under firm working strokes. Therefore, this instrument is indicated for times when light scaling and root planing are needed.

Like the universal curets, the Gracey curets are made by many different manufacturers, and the quality and type of metal and design vary somewhat between them. The dental hygienist must be knowledgeable about instrument differences and make decisions on that knowledge because it affects operator performance and care outcomes.

The basic modified pen grasp and fulcrum placement techniques used with the universal curet are also used with Gracey curets. Instrumentation in deep periodontal defects

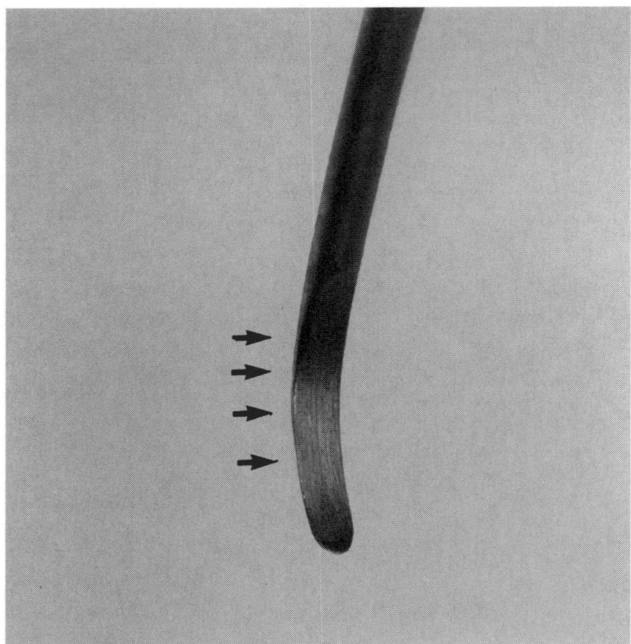

FIGURE 18-47
The longer curved side of the Gracey curet blade is the cutting edge.

or when using elongated, specialized Gracey curets requires the use of extended fulcrums and reinforcement scaling techniques.

Sharpening Techniques

The major difference between sharpening the Gracey and the universal curet is that the Gracey curet blade is offset. Both instruments may be sharpened with movement of the instrument or the stone. Grasp positions, angulation of 100 to 110 degrees, as well as movement across the blade are the same for the Gracey and universal curets. The Gracey curet blade face is offset at 60 to 70 degrees to the shank (as opposed to 90 degrees for the universal curet) which opens the angle of the stone on the Gracey when the lower shank of each is held perpendicular to the floor. When the Gracey curet blade face is held parallel with the floor (like the universal curet), the stone is positioned like the universal curet, but the handle and shank of the Gracey curet are tilted away from the stone and not perpendicular to the floor. Figure 18-50 shows a comparison of stone and handle when the face of a Gracey and a universal curet are held parallel to the floor. On the Gracey curet, only the lower, longer cutting edge from the area where blade sharpness begins and occasionally around the toe is sharpened. Following sharpening procedures, the blade should be tested for sharpness and wiped clean prior to instrumentation.

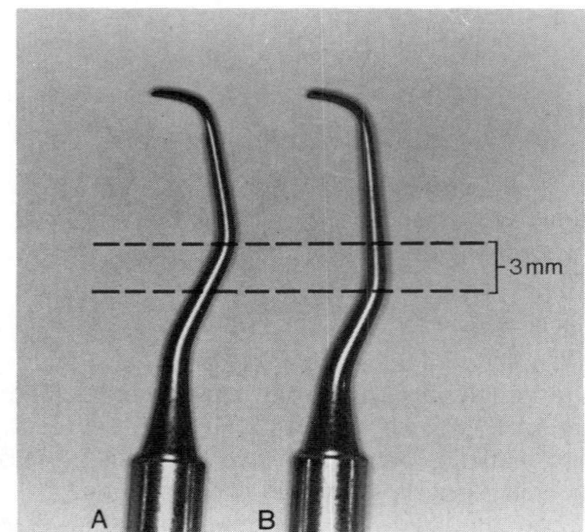

FIGURE 18-48
Gracey curet (A). Gracey After-Five with the elongated shank (B).

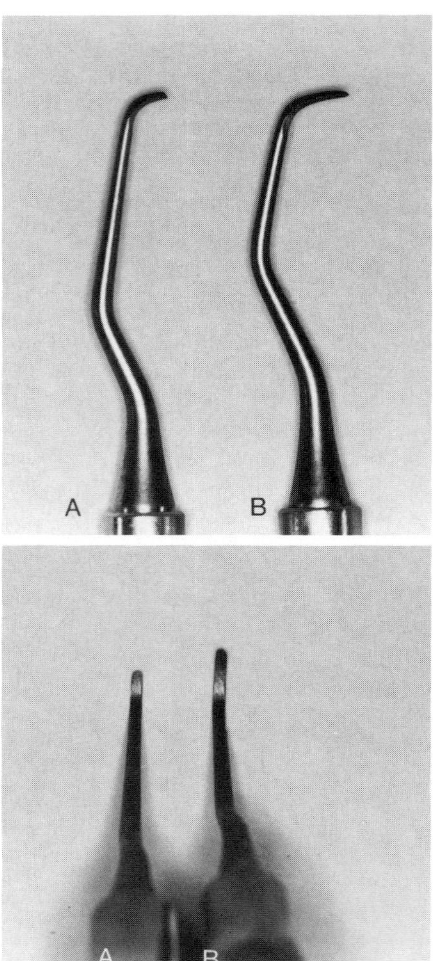

FIGURE 18-49
Top and *Bottom,* The Mini-Five with a shorter working blade (A), compared with the traditional Gracey curet (B).

HOE SCALER

Design and Use

The hoe scaler is used for heavy supragingival calculus removal. Because of design limitations, it is best used in subgingival areas where access is easy, such as facial and lingual surfaces (as opposed to interproximal surfaces), and

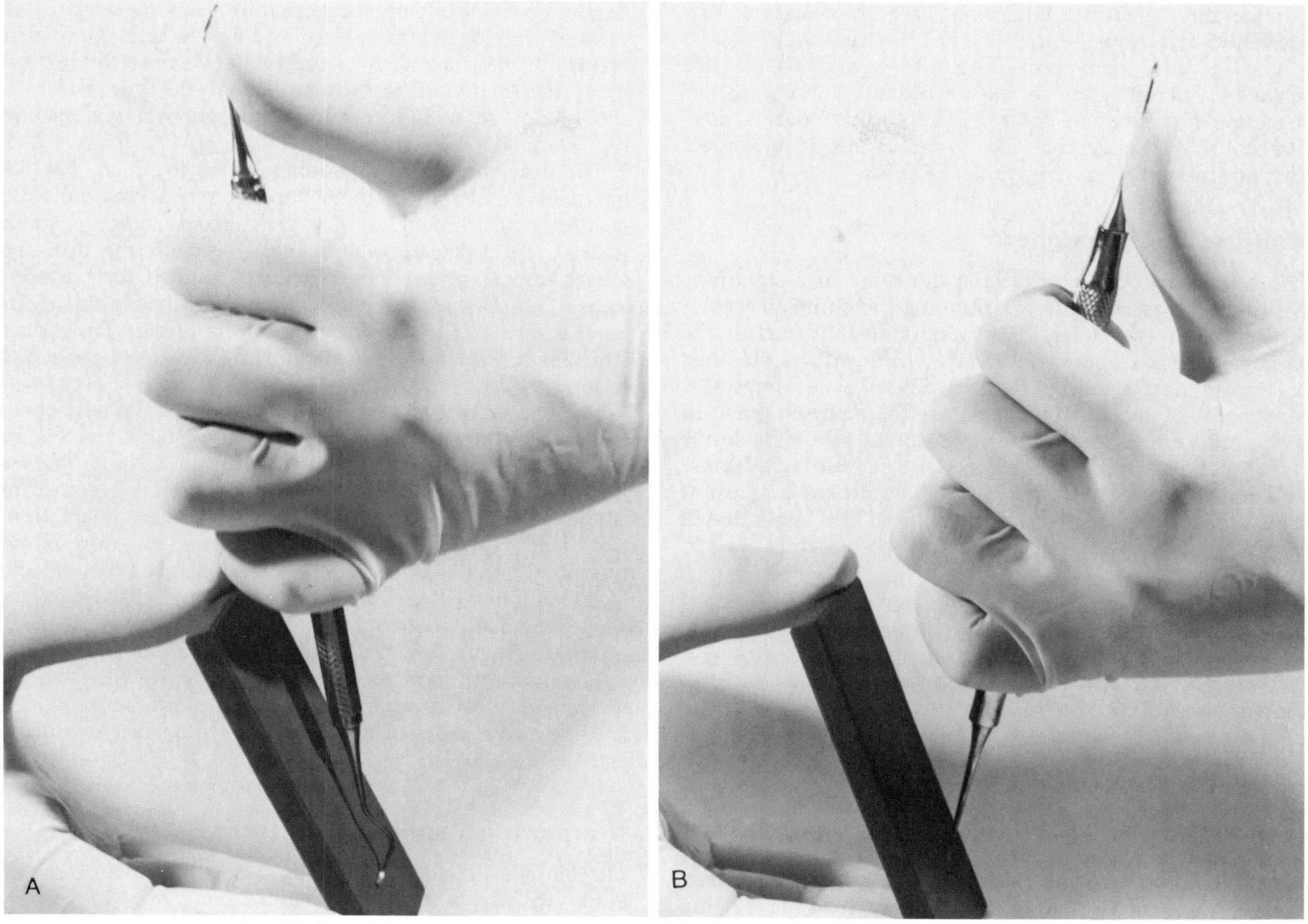

FIGURE 18–50
Comparison of handle position of a universal curet *(A)* and a Gracey curet *(B)* when the face of the blade is held parallel to the floor for sharpening.

when tissue tone is loose and edematous. It is not well suited for fine subgingival scaling and root planing.

The hoe scaler may be double- or single-ended. The hoe has paired working ends, and a set of four working ends is needed to instrument each surface of a tooth. Shank length on a hoe may vary from long to short and may also be bowed from slight to more acute angles (Fig. 18–51). These variations in shank length and angle help determine the best areas in which to use the hoe scaler. The longer and more angled the shank, the better suited the instrument for posterior areas. The shorter, less acutely angled shank is better suited for anterior areas.

The terminal end of the blade is bent to a 99- to 100-degree angle and the tip is beveled at a 45-degree angle to form a single cutting edge. The upper edge forms the actual cutting edge because the hoe scaler is a pull instrument. The cutting edge is a straight, thick, short blade with two sharp corners on each end. These corners may be rounded with a sharpening stone to prevent grooving or gouging of tooth structure.

When the instrument is inserted subgingivally and the blade is well adapted to the tooth surface, the side of the shank should contact tooth surface to form a two-point contact. This improves stability and leverage during instrumentation.

The limitations of the hoe scaler begin with the bow or angle in the shank. This characteristic angle of hoe scalers seriously limits the ability of the dental hygienist to instrument to the base of pocket depth unless the tissue is very loose. The short, straight, bulky blade also poses a problem

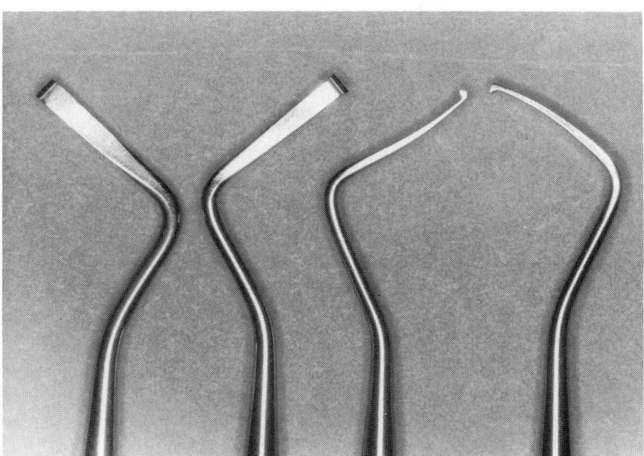

FIGURE 18–51
Hoe scaler.

of adaptation when instrumenting curved root surface. Tactile sensitivity also is limited.

The modified pen grasp should be used with the hoe scaler. A fulcrum close to the immediate working area is suggested for maximal control. The cutting edge is positioned under the deposit and a pull stroke in a vertical direction is applied to remove the calculus.

Sharpening Techniques

The hoe is sharpened by placing the stone in a stationary position on a tabletop and positioning the entire surface of the blade on the stone. It is important to maintain the 45-degree bevel. The instrument is held with a modified pen grasp and stabilized with a fulcrum on the stone. Movement of the instrument across the stone is made in short, moderate pull strokes. A push-pull or grinding stroke is not recommended. The corners at each cutting edge are occasionally rounded with light rolling strokes to prevent injury to soft tissue and tooth structure. The hoe is tested for sharpness on a testing stick and wiped of debris prior to instrumentation.

FILE SCALER

Design and Use

The file scaler is similar in design to the hoe scaler. It consists of a series of miniature hoe blades on a pad attached to the shank. Each blade is bent at an angle of between 90 to 105 degrees from the shank. Each blade possesses sharp corners that together pose somewhat of a hazard to tooth structure if adaptation is not maintained during stroke activation. These corners may be slightly rounded with a sharpening stone before the file is used (Fig. 18–52).

The file is a pull instrument. It may be used supragingivally or subgingivally for crushing or breaking up heavy subgingival calculus. The action of roughening up the surface of tenacious, burnished calculus helps to prepare the surface, making it easier for the curet to latch onto and break the piece away from the tooth. Because this instrument has many of the limitations of the hoe scaler, it should not be used for definitive subgingival scaling and root planing.

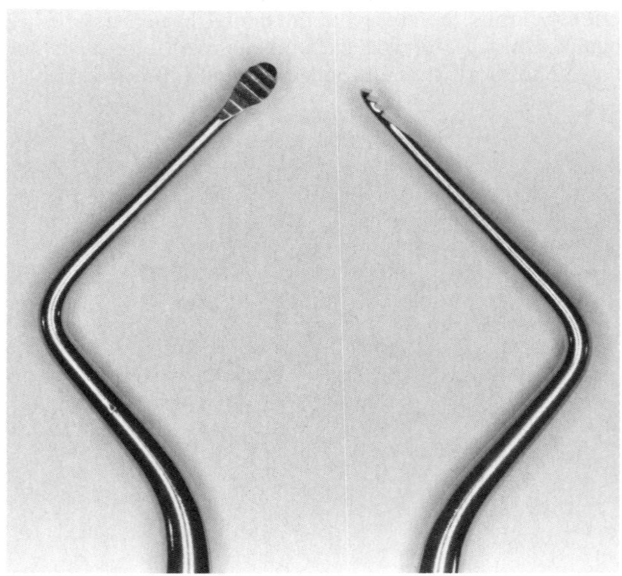

FIGURE 18–52
File scaler.

The instrument may be double- or single-ended. The file has paired ends, and like the hoe, four working ends are needed to instrument each of the four surfaces of a tooth (mesial, distal, facial, and lingual). As with the hoe, the longer, more angled shanks are better suited for posterior areas. The shorter, less angled shanks are better suited for anterior areas. The shank of the file is usually fairly rigid which is advantageous when applying pressure against the tooth.

The pad or base of the working end of the file may come in a variety of shapes (round, oval, or rectangular) and in numerous sizes depending on manufacturer. It is obvious that the larger the base, the more difficult it becomes in adapting to rounded root surfaces. The size, adaptation, and bend of the shank create problems for working in interproximal areas. Like the hoe, the easiest areas are the facial and lingual surfaces and mesial and distal surfaces where there are no contacts. Loose, edematous tissue is necessary for reaching areas close to the base of the pocket.

The modified pen grasp should be used with the file scaler with a fulcrum close to the immediate working area and the entire series of blades positioned against tooth surface.

Sharpening Techniques

The file is a difficult instrument to sharpen because of the miniature size of each blade. Sharpening may be accomplished with a tanged file sharpener positioned against each small, flat-bladed surface (Fig. 18–53). To begin the sharpening procedure, the instrument is stabilized on a firm surface (tabletop) and the practitioner stabilizes the working hand near the instrument on the tabletop to perform light, short, push-pull strokes across each blade. Consistently good results are difficult to achieve when sharpening this instrument.

CHISEL SCALERS

Design and Use

The chisel scaler is a double-ended instrument with either a straight or a curved shank. The blade is continuous with the shank, and the narrow cutting edge is formed with the tip beveled at a 45-degree angle (Fig. 18–54).

This instrument should be used only on heavy interproximal ledges of calculus, especially on lower anterior teeth. It should not be used for scaling and root planing procedures. The chisel is very limited and is not often used by dental hygienists because of the better versatility and advantages of other scaling instruments.

The chisel scaler is a push instrument. To avoid unnecessary trauma to soft tissues, it should be used only in a horizontal direction. The instrument should be stabilized against tooth structure and with a pushing motion used to dislodge heavy interproximal, facial, and lingual calculus from mandibular anterior teeth. Because the corners of the chisel are sharp, care should be taken to keep the blade

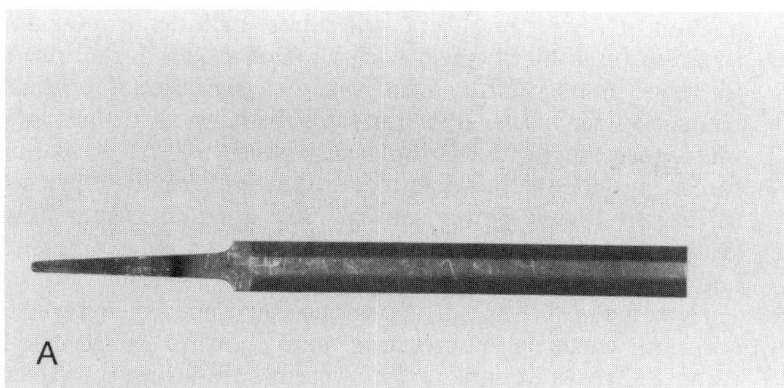

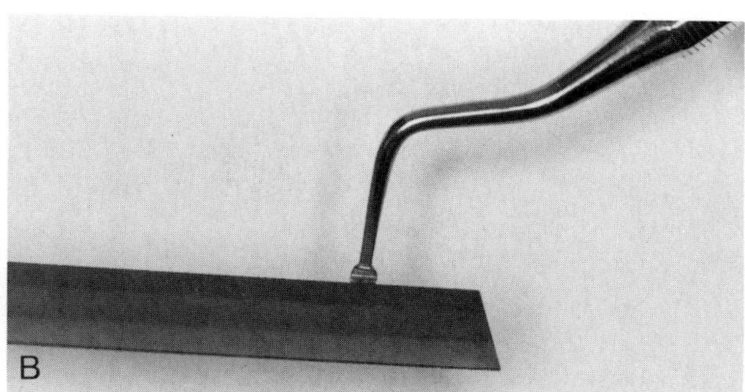

FIGURE 18–53
A and *B*, A tanged file for sharpening the file.

evenly on tooth structure during stroke activation. A modified pen grasp with an intraoral fulcrum close to the working area aids the practitioner in stabilizing this instrument. Sharpening objectives and procedures for the chisel scaler are similar to those of the hoe scaler.

ULTRASONIC AND SONIC SCALERS

Ultrasonic and sonic scaling instruments are electronically powered devices that produce vibratory motions to fracture deposits from tooth surfaces. They are important complements to manual scaling and root planing methods and traditionally have been used for initial scaling of extrinsic stain and supragingival and subgingival calculus followed by hand instrumentation. The advantages of ultrasonic and sonic scaling instruments are reduced time, improved operator comfort, and comparable results to hand scaling where access is possible for the operator. Several studies have reported ultrasonic instrumentation to be as effective as hand instrumentation in removing subgingival deposits,[15,16] whereas others have shown ultrasonic instrumentation to be less effective than hand instrumentation in producing smooth root surfaces.[17] Such inconclusive arguments for either method of instrumentation leave it to the individual dental hygienist to select the technique or combination of techniques that best meet the human needs of the client and the practitioner's ability.

Ultrasonic scaling units convert high-frequency electrical current into mechanical vibrations by either magnetostrictive or piezoelectric transducers. These scalers operate at high frequencies of 25,000 to 42,000 cycles per second, and it is this rapid vibratory action that is responsible for the removal of attached deposits.

The magnetostrictive unit operates by producing an alternating electromagnetic field in the handpiece insert (transducer) causing it to shorten and lengthen, thus producing ultrasonic vibrations with heat production (Fig. 18–55). The transportable unit attaches to electrical and water outlets, adjusts for manipulation of power and water, and is activated by foot control. The transducer is attached to the working tip and inserts into the handpiece of the unit. In conventional units, water is circulated through the handpiece of this unit and leaves the vibrating tip as a cavitation

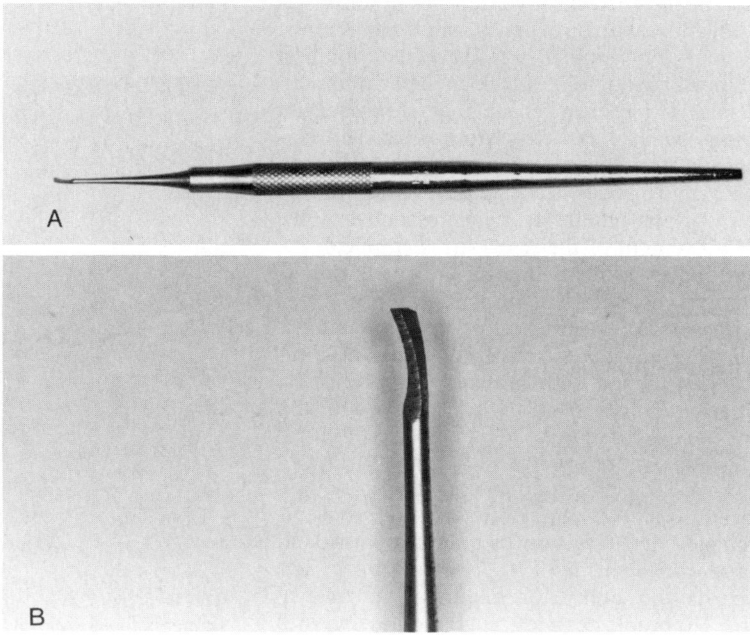

FIGURE 18–54
A and *B*, Chisel scaler.

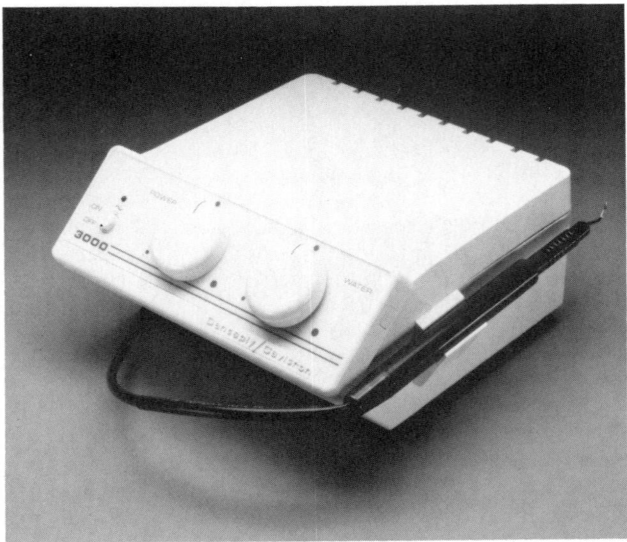

FIGURE 18-55
Dentsply magnetostrictive ultrasonic unit and handpiece.

of collapsing bubbles to cool the effects of the heat produced in the handpiece and at the tip. The cavitation of water at the tip acts as a gingival lavage to flush away debris as the vibratory motion of the insert tip loosens the deposit. Studies that have shown benefits of antimicrobial irrigants[18,19] have led to the development of designs of magnetostrictive handpieces that can deliver medicaments through hollow-tip inserts into the periodontal pocket during ultrasonic instrumentation. In one such model, one or two medicaments may be delivered individually or jointly and the flow rate is controlled at adjustable levels by a two-position foot switch (Fig. 18-56). The handpiece is cooled by a return-flow water cooling system that is separate from the delivery system for medicaments. Whether subgingival irrigation with ultrasonic instrumentation is the most efficacious mode of delivery is yet to be determined.

Earlier models of magnetostrictive ultrasonic units required manual adjustments of frequency and water supply. The higher the frequency applied, the faster the vibration and greater the heat production. Later models automatically adjust as load (or resistance, such as from heavier calculus) conditions change, and they are quieter than earlier models. Various tips that resemble a bulky, flattened periodontal probe, chisel scaler, sickle scaler, and curet are inserted into the working handle of magnetostrictive units. The direction of movement of the insert tip is elliptical.

Addressing the concerns of researchers and practitioners as to the limitations of hand instrumentation[20] and the effectiveness of ultrasonic instrumentation,[21-24] a manufacturer has introduced a magnetostrictive, manual-tuning ultrasonic unit with a modified P10 Dentsply/Cavitron insert (Dentsply International, Inc., York, PA).[24] Holbrook and Low suggest that their technique be used in place of curets rather than as an adjunct for scaling with curets (although the majority of oral health practitioners continue to rely on hand instrumentation).[24] The ultrasonic unit Holbrook selected is the Dentsply 660 Cavitron (a manually tuned ultrasonic unit) and the Dentsply P10 Cavitron tip.[24] The standard P10 tip is too bulky for definitive subgingival scaling; therefore, Holbrook has reduced the diameter with a series of stones and a fine grit rubber cylinder from shank to tip to resemble the size and shape of a periodontal probe for ease in negotiating deep, narrow periodontal pockets. Reduced-size insert tips also are bent with orthodontic pliers for ease of access into deep interproximal areas and furcations. The Holbrook technique requires the operator to use the lowest power setting, have adequate water flow, grasp the handle with a pen grasp, fulcrum on soft tissue, and use continuous back-and-forth scaling motions.

Herremans (1991), in an unpublished thesis, reported a scanning electron microscope study on extracted teeth using a three-split root surface design comparing the effects of no scaling and root planning, scaling with a curet, as well as ultrasonic instrumentation using Holbrook's modified P10 tip. Both the curet and Holbrook's modified P10 produced significantly smoother roots when compared to the control, but the modified P10 ultrasonic tip produced a higher percentage of smooth root surfaces compared to the curet. Such findings are significant and if replicable suggest a need for dental hygienists to reconsider the importance of ultrasonic instrumentation in therapeutic scaling and root planing. Not only is there benefit to the client, but the practitioner also may experience less physical stress and risk of injury than when using hand instrumentation.

The piezoelectric model operates by application of alternating electrical energy applied to piezoelectric crystals in the handpiece which produce ultrasonic vibrations through dimensional changes. Although there is less heat production with the piezoelectric transducer, commercial units are designed with a water-cooling system to lessen the effects of friction at the tip and to facilitate rinsing action. The unit is transportable with electrical and water attachments to the unit and a foot control (Fig. 18-57). Newer models are self-tuned for greater stability, regardless of changes in the tip and/or load. Various scaling tips are available for connection at the end of the handpiece. The scaling tip is designed to vibrate in a single plane to eliminate the lateral vibrations common to the magnetostrictive ultrasonics.

Sonic scalers are small power scaling devices that are air-driven handpieces (Fig. 18-58). There is no cumbersome electrical unit because the scaler fits directly into the handpiece lines of a dental unit where it derives its power.

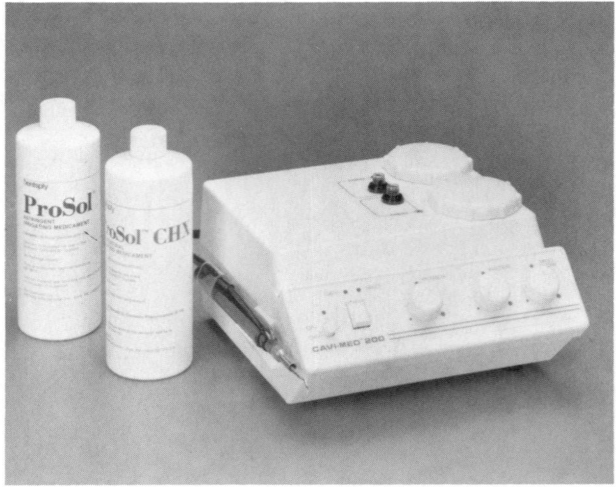

FIGURE 18-56
The Dentsply/Cavi-Med/ProSol system ultrasonic unit delivers medicaments to subgingival areas during ultrasonic instrumentation.

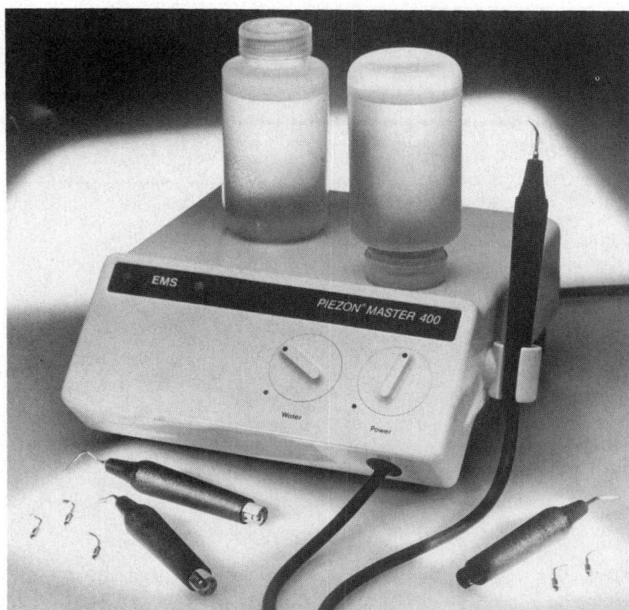

FIGURE 18–57
The Piezon Master 400 is a piezoelectric ultrasonic unit.

This feature gives the sonic scaler the advantage of easy mobility within the dental setting. Vibrations are produced by the passage of air over a metal rod contained within the handpiece. Unlike the ultrasonic scaling devices, the sonic scaler operates at a much lower audible range with an average of 6,000 cycles per second producing oscillation of the attached scaling tip in an elliptical motion. Compared to ultrasonic scalers, the sonic scaler is less powerful, and effectiveness has been shown to be influenced by the type of tip used, air pressure input, and the application load.[25] Like ultrasonic scalers, this device is supplied with different attachment tips that resemble basic scaling instruments.

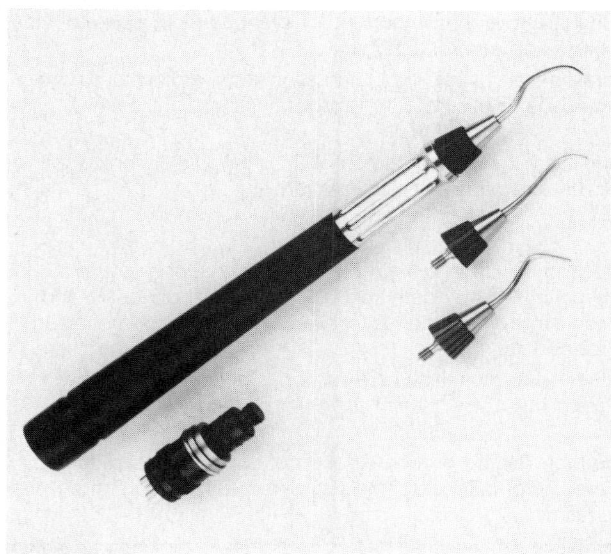

FIGURE 18–58
The Titan SW sonic scaler and insert tips is an air-powered mechanical scaler that runs at sonic frequency.

During operation of the sonic scaler, heat is not generated; however, water is passed through the handpiece to the tip to reduce whatever frictional heat may be generated at the tip-to-tooth interface and also to act as a lavage.

The client's health history is an important consideration in deciding to use the ultrasonic or sonic scaler. Magnetostrictive ultrasonic units may cause interference with cardiac pacemakers and should not be used on or near persons with such devices. The high degree of aerosolization from the water spray contraindicates the use of the ultrasonic scaler or sonic scaler in individuals with communicable diseases. Although administration of antimicrobial rinses (such as chlorhexidine) prior to treatment has been suggested, such medicaments do not have any effect on viruses such as the herpes virus(es) or hepatitis virus(es). Compliance with infection control protocols for the equipment, treatment area, and practitioner are essential when performing ultrasonic instrumentation (see Chapter 8).

The ultrasonic unit also is not advised for young children with their large pulps and who exhibit fear or sensitivity to the vibrating tip. In the adult, there may be actual sensitivity from the vibrating tip. Use of local anesthetics for pulpal and soft tissue block anesthesia prior to instrumentation is advised for the adult who may benefit from ultrasonic instrumentation but who has sensitive teeth.

The substantial amount of water that fills the mouth also may be uncomfortable for clients who are gaggers or who cannot tolerate breathing through their nose. In these situations, it is helpful to seat the client as upright as possible, provide adequate suction, and avoid continuous use of the instrument.

Although studies have shown that certain restorative materials such as composite resin and porcelain restoration may be damaged by ultrasonic instrumentation,[26] others have shown no detrimental effects.[27] The practitioner should be cautious and protective of the client's existing restorations by avoiding close and prolonged contact with ultrasonic instruments.

The procedure for use of ultrasonic and sonic instrumentation follows.

EXTRINSIC STAIN REMOVAL

Types of Stain

Intrinsic stain is an internal discoloration of the tooth that may be caused by exposure to medication (e.g., tetracycline or excessive fluoride ingestion) during tooth development. The dental hygienist must be able to identify and understand the etiology of such stains to recognize the limitations of professional care. Because it is impossible for the dental hygienist to alter intrinsic stains by scaling, root planing, or polishing procedures, it is important to educate clients about the cause of their stain and discuss possible cosmetic dental care options to meet the need for a wholesome body image.

Extrinsic stain is an external discoloration of the tooth that may be caused by certain foods, tobacco, chromogenic bacteria, metallic dust, or drug therapy. It may be removed through personal mechanical oral hygiene regimens, scaling, root planing, and/or polishing procedures. Because it is caused by external, often controllable factors, etiology should be discussed with the client and efforts made either to eliminate the cause and/or to improve oral hygiene pro-

PROCEDURE 18–1

ULTRASONIC AND SONIC INSTRUMENTATION

Equipment

Explorer
Sonic or ultrasonic instrument
Plastic drape
Protective barriers, including faceshield
Mouth mirror
Sterile tip insert
High-speed evacuation
Protection eyewear for the client

Steps	Rationale
1. Connect the ultrasonic unit to the water source on the dental unit and the electrical power source. For sonic scalers, attach the handpiece to the handpiece line on the dental unit.	Provides the power source to operate the equipment
2. Turn the ultrasonic unit on and allow the water to flow through the handpiece for 2 minutes by activating the foot control. Release the foot control.	Allows stagnant water and trapped air to flush through the handpiece.
3. Select a sterilized tip and insert into the water-filled handpiece of the ultrasonic unit. Attach a sterilized tip to the sonic scaler.	
4. Holding the handpiece over a water basin, adjust the water and power to the desired setting. The tip emits a mist of water without excessive dripping.	The practitioner selects the power setting by sensitivity level of the client, hardness of tooth structure to be scaled, and amount of calculus or stain to be removed. The higher the power setting, the more water needed to keep the tip properly cooled.
5. Seat the client in a semisupine position. Provide a plastic drape or additional paper toweling to control moisture around mouth and face.	A semisupine position helps to keep the water from pooling near the client's throat, keeping it at the floor of the mouth or in the buccal pocket areas where the suction is readily accessible.
6. Provide protective eyewear for the client.	When scaling large areas of heavy calculus, many times small pieces become airborne and could cause injury to the client's eyes.
7. In addition to the usual attire of protective clothing, glasses, mask, and gloves, the practitioner may desire to wear a protective shield over the face.	High aerosol contamination requires adequate barrier protection.
8. Position the aspirator (at high speed) comfortably on the side in which the water will pool.	Adequate suction is important for client comfort, operator visibility, and aerosol control.
9. Practitioner position, fulcrum position, and grasp are the same as for conventional scaling; however, fulcrum and grasp may be lighter than conventional scaling.	Ultrasonic and sonic instrumentation requires control to avoid damage to hard and soft tissues.
10. The side of the scaler tip is positioned against tooth surface. The pointed tip is only used for stain or calculus embedded in pit and fissures on enamel (usually occlusal) surfaces.	Working with the pointed tip of an ultrasonic or sonic scaler causes damage to tooth structure.
11. Activate the scaler by depressing the foot control. Keep the side of the tip in constant motion against tooth structure. The scaler also may be used in subgingival areas.	Allowing the tip to remain on one area too long causes grooving of the tooth surface. Subgingival ultrasonic and sonic instrumentation is followed by hand instrumentation for best results.
12. The operator occasionally releases the foot pedal to allow the suction to catch up water/debris aspiration or to allow the client a quick rest before continuing.	Water pools in areas where suction is not available. These areas must be aspirated for client comfort.
13. At the end of the appointment after ultrasonic or sonic instrumentation is completed, the dental hygienist follows current infection control protocol (see Chapter 8).	The high degree of aerosolization of contaminants requires the use of barrier techniques, surface disinfection, and sterilization.

cedures. Such dental hygiene intervention helps to meet the human need for a biologically sound dentition as well as a wholesome body image.

The majority of professional clinical interventions employed for stain removal cause some loss of tooth structure, whether it is in the outer fluoride-rich surface of enamel or the cementum of root structure.[28] For some individuals, stain removal may cause dentinal hypersensitivity during and after the appointment. When stain covers calculus, it must be removed along with the calculus. If stain is of aesthetic concern to the client, it should be removed to meet the individual's need for a wholesome body image. Heavy smokers may accumulate a thick, tarry stain that may resemble stain on calculus when evaluated with an explorer. This type of stain should be removed also because the thickness may irritate gingival tissues and attract bacterial plaque accumulation.

Selective Polishing

When stain is thin and undetectable to exploration, is not of aesthetic concern to the client, and is in an area where tooth structure must be conserved, the dental hygienist should apply the principle of **selective polishing.** This principle essentially eliminates polishing in areas where it fails to meet a human need related to oral health and when it could result in the loss of tooth structure. The dental hygienist may find resistance to selective polishing in clients who have become accustomed to polishing at the conclusion of each scaling appointment. Either the dental hygienist must educate the individual regarding the advantages of selective polishing when it is unnecessary, or choose a method of polishing that minimizes adverse affects, such as using the motor-driven handpiece with a very fine abrasive like a commercial toothpaste.

To increase efficiency during extrinsic stain removal, the dental hygienist should seek to remove stain in the same areas from which bacterial plaque and calculus are removed during instrumentation. In some instances, the stain is present without calculus. In these areas, the stain may be removed either before or after calculus removal. Generally, if the stain is thick and heavy, it should be removed with an ultrasonic scaler prior to hand instrumentation. If it is generalized but thin, stain may be removed at the conclusion of the appointment with the motor-driven handpiece.

Armamentarium for Extrinsic Stain Removal

The armamentarium for stain removal is quite varied and includes many of the instruments used in scaling and root planing. The instruments used in extrinsic stain removal include the following:

- Ultrasonic scaler
- Hand scaling instruments: hoes, sickles
- Scaling and root planing instruments: curets
- Motor-driven handpiece system
- Air-powder abrasive system (air polisher)
- Porte polisher
- Dental floss or tape and abrasive
- Finishing strip

Ultrasonic Scaler in Extrinsic Stain Removal

The ultrasonic scaler was described earlier as an initial scaling instrument. It also is useful in removing large areas of stain on all tooth surfaces including the occlusal surface. The advantages of the ultrasonic scaler are speed and energy conservation; the disadvantage lies in the aerosolization of blood, saliva, and tooth deposits. The health history should be used to rule out communicable diseases prior to using the ultrasonic scaler on a person. If the client has a communicable disease, other methods of polishing that produce less contamination must be used. Another disadvantage of the ultrasonic scaler is its potential to produce damage to tooth structure and excessive heat generation if the instrument tip rests too long on any one area or if the tooth structure is soft and of a malleable nature.

When using the ultrasonic scaler for stain removal, it is best to select a tip that is not too thin and pointed. A more rounded, broader tip causes less tooth damage and provides more coverage needed to remove broad areas of stain. The technique uses light, sweeping motions with more of the side of the tip to avoid letting any part of the instrument tip rest too long on enamel or root surfaces. A finer tip may be necessary for narrow fissures or occlusal pits.

The prosthetic component of dental implants may be cleaned and polished like any prosthesis; however, ultrasonic scaling devices are contraindicated for cleaning the titanium implant abutment cylinders because of the high probability of surface damage. Scratching the surface of the titanium abutment increases the likelihood of bacterial plaque retention and potential calculus accumulation.

Hand Instruments in Extrinsic Stain Removal

Hand scalers such as hoes and sickles may be used for stain removal but are of limited value because of poor adaptation to curved tooth surfaces. They may be used in flatter areas, but must be followed by the curet. The curet conforms well to tooth structure and should be used for stain removal, especially when time permits. The advantage of using the curet is not only the ability to perform complete stain removal, but also the ability to remove roughened cementum or light calculus to which the stain may be primarily attached. Unless the stain is particularly thick, a light, well-adapted root planing stroke should be used with all hand instruments during stain removal.

The Motor-driven Handpiece in Extrinsic Stain Removal

The **motor-driven handpiece** is probably the most common device used for extrinsic stain removal. The system consists of an air-driven, slow-speed handpiece, a prophylaxis angle, a rubber cup, and a brush (Fig. 18–59). The motor-driven handpiece and prophylaxis angle should be autoclavable with autoclavable or disposable prophylaxis angle, rubber cup, rubber tip, and brush attachments. Because operator injury may be aggravated from handling a heavy instrument such as a handpiece, the dental hygienist should use as small and lightweight a handpiece as possible to prevent long-term injury to the hand. A modified pen grasp with the handpiece resting in the rounded U of the hand (which is formed by the thumb and the index finger) and a built-up fulcrum with both the middle and index finger resting against the fulcrum finger are necessary for handling the weight of the dental handpiece. The fulcrum may be located intraorally (same arch or opposite arch) or extraorally.

Different grades of abrasives ranging from coarse to fine are used with the motor-driven handpiece system. Extrinsic

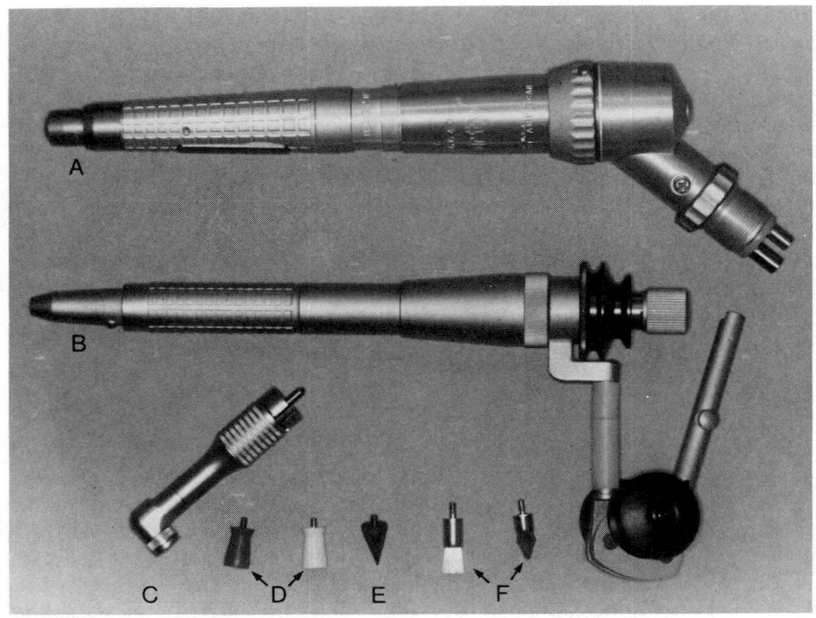

FIGURE 18–59
Motor-driven slow-speed handpiece (A), belt-driven slow-speed handpiece (B), prophylaxis angle (C), rubber cups (D), rubber tip (E), brushes (F).

stain removal may begin with a coarse-grade abrasive if stain is moderate and followed by use of fine polishing agents resulting in a smooth, shiny surface. If the stain is light from the beginning, only a fine polishing agent should be used. The abrasive is picked up with the rubber cup and moved along from the distal, facial or lingual, and mesial surfaces of the tooth. Small dabbing, circular strokes with light pressure are used, which allows the margin of the rubber cup to flare out slightly to reach subgingivally about 1 mm. The rubber tip may be used to polish the facial surfaces of orthodontically banded or bonded teeth when an arch wire is present. In addition, the rubber tip and brush may be used for polishing occlusal surfaces.

The handpiece speed is determined by the pressure of the operator's toes on the foot control or rheostat. The greater the number of revolutions per minute or the more the rheostat is depressed, the greater the heat generated on the tooth. The practitioner should attempt to keep an even, slow speed and a low temperature on the tooth surface by carefully depressing the rheostat when on tooth structure. Light-to-moderate, continuous pressure when putting the rubber cup on the tooth surface also reduces friction (temperature), potential injury to the pulp, and discomfort for the client. The dental hygienist should release the foot control when lifting the rubber cup off the tooth to stop the action and reduce the splatter back to the operator.

The advantage of using the motor-driven handpiece is the relative speed compared to hand instrumentation. It is especially advantageous when the stain is not bulky or thick such as light tea stain. The disadvantage lies mainly in heat generation, aerosolization, and splatter of contaminants.

In addition to the use of antimicrobial therapy, rubber cup polishing with a fine paste abrasive is recommended for individuals with a dental implant.[29] Consideration again is for maintenance of a smooth abutment that will deter bacterial plaque accumulation.

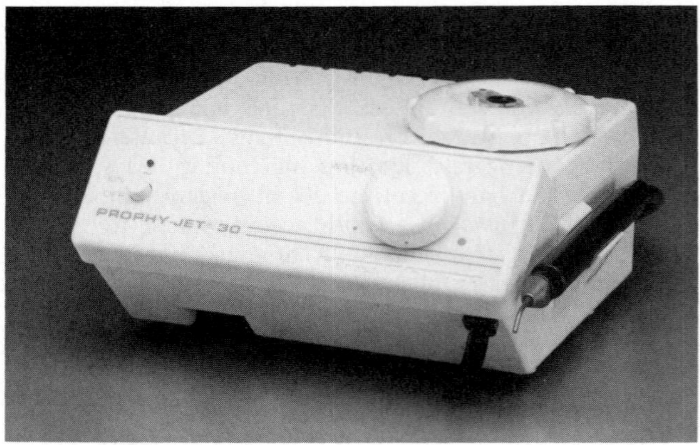

FIGURE 18–60
Prophy-Jet air polisher with separate sodium bicarbonate unit.

Air-Powder Abrasive System in Extrinsic Stain Removal

The **air-powder abrasive system** (air polisher) is a specially designed unit with a handpiece that delivers a spray of warm water and sodium bicarbonate under pressure; it has been shown to be particularly effective for stain removal.[30] The system is manufactured as (1) a console unit with a large, separate sodium bicarbonate unit, a lightweight handpiece, and attachments for air and water (Fig. 18–60), or (2) a multimodality console unit with ultrasonic scaling adaptability.

Because of the high aerosol delivery, care should be taken to screen the health histories for communicable diseases. If a communicable disease is present, another polishing technique should be used. The high-volume spray also is contraindicated for clients who may have respiratory problems and difficulty breathing if they cannot breathe through their mouths. The additional sodium uptake by individuals on sodium-restricted diets makes this instrument contraindicated for certain individuals (e.g., those with high blood pressure or on hemodialysis).

The fulcrum for the air polisher may be located intraorally (same arch or opposite arch) or extraorally. The practitioner should use a continuous circular motion with the spray angled away from the gingival margin to protect the free gingival tissues from trauma.[31] When used correctly, minimizing application time on tooth structure to just a few seconds, the air-powder abrasive system removes stain faster and results in less root surface removal than the curet.[30] Because of the abrasive potential, excessive air polishing of root surfaces should be avoided.[32] Barrier techniques and high-speed evacuation systems should be used to minimize aerosol contamination.

Porte Polisher in Extrinsic Stain Removal

The **porte polisher** is a hand-held straight instrument to which a wedge-shaped wooden tip (usually orangewood) is attached at a 90-degree angle (Fig. 18–61). It resembles the Perio-Aid so often prescribed for clients to control bacterial plaque. The handle is made of metal so that it can be autoclaved, and the disposable wooden tips come in a variety of sizes that are wider and more substantial than the toothpicks used with the Perio-Aid.

The porte polisher should be held with a modified pen grasp with the fulcrum point located intraorally or extraorally. A small amount of abrasive may be used to aid in the polishing process.

The porte polisher may be used on areas too sensitive for traditional modes of polishing (such as the motor-driven handpiece). It does not dispense the heat, create vibration, or cause significant structural damage seen with the motor- or air-driven instruments. The disadvantage of the porte polisher is that it is labor intensive, requiring an enormous amount of time and manual effort. The dental hygienist may find some areas too sensitive even for the porte polisher. When this occurs, the dental hygienist may meet the client's need for freedom from pain by anesthetizing the sensitive areas or leaving them alone. The decision should be based on the aesthetic versus the health-related value of removing the stain.

The porte polisher may be the only polishing instrument used when an individual is treated in an alternative setting such as an acute care or long-term care facility. The dental unit with attachments to water, electricity, and air compression frequently is not available in these types of settings which therefore does not allow the use of the ultrasonic scaler, the motor-driven handpiece, or the air polisher. Because there is no aerosolization, this instrument is particularly useful for medically high-risk persons.

Recently, the porte polisher has found a new niche in the maintenance of titanium implants. When used in conjunction with plastic or graphite scaling instruments, the porte polisher may safely remove bacterial plaque from the titanium implant abutment cylinder. For clients with dental implants, metallic scalers are not recommended because of the high probability of causing surface scratching, enhancing bacterial plaque retention (see Chapter 28).[33,34]

A

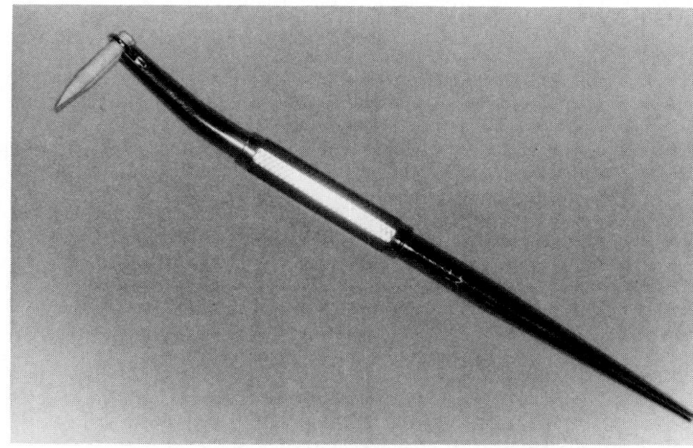

B

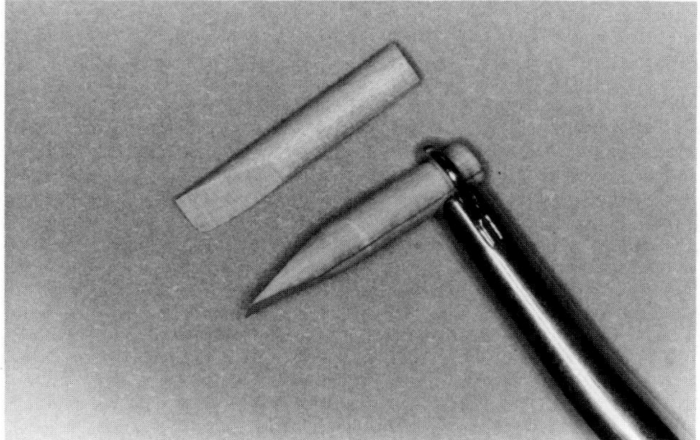

FIGURE 18–61
A and *B*, Porte polisher and wedge-shaped wooden tips.

Dental Floss and Tape With Abrasive in Extrinsic Stain Removal

The **dental floss or dental tape with abrasive** also may be used to remove stain from interproximal regions and around line angles. The floss or tape is wrapped around the tooth just as the client uses it for plaque control, but an abrasive is added to help with stain removal. Although this is particularly helpful in areas of tight contacts, it often can be frustrating because stain may be missed in the developmental depressions located interproximally on roots of teeth. The floss or tape also may be difficult to manipulate in tight areas and often tears or breaks before the stain is removed.

Finishing Strips in Extrinsic Stain Removal

The **finishing strip** is a thin plastic strip with abrasive agents bonded to one side. In theory it works like the dental tape with abrasive. Likewise, it is useful for anterior interproximal stain removal. However, in areas where there are long contacts and little interproximal space, the use of the thin plastic finishing strip may be particularly hazardous to the soft tissues. Selection of an appropriate width of strip for the area and tissue should be made. The dental hygienist should avoid using the finishing strip if it cannot be easily moved against the tooth in the interproximal space without impinging on the soft tissue.

OCCUPATIONAL INJURIES TO THE DENTAL HYGIENIST

Cumulative Trauma Injuries

Cumulative trauma disorder is a term used to identify the group of musculoskeletal disorders involving injuries to the tendons, tendon sheaths, and the related bones, muscles, and nerves of the hands, wrists, elbows, arms, feet, knees, and legs. Such injury may result from conditions in the workstation, tool design, and/or job tasks. Industrial engineers and healthcare workers concerned with occupational injury to employees have studied factors that contribute to worker injury and have offered suggestions to modify the workplace.[35,36]

Carpal tunnel syndrome (CTS), an identified cumlative trauma disorder, has recently been implicated as a significant occupational hazard in the clinical practice of dental hygiene.[37,38] For the dental hygiene clinician, this is particularly disheartening because of the difficulty of changing job assignment, modifying the workstation, or developing ergonomically safe instruments, as is often done in industry. The practice of dental hygiene requires whole body balance and routine physical use of the hand, wrist, arm, and most of the upper body. Unless nonsurgical periodontal therapy can be replaced by therapies that do not require repetitive, forceful hand movements resulting in nerve compression within the carpal tunnel (e.g., antimicrobial therapy), the dental hygienist must learn to incorporate protective strategies of positioning and instrumentation to prevent or lessen risk of injury. The term **"protective" scaling** (established by Tsutsui) is used to denote operator and client positioning, fulcrums, and reinforcements that seek to minimize practitioner injury. The following section of this chapter discusses the etiology and symptomology of CTS and examines strategies to reduce the risk of CTS and other related occupational injuries.

Carpal Tunnel Syndrome

Carpal tunnel syndrome occurs when the median nerve becomes compressed in the carpal tunnel. The carpal tunnel is a canal formed by the carpal bones in the wrist and

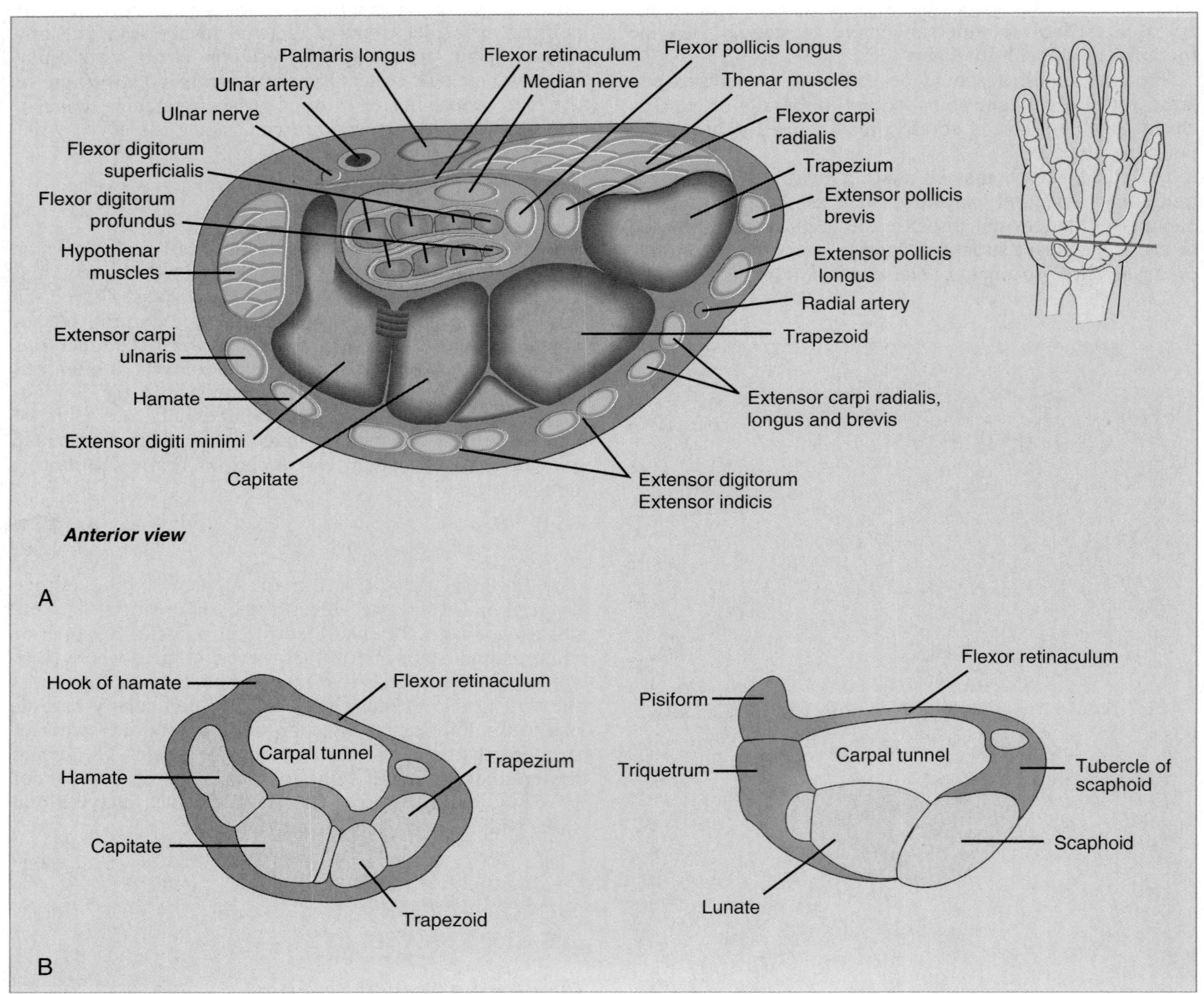

FIGURE 18–62

The carpal bones form a trough through which the flexor tendons and median nerve traverse into the hand. *A*, Transverse section of the wrist, carpal tunnel. *B*, Diagram of transverse section through the carpal tunnel. (Redrawn with permission from Agur, A. Grant's Atlas of Anatomy, 9th ed. Baltimore: Williams & Wilkins, 1991.)

the transverse carpal ligament. As illustrated in Figure 18–62, the carpal bones form a trough through which the eight flexor tendons and the median nerve traverse into the hand. When the flexor tendons swell, there is an increase in the volume of the contents of the canal, an alteration of the osseous trough, or a thickening of the transverse carpal ligament which places increased pressure on the median nerve.[39–41] The nerve compression initiates the carpal tunnel syndrome. The surveillance case definition for work-related carpal tunnel syndrome approved and reported by the National Institute for Occupational Safety and Health is shown in the chart on the following page. It is the definition to be used by physicians and other healthcare providers to facilitate healthcare provider surveillance activities and enhance uniformity of reporting work-related CTS. Underreporting of work-related injury, particularly carpal tunnel syndrome, is common, and increased surveillance of work-related CTS "can aid in identifying high risk workplaces, occupations, and industries and in directing appropriate preventive measures."[42]

Repeated exertions of flexion and extension movements of the wrist seem to aggravate the symptoms of carpal tunnel syndrome. When the wrist is flexed or hyperextended (Fig. 18–63), the contact forces of the tendons over the adjacent surfaces cause irritation of the synovial membrane, or synovitis.[39] The inflammation causes a thickening of the synovial membrane, which narrows the dimensions of the carpal tunnel causing compression of the median nerve. The nerve itself is stretched and, by repeated exertions, compressed between the walls of the carpal tunnel.

Nerve impairment results in reduced muscle control and atrophy. The thenar muscle, which is located at the base of the thumb and is responsible for most of the strength of the thumb, is commonly the muscle that atrophies.

Medical predisposition to CTS has been investigated with consideration given to pregnancy, arthritis, traumatic injury to the wrist, hypothyroidism, local tumor in the wrist, diabetes, endocrine disorders, hyperthyroidism, oral contraceptives, gynecological surgery, and wrist size. Osborn and colleagues indicated that the predisposing factors of arthritis and traumatic injury seem to put dental hygienists at risk for development of carpal tunnel symptoms.[37] Macdonald and colleagues noted that estrogen therapy and diabetes were significantly correlated with nocturnal pain and numbness.[38]

Repetitive wrist and hand movements used in knitting, crocheting, playing musical instruments, painting, woodworking, and gardening have long been associated with carpal tunnel syndrome. Macdonald and colleagues found a correlation between working conditions of dental hygiene practice and CTS.[38] The number of clients with heavy calculus treated per day, number of days practiced per week, and years working as a dental hygienist were all significant factors in the development of CTS symptomology.

A tingling feeling in the thumb, index, middle, and ring fingers is usually an early symptom. The little finger is rarely involved. Other associated symptoms that have been reported in studies of dental hygienists in California[38] and Minnesota[37] include nocturnal pain or numbness, paresthesia, hypesthesia, hand clumsiness, hand weakness, pain, and burning. The loss of sensory feedback from the hand is an extremely significant factor influencing a dental hygienist's ability to grasp, hold, and manipulate instruments.

Without intervention, CTS can lead to marked discomfort, impaired hand function, and disability (Fig. 18–64).

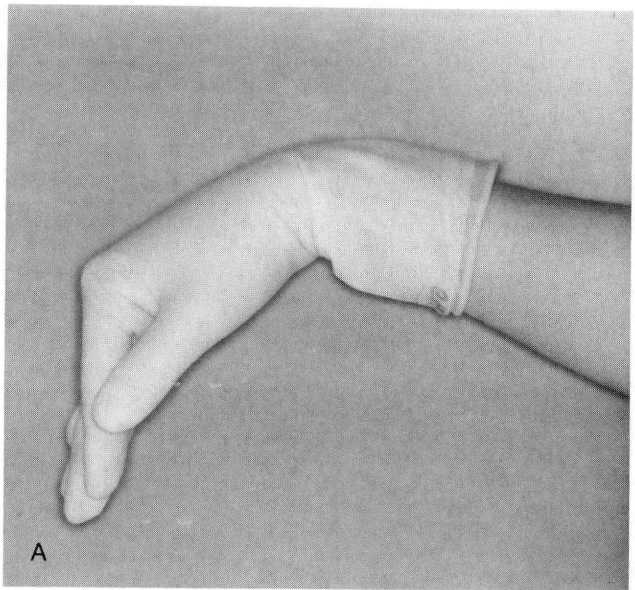

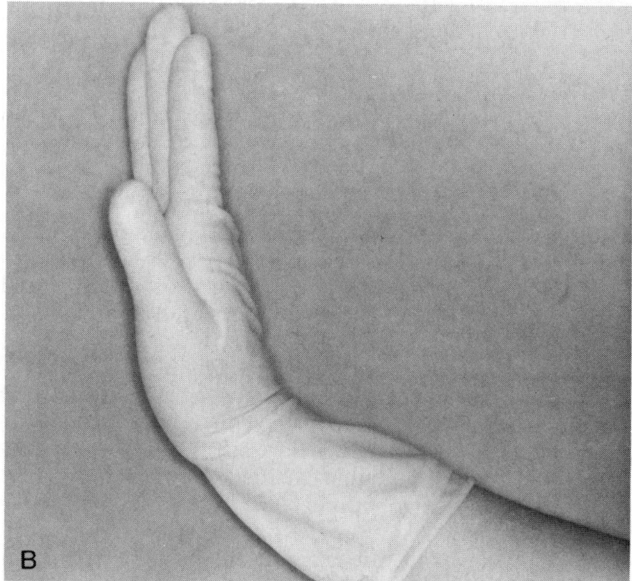

FIGURE 18–63
A, Flexion of the wrist. *B*, Hyperextension of the wrist.

Therapy includes limiting activities causing symptoms, splinting, physical therapy, oral antiinflammatory medications, cortisone injections, and surgery. Success is largely dependent on the reduction of contributory factors and therapy resulting in decompression and reduced irritation of the median nerve.

It may be beneficial for prospective dental hygiene students to be advised of the association of cumulative trauma disorders with the practice of dental hygiene, but there is little information on prevention for the asymptomatic clinician who would like to limit or minimize injury or for the student or practitioner who may be experiencing early symptoms of CTS. Without scientific information measuring the force of exertion created by the muscles during scaling (electromyography), identification of muscles and nerves stressed by the repetitive action of scaling and root planing using various techniques is only theoretical. Re-

SURVEILLANCE CASE DEFINITION FOR WORK-RELATED CARPAL TUNNEL SYNDROME (CTS)

One or more of the following symptoms suggestive of CTS is present*: paresthesias, hypoesthesia, pain, or numbness affecting at least one part of the median nerve distribution† of the hand(s).

Objective findings consistent with CTS are present in the affected hand(s) and wrist(s). EITHER:

Physical examination findings—Tinel's sign§ present or positive Phalen's test¶ or diminished or absent sensation to pin prick in the median nerve distribution of the hand. OR

Electrodiagnostic findings indicative of median nerve dysfunction across the carpal tunnel.**

Evidence of work-relatedness—a history of a job involving *one or more* of the following activities before the development of symptoms††:

Frequent, repetitive use of the same or similar movements of the hand or wrist on the affected side(s).

Regular tasks requiring the generation of high force by the hand.

Regular or sustained tasks requiring awkward hand positions of the affected side(s).§§

Regular use of vibrating hand-held tools.

Frequent or prolonged pressure over the wrist or base of the palm on the affected side(s).

* Symptoms should have lasted at least 1 week or, if intermittent, have occurred on multiple occasions. Other causes of hand numbness or paresthesias, such as cervical radiculopathy, thoracic outlet syndrome, and pronator teres syndrome, should be excluded by clinical evaluation.[1]

† Generally includes palmar side of thumb, index finger, middle finger, and radial half of ring finger; dorsal (back) side of same digits distal to PIP joint; and radial half of palm. Pain and paresthesias may radiate proximally into the arm.

§ Paresthesias are elicited or accentuated by gentle percussion over the carpal tunnel.

¶ Paresthesias are elicited or accentuated by maximal passive flexion of the wrist for 1 minute.

** Criteria for abnormal electrodiagnostic findings are generally determined by the individual laboratories (see, for example, references 1 and 2).

†† A temporal relationship of symptoms to work or an association with cases of CTS in co-workers performing similar tasks is also evidence of work-relatedness.

§§ Awkward hand positions predisposing to CTS include the use of pinch grip (as when holding a pencil), extreme flexion, extension, or ulnar deviation of the wrist, and use of the fingers with the wrist flexed.

From National Institute for Occupational Safety and Health, Centers for Disease Control, 1989.

search is needed on the modification of job tasks, ergonomic design of the workstation, instrumentation theory, and instruments for the dental hygienist. Presently, "protective" techniques of operator and client positioning and instrumentation process offer the most viable solutions to the problems of occupational injury to dental hygienists.

Conclusions from Macdonald,[38] Osborn,[37] and others[36] are valuable in examining dental hygienists' injuries and can be applied in developing preventive or protective instrumentation strategies. To reduce the possibility of developing a cumulative trauma disorder, the dental hygienist must look at the ergonomics of instrumentation and, beginning with basic operator positioning, client positioning, grasp, and fulcrum, must examine the effect instrumentation has on the practitioner's hand, wrist, elbow, shoulder, and back movement. The dental hygienist uses repeated flexion and extension at the wrist in addition to forceful exertions during scaling and root planing. Performing instrumentation related to dental hygiene care is a physical exercise. It involves significant pressure with an instrument in a confined area without causing undue trauma on the client's tissues. Even without force applied during instrumentation, there is always some tension in the fingers, thumb, and wrist to control the instrument, the client's head, or the jaw position. The dental hygienist must be able to work in positions that are comfortable for the client (i.e., respecting the human need for territoriality), allow access for scaling and/or root planing, and also maintain a

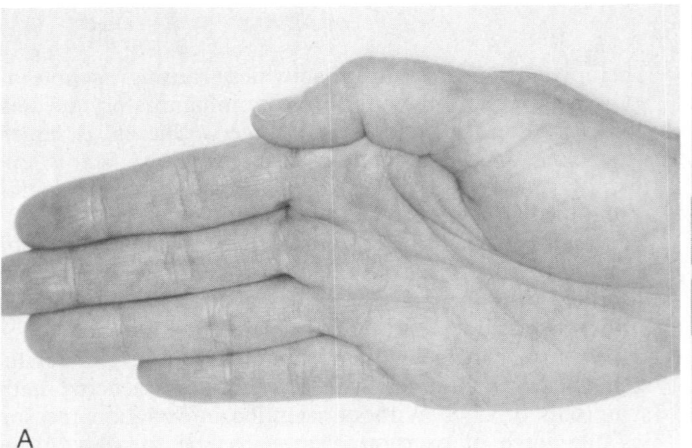

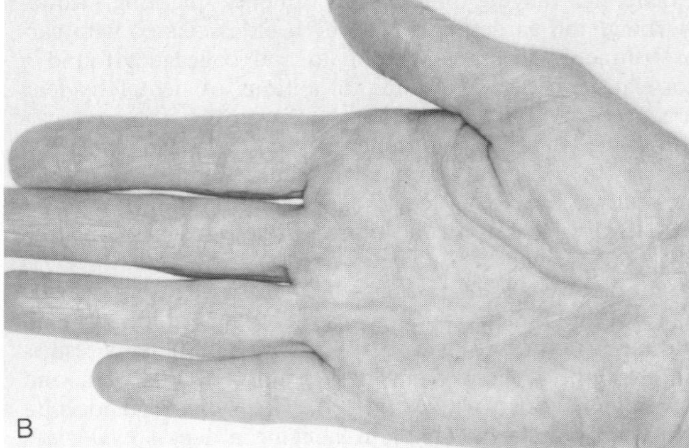

FIGURE 18–64
A, Normal hand of a dental hygienist with well-developed thenar muscle. *B*, Hand of a dental hygienist with CTS showing marked thenar atrophy.

comfortable operator position. In achieving such objectives, a compromise in instrument control may be made too frequently, resulting in additional stress to the working hand or wrist to avoid injury to the client with the instrument. In these situations it helps to use as many supportive mechanisms as possible, such as operator and client positioning and reinforcements to reduce the effort of exertion from the hand or wrist and still produce an effective, controlled stroke.

Industrial biomechanical studies suggest that the most protective position for the wrist is the position it is in when the arm is hanging relaxed at the side of the body.[35,36] Because a straight hand-to-wrist-to-arm position is almost impossible to maintain during all phases of scaling, it is necessary to attempt to simulate it as often as possible or minimize exertions coming from angles of flexion or hyperextension of the wrist. For example, using an extraoral fulcrum that allows some of the pulling action and lateral pressure to come from the arm as it pulls the instrument through the stroke and against the tooth (rather than total use of finger flexion and wrist action) decreases the effort required from the hand and wrist. Techniques of extended fulcruming and reinforcement scaling discussed and illustrated in the next section minimize flexion and hyperextension of the wrist.

Flexion of the wrist also is minimized when attention is given to client positioning. When instrumenting the mandible, it is most advantageous for the operator to seat the client in a slightly supine position with the mandible parallel to the floor. The client may aid the practitioner by lowering his chin and opening widely. Using this position, the practitioner maintains a straighter wrist than when the client is in a supine position. Or the clinician may stand at various clock positions around the client's chair and adjust the level of the client's mouth to her elbow level to encourage the use of the hygienist's arm with the hand and wrist rather than the hand and wrist alone during instrumentation. Conversely, when performing instrumentation on the maxilla, it is advantageous for the operator to assume a sitting position and to position the client in a supine position with chin tilted upward for access and use of a straighter arm during instrumentation. The dental hygienist may be comfortably seated or assume a standing position depending on the instrumentation area and/or the fulcrum position.

Table 18–15 offers suggestions on "protective" scaling techniques in operator positioning. The practitioner may wish to begin self-evaluation of comfort level during instrumentation by examining the effects after using various operator positions (see Evaluation of Basic Operator Tech-

TABLE 18–15
BASIC OPERATOR POSITIONING STRATEGIES OF "PROTECTIVE SCALING" FOR THE DENTAL HYGIENIST

Strategy	Rationale
1. Position self comfortably in chair with weight distributed evenly on the seat 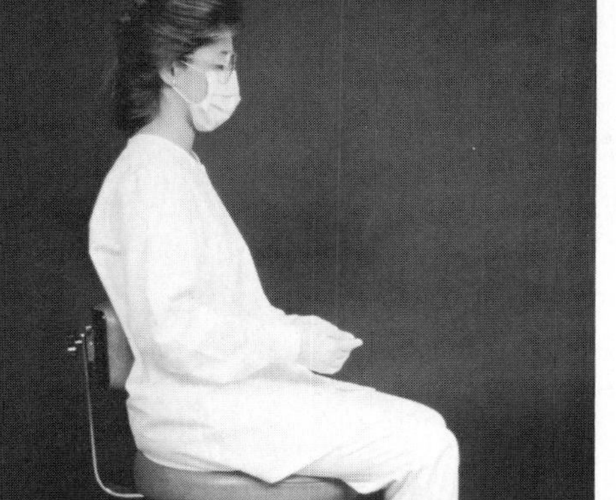	All dental operator chairs are small and tip over or move if operator's weight is not evenly distributed over the seat

Table continued on following page

TABLE 18–15

BASIC OPERATOR POSITIONING STRATEGIES OF "PROTECTIVE SCALING" FOR THE DENTAL HYGIENIST *Continued*

Strategy	Rationale
2. Lower back should be straight but does not have to be against the back of the seat. At times, when speaking with the client, (e.g., reviewing the health history) or if a moment of relaxation is required, the backrest may be used for support	It is impossible to keep the lower back against the backrest during scaling as one needs to lean over the client to distribute body weight over scaling arm to transfer some of the workload to the upper arm and shoulder. However, it is possible to maintain a straight lower back for much of the time during the appointment. This reinforces good postural habits and minimizes possible back injury
3. Knees should be bent in a sitting position. They should not be crossed or straight 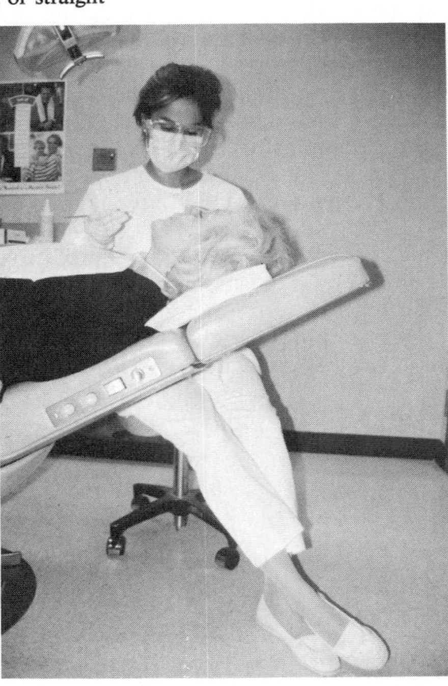	It is easier to control the moveable operator's stool when knees are bent to lessen the chance that the chair will flip out from under the operator. From this position, it is then easier to lean over the client, concentrating more total body effort to control scaling actions
4. Legs do not have to be kept together (i.e., they may straddle the chair). Pant dressing is essential 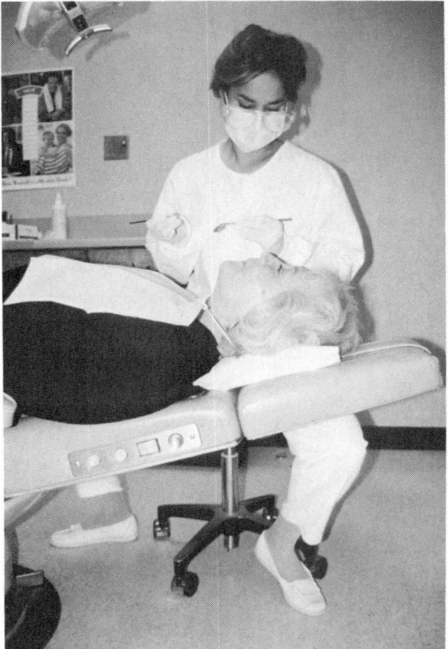	If a right-handed operator were to work on the client's left side, he would need to lean over the client to distribute weight to use the upper arm and shoulder in scaling. This is best accomplished by straddling the chair at 8:00 to 9:00 rather than sitting beside the chair and leaning over from operator's right side

TABLE 18–15

BASIC OPERATOR POSITIONING STRATEGIES OF "PROTECTIVE SCALING" FOR THE DENTAL HYGIENIST *Continued*

Strategy	Rationale
5. Both feet do not have to be positioned squarely on the floor. Either or both knees may be dropped, which changes the foot position to a side or toe placement instead of feet flat on the floor 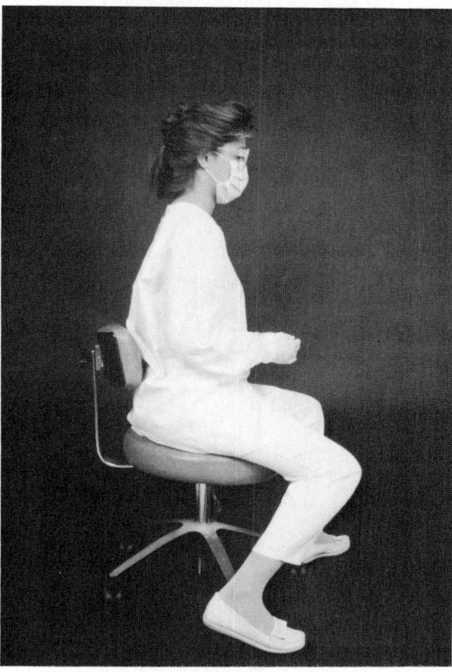	When both feet are planted squarely on the floor, the knees are in a right-angle position. This limits the ability of the operator to move around the client lying in a low supine position. Consequently, the operator must stretch and scale with the major effort coming from the fingers and particularly the wrist
6. The right- or left-handed operator may move anywhere from an 8:00 to a 4:00 seated position around the client	Some areas of the mouth are easier to reach from different angles
7. A standing approach is useful in all positions from 8:00 to 4:00	When seated, operator is unknowingly balancing the body on a moveable stool. The standing position is easier in some areas of the mouth (e.g., mandibular posterior mesial surfaces) because it allows traction and versatility to move over a client. Operator may use the upper arm and shoulder while scaling without the risk or need to control a moveable stool
8. The standing position is useful when it becomes difficult to see (e.g., in situations where the client is seated slightly upright, the mouth is small, or the client's chair does not drop low enough) 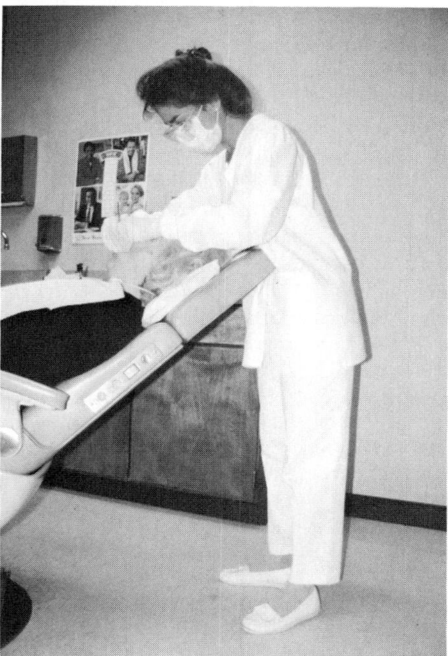	With the client seated upright and the operator in a seated position, it is necessary to reach up and subsequently flex and extend the wrist to perform instrumentation. In the standing position, the operator is simply able to reach down and use a pull stroke while keeping the wrist and arm in line with the shoulder

Table continued on following page

TABLE 18–15
BASIC OPERATOR POSITIONING STRATEGIES OF "PROTECTIVE SCALING" FOR THE DENTAL HYGIENIST *Continued*

Strategy	Rationale
9. In the standing position, the feet may be positioned squarely on the floor but may lift off onto the ball of the left foot (right-handed clinician) with the right hip leaning against the client's chair 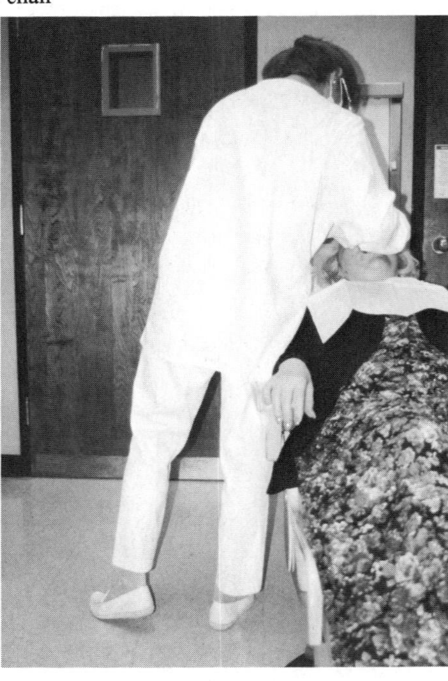	By lifting slightly up on toes and bracing the lower body against the client's chair, the operator may lean across the client and work with maximal control

EVALUATION OF BASIC OPERATOR TECHNIQUE

Problem	Solution
■ Did you rely on your legs and feet to stay in your seat at any point during the appointment?	■ You may have been sitting too close to the edge of the seat and even if the chair is of an anti-tip design, you unnecessarily used your lower body for stability when it may have been more efficient to conserve energy or direct it towards control during scaling.
■ At the end of the appointment or day of work, straighten your lower back. Does it feel stiff, tight, or sore?	■ If your back feels tight or achy, you have bent over from the lower back too often for long periods during the day (instead of keeping it straight as often as possible).
■ Does your right side around the waistline feel sore or stiff?	■ Indicates a scaling posture which utilizes an excessive leaning position for long periods of time. It would have been better to straddle the chair or stand, lean hip against the chair and work over the client.
■ Are your wrist, hand, or fingers and shoulders unusually tired and aching after scaling?	■ Indicates one or more of the following: Need to change operator from standard 8:00–9:00 o'clock approach to another angle Client position too high. Either lower dental chair and or operator chair or stand during instrumentation. Operator's body position should have been in better alignment with scaling hand to eliminate exertion at hand and wrist level Possibility of cumulative trauma disorder

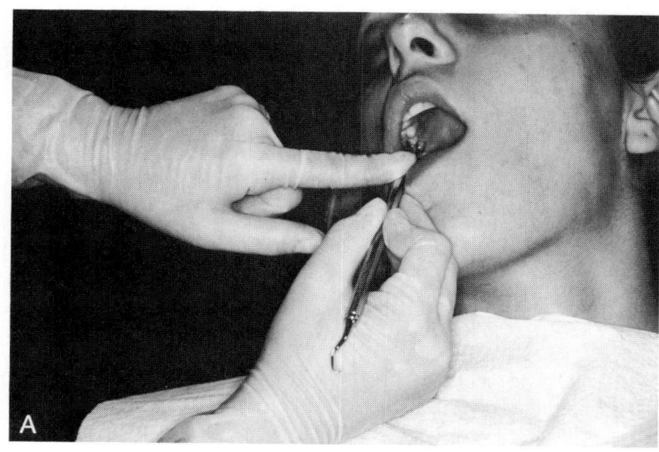

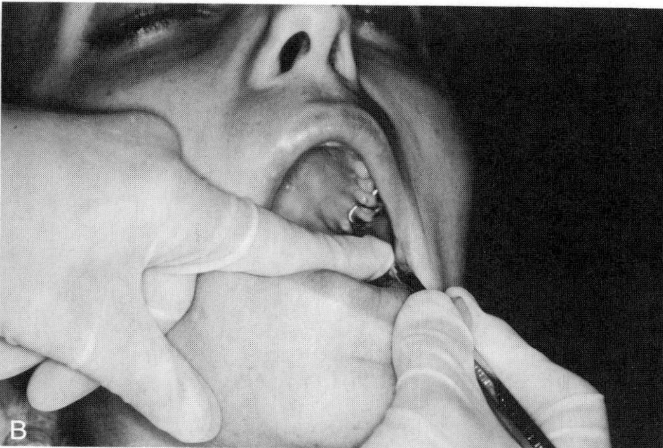

FIGURE 18–65
Index finger reinforcement. *A*, Right maxillary posterior mesial surface from lingual approach. Operator is at the 8:00 to 9:00 position. The Gracey curet 11–12 is being used. Position of the working hand is extraoral fulcrum, palm up. The position of the reinforcement hand shows the index finger on instrument applying pressure in the same direction of lateral pressure in which the dominant hand is working. *B*, Left maxillary mesial surface from lingual approach. Operator is at the 8:00 to 9:00 position. The Gracey curet 11–12 is being used. Position of the working hand is extraoral fulcrum, palm down. The position of the reinforcement hand shows the index finger on instrument applying pressure in the same direction of lateral pressure in which the dominant hand is working.

nique chart). Such self-evaluation also may be done at any time during the instrumentation process. It requires only that the practitioner be aware of where the area of stress is in the working hand or arm. If it is possible to transfer or equalize the stress of working from the hand and wrist to include the arm or even the shoulder, the dental hygienist minimizes injury to the median nerve. Table 18–15 outlines positioning techniques for protective scaling.

REINFORCEMENT SCALING TECHNIQUES

Reinforcement scaling has been used to gain additional stability and control of the instrument when scaling with both the intraoral and extraoral fulcrum.[1,6] In most cases, the use of reinforcement scaling means that the nondominant

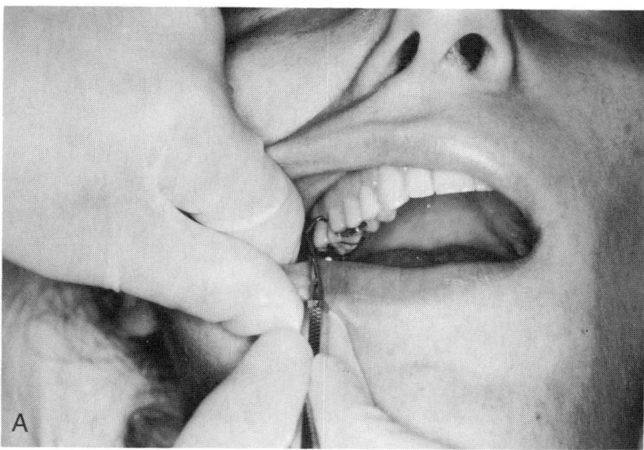

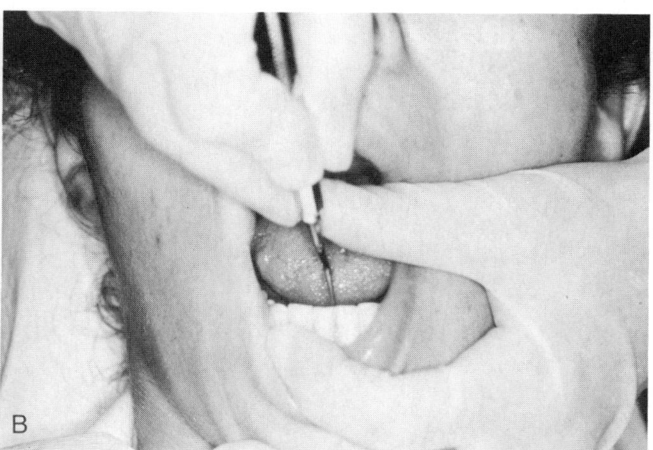

FIGURE 18–66
Thumb reinforcement. *A*, Right maxillary posterior distal surface from facial approach. Operator is at the 8:00 to 9:00 position. The Gracey curet 13–14 is being used. Position of the working hand is extraoral fulcrum, palm up. The position of the reinforcement hand shows the index finger retracting buccal mucosa, and the thumb on instrument applying pressure in the same direction of lateral pressure in which the dominant hand is working. *B*, Mandibular anterior lingual interproximal surface. Operator is at the 12:00 position. The Gracey curet 5–6 is being used. Position of the working hand is opposite arch fulcrum. The position of the reinforcement hand shows the index finger retracting the lower lip, and the thumb applying pressure in same direction of lateral pressure in which the dominant hand is working or supports in upward movement.

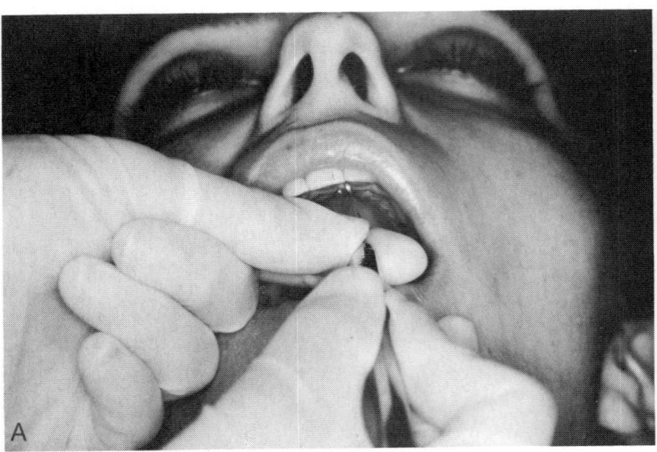
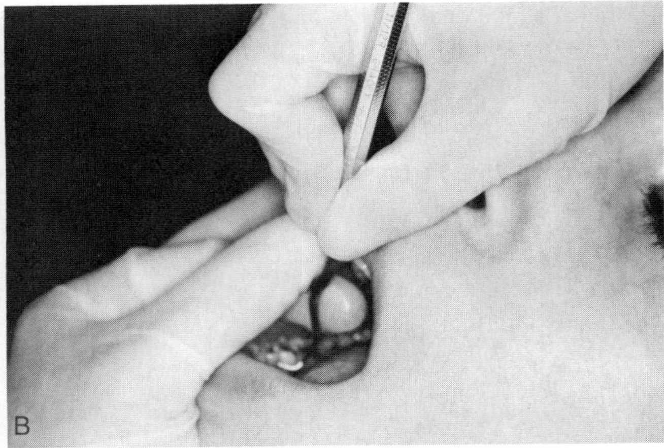

FIGURE 18–67
Index finger–thumb reinforcement. *A*, Maxillary anterior lingual interproximal surface. Operator is at the 8:00 to 9:00 position. The Gracey curet 5–6 is being used. Position of the working hand is extraoral fulcrum, palm up. The position of the reinforcement hand shows the index finger under instrument, thumb on top of instrument in pinch-like grasp. *B*, Mandibular right posterior mesial surface from lingual approach. Operator is at the 1:00 position. The Gracey curet 11–12 is being used. Position of the working hand is opposite arch fulcrum. The position of the reinforcement hand shows the index finger under instrument, thumb on top of instrument in pinch-like grasp.

hand is used for additional support of the instrument instead of holding the mouth mirror. In some cases (as illustrated in Figure 18–30), it is still possible to hold the mouth mirror and provide reinforcement with the nondominant hand. Reinforcement scaling is "protective" to the dental hygiene practitioner.

The added support from reinforcement may come from the index or thumb or thenar region (radial palm or fleshy mass on lateral side of palm) of the nondominant hand. The dominant hand must continue to play the major role in adapting and angulating the blade against the tooth surface. It also must exert control over the direction in which the instrument is pulled over the tooth. Reinforcement is used to:

- Provide additional lateral pressure in the same direction to which the dominant hand's fingers are directing pressure
- Guide the instrument in a longer pull stroke when an extended extraoral fulcrum is used
- Support the thenar region of the dominant hand which provides protective qualities during often strenuous and intensive instrumentation processes

The beneficial aspects of reinforcement scaling are found

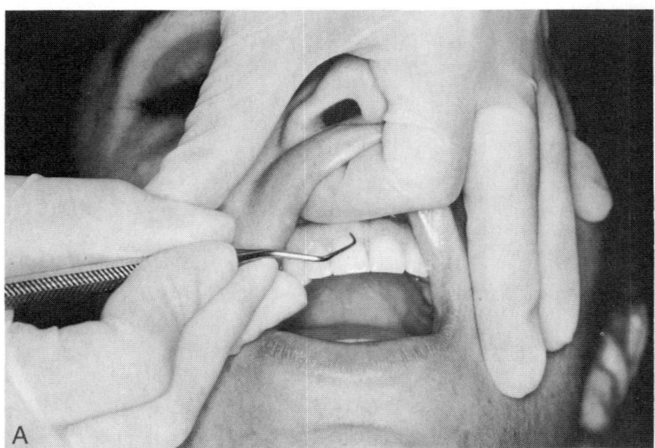
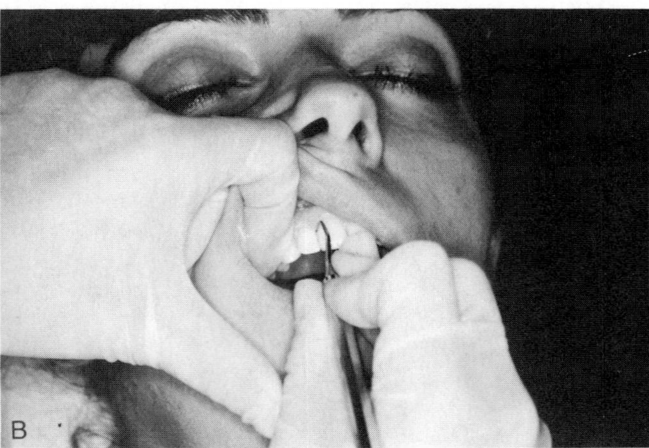

FIGURE 18–68
Thenar support reinforcement. *A*, Maxillary anterior facial surface from labial approach. Operator is at the 12:00 position. The Gracey curet 7–8 is being used. Position of the working hand is intraoral fulcrum close to working area. Position of the reinforcement hand shows the index finger retracting the lip, and thumb supporting working thumb to thenar area. *B*, Maxillary anterior interproximal surface from labial approach. Operator is at the 8:00 to 9:00 position. The Gracey curet 5–6 is being used. Position of the working hand is intraoral fulcrum close to the working area. The position of the reinforcement hand shows the index finger retracting the upper lip, and thumb supporting working thumb near thenar area.

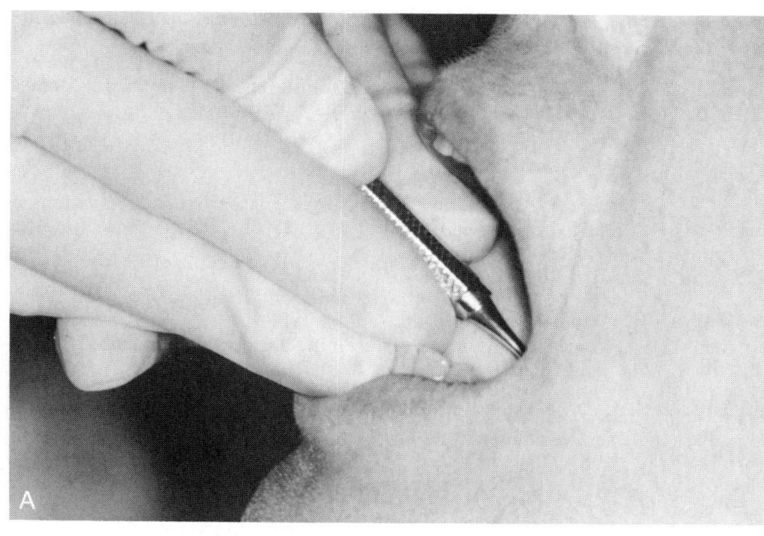

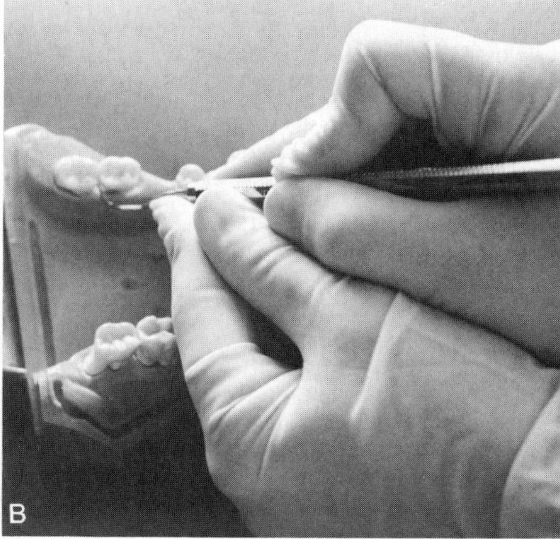

FIGURE 18–69
A and *B*, Index (thumb) thenar reinforcement. Mandibular right posterior distal line angle from lingual approach. Operator is at the 8:00 to 9:00 position. The Gracey curet 13–14 is being used. Position of the working hand is fulcrum same quadrant as area being scaled. Position of the reinforcement hand is index finger on instrument, and thumb (or thenar) of reinforcement hand on thumb (or thenar) of working hand.

only when the operator uses both intraoral and extraoral fulcrum techniques. Pattison and Pattison have illustrated the **index finger** and **thumb reinforcement** on the instrument.[6] Two additional reinforcements are introduced. These reinforcements are the **index finger–thumb reinforcement** and **thumb-to-thumb (or thenar) reinforcement.** The names of the reinforcements tell the operator where the reinforcements originate from. The placement of the index finger and thumb may be on or around the instrument between the working end and the dominant hand. The position of the reinforcing thumb also may be positioned against the dominant thumb or thenar region for support and comfort to the operator. Examples of reinforcement scaling in selected areas of the mouth are shown in Figures 18–65*A* to 18–69*B*.

References

1. Wilkins, E. Clinical Practice of the Dental Hygienist, 6th ed. Philadelphia: Lea & Febiger, 1989, p. 430.
2. Canis, M. F., Kramer, G. M., and Pameijer, C. M. Calculus attachment: Review of the literature and new findings. Journal of Periodontology 50:406, 1979.
3. Tal, H., Koslovsky, A., et al. Scanning electron microscope evaluation of wear and stainless steel and high carbon steel curettes. Journal of Periodontology 60(6):320, 1989.
4. Lindhe, J. Evaluation of periodontal scalers. II. Wear following standardized othogonal cutting tests. Odontologisk Revy 17:121, 1966.
5. Parkes, R., and Kolstad, A. Effects of sterilization on periodontal instruments. Journal of Periodontology 53(7):434, 1982.
6. Pattison, A., and Pattison, G. Periodontal Instrumentation, 2nd ed. Norwalk: Appleton & Lange, 1992, pp. 167–168.
7. Socransky, S. S., Haffajee, A. D., Goodson, J. M., and Lindhe, J. New concepts of destructive periodontal disease. Journal of Clinical Periodontology 11:21, 1984.
8. Lindhe, J. Textbook of Clinical Periodontology. Philadelphia: W. B. Saunders, 1983, p. 301.
9. Proceedings of the World Workshop in Clinical Periodontics, July 23–27, 1989. Chicago: American Academy of Periodontology, 1989, p. 123.
10. Armitage, G. C., Dickinson, W. R., et al. Relationship between the percentage of subgingival spirochetes and the severity of periodontal disease. Journal of Periodontology, 53:550, 1982.
11. Hancock, E. B., Cray, R. J., and O'Leary, T. J. The relationship between gingival crevicular fluid and gingival inflammation. A clinical and histologic study. Journal of Periodontology, 50:13, 1979.
12. Shapiro, L., Goldman, H., and Bloom, A. Sulcular exudate flow in gingival inflammation. Journal of Periodontology, 50:301, 1979.
13. Brouwsma, O., Caton, J., et al. Effect of personal oral hygiene on bleeding interdental gingiva. Histologic changes. Journal of Periodontology, 59:80, 1988.
14. Proye, M., Caton, J., and Polson, A. Initial healing of periodontal pockets after a single episode of root planing monitored by controlled probing forces. Journal of Periodontology, 53:296, 1982.
15. Stende, F. W., and Schaffer, E. M. A comparison of ultrasonic and hand scaling. Journal of Periodontology, 32:312, 1961.
16. Stewart, J. L., Drisko, R. R., and Herlach, A. D. Comparison of ultrasonic and hand instruments for the removal of calculus. Journal of the American Dental Association 75:153, 1957.
17. Hunter, R. K., O'Leary, T. J., and Kafrawy, A. H. The effectiveness of hand versus ultrasonic instrumentation in open flap root planing. Journal of Periodontology 55:697, 1984.
18. Silverstein, L., Bissada, M., et al. Clinical and microbiological effects of local tetracycline irrigation on periodontitis. Journal of Periodontology, 59:864, 1988.
19. Lang, N. P., and Ramseier-Grossman, K. Optimal dosage of chlorhexidine digluconate in chemical plaque control when applied by the oral irrigator. Journal of Periodontology, 8:189, 1981.
20. Moskow, B. S., and Bressman, E. Cemetal response to ultrasonic and hand instrumentation. Journal of the American Medical Association, 68:698, 1964.
21. Jones, S., Lozdan, J., and Boyde, A. Tooth surfaces treated in situ with periodontal instruments. British Dental Journal, 132:57, 1972.
22. Badersten, A., Nilveus, R., and Egelberg, J. Effect of nonsurgical periodontal therapy. I. Moderately advanced periodontitis. Journal of Clinical Periodontology, 8:57, 1981.

23. Badersten, A., Nilveus, R., and Egelberg, J. Effect of nonsurgical periodontal therapy. II. Severely advanced periodontitis. Journal of Periodontology 11:63, 1984.
24. Holbrook, T., and Low, S. Power-driven scaling and polishing instruments. In Clark, J. (ed.). Clinical Dentistry, vol. 3. Philadelphia: J. B. Lippincott, 1989, p. 1.
25. Gankerseer, E., and Walmsley, A. Preliminary investigation into the performance of a sonic scaler. Journal of Periodontology 58(11):780, 1987.
26. Patterson, C. J. W., and McLundie, A. C. A comparison of the effects of two different prophylaxis regimens in vitro on some restorative dental materials. British Dental Journal 157:166, 1984.
27. Gorfil, C., Nordenberg, D., et al. The effect of ultrasonic cleaning and air polishing on the marginal integrity of radicular amalgam and composite resin restorations: An in vitro study. Journal of Clinical Periodontology 16:137, 1989.
28. Tinanoff, N., Wei, S. H., and Parkins, F. M. Effect of pumice prophylaxis of fluoride uptake in tooth enamel. Journal of the American Dental Association 88:3849, 1974.
29. Thomson-Neal, D., Evans, G., and Meffert, R. M. Effects of various prophylactic treatment on titanium, sapphire, and hydroxyapatite-coated implants: An SEM Study. International Journal of Periodontics Restorative Dentistry 9(4):301, 1989.
30. Berkstein, S., Reiff, R. L., et al. Supragingival root surface removal during maintenance procedures utilizing air-powder abrasive system or hand scaling. An in vitro study. Journal of Periodontology 58:327, 1987.
31. Mishkin, D. J., et al. A clinical comparison of the effect on the gingiva of the Prophyjet and the rubber cup and paste techniques. Journal of Periodontology 57:151, 1986.
32. Galloway, S. E., and Pahley, D. H. Rate of removal of root structure by use of Prophy-Jet device. Journal of Periodontology 58:464, 1987.
33. Newman, M. G., and Fleming, T. F. Periodontal considerations of implants and implant-associated microbiota in dental implants. NIH Consensus Development Conference. National Institute of Dental Research, the Office of Medical Applications of Research, National Institutes of Health, and the Food and Drug Administration, Washington, D.C., June 13–15, 1988, p. 57.
34. Meffert, R. M. The soft tissue interface in dental implantology in dental implants. NIH Consensus Development Conference. National Institute of Dental Research, the Office of Medical Applications of Research, National Institutes of Health, and the Food and Drug Administration, Washington, D.C., June 13–15, 1988, p. 107.
35. Tichauer, E. Some aspects of stress on forearm and hand in industry. Journal of Occupational Medicine 8(2):63, 1966.
36. U.S. Department of Health and Human Services, Public Health Service, Centers for Disease Control, National Institute for Occupational Safety and Health. Carpal Tunnel Syndrome: Selected References, March, 1989.
37. Osborn, J., Newell, K., et al. Carpal tunnel syndrome among Minnesota dental hygienists. Journal of Dental Hygiene 64(2):79, 1990.
38. Macdonald, G., Robertson, M., and Erickson, J. Carpal tunnel syndrome among California dental hygienists. Journal of Dental Hygiene 62(7):322, 1988.
39. Armstrong, T., Castelli, W., et al. Some histological changes in carpal tunnel contents and their biomechanical implications. Journal of Occupational Medicine 26(3):197, 1984.
40. Tountas, C., Macdonald, C., et al. Carpal tunnel syndrome. Minnesota Medicine 66:479, 1983.
41. Phalen, G. The carpal-tunnel syndrome. Journal of Bone and Joint Surgery 4S-A(2):211, 1966.
42. Centers for Disease Control: Occupational disease surveillence: Carpal tunnel syndrome. Journal of the American Medical Association 262(7):886, 1989.

Suggested Readings

Badersten, A., Niveus, R., and Egelberg, J. 4-year observations of basic periodontal therapy. Journal of Clinical Periodontology 14:438, 1987.

Caffesse, R. G., Sweeney, P. L., and Smith, B. A. Scaling and root planing with and without periodontal flap surgery. Journal of Clinical Periodontology 13:205, 1986.

Conrad, J., Osborn, J., et al. Peripheral nerve dysfunction in practicing dental hygienists. Journal of Dental Hygiene 10(8):382, 1990.

Eaton, K. A., Kieser, J. B., and Davies, R. M. The removal of root surface deposits. Journal of Clinical Periodontology 12:141, 1985.

Garrett, J. S. Root planing: A perspective. Journal of Periodontology 48:553, 1977.

Haffajee, A. D., Socransky, S. S., and Goodson, J. M. Clinical parameters as predictors of destructive periodontal disease activity. Journal of Clinical Periodontology 10:257, 1983.

Herremans, K. L. Effects of ultrasonic scaling and hand scaling on root topography. Masters thesis submitted to the faculty of Old Dominion University, 1991.

Huntley, D., and Shannon, S. Carpal tunnel syndrome: A review of the literature. Journal of Dental Hygiene 62(7):316, 1988.

Knowles, J. W., Burgett, F., et al. Results of periodontal treatment related to pocket depth and attachment level. Eight years. Journal of Periodontology 50:225, 1979.

Lindhe, J., and Jacobson, L. Evaluation of periodontal scalers. I. Wear following clinical use. Odontologisk Revy 17:1, 1966.

Lindhe, J., Westfelt, E., et al. Long-term effect of surgical/non-surgical treatment of periodontal disease. Journal of Clinical Periodontology 11:448, 1984.

Loos, B., Kiger, R., and Egelber, J. An evaluation of basic periodontal therapy using sonic and ultrasonic scalers. Journal of Clinical Periodontology 14:29, 1987.

Lovhal, A., Arno, A., et al. Combined effects of subgingival scaling and controlled oral hygiene on the incidence of gingivitis. Acta Odontologica Scandinavica 19:537, 1961.

Nield, J., and Houseman, G. Fundamentals of Dental Hygiene Instrumentation, 2nd ed. Philadelphia: Lea & Febiger, 1988, p. 369.

Nishimine, D., and O'Leary T. J. Hand instrumentation versus ultrasonics in the removal of endotoxins from root surfaces. Journal of Periodontology 50:345, 1979.

Oosterwaal, J. J. M., Matee, M., et al. The effect of subgingival debridement with hand and ultrasonic instruments on the subgingival microflora. Journal of Clinical Periodontology 14:528, 1987.

Ramfjord, S. P. Root planing and curettage. International Dental Journal 30:93, 1980.

Ramfjord, S. P., Caffesse, R. G., et al. Four modalities of periodontal treatment compared over 5 years. Journal of Periodontology Research 22:222, 1987.

Tsutsui, P. Unpublished handout to senior dental students at the University of Southern California, 1992.

Waerhaug, J. Healing of dento-epithelial junction following subgingival plaque control (II). As observed on extracted teeth. Journal of Periodontology 49:119, 1978.

19

Root Morphology

OBJECTIVES

Mastery of the content in this chapter will enable the reader to:

- Define the key terms used
- Discuss the significance of root morphology to the dental hygiene process
- Identify all multirooted teeth in the permanent dentition
- Describe axial positioning and its importance in instrumentation
- Define trifurcation and name the teeth that are trifurcated
- Differentiate between the curve of Spee and the curve of Wilson
- Discuss the anatomical features of a permanent root form by listing a minimum of two characteristics of any tooth in the dentition
- Describe the challenges in the instrumentation of a maxillary first molar
- Identify two common root traits found on all permanent teeth
- List two prime challenges of instrumenting in furcations

INTRODUCTION

Careful root planing is a technically difficult procedure that is universally employed in the dental hygiene care of persons with periodontitis. The objective of root planing is to produce a root that is clean, smooth, and hard, making it more biologically acceptable to connective tissue reattachment. Understanding the topography and morphology of the roots is essential for therapeutic scaling and root planing. Root furcations, concavities, positioning, and anomalies influence the dental hygienist's choice of instruments and their adaptation for effective root instrumentation. Thorough root planing also requires that the dental hygienist have the ability to evaluate the degree of smoothness and hardness of the root surface and the ability to make a decision as to when the procedure is completed. To make a good clinical decision the dental hygienist must combine knowledge of root morphology with technical skills. Knowledge of root morphology provides the dental hygienist with a road map for performing therapeutic scaling and root planing as part of the dental hygiene process of care. In addition, in meeting the client's need for problem solving and self-determination, aspects of root morphology may need to be pointed out to the client, who on a daily basis must master oral hygiene techniques for keeping exposed root surfaces free from bacterial plaque.

Root morphology is the study of the topography of the root surfaces of the human dentition. Because teeth are not uniform or simple cylinders, they offer the dental hygienist a challenge during root instrumentation and the client a challenge in daily plaque control. Understanding the topography of the root surfaces is essential to mastering the skills of scaling and root planing and essential for effective client education. The clinician must be familiar with normal root structures to be able to distinguish them from calculus, altered cementum, and overhanging restorations. Proper adaptation of instruments depends on knowledge of root morphology and allows for optimal access to root surfaces for evaluation and care. Proper instrument adaptation and angulation decreases potential damage to the root structure and surrounding tissues and facilitates the hygienist's ability to instrument completely.

Roots have indentations, or **concavities,** as well as more rounded surfaces, or **convexities.** These anatomical features are considered by the dental hygienist before root instrumentation is done. The purpose of this chapter is to aid the dental hygienist in understanding root structures of teeth and to facilitate detection and instrumentation of acquired deposits and rough root surfaces as well as the general evaluation of the topography of root surfaces. Shapes of roots, their curvatures, angulations, and structures are discussed.

GENERAL MORPHOLOGICAL CONSIDERATIONS

Shapes of Roots

Each tooth in the permanent dentition is unique and differs from person to person in size and length. Teeth do, however, have the following common traits:[2,3]

- Roots are widest at the neck or cervical area of the tooth and taper toward the apex of the tooth

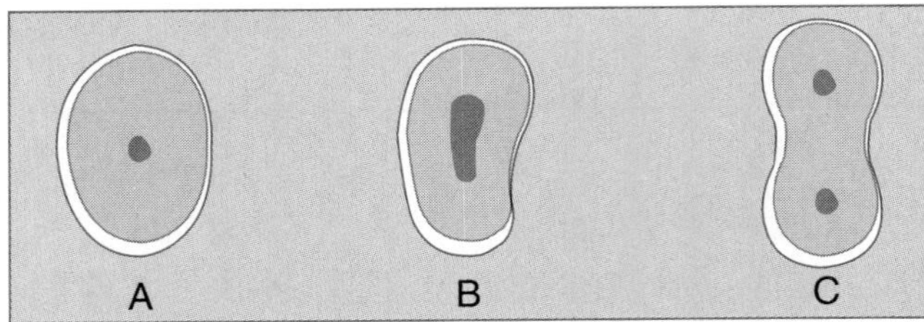

FIGURE 19-1
Examples of convex surface *(A)*, concave surface *(B)*, and ribbon effect *(C)* (view: midroot sections of teeth).

- Roots have more bulk on the facial surface than on the lingual surface. There is more tapering of the root on the lingual surface
- Single-rooted teeth include central incisors, lateral incisors, canines, maxillary second premolars, mandibular first and second premolars
- Double-rooted teeth include mandibular first, second, and third molars (one mesial and one distal root), maxillary first premolars (one facial and one lingual root)*
- Triple-rooted teeth include maxillary first, second, and third molars (one lingual, one mesiofacial, and one distofacial root)

Root Curvatures

Roots have rounded curvatures that form *convex* surfaces and indented curvatures that form *concave* surfaces. When a root has a concave curvature on the mesial and distal surfaces, the root may give a double-rooted appearance, although the tooth is actually single-rooted. This pseudo-double-rooted effect is known as a **ribbon effect.** It is important that the dental hygienist anticipate these anatomical changes for effective instrument adaptation (Fig. 19-1).

* The maxillary first premolar also may be a single-rooted tooth.

Root Angulations

Understanding root angulation is essential for proper adaptation of instruments and for careful evaluation of root morphology. The tooth's **axial positioning** is the vertical inclination of a tooth. Described in terms of root inclination, most teeth have a slight mesial, distal, facial, or lingual root inclination. These root inclinations are physiologically necessary for proper occlusal and incisal function of the teeth. Figure 19-2 shows the axial positioning of the permanent dentition.[4]

Roots of the maxillary anterior teeth have a great lingual and slight distal inclination. Premolar roots have a slightly lingual and distal inclination. Roots of the maxillary molars have a great lingual and moderate distal inclination.

In the mandibular arch, the angulations of the roots of the anterior teeth vary from nearly vertical to a great lingual inclination. Canines and premolars may have a slight distal root inclination. Mandibular molars have a great to moderate distal root inclination.[2,4]

Other angulations important to the positioning of the teeth are the curve of Spee and the curve of Wilson. The **curve of Spee** is the curvature of the occlusal surfaces of the posterior teeth. The curve is two-dimensional and curves upwards from the canines to the molars when viewed from the facial aspect (Fig. 19-3).

The **curve of Wilson** is the curvature of the occlusal plane of posterior teeth. The curve becomes deeper as one moves more posterior. The crowns of the mandibular molars tip lingually and the crowns of the maxillary molars tip facially (Fig. 19-4).[3]

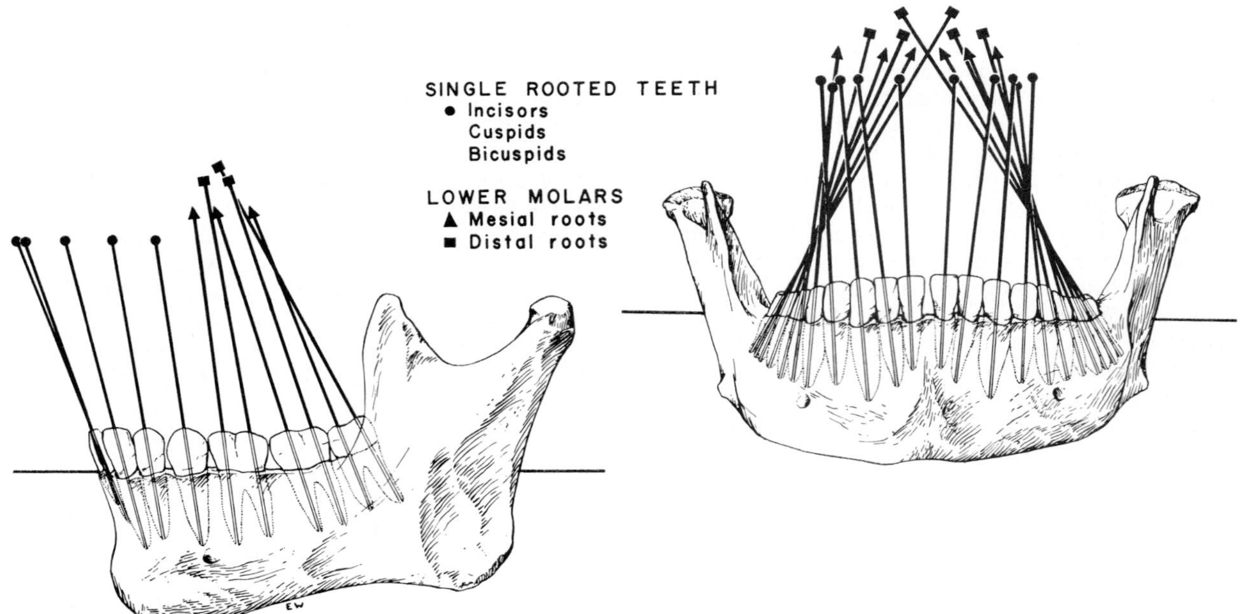

FIGURE 19-2
Axial positioning of permanent teeth. (Modified from Dempster et al., 1963; copyright by the American Dental Association. Reprinted by permission of *The Journal of the American Dental Association.*)

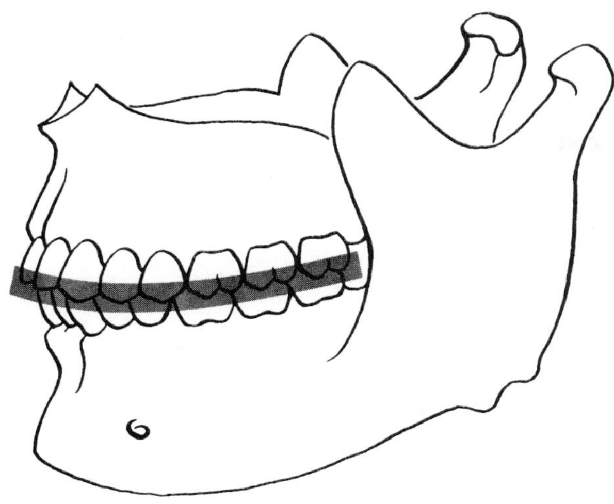

FIGURE 19–3
Curve of Spee. (With permission from Torres, H. O., and Ehrlich, A. Modern Dental Assisting, 5th ed. Philadelphia: W. B. Saunders, 1995.)

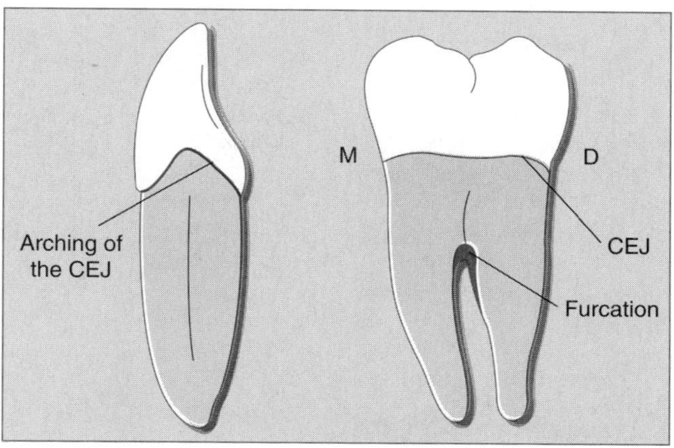

FIGURE 19–5
Appearance of cementoenamel junction (CEJ) on anterior and posterior teeth. Note how the CEJ arcs interproximally on the anterior tooth and the furcation area of the posterior tooth. *Left,* Anterior tooth, mandibular central incisor, mesial view. *Right,* Posterior tooth, mandibular right second molar, lingual view.

ROOT STRUCTURES

Cementoenamel Junction

The **cementoenamel junction** (CEJ) is an important root structure that the dental hygienist should be able to identify subgingivally with an instrument. Not only is the CEJ a key anatomical landmark when measuring periodontal attachment loss in clients who have had periodontitis, but it also may be a specific target area for client instruction if it involves a root irregularity that collects bacterial plaque and dental calculus.[5]

At the CEJ, the cementum overlaps the enamel in approximately 60 to 65% of the teeth. In roughly 30% of the teeth the enamel meets the cementum, and in 5 to 10% of the teeth there may be a small area of exposed dentin. The CEJ usually feels smooth or has a slight groove.[6]

On many posterior teeth, the CEJ is somewhat uniform in appearance and easily followed with an explorer. However, on anterior teeth the CEJ arcs interproximally. As a result, the area is difficult to instrument because of limited accessibility and the close proximity of teeth. Improper instrument adaptation in these areas may result in incomplete scaling and root planing (Fig. 19–5).

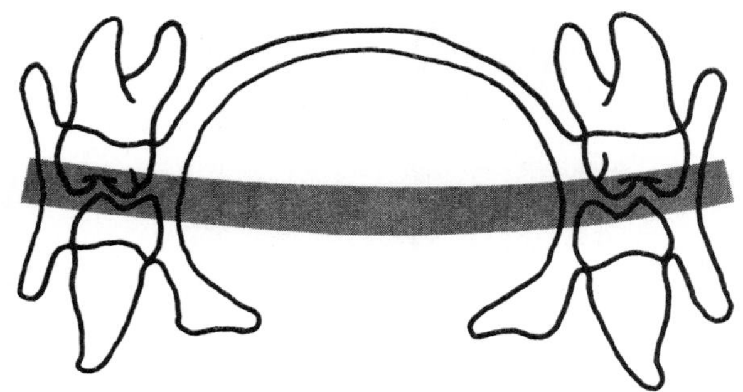

FIGURE 19–4
Curve of Wilson. (With permission from Torres, H. O., and Ehrlich, A. Modern Dental Assisting, 5th ed. Philadelphia: W. B. Saunders, 1995.)

Furcations

For effective root instrumentation, the clinician must take into account the number of roots each tooth has as well as the location of its roots. If a tooth is multirooted, special instrumentation considerations must be made for scaling and root planing the furcations. Furcations are the areas between the roots of teeth where the root trunk divides into separate roots (see Fig. 19–5). Furcations are narrow and difficult to reach with personal oral hygiene devices and scaling and root planing instruments. Therefore, personal bacterial plaque control and professional instrumentation in furcations is a challenge to master.[5,7]

Nevertheless, knowing the number of the furcations on each tooth and the location and configuration of each enables the dental hygienist to assess whether the furcation crotch or space between roots is accessible to instrumentation. Teeth that have two roots have two furcation crotches, and teeth with three roots have three furcation crotches (Fig. 19–6). Such furcation crotches can be either facial and lingual or mesial and distal, each with a slightly different configuration. Figure 19–7 shows the mandibular first molar, from both a facial and lingual perspective, to allow viewing of the tooth's facial and lingual furcations. Note that the facial furcation crotch is narrower than the lingual furcation crotch. Furcation crotches may be located far from the CEJ of the tooth or may be in close proximity. The facial and lingual furcation crotches of the mandibular first molar shown in Figure 19–7 are well removed from the neck of the tooth. In contrast, the facial and lingual furcations of the maxillary first premolar shown in Figure 19–8 are in close proximity to the CEJ.[5,7]

Maxillary first and second molars have three roots. As a result they are **trifurcated** with three furcation crotches, each with a slightly different configuration. Figure 19–6 shows a maxillary first molar from the facial, lingual, mesial, and distal perspectives. The maxillary first molar is triple-rooted with mesiofacial, distofacial, and lingual roots. The lingual root is the longest of the three and has a curvature. This curvature of the lingual root gives it a look similar to that of a banana. The other two roots are the mesiofacial root and the distofacial root. These roots have

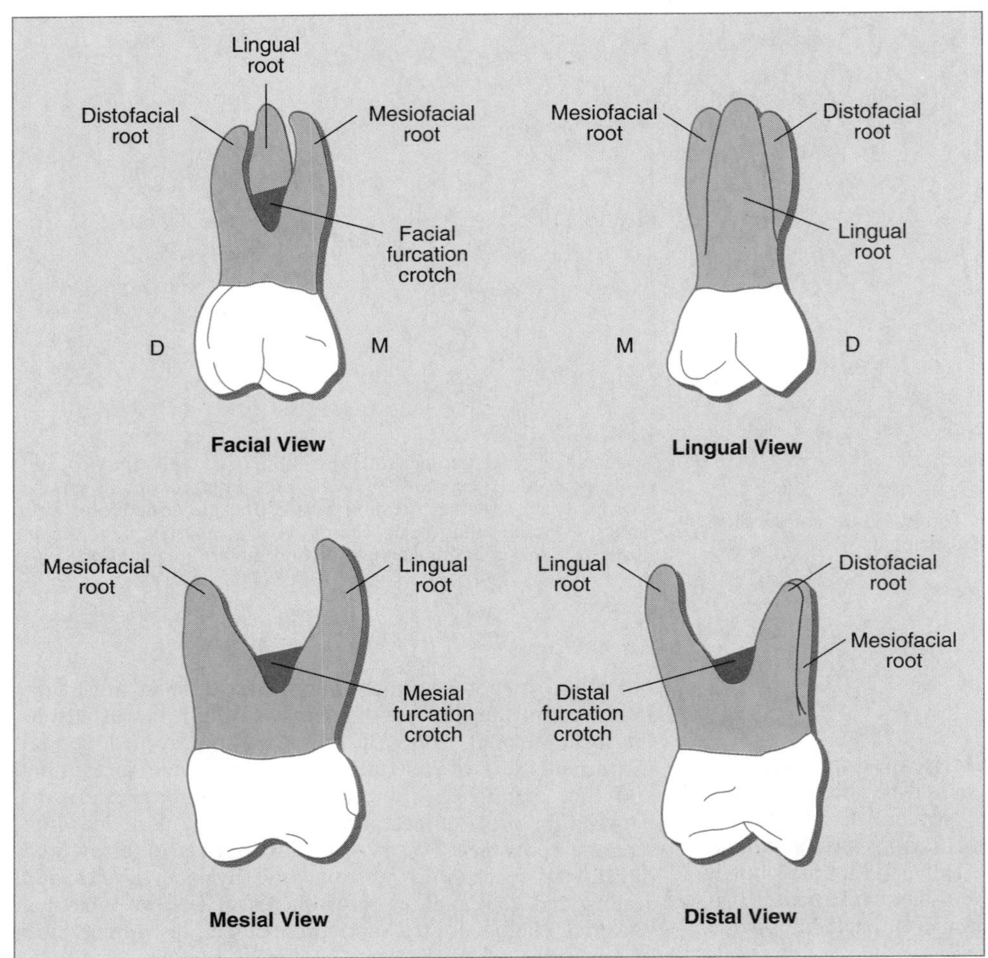

FIGURE 19–6
Trifurcated maxillary first molar shown from facial, lingual, mesial, and distal views.

an extreme curvature that makes them look like a handle from a pliers (see Fig. 19–6). The roots are widely separated and the furcations are well removed from the cervical area of the tooth.[3,4] Each of the three furcation crotches has an individual shape, which challenges the most adept clinician. The distal furcation crotch is wider than the mesial crotch. The mesial furcation is more easily assessible from the lingual aspect as a result of the pronounced convexity on the mesiofacial aspect of the molar. The mesiofacial root also is quite broad from this aspect and the furcation is therefore more easily reached from the lingual surface.

The ability to picture roots viewed from facial, lingual, mesial, and distal perspectives assists the dental hygienist with instrumentation on specific root surfaces and in furca-

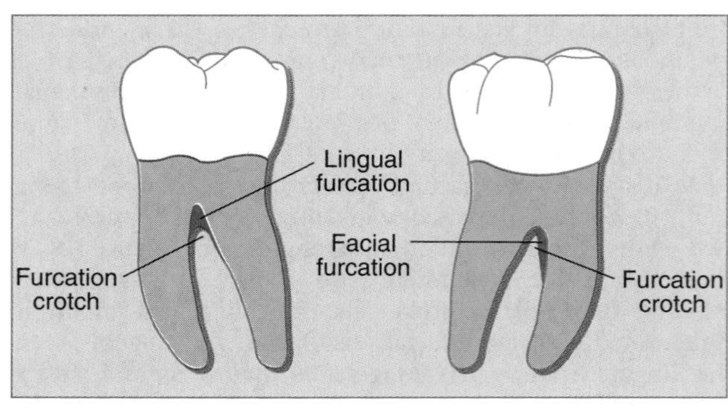

FIGURE 19–7
Mandibular first molar. *Left,* Lingual view. *Right,* Facial view. Note how crotches are well removed from the CEJ.

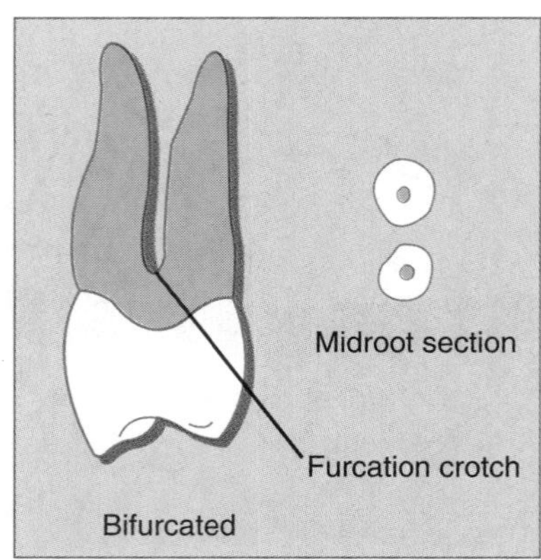

FIGURE 19–8
Mesial view of the maxillary first premolar. Note that the furcation crotches are in close proximity to the CEJ.

tions. Table 19–1 summarizes characteristics of roots associated with specific teeth and illustrates each from facial, lingual, mesial, and distal views.

ROOT ASSESSMENT

Use of Radiographs for Root Assessment

Prior to root instrumentation, the dental hygienist should assess the client's radiographs to determine the presence of root anomalies and normal variations in root form. Although radiographs do not reveal finite root topography, they assist the dental hygienist in determining the extent of bone loss, furcation involvement, and root abnormalities that affect instrumentation. Radiographs provide a guide for root topography and serve as a road map for instrumentation. Radiographs should be kept on the viewbox and referred to during client care.

TOOTH ANOMALIES WITH VARIATION IN ROOT FORM

Common anomalies that may be present on root surfaces are illustrated in Figure 19–9. Important variations in root form include

- Enamel pearls
- Dilaceration
- Flexion
- Fusion
- Concrescence
- Dwarfed roots
- Accessory roots
- Hypercementosis

It is important for the dental hygienist to recognize the presence of anomalies and take them into consideration when developing the dental hygiene care plan. Because

Text continued on page 545

TABLE 19–1
CHARACTERISTICS OF ROOTS

Tooth	Root Topography and Morphology
Maxillary Arch	
Central and lateral incisor	Single-rooted, conical shape May have moderate to deep proximal, vertical root concavities Bulbous and pronounced crowns create deep mesial and distal concavities at the CEJ Lingual aspect of roots is more tapered than facial aspect Lingual marginal groove may extend from crown to root
Canines	Single-rooted May have proximal root concavities Distal prominence of crown is at the CEJ, may cause instrumentation difficulties Root is long and narrow and lingual aspect is tapered Cross section is ovoid in shape

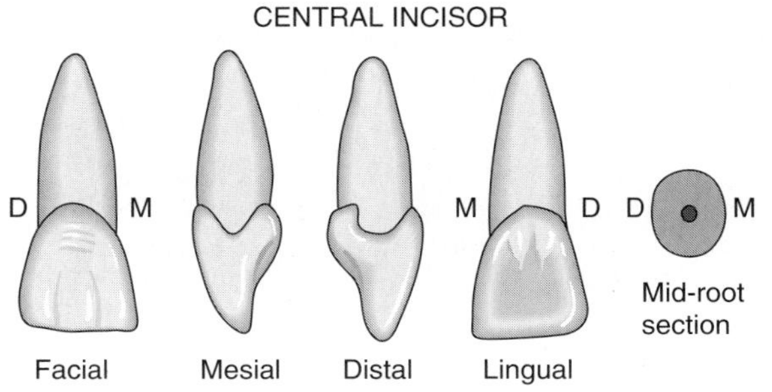

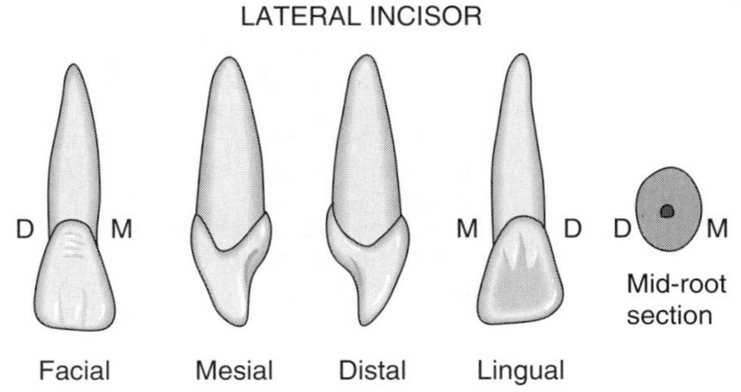

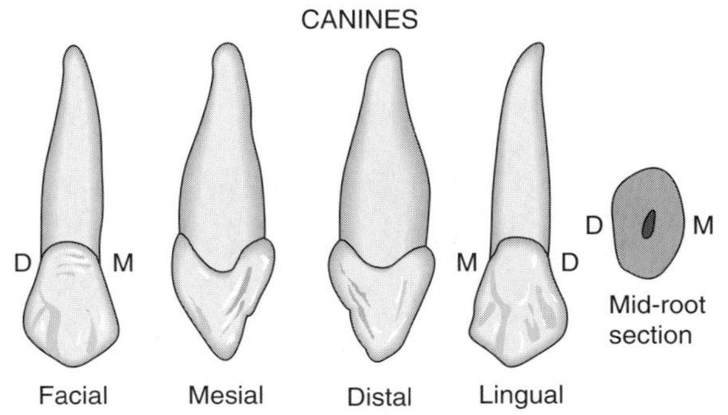

Table continued on following page

TABLE 19–1
CHARACTERISTICS OF ROOTS *Continued*

Tooth	Root Topography and Morphology	
Maxillary Arch		
First premolar	Classically double-rooted Mesial concavity Usually bifurcated at the apical third	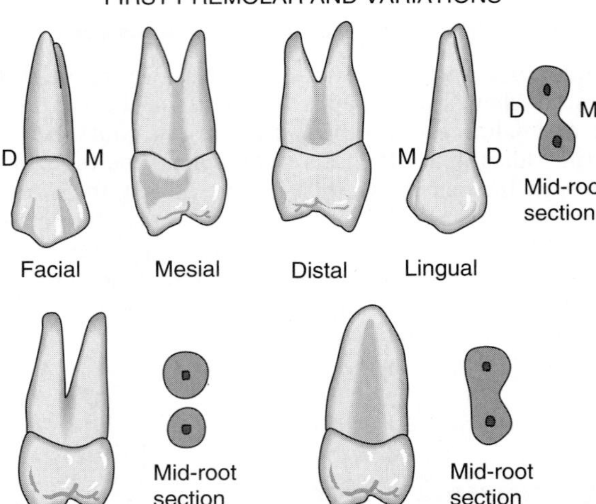
Second premolar	Single-rooted Mesial concavity not as pronounced as in first premolar	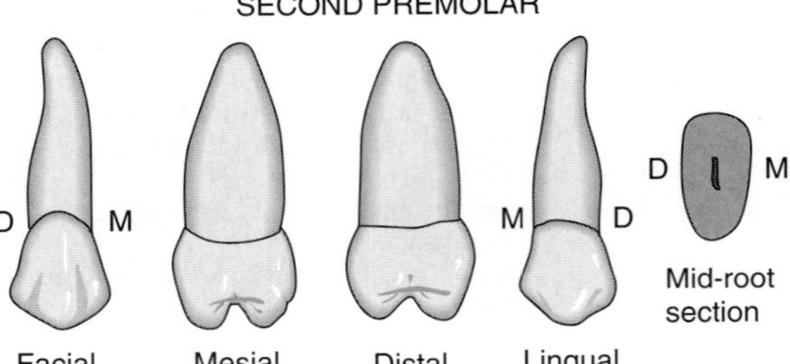
First molar	Triple-rooted—lingual, mesiofacial, and distofacial Lingual root longest; curves like a banana May have a vertical depression on the palatal surface MF and DF roots may have extreme curvature which gives them a look of a pliers handle Distal furcation crotch is wider than the mesial furcation crotch Mesial furcation may be more easily reached from the lingual aspect	FIRST MOLAR D M Facial 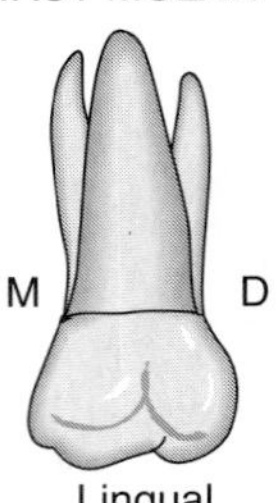 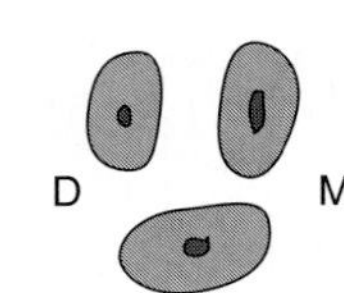 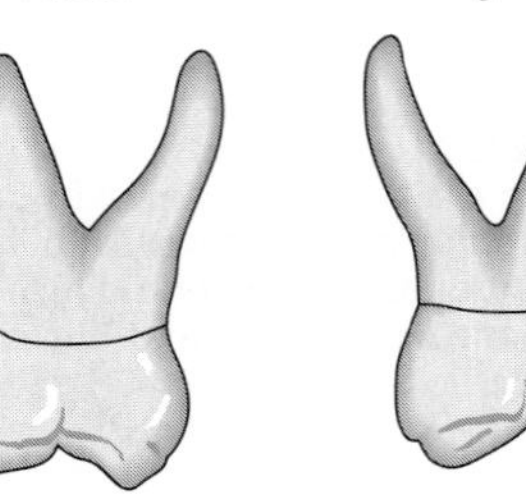

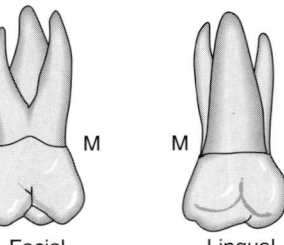

TABLE 19–1
CHARACTERISTICS OF ROOTS *Continued*

Tooth	Root Topography and Morphology
Maxillary Arch	
Second molar	Triple-rooted—lingual, mesiofacial, and distofacial Roots more parallel than in first molar Roots may show partial fusion Furcation crotch narrower than that in first molar
Third molar	Varies greatly May be triple-rooted Roots normally fused
Mandibular Arch	
Central and lateral incisors	Root is usually straight, converging gradually at the apex Proximal grooves may be deep, giving the teeth a double-rooted appearance Central roots are often grooved, which extends into the crown

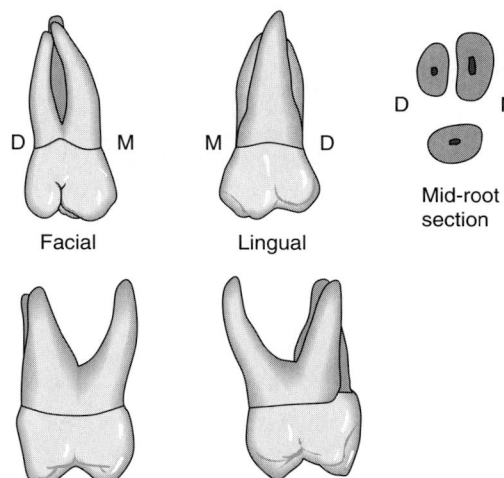

SECOND MOLAR

D M M D D M

Facial Lingual Mid-root section

Mesial Distal

THIRD MOLAR

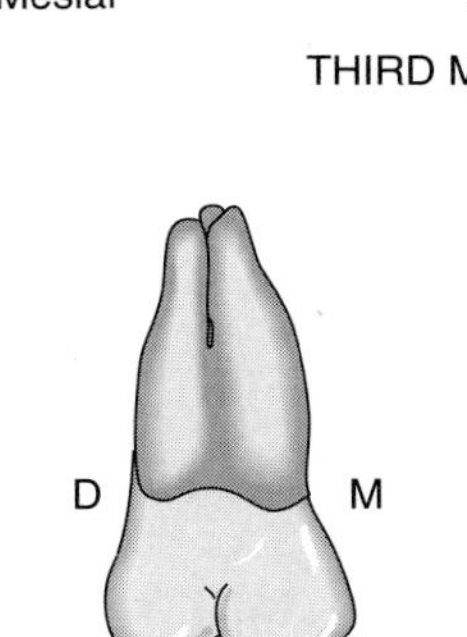

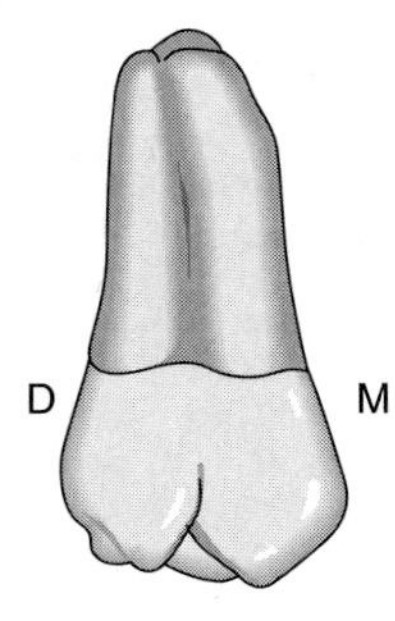

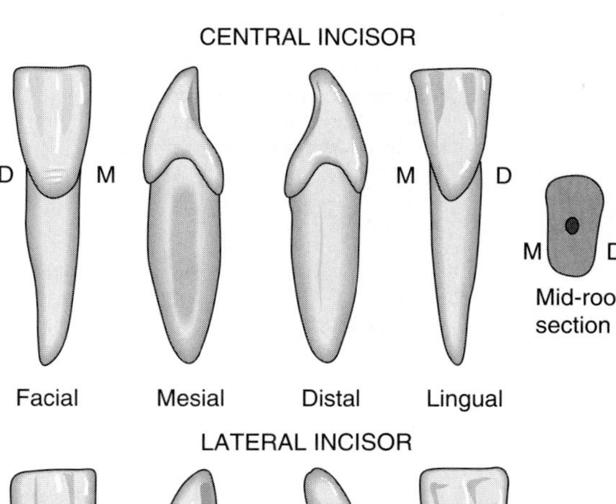

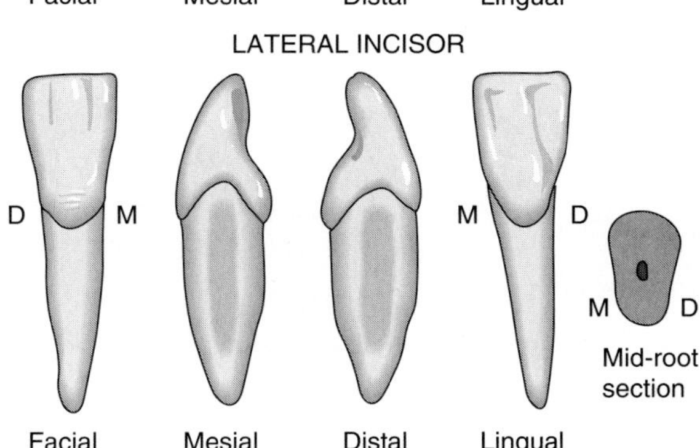

Table continued on following page

TABLE 19–1
CHARACTERISTICS OF ROOTS *Continued*

Tooth	Root Topography and Morphology
Mandibular Arch	
Canines	Conical in shape Taper from the cervix to the apex Slight mesial inclination Occasionally bifurcated Pronounced proximal concavity may give a double-rooted appearance
First premolar	Facial aspect more conical in shape The lingual aspect tapers May have deep groove on the distal root surface
Second premolar	Generally single-rooted Pronounced proximal concavities Roots are shorter and more blunt than those of maxillary premolars

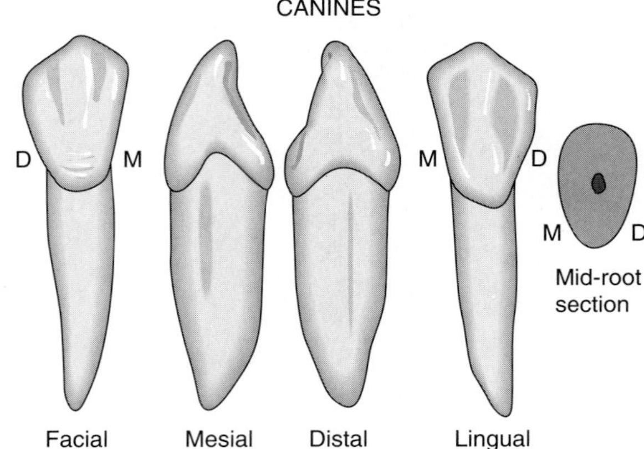

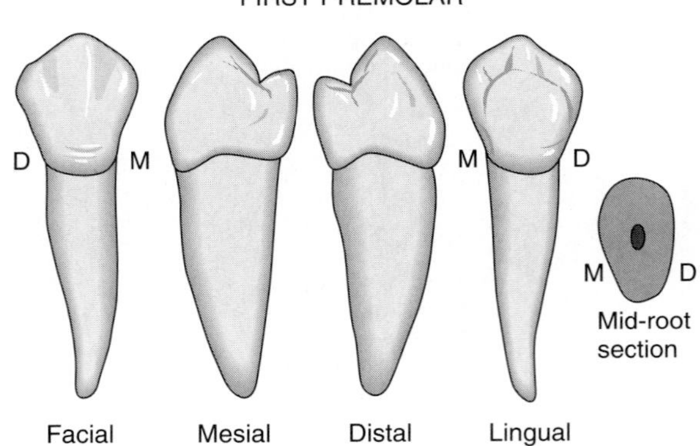

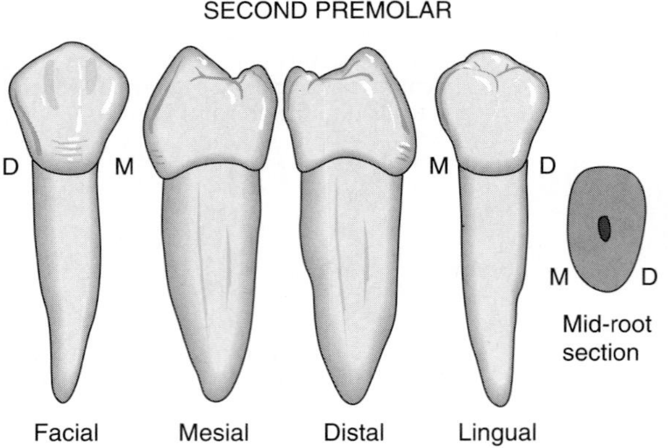

TABLE 19–1
CHARACTERISTICS OF ROOTS *Continued*

Tooth	Root Topography and Morphology
Mandibular Arch	
First molar	Double-rooted—mesial root and distal root Broad shallow concavity on the mesial root that runs down almost the entire length of the mesial root Distal root narrower than mesial root Widely separated roots (from the facial aspect) Furcations are well removed from the neck of the teeth Grooving may approach CEJ Facial furcation entrance diameter seems to be smaller than that of the lingual furcation Enamel projections into furcation area may cause problems 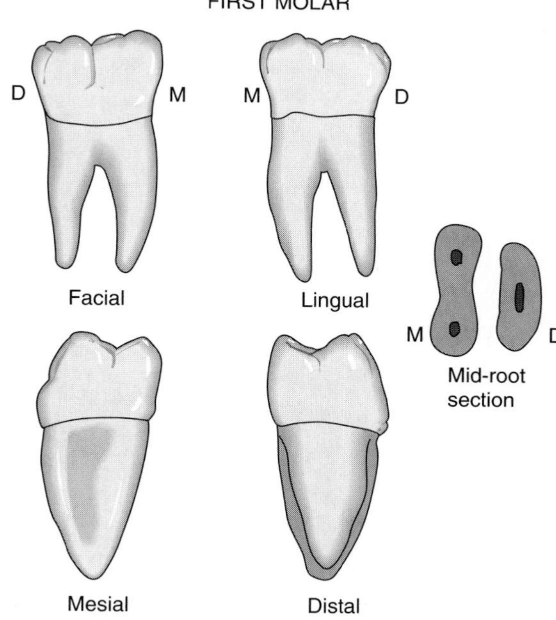
Second molar	Double-rooted mesial and distal roots are closer together than those of first molar Mesial root not as broad as in first molar Furcation is not as wide as in the first molar Furcation is closer to the CEJ 35% occurrence of cervicoenamel projections 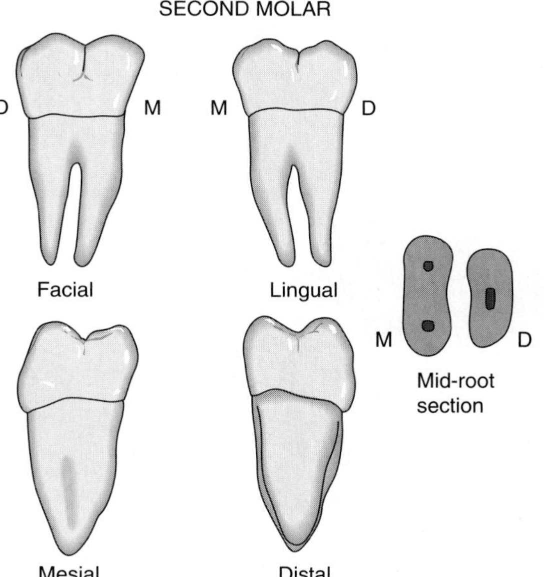

Table continued on following page

TABLE 19–1
CHARACTERISTICS OF ROOTS *Continued*

Tooth	Root Topography and Morphology
Mandibular Arch	
Third molar	Varies greatly Usually double-rooted Roots are short, usually fused

THIRD MOLAR

D M M D

Facial Lingual

Mesial Distal

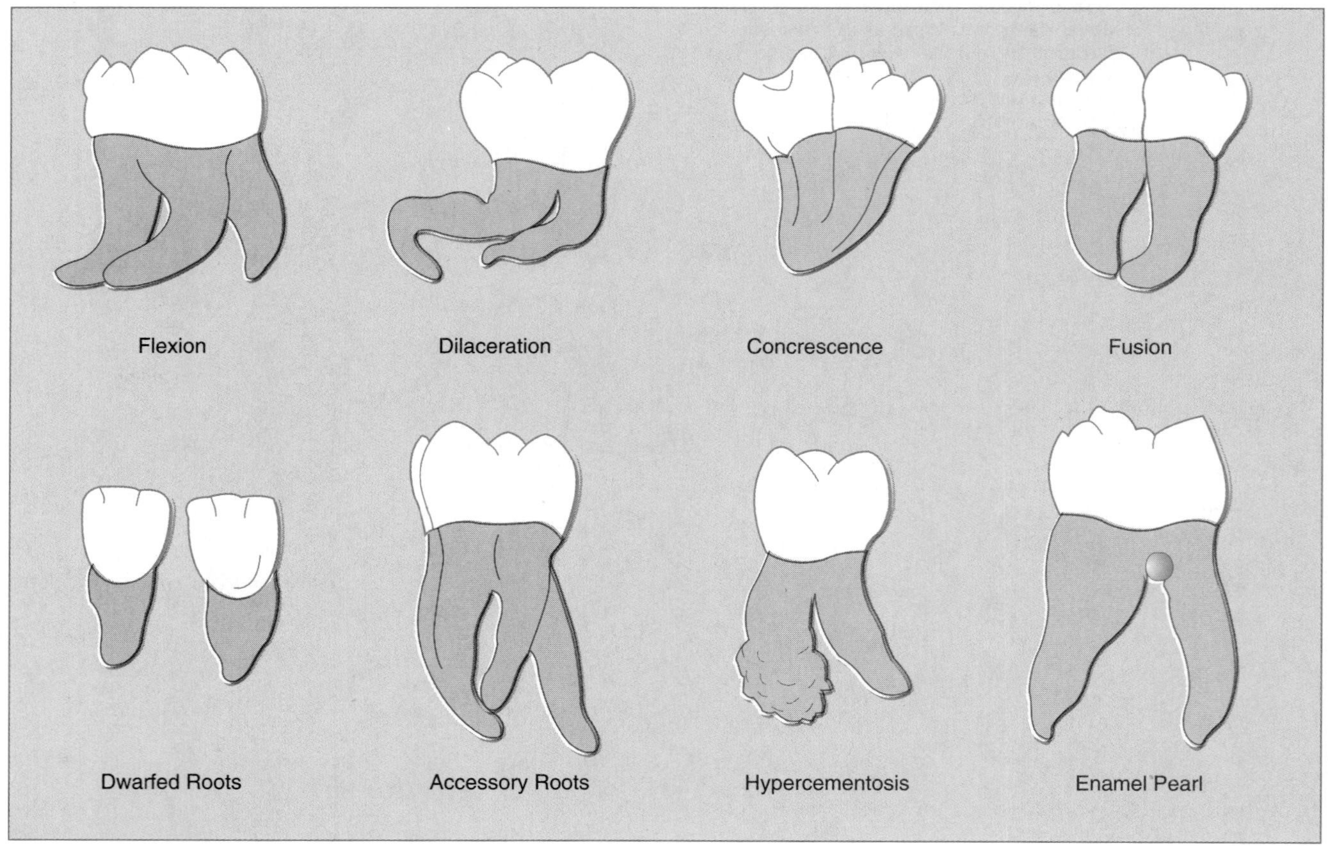

FIGURE 19–9
Tooth anomalies with variations in root form.

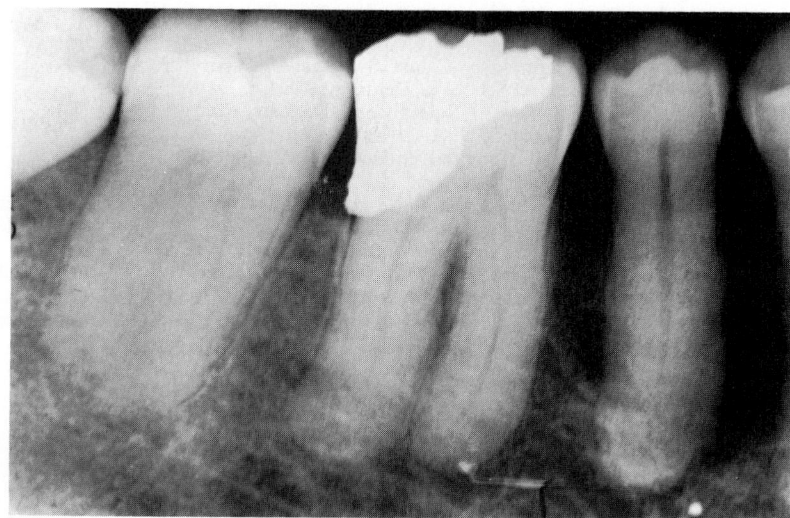

FIGURE 19–10
Hypercementosis. (With permission from Regezi, J. A., and Sciubba, J. J. Oral Pathology: Clinical-Pathologic Correlations, 2nd ed. Philadelphia: W. B. Saunders, 1993, p. 460.)

these anomalies affect root instrumentation strategies, each is discussed briefly below.

Enamel Pearl

The **enamel pearl** is an apical extension of enamel at the CEJ onto the root surface. The degree of enamel projection may vary from a slight dip in the enamel to a severe projection that may extend into the furcation. Periodontal problems associated with enamel pearls are related to the fact that gingival fibers must be embedded into the cementum of the roots to be anchored to the tooth structure. Consequentially, there is no gingival attachment over enamel projections and therefore the area is more vulnerable to advancing periodontal disease.[4,8] In instances when significant attachment loss is noted, referral of the client to a periodontist should be considered.

Dilaceration and Flexion

Dilaceration is a distortion of the root and the crown from their normal vertical position. Dilaceration is caused most commonly by trauma to or pressure on the developing tooth resulting in the displacement of the root. **Flexion,** a sharp bend or curvature of a root, is similar to dilaceration; however, it affects only the root portion of the tooth. It occurs later in the development of the tooth than does dilaceration and it too is the result of trauma or pressure to the tooth.[2,3] The dental hygienist must modify instrumentation to reach the root's topography.

Fusion

Fusion is the formation of a single tooth from the union of two adjacent tooth buds. The two buds are united through the enamel, dentin, and occasionally the pulp. Thus, radiographs are very helpful in distinguishing between fusion and gemination (see Chapter 12). For example, a fused tooth appears with two separate root canals, whereas a geminated tooth appears with a single canal. Fusion is thought to be caused by pressure or force during the development of adjacent roots.[2,3] Presence of a fused tooth should be noted on both the periodontal and tooth assessment charts. Because they are anatomically unique, careful attention should be paid to the assessment and instrumentation of these teeth.

Concrescence

Concrescence is the fusion of two teeth at the root through the cementum only. The teeth involved originally were separated but later joined from excessive cementum deposition. Concrescence occurs following the eruption of the teeth and is most commonly seen in maxillary molars of the permanent dentition.

Dwarfed Roots

Dwarfed roots are abnormally short roots of teeth that have normal-sized crowns. Dwarfed roots are hereditary and are most commonly seen in maxillary teeth. They also may occur in clients who have undergone orthodontic treatment with rapid tooth movement.

Accessory Roots

Accessory roots are extra roots that form on teeth after birth. These extra roots may be caused by trauma, pressure, or metabolic dysfunction.[2] Careful assessment of radiographs may assist the dental hygienist in determining if accessory roots are present. If present, the hygienist must document the root's presence and instrument appropriately.

Hypercementosis

Hypercementosis is the excessive formation of cementum around the root of a tooth after the tooth has erupted. It is often associated with the roots of permanent molars. Hypercementosis may be caused by trauma, chronic inflammation of the pulp, or a metabolic disturbance (i.e., Paget's disease).[2,3] The cemental thickening is irregular and this enlargement can obliterate the periodontal ligament, causing loss of the bony lamina dura (Fig. 19–10).

References

1. Armitage, G. C. Periodontology Course Syllabus. University of California, San Francisco, School of Dentistry, 1991.
2. Woefel, J. Dental Anatomy: Its Relevance to Dentistry, 4th ed. Philadelphia: Lea & Febiger, 1990.
3. Fuller, J., and Denehy, G. Concise Dental Anatomy, 2nd ed. St. Louis: Mosby-YearBook, 1984.
4. Kraus, B., Jordan, R., and Abrams, L. Dental Anatomy and Occlusion. Baltimore: Williams & Wilkins, 1969.
5. Pattison, A., and Pattison, G. Periodontal Instrumentation: A Clinical Manual. East Norwalk, CT: Appleton & Lange, 1991.
6. Wilkins, E. M. Clinical Practice of the Dental Hygienist, 6th ed. Philadelphia: Lea & Febiger, 1983, p. 183.
7. Wasserman, B. Root Scaling and Planing: A Fundamental Therapy. Chicago: Quintessence Books, 1986.
8. Masters, D. H., and Hoskins, S. W. Projection of cervical enamel into molar furcations. Journal of Periodontology 35:49, 1964.

Suggested Readings

Fuller, J., and Denehy, G. Concise Dental Anatomy, 2nd ed. St. Louis: Mosby-YearBook, 1984.

Woefel, J. Dental Anatomy: Its Relevance to Dentistry, 4th ed. Philadelphia: Lea & Febiger, 1990.

Zeisz, R., and Nuckolls, J. Dental Anatomy: The Form and Function of the Permanent Teeth. St. Louis: C.V. Mosby, 1949.

20

Dental Hygiene Care for Acute Gingival and Periodontal Conditions

OBJECTIVES

Mastery of the content in this chapter will enable the reader to:

- Define the key terms
- Explain the etiology, oral signs and symptoms, and treatment of clients with periodontal, gingival, and periapical abscesses
- Explain the etiology, oral signs and symptoms, and treatment of acute herpetic gingivostomatitis, acute periocoronitis, and acute necrotizing ulcerative gingivitis
- Discuss the emergency protocol used in the event of an avulsed tooth
- Discuss the rationale for the wearing of athletic mouthprotectors by at risk clients
- Outline the procedure for constructing a custom-made mouthprotector
- Describe the collaborative role of the dental hygienist in caring for clients with common periodontal and dental emergencies
- Educate clients about the prevention of common periodontal and dental emergencies
- Educate clients about the nature and expected outcome of periodontal and dental emergency care

INTRODUCTION

The dental hygienist frequently is in a position to identify deficits related to human needs that evolve from emergency periodontal conditions. Deficits may be related to the needs for freedom from pain and stress, for safety, for integrity of the mucous membranes of the head and neck, for self-determination, for conceptualization and problem solving, and for a value system. In these situations, it is essential for the dental hygienist to facilitate referral of the client to a dentist for emergency treatment. Postponement of palliative and therapeutic care can result in continued human needs deficits with possible consequences of prolonged pain, increased loss of bone, and further periodontal tissue destruction. The purpose of this chapter is to discuss common periodontal emergencies and the role of the dental hygienist in facilitating timely and appropriate care.

PERIODONTAL LESIONS

Acute Herpetic Gingivostomatitis

Acute herpetic gingivostomatitis represents the oral manifestations of primary infection with the herpesvirus, usually herpes simplex virus 1 **(HSV-1).** Historically, primary herpetic gingivostomatitis has been seen predominantly in infants and children. However, in recent decades the disease has been commonly found in young adults in their 20s and 30s. Primary herpetic gingivostomatitis in teenagers and adults is most likely HSV-1 but may be the initial manifestation of herpes simplex virus 2 **(HSV-2),** the form of the virus more commonly transmitted sexually, possibly explaining the increase in incidence in those age groups. Many clients presenting with primary herpetic infections become carriers of the disease and experience recurrent expressions of the virus as herpes labialis.[1]

The painful herpetic ulcers in the mouth associated with primary infection often cause reduction in food and fluid intake, creating a human need deficit in the area of nutrition, which can be critical with children and infants. Serious dehydration is not uncommon and can lead to hospitalization for infants.

Signs and Symptoms

Acute herpetic gingivostomatitis is recognized by a set of characteristic systemic and intraoral signs and symptoms. The disease is commonly associated with prodromal symptoms of rapid onset:

- Fever
- Malaise
- Headache
- Irritability
- Lymphadenopathy[2]

These prodromal symptoms should be investigated during client assessment by adequate questioning when suspicious oral lesions are observed. Questions such as "Have you been feeling very tired lately, or feverish?" help the dental hygienist glean information that may suggest viral infection.

Oral manifestations of primary herpetic gingivostomatitis begin as small, yellowish vesicles. These vesicles coalesce to form larger, round ulcers with grayish centers and very bright red borders. The vesicles and ulcers can be present on any of the oral mucous membranes, including the lips, tongue, gingiva, and buccal mucosa.[1] The infected client has serious, even extreme pain.

Recognition of primary herpetic gingivostomatitis is based on knowledge of the appearance of the ulcers and assessment of systemic manifestations. Diagnostic tests, such as culturing for herpesvirus by the client's physician, can be conducted for confirmation of the presence of the virus but are not routine. In addition, this is a highly infectious disease; therefore, the dental hygienist and client must work together to prevent transmission to family members and other members of the oral healthcare team.

Treatment

Referral of a client to the dentist for definitive dental diagnosis is the appropriate initial dental hygiene intervention (Fig. 20–1; see color section). Treatment for acute herpetic gingivostomatitis is primarily supportive because the disease runs its course in 7 to 10 days. Gingival inflammation can be reduced by bacterial plaque removal using a toothbrush only if the client can tolerate the discomfort. Instrumentation and local anesthesia should not be attempted because of the possibility of transmission of the virus to the dental hygienist and other workers. Even if the hygienist was previously exposed to herpesvirus, had an episode of initial infection, and had recurrent lesions, the possibility of initiating herpetic whitlow from an inadvertent finger puncture with an HSV-contaminated instrument exists. **Herpetic whitlow** is a recurrent lesion of the finger initiated by puncture from a herpesvirus-contaminated instrument. The lesions are often debilitating and can last many weeks longer than the usual 2-week course of herpesvirus in the oral tissues.[3]

The dental hygienist should educate the client about consuming adequate fluid and nutritious foods, performing oral hygiene as much as possible, and using over-the-counter topical anesthetics to help control discomfort. Topical anesthetics should be used cautiously with children so as not to anesthetize the throat, which can be frightening. Topical anesthetics can be swabbed onto the lesions by the client for more controlled local delivery.

Acute Pericoronitis

Acute pericoronitis is an abscess associated with a partially erupted tooth or fully erupted tooth that is covered completely or partly by a flap of tissue called an **operculum.** The most commonly affected tooth is the mandibular third molar, but maxillary third molars and other teeth that are the most distal in the arch have been associated with the disease. As bacteria accumulate under the gingiva next to the tooth, the tissue responds by becoming extremely inflamed and painful.[4] This disease is a common problem associated with young adults and has been considered to be a serious problem for military personnel, most of whom are in the 17- to 26-year-old group. In fact, 20% of dental emergencies reported by the military in World War II and 16% of those from the Viet Nam conflict were acute pericoronitis. In addition, a study reported an incidence of 1.9 cases of pericoronitis per 100 naval recruits (Fig. 20–2; see color section).

Signs and Symptoms

Oral areas that have an operculum are predisposed to pericoronitis. The signs and symptoms of acute pericoronitis include swelling of the operculum and other gingiva associated with the most distal tooth in the arch, redness, and extreme pain. The tissue may be so swollen that it interferes with mastication, and it may be traumatized during mastication. Trismus, or spasm of the muscles of mastication, may occur, and the client may have a fever.[4] Purulent exudate has been reported in half the cases in a military study of 359 recruits; however, few cases bled on palpation, and none of that population presented with a fever. Pain, swelling, and redness were present in every instance. In

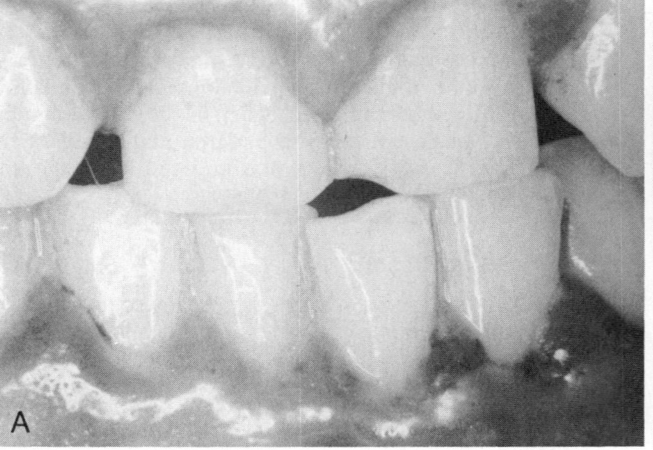

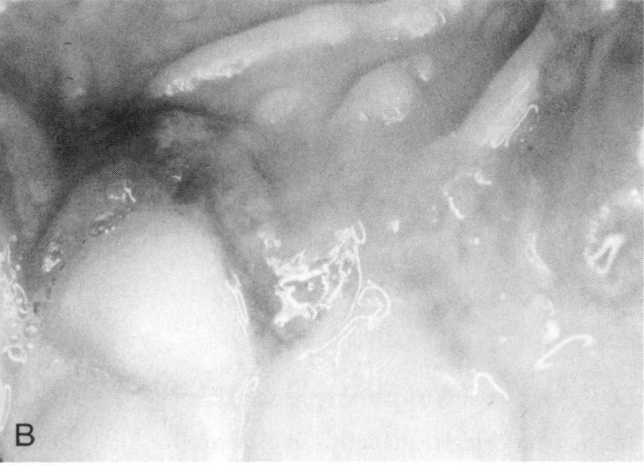

FIGURE 20–1
Primary herpetic infection of the mouth is characterized by bright red gingiva, vesicles, and pain. *A*, Facial gingiva showing swelling and color change. *B*, Lingual view of premolar and anterior teeth showing coalesced vesicles. (Courtesy of Philip R. Melnick, D.D.S.)

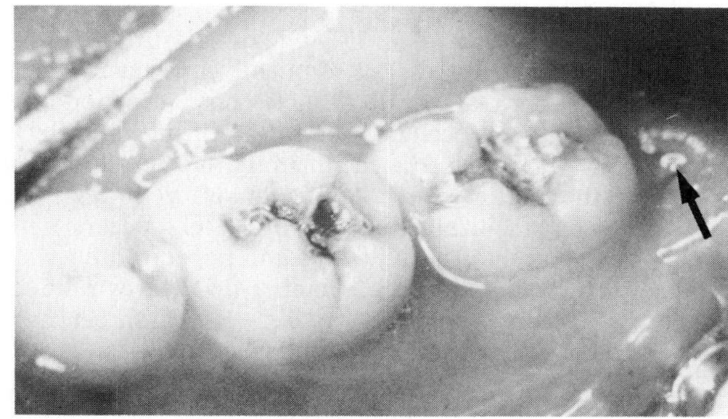

FIGURE 20–2
Acute pericoronitis is usually localized to the third molar region and can be extremely painful. Note the swelling and color change present at the distal side of the second molar. (Courtesy of Edward J. Taggart, D.D.S., M.S.)

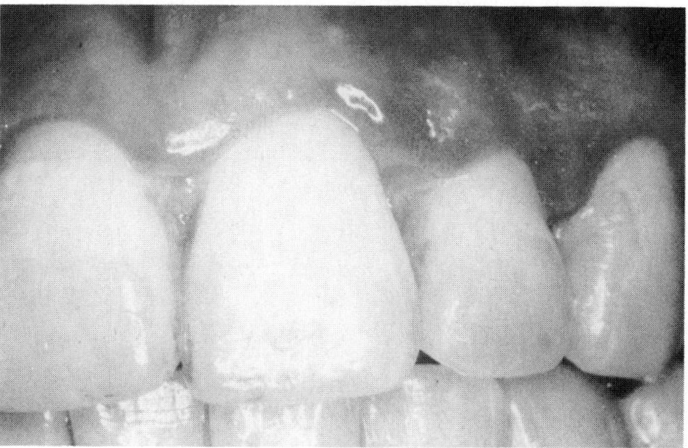

FIGURE 20–3
Acute necrotizing ulcerative gingivitis throughout the anterior area. (Courtesy of Philip R. Melnick, D.D.S.)

addition, two-thirds of the 25 cases in the naval population reported previous episodes of pericoronitis, suggesting that pericoronitis is often a recurrent problem.[5]

Treatment

A number of considerations are involved in treating pericoronitis, including the severity of the case, whether it is a recurrence, and possible systemic complications. The dentist may ask the dental hygienist to participate in the care of the client with pericoronitis. Treatment requires multiple visits.

Initial dental management is aimed at treating symptoms, with the goal of making the client more comfortable. The infected area is débrided, usually by gentle flushing with warm water or dilute hydrogen peroxide delivered in a disposable irrigating syringe with a blunt needle. Topical anesthetic should be applied first. Much manipulation of the tissue may not be possible, and débridement with instruments may not be tolerable at first. After this initial débridement, the client should be instructed to rest at home, use warm saltwater rinses, and drink fluids to avoid dehydration. The dentist may prescribe antibiotics if the client is febrile. Sometimes drainage is augmented by placement of a single thickness of iodoform gauze under the operculum for the first day or two.[6]

The client should be asked to return the next day. At the second visit, the area should be irrigated again and instrumented if possible, and more thorough home care should be initiated. A marked improvement is usually observed at the second appointment.

After the acute condition has resolved, the client should be evaluated by the dentist for further treatment. Dental treatment might include extraction of the offending third molar, or operculum removal to produce a more normal gingival contour if the tooth is to be retained.[3]

Acute Necrotizing Ulcerative Gingivitis

Acute necrotizing ulcerative gingivitis (ANUG) is an opportunistic infection of the gingiva that is associated with stress, lifestyle, and some chronic conditions such as blood dyscrasias, acquired immunodeficiency syndrome (AIDS), and Down syndrome. The disease was first described by Vincent in the late 19th century and was seen so commonly among troops fighting in Europe during World War I that the name **"trench mouth"** was adopted. It is seen primarily in young adult individuals and is no longer thought to be a communicable disease.[7] ANUG is a recurring disease with a complex bacteriology consisting of a large proportion of spirochetes and gram-negative organisms. These organisms invade the tissue, causing the characteristic appearance of the disease.[8]

Signs and Symptoms

ANUG has specific clinical characteristics that distinguish it from other forms of acute oral infections. The clinical appearance of the disease is one of cratered, or **"punched-out," papillae,** very reddened gingiva, often with a gray **pseudomembrane,** and pain. The gingival lesions may be localized to specific areas or generalized throughout the mouth. Clients frequently exhibit an extremely offensive breath odor that can be smelled anywhere in the room occupied by the client. In addition, the acute lesions can be extensive, covering parts of the face, as seen in Third World countries and associated with malnutrition (Fig. 20–3; see color section).

The three most reliable criteria for recognizing the disease as identified by Stevens and associates[9] are:

- Acute necrosis and ulceration of the interproximal papillae
- Pain
- Bleeding

In addition, several other symptoms have been recognized as strongly associated with the disease, and their relative frequency of occurrence is listed in Table 20–1.

Stress is often related to both initial occurrence and recurrence of this disease. The role of psychological factors involved with stress is not well understood, but it has been postulated that changes in the immune system occurring at stressful times predispose certain individuals to an exuberant bacterial response, resulting in ANUG.

Treatment

The course of an ANUG episode is usually short but painful. Clients come to the oral healthcare practitioner most often because of pain. Treatment focuses on microbial con-

TABLE 20–1
SYMPTOMS OF ACUTE NECROTIZING ULCERATIVE GINGIVITIS

Symptom	Occurrence (%)
Necrosis of interproximal papillae	100
Bleeding	100
Pain	100
Fetid odor	97
Pseudomembrane	85
Tobacco use	83
Lymphadenopathy	61
Fever	39

Adapted from Stevens, A. W., Cogen, R. B., Cohen-Cole, S., and Freeman, A. Demographic and clinical data associated with acute necrotizing ulcerative gingivitis in a dental school population. Journal of Clinical Periodontology 11:487, 1984. © 1984 Munksgaard International Publishers Ltd., Copenhagen, Denmark.

trol through mechanical débridement by both client and clinician because of the cyclic and recurring nature of the disease.[7] Treatment should progress on a daily basis during the acute phase of the disease because the pain often inhibits thorough cleaning by the client or the dental hygienist at the beginning of treatment. The recommended treatment sequence is described in Table 20–2.

Dental hygiene care focuses on meeting the unmet human needs identified during client assessment. Given the signs and symptoms, most clients with ANUG have unmet human needs in the areas of freedom from pain and stress, skin and mucous membrane integrity of the head and neck, nutrition, conceptualization and problem solving, and/or self-determination and responsibility. Client health and oral health and well-being are the keys to successful treatment of ANUG. The client must be knowledgeable about the roles of stress, bacteria, and nutrition in the disease process and encouraged to take control over his personal oral health and lifestyle behaviors. Suggestions to identify stress management techniques and improve nutrition are necessary components of dental hygiene care practiced within a human needs framework.

Acute Periodontal Abscesses

Acute periodontal abscesses, frequently associated with preexisting periodontal disease, usually occur in periodontal pockets that become occluded for some reason, often by a foreign body.[10] An exacerbated inflammatory reaction then occurs. If the pocket can continue to drain through the sulcus, it can stabilize, although this rarely occurs with foreign objects such as peanut skins and popcorn hulls.

Incomplete scaling and root planing that leaves residual calculus at the base of treated pockets also has been suggested as a cause of periodontal abscesses.

Signs and Symptoms

Acute periodontal abscesses may be associated with any tooth in the mouth and appear as shiny, red, raised, and rounded masses on the gingiva or mucosa. Abscesses can point and drain through the tissue or simply drain through the pocket opening. Purulent exudate is usually apparent around the opening of the abscess or can be expressed by finger pressure.[3] The signs and symptoms include any of the following:

- Throbbing pain
- Swelling
- Deep-red to bluish color of the affected tissue
- Tooth sensitivity to pressure
- Tooth mobility

The client also may report that the tooth "feels high," because it may become slightly extruded.[10] Radiographs may be helpful in locating a preexisting area of bone loss that looks like the origin of the abscess. However, the infection moves through the tissue in the direction of least resistance, so the external features may appear at some distance from the affected tooth[3] (Fig. 20–4; see color section).

Treatment

Treatment consists mainly of drainage and appropriate use of antimicrobial agents. The acute phase of the disease

TABLE 20–2
TREATMENT REGIMEN FOR ANUG

Day 1	First visit	Scale and débride as much as possible, use ultrasonic instruments and topical anesthetics. Instructions on bacterial plaque control and rinsing four or more times per day with oxygenating agents should be given
Day 1	Systemic therapy	The use of antibiotics such as penicillin or metronidazole is indicated if the client has fever and lymphadenopathy
Day 2	Second visit	Within a day or two, condition should be much less painful, so the dental hygienist can begin therapeutic scaling and root planing. Oral hygiene instructions should be reinforced
Day 3	Third visit	Two to five days later, therapeutic scaling should be completed, and oral hygiene reinforced. As many appointments as necessary to thoroughly scale and root plane should be planned and executed. Margination of defective amalgam restorations should be performed
Week 1	Evaluation after initial care	Cratering frequently occurs and can result in significant gingival defects that should be evaluated by the dentist for possible surgical correction
Month 1	Continued care	The first follow-up visit should be in 1 month to reinforce oral hygiene and scale and root plane, if necessary. Meticulous and regular débridement by the client and the dental hygienist to control bacterial pathogenicity is required
Month 3	Maintenance	The client should be encouraged to come to the dental hygienist for regular professional mechanical dental hygiene care to minimize the risk of recurrence

Data from Carranza F. A., Jr. Glickman's Clinical Periodontology, 7th Ed. Philadelphia: W. B. Saunders, 1990, and Cogan R. B. Acute necrotizing ulcerative gingivitis. In Genco, R. J., Goldman, H. M., Cohen D. W. (eds.). Contemporary Periodontics. St. Louis: C. V. Mosby, 1990.

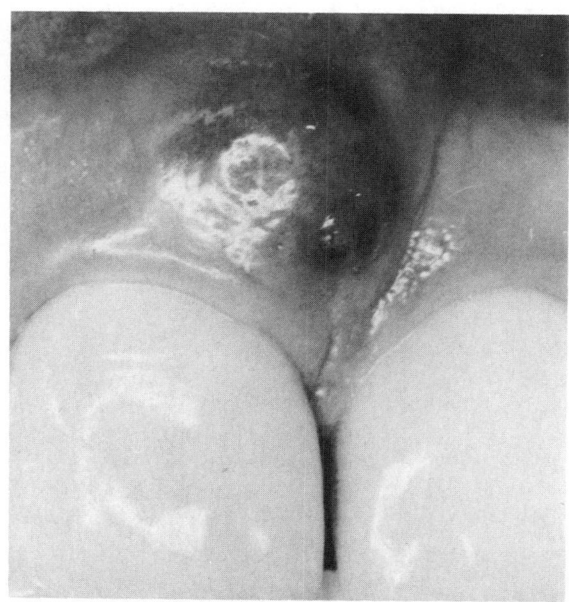

FIGURE 20–4
Acute periodontal abscess associated with tooth no. 8, characterized by redness and swelling. (Courtesy of Philip R. Melnick, D.D.S.)

must be managed to alleviate pain and prevent the spread of infection. The abscess must be drained, either through the pocket opening or through an incision. Drainage through the pocket opening is preferable. The tooth or teeth in the affected area are anesthetized, scaled, and root planed, and then gingival curettage is performed to remove granulation tissue. Postoperative instructions call for rest, fluid intake, and warm saltwater rinses to help reduce swelling. The client may require follow-up treatment usually involving periodontal surgery to eliminate the problem area. Following professional mechanical care, local irrigation with 10% povidone-iodine or 3% hydrogen peroxide, provided in the oral healthcare facility, has been recommended to help kill the pathogenic bacteria and flush the abscess area.[10]

The initial treatment of the abscess through the pocket is often delegated by the dentist to the dental hygienist. However, sometimes the procedure requires that the dentist perform a surgical flap procedure during the initial appointment for access to complete the débridement. If the client is febrile or lymphadenopathy is present, the dentist may prescribe antibiotic therapy. The antibiotic usually recommended, tetracycline, is a broad-spectrum drug with the unique ability to create a high titer in the gingival sulcus and inhibit collagenase in the host. These characteristics ensure maximal drug effect at the site of the infection.[3]

The repair potential for acute periodontal abscesses is excellent. Bone is lost rapidly during the acute phase, but with immediate recognition of the problem and proper mechanical and antimicrobial treatment, the lost tissue can be largely regained.[10]

Chronic Periodontal Abscess

Chronic periodontal abscess resembles acute periodontal abscess in that there is an overgrowth of pathogenic organisms in a periodontal pocket that drains inflammatory exudate. Chronic abscesses have communication to the oral cavity, either through the opening of the pocket or through a sinus tract that permits regular drainage. The chronic periodontal abscess is usually painless; however, the client may recount previous episodes of painful acute infection (Fig. 20–5).[3]

Signs and Symptoms

The chronic periodontal abscess exhibits inflammatory exudate seeping into the oral cavity without inducement or when digital pressure is applied to the pocket or sinus tract. The associated gingival tissue is reddened and swollen. As long as the chronic abscess is draining, it is rarely painful. The dental hygienist must assess exudate associated with the periodontium as indicative of possible chronic abscess so appropriate dental referral and treatment can be provided.

Treatment

Treatment of chronic periodontal abscess is similar to treatment of acute periodontal abscess. Scaling, root planing, and gingival curettage must be performed, usually requiring local anesthesia in the abscess area. Local antimicrobial therapy, usually irrigation with 10% povidone-iodine or 3% hydrogen peroxide delivered with a disposable syringe, is often provided immediately after scaling and root planing. The client must be seen by the dentist for follow-up care to diagnose the existing condition and to determine the need for more periodontal treatment to reduce pocket depth. This additional treatment usually includes pocket reduction periodontal surgery but may also include tooth extraction and/or more frequent supportive periodontal maintenance visits.[3]

The dental hygienist plays a major role in educating the client about the chronic nature of this condition, the possibility of future acute episodes if no further treatment is performed, and the need for meticulous supportive periodontal care including scaling, root planing, and control of bacterial plaque. Often, discussing the risk of rapid bone loss during acute episodes of abscess helps the client value the need to seek further care in order to better preserve the teeth.

Gingival Abscess

Gingival abscess usually occurs in previously disease-free areas and can often be related to forceful inclusion of some foreign body into the area. Most frequently, gingival abscesses are found on the marginal gingiva and are *not* associated with pathology of the deeper tissues.[10]

Signs and Symptoms

The gingival abscess can be observed on the marginal gingiva as a reddened, raised area of acute inflammation that is quite painful. A pus-filled lesion is clearly seen that is not associated with the sulcular epithelium (Fig. 20–6; see color section).

Treatment

The gingival abscess must be drained and irrigated by the dentist or periodontist. The acute lesion is incised, drained,

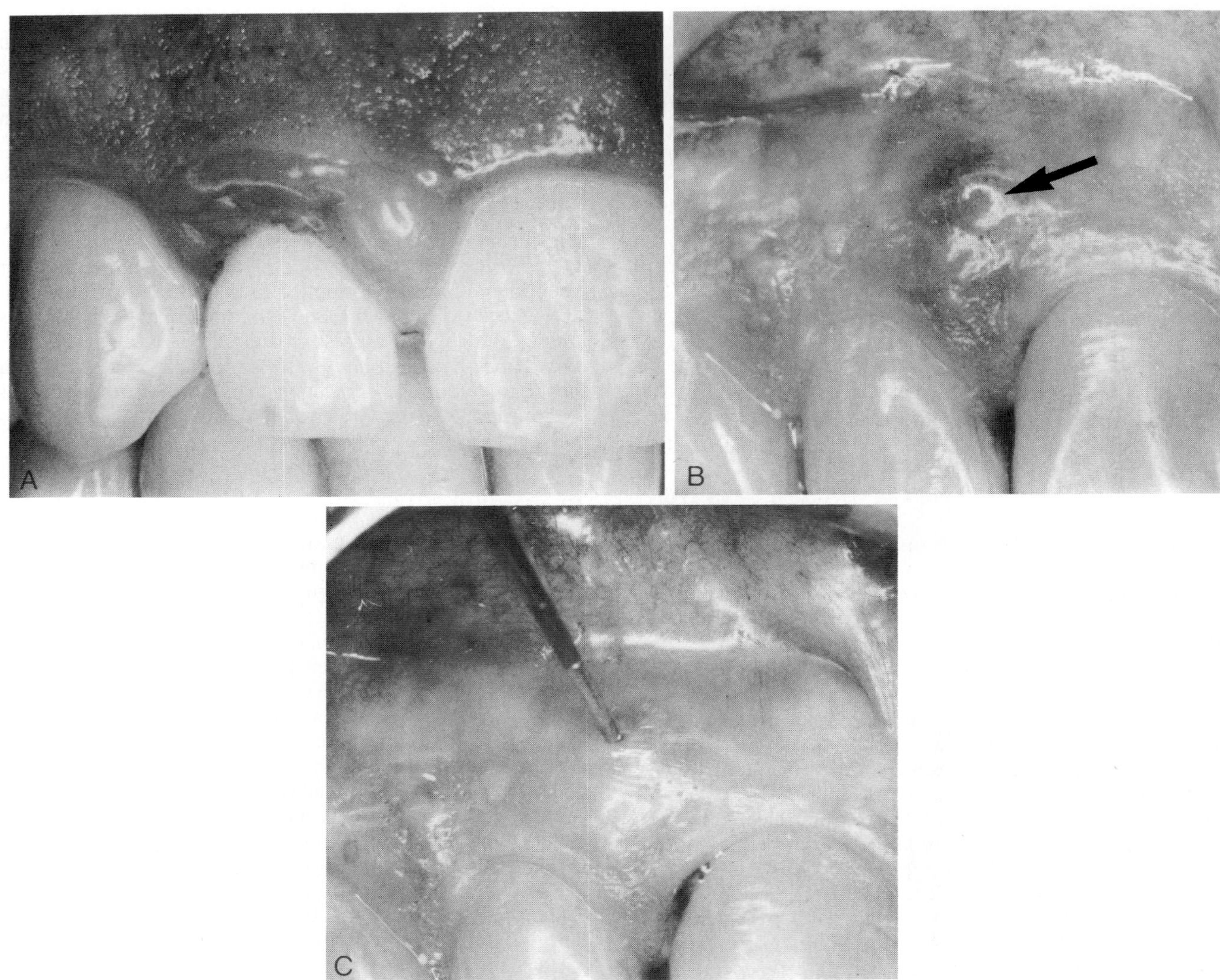

FIGURE 20–5
Chronic periodontal abscess. *A*, Draining through the periodontal pocket. *B*, Draining through a sinus tract. *C*, Probe inserted to show communication to periodontal pocket. (Courtesy of Philip R. Melnick, D.D.S.)

and irrigated with locally administered antimicrobials such as 3% hydrogen peroxide or 10% povidone-iodine. Warm saltwater rinses are recommended for postoperative therapy. Subsequent to the acute treatment of the gingival abscess, the reduced lesion may need to be excised. Also, subgingival instrumentation of the tooth is recommended to improve periodontal health in the area.[3]

PERIAPICAL (ENDODONTIC) ABSCESS

The **periapical** or **endodontic abscess** is sometimes difficult to distinguish from the acute periodontal abscess. The facial pain and tenderness to the tooth are similar. The endodontic abscess is the result of infection through caries, traumatic fracture of the tooth, or the trauma of a dental procedure. In addition, pulpal infection to a tooth can be spread laterally to the pulp from an adjacent infected tooth, through the lateral canals.[11] Most commonly, microorganisms spread into the pulp through the dentinal tubules from a carious lesion. The microorganisms colonize in the pulp and produce a variety of toxins that result in pulp cell death. Bacteria and their metabolic products then exit the apical foramen and can cause abscess formation.[12]

Signs and Symptoms

Often the periapical abscess is identifiable on radiographs as a rounded radiolucency at the apex of the tooth. However, early in the abscess formation, the radiographic changes are not evident. In addition, some abscesses drain through a sinus duct through the cortical bone, and some drain through the periodontal ligament, making them less identifiable on radiographs. These abscesses can resemble acute periodontal abscesses because their symptoms are identical (Fig. 20–7).

In assessing an abscess to determine its origin, it is help-

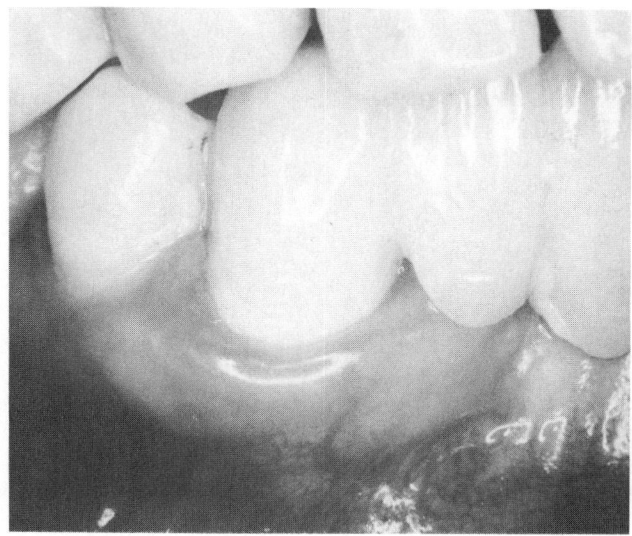

FIGURE 20-6
Gingival abscess associated with the marginal gingiva; note swelling and color change. (Courtesy of Philip R. Melnick, D.D.S.)

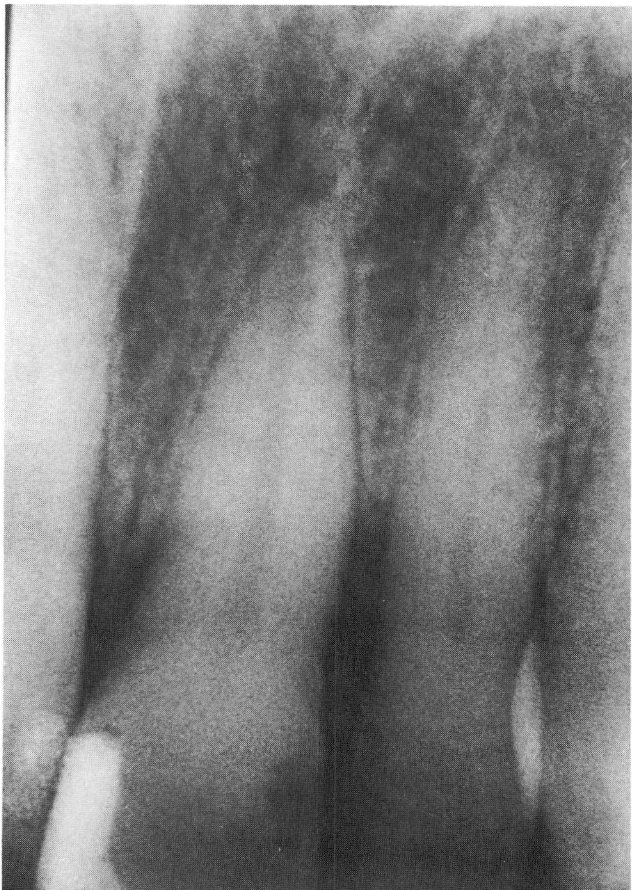

FIGURE 20-7
Radiographical appearance of an endodontic abscess associated with tooth no. 9, showing radiolucency at the apex. (Courtesy of Edward J. Taggart, D.D.S., M.S.)

ful to know that 85% of tooth pain is pulpal, and 15% periodontal. In addition, many periapically abscessed teeth are nonvital, which is a good distinguishing clue. However, some populations of clients, such as those being treated in the periodontal practice, are much more likely to have periodontal abscesses than pulpal ones. According to Killoy,[10] pain may be the distinguishing feature in differentiating between periapical and periodontal abscesses. Periapical pain is characterized as sharp, severe, intermittent, and hard to localize. In contrast, periodontal pain tends to be constant, localized, and less severe.[10]

Treatment

Treatment of periapical or endodontic abscesses requires either endodontic treatment, to remove the pulp of the tooth and replace it with inert material, or extraction of the tooth. Untreated endodontic abscesses can lead to severe cases of brain abscess[13] or fasciitis of the neck or chest wall that can be life-threatening.[12]

Combination Abscesses

An abscess can spread from the pulp to the periodontium or from the periodontal pocket to the pulp. Sometimes an abscess involves both of these routes of infection, resulting in a **combination periapical** and **periodontal abscess.**[3]

Signs and Symptoms

Combination abscesses present with some combination of the signs and symptoms mentioned, separately for periapical and periodontal abscesses. They are sometimes difficult to diagnose, and can result in extensive damage to the surrounding periodontium because of the intermittent nature of symptoms. Combination abscesses are diagnosed by the dentist when symptoms of both pulpal and periodontal infection are identified.

Treatment

These abscesses require extensive dental therapy, both periodontal and endodontic. Destruction of the bone and periodontium can be great and sometimes results in tooth loss (Fig. 20-8).

AVULSED TEETH

An avulsed tooth is one that is separated from the alveolar bone by trauma. **Avulsed teeth,** though not strictly a periodontal emergency, are traumatized teeth that can be replanted successfully if managed properly. Avulsion is the most common dental injury to children younger than 15 years of age as reported in the consumer product-related injuries survey of United States hospitals from 1979 to 1987.[14] Krasner[15] has stated that the situation occurs in as many as 1 in every 200 American children, approximately 2 million occurrences per year. In order to meet the client's human need for a biologically sound dentition, it is incumbent on dental hygienists to respond to this dental emergency because time lost and improper handling of the avulsed tooth after the injury can substantially reduce the chance for long-term success of replantation. Moreover, the dental hygienist, as an educator and oral health promoter,

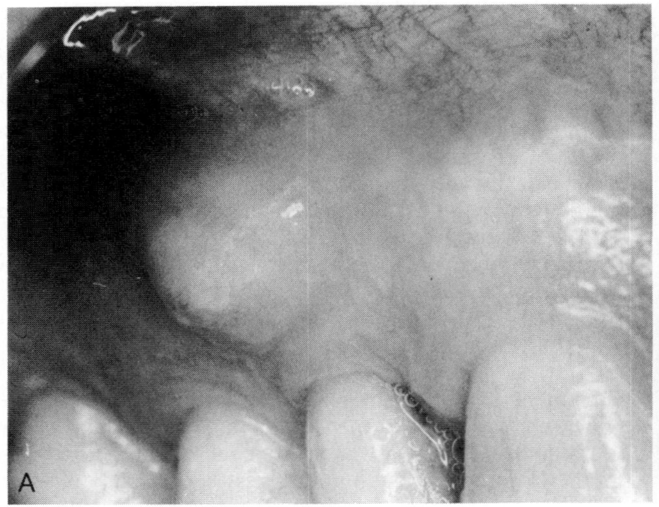

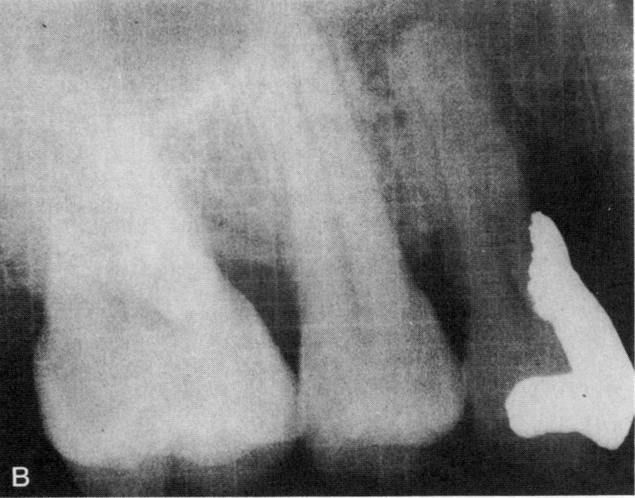

FIGURE 20–8
Combination periapical and periodontal abscess, probably occurring from spread of infection from the periodontium to the tooth. *A*, Pointed swelling is a common clinical characteristic. *B*, Radiolucency at the apex and significant bone loss may appear on the radiograph. (Courtesy of Philip R. Melnick, D.D.S.)

PROCEDURE 20–1

MAKING A CUSTOMIZED MOUTHPROTECTOR

Equipment

- Alginate impression of maxillary arch
- Stone mouth model
- Model vibrator
- Model trimmer
- Sheet of polyvinyl acetate-polyethylene
- Vacuum unit
- Sharp scissors
- Water
- Paper towels
- Cherry stone
- Scissors
- Alcohol torch
- Metal spatula
- Wet pumice
- Rag wheel

Procedure	Rationale
1. Make an alginate impression of the maxillary arch only	The custom-made mouthprotector covers only the maxillary teeth
2. Pour stone model immediately	Pouring the model immediately ensures a more accurate stone model
3. Assemble proper armamentarium for fabrication of mouthprotector	This provides for a more efficient utilization of the dental hygienist's time
4. Check trimming of maxillary mouth model for adequate thinness in palatal and mucobuccal regions	Accurate model trimming contributes to a properly fitted and comfortable mouthprotector
5. Drill hole in maxillary palatal region of the stone model	The hole facilitates the flow of air when the vacuum is created
6. Draw line one-quarter of an inch cervical to gingival margin of teeth at palatal side of study model	The line is used as a guide when cutting and trimming the mouthprotector
7. Draw line one-half of an inch short of frenula attachments on the buccal side	This line ensures that the mouthprotector does not impinge on the muscle attachments in the oral cavity
8. Connect lines on maxillary tuberosities	The line is used as a guide when cutting and trimming the mouthprotector

CONTINUED ON FOLLOWING PAGE

Procedure	Rationale
9. Wet the maxillary model with cool water	Wetting the model facilitates removal of the polyvinyl acetate–polyethylene material after the vacuum process is complete
10. Place polyvinyl acetate–polyethylene on a heating vacuum unit. Follow directions in vacuum unit manual and proceed	This begins the warming of the polyvinyl acetate–polyethylene material by the vacuum unit. The manufacturer's directions should be followed closely to create the heat and the vacuum necessary for an accurate fit of the material to the model
11. Hand-adapt the polyvinyl acetate–polyethylene over the model with a wet paper towel	This step improves the fit of the material to the model
12. Remove the mouthprotector from the model after it has cooled	Proper cooling prevents distortion of the mouthprotector
13. Trim excess material with sharp scissors. Remove rough edges with a cherry stone	Scissor trimming expedites the procedure. Using the stone rounds the sharp edges of the material created by the scissors
14. Remove rough edges with careful flaming of an alcohol torch	Flaming the borders rounds and smooths the edges of the mouthprotector
15. Smooth the mouthprotector with wet pumice and a rag wheel	This procedure ensures smooth edges of the mouthprotector
16. Place the mouthprotector intraorally, and allow the client to close gently on softened material	This step enables the dental hygienist to assess the fit
17. Make final adjustments by removing occlusal interferences with the flaming alcohol torch	This step improves the comfort and fit of the mouthprotector
18. Remove/smooth any edges that impinge on the oral tissue	This step improves the comfort and fit of the mouthprotector
19. Ascertain the client's comfort with the mouthprotector in position	This feedback ensures client satisfaction with the mouthprotector
20. Evaluate for disruption of breathing or speech while the mouthprotector is in the client's mouth	To increase compliance, it is important for the client to be able to breathe and communicate when the mouthprotector is in place
21. Label the mouthprotector with the client's name. Remove a small amount of material in the facial area of the first molar with a small stone. Place a name tag (3 × 6 mm) into the shallow indentation after it has been heated	This step provides for rapid identification of lost mouthprotectors
22. Overlay a thin piece of vinyl, and heat with the alcohol torch. Seal edges with a hot spatula.	This step contributes to quick identification of lost mouthprotectors
23. Provide the client with instructions on proper cleaning and storage	This step ensures longevity and infection control

should inform parents and teachers of the procedure so increased awareness can improve the opportunity for successful replantation when injuries involving avulsed teeth occur.

In addition, during the assessment phase of the dental hygiene process, clients who play contact sports should be identified as having a potential deficit in the human need for safety. The appropriate intervention would be education of the client and parent, and construction of a mouthprotector to prevent tooth avulsion and other oral injuries. The procedure for constructing a custom-made athletic mouthprotector is described in Procedure 20–1.

Treatment

Because an avulsed tooth is one that is traumatically separated from the alveolus, typically there is a layer of periodontal ligament cells remaining on the cemental surface, and a layer of periodontal ligament cells remaining on the bone in the socket. Treatment of avulsed teeth is dependent on rejoining intact periodontal ligament cells covering the cementum of the tooth to those remaining in the socket.

The object of this emergency treatment is to promote healing of the periodontal ligament once the tooth is replanted in the socket. To maximize the chances of healing, the tooth must be handled only by the crown so as not to further kill or damage the remaining periodontal ligament cells. It is essential that the avulsed tooth not be allowed to dry and that it not be débrided in any way. It has been reported that as little as 1 hour of dry storage prior to replantation negatively affects the success rate of the procedure.[16]

The ideal place to store and transport the avulsed tooth is in the socket, if it can be gently placed and held there while the client is taken to an oral healthcare setting or a hospital emergency room. The socket provides the most nutritious environment for the cells of the periodontal ligament, thereby increasing their survival rate. If it is not possible to replace the tooth temporarily in the socket because of other injuries associated with the trauma, physio-

TABLE 20–3
STORAGE OF AVULSED TEETH DURING TRANSPORTATION FOR TREATMENT

Choice	Transportation Medium
First	Replace in socket
Second	Store in physiological saline
Third	Store in cold, fresh milk
Fourth	Place in the client's mouth, under the tongue or in the cheek
Fifth	Store in warm saltwater

logical saline is a safe alternative but may not be handy. Milk is a good medium because it has physiological osmolality and relatively few bacteria. Saliva has more bacteria, and the client may be too upset or too young to hold the tooth in the mouth. Warm saltwater can prevent dehydration but cannot keep the cells alive long. Air-drying or wrapping the tooth in gauze or other materials, even for a short time, kills many of the periodontal ligament cells.[15] Alternatives may have to be thought through quickly, and a decision made during a stressful situation to avoid allowing the cells to dehydrate and die (Table 20–3).

Once at the emergency treatment facility, often a dentist's office, or possibly a hospital emergency room, the tooth should be removed from its transport medium, gently washed if necessary, replanted in the socket after the blood clot is removed, and splinted into place. Endodontic procedures need to be performed at a later time to avoid inflammatory root resorption.[17]

References

1. Balciunas, B. A., and Overholser, C. D. Diagnosis and treatment of common oral lesions. American Family Physician 35(5):206, 1987.
2. Balciunas, B. A., Kelly, M., and Siegel, M. A. Clinical management of common oral lesions. Cutis 47:31, 1991.
3. Carranza, F. A., Jr. Glickman's Clinical Periodontology, 7th ed. Philadelphia: W. B. Saunders, 1990, p. 666.
4. Genco, R. J. Periodontal diagnosis, prognosis, and treatment planning. In Genco, R. J., Goldman, H. M., and Cohen, D. W. (eds.). Contemporary Periodontics. St. Louis: C. V. Mosby, 1990, p. 357.
5. Leone, S. A., and Edenfield, M. J. Third molars and acute pericoronitis: A military problem. Military Medicine 152(3): 146, 1987.
6. Grant, D. A., Stern, I. B., and Listgarten, M. A. Periodontics, 6th ed. St. Louis: C. V. Mosby, 1988, p. 423.
7. Cogan, R. B. Acute necrotizing ulcerative gingivitis. In Genco, R. J., Goldman, H. M., Cohen D. W. (eds.). Contemporary Periodontics. St. Louis: C. V. Mosby, 1990, pp. 460–461.
8. Caton, J. Periodontal diagnosis and diagnostic aids. In Nevins, M., Becker, W., Kornman, K. S. (eds.) Proceedings of the World Workshop in Clinical Periodontics. Chicago: American Academy of Periodontology, 1989, pp. 1–2.
9. Stevens, A. W., Cogen, R. B., Cohen-Cole, S., and Freeman, A. Demographic and clinical data associated with acute necrotizing ulcerative gingivitis in a dental school population. Journal of Clinical Periodontology 11:487, 1984.
10. Killoy, W. J. Treatment of periodontal abscesses. In Genco, R. J., Goldman, H. M., Cohen D. W. (eds.). Contemporary Periodontics. St. Louis: C. V. Mosby, 1990, p. 475.
11. Kureishi, A., and Chow, A. W. The tender tooth: Dentoalveolar, pericoronal, and periodontal infections. Infectious Disease Clinics of North America 2(1):163, 1988.
12. Macfarlane, T. W. Plaque-related infections. Journal of Medical Microbiology 29:161, 1989.
13. Saal, C. J., Mason, J. C., Cheuk, S. L., and Hill, M. K. Brain abscess from chronic odontogenic cause: Report of a case. Journal of the American Dental Association 117(9):453, 1988.
14. Bhat, M., and Li, S.-H. Consumer product–related tooth injuries treated in hospital emergency rooms: United States 1979–87. Community Oral Health and Epidemiology 18:133, 1990.
15. Krasner, P. R. The treatment of avulsed teeth. Journal of Pediatric Health Care 4(2):86, 1990.
16. Andersson, L., Bodin, I., and Sorensen, S. Progression of root resorption following replantation of human teeth after extended extraoral storage. Endodontic Dental Traumatology 5:38, 1989.
17. Sidley C. G. Endodontic management of the avulsed tooth and tooth transplantation. Alpha Omegan 83:60, 1990.

Suggested Readings

Nevins, M., Becker, W., and Kornman, K. Consensus Report. Proceedings of the World Workshop in Clinical Periodontics, Chicago: American Academy of Periodontology, 1989.

Newman, M. G., and Sims, T. N. The predominant cultivable microbiota of the periodontal abscess. Journal of Periodontology 50:350, 1978.

Rose, L. F. Infective forms of gingivostomatitis. In Genco, R. J., Goldman, H. M., Cohen D. W. (eds.). Contemporary Periodontics. St. Louis: C. V. Mosby, 1990.

A

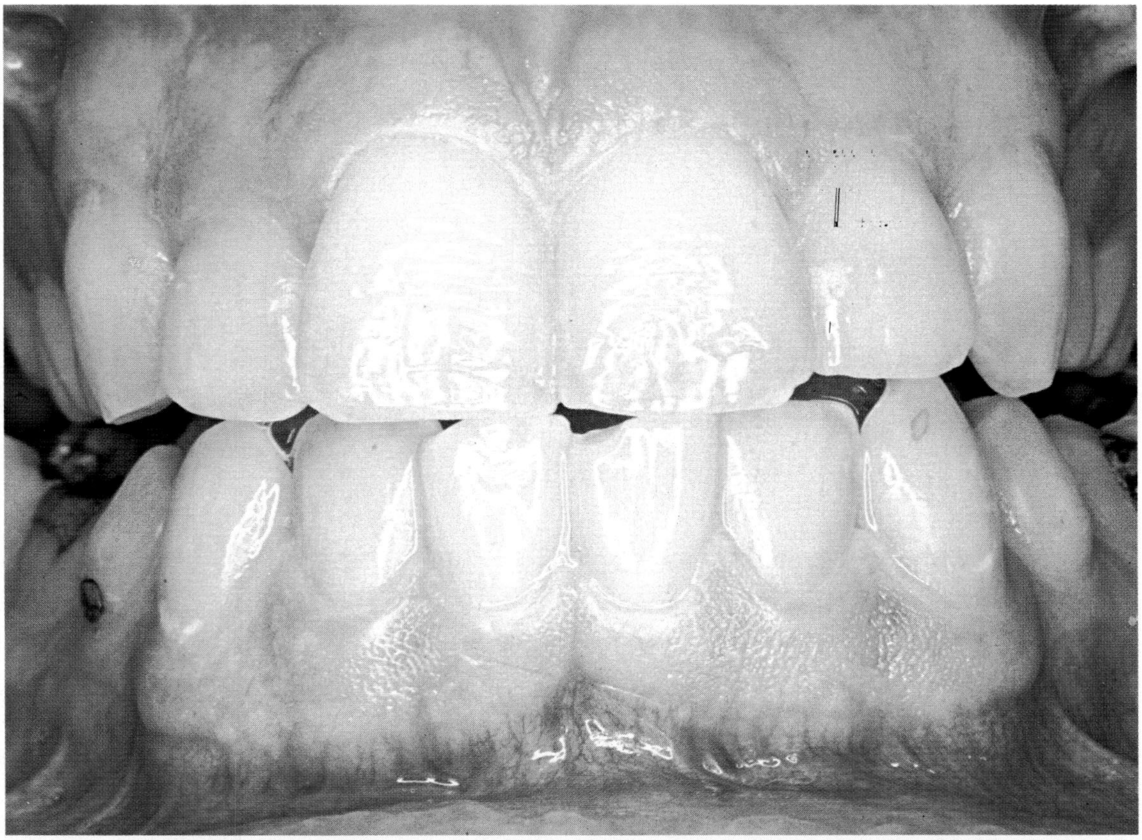

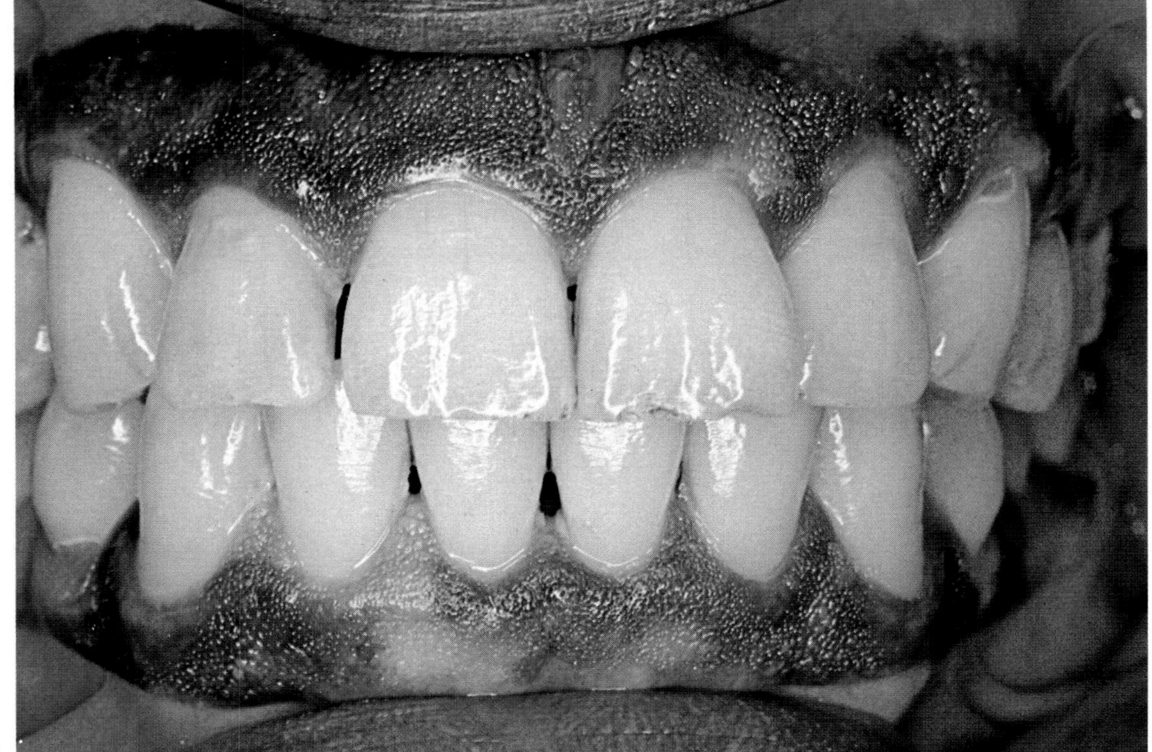

B

FIGURE 13–6
A, Clinically normal gingiva in light-skinned individuals. *B*, Clinically normal pigmented gingiva in dark-skinned individuals. (With permission from Glickman, I., and Smulow, J. B. Periodontal Disease: Clinical, Radiographic, and Histopathologic Features. Philadelphia: W. B. Saunders, 1974, p. 3.)

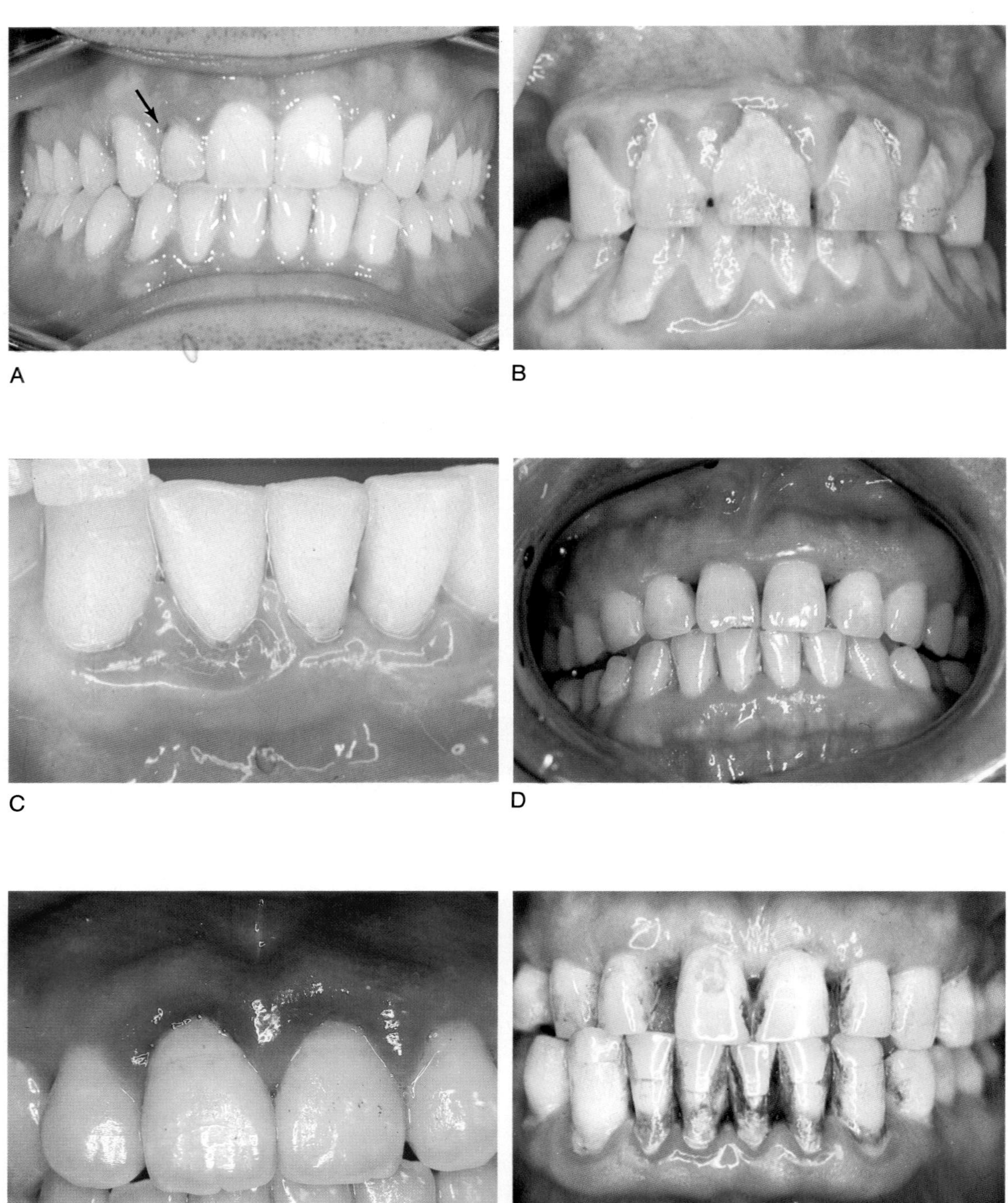

FIGURE 13–10
A, Incipient marginal gingivitis. Note slight puffiness and bleeding (*arrow*) around upper right lateral incisor. *B*, Edematous type of gingival inflammation. Note loss of stippling, increase in size, abundant plaque and materia alba, and change in color. *C*, Close-up view of edematous type of gingival inflammation. Note the red, shiny, smooth gingiva. *D*, Fibrotic type of gingival inflammation. Pockets of moderate depth are present, but the gingiva retains its stippling in some areas. *E*, Severe generalized gingival inflammation and inflammatory gingival enlargement. *F*, Fibrotic gingival inflammation. Note the abundant calculus and the gingival recession. The patient has pockets of moderate to severe depth in the mandibular anterior teeth and shallower pockets in the maxillary teeth. (With permission from Carranza, F. Glickman's Clinical Periodontology, 7th ed. Philadelphia: W. B. Saunders, 1990, p. 492.)

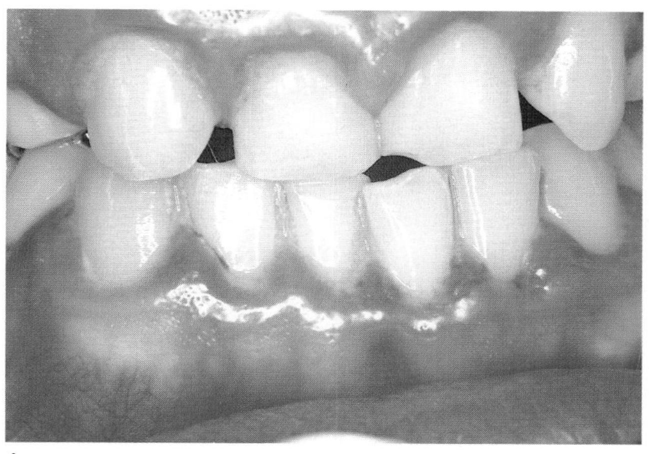
A

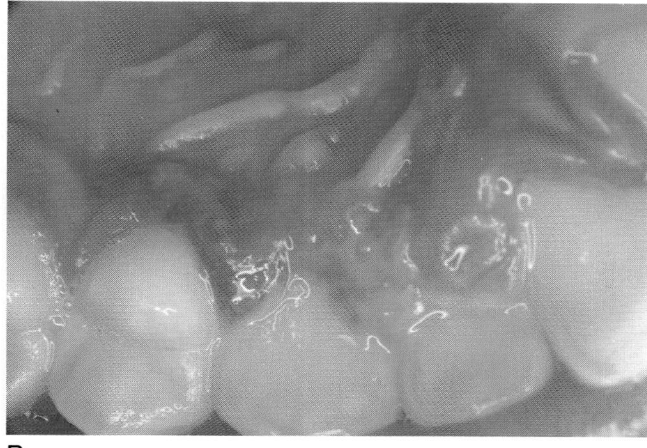
B

FIGURE 20-1
Primary herpetic infection of the mouth is characterized by bright red gingiva, vesicles, and pain. *A*, Facial gingiva showing swelling and color change. *B*, Lingual view of premolar and anterior teeth showing coalesced vesicles. (Courtesy of Philip R. Melnick, D.D.S.)

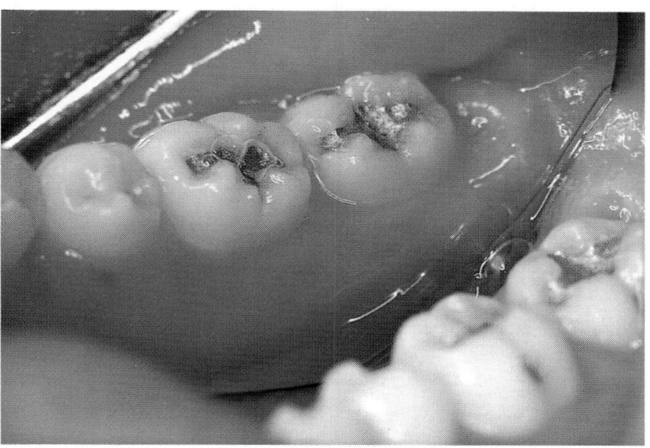

FIGURE 20-2
Acute pericoronitis is usually localized to the third molar region and can be extremely painful. Note the swelling and color change present at the distal side of the second molar. (Courtesy of Edward J. Taggart, D.D.S., M.S.)

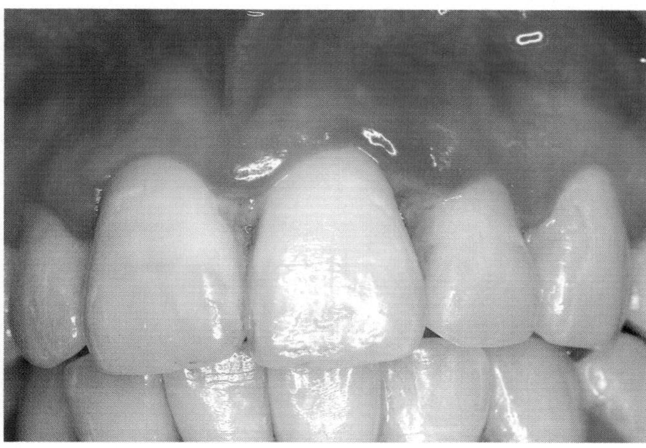

FIGURE 20-3
Acute necrotizing ulcerative gingivitis throughout the anterior area. (Courtesy of Philip R. Melnick, D.D.S.)

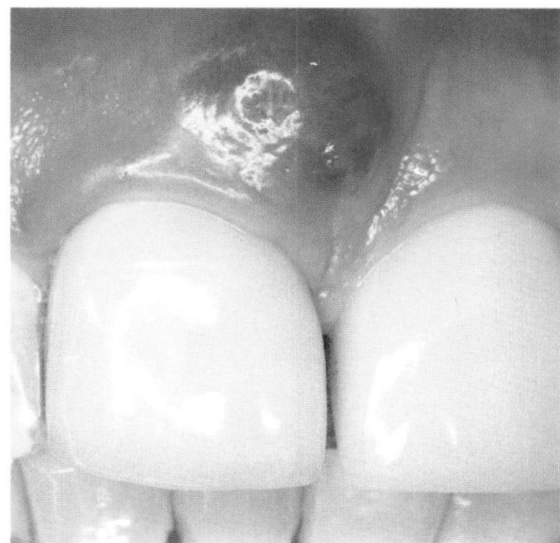

FIGURE 20-4
Acute periodontal abscess associated with tooth no. 8, characterized by redness and swelling. (Courtesy of Philip R. Melnick, D.D.S.)

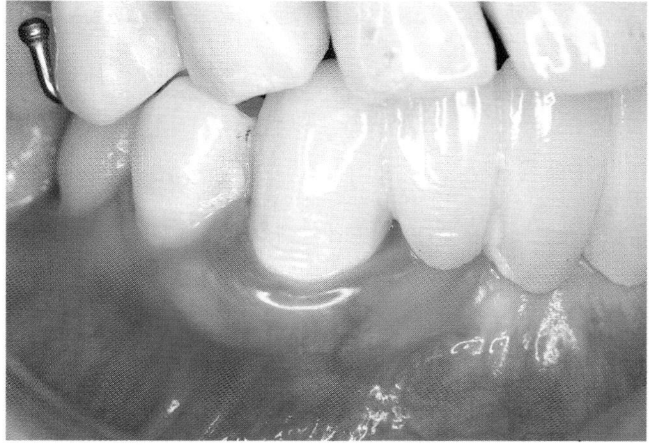

FIGURE 20-6
Gingival abscess associated with the marginal gingiva; note swelling and color change. (Courtesy of Philip R. Melnick, D.D.S.)

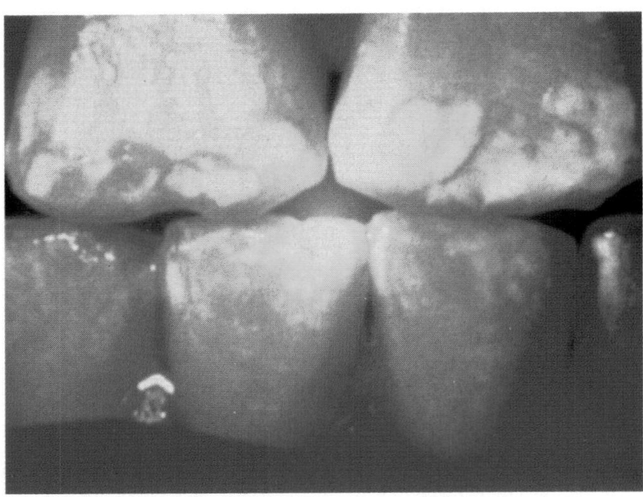

FIGURE 21-12
Fluorosis. (Courtesy of *Dental Hygienist News* funded by an educational grant from Procter and Gamble and published by Harfst Associates, Inc., Troy, Michigan.)

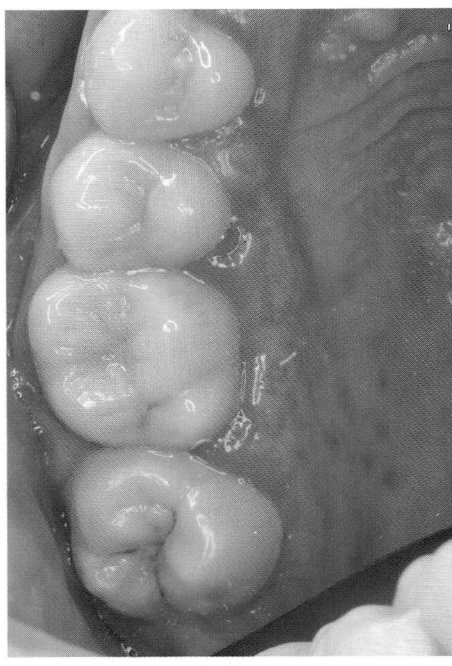

FIGURE 23-84
Herpes simplex virus lesions on the palate following quadrant scaling and root planing with local anesthetic injections.

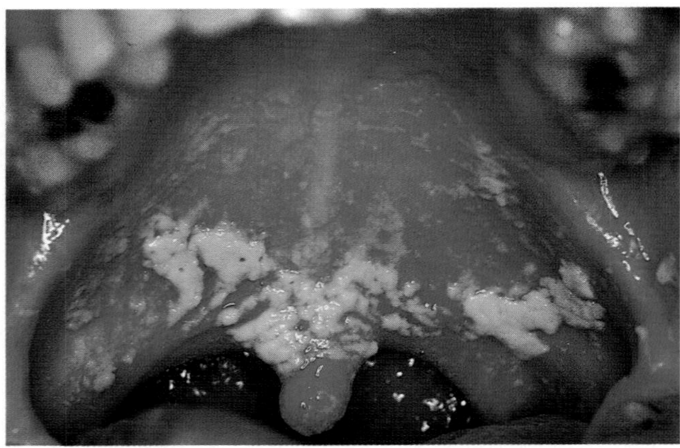

FIGURE 33-1
Pseudomembranous candidiasis in an individual with AIDS manifested as white plaques on the palate. (Courtesy of James R. Winkler, D.D.S., Switzerland.)

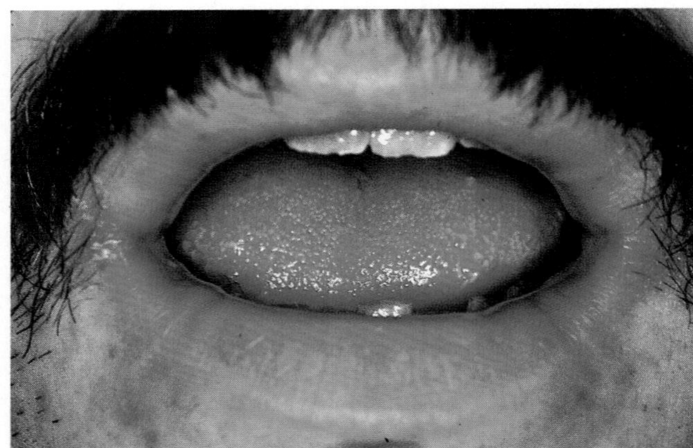

FIGURE 33-2
Angular cheilitis in a person with AIDS seen as cracked sores at the right corner of his mouth. (Courtesy of James R. Winkler, D.D.S., Switzerland.)

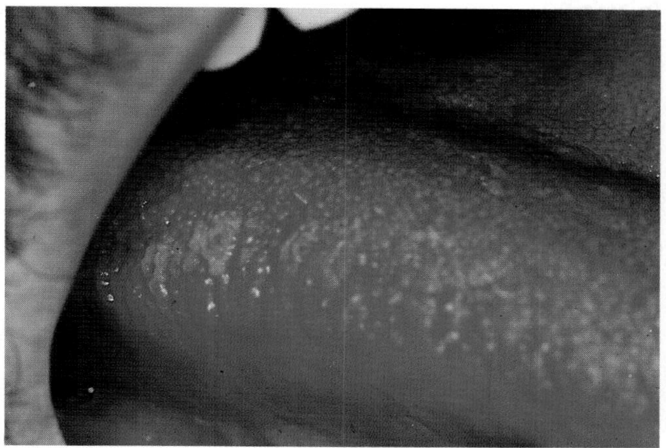

FIGURE 33–3
Hairy leukoplakia in an individual with AIDS located on the right lateral border of the tongue. (Courtesy of James R. Winkler, D.D.S., Switzerland.)

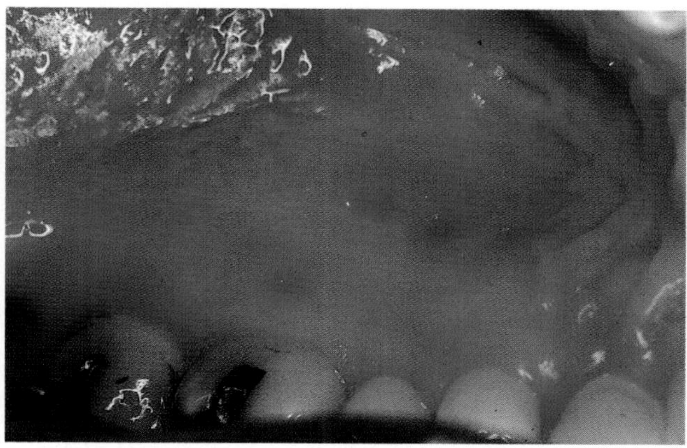

FIGURE 33–4
Oral Kaposi's sarcoma lesions on the palate of an individual with AIDS. (Courtesy of James R. Winkler, D.D.S., Switzerland.)

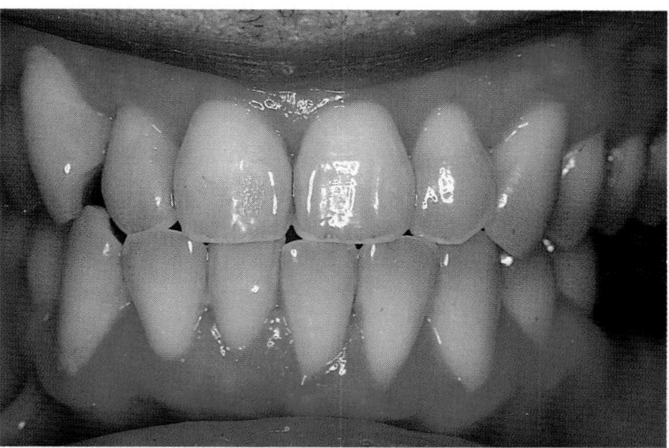

FIGURE 33–5
Necrotizing ulcerative gingivitis associated with HIV infection prior to care: The gingival margin shows color change to bright red that may extend onto the alveolar mucosa. (Courtesy of James R. Winkler, D.D.S., Switzerland.)

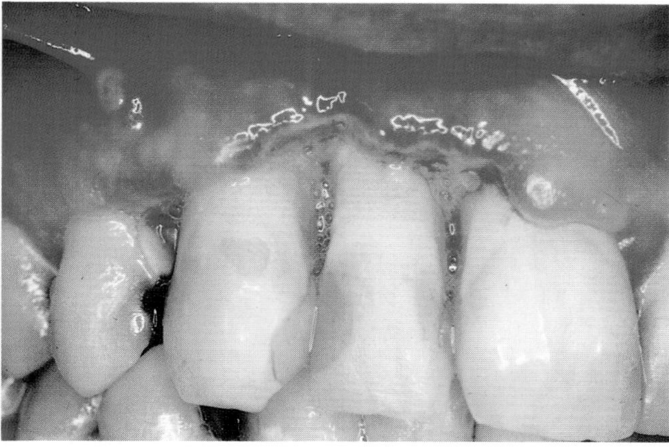

FIGURE 33–6
Necrotizing ulcerative periodontitis in an individual with AIDS showing color change, necrosis, and sloughing of the periodontal tissues. (Courtesy of James R. Winkler, D.D.S., Switzerland.)

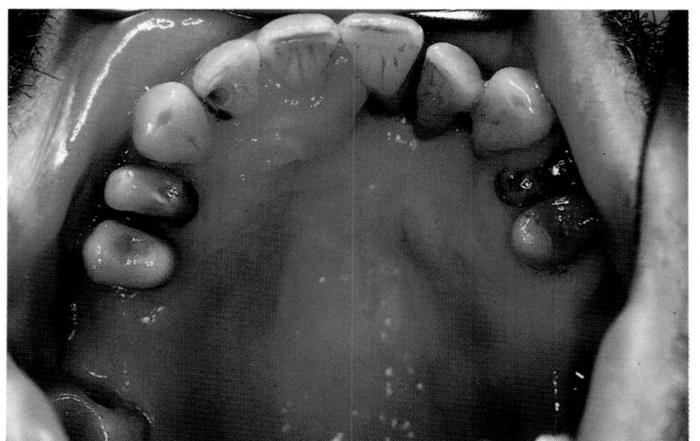

FIGURE 33–7
Kaposi's sarcoma associated with the teeth before treatment; dark lesions are present around the teeth and on the palate. (Courtesy of James R. Winkler, D.D.S., Switzerland.)

XYZ Dental Group, Ltd.
Dr. John Doe, DDS

PERIODONTAL CHART

Name: Newman, Paul Prov: Dr. Philip McKenzie	Pat#: NEWMPA	SSN: 127-21-6697 Date: 02-24-1992
Provider's Signature		Date
Notes: This is an actual printout from ** Chart-It ** For more information, please contact: SINGER Professional Services, Inc. 8401-K Mayland Drive Richmond, VA 23294 (804) 747-5289		

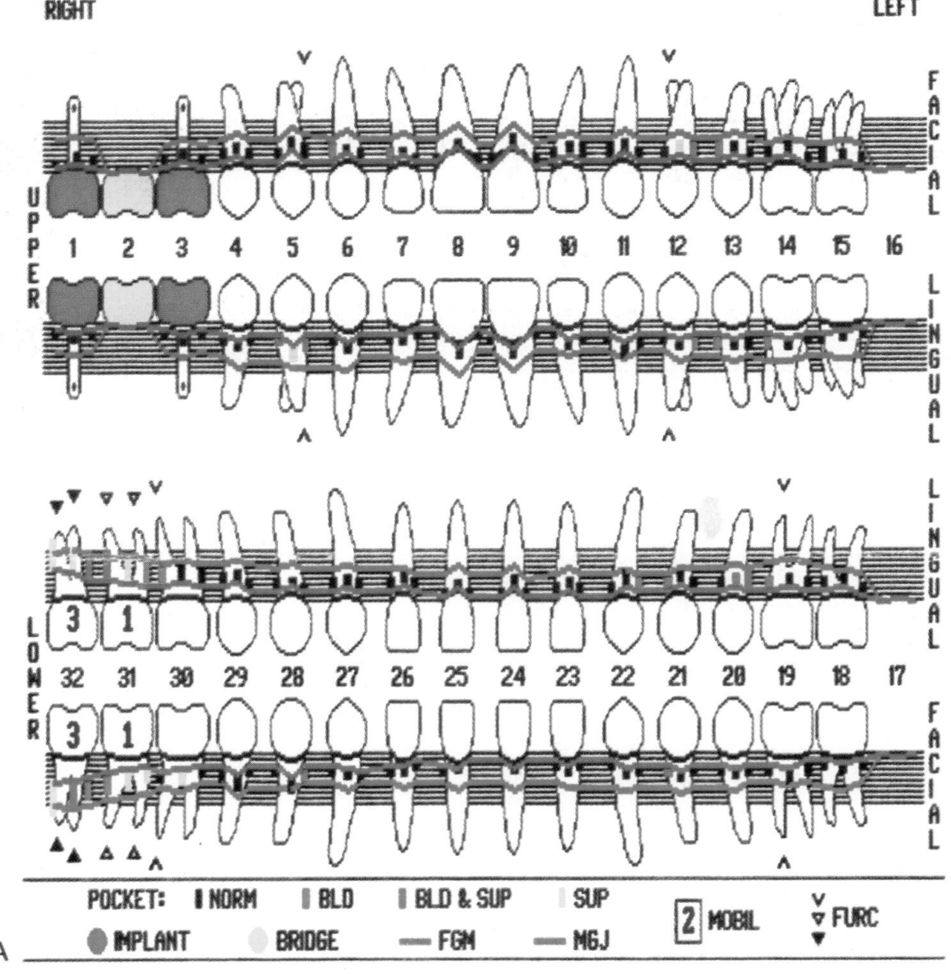

FIGURE 38–23
A, Computerized dental chart (CHART-IT). (Courtesy of Singer Professional Services, Inc. Copyright 1991, Singer Professional Services, Inc.)

21 Dental Hygiene Care: Caries Prevention and Control

OBJECTIVES

Mastery of the content in this chapter will enable the reader to:

- Define the key terms used
- Identify the roles of fluoride, pit and fissure sealants, and nutritional counseling in the prevention of dental caries
- Discuss the advantages and disadvantages of the three types of fluorides available for professional application (NaF, SnF_2, APF)
- Correctly administer an APF gel treatment using the tray method
- Identify and evaluate the degree of dental fluorosis on a client
- Explain how the ADA Seal of Acceptance can protect the consumer in the sale of dental products
- Perform the steps necessary to place either a light-curing or self-curing sealant when presented with a client who has explorer-detectable deep pits and fissures
- Describe the signs, symptoms, and treatment associated with acute fluoride toxicity
- Identify individuals in need of nutritional counseling
- Assess a client's diet for adequacy of intake from the five food groups/food pyramid
- Provide nutritional counseling to help the client achieve optimal oral and general health

INTRODUCTION

All persons have a human need for a biologically sound dentition that defends against harmful microbes and provides for adequate function and esthetics. Dental hygienists assist individuals in meeting this basic need by focusing on oral disease prevention and oral health promotion. In the area of caries prevention, the dental hygienist applies caries-preventive agents and counsels individuals as well as groups on the relationship between preventive measures and dental caries.

The use of fluorides provides the most effective method for the prevention and control of dental caries. In addition, plaque control, pit and fissure sealants, and nutritional counseling are important preventive measures to supplement the use of fluorides for caries control. The purpose of this chapter is to describe the use of fluorides, pit and fissure sealants, and nutritional counseling as they relate to caries prevention. (Personal plaque control techniques are presented in detail in Chapter 16.)

COMPREHENSIVE FLUORIDE THERAPY

Comprehensive fluoride therapy includes the use of systemic and topical fluoride at an optimal amount to maintain a caries-free oral environment. Fluoride can be delivered to the tooth in two ways:

- **systemically** (by entry into the blood supply of developing teeth
- **topically** (by direct contact on exposed surfaces of teeth)

Systemic Fluoride

The systemic administration of fluoride is delivered via the community water supply or by dietary supplements. To a lesser extent, fluoride can be consumed in certain foods and beverages such as fish, tea, and wine.[1] Water fluoridation and fluoride dietary supplements have been shown to decrease caries incidence by 50 to 60%.

The absorption of fluoride takes place mainly in the stomach and the intestines. Fluoride then circulates through the bloodstream and is incorporated into the developing teeth. Specifically, fluoride that is ingested as the teeth are forming is incorporated into the enamel structure by replacing hydroxyapatite crystals with fluorapatite crystals. This incorporation of fluorapatite into the enamel makes the tooth more resistant to erosion from acids. This resistance to erosion makes the tooth less likely to decay.

Use of systemic fluoride therapy is most effective from birth to 14 years of age. However, after the teeth erupt, systemic fluoride has a topical effect on the enamel when it comes into contact with the teeth directly through the salivary secretions.

Water Fluoridation

The most convenient and effective manner to reduce the incidence of dental caries on a large scale is to add fluoride to the community drinking water supply. Water fluoridaton should be done if the water does not contain adequate amounts of natural fluoride. Studies conducted during the 1930s and 1940s in the midwestern United States indicated that a 50% reduction of caries occurred at a fluoride concentration of 1 part per million (1 ppm) in the water.[2]

Water fluoridation is the most economical method of caries prevention. The annual cost for fluoridation of community water to optimal levels for caries prevention varies from 10 cents to 25 cents per person per year, depending upon the size of the community and the cost of the installation and running of a water fluoridation plant. Compared to the cost of the pain and discomfort from decayed teeth and the associated loss of time from school or work, the annual cost per capita for water fluoridation is economical, as well as valuable, as a public health measure.

Prenatal Fluoride Supplements

Prescribing prenatal fluoride supplements to pregnant women living in nonfluoridated areas ensures that fluoride is available to the developing tooth buds. Currently, many researchers agree that fluoride crosses the placenta and is absorbed in the developing hard and soft tissues of the fetus.[3] However, data on actual caries reduction in offspring is inconclusive.

Infant and Early Childhood Fluoride Supplements

Another source of systemic fluoride delivery is through dietary supplements prescribed by the dentist or pediatrician. Liquid drops, tablets, lozenges, and oral rinses are all acceptable methods of delivery. The fluoride supplement can be chewed or held in the mouth for 1 minute before swallowing it to obtain a localized effect on the enamel surface. The client should be advised not to eat, drink, or brush for 30 minutes to ensure maximal topical effect.

Control-release fluoride tablets contain small amounts of available fluoride on the surface for an immediate intraoral effect. The bulk of the fluoride is absorbed slowly after ingestion of the tablet. These control-release fluoride supplements are designed to prevent a high plasma fluoride peak.[4]

In areas where the community water supply is not fluoridated, dietary fluoride supplements should be prescribed for children from birth to 14 years of age. These supplements also should be prescribed if the water supply contains less than 0.7 ppm of the recommended amount of fluoride.[5]

Currently, dietary supplements are not recommended for infants who are breast fed and who reside in optimally fluoridated communities.[4] Breast milk contains 0.004 ppm fluoride. The reduction in caries observed clinically in thousands of children living in naturally fluoridated communities has occurred without supplementation of the children's diets during breastfeeding.

Dental fluorosis is defined as changes in the structure and composition of the enamel surface as a result of excessive fluoride ingestion. To prevent dental fluorosis, it is important to determine the level of fluoride in the drinking water before dietary supplements are prescribed. In different parts of the country, the quantity of fluoride in drinking water varies. For example, the midwestern United States has 74% of its water fluoridated as compared to the Pacific Coast, where only 19% of the population is provided with optimally fluoridated water.[4]

Dietary supplements should be adjusted in areas with very hot, dry climates. These areas may show an increase in the consumption of tap water as well as beverages mixed with tap water. These hot and humid areas potentially increase perspiration. Concentrations of 0.3 to 0.4 ppm fluoride are contained in the perspiration under normal conditions. When the temperature rises to 85°F, 15% of the excreted fluoride may be found in the perspiration. At elevated temperatures, as much as 50% of the fluoride may be excreted.[1]

Fluoride may be present naturally or it may be added by a municipal water department. A telephone call to the local water department is an easy way to determine the level of fluoride in your local water supply. Bottled water may or may not contain fluoride. When this information is not readily available on the label, consumers may contact the supplier of the bottled water to obtain the fluoride content. For those individuals who own private wells, individual samples of well water must be assayed to determine their fluoride concentration. These assay services are provided by many state health departments, dental schools, and commercial laboratories. A fluoride dosage schedule, adjusted to fluoride concentration of drinking water, can be used to determine the amount of fluoride supplements from birth through adolescence (Table 21–1).

Topical Fluoride

Studies have shown that a combination of fluoride therapies should be used to ensure optimal oral health.[1] The most beneficial caries prevention care plan incorporates the use of both systemic and topical fluoride. There are three categories of topically applied fluorides:

- Professionally applied in the oral healthcare environment
- Self-applied by the client at home and available over-the-counter
- Self-applied by the client at home, available by prescription only

Topical fluoride application is thought to work as an anticarious agent in several ways. One mechanism involves the continued maturation of enamel after the eruption of the teeth. The continued maturation of enamel involves the incorporation and concentration of fluoride in the form of fluorapatite crystals at the enamel surface.

TABLE 21–1
SUPPLEMENTAL FLUORIDE DOSAGE SCHEDULE (IN MILLIGRAMS F PER DAY*) ACCORDING TO FLUORIDE CONCENTRATION OF DRINKING WATER

	Concentration of Fluoride in Water (ppm)		
Age	**Less than 0.3**	**0.3 to 0.6**	**Greater than 0.6**
6 mon to 3 yr	0.25	0	0
3 to 6 yr	0.5	0.25	0
6 to 16 yr	1.0	0.5	0

* 2.2 mg NaF contain 1 mg F
Adapted with permission from Jakush, J. CDT to consider fluoride dosage. ADA News, February 21, 1994, p. 16.

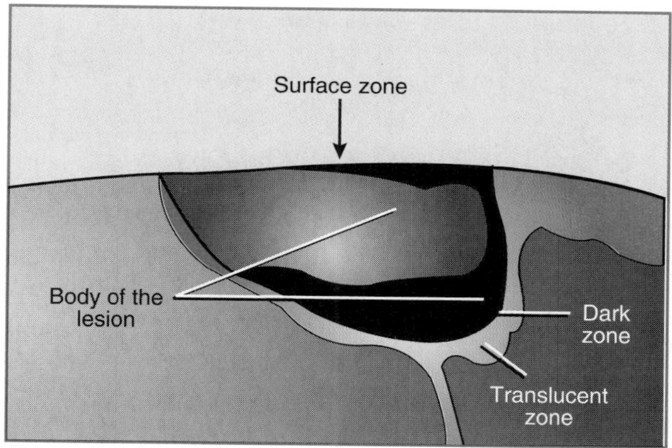

FIGURE 21–1
Zones of the carious lesion.

Another mechanism of topical fluoride action is the delay of demineralization by the remineralization process. Research supports the conclusion that small carious lesions can be arrested or reversed by remineralization.[6,7]

Remineralization

Remineralization is the deposition of minerals into previously damaged areas of a tooth. It is a reparative process by which enamel crystals are rebuilt. Fluoride delivered in low concentrations and with high frequency increases the rate of growth and size of crystals that are formed.[8] These larger crystals are more resistant to acid attack.

When acids from plaque diffuse through the enamel surface to produce a subsurface lesion, there is a loss of minerals from the tooth; this is referred to as "demineralization." Viewed histologically, the carious lesion contains four distinct zones (Fig. 21–1):

- Translucent zone
- A dark zone
- Body of the lesion zone
- Surface zone

These zones are believed to be formed through a continuous exchange of minerals between the tooth and its environment. The surface and dark zones are formed as a result of remineralization. The body of the lesion and the translucent zone are produced as a result of demineralization. Fluoride in toothpaste, gels, and rinses offers the client frequent exposures of low concentrations of fluoride and supports the remineralization process by accelerating the growth of enamel crystals.

A final mechanism of action of topical fluoride is its antibacterial effect on plaque. Specifically, there is growing evidence that stannous fluoride has antiplaque properties. Initially these antiplaque effects were considered nonspecific, but later studies have shown that *Streptococcus mutans,* the oral bacteria most often associated with dental caries, is reduced to a greater extent than other microorganisms.[9]

Professionally Applied Fluoride

There are three types of topical fluoride available for professional application:

- Sodium fluoride (2% NaF)
- Stannous fluoride (8% SnF_2)
- Acidulated phosphate fluoride (1.23% APF)

Table 21–2 presents the advantages, disadvantages, and criteria for administration for these professionally applied topical fluoride agents. All three types appear to be equally effective in the prevention of caries, but they differ in application, frequency, taste, cost, stability, gingival tissue acceptance, and staining tendency.[10] Professionally applied

TABLE 21–2
PROFESSIONALLY APPLIED TOPICAL FLUORIDE AGENTS

Type	Advantages	Disadvantages	Administration
2% sodium fluoride	Stable Acceptable taste	Four treatments are required over a short period of time	Gel form placed on teeth via intraoral tray for 4 minutes Series of four applications 1 week apart
8% stannous fluoride	Bacteriostatic Frequency of application conforms to 6-month recalls	Unstable Unacceptable taste	Operator must continually apply fluoride solution with cotton applicator for 4 minutes
1.23% acidulated phosphate fluoride	Easy to apply Stable Acceptable taste Does not stain teeth Does not irritate tissue	May be inappropriate for clients with porcelain or composite restorations	Gel form placed on teeth via intraoral tray for 4 minutes

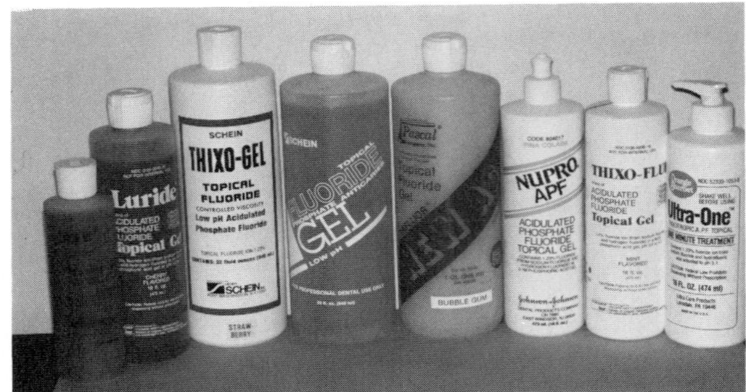

FIGURE 21–2
Topical fluoride gel for professional applications. (Courtesy of Oral-B Laboratories.)

topical fluorides have been shown to decrease caries incidence by 30 to 40%.

Sodium Fluoride

Sodium fluoride is an aqueous solution applied to clean, dry teeth for 3 to 4 minutes. Four applications are given 1 week apart in children at the ages of 3, 7, 10, and 13. The ages chosen coincide with the tooth eruption pattern of children. Sodium fluoride has an acceptable taste, it does not discolor the teeth, and it does not cause gingival irritation. The only disadvantage to the sodium fluoride application is the need to see the client weekly for 4 consecutive weeks.

Stannous Fluoride

Stannous fluoride has a pH level of 2.1 to 2.3, has an unpleasant taste, and may cause staining in demineralized areas of the teeth. In addition, it can irritate the tissues and cause gingival sloughing. Because stannous fluoride is unstable and cannot be stored, a fresh solution must be prepared for each application.

Acidulated Phosphate Fluoride

The most common professionally applied topical fluoride is the acidulated phosphate fluoride (APF). It is available as an aqueous solution or gel in a thixotropic base (Fig. 21–2). A **thixotropic** gel is able to liquefy when agitated and revert to a gelatinous state upon standing. Gels of this type can flow into interdental spaces. The APF gel is easy to apply and stable when stored properly. The solution does not cause tooth discoloration or gingival irritation, and the taste is acceptable by the addition of flavoring agents. Four minutes is the recommended length of time for an APF treatment.

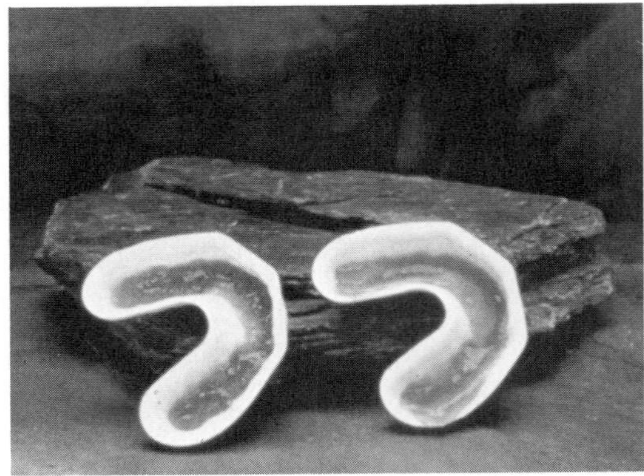

FIGURE 21–3
Single-arch trays. (Courtesy of *Dental Hygienist News* funded by an educational grant from Procter and Gamble and published by Harfst Associates, Inc., Troy, Michigan.)

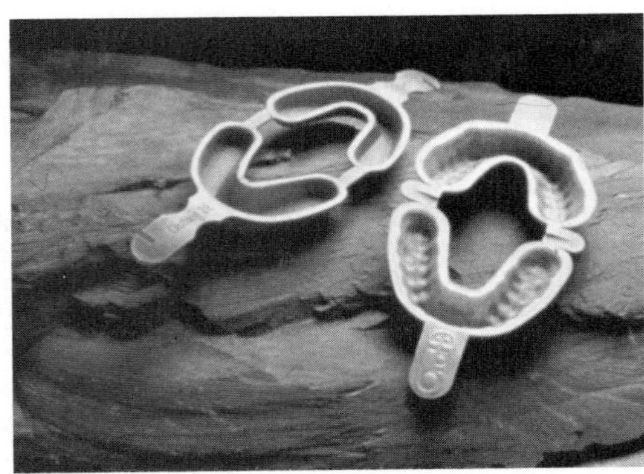

FIGURE 21–4
Dual-arch trays. (Courtesy *Dental Hygienist News* funded by an educational grant from Procter and Gamble and published by Harfst Associates, Inc., Troy, Michigan.)

It was once believed that professionally applied fluoride should be preceded by a rubber cup polishing of the teeth. The polishing procedure was to ensure removal of the pellicle so greater fluoride absorption could take place at the enamel surface. Research has shown that rubber cup polishing of the teeth is no longer indicated, and fluoride uptake is not inhibited by the presence of materia alba or the pellicle layer.[11] However, heavy calculus surrounding the root and crown should be removed prior to any fluoride therapy.

The APF gel tray method of fluoride application is comfortable for the client and convenient for the operator. Fluoride gel trays are available in small, medium, and large sizes as well as single-arch (Fig. 21–3) or dual-arch trays (Fig. 21–4). For optimal coverage of the teeth, a fluoride tray should be used that is deep enough to reach the entire vertical height of the crowns and exposed roots of the teeth (see Guidelines for Tray Selection for Fluoride Gels chart.)

GUIDELINES FOR TRAY SELECTION FOR FLUORIDE GELS

- Coverage of all tooth surfaces. If a tray is not deep enough to cover the root surfaces, a custom-made tray is needed
- Anatomical contours allow gel to flow into the interproximal spaces
- A positive seal and adequate distal dam (to prevent salivary dilution of the gel and to prevent accidental ingestion)
- Soft edges for client comfort
- Size selections in small, medium, and large
- Sturdy construction

Adapted from McCall, et al. Fluoride ingestion following APF gel application. British Dental Journal 155:333, 1983.

Research has cautioned the use of APF gels on clients with porcelain and composite restorations. A 4-minute application time of an acidic fluoride gel preparation may create dullness or loss of surface reflection to the restoration. To prevent this adverse effect, petrolatum should be placed over the restoration prior to APF fluoride tray administration.

Time-saving fluoride gels have been introduced to require a 1-minute application rather than the usual 4-minute treatment. A shorter treatment time helps prevent gel ingestion and lessens the possibility of etching or dulling the restorations. Wei and Hattab have indicated, however, that fluoride uptake in sound enamel is time-dependent.[12] A 1-minute fluoride application may result in a 2.5-fold decrease of enamel fluoride uptake when compared to the 4-minute application.

The clinical application for the administration of fluoride gel appears in Procedure 21–1.

PROCEDURE 21–1

APPLYING APF GEL METHOD

Equipment

Mouth mirror	Timer
Cotton forceps	Saliva ejector
Fluoride tray(s)	2 × 2 gauze
Cotton rolls	Tissues
APF gel	2 oz cup
Air syringe	Protective barriers

Steps	Rationale
1. Assemble equipment	Assembling equipment prior to seating the client promotes efficiency and infection control
2. Seat client in upright position	Prevents gagging and accidental ingestion of fluoride gel

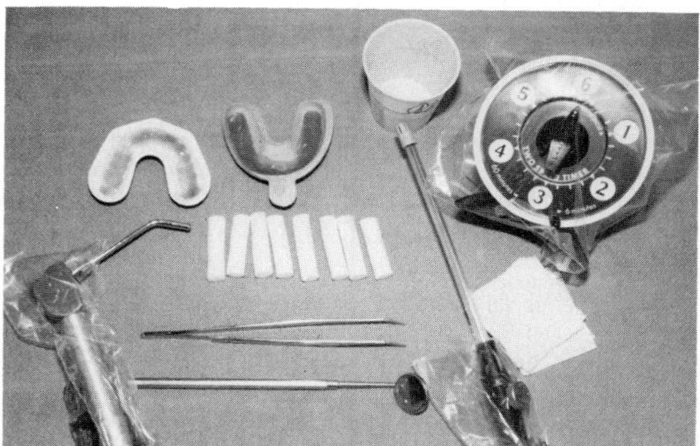

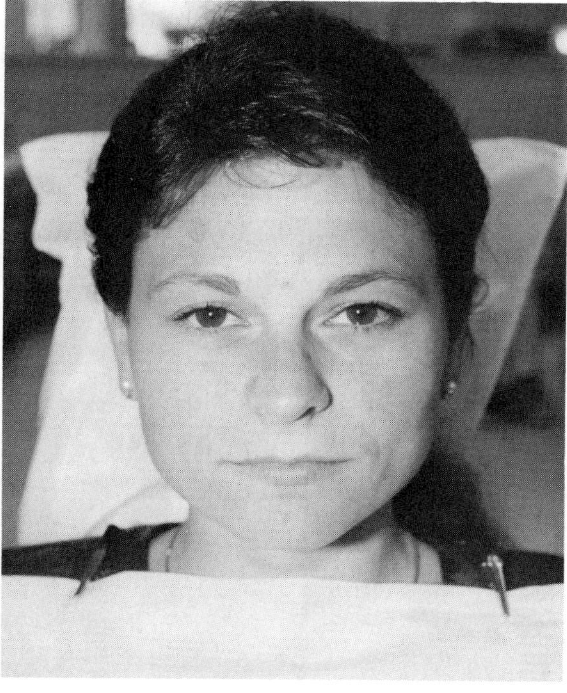

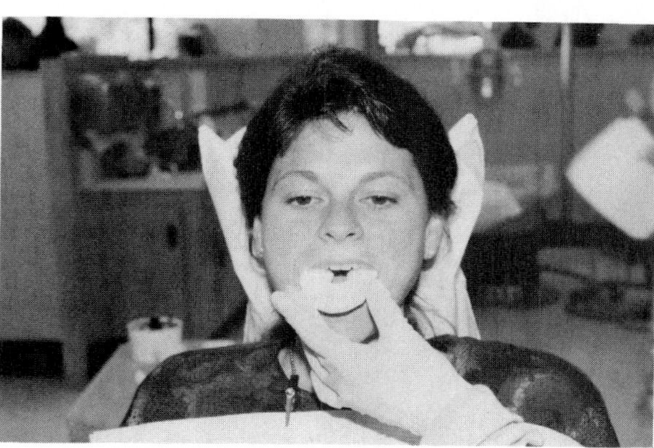

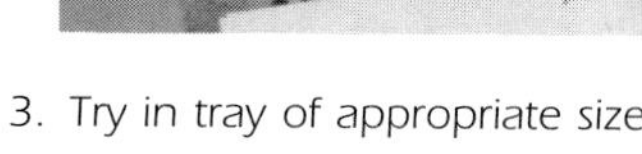

Steps	Rationale
3. Try in tray of appropriate size	Trays must be pliable, comfortable, and deep enough to cover all surfaces

CONTINUED ON FOLLOWING PAGE

PROCEDURE 21–1

APPLYING APF GEL METHOD *Continued*

Steps	Rationale
4. Load fluoride gel into trays 2 ml maximum for children 2.5 ml maximum for adults	Recommendations by the American Academy of Pediatric Dentistry Trays deliver fluoride to the exposed surfaces of the teeth

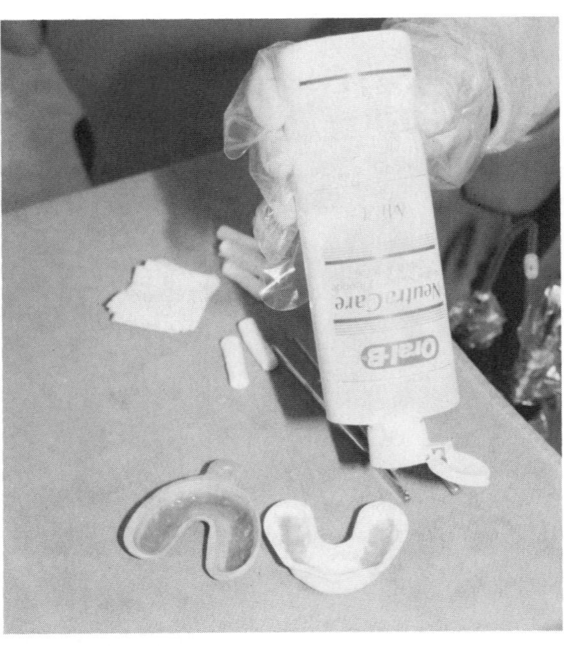

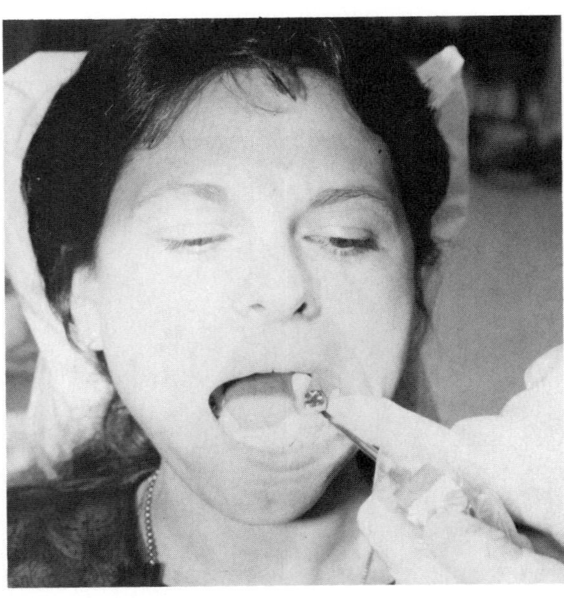

Steps	Rationale
5. Isolate teeth with cotton rolls. Dry with air syringe	A dry field is necessary for maximum fluoride uptake
6. Insert mandibular tray	The tray delivers the fluoride to the mandibular teeth; mandibular tray stays in place more easily than does the maxillary tray

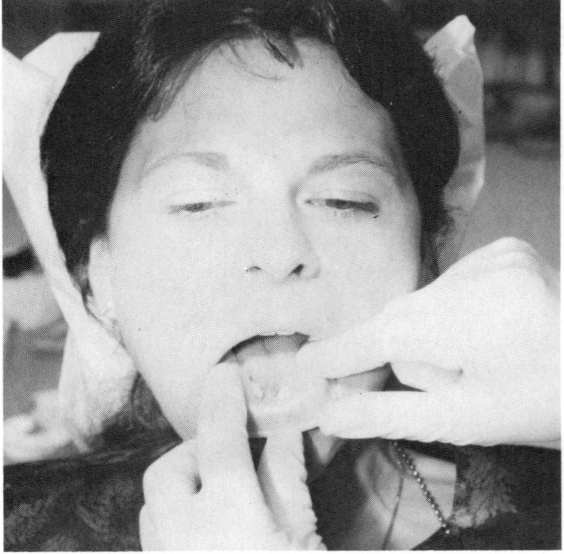

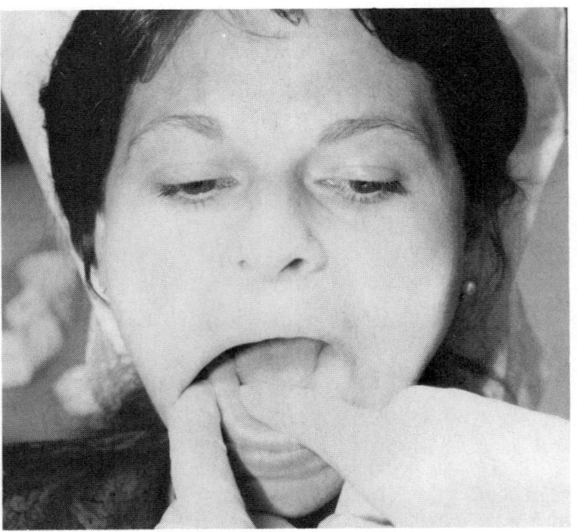

Steps	Rationale
7. Press tray against teeth	Forcing the gel between teeth ensures coverage into interproximal spaces

Steps	Rationale
8. Air dry maxillary arch and insert maxillary tray	Maintaining a dry field ensures efficacy of undiluted fluoride
9. Press tray against teeth and ask client to close the mouth and bite gently on trays or cotton rolls	Slight pressure from biting helps force the fluoride gel to surround all surfaces
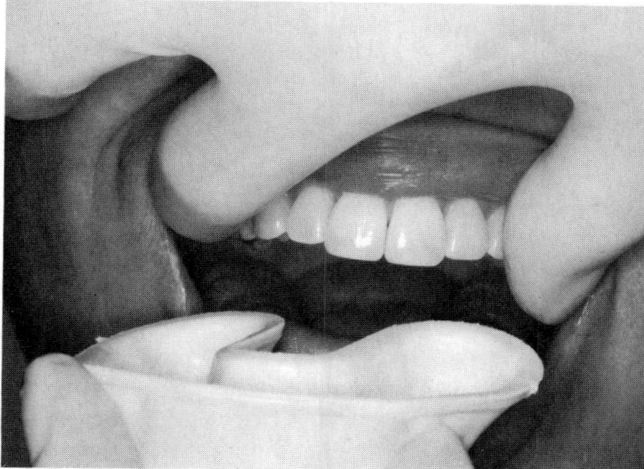	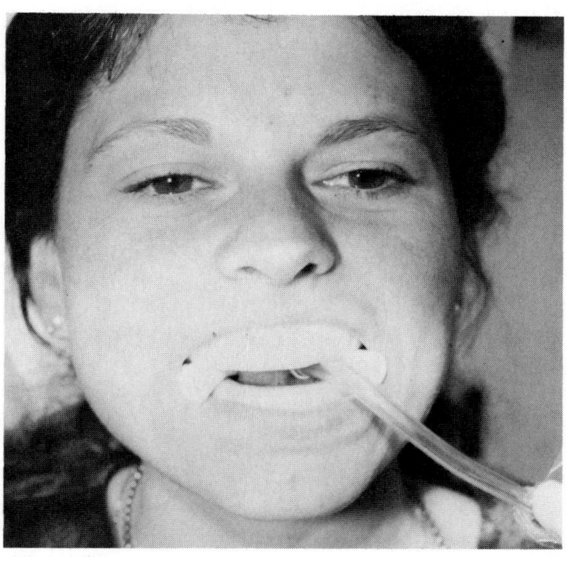
10. Place saliva ejector over the mandibular tray. Set timer for 4 minutes. Never leave the client unattended during the fluoride procedure	Removal of excess saliva prevents the saliva from diluting the fluoride. Four minutes are required for maximum fluoride exposure. Supervision is necessary to prevent accidental ingestion of fluoride or to aid if gagging results
11. Tilt chin down to remove trays	Tilting the chin allows fluids to flow to anterior region of mouth
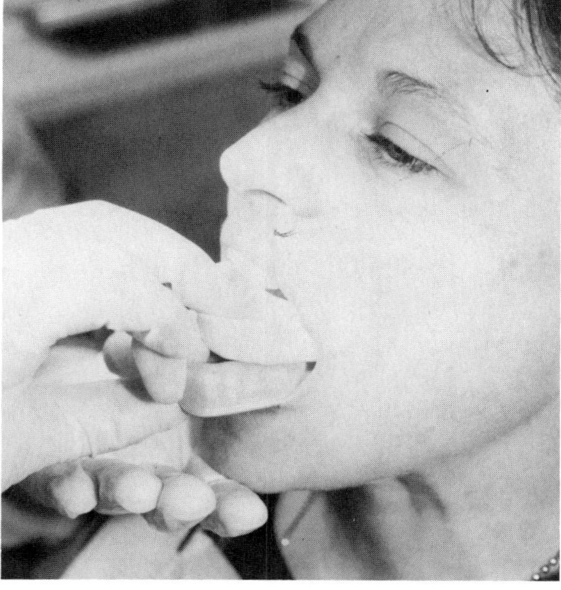	

CONTINUED ON FOLLOWING PAGE

PROCEDURE 21-1

APPLYING APF GEL METHOD *Continued*

Steps	Rationale
12. Request client to expectorate; suction excess fluoride from the mouth with saliva ejector	Prompt removal of fluoride gel from the mouth eliminates swallowing of excess gel
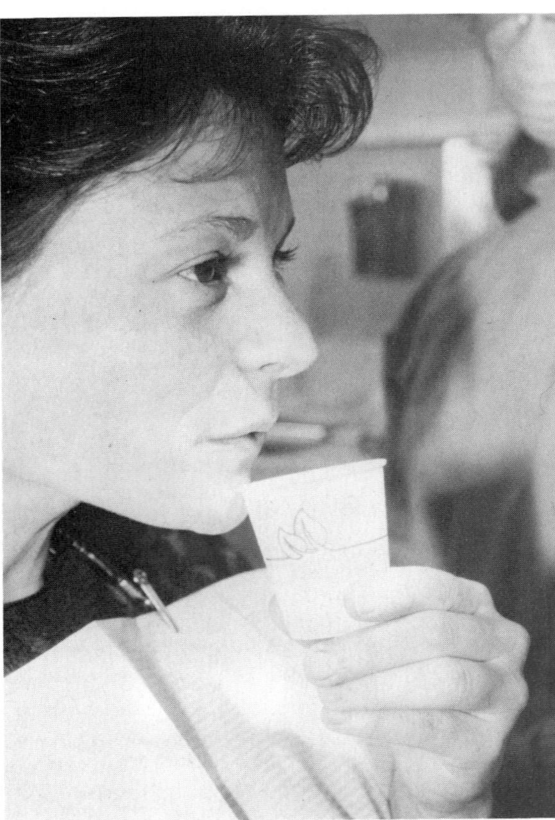	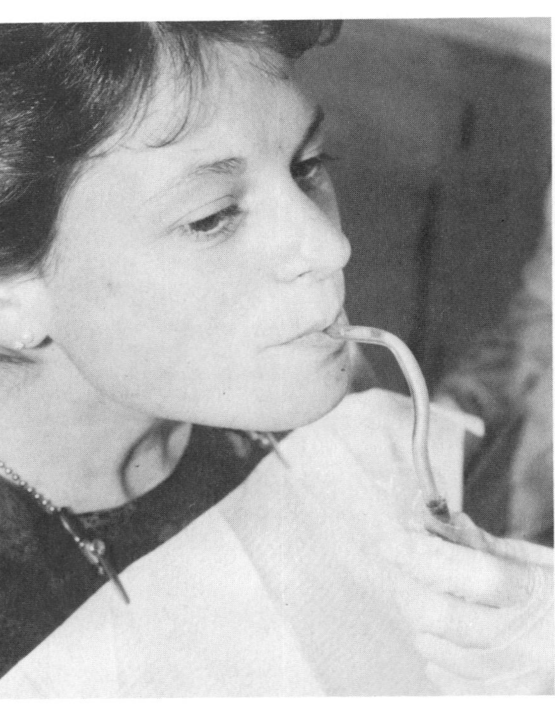
13. Instruct the client not to eat, drink, or rinse for 30 minutes	The delay allows residual fluoride to remain in contact with the teeth

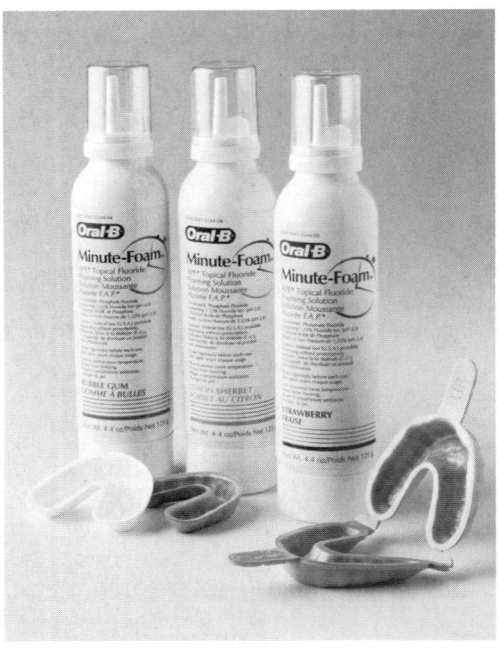

FIGURE 21-5
Fluoride foam. (Courtesy of Oral-B Laboratories.)

Fluoride Foams

Fluoride foam was introduced in 1993 (Fig. 21–5). It is a 1.23% liquid acidulated phosphate fluoride which, when mixed with aerosols, creates a foam. Because it is applied as a foam, the total mass of fluoride in the tray is actually less than that in the gel applications, yet the fluoride concentration itself remains identical to that of the gels. The advantage of the foam-based APF agent is that it is much lighter than a conventional gel and therefore only a small amount of the agent is needed for topical application (e.g., the amount of conventional gel needed to treat the teeth is about 4 g, whereas less than 1 g of foam-based APF fills a disposable upper and lower gel tray).[12] Therefore, the fluoride foam method of delivery in properly fitting trays may reduce the risk of accidental fluoride ingestion and systemic toxicity. Enamel fluoride uptake for the topical fluoride foam has been reported to be comparable to that of APF topical gel in sound enamel.[13]

Self-Applied Fluorides

Three types of self-applied fluorides are available for home use:

- Dentifrices
- Rinses
- Gels

Dentifrices

Dentifrice formulations usually are comprised of active fluoride salts, humectants (a substance to help retain moisture), and abrasive systems. According to the American Dental Association (ADA), Council on Dental Therapeutics, to establish the efficacy of fluoride dentifrices for caries prevention, dentifrice manufacturers need to evaluate the following: the effect of fluoride dentifrices in animal caries studies, fluoride availability and stability in dentifrices, fluoride bioavailability, and the ability of fluoride to enhance remineralization and delay demineralization. Dentifrices that have the ADA's seal of acceptance for caries prevention have support from such studies, the results of which indicate clinically significant anticaries effects (Fig. 21–6). The ADA seal is always displayed on the outside of the dentifrice package, indicating to the consumer that the anticaries claim is valid (Fig. 21–7).

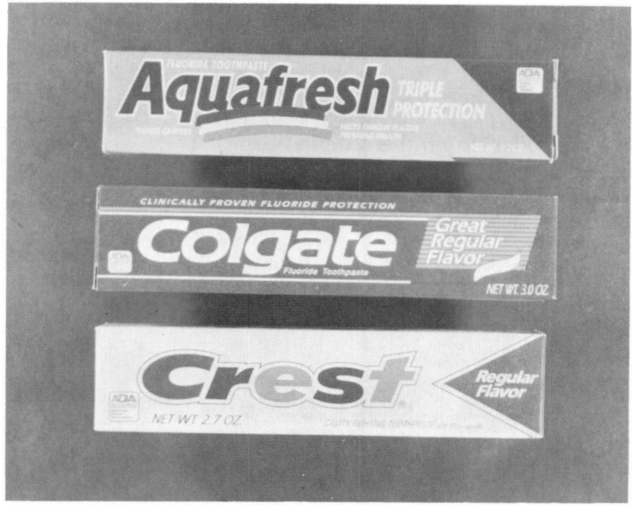

FIGURE 21–6
Sample dentifrices that have the ADA's Seal of Acceptance for caries prevention.

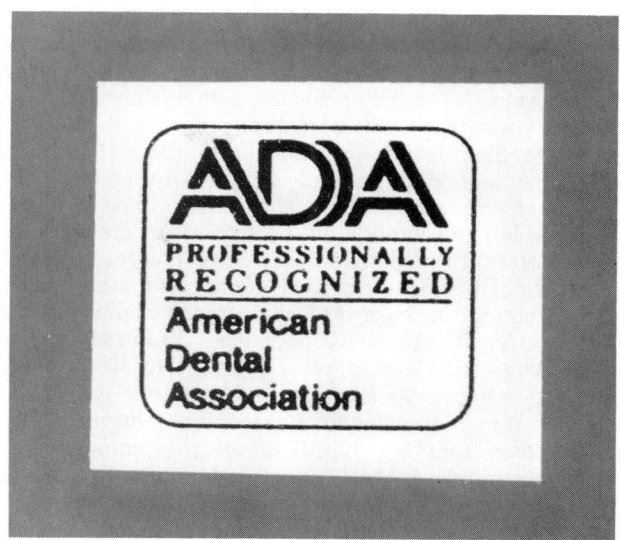

FIGURE 21–7
The ADA Seal of Acceptance for having significant anticaries effect.

Daily brushing with fluoride dentifrices proven effective by the ADA has shown to decrease caries incidence by 15 to 30%.[14] They are of benefit to individuals of all age groups. Children under the age of 6 or 7 years should be supervised, because ingestion of the fluoride-containing dentifrice may cause dental fluorosis.[14] In addition to having anticaries effects, some dentifrices remove topical stains, freshen breath, and may have tartar-controlling and desensitizing qualities.

The first clinical evaluation of dentifrices containing fluoride was done by Bibby in 1945. The studies evaluated dentifrices that had sodium fluoride incorporated into their existing formulations. None of the early sodium fluoride dentifrice formulations studied demonstrated a significant reduction in the incidence of dental caries. The probable reasons for these results were the incompatibility of the sodium fluoride ion with other dentifrice ingredients.[15] The abrasive used in these early studies reacted with the sodium fluoride to form calcium fluoride. Calcium fluoride is not able to react with enamel. Therefore, the lack of availability of a reactive fluoride ion was the major reason for failure of these dentifrices to prevent dental caries.[16]

A study by Fogels in 1979 showed a statistically significant decrease in caries activity when stannous fluoride dentifrices were compared to nonfluoride dentifrices. Shortly thereafter, stannous fluoride–silica dentifrice was accepted by the ADA and marketed for several years. Since then, numerous studies have been conducted on the efficacy of stannous, sodium, and monofluorophosphate fluoride systems in dentifrices. All three have been proven to reduce the incidence of dental caries when tested against placebo products.[17]

In a 2-year clinical study, an attempt was made to determine the most effective fluoride dentifrice preparation. A sodium fluoride dentifrice with acrylic particles was tested against a sodium monofluorophosphate dentifrice with calcium carbonate. The sodium fluoride–acrylic particle dentifrice was shown to be significantly superior in its caries-inhibiting effect.[18] Later a 3-year clinical study produced similar results.[19] The reason for the sodium fluoride (NaF) superiority was that upon immediate contact with water or saliva, the fluoride ion separated from the sodium ion, making the fluoride ion instantly available for reaction with the enamel surface. The strong chemical bond between the phosphate ion and fluoride ion in the sodium monofluorophosphate (MFP) preparation led to the failure of overall acceptance of this dentifrice. This ionic bond is broken by enzymes present in saliva through a process known as *acid hydrolysis.* Acid hydrolysis does not completely occur within the average toothbrushing time (15 to 30 seconds). Therefore, significantly less amount of fluoride is released from the monofluorophosphate preparations during toothbrushing than from the sodium fluoride preparations.[20]

In two clinical studies conducted by Zacherl, a direct comparison was made between a neutral sodium fluoride–silica dentifrice and a stannous fluoride–calcium pyrophosphate dentifrice.[21] The results showed that the sodium fluoride preparation was significantly more effective than the stannous fluoride preparation against caries. Moreover, stannous fluoride is seldom used in dentifrices because of its potential for staining the teeth and the high cost to formulate a compatible stannous fluoride abrasive system.[1]

Fluoride dentifrice can be obtained in a paste or gel form over the counter without a prescription. The percentage of fluoride concentration currently used in dentifrices is 0.22% in sodium fluoride and 0.4% in monofluorophosphate preparations. Toothbrushing with a fluoride dentifrice should be done at least once daily; however, two times per day is commonly recommended. A small amount of the fluoride dentifrice (a pea-size portion) should be placed on a soft-bristled toothbrush. Individuals are advised to brush for 2 to 3 minutes in a prescribed manner as directed by the dental hygienist, and to rinse thoroughly and expectorate after brushing.

Fluoride Rinses

Fluoride mouthrinses have been proven to be a simple, safe, and cost-effective method of providing caries protection. Over-the-counter 0.05% sodium fluoride rinses used daily (7 to 10 ml for 1 minute) (Fig. 21–8), and weekly rinses of prescribed 0.2% sodium fluoride in school-based programs (10 ml for 1 minute) have been shown to decrease the caries rate by 30 to 40%.[22] The mechanism of action of these rinses is believed to be remineralization of early, carious lesions through the frequent delivery of NaF in low concentrations.

Prescribed stannous fluoride mouthrinses (0.63% SnF_2), are better known for their antiplaque properties. The mechanism of action of stannous fluoride rinses appears to have an effect on the growth and adherence properties of certain bacterial plaque.[23] In addition to the effect on bacteria, many clinicians report that stannous fluoride is effective in decreasing dental hypersensitivity.

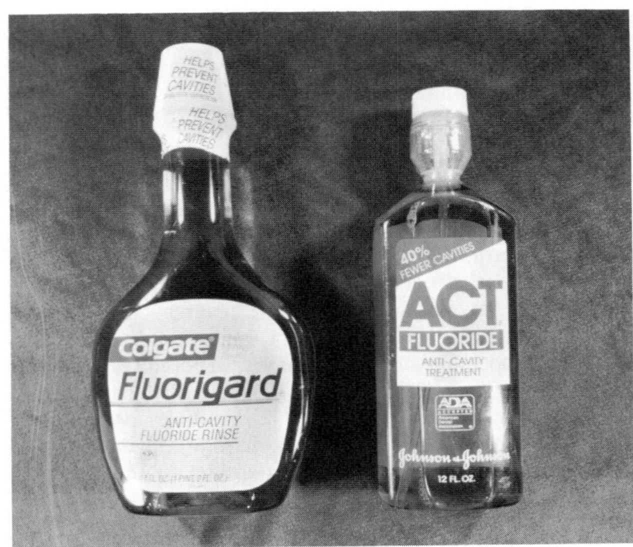

FIGURE 21–8
Sample of over-the-counter 0.05% sodium fluoride rinses with the ADA Seal of Acceptance.

The use of fluoride mouthrinses, in combination with daily brushing and flossing, should be part of a comprehensive preventive measure and should not be considered a substitute for any type of plaque control program. Table 21–3 summarizes the types of fluoride mouthrinses and conditions under which they are recommended.

Fluoride mouthrinses have maximal benefit when used after flossing and brushing. Approximately 10 ml of solution should be swished vigorously for 1 minute, then expectorated. The client should be instructed not to eat or drink for 30 minutes. Children under 6 years of age should not use a fluoride rinse because they may accidentally swallow it. Young children over the age of 6 years who may not have sufficient control to expectorate should have adult supervision to prevent accidental ingestion.

Self-Applied Fluoride Gels

Self-applied fluoride gels are recommended for clients who are susceptible to rampant dental caries. These are individuals who:

- Have a high caries rate after using a fluoride rinse for 1 year
- Are adults with a high incidence of root caries

TABLE 21–3
SELF-APPLIED FLUORIDE RINSES

Frequency	Concentration	Access	Indication
Daily	0.05% NaF	Over-the-counter (OTC)	Children over 6 years of age and adults with caries susceptibility
Weekly	0.2% NaF	Prescription	School-based programs
Daily	0.63% SnF_2	Prescription	High susceptibility to root surface caries Dentinal hypersensitivity

TABLE 21–4
SELF-APPLIED FLUORIDE GELS

Concentration	F Availability	Mode of Delivery	Indication	Access
1.19% NaF	5,000 ppm	Tray	Rampant caries Radiation therapy	Prescription
0.4% SnF_2	1,000 ppm	Brush on	High caries Hypersensitivity Xerostomia	Over-the-counter
0.5% APF	5,000 ppm	Tray Brush on	Rampant caries	Prescription

- Wear orthodontic appliances
- Have a full or partial reduction of salivary gland function from radiation therapy or degenerative diseases such as Sjögren's syndrome

When used daily, prescription gels of 1.19% NaF and 0.5% APF (5,000 ppm) have been shown to decrease caries incidence by 75 to 80%.[5] Recently, 0.4% stannous fluoride gel (1,000 ppm) has been granted over-the-counter status by the Food and Drug Administration (FDA) because it delivers the same amount of fluoride that is present in most fluoride dentifrices (1,000 ppm). Self-applied fluoride gels act to protect the tooth by reducing enamel solubility and oral bacteria. Self-applied fluoride gels and indications for use are presented in Table 21–4.

Self-applied fluoride gels can be delivered by the tray method or the brush-on method.

Tray Method Teeth should be flossed and brushed prior to self-application of the fluoride gel. When using the tray method, a layer of the gel is placed in a custom-fitted polyvinyl tray, placed in the mandibular and maxillary arch, and held in place for 4 to 6 minutes (Fig. 21–9). Excess gel should be expectorated, and the client should not eat, drink, or rinse for at least 30 minutes.

Brush-On Method After flossing and brushing, about 2 mg of the fluoride gel should be placed on the toothbrush (Fig. 21–10). The client should then brush again for 1 minute and expectorate. The brush-on fluoride gel should not be used in place of the fluoride dentifrice. Fluoride gels do not contain abrasive particles to control the deposition of pellicle, and their use in place of a dentifrice results in the accumulation of stained pellicle.[24]

ROOT CARIES

By the year 2000, individuals over the age of 65 will represent 13% of our population. This age group is the most rapidly growing sector in North America. Dental hygienists have witnessed the increased utilization of oral healthcare by the elderly and have incorporated into their appointment schedules personalized oral hygiene instructions to meet their specialized needs. A dental hygienist must be sensitive to this population's decreased manual dexterity, hearing loss, and impaired vision.

The intraoral findings in an aged mouth include furcation involvement, salivary gland dysfunction or xerostomia (dry mouth), a large number and variety of restored teeth, and gingival recession with concomitant root exposure. These findings can lead to a greater root caries incidence. It is estimated that by the year 2000, one-half of the population 50 years or older will have at least one surface of root caries.[24]

The clinical appearance of root caries is dark yellow, brown, or black. They may have a soft leathery texture when explored and appear immediately below the cementoenamel junction, undermining but not involving the enamel. In a study of 810 adults aged 54 and older, root caries were reduced 67% by use of 1,100 ppm sodium fluoride dentifrice.[25] Because exposed roots are more vulnerable to caries than the crowns of the teeth, continuous exposure to self-applied fluorides significantly helps to reduce the incidence of root caries.

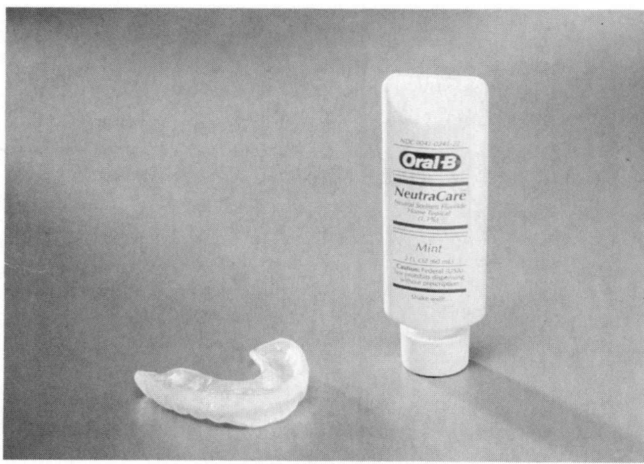

FIGURE 21–9
Tray method of fluoride gel. (Courtesy of Oral-B Laboratories.)

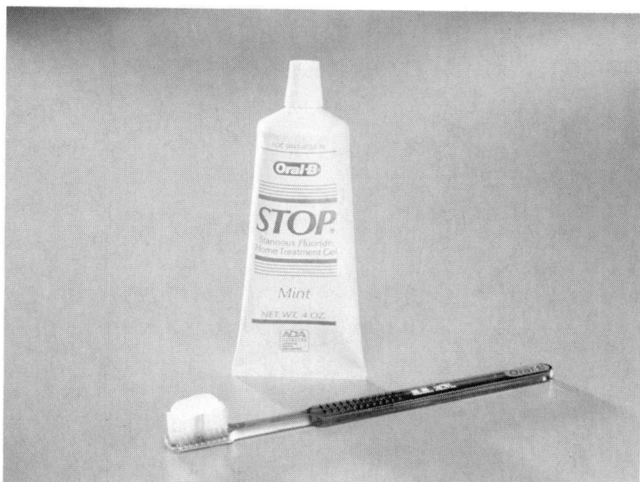

FIGURE 21–10
Brush-on method of fluoride gel. (Courtesy of Oral-B Laboratories.)

XEROSTOMIA

Xerostomia, or dryness of the mouth, varies from individual to individual. It is permanent if caused by biological aging, Sjögren's syndrome, or diabetes. Xerostomia is temporary if it is induced by radiation or drug therapy. Common drugs that cause xerostomia are decongestants, diuretics, antidepressants, antihistamines, antihypertensives, and antipsychotics.

The symptoms of xerostomia range from a burning sensation of the tongue and mucosa to difficulty in speech and in swallowing. Frequent sips of water and water rinses are essential for partial control of xerostomia. Sugarless chewing gum may be helpful in stimulating the salivary flow. Snythetic saliva solutions, saliva substitute lubricants, and moisturizing gels have been of limited help in the majority of individuals with dry mouth, although some favorable reports have been published.[26]

The lack of salivary flow creates an increased risk for dental caries, particularly root caries. Xerostomia is a primary factor in the initiation of rampant decay. Changes in the quantity and viscosity of saliva decrease its lubrication and cleansing abilities. There also is a loss in the buffering effects of the saliva (its ability to neutralize acids) and a decrease in remineralizing effects.[27] It is therefore essential that individuals with xerostomia, no matter how severe, use some type of fluoride therapy in combination with daily oral hygiene practices.

FLUORIDE TOXICITY

There are numerous studies that document the safety of water fluoridation at optimal levels.[4] Based on misinterpretation of data from a study in 1990 by the National Toxicology Program (NTP), the press published articles that led consumers to believe that water fluoridation was responsible for osteosarcoma or bone cancer among male rats. One male rat in a high-dose group (79 ppm) had osteosarcoma of bone. There were no such tumors in the female rats nor in the male or female mice. Because a chemical, in this case fluoride, must unequivocally cause cancer in at least two species to be classified as a carcinogen, the latest NTP catalog of carcinogens does not list fluoride.[28] Although the final results indicate that water fluoridation remains a safe means of fluoride delivery, possible toxic effects caused by other fluoride products deserve our attention.

TABLE 21–5
CLDS AND STDS OF FLUORIDE FOR SELECTED AGES

Age	Weight (lbs)	CLD (mg)	STD (mg)
2	22	320	80
4	29	422	106
6	37	538	135
8	45	655	164
10	53	771	193
12	64	931	233
14	83	1,206	301
16	92	1,338	334
18	95	1,382	346

From Heifetz, S. B., and Horowitz, H. S. The Amounts of Fluoride in Current Fluoride Therapies: Safety Considerations for Children, ASDC Journal of Dentistry of Children 51:257, July–August, 1984.

Prior to initiating a fluoride care plan, it is the responsibility of the dental hygienist, the dentist, or the pediatrician to determine total fluoride intake from all sources to avoid fluoride toxicity. The lethal doses (CLD) and safely tolerated doses (STD) of fluoride for selected ages are listed in Table 21–5, and Fig. 21–11 shows how to calculate the total fluoride ingested by a client.

Acute Fluoride Toxicity

The signs of acute fluoride toxicity are nausea, vomiting, hypersalivation, abdominal pain, and diarrhea. In more severe cases, symptoms may be cramping of the arms and legs, bronchospasm, cardiac arrest, ventricular fibrillation, fixed and dilated pupils, hyperkalemia, and hypocalcemia.[28]

The initial treatment for acute fluoride toxicity is to in-

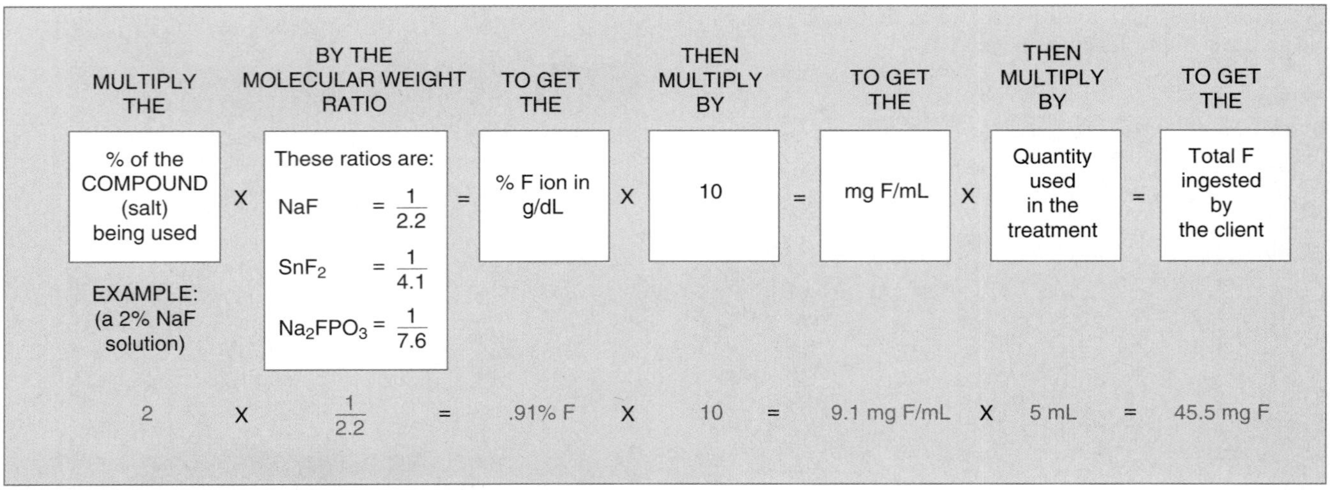

MULTIPLY THE		BY THE MOLECULAR WEIGHT RATIO		TO GET THE		THEN MULTIPLY BY		TO GET THE		THEN MULTIPLY BY		TO GET THE
% of the COMPOUND (salt) being used	X	These ratios are: NaF $= \frac{1}{2.2}$; SnF_2 $= \frac{1}{4.1}$; $Na_2FPO_3 = \frac{1}{7.6}$	=	% F ion in g/dL	X	10	=	mg F/mL	X	Quantity used in the treatment	=	Total F ingested by the client
EXAMPLE: (a 2% NaF solution) 2	X	$\frac{1}{2.2}$	=	.91% F	X	10	=	9.1 mg F/mL	X	5 mL	=	45.5 mg F

FIGURE 21–11
Flow chart depicts method for calculating the amount of fluoride ingested by a client from a compound used in professional care. (Redrawn and adapted with permission from Wilkins, E. M. Clinical Practice of the Dental Hygienist, 6th ed. Philadelphia: Lea & Febiger, 1989, p. 455.)

duce vomiting with ipecac syrup or by digital stimulation. Following that, fluoride-binding liquids such as lime water, liquid or gel antacids containing aluminum or magnesium hydroxide, or milk should be administered. The client should be taken to the hospital for further evaluation.

To ensure that all precautions are taken, fluoride-containing items such as toothpaste, gels, and rinses should be kept out of reach of children. Parents and oral healthcare professionals should be familiar with the signs, symptoms, and treatment of acute fluoride toxicity.

Chronic Fluoride Toxicity

Chronic fluoride toxicity can cause dental fluorosis, skeletal fluorosis, and kidney damage. Factors that increase the severity of chronic fluoride toxicity are:

- An increase in the consumption of naturally fluoridated water
- An elevated intake of fluoride in the food
- Nutritional diseases
- Low calcium diets[24]

Dental fluorosis is the result of ingestion of excessive amounts of fluoride during the early phase of tooth development. Fluorosis is caused by the disruption of enamel formation.

Clinically, dental fluorosis can range from mild to severe. Mild dental fluorosis appears as white flecks commonly seen on the maxillary anterior teeth (Fig. 21–12; see color section). Modest dental fluorosis appears as a slightly dark brown stain on the teeth where all enamel surfaces are affected. Severe dental fluorosis is evidenced by pitting and staining of the enamel surfaces. The entire enamel surface may not be intact, and the normal morphology of the teeth may be modified. This condition is commonly known as "mottled enamel." Table 21–6 gives classification and descriptions of the various degrees of dental fluorosis.

Individuals on kidney dialysis can be exposed up to 500 l of water per week.[24] In areas with high levels of natural fluoride in the water, individuals who are on kidney dialysis should use mineral-free water rather than tap water.

The need to fluoridate water supplies to prevent dental

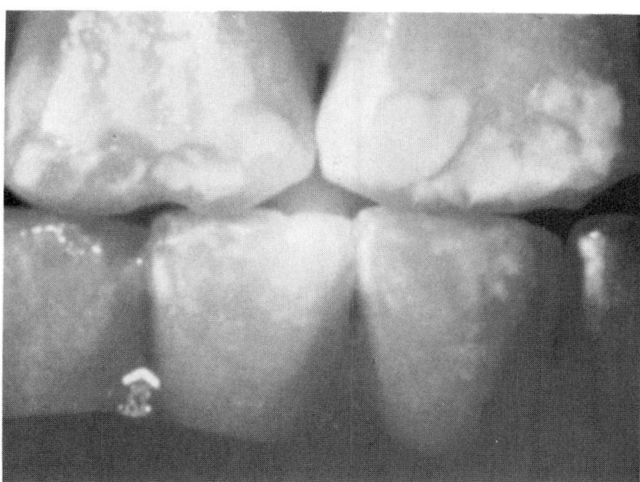

FIGURE 21–12
Fluorosis. (Courtesy of *Dental Hygienist News* funded by an educational grant from Procter and Gamble and published by Harfst Associates, Inc., Troy, Michigan.)

TABLE 21–6
CLASSIFICATION OF DEGREE OF DENTAL FLUOROSIS

Grade of Fluorosis	Description
Normal	None
Questionable	A few white flecks or white spots
Very mild	Small opaque, paper white areas involving less than 25% of the surface
Mild	White opacities are more extensive but do not involve as much as 50% of the surface
Moderate	All enamel surfaces affected, frequent brown staining
Severe	Discrete or confluent pitting, brown stains are widespread, all enamel surfaces are affected

From Newbrun, E., Fluorides and Dental Caries. Springfield, IL: Charles C Thomas, 1986.

caries is balanced by a similar need to remove excess fluoride in the water to avoid its toxic effects. Defluoridation of water is more expensive than the fluoridation of water. It is estimated to cost $1.50 per person per year. Defluoridation can be accomplished by one of two methods: additive methods and adsorption methods.[24] The additive method involves the addition of chemicals such as lime, magnesium, and aluminum to precipitate the fluoride. The adsorption technique involves the running of fluoride water over contact beds of synthetic hydroxyapatite or activated alumina. The fluoride is removed by ion exchange with the agent comprising the bed matrix.

In summary, a myriad of fluoride products are available for professional application and at-home client use; however, the selection of the most appropriate fluoride regimen often is confusing. Figure 21–13 presents a decision tree that may be helpful in matching the client's need with the appropriate fluoride therapy.

PIT AND FISSURE SEALANTS

Topically applied fluorides are most effective for preventing dental caries formation on the smooth surfaces of teeth and least effective in the pits and fissures. Consequently, the dental hygienist should consider the placement of pit and fissure sealants in planning dental hygiene care for the maximum prevention of dental caries. Dental hygienists can place sealants as an integral part of a comprehensive caries prevention program, along with providing fluoride therapy and nutritional counseling.

A **pit and fissure sealant** is a thin plastic coating placed in the pit and fissures of teeth to act as a physical barrier to decay (Fig. 21–14). Research has shown that the incidence of caries can be reduced 17 to 54% by applying sealants to the occlusal surfaces of posterior teeth.[29] The sealant material is made of a resin monomer (liquid plastic) that bonds directly to an etched tooth surface. Sealants can be white, clear, or opaque in color, and they feel smooth when touched with the tip of the explorer.

Pit and fissure sealants are of greatest benefit to children. Ages 3 and 4 years are the most important times for sealing the eligible primary teeth, ages 6 to 7 years for the first permanent molars, and ages 11 to 13 for the second permanent molars and premolars.[24] No toxic effects are appar-

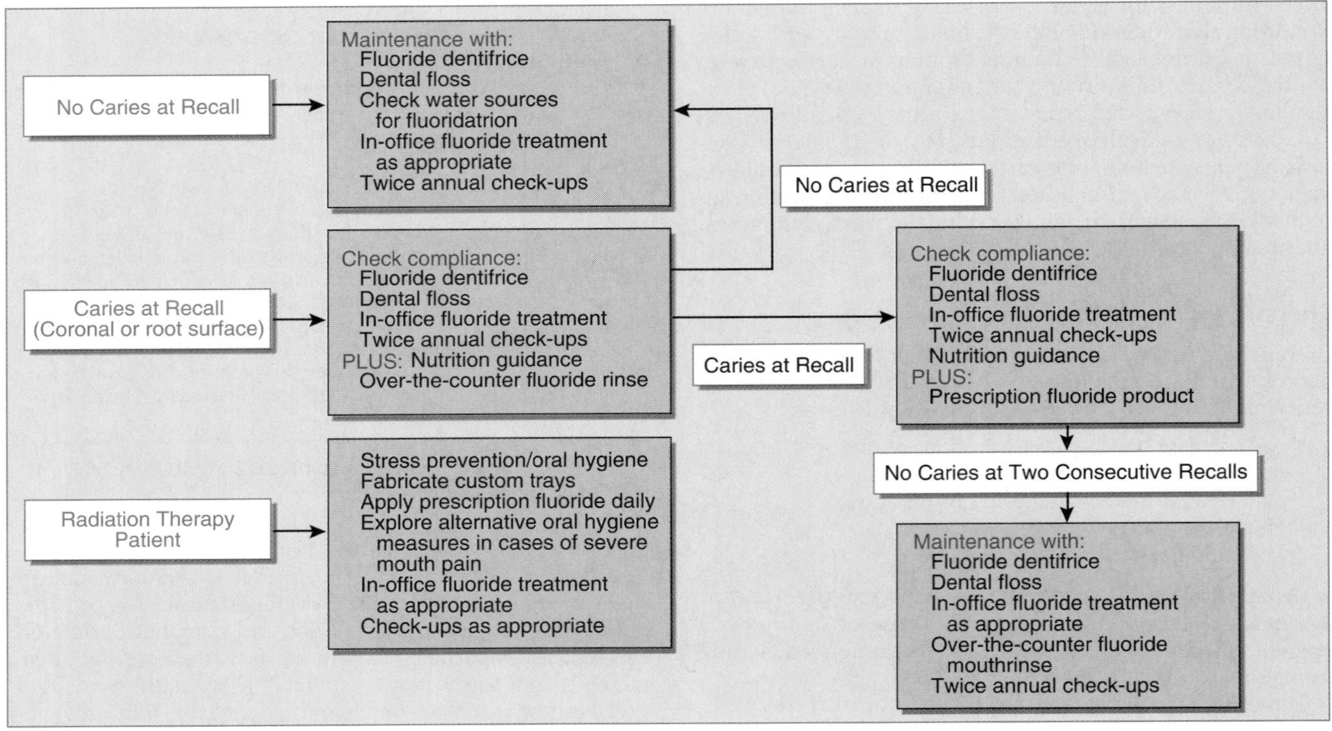

FIGURE 21–13
Decision tree for matching client need with fluoride therapies. (Courtesy of *Dental Hygienist News,* funded by an educational grant from Procter and Gamble and published by Harfst Associates, Inc., Troy, Michigan.)

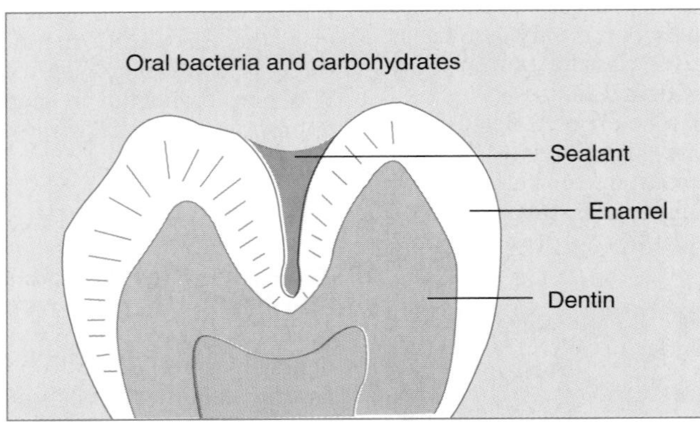

FIGURE 21–14
Sealant acts as a physical barrier. (Redrawn with permission from Preventing Pit and Fissure Caries: A Guide to Sealant Use. Massachusetts Department of Public Health and Massachusetts Health Research Institute, Inc., 1986, p. 3.)

TABLE 21–7
COMPARISON OF DENTAL SEALANT SYSTEMS

Type of Sealant System	Photopolymerization	Autopolymerization
Advantages	Operator initiates polymerization process No mixing or measuring necessary Available in unit dose cartridges Short polymerization time (20–30 sec)	Lower initial cost (light-curing light not needed)
Disadvantages	Higher initial cost (purchase of a curing unit and light-filtered protective eyewear) Critical placement of light wand	Setting time cannot be controlled once catalyst is added Long polymerization time (1–3 min)

ent from the chemical use of sealants, and sealant application is painless. Only sealant materials approved by the ADA Council on Dental Materials, Instruments, and Equipment should be used.

Prior to placing a dental sealant, the enamel surface of the tooth is acid-etched to create surface irregularities. The operator prepares the sealant and allows it to flow into the newly created enamel micropores. When the sealant hardens it forms a barrier to decay-producing bacteria.

Types of Sealant Materials

Most sealants used today are made of bisphenol A-glycidyl methylacrylate (BIS-GMA). Some sealants contain fillers such as microscopic glass beads and quartz rods to make them more resistant to occlusal forces. The fillers are coated with silane to facilitate their combination with the BIS-GMA plastic.[24]

Sealants can be categorized by the type of method required to convert them from the liquid to the solid state. This process by which sealants harden is known as polymerization. Polymerization can be accomplished by light curing with an ultraviolet or visible blue light *(photopolymerization)*, or by self-curing, where a monomer and a catalyst when mixed together create strong chemical bonds *(autopolymerization)*. The light-curing and the self-curing products appear to be equally effective in their retention in pits and fissures.[24] A comparison of the advantages and disadvantages of the type of sealant systems are listed in Table 21–7.

Application Principles and Methods

Although manufacturer's directions may differ, the success of a dental sealant is dependent upon the clinician's ability to:

- Maintain a dry field
- Properly etch and rinse the enamel surface
- Correctly place the sealant
- Accurately time the polymerization process

PROCEDURE 21–2

APPLYING SEALANTS

Equipment

Mouth mirror	High speed evacuation tube
Explorer	Slow speed handpiece
Saliva ejector	Bristle brush
Sealant kit	Pumice
Gauze	Floss
Cotton rolls/rubber dam	Face shield
Air/water syringe tip	Protective eyewear for client
Dri-Angles	Protective barriers

Optional Equipment Depending on Sealant System

Fiberoptic light unit	Finishing burs
Protective shield	Articulating paper

Steps	Rationale
1. Select fully erupted primary and permanent teeth with narrow pits and fissures that are caries-free or have only questionable carious surfaces. Evaluate deep buccal pits and cingulums	Erupted teeth promote visibility and the maintenance of a dry field Deep, narrow pits and fissures are prone to dental caries
2. Provide client with protective eyewear	Standard infection control procedures
3. Perform a preventive oral prophylaxis. Polish the intended surface with a slurry of pumice and water. Rinse with water. Use a bristled brush attached to a slow-speed handpiece	Surfaces to be sealed must be free of deposits and organic debris. Commercial pastes contain coloring and/or flavoring agents, glycerin, and/or fluoride interfere with the bonding process. A bristle brush efficiently cleans the occlusal surface
4. Isolate the teeth with a rubber dam or cotton rolls. Place Dri-Angle over Stensen's duct	Treatment site should be visible, accessible, and dry for proper sealant placement and retention
5. Dry the site to be sealed with compressed air, which is free of oil and moisture.	Oil or moisture interferes with bonding
6. Apply phosphoric acid to the clean, dry surface: Liquid etch—apply liquid with a brush Gel etch—apply gel and leave undisturbed	Acid etches the enamel to produce micropores into which the sealant flows, hardens, and is locked into place Success of sealant retention is dependent upon proper etching technique

CONTINUED ON FOLLOWING PAGE

PROCEDURE 21-2

APPLYING SEALANTS *Continued*

Steps	Rationale
	Rubbing the gel acid burnishes the enamel surface and causes it to become smooth again, which decreases retention and adversely affects bond strength
7. Rinse etched surfaces for 10–15 seconds using a water syringe and high-speed evacuation If gel etch is used, rinse for an additional 30 seconds	Rinsing removes the acid
8. Replace cotton rolls as they become wet	Moisture interferes with bonding
9. Dry the treatment site for 10 seconds. Evaluate etched surface	A properly etched area appears white, dull, and frosty
10. Apply liquid sealant over the pits, fissures, and inclined planes	Allow the sealant to flow into the etched surfaces. A low viscosity sealant prevents air entrapment
11. With photopolymerized sealants apply light to each portion of the sealant for 20–30 seconds as per manufacturer instructions before advancing the light to another area	The hardening of the sealant is initiated by the light source
12. With autopolymerized sealants prepare a separate mix for every two teeth sealed	If a mix is prepared for more than two teeth, the mix may begin to set and the liquid will become viscous. A viscous sealant does not allow for maximum flow into the pits and fissures and compromises the bond
13. After the polymerization process, evaluate the sealant with an explorer	A successful sealant feels hard and smooth. Air bubbles should not be present. Check for sealant retention
14. If imperfections are noted (e.g., incomplete coverage, air bubbles), reapplication of sealant is necessary. Re-etch tooth for 10 seconds, wash and dry, and apply additional sealant	Proper placement provides for effectiveness and retention of sealant
15. If a sealant containing filler particles has been used, check occlusion with articulating paper	Remove overfilled areas so they do not interfere with normal occlusion
16. Apply topical fluoride	Encourages remineralization

Tooth Selection for Sealant Placement

Teeth selected for sealant placement should be chosen in collaboration with the dentist. Sealants are indicated for primary and permanent teeth with deep, narrow pits and fissures that are caries-free or have only questionable carious surfaces. Not only are occlusal surfaces considered, but buccal pits and cingulum pits should be examined as well. A sharp explorer and compressed air aid in the determination of whether a tooth should be sealed. Once the tip of the explorer is retained, or "sticks" for a brief instant in the pit and fissures, and there is no evidence of decay penetrating into the dentinoenamel junction (DEJ), placing a sealant is preferable.[24] Questionable carious surfaces are ideal candidates for sealants because a sealant prevents the surface from advancing from a questionable status to definitive caries.[30] Pit and fissure sealants are contraindicated where the proximal surfaces are carious. These areas should be diagnosed by a dentist and restored using traditional operative procedures (Table 21–8).

Extrinsic Stain and Plaque Removal

In preparation of teeth for sealant placement, heavy stains, hard and soft deposits, and other organic debris must be removed from the tooth surface. To facilitate the removal of heavy stains, a bristle brush is placed on a slow-speed handpiece and used in conjunction with a slurry of pumice and water to polish the tooth surface (Fig. 21–15). Because this process creates a high level of aerosol droplets, dental hygienists should wear a face shield in addition to a face mask and protective eyewear. In addition, protective eyewear should be worn by the client throughout the procedure. Use of commercial polishing agents is contraindicated

TABLE 21–8
INDICATIONS AND CONTRAINDICATIONS FOR THE USE OF PIT AND FISSURE SEALANTS

Clinical Condition	Indications	Contraindications
Sound or Questionable Enamel		
pH and fissure morphology	Deep, narrow pits and fissures	Broad, well-coalesced pits and fissures
Status of proximal surfaces	Sound	Frank caries
Occlusal morphology	If pits or fissures are separated by a transverse ridge, a sound pit or fissure may be sealed	Pits or fissures with frank lesions

Adapted with permission from Preventing Pit and Fissure Caries: A Guide to Sealant Use. Massachusetts Department of Public Health and Massachusetts Health Research Institute, Inc., 1986.

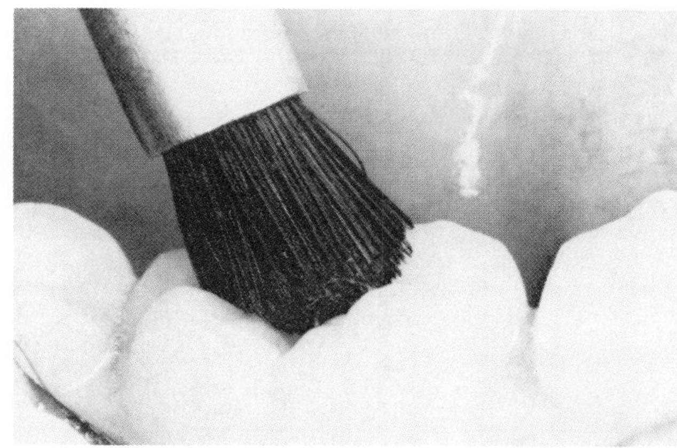

FIGURE 21–15
Placement of bristle brush to polish the occlusal surface. (With permission from Preventing Pit and Fissure Caries: A Guide to Sealant Use. Massachusetts Department of Public Health and Massachusetts Health Research Institute, Inc., 1986, p. 16.)

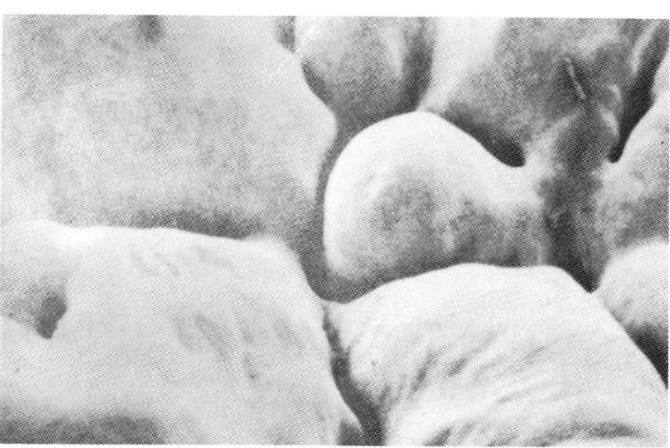

FIGURE 21–17
Electron micrograph of microscopic pores created on the enamel surface as a result of acid etching. (Preventing Pit and Fissure Caries: A Guide to Sealant Use. Massachusetts Department of Public Health and Massachusetts Health Research Institute, Inc., 1986.)

because they often contain oil, glycerin, and fluoride, all of which interfere with the etching process.

After extrinsic stain and plaque removal, the teeth should be thoroughly rinsed for 10 seconds.

Isolation and Drying

The proper placement of a sealant requires that the tooth be isolated and dry, so that the treatment site is visible and accessible. A rubber dam is effective for isolation when working on several teeth in the quadrant; however, Dri-Angles (Fig. 21–16) placed over the Stensen's duct and proper placement of cotton rolls in the vestibules and sides of the tongue are as effective and promote moisture control. It is critical to keep the working site free of water and saliva. The saliva ejector should be used to aid in moisture control, and the area should be dried with compressed air. Prior to drying the teeth with an air syringe, the air stream should be checked to ensure that it is not moisture-laden. A check for moisture can be accomplished by directing the air stream onto a cool mouth mirror; fogging indicates the presence of moisture.[24]

Acid Conditioning

An acid-etching solution is applied to the tooth, and the application timed according to the manufacturer's instructions. The acid supplied by most manufacturers is 35 to 50% phosphoric acid. This acid creates microscopic pores on the enamel surface to increase surface irregularities for sealant retention (Fig. 21–17). It is best to apply the liquid acid with a fine plastic-bristled brush (supplied by the manufacturer) and to use a continuous dabbing motion. Total application time is usually 1 minute for permanent teeth and 1.5 minutes for primary teeth. Fluorosed teeth require up to 1.75 minutes because of the enamel's resistance to acid. If the acid-etching solution is supplied as a gel (Fig. 21–18), it should be placed on the tooth surface and left undisturbed (Fig. 21–19). The gel should not be applied in a rubbing motion, because rubbing burnishes the enamel surface and causes it to become smooth again. A special note of caution is required for the handling of the enamel etching solution or gel. Contact of this material with eyes, oral tissues, and skin should be avoided. If accidental contact occurs, the area contacted should be flushed with copious amounts of water.

Rinsing and Drying

The areas etched by the phosphoric acid solution are rinsed for 10 to 15 seconds by the use of a water syringe and high-speed suction (Fig. 21–20). If a gel acid is used, a second rinse of 30 seconds is recommended.

Cotton rolls should be replaced as they become wet. It is

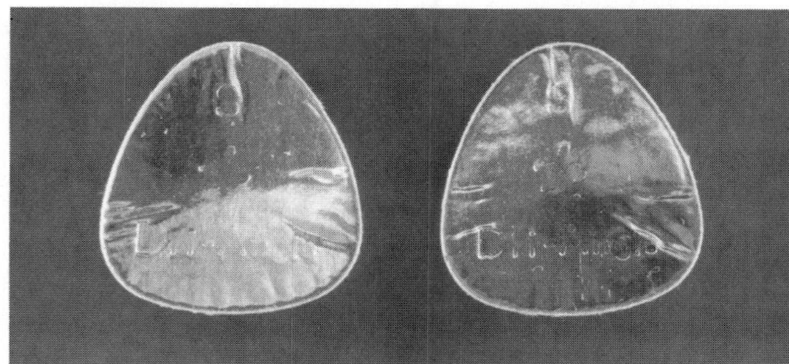

FIGURE 21–16
Dri-Angles for placement over Stensen's duct for isolation and moisture control.

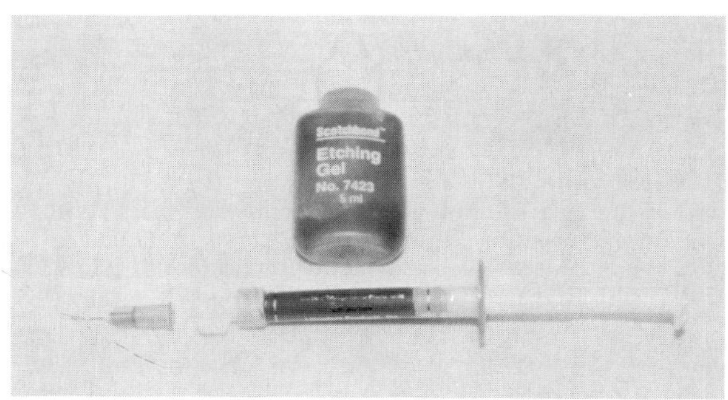

FIGURE 21–18
Acid etching solution in gel form.

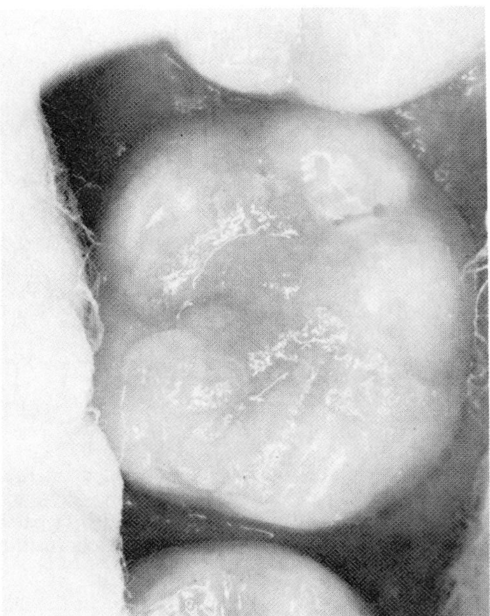

FIGURE 21-19
Placement of acid etching gel on the enamel surface. (With permission from Preventing Pit and Fissure Caries: A Guide to Sealant Use. Massachusetts Department of Public Health and Massachusetts Health Research Institute, Inc., 1986, p. 17.)

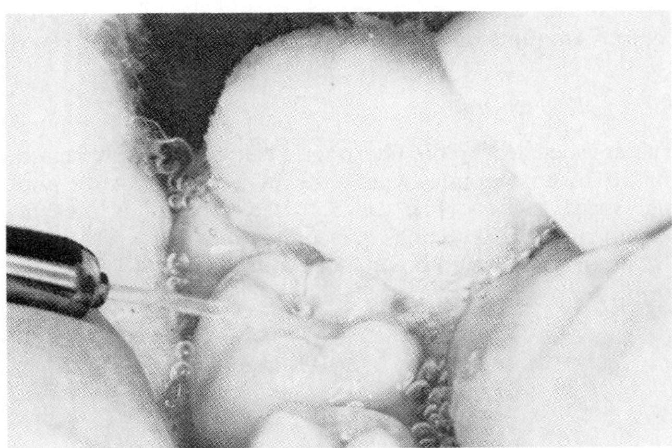

FIGURE 21-20
Rinsing of the acid solution from the enamel surface. (With permission from Preventing Pit and Fissure Caries: A Guide to Sealant Use. Massachusetts Department of Public Health and Massachusetts Health Research Institute, Inc., 1986, p. 17.)

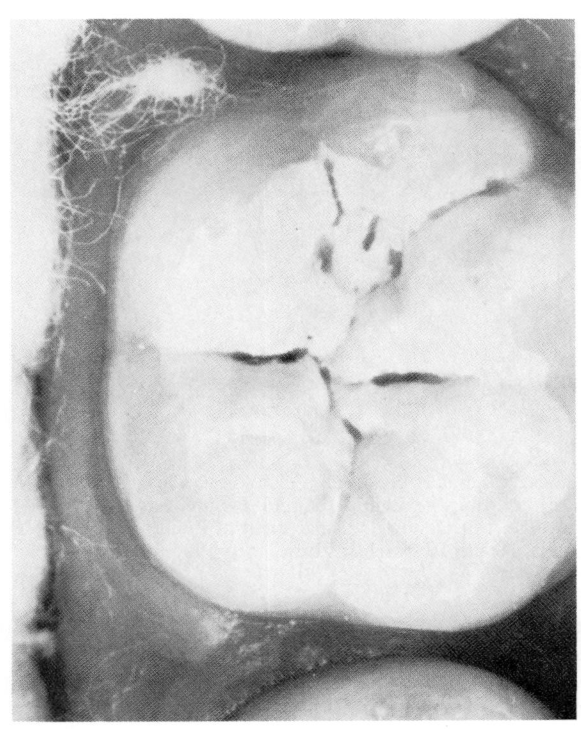

FIGURE 21-21
Frosty appearance of etched enamel surface. (With permission from Preventing Pit and Fissure Caries: A Guide to Sealant Use. Massachusetts Department of Public Health and Massachusetts Health Research Institute, Inc., 1986, p. 18.)

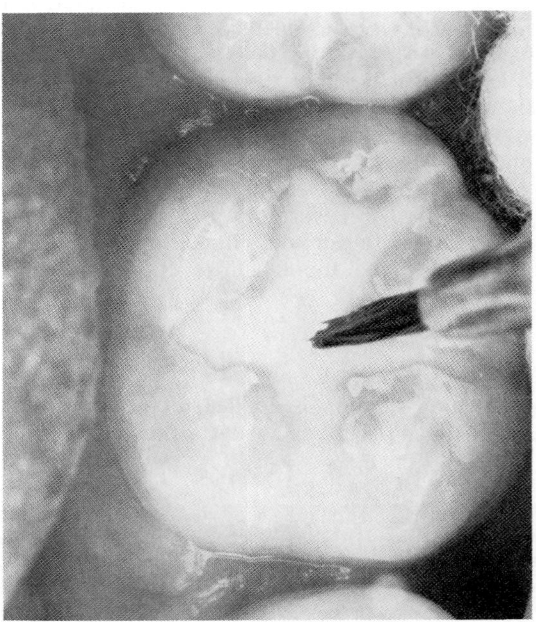

FIGURE 21-22
Application of sealant to enamel surface with a disposable brush. (With permission from Preventing Pit and Fissure Caries: A Guide to Sealant Use. Massachusetts Department of Public Health and Massachusetts Health Research Institute, Inc., 1986, p. 18.)

important to prevent saliva or other contaminants from flowing onto the treated area. If contamination occurs, the newly opened pores become occluded and the resin does not penetrate and bond with the enamel surface. Thus, if the etched surface becomes contaminated, the area must be reetched for 10 seconds, rinsed and thoroughly dried. A properly etched enamel surface appears white, dull, and frosty when compared to adjacent, normal enamel (Fig. 21–21).

Sealant Placement

With either the autopolymerized or the photopolymerized sealant system, the liquid sealant should be allowed to flow freely onto the etched enamel surface. The sealant should be placed into the deep pits and fissures, but marginal ridges and cusp tips should be avoided. The sealant is applied quickly with a plastic applicator or disposable brush and reapplied to add the desired thickness and bulk (Fig. 21–22).

Autopolymerization, or self-curing, requires mixing of the monomer and catalyst. Two drops from each vial are required for sealing two teeth. If more than two teeth are treated at one time, separate mixes should be prepared. If this is not done, the mix may begin to set and the liquid becomes viscous. This viscosity does not allow for maximal flow into the pits and fissures, and the bond with the enamel is compromised. Once polymerization begins, the sealant should not be disturbed.

Photopolymerization requires a high-intensity light-emitting unit with a fiberoptic light (Fig. 21–23). Protective glasses or a shield should be used by the clinician and client to assure eye protection from the light source (Fig. 21–24). To activate the polymerization process, the light source is held 2 mm from the sealant. Most light units have automatic timers that switch off after the time interval has been reached. The required time is set by the manufacturer and varies from 20 to 30 seconds. Each portion of the sealant must receive an appropriate amount of light before advancing the light to another area of the tooth.

Post-Application Inspection

The operator should evaluate the sealant with an explorer and feel for a hard, smooth surface (Fig. 21–25). If imperfections such as incomplete coverage or air bubbles are detected, a reapplication of the sealant material is necessary. The tooth must be reetched for 10 seconds, rinsed, dried, and resealed. Once a sealant has been successfully applied, the surface of the tooth should be wiped with a piece of gauze to remove any residual or unpolymerized sealant material. The client may rinse when the procedure is completed.

The treated area should be flossed to make certain that the sealant has not blocked contacts between the teeth. If this occurs, the residual sealant is scaled from the tooth. The occlusion should be checked with articulating paper to detect **high spots**—areas with excess sealant material that interfere with normal occlusion. Minor discrepancies with an unfilled sealant are eliminated by normal masticatory

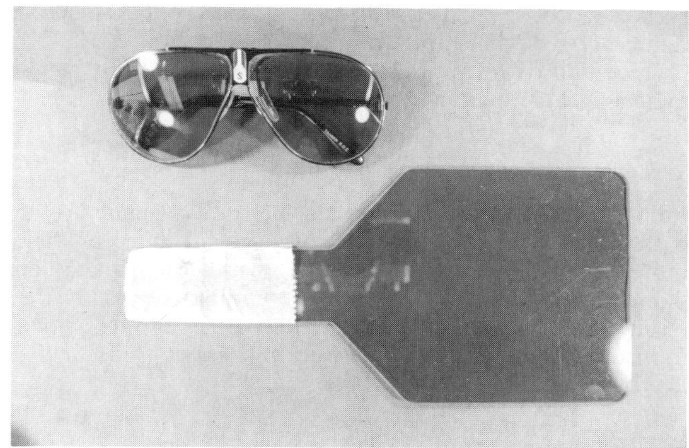

FIGURE 21–24
Protective glasses and shield used by the clinician for eye protection from the high-intensity light.

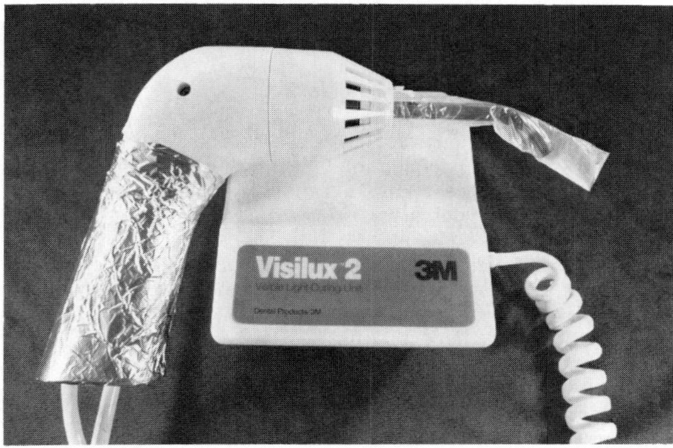

FIGURE 21–23
High-intensity light unit used for photopolymerization.

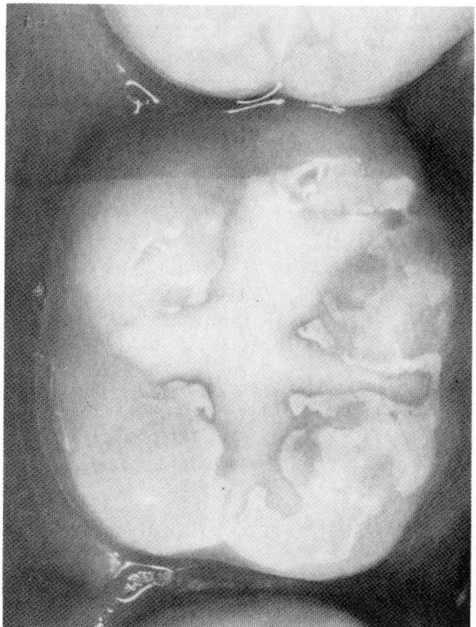

FIGURE 21–25
Postapplication inspection. (With permission from Preventing Pit and Fissure Caries: A Guide to Sealant Use. Massachusetts Department of Public Health and Massachusetts Health Research Institute, Inc., 1986, p. 19.)

processes; however, filled sealants with high spots should be removed with a finishing-type burr.

Once the sealant procedure is successful and complete, a topical fluoride treatment should be provided.

Retention of Sealants

Properly sealed teeth should retain their sealant material for 6 to 7 years. Sealants usually are retained better on first molars than on second molars, and better on mandibular than on maxillary teeth. This latter finding is possibly the result of the fact that the lower teeth are more accessible, the isolation of the teeth is easier, and gravity aids in the flow of the sealant into the fissures.[24]

Follow-Up Evaluation

Follow-up evaluation on the condition of the dental sealant should be performed every 6 months. If the site was contaminated from faulty techniques, partial or complete loss occurs within 6 to 12 months. The failure rate of sealants range from 5 to 10% within the first year of placement.[27] Complete retention of sealants has been documented up to 10 years.[24]

DIET ASSESSMENT AND NUTRITIONAL COUNSELING

Proper nutrition is important in the prevention of many diseases, including dental caries. The dental hygienist as a preventive specialist can be instrumental in preventing and detecting nutritional deficiencies, providing nutritional counseling, and identifying individuals in need of referral to a nutritionist. Nutritional counseling that promotes the oral health and general health of an individual is an integral component of comprehensive dental hygiene care. It constitutes much more than making recommendations for dietary change. Nutritional counseling involves motivating an individual to change his eating habits, behavior, and attitudes about food. This process is challenging because there are many factors that influence an individual's selection of food including:[31]

- Age of the individual
- Ethnicity and culture
- Income level
- Formal education received

Successful nutritional counseling requires knowledge of communication and motivational techniques, an understanding of the teaching-learning process, and a foundation in the science of nutrition.

Communication theory was discussed in Chapter 5. This section focuses on the role of the dental hygienist in identifying nutritional deficiencies and methods for dietary assessment and nutritional counseling that the dental hygienist can employ in practice. Nutritional counseling, together with fluoride therapy and sealants, promotes the oral health as well as the general well-being of the client.

Identifying Nutritional Deficiencies

Nutritional problems manifest themselves both orally and systemically (Tables 21–9 and 21–10). A **primary nutritional deficiency** is caused by inadequate dietary intake of a nutrient.[32] Once identified, this type of deficiency can be

TABLE 21–9
DIETARY SOURCES AND FUNCTIONS OF VITAMINS

Vitamin	Dietary Sources	Major Body Functions	Deficiency	Excess
Water Soluble				
Vitamin B_1 (thiamin)	Meat (especially pork and organ meats), grains, dry beans and peas, fish, poultry	Coenzyme (thiamine pyrophosphate) in reactions involving the removal of carbon dioxide in carbohydrate metabolism	Beriberi (peripheral nerve changes, edema, heart failure)	Nervous system hypersensitivity reaction
Vitamin B_2 (riboflavin)	Widely distributed in both animal and vegetable foods	Constituent of two flavin nucleotide coenzymes involved in energy metabolism (FAD and FMN)	Cracks at corner of mouth (cheilosis), inflammation of lips, glossitis, photophobia	None reported
Niacin (can be formed from tryptophan)	Liver, meat, fish, grains, legumes, poultry, peanut butter	Constituent of two coenzymes involved in oxidation-reduction reactions (NAD and NADP)	Pellagra (skin and gastrointestinal lesions, nervous, mental disorders, glossitis)	Flushing, burning and tingling around neck, face and hands
Vitamin B_6 (pyridoxine)	Meats (liver), vegetables, whole-grain cereals, egg yolks	Coenzyme (pyridoxal phosphate) involved in amino acid metabolism	Irritability, convulsions, muscular twitching, kidney stones, microcytic hypochromic anemia, glossitis, cheilosis	Severe impairment of the sensory nerves
Pantothenic acid	Widely distributed in all foods; organ meats and whole-grain cereals	Constituent of coenzyme A, which plays a central role in energy metabolism	Fatigue, sleep disturbances, impaired coordination, nausea (rare in man), GI distress	None reported

TABLE 21–9
DIETARY SOURCES AND FUNCTIONS OF VITAMINS *Continued*

Vitamin	Dietary Sources	Major Body Functions	Deficiency	Excess
Water Soluble				
Folacin	Liver, kidney, yeast, mushrooms, green vegetables	Coenzyme (reduced form) involved in transfer of single-carbon units in nucleic acid and amino acid metabolism	Macrocytic anemia; gastrointestinal disturbances, diarrhea, glossitis	None reported
Vitamin B_{12} (cobalamin)	Muscle and organ meats, eggs, dairy products (not present in plant foods)	Coenzyme involved in synthesis of single-carbon units in nucleic acid metabolism	Pernicious anemia, neurological disorders, glossitis	None reported
Biotin	Liver, kidney, milk, egg yolk, yeast	Coenzymes required for synthesis and oxidation of fats, carbohydrates, and deamination	Fatigue, depression, nausea, dermatitis, muscular pains, loss of hair	Not reported
Vitamin C (ascorbic acid)	Citrus fruits, tomatoes, green peppers, broccoli, spinach, strawberries, melon	Maintains intercellular matrix of cartilage, bone and dentin. Important in collagen synthesis, utilization of iron, calcium, and folic acid	Scurvy (degeneration of skin, teeth, blood vessels, epithelial hemorrhages), delayed wound healing, anemia	Induced scurvy, nausea, abdominal cramps, diarrhea; possible kidney stones
Fat Soluble				
Vitamin A (retinol)	Provitamin A (beta-carotene) widely distributed in green and yellow vegetables and fruits. Retinol present in milk, butter, cheese, fortified margarine, egg yolk	Constituent of rhodopsin (visual pigment). Maintenance of epithelial tissues. Role in mucopolysaccharide synthesis, bone growth, and remodeling	Xerophthalmia (keratinization of ocular tissue), night blindness, folliculosis, respiratory infections	Headache, vomiting, peeling of skin, anorexia, swelling of long bones, resorption of bones
Vitamin D	Fish-liver oil, eggs, dairy products, fortified milk, and margarine	Promotes growth and mineralization of bones and teeth, increases absorption of calcium in intestines	Rickets (bone deformities) in children. Osteomalacia in adults	Vomiting, diarrhea, loss of weight, kidney damage, hypercalcemia
Vitamin E (tocopherol)	Vegetable oils and seeds, green leafy vegetables, margarines, shortenings	Functions as an antitoxidant, in cellular respiration, synthesis of body compounds	Possibly anemia	Relatively nontoxic; possible GI disturbances
Vitamin K (phylloquinone)	Green and yellow vegetables. Small amount in cereals, fruits, and meats	Important in blood clotting (involved in formation of active prothrombin)	Conditioned deficiencies associated with severe bleeding, internal hemorrhages	Relatively nontoxic. Synthetic forms at high doses may cause jaundice

From Lee M., Stanmeyer W., and Wight A: Nutrition and dental health, Part I, Assessment of human nutrition requirements. Chapel Hill, NC, Health Sciences Consortium, 1982.

corrected by completion of a dietary assessment followed by nutritional counseling that promotes proper selection and adequate intake of nutrients. A **secondary nutritional deficiency** is caused by a systemic disorder that interferes with the ingestion, absorption, digestion, transport, and use of nutrients.[32] This type of deficiency is more complex and may best be treated by referral to a physician and a nutritionist.

Information collected during the assessment phase of the dental hygiene process can assist the dental hygienist in identifying nutritional problems and making the appropriate recommendations and referrals. The client's personal and cultural history can reveal information regarding personal, financial, and environmental influences on food intake. The health history can identify health factors and medications that interfere with an individuals' ability to eat or the body's inability to use nutrients. The dental history can provide information about an individual's caries susceptibility and use of fluoride; and the extraoral and intraoral examination may reveal the physical results of any nutritional excesses or deficiencies. These findings, along with a dietary assessment, direct dental hygienists in their role as dietary counselor.

Dietary Assessment

Oral health affects general health, yet not all individuals are in need of nutritional counseling. Screening a client's diet

TABLE 21-10
ORAL MANIFESTATIONS OF NUTRITIONAL DEFICIENCIES AND TOXICITIES

Tissue	Nutrient	Deficiency Symptoms	Toxicity Symptoms
Tongue and lips	Vitamin A	None	Cracking and bleeding of lips
	Thiamin (B_1)	Painful or burning tongue; loss of taste acuity	None
	Riboflavin (B_2)	Inflammation, fissures and ulcers at the corner of the lips (angular cheilitis); dry, scaly lips; red to purple color tongue; atrophy and inflammation of tongue papillae; enlarged fungiform papillae giving the tongue surface a pebbly appearance	None
	Niacin	Atrophy of tongue papillae resulting in a fiery, red, smooth, shiny surface; edematous or enlarged tongue; ulcerations of tongue on central surface; angular cheilitis; loss of appetite	None
	Pyridoxine (B_6)	Inflamed and atrophic tongue with a red, smooth appearance; angular cheilitis	None
	Vitamin B_{12}	Atrophy and inflammation of tongue; bright red, painful, edematous tongue with glossy appearance; altered taste sensations and decreased appetite	None
	Folic acid	Smooth, bright red tongue; patchy surface of tongue as papillae atrophy; ulcerations along edges of tongue; angular cheilitis	None
	Iron	Angular cheilitis; burning, painful tongue with atrophy of papillae; redenning at tip and around margins of tongue; ulcerations of tongue; pallor to ashen grey color of lips and tongue	None
	Zinc	Impaired taste; thickening and parakeratotic tongue with underlying muscle atrophy	None
	Protein	Red, smooth, edematous tongue; angular cheilitis; fissures on lower lip; depigmentation along buccal border of lips	None
Skin, eyes, salivary glands	Vitamin A	Drying of conjunctiva and cornea of eyes; decreased salivary flow	Dry, scaly skin lesion; a high carotene intake results in a yellow color skin
	Riboflavin (B_2)	Greasy, scaly dermatitis of nasolabial folds; keratinizing of corneal surface of eyes, resulting in opacities and ulcerations	None
	Niacin	Scaly and inflamed skin; skin thickening with dark pigmentation of sunlight-exposed skin	None
	Pyridoxine (B_6)	Seborrheic lesions of face	None
Bone	Vitamin D and calcium	Failure to mineralize bone matrix resulting in soft, fragile bones with pathological fractures and skeletal deformities; thinning of cortical bone, resorption of cancellous bone, and enlargement of medullary cavity resulting in overall bone loss; osteomalacia manifested in loss of lamina dura around roots of tooth and increased width of cortical bone	Calcium deposits in bone
	Vitamin C	Defect in collagen formation of osteoid matrix resulting in resorption of alveolar bone	None
Teeth	Fluoride	Less resistant tooth structure to oral irritants	Fluorosis
	Refined carbohydrate	None	Dental caries Bacterial formation
	Vitamin A	Abnormal formation of ameleoblasts and odontoblasts during early stages of tooth formation; results in hypoplastic enamel and dentin	None
	Vitamin D, calcium	Abnormal calcification of enamel and dentin	None

From Lee M., Stanmeyer W., and Wight A: Nutrition and dental health. Chapel Hill, NC: Health Sciences Consortium, 1982.

can provide meaningful information about the quality of the diet.[33] A practical assessment for identifying clients who would benefit from nutritional counseling is the following:

- A client's diet in terms of daily sugar exposures
- The adequacy of intake of foods from the five food groups/food pyramid

These assessments can be done by scoring the amount of sweets ingested by the individual to calculate the cariogenic potential of the diet and by performing a 24-hour dietary analysis to calculate the dental health diet score.

Evaluation of the Cariogenic Potential of the Diet

To assess the cariogenic potential of the diet, instruct the client to record a 24-hour diet that is representative of his

24-HOUR DIET FORM

Instructions to Client

1. List everything you eat and drink on an ordinary weekday, including snacks
2. Record when foods or snacks:
   (1) Were eaten
   (2) Amount ingested (examples: 4 oz tomato juice, 1 cup coffee with 1 tsp sugar, 3 oz chicken sandwich, 2 bread slices)
   (3) How food was prepared
   (4) Teaspoons of sugar added

Breakfast

Snacks

Lunch

Snacks

Dinner

Snacks

Instructions for Clinicians

1. Circle foods sweetened with added sugars or concentrated natural sweets (honey, figs, etc.), saturated fats, or alcohol
2. Place uncircled foods into one of the pyramid food groups on the form to calculate the dental health diet score (Figs. 22–28 to 22–30)
3. For each serving place a mark in food group block
4. Add number of checks and multiply by number shown
5. Add total and determine need for general nutritional counseling, then, complete steps for sugar evaluation and need for nutritional counseling for the prevention of dental caries

FIGURE 21–26
Twenty-four–hour diet form. (Adapted with permission from Nizel, A. E., and Papas, A. S. Nutrition and Clinical Dentistry, 3rd ed. Philadelphia: W. B. Saunders, 1989.)

typical eating patterns (Fig. 21–26). The type and amount of each food eaten, way that the food was prepared, and time of day the food was eaten must be included. This 24-hour recall diet is then used to calculate the cariogenic potential of the diet. The sugar ingested reported on the 24-hour diet form is categorized according to (1) liquid sugars, (2) solid and sticky sugars, and (3) slowly dissolving sugars. The frequency with which each sugar is ingested is tallied and multiplied by 5, 10, or 15 depending upon the sugar source (Fig. 21–27). A sweet score of 15 or more indicates that the individual is in need of nutritional counseling to reduce the cariogenic potential of his diet.

Evaluating the Adequacy of the Overall Diet

The same 24-hour diet form used to calculate the cariogenic potential of the diet (see Fig. 21–27) can be used to

Using the dietary recall of an ordinary weekday:

- Classify each sweet into liquid, solid and sticky, or slowly dissolving
- For each time a sweet was eaten, either at the end of a meal or between meals (at least 20 minutes apart), place a check in the frequency column
- In each group add the number of sweets eaten and multiply by the number provided. Write down the number of points
- Add all the points for the total score

EXAMPLE: 10:00 A.M. 1 jelly donut
12:00 Noon ham and cheese sandwich
1 C milk
1 cupcake
3:00 P.M. 1 coke
5:00 P.M. 1 cough drop

Form	Frequency	Points
Liquid	✓ × 5 =	5
Solid and sticky	✓✓ × 10 =	20
Slowly dissolving	✓ × 15 =	15

TOTAL SCORE = 40

Decay-Promoting Potential

Form	Frequency	Points
Liquid: soft drinks, fruit drinks, cocoa, sugar and honey in beverages, nondairy creamers, ice cream, sherbet, gelatin dessert, flavored yogurt, pudding, custard, popsicles	____ × 5 =	
Solid and Sticky: cake, cupcakes, donuts, sweet rolls, pastry, canned fruit in syrup, bananas, cookies, chocolate candy, caramel, toffee, jelly beans, other chewy candy, chewing gum, dried fruit, marshmallows, jelly, jam	____ × 10 =	
Slowly Dissolving: hard candies, breath mints, antacid tablets, cough drops	____ × 15 =	

TOTAL SCORE = ______

Sweet Score: ______
5 or less Excellent
10 Good
15 or more "Watch Out" Zone
* 15 or more—nutritional counseling needed for reducing sugar intake

FIGURE 21–27
Form to calculate the cariogenic potential of the diet from a 24-hour food diary. (Adapted with permission from Nizel, A. E., and Papas, A. S. Nutrition and Clinical Dentistry, 3rd ed. Philadelphia: W. B. Saunders, 1989.)

calculate the dental health diet score. Foods reported on the 24-hour dietary survey are placed into one of the pyramid food groups on the appropriate form used to calculate the dental health diet score (see Figs. 21-28 to 21-30). This information is useful in identifying individuals in need of general nutritional counseling. Nutritional requirements vary depending on the age, sex, and activity level of the individual. Because of these variations, a separate form should be used to calculate the dental health diet score for each of the following groups:

- Women and older adults (Fig. 21-28)
- Most men, children, teen girls, active women (Fig. 21-29)
- Teen boys and active men (Fig. 21-30)

Daily servings for each of the five food groups are tallied and multiplied by the number of servings represented on the form to calculate the dental health diet score. A food group score is calculated for each of the five food groups, and summed to provide a total score ranked accordingly: excellent, adequate, barely adequate, and not adequate. A total score of 91 or less for women and older adults is barely adequate and indicates that nutritional counseling is needed. Once an individual is identified as needing nutritional counseling, a more comprehensive dietary assessment must be completed. This assessment is accomplished by instructing the client to keep a 5-day food diary and then evaluating it.

A 5-day food diary should include a weekend to ensure that it is a representative sample of the individual's normal eating habits. All foods consumed in a 24-hour period should be recorded. It is important that the type of food eaten, the manner in which it was prepared, the exact amount of each food eaten, and the time of day in which it was eaten be recorded in detail (Fig. 21-31). The client should be encouraged to adhere to his normal dietary regime during this week.

The procedure for recording a 5-day food diary can be reviewed with the client by asking him to recall his diet from the previous 24 hours. Using this as a sample, the dental hygienist and the client review the procedure for completing a food diary. The following portions are considered one serving size and can assist the client in recording a detailed food diary:[34]

1 glass of milk
1 carton of yogurt
2 slices of cheese
3 scoops of cottage cheese
2 ounces of meat (e.g., a beef patty, chop, piece of fish,

Text continued on page 585

Food Group	Recommended Servings	Portion Size Considered One Serving	Number of Servings	Points
Bread, cereal, rice, beans	6	1 slice of bread 1/2 C cooked rice or pasta 1 oz ready to eat cereal 1/2 C cooked cereal	___ × 4 =	______ (highest possible score = 24)
Vegetable group	3	1 C raw leafy vegetable 3/4 C vegetable juice 1/2 C other vegetable cooked or raw	___ × 8 =	______ (highest possible score = 24)
Fruit group	2	1 medium apple, orange or banana 3/4 C fruit juice 1/2 C chopped, cooked, canned fruit	___ × 12 =	______ (highest possible score = 24)
Milk, cheese, yogurt group	2	1 C milk or yogurt 1 1/2 oz natural cheese 2 oz process cheese	___ × 12 =	______ (highest possible score = 24)
Meat, poultry, fish, dry bean, egg, nut group	2 or 5 oz	2 to 3 oz lean meat, poultry, fish cooked 1 egg 1/2 C cooked dry beans 2 tbsp peanut butter	___ × 12 =	______ (highest possible score = 24)

Food Group Score ______
102–120 Excellent
92–101 Adequate
75– 91 Barely adequate
0– 74 Not adequate
* Score of 91 or less—nutritional counseling needed

TOTAL SCORE = ______
(highest possible score = 120)

FIGURE 21-28
Form to calculate the dental health diet score for women and older adults. (Prepared by Lynn Tolle Watts, BSDH, MS, School of Dental Hygiene and Dental Assisting, Old Dominion University. Adapted from Nizel, A. E., and Papas, A. S. Nutrition and Clinical Dentistry, 3rd ed. Philadelphia: W. B. Saunders, 1989.)

Food Group	Recommended Servings	Portion Size Considered One Serving	Number of Servings	Points
Bread, cereal, rice, beans	9	1 slice of bread 1/2 C cooked rice or pasta 1 oz ready to eat cereal 1/2 C cooked cereal	___ × 3 =	______ (highest possible score = 27)
Vegetable group	4	1 C raw leafy vegetable 3/4 C vegetable juice 1/2 C other vegetable cooked or raw	___ × 6 =	______ (highest possible score = 24)
Fruit group	3	1 medium apple, orange or banana 3/4 C fruit juice 1/2 C chopped, cooked, canned fruit	___ × 8 =	______ (highest possible score = 24)
Milk, cheese, yogurt group	2	1 C milk or yogurt 1 1/2 oz natural cheese 2 oz process cheese	___ × 12 =	______ (highest possible score = 24)
Meat, poultry, fish, dry bean, egg, nut group	2 or 6 oz	2 to 3 oz lean meat, poultry, fish cooked 1 egg 1/2 C cooked dry beans 2 tbsp peanut butter	___ × 12 =	______ (highest possible score = 24)

Food Group Score ______
106–123 Excellent
96–105 Adequate
80– 95 Barely adequate
0– 79 Not adequate
* Score of 95 or less—nutritional counseling needed

TOTAL SCORE = ______
(highest possible score = 123)

FIGURE 21–29
Form to calculate the dental health diet score for most men, children, teen girls, and active women. (Prepared by Lynn Tolle Watts, BSDH, MS, School of Dental Hygiene and Dental Assisting, Old Dominion University. Adapted from Nizel, A. E., and Papas, A. S. Nutrition and Clinical Dentistry, 3rd ed. Philadelphia: W. B. Saunders, 1989.)

Food Group	Recommended Servings	Portion Size Considered One Serving	Number of Servings	Points
Bread, cereal, rice, beans	11	1 slice of bread 1/2 C cooked rice or pasta 1 oz ready to eat cereal 1/2 C cooked cereal	___ × 2 =	_____ (highest possible score = 22)
Vegetable group	5	1 C raw leafy vegetable 3/4 C vegetable juice 1/2 C other vegetable cooked or raw	___ × 5 =	_____ (highest possible score = 25)
Fruit group	4	1 medium apple, orange or banana 3/4 C fruit juice 1/2 C chopped, cooked, canned fruit	___ × 6 =	_____ (highest possible score = 24)
Milk, cheese, yogurt group	2	1 C milk or yogurt 1 1/2 oz natural cheese 2 oz process cheese	___ × 12 =	_____ (highest possible score = 24)
Meat, poultry, fish, dry bean, egg, nut group	2 or 7 oz	2 to 3 oz lean meat, poultry, fish cooked 1 egg 1/2 C cooked dry beans 2 tbsp peanut butter	___ × 12 =	_____ (highest possible score = 24)

Food Group Score ___________
101–119 Excellent
91–100 Adequate
73– 90 Barely adequate
0– 72 Not adequate
* Score of 95 or less—nutritional counseling needed

TOTAL SCORE = _____
(highest possible score = 119)

FIGURE 21–30
Form to calculate the dental health diet score for teen boys and active men. (Prepared by Lynn Tolle Watts, BSDH, MS, School of Dental Hygiene and Dental Assisting, Old Dominion University. Adapted from Nizel, A. E., and Papas, A. S. Nutrition and Clinical Dentistry, 3rd ed. Philadelphia: W. B. Saunders, 1989.)

Instructions: Please record everything you eat or drink for a five-day period which includes either *a weekend or a holiday.* Don't forget to include all snacks, gum, candies, soft drinks, etc.

Be Specific! It is very important to write down the following:

Amount
- 1/2 cup string beans
- 1 tablespoon butter
- 6 ounces steak

How food was prepared
- 1/2 cup string beans—boiled
- 6 ounces steak—fried
- 1 orange—fresh
- 1 peach—canned

What was added to the food/drink
- 1 cup coffee—1 tsp milk
- 1/2 grapefruit—1 tsp sugar

Time of day
- Lunch—12:30 P.M.
- Snack—3:00 P.M.

Also include the order in which the solids or liquids are eaten. If you want to use additional paper please feel free to do so.

____

Client Name

First Day		Second Day		Third Day	
Food	Quantity Prepared	Food	Quantity Prepared	Food	Quantity Prepared
Breakfast		Breakfast		Breakfast	
10:00 A.M.		10:00 A.M.		10:00 A.M.	
Lunch		Lunch		Lunch	
3:00 P.M.		3:00 P.M.		3:00 P.M.	
Dinner		Dinner		Dinner	
Extras		Extras		Extras	

Fourth Day		Fifth Day	
Food	Quantity Prepared	Food	Quantity Prepared
Breakfast		Breakfast	
10:00 A.M.		10:00 A.M.	
Lunch		Lunch	
3:00 P.M.		3:00 P.M.	
Dinner		Dinner	
Extras		Extras	

FIGURE 21–31
Five-day food diary form. (Prepared by Lynn Tolle Watts, BSDH, MS, School of Dental Hygiene and Dental Assisting, Old Dominion University. Adapted from Nizel, A. E., and Papas, A. S. Nutrition and Clinical Dentistry, 3rd ed. Philadelphia: W. B. Saunders, 1989.)

Instructions: For each food item, place a check mark (✓) in the appropriate block

Food Group	Portion Size Considered One Serving	1st Day	2nd Day	3rd Day	4th Day	5th Day	Average	Suggested Daily Amount: Women and Older Adults	Most Men Children Teen Girls Active Women	Teen Boys and Active Men	Difference
Bread, cereal, rice, pasta	1 slice bread 1/2 C cooked rice or pasta 1 oz cereal							6	9	11	
Vegetable group	1 C raw leafy vegetable 3/4 C vegetable juice 1/2 C other vegetable cooked or raw							3	4	5	
Fruit group	1 medium apple, orange, banana 3/4 C fruit juice 1/2 C chopped, cooked, canned fruit							2	3	4	
Milk, yogurt, cheese, group	1 C milk or yogurt 1/2 oz natural cheese 2 oz process cheese							2–3*	2–3*	2–3*	
Meat, poultry, fish, dry beans, egg, nut group	2 to 3 oz lean meat, poultry, fish cooked 1 egg 1/2 C cooked dry beans 2 tbsp peanut butter							2 total of 5 oz	2 total of 6 oz	3 total of 7 oz	
Fats, oils, sweets	1 tbsp margarine 1 tbsp salad dressing 1 can soft drink 1/2 C ice cream 1 slice cake							Sparingly	Sparingly	Sparingly	

* To age 24 need 3 servings; or if pregnant or breast feeding

FIGURE 21–32
Foundation foods. (Prepared by Lynn Tolle Watts, BSDH, MS, School of Dental Hygiene and Dental Assisting, Old Dominion University. Adapted from Nizel, A. E., and Papas, A. S. Nutrition and Clinical Dentistry, 3rd ed. Philadelphia: W. B. Saunders, 1989.)

chicken breast, two hot dogs), 4 tablespoons of peanut butter (enough for 2 sandwiches), two eggs, one bowl of soup or cooked dried beans, two handfuls of nuts or seeds

It is important that the dental hygienist remain nonjudgmental during this review process. Questions such as "What was the first thing you ate yesterday?" can elicit information about the client's diet without assuming that breakfast was the first meal of the day. The purpose of the 24-hour diet recall is to give the client guidance in completing a food diary. This process of recalling foods consumed in a 24-hour period is not a nutritional counseling session. Given the proper instructions, the client is able to record in detail a 5-day food diary. The information obtained from a 5-day food diary provides the basis for future nutritional counseling sessions.

Evaluating the 5-Day Food Diary

Upon completion of the 5-day diary, the dental hygienist and the client evaluate the diet for adequacy of intake from the five food groups (Fig. 21–32). Foods consumed by the client are categorized into each of the five food groups. The average number of servings for a 5-day period are calculated and recorded. The servings from the client's diet are compared to the suggested daily servings recommended by the USDA food pyramid (Fig. 21–33), and deficiencies or excesses are noted.

In addition to evaluating the diet for adequacy of intake from the five food groups, the cariogenic potential of the diet also must be analyzed. This analysis is accomplished by calculating the amount of acid produced in the diet (Fig. 21–34). Each sugar exposure is circled in red. A sugar exposure is defined as any sweet or sugar-sweetened food or liquid. The total number of liquid and solid sugar exposures ingested over a 5-day period are tallied and multiplied by the appropriate time interval. The number of liquid sugar exposures ingested over the 5-day period is multiplied by 20 minutes, and the number of solid sugar exposures ingested over the 5-day period is multiplied by 40 minutes. This figure is divided by five, and the resulting figure indicates the amount of time per day that the teeth are subjected to an acid exposure. The total daily acid production is calculated by adding the daily acid production from both liquid and solid sugars. Sugars consumed at the same time are considered one acid exposure (i.e., ice cream and cake

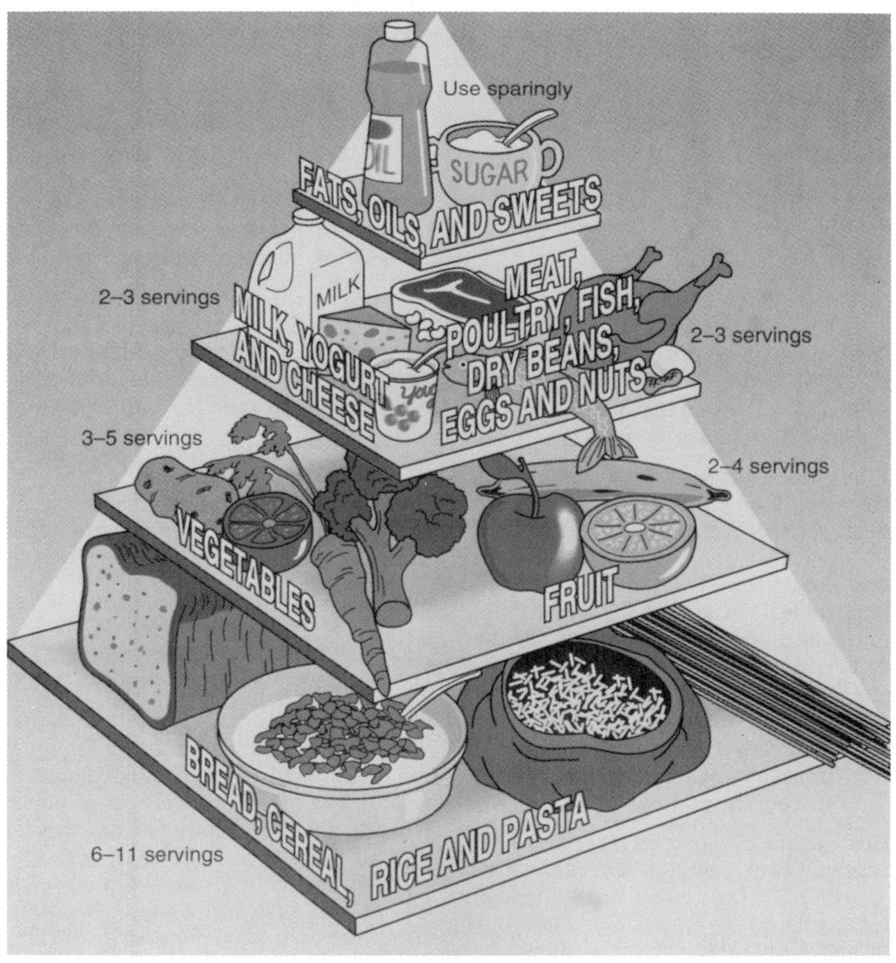

FIGURE 21–33
The Food guide pyramid. (With permission from Polaski, A., Warner, J. Saunders Fundamentals for Nursing Assistants. Philadelphia, W. B. Saunders, 1994, p. 527.)

Form of Sugar		When Eaten	1st Day	2nd Day	3rd Day	4th Day	5th Day	Total
Liquid	(soda, sugar in coffee, etc.)	With meals						
		Between meals						
Solid	(cookie, candy)	With meals						
		Between meals						

Grand total = ______ (Sugar in liquid form)

Grand total = ______ (Sugar in solid form)

$$\frac{\quad}{\text{Liquid Exposure}} \times \frac{\text{20 minutes}}{\text{pH below 5.5}} = \frac{\quad}{\text{Acid Production}} \div \text{5 DAYS} = \frac{\quad}{\text{Daily liquid acid production}}$$

$$\frac{\quad}{\text{Solid Exposure}} \times \frac{\text{40 minutes}}{\text{pH below 5.5}} = \frac{\quad}{\text{Acid Production}} \div \text{5 DAYS} = \frac{\quad}{\text{Daily solid acid production}}$$

$$\text{Total daily acid production} = \frac{\quad}{\text{Liquid acid production total}} + \frac{\quad}{\text{Solid acid production total}} = \frac{\quad}{\text{Total time tooth is exposed to acid daily (demineralization)}}$$

FIGURE 21–34
Form to calculate the cariogenic potential of the diet from a 5-day food diary. (Adapted with permission from Nizel, A. E., and Papas, A. S. Nutrition and Clinical Dentistry, 3rd ed. Philadelphia: W. B. Saunders, 1989.)

eaten for dessert equals one acid exposure). Sweet foods or liquids eaten 20 minutes apart are recorded as two acid exposures. Calculating the number of acid exposures illustrates to the client the cariogenic potential of the diet.

NUTRITIONAL COUNSELING

Once the dietary deficiencies and excesses are identified, the dental hygienist together with the client can develop a dietary program that best meets the nutritional needs of the individual. Nizel and Papas maintain that the following four rules should be adopted when making dietary modifications:[35]

- Maintain overall nutritional adequacy by conforming to the USDA Daily Food Guide for at least the recommended number of servings from each of the food groups
- The prescribed diet should vary from the normal diet pattern as little as possible
- The diet should meet the body's requirements for the essential nutrients as generously as the diseased condition can tolerate
- The prescribed diet should take into consideration and accommodate the individual's likes and dislikes, food habits, and other environmental factors as long as they do not interfere with the objectives

A diet that provides adequate nutrients to the whole body promotes the optimal well-being of an individual. When developing a nutritional program for an individual, the dietary guidelines developed by the USDA and the Department of Health and Human Services also should be considered. These recommendations are to:

- Eat a variety of foods
- Maintain healthy weight
- Choose a diet low in fat, saturated fat, and cholesterol
- Choose a diet with plenty of vegetables, fruits, and grain products
- Use sugars only in moderation
- Use salt and sodium only in moderation
- Drink alcoholic beverages in moderation

These guidelines in conjunction with the USDA food pyramid can assist in making the necessary diet modifications. It is important that the dental hygienist and the client work together in this process to develop a nutritional program that meets the specific needs of the individual.

Nutritional Counseling for the Prevention of Dental Caries

Sugar consumption is an important factor in the etiology of dental caries. However, three factors must be present for dental caries to occur:

- Acid-producing microorganisms
- A fermentable carbohydrate
- A susceptible tooth surface

Bacteria use the carbohydrate to form an organic acid. It is the production of this acid that draws minerals from the enamel in a process called **demineralization.** Nutritional counseling for the prevention of dental caries should target the elimination of fermentable carbohydrates from the diet. If this is not possible, then dietary recommendations to reduce the cariogenic potential of the individual's diet should be made. The goal is to limit the number of acid exposures per day. Frequent consumption of fermentable carbohydrates subjects the tooth enamel to repeated acid exposures. This demineralization process weakens the tooth and leads to the formation of dental caries. (See Chapter 12

TABLE 21–11
CURRENT ESTIMATES OF CARIOGENICITIES

Rank	Food	Substances
11	Items with added sugars: baked goods, candies	Sucrose/other sugars
10	Sugars, gums and beverages, honey, raisins, chocolate	Sucrose
8	Highly refined bread/cereals	Glusose, fructose, some cooked starches
5	Pastas, chips, some fruits, some breads/cereals	Other cooked starches, lactose
Safe		
2	Processed vegetables/fruits	Raw starch
1	Raw vegetables/fruits, milk, whole grains, legumes	Sorbitol, mannitol
0	Meats, eggs, cheese, olives, popcorn, peanuts, seeds	Xylitol, noncarbohydrates

Instructions for using hazardous carbohydrates

1. Use items 5 through 11 no more than four times a day, either at mealtime or as a snack
2. Select items that can be quickly consumed; avoid continual sipping, sucking, or nibbling, whether of food or nonfood hazardous items
3. Follow use of a cariogenic item or meal with a safe item, such as cheese or peanuts, with oral hygiene, or at least with a water rinse of the mouth
4. If items ranked 5–11 are ingested more than four times a day the use of fluoride products (e.g., fluoride mouth rinses and fluoride dentifrices) should be increased proportionately.

From Harris, N., and Madsen K. Nutrition and the plaque diseases. In Harris N., and Christen A. *Primary Preventive Dentistry,* 3rd ed. East Norwalk, CT: Appleton-Lange, 1991

for a review of the caries process.) Table 21–11 illustrates the relative cariogenicity of certain foods. Foods ranked 0 to 2 are considered noncariogenic, provided that sugar is not added to them. This information can be useful for suggesting foods for reducing the cariogenic potential of an individual's diet.

The following is a list of dietary recommendations for the reduction of dental caries:

- Limit the use of fermentable carbohydrates to mealtime. Foods other than carbohydrates serve as buffers to help neutralize plaque acids
- Omit sweet foods even with meals if the client is susceptible to caries
- Between-meal snacks should consist of protective, noncariogenic foods such as raw vegetables. Raw unrefined foods in the vegetable and fruit group require chewing. The chewing action increases the salivary flow thus aiding in the removal and dilution of sugars and their harmful byproducts
- Use as little concentrated sweets in the preparation of foods as possible
- Do not eat sweets before bedtime unless the teeth are brushed. Salivary flow decreases at night and foods are not readily cleared from the mouth as they are during waking hours. Acid left undisturbed remains in the mouth for 1½ to 2 hours
- Avoid natural sugars, since they are as detrimental to the tooth surface as refined sugars
- Avoid sticky foods, since they are retained in the mouth longer than nonsticky foods

The correlation between sugar consumption and dental caries is well documented.[36,37] Nutritional counseling for the prevention of dental caries must emphasize decreasing the frequency with which sugar is consumed and replacing cariogenic foods with nutritionally sound foods.

Nutritional counseling involves all phases of the dental hygiene process: assessment, diagnosis, planning, implementation, and evaluation. The dental hygienist assesses the client's diet for deficiencies or excesses. Once problems are identified, the client and the dental hygienist work together to plan a nutritionally sound diet. The client then follows through with the recommendations and implements the new diet, and the dental hygienist continually evaluates his progress. Through nutritional counseling, the dental hygienist helps individuals meet their human needs for nutrition and for a biologically sound dentition, thus assisting them to achieve optimal oral and general health.

References

1. Newbrun, E. Fluoride and Dental Caries, Springfield, IL: Charles C Thomas, 1986.
2. Blayney, J. R., and Hill, I. N. Fluorine and dental caries. Journal of the American Dental Association 74:233, 1967.
3. Clinical Research Associates Newsletter. 14(5):May, 1990.
4. Newbrun, E. Current regulations and recommendations concerning water fluoridation, fluoride supplements, and topical fluoride agents. Workshop on Changing Patterns of Fluoride Intake. University of North Carolina, Chapel Hill, April 23–25, 1991.
5. Ripa, L. W., Bohannon, H. M. et al. Preventing Pit and Fissure Caries: A Guide to Sealant Use. Massachusetts Department of Public Health, 1986.
6. Silverstone, L. M. Remineralization phenomena. Caries Research 11 [Suppl 1]:59, 1977.
7. Silverstone, L. M. Insights into the caries process and the role of fluorides. Symposium, San Diego, CA, 1982.
8. Featherstone, J. B. Insights into the caries process and the role of fluorides. Symposium, San Diego, CA, 1982.
9. Wei, S. (ed.). Clinical Uses of Fluorides, A State of the Art Conference on the Uses of Fluorides in Clinical Dentistry. Philadelphia: Lea & Febiger, 1985.
10. Ripa, L. W. Professionally (operator) applied topical fluoride therapy: A critique. Cinical Preventive Dentistry 4:3, 1982.
11. Ripa, L. W. Open Questions and Forum. In Wei, S. (chairman): Clinical Uses of Fluoride. Conference, San Francisco, May, 1984.
12. Wei, S., and Hattab, F. Relationship between enamel fluoride uptake and time of topical application. Journal of Dental Research 66:242, 1987.
13. Schemehorn, B. R. Indiana University School of Dentistry Oral Health Research Institution, 1991 findings. Quoted in: Rediscover Fluoride Foams versus Gels. Gardena, CA: Laclede Professional Products. 1993.
14. Heifetz, S. B., and Horowitz, H. S. Fluoride dentifrices. In Newbrun, E. (ed.). Fluoride and Dental Caries. Springfield, IL; Charles C Thomas, 1986.
15. Gron, P., and Brundevold, F. The effectiveness of NaF dentifrices. Journal of Dentistry for Children 34:122, 1967.
16. Stookey, G. K. Are all fluorides the same? In Wei, S. (ed.). Clinical Uses of Fluorides. Philadelphia: Lea & Febiger, 1985.
17. Edlund, K., and Koch, G. Effect on caries of daily supervised toothbrushing with sodium monofluorophosphate and sodium fluoride dentifrices after 3 years. Scandinavian Journal of Dental Research 85:41, 1977.

18. Gerdin, P. O. Studies in dentifrices on dental caries. Swedish Dental Journal 65:521, 1972.
19. Koch, G., Peterson, L. G., and Kling, L. Effect of 250 and 1,000 ppm fluoride dentifrice on caries: A three-year clinical study. Swedish Dental Journal 6:233, 1982.
20. Heifetz, S. B., and Horowitz, H. S. The amounts of fluoride in current fluoride therapies: Safety considerations for children. ASDC Journal of Dentistry for Children 51:257, 1984.
21. Zacherl, W. A. A three-year clinical caries evaluation of the effect of a sodium fluoride–silica abrasive dentifrice. Pharmacology of Therapeutic Dentistry 6:1, 1981.
22. National Fluoride Task Force of NFDH. A guide to the use of fluorides for the prevention of dental caries. Journal of the American Dental Association 113:503, 1986.
23. Tinanoff, N. Stannous fluoride in clinical dentistry. In Wei, S. (ed.). Clinical Uses of Fluorides. Philadelphia: Lea & Febiger, 1985.
24. Harris, N., and Christen, A. Primary Preventive Dentistry. Englewood Cliffs, NJ: Prentice-Hall, 1991.
25. Jensen, M. E., and Kahout, F. The effect of a fluoridated dentifrice on root and coronal caries in an older adult population. Journal of the American Dental Association 117(7):829, 1988.
26. Silverman, S. Oral Cancer, 3rd ed. Atlanta: American Cancer Society. 1990.
27. Woodall, I. R. Comprehensive Dental Hygiene Care. St. Louis: Mosby-Year Book, 1993.
28. Whitford, G. M. Acute and chronic fluoride toxicity. Workshop on Changing Patterns of Fluoride Intake. University of North Carolina, Chapel Hill, April 23–25, 1991.
29. Horowitz, H. S., Heifetz, S. B., et al. Retention and effectiveness of a single application of an adhesive sealant in preventing occlusal caries: Final report after five years of a study in Kalispell, Montana. Journal of the American Dental Association 95:1133, 1977.
30. Miers, J. C., and Jensen, M. E. Management of the questionable caries fissure: Invasive vs. noninvasive techniques. Journal of the American Dental Association 108:64, 1984.
31. Kant, A., Schatzkin, A., et al. Food group intake patterns and associated nutrient profiles of the U.S. population. Journal of the American Dietetic Association 91(12):1532, 1991.
32. Whitney, E. N., and Rolfes, S. R. Understanding Nutrition, 6th ed. St. Paul, MN: West Publishing, 1993.
33. Kant, A., et al. Dietary diversity in the U.S. population, NHANES II, 1976–1980. Journal of the American Dietetic Association 91(12), 1991.
34. Dairy Council of California. Big Ideas in Nutrition, 1980.
35. Nizel A., and Papas, A. Nutrition in Clinical Dentistry, 3rd ed. Philadelphia: W. B. Saunders, 1989.
36. Gustaffson, B. E., Quensd, C. E., et al. The Vipeholm dental caries study. The effects of different levels of carbohydrate intake on caries activity in 436 individuals observed for five years. Acta Odontologica Scandinavica 11:232, 1954.
37. Sreenby, L. M. Sugar availability, sugar consumption and dental caries. Community Dentistry and Oral Epidemiology 10:1, 1982.

Suggested Readings

American Dental Association. Perspectives on the use of prenatal fluorides, a symposium. Journal of Dentistry for Children 101:1, 1981.

Aronson, E., Turner, J. A., and Carlsmith, J. M. Communicator credibility and communicator discrepancy as determinants of opinion change. Journal of Abnormal and Social Psychology 67:31, 1963.

Beiswanger, B. B., Gish, C. W., and Mallatt, M. E. A three-year study of the effect of a sodium fluoride-silica abrasive dentifrice on dental caries. Pharacology of Therapeutic Dentistry 6:16, 1981.

Bibby, B. G. A test of the effect of fluoride-containing dentifrices on dental caries. Journal of Dental Research 24:297, 1945.

Brown, L. R. Insights into the caries process and the role of fluorides. Symposium, San Diego, CA, 1982.

Cacioppo, J. T., Petty, R. E., and Morris, K. J. Julius Streicher and the rhetorical foundations of the Holocaust. Paper presented to the Central States Speech Association Convention, 1983.

Campbell-Smith, R. Is fluoride just for kids? Prophyplus 2:6, 1989.

Carlos, J. P. Fluoride mouthrinses. In Wei, S. (ed.). Clinical Uses of Fluorides. Philadelphia: Lea & Febiger, 1985.

Chaiken, S., and Eagley, A. H. Communication as a determinant of message persuasiveness and message comprehensibility. Journal of Personality and Social Psychology 34:605, 1978.

Chaiken, S., and Eagley, A. H. Communication modality as a determinant of persuasion: The role of communicator salience. Journal of Personality and Social Psychology 45:241, 1983.

Erickson, B., Lind, E. A., Johnson, B. C., and O'Barr, W. M. Speech style and impression formation in a court setting: The effects of powerful and powerless speech. Journal of Experimental and Social Psychology 14:266, 1978.

Feagin, F. F. Insights into the caries process and the role of fluorides. Symposium, San Diego, CA, 1982.

Fogels, H. R. The relative caries-inhibiting effects of a stannous fluoride dentifrice in a silica gel base. Journal of the American Dental Association 99:456, 1979.

Food and Drug Administration. Statement of general policy or interpretation, oral prenatal drugs containing fluorides for human use. Federal Register, October 20, 1966.

Hemsley, G. D., and Doob, A. N. The effect of looking behavior on perceptions of a communicator's credibility. Journal of Applied Social Psychology 8:136, 1978.

Hoppenbrouwers, P. M. M., et al. The vulnerability of unexposed human dental roots to demineralization. Journal of Dental Research 65(7):957, 1986.

Hormati, A. A., Fuller, J. L., and Denehy, G. E. Effects of contamination and mechanical disturbances on the quality of acid-etched enamel. Journal of the American Dental Association 100:34, 1980.

Horowitz, H. S., and Chamberlain, S. R. Pigmentation of teeth following topical applications of stannous fluoride in a nonfluoridated area. Journal of Public Health Dentistry 31:32, 1971.

Hovland, C. I., Lumsdaine, A. A., and Sheffield, F. D. Experiments on mass communication. Studies in social psychology in World War II, vol. III. Princeton, NJ: Princeton University Press, 1949.

Ingersoll, B. D. Behavioral Aspects in Dentistry. New York: Appleton-Century-Crofts, 1982.

Koulourides, T. Insight into the caries process and the role of fluorides. Symposium, San Diego, CA, 1982.

Kula, K., Nelson, S., and Thompson, V. In vitro effect of APF gels on three composite resins. Journal of Dental Research 62:846, 1983.

Love, W. Fluoride therapy in clinical practice. Dental Clinics of North America 28(3):611, 1984.

McCann, D. Fluoride and oral health; A story of achievement and challenges. Journal of the American Dental Association 118(5):533, 1989.

Mertz-Fairhurst, E. J., Fairhurst, C. W., et al. A comparative study of two pit and fissure sealants: 7-year results in Augusta, GA. Journal of the American Dental Association 109:252, 1984.

Mintzer, M. A. Insights into the caries process and the role of fluorides. Symposium, San Diego, CA, 1982.

Miura, F., Naakagawa, K., and Ishizaki, A. Scanning electron microscopic studies of the direct bonding system. Bulletin of the Tokyo Medical-Dental University 20:245, 1973.

Myers, D. G. Social Psychology, vol 2. New York: McGraw-Hill, 1987.

National Institutes of Health. Dental Sealants in the Prevention of Tooth Decay. Consensus of Health and Human Services, Public Health Service, 1983.

National Research Council. Health Effects of Ingested Fluoride. Washington, DC: National Academy Press, 1993.

Newbrun, E. Insights into the caries process and the role of fluorides. Symposium, San Diego, CA, 1982.

Olson, J. M. and Cal, A. V. Source credibility, attitudes, and the recall of past behaviors. European Journal of Social Psychology 14:108, 1984.

Oral B Laboratories. Fluoride Usage Guide, 1986.

Ripa, L. W. The current status of pit and fissure sealants. A review. Canadian Dental Association Journal 5:367, 1985.

Shannon, I. Antisolubility effects of acidulated phosphate fluoride and stannous fluoride in the treatment of crown and root surfaces. Australian Dental Journal 16:240, 1971.

Sherman, S. J., Cialdini, R. B., Scwartzman, D. F., and Reynolds, K. D. Imagining can heighten or lower the perceived likelihood of contracting a disease: The mediating effect of ease of imagery. Personality and Social Psychology Bulletin 11:118, 1985.

Silverstone, L. M. Fluorides and remineralization. In Wei, S. (ed.). Clinical Uses of Fluorides. Philadelphia: Lea & Febiger, 1985.

Swango, A. The use of topical fluorides to prevent dental caries in adults: A review of the literature. Journal of the American Dental Association 107(3): 447, 1983.

Tinanoff, N., Brady, J. M., and Gross, A. The effect of NaF and SnF_2 mouthrinses on bacterial colonization of tooth enamel: TEM and SEM studies. Caries Research 10:415, 1976.

Tinanoff, N., Wei, S. H. Y., and Parkins, F. M. Effects of a pumice prophylaxis on fluoride uptake in tooth enamel. Journal of the American Dental Association 88:384, 1974.

Vehkalahti, M. M., and Paunio, I. K. Occurence of root caries in relation to dental health behavior. Journal of Dental Research 67(6):911, 1988.

Walsh, M. M., and Woodall, I. The Philosophy, Psychology and Practice of Preventive Care. In Clark's Clinical Dentistry. Philadelphia: J. B. Lippincott, 1988.

Webster's New World Dictionary, Third College Edition. Cleveland and New York, Simon & Schuster, 1988.

Woodall, I. R. Patient home care and plaque control: A behavioral approach. Compendium of Continuing Education in Dentistry 5:65, 1984.

Zacherl, W. A. A three-year clinical caries evaluation of the effect of a sodium fluoride–silica abrasive dentifrice. Pharmacology of Therapeutic Dentistry 6:1, 1981.

22 Restorative Therapy and the Dental Hygiene Process

OBJECTIVES

Mastery of the content of this chapter will enable the reader to:

- Describe the rationale for restorative therapy
- Discuss the role of the dental hygienist in restorative therapy
- Discuss the continuous role of assessment in the delivery of restorative therapy
- Describe an acceptable technique for rubber dam application
- State the rationale for rubber dam isolation
- Describe the qualities of a properly placed rubber dam
- Describe the proper sequence of steps in the removal of a rubber dam
- State the function of the matrix
- Describe the qualities of a properly placed matrix
- Compare the advantages and disadvantages of restorative materials
- Describe the preparation, condensation, and carving of dental amalgam
- Describe an acceptable amalgam-polishing technique
- List the procedures necessary for proper mercury hygiene in a dental office
- Describe the placement and finishing of composite resin
- Describe the preparation, placement, and finishing of glass ionomer cements
- Describe the rationale for using liners and bases
- State the rationale for and function of temporary or interim restorations
- Describe the technique for preparing zinc phosphate cement to both luting and base consistencies

INTRODUCTION

When a client's human need for a biologically sound dentition is in deficit, it is necessary to intervene with therapies that restore the oral cavity to a state of health. Restorative therapies are the dental services that restore the dentition to a state of health, support the maintenance of health, and provide aesthetic modifications to the dentition.

The modified patterns of dental disease are best exemplified by the documented reduction of dental caries in the United States and Canada.[1-5] Of additional significance is the documented increase in life expectancy and retention of the natural dentition, and the decrease in the number of individuals reported to be edentulous. In the recent past, the focus of restorative therapies was on the child and young adult. A shift in focus toward the adult and elderly is now apparent. With this shift in focus comes an increased concern for replacement therapy, the maintenance of the restored dentition, and care of root caries.[6]

Although the number of dental hygienists who actually perform the full range of restorative therapies presented in this chapter may be low, all dental hygienists are expected to perform tooth assessments and provide educational information about restorative therapies. Therefore, it is important for all dental hygienists to understand the rationale and goals of restorative therapy, the types of restorations, and the procedures involved in the restorative process.

RATIONALE FOR RESTORATIVE THERAPY

Restorative therapy includes the restoration of damaged tooth structure, defective restorations, aesthetic inconsistencies, and anatomical and physiological abnormalities. In many cases, restorative therapy prevents tooth loss by halting the progression of a disease process.

Restorative therapy requires a licensed dentist's diagnosis and dental treatment planning. In some states and provinces, some restorative dental treatment may be legally delegated by the dentist to the licensed dental hygienist.

Human beings have a need for a biologically sound dentition, which includes such factors as intact teeth, comfort, adequate function, and acceptable aesthetic appearance. Deficits in this human need may be indicated by tooth damage, defective restorations, and aesthetic, occlusal, or masticatory needs. Because many restorative procedures enhance the aesthetic appearance as well as the function of the dentition, the relationship of these procedures to the individual's human needs for a wholesome body image and nutrition also is addressed.

The restoration process requires the surgical removal of dental tissues such as enamel and dentin. Unlike most other body tissues, these structures do not regenerate and their removal is permanent. The replacement of the natural dental tissues with restorative materials of metals, resins, cements, and porcelain presents a compromise of the original form and function of the tooth. This concession requires thorough consideration of the human needs and well-being of the client and provision of the highest quality of care.

Tooth Damage

Acquired tooth damage is one of the main reasons for restorative therapy. The types of acquired tooth damage are discussed in Chapter 12.

Aesthetic Appearance

Appearance can be a key element in the motivation of clients toward improved health and well-being. A focus on sexuality and self-image is predominant in the media and thus further influences the consciousness of appearance and aesthetics. Because the smile speaks a thousand words, the appearance of the dentition and dental restorations is increasingly important in our image-conscious society and is an important factor in meeting a person's human need for a wholesome body image. Missing, broken, or obviously decayed teeth are often the reasons for individuals to seek oral healthcare. Dental anomalies such as diastemas, mottled enamel, congenital tooth defects, and intrinsic tooth discolorations such as tetracycline staining also may require restorative interventions to improve appearance. In many cases, the individual's primary goal in seeking dental treatment is to meet the need for a wholesome body image, that is, the improvement of appearance.

One of the main disadvantages of metallic restorations has been their appearance (Fig. 22-1). Because metals do not have the appearance of natural teeth, many clients object to their use. The relatively recent changes in consumer demands for natural-appearing restorations are the result of an unprecedented promotion and availability of **tooth-colored restorative materials.** These materials include composite resin, porcelain, castable ceramics, and glass ionomer cements. All of these materials have distinct limitations, but they can be an answer for the client who is motivated by appearance.

Defective Restorations

Defective restorations are ones that no longer restore the dentition to an acceptable state of form and function. Although restorations are referred to as being temporary or permanent, no restoration can be considered truly permanent. The physical properties of the available restorative materials make them susceptible to alteration and deterioration. However, certain materials have withstood the test of time and are more readily recognized for their wearability. When properly used, gold restorations are the most durable and compatible in the oral environment. Their resistance to corrosion, nonirritating chemistry, and similarity to enamel in texture and wear resistance are qualities that other materials often lack. Amalgam is the most commonly used restorative material in dentistry because of its versatility, workability, and clinical longevity. However, the forces generated through mastication and tooth-to-tooth contact eventually wear the occlusal margins of most amalgam restorations (Fig. 22-2). Tooth-colored composite resin restorations abrade more easily and wear more readily, causing them to deteriorate more rapidly than metal restorations.[7] Cement materials dissolve in the oral environment and may cause the loosening of luted restorations or loss of form in restorations composed entirely of cement.

However, the reasons for defective restorations may not

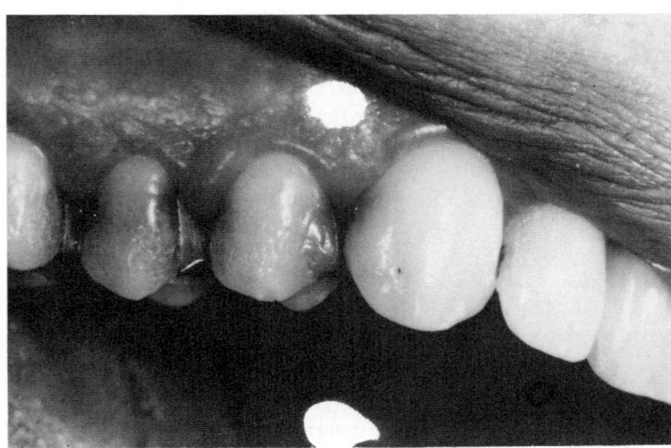

FIGURE 22-1
Tooth darkening due to the display of amalgam and associated internal staining.

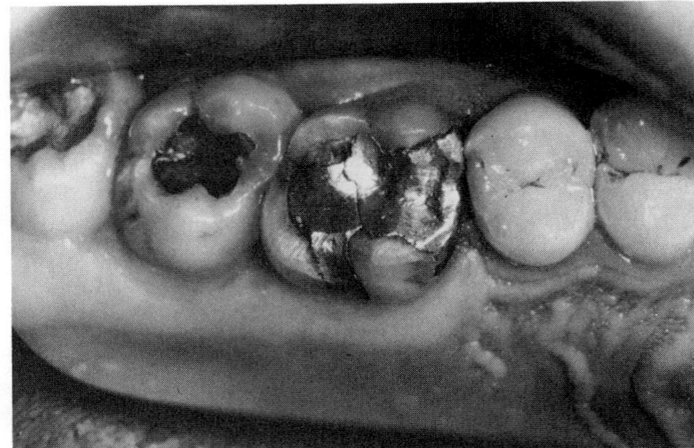

FIGURE 22-2
Large amalgam restoration, which has served for many years despite its poor design, exhibits fracture and defective margins.

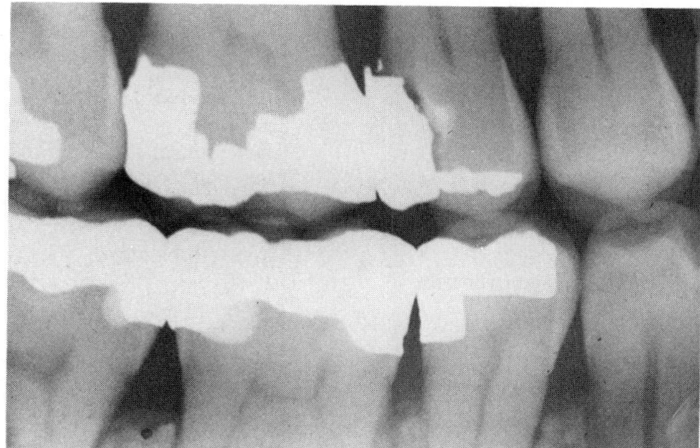

FIGURE 22–3
This radiograph shows poor proximal contour and a gingival overhang on the distal surface of the maxillary first molar. The maxillary second premolar exhibits amalgam fractures and dislodgement.

always be related to the restorative material. Rather, defective restorations can be the fault of the operator placing the restoration. Defects such as **overhangs,** open margins, short margins, poor contours, and open proximal contacts are the result of improper technique, poor judgment, and lack of attention to detail (Figs. 22–3 and 22–4). These are avoidable defects and are not considered acceptable standards of care.

Occlusion

The state of the occlusal relationship influences the function and health of the dentition. Various levels of restorative treatment can be provided to improve a person's occlusion. There are times when an occlusal adjustment, the selective reshaping of the dentition by grinding, improves the occlusion. This is especially true when previous restorations have been poorly shaped or contoured. When teeth become malaligned because of the loss of adjacent or opposing teeth, it may be necessary to recontour them to establish a stable and functional occlusion (Fig. 22–5). In some cases, complex restorations are necessary if this recontouring results in substantial tooth crown removal.

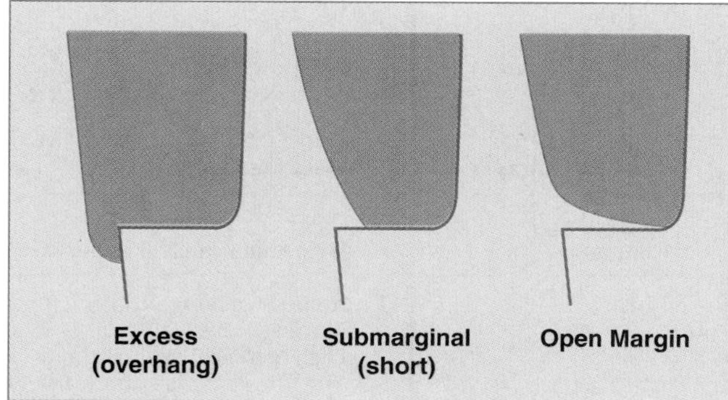

FIGURE 22–4
This illustration depicts possible defects at the gingival margins of restorations. It may be possible to remove an overhang without replacing the restoration; however, restorations with short and open margins require replacement.

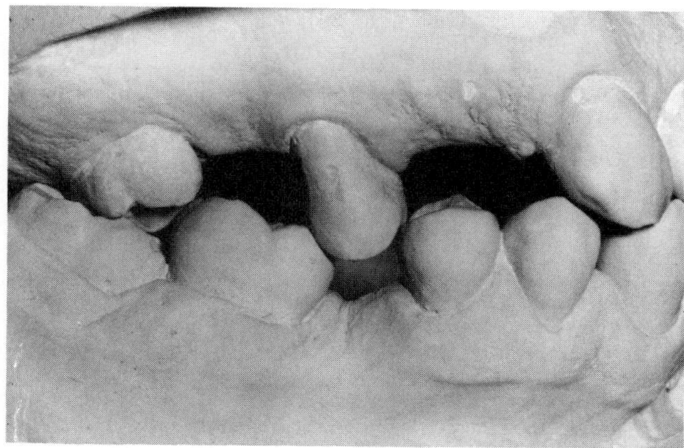

FIGURE 22–5
Tooth loss has resulted in pathological occlusion from tooth movement (tip, drift, and extrusion).

Complete coronal restorations (crowns) and even fixed partial dentures are necessary to restore occlusion in badly damaged dentitions.

Mastication

The most basic function of teeth is to chew food and thus begin the process of digestion. Early humans relied on their teeth much more than modern humans because primitive diets consisted of unrefined and coarse foods. The teeth and jaws served as valuable tools and their loss was crippling to survival.

Many modern food products require little or no chewing to provide adequate nutrition and digestion. Liquid foods and vitamins successfully supplement the diets of many people. Furthermore, many partially edentulous individuals seem to function well enough. It is not uncommon to hear of a person's ability to eat peanuts, crisp apples, or corn on the cob despite being partially or completely edentulous. For these individuals, functioning without replacements for the natural dentition is not a great hardship. A significant number of clients, however, have a chief complaint regarding their inability to chew adequately. Often frustration exists because certain favorite foods are difficult to chew. In addition to having favored foods, individuals have favored areas of the dentition with which they masticate. A missing tooth, defective restoration, or carious lesion can compromise an individual's eating pleasure and contribute to a deficit in his human need for nutrition.

CLASSIFICATIONS FOR CARIOUS LESIONS AND RESTORATIONS

Several classification systems are used to describe the type and location of dental caries and restorations. These classification systems are essential and expedite communication among the parties involved in the delivery of dental services. The classification of carious lesions and restorations varies, depending on the information to be conveyed: the type of caries or restorations, the location of the lesions or restorations, and the cavity preparation required to restore the tooth (see Chapter 12).

Carious lesions and restorations can be found on any of the surfaces of the tooth. As a result, the specific location

TABLE 22–1
DIRECT RESTORATIONS

Material	Primary Area of Use	Main Advantages	Main Disadvantages
Direct gold (foil, mat, and powder)	All Small cavities Avoid occlusal stress	Marginal seal Durability	High technical skill required Color
Silver amalgam	Posterior	Ease of placement Minimal leakage over time	Marginal breakdown Tarnish Color
Composite resin	All Avoid occlusal stress	Color Relative ease of placement	Occlusal wear Leakage
Glass ionomer cement	Class 5 (gumline cavities)	Ease of placement Bonds to enamel and dentin Fair color Releases fluoride	Easily abraded

on the tooth must be identified when completing tooth assessment and charting findings in the client's record. There are six tooth surfaces:

- Occlusal (O)
- Incisal (I)
- Mesial (M)
- Distal (D)
- Facial (F)
- Lingual (L)

TYPES OF RESTORATIONS

Restorations are categorized by the technique required for placement of the restorative material. These placement techniques have been classified as direct and indirect. **Direct restorations** are placed and formed directly in the cavity preparation. These restorations are typically placed in increments, adapted closely to the cavity walls, and shaped to the desired contours. The shaping is done with carvers when the materials are still in a soft or unset state and with rotating instruments such as burs and discs when the restorative materials are in a hard or set state. The materials used in direct restorations include moldable substances such as silver amalgam, composite resin, glass ionomer cement, and direct gold. The restorative procedures that have been legally delegated to dental hygienists fall within this direct restoration category. Table 22–1 outlines the uses, advantages, and disadvantages of direct restorative materials.

In contrast, **indirect restorations** are formed on reproductions (dies) of prepared teeth. The shaping of the restoration is done by preparing the desired form in wax and then casting this form in metal or ceramic. Porcelain restorations are formed by building the restoration to shape with porcelain powder and then solidifying the mass in a special "firing" oven. Gold inlays and porcelain crowns are typical indirect restorations. Because indirect restorations are rigid and solid objects, the cavity preparation must be specially designed to allow complete seating of the restoration at the time of permanent cementation. Table 22–2 outlines the uses, advantages, and disadvantages of indirect restorative materials.

CAVITY PREPARATION

A critical step in restoring the dentition is the preparation of the **cavity**. The form of the cavity preparation is dependent on the reason for restoration and the type of restoration. The intent of this section is not to discuss in detail the fundamentals of cavity preparation, but rather to present an overview of considerations essential to each member of the oral health team. Effective communication among dental practitioners supports the efficiency with

TABLE 22–2
INDIRECT RESTORATIONS

Material	Primary Area of Use	Main Advantages	Main Disadvantages
Gold alloy	Posterior (inlays and crowns)	Durability Contours	Color High technical skill required
Porcelain	All (inlays and crowns)	Color	Abrades opposing teeth Marginal seal High technical skill required
Castable ceramic	All (inlays and crowns)	Color	Marginal seal High technical skill required
Porcelain fused to metal	All (crowns)	Color Strength Marginal seal	Abrades opposing teeth High technical skill required

which oral health services are delivered. Essential to effective communication is a standardized nomenclature for cavity preparations. A basic understanding of the principles and instrumentation of cavity preparation supports the dental hygienist in the role of clinician, client advocate, and educator.

Nomenclature

The landmarks of prepared cavities require special description for the oral health team to communicate effectively. It is essential to consider two aspects when discussing the nomenclature of cavity preparations. First are the tooth surfaces to be involved in the preparation and second are the internal aspects of the preparation. When considering the tooth surfaces involved, it is important to remember that involvement may not be limited to those surfaces exhibiting carious lesions. For example, a tooth exhibiting a lesion on only the distal surface will likely require a cavity preparation involving the occlusal and distal surfaces. This cavity design is logically described as a "distoocclusal" (DO) preparation. When naming a cavity preparation with more than one involved surface, the "al" ending is dropped from and an "o" added to all surface names except the final identified surface (i.e., mesioocclusodistal—MOD). When communicating regarding the internal aspects of a cavity preparation, commonly used terms such as "top," "bottom," "side," and "left" are not very useful when referring to the minute details of a cavity preparation. A cavity nomenclature, a system of classifying the anatomical features of a cavity preparation, has been designed to facilitate communication. All cavity preparations have walls, angles, and margins. **Walls** are vertical or horizontal surfaces within the cavity preparation. They are usually named according to the closest tooth surface or approximating dental tissue. A simple occlusal cavity preparation (class 1) on a mandibular molar has five walls:

- Mesial (M)
- Distal (D)
- Facial (F)
- Lingual (L)
- Pulpal (P)

The mesial, distal, facial, and lingual walls appear as verti-

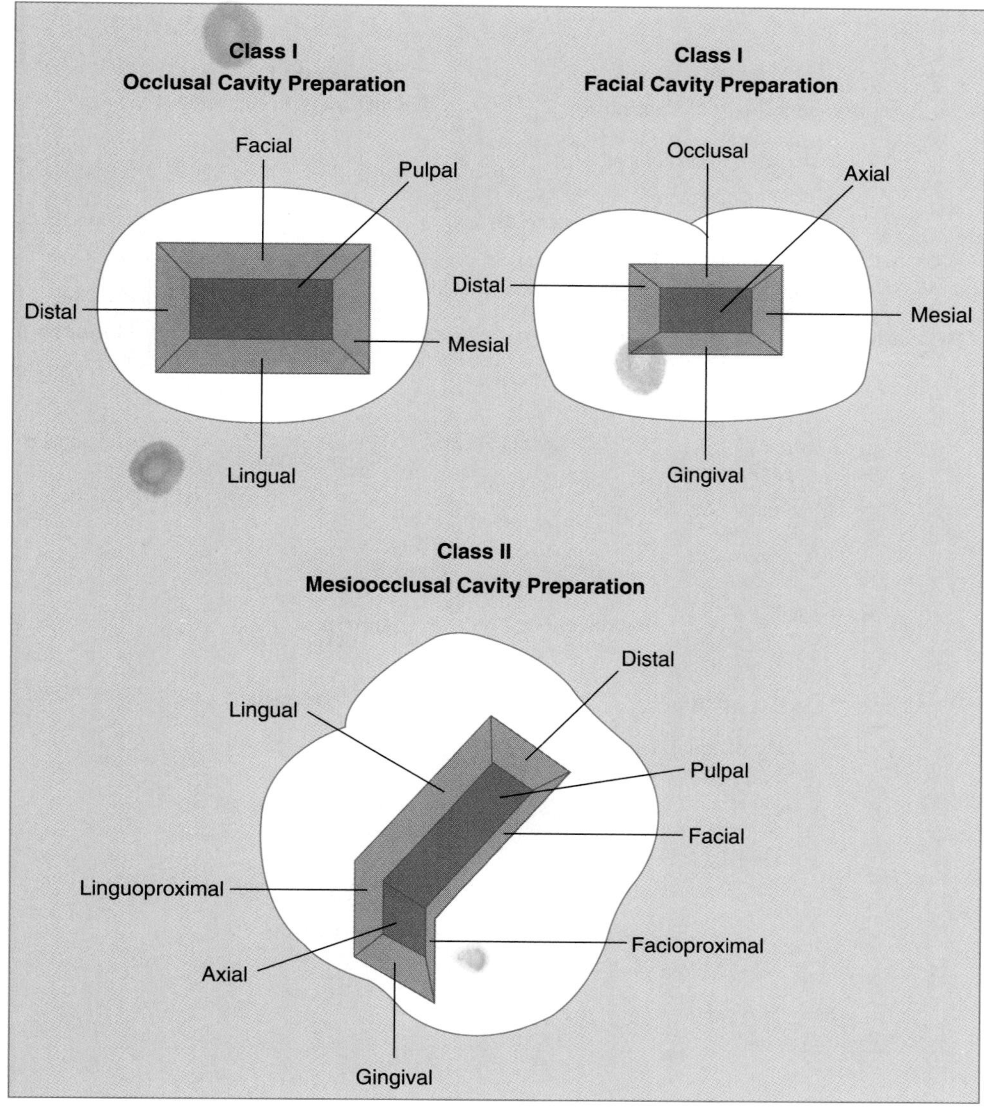

FIGURE 22–6
Schematic representation of the *walls* of class 1 and class 2 cavity preparations.

cal surfaces that closely approximate the corresponding tooth surfaces. The pulpal wall, named because of its proximity to the pulp, appears as a horizontal surface. Another term frequently associated with the pulpal wall is "pulpal floor." When visualizing a mandibular molar in a vertical position, it is easy to envision a floor surrounded by four walls. Another common area of reference is the long axis of the tooth. A wall aligned in the same general direction as the axis is termed an "axial (A) wall." A simple facial or lingual cavity preparation (class 1) on a mandibular molar also has five walls: mesial, distal, occlusal, gingival, and axial. The mesial, distal, occlusal, and gingival walls again are so named because of their proximity to specific tooth surfaces. The axial wall appears as a vertical surface in keeping with the long axis of the tooth (Fig. 22–6).

Line angles are formed by the meeting of two walls. They are usually named according to the walls involved. The naming of line angles follows the same procedure as naming carious lesions with multiple decayed surfaces; the "al" is dropped from and an "o" added to the first wall designation and the second wall name remains unchanged. For example, the mandibular molar with a simple occlusal cavity preparation and five walls has eight line angles formed by the meeting of the vertical and horizontal walls. These line angles are named:

- Mesiolingual (ML) line angle
- Distolingual (DL) line angle
- Mesiofacial (MF) line angle
- Distofacial (DF) line angle
- Mesiopulpal (MP) line angle
- Distopulpal (DP) line angle
- Faciopulpal (FP) line angle
- Linguopulpal (LP) line angle (Fig. 22–7)

The one exception to this rule for naming line angles is found in anterior proximal cavity preparations (class 3). Because the cavity form is typically a triangle, the line angle at the junction of the facial and lingual walls can be called the "faciolingual line angle." However, the more commonly accepted term is "incisal line angle" (Fig. 22–8). The walls and line angles meet the unaltered tooth surface at the **cavosurface** (cavity–tooth surface) **margin.**

The meeting of three walls results in a **point angle.** Point angles also are named according to the involved walls. When naming the point angles the "al" is dropped and an "o" is added to the first two walls with the name of the

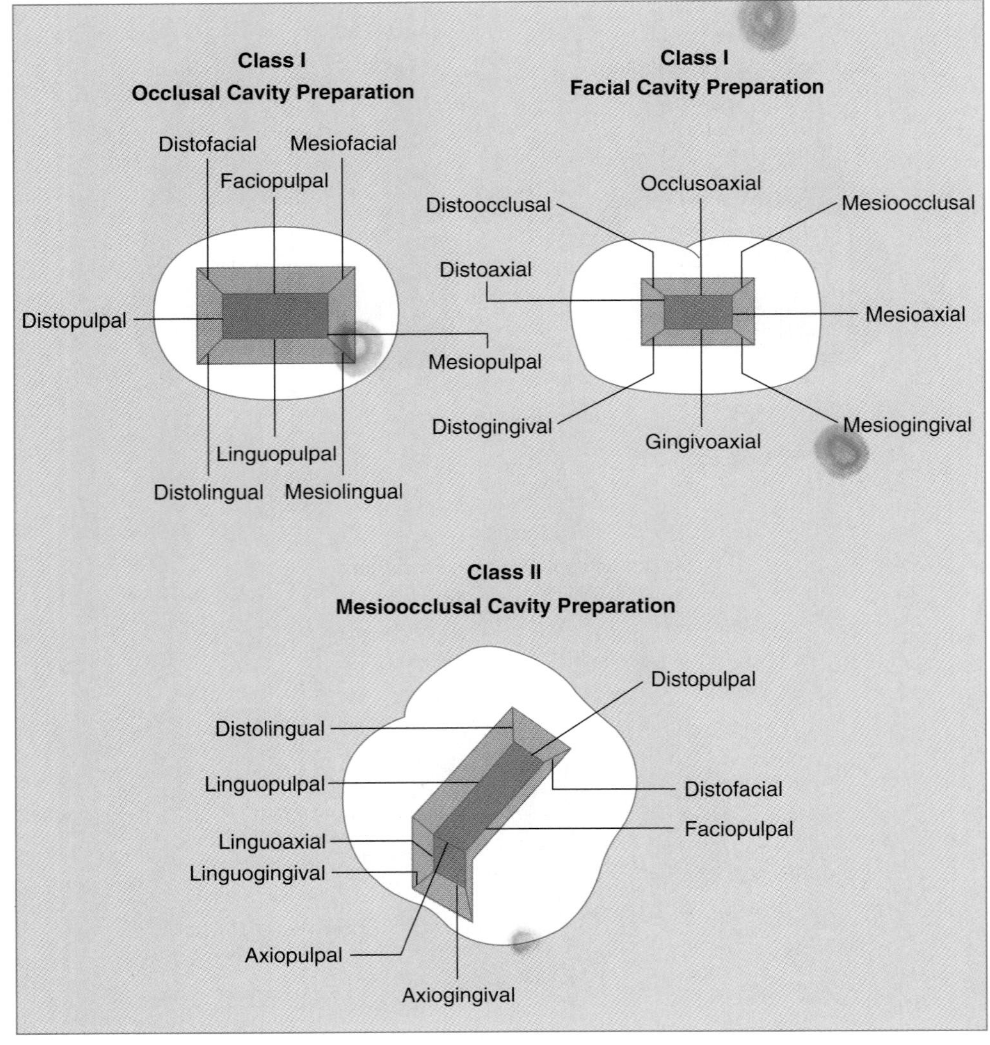

FIGURE 22–7
Schematic representation of the *line angles* of class 1 and class 2 cavity preparations.

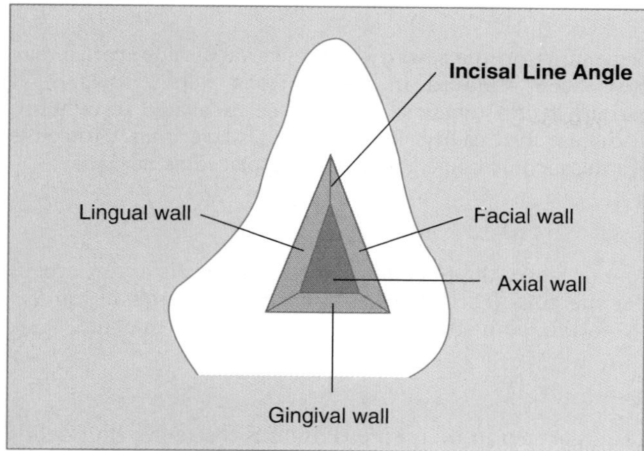

FIGURE 22–8
Schematic representation of the *incisal line angle* of a class 3 cavity preparation.

final wall left unchanged. The four point angles in the occlusal cavity preparation of the mandibular molar are:

- Mesiolinguopulpal (MLP) point angle
- Distolinguopulpal (DLP) point angle
- Mesiofaciopulpal (MFP) point angle
- Distofaciopulpal (DFP) point angle (Fig. 22–9)

More anatomical features are seen in posterior cavity preparations with proximal involvement. These are the proximal line angles and point angles, which also are named according to adjoining walls (see Figs. 22–7 and 22–9). Cavity preparations in anterior teeth have an incisal wall rather than an occlusal wall. The application of the appropriate names of the walls, line angles, cavosurface margins, and point angles defines specific locations within the cavity preparation that are not open to multiple interpretation. The distofaciopulpal point angle can be only one location. Familiarity with these basic landmarks of a cavity preparation enables the oral healthcare professional to spe-

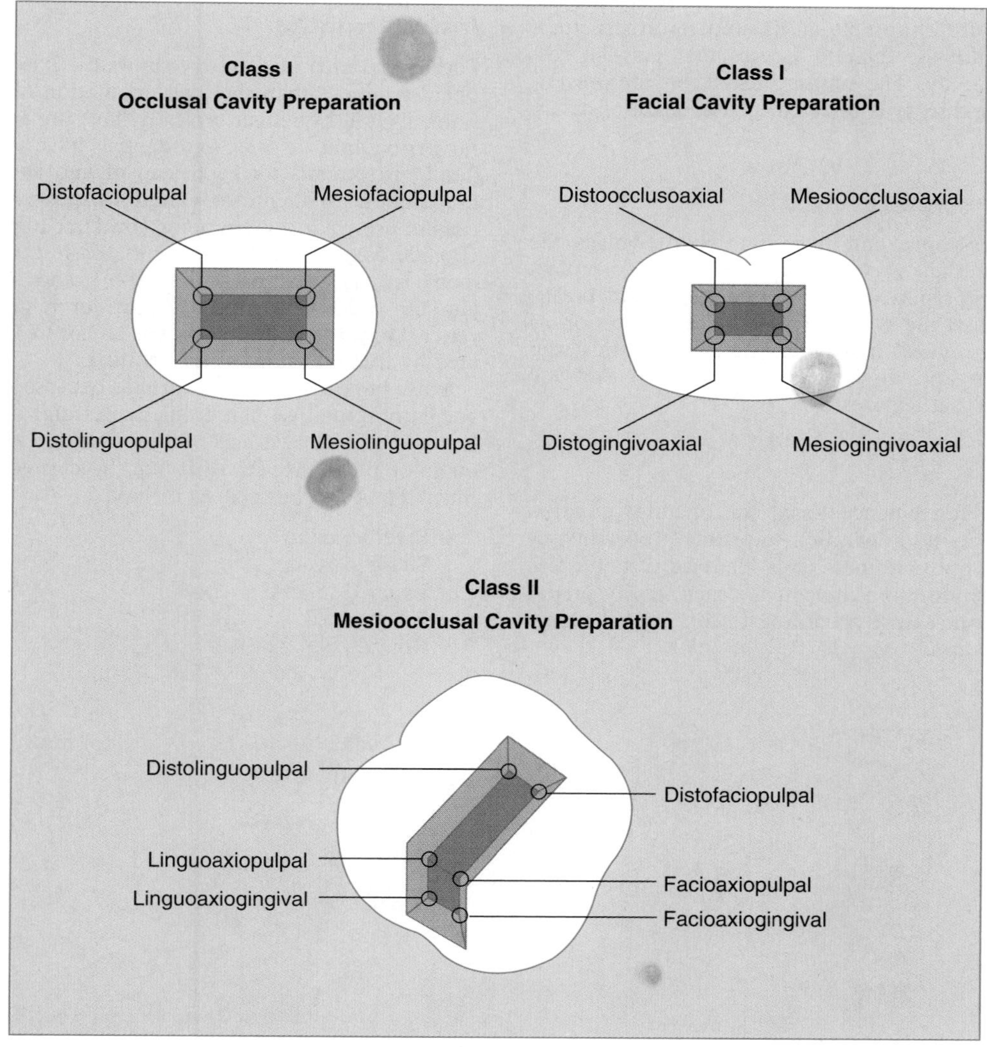

FIGURE 22–9
Schematic representation of the *point angles* of class 1 and class 2 cavity preparations.

cifically identify a location in a cavity preparation and communicate it exactly.

Principles

Although the dental hygienist is not responsible for cavity preparation, there is value in understanding that there is a systematic procedure of cavity preparation that is based on well-established biomechanical principles. Cavity preparation typically follows a series of six steps:

1. Establish the outline form
2. Obtain the resistance and the retention form
3. Obtain the convenience form
4. Remove caries
5. Finish the enamel
6. Debride the cavity

Outline Form

The establishment of an outline form provides the framework from which the remainder of the cavity preparation develops. This step includes the removal of weak or undermined enamel and existing defective restorative materials. The preparation margins should extend laterally beyond the decay or defect into cleansable and sound tooth structure. The outline should also include fissures that may be susceptible to new decay. The phrase "extension for prevention" of recurring disease is directed to this phase of cavity preparation.

Resistance and Retention Form

Obtaining the resistance and retention form involves the shaping of the internal aspects of the preparation to protect the tooth and restoration from forces that result in breakage. It also prevents the dislodgement of the restoration as a result of forces against it. Primary concerns in this step are the extension and direction of cavity walls and the refinement of internal features.

Convenience Form

In obtaining the convenience form, the operator enlarges and extends the cavity preparation to enable proper instrumentation for an optimal final result. Because certain areas of the dental arch are more difficult to reach, cavity preparations may vary in extent according to the needed access and visual field.

Caries Removal

Depending on the severity of the carious lesion, caries may have been removed in the previous steps. However, if carious dentin remains, it should be excavated to establish a disease-free cavity. It is at this stage that protective agents, such as liners and bases, are placed as needed.

Finish Enamel

At this stage, the operator smooths the walls and sharpens the margins. This supports the desired marginal seal between the tooth structure and the restorative material.

Débridement

The final step in cavity preparation is the removal of debris and moisture that compromise the restoration. This is typically accomplished with the water and air syringe.

Each tooth and cavity presents a unique challenge to the practitioner. The severity of the carious lesion influences the complexity of the cavity preparation process. However, these fundamental steps to cavity preparation result in a cavity ready for restoration.

Instrumentation

Perhaps no area of dentistry shows the individuality among operators more than the instrumentation of cavity preparations. Dental hygienists typically have preferred instruments for periodontal therapy, and dentists have favorite burs and hand instruments for each step of and situation in cavity preparation. With minor variations, however, most practitioners use rotary instruments (burs) at high speeds (above 100,000 rpm) to rapidly shape the basic cavity preparation. Slow speeds (up to 10,000 rpm) and medium speeds (10,000 to 100,000 rpm) are used for refinement. Air and water spray are commonly used to control the heat generated by friction during rotary cutting.

Most burs are made of carbide because of its durability and cutting ability. Bur head shapes and sizes are numerous and are selected according to the dental procedure and operator preference in achieving the desired internal cavity form. The basic bur shapes include:

- Inverted cone
- Straight fissure
- Tapered fissure
- Pear-shaped
- Round (Fig. 22–10)

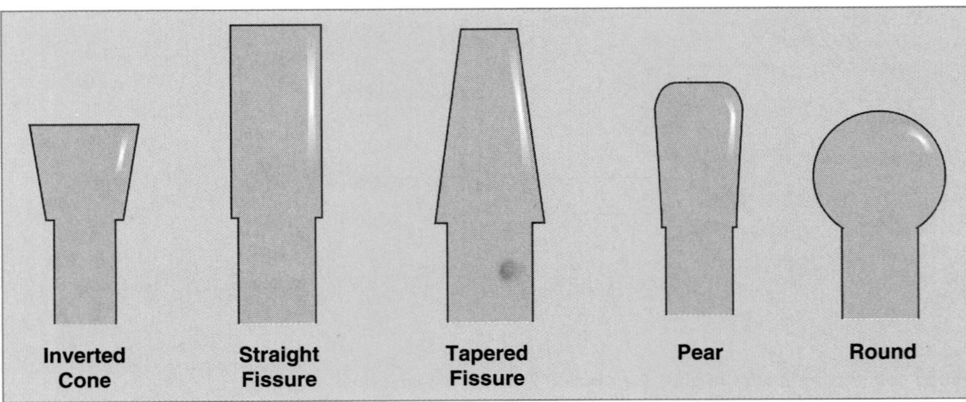

FIGURE 22–10
Profiles of common bur shapes.

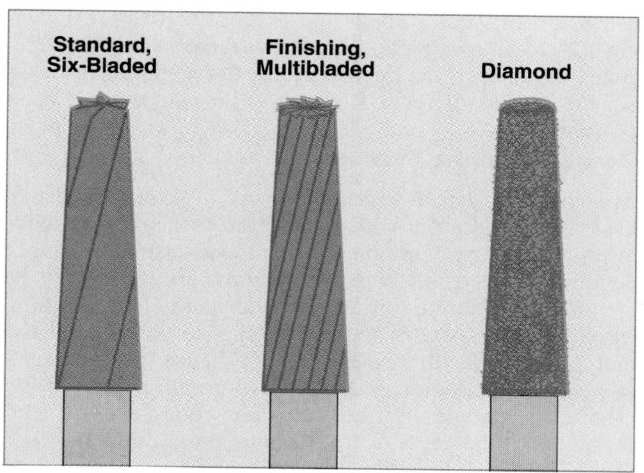

FIGURE 22-11
Comparison of burs.

The size of the bur is numerically indicated within each shape category, with the smaller numbers indicating a smaller bur head. Finishing burs are similar to standard burs except that they contain more blades. Other popular rotary instruments used for cavity preparation include diamond burs, which have diamond particle abrasives welded to the instrument head (Fig. 22-11). These also are available in numerous shapes, sizes, and grit configurations.

Hand instrumentation is used by many operators to provide exact detail to the inner cavity form and cavity margins. The hand-cutting instrument has three basic parts (Fig. 22-12):

- Blade
- Shank
- Handle or shaft

To deliver firm, controlled forces to the cutting edge, instruments must be designed to bring this area closely in line with the axis of the handle. Shank design can facilitate the desired control. Three common shank designs are (Fig. 22-13):

- Straight
- Monangle
- Binangle

Cutting instruments can be classified into two basic groups that describe their primary function. *Chisels* are chiefly used for planing enamel and include hatchets and gingival margin trimmers (Fig. 22-14). *Excavators* are primarily used for refining the internal cavity and include hoes and angle formers (Fig. 22-15). As with periodontal instruments, the efficient use of hand-cutting instruments requires very sharp cutting edges on the blade.

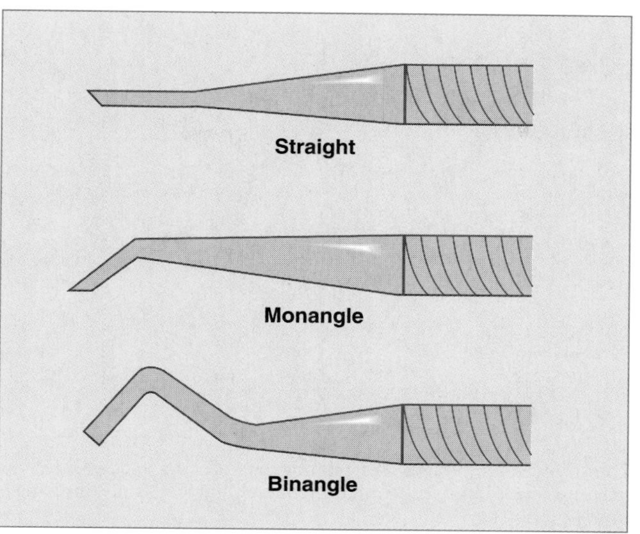

FIGURE 22-13
Hand instrument shank variations.

ROLE OF THE DENTAL HYGIENIST

The dental hygienist originally was chiefly responsible for the prevention of oral disease and thus the recognition today as an oral disease preventive and health promotion specialist. However, in the 1960s and 1970s, it was further theorized that the dental hygienist could play a significant role in supporting the health of the dentition through the delivery of restorative therapies. It was at this time that the primary focus of the dental profession was on improving the oral health of the public through the elimination and treatment of dental caries. Thus, the rationale for the initial delegation of restorative services was to provide a mechanism to respond to an expanding need and demand for dental care, and dental hygienists became responsible for **expanded functions.**

There is wide variability in the extent of delegation of restorative functions to the dental hygienist. In some legal jurisdictions, the dental hygienist is permitted to perform a broad range of restorative therapies including the placement and removal of the rubber dam; placement and removal of matrices and wedges; placement and removal of temporary restorations; placement of cavity liners and bases; placement, carving and finishing of permanent restorations; and amalgam polishing. In other jurisdictions the restorative scope of dental hygiene practice may be restricted to only amalgam polishing and placement and removal of the rubber dam. The restorative functions most commonly permitted for delegation to the dental hygienist include the placement and removal of the rubber dam,

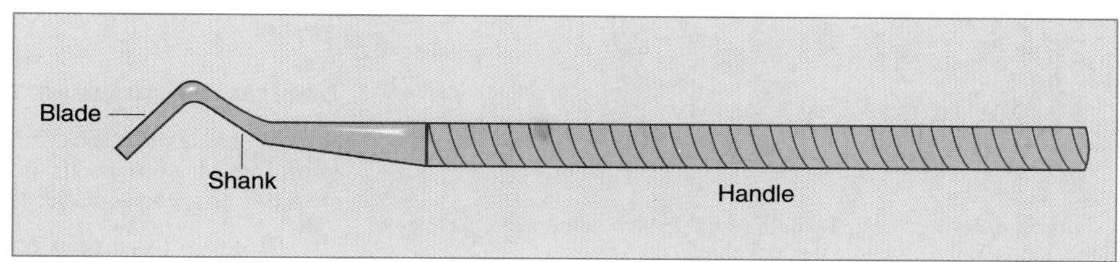

FIGURE 22-12
Basic hand instrument design.

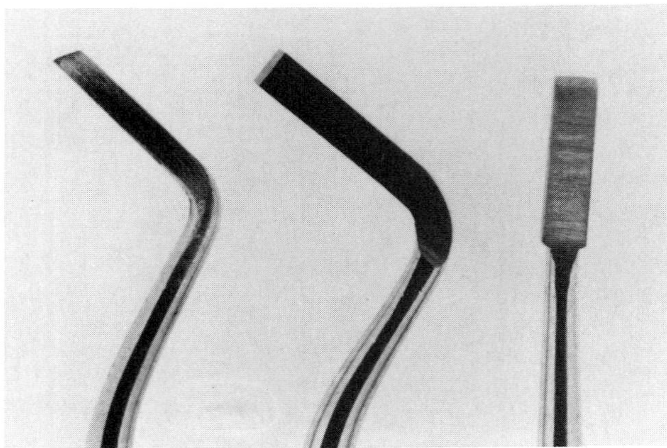

FIGURE 22–14
Common chisel designs for planing enamel. As pictured left to right, gingival margin trimmer, enamel hatchet, and monangle chisel.

placement and removal of matrices and wedges, placement of temporary restorations, and amalgam polishing.[8–10]

Because the scope of dental hygiene practice varies dramatically among states, provinces, and territories, not all educational programs prepare dental hygienists to practice in all locations in the United States and Canada. The procedures included in this chapter span the full range of restorative interventions delegated to the dental hygienist in the United States and Canada. It is the responsibility of the dental hygienist to be knowledgeable of the law pertinent to dental hygiene and to practice within the limits of that law. It is unacceptable to perform illegal functions at the directive of the dentist, client, or any other person. The dental hygienist has the legal and ethical responsibility to practice within the scope of the law at all times.

The participation of the dental hygienist in the delivery of restorative therapies affords a unique opportunity for the dentist and dental hygienist to fully utilize the knowledge and talents of the other as care providers. The efficient use of the dentist, dental hygienist, and dental assistant allows all members of the team to maximally use their expertise to deliver quality and cost-effective restorative treatment. Figure 22–16 illustrates the restorative care cycle that integrates the roles of the dentist and dental hygienist throughout the delivery of restorative care to the client.

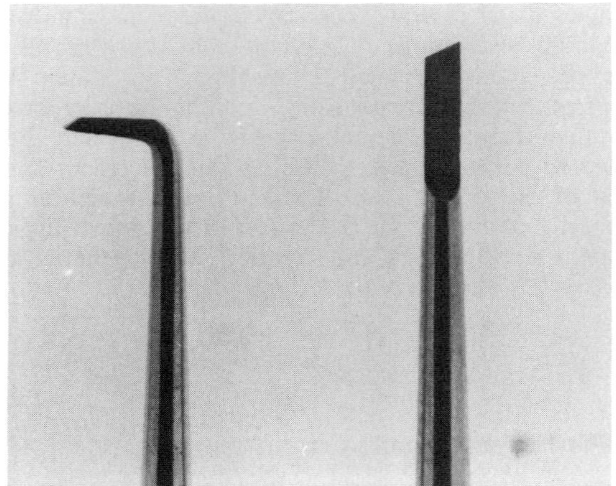

FIGURE 22–15
Common excavator designs for internal cavity refinement. As pictured left to right, hoe and angle former.

Dental Hygiene Process of Care

Applying the dental hygiene process of care, the dental hygienist collaborates with the dentist to achieve effective restoration of the dentition. During the assessment phase of dental hygiene care, tooth damage and its cause may be identified and communicated to the dentist. In addition, based on assessment of the client's oral hygiene status and oral health behaviors, the dental hygienist plans, implements, and evaluates oral disease prevention and health promotion strategies for the client. For example, client education about the cause of tooth damage and the removal of debris from the dentition are necessary to achieving and maintaining the desired quality of tooth restoration.

Definitive Restorative Examination and Dental Diagnosis

A definitive restorative examination by the dentist includes clinical and radiographic evaluation and other diagnostic indicators of disease. For example, certain features of the dentition may be assessed by evaluating accurately mounted casts or study models. Subtleties of the occlusion then may be examined without the interference of the lips, cheeks, and tongue. Interarch and interdental spaces can be measured and wear facets easily noted. A definitive restorative evaluation begins with the client's chief complaint. It integrates all information collected about the client and results in a dental diagnosis and care plan.

RESTORATIVE CARE PLANNING

The dentist is the oral healthcare professional responsible for the development of the restorative care plan. However, it is important that dental hygienists have an understanding of the restorative care planning process because of the important role they play in assessing and fulfilling human need deficits related to oral health and disease.

The restorative care cycle (see Fig. 22–16) includes the development of a care plan that outlines the design to be followed in the delivery of oral health services to the client. A comprehensive care plan should be all-encompassing and should include methods for preventing disease, eliminating disease, restoring health, and maintaining health. The restorative care plan is an essential component of the total care plan, but it is limited in that it focuses primarily on the restorative needs of the client. It is important to recognize that it cannot stand alone and must be integrated into the total care plan. The restorative care plan includes restorative operations that support the goal of the total care plan. The key elements of a restorative care plan are the goals of restorative therapy and the sequence of restorative care.

Goals of Restorative Therapy

Individuals always seek treatment because of some primary stimulus. Human needs that may be addressed through restorative therapy include, but are not limited to:

- Freedom from pain or discomfort from the dentition

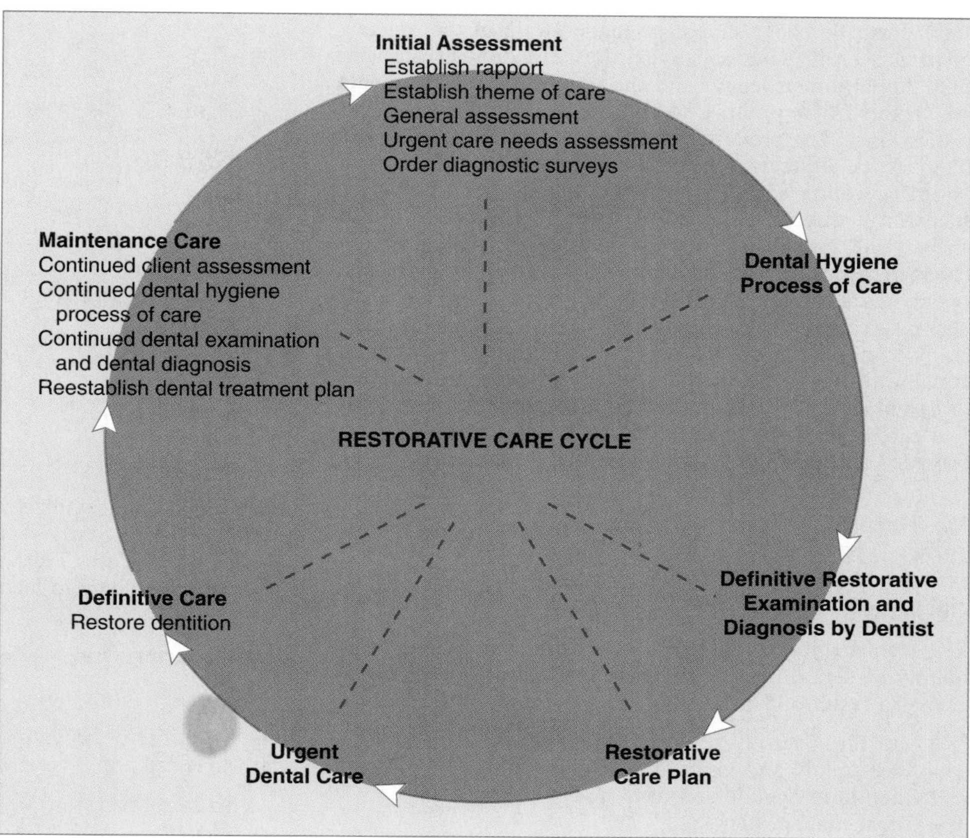

FIGURE 22–16
Comprehensive restorative care cycle.

- Difficulty in chewing (need for sound dentition)
- Dissatisfaction with appearance (need for wholesome body image)
- Desire to prevent dental problems (need for self-determination and responsibility)

Every good restorative care plan has a focus that addresses the client's overriding concern (or human need) for dental care. A client's goal for treatment may also be precipitated by exposure to information from the media. The accuracy and validity of the information vary depending on the source and how it specifically applies to the individual client. As consumer advocates, dental hygienists encourage individuals to be discriminating consumers of oral healthcare and support them in the informed healthcare decisions they make. Oral healthcare professionals, because of their knowledge and expertise, must play a key role in disseminating accurate information to the client. Misinformation, from whatever source, often leads to unrealistic expectations. Thus, based on an individual assessment of the client, the oral healthcare professional meets the client's human need for conceptualization and problem solving by providing education regarding the possibilities and limitations of restorative care.

The final plan of restorative treatment must reflect an agreement between the dentist and an educated client. Restorative materials are selected to best meet the goals of therapy, but they also must be consistent with the client's ability or willingness to pay for service. In cases when the dentist is unable to render the restorative service of choice, there is an ethical obligation to refer the client to a dentist who has the necessary skills and expertise. All plans are subject to change as a result of the development of unknowns; however, these changes are usually minor if the initial plan is based upon a thorough assessment of the restorative needs. The principle of informed consent should be applied and the individual informed of possible modifications to the plan. When properly developed and presented, the restorative care plan builds trust in the client-provider relationship and enables oral healthcare professionals to proceed efficiently with the delivery of care.

Sequence of Care

An essential element in the development of a restorative care plan is the establishment of a sequence of care. The sequence of care, established by the dentist, is the order in which the restorative treatment is placed to achieve the goals of therapy. Having been informed of their restorative needs, it is not unusual for individuals to inquire regarding the length of treatment or the number of appointments required to complete the treatment. Once the focus of treatment has been established and the restorative materials selected, it is possible to proceed with the establishment of a mutually agreed upon schedule of care.

The delivery of care is influenced by factors that are not simply technical in nature. Appointments must be designed to best meet the needs of the client and oral healthcare professionals, in order to achieve expeditiously the goals of therapy. It is sometimes wise to begin with the simplest, least threatening operation as long as the client's welfare is best served. Such an approach can help build client confidence and meet the human need for freedom from stress. However, when early intervention is required to prevent tooth loss, the client should be made aware of the urgency of care, even if it means solving the most difficult problem first. Appointment length and the number of appointments are factors of importance to the client and oral healthcare professional. The preferred sequence and schedule of care is likely to be different for the chronically ill elderly person and the young, healthy college student. Sequencing or scheduling care is designed to meet the needs of each client. The establishment of a positive rapport with the client demands that the concerns and needs of all parties be openly discussed and plans mutually agreed upon. Once the client agrees to the care plan, the oral healthcare team is ready to begin the delivery of care as outlined in the plan. Because of the numerous factors that influence the delivery of dental care, it is important to remember that the restorative care plan should be continuously reassessed as care is provided and new information is made available.

IMPLEMENTATION — RUBBER DAM ISOLATION

Rationale

The primary purpose of the rubber dam is to improve the quality of dental treatment. The effectiveness of the rubber dam is a result of four attributes:

- Moisture control
- Accessibility and visibility
- Client and operator protection
- Client management

The **moisture-control** property of the rubber dam ensures the essential dryness of the operating field and limits contamination by the oral fluids. Furthermore, the properties of the restorative material are preserved and protected in an environment free of moisture. The rubber dam provides accessibility and visibility by retracting the gingival tissue surrounding the site of restoration. The retraction of the cheeks, lips, and tongue from the field of operation also can be achieved with the rubber dam. The background of the dark rubber dam provides excellent contrast with the tooth structure. In addition, the rubber dam reduces glare from the moist surfaces of the tissues of the oral cavity. The client is protected by the rubber dam because it limits the possibility of aspirating or swallowing debris and materials associated with cavity preparation and restoration. The rubber dam also may protect the oral tissues from instruments and medications that may be injurious or distasteful. Additional protection may occur by the isolation of a tooth from contamination by saliva if pulp exposure occurs and the isolation of the oral cavity from exposure to noxious materials during an endodontic procedure. The client's and the practitioner's human need for safety is facilitated by the rubber dam because of its barrier properties, which limit the spread of microorganisms during dental treatment.[11] Client management is facilitated by promoting relaxation and discouraging conversation.

The disadvantages of the rubber dam most often cited are time consumption and client objection; however, objections are not universally accepted.[12] The efficient practitioner overcomes the perception of the procedure as time-consuming. The quality of restorations completed with the rubber dam should outweigh any perceived inconvenience. Client objection can usually be overcome with education, although there are certain instances when rubber dam application is contraindicated because of medical complications such as secondary herpetic lesions, cracks or fissures of the commissures, respiratory congestion, claustrophobia, asthma, and allergy to latex.

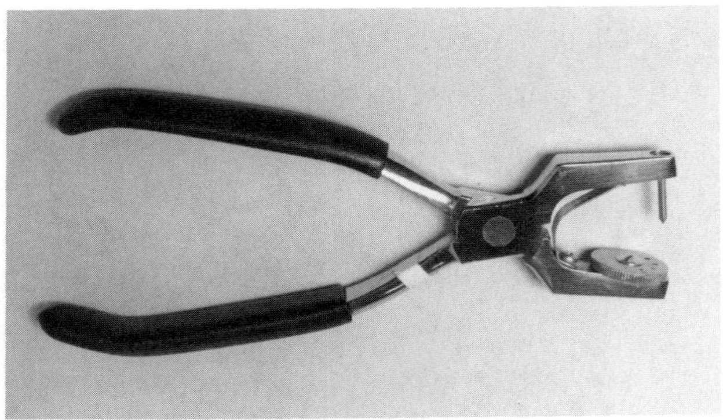

FIGURE 22–17
Rubber dam punch.

Armamentarium

Rubber Dam Material

The features to be considered in the selection of rubber dam material are

- Size (in inches)
- Weight
- Color

The rubber dam material is typically marketed as a sheet of latex in 5- × 5-inch or 6- × 6-inch dimensions. The 5 × 5 size is recommended for the child, and the 6 × 6 size is recommended for the adult. Rubber dam material is also available in rolls so that the rubber dam may be cut to the dimensions desired by the operator. The available weights of rubber dam material are light, medium, heavy, and extra heavy. The lighter weight, thinner dams are easier to apply because of their flexibility and comfort to the client, whereas the heavier weight, thicker dams provide better retraction of tissues and protection from revolving instruments. The medium and heavy weights are most commonly used for restorative procedures. The rubber dam material is available in an assortment of colors: black, gray, green, blue, and pastels. Many of these materials now are pleasantly scented. Although the color selection is based on operator preference, the main issues to consider in color

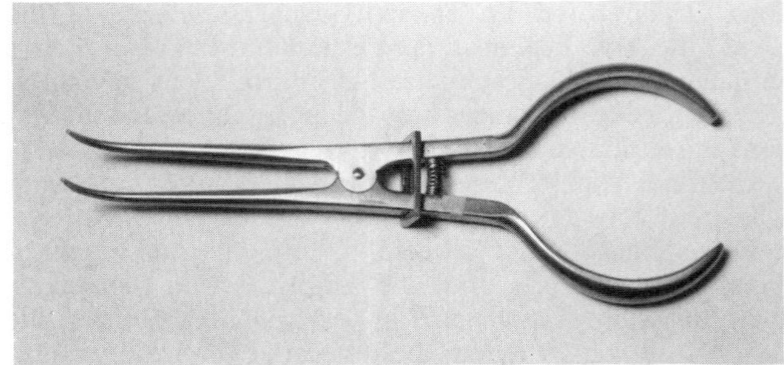

FIGURE 22–18
Rubber dam forceps.

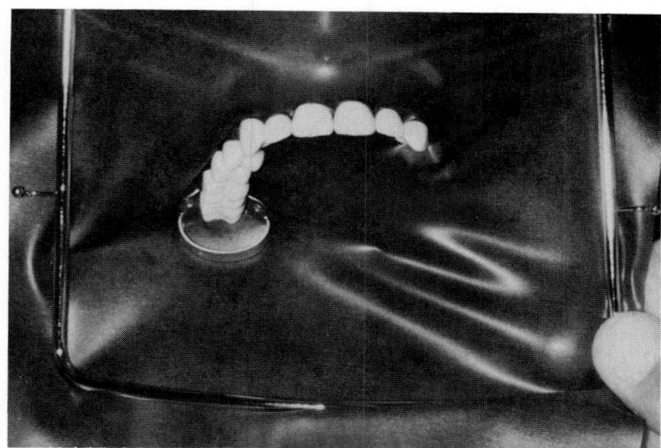

FIGURE 22-19
The rubber dam frame is used to secure the edges of the rubber dam.

selection are the contrast with the teeth and the comfort to the eye.

Rubber Dam Punch

The rubber dam punch is used to punch the tooth holes in the rubber dam material (Fig. 22-17). The rubber dam punch typically has five to six hole sizes. The punch requires regular maintenance, which includes oiling of the movable parts and dry or chemical sterilization rather than autoclaving for infection control.

Rubber Dam Forceps

The rubber dam forceps are used to place the rubber dam clamp on the anchor tooth (Fig. 22-18). The instrument is a pliers-like forceps that expands the rubber dam clamp for placement on the tooth. The beaks of the forceps are placed into the holes of the clamp, and by squeezing the handles of the forceps, the beaks are separated and the clamp expanded. The rubber dam forceps have a locking device that may be engaged by squeezing the handles, turning the forceps upside down, thus dropping the locking device into position, and releasing the handles.

Rubber Dam Frame

The rubber dam frame is used to secure the extraoral rubber dam material (Fig. 22-19). There are several styles of frames available for operator preference. However, the frames of choice must be able to be sterilized. The rubber dam frame is most commonly stainless steel and U shaped with small projections for securing the edges of the rubber dam sheet.

Rubber Dam Clamp

The rubber dam clamp provides the intraoral stabilization of the rubber dam material by anchoring the material securely in place. The rubber dam clamp is produced in winged and wingless design. The parts of the rubber dam clamp include the jaws, prongs, bow, and forceps holes (Fig. 22-20). The prongs of the clamp contact the clamped tooth and the bow joins the two jaws. The forceps holes are the insertion point for the rubber dam forceps during the placement and removal of the clamp.

Clamp designs are identified by number. Winged and wingless clamps of the same number are identical in shape, however, the letter W is used to designate the wingless clamp. The wings of a clamp provide additional retraction of the rubber dam material away from the clamped tooth. Clamps come in numerous shapes and sizes to take into consideration various factors such as the specific tooth to be clamped (permanent or primary), the stage of eruption of the tooth to be clamped, and the access needed for the operation (Fig. 22-21). The success of the rubber dam isolation depends largely on the stability of the rubber dam clamp.

Rubber Dam Material Preparation

The operator is encouraged to custom punch the rubber dam for each client in order to best achieve the goals of isolation. The mandibular rubber dam should be divided into sixths by:

- Dividing the dam in half horizontally
- Dividing the dam into thirds vertically

The **key punch** (the hole that guides the placement of all remaining holes) for the mandibular posterior dam is the hole for the most distal tooth to be isolated. Figure 22-22

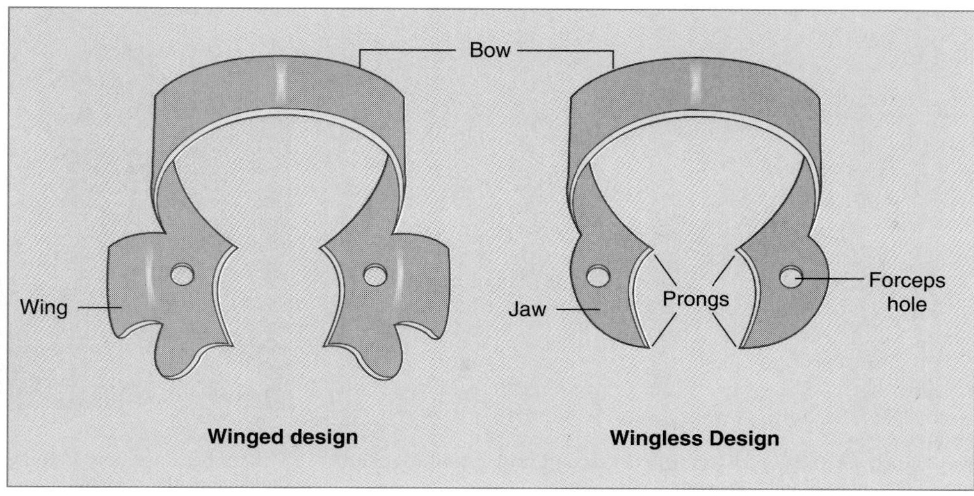

FIGURE 22-20
Rubber dam clamp basic design and parts.

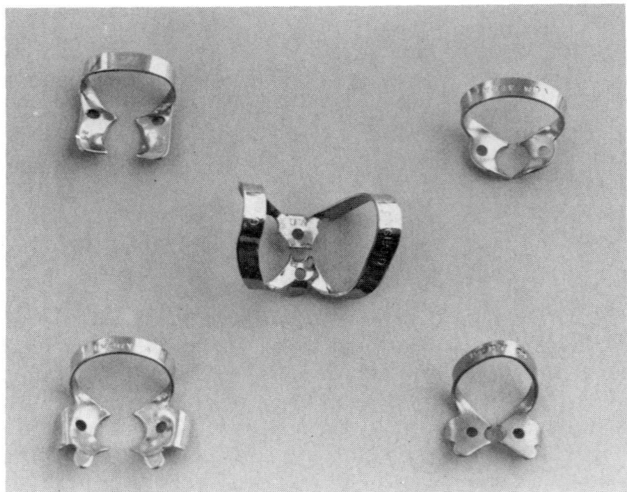

FIGURE 22–21
Rubber dam clamp variations. *Upper left and right,* Wingless molar clamps. *Lower right,* Winged premolar clamp. *Lower left,* Winged molar clamp. *Center,* Anterior clamp.

illustrates the placement of the key punch for first, second, and third molars. The key punch for the mandibular anterior rubber dam is for a mandibular central incisor. The placement is at the midsection of the lower half of the dam and 1.5 to 2.0 mm left or right of the center of the dam (Fig. 22–23). The maxillary rubber dam should be divided into fourths by:

- Marking the horizontal line approximately 1 inch below the top of the dam (when the rubber dam punch is positioned as seen in Figure 22–24, it is a handy guide for determining the location of the horizontal line)
- Dividing the dam in half vertically

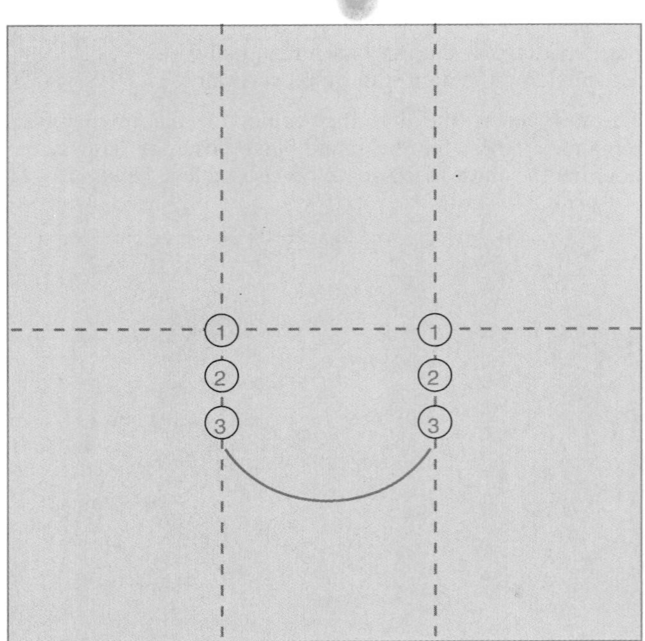

FIGURE 22–22
Key punch for the (1) first molar, (2) second molar, and (3) third molar in a mandibular posterior rubber dam.

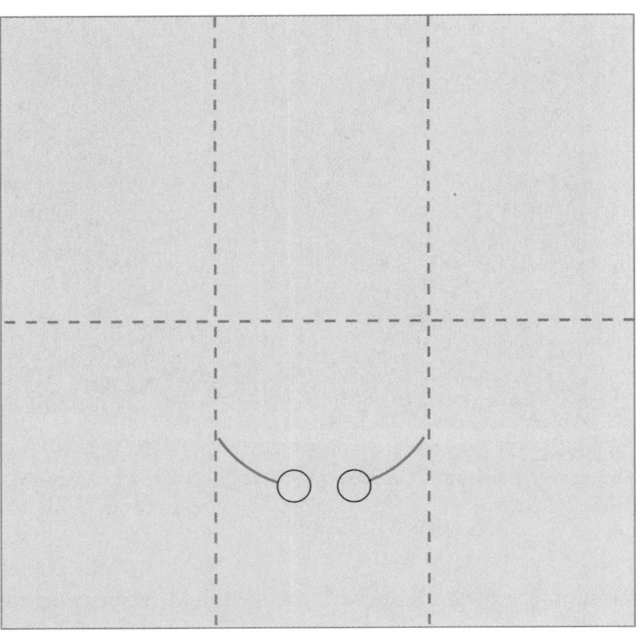

FIGURE 22–23
Key punch for the left or right central incisor in a mandibular anterior rubber dam.

The key punch for maxillary posterior and anterior rubber dams is the central incisor. Generally, there are 3 to 4 mm between the holes for the right and left central incisors, and they are placed at the center of the dam on the horizontal line (Fig. 22–25).

Following the placement of the key punch, the remainder of the holes are placed according to tooth position (and other factors identified in the dental assessment) and a few general guidelines. The size of the hole should correspond with the size of the tooth. The tooth to be clamped may require a double or triple hole (Fig. 22–26). Because the number of holes in a rubber dam punch vary, specific

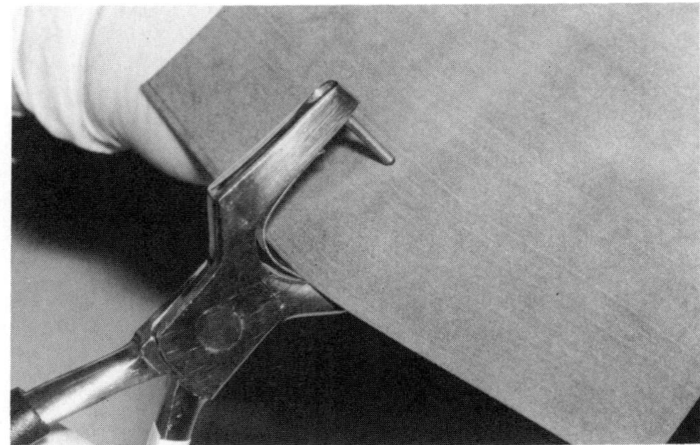

FIGURE 22–24
The rubber dam hole is being punched approximately 1 inch from the edge of the material.

guidelines cannot be provided; however, the smallest hole is generally too small to be of value for any permanent tooth. A hole that is too small may tear during placement. On the other hand, a hole that is too large may inadequately seal the tooth and may permit leakage. When the dentition is normally spaced and aligned, 3 to 4 mm should be left between holes (not between centers). Holes that are punched too close together cause stretching and inadequate seal around the tooth, whereas holes that are punched too far apart result in excess material and a bunching effect (Fig. 22–27). The placement of the holes should take into consideration the labiolingual positioning of the teeth. Additional space should be allowed for areas with missing teeth. This can be accomplished by measuring the space between the teeth adjacent to the edentulous area and adding 1 to 2 mm. The arrangement of punched holes should correspond with the shape of the client's arch. Hole arrangements that are punched too straight or curved produce folds and stretching that may hinder the operator's ability to attain an optimal seal. The holes must be punched precisely without leaving tags and tears. To punch clean holes, the rubber dam punch must be well maintained and free of lodged rubber dam material. In addition, the action of punching the dam must be sharp and determined, not uncertain and hesitant. During the punching process it is also important that the punch device be centered directly above a hole to avoid damaging the instrument.

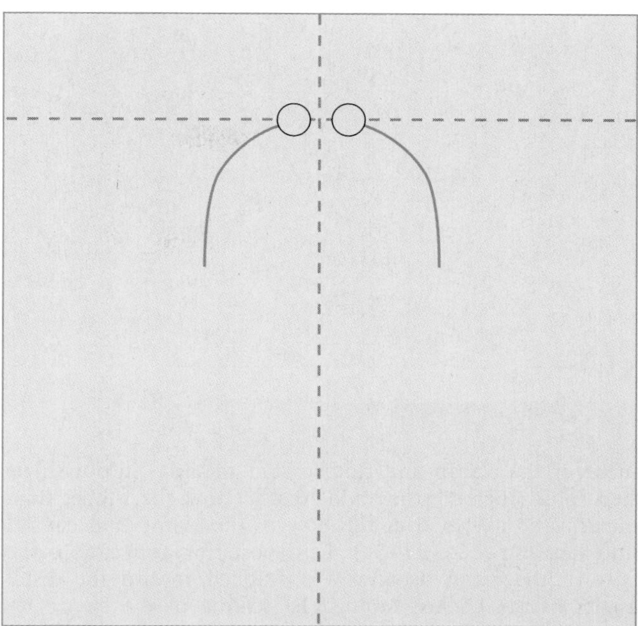

FIGURE 22–25
Key punch for the left or right central incisor in a maxillary posterior and anterior rubber dam.

Clamp Selection

The selection of the rubber dam clamp is the next step in the application of the rubber dam. The **anchor tooth** is the tooth to be clamped and is also the most distal tooth to be isolated. There are four points of consideration when selecting the clamp for the anchor tooth:

- Mesiodistal width at the cementoenamel junction (CEJ)
- Mesiodistal curvature at the CEJ
- Faciolingual width at the CEJ
- Height from CEJ to occlusal plane

The mesiodistal width between the prongs of the clamp jaws should be slightly narrower than the mesiodistal width of the anchor tooth at the CEJ. The mesiodistal curvature of the clamp jaws must be greater than the mesiodistal curvature of the anchor tooth at the CEJ. The faciolingual width between the prongs of the clamp jaws should be narrower than the faciolingual width of the anchor tooth at the CEJ. The bow of the clamp must arch high enough to clear the occlusal surface of the anchor tooth when the clamp is appropriately seated. These criteria are illustrated in Figure 22–28. Each of these criteria permits the correct and stable seating of the jaw prongs on the anchor tooth. Usually in the anterior aspects of the arches, the rubber dam can be successfully retained without clamps. Small pieces of rubber dam, or other devices such as wooden wedges and floss, can be inserted between teeth to hold the dam in position.

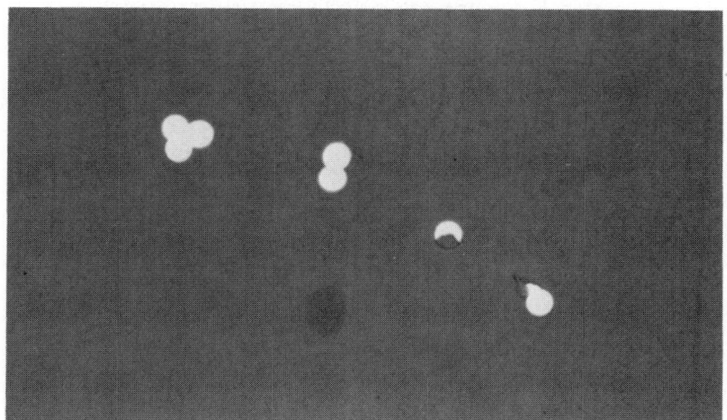

FIGURE 22–26
As pictured left to right, triple hole, double hole, tag, and tear.

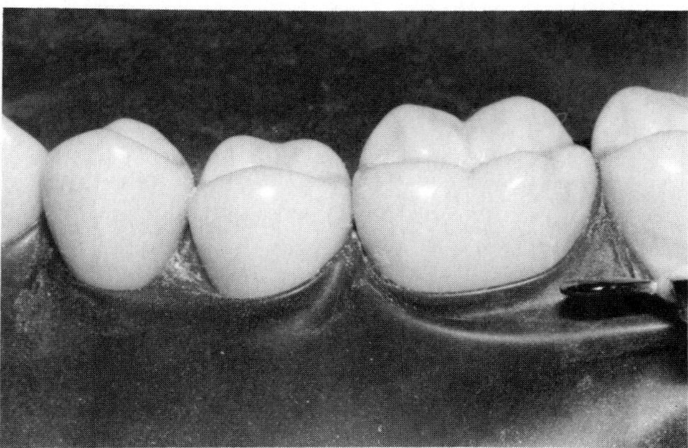

FIGURE 22–27
Rubber dam problems: (1) Dam is not through proximal contact between no. 18 and no. 19; (2) bunching of the dam between no. 19 and no. 20; and (3) stretching of the dam exposing the gingiva between no. 20 and no. 21.

Rubber Dam Placement Technique

There are two techniques for the placement of the clamp and rubber dam material. The first technique involves a two-step process of placing the clamp and then the rubber dam material. The second technique combines the place-

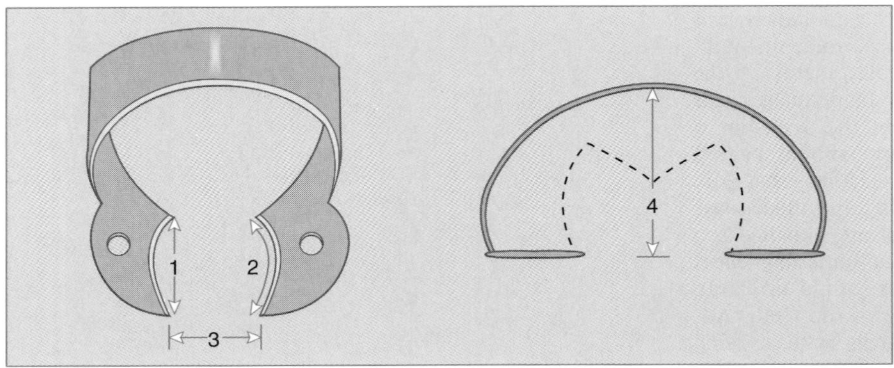

FIGURE 22–28
Clamp selection criteria: *1*, Mesiodistal width of the clamp. *2*, Mesiodistal curvature of the clamp. *3*, Faciolingual width of the clamp. *4*, Height of the clamp.

ment of the clamp and rubber dam material into a single step. This single-step method requires that the rubber dam material be placed over the bow of the clamp and carried into location (Fig. 22–29). In a posterior application, the bow of the clamp is always positioned toward the distal aspect of the anchor tooth. The seating of the clamp requires that the beaks of the rubber dam forceps be placed in the forceps holes. Using a palm grasp, the handles of the forceps are squeezed to separate the jaws of the clamp. The lingual jaw of the clamp is seated first, assuring that both prongs are in contact with the tooth. While continuing to squeeze the forceps and separate the jaws, the facial jaw is rotated over the occlusal surface of the anchor tooth. The jaw is then seated on the facial surface of the anchor tooth by releasing the pressure on the forceps handles (Fig. 22–30). The seating of a stable clamp requires that all four prongs be in contact with the tooth. Having obtained this status, the rubber dam forceps are removed and the stability of the clamp checked by applying pressure to the bow and the lingual and facial jaws of the clamp. There should be no rocking or shifting of the clamp.

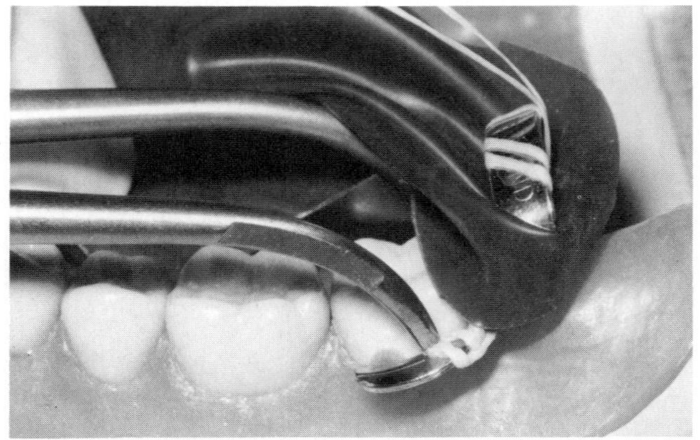

FIGURE 22–29
The clamp is seated and the rubber dam carried-in in a single step.

The advantage of the one-step procedure is the elimination of the necessity to stretch the rubber dam over the bow and risk springing the clamp from the anchor tooth. On the other hand, the two-step procedure improves visibility when seating the clamp. The selection of a technique is best left to operator preference and experience. The remainder of the placement steps are identical for both techniques. The hole is then stretched to the lingual side and spread over the lingual jaw and this procedure is then repeated for the facial side. The anchor tooth is now the only tooth isolated in the rubber dam (Fig. 22–31).

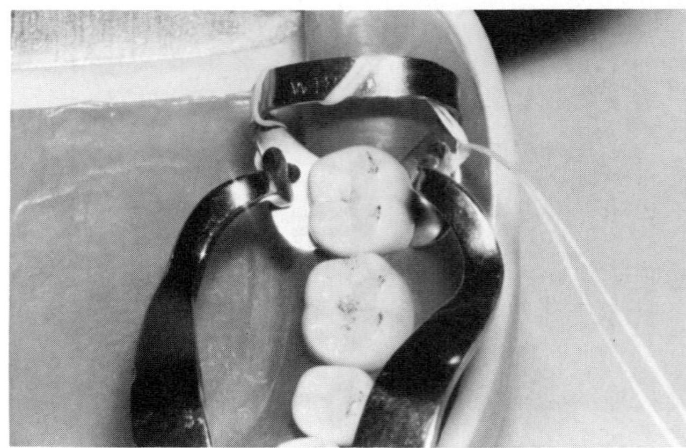

FIGURE 22–30
The clamp is positioned with rubber dam forceps.

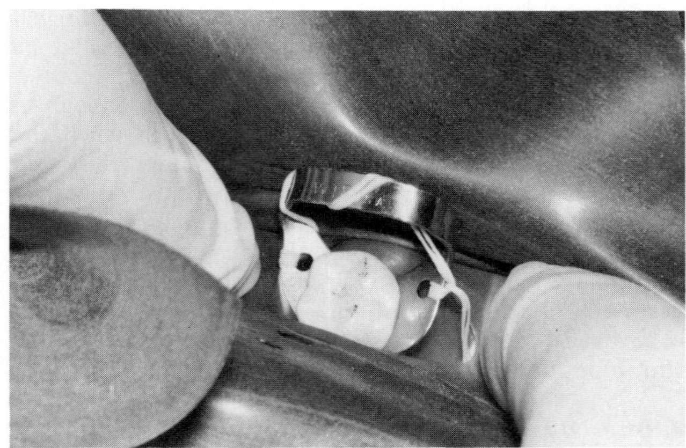

FIGURE 22–31
The rubber dam hole is stretched to enclose and isolate the clamp and anchor tooth.

PROCEDURE 22–1

APPLYING A RUBBER DAM

Equipment

Rubber dam material	Rubber dam frame	Water-soluble lubricant
Rubber dam punch	Rubber dam napkin	Spoon excavator
Rubber dam clamps	Dental floss or tape	Air/Water syringe
Rubber dam forceps	Petrolatum	Mouth mirror

Steps	Rationale
1. Explain the procedure to the client. One of the most threatening sensations produced by the rubber dam is the inability to breathe through the mouth. To meet the client's need for freedom from stress, the individual should be instructed to breathe through the nose after application of the rubber dam. It is also important for the individual to maintain an open mouth after placement of the rubber dam clamp, because biting on the bow of the clamp could cause it to become dislodged. A bite block can be used to support the jaws in maintaining an open position when individuals are unable to do this unassisted	The client who is unfamiliar with the procedure is more apprehensive and unable to appreciate the value of the rubber dam to the ultimate success of the restorative treatment
2. Put on protective eyewear and mask; wash your hands and put on gloves	Infection control procedures prevent the transmission of microorganisms
3. Place protective eyewear on the client	Protective eyewear prevents injury to the client by airborne objects
4. Assess the condition of the client's dentition and soft tissues. This assessment should begin with a confirmation of the tooth or teeth to be restored	These factors influence the operator's application of the rubber dam
5. Prepare the client as determined to be necessary from the oral assessment: remove bacterial plaque, debris, and supragingival calculus	The removal of oral debris simplifies the application process
6. Lubricate the client's lips with petrolatum	This prevents the lips from becoming chapped during isolation
7. Deliver supplemental anesthesia if determined to be necessary. Routine injections for pulpal anesthesia may not provide soft tissue anesthesia in areas where clamps must retract the free gingiva. Often, the lingual gingiva of maxillary molars and the facial gingiva of mandibular molars will require supplemental anesthesia. These areas are easily anesthetized by infiltrating a small amount of anesthetic solution adjacent to the area of clamp placement. The anterior soft tissue is typically not a concern because anterior rubber dams can be successfully retained without clamps	Routine injections for pulpal anesthesia may not anesthetize the areas where the clamp retracts the gingiva
8. Select the correct size, color, and weight rubber dam material for the procedure	Thinner dams tear more easily, but can be applied more rapidly; heavier dams provide better retraction and protection of the oral tissues
9. Mark the key punch for the rubber dam	The key punch provides a guide for the placement of all the remaining holes
10. Mark the remainder of the holes based on the individual client specifications	The individual placement of holes permits the operator to take into consideration factors such as missing teeth, extra teeth, tight contacts and malaligned teeth
11. Punch the holes as marked with a sharp and determined punching action	It is essential to obtain clean holes free of tears and tags that hinder the operator's ability to obtain the desired seal
12. Lubricate the punched rubber dam with a water-soluble solution such as shaving cream	The lubrication helps slip the dam through the contacts and prevent the dam from tearing during application
13. Select the appropriate rubber dam clamp for the anchor tooth	The placement of a stable rubber dam requires the selection of a clamp that securely adapts to the tooth

CONTINUED ON FOLLOWING PAGE

PROCEDURE 22–1

APPLYING A RUBBER DAM *(Continued)*

Steps	Rationale
14. Tie 18 inches of dental floss to the clamp; the floss should be tied through the lingual forceps hole, wrapped around the bow, and then tied through the facial forceps hole to ensure that both sides of the clamp are secured in the event of clamp breakage (Fig. 22–32)	This safety ligature permits the operator to recover the clamp in the event of dislodgement or breakage to prevent aspiration of the clamp

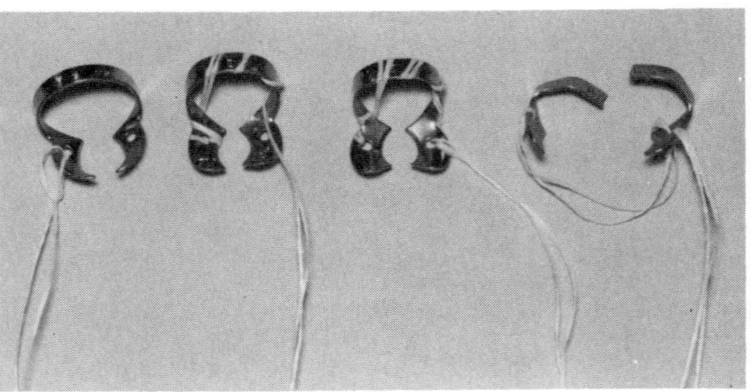

FIGURE 22–32
Clamp ligation progressing from lingual *(left)* to facial *(right)*, and a broken ligated clamp at far right.

Steps	Rationale
15. Seat the rubber dam clamp with the rubber dam forceps; when the anchor tooth has been restored with a gold or porcelain crown, the jaws of the clamp should be covered with a protective tape (autoclave tape is handy) to prevent scratching or gouging the margins of the crown (Fig. 22–33)	A properly seated clamp has four prongs in contact with the anchor tooth and provides stabilization for the rubber dam

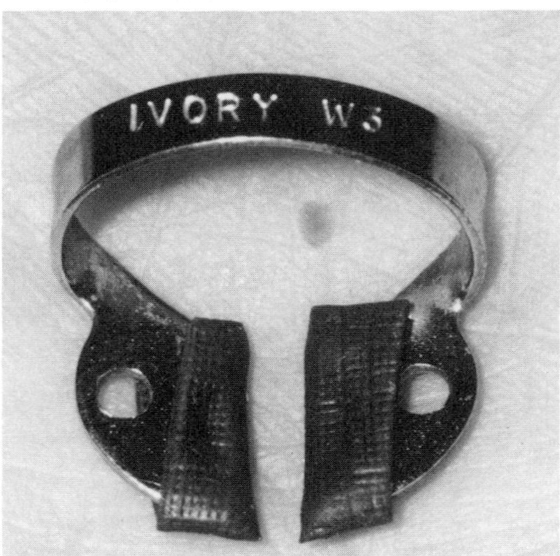

FIGURE 22–33
Jaws of a clamp covered with protective tape prior to being seated on a gold or porcelain crown.

Steps	Rationale
16. Stretch and place the anchor tooth hole over the bow of the clamp (unless the "one-step" technique was used during clamp placement) (see Fig. 22–34)	The clamp secures the rubber dam in place to expedite the placement of the remainder of the dam
17. Reveal most forward tooth to be isolated through the appropriate hole (Fig. 22–34); a piece of floss or dam can be used to help seat the dam and secure the isolation (Fig. 22–35) Place the rubber dam napkin between the rubber dam material and the client's face	This sequence ensures that the beginning and ending holes are appropriately placed and simplifies the isolation of the remaining teeth
18. Place the rubber dam frame	This removes the edges of the rubber dam from the isolation site

Steps	Rationale

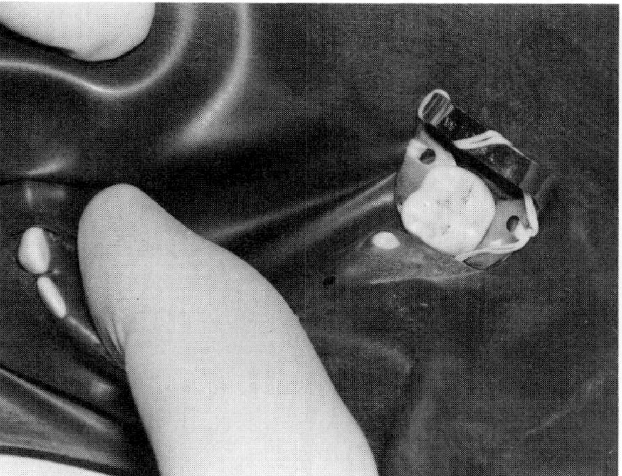

FIGURE 22–34
The rubber dam is stretched over the most forward tooth to be isolated.

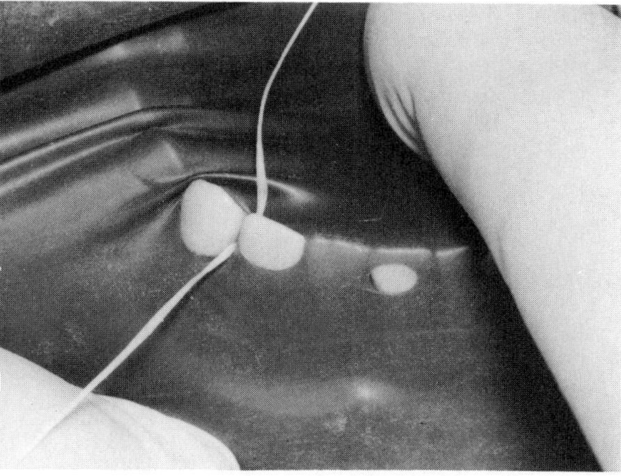

FIGURE 22–35
Dental floss is used to help seat the rubber dam around the most forward tooth.

19. Isolate the remainder of the teeth, working from front to back, through the holes; pass floss through the contacts to assist in positioning the rubber dam material through the **proximal contacts** (Figs. 22–36 and 22–37)

This sequence provides an established regimen that provides for the isolation of the easiest teeth first

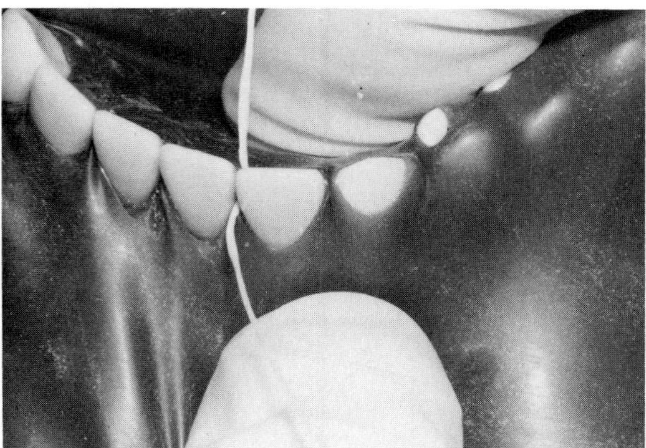

FIGURE 22–36
Dental floss is used to carry the septa between the teeth.

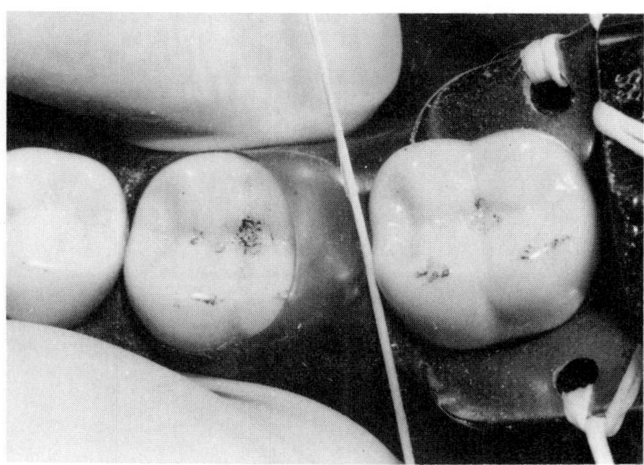

FIGURE 22–37
Dental floss is positioned to pull the rubber dam through the contact.

20. Invert rubber dam material when all teeth are completely isolated and the rubber dam is between all contacts
Several instruments can be used to invert, or tuck, the dam; however, the spoon excavator is the instrument of choice
An air stream is used to support the inversion process (Figs. 22–38 and 22–39)
When the teeth are properly isolated, the floss safety ligature should be secured to the frame

21. Center the rubber dam frame on the client's face, with the upper lip covered and nose revealed
If the nose is inadvertently covered, the rubber dam at the top of the frame can be folded or cut to uncover the nose. If client is experiencing nasal con-

A well-positioned dam and frame best isolates the surgical site from the oral cavity while still allowing comfortable breathing

CONTINUED ON FOLLOWING PAGE

PROCEDURE 22–1

APPLYING A RUBBER DAM *(Continued)*

Steps	Rationale

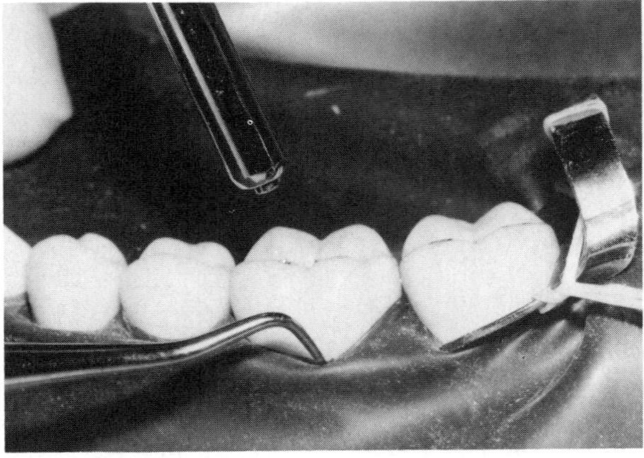

FIGURE 22–38
The spoon excavator is supported by an air stream to invert the dam and create a seal.

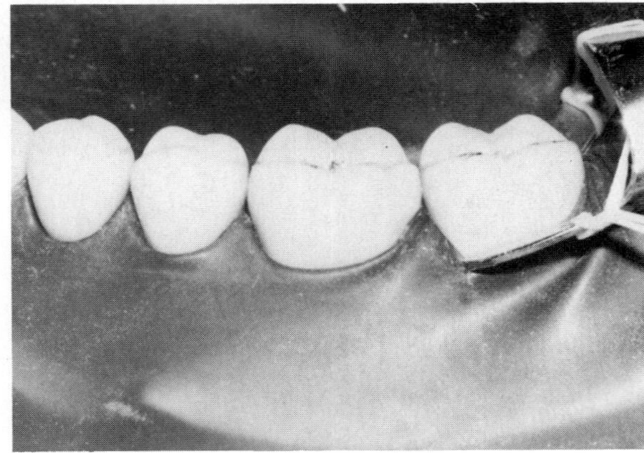

FIGURE 22–39
A well-sealed, properly inverted rubber dam.

Steps	Rationale
gestion or difficulty in breathing through the nasal passage, an incision can be cut in the rubber dam away from the surgical site to allow air passage	
22. Place a saliva ejector under the rubber dam if the client reports or exhibits signs of difficulty in swallowing	The supplemental evacuation supports the client's efforts to remove saliva from the oral cavity

PROCEDURE 22–2

REMOVING A RUBBER DAM

Equipment

Scissors
Rubber dam forceps
Dental floss or tape

Steps	Rationale
1. Cut the safety ligature and remove the rubber dam clamp with the rubber dam forceps The beaks of the rubber dam forceps should be replaced in the clamp forceps holes to spread the jaws and remove the clamp The facial jaw of the clamp should be raised over the contour of the tooth followed by the lingual jaw (Fig. 22–40)	The removal of the clamp provides improved access to cut the septa
2. Cut each septum between teeth with sharp, blunt scissors The operator should stretch the septa facially to improve access for cutting and protect the soft tissues of the oral cavity (Fig. 22–41)	Expedites the removal of the dam without concern for passage through the contacts
3. The dam, napkin, and frame are removed together	Done when possible in an efficient movement
4. Wipe the client's lips to remove excess saliva and debris; rinse and evacuate the mouth	Enhances client comfort
5. Briefly massage the client's facial muscles	This relieves the tension in the muscles from prolonged opening; many clients appreciate the show of concern for their comfort

CONTINUED ON FOLLOWING PAGE

Steps	Rationale
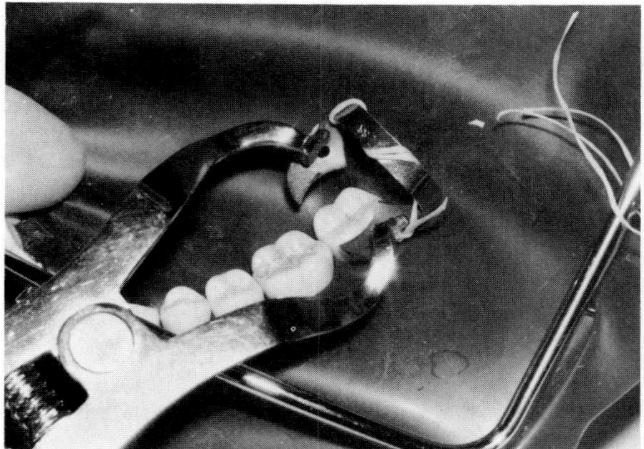 FIGURE 22–40 The safety ligature is released from the frame, and the clamp is removed from the tooth with forceps.	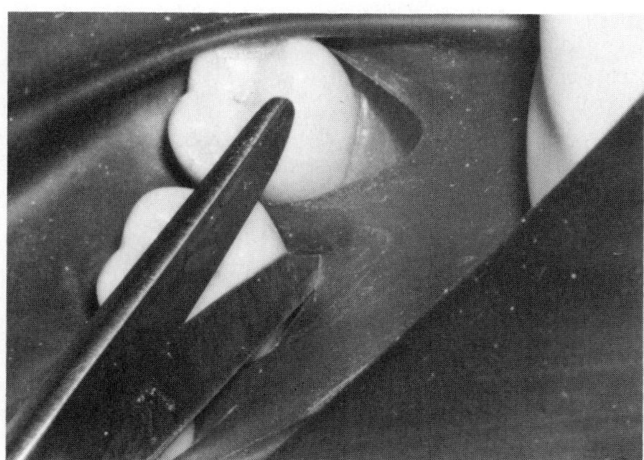 FIGURE 22–41 Rubber dam is stretched, and septa are cut with scissors.
6. Examine the rubber dam to ensure the removal of all rubber dam fragments and septa	Small fragments can go undetected and if left between teeth can produce discomfort and inflammation
7. Floss dental contacts to remove any dam fragments as necessary	Done if necessary to remove fragments

IMPLEMENTATION — PERMANENT RESTORATIONS

Amalgam

Rationale

Dental amalgam remains the standard restorative material for posterior teeth.[13] Its reputation is based upon decades of clinical evaluation during which it has proven to be a durable material even when placed in some highly compromised circumstances. Its longevity is directly related to proper cavity preparation and attention to basic principles of manipulation and condensation in a moisture-free environment.

Material

Dental amalgam is a compound of an **alloy,** a mixture of metals composed mainly of silver, copper, and tin, with mercury. The function of the mercury is to wet the alloy particles causing the mass to undergo metallurgical changes. These changes result in a hardened metallic mass that functions well in the oral environment. Early amalgams were unpredictable in their clinical longevity and were particularly subject to delayed expansion (creep), corrosion, and **margin deterioration.** These drawbacks have been attributed to a weak tin-mercury component or gamma-2 phase in the metal. Modern amalgam materials have been specially developed to virtually eliminate this phase in the metal. Accordingly, today's amalgams show marked improvement in stability, strength, and **margin integrity.** Amalgam alloy powders are available with spherical particle shapes or with a blend of spherical and lathe-cut particles. Spherical particle alloys handle differently when condensed into cavity preparations. These rounded particles do not resist condensation pressures as do the irregularly shaped, lathe-cut particles. Because the resulting amalgam restorations from both are quite similar, the selection of an alloy particle type is a matter of personal choice.

Armamentarium

Triturator. The **triturator** or amalgamator is the mechanical device used to mix the encapsulated alloy and mercury (Fig. 22–42). It is adjustable for speed and time of trituration to achieve the correct amalgam mix.

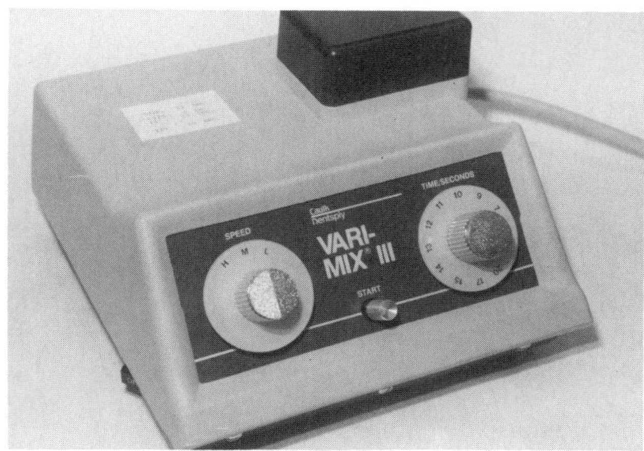

FIGURE 22–42
A typical amalgam triturator with dials for speed and time selection.

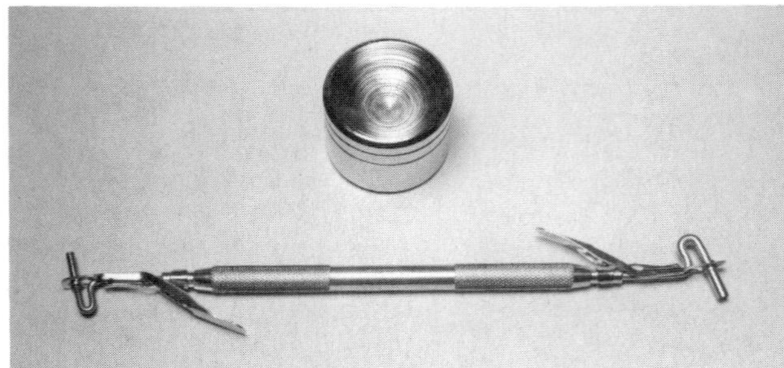

FIGURE 22-43
Amalgam well and carrier.

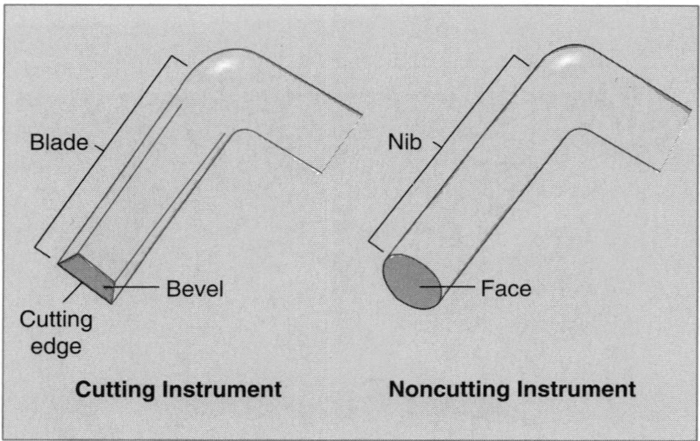

FIGURE 22-45
Comparison of the working end of a cutting hand instrument with a noncutting hand instrument.

Amalgam Well. The amalgam well is a small, heavy, stainless steel "dish" with a cup-like recess that confines the mixed amalgam to facilitate pick-up with the amalgam carrier (Fig. 22-43). The mixed amalgam is transferred immediately from the amalgam capsule to the amalgam well.

Amalgam Carrier. The amalgam carrier is used to carry and dispense amalgam into the cavity preparation (see Fig. 22-43). Amalgam is loaded into the barrel (cylinder) by pressing the barrel tip into the amalgam mass contained in the amalgam well. When pushed, the instrument lever forces a plunger to dislodge the contained restorative material from the barrel.

Condensing Instruments. Condensing instruments are used to pack amalgam and other restorative materials firmly into a cavity preparation. There are numerous shapes and sizes of condensers (Fig. 22-44). Noncutting hand instruments are similar in design to cutting instruments except that the nib replaces the blade and a face replaces the cutting edge (Fig. 22-45). Selection of an instrument is based on the size and configuration of the cavity preparation and the amount of material to be condensed.

Carving Instruments. Carving instruments are used to remove excess restorative material and refine the margins of the restoration. All carvers are sharp cutting instruments. There are numerous blade shapes and sizes that are selected for use based on the carving action to be completed and personal preference (Fig. 22-46).

Tofflemire Matrix System. The Tofflemire matrix system is comprised of a Tofflemire retainer, matrix bands, and wedges. The Tofflemire retainer is a stainless steel mechanical device used to hold the matrix band. There are two styles of retainers

- Straight
- Contraangle

The matrix band is a stainless steel, boomerang-shaped strip that comes in various sizes and adaptations (Fig. 22-47). Wedges are typically triangular (in cross-section) pieces of wood that also come in numerous sizes and adaptations.

Occlusal Analysis and Tooth Preparation

An analysis of the occlusion is done to help determine the final morphology of the planned restoration(s). In addition to examining wear facets, it may be useful to mark centric stops (tooth contacts in centric occlusion) and eccentric contacts (tooth contacts during mandibular movement) with articulating ribbon (Fig. 22-48). The dentist may choose to modify the cavity shape based on occlusal contacts.

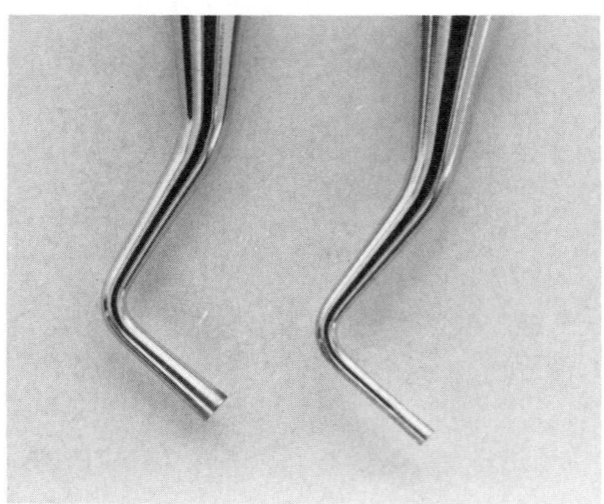

FIGURE 22-44
Large and small amalgam condensers.

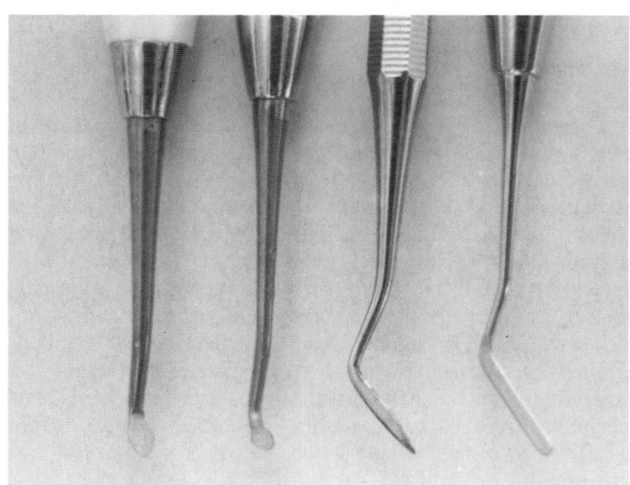

FIGURE 22-46
Common amalgam carvers. As pictured left to right, cleoid, discoid, 1/2 Hollenback, and Baum interproximal carver.

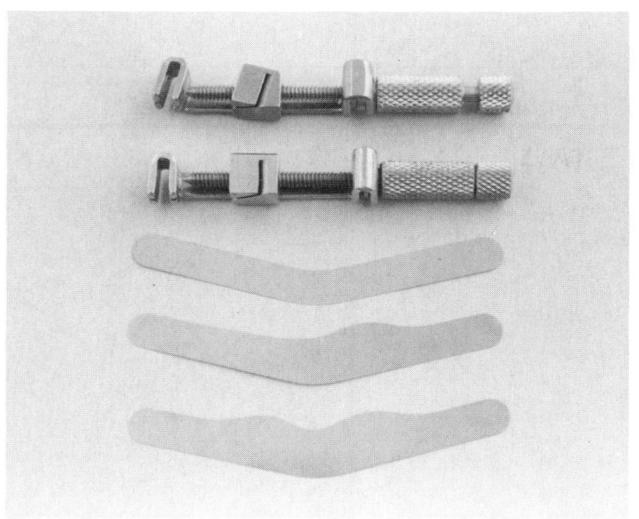

FIGURE 22–47
Tofflemire retainers and bands. As pictured top to bottom, contraangle retainer, straight retainer, and modified bands that fit either retainer.

Following this analysis, anesthesia, rubber dam isolation, and cavity preparation are completed to the specifications previously outlined. The cavity preparation is then assessed for the need for liners and bases. When determined to be necessary, placement is simplified if it precedes the positioning of the matrix band. A detailed discussion of liners and bases is included in a separate section of this chapter.

Matrix and Wedge Placement

A matrix is an artificial wall that is needed whenever a lateral wall is missing in a cavity preparation. Typically, a mesial or distal wall is absent in complex posterior cavities. The matrix serves to:

- Confine the amalgam material during insertion and condensation

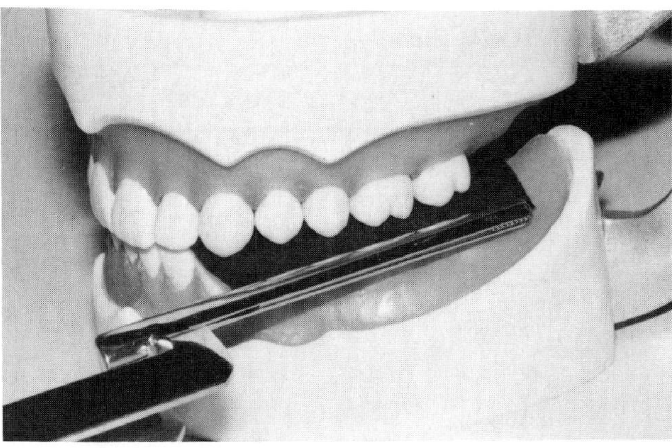

FIGURE 22–48
Occlusal contacts being registered with articulating ribbon.

- Provide a framework for reconstruction and contouring of the missing tooth part
- Support the establishment of proper proximal contacts
- Prevent amalgam overhangs

For these reasons, the matrix must be rigid, contoured, and stable. Numerous matrix techniques are available but by far the most popular and versatile is offered by the Tofflemire matrix system.

A wooden wedge is often necessary to adequately form the matrix band. The properly shaped and positioned wedge:

- Gently displaces rubber dam and gingival papilla in an apical direction
- Supports the matrix band in the proximal space without encroaching on the contact area
- Adapts the band to the gingival cavity margin
- Provides slight tooth separation that supports the attainment of a positive proximal contact after the removal of the matrix band

Numerous pretrimmed wedges are available for selection.

PROCEDURE 22–3

TOFFLEMIRE MATRIX SYSTEM

Equipment

Tofflemire retainer
Matrix bands
Wooden wedges
Metal cutting scissors
Cotton forceps
Modeling compound
Burnishing instrument

Steps	Rationale
1. Evaluate the prepared tooth	Helps to create a mental picture to aid in the selection of a matrix band
2. Select a matrix band that (1) best encloses all lateral aspects of the cavity and (2) extends 1 to 2 mm above the adjacent marginal ridge and 1 mm beyond the gingival margin	The selection of a band that needs little or no modification simplifies the procedure: (1) Class 2 cavities that have short proximal boxes can be enclosed with a standard band, (2) tall proximal boxes may require a band with gingival ex-

CONTINUED ON FOLLOWING PAGE

PROCEDURE 22–3

TOFFLEMIRE MATRIX SYSTEM *(Continued)*

Steps	Rationale
Trim the band with metal-cutting scissors as necessary (Fig. 22–49)	tensions, and (3) a single tall box may need a band with one gingival extension In any case, all gingival margins must be sealed against the band and the band must extend occlusally high enough to enclose missing ridges and cusps

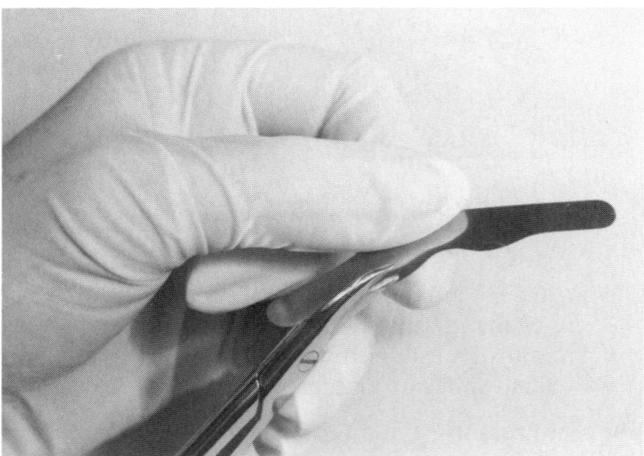

FIGURE 22–49
Metal-cutting scissors used to modify a matrix band.

Steps	Rationale
3. Select a matrix retainer	The contraangle Tofflemire retainer fits most situations; its design allows it to be positioned from the lingual if necessary The straight Tofflemire retainer is usually limited to facial applications
4. Loop the band in your fingers so that the ends are matched. The convergent opening (smaller) of the loop should be positioned next to the gingiva (rubber dam) (Fig. 22–50)	The convergent opening is smaller and matches the converging area of the crown (CEJ)

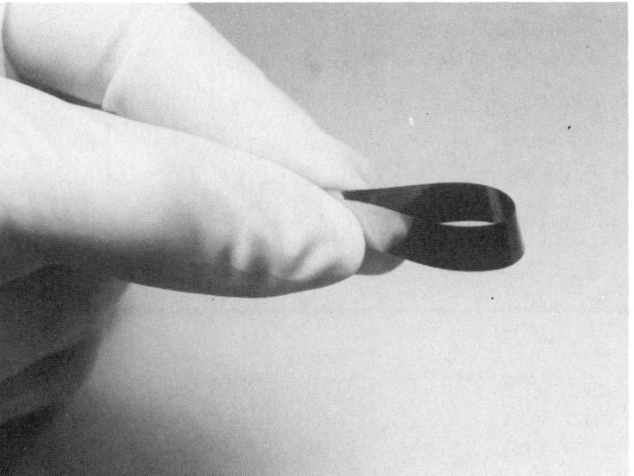

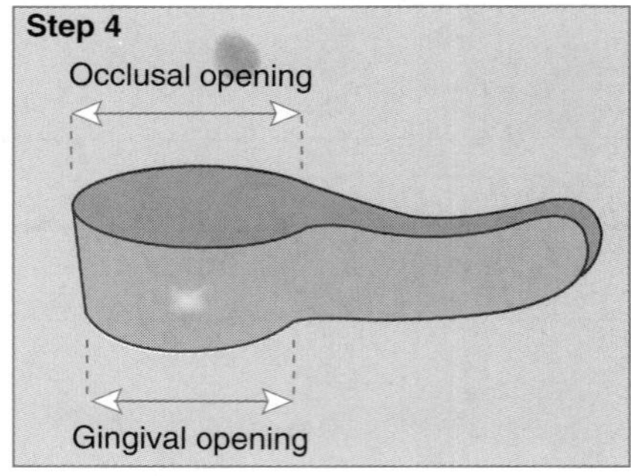

FIGURE 22–50
The ends of the band are placed evenly together to form a loop *(left)*. The loop is tapered to permit adaptation at the gingival aspect *(right)*.

Steps	Rationale
5. Position the locking vise approximately $\frac{1}{4}$ inch from the end of the retainer and free the locking screw (spindle) from the band slot in the locking vise (Fig. 22–51)	This prepares the retainer to receive the matrix band
6. Position the loop in the retainer (leading with the occlusal edge of the band) by inserting the matched ends into the slots in the locking vise and the loop into the appropriate guide channel When positioned, the guide channels of the retainer open toward the gingiva	The guide channel orientation allows the retainer to be lifted occlusally when the matrix is being disassembled If the retainer is inverted (guide channels open occlusally) the retainer is trapped because it cannot be removed in a gingival direction

Steps	Rationale

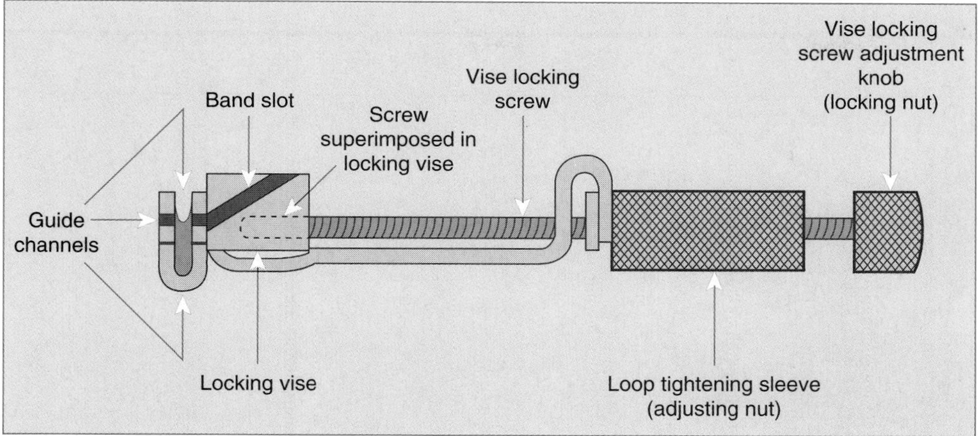

FIGURE 22–51
Diagram of the Tofflemire retainer.

The loop of the band should exit the guide channel to allow the loop to be positioned from the preferred side of the tooth (usually the facial side)

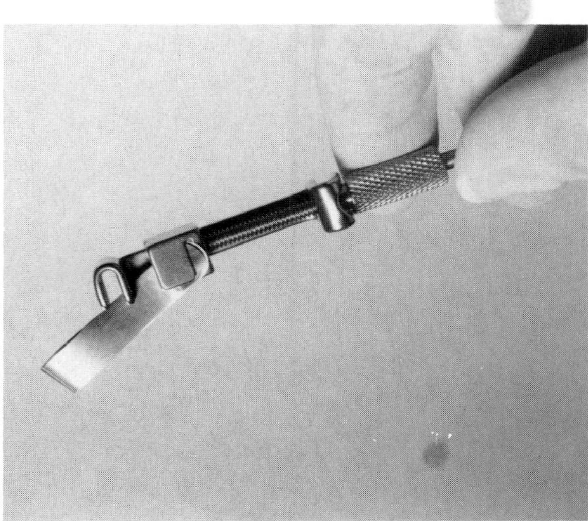

FIGURE 22–52
The initial placement of the band in the retainer slot with the occlusal aspect of the loop being inserted first.

Assuming that the seated retainer will be most commonly positioned on the facial aspect of the prepared tooth, the left channel guide is used for dentition in the maxillary left and mandibular right, and the right channel guide is used for dentition in the maxillary right and mandibular left

When inserting the band into the retainer, the wider occlusal aspect of the band should be inserted first, because the retainer is seated with the slots of the retainer toward the gingiva (Fig. 22–52)

Steps	Rationale
7. Secure the matrix band by advancing the locking screw (Fig. 22–53)	The band must be secured in the retainer, or it may loosen during condensation, ruining the restoration

CONTINUED ON FOLLOWING PAGE

PROCEDURE 22–3

TOFFLEMIRE MATRIX SYSTEM *(Continued)*

Steps	Rationale

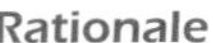

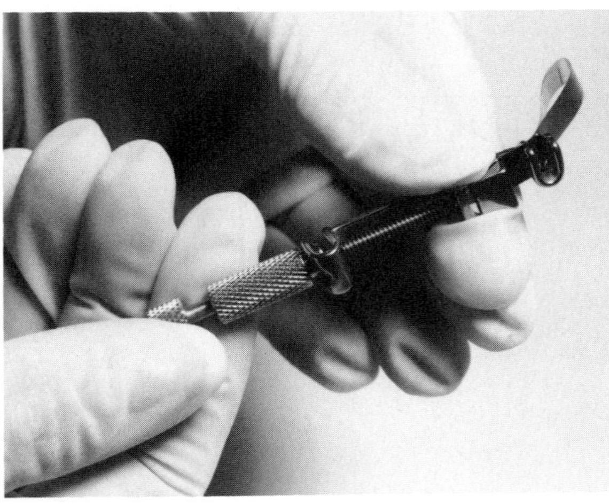

FIGURE 22–53
The locking nut is tightened to secure the band in the retainer.

Steps	Rationale
8. Shape the matrix loop into a rounded form: (1) insert an instrument handle through the loop, (2) pinch the band between the instrument handle and your thumb, and (3) rotate your wrist as you pinch the band (Fig. 22–54)	The opened loop slips over the tooth easily

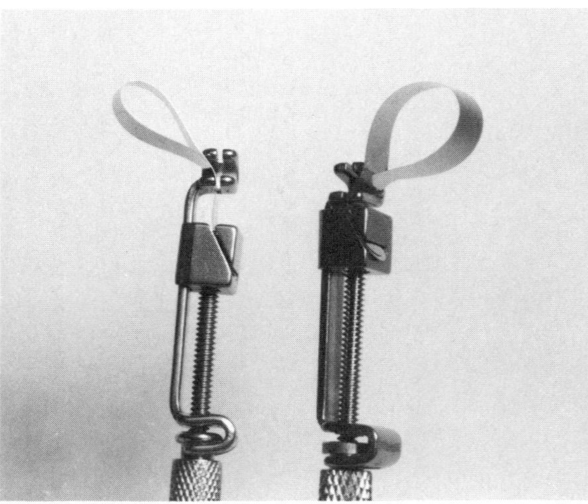

FIGURE 22–54
Inserted band before shaping *(left)* and band shaped to rounded form to facilitate placement *(right)*.

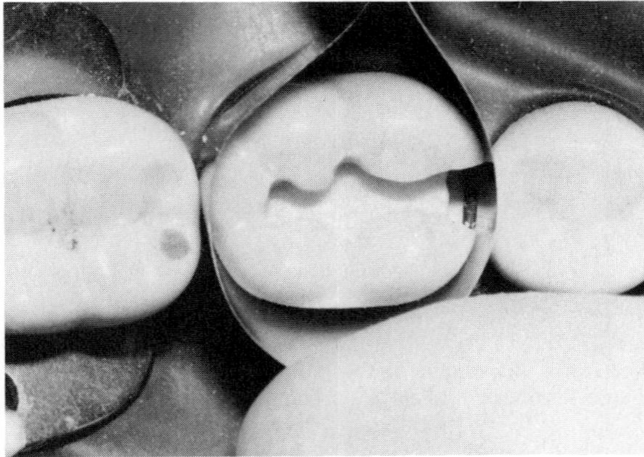

FIGURE 22–55
Initial placement of band over prepared tooth. Finger pressure supports the lingual aspect of the band.

Steps	Rationale
9. Position the loop around the tooth with the slots of the retainer and the narrow aspect of the band toward the gingiva (Fig. 22–55); brace the lingual aspect of the loop with the thumb of your opposite hand; gently tighten the band by rotating the adjusting nut An examination of the placement of the band should ensure that the band extends occlusally 1 to 2 mm beyond the adjacent marginal ridge; it should also extend apically approximately 1 mm beyond the gingival margin without impinging on the soft tissue	The opposite thumb adapts the band against the lingual aspect of the tooth Extreme tightening of the band tends to pull it away from the adjacent teeth, which could result in open proximal contacts
10. Place wedge(s) into the lingual embrasure between the band and the adjacent tooth, slightly beyond the gingival margin (Fig. 22–56)	Wedge(s) adapt the band at the gingival margin(s); the wedge should not encroach on the proximal contact area, or (1) an open contact may result, or (2) the proximal sur-

Steps | **Rationale**

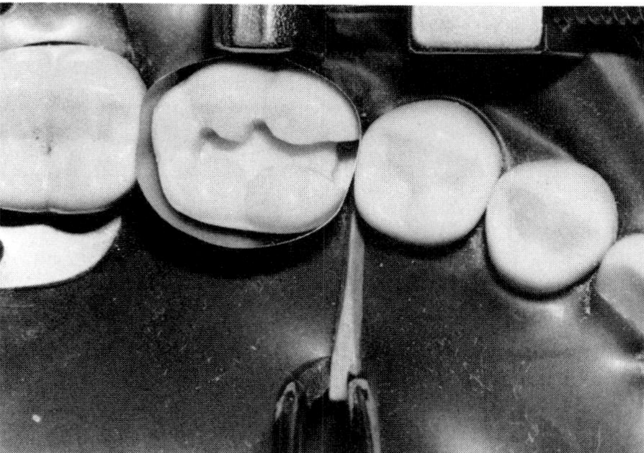

FIGURE 22–56
Wedge is inserted into the lingual embrasure between the band and the adjacent tooth using cotton forceps.

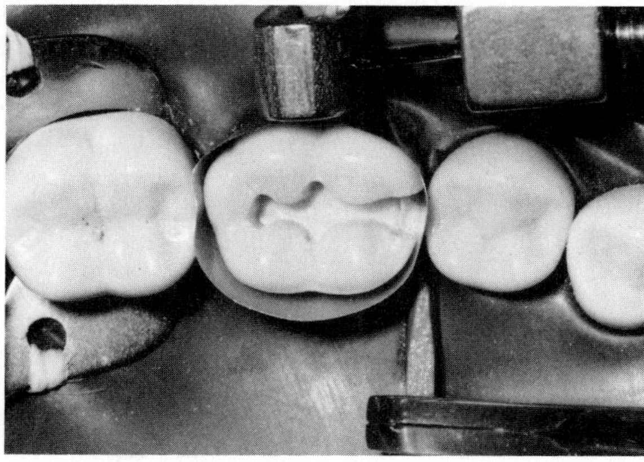

FIGURE 22–57
The handle of the cotton forceps is used to firmly position the wedge.

Steady pressure on the base of the wedge moves it in a facial direction and to the desired position (Fig. 22–57)
Wedges tend to be more stable when moistened before being positioned; trim the wedge(s) as necessary
With a custom-trimmed wedge, trimming can be accomplished by removing the necessary height or width with a knife or rotary instrument (Fig. 22–58). Numerous pretrimmed wedges are available for selection

face will be undercontoured; these defects could result in food impaction and gingival irritation (Fig. 22–59)

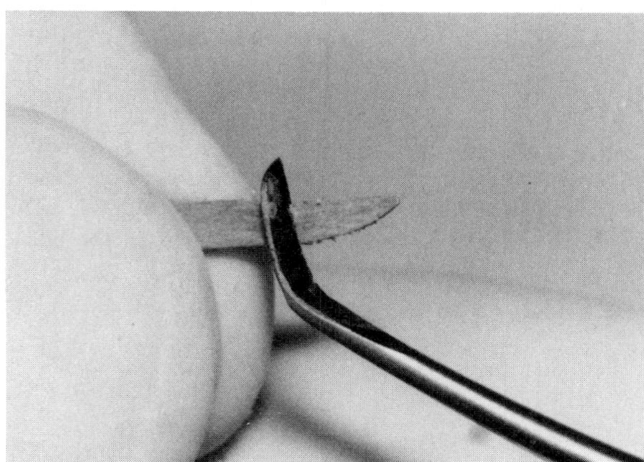

FIGURE 22–58
Trimming a wooden wedge with a gold knife.

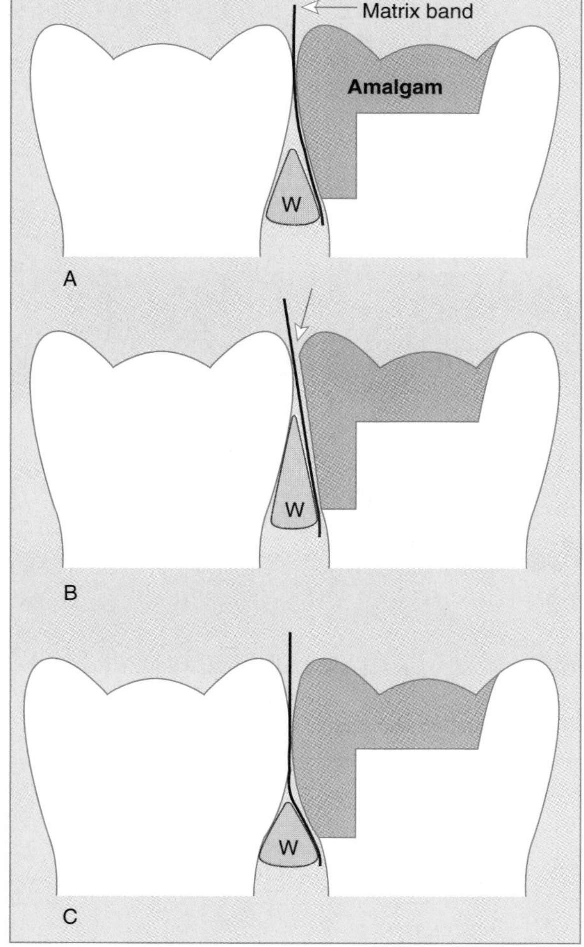

FIGURE 22–59
***A*, Proper selection and positioning of wedge (W) results in normal contour of the proximal surface amalgam. *B*, Untrimmed wedge encroaches on proximal contact area, causing flat, undercontoured surface. High wedge interferes with burnishing/contouring of the matrix band. Proximal contact is likely to be open, inviting food impaction *(arrow)*. *C*, Diminutive wedge may lead to overcontouring of proximal surface and gingival inflammation. The amalgam can be carved to contour, but with difficulty.**

CONTINUED ON FOLLOWING PAGE

PROCEDURE 22-3

TOFFLEMIRE MATRIX SYSTEM *(Continued)*

Steps	Rationale
11. Burnish the internal aspect of the band against the adjacent tooth (teeth) with a thin but rigid instrument (Fig. 22-60)	Facilitates achieving proximal contact(s) and proper proximal contour in the final restoration

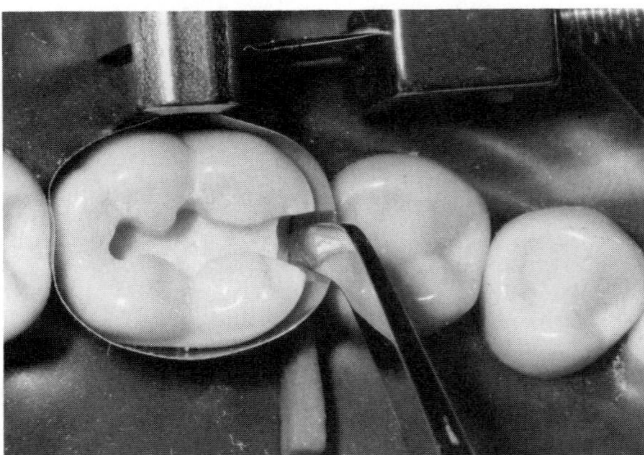

FIGURE 22-60
The band is firmly burnished against the adjacent tooth.

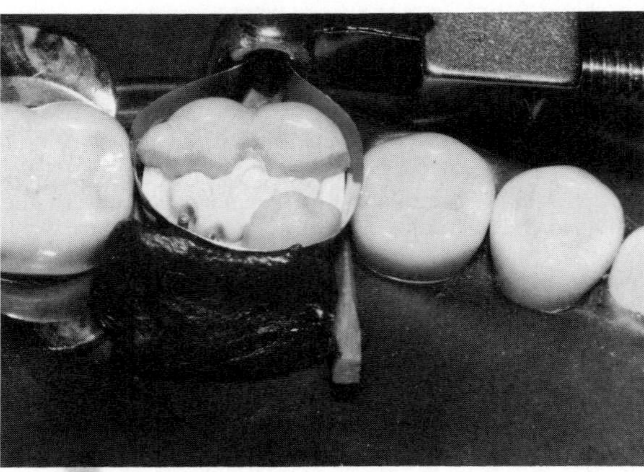

FIGURE 22-61
Modeling compound is used to stabilize the matrix in this complex cavity preparation.

Steps	Rationale
12. Evaluate the matrix for stability; add warmed modeling compound to the outside of the band as necessary	An insecure matrix is likely to move during condensation, resulting in fractures throughout the material Thorough condensation of the amalgam is not possible against a flexible matrix; warmed compound can be easily applied against the band for support (Fig. 22-61)
13. Conduct a final evaluation of the cavity preparation with the matrix system in place (Fig. 22-62)	Verifies that the preparation for a quality restoration has been completed

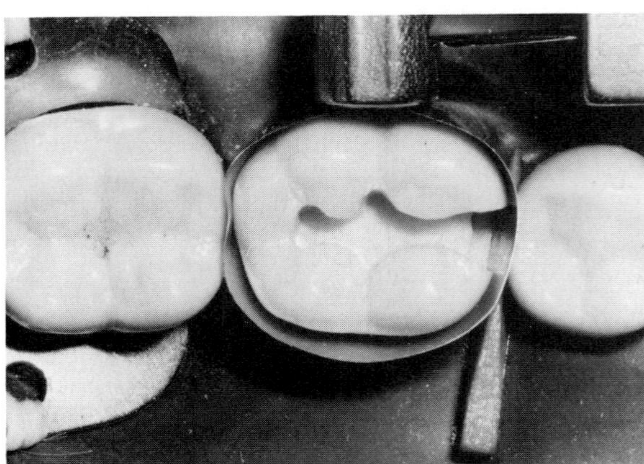

FIGURE 22-62
Final preparation and matrix system.

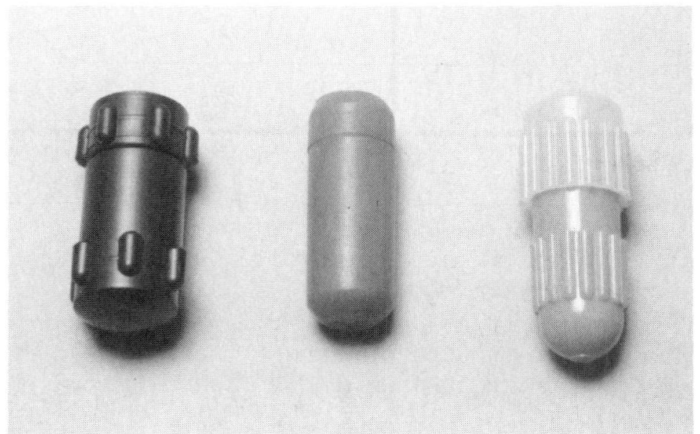

FIGURE 22-63
Common preencapsulated amalgam capsules.

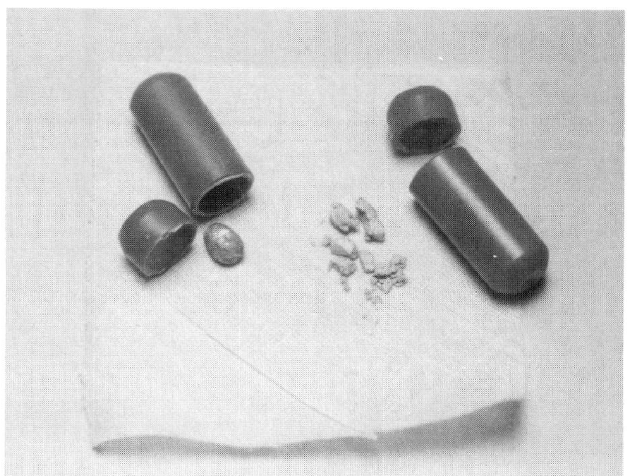

FIGURE 22-64
Soft, shiny proper amalgam mix *(left)* and dry, crumbly overtriturated mix *(right)*.

Trituration

Modern amalgam materials are preencapsulated to prevent mercury spills and provide consistent quality of mixes (Fig. 22-63). Capsules contain small and large quantities for selection according to the cavity size. Within each capsule is a plastic diaphragm that separates the mercury from the alloy. At the start of trituration, the diaphragm ruptures, allowing **amalgamation** (trituration) to begin. Thorough mixing occurs within a few seconds, according to the metallurgy of the mass and the speed of the amalgamator. The operator determines the proper setting of the instrument based on the manufacturer's recommendation, the amalgam material, and the desired mix. Following amalgamation, the mass is transferred to the amalgam well. Generally, a proper mix of amalgam is shiny and homogeneous and is easily manipulated with the amalgam carrier and condensers (Fig. 22-64).

Condensing and Carving the Amalgam

Condensation is the process of packing the amalgam into the prepared cavity preparation. Carving is the process of using hand instruments to shape the freshly placed amalgam into the anatomical form that will restore the tooth to function.

PROCEDURE 22-4

AMALGAM RESTORATION

Equipment

Isolation materials	Amalgam capsules	Articulating paper
Triturator	Condensing instruments	
Amalgam well	Tofflemire matrix system	
Amalgam carrier	Carving instruments	

Steps	Rationale
1. Pretest access to the cavity by holding condenser nibs in the confined areas of the preparation to verify accurate condenser selection	Condensers that are too large cannot adapt the amalgam to the internal aspects of the cavity
2. Adjust triturator settings for speed and time of mix, according to manufacturer's recommendations	Triturators vary in speeds; amalgam alloys also vary in composition and mixing requirements
3. Secure the amalgam capsule in the triturator locking device and close the protective lid	If not securely placed, the capsule may be propelled from the locking device, injuring someone or breaking open
4. Mix the amalgam and remove the capsule; open it over a catch tray and dispense the mix into the amalgam well	The tray catches loose fragments of amalgam; on occasion, amalgamation does not occur and free mercury spills out when the capsule is opened
5. Examine the mixed amalgam; note the time, or set a timer for 3 minutes	The amalgam should be a soft, round, shiny ball of material A dry, crumbly mix should be placed in the scrap container and a new mix prepared

CONTINUED ON FOLLOWING PAGE

PROCEDURE 22–4

AMALGAM RESTORATION *(Continued)*

Steps	Rationale
	Even proper mixes should be discarded after 3 minutes Such amalgam cannot be properly condensed and will not produce a homogeneous mass
6. Load the small end of the amalgam carrier; dispense a portion of this into the most confined area of the preparation (Fig. 22–65)	Attempting to rapidly fill the cavity with large increments produces voids in critical parts of the restoration; voids at margins invite leakage, sensitivity, and recurrent caries

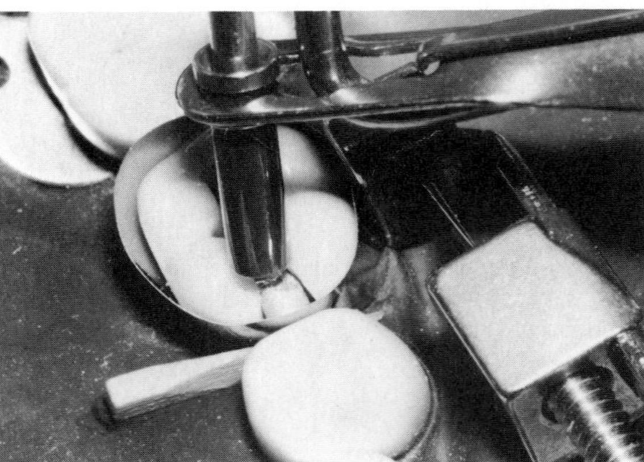

FIGURE 22–65
A small increment of amalgam is expressed into the proximal box of the cavity preparation.

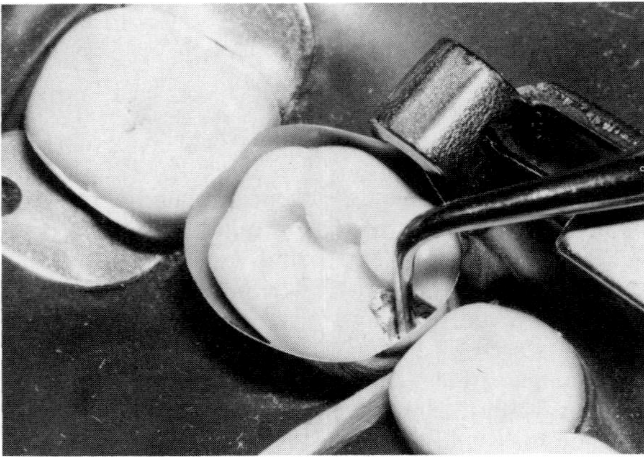

FIGURE 22–66
Initial condensation is begun with a small condenser in the proximal box.

Steps	Rationale
7. Using small condensers and stable hand position, firmly adapt the amalgam into all internal cavity features and over the margins (Fig. 22–66)	Firm pressure with smaller condensers is less likely to produce voids in confined areas Firm condensation is intended to (1) adapt the material intimately to cavity walls, (2) eliminate voids, and (3) express excess mercury from the mass
8. Continue to add increments; gradually increase condenser size; remove any "mercury-rich" surface by lateral scooping motions of the condenser nib	Firm condensation expresses mercury from the mass; its removal creates a dense, more durable restoration
9. Triturate fresh amalgam as needed; continue to add increments and condense, to build a moderate excess over the cavity margins (Figs. 22–67 and 22–68)	Larger cavities may require several mixes; if the mix begins to harden, discard it Overpacking ensures coverage of all margins and, when the material is heavily burnished, draws excess mercury to the surface so it can be readily carved away

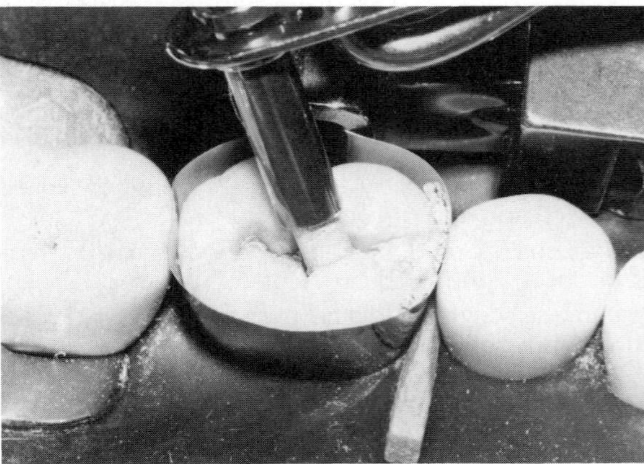

FIGURE 22–67
Additional increments of amalgam are carried to the cavity preparation.

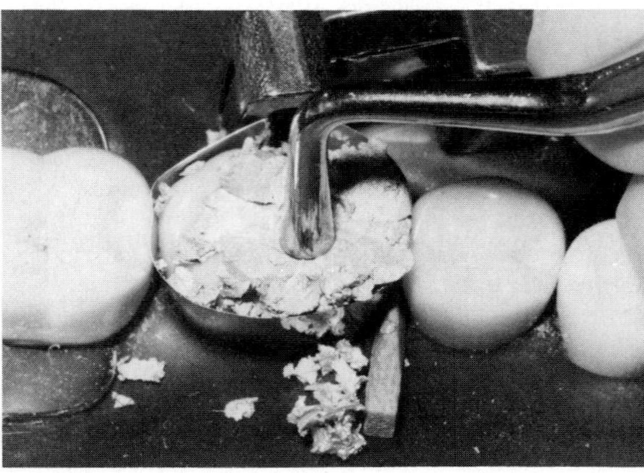

FIGURE 22–68
The cavity is overfilled with amalgam, and a large condenser is used to complete condensation.

Steps	Rationale
10. Rub and grossly shape the occlusal surface with a few firm strokes using a large ball or egg-shaped burnisher (Fig. 22–69)	Excess mercury is brought to the surface for easy removal

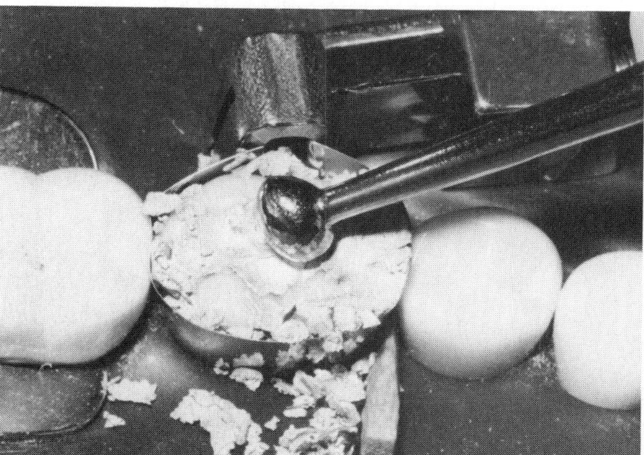

FIGURE 22–69
Burnishing of the overpacked amalgam.

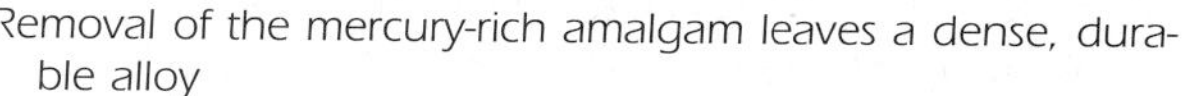

Steps	Rationale
11. Quickly carve and suction away all gross excess amalgam	Removal of the mercury-rich amalgam leaves a dense, durable alloy
12. Establish the marginal ridge height and outer contours next to the matrix band by carving with an explorer or similar fine, sharp instrument The excess amalgam is rapidly carved away, and occlusal margins are recovered (Figs. 22–70 to 22–72)	Marginal ridge contours are the most difficult to form and so should be shaped while the amalgam is carvable and while the matrix is in place

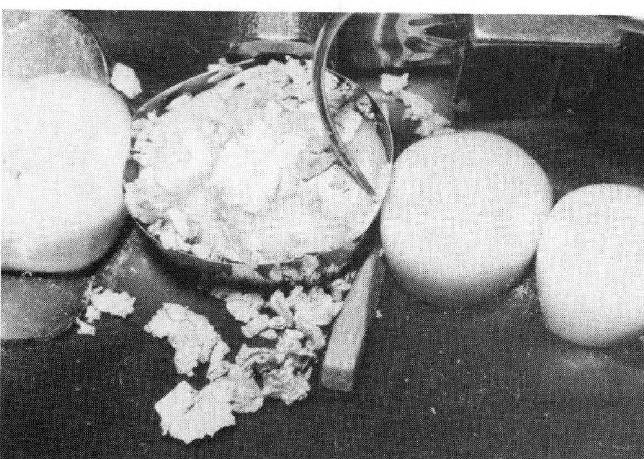

FIGURE 22–70
Marginal ridge height and outer contours are established with an explorer.

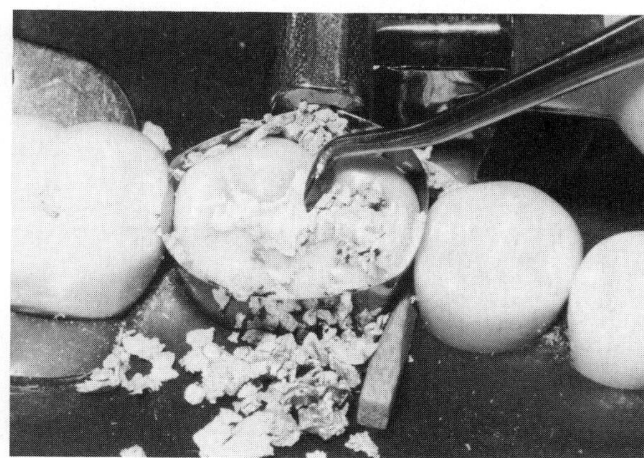

FIGURE 22–71
Excess amalgam is removed with a carver.

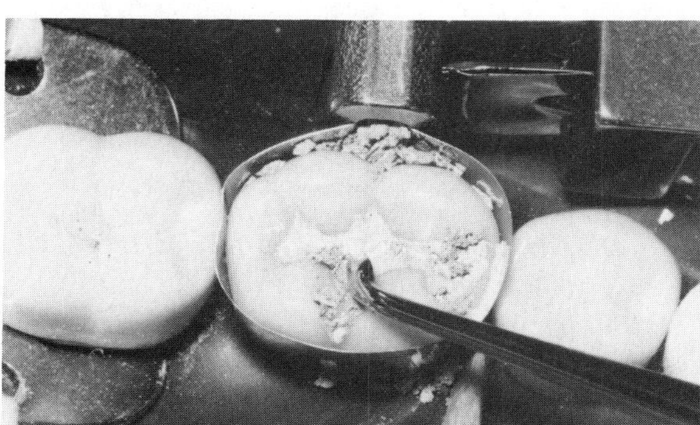

FIGURE 22–72
Occlusal margins are recovered.

CONTINUED ON FOLLOWING PAGE

PROCEDURE 22–4

AMALGAM RESTORATION *(Continued)*

Steps	Rationale
13. Release the matrix band from the retainer by loosening the band tightener and locking nut; remove wedges (Fig. 22–73)	Removal of the matrix system en masse is difficult and may fracture the amalgam

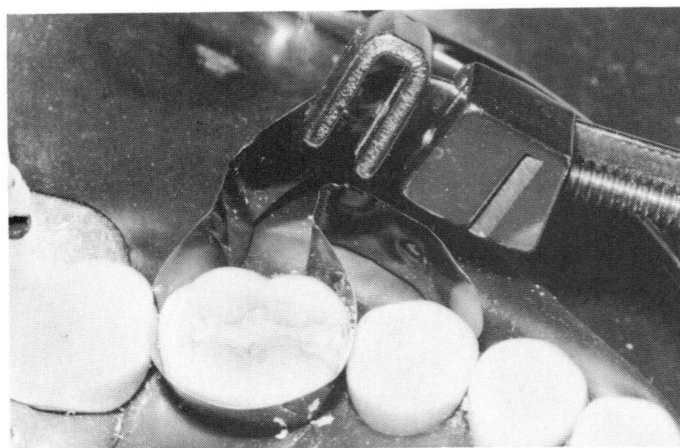

FIGURE 22–73
The wedge has been removed, and the retainer loosened from the band.

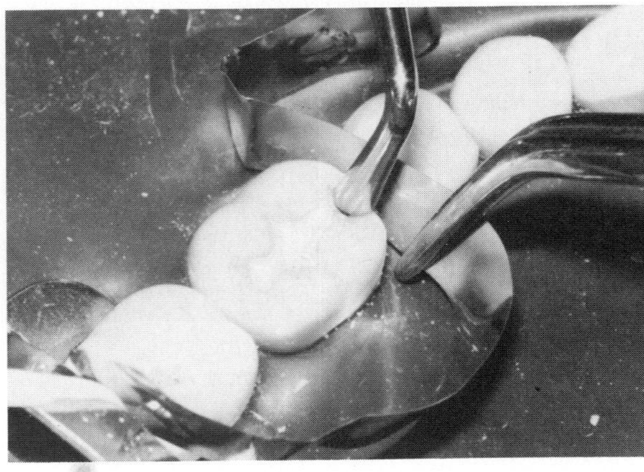

FIGURE 22–74
An amalgam condenser is used to stabilize the marginal ridge during the removal of the band.

Steps	Rationale
14. While maintaining gentle pressure on the marginal ridge with a large amalgam condenser, lift the matrix band from the unrestored proximal area first, then finally from the restored area (Fig. 22–74)	The apically directed force of the condenser resists the occlusally directed removal of the matrix band, preventing marginal ridge fracture; removing the band from the unrestored area first reduces pressure on the restored proximal contact
15. Explore the gingival margin for excess (overhang); carve away any excess with a fine-bladed instrument (such as the 1/2 Hollenback carver) (Figs. 22–75 and 22–76)	The gingival margin is the least accessible margin; it should be finalized before the amalgam becomes too hard

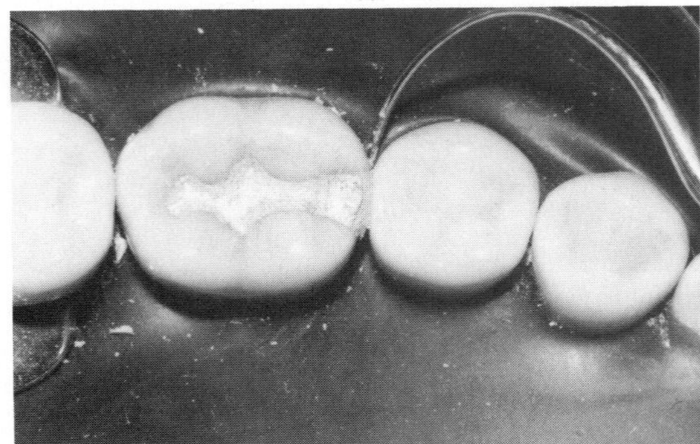

FIGURE 22–75
Gingival margin is checked for excess amalgam with an explorer.

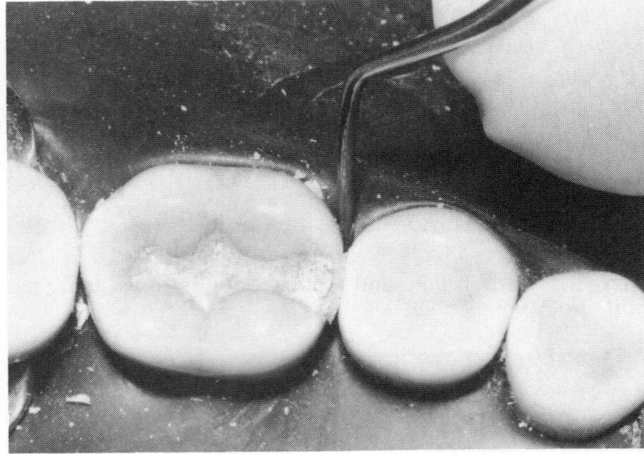

FIGURE 22–76
Excess amalgam at the gingival margin is carved away.

Steps	Rationale
16. Carve all proximal and outer contours to final form Recover all margins. At the margins, all cutting strokes should be directed parallel to the margins to maintain a seal and to avoid overcarving The tooth surface should be used as a guide by resting the carving edge on it as shaving strokes are made Carve occlusal anatomy to general form keeping pits and grooves shallow (Fig. 22–77)	Steep anatomy in amalgam leads to marginal breakdown

Steps	Rationale

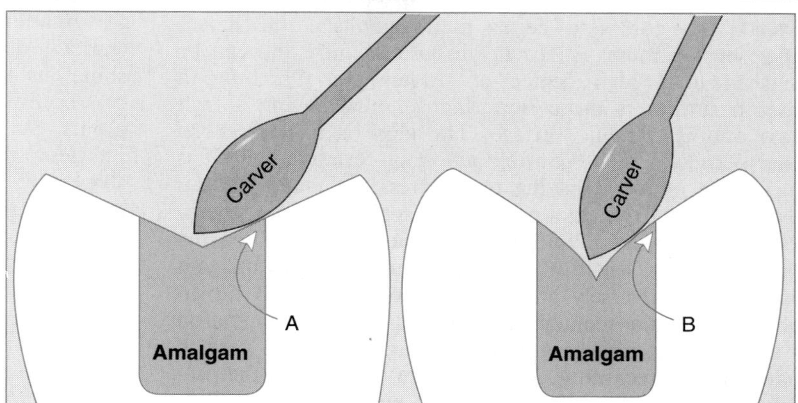

FIGURE 22–77
Amalgam anatomy should be carved to shallow form whenever possible. Doing so produces stronger margins *(A)*. Thin angles seen in *(B)* will eventually fracture from occlusal stress.

Steps	Rationale
17. Remove the rubber dam; caution the client against biting at this time	Inadvertent biting will likely fracture the amalgam because the occlusal surface has not yet been refined
18. Wipe lips carefully and suction the mouth to remove saliva; isolate the operating site with cotton rolls	Occlusal marking ribbon (articulation paper) does not mark well on wet surfaces
19. Insert articulating paper over the area and have the client "gently tap the back teeth together"	Forceful biting on fresh amalgam will cause fracture; tapping is done to examine centric occlusion
20. Carve away marking spots on the amalgam until centric occlusion is reestablished as it was before the operation; re-mark the occlusion as necessary, carving away **"high spots"** each time with a carver or round bur (Fig. 22–78)	Centric occlusion is reestablished

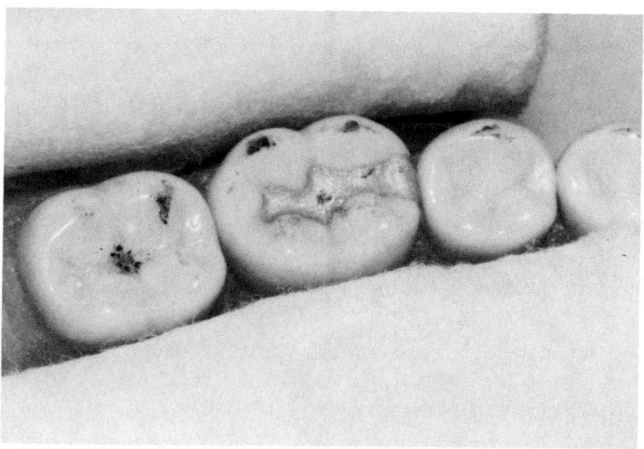

FIGURE 22–78
The occlusal markings show that the contact on amalgam, while present, is lighter than that on the natural tooth. As a result, the operator does not need to further reduce the occlusal contact.

Steps	Rationale
21. Insert the ribbon and have the client "gently grind the back teeth" Remove markings until presurgical contacts are restored	Eccentric contacts are reestablished
22. Finalize the carving, rinse and suction away all debris, caution the client not to chew on the restored tooth until the following day	Amalgam requires several hours to achieve its maximal hardness
23. Also caution the client that discernible "high spots" should be adjusted to avoid fracture	The client may later be aware of a "high spot" when the anesthesia is gone; also, a shift from the prone position of the dental chair to an upright position can produce a different bite sensation because the mandible changes position

Finishing and Polishing

Polished amalgam retains less bacterial plaque and resists **tarnish** and corrosion better than unpolished amalgam. After several hours, the amalgam hardens fully and can be polished to a high degree of smoothness. Obtaining a smooth surface is more important than achieving a high gloss on the metallic surface. The gloss is usually short-lived because of the scouring action of certain foods. It is imperative in the polishing procedures that *undue heat is not generated* from rotating rubber cups and points as they contact the amalgam. Such heat can harm the pulp, leaving the tooth very sensitive. The metallurgy of the amalgam also can be adversely affected. Air coolant should be directed against the metallic surface whenever heat generation is a possibility. Finishing and polishing procedures vary in materials and technique. However, the first step in the procedure is to recheck the occlusion to ensure that in polishing the operator does not destroy important occlusal contacts. If the carving has left a smooth amalgam, polishing proceeds simply and rapidly. In most cases, it is not realistic to attempt a polish of the proximal surface. If it is smooth, it should be left alone except for a brief "shoeshine" using wet flour pumice and dental tape. Other areas can be finished with discs, brushes, and rubber cups and points. A flour of pumice slurry and other polishing powders are used by many operators. More recently, abrasives were incorporated into special rubber polishing cups and points. After the amalgam margins have been refined with a sharp carver or finishing bur, these polishing cups and points are excellent for producing a smooth metallic surface. Using a light intermittent touch and rotary speeds in the slow-to-moderate range, the operator can rapidly produce an excellent finish. A periodic reshaping of the rubber points, rounded from wear, against an abrasive disc enables the operator to properly polish grooves and fossae.

PROCEDURE 22-5

FINISHING AND POLISHING AMALGAM

Equipment

Isolation materials
Finishing burs
Carving instruments
Handpiece
Rubber polishing cups and points (or flour of pumice and polishing powders)
Air and water syringe

Steps	Rationale
1. Question the client regarding occlusion and tooth sensitivity since the operation	Sensitivity may indicate premature centric and/or eccentric contacts; polishing should be delayed for very sensitive teeth
2. Explain the value of polished versus unpolished restoration to the client	The polished amalgam resists plaque retention, corrosion, and tarnish
3. Isolate and dry the area	For a simple polish, cotton roll isolation is adequate; several adjacent polishes or polishes in conjunction with new restorative treatment are best done under rubber dam isolation for improved visibility and control of polishing debris
4. Examine the amalgam for burnish marks; adjust occlusion as necessary with a round finishing bur	Burnish marks indicate occlusal contacts; large areas and areas on inclines should be reduced, consistent with the person's natural occlusion
5. Refine the occlusal margins with a sharp discoid carver, drawn in shaving strokes parallel to the margins (Fig. 22–79)	Minute excess amalgam is shaved flush with the margins, preventing fracture; parallel strokes reduce the possibility of enamel microfractures and overcarving the amalgam

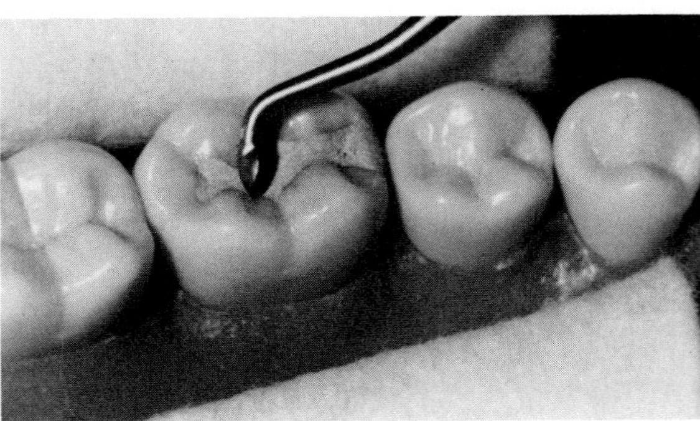

FIGURE 22–79
Using a stroke parallel to the margin, a sharp carver refines occlusal margins of the amalgam.

Steps	Rationale
6. Using slow-to-moderate speeds and intermittent brief strokes, polish the amalgam with abrasive-impregnated rubber cups and points (Figs. 22–80 and 22–81)	Rotary rubber instruments rapidly generate heat due to friction; this can create pulpal sensitivity and damage the amalgam restoration

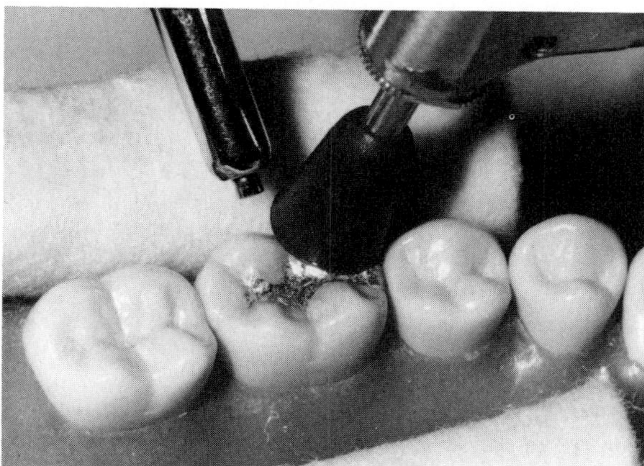

FIGURE 22–80
A rubber polishing cup is used to polish the marginal ridge and cusp slopes. An air stream is used as a coolant.

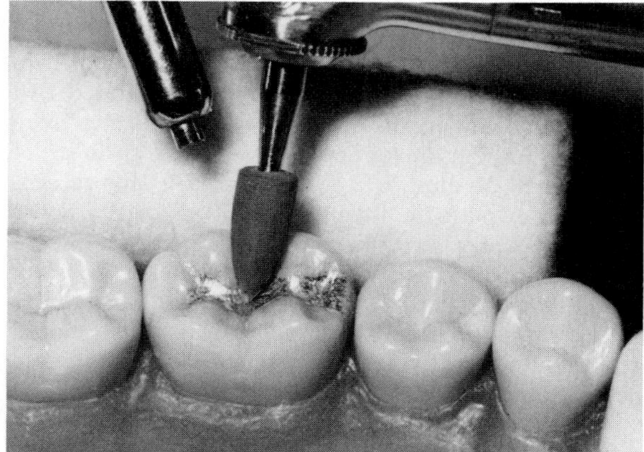

FIGURE 22–81
A rubber polishing point is used to polish pits and grooves.

Steps	Rationale
Begin with the most abrasive and end with the least abrasive; direct a gentle stream of air onto the amalgam during polishing procedures; avoid overpolishing established occlusal contacts	Once proper occlusal contacts are established, they should be maintained
7. Remove isolation materials and rinse the mouth of debris	Debris and excess saliva are annoying to the client
8. Show the client the polished restoration(s) and reiterate the value of the procedure (Fig. 22–82)	This helps to further instill confidence; clients may be motivated to take better care of their teeth; they appreciate professionalism and pride in extra effort

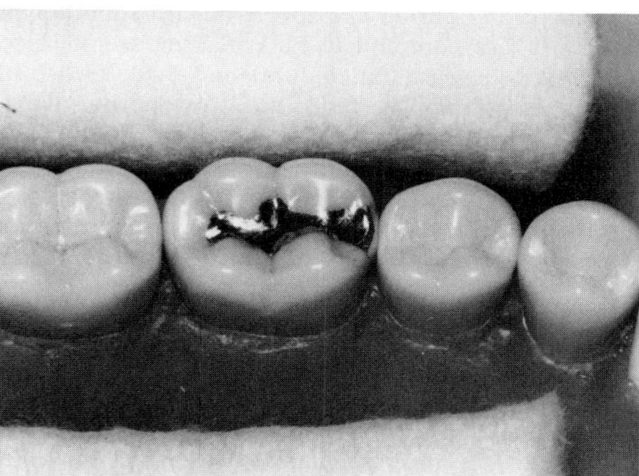

FIGURE 22–82
A polished amalgam.

Mercury Hygiene

In dentistry, the care exercised in preventing bodily harm from mercury ingestion or inhalation is termed **mercury hygiene.** There is little question that disregard for mercury's potential to cause disease may produce injury. However, in decades of use, careful handling of mercury has made it and dental amalgam safe.[14] Practitioners may routinely restore teeth with amalgam with the assurance that by exercising reasonable care, no harm will come to the professional staff or their clients. Alarmists have attempted to discredit not only the benefits of amalgam, but also the virtues of dentists who recommend amalgam. Many of their claims are based on half truths and are motivated by reasons that are unclear.

The individuals primarily at risk from mercury exposure are dental personnel. It has been shown repeatedly that good ventilation, avoidance of mercury spills, and proper handling of amalgam scrap remove virtually all the risks of mercury exposure.[15] In busy restorative practices, common sense provides a more than adequate margin of safety. This begins with work and storage spaces that are well ventilated. Special filters and detectors are available to monitor mercury vapors. In addition, a periodic monitoring service for mercury air levels is available through dental societies. Bulk stores of mercury are not recommended. Amalgam should be used as premeasured mercury and alloy and mixed in sealed capsules. Triturators are available that provide enclosed spaces for the capsules being triturated. All handling of amalgam mixes should be done over a deep tray to contain loose particles and promote easy clean-up of scrap amalgam. Carpeting in the work area is not recommended because periodic vacuuming of amalgam scrap may release mercury vapors. Scrap amalgam should be stored in air-tight containers and covered with x-ray fixer (sulfide) solution or other inactivating solutions. Disposal of amalgam capsules and other contaminated materials should be done in compliance with state and local environmental and safety policies.[13] Careful examination and cleaning of trays, amalgam wells, chair seams, and other susceptible areas may reveal small scrap particles that should be recovered safely and stored. In addition, evacuation traps should be cleaned routinely and amalgam scrap properly stored. Amalgam carriers should be checked for residual amalgam. The practice of heating a carrier over a flame to soften and remove clogged amalgam should be avoided because the release of mercury fumes may be toxic.

Client exposure to mercury is negated by the brevity of the dental appointment and by controlled and clean placement of the amalgam. Rubber dam isolation provides the best control of the surgical site. All scrap is readily removed when the dam is in place. Careful and thorough suctioning of particles is recommended. The combining of the mercury with the alloy prevents the release of mercury in a significant quantity. The claim by a few individuals that dentists are poisoning their clients has not been demonstrated scientifically or proven. Except in cases of client allergy to mercury, which is rare, oral healthcare professionals may continue to render fine restorative care using amalgam.

Composite Resins

Rationale

Resin materials have been used for several decades to address the client's desire for tooth-colored anterior restorations. Modern resins have been so vastly improved that their use in anterior teeth, to meet client aesthetic desires, has become routine. Small resin restorations that do not support occlusion last for many years and are an excellent restorative service. Their success has caused intense research for resins that can provide similar stability and durability in posterior teeth. When clinically compared to amalgam, the wear resistance of tested composite resins is inadequate to justify their routine use in areas of high occlusal stress.[7,16–19] Advancements in this area can be expected in the near future as intense research efforts continue.

Material

One of the great advances in operative dentistry was the development of a new, highly stable resin (BIS-GMA) by Bowen.[20] This complex organic resin has become the basis for the remarkable influx of new and steadily improving direct tooth-colored materials. The addition of special inorganic particles of glass, quartz, or silica to this resin can produce natural-appearing restorations when correctly shaped and polished. These **composites** are produced in a wide range of shades and vary in their abrasion resistance and polishability. The first of these newer resins hardened by joining chemicals via mechanical (spatulation) mix. The latest and best materials are activated and hardened by exposing the material to a special light. The light-activated materials are denser and more color stable. Incremental placement and curing overcomes much of the polymerization shrinkage common to bulk placement and allows the operator to develop the contours and shade blends of each restoration. Composite resins are provided by manufacturers in handy dispensing devices (Fig. 22–83).

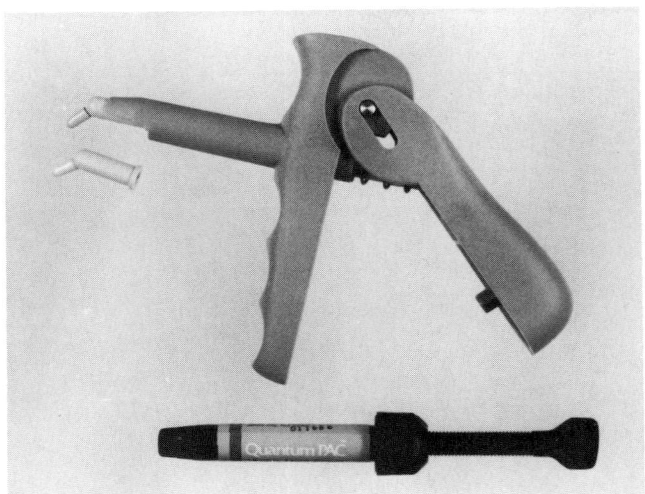

FIGURE 22–83
Two dispensing devices used to express limited quantities of composite resin. These containers are opaque to prevent polymerization due to exposure to sunlight.

Composite resin procedures and cavity design are unique. The research of Buonocore has provided a means for conserving tooth structure by his discovery that retention and resistance form for resins could be created on enamel.[21] This concept, known as **enamel bonding,** has become the basis for the routine placement of modern direct resin restorations and for such popular procedures as pit and fissure sealants and bonded veneers. As long as the prepared tooth presents an adequate enamel surface area, significant retention can be achieved via a careful technique. The enamel surface is shaped with instruments such as rotary burs or diamonds to establish the desired design. Then, the controlled application of acid (approximately 37% phosphoric acid) to the prepared enamel roughens the surface **(acid etching).** Thorough rinsing and forced-air drying displays the etched enamel (frosty appearance), which is ready to receive a bonding resin and thereby retain a resin restoration.

Compared to enamel bonding, **dentin bonding** is far less predictable. Obtaining dependable, biocompatible adhesion of resin to dentin has been the subject of intense research and debate in recent years. The composition of dentin presents special challenges for those attempting to bond to it. Dentin is more organic than enamel and, when instrumented, leaves a surface covered with microscopically observable debris. This **smear layer** may interfere with strong bonding at the dentin-resin interface. In addition, a trace amount of moisture emanating from the vital pulp is present on the dentin surface. Because restorative resins are incompatible with moisture (hydrophobic), numerous adhesive systems (hydrophilic) have been developed to chemically unite the resin with the moist dentin surface. Most of these adhesives are tested in laboratory settings using extracted teeth. Although manufacturers promote their respective products as being highly efficacious, oral health professionals have little assurance that they will be as successful when used clinically.

Perhaps the most important concern regarding dentin bonding is the potential for harming the vital pulp. This concern centers around cleansing or "conditioning" procedures that precede the application of the bonding resin. Shallow cavities limited to enamel can be acid-etched with impunity, because enamel is inert and virtually free of vital tissue. However, most cavities extend into dentin and it is the treatment of this tissue surface that is in question. A few manufacturers promote leaving the dentinal smear layer in place and modifying it via chemical agents to gain retention. Most, however, advocate its removal. The removal of the smear layer by conditioning agents (usually acids) risks opening the dentinal tubules leading to the pulp. Although mechanical retention is gained when resin flows into the open tubules, the pulp may be harmed in the process. Open tubules may allow the ingress of microorganisms and chemicals via leakage beneath the restoration. Many manufacturers promote their products by claiming that true adhesion occurs without pulp damage. Long-term clinical testing is needed to determine the efficacy of dentin conditioning in view of the potential harm. Recently, techniques have been promoted that utilize weaker acids, which theoretically reduce the potential for pulp damage and yet still adequately etch the enamel. Regardless of the technique, record entries should indicate accurately the details of any procedure for the subsequent evaluation of untoward symptoms or radiographic diagnoses by the dentist. At this time, it can be said that no reliable and safe dentin bonding system has a proven *clinical* track record.[22]

With such limitations, composite resin is the best material for conservative tooth-colored restorations. Its use is generally limited to the anterior teeth and nonstressbearing areas of posterior teeth. Where inadequate enamel remains for resistance and retention, special locking grooves can be designed into the preparation.

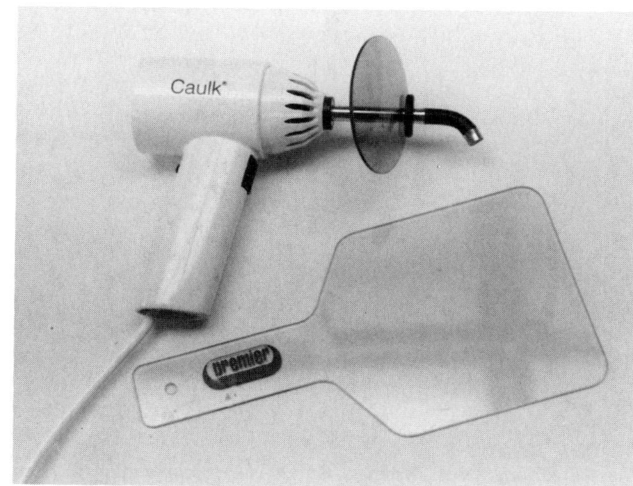

FIGURE 22-85
Protective shields: a hand-held paddle-shaped shield and a disc-shaped shield that encircles the light wand close to the tip.

Armamentarium

Curing Light. The curing light is required to initiate **polymerization** of the resin matrix. The light is in the blue range and is transmitted from its electrical source via a fiberoptic bundle to the tip of a small wand that is positioned on the tooth surface (Fig. 22-84).

Protective Shields. Protective shields are available to prevent eye injury and meet the human need for safety. The wave lengths produced by the curing light have been shown to damage the retina and must be screened to protect operator, assistant, and client. Protective shields may be hand-held, attached to the wand, or incorporated in specially made eyeglasses (Fig. 22-85).

Plastic Instruments. Plastic instruments are conven-

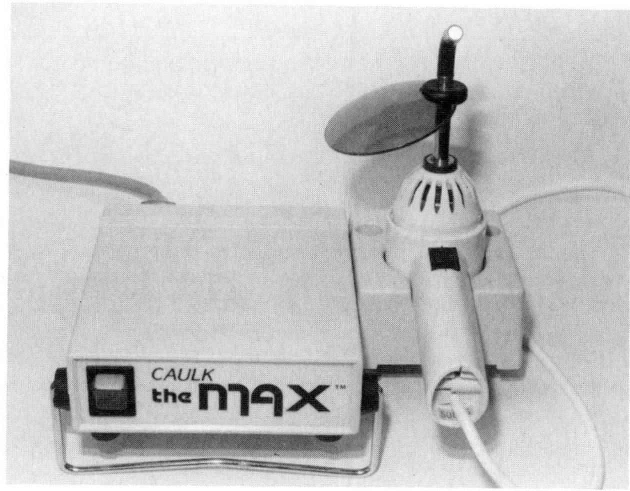

FIGURE 22-84
A light source for polymerization.

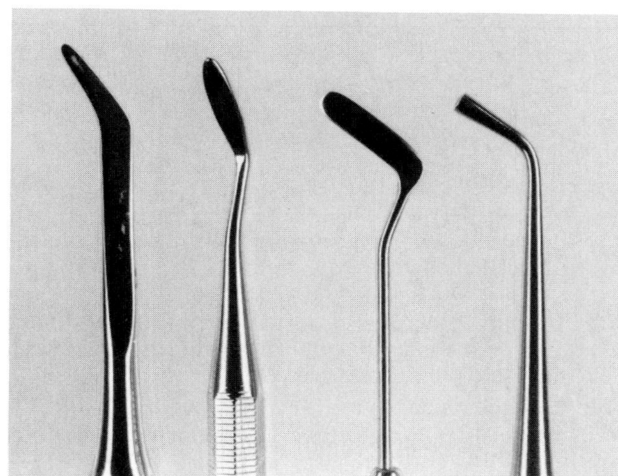
FIGURE 22-86
Common plastic instruments.

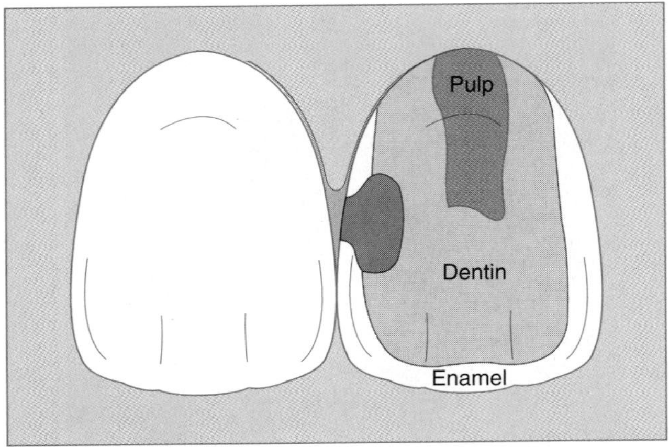

FIGURE 22–87
Class 3 carious lesion depicted. Caries is shown invading the dentin, but the cavity does not endanger the incisal corner.

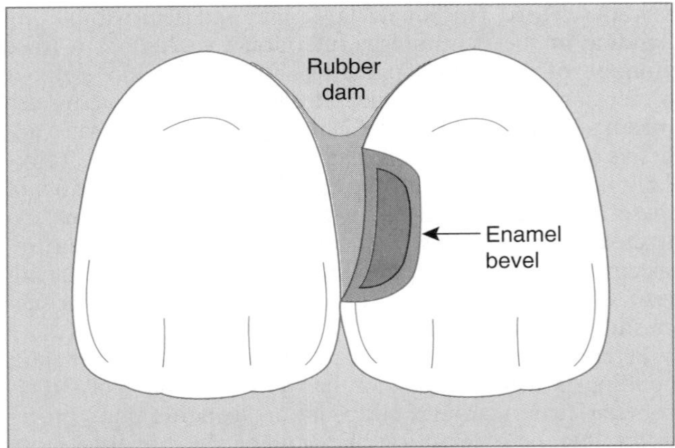

FIGURE 22–88
Lingual view of the completed class 3 cavity preparation. The dentin is protected by a cavity liner, an enamel bevel has been placed, and the rubber dam retracts the gingiva to provide access.

iently designed to carry, shape, and mold soft (plastic) materials. They are blunt-ended instruments not intended for firm condensation or cutting. Selection of instruments is based on the location of the cavity preparation and personal preference (Fig. 22–86).

Class 3 Restoration Placement and Finishing

Before applying the rubber dam, small samples of composite resin should be placed on the tooth surface and cured for 20 to 30 seconds. Matching the tooth shade before it becomes dry (and lighter in shade) under isolation ensures a closer shade match in the final restoration. Resin also tends to change slightly in shade as a result of curing. Removal of this sample resin is simple because the tooth surface has not been etched.

A typical class 3 carious lesion is illustrated in Figure 22–87. The preparation is made to satisfy all principles but with emphasis on conservatism in outline form. The plastic nature of the material allows it to be placed under virtually no force, and specially designed delicate instruments are available for placement and finishing. In the maxillary anteriors, access is usually from the lingual direction and care is taken to preserve the marginal ridge whenever possible. Following complete caries removal, liners are placed to protect the pulp. Complete dentin coverage with a glass ionomer cement or calcium hydroxide liner prevents acid irritation to the pulp. An enamel bevel enhances mechanical retention by exposing the ends of enamel rods, which are highly susceptible to etching (Fig. 22–88; see Procedure 22–6.)

PROCEDURE 22–6

COMPOSITE RESIN RESTORATION

Equipment

Isolation materials	Composite resin	Finishing burs and discs
Cavity liner	Matrix system	Spoon excavator
Acid gel	Curing light	Air and water syringe
Bonding resin	Plastic instruments	Articulating paper

Steps	Rationale
1. Query the client regarding expectations, explain the nature of composite resins	All restorative materials have limitations; composite resins may stain and fracture resulting in the need for replacement in time; shades may not be perfect
2. Select the composite shade, place a small amount of material on the tooth near the lesion and cure it, involve the client in the shade selection	Cured resin may have a slight shade difference from the shade guide, and patient preapproval is always a good idea, especially where aesthetics is concerned
3. Place the rubber dam	A dry operating field is essential
4. Following cavity preparation, apply cavity liners as indicated	Vital dentin should be protected from the acid in the etching procedure

Steps	Rationale
5. Position a clear, plastic matrix strip between the preparation and the adjacent tooth	This prevents acid from etching the adjacent tooth surface
6. Dry the tooth and apply etchant (37% phosphoric acid) to the peripheral, beveled enamel for at least 15 seconds; rinse with an air-water spray for at least 15 seconds; dry with forced-air drying Reposition the matrix as necessary and position a wedge interproximally	Enamel etching is the primary retentive feature of most composite resin cavity preparations; the wedge stabilizes the matrix and adapts it to the gingival margin, preventing overhangs
7. Inspect the peripheral etched pattern	A chalky appearance over the entire bevel identifies adequate etching; if not present, repeat the etching procedure
8. Apply a thin coat of bonding resin to the preparation; spread the resin over the etched enamel with a small brush or sponge and a gentle stream of air (Fig. 22–89)	The fluid resin flows into the minute irregularities of the enamel The stream of air evenly spreads the resin over the preparation, prevents pooling of the resin, and ensures a more uniform coating

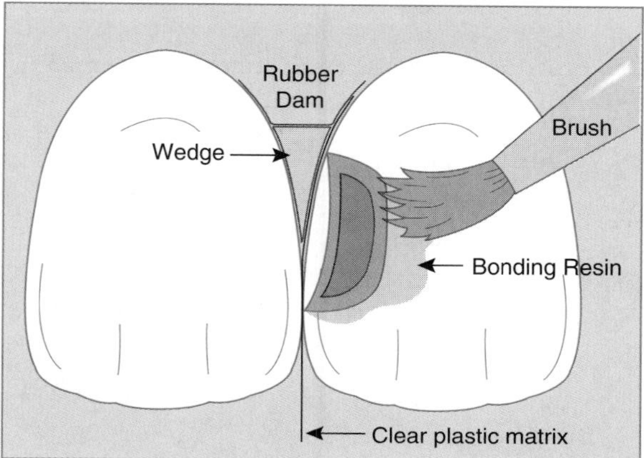

FIGURE 22–89
The etched enamel receiving a coating of bonding resin. A matrix separates the cavity from the adjacent tooth and is contoured and stabilized by a wedge placed interproximally.

Steps	Rationale
9. Place a special protective eyeshield on operator, assistant, and client to avoid eye damage during the curing that is about to start	The eyes must be protected from the damaging effects of the blue curing light
10. Polymerize the bonding resin with the curing light for 15 to 20 seconds; light wand should be as close as possible without direct contact. Careful inspection of the cured bonding resin will reveal a slightly tacky surface. This very thin layer of resin is unable to completely polymerize because of the influence of air. It will rapidly polymerize once covered by composite resin or a matrix strip and reexposed to the curing light	Establishes the bond of composite resin to enamel
11. Remove the cap from the composite resin dispensing device and express a small amount of the selected composite resin onto a small paper pad; replace the cap	The pad is convenient for loading the placing instrument. It can also be covered with an opaque lid to protect the resin from sunlight; replacing the cap prevents the material in the dispensing device from polymerizing
12. With a plastic instrument, place an increment of resin in the preparation and adapt it to the walls and margins; cure this first increment for 20 to 30 seconds (Fig. 22–90)	Careful adaptation eliminates voids and enhances retention and marginal seal; larger increments require longer curing times to ensure penetration of the light waves into the mass
13. Continue to add and cure increments, building the form to a slight excess in contour In small cavities final form may be achieved by firmly wrapping the clear matrix against the tooth and curing through it (Fig. 22–91) Remove the wedge and matrix	Slight overcontouring allows finishing without leading to undercontouring

CONTINUED ON FOLLOWING PAGE

PROCEDURE 22–6

COMPOSITE RESIN RESTORATION *(Continued)*

Steps	Rationale

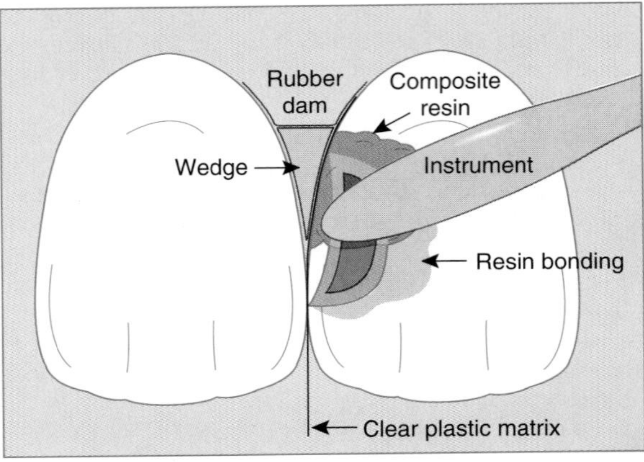

FIGURE 22–90
The placement of increments of composite resin into the preparation. The resin must be adapted into the recesses of the cavity and built against the matrix and cavity walls.

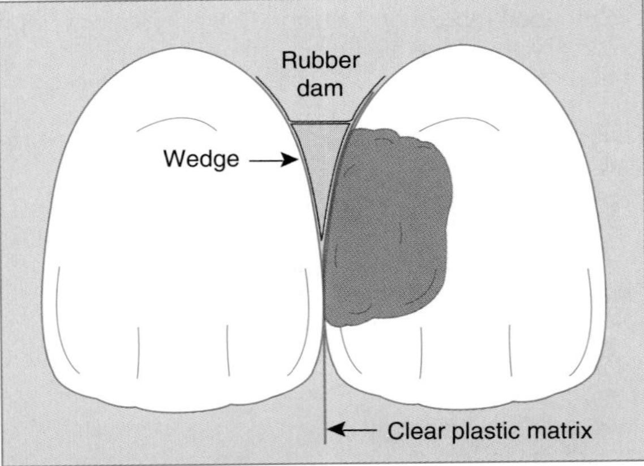

FIGURE 22–91
The cavity filled to slight excess, cured and prepared for finishing.

14. Contour the restoration with finishing burs and discs, exercising care to avoid tooth damage (Figs. 22–92 and 22–93

Rotary instruments can rapidly remove tooth structure

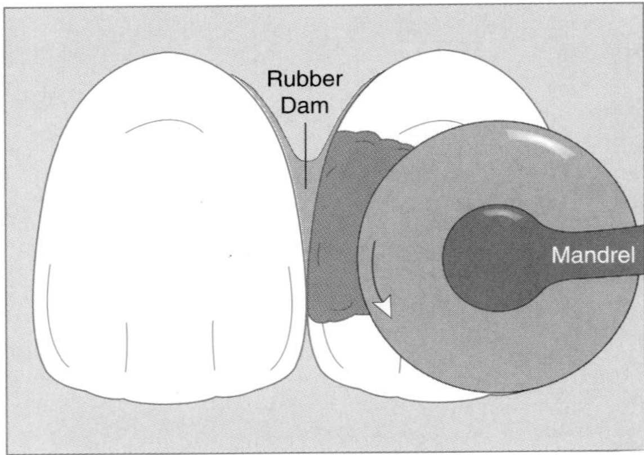

FIGURE 22–92
Contouring the composite resin with a disc to achieve the final form. The wedge and matrix have been removed.

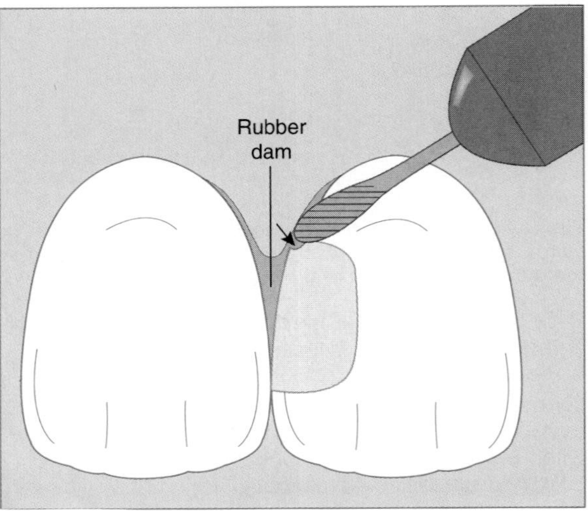

FIGURE 22–93
Damage to the tooth structure if due caution is not exercised with the use of a bur in the finishing procedure.

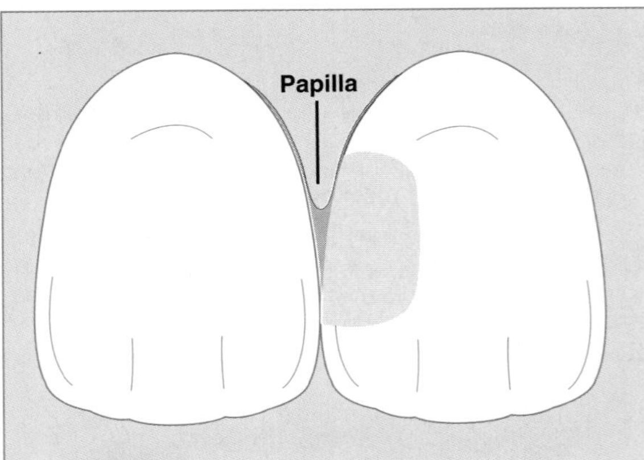

FIGURE 22–94
Finished class 3 composite resin restoration.

Steps	Rationale
15. Remove the rubber dam and check for occlusal prematurities on the restoration High spots can be carefully reduced with a large rounded finishing bur	In particular, lingual aspects of maxillary class 3 restorations may require occlusal adjustment
16. Polish all accessible parts of the restoration with polishing discs; examine the gingival sulcus and remove debris	Polishing enhances oral hygiene and reduces plaque accumulation
17. Show the client the restoration; explain shade discrepancies (Fig. 22–94)	Teeth isolated by the dam appear lighter because of their being dry; as moisture returns they appear more natural, blending with the new resin restoration

Class 5 Restoration Placement and Finishing

One of the most perplexing problems in restorative dentistry is the course and treatment of lesions at the gingival margin. Abrasion, erosion, dental caries, or combinations of these can create defects that are difficult to properly restore. They often require isolation with special rubber dam clamps, because they frequently extend into the gingival sulcus. The most durable material for restoring these lesions is direct gold; amalgam is a satisfactory compromise. But these metals are often unacceptable to the client because of their unnatural color. Composite resin is a reasonable alternative, offering a natural appearance with fair longevity.

Shade selection is accomplished prior to the rubber dam placement. The rubber dam is placed in a routine manner. To properly isolate the lesion, it may be necessary to retract the free gingiva to expose the gingival margin of the cavity. Several rubber dam clamps work well for this purpose. Perhaps the most versatile is the Ferrier 212 clamp, which was specifically designed to gain access for class 5 cavities. It should be stabilized with modeling compound to prevent it from moving during the operation.

Enamel, again, is the key to retention and margin seal. Because enamel is absent on the root, the dentist may place a supplemental retention groove in the gingival wall. Deep areas within the cavity are covered with a protective liner such as calcium hydroxide or glass ionomer cement. An enamel bevel is created with a rotary instrument and is then etched with acid gel. If there is any danger that the gel placement will extend onto dentin, a protective liner should be placed over all the dentin. After etching, rinsing and drying, the preparation is coated with bonding resin that is spread gently with a stream of air and cured for 15 seconds. This is followed by incremental placement and curing of the composite resin. Contour can be developed by tamping the final increments into place with an instrument tip that has been dipped in bonding resin. This procedure produces a smooth contoured surface that requires a minimum of finishing. After final curing, careful shaping and polishing are accomplished with finishing burs and discs. The gingival sulcus should be cleansed of any debris before dismissing the patient.

Class 1 (Occlusal) and Class 2 Restorations

Clients' demands for naturally appearing teeth have also resulted in the use of composite resins for restoring posterior teeth. However, these materials have not found acceptance for all such cases. To date, wear resistance properties have not proved adequate when compared with dental amalgam, the time-honored standard.[17] Accordingly, the use of composite resins in posterior teeth should be limited to small lesions and conservative preparations, to minimize wear and direct occlusal contact. As these materials are acceptably improved, their use may become routine for more complex restorations.

Class 2 composite restorations have an additional drawback: marked technique sensitivity. In addition to the need for very careful isolation and moisture control, manipulation of the matrix is critical. Establishing a positive proximal contact that is physiologically contoured is one of the biggest challenges facing the operator. Since composite resin cannot be forcibly condensed against the matrix (as with amalgam), developing the proximal contact necessary to prevent food impaction and tooth drift is difficult. The placement, curing, and finishing of composite resins for other than the simplest posterior restorations demand the utilization of four-handed dentistry at its best. The inclusion of this area is not ruled out as a legitimate consideration under expanded functions, but specific procedures will not be covered in this chapter.

Glass Ionomer Cements

Rationale

These materials have been improved in recent years and are available as cavity liners as well as definitive restorative

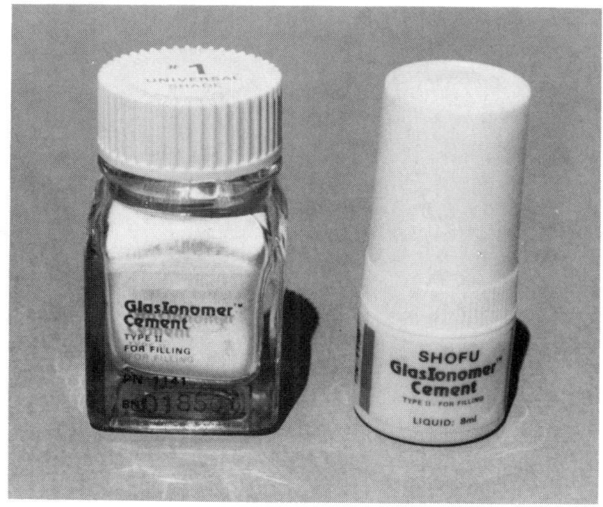

FIGURE 22–95
A typical glass ionomer cement product.

materials. Like all cements, they undergo dissolution when exposed to saliva. However, these restorative cements dissolve slowly and release fluoride ions in the process. As a result, recurrent caries are rarely seen at the margin of a glass ionomer cement restoration. Glass ionomer cements are composed of aluminosilicate glass (powder) and polyacrylic acid (liquid) (Fig. 22–95). Although somewhat opaque, the cements have been improved both in their transparency and shades through the incorporation of special glass particles in the powder. A great benefit of this material is that it apparently truly adheres **(chemical bonding)** to prepared tooth structure.[23] Glass ionomer restorative cements are brittle and should not be used in areas of direct occlusal stress. Root caries are one of the more perplexing decay patterns, often presenting as nearly impossible restorative challenges. Access and detailed cavity design can be extremely difficult. In these cases, caries excavation and restoration with glass ionomer cement can provide the solution. As compared to amalgam, which requires specific retention design and a rigid matrix to withstand condensation, glass ionomer cements adhere to the tooth and flow into the recesses of the cavity. Another excellent use of glass ionomer cements is for the restoration of abrasion and erosion (gingival margin) lesions. The ability to truly adhere to the "notched" dentin enables the operator to restore these frequently sensitive lesions atraumatically.

Class 5 (Abrasion Lesion) Placement and Finishing

Because surgery of the teeth is not necessary in many abrasion lesions, it is possible to accomplish these restorations without anesthesia unless the lesion is substantially below the gingival margin. If these lesions are *not* carious, and therefore require no operative preparation, restoration can be completed at the oral prophylaxis appointment. Once placed, at subsequent appointments, care should be taken to prevent dehydration of the glass ionomer cement restorations.

PROCEDURE 22–7

GLASS IONOMER CEMENT RESTORATION OF CLASS 5 ABRASION LESIONS

Equipment

Isolation materials	Polishing cup	Curing light
Glass ionomer cement	Plastic instruments	Matrix system
Polyacrylic acid	Carving instrument	Protective barriers
Flour of pumice	Bonding resin	

Steps	Rationale
1. Examine the lesions and assess the need for local anesthesia	Nonsensitive, noncarious lesions that are easily accessible may not require anesthesia
2. Select the shade of restorative material to be used; involve the client in the selection	Client preapproval is always a good idea, especially where aesthetics are concerned
3. Place the rubber dam (Fig. 22–96)	The rubber dam is the best device to control contamination of the cavity

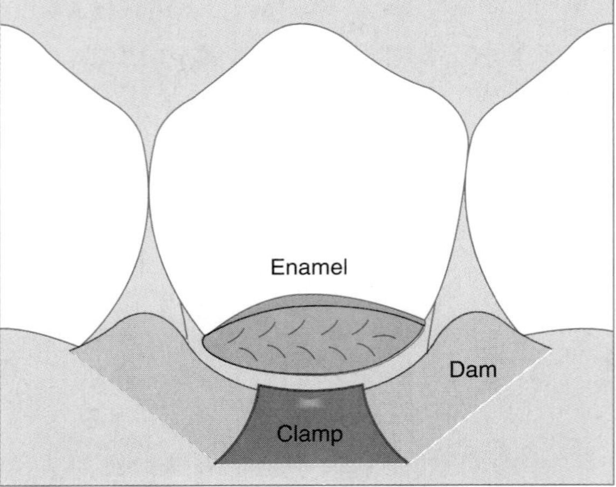

FIGURE 22–96
A typical abrasion lesion isolated with a rubber dam and retracting clamp.

Steps	Rationale
4. Briefly, débride the cavity and adjacent tooth structure with a flour of pumice and water slurry in a rubber polishing cup; rinse thoroughly and dry (Fig. 22–97)	Plaque and debris compromise the adherence of the restorative material

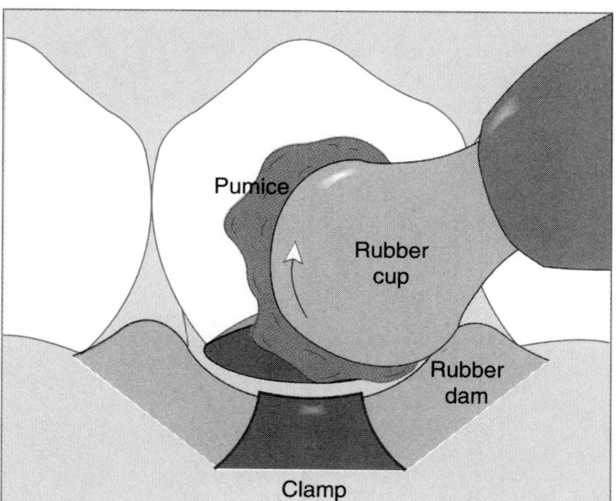

FIGURE 22–97
The débridement of the lesion with a flour of pumice slurry and rubber cup.

Steps	Rationale
5. Select a matrix that matches the tooth contour in the cervical area	A cervical matrix greatly facilitates the management of this runny material
6. According to the manufacturer's instructions, apply polyacrylic acid to the abrasion lesion (approximately 15 seconds); rinse thoroughly for 15 seconds with a strong air-water spray, and dry but do not desiccate (Fig. 22–98)	Brief exposure to polyacrylic acid removes microscopic debris (smear layer) without opening dentinal tubules; desiccation of the dentin may upset the adherence of the cement, which is very sensitive to moisture changes

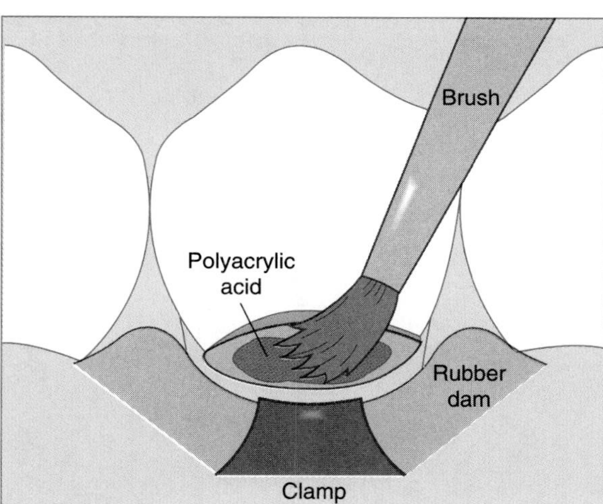

FIGURE 22–98
The application of polyacrylic acid to cleanse the dentin.

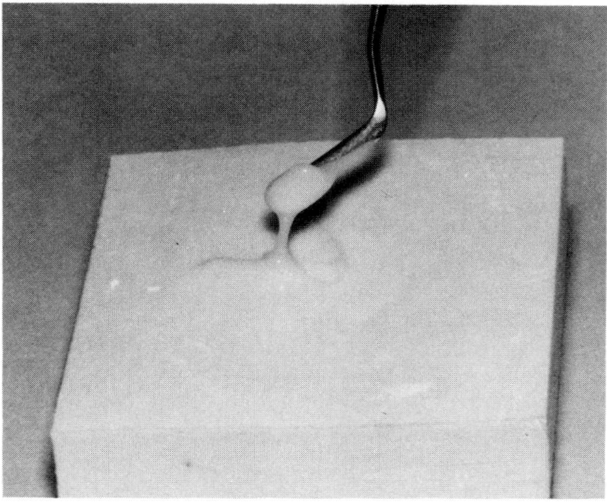

FIGURE 22–99
A proper mix of glass ionomer cement.

Steps	Rationale
7. According to the manufacturer's directions, prepare a creamy mix of restorative cement (Fig. 22–99)	Directions should be followed closely because ratios of powder and liquid, as well as mixing times, are critical
8. Rapidly fill the cavity to slight excess using a plastic instrument to place the material (Fig. 22–100); position the cervical matrix over the cavity to hold the cement against the tooth (Fig. 22–101)	The cement may begin to harden so expeditious placement is important; the matrix prevents the material from slumping or running out of the cavity; it also prevents the material from drying out and crazing as it hardens

CONTINUED ON FOLLOWING PAGE

PROCEDURE 22-7

GLASS IONOMER CEMENT RESTORATION OF CLASS 5 ABRASION LESIONS *(Continued)*

Steps	Rationale

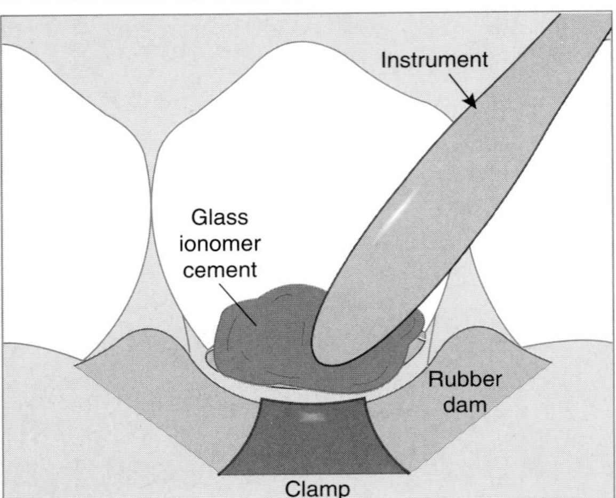

FIGURE 22-100
The placement of the glass ionomer cement to slightly overfill the cavity.

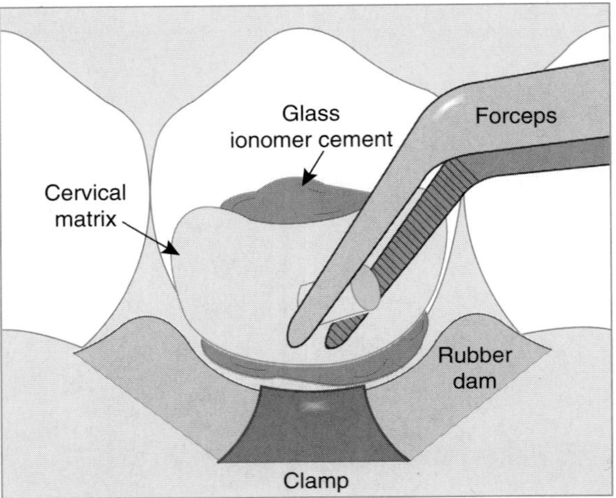

FIGURE 22-101
The positioning of the clear cervical matrix over the cavity and expressing excess glass ionomer cement at the edges of the matrix.

Steps	Rationale
9. If it is stable, pressure on the matrix may be released after 1 minute; coat the excess cement at the matrix periphery with bonding resin or special cement varnish	The coating of bonding resin prevents dehydration of the cement
10. After 4 to 5 minutes, remove the matrix; shave off the gross excess cement with a sharp, chisel-like instrument (Fig. 22-102); recoat with bonding resin or special varnish; cure the bonding resin for 15 seconds	The cement can still be easily shaped Final contouring is delayed until it has fully hardened; it is not necessary to cure the resin to protect against dehydration of the cement, however, uncured resin is messy

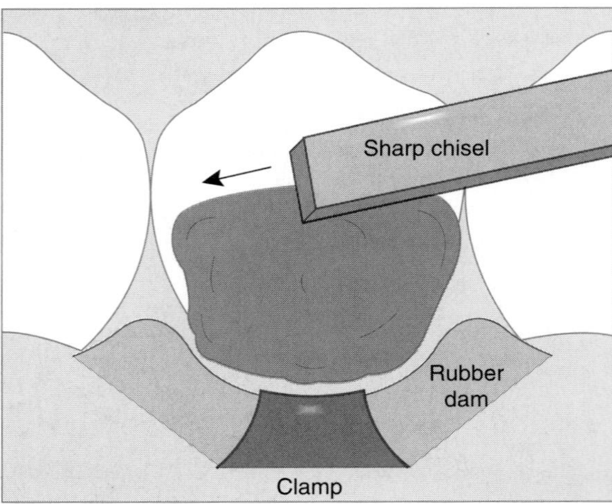

FIGURE 22-102
The trimming of the gross excess with a sharp instrument such as a chisel.

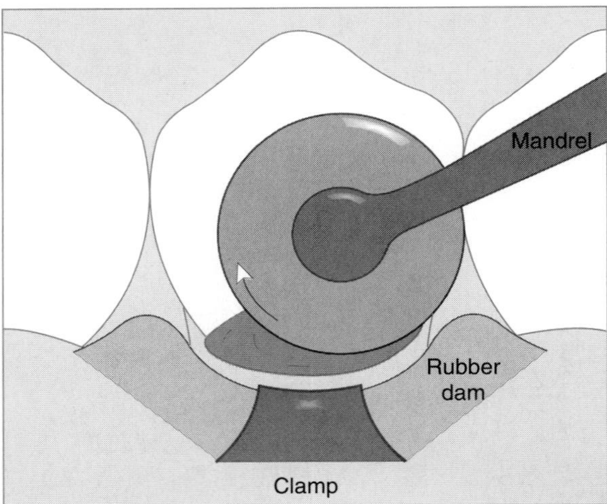

FIGURE 22-103
The final contouring of the restoration with a disc.

Steps	Rationale
11. After approx. 10 more minutes, contour the restoration with finishing burs and discs (Fig. 22-103); take care to avoid damage to the tooth root (Fig. 22-104)	Most glass ionomer cement restorations can be finished after this length of time Rotary instruments can rapidly score the root (Fig. 22-104)
12. Apply a thin coat of bonding resin to the cement restoration surface and cure the resin for 15 to 20 seconds	The cured resin coating will protect the cement from excess moisture or drying for several hours
13. Remove the rubber dam; examine the gingival sulcus and remove debris	Cured bonding resin debris is very difficult to see because it is transparent

Steps	Rationale

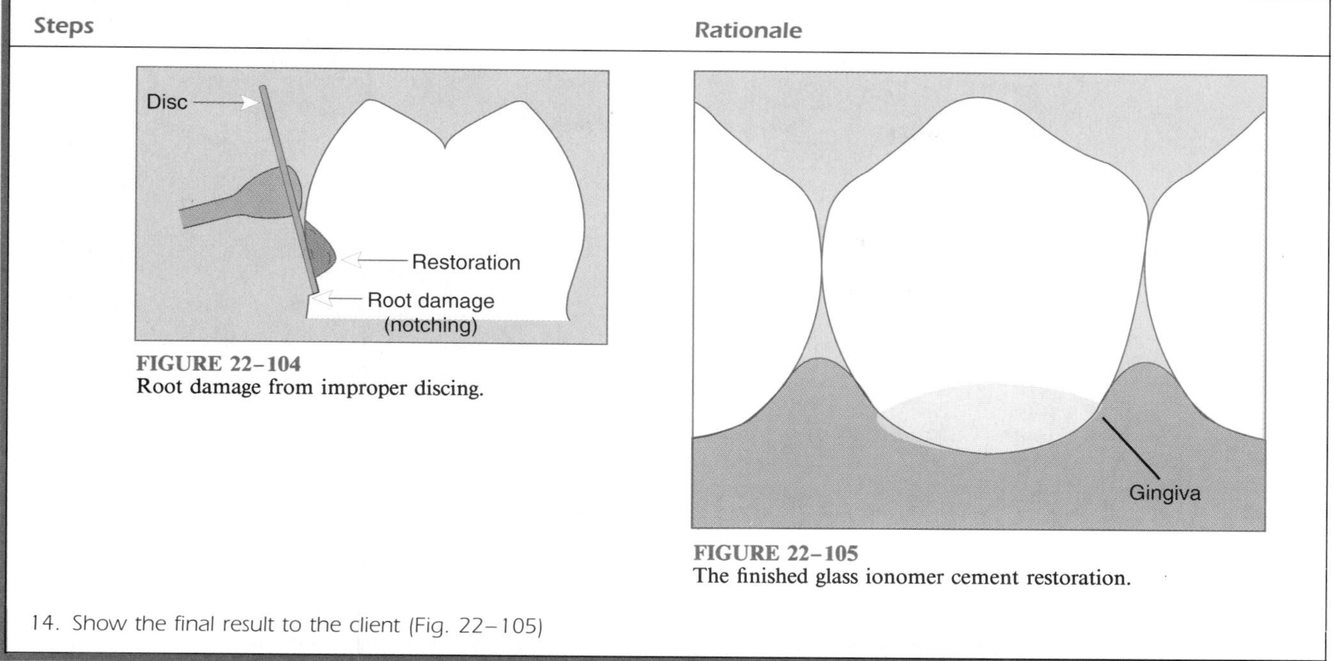

FIGURE 22-104
Root damage from improper discing.

FIGURE 22-105
The finished glass ionomer cement restoration.

14. Show the final result to the client (Fig. 22-105)

Liners and Bases

Rationale

Preserving and protecting the dental pulp is a concern in every restorative procedure on vital teeth. Some pulps seem to survive numerous insults whereas others degenerate and die from what appears to be minor trauma. The insults of dental caries followed by drilling procedures, chemical and thermal shock, and microleakage around restorations, individually or collectively, can cause pulpal damage and discomfort to the client. It should be the goal of each therapist to perform procedures in the most atraumatic manner possible so as to promote **pulp protection.**

Vital dentin is a dynamic tissue. The tubules with which it is constituted connect with the pulp and contain fluid and cellular components that are adversely affected by surgical procedures. At a microscopic level it is easy to understand how a gentle stream of air may be injurious to a delicate pulp that is covered by a paper-thin thickness of dentin. Deep cavities in particular must be specially treated to protect the pulp from further insult. Liners and bases are intended to provide such protection.

Liners

No clear distinction exists between liners and bases. However, it can generally be concluded that liners are liquid-like materials applied in thin coatings (< 0.5 mm) to heal the pulp or seal the dentinal tubules against chemical insult. Calcium hydroxide preparations are commonly used to protect the pulp in deep cavity preparations. They also are used in situations when the pulp has been exposed to stimulate the vital pulp to heal if the wound is small and clean. These liners are easily prepared and are usually supplied by manufacturers in small tubes (Fig. 22-106). Equal amounts of base and catalyst are expressed onto a small pad, quickly mixed, and then specifically placed on the dentin or over the pulp exposure (Figs. 22-107 and 22-108). Because these materials typically do not resist compressive forces, an additional hard protective base material is often used for protection.

Cavity varnish is another example of a liner (Fig. 22-109). Varnishes are composed typically of resins dissolved

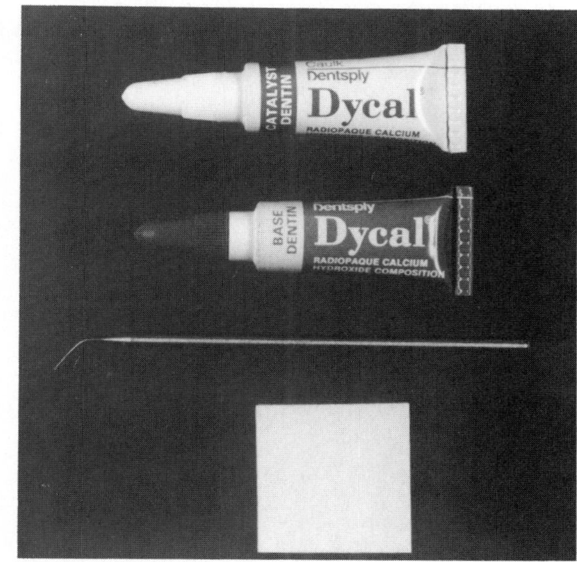

FIGURE 22-106
A popular calcium hydroxide product, an applicator, and a mixing pad.

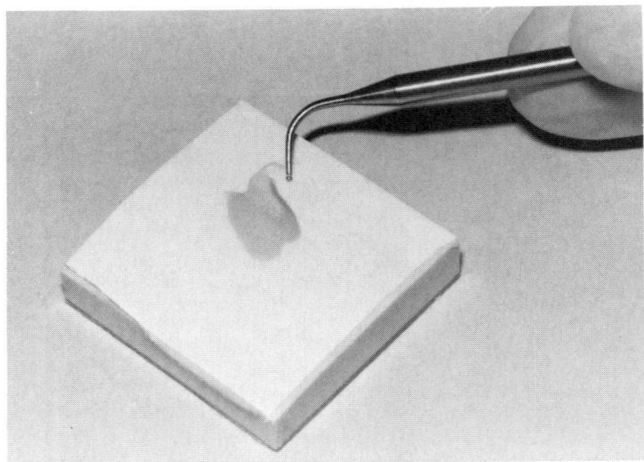

FIGURE 22-107
Equal amounts of the calcium hydroxide base and catalyst have been mixed.

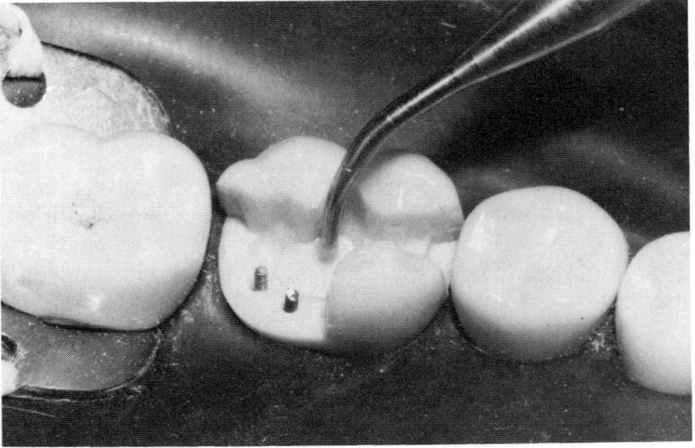

FIGURE 22-108
Placement of the mixed calcium hydroxide in the deeper areas of the cavity preparation.

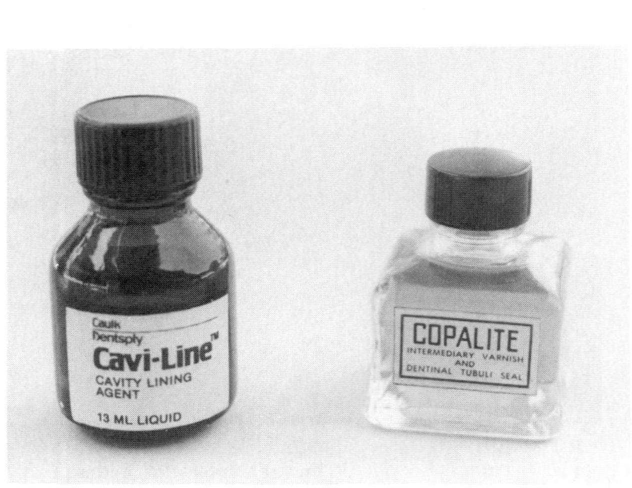

FIGURE 22-109
Two popular cavity varnishes.

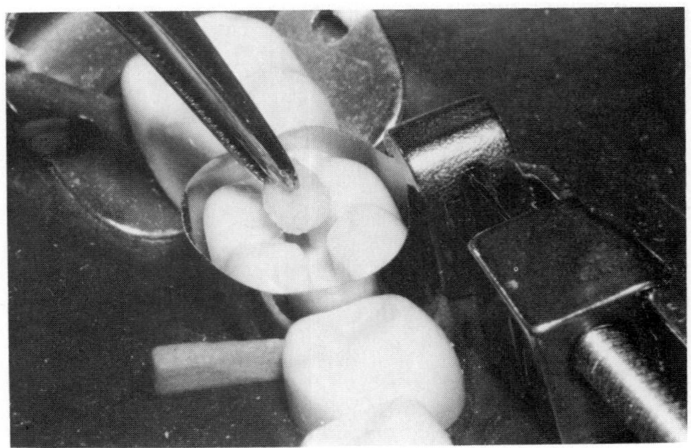

FIGURE 22-110
Application of cavity varnish using a small cotton pellet.

in an organic solvent such as ether. Their function is to seal dentinal tubules to protect the pulp from chemical irritation. Varnishes provide coatings of only a few microns in thickness and therefore offer little thermal insulation. They are usually applied via very small cotton pellets (Fig. 22-110). At least two applications are made to ensure that a uniform coating is obtained.

Bases

Bases are materials placed to provide thermal insulation and support under metallic restorations. They must be strong enough to resist occlusal forces and, in the case of amalgam, resist firm condensation. This category includes zinc phosphate and glass ionomer cements.

Bases of zinc phosphate cement have served dentistry well, providing dependable support and insulation under metallic restorations (Fig. 22-111). The proper preparation of zinc phosphate cement, however, requires attention to detail.

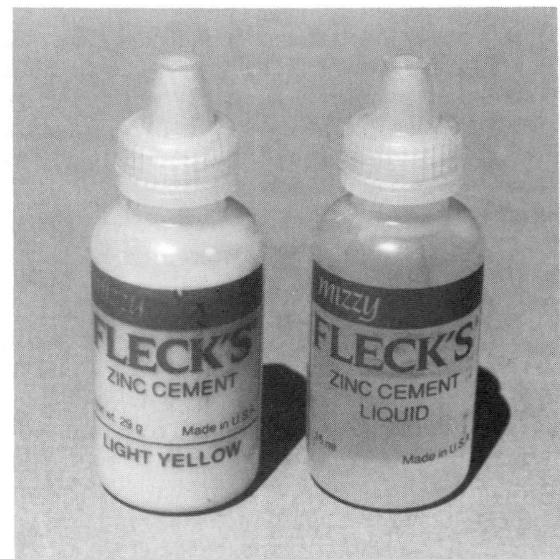

FIGURE 22-111
A popular zinc phosphate cement.

PROCEDURE 22-8

USING ZINC PHOSPHATE CEMENT—LUTING AGENT AND BASE

Equipment

Isolation materials
Cool glass slab
Zinc phosphate cement
Stainless steel spatula
Plastic instruments
Protective barriers

Steps	Rationale
1. Cool a thick glass mixing slab or tile to approximately 70°F	The chemical reaction and set of zinc phosphate cement are strongly influenced by heat
2. According to the manufacturer's instructions, measure the powder and place it at one end of the cool, dry slab Divide it into several convenient portions, some of which are small; place a small amount of extra powder in one corner of the slab	The extra powder can be used to coat the nib of the plastic instrument to prevent the cement from adhering
3. Dispense the recommended amount of liquid (acid) toward the opposite end of the slab (Fig. 22–112)	The liquid is not dispensed until just before the mixing is begun It absorbs moisture from the air which may affect the properties of the cement

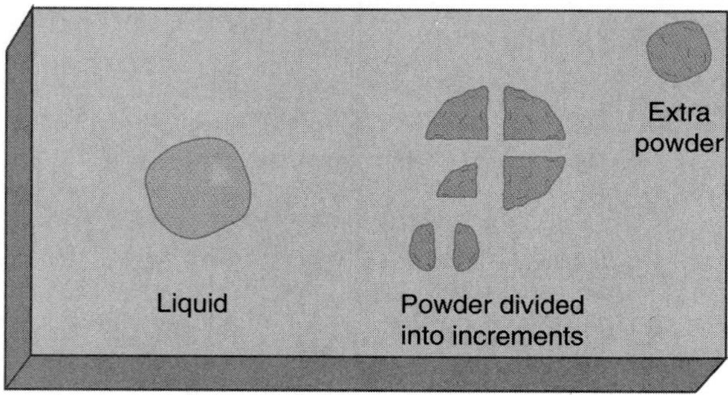

FIGURE 22–112
Zinc phosphate cement components dispensed on a mixing slab. The powder has been divided into increments for mixing.

Steps	Rationale
4. In a timed procedure, draw a small increment of powder into the liquid with the cement spatula Using smooth strokes, spread the mix over approximately $\frac{1}{2}$ of the slab; mix for 10 to 15 seconds (Fig. 22–113)	The reaction is slowly initiated with the small increment; the large area of the cool slab further slows the reaction By slowing the reaction, more powder can be incorporated, providing a stronger, less acidic cement

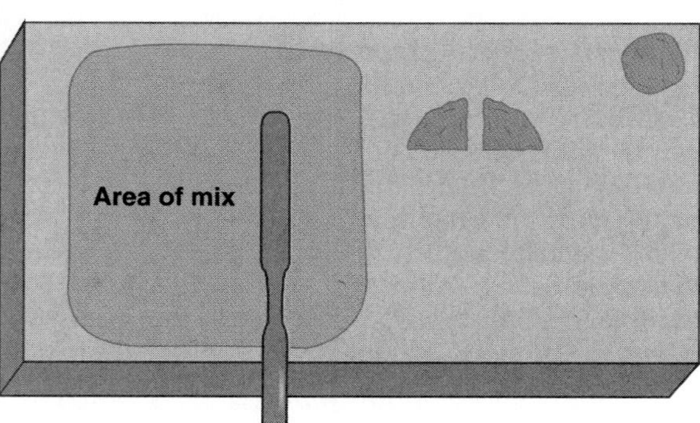

FIGURE 22–113
The incorporation of powder into the liquid as it is mixed over a large portion of the slab.

CONTINUED ON FOLLOWING PAGE

PROCEDURE 22–8

USING ZINC PHOSPHATE CEMENT—LUTING AGENT AND BASE *(Continued)*

Steps	Rationale
5. Continue to add increments, gradually increasing the amount of powder; mix each increment for approximately 20 seconds As the cement thickens, test it for consistency	A controlled technique is important to obtain a consistent result; after approximately 90 seconds the mix should be near *LUTING* consistency and should string out $1\frac{1}{2}$ inches when suspended from the spatula (Fig. 22–114)

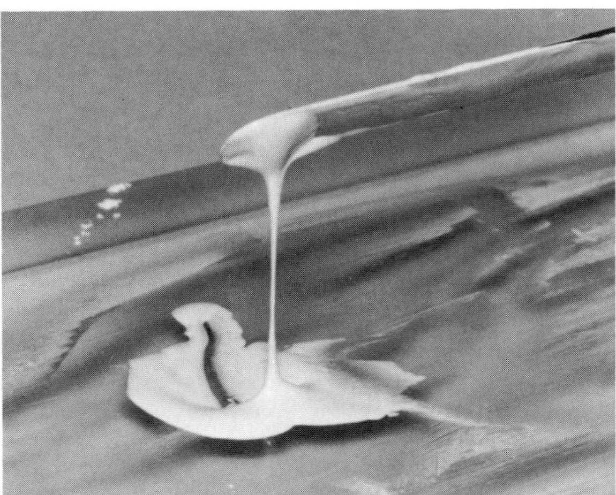

FIGURE 22–114
Zinc phosphate cement is of proper cementation consistency.

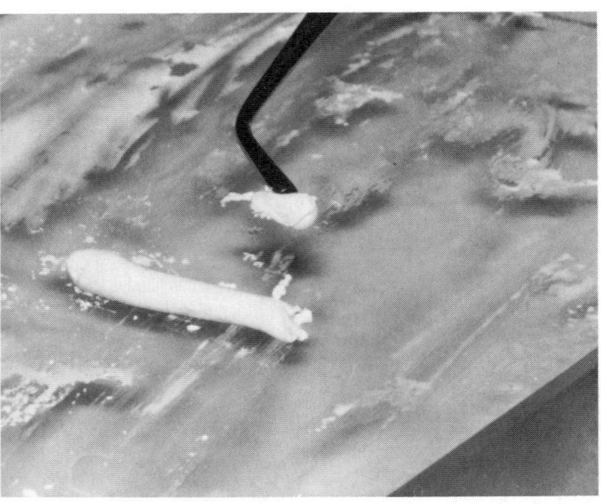

FIGURE 22–115
Zinc phosphate cement is of proper base consistency.

Steps	Rationale
6. Continue to add powder and mix the thickening mass When it can be gathered and rolled into a rope form, the mix is nearly complete (Fig. 22–115) The surface of the cement should be tacky	After approximately 2 minutes of mixing, *BASE* consistency is reached; the tacky surface causes it to stick to the cavity walls
7. Using a plastic instrument, pick up an increment of the cement estimated to be slightly in excess of that required to form the base, adapt it against the cavity walls (Figs. 22–116 and 22–117)	Separate increments may not adhere well to each other, resulting in a weak base; the irregular features of the cavity walls help retain the base

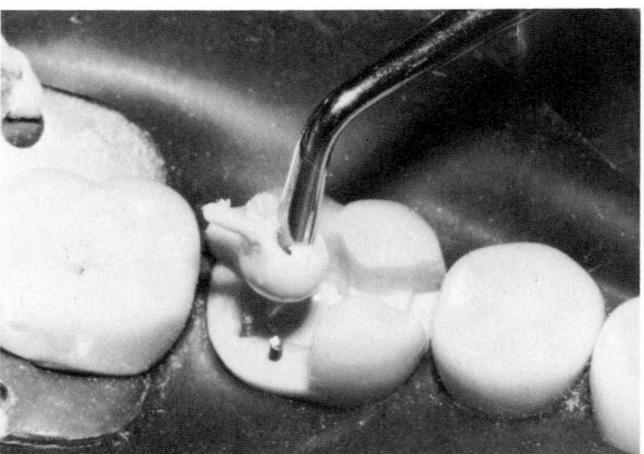

FIGURE 22–116
Zinc phosphate cement base is placed in cavity preparation.

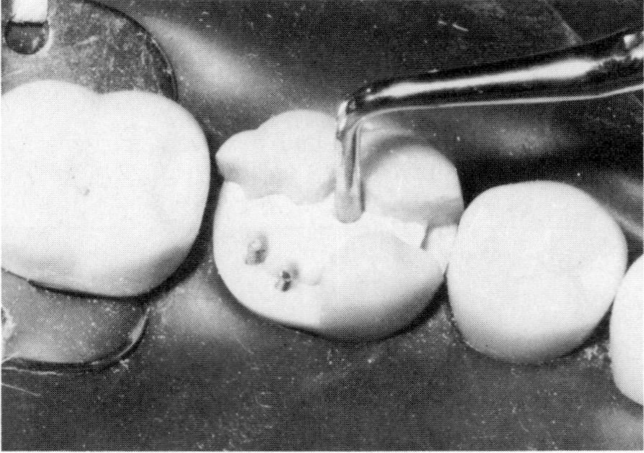

FIGURE 22–117
The base is brought to final form and allowed to harden.

Steps	Rationale
8. Wipe off the instrument nib and dip it in the extra powder kept in the corner of the slab; form the base with the nib The base should generally be formed to simulate a cavity preparation of ideal pulpal and axial wall depth (Fig. 22–118)	The powder coating on the nib prevents the cement from sticking to it; a base built to ideal cavity form gives maximal thermal protection without compromising sufficient thickness of the overlying restoration

Steps	Rationale
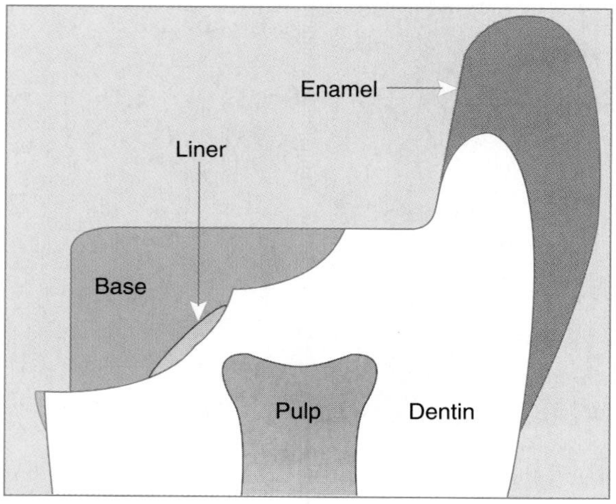 FIGURE 22–118 Cross-section of cavity preparation with liner and cement base.	
9. After the base has reached final form, immerse the spatula and slab in water or sodium bicarbonate (baking soda) solution	This facilitates the cleaning of the slab and spatula
10. Allow the cement to harden (approximately 2 additional minutes); clean cement from walls and margins The base is now ready to support a restoration	Cement base at a margin can be expected to gradually dissolve, resulting in leakage beneath the restoration

When compared with zinc phosphate cement, glass ionomer cements require less time to prepare and also to truly bond to dental tissue. However, mixing and manipulation times are more critical. Glass ionomer cements may be mixed on a nonabsorbent pad, according to the manufacturer's directions. Some products are available in cartridge form and can be mixed mechanically in a few seconds. For best adhesion, the cavity is cleansed with a 10- to 20-second application of polyacrylic acid to remove microscopic debris (smear layer). Following rinsing and gentle drying of the cavity, the mixed cement is rapidly brought into the cavity on a suitable instrument and molded to the desired form while it is in a gel state. In a few minutes, the material hardens at which time it should be coated with a special varnish to prevent moisture loss or gain. Depending on the specific product, amalgam can be condensed on the set base within 4 to 10 minutes from the start of the mix.

IMPLEMENTATION—TEMPORARY OR INTERIM RESTORATIONS

Rationale

Frequently, a significant span of time elapses between the initial or final tooth preparation and the restoration placement. The reasons for this lapse in time vary but may include the need to prepare or cast the final restoration, the desire to allow the tooth to respond to a medication, or the lack of time in a given appointment to complete a procedure. In these situations, protection of the prepared tooth and associated dentition may be imperative to prevent client discomfort and technical complications. Temporary restorations can provide the protective function required during this interim phase in restorative treatment. The primary factors to be considered when determining the need for temporary restorations include:

- Client comfort
- Tooth protection
- Gingival protection
- Tooth movement

Client Comfort

Vital, freshly cut dentin is very sensitive to thermal and chemical insults. As a result, all vital dentin should be covered and sealed from salivary contamination. This protection also prevents the pulp from being exposed to undue insults that may threaten the vitality of the tooth. The temporary restoration also can permit the individual to chew normally.

Tooth Protection

The protection of cusps and cavity margins from fracture after the final tooth preparation is extremely important. The unprotected tooth may break irreparably. Even small fractures to a cavity preparation may require that the tooth be reprepared prior to the placement of a final restoration. A proper temporary restoration protects the prepared tooth from mechanical insult prior to the placement of the final restoration.

Gingival Protection

Unsupported gingival papillae and free gingival margins tend to grow into open and unsealed cavity preparations. It is difficult for the client to maintain a bacterial plaque-free environment with the presence of gingival overgrowth. These factors result in gingival irritation and bleeding that may compromise the quality and success of the final restoration. A restoration must provide proper contour and proximal contact to support the gingiva and prevent food impaction and bacterial plaque retention that can injure the periodontium and cause discomfort to the client. The temporary restoration can provide this necessary anatomical form for an interim period.

Tooth Movement

Without a temporary restoration or unless the temporary restoration is durable and properly contoured, the prepared tooth may **drift** or move slightly in a mesial or distal direction. The prepared tooth may also **extrude** or move in an occlusal direction. In addition, adjacent teeth may drift toward the prepared tooth and opposing teeth may extrude. These situations may complicate the fabrication of a successful restoration. The temporary restoration prevents the occurrence of tooth movement and maintains the occlusal relationship.

Temporary Materials and Placement Techniques

Temporary Stopping

Temporary stopping is a thermoplastic compound that is quickly and easily prepared and placed (Fig. 22–119). It is best used to seal *small,* shallow cavities requiring temporary restoration for periods of *not more than* 2 weeks in length. Temporary stopping rapidly develops leakage because of expansion and contraction in response to thermal changes, limiting its use to short durations.

The placement of the temporary stopping requires that the end of a stick of material be slowly warmed over an alcohol flame until it softens. It is then allowed to cool until it can be handled by the operator. Small increments are rapidly molded in the fingers and positioned on the tip of a placing instrument (Fig. 22–120). These increments are rapidly and firmly packed into the cavity until the material fills the preparation. The criterion for determining the amount of material required to fill a cavity preparation is that the margins be secured and sealed. Minor shaping of the restoration, to restore the tooth as close as possible to the original occlusion or anatomy, is done with a warm, not hot, instrument tip.

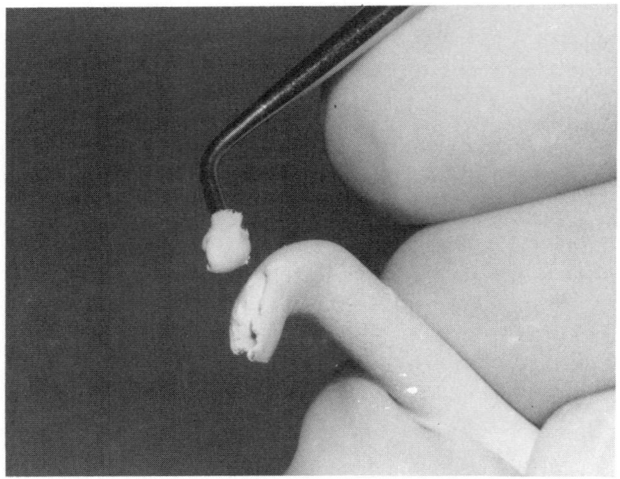

FIGURE 22–120
Temporary stopping material has been warmed over an alcohol flame until soft and then positioned on the tip of a placing instrument.

Reinforced Zinc Oxide With Eugenol

Reinforced zinc oxide with eugenol readily restores intermediate-size cavities that require a more durable material. It is prepared with a mixture of zinc oxide powder and eugenol liquid (Fig. 22–121). The insulating properties of the hardened zinc oxide mass and the obtundent effect of

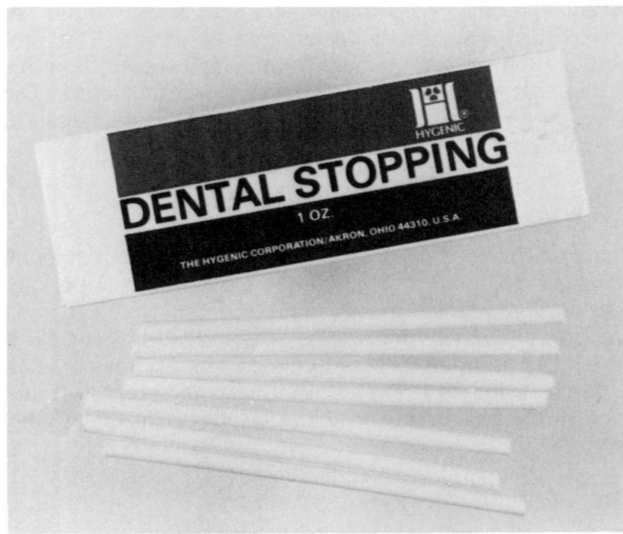

FIGURE 22–119
A popular temporary stopping product.

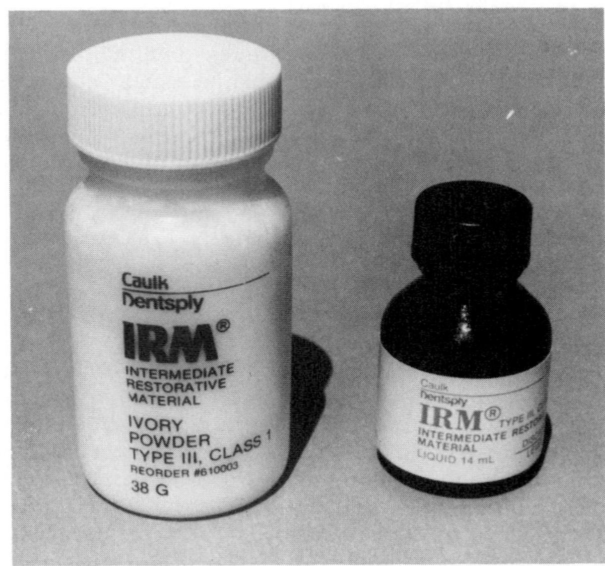

FIGURE 22–121
A popular reinforced zinc oxide with eugenol material.

the eugenol result in a material that dependably protects the vital pulp against chemical and thermal insults. Reinforced zinc oxide with eugenol is relatively easy to prepare and place and is reliable for interim periods of a few months.

The powder and liquid are mixed on a nonabsorbent pad according to the manufacturer's instructions. Firm pressure on the spatula is needed to thoroughly mix the material. When properly mixed, the consistency of the material is thick and clay-like. The material is then rolled with the finger tips (on the pad) into a cylindrical form. Increments can be pinched off the end of the mass with a placing instrument and firmly packed into the preparation until it is full.

PROCEDURE 22-9

PREPARING REINFORCED ZINC OXIDE AND EUGENOL TEMPORARY RESTORATIONS (CLASS 2 CAVITY PREPARATION)

Equipment

Isolation materials
Tofflemire matrix system
Petrolatum
Reinforced zinc oxide and eugenol
Nonabsorbent mixing pad
Plastic instruments
Cotton pellets and rolls
Finishing burs
Carving instruments
Articulating paper
Protective barriers

Steps	Rationale
1. Isolate operating site as appropriate	Isolation varies, depending on goals of therapy. Cotton roll isolation may be sufficient
2. Prepare a Tofflemire matrix system. Apply a thin coat of petrolatum, with a cotton pellet, or cotton swab, on the inside of the matrix band; position the matrix, secure it, and place interproximal wedges as needed	A matrix is needed to contain the material in the cavity preparation because the walls are missing. The petrolatum prevents the material from sticking to the band; excess material may be expressed into the gingival sulcus if the band is not supported interproximally
3. Review the manufacturer's instructions for measuring and mixing	Products vary
4. Prepare the mix; when the material has reached the consistency of firm clay, carry an ample amount to the cavity with a plastic instrument Firmly adapt the rubbery material to all walls of the cavity with a placing instrument (Figs. 22-122 and 22-123)	If the material is too soft, it will not adapt well and it will stick to the instrument; if the material is too firm, it will not condense adequately to prevent voids and will result in leakage

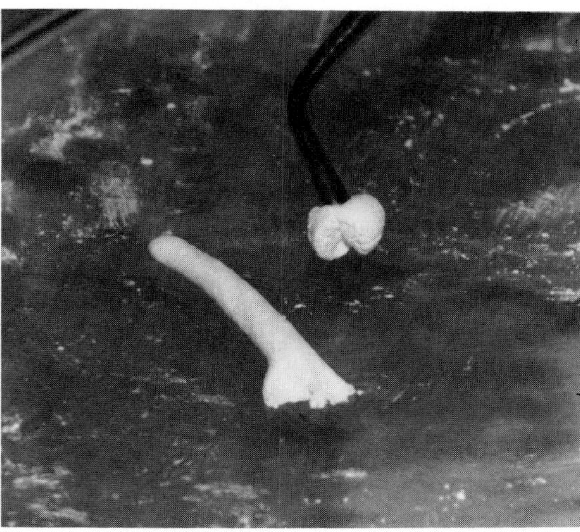

FIGURE 22-122
Properly mixed reinforced zinc oxide with eugenol ready for placement.

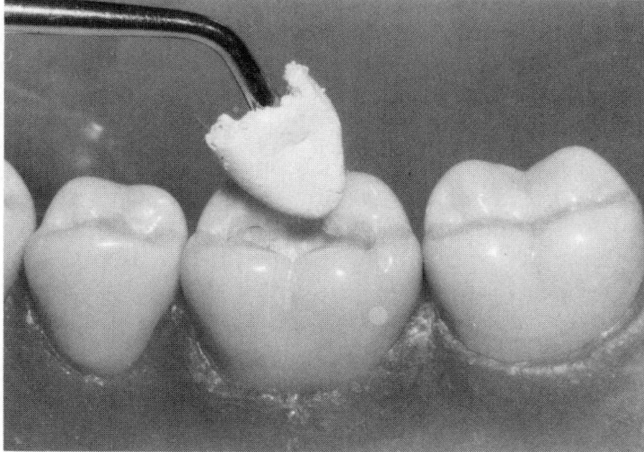

FIGURE 22-123
Reinforced zinc oxide with eugenol being placed in cavity preparation.

Steps	Rationale
5. Fill the cavity to slight excess; shape the occlusal anatomy by using a moist cotton pellet in cotton forceps to create a general anatomical form	Excess material ensures margin coverage; moisture hastens the set of zinc oxide-eugenol materials Detailed anatomy is not needed

CONTINUED ON FOLLOWING PAGE

Steps	Rationale
6. When the material has hardened, remove wedge(s), retainer, and matrix band; apply pressure apically on the temporary restoration to counteract the removal of the band	Removing the band before the material has set may break the marginal seal and dislodge the temporary restoration
7. Check the proximal and gingival margins for excess material and remove with a sharp, narrow-bladed carving instrument	Excess material at the gingival margins (overhang) could result in gingival irritation and hinder the client's ability to maintain a plaque-free environment

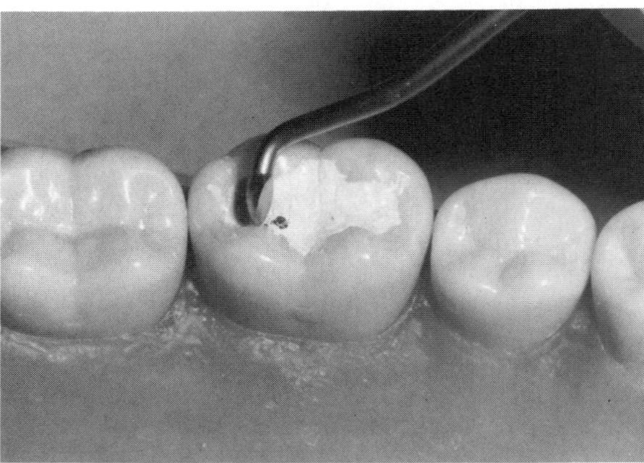

FIGURE 22–124
Final adjustment to the occlusal aspect of the temporary restoration with a carver.

Steps	Rationale
8. Remove isolation materials; evaluate premature occlusion on the temporary restoration with articulating paper and adjust as necessary with a large round bur and carving instruments (Fig. 22–124)	Premature occlusion is very likely to fracture the temporary restoration
9. Examine the gingival sulcus for debris and remove as necessary; excess material at the gingival margin can be removed using a bladed instrument such as the 1/2 Hollenback carver	Debris from the restorative procedure can irritate the gingival tissues

Custom-made Acrylic Resin

The custom-made acrylic resin temporary restoration is recommended for complex restorations such as inlays and partial or complete veneer crowns. The main advantage of this type of temporary restoration is that the technique permits the reproduction of the client's tooth anatomy. The material used in the construction of this temporary restoration is an autopolymerizing acrylic resin. The acrylic is composed of a liquid (monomer) and a powder (polymer) that are mixed together and polymerize through a chemical reaction resulting in a hardened resin mass. Because of the numerous steps involved in the preparation of a custom-made acrylic resin restoration, the main disadvantage of this type of restoration is the time required for production. A limitation of this technique is the requirement that the tooth to be restored be intact or nearly intact. However, the final product is durable, smooth, and comfortable and can serve for several months.

PROCEDURE 22–10

MAKING A CUSTOM ACRYLIC RESIN TEMPORARY CROWN

Equipment

Isolation materials and protective barriers	Petrolatum	Articulating paper
Irreversible hydrocolloid material	Dappen dish	Polishing wheel
Disposable impression tray	Acrylic resin	ZOE temporary cement
Scalpel	Finishing burs and discs	Cotton pellets and rolls

Steps	Rationale
1. Since it has been decided to reproduce the client's tooth form in the temporary restoration, make an impression of the tooth and of those adjacent; use irreversible hydrocolloid material in a sectional disposable tray (Figs. 22–125 and 22–126)	The impression records the exact tooth form; irreversible hydrocolloid is inexpensive and compatible with resin; a sectional tray (quadrant size) works best and disposable ones are inexpensive

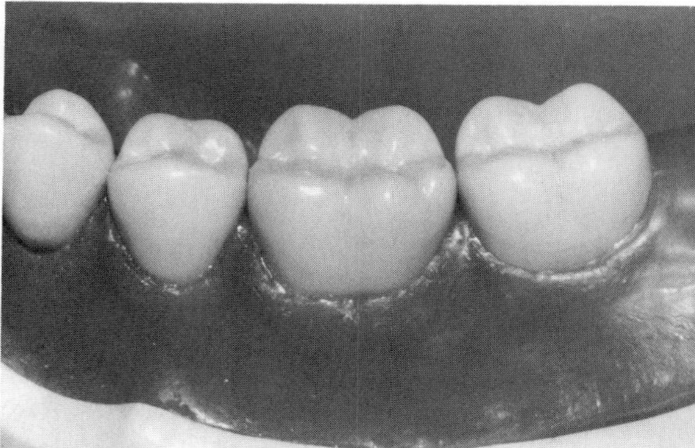

FIGURE 22–125
Intact mandibular first molar.

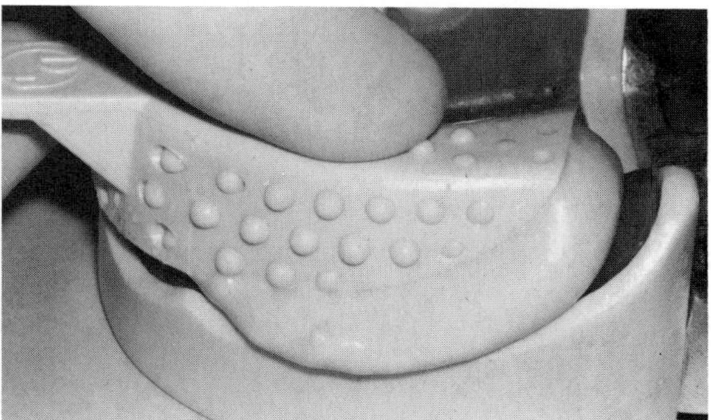

FIGURE 22–126
Irreversible hydrocolloid impression of the intact tooth and operating area.

Steps	Rationale
2. With a sharp blade (scalpel) cut out V-shaped notches in the impression to extend from its periphery into the facial and lingual crown area of the tooth to be prepared (Fig. 22–127); loosely wrap the impression in a moist paper towel and set it aside	The notches serve as sluiceways into which excess resin can flow; the moist towel prevents the impression from drying out and distorting

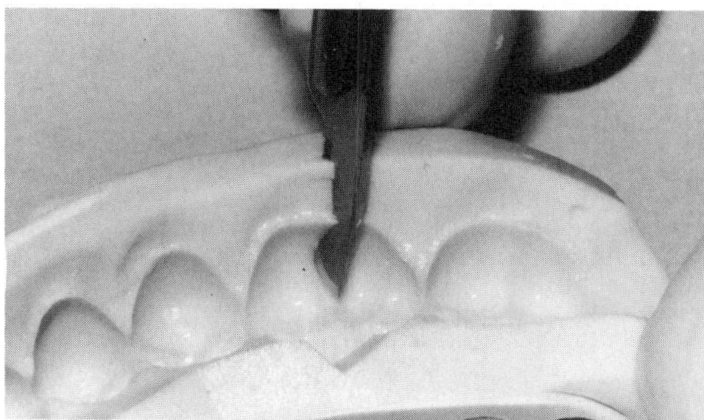

FIGURE 22–127
Scalpel is used to cut V-shaped notches in impression to permit the escape of excess acrylic resin.

Steps	Rationale
3. After the tooth has been prepared by the dentist (Fig. 22–128), coat it and adjacent teeth with petrolatum using cotton pellets or a cotton swab (Fig. 22–129)	Petrolatum reduces the irritating effects of the resin and facilitates the removal of the hardening resin from the tooth

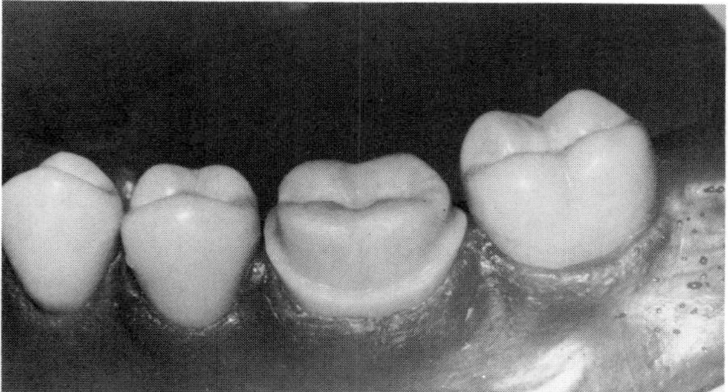

FIGURE 22–128
Crown preparation for the mandibular first molar.

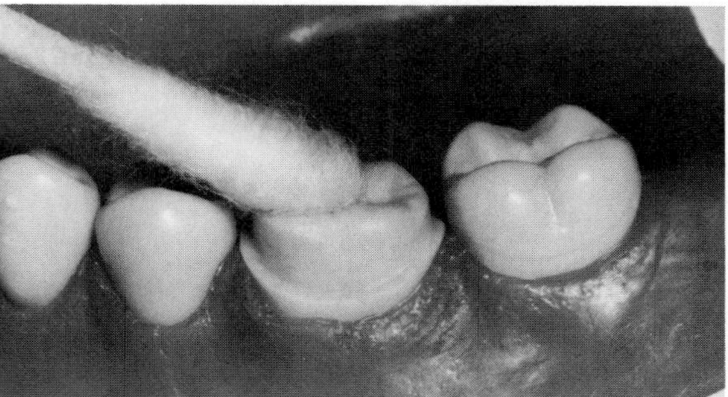

FIGURE 22–129
The prepared tooth is coated with petrolatum to protect the tooth and facilitate removal of the setting resin.

CONTINUED ON FOLLOWING PAGE

PROCEDURE 22–10

MAKING A CUSTOM ACRYLIC RESIN TEMPORARY CROWN *(Continued)*

Steps	Rationale
4. In a dappen dish, prepare autopolymerizing resin by mixing monomer (liquid) and polymer (powder) to a runny consistency (Fig. 22–130); as the mix appears to lose its sheen (approximately $1\frac{1}{2}$ minutes after mixing), fill the crown area in the impression with the runny polymerizing resin (Fig. 22–131)	If the resin is placed in the mouth too soon, it will stick to the teeth; if it is placed too late, it will not flow and adapt well to the prepared tooth

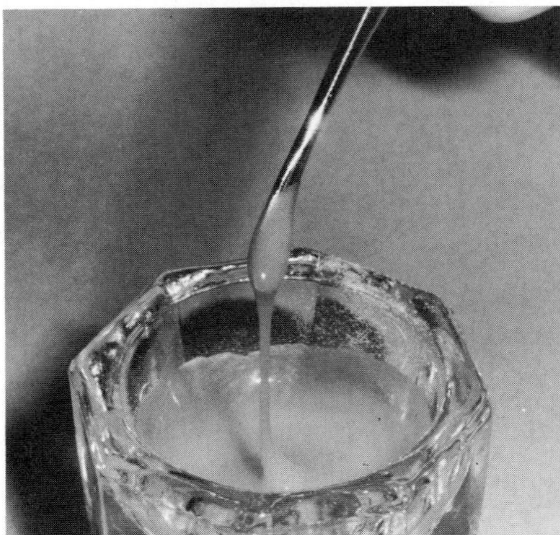

FIGURE 22–130
A runny mix of acrylic resin is prepared in a dappen dish.

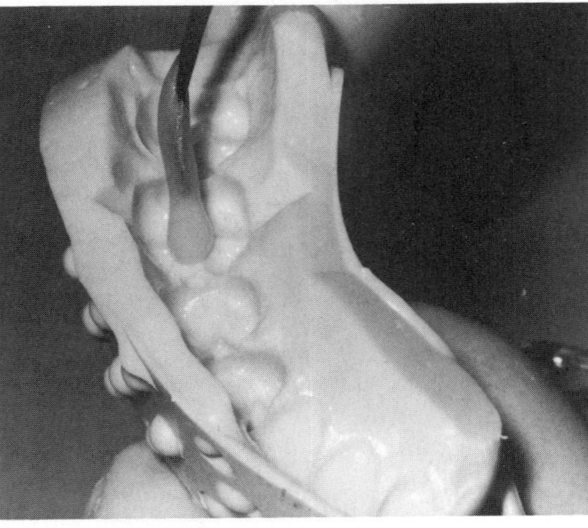

FIGURE 22–131
The flowing acrylic mix is transferred to the first molar area of the impression.

Steps	Rationale
5. Return the impression tray to the mouth and firmly seat it to its original position (Fig. 22–132)	The pressure within the impression forces the resin to flow around the prepared tooth and into the sluiceways; the soft acrylic molds itself to the lubricated preparation

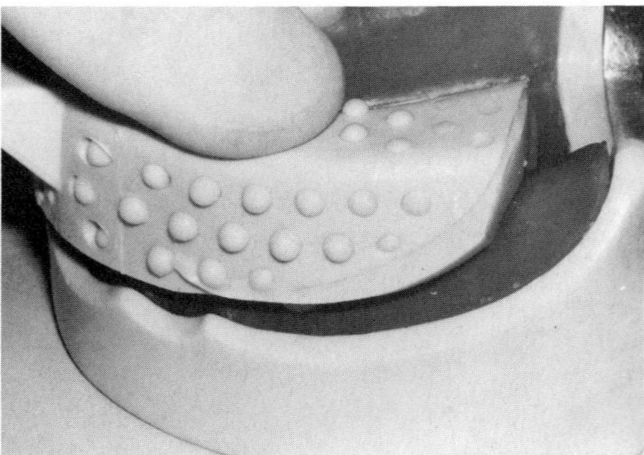

FIGURE 22–132
The impression tray is seated back to its original position over the teeth.

Steps	Rationale
6. After holding the tray in position for approximately 2 minutes, *slightly* dislodge it and immediately reseat it; repeat this three to four times over the next 2 minutes	The resin is polymerizing to firmness; unseating and reseating it as it hardens ensures its ready removal when it has set
7. Remove the impression from the mouth; the resin almost always is held in place by the impression material and is automatically removed at the same time; immerse the impression containing the resin in warm water for 2 min.	The warm temperature completes the polymerization (hardening) reaction

Steps	Rationale
8. Remove the resin crown from the impression with a pointed instrument (Fig. 22–133); trim away excess resin (Fig. 22–134); place the temporary crown on the tooth and check it for fit	The fit is usually very good, but the crown may have slightly distorted; if the fit is poor, the impression can be relined and a new temporary crown made

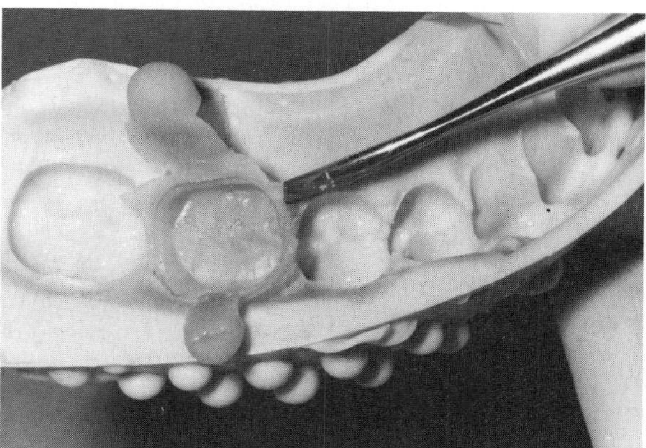

FIGURE 22–133
The acrylic restoration is removed from the impression.

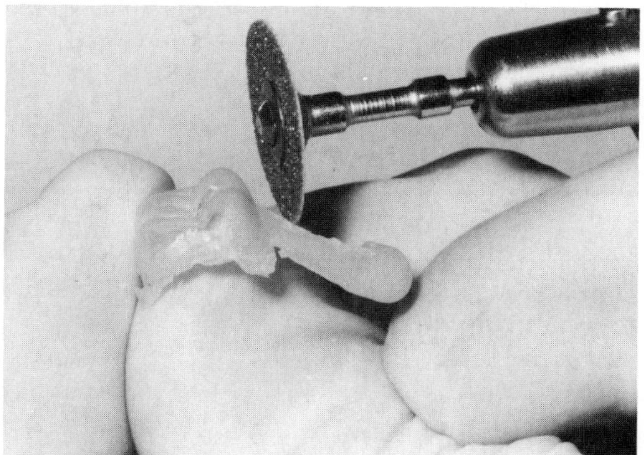

FIGURE 22–134
Excess acrylic is trimmed away with a disc.

Steps	Rationale
If internal aspects of the crown are binding, preventing the crown from seating, relieve them with a large round bur	
9. Check the seated crown for margin fit and occlusion; excess at the margins can be disced; occlusal prematurities can be reduced with a large round bur	Some adjustments are always necessary
10. Polish the temporary resin crown with a handpiece polishing wheel or use flour of pumice on a lathe rag wheel (Fig. 22–135)	A polished crown is comfortable to the client and is easily cleaned

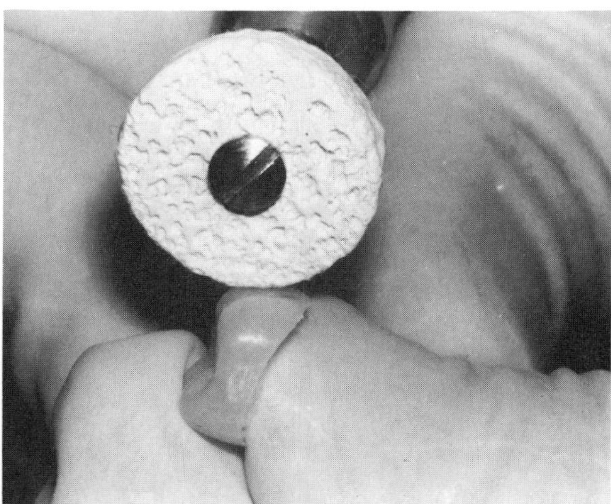

FIGURE 22–135
The trimmed resin crown is polished.

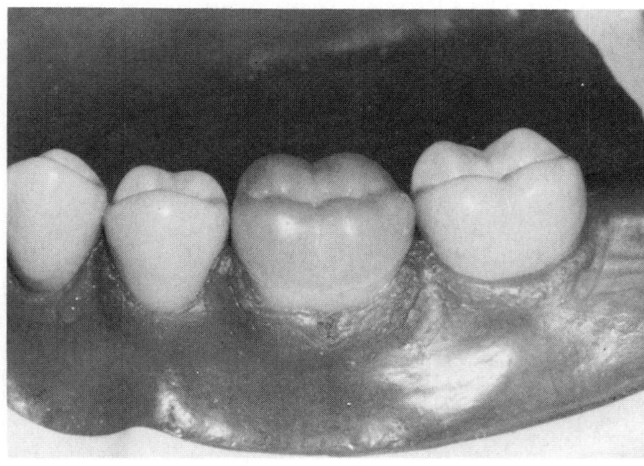

FIGURE 22–136
The finished custom acrylic resin temporary crown is temporarily cemented.

Steps	Rationale
11. Isolate the tooth with cotton rolls; prepare a zinc oxide–eugenol temporary cement and coat the inside of the crown with it; briefly dry the tooth with a gentle stream of air and seat the temporary crown with firm finger pressure Hold the crown in position for 2 minutes	Zinc oxide–eugenol has a sedating effect on freshly cut dentin; the tooth should be free of debris and saliva when the temporary crown is seated; after 2 minutes the temporary cement has usually hardened
12. Remove the hardened cement expressed from under the temporary crown with an explorer or curet-like instrument; examine the gingival sulcus and remove debris (Fig. 22–136)	Retained cement and debris irritate the gingiva

Preformed Stock Crown (Metal or Polycarbonate)

Preformed stock crowns make handy and useful temporary crowns. These crown forms are readily trimmed and modified for fit and provide a satisfactory alternative to the custom-made acrylic crown previously discussed. The final product is extremely durable; however, it is a compromise in both form and shape. These temporary crowns are usually comfortable for the client, but on occasion, the metal crowns present an objectionable metallic taste. This technique is useful primarily for complete veneer crowns.

A suitable crown form is selected after the completion of the tooth preparation. Preformed stock crowns come in an assortment of sizes for each tooth within the dentition. The size of the desired temporary crown is based on the space present in the area of the preparation.

PROCEDURE 22–11

PREPARING A METAL (ALUMINUM) TEMPORARY CROWN

Equipment

Isolation materials	Petrolatum	Articulating paper
Metal temporary crowns	Dappen dish	Polishing wheel
Metal cutting scissors	Cotton pellets and rolls	ZOE temporary cement
Acrylic resin	Finishing burs and discs	Protective barriers

Steps	Rationale
1. Select a metal (aluminum) crown with greatest mesiodistal width matching the distance between the adjacent teeth	The completed temporary crown should contact the adjacent teeth, preventing food impaction
2. Using metal-cutting scissors, cut away the gingival portion of the temporary crown (Fig. 22–137); the trimmed periphery should generally follow the contour of the margins of the tooth preparation, but should be 1 to 2 mm short of the margins Place the crown over the prepared tooth to confirm fit	Because acrylic resin will line the metal crown and provide the fit at the margins, the metal trimming can be liberal Sharp edges should be smoothed with polishing wheels to improve client comfort

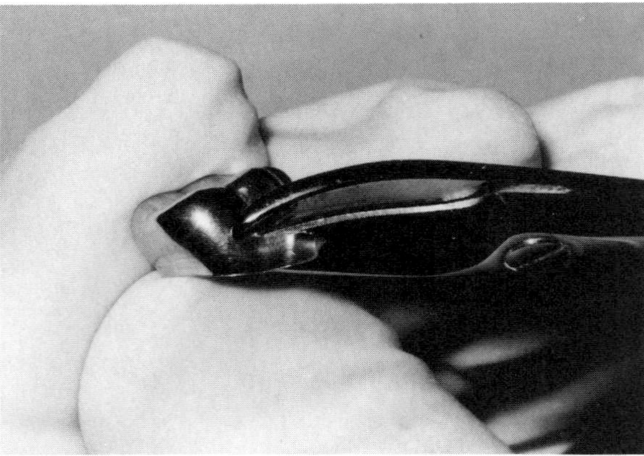

FIGURE 22–137
Gingival margins of crown are trimmed with metal-cutting scissors.

Steps	Rationale
3. Prepare a mix of autopolymerizing acrylic resin as described in Procedure 22–10	The acrylic liner provides customized internal fit
4. While the resin begins to polymerize, place cotton rolls for isolation, dry the prepared tooth, and coat it with petrolatum	Petrolatum does not adhere to wet teeth; this lubricant facilitates the removal of the resin-lined crown
5. As the mixed resin begins to lose its sheen, fill the trimmed crown form Seat it on the prepared tooth with finger pressure guiding it into position to match adjacent marginal ridges and crown contours as much as possible (Fig. 22–138)	As the crown is seated the excess acrylic is expressed to cover the margins; this forms a collar of acrylic as well as a lining inside the metal crown No preformed crown exactly matches natural tooth form

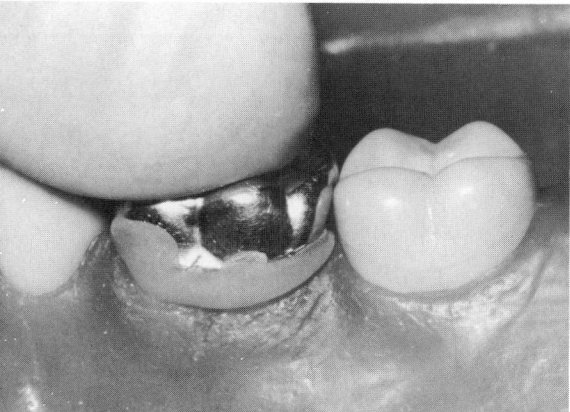

Steps	Rationale
FIGURE 22–138 **Lined crown form is seated to place over the prepared tooth.**	
6. After 2 minutes *slightly* lift the crown free from its seat on the preparation; reseat the crown Repeat this procedure three to four times over the next 2 minutes	The "on and off" movement facilitates removal of the lined crown after the acrylic becomes firm
7. Carefully remove the crown and immerse it in warm water for 2 minutes; remove cotton rolls	Careful removal guards against distortion; warm water speeds polymerization
8. Trim the excess acrylic back to the margin and contour the acrylic "collar" with abrasive discs (Fig. 22–139) Reseat the crown and verify marginal fit	Discing is an efficient and handy technique for recontouring undesirable acrylic bulk
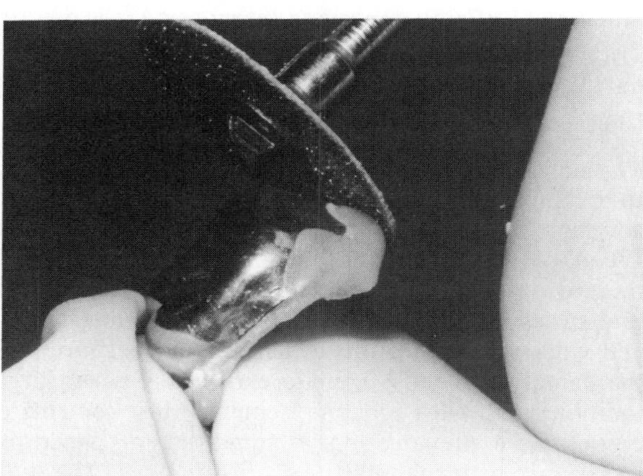 **FIGURE 22–139** **The excess acrylic is trimmed with a disc.**	
9. Evaluate the occlusion; mark prematurities using articulating paper; liberally reduce "high spots" with large round finishing burs	These crowns are usually premature in occlusion; it does not matter if the metal is perforated in adjusting the occlusion because the hard acrylic liner is present to protect the prepared tooth
10. Smooth the acrylic collar and rough occlusal areas with a polishing wheel in a handpiece	Smooth margins and contours are more comfortable to the patient and are more cleansable
11. Isolate the tooth with cotton rolls Prepare a zinc oxide–eugenol temporary cement and coat the inside of the crown with it Briefly dry the tooth with a gentle stream of air and seat the temporary crown with firm finger pressure; hold the crown in position for 2 minutes	Zinc oxide–eugenol has a sedating effect on freshly cut dentin The tooth should be free of debris and saliva when the temporary crown is seated; after 2 minutes the temporary cement usually has hardened

CONTINUED ON FOLLOWING PAGE

PROCEDURE 22–11

PREPARING A METAL (ALUMINUM) TEMPORARY CROWN *(Continued)*

Steps	Rationale
12. Remove the hardened cement expressed from under the temporary crown with an explorer or curet-like instrument. Examine the gingival sulcus and remove debris (Fig. 22–140)	Retained cement and debris irritate the gingiva

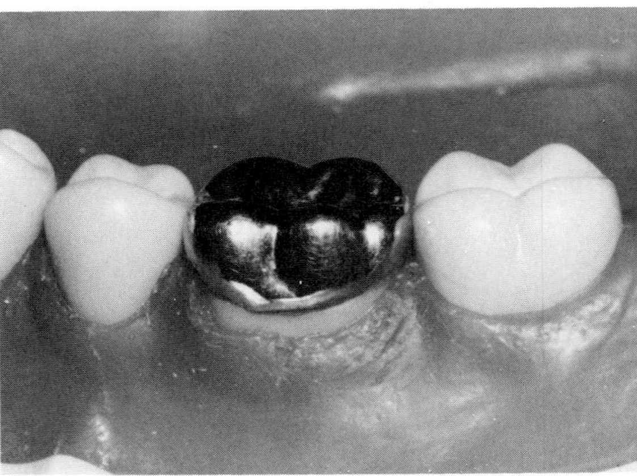

FIGURE 22–140
The finished preformed stock temporary crown is temporarily cemented.

Luting Agents

Rationale

Indirect restorations are fabricated in the dental laboratory on dies made from impressions of prepared teeth. These restorations include crowns and inlays made of rigid substances such as metal, cast ceramic, or porcelain. Because these materials cannot be incrementally built inside the actual cavity preparation, their fit is less precise when compared to direct restorations.

The design of indirect restorations and the preparations that receive them includes tapering features. This allows the rigid restoration to be seated under controlled pressure, in or on the tooth. When these restorations are completely seated, all margins should intimately fit. Softer cast metals can have near perfect margins, because the dentist can disc and burnish them to fit. However, between the restoration and the cavity walls exists a minute space. This space is filled with a luting agent which, when set, prevents the indirect restoration from loosening. Dislodging forces of occlusion and mastication are resisted by this firm interface of cement. Without a proper luting agent, castings leak and loosen and therefore fail.

Zinc Phosphate Cement

Zinc phosphate is the oldest of the luting agents. It has stood the "test of time" and remains the standard for cementation of most indirect restorations. Because it is quite acidic, vital pulps should be protected by a varnish barrier before the cement contacts the dentin. When properly mixed, the set is extended, allowing the operator ample time to adapt and seal the margins of the restoration. The preparation of zinc phosphate luting cement is described in the section on liners and bases.

Glass Ionomer Cement

The adhesion of this material to the tooth surface has led to its more routine use as a luting agent. To gain this adhesion, no protective varnish is used to coat the dentin. When compared to zinc phosphate, it is less acidic and more compatible with the dental pulp and it inhibits recurrent caries through the slow release of fluoride. The mixing and working times of this cement are quite short, and thus the dental team must exercise expediency when luting restorations with glass ionomer cement. Most cements of this type can be prepared on a nonabsorbent paper pad, in accordance with manufacturer's instructions. The luting cement is much less viscous than the glass ionomer cement base material previously described.

Zinc Oxide and Eugenol

The primary materials for temporary **cementation** of restorations are preparations of zinc oxide with eugenol. These materials vary in their hardness and retaining abilities and should be selected accordingly. Temporary cements are most commonly contained in small tubes and have a fluid-paste consistency. Equal amounts of base and catalyst are expressed onto a small pad and rapidly mixed. The cement is applied to cover the inside of the restoration (usually a temporary restoration), which is then seated and held in place until the cement has hardened. The excess, hard cement is removed carefully with an appropriate instrument such as a periodontal curet or an explorer. Finally, smudges can be wiped away with a cotton pellet moistened in alcohol or orange solvent. The gingival sulcus should be examined carefully and all debris removed.

EVALUATION

The ultimate success of restorative treatment requires thorough evaluation of the therapies delivered to the client. The evaluation should be both process- and outcome-oriented. The process evaluation requires a focus on detail as outlined in the procedure tables. An outcomes evaluation looks at the success of the final product (achievement of the client goals) in both a short-term and long-term time frame. Evaluation must take into consideration the technical quality of the restoration as well as the ability of the treatment to achieve the goal of therapy. As previously discussed, restorative therapy meets the client's human needs for a wholesome body image and a biologically sound dentition that might be in deficit because of damaged tooth structure, defective restorations, aesthetic inconsistencies and anatomical or physiological abnormalities. Outcomes evaluation can be done at the time of treatment and during the maintenance phases of care. The continuity of the **restorative care** cycle demands an ongoing assessment and evaluation regimen. A continuous cycle of evaluation is essential to the delivery of appropriate restorative treatment.

The appropriateness of treatment must be judged from the perspectives of both the professional and the client. The professional must be responsible for paying attention to detail and evaluating the technical qualities of the restoration, whereas the client is best prepared to address issues such as comfort, function, and acceptance. Thus, the oral healthcare professional and the client participate as a team in the outcomes evaluation of restorative treatment.

DOCUMENTATION

All restorative treatment must be accurately documented in the client's record. In addition to addressing medicolegal considerations, this practice benefits the members of the oral health team as well as the client. The documentation must include all procedures in the delivery of restorative treatment and may include, but is not limited to, the teeth and locations of restoration, anesthetic agents and medications, tooth isolation procedures, restorative materials, complications, and client education. When restorative treatment may dictate special precautions for future treatment, specific details should be provided in the record. For example, lesions restored with glass ionomer cement should be protected against dehydration. When these lesions require prolonged rubber dam isolation that results in dehydration, a special varnish can be used to prevent damage to the restoration. However, unless specifically noted, this preventive measure could go unaddressed. A special section in the client record can be designed to summarize restorative treatment precautions for all members of the oral health team. When establishing mechanisms of documentation, it is imperative that the impact of restorative therapies on the delivery of comprehensive care be considered and record-keeping practices be appropriately designed to address the needs of all members of the oral healthcare delivery team.

MAINTENANCE OR CONTINUED CARE

Assessment is an ongoing element in the delivery of restorative care. For example, the dental hygienist may have primary responsibility for the maintenance care programs. During the maintenance care appointment, the dental hygienist thoroughly reviews the health and personal status of the client, assesses the outcomes of dental hygiene care and dental treatment, and evaluates the client's current tooth and oral health status. These assessments, when regularly communicated to the dentist, support a continued plan of care.

The authors of this chapter wish to acknowledge James R. Clark for the photography provided for this chapter.

References

1. Johnston, D. W., Grainger, R. M., and Ryan, R. K. The decline of dental caries in Ontario school children. Journal of the Canadian Dental Association 53(5):411, 1986.
2. Lizaire, A. L., Hargreaves, J. A., et al. Oral health status of 13-year-old school children in Alberta, Canada. Journal of the Canadian Dental Association 53(11):845, 1987.
3. National Institute of Dental Research. Oral health of United States adults. The National Survey of Oral Health in U.S. Employed Adults and Seniors, 1985–86: National findings. Bethesda, Maryland, 1987, U.S. Department of Health and Human Services, Public Health Service, NIH Publication No. 87-2868.
4. National Institute of Dental Research. Oral health of United States children. The National Survey of Dental Caries in U.S. School Children, 1986–87: National and regional findings. Bethesda, Maryland, 1989, U.S. Department of Health and Human Services, Public Health Service, NIH Publication No. 89-2247.
5. Payette, M., Plante, R., and L'Heureux, J. B. Comparison of dental caries and oral hygiene indices for 13–14 year old Quebec children between 1977 and 1984. Journal of the Canadian Dental Association 54(3):183, 1988.
6. Meskin, L. H., Dillenberg, J., et al. Economic impact of dental service utilization by older adults. Journal of the American Dental Association 120:665, 1990.
7. Leinfelder, K. F. Criteria for clinical evaluation of composite resin restorations. In Anusavice, K. (ed.). Quality Evaluation of Dental Restorations: Criteria for Placement and Replacement. Chicago: Quintessence Publishing, 1989, pp. 139–146.
8. American Dental Association. Legal Provisions for Delegating Functions to Dental Assistants and Dental Hygienists. Chicago: American Dental Association, 1987.
9. American Dental Hygienists' Association. A Comparative Overview of 51 Practice Acts. Chicago: American Dental Hygienists' Association, 1989.
10. Canadian Dental Hygienists' Association. Dental Hygiene in Canada: Portability, Placement, Practice-licensure. Ottawa: Canadian Dental Hygienists' Association, 1990.
11. Cochran, M. A., Miller, C. H., and Sheldrake, M. A. The efficacy of the rubber dam as a barrier to the spread of microorganisms during dental treatment. Journal of the American Dental Association 119:141, 1989.
12. Gergely, E. J. Rubber dam acceptance. British Dental Journal 167:249, 1989.
13. O'Brien, W. J. Dental Materials: Properties and Selection. Chicago: Quintessence Publishing, 1989.
14. Langan, D. C., Fan, P. L., and Hoos, A. A. The use of mercury in dentistry: A critical review of the recent literature. Journal of the American Dental Association 115:867, 1987.
15. American Dental Association, Council on Dental Materials, Instruments and Equipment. Recommendations in dental

mercury hygiene, 1984. Journal of the American Dental Association 109:617, 1984.
16. Ferracane, J. L. Using posterior composites appropriately. Journal of the American Dental Association 123:53, 1992.
17. Johnson, G. H., Bales, D. J., et al. Clinical performance of posterior composite resin restorations. Quintessence International 23(10):705, 1992.
18. Leinfelder, K. F. Wear patterns and failure mechanisms. Posterior Composites: Proceedings of the International Symposium on Posterior Composite Resin, Chapel Hill, NC, 13–14 October 1982; published in 1984 by Duane F. Taylor.
19. Leinfelder, K. F., and Lemons, J. E. Clinical Restorative Materials and Techniques. Philadelphia: Lea & Febiger, 1988, p. 85.
20. Bowen, R. L. Dental filling material comprising vinyl-silane treated fused silica and a binding of the reaction product of bis-phenol and glycidyl acrylate. U.S. Patent 3, 006, 112, November 27, 1962.
21. Buonocore, M. G. A simple method of increasing adhesion of acrylic filling materials to enamel surfaces. Journal of Dental Research 34:849, 1955.
22. Retief, D. H. Dentin bonding agents: A deterrent to microleakage? In Quality Evaluation of Dental Restorations: Criteria for Placement and Replacement. Chicago: Quintessence Publishing, 1989.
23. Wilson, A. D., and McLean, J. W. Glass-ionomer Cement. Chicago: Quintessence Publishing, 1988.

23 Local Anesthesia

OBJECTIVES

Mastery of the content in this chapter will enable the reader to:

- Define the key terms used
- Describe the physiological mechanism of nerve conduction
- Describe each of the anesthetic agents and vasoconstrictors used in dentistry and discuss the rationale behind the selection of a particular agent when providing dental hygiene care
- Calculate the maximal safe dose of each local anesthetic agent and vasoconstrictor for each client
- Assess each client's health history to determine his suitability to receive local anesthetics or vasoconstrictors, and determine if modifications to the dental hygiene care plan are required
- Assemble, disassemble, and properly maintain the armamentarium required for the administration of local anesthetic agents
- Identify the anatomical landmarks on both a skull and a client for the following injections: supraperiosteal, anterior superior alveolar nerve block, infraorbital nerve block, middle superior alveolar nerve block, posterior superior alveolar nerve block, greater palatine nerve block, nasopalatine nerve block, inferior alveolar nerve block, lingual nerve block, buccal nerve block, mental nerve block, incisive nerve block
- Identify which nerve, teeth, and soft tissue structures are anesthetized with each of the preceding injections
- Identify the local complications that may result from the administration of anesthetic agents and the proper management of these complications
- Recognize and assist in the management of systemic complications that may result from the administration of anesthetic agents

INTRODUCTION

In the 1960s, projections of inadequate availability of dental care provided the impetus for educating dental hygienists in expanded responsibilities.[1] From the success of these educational programs[2] and the recurring predictions of a shortage of dentists, the following jurisdictions amended their dental practice acts to allow delegation of expanded functions to dental hygienists: Alaska, Arizona, California, Colorado, Hawaii, Idaho, Kansas, Missouri, Montana, Nevada, New Mexico, Oklahoma, Oregon, South Dakota, Utah, Vermont, Washington, Wyoming, and the provinces of British Columbia and Saskatchewan.[3]

Not all individuals require local anesthesia. Clients receiving a preventive oral prophylaxis or even periodontal maintenance care may experience little or no discomfort. However, local anesthetic administration usually is required if the dental hygiene care plan includes therapeutic scaling and root planing, gingival curettage, or if a client is simply experiencing undue tooth or soft tissue sensitivity. Additionally, a dental hygienist working in collaboration with a dentist may be called upon to anesthetize individuals for the dentist in preparation for them to receive restorative therapy or periodontal surgery.

The purpose of this chapter is to discuss the physiology of nerve conduction, the properties of local anesthetic agents and vasoconstrictors, the preanesthetic client evaluation, the armamentarium, the procedures for a successful injection, the injection techniques, and the prevention of local and systemic complications.

PHYSIOLOGY OF NERVE CONDUCTION

Local anesthesia is the loss of sensation in a circumscribed area of the body as a result of the depression of excitation in nerve endings or the inhibition of the conduction process in peripheral nerves.[4] Local anesthetic agents used in clinical practice today prevent both the generation and conduction of a nerve impulse. Essentially, the local anesthetic agent provides a chemical roadblock between the source of the **impulse** (e.g., a periodontal abscess) and the brain. The impulse is unable to reach the brain and is, thus, not interpreted as pain or discomfort by the client.

To understand how local anesthetic agents work, the dental hygienist needs to be familiar with the physiology of **nerve conduction.** Two principal ions are needed for nerve conduction: potassium (K^+) and sodium (Na^+). Because these two molecules are positively charged they normally exist in equal concentration across a membrane. However, in a nerve cell this equilibrium does not exist (Fig. 23–1, phase 1). Because of a sodium pump located within the cell membrane, the positively charged sodium molecules are forced outside the nerve cell. As the sodium leaves the intracellular fluid, a state of negativity is created inside the nerve cell. At the same time, the extracellular fluid, which has received the sodium, becomes positive. Once the sodium ion is transported out of the cell, it is not able to diffuse back into the intracellular fluids because of the relative impermeability of the nerve membrane to this ion. Conversely, although the nerve membrane is freely permeable to the potassium, this ion remains within the nerve cell because the negative charge of the nerve membrane restrains the positively charged ion by electrostatic attraction. The nerve is **polarized** or in a **resting state** or at **resting potential** when this balance exists between positive sodium ions on the outside of the nerve membrane and negative potassium ions on the inside of the membrane. Polarization of the membrane continues as long as the nerve remains undisturbed.

A stimulus, which may be chemical, thermal, mechanical, or electrical in nature (such as pain), produces excitation of the nerve fiber and thus a change in the ion balance (see Fig. 23–1, phase 2). During this phase, referred to as **depolarization,** the nerve membrane becomes more permeable to the sodium ion. Consequently, the positive sodium ions move rapidly across the nerve membrane to the inside of the nerve cell. During this influx of sodium, the potassium ions diffuse from the inside to the outside of the nerve membrane. Thus, during depolarization there is a reversal in the ion balance of the nerve cell. The interior of the nerve membrane contains the positive sodium ions whereas on the exterior of the nerve cell are the potassium ions. The inside of the nerve is now electrically positive compared to the outside of the nerve.

Immediately after depolarization, the permeability of the membrane to the sodium ion once again decreases (see Fig. 21, phase 3). This is referred to as **repolarization.** During this phase, the sodium pump actively transports the sodium ion out of the nerve cell while potassium ions diffuse and are pumped to the inside of the nerve cell. Thus, the nerve's resting potential is reestablished, whereby the interior of the nerve membrane contains the negative potassium ions while the exterior of the nerve cell consists of the positive sodium ions. This rapid sequence of changes, depolarization and repolarization, is termed **action potential.**

Once the resting potential of the nerve membrane is disrupted by a stimulus, such as pain, and depolarization occurs, the impulse must be transmitted along the nerve fiber. This impulse propagation is achieved when the ion changes during depolarization produce a new electrical equilibrium (the interior of the cell changing from negative to positive, the exterior of the cell changing from positive

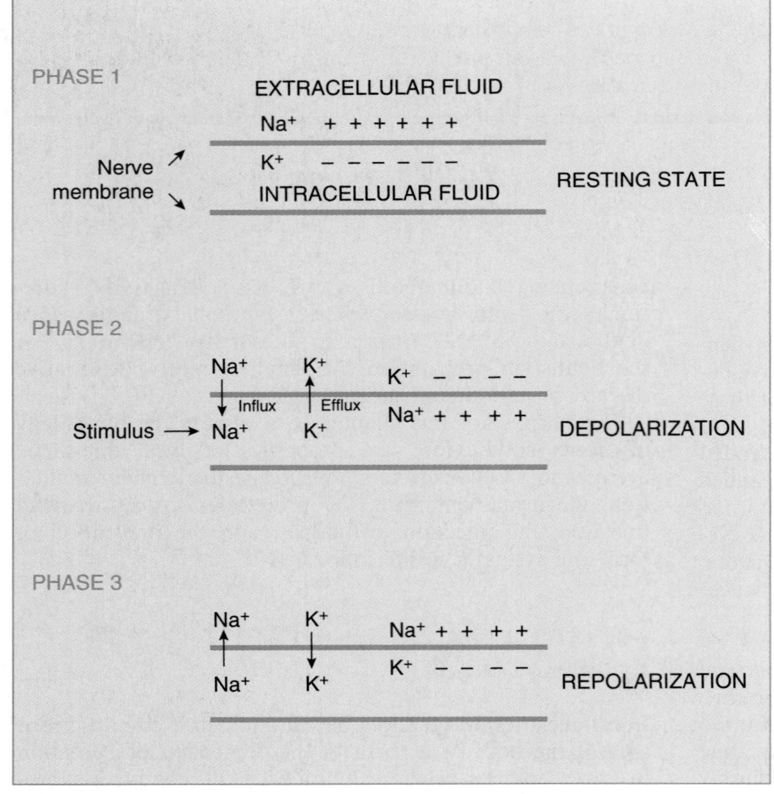

FIGURE 23–1
Action potential.

to negative). This in turn produces local currents that flow from the depolarized segment of the nerve to the adjacent resting area. As a result of this electrical current flow, depolarization begins in this previously resting area and continues propagating itself the entire length of the nerve fiber. Thus, the depolarization step begins a chain reaction that continues the action potential along the nerve. It is in this manner that the impulse is propelled along the nerve fiber to the central nervous system.

Mechanism of Action of Local Anesthetic Agents

Although there are several theories on how local anesthetics work, it has been established that the primary action of these drugs is in reducing the nerve membrane permeability to the sodium ions (Na^+). The nerve membrane remains impermeable to the sodium ions despite the introduction of a stimulus to the nerve. Because the sodium ions remain on the outside of the nerve cell and are unable to enter the nerve membrane, an action potential never occurs. The nerve cell remains in a polarized state (resting state) because the ionic movements responsible for the action potential do not develop. Thus, the action of depolarization that is required to initiate or to continue nerve impulse transmission (propagation) is blocked. An impulse that arrives at the blocked nerve segment is unable to be transmitted to the brain and is, therefore, not interpreted as pain or discomfort by the client.

LOCAL ANESTHETICS

Chemical Properties of Local Anesthetics

Chemically, all injectable local anesthetic agents used in oral healthcare today have three components:

- Aromatic lipophilic group
- Intermediate chain
- Hydrophilic amino group (Fig. 23–2)

The **lipophilic** group, composed of the aromatic ring structure, ensures that the anesthetic agent is able to penetrate the lipid-rich nerve membrane where impulse conduction is blocked. The **hydrophilic** portion, when combined with hydrochloric acid, allows the anesthetic to diffuse

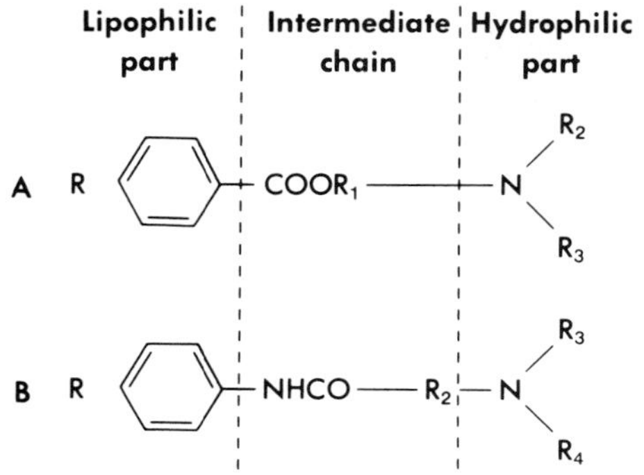

FIGURE 23–2
Typical local anesthetic. *A,* Ester type. *B,* Amide type. (With Permission from Malamed, S. F. Handbook of Local Anesthesia, 3rd ed. St. Louis: Mosby–Year Book, 1990, p. 15.)

TABLE 23–1
ESTER LOCAL ANESTHETICS

Generic Name	Proprietary Name
Procaine	Novocaine
Proproxycaine	Ravocaine
Benzocaine (topical)	
Tetracaine (topical)	

through the interstitial fluid in the tissues to reach the nerve.

The third component of the chemical structure of local anesthetics is the **intermediate chain linkage.** This linkage determines whether the local anesthetic agent is classified as an ester or an amide. The nature of the intermediate linkage is important in defining several properties of the local anesthetic, including possible allergic response (discussed in Preanesthetic Client Assessment) and metabolism (biotransformation).

Metabolism (Biotransformation) and Excretion of Local Anesthetics

The mechanism by which local anesthetic agents are metabolized is important because the overall toxicity of an agent is dependent on the balance between the agent's rate of absorption into the bloodstream at the injection site and the rate of the agent's removal from the blood through the processes of tissue uptake and metabolism. An important difference between the two classifications of local anesthetic drugs is the process by which they are metabolized. **Ester** local anesthetics are metabolized by hydrolysis (splitting of the compound into fragments by the addition of water) (Table 23–1). The hydrolysis process occurs primarily in the plasma and to a lesser extent in the liver, and is activated by the enzyme pseudocholinesterase. Concern about the metabolism of ester local anesthetics arises regarding persons with genetically determined atypical plasma cholinesterase, which is found in approximately 1 out of every 2800 individuals.[5] These individuals have an increased potential for toxicity because they are unable to inactivate the ester agents at the normal rate and therefore, develop high blood levels of the anesthetic (see Preanesthetic Client Assessment and Systemic Complications).

Amide local anesthetics undergo biotransformation in the liver by microsomal enzymes (Table 23–2). Therefore, the liver function of a client influences the rate of biotransformation of an amide drug. Those clients with impaired liver function are unable to metabolize amide local anesthetics at a normal rate, thereby leading to excessive levels of the

TABLE 23–2
AMIDE LOCAL ANESTHETICS

Generic Name	Proprietary Name
Articaine	Ultracaine (not available in USA)
Bupivacaine	Marcaine
Etidocaine	Duranest
Lidocaine	Xylocaine, Alphacaine, Octocaine
Mepivacaine	Carbocaine, Arestocaine, Isocaine, Polocaine
Prilocaine	Citanest

agent in the blood, which increases the potential for toxic overdose (see Preanesthetic Client Assessment and Systemic Complications).

The metabolic products of both the ester and amide local anesthetics are almost entirely excreted by the kidneys. In addition, a small amount of a given dose of local anesthetic agent is excreted unchanged in the urine. Because the esters are metabolized almost completely in the plasma, this agent appears in only small amounts in an unchanged form in the urine. Because of their more complex process of biotransformation, amides are usually excreted in their original form in larger amounts than the esters. Despite this, only small concentrations of the amides are found unchanged in the urine. Clients with significant renal impairment or those undergoing renal dialysis may be unable to remove efficiently the unchanged form of the local anesthetic compound or its breakdown products from their blood, leading to elevated local anesthetic levels and an increased potential for toxicity (see Preanesthetic Client Assessment and Systemic Complications).

VASOCONSTRICTORS

All local anesthetic agents presently used in dentistry produce **vasodilation.** After their injection into the tissues the following reactions occur:[5]

- Increased blood flow to the injection site as the local anesthetic agents dilate the blood vessels
- Accelerated rate of absorption of the local anesthetic into the bloodstream, causing the anesthetic to be carried away from the injection site
- Higher amounts of local anesthetic in the blood with the attendant greater risk of an overdose reaction
- Decreased duration of action and decreased effectiveness of the local anesthetic because it diffuses away from the site of administration more rapidly
- Increased bleeding at the injection site because of the increased blood flow to the area

To counteract the vasodilating properties of the local anesthetic agents, **vasoconstrictors** are added to the local anesthetic solution. These drugs constrict the blood vessels, and thus control bleeding in the area of the injection. This vasoconstriction in turn leads to:

- Decreased blood flow to the injection site as the vasoconstrictors constrict the blood vessels
- Slowed rate of absorption of the local anesthetic into the bloodstream, thus keeping it at the injection site longer and producing lower levels in the bloodstream
- Lower amounts of local anesthetic in the blood, thereby decreasing the risk of an overdose reaction (or reducing the potential for systemic toxicity)
- Increased duration of action and increased effectiveness of the local anesthetic as higher concentrations of the agent remain in and around the nerve for a longer period
- Decreased bleeding at the injection site **(hemostasis)** from the decreased blood flow to the area

Vasoconstrictors are an important addition to a local anesthetic solution because they decrease the potential toxicity of the anesthetic solution while simultaneously increasing the duration and effectiveness of pain control.

Mechanism of Action of Vasoconstrictors

The **sympathetic nervous system** component of the **autonomic nervous system,** in addition to other functions, controls the dilation and constriction of various blood vessels throughout the body. **Adrenalin,** also known as **epinephrine,** is one of the naturally occurring agents responsible for sympathetic nervous system activity.[6] The vasoconstrictors used with local anesthetics are chemically identical to or very similar to those agents produced naturally during sympathetic nervous system stimulation. Thus, because the actions of the vasoconstrictors so closely mimic the action of the sympathetic autonomic nervous system they are referred to as **sympathomimetic** or **adrenergic agents.**

Throughout the tissues of the body **adrenergic receptors** are found that are stimulated by the chemicals released by the sympathetic nervous system or a sympathomimetic agent (drug). These receptor sites are divided into two major categories, alpha and beta. Activation of the **alpha** (α) receptors by a sympathomimetic agent (drug) results in contraction of the smooth muscle in blood vessels. This contraction produces a constriction of the vessels referred to as **vasoconstriction.** The primary reason sympathomimetic agents are added to local anesthetic solutions is to produce this vasoconstriction. As discussed previously, the addition of vasoconstrictors to local anesthetic solutions decreases the potential of systemic toxicity by slowing the rate of absorption of the local anesthetic into the bloodstream while prolonging the duration of local anesthetic activity and producing hemostasis at the site of the injection.

Activation of the **beta** (β) receptors by a sympathomimetic agent (drug) produces smooth muscle relaxation and cardiac stimulation. Beta receptors have been further characterized as beta$_1$ and beta$_2$. Activation of **beta$_1$ receptors** increases cardiac rate and force, whereas **beta$_2$ receptors** are responsible for bronchodilation and vasodilation. Those changes resulting from beta receptor stimulation are not required in oral healthcare and are undesirable "side effects" of sympathomimetic drug incorporation into local anesthetic solutions. Therefore, the vasoconstriction produced by alpha receptor activation is the primary effect for which sympathomimetic agents are used in oral healthcare. The beta effects are both undesirable and potentially hazardous.

Concentrations of Vasoconstrictors

Vasoconstrictor concentrations are most often expressed as a ratio such as 1 part per 100,000. This ratio appears as 1 : 100,000 in a written format.

Table 23–3 lists the vasoconstrictors and their concentra-

TABLE 23–3
VASOCONSTRICTORS EMPLOYED IN DENTAL LOCAL ANESTHETIC SOLUTIONS

Generic Name	Proprietary Name	Concentrations
Epinephrine	Adrenalin	1:50,000; 1:100,000; 1:200,000
Levonordefrin	Neo-Cobefrin	1:20,000
Norepinephrine (levarterenol)	Levophed	1:30,000

tions that are incorporated into dental local anesthetic solutions in the United States.

Whereas a variety of vasoconstrictors are used presently in oral healthcare, epinephrine is the most potent and widely employed, and is the standard by which all other vasoconstrictors are compared. Epinephrine 1:100,000 is the most commonly used concentration; however, it is thought that the optimal concentration for prolongation of pain control is 1:200,000[7] or even 1:250,000.[8] *The use of 1:50,000 epinephrine for pain control is neither necessary nor recommended.*[8] The 1:50,000 dilution contains twice the epinephrine per milliliter as a 1:100,000 dilution and four times that contained in a 1:200,000 concentration, and does not add any positive attributes to the solution with regard to pain control for the client. A concentration of 1:50,000 epinephrine provides no advantage in the quality or duration of pain control, but it may be more effective than the less concentrated solutions in the control of bleeding during dental hygiene instrumentation.[5] However, effective hemostasis also may be obtained with concentrations of 1:100,000 epinephrine and, indeed, the dental hygienist should consider the use of the less concentrated solution, particularly with clients known to be cardiovascularly compromised.[5] (Refer to Preanesthetic Client Assessment for further guidelines.)

Levonordefrin and **norepinephrine (levarterenol)** also are proven effective **vasopressors.** Levonordefrin is approximately one-sixth (15%) as potent a vasoconstrictor as epinephrine and as such is used in a greater concentration of 1:20,000. At this concentration, levonordefrin possesses the same clinical capabilities as epinephrine 1:100,000. Similarly, norepinephrine is approximately 25% as effective a vasopressor as epinephrine and is used clinically in a 1:30,000 dilution.

SELECTION OF AN APPROPRIATE AGENT

Selection of a Local Anesthetic Agent

As detailed in Table 23-1 and Table 23-2 there are several local anesthetic agents available to the dental hygienist when providing pain control. Table 23-4 lists those local anesthetics and the combinations of vasoconstrictors that currently are available in the United States and Canada.

The dental hygienist must weigh several factors when determining the appropriate anesthetic agent to use during dental hygiene care:

- The duration of action of the local anesthetic agent and the length of time that pain control is needed
- The need for pain control after treatment
- The health status of the client
- Current medications being taken by the client
- A local anesthetic allergy

Discussion of both duration of action and length of time that pain control is needed and the requirement for pain control after treatment will be discussed here. Those remaining factors influencing the dental hygienist's choice of a local anesthetic agent are reviewed in the section on preanesthetic client evaluation.

Duration of Action of the Local Anesthetic Agent and Length of Time That Pain Control Is Needed

An important consideration when selecting a local anesthetic agent for pain control during dental hygiene care is

TABLE 23-4

LOCAL ANESTHETIC AGENTS AND DURATION OF PULPAL AND SOFT TISSUE ANESTHESIA

Agent	Category	Duration (approx. minutes)	
		Pulpal	Soft Tissue
Short Duration			
Lidocaine 2%	Amide	5–10	60–120
Prilocaine 4% (infiltration)	Amide	5–10	90–120
Mepivacaine 3%	Amide	20–40	120–180
Intermediate Duration			
Articaine 4%, epinephrine 1:200,000*	Amide	45	180–240
Mepivacine 2%, epinephrine 1:200,000*	Amide	45	120–240
Procaine 2%, propoxycaine 0.4%, levonordefrin 1:20,000	Ester	30–60	120–180
Lidocaine 2%, epinephrine 1:50,000	Amide	60	180–240
Lidocaine 2%, epinephrine 1:100,000	Amide	60	180–240
Mepivacaine 2%, levonordefrin 1:20,000	Amide	60	180–240
Prilocaine 4% (block)	Amide	60	120–240
Articaine 4%, epinephrine 1:100,000*	Amide	75	180–300
Prilocaine 4%, epinephrine 1:200,000	Amide	60–90	120–240
Long Duration			
Bupivacaine 0.5%, epinephrine 1:200,000	Amide	>90	240–540
Etidocaine 1.5%, epinephrine 1:200,000	Amide	>90	240–540

Short-duration agents provide pulpal anesthesia for 30 minutes or less; intermediate-duration agents for approximately 60 minutes; long-duration for longer than 90 minutes. The classification of duration is approximate. Variations may be noted.

* Not available in the United States of America (January 1994)

Adapted from Malamed, S. F. Handbook of Local Anesthesia, 3rd ed. St. Louis: Mosby-Year Book, 1990, p. 47.

the approximate duration of action of the local anesthetic agent coupled with the length of time that pain control is needed. Table 23–4 lists the local anesthetic agents and their approximate duration of pulpal and soft tissue anesthesia. The anesthetics are categorized as:

- Short duration local anesthetics that provide approximately 30 minutes of pulpal anesthesia
- Intermediate duration local anesthetics that provide approximately 60 minutes of local anesthesia
- Long duration local anesthetics that provide approximately 90+ minutes of local anesthesia.

These times are approximations, and the actual duration of clinical anesthesia may vary. In addition to the presence or absence of a vasoconstrictor (see Selection of a Vasoconstrictor), several other factors may affect both the duration and depth of the anesthetic agent's action either increasing or, more commonly, decreasing the drug's effectiveness, including:[5]

Variation of the individual's response to the agent administered. While most individuals respond predictably to an anesthetic agent (e.g., the duration of pulpal anesthesia after administering 2% lidocaine with epinephrine 1:100,000 is approximately 60 minutes), some clients exhibit either a longer or shorter duration of action than anticipated. This variation in response is normal and is simply a variation in the individual's reaction to the anesthetic agent.

Accuracy of the administration of the agent. This factor becomes significant when a substantial amount of soft tissue must be penetrated to reach the nerve to be anesthetized. For example, the inferior alveolar nerve block involves advancing through 20 to 25 mm of soft tissue before reaching the nerve, thereby influencing the accuracy of the injection. On the other hand, when injecting where it is not necessary to penetrate a large amount of tissue to block the nerve, such as with an infiltration, accuracy is seldom a problem.

Condition of the soft tissues at the site of drug deposition. Anesthetic duration is increased in areas of decreased vascularity. Conversely, the presence of inflammation or infection often decreases the anesthetic agent's duration of action from the increased vascularity. This response is caused by a more rapid absorption of the anesthetic agent than found in healthy tissues.

Anatomical variation. The injection techniques described in this chapter are based on a "normal" anatomy. Of course, anatomic variations from this "norm" exist and can cause a decrease in the duration of local anesthetic action. Those variations in the maxilla that may account for failed effectiveness and duration include:

- Extra dense alveolar bone
- Palatal roots of maxillary molars that flare more than normal to the midline of the palate, thus affecting the anesthetic's action on these roots
- An unusually low zygomatic arch common in children, thereby preventing anesthesia or lessening its duration in the first and second molars

Those anatomical variations in the mandible that are cause for concern include,[5,9,10]

- The height of the mandibular foramen
- A wide flaring mandible
- A wide ramus in the anterior-posterior direction
- A long ramus in the superior-inferior direction
- Bulky musculature or excess adipose tissue
- Accessory innervation to the mandibular teeth

Suggestions for overcoming these variations in anatomy when administering anesthetic solution are discussed in the section on injection techniques.

Type of injection administered. For any anesthetic solution administered, both pulpal and soft tissue anesthesia are sustained for a longer period when a nerve block rather than a supraperiosteal/infiltration injection has been employed. For example, if administering 2% lidocaine with 1:100,000 epinephrine, a posterior superior alveolar nerve block provides approximately 60 minutes of pulpal anesthesia, whereas a supraperiosteal injection allows only 40 minutes' duration. Of course, to achieve the desired duration, the recommended minimal volume of anesthetic must be administered.

Need for Pain Control After Treatment

Although the need for pain control after dental hygiene care may be limited, the dental hygienist should be advised that long-duration agents may be administered if posttreatment discomfort is a factor. Anesthetic agents such as 4% prilocaine with 1:200,000 epinephrine can provide 5 to 8 hours of soft tissue anesthesia, whereas 0.5% bupivacaine or 1.5% etidocaine with 1:200,000 epinephrine can alleviate posttreatment discomfort for 8 to 12 hours. These agents can be administered prior to beginning dental hygiene care or even at the end of the care to allow for maximal posttreatment anesthesia. These drugs should not be given to children or people who are mentally or physically disabled because they may accidently chew or bite their lip or tongue.

Selection of a Vasoconstrictor

Currently, there are three vasoconstrictors available in local anesthetic solutions in the United States (see Table 23–3):

- Epinephrine
- Levonordefrin
- Norepinephrine (levarternol)

Norepinephrine is rarely used, however, and there are actually only two vasoconstrictors from which to choose when administering local anesthetics during dental hygiene care.

Five factors need to be considered when deciding if a vasoconstrictor is indicated and, if so, selecting the most appropriate agent:

- The length of the dental hygiene procedure
- The need for hemostasis
- The health status of the client
- Current medications being taken by the client
- An allergy to sodium bisulfite/metabisulfite

Both the length of the dental hygiene procedure and the need for hemostasis are reviewed here, whereas the health status of the client, current medications being taken by the client, and an allergy to sodium bisulfite/metabisulfite are discussed in Preanesthetic Client Assessment.

Length of the Dental Hygiene Procedure

Local anesthetics currently used in oral healthcare are vasodilators, and, as such, they increase their own rate of absorption. The addition of a vasoconstricting agent slows the rate of absorption of the local anesthetic and consequently increases the duration of clinically effective pulpal and soft tissue anesthesia. Thus, it becomes important to include a vasoconstrictor in the local anesthetic solution to provide pain control of sufficient length during dental hygiene care. For example, the addition of 1:100,000 or 1:200,000 epinephrine to 2% lidocaine increases the duration of pulpal and hard tissue anesthesia from approximately 10 minutes to 60 minutes. Dental hygiene appointments are frequently 45 to 60 minutes in length, and thus vasoconstrictors are necessary to provide a pain-free state for clients during completion of dental hygiene care.

Need for Hemostasis

Dental hygiene care often involves soft tissue manipulation, and hemorrhage is a frequent result, especially when inflammation is present. The use of local anesthetics without vasoconstrictors is problematic because the vasodilating properties of the anesthetic actually increase bleeding at the site of the injection. Vasoconstrictors are added to the anesthetic solution to counteract this unwanted action, and thus they prevent or minimize bleeding during dental hygiene care.

Epinephrine is the preferred agent for hemostasis. Levonordefrine is thought to be less effective in providing hemostasis, and norepinephrine can cause tissue ischemia leading to necrosis and sloughing, particularly on the palate. Therefore, norepinephrine should not be considered for vasoconstricting purposes. Indeed, many authorities recommend that it be excluded from all local anesthetic agents.[5]

Epinephrine is frequently used for hemostasis in a concentration of 1:50,000. However, a concentration of 1:100,000 epinephrine also provides excellent hemostasis and many dental professionals claim, with regard to hemostatic benefits, that there is no discernible clinical difference between the two. Because there is always the concern of systemic effects, such as alteration in cardiac function, it is recommended that the least concentrated form of epinephrine that provides clinically effective hemostasis be used.

For pain control, nerve blocks, such as the posterior superior alveolar or inferior alveolar nerve blocks, are frequently the technique of choice when providing dental hygiene care. However, to derive the benefits of bleeding control from the vasocontrictor, the drug must be administered, via local infiltration, directly into the area where the bleeding is occurring or is expected to occur. For example, to provide pain control to the maxillary molars and the buccal tissue over these teeth, a posterior superior alveolar nerve block is administered. The anesthetic agent is deposited posterior and superior to the posterior border of the maxilla, some distance from the area being anesthetized. However, if hemostasis is needed on the buccal tissue over any of the molars, the administration of a local infiltration into the area is necessary even though the anesthesia may be profound. Fortunately, only small volumes of solution are required (approximately 1 mL) for hemostatic purposes.

Maximal Safe Doses of Local Anesthetics

All drugs, if administered in excess, are capable of producing an overdose reaction. The exact dosage or the blood level at which a toxic reaction occurs is impossible to predict because biological variability greatly influences how individuals respond to a drug. However, maximal dosages can be calculated to serve as a guideline for the dental hygienist. A maximal safe dose is the maximal amount of a drug that can be safely administered to a healthy individual. Maximal doses of injectable local anesthetics should be determined after consideration of the following factors:[5]

Client's age. Individuals on both ends of the age spectrum (i.e., the young child or the elderly adult) may be unable to tolerate normal dosages. Therefore, the dosage of local anesthetic should be decreased accordingly.

Client's physical status. The calculated dosage must be adjusted for clients with compromised health. For example, a client with significant liver or renal dysfunction may be given a reduced dosage of local anesthetics.

Client's weight. The larger the individual (within limits), the greater the drug distribution. When administering a normal dosage of local anesthetic to a large individual, the blood level of the drug is lower than that in a small person. Thus, a larger dose can be safely given. Although this rule is generally true, there may be exceptions, and care must always be exercised.

Table 23–5 lists the recommended maximal safe dose and the milligrams of local anesthetic per cartridge of available local anesthetic agents. It is important to note that the

TABLE 23–5
RECOMMENDED MAXIMAL SAFE DOSES FOR AVAILABLE LOCAL ANESTHETICS

Local Anesthetic Agent	Anesthetic Dose per Cartridge (mg)	Maximal Safe Dose	
		Mg/lb of Body Weight	Maximum (mg)
Articaine 4%—Adults	72	3.2	500
Children	72	2.3	500
Bupivacaine 0.5%	9	0.6	90
Etidocaine 1.5%	27	3.6	400
Lidocaine 2% with or without vasoconstrictor	36	2	300
Mepivacaine 2% or 3% with or without vasoconstrictor	2% = 36 3% = 54	2	300
Prilocaine 4% with or without vasoconstrictor	72	2.7	400
Propoxycaine 0.4% + Procaine 2%	43.2	2.7	400 mg of **total** amine (propoxycaine + procaine)

maximal dosages are expressed in terms of milligrams per pound of body weight. Therefore, the dental hygienist must be familiar with the relationship between solution percentage and the amount of milligrams contained in that solution.

A 1% solution of local anesthetic contains 10 mg/mL of solution. A 2% solution contains 20 mg/mL, 3% contains 30 mg/mL, 4% contains 40 mg/mL, and so on. The number of milligrams of anesthetic in a cartridge is derived by multiplying the number of milligrams per milliliter of solution (e.g., 20 in a 2% solution) and the amount of solution (1.8 mL in a dental cartridge). The computation $20 \times 1.8 = 36$ gives the dental hygienist the number of milligrams of anesthetic in the dental cartridge.[8] Table 23–5 provides the computed number of milligrams of local anesthetic per cartridge for anesthetic agents.

Table 23–6 provides recommended maximal doses based on body weight for more commonly used local anesthetic agents. The guidelines provided in Tables 23–5 and 23–6 are helpful when working with healthy clients. Unfortunately, there are no set guidelines to determine the amount of dosage reduction needed for an elderly adult or medically compromised individual. It is suggested that the dental hygienist carefully assess the client's dental hygiene care needs and formulate a care plan that takes into account that individual's requirement for a decreased dose of local anesthetic at each appointment.

Fortunately, it is not likely that the dental hygienist will need to approach the maximal doses listed, especially in adult clients. If the dental hygiene care plan involves scaling and root planing a quadrant, the administration of one to two cartridges often suffices. Indeed, seldom is there a need to administer more than three or four cartridges during any appointment involving dental hygiene care.

In addition to considering the recommended maximal safe doses, the dental hygienist must follow other procedural guidelines to increase safety during administration of local anesthetics and prevent an overdose reaction. These include:

- Careful evaluation of the client's health history
- Use of a vasoconstrictor whenever possible
- Aspiration prior to deposition
- Slow injection
- Use the smallest amount of drug necessary

A more detailed discussion of these guidelines can be found in Procedures for a Successful Injection and Systemic Complications.

Maximal Safe Doses of Vasoconstrictors

Currently, vasoconstrictors commonly are used in local anesthetic solutions. Epinephrine has proven to be the most effective agent and is most frequently employed. Overdose reactions, although possible, are uncommon with vasoconstrictors other than epinephrine because of the lesser potency of these agents.[8] Table 23–7 outlines the recommended maximal safe doses in milligrams and number of cartridges per appointment of epinephrine, levonordefrin, and levarterenol for healthy clients and for clients with significant cardiovascular impairment. (Refer to Selection of a Vasoconstrictor and Preanesthetic Client Assessment for further discussion.)

It is important to note that in any local anesthetic solution containing a vasoconstrictor, the maximal safe dose of the solution may be determined by either the anesthetic agent or the vasoconstricting agent. For example, the maximal safe dose for 2% lidocaine may be reached before the maximal safe dose of the 1:100,000 epinephrine, included in the solution, is reached. Thus, it is the anesthetic agent that limits the total amount of solution to be administered. Conversely, the maximal safe dose for epinephrine

TABLE 23–6
RECOMMENDED MAXIMAL SAFE DOSES OF COMMONLY USED LOCAL ANESTHETICS*
(BASED ON BODY WEIGHT)

	Lidocaine 2% with/without Vasoconstrictor		**Mepivacaine 2% or 3%**			**Prilocaine 4% with/without Vasoconstrictor**		**Articaine 4% with Vasoconstrictor**			
	2 mg/lb, 300 mg max		**2 mg/lb, 300 mg max**			**2.7 mg/lb, 400 mg max**		**Adult 3.2 mb/lb, 500 mg max**		**Child 2.3 mg/lb, 500 mg max**	
Patient Weight (lb)	mg	No. of Cartridges	mg	No. of Cartridges (2%)	(3%)	mg	No. of Cartridges	mg	No. of Cartridges	mg	No. of Cartridges
20	40	1.1	40	1.1	0.8	54	0.75	64	0.9	46	0.6
40	80	2.2	80	2.2	1.5	108	1.5	128	1.8	92	2.3
60	120	3.3	120	3.3	2.0	162	2.25	192	2.7	138	1.9
80	160	4.4	160	4.4	3.0	216	3.0	256	3.6	184	2.5
100	200	5.5†	200	5.5	3.5	270	3.75	320	4.4	230	3.0
120	240	6.5	240	6.5	4.0	324	4.5	384	5.33		
140	280	7.5	280	7.5	5.0	378	5.0	448	6.2		
160	300	8.0	300	8.0	5.5	400	5.5	500	7.0		
180	300	8.0	300	8.0	5.5	400	5.5	500	7.0		
200	300	8.0	300	8.0	5.5	400	5.5	500	7.0		

* These are for normal healthy patients. They should be decreased for debilitated or elderly persons.
† The limiting factor for 1:50,000 epinephrine is the 0.2 mg dose.
From Malamed, S. F. Handbook of Local Anesthesia, 3rd ed. St. Louis: Mosby–Year Book, 1990, p. 264.

TABLE 23–7
RECOMMENDED MAXIMAL SAFE DOSE OF VASOCONSTRICTOR FOR HEALTHY AND CARDIAC CLIENTS

Agent	Concentration	Mg/mL	Mg per Cartridge (1.8 mL)	Maximal Dose (mg)		Max. Number of Cartridges
Epinephrine	1:50,000	0.02	0.036	Healthy adult client	0.2	5
				Cardiac client	0.04	1
Epinephrine	1:100,000	0.01	0.018	Healthy adult client	0.2	10
				Cardiac client	0.04	2
Epinephrine	1:200,000	0.005	0.009	Healthy adult client	0.2	20
				Cardiac client	0.4	4
Levonordefrin (Neo-Cobefrin)	1:20,000	0.5	0.09	Healthy adult client	1.00	10
				Cardiac client	0.2	2
Norepinephrine/levarterenol (Levophed)	1:30,000	0.034	0.06	Healthy adult client	0.34	5
				Cardiac client	0.14	2

Adapted from Malamed, S. F. Medical Emergencies in the Dental Office, 4th ed. St. Louis: C. V. Mosby, 1993.

1:50,000 may be reached before the maximal safe dose of the 2% lidocaine in which it is incorporated. In this case, it is the epinephrine that limits the total amount of solution to be administered. Therefore, the dental hygienist must be familiar with the maximal safe doses of both the local anesthetic agent and the vasoconstricting agent to determine which drug limits the total amount of solution that can be administered to a client.

PREANESTHETIC CLIENT ASSESSMENT

To meet the human need for safety, an evaluation of the client's health history and current health status is an essential prerequisite to dental hygiene care. The dental hygienist must ascertain if there are conditions that represent contraindications or require alterations to the dental hygiene care plan to eliminate or decrease the risk presented to the client. The administration of local anesthetic and vasoconstricting agents provides an additional rationale for a thorough health history and health status review. Local anesthetics and vasoconstrictors, like all drugs, exert actions on multiple body systems. It is important to evaluate, through the health history, the client's ability to physically tolerate the administration of a local anesthetic or vasoconstrictor, a history of allergic responses, and current medications. Collection of these data guides the dental hygienist in determining the appropriateness of administering a local anesthetic or vasoconstrictor, of seeking medical consultation, and of modifying the dental hygiene care plan. Thus, a thorough preanesthetic client assessment helps prevent or minimize complications and emergencies.

Contraindications to local anesthetics and vasoconstrictors are divided into two categories:

- Absolute
- Relative

Absolute contraindications require that the offending drug not be administered to the individual under any circumstances.[5] The administration of such a drug is contraindicated in all situations because it substantially increases the possibility of a life-threatening risk for the client. An example is a documented local anesthetic allergic reaction.

Relative contraindications signify that it is preferable to avoid administration of the suspected drug because there is the increased possibility that an adverse reaction may occur. However, if an acceptable substitute is not available, the drug may be used judiciously (i.e., administration of a minimal dose that still produces sufficient pain control).

Health Status of the Client

Although local anesthetics and vasoconstrictors are considered relatively safe drugs when administered properly, there are certain health conditions that require limiting or eliminating their use. Table 23–8 summarizes those health conditions that may affect the selection of a local anesthetic or vasoconstrictor and appropriate actions that the dental hygienist may follow. Those conditions include:

- Hypertension
- Cardiovascular disease
- Hyperthyroidism
- Atypical plasma cholinesterase
- Methemoglobinemia
- Malignant hyperthermia
- Significant liver dysfunction
- Significant renal dysfunction
- Pregnancy

There are few health conditions that are absolute contraindications to vasoconstrictors in the concentrations found in local anesthetic solutions used in oral healthcare. However, the dental hygienist must carefully consider the benefits versus the risks of administering a vasoconstrictor to clients with a history of hypertension, cardiovascular disease, or hyperthyroidism.

Hypertension and Cardiovascular Disease

The guidelines for assessing clients with hypertension and cardiovascular disease for dental hygiene care are the same as the guidelines used when assessing clients for administration of local anesthetics and vasoconstrictors. The following medical conditions preclude any dental hygiene care, and thus the administration of a local anesthetic and vasoconstrictor.[5]

- Clients with blood pressure in excess of 200 mm of Hg systolic or 115 mm of Hg diastolic.
- Clients with severe cardiovascular disease
  - Less than 6 months after a myocardial infarction
  - Less than 6 months after a cerebrovascular accident

TABLE 23–8
HEALTH CONDITIONS THAT AFFECT THE SELECTION OF LOCAL ANESTHETIC AGENTS AND VASOCONSTRICTORS

Health Condition	Type of Contraindication	Drugs to Avoid	Potential Problem(s)	Action/Alternative Drug
Uncontrolled hypertension (>200 systolic/ >115 diastolic)	Relative	—	May not be able to tolerate increased stress caused by anxiety or pain	Should not receive elective oral healthcare
Myocardial infarction or cerebrovascular accident within last 6 months	Relative	—	"	"
Unstable angina	Relative	—	"	"
Uncontrolled cardiac arrhythmias	Relative	—	"	"
Significant cardiovascular disease but able to receive oral healthcare	Relative	High concentrations of vasoconstrictors	Potential for increased stress on cardiovascular system	Use epinephrine concentrations of 1:200,000 or 1:100,000 or use 3% mepivacaine or 4% prilocaine (see Table 23–7 for maximal doses of vasoconstrictors for cardiac clients)
Hyperthyroidism (uncontrolled)	Relative	High concentrations of vasoconstrictors	Exaggerated response to vasoconstrictors	Avoid or limit use of vasoconstrictors; use 3% mepivacaine or 4% prilocaine
Atypical plasma cholinesterase	Relative	Esters	Toxic overdose	Use amide local anesthetics
Methemoglobinemia (idiopathic or congenital)	Relative	Prilocaine and articaine	Cyanosis-like state, respiratory distress, lethargy	Use other amides or esters
Malignant hyperthermia (malignant hyperpyrexia)	Relative	—	Life-threatening syndrome caused by administration of certain drugs in combination with amides	Amides or esters in normal doses/medical consultation
Significant liver dysfunction	Relative	Amides	Difficulty metabolizing amides, potential for toxic overdose	Use amides or esters judiciously
Significant renal dysfunction	Relative	Amides and esters	Difficulty eliminating local anesthetics, potential for toxic overdose	Use amides or esters judiciously
Pregnancy	Relative	—	Complications with pregnancy	Use local anesthetics and vasoconstrictors judiciously; avoid elective treatment in first trimester

Daily episodes of angina pectoris or unstable (preinfarction) angina

Cardiac dysrhythmias despite appropriate therapy

Guidelines for the oral healthcare management of clients according to the level of blood pressure can be found in Chapter 10. Clients with mild to moderate elevations in systolic or diastolic pressure may receive dental hygiene care including the administration of local anesthetics with vasoconstrictors.[5] Blood pressure should be routinely monitored and the client's care should be managed according to the most recent values. The dental hygienist's adherence to these guidelines minimizes the development of acute complications associated with elevated blood pressure.

If a client has a history of mild to moderate cardiovascular disease and is able to receive dental hygiene care, local anesthetics for pain control are considered safe. However, the effects that vasopressors may have on the cardiovascular system from $beta_1$ receptor stimulation often raises the concern of local anesthetic solutions with vasoconstrictors being administered to clients with a history of cardiovascular disease. The amount of vasoconstrictor used in anesthetic solutions is considerably less than that introduced by the stimulation of the individual's own sympathetic nervous system brought on by stress and fear. The anxiety and stress associated with discomfort and pain because of inadequate or premature termination of the local anesthetic agent stimulate the release of **endogenous** (systemically generated) **catecholamines** (epinephrine and norepinephrine), provoking an increase in the cardiovascular workload. An increased workload on an already compromised cardiovascular system may lead to an acute exacerbation of the condition, possibly with anginal pain, acute myocardial infarction, heart failure, or cerebrovascular accident.[8]

Thus, the dental hygienist's goal is to minimize the endogenous release of catecholamines during dental hygiene care by reducing or eliminating anxiety and stress and providing effective pain control of adequate duration. A local anesthetic with a vasoconstrictor provides more profound anesthesia of longer duration than the same agent without a vasoconstrictor. Therefore, the client is less likely to experience pain and an exaggerated stress response during dental hygiene procedures.

The maximal safe dose for each of the vasoconstrictors is reduced for individuals with cardiovascular disease as compared to the maximal dose recommended for healthy clients. Furthermore, it is recommended that minimal concentrations of vasoconstrictors be administered to cardiac risk persons (e.g., epinephrine 1:100,000 or 1:200,000). These guidelines are presented in Table 23–7. In addition to dosage limitations and minimal concentrations, it is recommended that the solution be administered slowly and after negative aspiration has been ensured. Observation of these guidelines when administering local anesthetic solutions with vasoconstrictors will most likely avoid complications.

Should there be any question about the use of a vasoconstrictor for a specific individual, the person's physician should be consulted prior to dental hygiene care. It is important to communicate to the physician the type, concentration, and amount of vasoconstrictor to be used and the time frame of use. This consultation assists the physician in assessing the appropriateness of a vasoconstrictor for the person. If the physician advises against the use of a vasopressor during dental hygiene care, local anesthetic solutions without vasoconstrictors are available and have proven satisfactory. Local anesthetics used in oral healthcare are listed by their duration of action in Table 23–4.

Hyperthyroidism

Uncontrolled **hyperthyroidism** is a condition characterized by increased nervousness and sweating, hypersensitivity to heat, fatigue, weight loss, heart palpitation, and tachycardia.[8] Although individuals with uncontrolled hyperthyroidism are able to receive local anesthetics, vasoconstrictors are contraindicated. Administration of epinephrine to people with uncontrolled hyperthyroidism may precipitate an exaggerated response to the vasopressor, resulting in cardiac stimulation. Persons who have surgically corrected or medication-controlled hyperthyroidism do not exhibit a magnified response to epinephrine and thus may receive local anesthetics with vasoconstrictors.

Atypical Plasma Cholinesterase

Atypical plasma cholinesterase is an inherited condition in which the individual produces an atypical form of the enzyme plasma cholinesterase. Subsequently, these individuals are unable to metabolize effectively ester local anesthetics that are inactivated in the plasma by the cholinesterase enzyme (see Table 23–1). Signs and symptoms of a local anesthetic overdose may develop despite administration of "normal" amounts. It is recommended that amide anesthetics (see Table 23–2), which are metabolized in the liver, be used instead.

Methemoglobinemia

Methemoglobinemia is a condition marked by the development of a cyanosis-like state in the absence of cardiac or respiratory abnormalities.[5] It can be hereditary, congenital, or acquired. During an incident of methemoglobinemia, more than 1% of the individual's hemoglobin is oxidized to the ferric form. Signs and symptoms of the condition vary with the blood levels of methemoglobin and may include lethargy, cyanosis of the nailbeds and mucosa, a pale gray appearance of the skin, and respiratory distress.[5] High doses of the local anesthetic agents prilocaine and articaine have been cited in triggering an episode.[5,11] (Acetanilid, aniline derivatives, benzene derivatives, cyanides, methylene blue, nitrates, para-aminosalicylic acid, and sulfonamides found in other substances also have been implicated.) Thus, the presence of methemoglobinemia is a relative contraindication to the administration of prilocaine and articaine. Because this condition is dose-related, it is recommended that minimal amounts of these agents be administered or an alternate local anesthetic be employed.

Malignant Hyperthermia

Malignant hyperthermia is a life-threatening complication associated with the administration of general anesthesia.[5,12] The syndrome is transmitted genetically, and reports of its occurrence in North America appear to be clustered in Wisconsin, Nebraska, and Toronto, Canada. Most of the affected individuals are functionally normal. Indeed, the presence of malignant hyperthermia becomes known only after exposure to a triggering agent or through specific testing. An incident is characterized by tachycardia, tachypnea, cardiac dysrhythmias, muscle rigidity, and extreme rise in body temperature. The mortality associated with malignant hyperthermia is 53%. Two drugs, halothane and succinylcholine, are considered to be the primary causative agents.[13] The significance to oral healthcare is that lidocaine and mepivacaine (both amides) were administered with other agents in cases in which malignant hyperthermia developed. Originally it was thought that a history of malignant hyperthermia should be an absolute contraindication to amide local anesthetics. However, recent findings and publications by the Malignant Hyperthermia Association of the United States have indicated that amide local anesthetics administered in the usual dosages employed in oral healthcare appear to be safe for malignant hyperthermia-susceptible individuals.[14] Malignant hyperthermia is classified as a relative contraindication to amide anesthetics. However, when the presence of malignant hyperthermia is disclosed, consultation with the individual's physician is recommended prior to administering local anesthetics.[5]

Current Medications Being Taken by the Client

A *drug interaction* occurs when one drug modifies the action of another drug. A drug may potentiate or diminish the action of another drug and may alter the way in which another drug is absorbed, metabolized, or eliminated from the body.[15] Although local anesthetics and vasoconstrictors exhibit few interactions with other drugs, the dental hygienist should consult the *Physicians' Desk Reference* or another comparable reference when a client reports being treated with any medication. This practice enables the clinician to assess both the drug's activity and the drug-to-drug interactions between the local anesthetic and vasoconstrictor and the prescribed medication and thereby meet the client's human need for safety. If further questions remain

TABLE 23–9
MEDICATIONS THAT AFFECT THE SELECTION OF LOCAL ANESTHETIC AGENTS OR VASOCONSTRICTORS

Medication	Type of Contraindication	Drugs to Avoid	Potential Problem(s)	Action/Alternative Drug
CVS depressants CNS depressants	Relative	Large doses of local anesthetics	Increased depression of CVS or CNS	Minimize dose of local anesthetic
Tricyclic antidepressants	"	Large doses of vasoconstrictors	Potentiate the action of epinephrine and ↑ blood pressure	Epinephrine concentrations of 1:200,000 or 1:100,000 used judiciously or mepivacaine 3% or prilocaine 4%
Phenothiazines	"	"	"	"
Beta-receptor blockers	"	"	"	"
Adrenergic neuron blockers	"	"	"	"
Sulfonamides	"	Esters	Esters inhibit action of sulfonamides	Amides

regarding the use of a local anesthetic or vasoconstrictor while a prescribed medication is being taken, the dentist or the individual's physician should be consulted.

Table 23–9 summarizes those medications that may affect the selection of a local anesthetic or vasoconstrictor and appropriate actions the dental hygienist may choose.

Local anesthetics have proven to have few interactions with other prescribed drugs. Procaine has been cited as interfering with the action of antiinfective **sulfonamide** drugs.[7] When **central nervous system (CNS) depressants** or **cardiovascular system (CVS) depressants** are being taken by an individual, it is recommended that doses of local anesthetics be kept at a minimum because they may cause further depression.[5]

There are many conflicting reports of drug-to-drug interactions between vasoconstrictors and prescribed medications, but it is recommended that the dental hygienist proceed cautiously when administering a vasopressor to a person who is being treated with any of the following groups of drugs:

- Tricyclic antidepressants
- Phenothiazines
- Beta-receptor blockers
- Adrenergic neuron blockers

Tricyclic antidepressants are antidepressant medications. These medications have been cited as possibly potentiating the action of epinephrine and norepinephrine and resulting in an increase in blood pressure.[16] **Phenothiazines** such as prochlorperazine are categorized as antipsychotic drugs but also are often prescribed for treatment of nausea. There is concern that these drugs, when combined with vasoconstrictors, may cause an exaggerated response to the vasopressor. **Beta-receptor blockers** and **adrenergic neuron blockers** are both categorized as cardiovascular drugs. Beta-receptor blockers such as propranolol decrease systolic and diastolic blood pressures.[6] However, when combined with epinephrine from a local anesthetic injection, significant increases in blood pressure may result. Adrenergic neuron blockers such as guanethidine and reserpine also are used to lower blood pressure through the interference in the normal release of norepinephrine.[6] When these drugs are combined with a vasoconstrictor, the effects of the vasopressor may be exaggerated, resulting in an increase in blood pressure.

Currently, none of these drugs pose an absolute contraindication to the administration of a vasoconstrictor. However, it is recommended that the dental hygienist exercise caution by administering the smallest dose that is clinically effective (such as that recommended for persons at cardiovascular risk) or eliminating the vasopressor entirely. If the dental hygienist is uncertain about the inclusion of a vasoconstrictor in the local anesthetic solution, consultation with the client's physician is advisable.

Allergies

An **allergy** is a hypersensitive reaction acquired through exposure to a specific substance (allergen); reexposure to the allergen increases one's potential to react. Approximately 1% of all reactions that occur during local anesthetic administration are true allergic reactions.[7] A documented local anesthetic allergy, however, represents an absolute contraindication and must be investigated for authenticity. Table 23–10 summarizes allergies that affect the selection of a local anesthetic agent or vasoconstrictor and appropriate alternative drugs the dental hygienist may choose.

One of the breakdown products of the ester local anesthetics is **para-aminobenzoic acid (PABA).** This substance induces allergic reactions in a small percentage of the population.[5] Allergic reactions that occur in response to ester local anesthetics are probably not reactions to the ester local anesthetic agent itself but rather to the PABA.

Allergic response to ester local anesthetics is well documented; however, substantiation of a true allergic response to a *pure* amide drug is extremely rare. The potential for a true allergic reaction to amides may exist; however, a verifiable occurrence is virtually nonexistent.

Allergic reactions are specific to the two chemical classifications of local anesthetic agents—amides and esters.[7] An individual who is allergic to an ester local anesthetic should not be allergic to an amide drug, and vice versa. Therefore, if a client reports a previous allergic response to a local anesthetic, it is imperative that the dental hygienist determine the specific agent responsible for the allergic response and the chemical group to which it belongs (see Systemic Complications).

Allergic reactions have been documented for various contents of the dental cartridge. **Sodium bisulfite** or **metabi-**

TABLE 23–10
CLIENT ALLERGIES THAT AFFECT THE SELECTION OF LOCAL ANESTHETIC AGENTS OR VASOCONSTRICTORS

Reported Allergy	Type of Contraindication	Drugs to Avoid	Potential Problem(s)	Alternative Drug
Local anesthetic allergy, documented	Absolute	All local anesthetics in same chemical class (esters vs. amides)	Allergic response, mild (e.g., dermatitis, bronchospasm) to life-threatening reactions	Local anesthetics in different chemical class (esters vs. amides)
Sulfa	"	Articaine	Allergic response	Non-sulfur-containing local anesthetic
Sodium bisulfite/metabisulfite	"	Local anesthetics containing a vasoconstrictor	Severe bronchospasm, usually asthmatics	Local anesthetic without vasoconstrictor
Methylparaben	"	Excluded from all local anesthetic cartridges manufactured in USA after January, 1984	Dermal reactions	

sulfite are antioxidants that are incorporated into local anesthetic solutions to act as a preservative for the vasoconstrictor. In addition to their use in local anesthetic cartridges, these agents are often sprayed on fruits and vegetables to keep them appearing "fresh." They also are included in a variety of canned foods. Allergy to the bisulfites has been reported.[17,18] Clients with a history of asthma may be particularly susceptible to an allergic response. The Food and Drug Administration (FDA) estimates that 5% of the 9 million allergy sufferers in the United States may be hypersensitive to sulfites.[19,20] The FDA has recently enacted regulations limiting the use of bisulfites on food. If a client reports a history of sulfite sensitivity, the dental hygienist should be alerted to the possibility of a similar response if a sulfite is included in the dental cartridge. Although sodium bisulfite or metabisulfite is found in all dental cartridges containing a vasoconstrictor, these agents are not included in solutions in which there is no vasopressor. Thus, it is recommended that the dental hygienist administer local anesthetics containing no vasoconstrictor to clients with a history of sulfite sensitivity.[21]

Of special note with regard to allergy is the preservative **methylparaben.** Prior to January 1, 1984, this agent was used as a preservative in cartridges of local anesthetics. It was considered to be the agent responsible for allergic responses when amide anesthetics were administered. However, since 1984 methylparaben has been excluded from all dental cartridges manufactured in the United States.

ARMAMENTARIUM

The components essential for the administration of a local anesthetic agent are the following:

- Syringe
- Needle
- Cartridge of local anesthetic agent
- Supplementary armamentarium

Each of these components is reviewed including care and handling, potential problems, and preparation of the armamentarium.

The Syringe

The syringe is that component of the local anesthetic armamentarium that holds the needle and cartridge of anesthetic (thus allowing the solution to be delivered to the client). There are several types of syringes that may be used for local anesthetic administration.[5,7]

1. Reusable
   a. Breech-loading, metallic, cartridge-type
      1. Aspirating
      2. Nonaspirating
   b. Breech-loading, metallic, self-aspirating, cartridge type
   c. Pressure type
   d. Jet injector
2. Disposable

Those syringes most often employed in oral healthcare are the reusable aspirating syringe and the self-aspirating syringe.

Reusable Breech-Loading, Metallic, Cartridge-Type Aspirating Syringe

This is the most commonly used syringe for the administration of an intraoral local anesthetic agent (Fig. 23–3). The needle is affixed to the threaded portion (or needle adaptor) at one end of the syringe. At the other end, a thumb ring and finger rest provide the dental hygienist with a means to grasp and control the syringe. The body of the syringe holds the cartridge of anesthetic solution. The aspirating syringe is characterized by a barbed piston also referred to as the **harpoon.** The harpoon engages the rubber or silicone stopper of the cartridge of anesthetic. The harpoon allows the dental hygienist to exert negative pressure

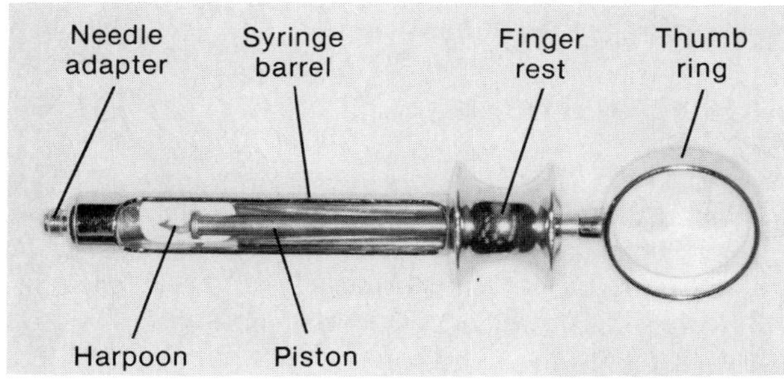

FIGURE 23–3
Breech-loading, metallic, cartridge-type aspirating syringe.

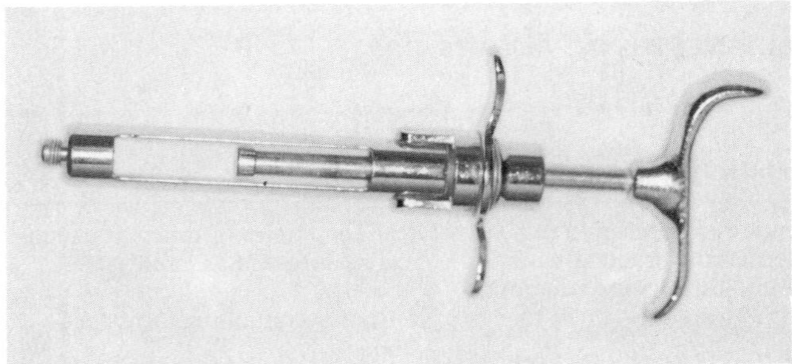

FIGURE 23-4
Nonaspirating syringe.

on the thumb ring to assess the location of the lumen of the needle, a procedure referred to as **aspiration.** If the needle lumen rests within a blood vessel, blood appears in the cartridge after applying negative pressure to the thumb ring. If this should occur, the dental hygienist needs to withdraw the needle, replace the cartridge of anesthetic solution, and repeat the procedure. Positive pressure on the thumb ring injects the anesthetic solution into the tissues.

Breech-Loading, Metallic, Cartridge-Type Nonaspirating Syringe

This syringe does not have a harpoon on the end of the piston, and thus the dental hygienist is unable to aspirate prior to depositing the anesthetic solution (Fig. 23-4). It is impossible for the dental hygienist to ascertain the precise location of the needle tip with a nonaspirating syringe, and thus this type of instrument should *never* be employed when administering local anesthetic during dental hygiene care.

Reusable, Breech-Loading, Metallic, Cartridge-Type, Self-Aspirating Syringe

The importance of aspirating prior to injecting an anesthetic solution is widely accepted, and the self-aspirating syringe was developed to aid the oral healthcare provider in completing this important step. This type of syringe achieves the negative pressure necessary for aspiration via the elasticity of the rubber diaphragm in the cartridge of anesthetic (Fig. 23-5). When the cartridge is placed in the syringe, the diaphragm rests against a metal projection inside the syringe; this projection also directs the needle into the cartridge (Fig. 23-6). Pressure exerted by the dental hygienist on the thumb disc (Fig. 23-7) or on the plunger by way of the thumb ring moves the cartridge slightly toward the metal projection, thereby stretching the rubber diaphragm. When the pressure is released, the cartridge rebounds slightly, thus producing enough negative pressure within the cartridge to achieve aspiration. Therefore, the dental hygienist does not need to pull back on the thumb ring to aspirate, as is necessary with an aspirating syringe.

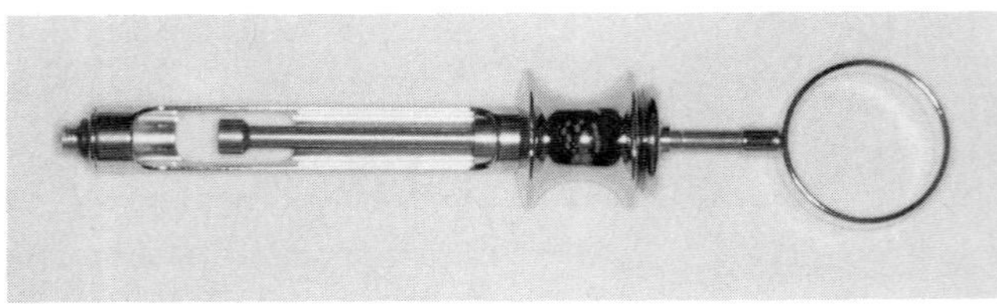

FIGURE 23-5
Self-aspirating syringe.

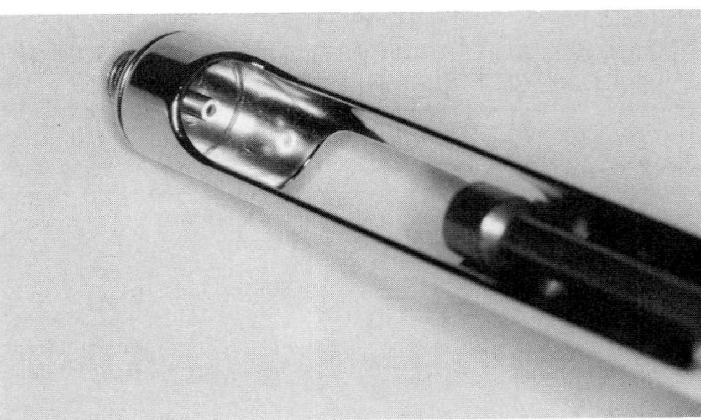

FIGURE 23-6
Metal projection of a self-aspirating syringe that directs the needle into the cartridge and depresses the cartridge diaphragm.

As noted, there are two methods to achieve aspiration with the self-aspirating syringe. First, the dental hygienist need only depress and release the thumb ring (and thus the plunger). This way, aspiration is achieved whenever the dental hygienist stops applying positive pressure to the thumb ring. A second method involves moving the thumb off the thumb ring and onto the thumb disc (see Fig. 23-7). Pressure is applied to the thumb disc, thereby increasing the pressure within the cartridge. Pressure on the thumb disc is then released and aspiration is accomplished. At this point the thumb is placed back into the thumb ring to deliver the anesthetic solution. This is the best technique to assure satisfactory aspiration with the self-aspirating syringe, but adequate aspiration also may be obtained by the first method of simply pressing and releasing the thumb ring.[5]

Pressure-Type Syringe

Another type of syringe that the dental hygienist may encounter is a pressure-type syringe (Fig. 23-8). This type of instrument is presently used when administering a peri-

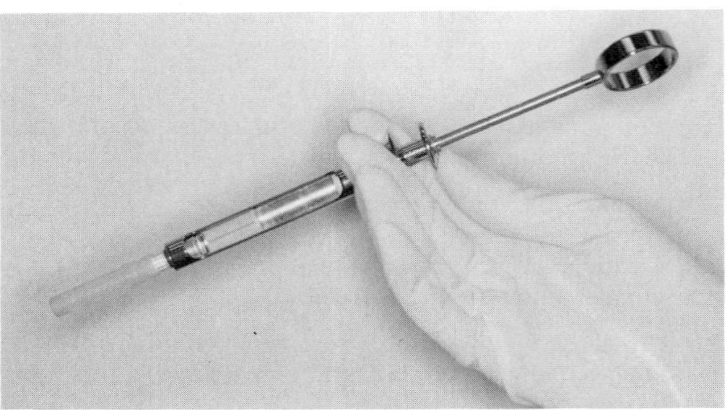

FIGURE 23-7
Pressure exerted on the thumb disc (as shown in illustration), or the thumb ring increases pressure within the cartridge. Aspiration occurs when the pressure is released.

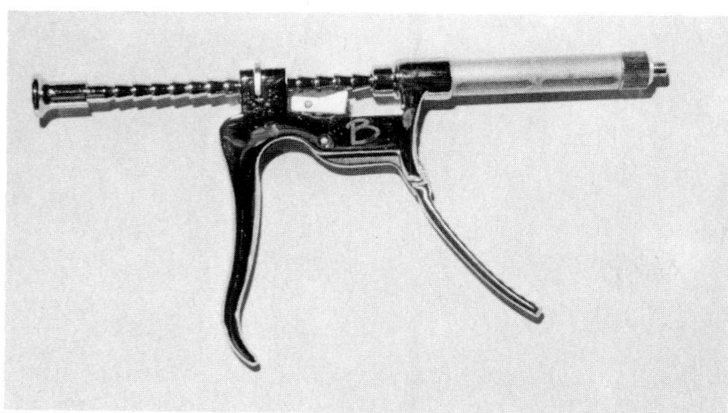

FIGURE 23–8
Pressure-type syringe.

odontal ligament (PDL) or intraligamentary injection (ILI), which provides pulpal anesthesia to one tooth on the mandible. A standard aspirating syringe can be used for this type of injection, but the pressure-type syringe is equipped with a trigger mechanism that delivers a measured dose (0.2 mL) of anesthetic solution and allows the administrator to more easily express the solution despite significant tissue resistance. This type of syringe permits easy administration of the solution; however, the dental hygienist must take care to slowly inject even this small measured dose of anesthetic agent. If deposition of the agent is done too rapidly, client discomfort may ensue during the injection and after the anesthesia has worn off.

Jet Injector

The jet injector syringe delivers 0.05 to 0.2 mL of anesthetic agent to the mucous membranes at a high pressure (2,000 psi) via small openings called jets (Fig. 23–9). The jet injector is used primarily to obtain topical anesthesia prior to insertion of a needle or to achieve soft tissue anesthesia of the palate. To acquire complete anesthesia, nerve blocks or supraperiosteal injections also must be administered with a conventional syringe and needle. With the jet injector, the anesthetic solution is delivered without the use of a needle, hence it becomes a "needleless injection." However, clients may dislike the "jolt" of the jet injection, and postinjection discomfort may follow. Properly applied topical anesthetics accomplish the same objectives as the jet injector.

Disposable Syringe

Disposable plastic syringes are most often used for intramuscular or intravenous drug administration, but they may

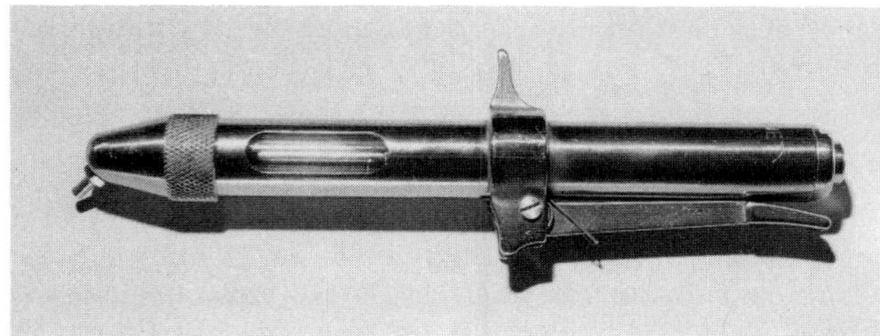

FIGURE 23–9
Jet injector syringe.

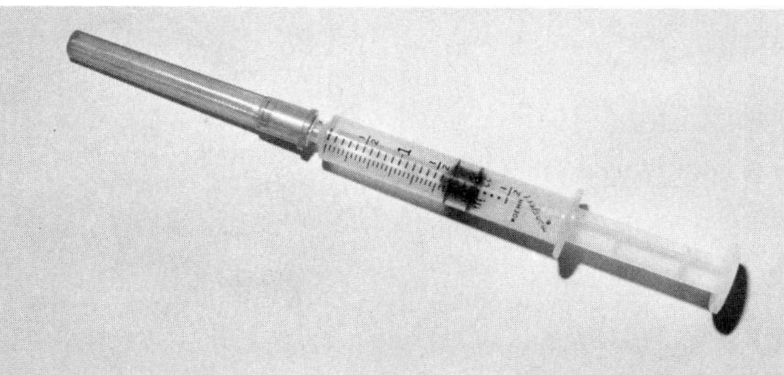

FIGURE 23–10
Disposable plastic syringe.

be employed during intraoral injections (Fig. 23–10). These syringes do not accept standard dental cartridges, and thus it is necessary to insert the attached needle into a vial or cartridge of local anesthetic drug and eject the appropriate amount of solution. Furthermore, because these syringes have no thumb ring, aspiration is difficult and may require two hands. Because the disadvantages of the disposable syringe far outweigh the advantages, this type of syringe is not recommended for routine use.

Care and Handling of the Syringe

Recommendations for the care of reusable syringes used for local anesthetic administration follow:[5,7]

- The syringe should be sterilized after each use following the appropriate infection control protocol. Deposits resembling rust may accumulate on the syringe and interfere with function and appearance. They may be removed by ultrasonic cleaning or scrubbing (see Chapters 8 and 9)
- After several autoclavings, the hygienist should dismantle the syringe and lubricate all the threaded joints
- The piston and harpoon may be replaced if the harpoon loses its sharpness and fails to engage the rubber stopper of the cartridge

Problems with the Syringe

Bent harpoon. The syringe harpoon must be sharp and straight to embed the rubber stopper of the cartridge. If the harpoon becomes bent, it may fail to engage the rubber stopper of the cartridge accurately. Consequently, aspiration may be unreliable.

Disengagement of the harpoon from the rubber stopper of the cartridge during aspiration. Disengagement may ensue if the harpoon is dull or if the dental hygienist applies excessive pressure to the thumb ring during aspiration. With regard to aspiration, only a gentle retraction of the thumb ring is needed; forceful action is not required.

Difficulty aspirating because of practitioner's hand size. When using an aspirating syringe, the dental hygienist must be able to stretch her fingers and thumb to retract the thumb ring of the syringe. If this cannot be done effectively, reliable aspiration does not occur. Thus, it becomes important that the syringe "fit" the practitioner's hand. Most syringes are similar in their dimensions, but variations do exist. Therefore, when selecting an aspirating syringe, it is beneficial to hold

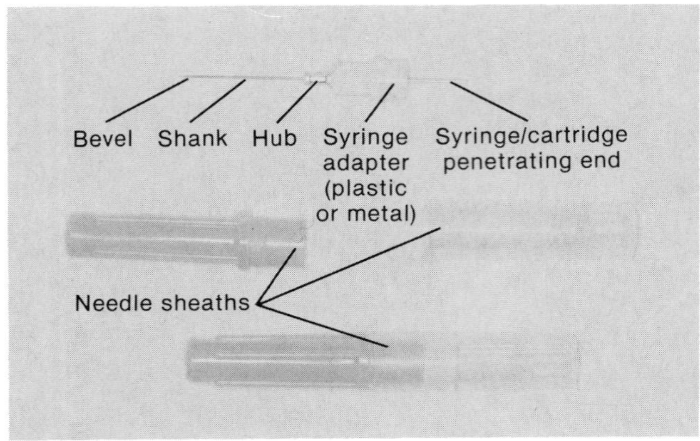

A

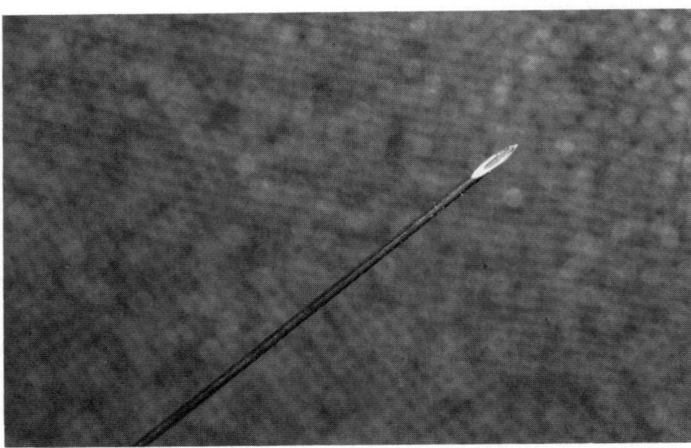
B

FIGURE 23–11
A, Parts of the needle. *B*, Bevel of the needle.

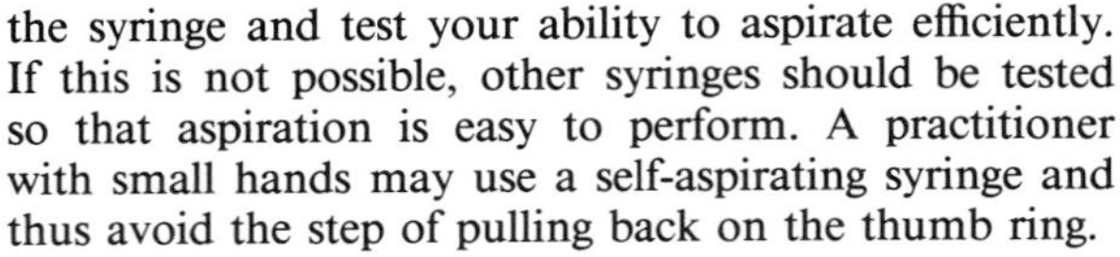

the syringe and test your ability to aspirate efficiently. If this is not possible, other syringes should be tested so that aspiration is easy to perform. A practitioner with small hands may use a self-aspirating syringe and thus avoid the step of pulling back on the thumb ring.

The Needle

The needle is that component of the armamentarium that delivers the anesthetic agent from the cartridge to the tissues surrounding the needle tip. Virtually all needles used in oral healthcare today are made of stainless steel, are presterilized by the manufacturer, and are disposable.

Parts of the Needle

Needles used for local anesthetic administration have several components (Fig. 23–11). The **bevel** is the angled surface of the needle point that is directed into the tissues. The **shank** refers to the length of the needle from the point to the hub. The **hub** or **syringe adaptor** is a plastic or metal piece that attaches the needle onto the syringe. The interior surface of metallic syringe adaptors is prethreaded. Plastic syringe adaptors are not prethreaded. Consequently, to attach a plastic-hubbed needle to a syringe, the dental hygienist must concurrently push and screw the needle onto the syringe. The **syringe/cartridge–penetrating end** enters the needle adaptor component of the syringe and engages the rubber diaphragm of the local anesthetic cartridge. This sterile needle is packaged in a plastic encasement consisting of two protective shields. A colored shield protects the part of the needle that is inserted into the tissues and a clear or white shield covers the syringe and cartridge end of the needle.

Gauge

Gauge is the diameter of the lumen of the needle. The higher the gauge number, the smaller the diameter of the lumen. Thus, a 30-gauge needle has a smaller internal diameter than a 27-gauge needle. The most commonly employed needles in oral healthcare are the 25-, 27-, and 30-gauge.

A common assumption is that a larger-diameter needle (e.g., 25-gauge) is more uncomfortable to the client upon insertion than a smaller-diameter needle (e.g., 30-gauge). However, this assumption is untrue. Research suggests that people cannot distinguish between a 25-, a 27-, or a 30-gauge needle when injected with each.[5]

Actually, larger gauge needles (i.e., 25-gauge) have several advantages over smaller gauge needles. Less deflection occurs when the larger gauge needle passes through the tissues. Because it is larger and more rigid, it can be guided to the deposition site with minimal deviation, thus ensuring greater accuracy and a higher rate of injection success. This needle rigidity is particularly important with injections requiring significant penetration of the soft tissues, such as the inferior alveolar nerve block. Although needle breakage is uncommon with disposable needles, it is less likely to occur with a larger gauge needle. Another advantage of larger gauge needles is the ability to aspirate and thereby reduce the possibility of intravascular injections. Opinions vary, but many authorities conclude that aspiration is easier and more reliable through the larger lumen, and smaller gauge needles (i.e., 30-gauge) have diameters too narrow to adequately aspirate.[5,7,22] Blood may be aspirated through a 25-, 27- or 30-gauge needle, but more pressure is required when a smaller gauge needle is employed. This difficulty in aspirating may decrease the reliability of the aspiration and increase the likelihood of the harpoon of the aspirating syringe becoming disengaged from the rubber stopper. Therefore, it is recommended that the dental hygienist use a 25-gauge needle for those injections that pose a high risk of aspiration or when a significant depth of soft tissue must be penetrated (e.g., inferior alveolar, posterior superior alveolar, or mental/incisive nerve blocks). The 27-gauge needle may be used for all other injections, provided the possibility of aspiration and the depth of tissue penetration are minimal. The 30-gauge needle is not recommended.

Length

The most common needle lengths used in oral healthcare are the "short" (approximately 1 inch or 25 mm) and the "long" (approximately 1⅝ inches or 40 mm) as measured from the hub to the needle tip (Fig. 23–12). Choice of needle length is dependent on accessibility of the area to be anesthetized. Long needles are preferred for those injections

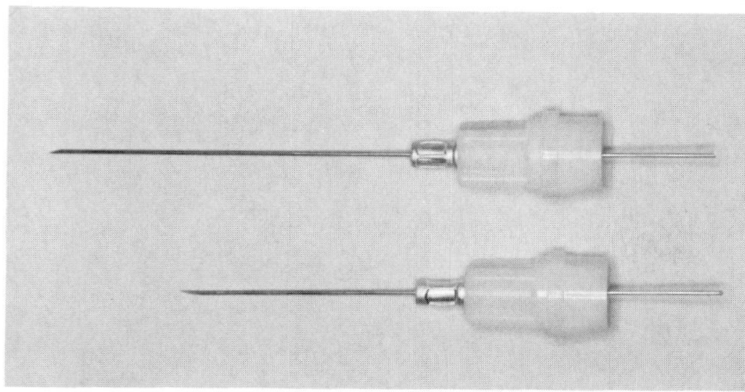

FIGURE 23-12
Long and short needles.

that require penetration of a significant thickness of soft tissue (e.g., inferior alveolar and the infraorbital nerve blocks). Short needles are indicated for injections in which smaller amounts of tissue are to be entered.

Care and Handling of the Needle

Recommendations for the care and handling of disposable needles used for local anesthetic administration follow:[5]

- Never use a needle for more than one client
- The needle should be changed after the administration of approximately three to four injections on the same client. The stainless steel becomes dull after several injections, causing each succeeding tissue penetration to be potentially traumatic and causing postinjection soreness
- The needle should be covered with a protective sheath when it is not being used—both before the injection and immediately upon completion of the injection
- The position of the uncovered needle tip should be watched at all times to prevent needle injury to both the client and the operator
- Needles should be disposed of in an approved sharps container. These rigid, puncture proof, leak resistant containers should be disposed of in accordance with federal, state, and local regulations (see Chapter 8).

Problems with the Needle

The following are problems the dental hygienist may encounter with the needle when administering local anesthetic agents:

Pain on insertion. Clients may experience discomfort of the tissues during insertion if the needle is dull; therefore, the clinician should change the needle after three or four insertions if reinjection is necessary

Pain on withdrawal. Client discomfort may occur when the needle is being withdrawn from the tissues if any barbs are on the needle tip. Barbs may be a result of the manufacturing process; however, they are more likely to occur if the needle tip contacts bone or any hard surface with too much force. To check for needle sharpness during preparation of the armamentarium, the needle tip may be drawn backward across a sterile piece of gauze. A needle barb snags the gauze, indicating the need for replacement with a new needle. Additionally, a needle should never be pushed forcefully against bone

Needlestick exposure to the administrator. To prevent an accidental needlestick injury, the needle should remain capped with a protective shield prior to being used and immediately upon termination of the injection. Should a needlestick exposure occur, follow the percutaneous exposure protocol and postexposure evaluation outlined in Chapter 7

Needle breakage. Refer to Local Complications

The Cartridge

The cartridge is that component of the armamentarium which contains the local anesthetic drug in addition to other ingredients. The local anesthetic cartridge is often referred to as a "carpule" by oral health professionals. However, this term is a registered trademark name for the anesthetic cartridge manufactured by Cook-Waite Laboratories.[5]

Parts of the Cartridge

The cartridges used for local anesthetic administration have four components (Fig. 23-13). The **rubber stopper/plunger** is located on one end of the cartridge and is the part in which the harpoon of an aspirating syringe is embedded. It is this component that is pushed into the glass cylinder by pressure on the thumb ring of the syringe, thereby ejecting the local anesthetic solution through the needle. During manufacturing, the rubber stopper is often treated with silicone to allow it to transverse the glass cylinder without "sticking." In an unused local anesthetic cartridge the end of the rubber stopper is slightly indented from the rim of the glass cylinder. Cartridges that do not exhibit this characteristic should not be used because it is an indication that the solution has been contaminated. This will be discussed more fully under Problems.

On the opposite end of the cartridge is a **diaphragm** into which the needle penetrates. The diaphragm is made of a semipermeable material, usually rubber, that allows solutions to diffuse into the cartridge if it is stored improperly. An **aluminum cap** fits securely around the neck of the cartridge, holding the diaphragm in place. The **glass cylinder** makes up the body of the cartridge on which the contents of the cartridge, the amount of solution and the manufacturer's name are imprinted. Also, several manufacturers now place a color-coding band around the glass cylinder to aid in identification of the drug.

Ingredients

There are several ingredients that collectively form the anesthetic solution. The **local anesthetic drug** or combination

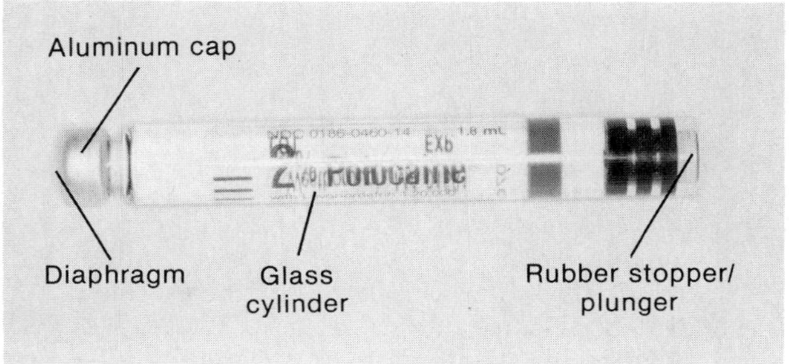

FIGURE 23-13
Components of the local anesthetic cartridge.

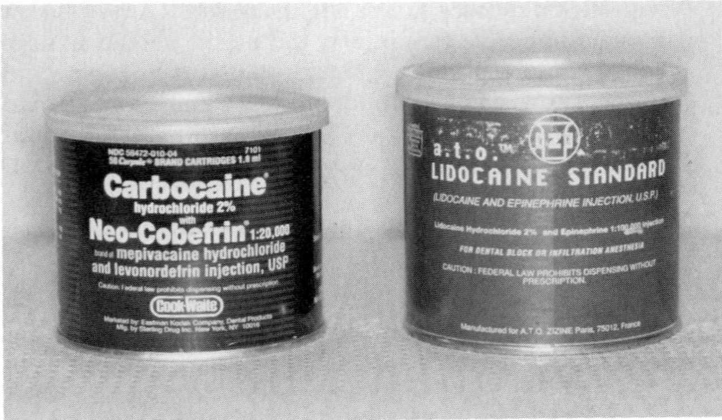

FIGURE 23–14
Local anesthetic cartridges packaged in metal canisters.

of drugs is, of course, the primary reason for the dental cartridge. The local anesthetic molecule is very stable and can withstand being boiled or autoclaved without breaking down. Unfortunately, other ingredients and components of the dental cartridge are more fragile.

A **vasoconstricting drug** in various concentrations is included in some anesthetic cartridges. This component increases the safety and duration of action of the local anesthetic agent. Those cartridges that include a vasoconstrictor also contain a **preservative for the vasoconstrictor.** The agent most often employed is sodium bisulfite, which prevents biodegradation of the vasoconstrictor by oxygen.

Sodium chloride is added to the dental cartridge to make the solution isotonic with the body tissues. Finally, **distilled water** is incorporated to produce a sufficient volume of solution in the cartridge. Cartridges available in the United States contain a total of 1.8 mL of solution.

Care and Handling of the Cartridge

Local anesthetic cartridges are packaged either in a vacuum-sealed metal canister containing 50 cartridges (Fig. 23–14) or in boxes that include 10 sealed units of 10 cartridges each, referred to as a "blister pack" (Fig. 23–15). Regardless of how the cartridges are packaged, it is recommended that the cartridges be stored in their original container at room temperature in a dark place. Exposure to

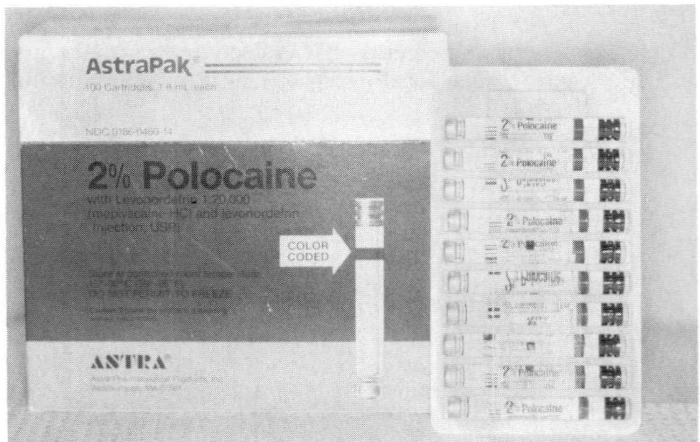

FIGURE 23–15
Local anesthetic cartridges packaged in a blister pack.

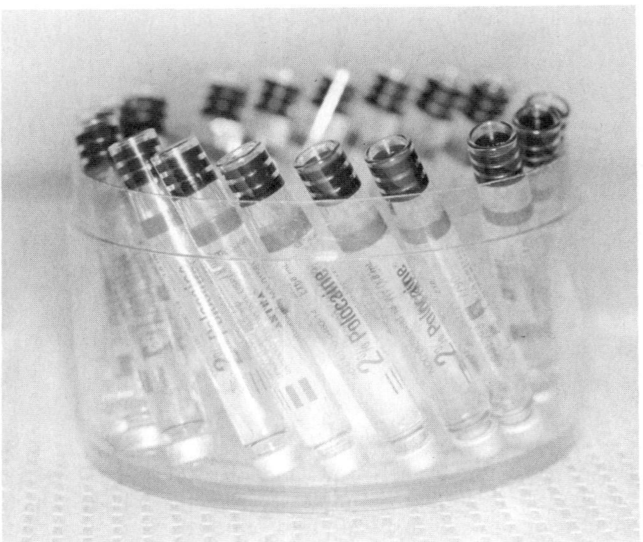

FIGURE 23–16
Local anesthetic cartridge dispenser.

prolonged heat or direct sunlight results in an accelerated deterioration of the solution, particularly the vasoconstrictor. In addition, if kept in these original containers the cartridges remain clean and uncontaminated.

Indeed, it is not necessary to prepare a cartridge prior to its being used. The local anesthetic solution itself is sterilized during the manufacturing process, and bacterial cultures taken from exterior cartridge surfaces immediately after opening a container usually fail to produce bacterial growth.[5] However, if the oral healthcare provider is concerned about the exterior of the cartridge, all components may be wiped with a disinfectant approved by the American Dental Association (ADA) and Environmental Protection Agency (EPA). Plastic cartridge dispensers also are available to aid in disinfecting cartridges (Fig. 23–16). They can hold one day's supply of cartridges with the diaphragm/aluminum cap placed downward. Gauze moistened with a disinfectant is placed in the center. When assembling the armamentarium for local anesthetic administration, the oral healthcare provider may wipe the diaphragm end of the cartridge against the moistened gauze (Fig. 23–17).

Cartridges should never be immersed in liquid disinfectant or sterilant. These solutions may diffuse through the semipermeable material of the diaphragm and contaminate the contents of the cartridge or may corrode the aluminum cap. In addition, local anesthetic cartridges should not be autoclaved. Both the labile vasoconstrictor and the seals of the cartridge cannot withstand the extreme temperatures.

Cartridge warmers that bring the local anesthetic solution to "body temperature" to promote client comfort during administration are commercially available. However, they are neither necessary nor recommended.[5,7] Local anesthetics stored and injected at room temperature are not uncomfortable to clients. Indeed, an overheated cartridge may cause a burning sensation during the injection and may destroy the heat-sensitive vasoconstrictor, thus producing a shorter duration of anesthesia.

Each box or canister is marked with an expiration date by the manufacturer. This expiration date also appears on the individual cartridges. Cartridges should not be used

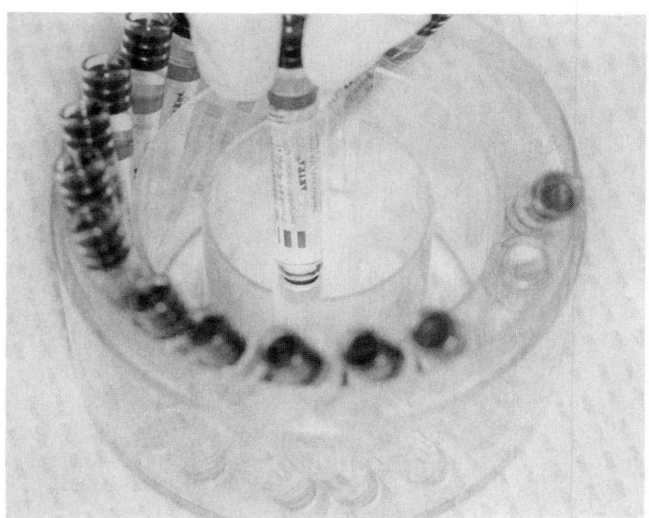

FIGURE 23-17
When assembling the armamentarium the diaphragm end of the cartridge may be wiped against gauze moistened with a disinfectant.

beyond the expiration date because injection with an outdated local anesthetic solution may result in client discomfort and unreliable anesthesia.

A product identification package insert is placed in all local anesthetic containers. It includes important information about the local anesthetic agent including dosages, contraindications, warnings, care and handling, and more. It is imperative that the dental hygienist be familiar with this material to assure client safety and comfort.

Problems

Problems are seldom encountered with cartridges, but the following may be noted:[5,7]

Bubble in the cartridge. Small bubbles (1 to 2 mm in diameter) may at times be seen in a cartridge. It is nitrogen gas that was bubbled into the anesthetic solution during the manufacturing process to preclude oxygen, which destroys the vasoconstrictor, from being trapped in the cartridge. These bubbles are harmless and may be ignored. However, a larger bubble (larger than 2 mm) in the cartridge is an indication that the solution has been frozen. This may be accompanied by a stopper that extends beyond the end of the cartridge (extruded). Because sterility of the solution is no longer guaranteed, the cartridge should not be used.

Extruded stopper. As noted previously, an extruded rubber stopper accompanied by a large bubble in the cartridge is an indication the solution has been frozen. Having a stopper that extends beyond the rim of the glass cylinder with no bubble present is often a sign that the cartridge was stored in a disinfectant and the solution has diffused through the diaphragm into the cartridge. When this occurs, the contents are contaminated and the cartridge should be discarded.

Sticky stopper. A "sticky" stopper does not advance smoothly through the glass cylinder when pressure is applied to the thumb ring of the syringe. Because rubber stoppers are more frequently being treated with silicone during manufacturing, this has become less of a problem. If, however, paraffin is being employed by the manufacturer, difficulty may be encountered. To minimize the problem, it is recommended that cartridges be stored at room temperature. If the problem persists, the healthcare provider should consider using only cartridges that have a silicone-treated stopper to facilitate a smooth, even deposition of solution.

Corroded cap. Corrosion of the aluminum cap may be observed if it has been immersed in quartenary compounds such as benzalkonium chloride. If disinfecting the cartridge is necessary, an ADA/EPA–approved disinfectant is recommended. Cartridges exhibiting corrosion should not be used.

Rust on the aluminum cap. The presence of rust signifies that a cartridge has broken or leaked in the metal container. The metal container rusts and deposits appear on the cap of the cartridge. A cartridge that has a rust deposit should not be used, and each cartridge in the container should be carefully inspected.

Broken cartridge. Cartridge breakage may occur if the cartridge has been fractured during handling. Damaged containers should be returned to the supplier. Prior to being used, each cartridge should be checked for signs of cracked or chipped glass. The area surrounding the stopper and the cylinder/cap interface need to be carefully examined. If a fractured cartridge is subjected to the pressure of an injection, it may shatter. Fortunately, the introduction of the color-coding band around the glass cylinder has minimized such an occurrence by reinforcing the glass.

A broken cartridge may result if excessive force is used when the dental hygienist engages the harpoon of an aspirating syringe. The harpoon is engaged by gently pressing the thumb ring and piston into the rubber stopper. If it is necessary to use more pressure to embed the harpoon, the dental hygienist should use one hand to cover the glass cartridge (see Procedure 23-1).

Pressure on the thumb ring of the syringe may cause the cartridge to break if the syringe harpoon is bent or the needle is bent and not perforating the cartridge diaphragm. Thorough examination and proper preparation of the armamentarium prior to use prevents this from occurring. One should never apply excessive pressure on the dental cartridge if significant resistance is met.

Leakage during injection. An off-center perforation of the needle into the diaphragm of the cartridge produces an oval-shaped puncture. When positive pressure is applied to the plunger, anesthetic solution may leak through the perforation. It is important to carefully insert the needle into the cartridge diaphragm so a centric perforation occurs and leakage during the injection is prevented (see Procedure 23-1).

Burning on injection (refer to Local Complications).

Supplementary Armamentarium

In addition to the syringe, needle, and cartridge, other items are needed to effectively administer local anesthetics. These include topical antiseptic, topical anesthetic, applicator sticks, gauze, and hemostat or cotton pliers.

Topical Antiseptics

Topical antiseptics may be applied to the surface of the mucosa at the injection site to reduce the risk of introduc-

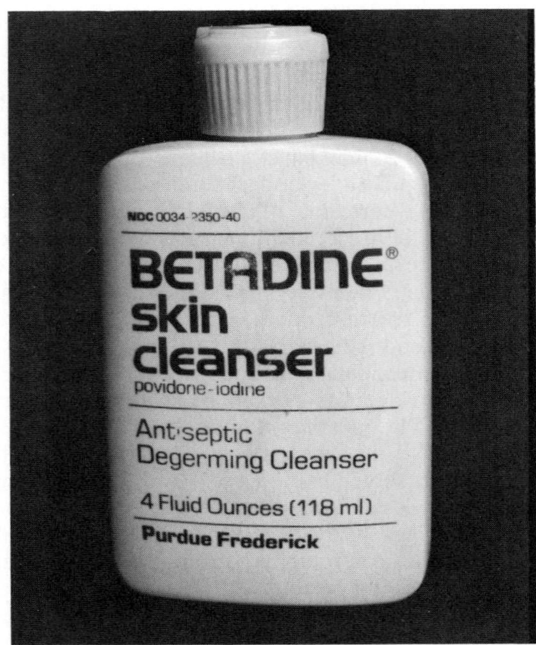

FIGURE 23-18
Topical antiseptic.

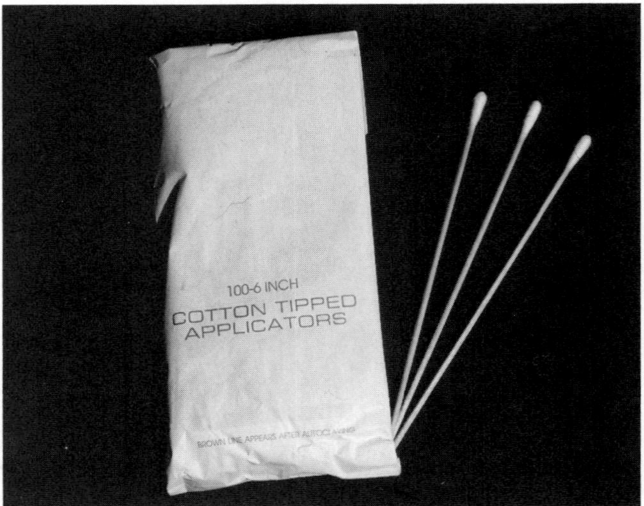

FIGURE 23-20
Cotton-tipped applicator sticks.

ing surface microorganisms into the tissue, which could result in inflammation and infection. (Fig. 23-18). Betadine (providone-iodine and Merthiolate (thimerosal) are agents commonly used for this purpose.[5] A small quantity of the agent is placed at the site of the injection for 15 to 30 seconds prior to placement of the topical anesthetic and the initial needle penetration. The use of sterile gauze for wiping the surface has been suggested as an adequate alternative, with topical antiseptic application as an option for further microbe reduction.[5] However, because postinjection infections may occur, the use of a topical antiseptic should be considered especially when administering local anesthetic agents to individuals who may be immunosuppressed.

Topical Anesthetic Agents

Topical anesthetic agents are applied to the mucous membrane prior to the initial needle penetration to anesthetize the terminal nerve endings, and thus promote client comfort during the injection procedures (Fig. 23-19). For maximal effectiveness, the topical anesthetic agent should be placed at the penetration site for 1 to 2 minutes.

The concentration of agents used for topical application is high to facilitate diffusion of the drug through the mucous membranes (usually 2 to 3 mm). Therefore, only small amounts applied to a limited area should be used to avoid toxicity. Both ester and amide topical anesthetic agents are available. They are prepared in the form of gels, ointments, solutions, or sprays. Topical anesthetic sprays that, when activated, deliver a continuous stream until deactivated may potentially deliver a very high dose of the anesthetic agent and are therefore not recommended. Those sprays that deliver a measured dose limit the amount that can be expelled and are much preferred.

Cotton-Tipped Applicator Sticks

Cotton-tipped applicator sticks are needed for topical antiseptic and anesthetic agent application (Fig. 23-20). They

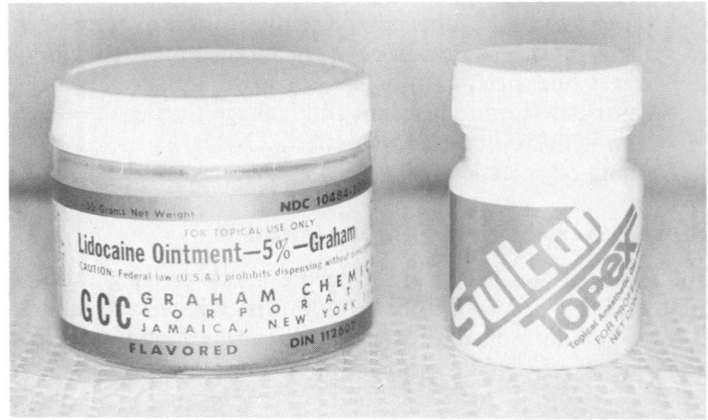

FIGURE 23-19
Topical anesthetics.

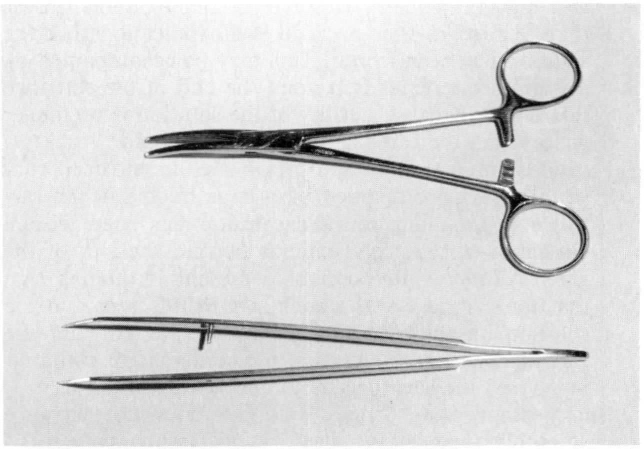
FIGURE 23-21
Hemostat and forceps.

also may be used to apply pressure to the tissue before and during palatal injections.

Gauze

Gauze is used to wipe the tissue at the injection site prior to applying the topical antiseptic and anesthetic agents and again prior to inserting the needle. This removes the saliva and debris from the injection site. It also may serve as a suitable, though not as effective, replacement for the topical antiseptic (see Topical Antiseptic). In addition, the gauze aids in retraction, visibility, and stability during the injection procedures.

Hemostat, Forceps, Cotton Pliers

Hemostat, forceps, or cotton pliers should be a component of the armamentarium in the unlikely event a needle breaks during administration and must be retrieved from the soft tissues (Fig. 23–21).

Preparation of the Armamentarium

Proper preparation of the armamentarium is essential to prevent complications associated with the syringe, cartridge, and needle, and to assure client safety and comfort during local anesthetic administration (Procedure 23–1).

PROCEDURE 23–1

LOADING THE SYRINGE

Equipment

Syringe
Anesthetic cartridge
Needle
Gauze
Protective barriers

Step	Rationale
1. Inspect each component of the armamentarium prior to assembly	Ensures armamentarium is free of defects and in proper working order
2. Retract the piston of the syringe by pulling back fully on the thumb ring (Fig. 23–22)	Allows room for the cartridge to fit into the syringe

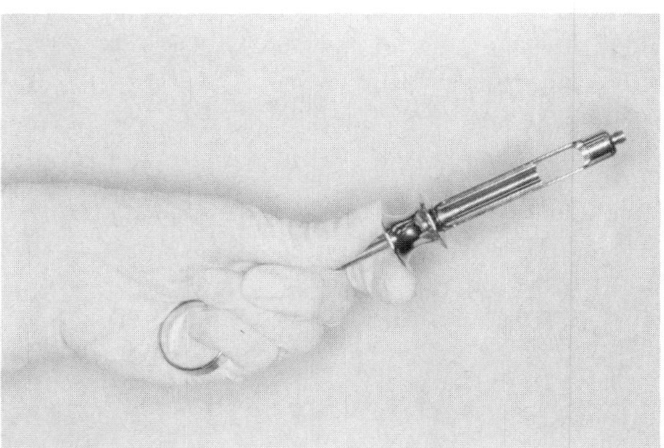

FIGURE 23–22
Retract the piston of the syringe.

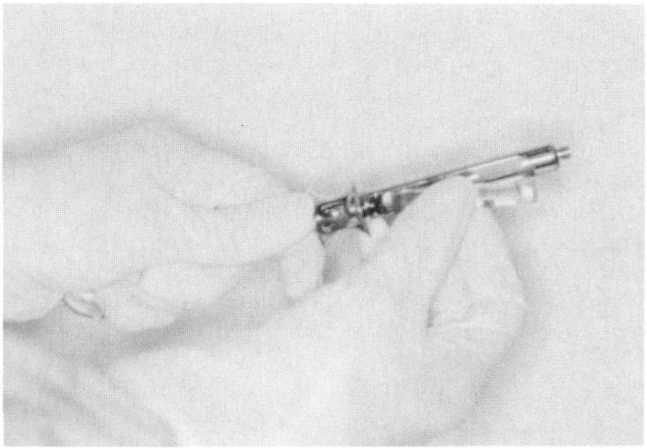

FIGURE 23–23
Insert the cartridge while continuing to retract the piston.

Step	Rationale
3. Insert the cartridge, rubber stopper end first, while continuing to retract the piston (Fig. 23–23). The cartridge should lie flat within the barrel of the syringe	Cartridge fits into the syringe without being damaged
4. Release the piston of the syringe	Secures the cartridge in the barrel of the syringe
5. Engage the harpoon by gently pressing on the thumb ring until the harpoon is embedded into the rubber stopper of the cartridge. Excessive force is not necessary (Fig. 23–24). This step is unnecessary when loading a self-aspirating syringe	The harpoon must engage into the rubber stopper for the dental hygienist to aspirate. Too much force on the thumb ring of the syringe may cause the cartridge to break

CONTINUED ON FOLLOWING PAGE

PROCEDURE 23-1

LOADING THE SYRINGE *Continued*

Step	Rationale
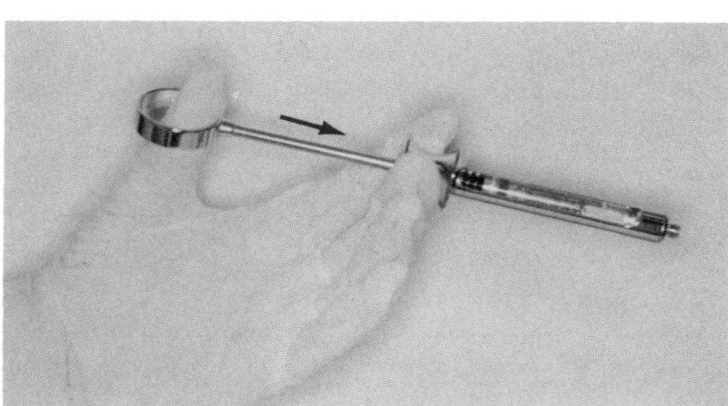 FIGURE 23-24 Engage the harpoon by gently pressing on the thumb ring.	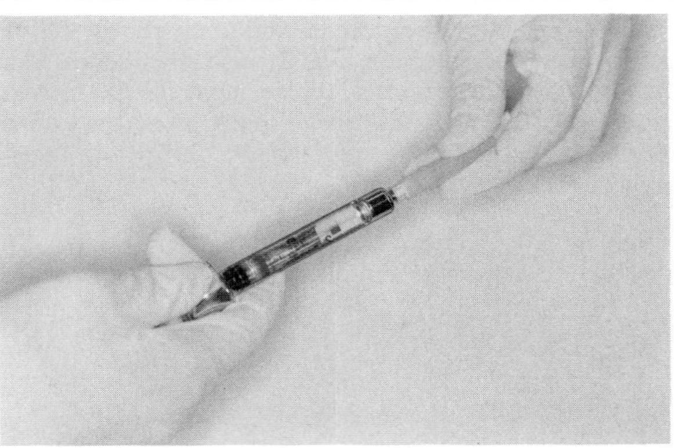 FIGURE 23-25 Attach the needle to the syringe.
6. Attach the needle to the syringe by removing the clear or white plastic cap from the syringe end of the needle and screwing the needle onto the syringe (Fig. 23-25). Needles with a plastic hub need to be pushed and screwed onto the syringe. Metal hub needles have threading. Do not dispose of the cap, it will be needed when unloading the syringe. **Safety Note:** The sequence of inserting the cartridge and engaging the harpoon (of an aspirating syringe) prior to attaching the needle is preferred. This prevents having to hit the thumb ring and piston with force to engage the harpoon when the needle is already attached. This may lead to a broken cartridge or anesthetic solution leaking from the needle prior to the injection. The sequence described above also prevents the needle from being bent when perforating the diaphragm of the cartridge	Secures the needle onto the syringe
7. Check for needle sharpness by removing the colored plastic cap from the needle and drawing the needle tip across sterile gauze (optional). A needle barb would snag the gauze and the needle should be replaced (Fig. 23-26) 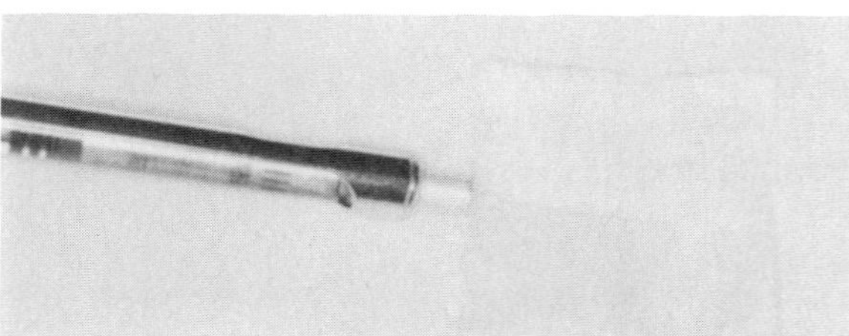 FIGURE 23-26 Check the needle sharpness by drawing the needle backward on sterile gauze. If there is fear of needle contamination, this step may be omitted.	Checks for needle sharpness to ensure an atraumatic insertion and withdrawal
8. Expel a few drops of anesthetic solution	Ensures the syringe, needle, and cartridge are properly prepared and functional
9. Resheath the needle using a one-handed "scoop" technique or an approved mechanical device for needle capping (See Procedure 23-3)	Keeps the needle in a sterile field and prevents needlestick exposure

At the completion of the dental hygiene care appointment, local anesthesia armamentarium needs to be dismantled. Procedure 23–2 describes the sequence of properly unloading the syringe and the rationale for each step.

During the course of administering local anesthetics during dental hygiene care, it may be necessary to replace an empty cartridge. Malamed recommends totally unloading the syringe, placing a new cartridge in the syringe, and reattaching the needle to prevent potential cartridge breakage or anesthetic solution leaking from the needle prior to the injection.[5] This sequence of loading the syringe prior to securing the needle is preferred when initially preparing the armamentarium. However, the risk of removal and increased handling of a contaminated needle and potential for a needlestick exposure needs to be weighed against the risk of cartridge breakage and leakage. In any case, the dental hygienist should use extreme care when handling the local anesthetic armamentarium to prevent injury to both client and self.

PROCEDURE 23–2

UNLOADING THE SYRINGE

Equipment

Syringe
Anesthetic cartridge
Needle
Sharps container
Protective barriers

Step	Rationale
1. Resheath the needle utilizing the one-handed "scoop" technique or an approved mechanical device for needle capping (see Procedure 23–3)	Prevents a needlestick exposure while unloading the syringe
2. Retract the piston of the syringe by pulling back fully on the thumb ring	Allows room for the cartridge to be disengaged from the syringe
3. While retracting the piston, remove the cartridge by pulling it away from the needle and disengaging the rubber stopper from the harpoon (Fig. 23–27). Turn the window of the syringe downward to aid in removal. With a self-aspirating syringe there is no harpoon disengagement	Frees the cartridge from the barrel of the syringe

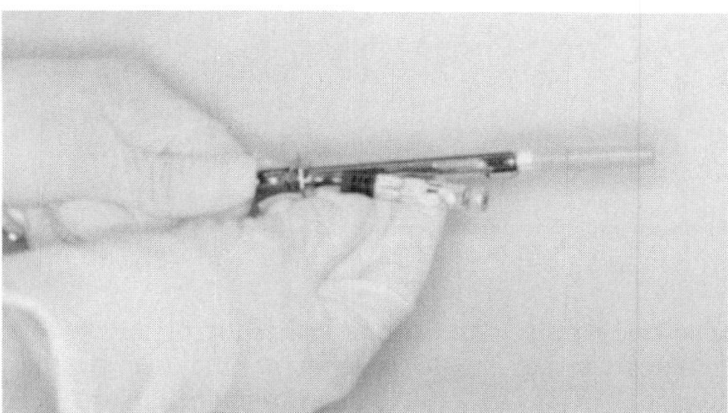

FIGURE 23–27
Retract the piston, and remove the cartridge.

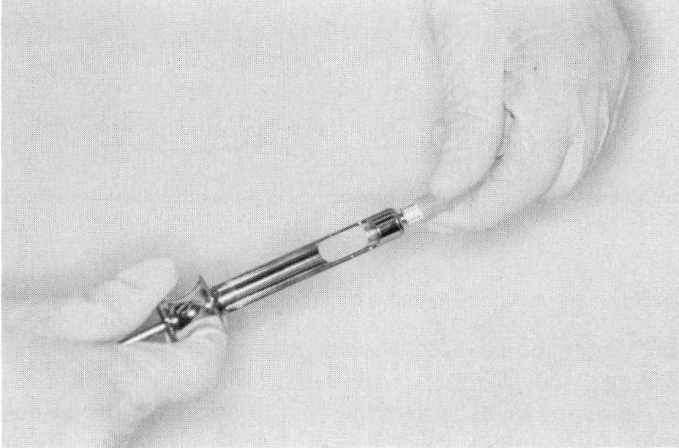

FIGURE 23–28
Unscrew and remove the sheathed needle from the syringe.

Step	Rationale
4. Unscrew and remove the needle from the syringe (Fig. 23–28)	Frees the needle from the syringe
5. Resheath the syringe end of the needle using the one-handed "scoop" technique or an approved mechanical device for needle capping (see Procedure 23–3)	Protects the dental hygienist from needlestick exposure during disposal

CONTINUED ON FOLLOWING PAGE

PROCEDURE 23–2

UNLOADING THE SYRINGE *Continued*

Step	Rationale
6. Directly dispose of the needle and cartridge in a sharps container (Fig. 23–29)	Used needles and cartridges are considered infectious. Sharps must be discarded in a rigid, puncture proof, leak-resistant container (see Chapter 9)

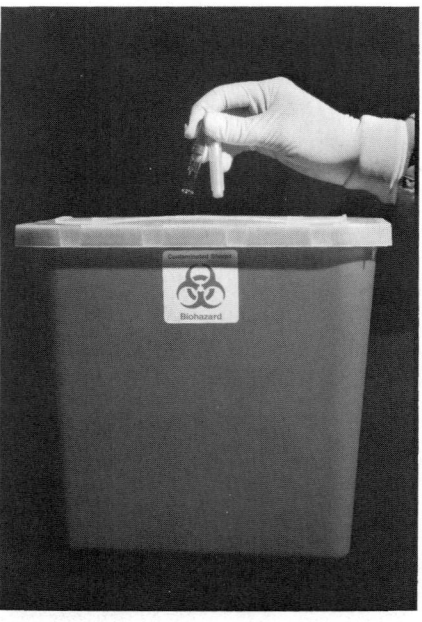

FIGURE 23–29
Dispose of the needle and cartridge in a sharps container.

Safety Note: Needles should not be bent, broken or cut prior to disposal in a sharps container.[27] This minimizes the possibility of a needlestick exposure

Step	Rationale
7. The syringe should be sterilized following the appropriate protocol	Syringe is available for subsequent utilization

Unsheathing and Resheathing the Needle

A needle should be covered with a protective shield when it is not being used. Concerns over the possibility of a needlestick exposure have led to the formulation of guidelines for resheathing needles. Oral healthcare providers are most often injured with needles when the needle is being resheathed following an injection.[23] At this time the needle is contaminated with blood, saliva, and debris and the potential for disease transmission exists. A variety of techniques have been suggested, but currently a one-handed "scoop" technique for sheathing the needle is recommended. Procedure 23–3 describes each step for unsheathing and resheathing the needle using the one-handed "scoop" procedure.

Mechanical devices such as shields and needle sheath props are available to aid in the prevention of an accidental needlestick exposure (Fig. 23–30). Dental hygienists should be familiar with the devices available and determine which technique or mechanical device is most acceptable to them.

The one-handed resheathing technique or an approved mechanical device should be consistently used by the dental hygienist regardless of whether the needle has been contaminated.

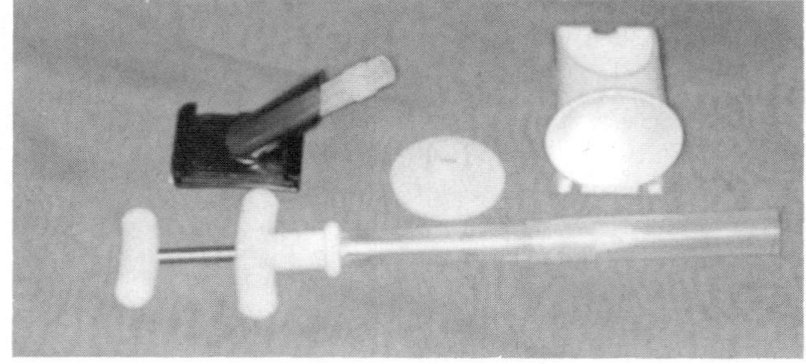

FIGURE 23–30
Devices such as shields and needle sheath props are available to aid in the prevention of an accidental needlestick exposure.

PROCEDURE 23-3

UNSHEATHING AND RESHEATHING THE NEEDLE—ONE-HANDED "SCOOP" TECHNIQUE

Equipment

Syringe
Anesthetic cartridge
Needle
Gauze
Protective barriers

Unsheathing the Needle

Step	Rationale
1. Disengage the colored plastic cap while directing the needle away from the body or hand	Decreases the likelihood of a puncture injury
2. Keeping the hand at the needle hub, gently loosen the cap (Fig. 23–31). Avoid disengaging the cap while holding onto the needle tip end of the plastic sheath	Removing the cap by pulling on the needle tip end may cause the hand to "bounce back," leading to a needlestick exposure

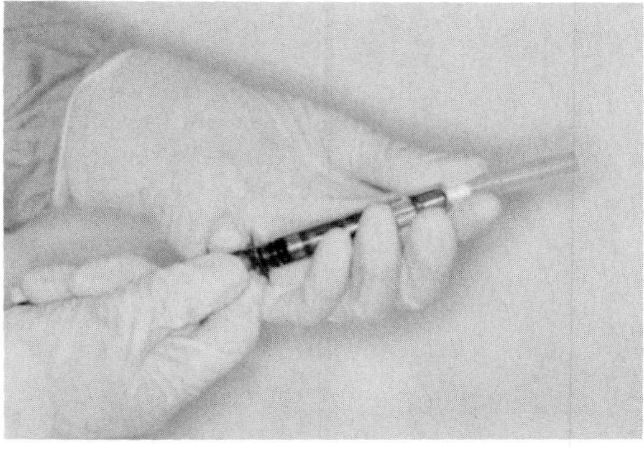

FIGURE 23–31
Directing the needle away from the body, keep the hand at the needle hub and loosen the cap.

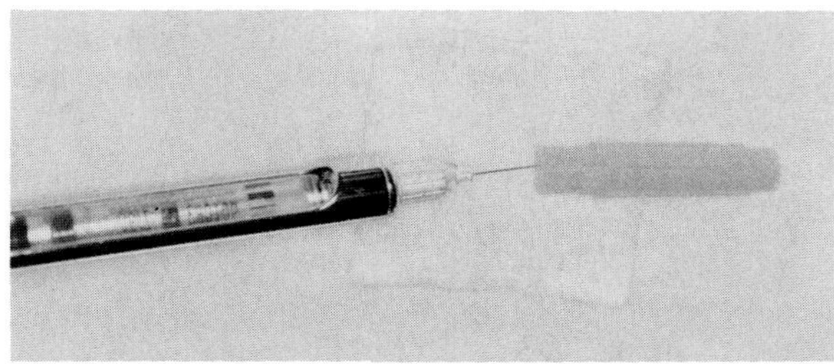

FIGURE 23–32
Let the cap slide off the needle and onto a piece of sterile gauze.

Step	Rationale
3. Let the cap slide off the needle and onto a piece of sterile gauze lying on the instrument tray (Fig. 23–32)	Minimizes the likelihood of a puncture injury

Resheathing the Needle–One-handed "Scoop" Technique

Step	Rationale
1. Hold the syringe with one hand and glide the needle into the colored plastic cap lying on the instrument tray (Fig. 23–33).	Prevents the dental hygienist from self-inflicting a puncture wound

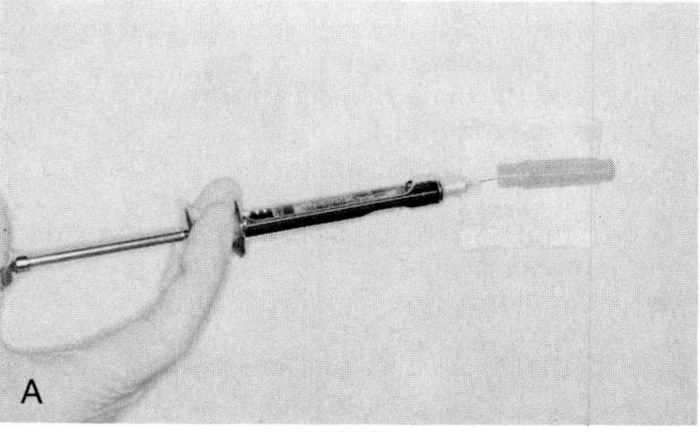

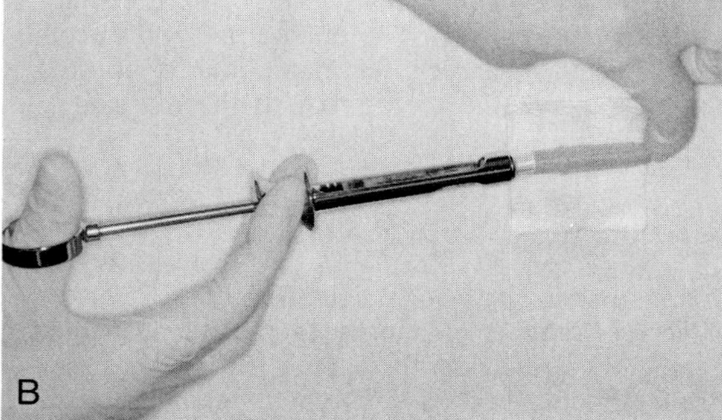

FIGURE 23–33
***A,* Glide the needle into the cap lying on the instrument tray. *B,* Secure the cap to the hub of the needle.**

CONTINUED ON FOLLOWING PAGE

PROCEDURE 23–3

UNSHEATHING AND RESHEATHING THE NEEDLE—ONE-HANDED "SCOOP" TECHNIQUE *Continued*

Resheathing the Needle–One-handed "Scoop" Technique

Step	Rationale
Never attempt to hold cap with other hand. As an alternative, forceps may be used to hold cap on tray. This provides more control over cap and keeps dental hygienist's hand a safe distance from needle	
2. Tilt the syringe upward to allow the cap to slide down to the hub and cover the needle. If the cap starts to slip off the needle, do not attempt to stop it with the other hand because this may lead to an accidental needlestick exposure. Instead, let the cap fall on the instrument tray and begin the process again	Prevents the dental hygienist from an exposure incident
3. Secure the cap to the hub of the needle (see Fig. 23–33)	Creates a barrier between the outside environment and the contaminated needle

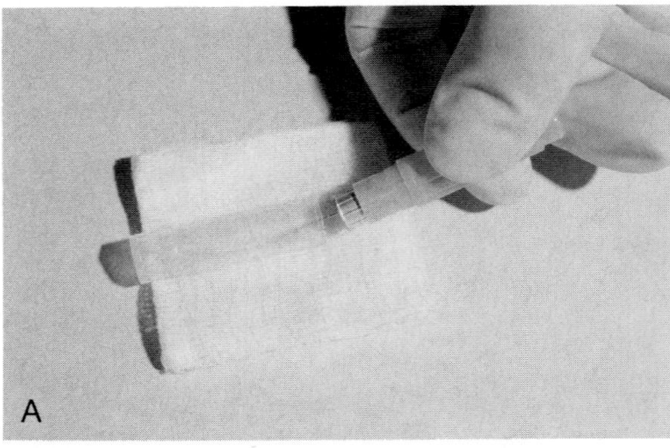

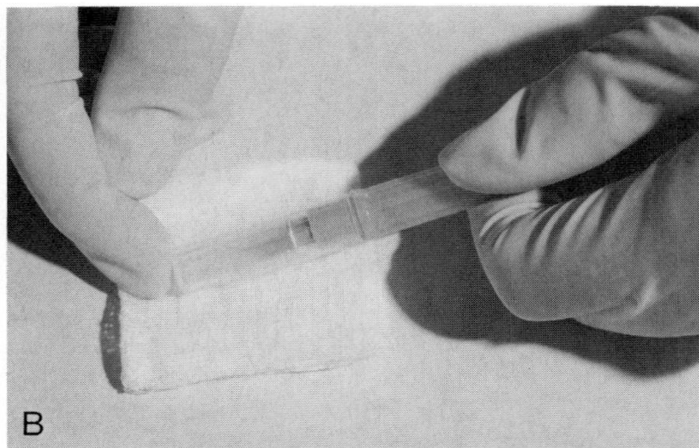

FIGURE 23–34
A, After removing the needle from the syringe, glide the syringe end of the needle into the sheath lying on the instrument tray. *B,* Secure the cap to the hub of the needle.

Step	Rationale
4. When removing the needle from the syringe, the colored plastic cap should remain on the needle. The syringe end of the needle should be resheathed using the one-handed "scoop" technique described above (Fig. 23–34) or an approved mechanical device for needle capping	Prevents an accidental needlestick exposure

THE TRIGEMINAL NERVE

The **trigeminal nerve** is the fifth and largest of the 12 cranial nerves (Fig. 23–35*A*). The three divisions of the trigeminal nerve include: the ophthalmic (V_1), the maxillary (V_2), and the mandibular (V_3). The ophthalmic and maxillary divisions are totally sensory; the mandibular division is sensory and also carries the motor root to the muscles of the mandible.

Ophthalmic Division (V_1)

The **ophthalmic nerve,** the first and smallest division of the trigeminal nerve, branches off the trigeminal (semilunar or gasserian) ganglion and forms three branches, the nasociliary nerve, the frontal nerve, and the lacrimal nerve. This division of the trigeminal nerve innervates tissues superior to the oral structures including the eye, nose, and frontal cutaneous tissues. It has only sensory function. Of the three divisions of the trigeminal nerve, the ophthalmic is the least important to intraoral local anesthetic administration.

Maxillary Division (V_2)

The **maxillary division** of the trigeminal nerve, entirely sensory in function, arises from the trigeminal (semilunar or gasserian) ganglion, exits the cranium via the foramen rotundum and then passes into the pterygopalatine fossa where it gives off a number of branches (see Fig. 23–35*B* and *C*). Only those branches pertinent to intraoral local anesthesia are discussed.

Pterygopalatine Nerves

Two branches pass through the pterygopalatine ganglion and form the **greater (anterior) palatine nerve** and the **nasopalatine nerve** (see Fig. 23–35*B*). The greater palatine nerve enters the oral cavity on the hard palate via the greater palatine foramen and innervates the palatal soft tissues and bone of the posterior teeth. The nasopalatine nerve leaves the pterygopalatine ganglion and passes forward and downward, entering the oral cavity through the incisive foramen. This nerve provides sensory innervation to the lingual bone and soft tissues in the premaxilla (canine to canine).

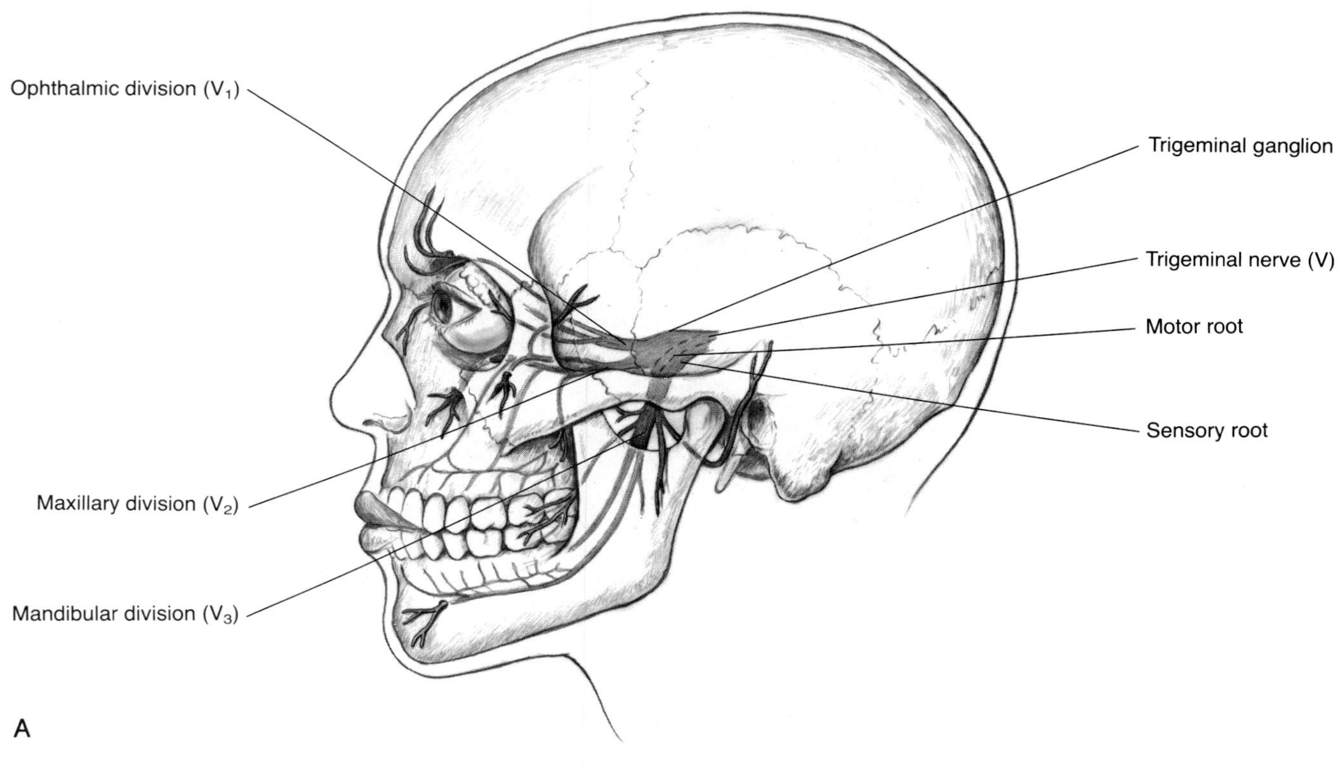

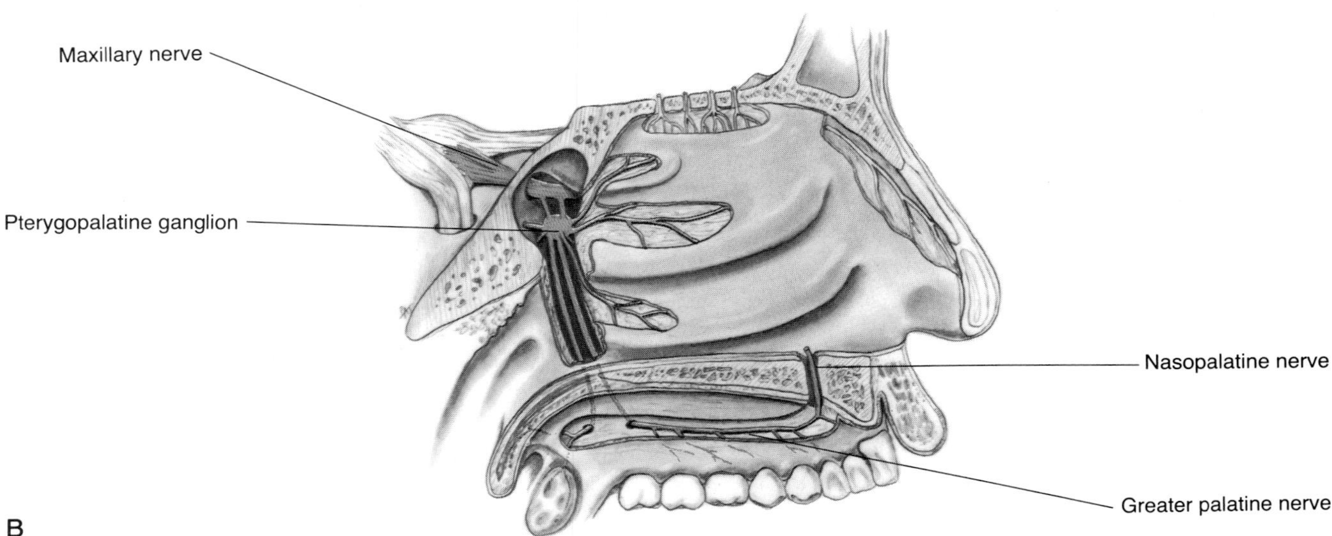

FIGURE 23–35
A, Trigeminal nerve distribution. *B*, Palatal branches of the maxillary division (V_2). *C*, Distribution of the maxillary division (V_2). *D*, Distribution of the mandibular division (V_3). (*A to D* from Fehrenbach, M. J. Illustrated Anatomy of the Head and Neck. Philadelphia: W. B. Saunders [in press].)

Illustration continued on following page

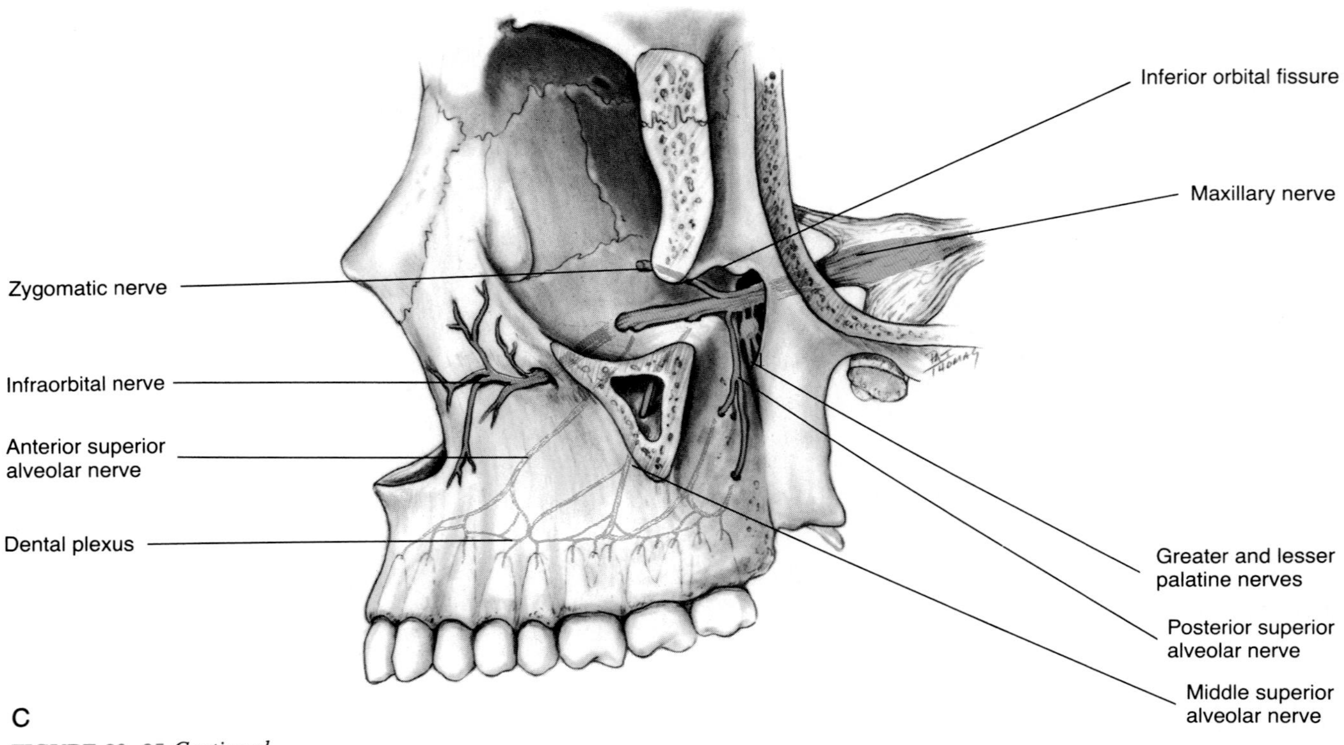
Inferior orbital fissure
Maxillary nerve
Zygomatic nerve
Infraorbital nerve
Anterior superior
alveolar nerve
Dental plexus
Greater and lesser
palatine nerves
Posterior superior
alveolar nerve
Middle superior
alveolar nerve
C

FIGURE 23-35 *Continued*

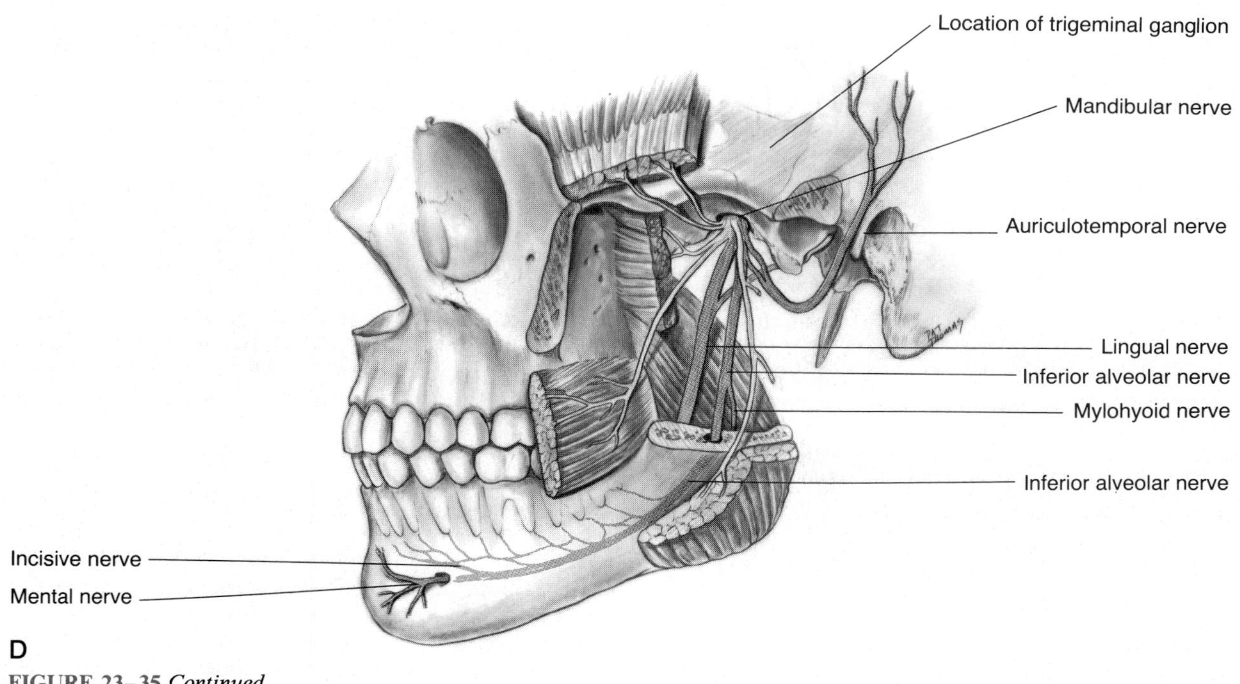

FIGURE 23-35 *Continued*

Posterior Superior Alveolar Nerve

The **posterior superior alveolar nerve** (PSA) (see Fig. 23-35*C*) descends from the main trunk of the maxillary nerve just before it enters the infraorbital canal. Most often there are two PSA branches that pass downward on the posterior surface of the maxilla. An internal branch enters the posterior superior alveolar foramen located on the superior portion of the maxillary tuberosity. This branch provides sensory innervation to the pulpal and osseous tissues and the periodontal ligaments of the maxillary third, second, and first molars (usually with the exception of the mesiofacial root of the first molar). An external branch of the posterior superior alveolar nerve remains on the outer surface of the maxilla and continues downward to innervate the facial gingiva of the maxillary molars and the adjacent vestibular mucosa.

Branches of the Infraorbital Nerve

The maxillary nerve continues anteriorly after having given off the posterior superior alveolar nerve and enters the infraorbital canal. At this point the maxillary nerve is referred to as the "infraorbital nerve" (see Fig. 23-35*C*). Two branches may descend from the infraorbital nerve: the middle superior alveolar and the anterior superior alveolar nerves.

The **middle superior alveolar nerve** (MSA) branches off the infraorbital nerve within the infraorbital canal. This nerve provides sensory innervation to the maxillary premolars, the mesiofacial root of the first molar, the periodontal tissues, and the facial soft tissue and bone in the premolar area. The MSA nerve is not present in approximately 60% of individuals.[24] In its absence, these areas are innervated by the posterior superior alveolar nerve, or more frequently, the anterior superior alveolar nerve.

The **anterior superior alveolar nerve** (ASA) descends from the infraorbital nerve just prior to the latter's exit from the infraorbital foramen. The ASA nerve provides innervation to the central and lateral incisors, the canine, the periodontal tissues, and facial soft tissue and bone over these teeth. In those individuals without an MSA nerve, the ASA nerve most often provides innervation to the premolars and possibly the mesiofacial root of the first molar.

Mandibular Division (V_3)

The **mandibular nerve,** the third and largest division of the trigeminal nerve, has both a sensory root and carries the motor root for the trigeminal nerve (see Fig. 23–35*D*). The sensory root arises from the trigeminal ganglion after which it is joined by the motor root. Both roots emerge from the cranium via the foramen ovale, and at this point, they unite to form the main trunk of the mandibular nerve. The trunk then divides into an anterior branch and a posterior branch. Those nerves arising from these branches that relate to intraoral local anesthesia are the following:

Branches of the Anterior Division

The anterior division is smaller than its posterior counterpart and contains primarily motor fibers. The motor component innervates the muscles of mastication: the masseter, the temporalis, and the lateral and medial pterygoid. The sensory component of the anterior division is the **buccal nerve.** At the level of the occlusal plane of the mandibular molars, it crosses the anterior border of the ramus and branches to innervate the buccal gingiva of the mandibular molars.

Branches of the Posterior Division

The posterior division of the mandibular nerve is primarily sensory, but it also has a small motor component. The branches of the posterior division related to mandibular anesthesia are the lingual and inferior alveolar nerves.

The **lingual nerve** emerges between the lower head of the lateral pterygoid and medial pterygoid muscles and lies between the ramus and the medial pterygoid muscle in the pterygomandibular space. It turns anteriorly where it enters the oral cavity and innervates the anterior two-thirds of the tongue, the mucous membranes of the floor of the mouth, and the lingual gingiva of the mandible.

The **inferior alveolar nerve** runs posterior and parallel to the lingual nerve within the pterygomandibular space where it enters the mandibular foramen. Within the mandible the inferior alveolar nerve travels in the mandibular canal and innervates the pulpal and osseous tissues of the mandibular teeth in the quadrant and facial soft tissues anterior to the first molar. Throughout its course the inferior alveolar nerve is accompanied by the inferior alveolar artery and vein.

As the inferior alveolar nerve reaches the mental foramen, it divides into two terminal branches. The **incisive nerve** is a direct extension of the inferior alveolar nerve continuing anteriorly within the mandibular canal. It innervates the pulpal and osseous tissues of the mandibular first premolar, canine, lateral and central incisors, and the facial periodontal tissues of the teeth.

The **mental nerve** branches from the inferior alveolar nerve and exits the mandible via the mental foramen and provides sensory innervation to the mucous membranes and skin of the lower lip and chin.

The **mylohyoid nerve** branches from the inferior alveolar nerve before the latter enters into the mandibular foramen. It advances downward and forward in the mylohyoid groove on the medial side of the ramus and provides motor innervation to the mylohyoid and anterior digastric muscles. In some individuals the mylohyoid nerve may supply accessory sensory innervation to the mandible in the premolar and molar area.

LOCAL ANESTHESIA TECHNIQUES

When choosing the appropriate injection to be administered, the dental hygienist needs to consider the area to be treated, the procedure to be performed, the extent of anesthesia necessary, and the client's needs and comfort. In oral healthcare there are three major types of injections used to obtain local anesthesia:

- Local infiltration
- Field block
- Nerve block

These are differentiated by the site of anesthetic solution deposition relative to the area to receive treatment.

Local Infiltration

This injection refers to the placement of the anesthetic solution close to the smaller terminal endings of the nerve fibers in the immediate area to be treated (Fig. 23–36). An example would be the injection of anesthetic solution into an interproximal papilla prior to therapeutic scaling and root planing.

Field Block

This method of obtaining anesthesia refers to the deposition of solution near large terminal nerve branches (Fig.

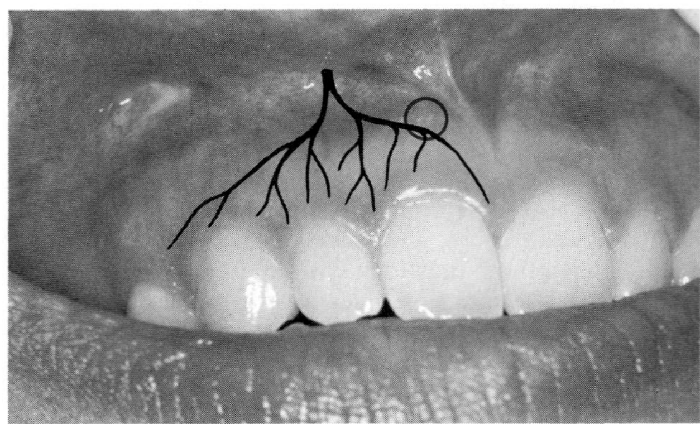

FIGURE 23–36
Local infiltration. The local anesthetic is placed in the immediate area to be treated.

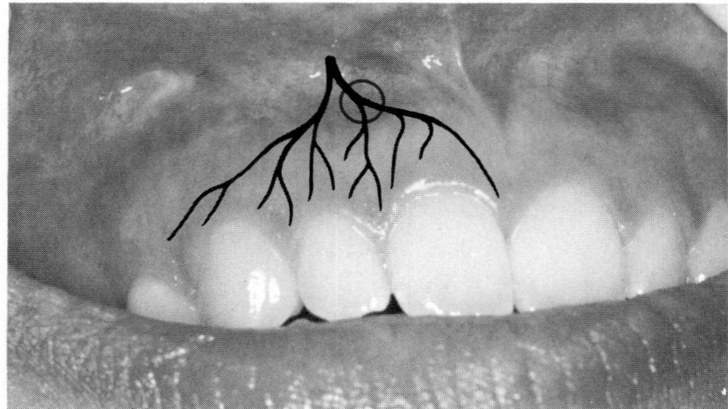

FIGURE 23–37
Field block. The local anesthetic is deposited near the larger terminal nerve endings. Treatment is away from the site of the injection.

23–37). The resulting anesthesia is more circumscribed, most often involving one tooth and the tissues surrounding the tooth. Treatment is away from the site of the injection. The deposition of anesthetic solution above the apex of a maxillary tooth, such as the maxillary right central incisor, is an example of a field block. In oral healthcare a field block is often incorrectly referred to as a "local infiltration."

Nerve Block

The nerve block refers to the deposition of anesthetic solution close to a main nerve trunk often at some distance from the treatment area (Fig. 23–38). This type of injection most often anesthetizes a larger area than that of a field block. Examples include a posterior superior alveolar nerve block and an inferior alveolar nerve block.

Thus, when providing dental hygiene care in a small, isolated area, infiltration anesthesia may be the best choice, whereas a field block is the injection of choice when one or two teeth are to be treated. When the dental hygiene care plan involves a sextant or quadrant, nerve block anesthesia is recommended.

The term "anesthesia" is often preceded by either the word *local* or *regional*. Either phrase is correct; each indicates that a specific area is anesthetized and that the client is conscious, unlike general anesthesia, in which the client is unconscious. Thus, the use of either term is appropriate and used interchangeably, although "local anesthesia" appears to be more commonly used.

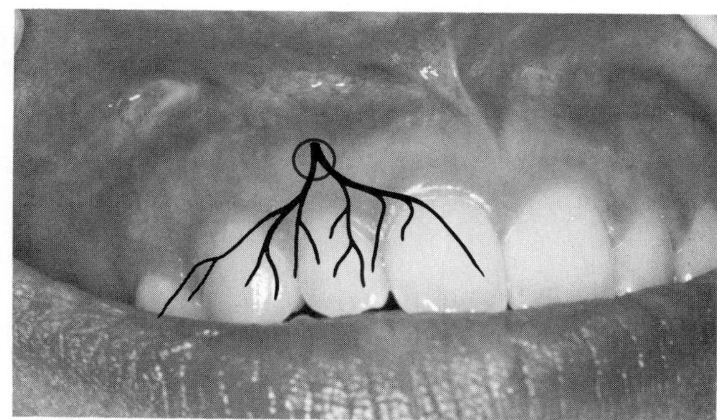

FIGURE 23–38
Nerve block. The local anesthetic is deposited near a main nerve trunk often located some distance from the site of treatment.

PROCEDURES FOR A SUCCESSFUL INJECTION

The goal for each administration of local anesthetic is, of course, to give a safe, comfortable injection for control and elimination of painful sensations during and after dental and dental hygiene care. It is ironic, however, that a procedure meant to control pain for the client is often reported to be the most dreaded by clients. Although the prospect of receiving an intraoral injection provokes fear and apprehension for many individuals, local anesthetic agent administration need not be painful. The dental hygienist strives to make all dental hygiene care free from pain and stress, and especially when administering intraoral local anesthetic agents. Such techniques as using a topical anesthetic prior to needle insertion, cautiously advancing the needle, and slowly depositing the anesthetic solution help to minimize or eliminate discomfort. Strategies used to minimize anxiety include communicating with the client about the progress of the procedure. Keeping clients informed of the procedures in a calm manner and using nonthreatening language helps to minimize apprehension and promote trust and cooperation. For example, telling clients "I'm applying the topical anesthetic to the tissue so the remainder of the procedure is more comfortable" or, "I don't expect you to feel this" when inserting the needle into the tissue places a "positive" idea in the client's mind regarding the injection and keeps the client informed of the impending procedure. Taking the extra time necessary to complete these steps results in a more comfortable procedure for the client, thus meeting the need for freedom from pain and stress.

Procedure 23–4 presents steps to ensure comfort, safety, and success common to all injections. Although each injection is unique with regard to anatomical considerations, these steps should be employed regardless of the injection being administered. Not every injection is successful and totally free of discomfort because the reactions of clients and the skills of the hygienist may vary. However, if the appropriate procedures are followed, the client and the dental hygienist will enjoy the benefit of the safest and least traumatic injection possible.

PROCEDURE 23–4

GIVING A SUCCESSFUL INJECTION

Equipment

Health history form
Sphygmomanometer
Stethoscope
Gauze
Topical anesthetic agent
Cotton-tip applicator
Syringe
Anesthetic cartridge
Needle
Protective barriers

CONTINUED ON FOLLOWING PAGE

PROCEDURE 23–4

GIVING A SUCCESSFUL INJECTION *Continued*

Step	Rationale
1. Assess the health history data	Assists the dental hygienist in determining if the client is physiologically and psychologically able to tolerate the proposed treatment and local anesthetic administration, and in modifying approach to care, if necessary, to decrease risks and prevent subsequent medical emergencies
2. Take vital signs. Minimal examination should include blood pressure, heart rate (pulse), and respiratory rate.[8]	Following guidelines for dental management of clients according to blood pressure level, heart rate, and respiratory rate minimizes medical complications
3. Confirm care plan	Verifies with the client the dental hygiene care indicated
4. Check armamentarium	Ensures that all materials are properly assembled, prepared, and functional so the procedure is efficient
5. Load the syringe and determine the syringe window and needle bevel orientation[5]	The large window of the syringe should face the operator so she is able to see the amount of anesthetic being administered and detect a positive aspiration. The bevel of the needle should face the bone, thus, if the needle contacts bone, the bevel deflects over the periosteum, minimizing discomfort and trauma. If the bevel faces away from the bone, the point of the needle may tear the sensitive tissues causing discomfort both during and after the injection
6. Check needle sharpness by pulling the needle tip across sterile gauze, and watching for snags (optional)[5]	A sharp needle free of barbs does not snag gauze and provides an atraumatic insertion and withdrawal
7. Check the flow of solution	Ensures the syringe, needle, and cartridge are properly prepared and functional so the procedure is efficient
8. Position the client in a supine position	Placing the client in a supine position provides better accessibility and visibility for the clinician and reduces the likelihood of syncope for the client. Position may vary with client's health status or clinician's preference
9. Communicate with the client. Do not use words with a negative connotation such as shot, injection, pain or hurt. Instead, speak in less threatening terms such as "administer the local anesthetic"[5]	Keeping clients informed of the procedures helps them anticipate the operator's actions. A calm approach minimizes client anxiety
10. Clinician positions self	Provides optimal accessibility and visibility for the clinician relative to the specific injection being administered
11. Visualize or palpate to locate the penetration site	Accurate injection of anesthetic requires insertion in correct site
12. Dry the penetration site with gauze	Removes saliva and debris from the penetration site, reducing the risk of infection
13. Apply topical antiseptic to the penetration site (optional)	Decreases microorganisms at the penetration site, reducing the risk of infection
14. Apply topical anesthetic to the penetration site for 1–2 minutes	Application of topical anesthetic results in a more comfortable penetration
15. In the case of palatal injections, when placing topical anesthetic on the injection site, apply considerable pressure with the cotton swab for a minimum of 1 minute prior to the injection. Move the swab immediately adjacent to the penetration site and maintain pressure at this site during the injection	Injections into the dense, tightly attached, palatal tissue can be extremely painful to the client. Pressure anesthesia provides for a more comfortable procedure by producing ischemia and blocking pain impulses arising from the needle penetration[5]
16. Redry the penetration site	Removes the saliva and excess topical anesthetic from the injection site
17. Make the tissue taut at the penetration site by retracting it (except the palate) utilizing sterile gauze	Gauze is used to aid in retraction and stability. Stretching the tissue tight at the penetration site provides maximal visibility and allows the needle to enter the tissue with minimal resistance and discomfort. Avoid jiggling the soft tissues or pulling the lip over the needle tip, which may impair visibility of the penetration site
18. Keep syringe and needle out of the client's line of vision	Minimizes client anxiety
19. Place the needle at the penetration site	Accurate injection of anesthetic agent requires insertion in the correct site
20. Utilize a handrest (Fig. 23–39)	Provides stability and control during the injection, thus ensuring greater client safety and comfort

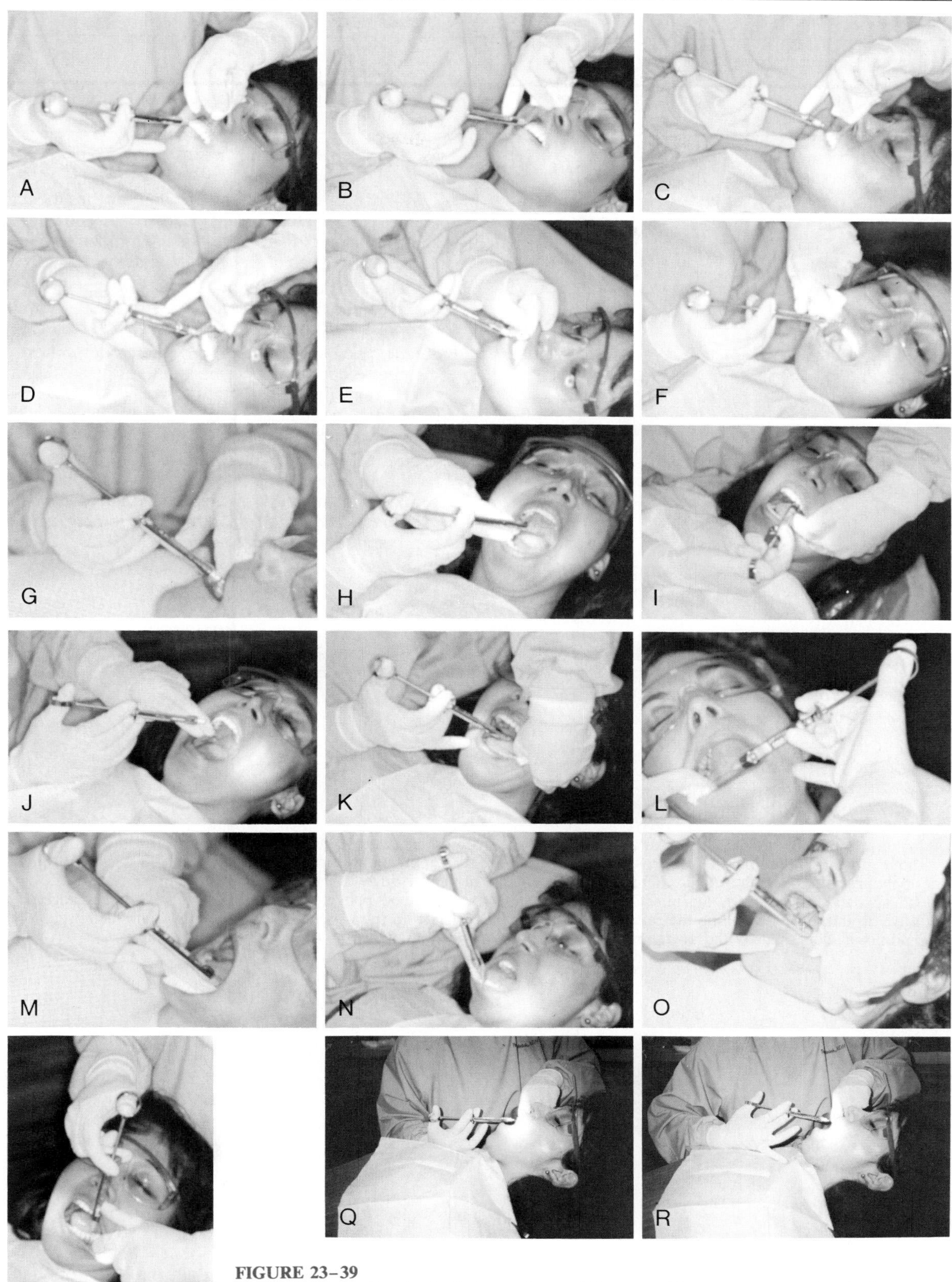

FIGURE 23–39
Handrests. *A–E.* Handrests that may be used for a maxillary supraperiosteal injection, anterior superior alveolar and middle superior alveolar nerve blocks. *A* and *E* may be used for the infraorbital nerve block. *F and G,* Handrests for a posterior superior alveolar nerve block. *H and I,* Handrests for a greater palatine nerve block. *J,* Handrest for the nasopalatine nerve block. *K and L,* Handrests for the inferior alveolar and lingual nerve blocks. *M,* Handrest for the buccal nerve block. *N–P,* Handrests for the mental and incisive nerve blocks. *Q,* When possible, hold the arms close to the body to increase stabilization. *R,* Do not use the client's arm or chest as a handrest.

CONTINUED ON FOLLOWING PAGE

PROCEDURE 23–4

GIVING A SUCCESSFUL INJECTION *Continued*

Step	Rationale
21. Gently insert the needle into the mucosa until the bevel is completely under the tissue	Initiates needle penetration with minimal discomfort
22. Observe and communicate with the client. Watch for any signs of discomfort or distress	Keeping clients informed of the procedures helps them to anticipate the operator's actions and minimizes anxiety. Careful observation of the client alerts the clinician to a potential behavioral problem, or medical emergency.
23. Deposit a few drops of anesthetic solution and pause for 5 seconds	Anesthetizes the tissues in front of the needle prior to its advancement, thus minimizing discomfort. Pausing for several seconds allows the anesthesia to develop
24. Slowly advance to the deposition site, injecting solution drop by drop in advance of the needle	Proceeding slowly and anesthetizing the tissues in front of the needle during advancement ensures greater client safety and comfort. At this point, aspiration is not necessary because of the small amount of solution being deposited over a changing injection site
25. Aspirate on arrival at the deposition site (Fig. 23–40)	Minimizes the possibility of an intravascular injection by ascertaining if the needle tip is located within a blood vessel. Aspiration of blood into the cartridge indicates intravenous placement of the needle and the need to replace the cartridge and repeat the procedure

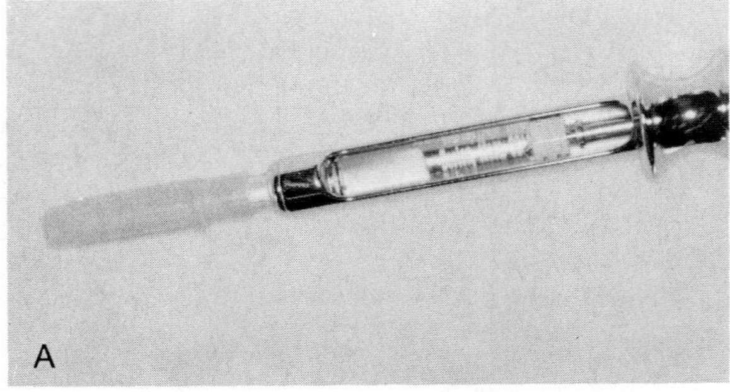

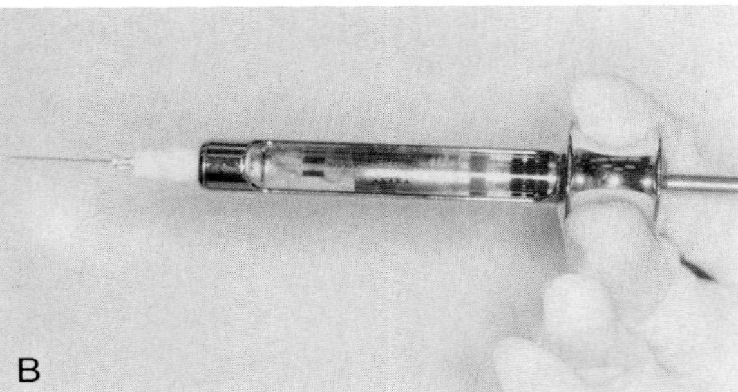

FIGURE 23–40
Prior to injecting anesthetic solution at the deposition site, with an aspirating syringe, gently pull back on the thumb ring without moving the needle tip. With a self-aspirating syringe stop applying pressure (pushing forward) on the thumb ring, or apply pressure to the thumb disc. Observe the needle end of the cartridge for signs of blood entering the cartridge. If no blood appears, proceed with the injection. *A,* Positive aspiration. Blood pooling at the needle end of the cartridge. *B,* Positive aspiration. Blood filling the cartridge. Both *A* and *B* indicate an intravascular penetration, and anesthetic solution should not be deposited. Withdraw the needle, replace the cartridge of anesthetic, and repeat the procedure.

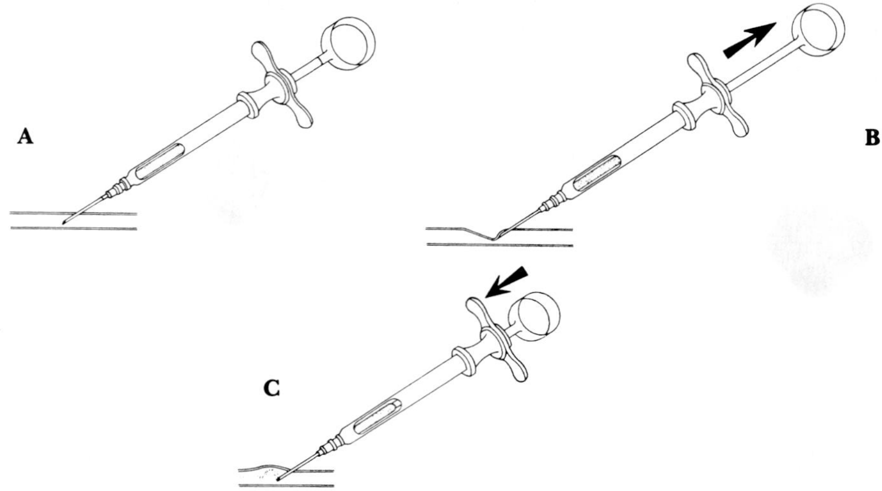

FIGURE 23–41
Intravascular injection of local anesthetic. *A,* Needle is inserted in lumen of blood vessel. *B,* Aspiration test is performed. Negative pressure pulls vessel wall against bevel of needle; therefore, no blood enters syringe (negative aspiration). *C,* Drug is injected. Positive pressure on plunger of syringe forces local anesthetic solution out through needle. Wall of vessel is forced away from bevel, and anesthetic solution is deposited directly into lumen of blood vessel. (With permission from Malamed, S. F. Medical Emergencies in the Dental Office, 4th ed. St. Louis: C. V. Mosby, 1993, p. 321.)

Step	Rationale
26. Perform multiple aspirations as indicated a. Rotate the syringe slightly (approximately 1/4 turn) between the index and third fingers b. Reaspirate c. Return the syringe to its original position d. Reaspirate (Optional; however, recommended for the posterior superior alveolar nerve block, inferior alveolar nerve block, and mental/incisive nerve blocks because of high percent of positive aspirations)	"False" negative aspiration may occur if the needle bevel is occluded by the inner wall of the blood vessel. Multiple aspirations with the needle bevel in different planes prevents this potential problem. (Fig. 23–41)
27. Slowly deposit the anesthetic solution over the indicated number of seconds. Solution should be introduced into the tissues at a rate of 1 ml/min or approximately 2 minutes for a full cartridge[5]	Aspirating several times while injecting helps the operator to slow down the deposition rate and reaffirms extravascular position of the needle tip. Slow deposition reduces the risk/severity of an overdose reaction in case of inadvertent intravascular injection and prevents tearing and necrosis of the tissue and subsequent discomfort. If, despite slow introduction of the solution, blood levels of anesthetic become elevated, the severity and duration of the toxic reaction will be reduced. Slow injection of the anesthetic solution is critical to preventing an adverse drug reaction
28. Observe and communicate with the client. Watch for any signs of discomfort or distress; Reassure the client with statements such as, "I'm depositing the solution slowly so this procedure is comfortable for you."	Keeping the client informed of the progress of the procedures helps them to anticipate the operator's actions and minimizes anxiety.
29. When the indicated amount of anesthetic has been deposited slowly withdraw the needle	Concludes the injection with minimal discomfort
30. Replace the needle sheath utilizing the "scoop" technique. (see Procedure 23–3)	Prevents inadvertent needlestick injury with contaminated needle to the hygienist and other oral healthcare personnel
31. Observe the client	Most adverse reactions, such as syncope, occur either during the injection or within 5–10 minutes after completion of administration, thus remaining with the client following the injection is imperative[5]
32. Rinse the client's mouth	Washes out any anesthetic solution that may have dripped into the client's mouth
33. Massage the tissue over the injection site when indicated	Gives the client a sense of well-being
34. Test for anesthesia by touching the rounded back of an explorer to both the area anesthetized and an area not anesthetized. The client should have little or no sensation in the anesthetized area	Assures that proper anesthesia is obtained prior to commencing treatment
35. Reassure the client that numbness, tingling and a sense of swelling or the tooth feeling different are normal responses	Gives the client a sense of well-being
36. Record the injection(s) in the client's chart including: a. Area anesthetized and specific injection(s) given b. Type of anesthetic used and type of vasoconstrictor and its concentration (ratio) c. Total amount of solution administered (in milliliters and/or total cartridges) d. Client reaction	Accurate documentation provides a reference for future appointments, essential information if the client exhibits any negative reactions, and provides your best line of defense if a client challenges the care received[25]

INJECTION TECHNIQUES OF THE MAXILLARY TEETH AND FACIAL HARD AND SOFT TISSUES

Oral healthcare professionals are fortunate to have several safe, technically easy alternatives available for anesthetizing structures on the maxilla. The thin, porous nature of the maxillary bone allows the anesthetic solution to diffuse easily from the deposition site through the bone to the apices of the maxillary teeth. Thus, one injection may be administered to anesthetize a single tooth and a small area of soft tissue. However, if a larger area is to be treated or if single-tooth anesthesia is contraindicated because of the presence of inflammation and infection, regional nerve block anesthesia can achieve the necessary pain control.

The injection techniques available to anesthetize the maxillary teeth and the facial hard and soft tissues include: supraperiosteal injection, anterior superior alveolar nerve block (ASA), middle superior alveolar nerve block (MSA), infraorbital nerve block, and posterior superior alveolar nerve block (PSA).

Supraperiosteal Injection

A **supraperiosteal injection,** more commonly referred to as a **local infiltration,** involves depositing anesthetic solution near the apex of a single tooth, thus providing anesthesia of the tooth and the immediate surrounding area. This injection is most often used to anesthetize maxillary teeth. The rather thin, porous nature of the bone in the maxilla facilitates diffusion of the anesthetic solution from the deposition site to the apex of the tooth to be treated. By contrast, the mandible consists of much denser bone that prevents diffusion of the anesthetic agent to the apices of the posterior teeth, therefore precluding the supraperiosteal injection in this area. A supraperiosteal injection may be used to anesthetize the central and lateral teeth in the mandible because the bone in this area is thinner and nutrient canals may be present.

Indications for this injection include the need for pulpal anesthesia of maxillary teeth when only a limited number of teeth are to be treated and for soft tissue procedures to be performed on a circumscribed area. Because the anesthetic and vasoconstrictor are deposited so near the area to be treated, this injection provides effective hemostasis that is often needed during dental hygiene care. Conversely, if there is infection or severe inflammation in the area, administration of the anesthetic solution at a distance from

TABLE 23–11
SUPRAPERIOSTEAL INJECTION (LOCAL INFILTRATION, PARAPERIOSTEAL INJECTION)

Nerves anesthetized	Large terminal branches of the dental plexus
Areas anesthetized	Entire region innervated by the large terminal branches of the plexus: pulp of the tooth, facial periosteum, connective tissue, and mucous membrane overlying the tooth (Fig. 23–42)

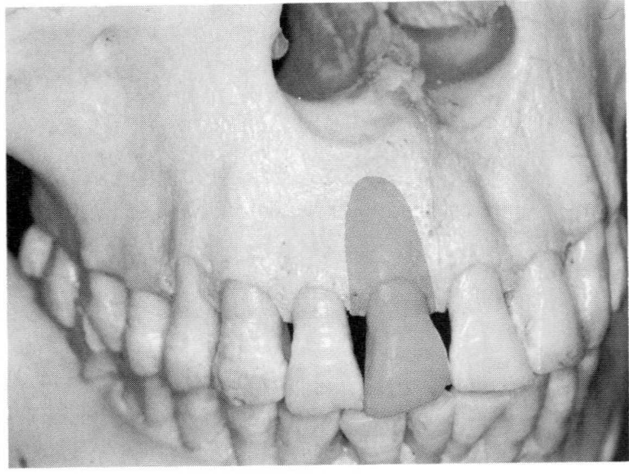

FIGURE 23–42
The anesthetic agent is deposited at the apical region of the targeted tooth.

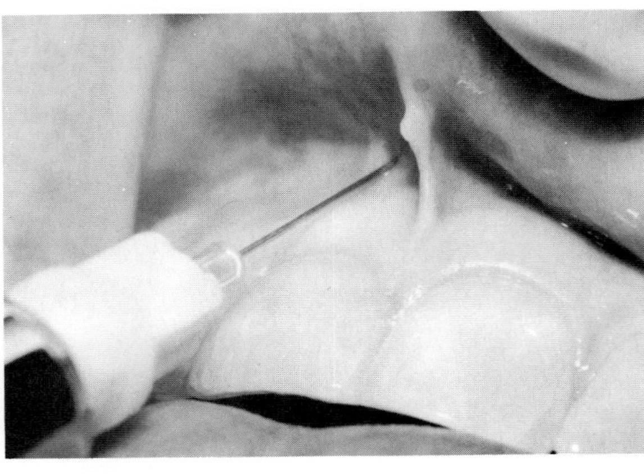

FIGURE 23–43
Penetration site for a supraperiosteal injection of the maxillary right central incisor.

Needle gauge/length	25- or 27-gauge short
Operator/client position	8 or 9 o'clock
Penetration site	Height of the mucofacial fold above the apex of the tooth to be anesthetized (Fig. 23–43)
Landmarks	Mucofacial fold, crown of the tooth, root contour of the tooth
Syringe orientation	Parallel to the long axis of the tooth (Fig. 23–44)

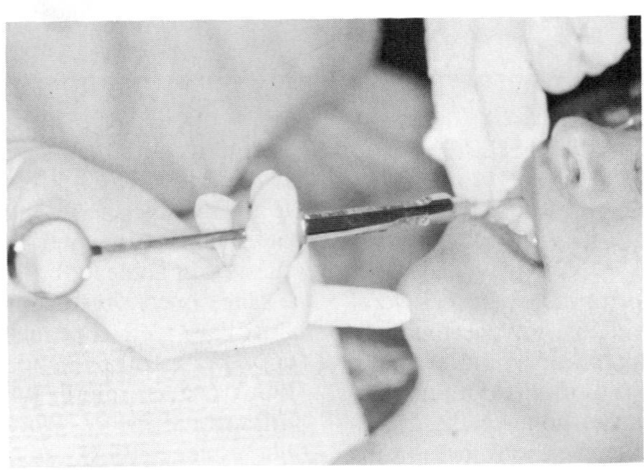

FIGURE 23–44

TABLE 23–11
SUPRAPERIOSTEAL INJECTION (LOCAL INFILTRATION, PARAPERIOSTEAL INJECTION) *Continued*

Handrests	Client's chin, forefinger, or wrist of the operator's opposite hand (see Fig. 23–39)
Deposition site	Apical region of the tooth to be anesthetized
Depth of penetration	Usually only a few millimeters, no more than 6 mm or 1/4 of the needle length; sometimes no advancement beyond the initial penetration is necessary
Amount of anesthetic deposited	0.6 mL or 1/3 of a cartridge
Length of time to deposit anesthetic	Approximately 20–30 seconds
Signs/symptoms of a successful injection	Numbness in the area of administration, absence of pain during dental hygiene care
Tips for Success	
Failure of anesthesia	To correct
1. Anesthetic deposition is below the apex of the tooth resulting in insufficient tooth anesthesia	Increase depth of penetration so the needle is at the apical region of the tooth
2. Needle too far from bone, and thus solution deposited into buccal soft tissue	Redirect the needle closer to the periosteum
3. Dense bone may cover teeth apices. Most often occurs on permanent maxillary first molars in children because the tooth apex is under the dense zygomatic bone. May occur on central incisors where the apex lies beneath the nose[5]	
Complications	To correct
Pain on insertion with the needle against the periosteum	Withdraw the needle and reinsert farther away (laterally) from the periosteum

the area of inflammation (i.e., nerve block) provides better and safer pain control because of the presence of more normal tissue conditions at the deposition site. Furthermore, if a large area involving several teeth needs to be treated, the supraperiosteal injection is not suitable because of the need for multiple needle insertions and the necessity of administering large volumes of anesthetic solution.

Table 23–11 summarizes the criteria pertinent to a supraperiosteal injection and provides tips for success. Procedure 23–4, Giving a Successful Injection, should be re-

TABLE 23–12
ANTERIOR SUPERIOR ALVEOLAR NERVE BLOCK

Nerves anesthetized	Anterior superior alveolar
Areas anesthetized	Pulps of the maxillary central incisor, lateral incisor and canine, facial periodontal tissues and bone overlying these same teeth (Fig. 23–45)

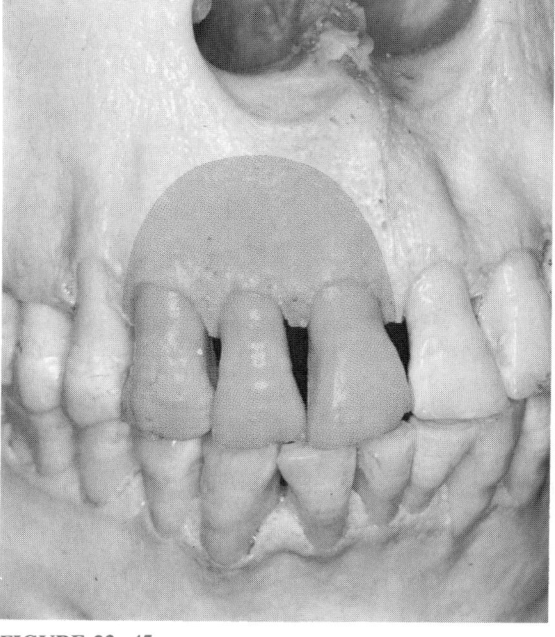

FIGURE 23–45

Table continued on following page

TABLE 23–12
ANTERIOR SUPERIOR ALVEOLAR NERVE BLOCK *Continued*

Needle gauge/length	25- or 27-gauge short
Operator/client position	8 or 9 o'clock
Penetration site	Height of mucolabial fold slightly mesial to the canine eminence (Fig. 23–46)
Landmarks	Mucolabial fold, canine and canine eminence, depression (fossa) located just anterior to the canine eminence

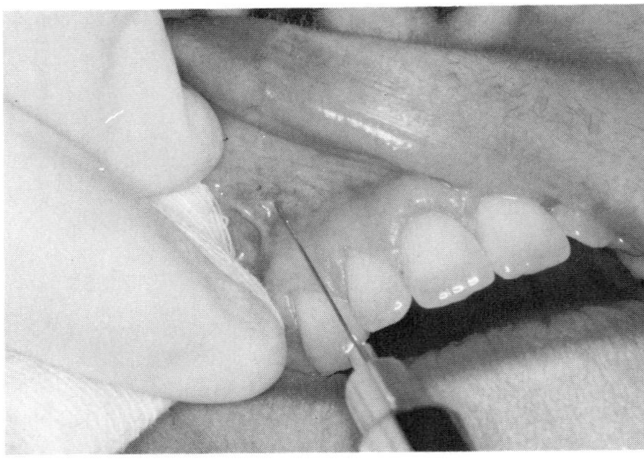

FIGURE 23–46

FIGURE 23–47

Syringe orientation	Parallel with the long axis of the canine (Fig. 23–47)
Handrests	Client's chin, forefinger, or wrist of the operator's opposite hand (see Fig. 23–39)
Deposition site	Apical region of the canine
Depth of penetration	Usually only a few millimeters, no more than 6 mm or 1/4 of the needle length; sometimes no advancement beyond the initial penetration is necessary
Amount of anesthetic deposited	0.6–0.9 mL or 1/3 to 1/2 of a cartridge
Length of time to deposit anesthetic	Approximately 20–30 seconds
Signs/symptoms of a successful injection	Numbness in the area of administration, absence of pain during dental hygiene care

Tips for Success

Failure of anesthesia	To correct
1. Anesthetic deposition is below the apex of the canine	Increase depth of penetration so the needle is at the apical region of the canine
2. Needle is too far from bone, and thus solution is deposited in the buccal soft tissue	Redirect the needle closer to the periosteum

Complications	To correct
Pain on insertion with the needle against periosteum	Withdraw the needle and reinsert farther away (laterally) from the periosteum

ferred to for those procedures common to all intraoral injections to ensure comfort, safety, and success.

Anterior Superior Alveolar Nerve Block

The **anterior superior alveolar nerve block (ASA)** is recommended for management of pain when treatment is to be done on the maxillary anterior teeth. This injection is not considered by some authorities because of the advantages of the infraorbital injection. However, if treatment is to be limited to anterior teeth or if the clinician is uncomfortable with the alternative techniques, this injection provides another choice. Table 23–12 describes the criteria specific to the anterior superior alveolar nerve block, including tips for success.

Middle Superior Alveolar Nerve Block

The **middle superior alveolar nerve block** (MSA) is the injection of choice when treatment involves only the premolars or if the infraorbital nerve block fails to provide pain control distal to the maxillary canine. Research indicates that the middle superior alveolar nerve is present in only 28 to 40% of the population, in which case this area is most often innervated by the anterior superior alveolar nerve.[24,26] Regardless of its presence or absence, this area can be anesthetized easily by means of the MSA technique described in Table 23–13. This table provides the guidelines for administering an MSA nerve block and suggestions to ensure success.

Infraorbital Nerve Block

While the ASA (see Table 23–12) and the MSA (see Table 23–13) are most often employed by oral healthcare professionals when they are anesthetizing the maxillary anterior and premolar teeth, the **infraorbital nerve block** is the injection of choice by many authorities when providing pain control to this area.[5,7] The infraorbital nerve block provides both pulpal and facial soft tissue anesthesia of the maxillary

TABLE 23–13
MIDDLE SUPERIOR ALVEOLAR NERVE BLOCK

Nerves anesthetized	Middle superior alveolar and terminal branches
Areas anesthetized	Pulps of the maxillary first and second premolars, mesiobuccal root of the first molar, buccal periodontal tissues and bone overlying these same teeth (Fig. 23–48)
Needle gauge/length	25- or 27-gauge short
Operator/client position	8 or 9 o'clock

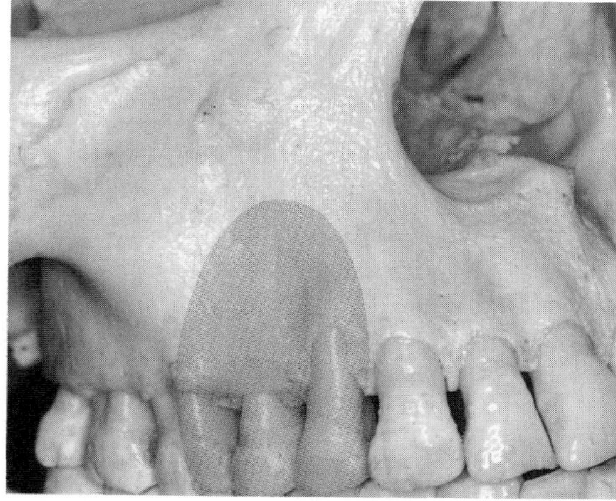

FIGURE 23–48
Area anesthetized by a middle superior alveolar nerve block.

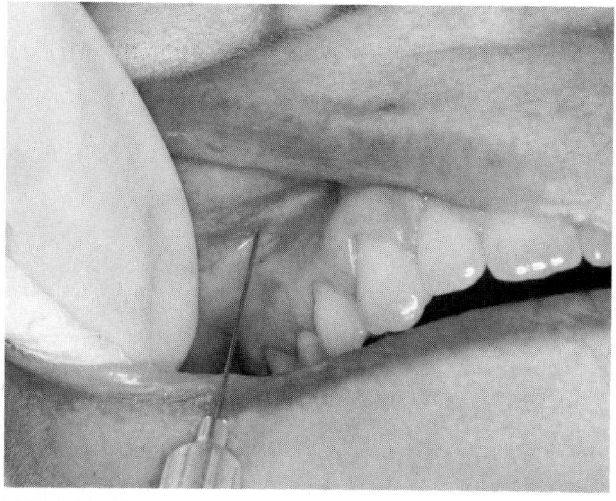

FIGURE 23–49
Penetration site for a middle superior alveolar nerve block.

Penetration site	Height of mucobuccal fold above the maxillary second premolar (Fig. 23–49)
Landmarks	Mucobuccal fold, second premolar
Syringe orientation	Parallel to the long axis of the second premolar (Fig. 23–50)

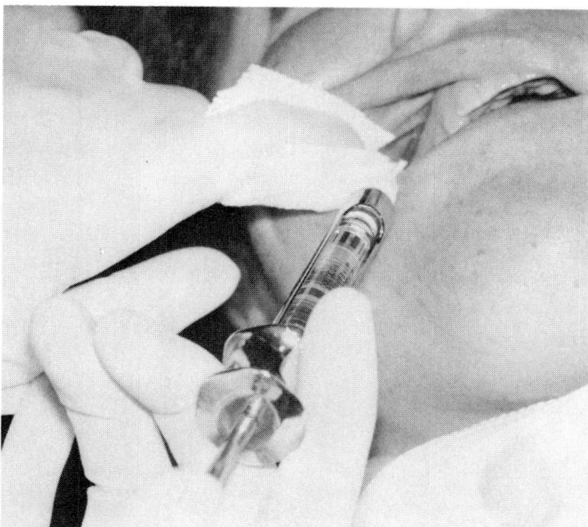

FIGURE 23–50
For a middle superior alveolar nerve block, the syringe is lined up parallel to the long axis of the maxillary second premolar.

Handrests	Client's chin or cheek, forefinger or wrist of the operator's opposite hand (see Fig. 23–39)
Deposition site	Above (3–5 mm) the apical region of the second premolar
Depth of penetration	Usually only a few millimeters, no more than 6 mm or 1/4 of the needle length; sometimes no advancement beyond the initial penetration is necessary
Amount of anesthetic deposited	0.9–1.2 mL or 1/2 to 2/3 of a cartridge
Length of time to deposit anesthetic	Approximately 30–45 seconds
Signs/symptoms of a successful injection	Numbness in the area anesthetized, absence of pain during dental hygiene care

Table continued on following page

TABLE 23-13
MIDDLE SUPERIOR ALVEOLAR NERVE BLOCK *Continued*

Tips for Success	
Failure of anesthesia	To correct
1. Anesthetic deposition is below the apex of the second premolar	Increase depth of penetration so the needle is above the apical region of the second premolar
2. Needle is too far from bone, and thus solution deposited in the buccal soft tissue	Redirect the needle closer to the periosteum
3. Bone of the zygomatic arch at the site of injection preventing diffusion of anesthetic	Use supraperiosteal, infraorbital, or PSA injection instead of the MSA
Complications	To correct
Pain on insertion with the needle against periosteum	Withdraw the needle and reinsert farther away (laterally) from the periosteum

TABLE 23-14
INFRAORBITAL NERVE BLOCK

Nerves anesthetized	Anterior superior alveolar, middle superior alveolar, branches of the infraorbital: inferior palpebral, lateral nasal, superior labial
Areas anesthetized	Pulps of the maxillary central incisor, lateral incisor and canine; in approximately 60% of clients, the pulps of the maxillary premolars and mesiobuccal root of the first molar; buccal and labial periodontal tissues and bone overlying these same teeth; lower eyelid; lateral aspect of the nose; upper lip (Fig. 23-51)

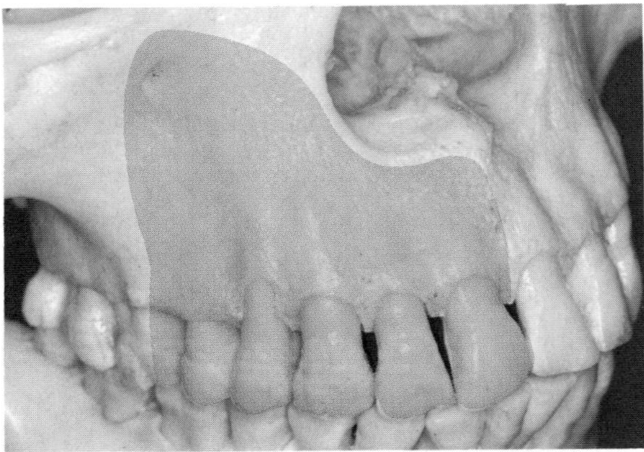

FIGURE 23-51
Area anesthetized by an infraorbital nerve block in approximately 60% of individuals.

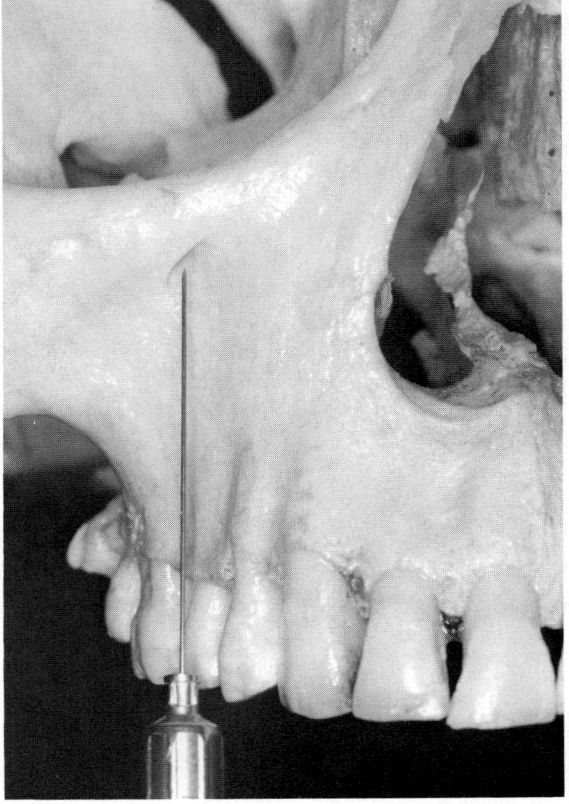

FIGURE 23-52
The needle is held parallel to the long axis of the first premolar to avoid hitting bone prematurely.

Needle gauge/length	25-gauge long; 25-gauge short for smaller clients
Operator/client position	8 or 9 o'clock
Penetration site	Height of mucobuccal fold above the first premolar
Landmarks	Mucobuccal fold, infraorbital notch, infraorbital ridge, infraorbital depression, infraorbital foramen
Syringe orientation	Parallel to the long axis of the first premolar while advancing toward the infraorbital foramen
Handrests	Client's chin or cheek, forefinger or wrist of the operator's opposite hand (see Fig. 23-39)
Deposition site	Upper rim of the infraorbital foramen; the needle should gently contact bone when reaching the deposition site (Fig. 23-52)

TABLE 23–14
INFRAORBITAL NERVE BLOCK *Continued*

Depth of penetration	Approximately 16 mm or 1/2 the needle length; approximation of the penetration depth can be made by estimating the distance between a finger placed on the infraorbital foramen and another on the injection site in the mucobuccal fold
Amount of anesthetic deposited	0.9–1.2 mL or 1/2 to 2/3 of a cartridge
Length of time to deposit anesthetic	Approximately 30–45 seconds
Signs/symptoms of a successful injection	Numbness of lower eyelid, side of the nose, and upper lip indicate anesthesia of the infraorbital nerve (develops almost immediately); numbness of the teeth and soft tissues along the distribution of the ASA and MSA nerves if pressure over the injection site is maintained; no pain during dental hygiene care

Tips for Success

Technique

1. Locate the infraorbital foramen: Feel the infraorbital notch. Move your finger downward from the notch, applying gentle pressure. The bone immediately below the notch is convex (appearing to bulge outward). This is the lower border of the orbit and the roof of the infraorbital foramen. As your finger continues inferiorly, the bone seems to "disappear"; however, it is simply concave in the area overlying the infraorbital foramen. Applying pressure, feel the outlines of the infraorbital foramen at the site. The patient senses a mild aching or sensitivity when the foramen is palpated (Fig. 23–53)

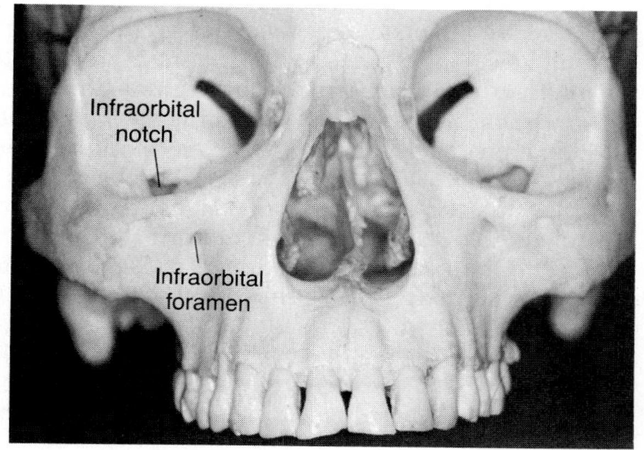

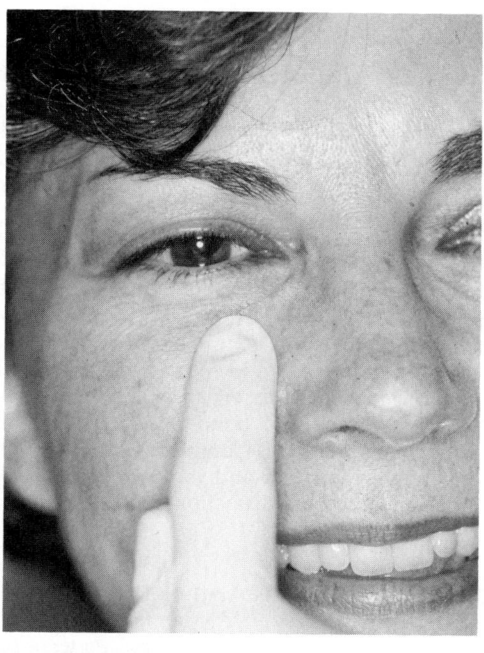

FIGURE 23–53
A, Location of the infraorbital notch and infraorbital foramen. *B,* Palpate to locate the infraorbital notch and foramen.

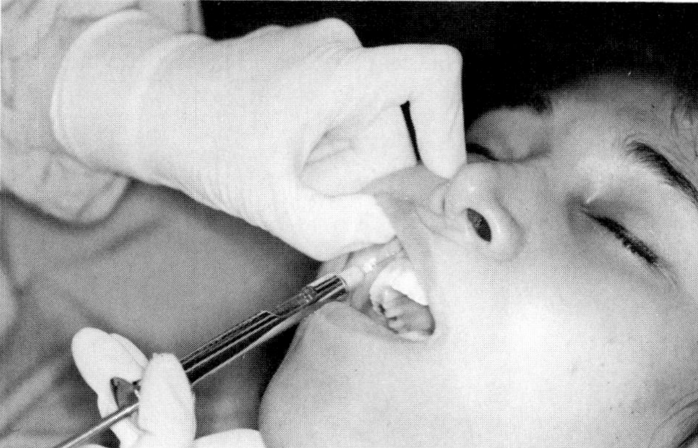

FIGURE 23–54
During the injection, keep a finger over the infraorbital foramen while retracting the lip.

2. Maintain pressure with your finger over the foramen during the injection. This helps direct the needle toward the foramen (Fig. 23–54)
3. Continue to maintain pressure with your finger over the foramen for 1–2 minutes following the injection. This aids the flow of solution into the foramen.

Table continued on following page

TABLE 23–14
INFRAORBITAL NERVE BLOCK *Continued*

Failure of anesthesia	To correct
1. Needle contacting bone below the infraorbital foramen; anesthesia of lower eyelid, nose or upper lip with little or no dental anesthesia; bolus of solution felt beneath the skin in the area of deposition. Each of these are common causes of anesthetic failure of the ASA nerve.	Keep needle in line with infraorbital foramen during penetration; estimate depth of penetration before injecting
2. Needle deviation medial or lateral to the infraorbital foramen	Orient needle toward the foramen before advancing through the tissue; check needle position before aspirating and depositing the solution.

central incisor through the premolars in approximately 60% of individuals.[24] Thus, one injection of 0.9 to 1.2 mL of solution provides pain control in a relatively large area, effectively minimizing needle penetrations and volume of solution administered. Despite these advantages, this injection is not used as often as indicated because many operators are fearful of injuring the client's eye. However, this fear is unfounded, and when the appropriate procedures are followed this injection is highly effective and safe. Table 23–14 describes the criteria applicable to the infraorbital nerve block and includes directions for locating the infraorbital foramen and directing the needle and anesthetic solution to the nerve.

Posterior Superior Alveolar Nerve Block

The **posterior superior alveolar nerve block** (PSA), employed to anesthetize the maxillary molars, is preferred to supraperiosteal (infiltration) injections because it minimizes both the number of injections required and the volume of anesthetic solution administered. Also, because the anesthetic solution is deposited into an area of soft tissue with no bony landmarks (hence no bone contact) it is a comfortable injection for the client. Complete pulpal anesthesia is obtained in the first, second, and third molars in at least 60% of persons.[24] However, dissection studies reveal that the MSA nerve, when present, may supply sensory innervation to the mesiofacial root of the first molar, therefore necessitating either a supraperiosteal injection, an MSA nerve block, or an infraorbital nerve block to anesthetize the remainder of this tooth. Furthermore, if access is difficult or if the third molar is missing and treatment is limited to only the first and second molars, supraperiosteal injections may be substituted.

Other considerations are safety and needle length. Frequently, a long 25-gauge needle is recommended for this injection. Problems associated with needle length, however, may result in an increased risk of hematoma formation. There are no anatomical safety features to prevent inadvertently inserting the needle too far posteriorly into the pterygoid plexus of veins and the facial artery, thereby causing a hematoma. Therefore, to minimize the risk of hematoma formation following the PSA nerve block, a short 25- or 27-gauge needle is recommended. Although depth of insertion with the long needle is 16 mm or one-half of its length, the short needle is inserted three-fourths of its length. Thus, the risk of overinsertion and hematoma formation decreases when using a short needle. Regardless of the needle length used, multiple aspirations and slow anesthetic deposition are imperative to assure a safe injection.

Table 23–15 provides the essential criteria for a PSA nerve block. Of particular significance to this injection is

TABLE 23–15
POSTERIOR SUPERIOR ALVEOLAR NERVE BLOCK

Nerves anesthetized	Posterior superior alveolar
Areas anesthetized	Pulps of the maxillary third and second molars, the first molar entirely anesthetized in 60% of clients while mesiobuccal root of the first molar not anesthetized in 40% of clients, buccal periodontal tissues and bone overlying these same teeth (Fig. 23–55)

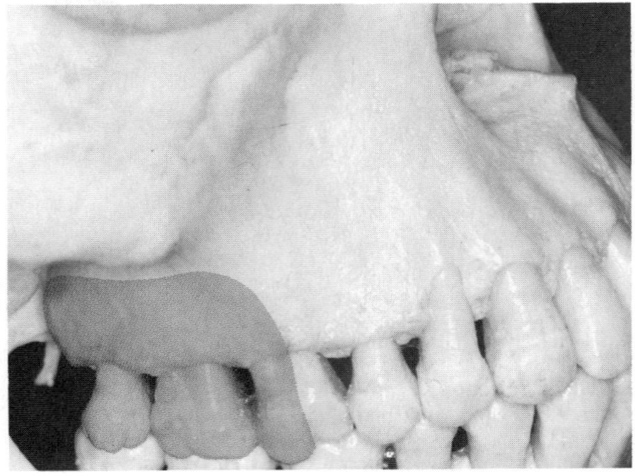

FIGURE 23–55

TABLE 23–15
POSTERIOR SUPERIOR ALVEOLAR NERVE BLOCK *Continued*

Needle gauge/length	25- or 27-gauge short, 25-gauge long on very large clients
Operator/client position	8 or 9 o'clock
Penetration site	Height of mucobuccal fold opposite the distal portion of the second molar (Fig. 23–56)
Landmarks	Mucobuccal fold, second molar, maxillary tuberosity, maxillary occlusal plane, midsagittal plane

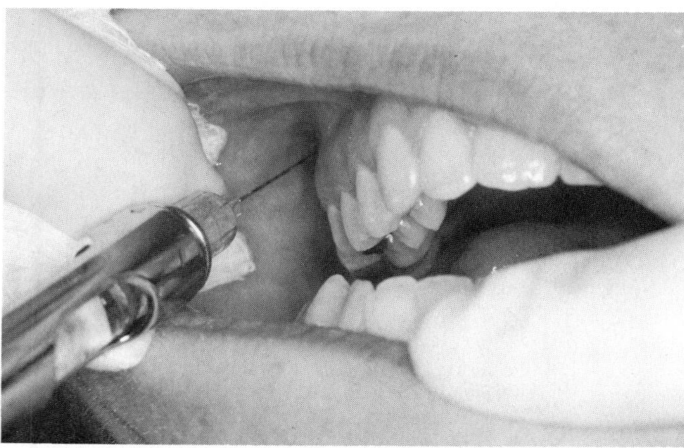

FIGURE 23–56

Syringe orientation	45 degrees to maxillary occlusal plane and 45 degrees to midsagittal plane (Fig. 23–57)
Handrests	Forefinger or thumb of opposite hand, which is retracting client's cheek (Fig. 23–39)

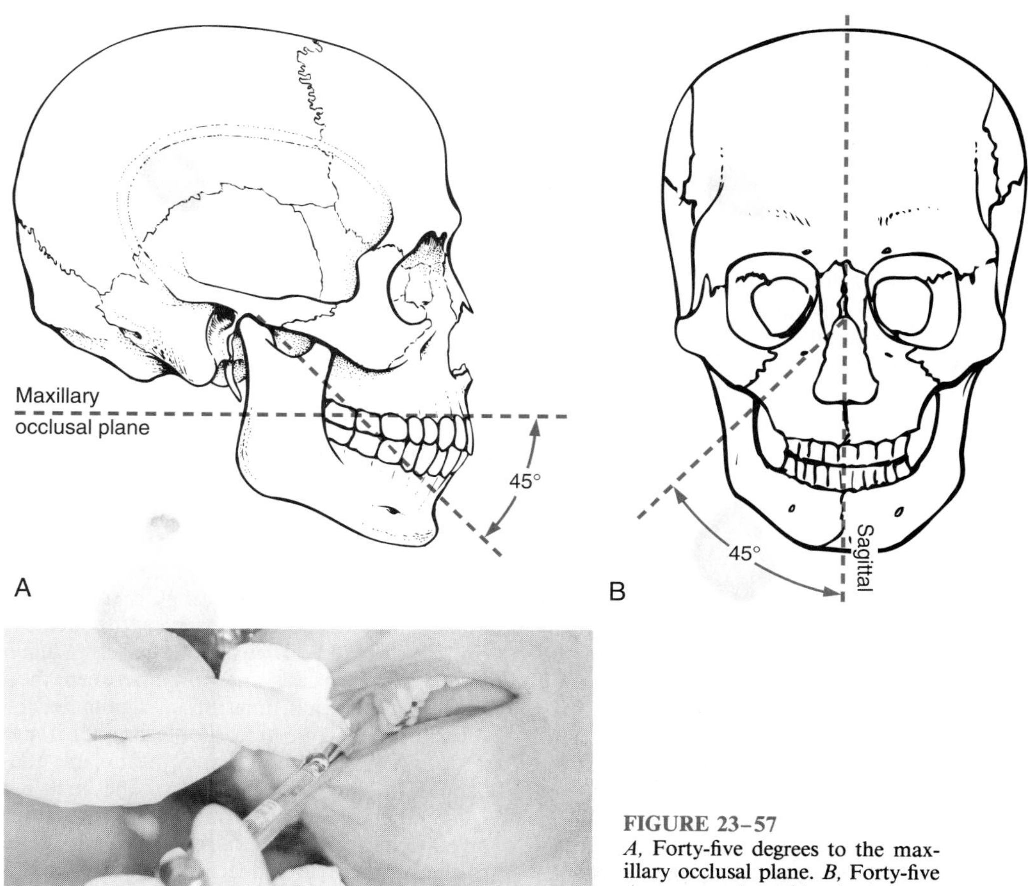

FIGURE 23–57
A, Forty-five degrees to the maxillary occlusal plane. *B*, Forty-five degrees to the midsagittal plane. *C*, Orientation of syringe during a PSA nerve block.

Table continued on following page

TABLE 23–15
POSTERIOR SUPERIOR ALVEOLAR NERVE BLOCK *Continued*

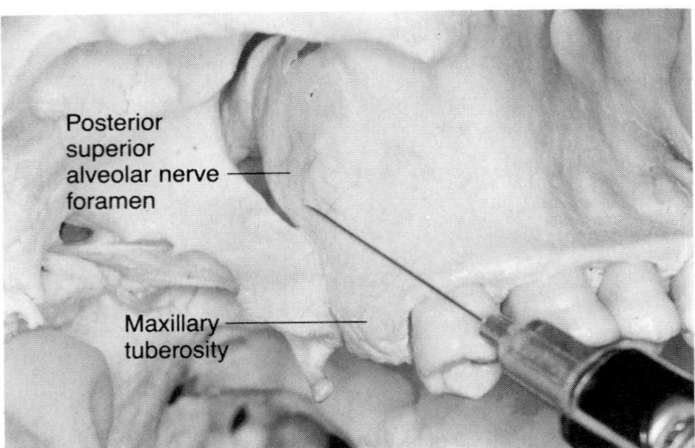

FIGURE 23–58

Deposition site	Posterior and superior to the posterior border of the maxilla at the PSA nerve foramina (Fig. 23–58)
Depth of penetration	Short needle—16 mm or approximately 3/4 of the needle length for normal sized adult, 10–14 mm or approximately 1/2 to 2/3 of the needle length for a small-boned client; long needle—16 mm or approximately 1/2 of the needle length
Amount of anesthetic deposited	0.9–1.8 mL or 1/2 to total cartridge
Length of time to deposit anesthetic	Approximately 30–60 seconds
Signs/symptoms of a successful injection	Numbness in the area anesthetized, absence of pain during dental hygiene care

Tips for Success

Complications	To correct
1. Bone is contacted. The angle of the needle with regards to the midsagittal plane is too great	Withdraw the needle and bring the syringe closer to the midline
2. Mandibular anesthesia. The mandibular division of the trigeminal nerve is lateral to the PSA nerves	Review landmarks and syringe orientation so as not to deposit anesthetic lateral to the PSA nerves

the syringe orientation of 45 degrees to the maxillary occlusal plane and 45 degrees to the midsagittal plane. This angulation, maintained throughout the injection, advances the needle around the maxillary tuberosity to reach the deposition site.

INJECTION TECHNIQUES OF THE PALATAL HARD AND SOFT TISSUES

When dental hygiene care involves the hard and soft tissues of the palate, such as during therapeutic scaling, root planing, and soft tissue curettage procedures, anesthesia of the palatal tissue may be needed. Unfortunately, for many clients these injections are traumatic. Yet palatal injections need not be painful if appropriate techniques are followed. Especially important to facilitate comfort during palatal injections is to:

- Provide topical and pressure anesthesia with a cotton swab at the penetration site both before and during the injection
- Deposit the solution slowly to avoid tearing the palatal tissue, which is dense and firmly attached to the bone
- Be confident that you, the dental hygienist, will administer the injection with minimal discomfort to the client

Injection techniques used to anesthetize the palatal hard and soft tissues are the greater palatine nerve block and the nasopalatine nerve block.

Greater Palatine Nerve Block

The **greater palatine nerve block** is used to anesthetize the hard and soft palatal tissues overlying the molars and premolars; no pulpal anesthesia is obtained. This nerve block provides anesthesia to a large area, thereby minimizing the number of needle penetrations and total amount of anesthetic solution needed. However, the greater palatine nerve can be blocked at any point after it emerges from the foramen and passes anteriorly between the hard and soft tissues. As a result, anesthesia is obtained only anterior to the site of the injection. For example, if treatment is limited to the first molar and premolars, the injection site should be slightly posterior to the first molar along the greater palatine nerve path. This practice ensures that the areas to be treated are anesthetized, but the posterior region of the palate is not unnecessarily anesthetized.

Table 23–16 provides the criteria pertinent for the administration of a greater palatine nerve block and includes suggestions for locating the greater palatine foramen and maximizing client comfort.

TABLE 23–16

GREATER PALATINE NERVE BLOCK (ANTERIOR PALATINE NERVE BLOCK)

Nerves anesthetized	Greater palatine
Areas anesthetized	Hard palate and overlying soft tissue from the maxillary third molar through the first premolar on the side injected (Fig. 23–59)

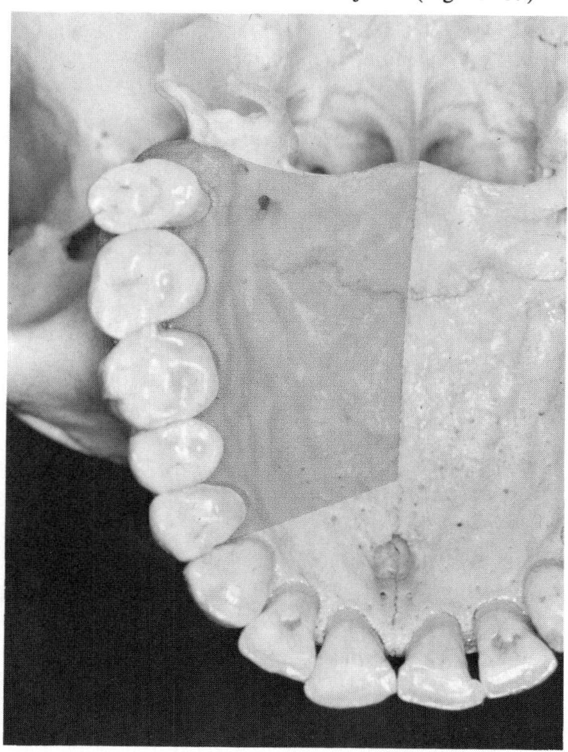

FIGURE 23–59

Needle gauge/length	25- or 27-gauge short
Operator/client position	8 or 9 o'clock
Penetration site	Slightly anterior to the greater palatine foramen
Landmarks	Greater palatine foramen located at the junction of the maxillary alveolar process and palatine bone distal to the maxillary second molar (may be anterior or posterior to this usual location) (Fig. 23–60)

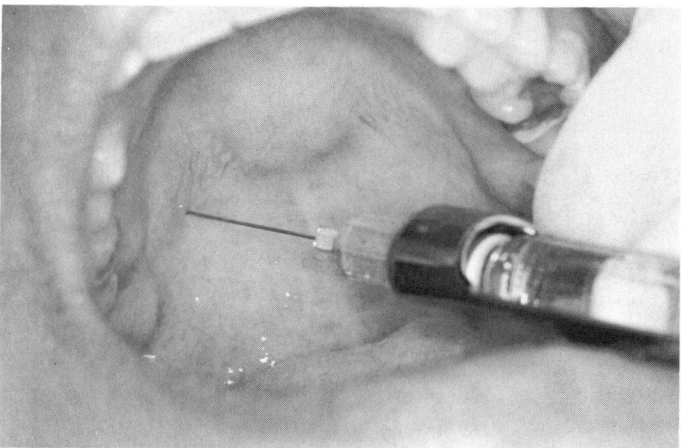

FIGURE 23–60

Syringe orientation	Approaching from the opposite side being injected with the needle at a right angle to the penetration site

Table continued on following page

TABLE 23–16
GREATER PALATINE NERVE BLOCK (ANTERIOR PALATINE NERVE BLOCK) *Continued*

Handrests	When injecting opposite side from operator position (e.g., right-handed operator is injecting client's left side) use back of opposite hand (Fig. 23–39). When injecting same side as operator position use finger of opposite hand (see Fig. 23–39). A handrest may not be used if the operator's opposite hand is used to apply pressure with a cotton swab during the injection. In this case the barrel of the syringe is stabilized by the corner of the mouth and teeth and/or a finger resting on the client's cheek (Fig. 23–61)

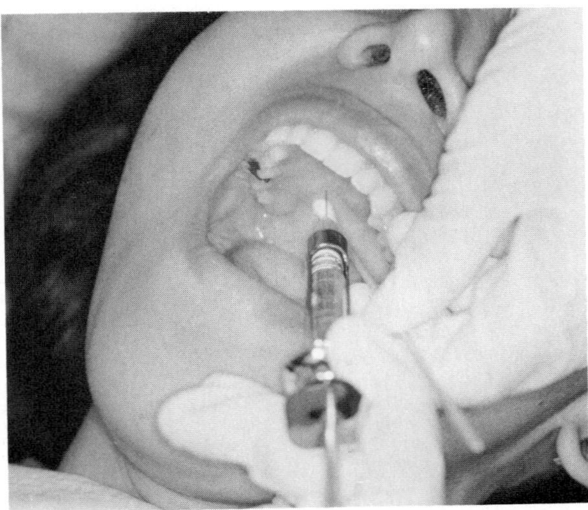

FIGURE 23–61

Deposition site	Greater palatine nerve located between soft tissue and bone of the hard palate
Depth of penetration	No more then 10 mm (usually only 3–6 mm) or until palate is lightly contacted
Amount of anesthetic deposited	Varies from several drops to 0.45 mL or 1/4 of a cartridge
Length of time to deposit anesthetic	Approximately 20–30 seconds
Signs/symptoms of a successful injection	Numbness in the area anesthetized, absence of pain during dental hygiene care

Tips for success

Technique
1. For better visability have the patient open wide and extend the neck
2. To locate the greater palatine foramen place a cotton swab or forefinger at the junction of the maxillary alveolar process and the hard palate in the region of the first molar. Palpate posteriorly until a depression is felt. This is the greater palatine foramen
3. For greater client comfort, when placing topical anesthetic on the injection site apply considerable pressure with the cotton swab for a minimum of 1 minute. Ischemia will develop. Move the swab posteriorly so it is directly over the greater palatine foramen. Maintain pressure at this site while injecting into the ischemic tissues slightly anterior to the swab (see Fig. 23–61)

Failure of anesthesia	To correct
1. Anesthetic is deposited too far anterior to the foramen and thus inadequate anesthesia in the posterior palatal tissues	Move needle posteriorly
2. Inadequate anesthesia at first premolar because of overlapping innervation from the nasopalatine nerve	Infiltrate palate in area of first premolar

Nasopalatine Nerve Block

The **nasopalatine nerve block** anesthetizes the palatal hard and soft tissues from the mesial aspect of the right premolar to the mesial aspect of the left premolar. As with the greater palatine nerve block, a minimal number of needle penetrations and a small amount of anesthetic solution are needed to anesthetize a wide area. However, because the soft tissue is dense, firmly attached to the bone, and very sensitive, this nerve block is potentially the most painful of all the injections unless the protocol for an atraumatic injection is closely followed.

Two techniques are available when giving this injection. The first involves only one needle penetration on the lateral side of the incisive papilla. The second technique includes giving one injection between the maxillary central incisors followed by a second penetration into the papilla between these same teeth. In some cases these two injections provide sufficient pain control for dental hygiene care. If not, an injection is made into the partially anesthetized palatal tissues on the lateral side of the incisive papilla to complete the nasopalatine nerve block. Each approach is acceptable and dental hygienists should select the procedure that they feel most comfortable with and that provides the most atraumatic injection possible for the client (Table 23–17).

TABLE 23–17
NASOPALATINE NERVE BLOCK

Nerve anesthetized	Nasopalatine
Areas anesthetized	Hard palate and overlying soft tissue of the maxillary anterior teeth bilaterally (Fig. 23–62)
Needle gauge/length	25- or 27-gauge short
Operator/client position	8 or 9 o'clock

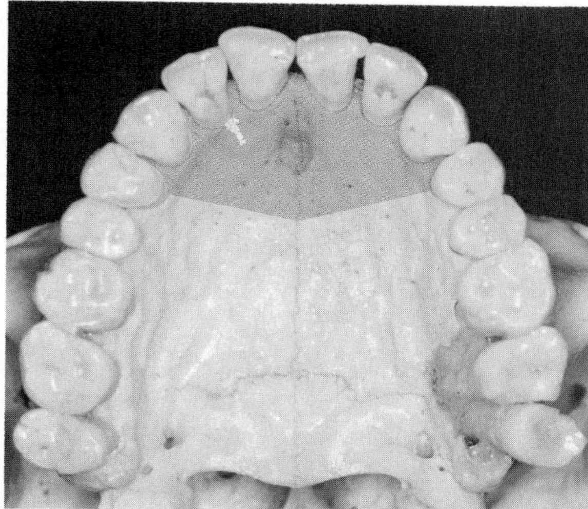
FIGURE 23–62

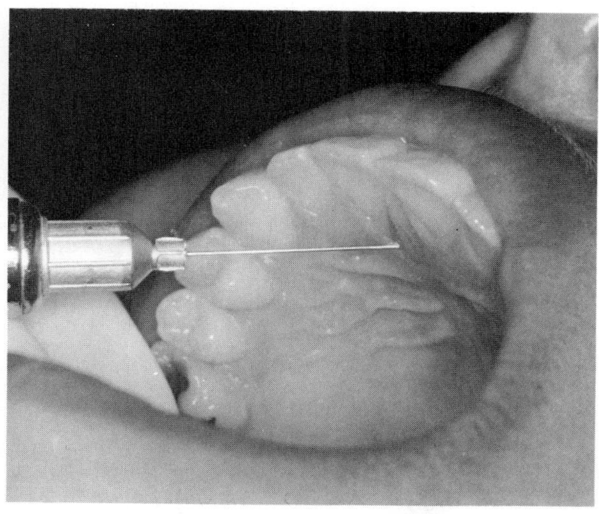
FIGURE 23–63

Penetration site	Lateral to the incisive papilla (at the base of the incisive papilla) (Fig. 23–63)
Landmarks	Central incisors, incisive papilla
Syringe orientation	Approaching from the canine/premolar area with the needle at a 45-degree angle to the incisive papilla
Handrests	Finger of opposite hand (see Fig. 23–39). A handrest may not be used if the operator's opposite hand is used to apply pressure with a cotton swab during the injection. In this case the barrel of the syringe is stabilized by the corner of the mouth and teeth and/or a finger resting on the client's cheek (Fig. 23–64)

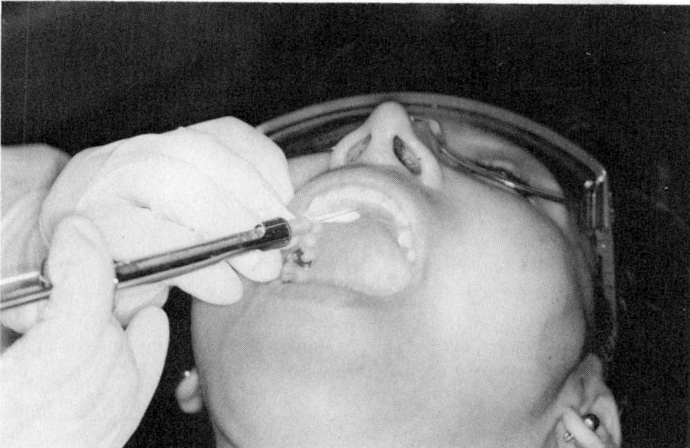
FIGURE 23–64

Deposition site	Incisive foramen beneath the incisive papilla
Depth of penetration	No more than 4–6 mm or until bone is lightly contacted
Amount of anesthetic deposited	Varies from several drops to 0.45 mL or 1/4 cartridge
Length of time to deposit anesthetic	Approximately 20–30 seconds
Signs/symptoms of a successful injection	Numbness in the area anesthetized, absence of pain during dental hygiene care

Tips for success

Technique
1. For better visability have the client open wide and extend the neck

Table continued on following page

TABLE 23–17
NASOPALATINE NERVE BLOCK *Continued*

2. For greater client comfort, when placing topical anesthetic on the injection site, apply considerable pressure with the cotton swab for a minimum of 1 minute. Ischemia will develop. Move the swab so it is directly over the incisive papilla. Maintain pressure at this site while injecting into the ischemic tissue lateral to the papilla and the swab (see Fig. 23–64)
3. Do not insert directly into the incisive papilla because this causes extreme client discomfort. Additionally, slow deposition of the proper amount of solution minimizes discomfort

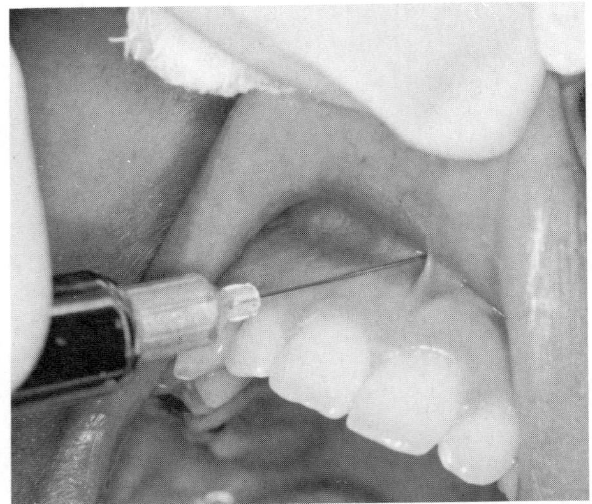
A

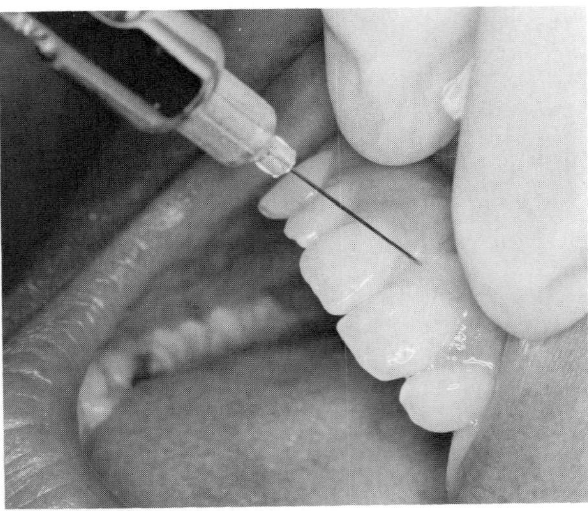
B

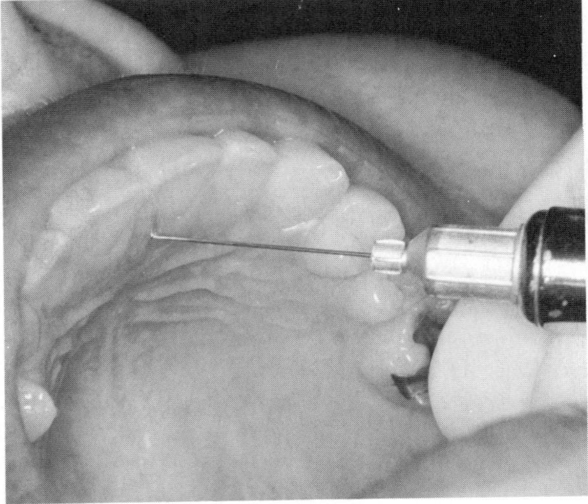
C

FIGURE 23–65

4. An alternative technique includes infiltrating (Fig. 23–65): (a) the labial frenum between the maxillary central incisors with 0.3 mL solution, (b) the interdental papilla between the central incisors with no more than 0.3 mL, and, if needed, (c) the tissue lateral to the incisive papilla

Failure of anesthesia	To correct
1. Unilateral anesthesia: Anesthetic solution deposited to side of incisive foramen	Reinsert the needle until it is directly over the incisive foramen
2. Inadequate anesthesia in the canine/first premolar area because of overlapping innervation from greater palatine nerve	Infiltrate palate in area of canine/first premolar

Complications	To correct
Because of the density of the tissues, anesthetic solution may appear (or squirt out) around the needle penetration site during administration	Completely insert the bevel under the tissue

INJECTION TECHNIQUES OF THE MANDIBULAR TEETH AND HARD AND SOFT TISSUES

In contrast to the maxilla, the mandible consists of dense bone that covers the apices of the teeth and effectively eliminates the possibility of supraperiosteal injections in the posterior teeth. Also, because of mandibular bone density, the dental hygienist must accurately deposit the solution within 1 mm of the target nerve to obtain pulpal anesthesia. However, in the case of the inferior alveolar nerve block, the most commonly used nerve block in the mandible, access is difficult and there is wide variation in anatomy. Although the incisive nerve is much easier to reach, pulpal anesthesia is obtained in only those teeth anterior to the mental foramen. The remaining three nerve blocks reviewed in this section anesthetize soft tissues only. Thus, administering injections in the mandible requires accuracy and proficiency to maximize the success rate.

Those five injections that can be used to anesthetize the mandibular teeth and hard and soft tissues include the inferior alveolar, lingual, buccal, mental, and incisive nerve blocks.

Inferior Alveolar Nerve Block and Lingual Nerve Block

The **inferior alveolar** and **lingual nerve blocks** are frequently employed when dental hygiene care involves the mandible. The biggest advantage is that one penetration anesthetizes the entire quadrant, with the exception of the facial soft tissue over the molars. However, the disadvantages are formidable, and the success rate of the inferior alveolar nerve block is considerably lower than many other injections, because of (1) the anatomical variation with regard to the height of the mandibular foramen on the medial side of the ramus; (2) accessory innervation by means of the mylohyoid nerve or a bifid inferior alveolar nerve; and (3) the considerable depth of soft tissue penetration needed to reach the nerve. In addition, the inferior alveolar nerve block has the highest rate of positive aspiration of all the intraoral injections.[5] Unfortunately, the density of the mandibular bone precludes using the easier supraperiosteal injection on any posterior teeth in the mandible, thus necessitating the dental hygienist to become proficient in administering the inferior and alveolar and lingual nerve blocks.

Appropriate care planning is important when anesthetizing the mandible. Bilateral inferior alveolar and lingual nerve blocks produce anesthesia of the client's entire tongue and lingual soft tissues, resulting in an inability to swallow and enunciate, and a lack of sensation. Thus, the optimal care plan is to provide therapy only to the entire right side or only the entire left side (maxilla and mandible) of the client's oral cavity at one appointment. Another alternative is to administer the inferior alveolar nerve block to that side which requires the most treatment (particularly involving lingual tissue) or has the greatest number of teeth, and administer the incisive nerve block (see Table 23–21) on the opposite side. Because the incisive nerve block does not provide pain control to the lingual tissues, a lingual infiltration may be given, if necessary.

Table 23–18 describes the criteria essential for administering the inferior alveolar and lingual nerve blocks. It is important to carefully follow the guidelines regarding the landmarks for the penetration and deposition sites. Many

TABLE 23–18
INFERIOR ALVEOLAR NERVE BLOCK AND LINGUAL NERVE BLOCK

Nerves anesthetized	1. Inferior alveolar nerve block: Inferior alveolar, incisive, mental 2. Lingual nerve block: Lingual
Areas anesthetized	1. Inferior alveolar nerve block: Mandibular teeth to the midline, body of the mandible and inferior portion of the ramus, facial tissue from the second premolar to the midline and the lower lip on the side being injected (mental nerve) (Fig. 23–66) 2. Lingual nerve block: All lingual gingival tissue to the midline, anterior ⅔ of the tongue and floor of the oral cavity (see Fig. 23–66)

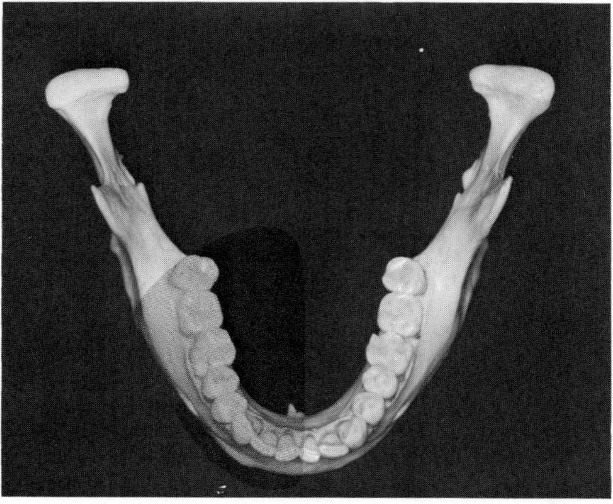

FIGURE 23–66

Table continued on following page

TABLE 23–18
INFERIOR ALVEOLAR NERVE BLOCK AND LINGUAL NERVE BLOCK *Continued*

Needle gauge/length	25-gauge long
Operator/client position	8 or 9 o'clock
Penetration site	Middle of the pterygomandibular triangle (formed by the pterygomandibular raphe on the medial side and the internal oblique ridge on the lateral side) at the height of the coronoid notch (6–10 mm above the occlusal plane of the mandibular molars) (Fig. 23–67)

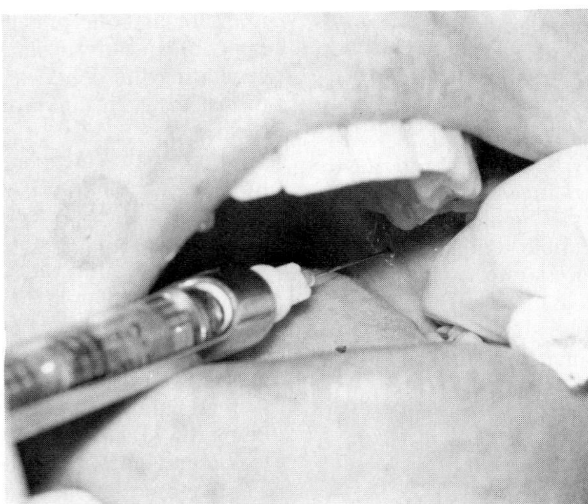

FIGURE 23–67

Landmarks	Anterior border of ramus, external oblique ridge, coronoid notch (greatest concavity on the external oblique ridge), internal oblique ridge, pterygomandibular raphe, pterygomandibular triangle, mandibular occlusal plane (Fig. 23–68)

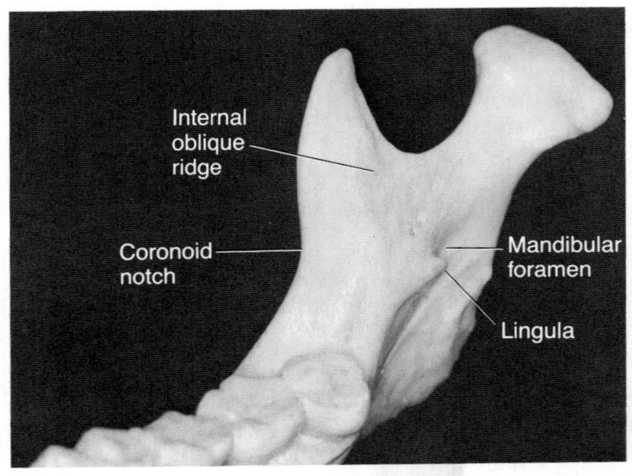

A

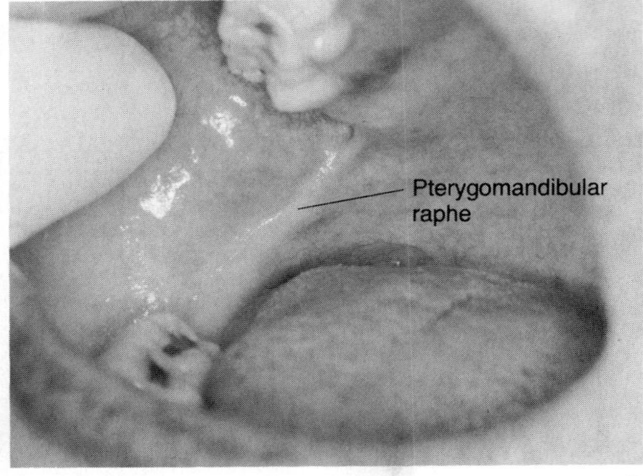

B

FIGURE 23–68
A, Landmarks on the mandible for the inferior alveolar and lingual nerve blocks. *B,* Intraoral landmarks, for inferior alveolar and lingual nerve blocks.

Syringe orientation	Over the opposite premolars parallel to the mandibular occlusal plane (Fig. 23–69)
Handrests	Small finger on client's chin (Fig. 23–39)
Deposition site	1. Inferior alveolar nerve block: Superior to the mandibular foramen at the inferior alveolar nerve before it enters the foramen (Fig. 23–70) 2. Lingual nerve block: After depositing solution for the inferior alveolar nerve block, withdraw the needle until half its length remains in the tissues. (Often this deliberate deposition for the lingual nerve is not necessary because solution from the inferior alveolar injection diffuses to the lingual nerve)

TABLE 23–18
INFERIOR ALVEOLAR NERVE BLOCK AND LINGUAL NERVE BLOCK *Continued*

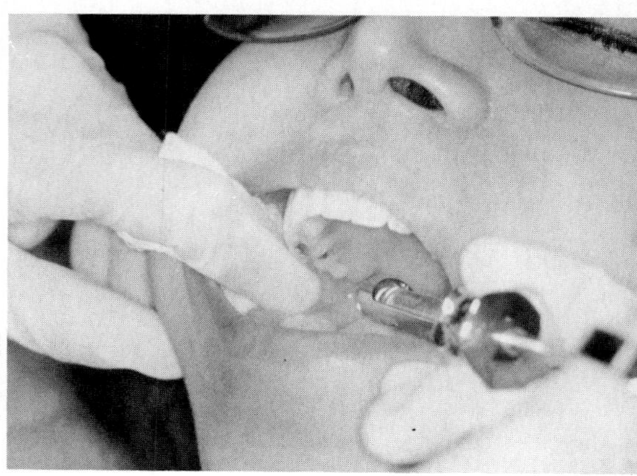

FIGURE 23–69

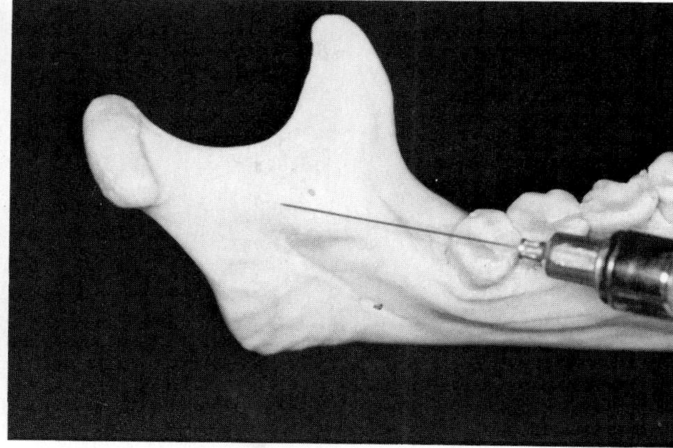

FIGURE 23–70

Depth of penetration	1. Inferior alveolar nerve block: Until bone is lightly contacted with approximately 20–25 mm or ⅔ to ¾ of the needle length inserted. Withdraw needle 1 mm 2. Lingual nerve block: After depositing solution for the inferior alveolar nerve block, withdraw the needle until half its length (approximately 16 mm) remains in the tissues
Amount of anesthetic deposited	1. Inferior alveolar nerve block: 0.9–1.8 mL. or ½ to all of a cartridge 2. Lingual nerve block: 0.45 mL. or ¼ of a cartridge or less (if given as a separate injection)
Length of time to deposit anesthetic	1. Inferior alveolar nerve block: Approximately 60 seconds 2. Lingual nerve block: Approximately 15–20 seconds if given as a separate injection
Signs/symptoms of a successful injection	1. Inferior alveolar nerve block: Tingling and numbness of the lower lip on the same side injected, absence of pain during dental therapy 2. Lingual nerve block: Tingling and numbness of the tongue on the same side injected, absence of pain during dental hygiene care

Tips for success

Technique

1. To locate the pterygomandibular triangle, place your thumb or index finger on the greatest depression on the anterior border of the ramus. This is the coronoid notch. Roll your finger medially to locate the internal oblique ridge. The point of penetration is between the internal oblique ridge and the pterygomandibular raphe (in the pterygomandibular triangle), 6–10 mm above the mandibular occlusal plane (see Fig. 23–67). While inserting, advancing and withdrawing the needle, it is important to place the thumb or index finger on the internal oblique ridge and at the same time grasp the posterior border of the mandible with the remainder of the hand. This technique provides stabilization and control in the event the client moves unexpectedly during the procedure.

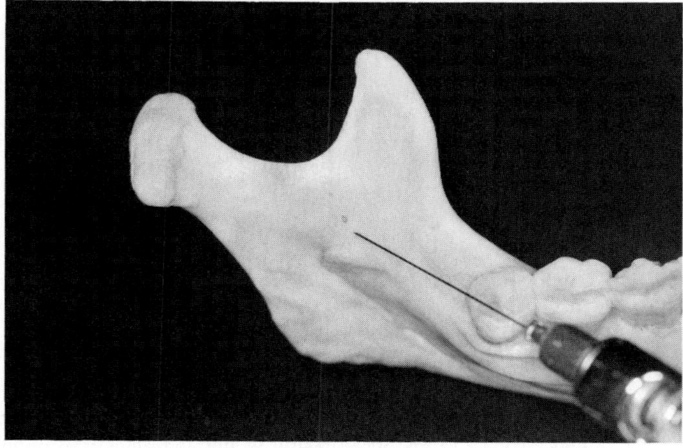

A

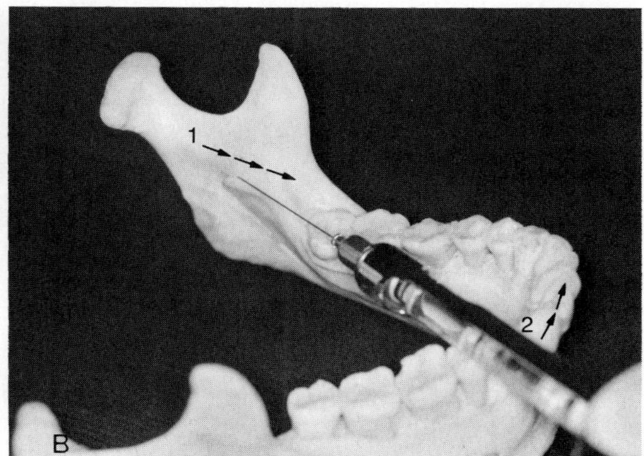

B

FIGURE 23–71

2. If bone is contacted with less than ½ needle length inserted, the needle tip is too far anterior (Fig. 23–71*A*). To correct: Withdraw needle but do not remove from the tissues. Bring the syringe toward the anterior teeth and insert the needle to a more appropriate depth. Return the syringe to the contralateral premolar area and continue insertion until bone is contacted (Fig. 23–71*B*).

Table continued on following page

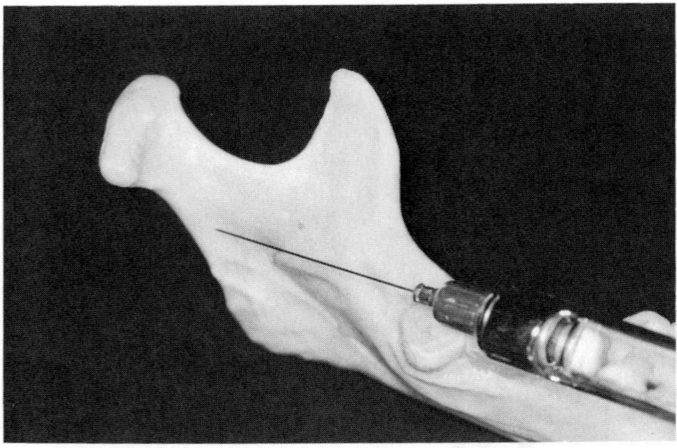

A

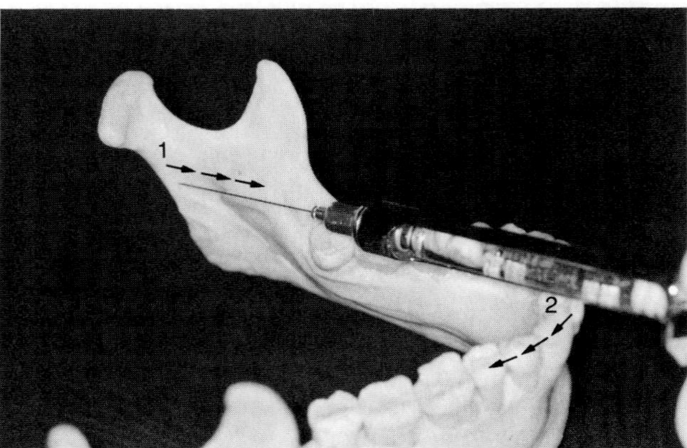

B

FIGURE 23–72

3. If bone is not contacted, the needle tip is too far posterior (Fig. 23–72*A*). To correct: Withdraw needle but do not remove from the tissues. Bring the syringe over the mandibular molars and continue insertion until bone is contacted (see Fig. 23–72*B*)
4. Sit client upright after injection to help obtain anesthesia

Failure of anesthesia	To correct
1. Deposition of anesthetic below the mandibular foramen	Reinject at a higher penetration site
2. Deposition of anesthetic too far anterior on the ramus indicated by bone being contacted with less than 1/2 needle length inserted. May have anesthesia at the injection site	See Tips for success, technique 2
3. Incomplete pulpal anesthesia on molars (often mesial of first molar) or premolars. Theorized that the mylohyoid nerve (which is not blocked by the inferior alveolar nerve block) provides accessory innervation to these areas	Using a 25-gauge long needle, direct syringe from opposite corner of mouth and penetrate the apical region of the tooth just distal to the unanesthetized tooth. Advance 3–5 mm and deposit 0.6 mL or 1/3 of a cartridge over 20 seconds (Fig. 23–73)
4. Incomplete anesthesia. Bifid inferior alveolar nerve may be detected on the radiographs.[9] A second mandibular foramen often exists in a more inferior position.	Reinject and deposit solution at a point lower than normal

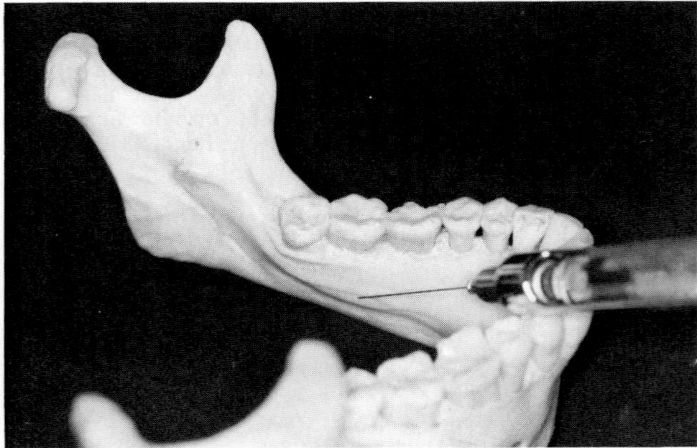

FIGURE 23–73

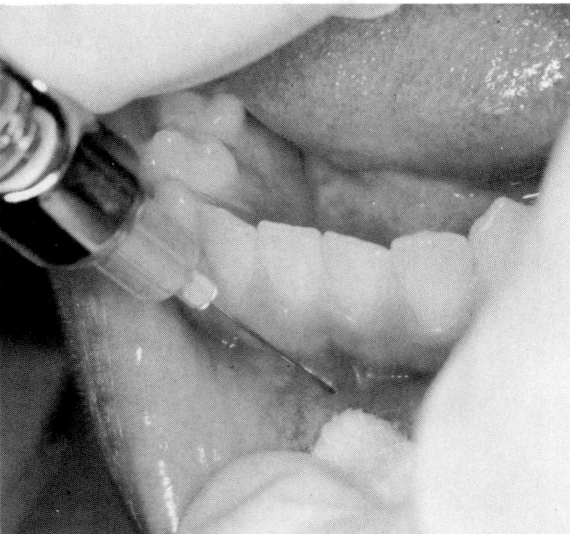

FIGURE 23–74

5. Incomplete anesthesia of the central or lateral incisors. May be the result of innervation by the mylohyoid nerve or cross innervation of the opposite side inferior alveolar nerve	Using a 27-gauge short needle, infiltrate the mucobuccal fold and advance to the apical region of the unanesthetized tooth. Deposit 0.6 mL or 1/3 of a cartridge over 20 seconds (Fig. 23–74)

Complications	To correct
Transient facial paralysis from deposition of anesthetic into parotid gland. Management of problem discussed in Local Complications	Contact bone prior to administration of anesthetic agent

oral health professionals encounter difficulty with the inferior alveolar nerve block, however, adherence to the recommendations help to assure a successful injection and minimize or eliminate complications.

In many instances the deliberate deposition of anesthetic solution to anesthetize the lingual nerve is unnecessary because solution deposited for the inferior alveolar nerve block diffuses and anesthetizes the lingual nerve. However, a separate technique for a lingual nerve block is described in Table 23–18 in the event deliberate deposition of anesthetic solution is needed.

Buccal Nerve Block

The **buccal nerve block** provides pain control to the soft tissues facial to the mandibular molars, thus this injection, along with the inferior alveolar and lingual nerve blocks, anesthetizes the entire quadrant in which they are given. If dental hygiene care involves manipulation of the buccal tissues of the molars, such as therapeutic scaling, root planing, and soft tissue curettage, this injection is indicated. However, if treatment does not include these tissues, the dental hygienist may simply forgo this injection. Unlike the other injections needed to anesthetize the mandible, the buccal nerve block is easy to administer and has a high success rate (Table 23–19).

Mental Nerve Block

At or near the apices of the premolars, the mental nerve exits the mental foramen and innervates the facial soft tissues anterior to the foramen, the lower lip, and the chin on

TABLE 23–19
BUCCAL NERVE BLOCK

Nerves anesthetized	Buccal
Areas anesthetized	Soft tissues buccal to the mandibular molars (Fig. 23–75)
Needle gauge/length	25-gauge long. This size is used because this injection is often administered immediately following the inferior alveolar nerve block. Also, the long needle facilitates access to the posterior penetration site

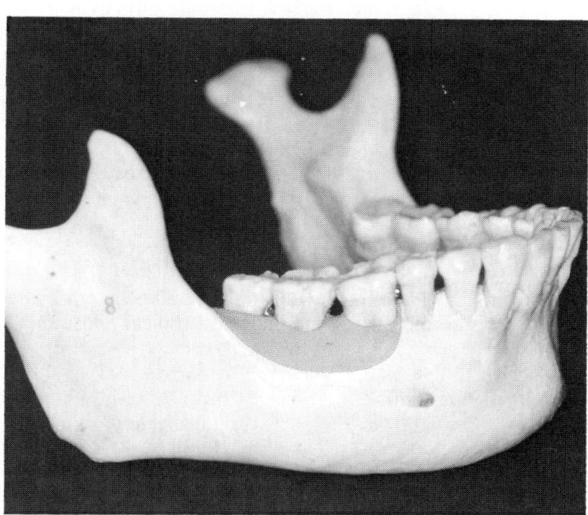

FIGURE 23–75

Operator/client position	8 or 9 o'clock
Penetration site	In the vestibule, distal and buccal to the most distal molar in the quadrant (Fig. 23–76)

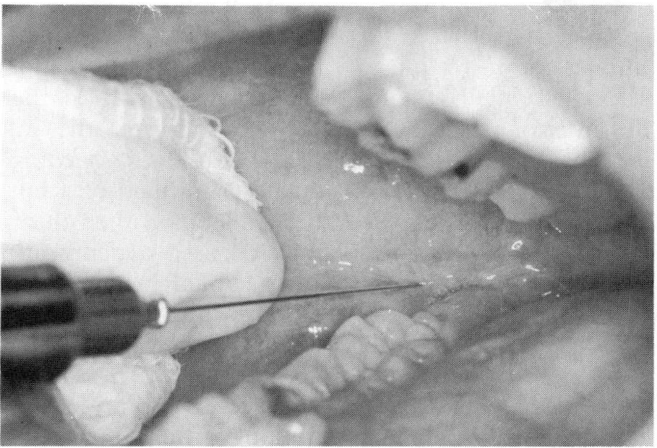

FIGURE 23–76

Table continued on following page

TABLE 23–19
BUCCAL NERVE BLOCK *Continued*

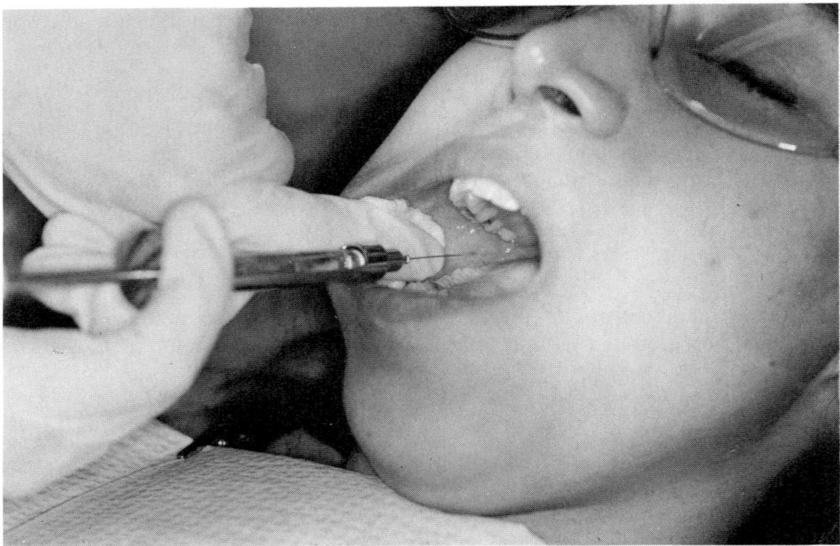

FIGURE 23–77

Landmarks	Mandibular molars, vestibule, mucobuccal fold
Syringe orientation	Parallel to the mandibular occlusal plane on the buccal side of the teeth (Fig. 23–77)
Handrests	Client's cheek or chin, back of operator's opposite hand (see Fig. 23–39)
Deposition site	Buccal nerve as it passes over the anterior border of the ramus
Depth of penetration	1–4 mm (usually 1–2 mm) or until bone is gently contacted
Amount of anesthetic deposited	0.3–0.45 mL or 1/8 to 1/4 cartridge
Length of time to deposit anesthetic	Approximately 10–20 seconds
Signs/symptoms of a successful injection	Numbness in the area anesthetized, absence of pain during dental hygiene care

Tips for success

Technique
The buccal nerve block can be administered immediately following the inferior alveolar and lingual nerve blocks. Thus, the penetration sites for both injections can be prepared with topical antiseptic (optional) and topical anesthesia at the same time

Complications	To correct
Solution appears around the injection site during deposition. (May also result in failure of anesthesia)	Completely insert the bevel under the tissue. Withdraw the needle and reinsert farther away (laterally) from the periosteum

the side of the injection. Because of the easy access of the anatomical landmarks, the **mental nerve block** is simple to administer, has a high success rate and is usually atraumatic.

Although this injection has limited application in restorative dentistry, it may be used more frequently by dental hygienists doing gingival curettage in the anterior portion of the mandible. Because the mental nerve block does not provide pain control to the lingual tissues, a lingual infiltration may be needed.

Table 23–20 indicates those criteria that are essential for the administration of the mental nerve block, including suggestions for locating the mental foramen.

Incisive Nerve Block

The incisive nerve block originates at the mental foramen and innervates those teeth anterior to the foramen. As a terminal branch of the inferior alveolar nerve, the incisive nerve is anesthetized when an inferior alveolar nerve block is successfully given. However, the **incisive nerve block** may be the injection of choice in several instances. Because bilateral inferior alveolar and lingual nerve blocks are contraindicated owing to client discomfort, an alternative may be to administer the inferior alveolar and lingual nerve blocks to the side needing the most treatment or having the greatest number of teeth, and to administer the incisive nerve block on the other side. The incisive nerve block also may be used concurrently on both the right and left sides when dental hygiene care requires anesthesia on only the anterior portion of the mandible. An infiltration of the lingual tissues may be needed because this area is not anesthetized by the incisive nerve block.

Table 23–21 presents the criteria necessary for administration of the incisive nerve block and suggestions for locating the mental foramen. Although some authorities rec-

TABLE 23–20
MENTAL NERVE BLOCK

Nerves anesthetized	Mental (terminal branch of the inferior alveolar)
Areas anesthetized	Facial soft tissues from the mental foramen (near the second premolar) anterior to the midline, lower lip, and skin of the chin (Fig. 23–78)

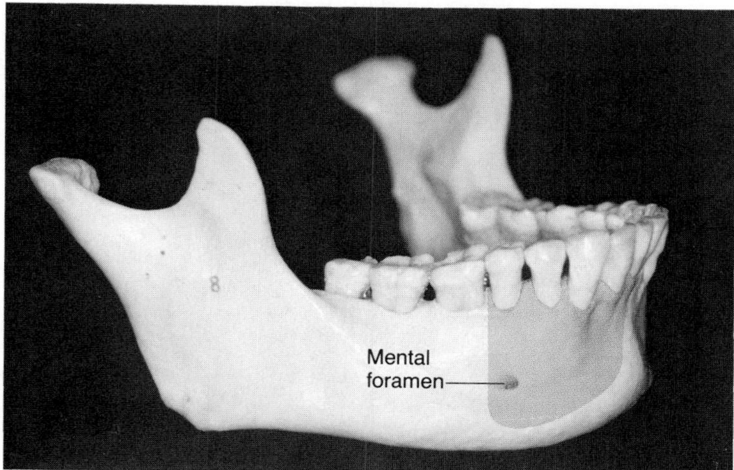

FIGURE 23–78

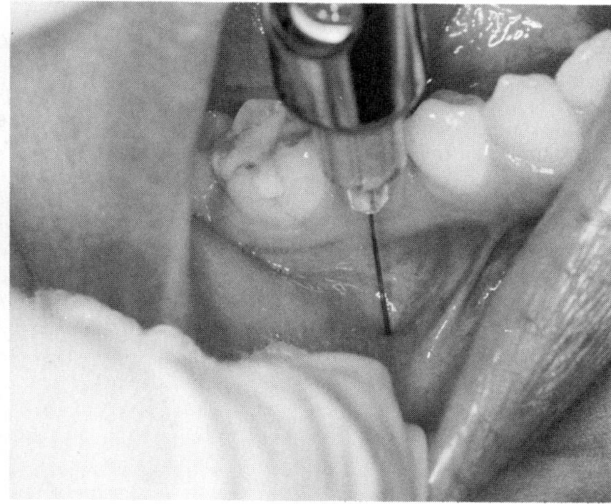

FIGURE 23–79

Needle gauge/length	25- or 27-gauge short
Operator/client position	8 or 9 o'clock or 11 or 1 o'clock
Penetration site	Mucobuccal fold directly over or just anterior to the mental foramen (Fig. 23–79)
Landmarks	Mucobuccal fold, mandibular premolars, mental foramen
Syringe orientation	Directed toward the mental foramen (Fig. 23–80)

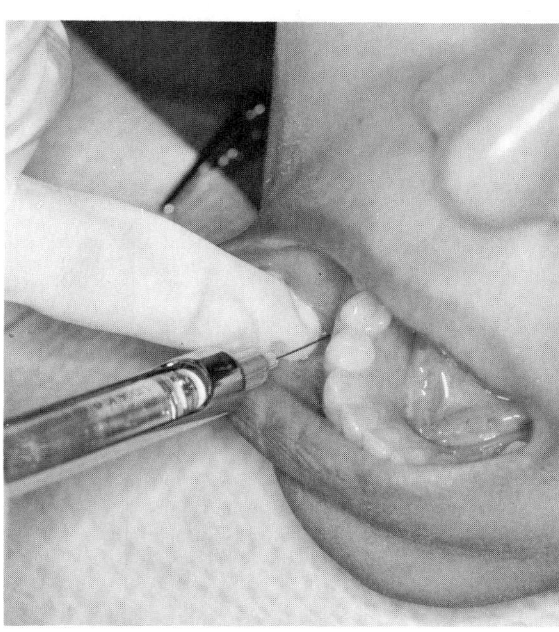

A

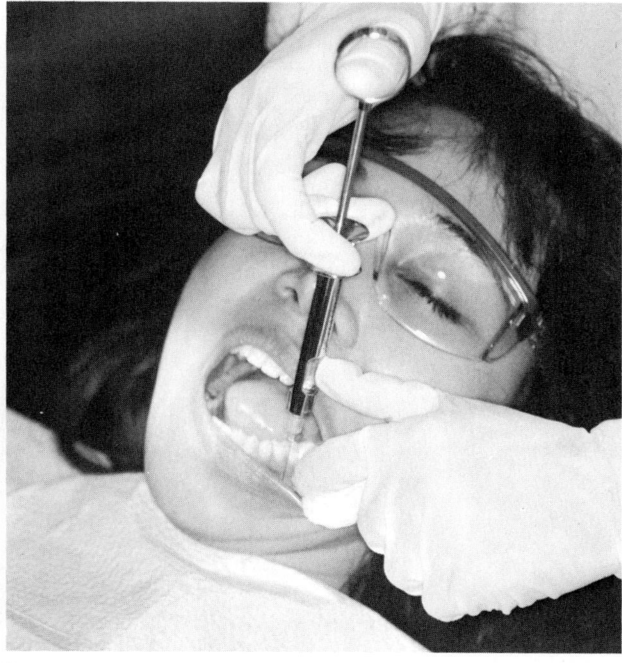

B

FIGURE 23–80
A, The administrator directs the syringe toward the mental foramen from a front-seated position. *B*, The syringe is directed toward the mental foramen from a back-seated position.

Handrests	Client's chin, forefinger, operator's opposite hand or wrist (see Fig. 23–39)
Deposition site	Directly over the mental foramen (usually between the apices of the first and second premolar)

Table continued on following page

TABLE 23–20
MENTAL NERVE BLOCK *Continued*

Depth of penetration	5–6 mm or 1/4 the needle length. (Do not enter the mental foramen)
Amount of anesthetic deposited	0.6 mL or 1/3 of a cartridge
Length of time to deposit anesthetic	Approximately 20 seconds
Signs/symptoms of a successful injection	Tingling and numbness of the lower lip, absence of pain during dental hygiene care

Tips for success

Technique

1. To locate the mental foramen place your forefinger in the mucobuccal fold against the body of the mandible near the first molar. Palpate anteriorly until a depression is felt or the bone feels irregular. This is the mental foramen, which most often is found between the apices of the first and second premolars

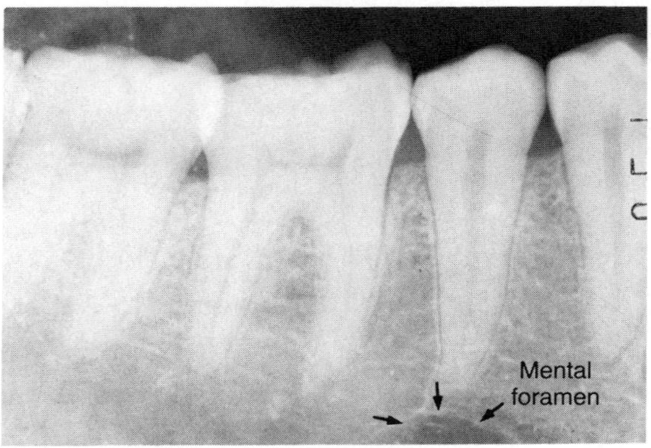

FIGURE 23–81

2. Palpation of the mental foramen produces tenderness for the client as the mental nerve is pressed against the bone
3. Use radiographs to assist you in finding the mental foramen (Fig. 23–81)

TABLE 23–21
INCISIVE NERVE BLOCK

Nerves anesthetized	Incisive and mental (terminal branches of the inferior alveolar)
Areas anesthetized	Mandibular second premolar anterior to the midline, facial soft tissues from the mental foramen to the midline, lower lip and skin of chin (Fig. 23–82)
Needle gauge/length	25- or 27-gauge short
Operator/client position	8 or 9 o'clock or 11 or 1 o'clock
Penetration site	Mucobuccal fold directly over or just anterior to the mental foramen (see Fig. 23–79)

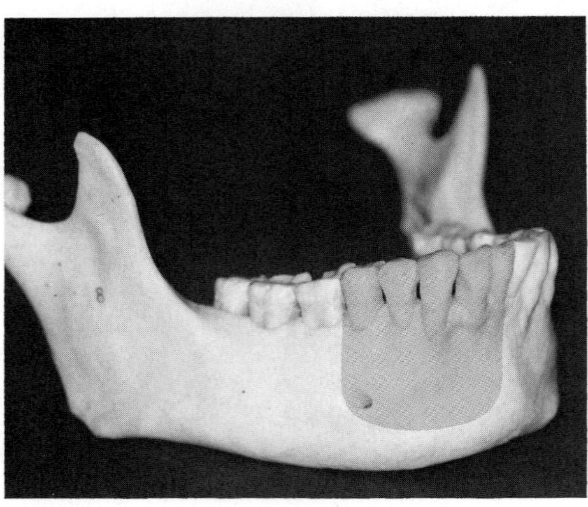

FIGURE 23–82

TABLE 23-21
INCISIVE NERVE BLOCK *Continued*

Landmarks	Mucobuccal fold, mandibular premolars, mental foramen
Syringe orientation	Directed toward the mental foramen (see Fig. 23-80)
Handrests	Client's chin, operator's opposite hand or wrist (see Fig. 23-39)
Deposition site	Directly over the mental foramen (usually between the apices of the first and second premolar)
Depth of penetration	5-6 mm or 1/4 the needle length. (Do not enter the mental foramen)
Amount of anesthetic deposited	0.6-0.9 mL or 1/3 to 1/2 of a cartridge
Length of time to deposit anesthetic	Approximately 20-30 seconds
Signs/symptoms of a successful injection	Tingling and numbness of the lower lip, absence of pain during dental hygiene care

Tips for success

Technique
1. To locate the mental foramen, place your forefinger in the mucobuccal fold against the body of the mandible near the first molar. Palpate anteriorly until a depression is felt or the bone feels irregular. This is the mental foramen, which most often is found between the apices of the first and second premolars
2. Palpation of the mental foramen produces tenderness for the patient as the mental nerve is pressed against the bone
3. Utilize radiographs to assist you in finding the mental foramen (see Fig. 23-81)
4. During deposition, apply gentle pressure (extraoral or intraoral) over the injection site with your finger to force solution to enter the mental foramen (Fig. 23-83)

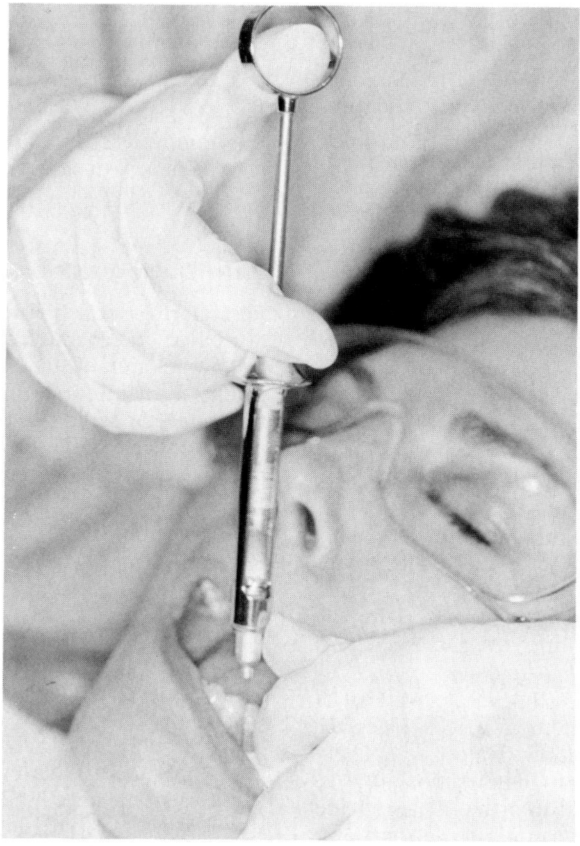

FIGURE 23-83

5. Maintain pressure over the mental foramen with your finger for 1-2 minutes following the injection. This aids the flow of solution into the foramen

Failure of anesthesia	To correct
1. Incomplete tooth anesthesia. Anesthetic solution did not reach incisive nerve inside mental foramen	Redirect needle toward mental foramen and maintain pressure over the deposition site
2. Incomplete anesthesia of the central or lateral incisors. May be the result of innervation by the mylohyoid nerve or cross innervation of the opposite side inferior alveolar nerve	Using a 27-gauge short needle, infiltrate the mucobuccal fold and advance to the apical region of the unanesthetized tooth. Deposit 0.6 mL or 1/3 of a cartridge over 20 seconds (see Fig. 23-74)

ommend penetrating the needle into the mental foramen to reach the incisive nerve, anesthesia can be obtained much more easily and safely by depositing the solution outside the foramen and using digital pressure over the site to direct the anesthetic into the foramen.[7]

LOCAL COMPLICATIONS

Local anesthesic agents are safe when used properly. However, despite careful preanesthetic client assessment and adherence to the recommended procedures for local anesthetic administration, complications may develop. Complications may be divided into those reactions that occur in the region of the injection (locally) and those that are manifested systemically.

Needle Breakage

The introduction of disposable stainless steel needles has significantly reduced the incidence of needle breakage, and, indeed, virtually all needle breaks are preventable. When breakage does occur, it is primarily caused by a sudden, unexpected movement by the client during needle insertion or poor injection technique.[5] If a needle does break during insertion and can be retrieved without surgical intervention, no emergency exists. Those needles that are not retrieved most often remain in place and become encased by scar tissue. Leaving the needle in the tissue often produces fewer difficulties than the surgery required for its removal.

Prevention

- Inform the client about the procedure both before and during the injection. Effective communication helps the individual to anticipate the dental hygienist's actions and control anxiety
- Use long, large-gauge needles (e.g., 25-gauge) when penetrating significant tissue depth. These are less likely to break than smaller needles
- Never bend the needle because this weakens the metal
- Advance the needle slowly. A forceful contact with bone may break the needle or may precipitate a quick movement by the client because of associated pain
- Never force a needle against firm resistance such as bone
- Do not change the direction of the needle while it is almost completely within the tissues. If it is necessary to redirect the needle, first withdraw almost completely out of the tissue and then modify the direction
- A needle should not be inserted into the tissues all the way to the hub. This juncture at the needle shaft and hub is the weakest part of the needle and is vulnerable to breakage. If needle breakage occurs at this point, a portion of the shaft must be exposed in order for the needle to be retrieved without surgery

Management

The following are recommendations made for management of a broken needle during local anesthetic agent administration.[28]

When a needle breaks:

- Remain calm; do not panic
- Instruct the client not to move. Do not remove your hand from the client's mouth and keep the client's mouth open. If possible, place a bite block in the client's mouth
- If the needle fragment is protruding, attempt to remove it with cotton pliers or a hemostat

If the needle is not visible and cannot be readily retrieved:

- Calmly inform the client; attempt to alleviate fears and apprehension
- Refer the client to an oral and maxillofacial surgeon for consultation
- Document the incident and the client's response in the client's chart. Keep the remaining needle fragment. Inform your insurance carrier immediately

When a needle breaks, surgical removal should be considered:

- If it is superficial and easily located through radiological and clinical examination, removal by an oral and maxillofacial surgeon is possible
- If, despite the superficial location, retrieval is unsuccessful, it is prudent to abandon the attempt and allow the needle fragment to remain in the tissue
- If the needle is located in deeper tissues or is difficult to locate, permit it to remain without an attempt at removal. There is considerable precedent to justify the retention of a broken needle if removal appears difficult

Pain During the Injection

Pain during local anesthetic agent administration may be attributed to several factors, including a careless injection technique and callous attitude toward the client, a dull needle from multiple injections, a barbed needle from hitting bone, or rapid deposition of the anesthetic solution. It is not possible to ensure that every injection is totally free from discomfort, because the reactions of clients vary. However, the dental hygienist should take every precaution to prevent pain during the injection or prevent its reoccurrence.

Prevention

- Adhere to the proper techniques of administration as described in Procedure 23–4 and Tables 23–11 to 23–21
- Use sharp, disposable needles
- Apply topical anesthetic prior to insertion of the needle
- Use sterile anesthetic agents
- Inject the anesthetic agent slowly
- Store anesthetic solutions at room temperature and avoid using cartridge warmers

Burning During the Injection

A burning sensation reported by the client during deposition of the local anesthetic agent may be caused by a local anesthetic with a vasopressor that is more acidic than the tissue in which it is deposited. The burning sensation, which lasts only a few seconds, disappears as anesthesia develops and is unapparent when the anesthesia fades. However, a more acute burning may occur if there is contamination of the local anesthetic solution from improper storage of the cartridge in a chemical disinfectant, if the cartridge is overheated in a cartridge warmer, if the expiration date of the solution has lapsed, or if the solution is deposited too rapidly, particularly on the palate. When burning occurs as a result of these factors, the tissue is damaged and subsequent postanesthetic trismus, edema, or possible paresthesia may develop.

Prevention

- Store the cartridges in a dark place at room temperature in the original container. Avoid storing cartridges in chemical disinfectants or using cartridge warmers
- Check the expiration date of each cartridge prior to usage. Anesthetic solution that has exceeded the expiration date should be discarded
- Inject the anesthetic solution slowly

Management

Most often, burning during an injection is a temporary condition and needs no specific treatment. However, if complications result, such as trismus, edema, or paresthesia, the dental hygienist must inform the dentist and treat these conditions as indicated.

Hematoma

A hematoma is a swelling and discoloration of the tissue resulting from the effusion of blood into the extravascular spaces. Hematomas occur subsequent to an inadvertent puncture of a blood vessel, particularly an artery, during local anesthetic administration. They appear most often following the administration of a posterior superior alveolar or inferior alveolar nerve block because the tissues associated with these injections are less dense and readily accommodate large volumes of blood. Bleeding continues until extravascular pressure exceeds intravascular pressure or until clotting occurs. A hematoma is less likely to develop after a palatal injection because of the density of the tissue in this area.

A hematoma that ensues following a posterior superior alveolar nerve block is the largest and most visible. The bleeding occurs in the infratemporal fossa, and the swelling and discoloration appear on the side of the face. Clinical manifestations of a hematoma following an inferior alveolar nerve block include intraoral tissue discoloration and swelling on the lingual aspect of the ramus. Other than the "bruise" which may or may not be visible extraorally, a hematoma may be accompanied by trismus and pain.

Prevention

- Be attentive to anatomical detail involved in each injection
- Modify the injection technique as indicated by the client's anatomy. For example, the depth of needle penetration for a posterior superior alveolar nerve block may be shallower for a client with small anatomical features
- Use a short needle for the posterior superior alveolar nerve block to minimize the risk of overinsertion and the potential for hematoma formation
- Minimize the number of needle insertions
- Observe the appropriate techniques for local anesthetic administration

Management

- If swelling appears, immediately apply direct pressure to the site of the bleeding for at least 2 minutes. For an inferior alveolar nerve block the pressure point is the medial side of the ramus. For the mental or incisive nerve blocks, pressure is applied over the mental foramen. If hematoma formation follows an infraorbital nerve block, the pressure point is the skin over the infraorbital foramen. Unfortunately, it is difficult to apply pressure directly to the site of bleeding after a posterior superior alveolar nerve block because the vessels are located posterior, superior, and medial to the maxillary tuberosity. Pressure may be applied to the tissues of the mucofacial fold as far distally as the client can tolerate.
- Apply ice to the region when hematoma formation begins. Ice constricts the blood vessels, minimizes the size of the hematoma and acts as an analgesic
- Inform the client about the possibility of soreness and limitation of movement. If soreness develops, analgesics may be taken. Beginning the next day, warm moist towels may be applied to the affected region for 20 minutes every hour. This provides comfort and helps blood resorption. However, heat therapy should not commence for at least 4 to 6 hours after hematoma formation. Prior to this, heat may produce further vasodilation and an even larger hematoma
- Advise the client that the swelling and discoloration will gradually disappear over 7 to 14 days
- Dismiss the client when the bleeding has stopped. Avoid further dental and hygiene care in the area until signs and symptoms of the hematoma have disappeared. Document the incident and the client's response in the client's chart

Facial Nerve Paralysis

Facial paralysis is a loss of motor function of the facial expression muscles. Unilateral facial nerve paralysis occurs when the local anesthetic solution is inadvertently deposited in the parotid gland, located on the posterior border of the ramus, during an inferior alveolar nerve block.

The loss of motor function is temporary and subsides in a few hours. However, during this time, the client is unable to control these muscles and the face appears "lopsided." It also may be impossible for the client to voluntarily close the eye on the affected side. Fortunately, the corneal reflex is functional and tears continue to lubricate the eye.

Prevention

Adhere to the techniques recommended for the inferior alveolar nerve block. The needle should contact bone (medial aspect of the ramus) prior to deposition of the local anesthetic solution. If bone is not contacted, withdraw the needle almost entirely out of the tissue, bring the barrel of the syringe more posterior (thereby directing the needle more anterior), and readvance the needle until bone is contacted. Following these steps precludes deposition of the solution into the parotid gland.

Management

Within a short time following deposition of the anesthetic solution into the parotid gland, the client senses a weakening of the facial muscles on the affected side. The inferior alveolar nerve is not anesthetized. Management includes:[5]

- Reassure the client. Explain that the paralysis lasts only a few hours and resolves with no residual effects
- Instruct the client to remove contact lenses
- Ask the client to close the eyelid manually to keep the cornea lubricated
- There are no contraindications to proceeding with treatment at this time, but it may be advisable to reschedule the client
- Document the incident and the client's response in the client's chart

Paresthesia

Prolonged anesthesia or paresthesia is a condition wherein the client experiences numbness for many hours or days following a local anesthetic injection. Paresthesia may be the result of irritation to the nerve after injection of an anesthetic agent that has been contaminated with alcohol or a disinfectant. The ensuing edema places pressure on the nerve, leading to paresthesia. Persistent anesthesia also may result from trauma to the nerve sheath caused by the needle contacting the nerve during an injection. Frequently, the client reports the sensation of an electric shock when this occurs. Finally, hemorrhage into or around the neural sheath may create pressure and subsequent paresthesia.

A complication of paresthesia is the client inadvertently precipitating a biting, thermal, or chemical injury from the diminished sensation in the area.

Prevention

- Store dental cartridges properly. Avoid placing cartridges in disinfectants
- Follow the proper injection protocol as recommended in Procedure 23–4 and Tables 23–11 to 23–21

Management

Most often paresthesia involves the lingual nerve or the inferior alveolar nerve. The sensory deficit usually is minimal and rarely is accompanied by permanent nerve damage. Fortunately, the majority of incidents resolve within 8 weeks. Recommendations for the management of a client with paresthesia follows:[5]

- Reassure the client. The client usually contacts the dental office the day after treatment to report continuing numbness. Explain that paresthesia following local anesthetic administration is not uncommon
- Arrange for an examination of the client by the dentist who will determine the location and extent of paresthesia. Explain to the client that paresthesia often continues for 2 months and may last longer
- Arrange to have the client examined every 2 months until cessation of the paresthesia. Consultation with an oral and maxillofacial surgeon is advisable if paresthesia persists after 12 months or sooner if the client and dentist consider it appropriate
- Record the incident, conversations with the client, and all clinical findings in the client's chart. Inform your liability carrier of the circumstances
- Dental and dental hygiene care may continue. Avoid injecting into the area of the traumatized nerve, employing alternative pain control techniques

Trismus

Trismus, a spasm of the muscles of mastication that results in soreness and difficulty opening the mouth, most often occurs as a result of trauma to the muscles in the infratemporal space following intraoral injections. This trauma may be the result of multiple needle insertions, administration of an anesthetic solution contaminated with a disinfectant, injection of large amounts of local anesthetic solution into a restricted area causing distension of the tissues, hemorrhage that leads to muscle dysfunction as the blood is resorbed, or a low-grade infection.

Prevention

- Store the local anesthetic cartridges properly. Avoid immersing the cartridges in a disinfectant
- Use sharp, sterile, disposable needles
- Follow appropriate infection control protocol. Needles that become contaminated should be replaced
- Use minimal effective amounts of local anesthetic solution and deposit the solution slowly
- Adhere to the recommended techniques of local anesthetic administration as outlined in Procedure 23–4 and Tables 23–11 to 23–21. Observe anatomical landmarks and strive to improve administration techniques. Each of these recommendations facilitates atraumatic injections and prevents repeated needle insertions.

Management

Often the client complains of soreness and difficulty in opening the mouth the day after the administration of an inferior alveolar or a posterior superior nerve block. Recommendations for the management of a client with trismus follow:[5,7]

- Arrange for an examination of the client by the dentist
- Heat therapy should be started immediately. This entails placing moist, hot towels to the affected area for 20 minutes every hour. Analgesics may be recommended to manage the discomfort. Codeine and muscle relaxants may be prescribed by the dentist if needed
- Direct the client to open and close and move the mandible from side to side (lateral) for 5 minutes every 3 to 4 hours. This may be accomplished by chewing gum.
- Continue steps 1 to 3 until the client is free of symptoms. Often improvement is reported within 48 hours and symptoms diminish gradually over several days
- If symptoms continue after 48 hours, the possibility of an infection exists. Antibiotic therapy (prescribed by the dentist) should be added to the recommended care regimen
- If severe pain and dysfunction continue despite therapy, the client should be referred to an oral and maxillofacial surgeon for consultation
- Record the incident, conversations with the client, the results of clinical examinations, and care recommended in the client's chart
- Avoid elective dental hygiene care until symptoms resolve and the client is more comfortable

Infection

Infection from local anesthetic administration occurs rarely with the introduction of sterile disposable needles and glass cartridges. However, postinjection infection may be precipitated by contamination of the needle prior to the injection, improper handling of the local anesthesia armamentarium, or improper tissue preparation prior to the injection. When a contaminated needle or local anesthetic solution is introduced into the deeper tissues, infection may occur. If infection is not recognized and treated, trismus may ensue.

Prevention

- Use sterile, disposable needles
- The needle should be sheathed prior to being used and resheathed after the injections have been administered. This prevents the needle from contacting nonsterile surfaces
- Use appropriate infection control protocol when handling the anesthetic cartridges. Store the cartridges in their original container, and, if necessary, wipe the diaphragm of the cartridge with a disinfectant prior to syringe assembly
- To reduce microorganisms at the penetration site, wipe the tissue with gauze and apply a topical antiseptic prior to the initial needle insertion

Management

When infection occurs, the client often reports pain and dysfunction, similar to trismus, a few days following dental hygiene care. At this point signs and symptoms of infection often are not obvious, and immediate treatment includes procedures for managing trismus (e.g., heat therapy, physiotherapy, analgesics, and muscle relaxants). If the client does not respond to therapy within 3 days, an infection most likely exists and antibiotic therapy should be prescribed by the dentist or physician. Document the recommended therapy and client progress in the client record.

Edema

Edema, a swelling of the tissues, is a clinical sign of a complication. It may be caused by trauma during the injection, administration of contaminated solutions, hemorrhage, an infection, or an allergic response. Most often edema manifests as localized pain and dysfunction. In the most severe case, edema precipitated by an allergic response may produce airway obstruction and represents a life-threatening emergency.

Prevention

- Follow appropriate infection control protocol when storing and handling components of the local anesthesia armamentarium
- Observe the guidelines for administering atraumatic injections, as described in Procedure 23–4
- Conduct an adequate preanesthetic client assessment prior to local anesthetic administration

Management

The course and treatment of edema is dependent on its etiology.[5] When produced by the administration of a contaminated anesthetic solution or traumatic injection, edema usually subsides in 1 to 3 days without treatment. Analgesics may be recommended. If edema is caused by hemorrhage, the tissue appears discolored and should be managed in the same manner as a hematoma. Resolution of the edema may take 7 to 14 days as the blood is resorbed into the tissues. Edema produced by infection often becomes progressively worse. If the pain and dysfunction do not subside in 3 days, antibiotic therapy may be instituted by the dentist or physician. The treatment of edema caused by an allergic reaction is dependent on the degree and location of the tissue swelling. If there is no airway obstruction, treatment involves the administration of intramuscular and oral antihistamines and consultation with an allergist/physician. If the edema occurs in an area where it compromises the airway, the recommendations outlined in the section on systemic complications should be followed.

Tissue Sloughing

Surface layers of epithelium may be lost because of tissue irritation caused by the application of topical anesthetic for an extended period or a client's heightened sensitivity to the local anesthetic. A sterile abscess, a form of tissue sloughing most frequently occurring on the hard palate, may develop after prolonged ischemia induced by the inclusion of a vasoconstrictor in the local anesthetic agent.

Prevention

- Use topical anesthetics appropriately. Apply a limited amount of topical anesthetic to the tissue for 1 to 2 minutes to minimize irritation and maximize effectiveness
- When using vasoconstrictors for hemostasis, avoid using high concentrations. Epinephrine 1:50,000 and norepinephrine (Levophed) 1:30,000 are the agents most likely to cause prolonged ischemia leading to a sterile abscess

Management

Tissue sloughing usually requires no treatment and disappears within a few days. A sterile abscess resolves in 7 to 10 days. Analgesics may be recommended for discomfort and topical ointment to minimize irritation. Document the progress and response of the client in the client's record.

Soft Tissue Trauma

Lip, tongue, or cheek trauma results when the client inadvertently chews or bites these tissues while they are still anesthetized. Trauma, most often observed in children or in mentally or physically disabled individuals, may lead to swelling and significant discomfort when the anesthesia subsides.

Prevention

- Select a local anesthetic agent with a duration that is appropriate for the length of the dental hygiene care appointment
- Warn the client not to eat, drink, or test the anesthetized area by biting until normal sensation has returned. The client's guardian also should be advised of the potential for injury

- If anesthesia is still present on dismissal, place a cotton roll between the teeth and soft tissues. The cotton roll can be held in position with dental floss wrapped around the teeth
- Warning stickers may be placed on children to serve as a reminder to the child and the guardian to be careful

Management

- Coat the lip with petrolatum to minimize irritation and discomfort
- Recommend warm saline rinses to help decrease swelling
- Recommend analgesics for pain
- If infection occurs, the dentist or physician may prescribe antibiotic therapy

Postanesthetic Intraoral Lesions

Intraoral lesions, such as those from aphthous stomatitis or herpes simplex virus, may develop following the administration of local anesthesia or trauma to the intraoral tissues. Aphthous stomatitis occurs on tissue not attached to bone, such as the mucofacial fold or inner lip. Herpes simplex virus lesions (Fig. 23–84; see color section) may develop intraorally where it manifests on tissues attached to bone, such as the hard palate, or extraorally. Trauma to the area by a needle or any equipment used during the dental hygiene care appointment may activate herpetic recurrence.

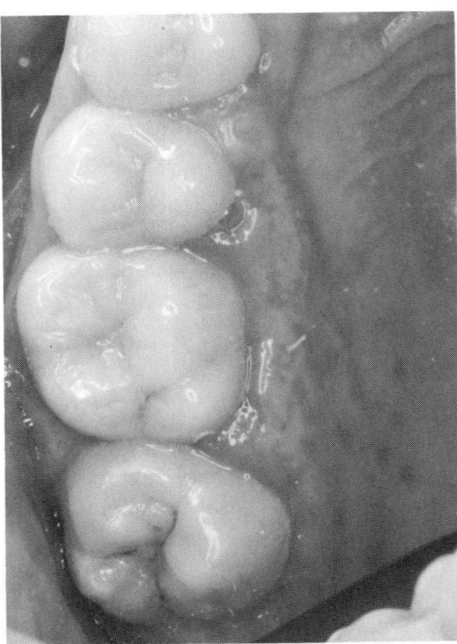

FIGURE 23–84
Herpes simplex virus lesions on the palate following quadrant scaling and root planing with local anesthetic injections.

Prevention

Preventing the development of postanesthetic intraoral lesions is impossible in susceptible clients. However, minimizing trauma during procedures for local anesthetic administration is advisable.

Management

Approximately 2 days following the dental hygiene care appointment, the client reports ulcerations and intense pain, usually near the injection site(s). If the discomfort is tolerable, no management is necessary. However, if the pain is acute, topical anesthetic solutions or protective pastes, such as Orabase, may provide relief. The lesions last for 7 to 10 days. Reassure the client and document the occurrence of the lesion in the client's record.

SYSTEMIC COMPLICATIONS

Client assessment is a key factor in preventing systemic complications associated with local anesthetic administration. It is estimated that a comprehensive health assessment of each client by the oral health professional will prevent approximately 90% of potential life-threatening situations.[29] The remaining 10% occur despite all preventive efforts.

If, despite careful assessment, a local anesthetic systemic complication occurs, the dental hygienist should be able to recognize the signs and symptoms of an adverse drug reaction and properly manage the emergency that may develop. To be adequately prepared for an emergency, the dental hygienist, as well as all members of the oral health team, should be trained in the recognition and management of medical emergencies, and be able to monitor vital signs, administer oxygen, and perform basic life support procedures by establishing an airway and performing basic cardiopulmonary resuscitation (Fig. 23–85). This enables the

PROTOCOL FOR RESPONSIBILITIES DURING A MEDICAL EMERGENCY FOR A THREE MEMBER TEAM IN THE HEALTH CARE SETTING

Team Member 1—Team Director

- Evaluate client's condition
- Initiate basic life support as indicated (Airway, Breathing, Circulation)
- Alert office personnel and direct emergency proceedings
- Stay with victim

Team Member 2

- Assist with basic life support
- Administer oxygen
- Monitor vital signs
- Assist as needed
- Record data

Team Member 3

- Bring emergency kit and oxygen to site of emergency
- Prepare emergency drugs for administration (or possibly administer them)
- Call for medical aid as directed
- Meet rescue team at building entrance
- Relieve others at CPR
- Assist as needed

Adapted from Malamed, S. F. Medical Emergencies in the Dental Office, 4th ed. St. Louis: C. V. Mosby, 1993; and Wilkins, E. M. Clinical Practice of the Dental Hygienist, 6th ed. Philadelphia: Lea & Febiger, 1989.

dental hygienist to administer care to reverse the emergency or to sustain the client until advanced life support systems arrive. Preparedness is further enhanced by regular reviews and rehearsals for emergencies by the dental team members, including emergency telephone contacts and maintenance of a well stocked emergency kit (Table 23–22). Organization is important in being prepared for an emergency. Team planning and individual responsibility promote efficiency and composure at the time of difficult circumstances (see Protocol for Responsibilities During a Medical Emergency for a Three Member Team in the Health Care Setting chart).

In this section causes, prevention, clinical manifestations, and management of local anesthetic overdose, epinephrine overdose, and local anesthetic allergy are reviewed. The information presented in this section is basic and intended to provide an outline for reference and review. It is not meant to replace training in emergency procedures and basic life support, which is required for preparation in an emergency.

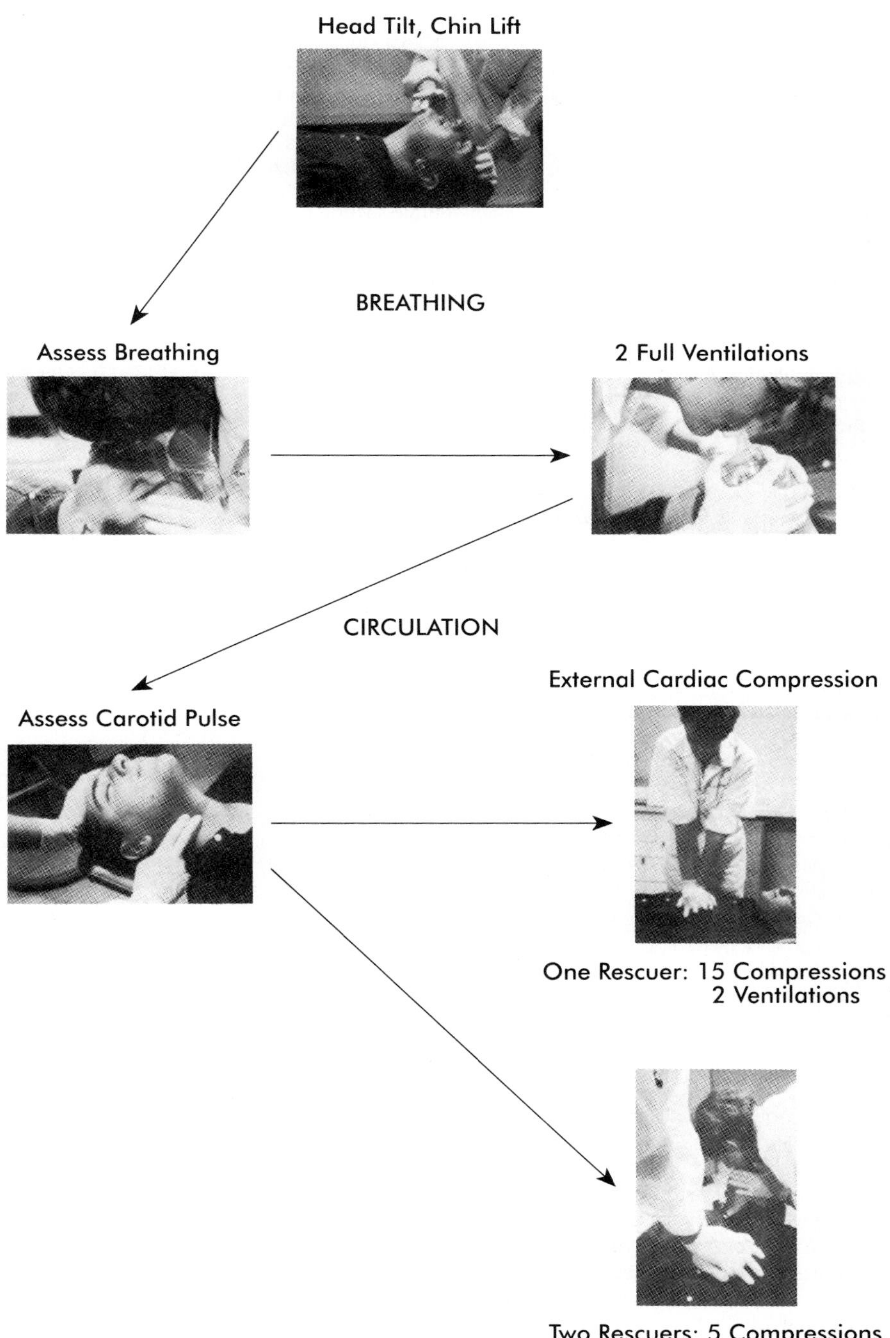

FIGURE 23–85
Summary of basic life support for an adult victim. (With permission from Malamed, S. F. Medical Emergencies in the Dental Office, 4th ed. St. Louis: C. V. Mosby, 1993, p. 429.)

TABLE 23–22
ESSENTIAL DRUGS AND EQUIPMENT FOR AN EMERGENCY KIT/CART FOR THE ORAL HEALTH CARE SETTING

	Primary Drug			Recommended for Kit	
Category	**Generic**	**Proprietary**	**Alternative**	**Quantity**	**Availability**
Injectables					
Antiallergy	Epinephrine	Adrenalin	None	1 preloaded syringe and 3–4 1-mL ampules	1:1000 (1 mg/mL)
Antihistamine	Chlorpheniramine	Chlor-Trimeton	Diphenhydramine	2–3 1–mL ampules	10 mg/mL
Noninjectables					
Oxygen	Oxygen	Oxygen	None	Minimum of 1 "E" cylinder	
Vasodilator	Nitroglycerin	Nitrolingual spray	Nitrostat tablets	1 spray bottle	0.4 mg/dose

Equipment	**Description**	**Quantity for Office**
Emergency Equipment		
Oxygen delivery system	Positive pressure/demand valve, *or* bag-valve-mask device and clear full face masks of various sizes	Minimum of one O_2 delivery system Minimum of 1 small (child) and 1 large (adult) mask
	Pocket mask is recommended for all office employees	1 pocket mask per employee
Suction and suction tips	High-volume suction system	Office suction system
	Large diameter, round-ended suction tips or tonsillar suction	Minimum of two
Syringes for drug administration	Disposable syringes	2–3 2–mL syringes with attached needle for parenteral drug administration
Tourniquets	Rubber or Velcro tourniquet, rubber tubing, or sphygmomanometer	Minimum of 1, up to 3
Magill intubation forceps	Magill intubation forceps	One forceps

From Malamed, S. F. Medical Emergencies in the Dental Office, 4th ed. St. Louis: C. V. Mosby, 1993.

PROCEDURE 23–5

BASIC LIFE SUPPORT

Step	Rationale
ONE PERSON	
1. Assess for unresponsiveness; observe for spontaneous respirations; palpate carotid pulse; ask victim "Are you OK?"	Prevents injury from attempted resuscitation of a person who has not suffered a cardiac or respiratory arrest.
2. Call for help: in a hospital setting, call a "code"; in a community setting, call an emergency phone number (usually 911).	Activates mechanism for additional personnel.
3. Place the victim supine on a hard surface, or use a backboard.	External compression of the heart is facilitated. The heart is compressed between the sternum and the hard surface.
4. Kneel at the level of the victim's shoulders.	This position allows performance of rescue breathing and chest compressions without moving knees.
5. Open victim's airway:	
a. Head-tilt/chin-lift maneuver (adults and children): place one hand on victim's forehead and apply firm, backward pressure with the palm to tilt the head back. Place the fingers of the other hand under the bony part of the jaw near the chin and lift to bring the chin forward and the teeth almost to occlusion, thus supporting the jaw and helping to tilt the head back (see illustration).	This maneuver is more effective in opening the airway than the previously recommended head-tilt/neck-lift. This maneuver removes the tongue or epiglottis as an airway obstruction.

Step	Rationale
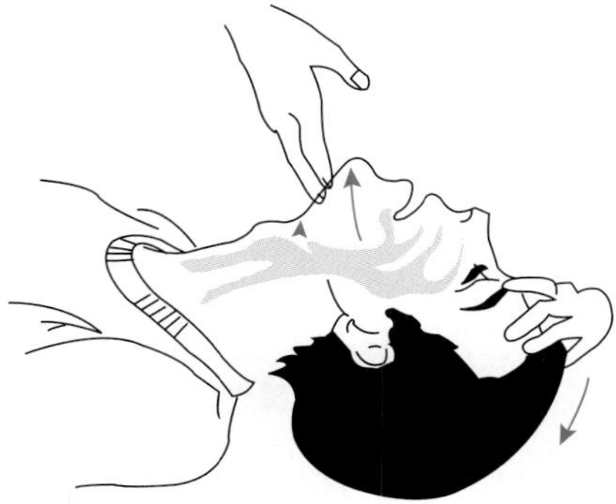 Step 5a	
b. Jaw thrust maneuver (adults and children): grasp angles of the victim's lower jaw and lift with both hands, thus displacing the mandible forward while tilting the head backward.	This technique without head-tilt is the safest first approach to opening the airway of the victim with suspected neck injury because it can usually be accomplished without extending the neck.
6. Check for breathing (3–5 seconds): a. Place your ear over the victim's mouth and nose while maintaining an open airway. b. Look at victim's chest to check for rise and fall; listen and feel for breathing.	Assesses the presence or absence of spontaneous breathing and the need to continue with rescue breathing.
7. Prepare for rescue breathing: For mouth-to-mouth resuscitation of an adult, pinch the victim's nose and occlude his mouth with yours. For an infant, place your mouth over the infant's nose and mouth.	An airtight seal is formed, and air is prevented from escaping from the nose.
8. Perform rescue breathing: a. For mouth-to-mouth resuscitation of an adult, blow two slow breaths into the victim's mouth. Adequate time for the two breaths (1½–2 seconds per breath) should be allowed to provide good chest expansion and decrease the possibility of gastric distention.	In most adults this volume is 800–1200 mL and is sufficient volume to make the chest rise. An excess of air volume and fast inspiratory flow rates are likely to cause pharyngeal pressures that exceed esophageal opening pressures, allowing air to enter the stomach and result in gastric distention, thereby increasing the risk of vomiting.
b. For mouth-to-mouth resuscitation of an infant or child, administer two slow breaths, 1–1½ seconds per breath with a pause between for rescuer to take a breath.	Since an infant's air passages are smaller with resistance to flow quite high, it is difficult to make recommendations about the force or volume of the rescue breaths. However, three factors should be remembered: (1) rescue breaths are the single most important maneuver in assisting a nonbreathing child, (2) an appropriate volume is one that makes the chest rise and fall, and (3) slow breaths provide an adequate volume at the lowest possible pressure, thereby reducing the risk of gastric distention.
9. Observe for rise and fall of the chest wall with each respiration. If lungs do not inflate, reposition the head and neck and try two more breaths. If still unsuccessful, suspect choking and proceed with foreign body airway obstruction procedures.	Observing chest wall movement ensures that artificial respirations are entering the lungs.
10. Assess for presence of the carotid pulse; pulse check should take 5–10 seconds. a. Carotid pulse is most central and accessible artery in children over 1 year. However, in an infant the short, chubby neck makes carotid difficult to palpate; brachial artery is recommended instead.	Carotid artery pulse will persist when the more peripheral pulses are no longer palpable. Performing external cardiac compressions on a victim who has a pulse may result in serious medical complications.
11. If victim is pulseless, begin external cardiac compressions: **Adult** a. Proper hand position (see illustration): (1) Using middle index finger of the hand nearest the victim's legs, locate lower margin of rib cage on the side next to rescuer.	Properly performed external chest compressions can produce systolic blood pressure peaks of 60–80 mm Hg, but the diastolic pressure is low, with the mean blood pressure in the carotid arteries seldom exceeding 40 mm Hg. Blood flow through the carotid artery is only one-fourth to one-third of normal.

CONTINUED ON FOLLOWING PAGE

BASIC LIFE SUPPORT *Continued*

Step	Rationale
(2) Move fingers up the rib cage to the notch where the ribs meet the sternum. Place middle finger on notch, and index finger next to it, on the lower end of the sternum.	Proper hand position results in maximal compression of the heart between the sternum and the vertebrae. If compressions occur over the xiphoid process, the victim's liver can be lacerated.
(3) Place long axis of the heel of the hand nearest victim's head on the long axis of the sternum next to the index finger.	
(4) Remove first hand from notch, place on top of the hand on the sternum so that the hands are parallel to each other.	
(5) Either extend or interlace fingers, but keep fingers off the chest.	Reduces risk of rib fracture during compression.

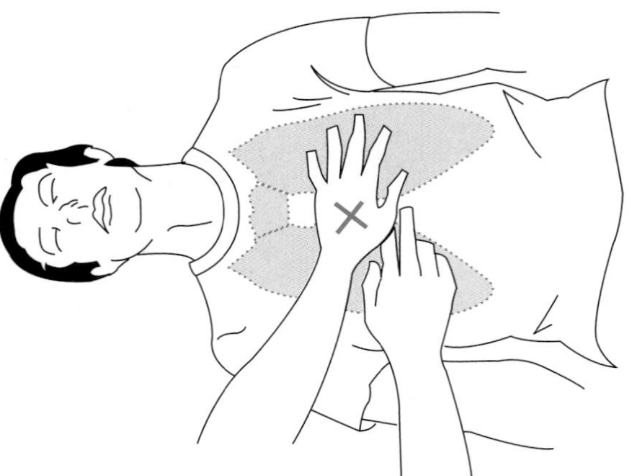

Step 11a (adult)

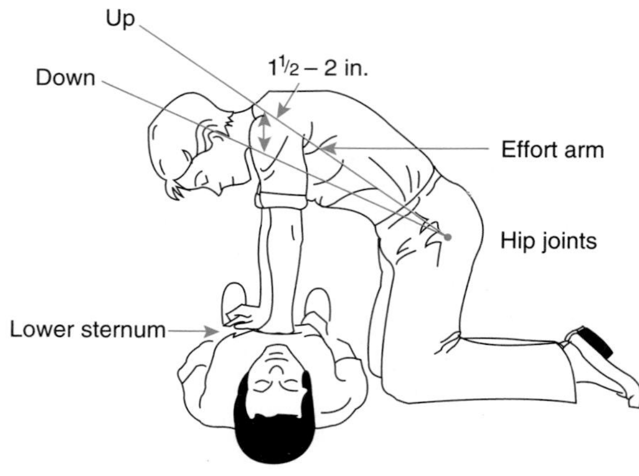

Step 11b (adult)

Step	Rationale
b. Lock elbows, maintain arms straight and shoulders directly over the hands on victim's sternum (see illustration):	In this manner the thrust for each compression is straight down on the sternum.
(1) Compress chest 3.8–5.0 cm (1½–2 in.).	
(2) Compress chest 80–100 times per minute. Perform 15 external compressions with the mnemonic "one and, two and, three and . . ." to 15.	Faster rate increases blood flow with an increased flow to the brain and heart. Faster rate also allows a pause for ventilation in two-rescuer CPR.
c. Ventilate lungs with two ventilations as in steps 7 and 8.	
d. Reassess victim after four cycles (15 compressions: 2 ventilations each cycle).	Determines return of pulse and respiration and the need to continue CPR.
Infant (1–12 months)	
a. Proper hand position:	Proper hand position results in maximal compression.
(1) Draw an imaginary line between the nipples over the breast bone (sternum).	
(2) Place the index finger of the hand farthest from the infant's head just under the intermammary line where it intersects the sternum.	The area of compression is one finger's width below this intersection at the location of the middle and ring fingers.
b. Using two fingers (middle and ring fingers) compress 1.3–2.5 cm (½–1 in.) at least 100 times per minute.	Promotes adequate cardiac output.
c. At the end of every fifth compression a pause should be allowed for a ventilation (1–1½ seconds).	Promotes adequate ventilation during CPR.
d. Reassess victim after ten cycles (5 compressions: 1 ventilation each cycle).	Determines return of pulse and respiration and the need to continue CPR.
Child (1–7 years)	
a. Proper hand position:	Proper position results in maximal compressions.
(1) Locate lower margin of the victim's rib cage on the side next to the rescuer with the middle and	

Step	Rationale
index fingers of the hand nearer the victim's feet. (2) Follow the margin of the rib cage with the middle finger to the notch where the ribs and breast bone meet. (3) Place index finger next to middle finger. (4) Place heel of same hand next to the index finger with long axis of the heel parallel to the sternum.	
b. Compress sternum with one hand 2.5–3.8 cm (1–1½ in.) at a rate of 80–100 times per minute.	Promotes adequate cardiac output.
c. At the end of every fifth compression a pause should be allowed for a ventilation (1–1½ seconds).	Promotes adequate ventilation during CPR.
d. Reassess victim after 10 cycles (5 compressions: 1 ventilation each cycle).	Determines return of pulse and respiration and need to continue CPR.
TWO PERSONS	
12. One person is positioned at the victim's side and performs external cardiac compression while the other remains at the victim's head, maintains an open airway, and monitors the carotid pulse. The compression rate is 80–100 per minute. The compression-ventilation ratio is 5:1 with a pause for ventilation (1½–2 seconds). When the compressor becomes fatigued, the rescuers should exchange positions as soon as possible.	

Adapted from Standards and guidelines for cardiopulmonary resuscitation (CPR) and emergency cardiac care (ECC). Journal of the American Medical Association, Vol. 268, No. 16, pp. 2172–2261, 1992; copyright 1992, The American Medical Association.

With permission from Potter, P. A., and Perry, A. G. Fundamentals of Nursing: Concepts, Process, and Practice, 2nd ed. St. Louis: C.V. Mosby, 1989, pp. 1016–1018.

Local Anesthetic Overdose

A **drug overdose reaction** or **toxic reaction** is defined as those signs and symptoms that result from overly high blood levels of a drug in various organs and tissues.[8] Normally, there is a continual absorption of the drug from its site of administration into the circulation. Concurrently, the drug is being removed from the blood as it undergoes redistribution and biotransformation. When this equilibrium exists, high blood levels of the drug seldom occur. However, if this equilibrium is altered, the elevation of the blood level of the drug may be sufficient to produce an overdose reaction.

Many factors have a profound impact on the rate at which a local anesthetic drug level is elevated and the length of time it remains elevated. The presence of one or more of these factors predisposes the client to the development of an overdose reaction. These factors are divided into predisposing client factors and drug factors. Client factors modify the response of an individual to the usual drug dosage (i.e., individual variation). Drug factors involve the drug and its site of administration. Table 23-23 describes how each of these factors influences the potential for an overdose reaction.

Causes and Prevention of a Local Anesthetic Overdose Reaction

High blood levels of local anesthetics may occur in one or more of the following ways:[5,7]

- Biotransformation of the anesthetic is unusually slow
- Elimination of the anesthetic from the body through the kidneys is unusually slow
- The total dose administered is too large
- Absorption of the anesthetic from the site of injection is unusually rapid
- The anesthetic is inadvertently administered intravascularly

The first two potential causes of an overdose—delayed biotransformation and elimination of the anesthetic agent—relate to the health of the client. Therefore, it is imperative that the dental hygienist carefully assess the client's health status, obtain medical consultation if necessary, and modify the dental hygiene care plan as indicated to prevent drug-related complications.

The three remaining causes of an overdose reaction—excessive dose, rapid absorption, and intravascular injection—may be prevented through adherence to proper technique of local anesthetic agent administration. Thus, careful assessment of the client prior to dental hygiene care and proper administration technique minimize the risk of a local anesthetic overdose.

Biotransformation and Elimination of the Anesthetic. Ester anesthetics are biotransformed primarily in the blood by the enzyme pseudocholinesterase which causes the drug to undergo hydrolysis to para-aminobenzoic acid. Clients with a familial history of atypical pseudocholinesterase may be unable to detoxify ester anesthetic agents at the usual rate. As a result, high blood levels of anesthetic may develop. Amide local anesthetics may be administered to these individuals without an increased risk of overdose.

Biotransformation of amide anesthetics occurs in the liver. A history of liver disease may indicate some hepatic dysfunction, and the ability of the liver to biotransform amide anesthetics may be compromised. Clients with a his-

TABLE 23–23
PREDISPOSING FACTORS TO LOCAL ANESTHETIC OVERDOSE REACTION

Client Factors	
Age	Biotransformation may not be fully developed in younger age groups and may be diminished in older age groups
Body weight	Lower body weight increases risk
Genetics	Genetic deficiencies may alter response to certain drugs (e.g., atypical plasma cholinesterase)
Disease	Presence of disease may affect the ability of the body to biotransform the drug into an inactive substance (e.g., hepatic or renal dysfunction, cardiovascular disease)
Mental attitude and environment	Psychological attitude affects response to stimulation; anxiety decreases seizure threshold
Gender	Very slight risk increase during pregnancy
Drug Factors	
Vasoactivity	Vasodilation increases risk
Drug dosage	Higher dose increases risk
Route of administration	Intravascular route increases risk
Rate of injection	Rapid injection increases risk
Vascularity of injection site	Increased vascularity increases risk
Presence of vasoconstrictors	Decreases risk
Other medications	Concomitant medications may influence local anesthetic drug levels

Adapted from Malamed, S. F. Medical Emergencies in the Dental Office, 4th ed. St. Louis: C. V. Mosby, 1993.

tory of liver disease who are ambulatory may still receive amide local anesthetics. However, only small amounts should be injected because average amounts may produce an overdose reaction.

Both ester and amide anesthetics are eliminated to some degree through the kidneys. Renal dysfunction may delay elimination of the local anesthetic from the blood, precipitating accumulated levels of local anesthetic and increased potential for an overdose. Those clients who have significant renal impairment or who require renal dialysis should receive the minimal amount of local anesthetic needed for effective pain control.

Excessive Total Dose of Anesthetic. If an excessive total dose of local anesthetic is administered to a client, toxic effects develop. Responses to drugs vary considerably, but guidelines exist for the dental hygienist to calculate maximal safe doses of local anesthetic agents based on body weight (see Tables 23–5 and 23–6). The dental hygienist also needs to factor in the client's age and physical status and adjust the dosage accordingly. A more detailed discussion can be found under Maximal Safe Doses of Local Anesthetics.

Rapid Absorption of Anesthetic Into the Circulation. The addition of a vasoconstricting drug in the local anesthetic solution reduces the systemic toxicity of the anesthetic agent by slowing its absorption into the cardiovascular system. Therefore, unless specifically contraindicated because of health status or limited duration of dental hygiene care, local anesthetic solutions containing a vasoconstrictor should be employed. A vasoconstrictor minimizes the potential for an overdose reaction and subsequently increases client safety.

Topical anesthetic agents applied to the oral mucosa are absorbed rapidly into the circulation. The concentration of these topical agents is much greater than that of injectable anesthetic solutions. When small amounts are used in a localized area, there is little chance of complications devel-

TABLE 23–24
COMPARISON OF PATTERNS OF LOCAL ANESTHETIC OVERDOSE

	Rapid Intravascular	Too Large a Total Dose	Rapid Absorption	Slow Biotransformation	Slow Elimination
Likelihood of occurrence	Common	Most common	Likely with "high normal" dosages if no vasoconstrictors are used	Uncommon	Least common
Onset of signs and symptoms	Most rapid (seconds); intraarterial faster than intravenous	3–5 minutes	3–5 minutes	10–30 minutes	10 minutes to several hours
Intensity of signs and symptoms	Usually most intense	Gradual onset with increased intensity; may prove quite severe		Gradual onset with slow increase in intensity of symptoms	
Duration of signs and symptoms	2–3 minutes	Usually 5 to 30 minutes; depends on dose and ability to metabolize or excrete		Potentially longest duration because of inability to metabolize or excrete agents	
Primary prevention	Aspirate, slow injection	Administer minimal doses	Use vasoconstrictor; limit topical anesthetic use or use nonabsorbed type (base)	Adequate pretreatment physical assessment of client	
Drug groups	Amides and esters	Amides; esters only rarely	Amides; esters only rarely	Amides and esters	Amides and esters

From Malamed, S. F. Medical Emergencies in the Dental Office, 4th ed. St. Louis: C. V. Mosby, 1993.

oping. However, if applied over a large area such as a quadrant or whole arch, a significant increase in blood level may occur, precipitating an overdose reaction.[8] To prevent complications with topical anesthetics, it is recommended to limit the area of application and avoid topical anesthetic aerosol sprays because of lack of dosage control and sterility concerns.

Intravascular Injection. The introduction of a local anesthetic solution directly into the bloodstream via an intravascular injection (intravenous or intraarterial) may produce an overdose response. An intravascular injection may result with any intraoral injection; however, it is more likely to occur during a nerve block, particularly an inferior alveolar, mental, incisive, or posterior superior alveolar nerve block.[30]

Fortunately, an overdose reaction from an intravascular injection can be prevented by having a complete knowledge of the anatomical features of the area to be anesthetized and adhering to careful injection technique. This includes using an aspirating syringe, a 25- or 27-gauge needle, aspirating in two planes prior to deposition, and slowly administering the anesthetic agent.

Clinical Manifestations and Management of a Local Anesthetic Overdose Reaction

The onset, intensity, and duration of a local anesthetic toxic reaction may vary depending on the original cause of the overdose. Table 23–24 compares the various patterns of local anesthetic overdose reactions.

Table 23–25 describes the clinical signs and symptoms that may occur during an overdose reaction (during minimal-to-moderate and moderate-to-high blood levels of anesthetic) and the procedures for managing a local anesthetic overdose response. Management of an overdose response depends upon the severity of the reaction. Most often, the reaction is mild and transitory with little or no specific treatment need.[5,7] However, a severe or longer duration reaction necessitates prompt recognition and immediate care.

TABLE 23–25
CLINICAL MANIFESTATIONS AND MANAGEMENT OF A LOCAL ANESTHETIC OVERDOSE REACTION

Signs/Symptoms	Management
Minimal to Moderate Blood Levels (Mild Overdose Reaction)	
Confusion	Terminate procedure
Talkativeness	Reassure client
Apprehension	Position client comfortably
Excitedness	Administer oxygen
Lightheadedness	Provide basic life support, as indicated
Dizziness	Monitor vital signs
Ringing in ears (tinnitus)	Summon medical assistance, if needed
Headache	Allow client to recover and discharge
Slurred speech	
Generalized stutter	
Muscular twitching and tremor of face and extremities	
Blurred vision, unable to focus	
Numbness of perioral tissues	
Flushed or chilled feeling	
Drowsiness, disorientation	
Elevated blood pressure	
Elevated heart rate	
Elevated respiratory rate	
Loss of consciousness	
Moderate to High Blood Levels (Severe Overdose Reaction)	
Tonic-clonic seizure, followed by:	Terminate procedure
CNS depression	Position client supine, legs elevated
Depressed blood pressure, heart rate, and respiratory rate	Summon medical assistance
Unconsciousness	Manage seizure—protect client from injury
	Provide basic life support, as indicated
	Administer oxygen
	Monitor vital signs
	Administer an anticonvulsant (prolonged seizure)
	Transport client to hospital after stabilization

Some data from Malamed, S. F. Medical Emergencies in the Dental Office, 4th ed. St. Louis: C.V. Mosby, 1993.

Epinephrine Overdose

Although several vasoconstrictors are currently used in oral health care (see Table 23–3), epinephrine is the most potent and widely employed. Consequently, overdose reactions occur more often with epinephrine than with other vasopressor agents because the latter agents are weaker and are used less frequently.

Causes and Prevention of an Epinephrine Overdose Reaction

An epinephrine overdose reaction is more likely to develop if concentrations of epinephrine greater than 1:100,000 are administered. Indeed, some authorities state that a concentration of 1:250,000 epinephrine provides adequate duration of action for dental procedures and minimal toxicity. Therefore, the use of a 1:50,000 concentration of epinephrine for pain control is unwarranted. The only benefit this concentration may have over lesser concentrations is its ability to control bleeding. If epinephrine is to be used for hemostasis, only small quantities of solution need be infiltrated into the immediate area. Overdose reactions under these circumstances are rare. Therefore, to avoid an epinephrine overdose reaction, it is recommended that the dental hygienist use the lowest effective concentration of epinephrine needed to produce the desired effect and carefully observe dosage guidelines (see Table 23–7).

There is a greater potential for epinephrine overdose in clients with cardiovascular disease. An increased workload on an already compromised cardiovascular system may precipitate further cardiac distress. Therefore, the total dose of vasoconstrictor must be reduced to avoid systemic complications (see Tables 23–7 and 23–8).

An intravascular injection also may produce an epinephrine overdose reaction.[7] Recommendations for prevention of an intravascular injection may be found in the Local Anesthetic Overdose section.

Clinical Manifestations and Management of an Epinephrine Overdose Reaction

Clinically, the signs and symptoms of epinephrine toxicity resemble the "fight or flight" response. Table 23–26 identifies those signs and symptoms of an epinephrine overdose

TABLE 23–26
CLINICAL MANIFESTATIONS AND MANAGEMENT OF A CLIENT WITH AN EPINEPHRINE OVERDOSE REACTION

Signs/Symptoms	Management
Fear, anxiety	Terminate procedure
Tenseness	Position client upright
Restlessness	Reassure client
Throbbing headache	Basic life support, as indicated
Tremor	Monitor vital signs
Perspiration	Summon medical assistance, if needed
Weakness	Administer oxygen, if needed
Dizziness	Allow client to recover and discharge
Pallor	
Respiratory difficulty	
Palpitations	
Sharp elevation in blood pressure, primarily systolic	
Elevated heart rate	
Cardiac dysrhythmias	

Some data from Malamed, S. F. Medical Emergencies in the Dental Office, 4th ed. St. Louis: C.V. Mosby, 1993.

reaction. The procedures for managing this complication also are included. Most cases of epinephrine overdose are of short duration and need little or no definitive management. However, if a prolonged reaction occurs, the dental hygienist must be prepared to respond accordingly.

Allergy

Allergic reactions are the result of an antigen-antibody response to a specific agent. Exposure to an initial dose of a medication causes an immunological response. The drug acts as an antigen, prompting antibodies to be produced. As a result, administration of a subsequent dose causes the client to develop an allergic response to the drug, its chemical preservative, or a metabolite.[15] Once clients manifest a specific drug allergy, they remain allergic to that drug indefinitely.[7]

Causes

Allergic reactions to local anesthetics occur most often in response to ester-type anesthetic agents (see Table 23–1). The incidence of such responses is extremely rare with the amide-type local anesthetics (see Table 23–2). As a result of their nonallergenic nature, amides are now used almost exclusively for pain control during dental and dental hygiene procedures.

Allergic responses to other contents of the dental cartridge have been demonstrated. Reports of allergy to sodium bisulfite and metabisulfite are numerous.[17–21] Bisulfites are incorporated in all dental cartridges containing a vasoconstrictor. However, they are not included in cartridges that contain no vasopressor. These agents are also sprayed on fruits and vegetables to prevent discoloration. A client with a history of bisulfite allergy (mostly asthmatic clients) should alert the dental hygienist to the possibility of a similar reaction if a local anesthetic containing a vasoconstrictor is administered. See the section on Preanesthetic Client Assessment/Allergies for further discussion.

Prevention

The preanesthetic client assessment is the primary measure for prevention of an allergic reaction. A client who has multiple allergies (e.g., asthma, hay fever, allergy to foods) has an increased potential for allergic reactions to medications.[5,7,29] Thus, the dental hygienist must proceed cautiously when considering the administration of local anesthetics to these clients.

If the client reports that he has experienced an allergic reaction to local anesthetics, it is important the dental hygienist assume that the client is truly allergic to the local anesthetic in question until proven otherwise. Unfortunately, any adverse drug reaction is often labeled an "allergy" by clients when actually overdose reactions occur much more frequently than allergic reactions.[31] Thus, it is imperative for the dental hygienist to seek as much information as possible from the client so that the exact nature of the reaction can be determined. This is done by means of a dialogue history whereby the dental hygienist asks the client a series of questions to ascertain the validity of the allergy[5] (see Dialogue to Evaluate an Alleged Allergic Reaction to Local Anesthetics chart). It is important that the anesthetic agent or any closely related agent to which the client claims to be allergic *not* be used until the allergy is disproved.

If, after the dialogue history, questions remain about the cause of the reaction, the dental hygienist should consult with the dentist and client's physician, and referral for allergy testing should be considered. Dental hygiene care requiring local anesthetics (topical or injectable) should be delayed until an evaluation of the client is complete. Dental hygiene procedures not requiring anesthesia may be performed during the interim.

For those clients who have a confirmed allergy to local anesthetics, management varies according to the nature of the allergy. Table 23–10 describes alternative drugs that may be employed in place of those agents that cause an allergic response.

Clinical Manifestations and Management

The amount of time that elapses between exposure to an allergenic agent and manifestation of signs and symptoms

DIALOGUE TO EVALUATE AN ALLEGED ALLERGIC REACTION TO LOCAL ANESTHETICS

Describe exactly what occurred
What treatment was given?
What position were you in during the injection?
What was the time sequence of events?
Were the services of a physician or emergency personnel needed?
What drug was used?
What amount of drug was administered?
Did the drug contain a vasoconstrictor?
Were you taking any other medications at the time of the incident?
What is the name and address of the doctor (dentist, physician, hospital) who was treating you when the reaction occurred?

Adapted from Malamed, S. F. Handbook of Local Anesthesia, 3rd ed. St. Louis: Mosby–Year Book, 1990.

is important. As a rule, the more rapid the onset of signs and symptoms following exposure, the more severe the ultimate reaction.[32] Conversely, the greater the time between exposure and onset of signs and symptoms, the less severe the reaction. This time factor helps the dental hygienist determine the appropriate management of the reaction.

The most common allergic reaction associated with local anesthetics is a dermatological reaction. A skin reaction that appears alone or after a considerable lapse of time (60 minutes or more) is usually not life-threatening; however, if a skin reaction develops rapidly, it may be the first indication of an ensuing generalized reaction.

An allergic reaction may manifest solely in the respiratory tract or may accompany other systemic responses. In slowly evolving generalized allergic reactions, respiratory distress follows skin and gastrointestinal reactions but occurs prior to cardiovascular signs and symptoms.

Generalized **anaphylaxis** is the most life-threatening allergic reaction. Most reactions develop quickly, reaching maximum intensity within 5 to 30 minutes of exposure, although delayed responses have been reported.[8]

Table 23–27 describes the signs and symptoms and the management of clients with dermatological and respiratory reactions and generalized anaphylaxis. The reaction types are further defined as delayed and immediate.

TABLE 23–27
CLINICAL MANIFESTATIONS AND MANAGEMENT OF AN ALLERGIC REACTION

	Signs/Symptoms	Management
Delayed	*Skin* Erythema Urticaria (hives) Pruritis (itching) Angioedema (localized swelling of extremities, lips, tongue, pharynx, larynx)	*Skin* Administer antihistimine Medical consultation
	Respiration Bronchospasm: Distress Dyspnea Wheezing Perspiration Flushing Cyanosis Tachycardia Anxiety	*Respiration* Terminate procedure Position client semierect Reassure client Basic life support, as indicated Summon medical assistance, if needed Administer epinephrine Monitor vital signs Administer antihistamine Allow client to recover and discharge
	Laryngeal Edema: Swelling of vocal apparatus and subsequent obstruction of airway Respiratory distress Exaggerated chest movements High-pitched sound to no sound Cyanosis Loss of consciousness	*Laryngeal Edema* Terminate procedure Position client supine Summon medical assistance Administer epinephrine Maintain airway Administer oxygen Additional drug management: antihistamine, corticosteroid Cricothyrotomy, if needed Transfer client to hospital
Immediate Anaphylaxis	*Skin:* Pruritus (itching) Flushing Urticaria (face and upper chest) Feeling of hair standing on end Conjunctivitis, vasomotor rhinitis *Gastrointestinal/genitourinary:* Abdominal cramps Nausea, vomiting Diarrhea *Respiratory:* Substernal tightness or chest pain Cough, wheezing Dyspnea Cyanosis of mucous membranes, nail beds Laryngeal edema *Cardiovascular:* Pallor Lightheadedness Palpitations, tachycardia Hypotension Cardiac dysrhythmias Unconsciousness Cardiac arrest	Terminate procedure Position client supine, legs elevated Basic life support, as indicated Summon medical assistance Administer epinephrine Administer oxygen Monitor vital signs Additional drug management: antihistamine, corticosteroid Transport client to hospital

References

1. Hollinshead, B. S. (ed.). Survey of dentistry, the final report. Commission of the Survey of Dentistry in the United States. Washington, D.C.: American Council on Education, 1961.
2. Sisty, N. L., Henderson, W. G., and Paule, C. L. Review of training and evaluation studies in expanded functions for dental auxilliaries. Journal of the American Dental Association 98:233, 1979.
3. American Dental Hygienists' Association. Personal communication, June, 1993.
4. Covino, B. G., and Vassallo, H. G. Local Anesthetics: Mechanisms of Action and Clinical Use. New York: Grune & Stratton, 1976.
5. Malamed, S. F. Handbook of Local Anesthesia, 3rd ed. St. Louis: C. V. Mosby, 1990.
6. Requa, B. S., and Holroyd, S. V. Applied Pharmacology for the Dental Hygienist. St. Louis: C. V. Mosby, 1982.
7. Bennett, C. R. Monheim's Local Anesthesia and Pain Control in Dental Practice, 7th ed. St. Louis: C. V. Mosby, 1984.
8. Malamed, S. F. Medical Emergencies in the Dental Office, 4th ed. St. Louis: C. V. Mosby, 1993.
9. Langlais, R. P., Broadus, R., and Glass, B. J. Bifid mandibular canals in panoramic radiographs. Journal of the American Dental Association 110:923, 1985.
10. Wong, M., and Jacobsen, P. L. Reasons for local anesthesia failures. Journal of the American Dental Association 123:69, 1992.
11. Warren, R. E., Van de Mark, T. B., and Weinberg, S. Methemoglobinemia induced by high doses of prilocaine. Oral Surgery 37:866, 1974.
12. Maseman, D. C., and Whetstone, S. D. Medical history review prior to local anesthesia administration. Dental Hygiene 62:131, 1988.
13. Scheitler, L. E., Getzendanner, L., et al. Malignant hyperthermia during oral surgery. Anesthesia Progress 31:170, 1984.
14. Malignant Hyperthermia Association of the United States. MHAUS Professional Advisory Council adopts new policy statement on local anesthetics. Communicator 3(4):1, 1985.
15. Potter, P. A., and Perry, A. G. Fundamentals of Nursing: Concepts, Process, and Practice, 2nd ed. St. Louis: C. V. Mosby, 1989.
16. Goulet, J., Perusse, R., et al. Contraindications to vasoconstrictors in denistry: Part III. Oral Surgery, Oral Medicine, Oral Pathology 74:692, 1992.
17. Schwartz, H. J. Sensitivity to ingested metabisulfites: Variations in clinical presentation. Journal of Allergy and Clinical Immunology 71:487, 1983.
18. Simon, R. A., Green, L., and Stevenson, D. D. The incidence of ingested metabisulfite sensitivity in an asthmatic population. Journal of Allergy and Clinical Immunology. 69:118, 1982.
19. Prenner, B. M., and Stevens, J. J. Anaphylaxis after ingestion of sodium bisulfite. Annals of Allergy 37:180, 1976.
20. Twarog, F. J., and Leung, D. Y. M. Anaphylaxis to a component of isoetharine (sodium bisulfite). Journal of the American Medical Association 248:2030, 1982.
21. Seng, G. F., and Gay, A. J. Dangers of sulfites in dental local anesthetic solutions: Warning and recommendations. Journal of the American Dental Association 113:769, 1986.
22. Wittrock, J. W., and Fischer, W. E. The aspiration of blood through small-gauge needles. Journal of the American Dental Association 76:79, 1968.
23. Miller, C. H. Reduced chance of exposure. RDH, 11(4):32, 1991.
24. DuBrul, E. L. Sischer and DuBrul's Oral Anatomy, 8th ed. St. Louis: Ishiyaku EuroAmerican, 1988.
25. Murrell, C. Record keeping: Its role in malpractice avoidance and defense. Dental Hygiene 60:324, 1986.
26. Loetscher, C. A., and Walton, R. E. Patterns of innervation of the maxillary first molar: A dissection study. Oral Surgery 65:86, 1988.
27. American Dental Association Council on Dental Materials, Instruments and Equipment; On Dental Practice, and On Dental Therapeutics. Infection control recommendations for the dental office and the dental laboratory. Journal of the American Dental Association 116:241, 1988.
28. Shira, R. B. Surgical emergencies. In McCarthy, F. M. (ed.). Emergencies in Dental Practice, 3rd ed. Philadelphia: W. B. Saunders, 1979.
29. McCarthy, F. M. Essentials of Safe Dentistry for the Medically Compromised Patient. Philadelphia: W. B. Saunders, 1989.
30. Barlett, S. Z. Clinical observations on the effects of injections of local anesthetics preceded by aspiration. Oral Surgery 33:520, 1972.
31. Caranasos, G. J. Drug reactions. In Swartz, G. R., Safar, P. et al. (eds.). Principles and Practice of Emergency Medicine, 3rd ed. Philadelphia: W. B. Saunders, 1992.
32. Kelly, J. K., and Patterson, R. Anaphylaxis: Course, mechanisms and treatment. Journal of the American Medical Association 227:1431, 1974.

Suggested Readings

Wilkins, E. M. Clinical Practice of the Dental Hygienist, 6th ed. Philadelphia: Lea & Febiger, 1989.

24 Nitrous Oxide–Oxygen Analgesia

OBJECTIVES

Mastery of the content in this chapter will enable the reader to:

- Define the key terms
- Discuss the indications and contraindications for use of this sedation modality
- Discuss the advantages, disadvantages, and complications associated with use
- Discuss the signs and symptoms of the baseline level of conscious sedation
- List safety features associated with gas cylinders and the gas machine
- Calculate the percentage of nitrous oxide and the percentage of oxygen from the tidal volume
- Safely administer nitrous oxide oxygen sedation by using titration to induce the proper level of sedation, monitoring the client during analgesia, and oxygenating the client at the completion of the sedation period

INTRODUCTION

Nitrous oxide (N_2O) delivered in combination with oxygen (O_2) is an inhalation method of conscious sedation. This conscious sedation method can significantly enhance the clinician's ability to meet the client's need for freedom from pain and stress in a safe and effective way. When used as the sole sedative, it suffices to relax individuals who are mildly apprehensive about the dental or dental hygiene experience and provides pain control for procedures that are only slightly or moderately painful. Such procedures include scaling hypersensitive root surfaces, removing periodontal sutures, cementing crowns or inlays, irrigating under an inflamed operculum, or administering a local anesthetic. If significant pain is anticipated during a dental or dental hygiene procedure, then nitrous oxide–oxygen (N_2O–O_2) conscious sedation is accompanied by local anesthesia. Although used in combination with other general anesthetics such as halothane and Demerol by oral surgeons to achieve surgical anesthesia, when used alone nitrons oxide–oxygen is a very weak anesthetic but an intense analgesic.[1] This pharmacological property of nitrous oxide–oxygen makes it ideal for use in dental hygiene care because clients often are mildly apprehensive and require minor pain control, but also must remain conscious and responsive.

A number of synonyms refer to nitrous oxide–oxygen conscious sedation, including[1]:

- Conscious sedation
- Inhalation sedation
- Nitrous oxide psychosedation
- Relative analgesia

Conscious sedation refers to the fact that during the administration of nitrous oxide–oxygen sedation the client is always awake and able to respond to verbal commands, breathe automatically, and cough so that aspiration is avoided.[2] **Inhalation sedation** reflects that the nitrous oxide and oxygen gases are inhaled through the nose. **Nitrous oxide psychosedation** refers to the fact that nitrous oxide acts on the "psyche" or the central nervous system in such a way that pain impulses are not relayed to the cerebral cortex or their interpretation is altered.[3] **Relative analgesia** refers to the state of sedation produced, which is relative analgesia that alters mood and increases the pain reaction threshold but does not totally block pain sensations. This chapter presents the principles and techniques of nitrous oxide–oxygen sedation, highlighting indications, contraindications, advantages, and disadvantages of its use as a sedation modality. Initially, however, a brief overview is presented of the history, chemistry, pharmacology, and physiology of nitrous oxide–oxygen, and the stages of anesthesia.

HISTORY

Nitrous oxide was discovered by Joseph Priestley in 1772. The first report of its use in dentistry was in 1844. Nitrous oxide was administered by Gardner Cotton, a traveling chemist, to a person having a tooth extracted by a dentist.

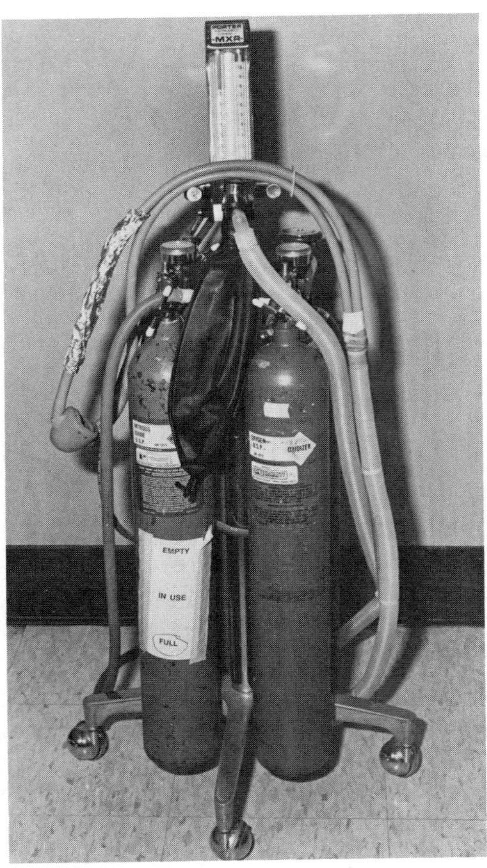

FIGURE 24–1
A portable gas machine with a green cylinder containing oxygen and a blue cylinder containing nitrous oxide, stored directly on the gas machine.

It was reported that no pain was observed. A year later, however, the same dentist unsuccessfully demonstrated its use for pain control during an extraction procedure at Harvard Medical School. It was not until 1863 that its usefulness for pain control was reestablished by Cotton, and in 1868 it was combined with oxygen for use in pain control.[4]

CHEMISTRY

Nitrous oxide is a colorless, tasteless, sweet-smelling, nonexplosive agent that supports combustion.[5] It is stored as a liquid at 650 to 900 pounds per square inch (psi) in a blue compressed gas cylinder (Fig. 24–1). Although it is stored as a liquid and vapor (gas) in equilibrium, it is delivered as a gas to the client. The pressure within the cylinder, indicated by the needle reading on the pressure gauge, reflects the pressure created by the gaseous state of nitrous oxide in the cylinder (Fig. 24–2). As long as one-eighth of the liquid nitrous oxide is present in the cylinder to convert to the gaseous state, the reading on the pressure gauge of 650 to 900 psi remains constant. Consequently, clinicians use their nitrous oxide for a considerable amount of time before the pressure gauge reads 500 psi, after which the pressure reading on the gauge precipitously drops, indicating that the cylinder is empty. Because the contents of the nitrous oxide cylinder cannot be determined by the pressure gauge reading until it is almost empty, it is important for the operator to keep a close eye on the nitrous oxide pressure gauge of portable gas machines. This monitoring allows the clinician to detect when the pressure begins to fall and to substitute a full nitrous oxide cylinder before the original cylinder is empty. In addition, each nitrous oxide cylinder should be marked with the date the full tank was opened and the dates and lengths of subsequent use to facilitate the monitoring process and to prevent the clinician from running out of the nitrous oxide before the client care procedure is completed.

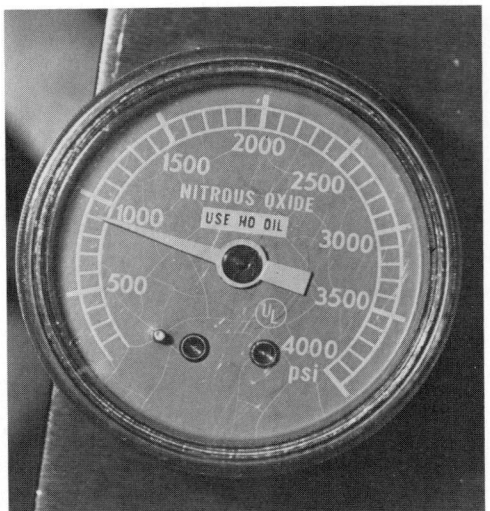

FIGURE 24–2
Pressure gauge for a nitrous oxide cylinder.

Oxygen is stored as a gas in green compressed gas cylinders and is delivered as a gas (see Fig. 24–1). The contents of the oxygen cylinder can be determined by the reading on the pressure gauge. A full tank of oxygen is reflected by a pressure gauge reading of 2,100 psi (Fig. 24–3). As the oxygen is depleted in the cylinder as a result of use, the pressure falls correspondingly as indicated by the needle

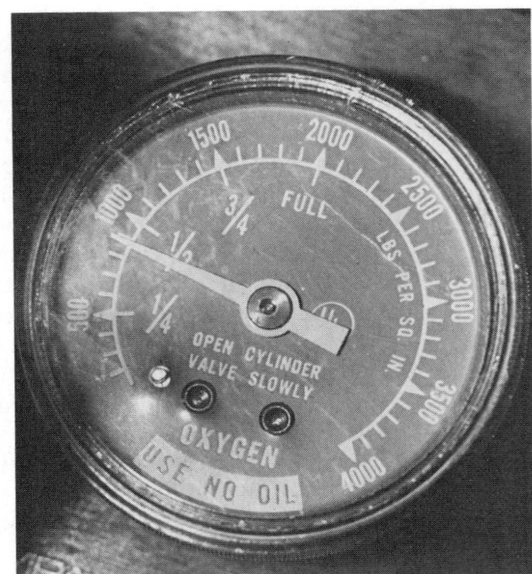

FIGURE 24–3
Pressure gauge for an oxygen cylinder.

Stage I	Stage II	Stage III	Stage IV
Analgesia Stage	Delirium (Excitement)	Surgical Anesthesia	Respiratory Paralysis
Plane 1, Plane 2, Plane 3		Plane 1, Plane 2, Plane 3, Plane 4	

FIGURE 24–4
Stages of anesthesia.

position on the oxygen pressure gauge. Consequently, one has an accurate assessment of how much oxygen is left in the cylinder at all times.

The blood/gas solubility coefficient of nitrous oxide is 0.47, meaning that 100 ml of blood dissolves 47 ml of nitrous oxide. This blood/gas solubility coefficient accounts for the rapid onset and rapid recovery from the analgesic effects of nitrous oxide sedation. Because nitrous oxide is 15 times more soluble in the blood than nitrogen, it displaces nitrogen in the blood. It does not compete with oxygen and carbon dioxide for combination with the hemoglobin molecule.[1,6]

PHARMACOLOGY

Nitrous oxide has no effect on the heart rate, blood pressure, liver, or kidney as long as an adequate amount of oxygen is delivered concurrently.[2,7] It does, however, have an effect on all sensations such as hearing, touch, pain, and warmth. With regard to hearing, clients report that they can hear distant sound better than close sounds. Consequently, clients under the influence of nitrous oxide may key in to background sounds such as music or the conversation in the next room rather than to what the operator is saying. In addition, nitrous oxide reduces the gag reflex but does not eliminate it. Therefore, if a client tends to gag, this sedation modality should be considered for use.[1]

PHYSIOLOGY

Nitrous oxide acts to depress the central nervous system. Specifically, it affects the cerebral cortex, thalamus, hypothalamus, and reticular activating system. The exact mechanism of action is unknown; however, it results in either altering the relay of nerve impulses to the cerebral cortex or causing them to be interpreted differently.[3] As a result, the individual experiences reduced anxiety and increased pain tolerance. Pain perception is not blocked, however, and nitrous oxide–oxygen must be used in combination with a local anesthetic for many procedures. Nitrous oxide does not combine with any body tissues, and it is the only anesthetic used that is not metabolized. The nitrous oxide molecule enters the blood through the lungs where it displaces nitrogen and eventually exits unchanged through the lungs.[1]

Nevertheless, there are toxic reactions associated with oversedation with nitrous oxide. Hypoxia (lack of oxygen to the tissues), characterized by a headache and nausea, is associated with receiving too much nitrous oxide and lack of a subsequent oxygenation period. In addition, bone marrow depression and white blood cell depression have been reported after prolonged administration of 2 to 4 days.

STAGES OF ANESTHESIA

The four stages of anesthesia are depicted in Figure 24–4. Stage I is the **analgesia stage.** In analgesia, the person feels pain, but does not care. The analgesia stage of anesthesia has three planes. The first two planes are relative analgesia, and these are the planes appropriate for dental hygiene care.

Stage II is the **delirium** or **excitement stage** of light anesthesia. This stage of anesthesia is characterized by hyperresponsiveness to stimuli, exaggerated inspirations, and loss of consciousness. For individuals receiving dental hygiene care, the immediate treatment of entry into the excitement stage of anesthesia is to increase the percentage of oxygen immediately to 100% and to turn the nitrous oxide off.

Stage III is **surgical anesthesia** and it has four planes. Oral and maxillofacial surgeons take their patients to this level of anesthesia and it is acceptable; dental hygienists never need to provide this level of anesthesia for their clients. Loss of consciousness by an individual receiving dental hygiene care indicates oversedation, and the immediate treatment is to increase the percentage of oxygen immediately to 100% and to turn the nitrous oxide off. The 0.47 blood/gas solubility coefficient for nitrous oxide promotes rapid recovery of the individual.

Stage IV anesthesia is **surgical anesthesia with respiratory paralysis.** This level of anesthesia is reserved for use when a person undergoes major surgery in a hospital setting.

As noted earlier, nitrous oxide produces intense analgesia, but it is a very weak anesthetic. In fact, usually one would need to give more than 80% nitrous oxide to achieve surgical anesthesia.[1] This pharmacological property makes nitrous oxide–oxygen a good pain and anxiety control modality for use in dental hygiene care.

INDICATIONS FOR USE

Nitrous oxide–oxygen sedation is recommended for use in the following situations[1,2,4,5,8].

- Mild apprehension
- Refusal of local and general anesthesia
- Allergy to local anesthetics
- Hypersensitive gag reflex
- Intolerance for long appointments
- Cardiac conditions
- Hypertension
- Asthma
- Cerebral palsy
- Mental retardation

Mild Apprehension

Individuals who are fearful of, or mildly anxious about, the oral healthcare experience are good candidates for nitrous oxide–oxygen sedation because it relaxes them and takes the edge off their apprehension.

Allergy to or Refusal of Other Anesthetics

Individuals who are allergic to all types of local anesthetics, those who refuse a local or general anesthetic for other reasons, or those who are unable to experience good local anesthesia because use of a vasoconstrictor is medically contraindicated are good candidates for nitrous oxide–oxygen analgesia.

Hypersensitive Gag Reflex

Individuals who are prone to gagging easily during oral healthcare procedures, such as those having impressions taken or their third molars scaled, are good candidates for nitrous oxide–oxygen sedation because this analgesic reduces the gag response.

Inability to Tolerate Sitting for Long Periods

Nitrous oxide–oxygen analgesia is recommended for persons with back problems or other conditions that make them unable to tolerate sitting in the dental chair for very long periods. This recommendation is based on the fact that nitrous oxide–oxygen analgesia makes one perceive that time is passing quickly.

Cardiovascular Disease and Hypertension

Individuals who have cardiovascular disease or hypertension are good candidates for nitrous oxide–oxygen analgesia because it decreases stress and exposes the individual to more oxygen than is normally available. For example, even at a gas ratio of 50:50, the client is receiving 50% oxygen compared with the 22% oxygen available in room air. This oxygen enrichment coupled with stress reduction is a major advantage of nitrous oxide–oxygen sedation for these medically complex clients.

Asthma

Individuals who have asthma are candidates for nitrous oxide–oxygen analgesia because during sedation they receive more oxygen than normally is available to them. This oxygen enrichment facilitates breathing and decreases stress.

Cerebral Palsy and Mental Retardation

Persons with cerebral palsy and mental retardation are candidates for nitrous oxide–oxygen sedation because they are sometimes difficult to manage in the oral healthcare setting and this analgesic relaxes them. The client, however, must be able to communicate with the operator, breathe through the nose, and cooperate by leaving the mask in place.

CONTRAINDICATIONS TO USE

There are no absolute medical contraindications to nitrous oxide–oxygen sedation, but there are some relative contraindications that make it a poor choice for certain clients. The following conditions contraindicate the use of nitrous oxide–oxygen sedation.[1,2,4,5,9]

- Pregnancy
- Communication difficulty
- Nasal obstruction
- Emphysema
- Multiple sclerosis
- Emotional instability
- Epilepsy
- Negative past experience

Pregnancy

Nitrous oxide–oxygen sedation is not recommended for individuals who are pregnant. Although there is no evidence that sufficient nitrous oxide crosses the placenta to produce depression of the fetal central nervous system, it is better to err on the side of caution with pregnant women given that long-term exposure to nitrous oxide is associated with spontaneous abortion.[1] In general, all unnecessary drugs are avoided during pregnancy, especially during the first trimester.

The Existence of a Communication Barrier

Individuals who have a language barrier or with whom communication is difficult should not be given nitrous oxide–oxygen sedation because communication between the client and the operator is essential for success with conscious sedation. The operator must question the client during the administration of nitrous oxide–oxygen to determine the appropriate level of sedation and the client's response to the drug. Communication barriers make it difficult or impossible for this monitoring to occur.

Nasal Obstructions

Individuals who have a cold, allergy, or other type of nasal obstruction are not good candidates for nitrous oxide–oxygen analgesia because the gas is inhaled. Nasal obstruction prevents the client from obtaining the benefit of the drug. Also, respiratory infections contaminate the tubing and reservoir bag.

Chronic Obstructive Pulmonary Disease

The respiratory systems of persons with emphysema, multiple sclerosis, or chronic bronchitis function on less oxygen than those of healthy individuals because these diseases affect the lung's capacity to exchange air. Consequently, they depend on a lowered blood oxygen level to stimulate respiration. The increased oxygen saturation of the blood made available with nitrous oxide–oxygen sedation removes the stimulus of the lowered oxygen blood level and may indicate to the brain that the individual need not perform as many inspirations, thus producing apnea.[8]

Emotional Instability

Nitrous oxide–oxygen is contraindicated for individuals who are emotionally unstable. Because this type of sedation causes a distortion of one's perception of reality, it can precipitate problems for clients with a history of schizophrenia or alcoholism. Moreover, individuals who have recently experienced the death of a loved one or who are going through a painful divorce often go through a period of emotional instability. It is, therefore, not recommended to use nitrous oxide–oxygen sedation because unpleasant feelings may surface under the influence of this drug and cause the client to cry uncontrollably.

Fear of Nitrous Oxide–Oxygen

Individuals who are fearful of having nitrous oxide–oxygen sedation or those with compulsive personalities who must always be in control may suddenly tear off the sedation mask from fear of the unknown or of becoming unconscious. In the dental hygiene care setting, a good rule of thumb is never to talk someone into being sedated with nitrous oxide. Individuals should be willing and wanting to try this sedation method.

Epilepsy

Nitrous oxide–oxygen sedation may trigger epileptic seizures in individuals with epilepsy. Therefore, its use is not recommended for clients with a history of epilepsy.

ADVANTAGES AND DISADVANTAGES OF USE

Advantages

- Excellent choice of sedation for the high-risk person with a history of cardiovascular disease
- Simple, relatively safe procedure to perform and not requiring the service of special personnel such as an anesthetist
- Equipment is not cumbersome and requires little maintenance
- Restraining straps and pharyngeal airways are not required
- Individual is awake and responsive at all times and the depth of sedation can be controlled moment to moment
- Onset and recovery are nearly always rapid
- Most adults being sedated do not have to be accompanied to their appointment by another responsible adult
- No need for preoperative laboratory tests or for food intake to be restricted prior to sedation, as is the case prior to having a general anesthetic
- No need for a special recovery room, or to monitor the person for a long time after recovery

Disadvantages

- Production of vertigo, nausea, or vomiting if too much nitrous oxide is given or if the operator fluctuates the levels of nitrous oxide too much during administration of the agent. (Aspiration is not a problem, however, because the client is awake and the gag reflex is not eliminated.)
- Individuals with extremely difficult behavior problems cannot always be managed
- When instrumenting teeth in the maxillary anterior region, the mask gets in the way

SIGNS AND SYMPTOMS OF NITROUS OXIDE–OXYGEN SEDATION

A "sign" is something that can be directly observed. A "symptom" is something that must be reported to one person by another. Thus, signs of nitrous oxide–oxygen sedation are observed objectively by the operator and symptoms of nitrous oxide–oxygen sedation are reported subjectively by the client.

Signs

Objective signs that clients have reached a desirable level of nitrous oxide–oxygen sedation are that they are awake but drowsy and relaxed in appearance (e.g., feet pointing out and hands limp). They have reduced reaction to painful stimuli, and respiration is normal and smooth. In contrast, if a client demonstrates hyperresponsiveness to stimuli and exaggerated inspirations, these are signs of oversedation and of the need to give 100% oxygen to the person and discontinue the nitrous oxide altogether.

Other signs that clients have reached a desirable level of nitrous oxide–oxygen sedation are that their blood pressure and pulse, eye reaction, and pupil size are observed to be normal.[2,7] Little or no gagging or coughing is observed. The client's speech is slow and tends to be guttural.[1] There may be some perspiration and tearing. Heavy perspiration and lacrimation, although possibly reflecting appropriate sedation for oral surgery treatment, are inappropriate for dental hygiene care and indicate a need to turn down the nitrous oxide. Likewise, uncontrollable laughing by the client indicates a need to turn the nitrous oxide level down. Following is a list of signs of baseline nitrous oxide–oxygen sedation appropriate for dental hygiene care.[1]

- Client awake
- Lessened pain reaction
- Drowsy, relaxed appearance
- Eye reaction and pupil size normal
- Respiration normal
- Blood pressure and pulse normal
- Minimal movement of limbs
- Flushing of skin
- Perspiration
- Lacrimation
- Little or no gagging or coughing
- Speech infrequent and slow

Symptoms

Subjective symptoms of nitrous oxide–oxygen sedation can be determined by direct questioning of the client as well as by observation. For example, asking "How do you feel?" or "Do you feel relaxed?" elicits desired information. If clients report that they are relaxed, that sounds seem distant, and if they indicate an indifference to their surroundings, these are symptoms that the desired level of sedation for dental hygiene care has been achieved. For instance, if the operator says to the client, "Shall I go ahead and numb up this area?" and the client replies "I don't care," indifference is apparent. Other desirable symptoms are client reports of lessened pain awareness during, for example, probing a previously sensitive tooth; and of feeling tingling, lightheadedness, a floating sensation, or waves of warmth over the entire body. A tingling sensation in the fingers and toes and then in the arms and the legs is usually one of the first symptoms reported, indicating a desirable level of sedation. The operator may begin by asking the client, "Do you feel any tingling in your fingers or toes or in your arms and legs?" Reported feelings of heaviness in the chest or of vibration or spinning, although reflecting appropriate sedation for oral surgery treatment, are not symptoms of appropriate sedation levels for dental hygiene care. Instead, they indicate a need to turn down the nitrous oxide. If the client does not respond to questioning, this indicates that he has sunk below the desirable level of sedation. The operator should immediately decrease the liter flow of nitrous oxide

TABLE 24–1
SIGNS AND SYMPTOMS IN RESPONSE TO NITROUS OXIDE AND OXYGEN CONSCIOUS-SEDATION

Concentration N_2O	Response
10% to 20%	Body warmth Tingling of hands and feet
20% to 30%	Circumoral numbness Numbness of thighs
20% to 40%	Numbness of tongue Numbness of hands and feet Droning sounds present Hearing distinct but distant Dissociation begins and reaches peak Mild sleepiness Analgesia (maximum at 30%) Euphoria Feeling of heaviness or lightness of body
30% to 50%	Sweating Nausea Amnesia Increased sleepiness
40% to 60%	Dreaming, laughing, giddiness Further increased sleepiness, tending toward unconsciousness Increased nausea and vomiting
50% and over	Unconsciousness and light general anesthesia

From Bennett, C.R. Conscious Sedation in Dental Practice, 2nd ed. St. Louis: C.V. Mosby, 1978.

and increase the oxygen by 2 L. If this does not produce a client response, 100% oxygen should be given.

The point at which a relaxed state of "floating sensation" is reported can be taken as the "baseline" level of sedation. *Baseline* is the ideal minimal amount of nitrous oxide with oxygen needed to relax the client. Once baseline is obtained, the person should then be maintained at a slightly reduced nitrous oxide level by reducing the nitrous oxide level by 1 to 2 L and increasing the oxygen level by 1 to 2 L. Following is a list of characteristic symptoms of a baseline level nitrous oxide–oxygen sedation appropriate for individuals receiving dental hygiene care.

- Mental and physical relaxation
- Indifference to surroundings and passage of time
- Lessened pain awareness
- Floating sensation
- Drowsiness
- Warmth
- Tingling or numbness
- Sounds seem distant

The percentage of nitrous oxide delivered to the lungs determines the sedative effect on the central nervous system. Although individual reactions at any given concentration of nitrous oxide may vary greatly from individual to individual, a range of responses may occur at given concentrations, as summarized in Table 24–1.

EQUIPMENT

Cylinders

Nitrous oxide and oxygen[1] are dispensed in steel containers called cylinders, which are colored green for oxygen and

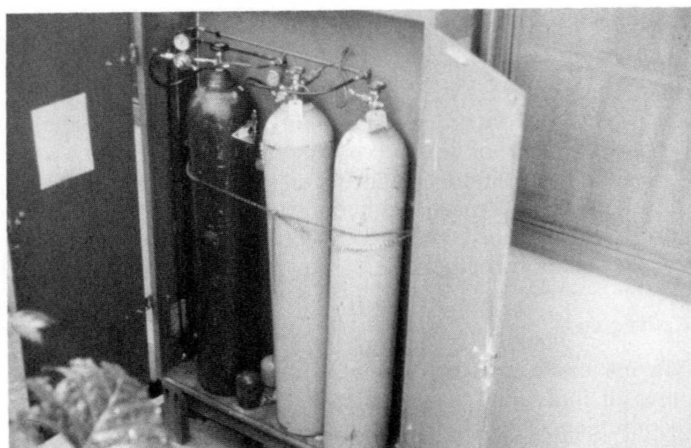

FIGURE 24–5
N_2O and O_2 cylinders stored in an area away from the gas machine.

blue for nitrous oxide (see Fig. 24–1). Cylinders should always be returned to the appropriate vendor for refilling. It is hazardous to refill a small cylinder from a larger one, and this should not be attempted by oral healthcare personnel. For quality control, cylinders are tested usually every 5 years by the manufacturer. The date of the test is permanently stamped on the cylinder. Cylinders should be stored in an upright position, away from a heat source, and chained to the wall to prevent them from falling on their cylinder valve stem, which could cause the cylinder to explode. In addition, at high pressures oxygen and nitrous oxide can form an explosive mixture in the presence of grease or oil. Therefore, grease or oil should never be used on cylinder valves and gauges on the gas machine.

Cylinders may be stored directly on the gas machine (see Fig. 24–1) or in an area away from the gas machine (Fig. 24–5). When cylinders are stored in an area away from the gas machine, regulation copper tubing with a ⅜-inch outside diameter is fed through drilled holes in the wall to a quick-coupling type of outlet. A quick-coupling type of outlet is ideal because it permits rapid hookup and disengagement of the machine (Fig. 24–6).

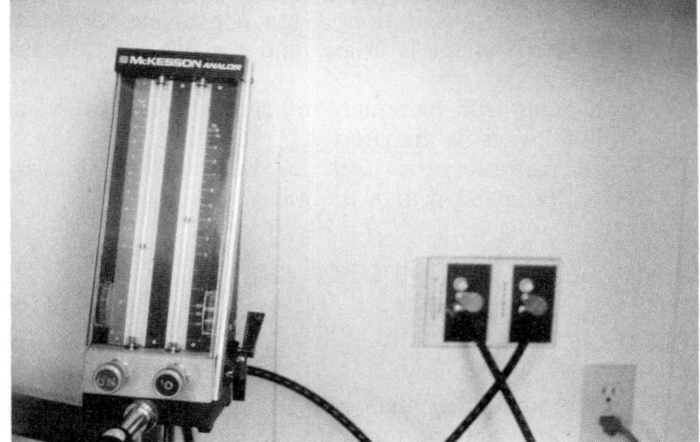

FIGURE 24–6
A quick-coupling type of outlet.

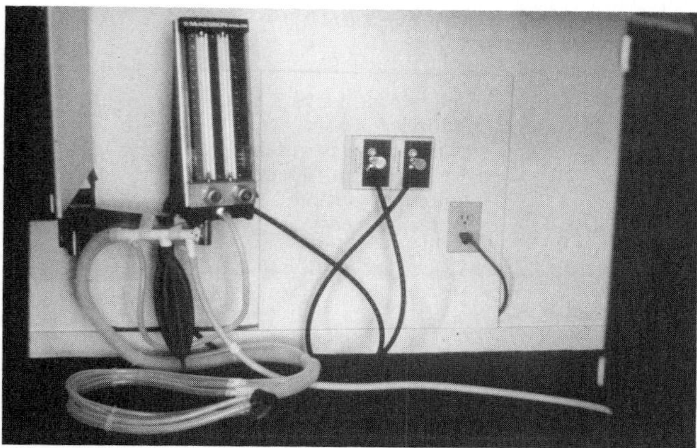

FIGURE 24–7
Gas machine with gas cylinder stored in an area away from the gas machine. Also shows quick-coupling outlet, reservoir bag, flow meter, and gas hose.

Gas Machine

Nitrous oxide–oxygen gas machines are available as a portable (see Fig. 24–1) or central system (Fig. 24–7). Components of gas machines are yokes, control valves, flow meters, pressure gauges, reservoir bag, and a gas hose. **Yokes** hold the cylinders in contact with the gas machine (Fig. 24–8). From each yoke, gas goes through an automatic pressure-reducing valve and then to a fine-control valve that allows the gas to be delivered to the client at 50 psi.

The **flowmeter** indicates the rate of flow of the gas. A small ball floats in the stream of gas that flows upward through a tapered tube. The greater the flow of volume of the gas used, the higher the ball rises. Separate color-coded flowmeters are used for nitrous oxide and oxygen, and each is calibrated to measure the volume of gas delivered (Fig. 24–9). Flowmeters show the exact volume and proportions of gas output from the gas machine.

The **pressure gauge** indicates the pressure of the cylinder contents (see Figs. 24–2 and 24–3). The **reservoir bag** (see Fig. 24–7) is attached to the gas machine and is the site where the gases (nitrous oxide and oxygen) are mixed and stored so that the client has a plentiful supply upon which to draw for breathing. The **gas hose** delivers the gas mixture from the reservoir bag to the client's mask continually at the volumes and proportions set by the clinician on the flowmeter (see Fig. 24–7).

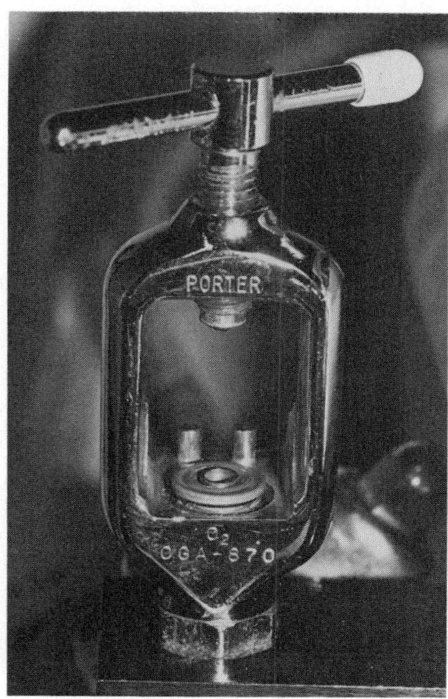

FIGURE 24–8
Yoke to hold cylinders in contact with gas machine. Note prongs that will insert into the valve stem of the gas cylinder.

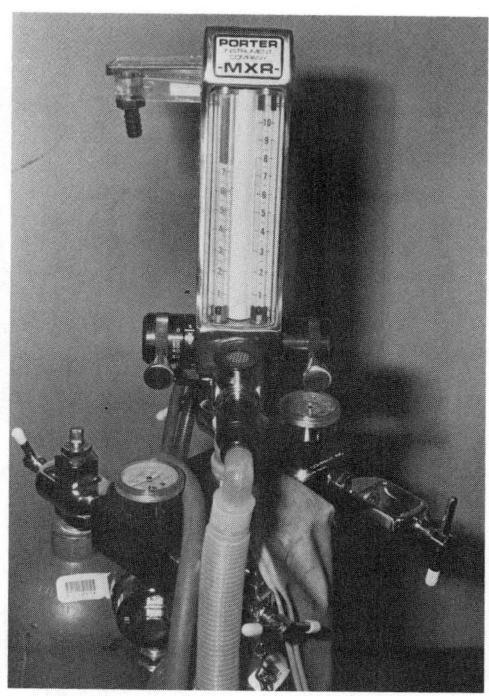

FIGURE 24–9
Flowmeter.

Mask

The mask is the nasal inhaler through which the client breathes the nitrous oxide–oxygen analgesic. Masks come with and without a scavenger system. If there is no scavenger system in place, the mask has only one hose coming off each side of it (Fig. 24–10). These two tubes carry the nitrous oxide–oxygen to the client. If there is a scavenger system in place, the mask has two hoses coming off each side of it (Fig. 24–11). One pair of hoses delivers the nitrous oxide–oxygen analgesic, and the other carries away the exhaled nitrous oxide–oxygen into the suction system. The purpose of a **scavenger system** is to reduce the nitrous oxide exhaled into the air by the client and thus breathed by the operator. Scavenger systems reduce the amount of nitrous oxide breathed into the environment from 900 parts per million (ppm) to 30 ppm. The ideal, maximal amount of nitrous oxide–oxygen allowable in the health-care environment is 50 ppm.

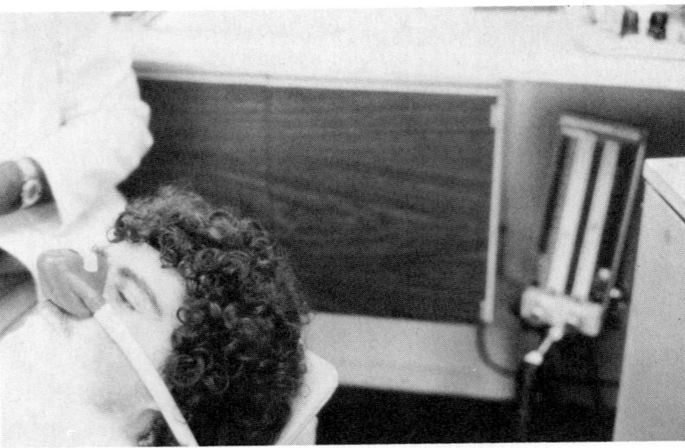

FIGURE 24–10
Mask with only one hose coming off each side of it, indicating there is no scavenger system in place.

SAFETY MEASURES

Safety features are built into cylinders and gas machines to prevent the inadvertent delivery of nitrous oxide when one is intending to deliver oxygen to the client. These fail-safe mechanisms are listed in Table 24–2 and explained below.[2,5,9]

Color Coding

Cylinders, quick coupling tubing, outlets, and pressure gauges are color coded according to the gas they contain and monitor. Green indicates oxygen and blue indicates nitrous oxide.

Pin Indexing System

Prongs (pins) on the yoke that hold the oxygen cylinder and the corresponding holes on the oxygen cylinder head are placed a specific distance apart, which is different from their counterparts on the nitrous oxide yoke and cylinder (Fig. 24–12; see Fig. 24–8). Thus, the nitrous oxide cylinder does not fit in the yoke that is to hold the oxygen cylinder and vice versa. Also, to prevent delivering nitrous oxide to an individual in the mistaken belief that oxygen is being delivered, the connection for the cylinders and hoses for nitrous oxide does not fit to the oxygen hookups, and vice versa.

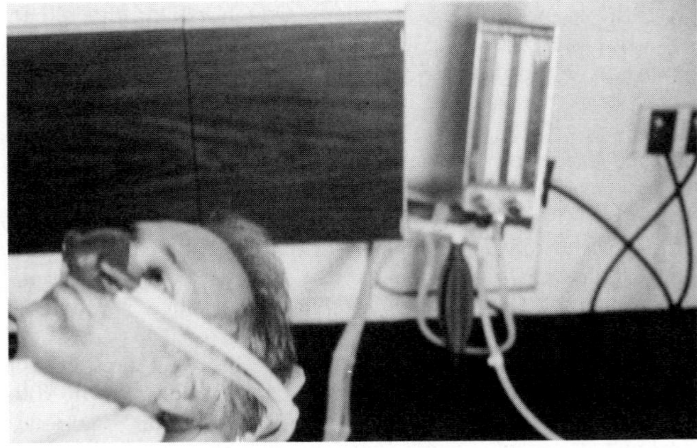

FIGURE 24–11
Mask with two hoses coming off each side of it, indicating that there is a scavenger system in place.

TABLE 24–2
SAFETY FEATURES

- Color-coded tanks
- Pin index system
- Diameter index system
- Audible alarm system
- Automatic turnoff
- O_2 maintained at 2 to 3 L
- O_2 flush

Diameter Indexing System

The diameter of the hole at the top of the oxygen cylinder and the corresponding diameter of the cylinder head that is inserted into the hole are different from the diameter of their counterparts on the nitrous oxide cylinder and cylinder head. Consequently, a cylinder head for a nitrous oxide cylinder does not fit into an oxygen cylinder. Thus, a diameter indexing system prevents an override of the pin indexing system, and is another protective mechanism for assuring that an adequate supply of oxygen always is delivered to the client.

Indicators That Oxygen Is Depleted

Many gas machines have an alarm that goes off when the oxygen runs out. Other machines simply turn off automati-

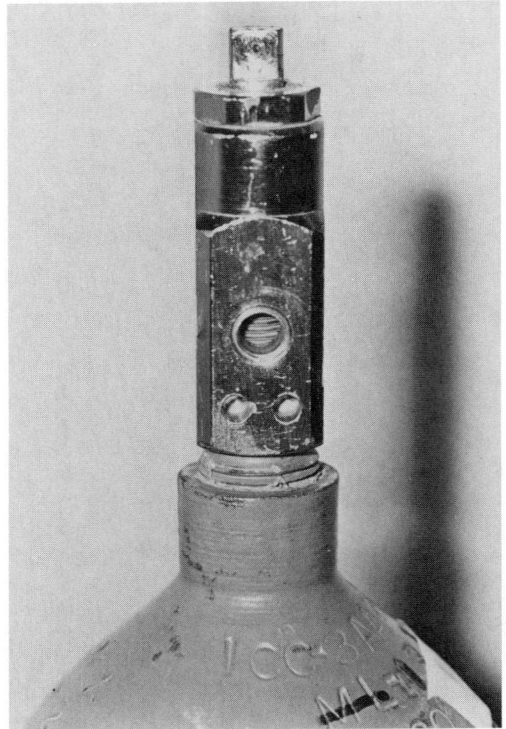

FIGURE 24–12
O_2 cylinder head, with holes placed at a specific distance apart to fit the prongs on the yoke that holds the O_2 cylinder.

cally when the oxygen is depleted. These features prevent the operator from administering 100% nitrous oxide to the client.

Automatic Maintenance of Minimal Oxygen Levels

On most gas machines, the oxygen flowmeter cannot go below 2 to 3 L of oxygen. When the machine is turned on, the oxygen volume automatically goes to 2 to 3 L. This constant flow of oxygen is provided at all times when the gas machine is on, thus preventing the possibility of providing 100% nitrous oxide to the client.

Oxygen Flush Button

All machines have an oxygen flush button that, when pushed, fills the reservoir bag with 100% oxygen and enables a high flow rate of oxygen to the client very quickly, if needed.

TECHNIQUE OF ADMINISTRATION

Administration of nitrous oxide–oxygen includes inducing the appropriate level of analgesia, monitoring the individual during the sedation, and oxygenating the individual for the appropriate amount of time upon completion of treatment. The office should have a quiet atmosphere throughout the sedation period. Specifics of technique are discussed below and summarized in Procedure 24–1.

All oral healthcare personnel who interact with clients should have experienced personally the sensations produced by nitrous oxide–oxygen sedation so that they can relate these feelings to the client. Preparation of armamentaria should be completed prior to seating the client. Upon seating clients ask them if they need to visit the restroom. If they wear contact lenses ask them to remove them because sometimes gas escaping from the mask can dry out the cornea and increase the risk of corneal abrasion.

After reviewing the health history and vital signs, the operator explains to the client that which is about to happen and describes the sensations of warmth and tingling that will be experienced. For example, the operator tells clients that they will feel very relaxed, as if they had had a couple of alcoholic drinks. The dental hygiene operator assures clients that they are in complete control in the sense that if they feel they are receiving too much nitrous oxide–oxygen sedation, they just need to inform the operator, who will turn down the nitrous oxide and turn up the oxygen.

The client's tidal volume is estimated. **Tidal volume** is the amount of air a person needs for one respiration cycle. For an average adult it could be from 6 to 8 L, depending on the size and metabolic rate of the individual. A flow of oxygen is introduced based on the estimated tidal volume. For example, if the tidal volume is estimated to be 8 L, the oxygen flowmeter is set to 8 L of oxygen and the nose mask is placed over the nose and centered on the face snugly to prevent leakage at the edges of the mask. If the mask is too big and gas is escaping at its edges, a gauze square may be used to contour around the mask to adapt it to the client's nose and plug some of the leakage spaces. Clients should be asked if they have enough air to breathe comfortably. If they do not, the tidal volume should be increased. If the air is reported to be blowing up their nose, the tidal volume should be decreased.

Once the correct tidal volume has been established and documented in the client's record, nitrous oxide is introduced at the rate of 1 L/min while decreasing the oxygen flow at a similar rate. A 1- to 2-minute pause is made between each adjustment until the baseline state is reached. Generally, for dental hygiene care, 50% nitrous oxide or less is effective for achieving baseline. Once baseline is reached, the operator should drop back on the nitrous oxide flow about 0.5 to 1 L, because with time the intensity of the sedation increases. This titration technique minimizes the risk of overshooting baseline and causing a problem by carrying the person too deeply into the excitement stage of general anesthesia.

Once baseline is reached, the dental hygienist should work efficiently and quietly, asking the client periodically how she is doing. Unnecessary talking should be avoided to allow the person to relate to the sedation and because client's talking expels nitrous oxide into the immediate environment of the practitioner. When scaling and root planing are completed, the nitrous oxide should be turned off and the oxygen increased to maintain the tidal volume. For every 15 minutes of exposure to nitrous oxide, the client must receive 5 minutes of 100% oxygen. Thus, if the client receives 45 minutes of nitrous oxide–oxygen sedation, she should receive 15 minutes of 100% oxygen. If an individual is sedated for less than 5 minutes, she still should be oxygenated for a minimum of 5 minutes. This oxygenation period is essential to prevent tissue hypoxia, characterized by headache and upset stomach, upon completion of the sedation procedure.

The tidal volume, the time baseline was reached, and the amount or percentage of gases administered should be recorded in the client's chart. To calculate the percentage of gases administered, the flow rate of a specific gas is divided by the tidal volume and multiplied by 100. For example, if the client's tidal volume (TV) is 7 L/min the oxygen flow is 5 L/min, and the nitrous oxide flow rate is 2 L/min, the percentage of nitrous oxide delivered is $2/7 \times 100$, which is 29% of total flow, and the percentage of oxygen delivered is $5/7 \times 100$, which is 71%.

$$TV = 7\ L$$

$$N_2O = 2 \qquad 2/7 \text{ or } 29\%$$

$$O_2 = 5 \qquad 5/7 \text{ or } 71\%$$

In addition to the tidal volume, the percentages of gases used, the duration of sedation, the length of the oxygenation period, the client's response, and the dental hygiene care delivered should all be documented in the client's chart (Fig. 24–13).

Text continued on page 738

Health Hx and vital signs WNL; TV = 7 L; N_2O = 2 L (29%); O_2 = 5 L (71%) for 45 minutes. Oxygenation period = 15 minutes. Client did well. Probing WNL scaled and polished. Excellent oral hygiene, no gingival inflammation observed throughout. Continued care interval 6 months.

FIGURE 24–13
Sample entry into client's record.

PROCEDURE 24–1

ADMINISTRATION OF NITROUS OXIDE–OXYGEN ANALGESIA

Equipment

Gas machine
Sterilized mask
Gauze
Saliva ejector

Steps	Rationale
1. Prepare the gas machine and related armamentaria prior to seating the client	Preparation of equipment when the client is seated may raise the anxiety level of the client
2. Check for adequate gas supply to complete the procedure	This check enables the operator to replenish the gas supply to ensure adequate gas is available for the procedure
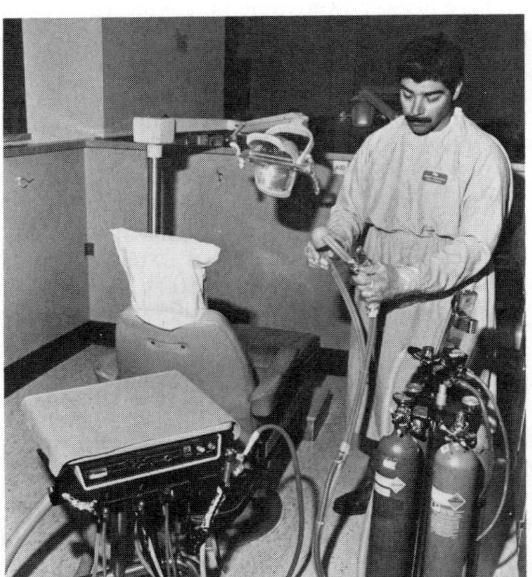	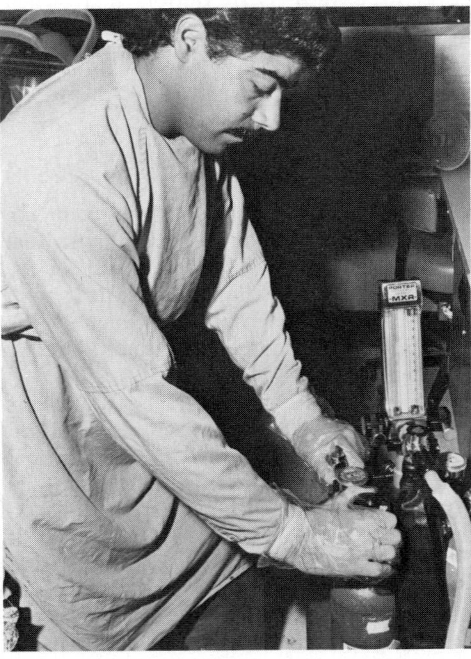
3. Obtain suction calibrator	Adjusting the suction calibrator allows the operator to obtain the optimal level of suction for the scavenger system
4. Attach the suction calibrator to the high-speed vacuum system and adjust the suction until the steel ball in the calibrator is made to float in the clear zone of the calibrator's window. Remove the suction calibrator from the high-speed suction system and tape the button used to adjust the suction in place.	Calibrating the degree of suction in the high-suction vacuum system assures that the suction removes the exhaled nitrous oxide–oxygen at an appropriate rate—not so fast that gas is removed before it has been inhaled, and not so slow that gas overaccumulates in the mask and leaks into the breathing zone of the operator. Taping the suction adjustment button in place prevents it from being moved and altering the degree of suction available.

Steps	Rationale

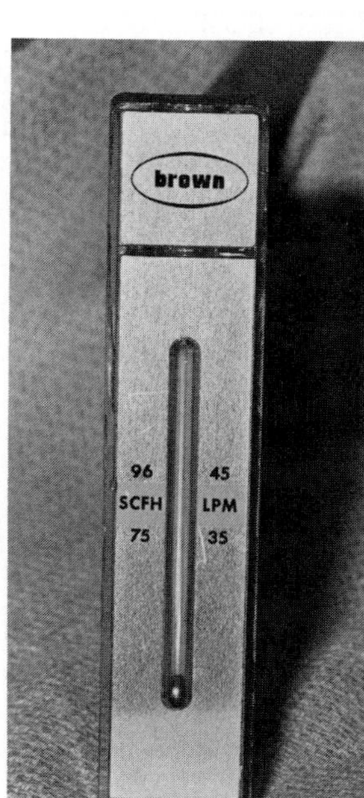

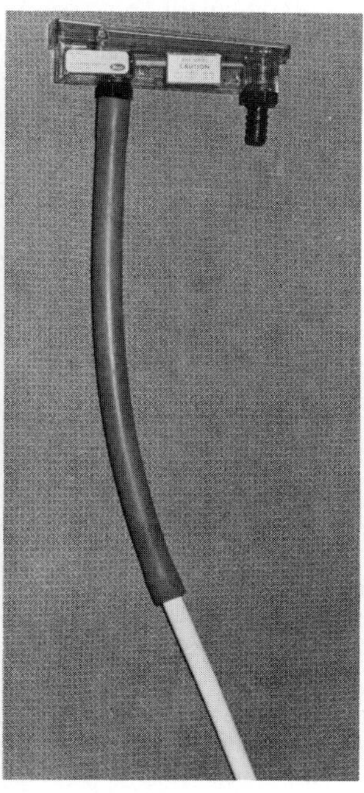

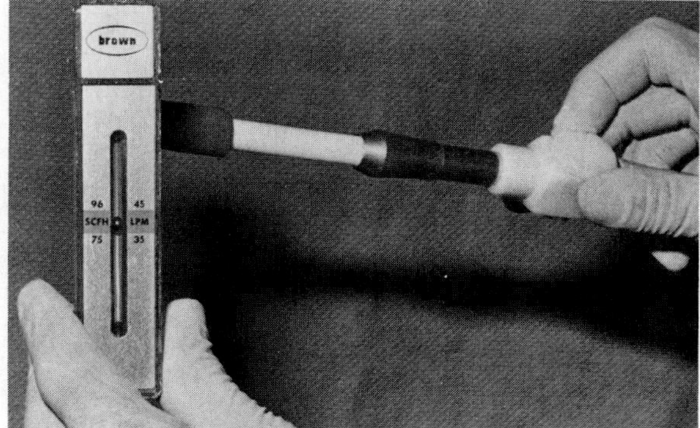

5. The sterilized nose mask has two hoses coming off each side of it. One pair delivers the N_2O-O_2 to the client and the other pair carries away the exhaled N_2O-O_2 into the suction system.

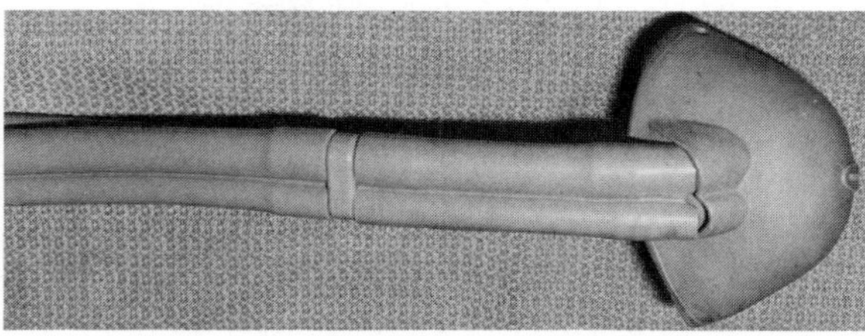

Each pair of hoses is joined by an adaptor. The larger adaptor connects to the gas machine. The smaller adaptor connects to the high-speed suction system.

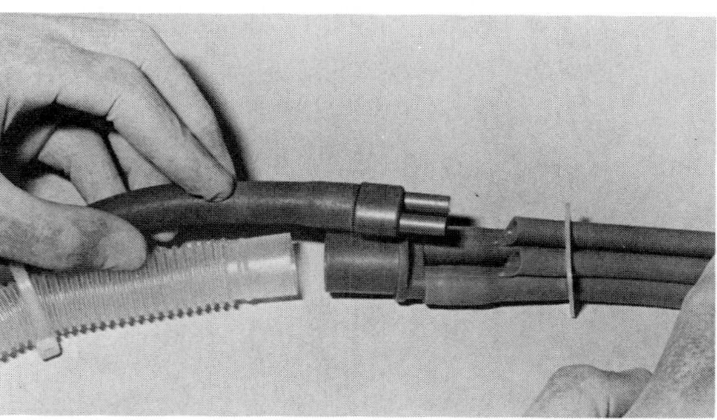

CONTINUED ON FOLLOWING PAGE

PROCEDURE 24–1

ADMINISTRATION OF NITROUS OXIDE–OXYGEN ANALGESIA *Continued*

Steps	Rationale
Attach the smaller adaptor on the nose mask to the calibrated high-speed vacuum system	This connection allows the exhaled N_2O-O_2 to be suctioned away, ensuring that nitrous oxide concentration breathed by the operator is reduced to 30 to 50 ppm from 900 ppm

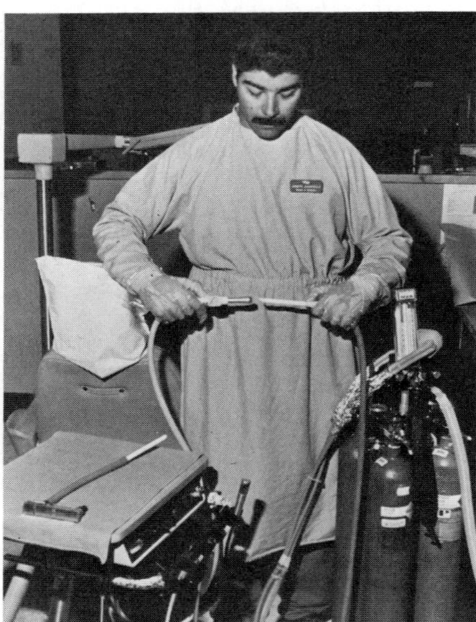

Steps	Rationale
6. Attach the larger adaptor of the sterilized nose mask to the gas machine. Turn on the gas machine.	This connection carries the gas mixture of preset proportions by the clinician to the client from the reservoir bag
7. Seat the client, check and record the health history, blood pressure and pulse	To meet the client's human need for safety, it is essential that her health and vital signs are within normal limits prior to providing dental hygiene care

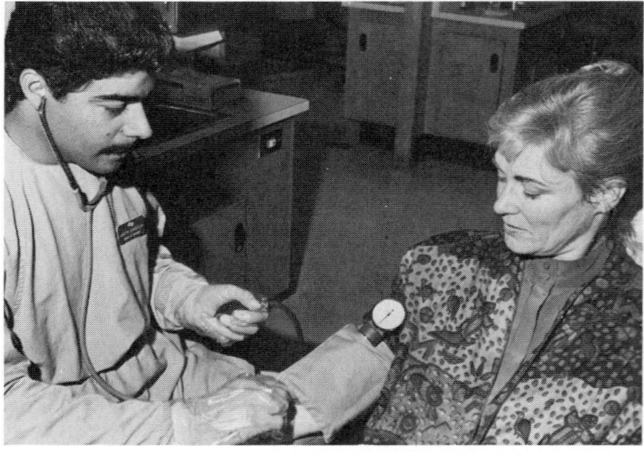

Steps	Rationale
8. Familiarize client with procedures; discuss nasal breathing and nose mask, and describe sensations of warmth and tingling that will be experienced; reaffirm the relaxing comfortable feeling the client will experience. Assure clients that they will be aware of and in control of their actions.	Informing clients about what they can expect to experience with nitrous oxide–oxygen sedation helps to prevent behavior problems based on the fear of the unknown, or of going unconscious. In addition, studies report that providing information to individuals receiving a drug increases pain thresholds and tolerance of pain. These findings suggest that influencing thought process in conjunction with giving analgesia can increase the depth of sedation.

Steps	Rationale
	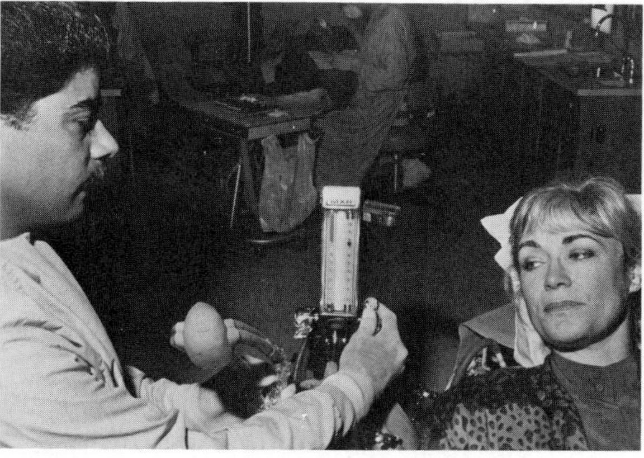
9. Start oxygen flow at estimated tidal volume (6 to 8 L/min)	This estimate provides a reasonable amount of oxygen as a basis for determining the exact tidal volume
10. Activate oxygen flush valve to fill the reservoir bag with oxygen	Filling the reservoir bag with oxygen ensures that there is enough oxygen available for the client's first couple of breaths
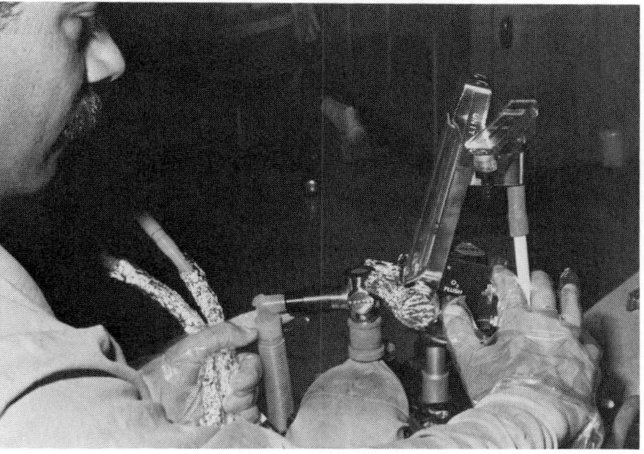	
11. Have client seat the nose mask on herself and adjust it so it is comfortable. Then, operator should adjust nose mask tubing to hold the mask in place, and confirm comfortable fit with the client.	Personal placement and adjustment of the mask by the client ensures a comfortable fit; adjustment of mask tubing holds nose mask in place and ensures a minimum amount of gas leakage from the mask
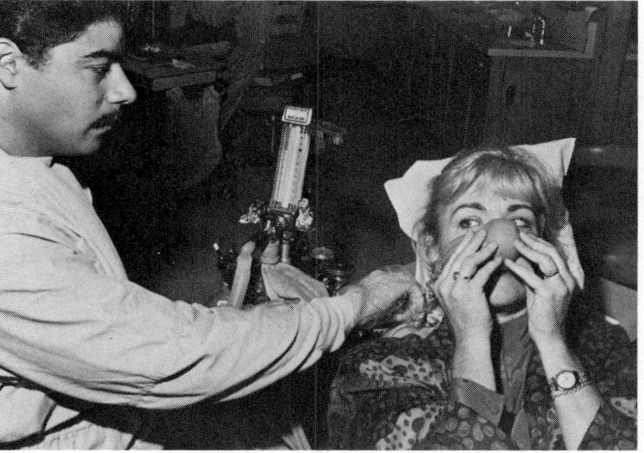	

CONTINUED ON FOLLOWING PAGE

PROCEDURE 24–1

ADMINISTRATION OF NITROUS OXIDE–OXYGEN ANALGESIA *Continued*

Steps	Rationale
12. If mask is impinging on a sensitive area on the face or if the mask is too big, place a gauze square under the edge of the mask	The gauze square makes the mask feel more comfortable if there is a sensitive area and closes any leakage if the mask is too big

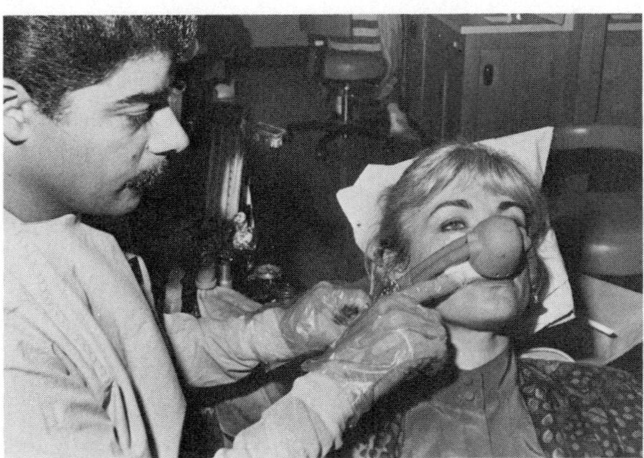

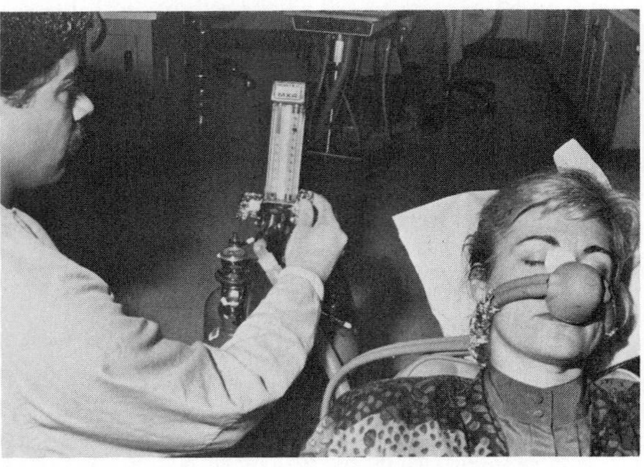

Steps	Rationale
13. Determine exact tidal volume by asking the client if he has enough air to breathe comfortably. Adjust volume of oxygen as per client response.	This determination provides the client with an adequate and comfortable amount of gas per respiration
14. Introduce nitrous oxide in increments of 0.5 to 1 L/min and reduce oxygen by a corresponding amount	Slow introduction of nitrous oxide allows the operator to find baseline for the individual and ensures that the client is not oversedated. Decreasing the oxygen the same amount that nitrous oxide is increased maintains the established tidal volume.

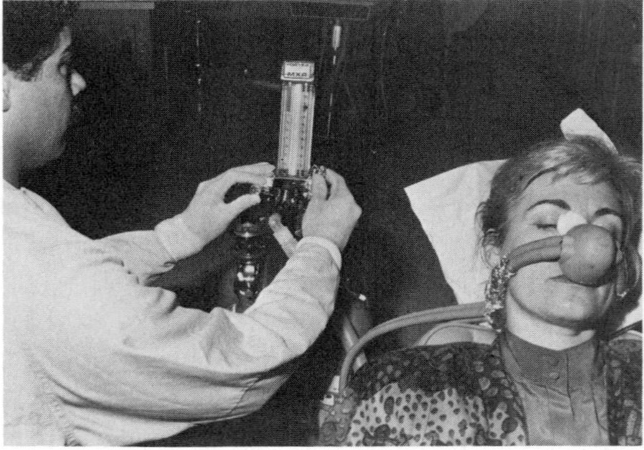

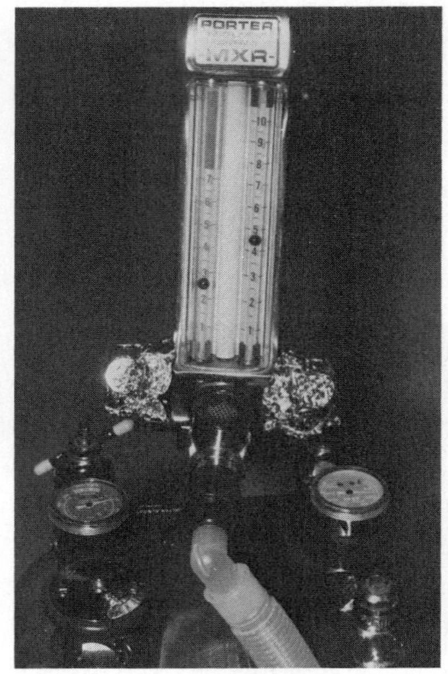

Steps	Rationale
15. Repeat step 14 at 60-second intervals until a baseline level is established. (This is called titration.)	There is a great deal of individual variation as to the amount of nitrous oxide one needs to achieve baseline. Usually the optimal concentration of nitrous oxide does not exceed 35%.
16. Determine client's baseline level using subjective symptoms and objective signs and document baseline nitrous oxide and oxygen volumes (or concentrations) as well as the time that baseline is established in the client record	Documenting baseline levels provides a reference for future nitrous oxide–oxygen sedation procedures. Noting time baseline is necessary to determine oxygenation period before dismissing the client.

Steps	Rationale
17. Monitor client and reassure as necessary; comment on how comfortable and relaxed the client seems	Checking with clients periodically about their comfort level allows the operator to reduce or increase nitrous oxide concentration as needed. The client should never be left alone while under nitrous oxide–oxygen sedation in case the level of sedation needs to be lowered or in case of emergency. Persons under nitrous oxide–oxygen sedation are very suggestible.
18. If nausea, sleepiness, dreaming, vertigo, repeated closing of the mouth, a rigid mandible, or restlessness is observed by the operator or reported by the client, reduce the percentage of nitrous oxide by 2 L/min to lighten the level of sedation	These signs and symptoms indicate that the concentration of nitrous oxide is too high and the client is no longer comfortable
19. When baseline is achieved, proceed with the care plan	At this level of sedation the client is relaxed and comfortable
20. Near the end of the appointment, discontinue the nitrous oxide and increase the oxygen concentration to 100%	Oxygenating clients 5 minutes for every 15 minutes of nitrous oxide exposure prevents diffusion hypoxia
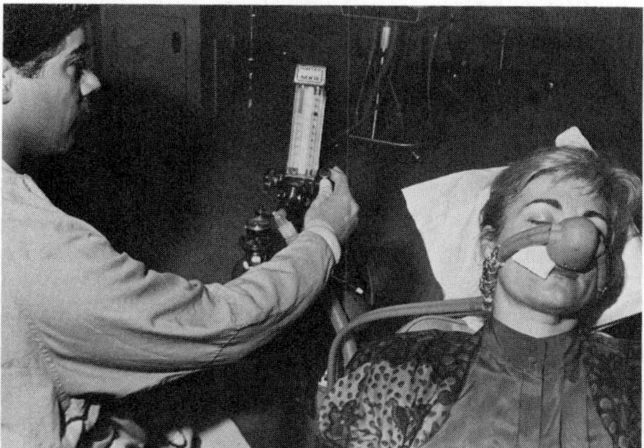	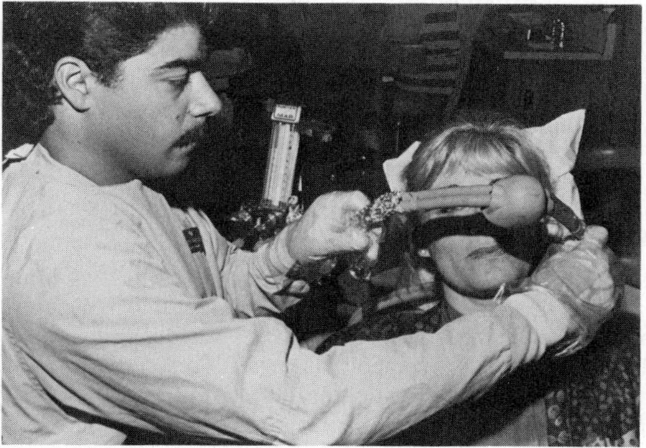
21. Remove the nose mask and slowly bring the client to an upright position	Bringing the client to an upright position in an abrupt manner may cause syncope
22. If the client feels normal, dismiss the client	After the appropriate oxygenation period, there is no additional recovery time needed if the individual states he feels normal
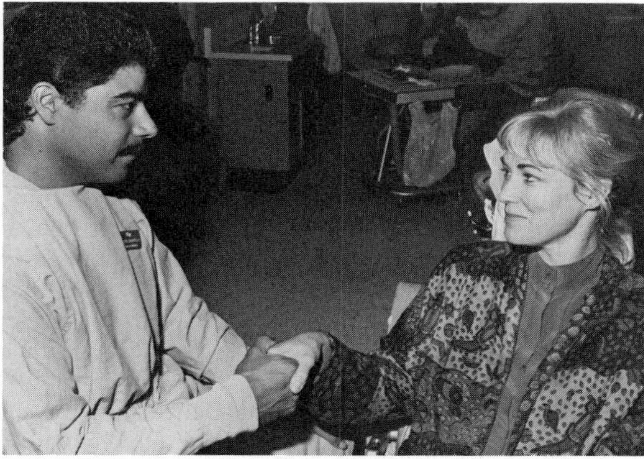	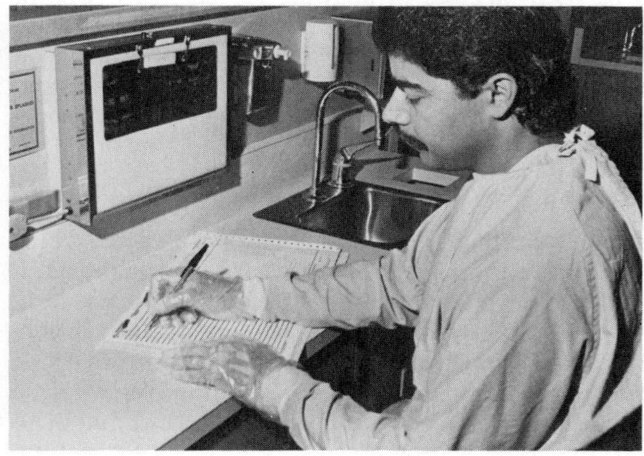
23. Document the experience in the client's record. Note vital signs, concentrations of nitrous oxide and oxygen administered, length of time of sedation and oxygenation, the care provided, and the client's response to the sedation	This documentation provides a legal record of care and also serves as a reference for future care and administration of nitrous oxide–oxygen conscious sedation

COMPLICATIONS[1]

Complications associated with nitrous oxide–oxygen analgesia can be mitigated by carefully selecting candidates based on their health and personal history, and by adopting the technique described above for the administration of this sedation modality. Specifically, inducing clients to an individualized baseline level by the process of titration and oxygenating them for an appropriate amount of time facilitate the avoidance of some complications with this somewhat innocuous agent. The following is a description of the complications associated with nitrous oxide–oxygen sedation.[1]

- Expectoration
- Nausea
- Vomiting
- Perspiration
- Behavior problems
- Airway obstruction
- Repeated closing of the mouth
- Rigid mandible
- Reluctance to awaken
- Emotional reaction
- Corneal irritation

Diffusion Hypoxia

Diffusion hypoxia, a lack of oxygen to the tissues, is characterized by headache, grogginess, nausea, and what generally may be described as a "hungover" feeling after exposure to nitrous oxide–oxygen analgesia. This complication is related to not being oxygenated an appropriate period of time following the completion of the sedation procedure.

Head Injury During Expectoration

A sedated client is at risk for bumping his head on the cuspidor if he attempts to expectorate while under sedation. Consequently, a saliva ejector or high-vacuum suction should be used in place of allowing the client to rinse or expectorate into a cuspidor. However, if such expectoration cannot be avoided, the clinician should place her hand on the client's forehead to guide the client to the cuspidor and prevent possible injury.

Nausea and Vomiting

Nausea and vomiting are associated with the client's being given too much nitrous oxide–oxygen sedation, although it also may occur when the client consumes a heavy meal prior to the dental hygiene care appointment. In addition, nausea can be brought on by seesawing the nitrous oxide levels during the titration process. For example, giving a client 3 L of nitrous oxide, then increasing the amount to 5 L and decreasing it back down to 4 L and then back up to 6 L in a short period can produce nausea. If a client indicates nausea (either verbally by self-report, or nonverbally by holding the stomach), the nitrous oxide should be turned down by 2 L and oxygen should be increased by 2 L. If the nausea persists, nitrous oxide should be discontinued and the client should be given 100% oxygen for an appropriate oxygenation period.

If vomiting occurs, the nitrous oxide must be turned off immediately, the mask removed, and the client's head tipped forward over the cuspidor to facilitate emesis. A high vacuum suction may be used to facilitate removal of vomitus. Give the client a cool wet towel to clean up and the treatment area should be cleaned as quickly as possible. Reassure the individual that he will feel better after breathing 100% oxygen.

Corneal Irritation

Leakage of gas from the mask can dry out the eyes and cause corneal abrasion in individuals wearing contact lenses. This problem can be prevented by having clients remove their contact lenses prior to administering the nitrous oxide–oxygen sedation to them.

Behavioral Problems

Several types of behavioral problems can be associated with nitrous oxide–oxygen sedation. Repeated closing of the mouth and a rigidity of the mandible are usually signs of too much nitrous oxide. Turning the nitrous oxide down by 2 L and increasing the oxygen by 2 L eliminates the problem.

Individuals who do not like to give up control are often threatened by the tingling and floating feelings characteristic of this mode of sedation. As a result, they may respond by suddenly sitting forward and taking off the mask because of fear of the unknown or of becoming unconscious. This problem can be prevented by carefully screening candidates for this sedation method, thoroughly explaining what they can expect to experience, and never talking clients into trying it unless they express a desire for this type of anxiety and pain control.

Individuals who are going through a period of emotional instability may be prone to crying under the influence of nitrous oxide–oxygen sedation. If this occurs, the nitrous oxide should be discontinued and 100% oxygen should be given for an appropriate oxygenation period. Careful screening of candidates prior to offering this sedation modality prevents this problem, which can be very embarrassing to both client and clinician.

Sexual fantasies and attempts at amorous behavior have been reported in individuals who have been given nitrous oxide concentration greater than 50% and who were sedated without an assistant as a witness in the room.[10] Decreasing the amount of nitrous oxide by at least 2 L and increasing the oxygen by a corresponding amount may solve the problem. If not, the nitrous oxide should be discontinued and 100% oxygen given to the client for an appropriate amount of time. Individuals who respond with this type of behavior problem should not be judged harshly, because they have placed themselves in the care of the clinician and have allowed their sense of reality to be altered based on the trust and confidence they have in the clinician. It is the responsibility of the clinician to protect the client while the client is under the clinician's care.

Equipment Malfunction

Contaminated nitrous oxide cylinders can contain nitrogen dioxide and on administration may produce nitric acid with serious consequences to a client. Valves on the nitrous oxide cylinders must be kept closed when not in use to prevent this dire circumstance from occurring.[1]

Hazards to Personnel

The effects of chronic exposure to nitrous oxide (1,000 to 15,000 ppm) reported in animal[11] and human studies of operating room personnel and of oral surgeons and others who used nitrous oxide in their practice[12–15] include:

- Spontaneous abortion
- Birth defects
- Bone marrow depression
- Anemia
- Hepatic and renal diseases
- Cancer

Hazardous concentrations of nitrous oxide in the oral healthcare setting can be reduced from 900 ppm to 30 ppm using a combination of the following methods:

- Use of a nitrous oxide scavenging system
- Fitting the nasal mask to the client as well as possible
- Discouraging client conversation and mouth breathing
- Venting the suction machine containing the exhaled gases outside the building
- Use of a fan to direct the nitrous oxide away from the breathing zone of the operator
- Maintaining the anesthetic equipment; testing for leakage, and inspecting the connectors at frequent intervals
- Monitoring nitrous oxide in the oral healthcare environment; a badge can be worn to detect nitrous oxide levels in the operator's breathing zone
- Opening a window in the treatment area to improve air circulation or using a nonrecycling air conditioning system
- Limiting the duration of nitrous oxide exposure for clients
- Shutting off and securing the equipment at the end of each day that it is used

References

1. Gordon, N. C., and Smith, R. Nitrous oxide/oxygen psychosedation for the general practitioner. Course syllabus, University of California, School of Dentistry, San Francisco, 1985.
2. Bennett, C. R. Conscious Sedation in Dental Practice, 2nd ed. St. Louis: C.V. Mosby, 1978.
3. Swepston, B. Dental phobia becomes euphoria: Advantages of nitrous oxide, parts 1 and 2. Dent Pract 1(5):60, 1(6):42, 1980.
4. Langa, H. Relative Analgesia in Dental Practice, Inhalation Analgesia and Sedation with Nitrous Oxide, 2nd ed. Philadelphia: W.B. Saunders, 1976.
5. Malamed, S. F. Sedation: A Guide to Patient Management, 2nd ed. St. Louis: C.V. Mosby, 1989.
6. Giovannitti, J. A. Nitrous oxide and oral premedication. Anesth Prog 31(2):56, 1984.
7. Roberts, G. J., Gibson, A., Porter, J., and DeZoysa, S. Physiological changes during relative analgesia—a clinical study. J Dent 10:55, 1982.
8. McCarthy, F. M. Essentials of Safe Dentistry for the Medically Compromised Patient. Philadelphia: W.B. Saunders, 1989.
9. DeMartina, B. K., and Garber, J. G. Analgesia in dental practice. Contin Dent Educ 2:5, 1979.
10. Jastak, J. T., and Yagiela, J. A. Nitrous oxide and sexual phenomena. *Dental Anaesthesia Sedation* 13(2):56, 1984.
11. Corbett, T. H., and Valeriote, F. Effects of low concentrations of nitrous oxide on rat pregnancy. Anesthesiology 39:299, 1973.
12. Cohen, E. N., Brown, B. W., Bruce, D. L., Cascorbi, A. F., et al. Occupational disease among operating room personnel: A national study. Anesthesiology 41:321, 1974.
13. Cohen, E. N., Brown, B. W., Bruce, D. L., Cascorbi, A. F., et al. A survey of anesthetic hazards among dentists. Journal of the American Dental Association 90:1291, 1975.
14. Eastwood, D. W. Effect of nitrous oxide on the white cell count in leukemia. New England Journal of Medicine 268:297, 1963.
15. American Dental Association Monograph Series on Dental Materials and Therapeutics: Safety and Infection Control in the Dental Office, 1st ed. Chicago: ADA, 1990.

25 Evaluation of Dental Hygiene Care

OBJECTIVES

Mastery of the content of this chapter will enable the reader to:

- Define key concepts used
- Define evaluation according to its purpose and relationship to other steps in the dental hygiene process
- Evaluate the achievement of client goals as established in the plan of care
- Explain the professional and legal rationale for the evaluation of care
- Explain the relationship between evaluation of care and quality assurance
- Discuss how participation in quality assurance programs contributes to the professionalization of dental hygiene

INTRODUCTION

During the fifth step of the dental hygiene process, **evaluation,** both the dental hygienist and the client measure the client's progress toward achieving the goals specified in the plan of care. At this time, the dental hygienist makes and records a determination of the client's goals and whether the goals have been met. A dental hygienist may perform an intervention competently, but if the action does not help the client achieve the desired goal, the action is ineffective and a new intervention must be implemented.

The evaluation of dental hygiene interventions directed at the achievement of client goals occurs periodically so that the dental hygienist can decide to:

- Modify the plan because the client is having difficulty in achieving the goal
- Continue the plan because the client needs more time to achieve the goal
- Terminate the plan of care because the client has achieved the goals (Fig. 25–1).

UNIQUE FOCUS OF EVALUATION IN THE DENTAL HYGIENE PROCESS

The aim of evaluation in the dental hygiene process is to ensure quality dental hygiene care that facilitates the client's human need fulfillment related to oral health and wellness. Dental hygienists are involved in the evaluation process from various perspectives, depending on their primary functional role. For example, dental hygienists use evaluative skills to measure:

- How well clients have achieved mutually established oral healthcare goals (clinician)
- The competence of fellow dental hygienists (manager)
- The quality of care provided within a facility (manager, consumer advocate)
- The degree to which various factors affect dental hygiene care and client oral wellness (research)

Because the unique focus of dental hygiene is to assist clients in meeting their human needs through the performance of those oral health behaviors and practices that lead to optimal wellness and quality of life, the client is always the primary concern during the evaluation phase. Failure to evaluate the client can lead to what has been referred to as **supervised neglect.** Supervised neglect of a client occurs when the client continues to require further dental hygiene care to achieve higher levels of oral wellness or to prevent or control the oral disease process, yet the client has been erroneously discharged from care thinking that a healthy state was achieved. Supervised neglect can occur in practices that have a "one approach fits all" philosophy. "Just do what you can in the time allotted," or "Do your best given the schedule," or "Everyone in this office gets a prophy and four bite-wings." In situations such as these, emphasis is on the mechanics of "doing," with too little regard for the human needs of the person and the impact of care on the client's needs and health status. Evaluation is always needed to determine whether the client's treatment goals have been attained, reactivating the cycle of the dental hygiene process of care. Evaluation does not meet every

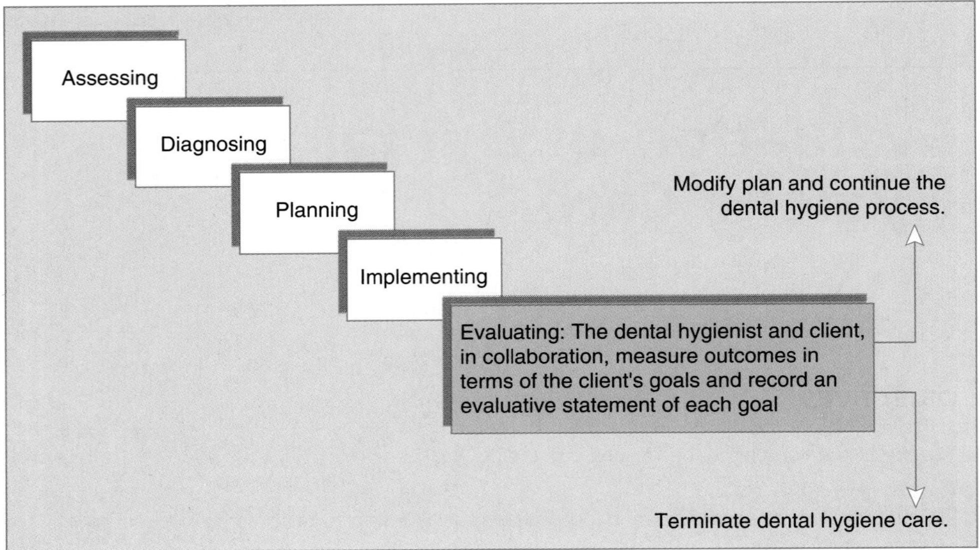

FIGURE 25-1
Evaluation phase of the dental hygiene process.

person's need, but it provides the assurance that human need deficits related to dental hygiene will not be overlooked or neglected.

THE EVALUATION PROCESS

Evaluation Criteria and Standards

The evaluation process determines the quality of dental hygiene care in relation to accepted criteria and standards. Although the terms "criteria" and "standards" are often used interchangeably, they have different meanings. **Criteria** are the qualities or characteristics by which knowledge, skills, or oral health status are measured. Criteria describe acceptable levels of performance by delineating the behaviors of the client or dental hygienist. The dental hygienist sets the criteria that are used to evaluate goal attainment. Examples of criteria reflected in client goals are:

- Client achieves a score of 1 on the Patient Hygiene Performance (PHP) index after using the toothbrush and floss
- Parent observes no more than three areas of gingival bleeding after flossing the child's teeth
- Probing attachment levels remain the same or are reduced by 1 mm
- Parent of client reports cleaning the child's teeth once each day
- Client uses gingival bleeding as an indicator of active oral infection for 1 month.

Standards are acceptable, expected levels of performance by the dental hygienist or other health professional that are established by national consensus. For example, the American Dental Hygienists' Association (ADHA) has published Standards of Applied Dental Hygiene Practice.[1] Each standard is further delineated by a number of components for measuring the quality of dental hygiene care provided (see Chapter 3, Introduction to the Dental Hygiene Process, Table 3-1). The ADHA standards are based on the dental hygiene process; therefore, evaluation of the quality of dental hygiene care is contingent on the use of the dental hygiene process. The standards and the dental hygiene process encourage dental hygienists to assess the client, analyze assessment data to formulate a dental hygiene diagnosis, develop a care plan that includes client goals and dental hygiene actions, and evaluate the client's response. Evaluation results in information that starts the dental hygiene process again.

In the dental hygiene process, criteria used during evaluation are the client goals developed during the planning phase. Because client goals reflect the desired outcomes in client oral health knowledge, behavior status, or values, and because dental hygiene interventions are directed toward the achievement of these goals, the goals are the evaluative criteria.

MEASURING CLIENT GOAL ACHIEVEMENT

Collecting Evaluative Data

The dental hygienist collects data during the assessment phase to identify client human needs deficits related to oral health; the dental hygienist collects data during the evaluation phase to determine whether the client goals have been achieved and the human need deficits related to oral health have been met.

Cognitive Goals

Knowing which data to collect is contingent on the types of goals established with the client. Several types of client goals may be established prior to dental hygiene intervention:

- Cognitive goals
- Psychomotor goals
- Affective goals
- Oral health status goals

Cognitive goals involve increases in the client's knowledge. Human needs related to dental hygiene care that provide the basis for cognitive goals are wholesome body image; nutrition; safety; and conceptualization and problem solving. Several cognitive goals may include:

- Mr. Smith will explain the relationship between bacterial plaque and gingival bleeding by August 17
- Mrs. Jones will verbalize the importance of fluoride supplements for her 1-year-old child by April 20
- Mrs. Thomas will verbalize the importance of removing her dentures at night before sleep by June 25
- John Smith will explain the effects of snuff (spit tobacco) use on the oral tissues by October 31
- Mary Jones will verbalize the relationship between sugar exposure in her dietary analysis and her dental caries activity by December 20

Methods used to evaluate cognitive goals may include having the client repeat information learned, apply the knowledge in a new situation, or share the information with significant others.

Psychomotor Goals

Psychomotor goals reflect the client's skill development. They can be evaluated by observing while the client demonstrates the newly acquired skill. The human need related to dental hygiene care that provides the basis for psychomotor goals is the human need for self-determination and responsibility. Psychomotor goals may include:

- Mrs. Allen will demonstrate the correct use of the interdental brush by September 10
- Mrs. Ross will demonstrate the desired toothbrushing technique that she uses on her disabled child by January 4
- Karen Long will demonstrate the use of an antimicrobial agent in an oral irrigator by October 1
- Mr. Ames will demonstrate the technique for oral cancer self-examination by November 23

Affective Goals

Desired changes in client values, beliefs, and attitudes are **affective goals.** Affective goals can be evaluated by observing the client's verbal and nonverbal behavior. Human needs that provide the basis for affective goals are the needs for a wholesome body image; freedom from pain and stress; safety; territoriality; and appreciation and respect. Affective goals may include:

- Mrs. Gordon states that the dental hygiene treatment has made her feel better about the way she looks by May 7
- Mr. Johnson says that he no longer feels anxious about seeking dental care by July 15
- Mrs. Damon indicated that her husband has noticed an improvement in her breath by November 9

Oral Health Status Goals

Desired changes in the client's oral health status, **oral health status goals,** reflect tangible outcomes and are the most definitive way of evaluating the effectiveness of dental hygiene care. Human needs that provide the basis for oral health status goals tend to be the human need for skin and mucous membrane integrity of the head and neck and the need for a biologically sound dentition. Oral health status goals may include:

- Ms. Lynch will reduce periodontal probe depths by 1 mm by December 15
- Mrs. Brangan will have no signs of gingival bleeding as measured by the gingival index by February 12
- Mr. Dunham will have no clinical gingival irritation from improper toothbrushing by October 15
- Dana Smith will have no new root caries by March 3

A reference chart for clarifying client goals and methods of evaluating goal attainment is presented in Table 25-1. Table 25-1 also presents the human needs related to the cognitive, psychomotor, affective, and oral health status goals.

Evaluation Statement

As demonstrated in the aforementioned examples, client goals also should reflect a time dimension. Clients need time to absorb information, integrate new knowledge, practice new skills, experience physical and attitudinal changes related to oral health and wellness, and assess the importance of these changes to their lifestyle. Time must be provided to the client to process information and to make lifestyle modifications. Therefore, a time frame is established and incorporated into the client goal for determining whether the specified change in the client has been observed. Client goals evaluated too early restrict the dental hygienist's (and the client's) ability to determine the impact of the care provided. Failure to evaluate client goals leaves the dental hygienist ignorant of the health status of the client and whether the care made any difference. From a legal perspective, failure to evaluate the status of the client after care may be grounds for negligence or malpractice charges because the client's oral health knowledge, behaviors, status, or values still may be contributing to an oral health deficit. When dental hygienists evaluate the **outcome** of dental hygiene care and record that outcome in the permanent record, it is an indication of willingness to assume responsibility for the quality of care provided.

During the evaluation phase of the dental hygiene process, the dental hygienist must record the degree to which the client goal has been achieved in an **evaluative statement** (Fig. 25-2). The evaluative statement contains the dental hygienist's decision on how well the goal was achieved and the defining characteristics that support the decision. Three possible decisions can be made about the client's level of goal attainment:

- Goal met
- Goal partially met
- Goal not met

One of these decisions, along with the supporting evidence, constitutes the evaluative statement that is written into the client's permanent record, signed, and dated by the dental hygienist. Samples of evaluative statements as they relate to the dental hygiene diagnosis and client goal are displayed in Table 25-2.

Factors Influencing Client Goal Attainment

Numerous variables interact in the healthcare setting to enhance or hinder goal attainment. The astute dental hygienist identifies both positive and negative factors that affect client goal attainment. Positive factors can be reinforced and negative factors can be resolved to facilitate the achievement of the desired oral health outcome.

TABLE 25–1
DATA NEEDED TO EVALUATE OUTCOMES OF CLIENT GOALS AND THE HUMAN NEEDS THAT PROVIDE THE BASIS FOR THE GOALS

Types of Client Goals	Related Human Needs	Examples of Client Goals	Evaluative Data Needed to Determine Goal Attainment
Cognitive goals: Reflect increases in client knowledge	Nutrition, safety, conceptualization, and problem solving	By 7/15, client explains why dental plaque contributes to his experience of root sensitivity By 9/10, client verbalizes the relationship between plaque and gingival bleeding	Have client repeat information in own words Have client apply knowledge in new situations Have client teach significant others new information
Psychomotor goals: Reflect the client's acquisition of a new skill	Self-determination and responsibility	By 5/7, parent demonstrates oral physiotherapy on the child (client). By 1/5, client demonstrates the proper use of the home oral irrigator By 2/7, client demonstrates removal of plaque from around dental implants	Have client demonstrate the skill Have primary caregiver demonstrate the skill
Affective goals: Reflect the client's acquisition of or change in values, beliefs, and attitudes	Wholesome body image, freedom from pain/stress, safety, territoriality, appreciation and respect, value system	By 1/15, client verbalizes that "flossing has become a ritual with me" By 2/10, client verbalizes that "daily flossing and toothbrushing have minimized the bad taste in my mouth"	Observe client's verbal and nonverbal behaviors Have primary caregiver share information about the client's response to the prescribed intervention
Oral health status goals: Reflect physical changes in the client	Wholesome body image, skin and mucous membrane integrity of the head and neck, biologically sound dentition	By 8/17, client will experience a reduction of 2 mm in pocket depths around tooth numbers 13, 14, and 30, 31 By 8/30, client will experience a 5-point decrease in the gingival bleeding index	Use physical examination techniques to collect data and compare to client's data recorded at an earlier time to determine change Use dental indices to monitor physical changes in bleeding, attachment levels, plaque

Positive factors might include:

- Client's interest in oral health, motivation, or sense of inquiry
- A family environment that values personal and professional oral healthcare and oral wellness
- A dental hygienist who keeps abreast of current knowledge in the discipline
- A work environment that values quality healthcare and offers incentives for dental hygiene care that meets or exceeds national standards

Table 25–3 presents common negative variables that can detract from quality dental hygiene care. Possible dental hygiene responses are presented to initiate thinking about overcoming variables that impede client goal attainment.

Modifying or Terminating the Dental Hygiene Care Plan

When the evaluation reveals that the client has made little progress toward goal attainment, the dental hygienist again initiates the dental hygiene process of care with the assessment (reassessment). New assessment data may be collected; dental hygiene diagnoses may be altered; goals may need modification; client's attitudes, beliefs, and practices must be considered; and dental hygiene interventions must be changed. On reassessment, the dental hygienist may find some common problems in how the dental hygiene process was used. Some common problems may include:

- Inaccurate, superficial, or incomplete data collected
- Invalid dental hygiene diagnoses

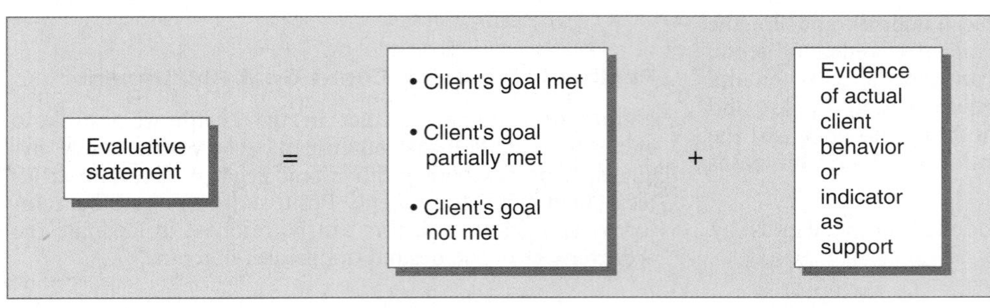

FIGURE 25–2
Components of an evaluative statement.

TABLE 25–2

SAMPLE OF EVALUATIVE STATEMENTS AS RELATED TO THE DENTAL HYGIENE DIAGNOSIS AND CLIENT GOAL STATEMENTS

Dental Hygiene Diagnosis	Goal Statement	Evaluative Statement
Deficit in self-determination related to impaired physical ability	Client will use a manual toothbrush modified with an enlarged, elongated handle at least one time each day by 11/1	11/2 Goal met. Client used modified toothbrush correctly two times each day
Deficit in wholesome body image related to wearing a denture and halitosis	Client will meet at least two other individuals who successfully wear dentures by 12/1	12/5 Goal partially met. Client met one person who successfully wears dentures and verbalized that the dentures looked natural
	Client will clean dentures, tongue, and oral cavity with appropriate brushes and dentifrice by 11/25	12/5 Goal met. Client cleaned mouth two times a day as directed and reported that spouse no longer complained about her bad breath
Value system: Potential to optimize oral wellness related to client's interest and enthusiasm about his mouth	Client will build on his already good toothbrushing and flossing technique and begin to use the perio aid on all molars present, at least one time every day by 5/15	5/20 Goal not met. Client felt that he was satisfied with the home care procedures that he was now using and did not want to regularly use the perio aid
Deficit in nutrition related to high sugar intake	Client will decrease her daily sugar exposure by following the recommended allowances of the four basic food groups by 10/15	11/1 Goal met. Client has decreased her daily exposures to sugar to once a day
Deficit in conceptualization and problem solving related to a knowledge deficit about the periodontal disease process	Client will verbalize the periodontal disease process and will identify plaque as a prime etiological agent by 9/20	9/20. Goal met. Client can describe the role of bacterial plaque and the periodontal disease process
Deficit in biologically sound dentition related to the signs of four carious lesions	Client will follow up on a referral made to the dentist of record and have the four carious lesions diagnosed and restored by 8/1	8/15. Goal met. Client has obtained needed dental care
Deficit in self-determination and responsibility due to an inability to perform dental flossing	Client will demonstrate the proper use of dental floss in all appropriate areas by 3/12	3/15. Goal partially met. Client can remove bacterial plaque with the dental floss in all areas except between 1–2, 2–3, 15–16, 17–18, 19–20, 30–31, 31–32

TABLE 25–3

CLIENT, DENTAL HYGIENIST, AND ENVIRONMENTAL FACTORS THAT MAY DETRACT FROM QUALITY DENTAL HYGIENE CARE

Variables/Factors	Possible Dental Hygiene Response
Client Variables	
Client who refuses to cooperate with therapeutic regimen	Determine underlying reason for the observed behavior; consider possible socioethnocultural factors Counsel and educate appropriately Communicate observation to colleagues to develop a consistent approach to care
Client who rarely communicates needs	Encourage client to communicate by asking questions Be nondirective in the educational approach Educate client to be an assertive healthcare consumer Consider need to involve primary caregiver, family, or interpreter in communication process
Dental Hygiene Variables	
Dental hygienist who gives 200% of self when others do not	Learn to leave work on time, avoid assuming work of others, leave work-related concerns at the workplace Work to positively resolve work-related problems; seek strategies that improve motivation and morale of colleagues and self Learn to view problems as challenges rather than insurmountable obstacles Develop a realistic sense of what can be accomplished in the given amount of time When resources do not permit quality care and strategies do not result in positive change, explore other employment options
Dental hygienist is bored	Seek avenues within the employment setting for growth and development; participate in staff development and continuing education programs; identify a project and become involved in it; initiate strategies to result in positive change Evaluate long-term career goals; seek advanced degrees Participate in professional associations Search for new position

Table continued on following page

TABLE 25–3
CLIENT, DENTAL HYGIENIST, AND ENVIRONMENTAL FACTORS THAT MAY DETRACT FROM QUALITY DENTAL HYGIENE CARE *Continued*

Variables/Factors	Possible Dental Hygiene Response
Dental Hygiene Variables *Continued*	
Dental hygienist is under stress from outside concerns, e.g., illness or death of significant others; marriage, childbirth, divorce, separation; conflict with roles as professional, parent, spouse; significant life changes	Evaluate whether this is the exception or the rule, and assess whether performance at work is less than optimal. May need to reduce work hours rather than "cheat" clients
Environmental Variables	
Inadequate supplies and equipment	Identify and document problems with supplies and equipment Talk with co-workers about their experiences Identify specific supply and equipment needs and discuss with employer
Inadequate time allotted to provide quality care	Identify and record the type of dental hygiene care required Relate client needs and outcomes to the level of care provided Demonstrate and document how more time can provide a difference in client outcomes Discuss with employer
Inadequate respect, recognition, and reward from employer	Identify and document incidents when respect, recognition, or reward were withheld Talk with employer about the specific incidents Give employer suggestions on how situation can be improved Search for new position Initiate cultural diversity training in the workplace

Adapted from Taylor, C., Lillis, C., and LeMone, P. Fundamentals of Nursing, 2nd ed. Philadelphia: J. B. Lippincott. 1993, p. 310.

- Improperly developed client goals; goals that, if achieved, do not guarantee a resolution of the problem
- Care plan that does not specifically address the client's goals and unique socioethnocultural characteristics; plan contains only general information
- Care plan has not been updated
- Failure to evaluate
- Inadequate documentation

Once the dental hygienist understands why the client has failed to achieve goals, the evaluative statement can be used to redirect the care plan. An example of a complete dental hygiene care plan and a sample dental hygiene diagnosis follow.

DENTAL HYGIENE CARE PLAN: YOUNG WOMAN WHO RECENTLY OBTAINED ORTHODONTIC APPLIANCE

OBJECTIVE DATA

1. No significant findings in the health history
2. Class II, div. II malocclusion
3. Generalized, moderate gingivitis
4. Recent rapid weight loss
5. Fair bacterial plaque control
6. PHP index = 1.7
7. GI index = 0.9
8. DMF index = 5.4
9. No active dental caries
10. Wears orthodontic appliances

SUBJECTIVE DATA

1. Ms. Smith verbalized that "Not very many 16-year-olds at my school wear braces." "I can't wait to get them off!" "I can't stand to look at myself in the mirror." "Food sticks to my braces, and I feel embarrassed if the braces retain food." "I can't eat in the cafeteria at school or when I go out with my friends on weekends."

Dental Hygiene Diagnosis	Due To or Related To	As Evidenced By	Goals/Expected Behavior
Deficit in the need for a wholesome body image	• Acquisition of orthodontic appliances	• Unwillingness to smile, constant negative referral to the appliances, anxiety about wearing appliances	• Increase in smiling behavior after 1 month • Verbalizes acceptance of appliances after 2 months

DENTAL HYGIENE CARE PLAN: YOUNG WOMAN WHO RECENTLY OBTAINED ORTHODONTIC APPLIANCE *Continued*

DENTAL HYGIENE INTERVENTIONS

1. Compliment client on appearance.
2. Assist Ms. Smith in visualizing her altered body image and the temporary status of the orthodontic appliances.
3. Emphasize that the altered body image is a normal part of wearing orthodontic appliances.

EVALUATIVE STATEMENTS

1. By 2/25, goal is met. Client readily smiles and verbalizes that she is used to the appliances.
2. By 3/30, goal is partially met. Client verbalizes that the braces aren't so bad after all.

Dental Hygiene Diagnosis	Due To or Related To	As Evidenced By	Goals/ Expected Behavior
Deficit in the need for nutrition	• Inability to eat and a lack of desire to eat	• Loss of weight and anxiety about wearing orthodontic appliances	• Client will experience adequate nutrition by 5/25 • Client's weight will become stabilized by 5/25

DENTAL HYGIENE INTERVENTIONS

1. Describe dietary needs of adolescents.
   - Explain use of food pyramid
   - Review a basic food plan
2. Instruct Ms. Smith in the process of keeping a food diary.
3. After 1 week, review food diary and lead Ms. Smith to identify areas of concern that may be contributing to undernutrition:
   - Discuss alternative food choices (e.g., foods that are less retentive)
   - Explain how good nutrition will enable her to cope better with the appliances
4. After 1 month, check with client about eating habits and body weight.
5. After 2 months check with client about eating habits and body weight.

EVALUATIVE STATEMENTS

1. By 5/25, goal has been met. Client is able to select healthy foods, as reflected in the diary. Client reports feeling better since the change in diet.
2. Goal has been met. Client has not lost any more weight since her first appointment.

When all the client goals have been achieved and no new problems have been identified, the dental hygienist and client have achieved the ultimate purpose of dental hygiene care—placing the responsibility for oral health maintenance under the full control of the individual. Throughout dental hygiene care, the client has been educated to assume control over his own oral health. Written and verbal instructions should be given to the client to take home, and signs and symptoms of any possible future problems should be fully understood. "The [client] and his family [or primary caregiver] should be able to verbalize the type of problems they should be avoiding and preventing, the correct management of their specific problems, and the resources that they may be planning to use to improve their health."[2]

PROGRAMS TO EVALUATE QUALITY DENTAL HYGIENE CARE

In addition to each dental hygienist's evaluation of client goal achievement, formal mechanisms exist to ensure quality dental hygiene care. Agencies such as the State Boards of Dentistry, State Committee on Dental Hygiene, American Dental Association (ADA) Commission on Dental Accreditation, and National Board Dental Hygiene Examination Committee are concerned with quality care and quality control. In 1982, the ADHA Commission for Assurance of Competence (1979) and Task Force to Develop Standards of Practice (1980) developed a detailed plan for the Competence Assurance Program that included components of assessment, postgraduate education, and recognition of achievement. Since that time, efforts are continuing toward development of the various aspects of the program. Most alternative healthcare delivery and financing systems, such as health maintenance organizations, prepaid healthcare plans, exclusive provider organizations, and preferred provider organizations, have quality assurance programs.

Methods of Evaluating Dental Hygiene Care

Evaluation of dental hygiene care has implications that extend to the entire dental profession. Factors such as the

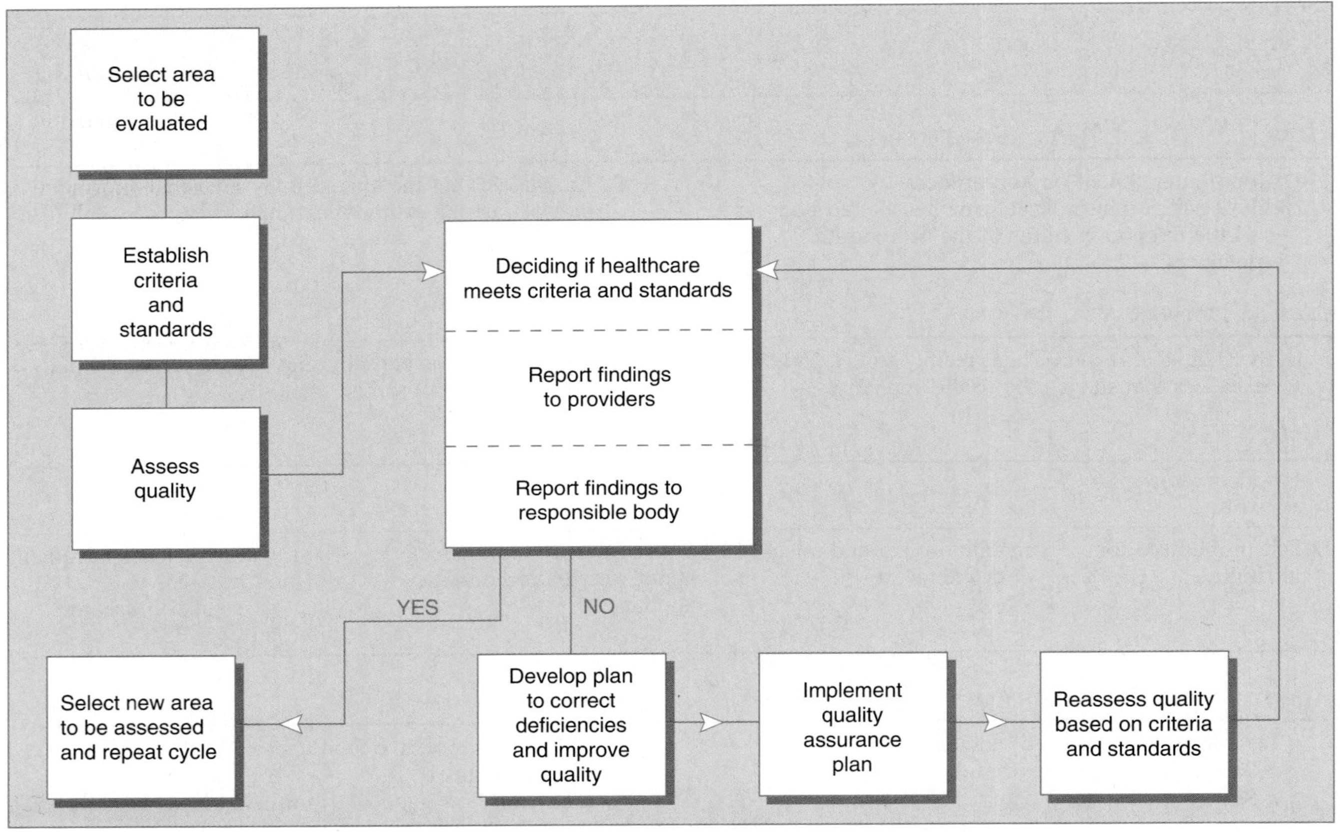

FIGURE 25–3
Basic elements of a quality assurance program. (Modified from DiAngelis, A. J. Quality assurance: Definitions and directions for the 1980s. Journal of Dental Education 48:27, 1984; as adapted from Bailit, N. L. Quality assurance in general dentistry. Part II. Compendium of Continuing Education in Dentistry 1:177, 1980.)

increase in healthcare costs, the proliferation of dental prepayment mechanisms to control cost, the implementation of Professional Standards Review Organization legislation aimed at controlling quality of care, the consumer demand for participation in healthcare, and the increase in litigation against healthcare providers all have influenced the expansion of quality assurance activities in the healthcare arena.

Quality assurance refers to all activities that are directed toward the maintenance or improvement of a standard of excellence in healthcare. A **quality assurance program** is a highly developed and coordinated structure of processes, criteria, and evaluation mechanisms implemented to determine quality of care provided and strategies for improving quality if necessary.

Healthcare is considered to be of quality if it is executed in a technically acceptable way, if it is available to clients, if it is appropriate for meeting the needs of the client, and if it is provided in a timely, cost-effective manner. Whereas a quality assurance program must be concerned with technical quality, client satisfaction, client access to care, cost, and timeliness, measurement of these factors is not enough.[3] To be effective, quality assurance must go beyond assessment to provide performance feedback to the healthcare providers, so that they can implement corrective action if necessary and periodically report results to responsible bodies.[4] The basic elements of a quality assurance program are diagrammed in Figure 25–3.

The evaluation of dental hygiene care and client outcomes may be determined during the process of care and is termed a **concurrent evaluation.** Concurrent evaluations use pretreatment review of services, review of appropriateness of care, direct observation of dental hygiene care, records review, and client interviews to determine whether specified evaluative criteria are met.

A **retrospective evaluation** of dental hygiene care occurs after the client care has been completed and may be conducted using client interviews to determine the level of client satisfaction, or may include chart reviews or questionnaires to collect data. A **dental hygiene audit** is a method of evaluating dental hygiene care by reviewing client records to assess the outcomes of dental hygiene care. The audit depends on appropriate documentation by the dental hygienist. These and other mechanisms to ensure quality of care are explained in more detail in Chapter 40.

SUMMARY

Evaluation is a critical component of the dental hygiene process to document dental hygiene success in achieving a desired outcome in the client's oral health status. Furthermore, it is a management strategy to minimize the risk of litigation. Without evaluation, a dental hygienist's contribution to the oral health of the client becomes invisible and undervalued.

Over the past few decades, evaluation of client care has branched into an expanded responsibility for all healthcare providers in the assurance of quality healthcare. Participation in a quality assurance program is an integral component of professional dental hygiene practice and meets the accountability requirements expected of a true profession. Evaluation, when carefully planned, executed, and documented, can result in benefits to the client, society, and the profession of dental hygiene.

References

1. American Dental Hygienists' Association. Standards of Applied Dental Hygiene Practice. Chicago: American Dental Hygienists' Association, 1985.
2. Alfaro, R. Application of Nursing Process: A Step-by-Step Guide. Philadelphia: J. B. Lippincott, 1986.
3. Atchison, K. A. The levels of quality assurance in dentistry. Journal of Dental Education 53(11):670, 1989.
4. Jerge, C. R., and Orlowski, R. M. Quality assurance and the dental record. Dental Clinics of North America 29(3):483, 1985.
5. Taylor, C., Lillis, C., and LeMone, P. Fundamentals of Nursing, 2nd ed. Philadelphia: J. B. Lippincott, 1993.

Suggested Readings

O'Hehir, T. Planning treatment. RDH 4(4):18, 1984.

Yura, H., and Walsh, M. The Nursing Process, 5th ed. Norwalk, CT: Appleton & Lange, 1988.

VI DENTAL HYGIENE CARE FOR INDIVIDUALS WITH SPECIAL NEEDS

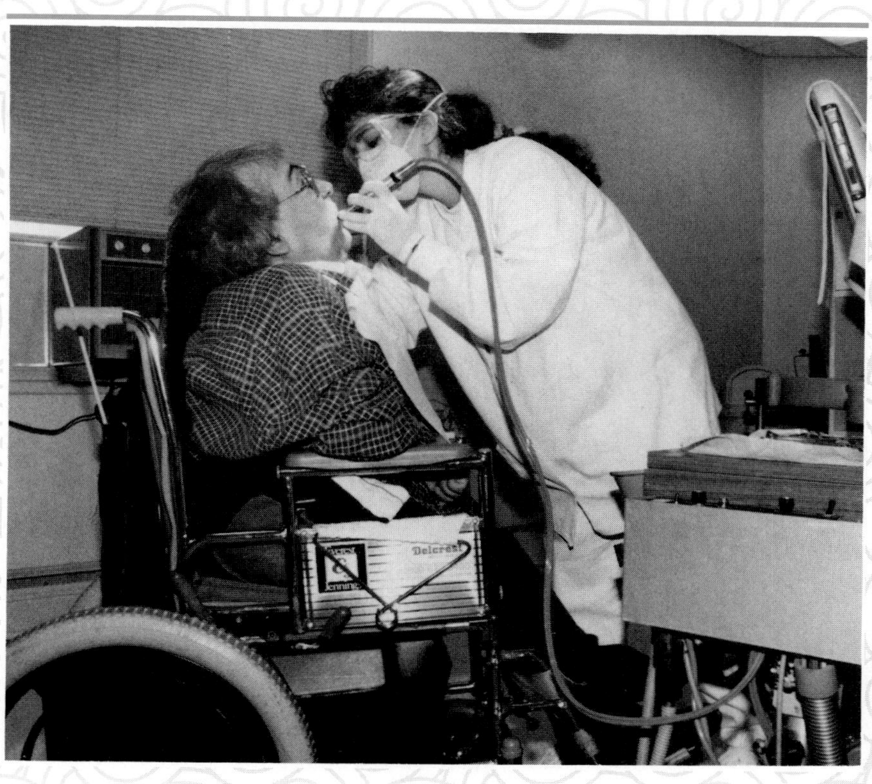

26 Basic Principles of Working with Clients with Special Dental Hygiene Care Needs

OBJECTIVES

Mastery of the content of this chapter will enable the reader to:

- Define the key terms used
- Discuss the historical development of the concept of rehabilitation
- Identify several barriers that limit access to healthcare services for clients with special needs
- Discuss the interrelationship between the concepts of normalization and mainstreaming, and describe how these concepts contribute to the process of deinstitutionalization
- Discuss the significance of the Education for All Handicapped Children Act of 1975, and the current impact that this law has on educational methods used today
- Appreciate how negative stereotypes and attitudes of the public have affected the acceptance of physically and mentally challenged persons into society
- Design a dental hygiene care facility that meets the federal barrier-free design standards for accessibility
- Contrast the terms "disability" and "handicap," and provide a correct example of use for each term
- Identify several examples of positive and negative portrayal issues associated with persons with special needs
- Discuss the significance of the Vocational Rehabilitation Act of 1973 and the Americans with Disabilities Act of 1992 in relationship to employment, healthcare, and educational opportunities for the disabled
- Distinguish between congenital disabilities, developmental disabilities, and acquired disabilities, and provide an example of each
- Discuss three ways in which disabilities can be categorized
- State the five activities of daily living
- Describe several types of devices available for clients to use to assist with accomplishing the activities of daily living
- Discuss the periodontal implications of long-term use of a mouthstick for the client who is paralyzed
- Describe assessment techniques used to determine the client's range of motion, grip strength, and finger closure when designing oral hygiene assistive devices
- Identify appropriate methods used to stabilize a client during dental hygiene care
- Differentiate between one-person and two-person wheelchair transfer techniques
- Identify the signs of autonomic dysreflexia, and describe dental hygiene management strategies associated with prevention and intervention of this condition
- Apply the dental hygiene process to the oral healthcare of persons with special needs
- Describe how the dental hygienist can serve as an advocate for clients with special needs

INTRODUCTION

The rising costs of healthcare and technological advances in medicine have resulted in an increased number of medically compromised and disabled individuals living within the community outside of institutional care settings. Consequently, dental hygienists practicing within the private sector have more opportunities to address the often complex medical, oral, and psychosocial needs of this ever-growing population group. The care of the client with special needs poses unique challenges in decision making for the dental hygienist.

Historically, disabilities have existed since the beginning of known civilization.[1] Medical descriptions of disabled people were recorded throughout ancient history. People were described as being afflicted or diseased and were generally treated as outcasts by the rest of the community. It was not until the turn of the eighteenth century that possible explanations for these disorders began to be addressed. Early medical scholars began to develop a model of how the human body worked, and they attempted to uncover clues as to how deficits and deformities occurred in human development.

Throughout the 1900s, tremendous advances in technology and research fostered a better understanding of human physiology and disease. Despite these advances, care of disabled and chronically ill people continued to focus on care delivery from a custodial perspective, promoting the segregation of those deemed as "different" or "sick" from the rest of the population. Institutionalization of those unable to care for themselves or of those requiring constant medical attention remained an adequate solution to the health problems presented by the disabled.

The advent of two world wars brought to medical science the new concept of **rehabilitation,** a process in which individuals with functional deficits could be retrained to live and work independently. Following World War II, numerous acts of legislation promoted the development of and access to rehabilitative programs to address the large numbers of veterans returning home after the war with disabilities. Many of these veterans were not "sick" but were permanently disfigured or impaired from their war injuries. The goal of rehabilitative medicine was to assist veterans with functional problems to relearn skills needed to return to their jobs and homes in their original contributing roles. The tremendous needs presented by the disabled veterans created an increased awareness of the needs of other disabled individuals, such as disabled children and elderly. As a result of this awareness, organizations were created that advocated specialized educational, occupational training, and social service programs for specific disabilities, many of which are still in existence today. Federal agencies were also developed to provide funds for financing the multiple care needs of the disabled population.

Although rehabilitation services for the disabled have markedly increased over the past 20 years, multiple barriers remain, preventing the acceptance of these individuals into the community and into the healthcare system. Often, human needs such as the need for a wholesome body image, for safety, for appreciation and respect, for self-determination and responsibility, and for freedom from pain or stress are in deficit in clients with special needs. This chapter addresses the psychosocial, economic, and legislative issues associated with overcoming barriers to care for clients with special needs. In addition, a thorough discussion of disability classification systems, assistive devices, and client management strategies used in the dental hygiene process follows.

LEGISLATION FOR DISABLED PERSONS

Disabled individuals confront numerous obstacles that limit their ability to have access to healthcare, education, and employment opportunities. Access to these services is essential for the person to function at an acceptable level of health and wellness and to maintain as much **independence** as possible. Other **barriers** include limited financial resources, lack of transportation, inadequate housing, poor environmental design of existing facilities, and limited access to personal and vocational rehabilitation services.

Awareness of the myriad needs required by the disabled population developed during the late 1960s when the term **"normalization"** was first introduced into the literature. Normalization referred to a process that enabled mentally retarded citizens to engage in normal patterns of everyday life. The outcome of this process was an attempt at **"mainstreaming"** these citizens into society.[2] This concept promoted **deinstitutionalization** of those mentally retarded persons capable of living and functioning independently with little or no assistance of a caregiver. It was hoped that these individuals could effectively interact within their environment while contributing to the community. Mainstreaming, a spinoff term from the normalization process, rapidly became the goal of many long-term care providers and educators associated with people with all types of disabilities.

Mainstreaming disabled people created a host of problems not frequently encountered by the general population —problems that demanded immediate attention and resources, most of which were either unavailable or nonexistent. It was really the cooperative efforts of groups of individuals with disabilities, for example, disabled veterans, who formed organizational networks to begin to address the needs of their specific population groups. Many of these organizations grew into nationwide networks, most of which are still in existence today (see Organizations Representing Clients with Disabilities chart). Their efforts greatly influenced the government in developing and setting standards to ensure equal opportunities for the disabled.

To mainstream disabled people into society, education was needed to prepare these individuals for their roles in the home and in the job market. In 1975, the Education for All Handicapped Children Act (Public Law 94-142) was passed to ensure all disabled children the right to an adequate education. This law was the culmination of years of **advocacy** via state and national legislation. Components of this law include mandated diagnostic testing to determine the extent of the child's disability, that the test be given in the native language of the child, that the child has the right to attorney representation for protection, and that the parents or legal guardians of the child have access to all information obtained through diagnostic testing. It is important to note that because there are certain societal stigmas attached to classifying a child as "handicapped" within the school system, classification and diagnostic standards are built into this law to promote accurate confirmation of a diagnosis of a learning or mental disability. In addition,

ORGANIZATIONS REPRESENTING CLIENTS WITH DISABILITIES

Alzheimer's Association
70 East Lake Street
Chicago, IL 60601

American Association of Retired Persons
1909 K Street, N.W.
Washington, D.C. 20049
202-872-4700

American Cancer Society
890 Park Avenue
New York, NY 10016

American Diabetes Association
Two Park Avenue
New York, NY 10016

American Heart Association
7320 Greenville Avenue
Dallas, TX 75231

Arthritis Foundation
1314 Spring Street, N.W.
Atlanta, GA 30309

Department of Veterans Affairs
Central Office
810 Vermont Avenue, N.W.
Washington, D.C. 20420
301-496-2883

National Association of Developmental Disabilities Councils
1234 Massachusetts Avenue, N.W.
Washington, D.C. 20005
202-347-1234

National Association of the Deaf
814 Thayer Avenue
Silver Spring, MD 20910
301-587-1788

National Citizens Coalition for Nursing Home Reform
1424 16th Street, N.W., Suite L2
Washington, D.C. 20036

National Council on the Handicapped
800 Independence Avenue, S.W.
Washington, D.C. 20024
202-267-3846

National Veterans Legal Services Project
2001 South Street, N.W.
Washington, D.C. 20009
202-265-8305

National Vietnam Veterans Coalition
3001 Veazey Terrace, N.W.
Washington, D.C. 20008
202-338-6882

Older Womens League
730 11th Street, N.W., Suite 300
Washington, D.C. 20004
202-783-6686

Parkinson's Disease Foundation
650 West 168th Street
New York, NY 10030

the diagnostic process must lead to the categorization of the child's disability to enable the child to be eligible for state and federal aid. It is unethical to classify a child as "disabled" without providing an educational opportunity to assist with the child's development. The programs designed for these children are required, by law, to be reviewed every year. This law greatly influenced access to and improvement of special educational services required by the disabled.

Discrimination in the Workplace

Mosher[3] identifies several barriers that exist to prevent the hiring of the disabled, such as **discrimination, attitudes** of employers and coworkers, and employer **prejudices.** In addition, the author states that those disabled persons who accept the negative societal **stereotypes** about their inability to succeed in the workforce fall into a self-fulfilling prophecy: those who believe that they are destined to fail will fail. Ironically, those who do succeed are viewed as superhumans, not as individuals who are able to overcome the attitudes that promote limitations on achievement. The United States Vocational Rehabilitation Act of 1973, Section 503, requires all employers with federal contracts over $2,500 to take affirmative action in employing and advancing qualified disabled employees. This law helps to prevent discrimination against hiring a disabled individual by enforcing the removal of job-related criteria that prohibit employing a disabled person and by demanding that the workplace be architecturally accessible.

It was Section 504 of the Rehabilitation Act of 1973, and the Americans with Disabilities Act of 1992, that resulted in the most significant and lasting effects in removing barriers for the disabled, by guaranteeing that:

> No otherwise qualified person shall, by reason of his/her handicap, be discriminated against in the areas of education, employment, or social services including healthcare.

Physical Barriers Related to Independent Living

The Americans with Disabilities Act of 1992 mandated the recognition of universal changes nationwide, perhaps most notably **barrier-free design,** which enabled wheelchair **accessibility** to public buildings. This law strengthened existing legislation for improved telecommunication systems for hearing- and speech-impaired people and the development of closed-captioned television programs, which were first developed under Section 504 of the Rehabilitation Act of 1973.[4]

The purpose of barrier-free design is to enable a person to function independently both within and outside of the home environment. Barrier-free oral healthcare environments facilitate the disabled person's human needs for safety and self-determination. Furthermore, such settings are an indication that the healthcare providers who staff the facility appreciate the needs of the disabled, respect them as human beings, and value them as clients. The concept of *continuous sequence* is used when constructing these facilities, meaning that all aspects of the design are interrelated without limiting the use of any parts of the facility.[5] For example, a building that contains elevators and accessible restrooms is not considered truly barrier-free if there are no ramps or electronically operated doors to gain entrance to the building.

Specific building codes and architectural standards for constructing a barrier-free facility are available from federal and state resources, and these may vary from state to state. These codes are summarized in the Basic Design Characteristics for a Barrier-Free Facility chart.[5,6]

These guidelines for barrier-free facility design are applicable to all types of buildings, whether in public or private domain. Additional standards are available for existing buildings that require only partial or modest renovations for accessibility. Also, temporary or removable accommodations can be made within a facility for use when needed by a disabled individual, such as removable seats in an auditorium.

Barrier-free design is critical if a disabled person is expected to function independently. One of the most difficult transitions that a disabled person must make upon leaving an institutional setting is adjusting to a home environment that is not adapted to that person's mobility and functional needs. For example, a one-story home with no stairs is preferable for those in a wheelchair, because stairs would prohibit easy movement from one floor to another. Wheelchair lifts are available for installation in homes with more than one floor, but the cost of construction and installation prohibits many from purchasing this luxury item. The cost of renovating a private home into an accessible environment is extremely high, and many individuals are forced to relocate into either a planned community or an alternative living setting, such as a group home. Section 231 of the Housing and Community Development Act of 1974 supports the provision of loans to nonprofit organizations and public agencies for the construction of specifically designed rental homes for disabled people. However, advocates for disabled people argue that building special housing facilities for groups of disabled people is too segregating and should be considered only as a temporary transition to permanent relocation in a private setting.[7]

BASIC DESIGN CHARACTERISTICS FOR A BARRIER-FREE FACILITY

Parking. One space per 25 spaces should be allotted for those who are disabled. Space width must be a minimum of 96 inches wide, and should be clearly marked with a sign posted 5 feet above street level. Spaces should be located closest to the nearest accessible ramp and/or building entrance.

Ramps. Ramps should be located at all curbs and should be close to the building entrance. Ramp elevation should not exceed 36 inches, with a slope not to exceed 1 : 12 inches. A minimum of one handrail should be present at a height of 32 inches and should extend for the length of the rampway. No lip should be present at the junction of the ramp with the platform or sidewalk. If outside, a nonskid surface must be used, preferably with a snow-melting device.

Doors. At least one accessible doorway with access to elevators should be present. Doors should be made of a clear material to permit viewing of the approach. Doorways must be a minimum of 32 inches wide to permit clear wheelchair passage, preferably with an additional 4 to 8 inches to limit bumping against the door frame. Door frames should be flush with the floor. Door weight should not exceed 8 pounds. Electronically operated doors are preferred, and may be constructed with either a sensing device that causes doors to open automatically, or with a wall-mounted button to operate the opening. Closure of the doors should be timed for adequate clearance through the doorway. Lever handles, as opposed to doorknobs, should be no higher than 48 inches above the floor.

Stairs. Outside stairs should have a nonskid surface, with a handrail at 32 inches of height. Riser height should not exceed 6 inches. Inside stair design is the same, although riser height may be as great as 7 inches. All stairwells should be clearly marked and lighted. No protrusions that may cause tripping should extend beyond the riser.

Elevators. Elevators must be installed in all buildings with two or more floors. The minimum size of the elevator cab is 5 feet deep and 5½ feet wide. Doors should allow for maximal clearance of a wheelchair, and should have a sensing device for safety of entering passengers. Buttons should be clearly marked and at a height no more than 4 feet from the floor. Controls should be marked with braille for blind clients and should have voice-activated announcements upon arrival at each floor.

Corridors. Hallways must be a minimum of 48 inches wide, preferably 64 inches wide to accommodate two passing wheelchairs. Adequate space should be available to allow a 360-degree turn in a wheelchair without bumping into the wall. Hallways should be clearly marked with signs no higher than 5 feet above the floor, and should always be lighted.

Signs. Signs should be easily read, and should contain bright, contrasting colors. Signs should be posted no higher than 5 feet above the floor. Braille and/or raised lettering is needed for blind clients. Alarms should contain both a visual and an audible warning announcement to accommodate both hearing and visually impaired clients.

Restrooms. Stall sizes should be a minimum of 3 feet wide by 5 feet deep, with an outswinging door of 32 inches clearance. Toilets should be wall-mounted with the seat no higher than 17 inches. Grab bars should be wall-mounted for easy access throughout the stall. Sinks should be wall-mounted with a 27-inch minimal clearance from the floor. Faucets should be of a lever type or have buttons with a slow, timed release of water. Soap and towel dispensers should be no more than 4 feet above the floor. Automatic sensors are available for toilet flushing and for water dispensing in the sink.

Floor coverings. Floors should be covered in a nonskid surface. Seamless linoleum floors are preferred; however, if carpeting is present, it should be a smooth, low pile to prevent snagging of wheels or other devices. Area rugs and doormats should be eliminated.

Water fountains. Fountains should be wall-mounted with a minimal clear space of 27 inches above the floor. Controls should be located at the front of the fountain with a pushplate or lever to operate.

Telephones. Telephones should not be placed in booths and should have a clearance of 27 inches above the floor. Controls should be located between 3 and 4 feet from the floor. Devices for raising and lowering the volume should be available for hearing-impaired people.

Barriers Related to Transportation

One aspect of accessibility frequently overlooked is the design of mass transportation services. Subways, buses, rail systems, and airplanes still provide only limited assistance to the disabled, despite federal regulations that require modifications for greater ease of use of services by disabled people. The Urban Mass Transportation Act of 1974, Section 16, states that disabled and elderly people have the same rights as others to use mass transportation facilities and services. This law also requires that federal programs providing assistance in the field of mass transportation support these rights by complying with plans for building accessible transportation services.

Attitudes of transportation companies and workers often downplay the significance of accessibility, and therefore modifications in the system remain a low priority. Many stations and transportation vehicles remain inaccessible today, partly because the ratio of disabled persons to nondisabled persons is low, and the time and efforts required to renovate the system seem unrealistic and too costly to justify the changes. When modifications are made, the expenses of renovation are frequently passed along to passengers, driving the costs of transportation services upward. The expense of traveling then becomes an additional barrier to disabled people, who are frequently on a fixed income and may not be able to afford transportation services anyway. Frequently, these persons rely upon others for transportation to and from their homes, which may not always be convenient for the driver or for the disabled person.

Use of public transportation services may be difficult and frustrating for everyone. Interpreting the schedule, finding the exact fare, waiting at a boarding stop during inclement weather, boarding the right vehicle, and tracking the number of stops can be extremely difficult for someone with a physical or mental **impairment.** Transportation officials who are not trained in basic concepts to assist the disabled are often ineffective in helping these individuals arrive at their destinations. It is not surprising then to find that many disabled people do not use mass transportation services; instead they choose to remain at home rather than risk an opportunity to travel. This behavior can become quite problematic, especially if the individual chooses to skip medical appointments or does not shop for groceries because it is "safer" to remain at home. To address this issue, many agencies and organizations offer a special van service providing travel opportunities to a variety of destinations for disabled individuals. However, these services are offered only in limited areas and can be quite expensive.

Other Barriers Related to Healthcare

Cost

Even though federal mandates have increased availability of services to disabled people, cost remains the primary barrier in limiting the utilization of most services. Financial resources are needed to obtain an education, to participate in rehabilitative programs, to train for a job, to find adequate housing, to utilize basic transportation services, and just to survive. State and federal funds are not sufficient to cover the costs of everyone's needs, and therefore many disabled people are forced to prioritize their spending according to their most immediate needs, often at the expense of other needs.

Most disabled people are on a fixed income and rely upon state and federal support, such as Social Security payments, to cover their daily living expenses. Those individuals who are able to work earn low wages, and unemployment rates remain relatively high.[4]

Without adequate funds for daily expenses, medical and dental care is often neglected. Most cannot afford private healthcare insurance and rely upon Medicare and Medicaid reimbursement for financial assistance. For those on a limited income without insurance, money spent for healthcare services is an out-of-pocket expense: frequently, healthcare is sought on an episodic basis, specifically for emergency intervention or for pain control. For those living in an institution, medical and limited dental services may be provided, but high fees may be associated with rendering these services, the cost of which is either passed on to the family or to the state. If a severely disabled person needs to be institutionalized, the costs to the family can be enormous and may drain the financial resources of the family. The costs associated with medical care for the person may exceed the money that the family has available to spend. Many families choose to care for a severely disabled individual at home, because the cost of long-term care is too great a burden for the family to manage.

The fact that more disabled persons now live outside of the institutional setting means that more of them need to be treated within the private sector. Some private medical and dental practitioners may choose not to treat disabled individuals, because reimbursement for services through Medicare and Medicaid is often not equivalent to the customary and reasonable fee schedules charged in the area. In fact, eligibility requirements for Medicare and Medicaid may actually limit access to oral care services for residents mainstreamed into group homes that otherwise would have been provided to residents in an institutional setting. In addition, extra time is often needed to treat these individuals, so that available time for treating others is lost, with a concomitant reduction in income earnings.

Attitudes of Health Professionals

Frequently, the attitudes of practitioners are an even greater barrier to adequate care. Fear of interacting with a disabled person and conflicting personal values about the disabled may make an individual avoid treating such a person.[8–11] To address this issue among dentists and dental hygienists, curriculum guidelines have been developed through the American Association of Dental Schools to prepare future oral healthcare practitioners to care for disabled clients and to sensitize practitioners about the special needs of this population group.[11,12]

Kimmelman[13] says that disabled Americans have been "shut out" from access to dental services as a result of failure on the part of the medical and dental communities to provide comprehensive healthcare to this population.[13] Kimmelman also states that oral care has a much greater significance among disabled clients, in that the oral cavity is frequently the "lifeline" for the client. The mouth is important not only for mastication and speaking, but for expressing personality, using **telecommunicative devices,** working at a job, and for portraying a positive self-image. A healthy, well-functioning mouth implies that the individual values health and physical appearance. This positive **portrayal** of the person can contribute to the client's sense of self-worth and self-esteem and of having a wholesome body image.

Client Factors

Self-esteem is an essential component of the disabled client's sense of **self-concept.** All people have periods of achievement that build confidence and periods of disappointment that lower confidence, and the disabled client copes with these normal life events with the same behaviors as the nondisabled individual. However, disabled clients have certain barriers that interfere with how others may view them, which in turn affects how they view themselves.

The physical positioning of the disabled person may cause the feeling of intimidation or self-consciousness when in proximity to other individuals. For example, people who use wheelchairs are physically lower than standing adults, which causes others to look down upon them while conversing. People who use assistive devices, such as canes, braces, or walkers, may be viewed as inept because they are unable to ambulate on their own. People who are hearing or visually impaired may have difficulty participating and following a conversation, and therefore may be excluded from the group, creating a deficit in their human need for appreciation and respect. People with tremors or other muscular disorders may take a longer time to speak and may be viewed as mentally impaired by those who are impatient or unwilling to listen.[14]

Counseling and group discussions may benefit the disabled client in promoting self-worth by providing an opportunity to discuss frustrations and a forum for objective self-evaluation of other capabilities. However, disabled clients should be encouraged to perform self-assessment independently so they do not become dependent upon others for approval. Disabled clients are individuals who have their own personal capabilities and limitations, and they adapt to life experiences in much the same way as others cope with these challenges. Therefore, clients should not be viewed as stereotypically "different" from their counterparts, but rather as individuals who can provide unique contributions to the community despite their disabilities and who have human needs similar to those presented by most clients.

DEFINING DISABILITIES

It is easy to encounter confusion when trying to select an appropriate term to describe a client with a disability. Derogatory or slang terms often come to mind, because most individuals are not taught the appropriate descriptors in their formal education unless their personal situations dictate the need for such knowledge. Unfortunately, contradictory terms also exist within the medical literature, which compounds the confusion.

The literature rarely differentiates between the terms "disabled" and "handicapped," except in government publications, wherein "handicapped" appears to be the preferred term.[15]

"Disability" is a term used to describe a condition that is either permanent or semipermanent and that interferes with an individual's ability to do something independently. This term can be used either as a noun or as an adjective, for example, as in "disabled clients."[16] An individual who has a disability is different from a "normal" person in some way, because of trauma, birth defects, accidents, or disease. These differences may be physical, mental, or psychological manifestations of the individual's ability to function.

"Handicap" is a term used to describe the feeling a person may have regarding adequacy of performance either generally or under a particular circumstance.[14] For example, when a person uses a computer for the first time, the lack of computer skills may "handicap" the person in the ability to adequately operate the computer. An individual who is unable to bend at the knees may be "handicapped" by stairs or by street curbs that are too high. Everyone is "handicapped" at some point or another, regardless of level of disability. Clearly, this term is not synonymous with "disability," and care should be taken when utilizing the word.

Frequently, there is a stigma attached to disabilities, such as an assumed level of inability or illness. Therefore, it is often difficult for a disabled person to become accepted as an individual with unique talents and limitations like any other person. Environmental influences such as **family values,** attitudes of peers, and the **cultural beliefs** of the community all affect how a person views the capabilities of those who are disabled.[14]

When describing or interacting with persons with disabilities, it is important to remember several key points associated with negative portrayal issues.[16] First, a person is not a disability; the client is a person who has a disability. Therefore, it is inappropriate to say, "She is my multiple sclerosis case." It is more appropriate to say, "This is my client, Mrs. Jones. She has multiple sclerosis." Second, the presence of a disability does not override all other characteristics of the client; therefore, the disability should be addressed only when necessary or relevant to the situation. Emphasizing the disability without reason should be avoided. Third, clients with disabilities are not superhuman; learning to function as a person despite the presence of a disability is survival, not a unique act that requires special talents or gifts. Sensationalizing goal attainment by disabled people is a common reaction, such as "he triumphed over his inability to walk," implying that the client was a "victim" of the disability. Fourth, sensationalizing terms that draw on the emotions, such as "relies on a cane" or "bound to a wheelchair," are inappropriate and may imply a false level of **dependency** on the part of the client. Fifth, people with disabilities are not necessarily sick, regardless of whether the disability was caused by an illness. It is inappropriate to describe a disabled client as a "patient" or a "case" unless that person is actively under medical care.

Other portrayal issues are encountered in everyday life, either through personal contact or through mass media. For example, many people express pity for a disabled person without knowing the individual, or they express disbelief when seeing a disabled person enjoying himself "despite his disability." Healthcare professionals who work primarily with disabled clients are often viewed as having special motivation or as "truly patient." Television portrayals of disabled people often tend to treat the disabled adult like a child or an inferior. A disabled adult may be addressed by first name or with a nickname when the situation dictates use of a more formal title. Other examples are speaking for another person in the presence of that person as if the individual was not there, and assuming that the individual cannot make decisions alone and requires assistance by another adult. Behaviors that reflect negative portrayal issues should be addressed and corrected to facilitate the client's human need for appreciation and respect. This lays the foundation for establishing a positive therapeutic relationship between the dental hygienist and the disabled client.

Classification of Disabilities

Several classification methods are used to categorize individuals with disabilities. Government classification standards are primarily based on the criteria delineated in Section 504 of the Vocational Rehabilitation Act of 1973.

These criteria state that an individual with a disability is one who:

- Has a physical or mental impairment that substantially limits one or more life activities such as caring for oneself, performing manual tasks, walking, seeing, hearing, speaking, breathing, learning, and working

TABLE 26–1
CLASSIFICATIONS OF DISABILITIES

Developmental Disabilities	
Mental retardation	Includes Down syndrome, and reflects difficulties with learning, critical thinking, and skill development
Cerebral palsy	Nonprogressive disorder caused by brain damage either at birth or before the central nervous system (CNS) reaches maturity
Epilepsy	Caused by a chemical imbalance in the brain; associated with head injury, infection, and developmental disorders
Autism	Lifelong neurological disability; associated with mental retardation
Sensory Impairments	
Visual impairments	Changes in visual acuity to blindness
Hearing impairments	Varying degrees of hearing loss to deafness
Orthopedic Disorders	
Paralysis	Most commonly associated with stroke
Spinal cord injury	Accidents or injury
Missing extremities	Injury, diabetes
Medical Disabilities	
Cardiovascular diseases	Hypertension, congestive heart disease, stroke, valvular disease
Arthritis	Lupus, gout, Sjögren's syndrome, scleroderma, rheumatoid arthritis, and osteoarthritis
Cancer	
Diabetes	
Respiratory diseases	
Renal disease	
Blood disorders	Bleeding disorders, platelet disorders, sickle cell anemia, other anemias
Alcoholism	
Drug abuse	
Cognitive Impairments/Mental Illness	
Anorexia and bulimia	
Depression	
Alzheimer's disease	
Dementia	
Cerebrovascular accident (CVA, stroke)	
Degenerative Nervous System Disorders	
Alzheimer's disease	Neuronal degeneration in the cerebral cortex resulting in loss of memory, critical thinking, and reasoning ability
Parkinson's disease	Degeneration of deep cerebral nuclei resulting in loss of control of voluntary movements; tremors, slowness of movement (bradykinesia); gradual onset of dementia
Huntington's disease	Autosomal dominant disorder that causes degeneration of the deep nuclei, cauda, and putamen; behavioral problems and constant muscle movement (chorea)
Cerebellar ataxias	Normal mental status; changes in gait and coordination
Motor neuron disease and amyotrophic lateral sclerosis (ALS)	Cell death in the motor neurons of the spinal cord and cerebral cortex; progressive muscle atrophy leading to respiratory failure; no loss of mental or sensory functions
Multiple sclerosis (MS)	Muscle weakness characterized by cyclical nature of progression
Myasthenia gravis	Muscle involvement around the eyes and throat; difficulty in swallowing
Neurofibromatosis	Genetic autosomal dominant disease; multiple benign tumors
Communication Disorders	
Dysarthria	Speech disorder from muscle weakness caused by damage to the central or peripheral nervous system or both; slurred speech patterns; associated with Parkinson's disease, ALS, MS, and CVA
Apraxia	Speech disorder caused by a lesion within the CNS; impaired capacity to position muscles to form speech; stuttering
Aphasia	Language disorder caused by neurological damage; inability to put thoughts into words or to comprehend words

- Has a record of such an impairment that limits major life activities
- Is regarded as having such an impairment

These criteria are used to determine eligibility for federal assistance under the Section 504 legislation. These definitions can be further delineated into developmental and acquired disabilities.

Developmental Disabilities

A **developmental disability** is one that occurs congenitally or occurs during the developmental period of the child, a period that lasts from birth to the age of 22 years. Developmental disabilities are generally chronic in nature, continue throughout the life of the person, and appear as either mental, physical, or combined impairments. Individuals with developmental disabilities may experience difficulties with many functions and may be limited in their abilities to care for themselves, communicate effectively, learn new concepts, ambulate, or live independently.[17]

Acquired Disabilities

Acquired disabilities are those that occur after the age of 22 years. They usually are caused by a disease or some type of trauma or injury to the body. Common types of acquired disabilities include spinal cord paralysis from sports injuries or automobile accidents, limb amputation because of cancer, and limitations in range of motion from arthritis. The amount of limitation experienced by the person is dependent upon the nature of the disability, areas of the body involved, and the severity of the condition or injury.

A second type of classification system groups types of disabilities into several major divisions, clustering impairments with similar manifestations together for ease of reference. Table 26–1 displays a list of disabilities grouped by division.[4,18–22] These categories are useful when studying a group of disorders or when attempting to classify the condition of a client who presents with symptomatology associated with a known disorder. However, this classification system mainly categorizes a person according to medical status, a system that provides little information about how

TABLE 26–2
FUNCTIONAL LEVELS FOR CATEGORIZING DISABILITIES BASED ON ABILITY TO CONDUCT ACTIVITIES OF DAILY LIVING

Level of Impairment	Communication	Movement	Mental Ability
Level I			
Near-normal function	May be difficult for the practitioner to understand the client and vice versa	Client may walk more slowly than normal	Extra effort for explanations and reassurance to client
Level II			
Simulation of normal function with adaptive equipment, medication, or methods	Client may use communication board, writing, or gesturing instead of speech	Office may need to be wheelchair accessible and have furniture rearranged to allow room for movement Client may need to make special arrangements for transportation Possible assistance in getting into treatment chair	Client may be using medications to maintain emotional equilibrium or need special approach in order to accept routine dental and dental hygiene care in office
Level III			
Simulation of normal function with aid of third party	Deaf person may need interpreter Client may bring friend, parent, or attendant to assist in communication Client consent may be needed to give information to third party	Attendant or other caregiver may be responsible for dental hygiene Obtain client consent to give information and education to third party Will need assistance in getting into treatment chair	Client may have legal guardian If so, practitioner should have guardian's consent and proof of guardianship
Level IV			
Simulation of normal function not possible	Client will have legal guardian Dental practitioner should have guardian's consent and proof of guardianship for care Residential caregiver responsible for dental hygiene should be given information and education	Home visit required for routine dental and dental hygiene care If practitioner cannot make one, refer to appropriate resource	Client will have legal guardian Must have guardian's consent and proof of guardianship for care

Modified from Shaffer, S., Margon, C., and Stiefel, D. J. Principles of rehabilitation (Project DECOD). Seattle: University of Washington School of Dentistry, 1985, p. 8.

well an individual can compensate for limitations in daily function as a result of the disorder.

Evaluating **functional status** is perhaps the most useful method for categorizing disabilities, because each disabled person presents with individual differences in abilities and limitations, regardless of medical diagnosis or degree of system involvement. Functional status describes how well the client can conduct his **activities of daily living** (ADLs): eating, speaking, bathing, dressing, toileting, and ambulation. The dental hygienist who is able to facilitate the client's human need for self-determination and responsibility by developing the client's preventive oral health behaviors (ADLs) also increases the client's functional status.

Impairments can affect five aspects of an individual's ability to function: communication, movement, mental ability, medical health, and vision.[4] However, these categories of function are limited in that they do not address the degree of severity or extent of involvement of the impairments, which may cause varying degrees of functional limitations. To further illustrate how functional limitations are related to the severity of impairment, classification into four levels of involvement is depicted in Table 26–2.

It is essential for the dental hygienist to understand the nature of disabling conditions, as well as the capabilities and limitations of disabled clients, in order to meet their dental hygiene care needs appropriately. Many clients present with complex oral care needs associated directly with their conditions or with medications taken to stabilize or control the symptoms of their conditions. In addition, these clients may require special assistance in accomplishing **self-care** behaviors necessary for oral health and awareness. Knowledge of how to assess functional status assists the hygienist in better serving the client's needs so that the client may remain as independent as possible while striving for an attainable level of wellness. (For significant factors related to the dental hygiene care of individuals with special needs, see Table 26–8.)

ASSISTIVE DEVICES FOR DISABLED CLIENTS

The extent of the client's disability may dictate the need to use some form of device to achieve independence in daily functions and communication. These are **assistive devices.** Many devices are available through area pharmacies and agencies; others are professionally or self-designed, specifically tailored for the needs of the client. It is important for the dental hygienist to be familiar with these devices because the indications for their use may affect client goals and decisions in the process of care.

Walking Devices

A variety of devices are available to assist the client who has difficulty with ambulation. Canes, leg braces, crutches, and walkers are all devices that assist the client by bearing the weight of the body during motion, for example, while walking (Figs. 26–1 and 26–2). These devices replace function either unilaterally or bilaterally and greatly increase the client's mobility. In addition to increasing mobility for ambulation, these devices also are used to support the individual while raising and lowering the body from a bed or chair. When a client uses this type of device, it must always

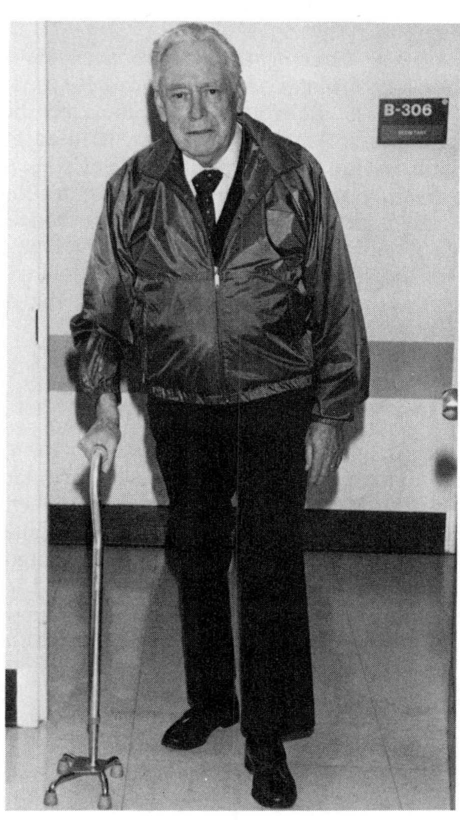

FIGURE 26–1
Use of a walker greatly increases the client's mobility.

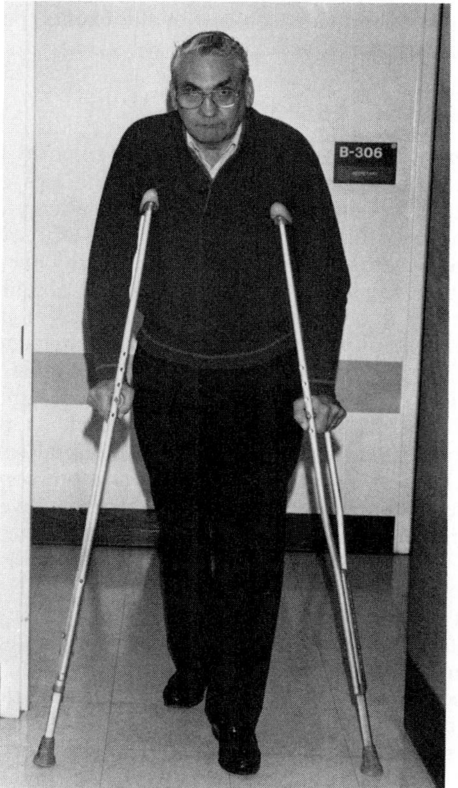

FIGURE 26–2
Crutches assist the client by bearing the weight of the body during motion.

remain close to the client for easy access when needed. For example, if the need arises for the dental hygienist to remove the device from the treatment area, the client must always be informed of the location of the device to reduce any apprehension of feeling "trapped" in the oral care environment. The dental hygienist must always retrieve the device when needed or at the client's request, and should hand the device directly to the client for use. It is not unusual for the anxious client to prefer to hold the device on his lap as a measure of security in the healthcare environment. Although not ideal, this behavior may be tolerated as long as the device does not interfere with the provision of care. As the client gains trust and confidence in the dental hygienist, the client may no longer feel the need to hold the device and may allow the hygienist to place the device within easy reach of the chair. These actions on the part of the dental hygienist help to meet the client's need for freedom from stress.

Wheelchairs

Wheelchairs also are devices that assist clients who have limited or no mobility in the legs for ambulation. Wheelchairs increase mobility for a client who may otherwise be confined to a bed or chair. Because of improvements in building design, many facilities are completely accessible to wheelchairs, thus enabling clients to move freely about without being inhibited by physical limitations in ambulation. Clients who arrive for dental hygiene care may be treated in the wheelchair or may be transferred into the dental chair for care (see section on wheelchair transfer techniques later in this chapter). Wheelchairs may be hand-operated or motorized, and vary in style and cost. Most clients prefer to operate the wheelchair themselves; assistance should be provided only with the clients' permission or at their specific request.

Prosthetic Devices

Clients may use *prosthetic devices* that enhance their appearance and improve function. Prosthetic legs often are fitted after amputation to improve ambulation, prosthetic arms are used to increase reach and range of motion, and prosthetic hands are used to improve grasp. Other devices may be used to replace structures or organs absent because of congenital anomalies or removed because of pathology or trauma. Prosthetic devices may be permanently fitted through surgical implantation or are removable and are worn only when needed for functional or cosmetic purposes. Clients with removable devices such as those designed for persons who have had maxillofacial surgery related to head and neck cancer may feel more comfortable when the prosthesis is in place; therefore, removal should occur only during assessment or when indicated during care. All devices should be replaced immediately after completion of the procedure to ensure client comfort and ease. To meet the client's need for respect, privacy must always be maintained when the prosthetic device is removed, preferably in a closed area or an examination room with no visual access by others. To meet the human need for safety, antibiotic premedication may be indicated for the client with a permanent surgical implantation device prior to dental hygiene care. Consultation with the client's physician is indicated to determine antibiotic premedication needs.

Assistive Listening Devices

Clients with hearing impairments may use one or more devices to detect sounds and to assist with understanding speech. Hearing aids are used to amplify sounds, and are effective only when some hearing capacity exists; hearing aids are not indicated for the client with complete hearing loss. Hearing aids may be worn in the outer ear to improve sound conduction or behind the ear for inner ear conduction. Because many people deny hearing loss, some clients may own a hearing aid but choose not to wear the device out of self-consciousness or embarrassment. These clients may appear unresponsive to questions or to conversation. Such behaviors should alert the dental hygienist to possible hearing impairment, and the client should be asked about the use of a hearing device.

The oral healthcare environment can create annoyances for the client who wears a hearing aid. Close operator proximity or incorrect placement of the hearing aid may cause the aid to "squeal," which is extremely unpleasant for the client. In addition, high-pitched noises, such as those caused by a dental handpiece or ultrasonic devices, also cause this reaction. The dental hygienist should instruct the client to turn down the hearing aid during some phases of dental hygiene care. Clients adapting to a new hearing aid often turn down the aid, complaining that "everything seems so noisy." Because all sounds are amplified, these clients may become aware of sounds that they have never heard before or have not heard in a long time, especially if the hearing loss was gradual and untreated. Most oral healthcare environments contain background noise, and clients may turn off the hearing aid before coming for their appointments. It is important for the hygienist to be sensitive to the needs of those wearing hearing aids and to discuss any issues or concerns with the client prior to the onset of care.

Other *assistive listening devices* are available to those with hearing impairments. Amplifiers can be used on telephones to increase the volume of sound for those with partial hearing loss. Amplifiers also can be used for televisions and for radios. Closed-captioned television programs assist the hearing impaired client with lip reading. Telecommunication devices for telephones reproduce sounds from a caller and convert them into written type that can be read by the hearing-impaired person from a monitor and who in turn can type a response into the device to transmit a message back to the caller.

Aids for the Visually Impaired

Clients who are visually impaired usually wear *corrective lenses* to improve vision. Glasses and/or contact lenses must always be worn by visually impaired clients when interacting with the dental hygienist. If oral healthcare instructions are given to a client who has forgotten his glasses, the instructions should be supplemented with written material to read at home after the appointment.

These materials should contain large print with adequate contrast to facilitate seeing the letters. Clients who are blind frequently wear dark glasses to protect the eyes from light rays that may cause sensitivity.

Blind clients may require guidance through the care setting, especially if the client is new to the environment. Clients should be greeted by grasping hands during introductions. To assist the client to the treatment area, the client's nondominant hand should be placed under the elbow of the hygienist, and the client should be asked to stand next to, but slightly behind, the hygienist. Specific directions should be given while guiding a client, such as "take three steps forward, then turn to the right. We're going to step down onto a smooth floor. There is only one step." When arriving in the treatment area, the client should be told about the location of objects in the room. "The chair is directly in front of you, about 1 foot away from where you are standing now." Allow the client to feel the location and direction of the chair by placing the client's hands onto the chair while giving verbal instructions. It is reassuring to the client for the dental hygienist to remain close by with a hand resting on the shoulder to ensure comfort and concern for the client's safety while he is getting settled into the chair. Again, guidance should be used only with the client's permission or when specifically requested.

Some blind clients may use a *cane* or a *dog guide* for assistance during ambulation and may actually prefer the use of these aids to assistance by another individual. Use of these aids adds to the client's feeling of independence and should always be respected when the client is brought to the oral healthcare environment. As with any device, canes should not be removed without the client's permission. If the cane is taken from the client, the client must be informed of its specific location, and it should be returned directly to the client upon request. Dog guides are permitted to remain with the client in the treatment area and should be encouraged by the client to sit close to or with a clear view of the client during all procedures. Dog guides should not be left alone in another area, because they may become extremely anxious in the absence of their owners.

Assistive Speaking Devices

Clients who are unable to speak have difficulty communicating their needs to others. Clients who have had surgical removal of the larynx, most often because of cancer, cannot make any sounds from the throat. Assistive devices for these individuals are used to recreate sounds that mimic normal speech patterns. *Electronic speech devices* that are held against the throat detect vibrations of air passing through the throat as the person mimics normal speaking activity. The device reproduces a noise that resembles an automated, robot-like speech. Use of this device greatly enhances verbal communication for the person. Speech therapists also can train clients with laryngectomies to use expelled air from the esophagus for sound formation to produce altered speech. When treating this type of client, the dental hygienist must listen carefully and repeat the message given by the client to ensure accuracy in understanding. With practice, it becomes relatively easy to understand these clients and to communicate effectively.

Assistive Devices for Paralyzed Clients

Elimination Devices

Clients who are paralyzed below the waist may experience difficulty with normal waste elimination, and may utilize a *catheter* for assistance with urination. Care must be taken when transferring a client with a catheter into the dental chair, because the catheter may become kinked or dislodged. Also, clients may have a bowel and bladder routine to regulate their waste elimination. Clients should be questioned regarding their waste elimination program during assessment so that necessary modifications can be made in the process of care.

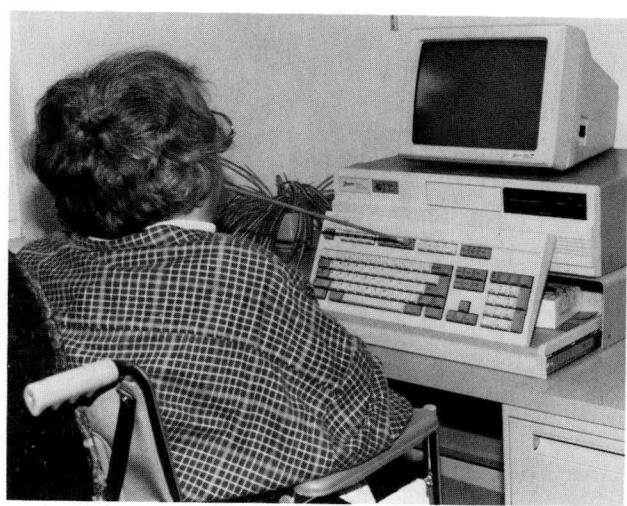

FIGURE 26–3
Mouthsticks are used mainly for communication, such as typing on a keyboard.

Communication Devices

Clients who are paralyzed below the neck use a variety of devices to accomplish daily activities, most of which are designed by occupational therapists for easy access and use. The mouth is needed to operate many of these devices, which alters the health and function of the oral structures. The most common device used by quadriplegic clients is the **mouthstick,** a simple rod with a rubber tip held in place by the teeth and lips (Fig. 26–3). Mouthsticks are used mainly for communication, such as typing on a keyboard or pressing the buttons to dial a telephone. Mouthsticks are used also to turn pages in a book, operate a computer, and operate appliances, such as microwave ovens and remote-controlled television sets.

Problems Associated with Use of a Mouthstick Typically, mouthsticks are made from ordinary balsa wood or plastic, and the client then holds the stick in place with the anterior teeth. The lips are closed around the mouthstick to provide added strength and stability. The anterior teeth are then subjected to occlusal trauma, which in the presence of inflammation may result in rapid periodontal ligament and bone destruction, and ultimately tooth loss. The need for a biologically sound dentition and skin and mucous membrane integrity is of great significance to these clients, because without healthy teeth and supporting structures, they may not be able to hold the stick in place and therefore may lose the ability to communicate and function independently (Fig. 26–4).

Other problems associated with mouthsticks of this basic design include muscle fatigue, oral tissue trauma from difficulty in inserting the stick, difficulty with insertion without assistance by a caregiver, unpleasant taste, temporomandibular joint discomfort, and gagging.[23] Numerous case reports appear in the literature that describe improved mouthstick design for disabled clients.[24–26] To meet the client's human need for a biologically sound dentition and for skin and mucous membrane integrity, key considerations in the fabrication of mouthstick appliances should be met[23] (see Key

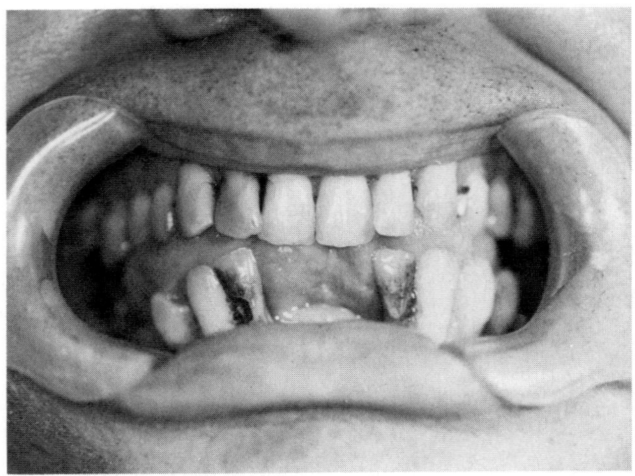

FIGURE 26-4
Use of a mouthstick subjects the anterior teeth to occlusal trauma, which, in the presence of inflammation, may lead to tooth loss.

Considerations in the Fabrication of a Mouthstick Appliance chart).

The dental hygienist easily can assess the client's need for a mouthstick appliance. In conjunction with the client's occupational therapist, the dental hygienist can determine a variety of uses for the mouthstick based upon the individual client's needs and the range of motion and stick length required to accomplish these functions. The dental hygienist then consults with a prosthodontist for the manufacture of the appliance to hold the mouthstick.

In manufacturing a mouthstick, first, an impression is taken of both arches for the fabrication of study casts. Next, an acrylic mouthguard is made to fit over the mandibular study cast. The mouthguard is adjusted in the client's mouth for fit and occlusal stability. A hole is made within the appliance and adapted for the mouthstick. Mouthsticks can be made of acrylic or another plastic, and should be of adequate thickness to limit breakage. The occupational therapist also can assist the prosthodontist with final evaluation of the length and design of the stick based upon the usage needs of the client. For clients who have multiple occlusal problems and/or limited range of motion, the team approach to assessment, appliance fabrication, and adjustment is in the best interest of the client. Prior to the insertion of the appliance, oral inflammation should be eliminated to prevent further periodontal tissue destruction. Careful monitoring of the fit and use of the appliance should be done on a routine basis by the dental hygienist to minimize periodontal trauma and to ensure optimal benefit for the client.

KEY CONSIDERATIONS IN THE FABRICATION OF A MOUTHSTICK APPLIANCE

The appliance must minimize occlusal trauma by equally distributing the biting forces across as many teeth within the arch as possible to minimize periodontal destruction and muscle fatigue.

- The appliance should not cause tooth movement and should be stable when held in place
- The device should be relatively inexpensive to make and should be made of a material that is easy to clean
- The device should also be designed to hold a variety of implements to best meet the client's needs
- The device should be comfortable, should not inhibit speech or swallowing, and the stick itself should be out of the client's line of vision[23]

Assistive Devices for Protection and Oral Function

Custom mouth protectors are devices used to prevent self-inflicted trauma by clients with behavioral problems.[27] The device is manufactured by a general dentist or prosthodontist from soft rubber, and it fits over both arches, covering the occlusal surfaces and a portion of the palate. The tongue is isolated away from the teeth by a lingual extension of the device made of soft rubber or metal. Use of a mouth protector prohibits the client from chewing on the lips and from biting the tongue. These types of self-inflicted oral injuries are commonly found in children with profound mental retardation and autism. The custom mouth protector serves two purposes. First, wearing the device provides a protective function by allowing traumatized tissues to heal without further injury. Second, the device is used in behavioral modification therapy to train the child to stop injuring the oral tissues with uncontrolled chewing habits. The devices are effective in controlling self-injurious behavior but should be used only in consultation with a behavioral specialist.

Clients with neuromuscular disorders such as Parkinson's disease and stroke or who have had surgery in which a portion of the throat or palate has been removed may present with difficulty in speaking and swallowing[28] and may require a device to assist with oral function. Neil and Saunders describe several devices that can be used to correct deficiencies in the palatal region, thus improving speech and swallowing.[28] Palatal lifts, palatal augmentation devices, and obturators are all devices that improve function by recreating normal physiologic movement of the oral tissues. The dental hygienist caring for the client with this type of device must evaluate the client for changes in speaking patterns and swallowing ability and for cleanliness of the device. If the dental hygienist determines the need for adjustment of this type of device, the client should be referred to a prosthodontist.

CREATING ORAL HYGIENE ASSISTIVE DEVICES FOR CLIENTS

Although many devices are available to assist the client with performing activities of daily living, few existing devices are available to help the client carry out oral health behaviors independently. The dental hygienist is capable of developing creative alternatives to the traditional oral hygiene devices used by clients without disabilities to promote better oral health among those with limitations in function. Successful use of these devices by disabled clients to a large extent depends upon the design of the device. All devices should be made to adapt to the individual client's needs after careful consideration has been made of the client's existing skill level and functional status.

Client Assessment

Prior to making a device, the dental hygienist should perform a complete assessment of the client's physical and

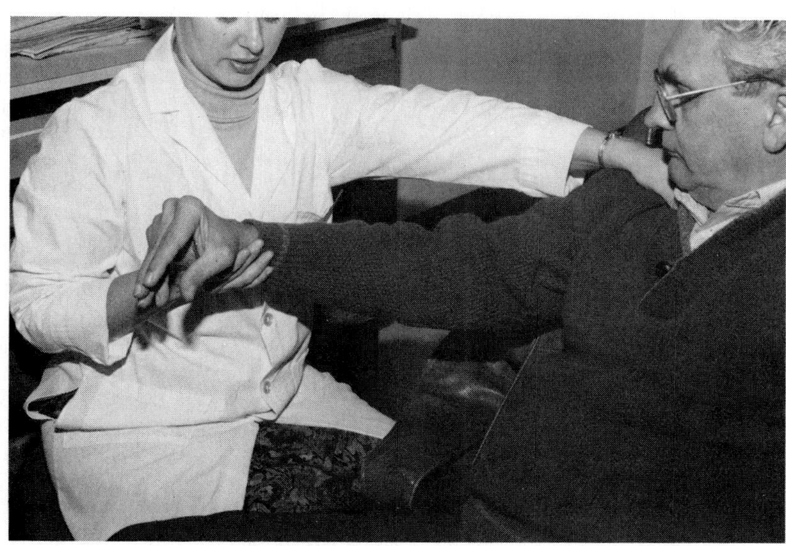

FIGURE 26–5
Assessing range of motion to determine the client's ability to reach and extend.

mental limitations that may affect how well the client adapts to using a device. First, the hygienist should evaluate the client's physical **range of motion** to determine the client's ability to reach the oral cavity with the arms and hands (Figs. 26–5 and 26–6). The extent of the range of motion reveals the length of the device required to accommodate for any physical limitations in reaching the mouth. For example, a client with a muscular impairment may be able to reach halfway across his body, yet can elevate the arm only to heart level. This client needs an extended length to compensate for the limited motion of reaching above heart level. Similarly, the client who is unable to bend at the elbows or wrists may have difficulty reaching certain areas of the oral cavity and may need a device that is angulated for improved reach to fit in all areas of the mouth.

Second, the hygienist should assess the client's **grip strength.** Clients with arthritis or neuromuscular disorders may experience difficulty in holding a device that is too narrow or small (Fig. 26–7). To assess the client's grip strength, have the client hold a variety of sizes of balls to determine the extent of **finger closure** around the ball (Fig. 26–8). The use of tennis balls, softballs, and golf balls is very helpful with this exercise. Another measure of grip strength includes assessing the client's ability to retain finger closure for an extended length of time (Fig. 26–9). Grasp the client's hand gently, and ask the client to squeeze with as much force as possible and hold this position for one minute. This assessment helps to determine the strength needed to hold the device for a given length of time. If the client is unable to keep the fingers closed for 1 minute, a Velcro strip may be needed to assist the client with holding the device in the hand.

Third, the hygienist must assess the skill level of the client in using a device to clean the mouth by determining dexterity and coordination. This skill level can be measured by watching the client simulate the motion used to brush the teeth, or by watching the client actually brush the teeth with his current technique. The client should be prompted to perform certain skills such as reaching into the upper right quadrant, brushing the tongue, cleaning the lingual surfaces, and brushing the facial surfaces of anterior teeth.

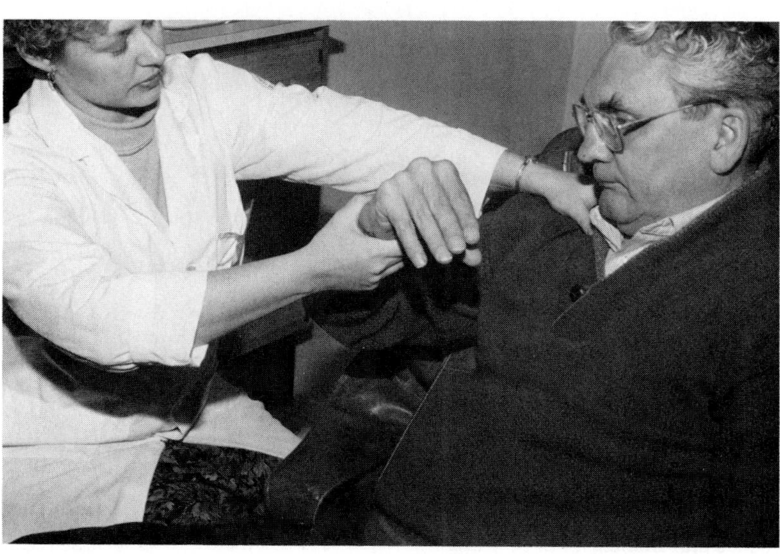

FIGURE 26–6
Clients who have difficulty in bending at the elbows may not be able to adequately reach the oral cavity.

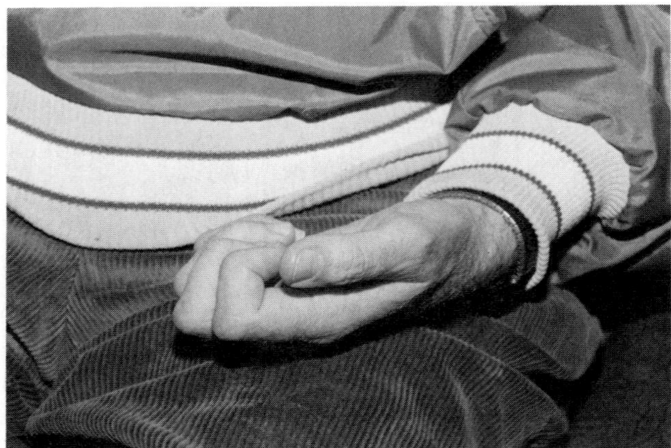

FIGURE 26-7
Clients with arthritis or neuromuscular disorders may experience difficulty in holding a device that is too narrow or small.

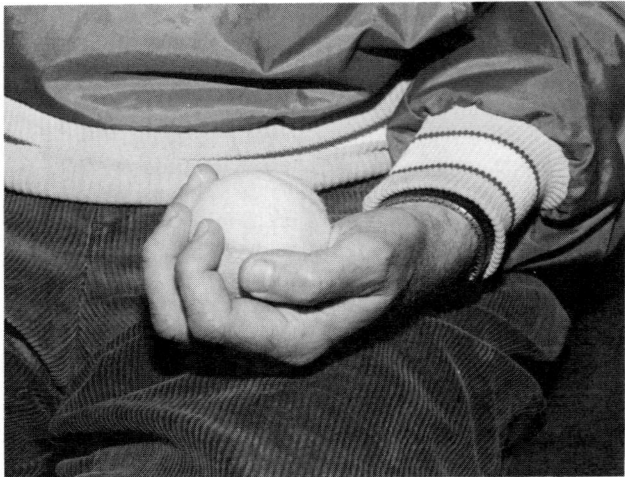

FIGURE 26-8
Use of a tennis ball may help determine finger closure capability.

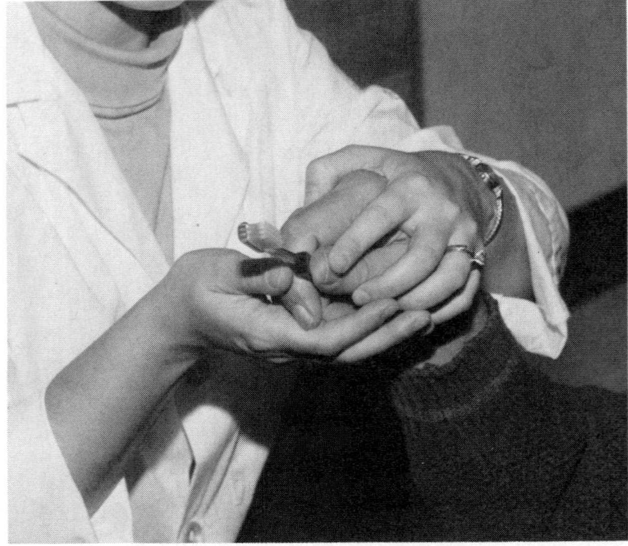

FIGURE 26-9
Retaining finger closure around a small device measures the client's grip strength.

It is important to note what the client is capable of performing with relative ease and which behaviors present the most difficulty or confusion to the client. These capabilities are important to consider when planning the overall design of the device.

Fourth, the client's ability to understand and follow directions is assessed. This assessment can be done during the grip strength assessment phase with the client. The hygienist should ask a sufficient number of questions to determine whether the client is capable of responding accurately to verbal commands and instructions. For example, the client who is cognitively impaired may have difficulty in producing a response on command and may require a device such as a powered toothbrush that accomplishes the task with very little effort from the client.

Fifth, the client is asked about what motions seem "easy" to accomplish versus what motions present the most difficulty. Direct feedback from the client is essential for a complete assessment, in that the client's perceptions may influence compliance with any device, whether well adapted for his needs or not. The client should understand his key role in the design of his device—a motivational strategy that promotes ownership of the responsibility to carry out oral self-care behaviors.

Sixth, a careful intraoral examination should be performed to assess the client's current self-care techniques. *The intraoral assessment should include an examination of hard and soft deposits, gingival structures, periodontal structures, and occlusal status.* In addition, the range of opening of the mouth and the activity of the musculature, especially the tongue, should be noted. This intraoral assessment provides valuable information about existing oral conditions that may dictate the need for certain design characteristics of oral physiotherapeutic aids.

These assessment measures work well with clients who have an existing range of motion and who are mentally capable of cooperating with learning new self-care techniques. However, some clients may not be able to move their upper extremities at all or may be severely cognitively impaired, and therefore rely upon a primary **caregiver** to perform their oral hygiene procedures. For clients who are uncooperative, conducting an intraoral assessment may be impossible, and an interview with the primary caregiver may be all that is available to obtain information about the client's needs. Caregiver inteviews are important to assess the willingness of the individual to provide oral healthcare for the client, determine the existing skill level of the caregiver, and identify any specific concerns that the caregiver may have in performing these procedures.

Customizing Personal Oral Hygiene Devices

After assessing the capabilities of the client, the hygienist must consider several design characteristics of the device. First, the device should be made of a lightweight material and should be easily constructed. Plastics are preferred in the construction of any device because they resist water damage and can be easily cleaned, rinsed, and dried. Second, the materials needed should be readily available and should be inexpensive. Third, the device should allow for interchangeable parts; for example, a constructed alternative handle on a device should adapt easily to changing worn-out toothbrushes without having to replace the handle. Fourth, the device should be easily used, and should not require special preparation or set-up time prior to use.

For clients with limited range of motion, extended handles are needed to promote better access to the mouth. Plastic rulers and plastic rods are available from most hardware stores. They can be attached to toothbrushes and floss holders with heavy electrical tape. The added length of the handle facilitates reach but may make placement of the working end of the device in the mouth difficult. To compensate for this problem, a small children's toothbrush or a toothbrush with a compact head size may be used for better intraoral fit. The existing plastic handle of the toothbrush can be bent to angulate the bristles of the brush against the curve of the arches. To bend the handle of a toothbrush, gently heat the handle above a flame or simply hold the handle under very hot tap water until pliable (Fig. 26–10).

To assist the client with weak grip strength, the handle of the device can be built up with a variety of materials. The size of the handle is determined by the client's finger closure capability. For the client with limited finger closure, a wide, bulky handle is needed to assist with grip. Bicycle grips, tennis balls, and styrofoam molds can be used for alternative handles, and they greatly improve the client's ability to hold the device (Figs. 26–11 and 26–12). Toothbrushes and floss holders can be inserted into these devices easily and can be changed when necessary. The disadvantage of using tennis balls and styrofoam molds is that they retain water and become damaged and dirty with time. In addition, styrofoam molds break easily for the client with a clumsy but strong grip because the material is very weak and porous. Clients who have difficulties with coordination may find that a lightweight handle is hard to manage and that a "weighted" end may be easier to find and to hold.

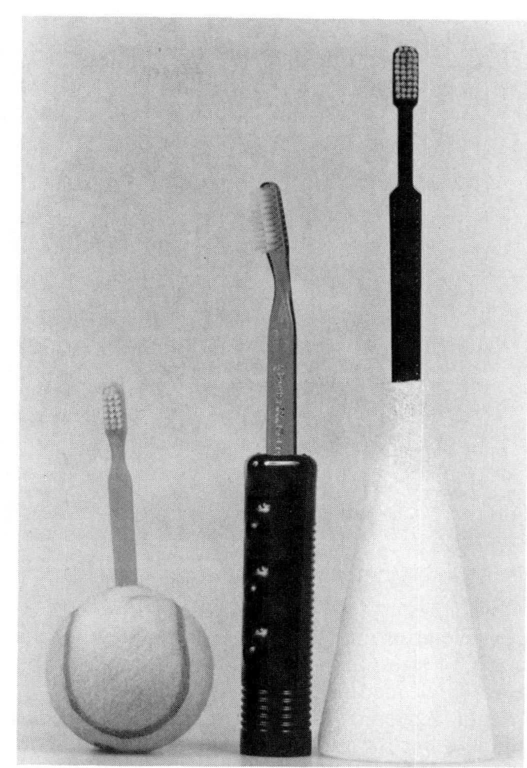

FIGURE 26–11
Bicycle grips, tennis balls, and Styrofoam molds can be used as alternative handles to improve the client's grasp.

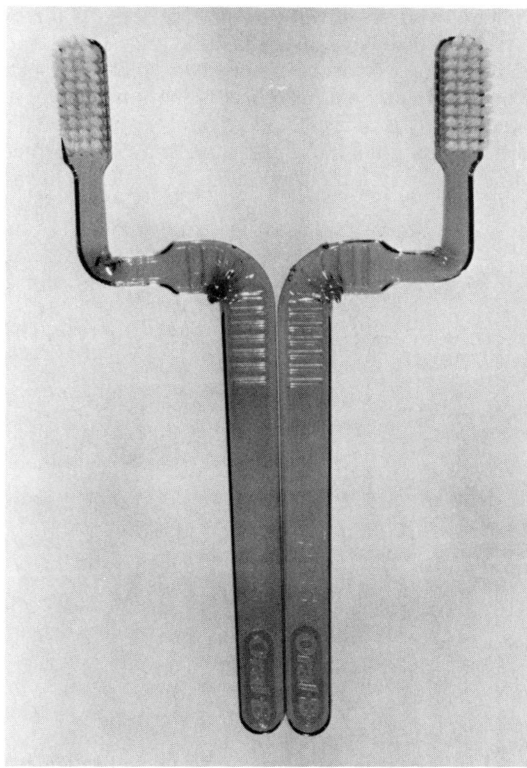

FIGURE 26–10
Plastic handles can be bent to better adapt the device to the arches.

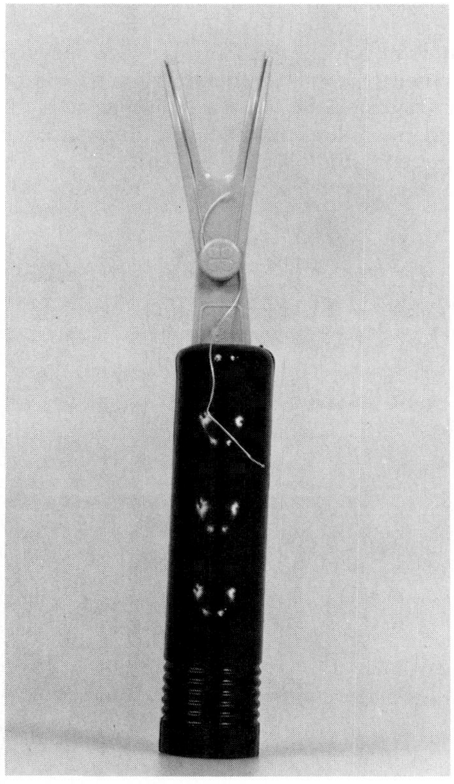

FIGURE 26–12
Floss holders can easily be inserted into an alternative handle.

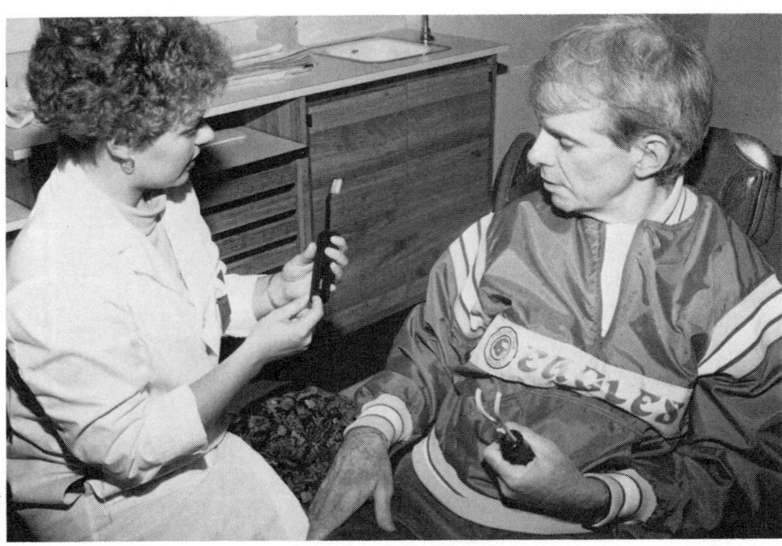

FIGURE 26-13
Client feedback is essential in evaluating compliance, efficacy, and ease of use of the device.

Plastic bicycle grips are preferred because they are available in a variety of sizes, textures, and weights; are inexpensive; and are easily cleaned and rinsed after use.

The dental hygienist is responsible for making these devices initially, but the caregiver may be trained to construct them thereafter. If delegating the responsibility to the caregiver, the hygienist should carefully monitor the construction of the devices for an extended period of time to ascertain whether the construction appropriately meets the client's needs. Any custom-made device should be brought in by the client at every dental hygiene appointment to assess design, usage, and the need for replacement. Client feedback is essential in evaluating compliance, efficacy, and ease of use of the device (Fig. 26-13).

Some devices are currently available on the market that are easily used by disabled clients. They should be considered when assessing the client's oral hygiene status. Many clients with poor dexterity and coordination benefit from using a powered toothbrush—a device that also can be easily manipulated by a caregiver (Fig. 26-14). Several manufacturers, such as John O. Butler Company, Oral B Laboratories, Pycopay, and Sensodyne, market toothbrushes that can be bent by hand without heating to promote better angulation and access into the client's mouth. Floss holders and toothbrushes with wide handles or with specific handle designs all promote improved grasping ability by the client. Toothpaste containers with alternative dispensers, such as flip-top lids and levers, should be recommended to clients with limited finger motion because minimal grip strength is needed to dispense the toothpaste. Oral irrigation devices are excellent supplementary aids for disabled clients for oral hygiene self-care and local delivery of antimicrobial agents.

For clients who are unable to hold devices on their own, a **universal strap** may be used for assistance. This strap fits around the arm or wrist and acts as a splint for stabilization. The strap contains Velcro adhesive on which various implements can be attached. Universal straps are valuable tools for occupational therapists and may be adapted for use with oral physiotherapy aids. The dental hygienist

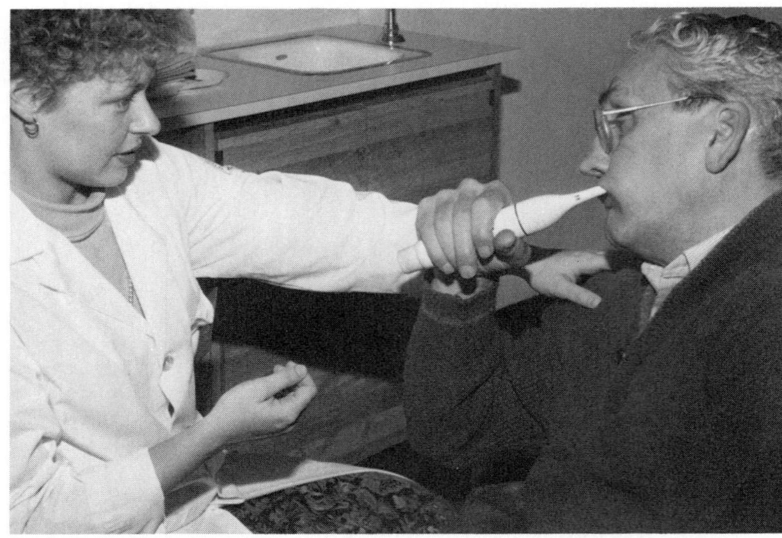

FIGURE 26-14
Clients with poor dexterity and coordination benefit from using a rotary toothbrush.

should consult with an occupational therapist when treating a client who could benefit from use of a universal strap for oral home care devices.

CLIENT POSITIONING AND STABILIZATION

Clients with disabilities may present physical demands on the hygienist throughout the process of care. Disabled clients frequently have problems with support and balance, and special considerations must be made to address these physical problems while in the oral care environment. A physical assessment of the client prior to dental hygiene care is critical to determine whether adaptations are needed to safely treat the client.

Clients with neuromuscular problems, such as tremors, muscle spasms, or hyperflexive responses, may require the use of a physical restraint, such as a seatbelt, to help remain in an upright and stable position. Other restraints such as wraps are available to use with clients who have extreme spasticity or severe behavioral problems, but these restraints should not be considered for use on a routine basis. Use of these restraints engenders distrust in the client and may actually make the problem worse. In addition, *physical restraints* have been associated with bruising, respiratory compromise, aspiration pneumonia, and cellulitis from limb restraint.[19] Pillows or rolled towels may be placed underneath the knees and neck of the client to prevent muscle spasms and to provide additional support during treatment. Restraint or **support devices** should be used with caution with a seizure-prone client, because these devices must be removed quickly in the event of a seizure.

Clients with involuntary muscle spasms or clients who exhibit aggressive behavior during a procedure require minimal restraint for the protection and safety of both the healthcare provider and the client. To prevent injuries during care, a dental assistant or caregiver may hold the client's arms and legs in a comfortable position. A dental assistant can easily rest the arm closest to the client across the client's chest, with the client's arms tucked underneath, so that in the event of a muscular reflex, the client's arms are prevented from moving into the working area. In the case of the disabled child who is difficult to keep still while in the dental chair, the child may lie on top of the parent, with the parent's arms around the child's body. This practice should be discontinued early in the course of care after behavioral management techniques and trust exercises have been conducted with the child (Table 26–3). Clients who are unable to remain still in the dental chair may be indicated for sedation to complete the plan of care.

At times, the dental hygienist may find the need for additional head support and *stabilization* for the client during care. Sitting at the twelve o'clock position, the dental hygienist should wrap his nondominant arm around the head and under the chin of the client. The hand may be used to gently, but firmly, cup the client's chin for stabilization. Small pillows also may be placed on either side of the client's head for additional support, as may a neck roll or a rolled bath towel.

Seat belts and handles are commonly used on wheelchairs to help keep the client positioned correctly in the chair (Fig. 26–15). Cushions are frequently used with paralyzed clients to provide additional support and to minimize the occurrence of pressure sores (**decubitus ulcers** or decubiti). Removable headrests are available for wheelchair adaptation, as are additional neck and back supports.

Occasionally, it may be difficult to teach the parent or caregiver of a severely disabled child how to perform oral hygiene techniques, especially if the child is uncooperative and resists sitting in the dental chair. Parents and caregivers should be encouraged to have the child lie on the floor, and by placing the child's head in the parent's lap, improved visual and physical access into the mouth may be

TABLE 26–3
BEHAVIORAL MANAGEMENT TECHNIQUES

Explanation and exposure (desensitization)	Use of graduated exposure to the oral healthcare setting instills client familiarity with the environment and others
Familiarization visit	Introducing the client to the oral healthcare environment prior to the initiation of care reduces anxiety and fear of unknowns
Demonstration (tell-show-do)	Use of demonstration exercises with the client reinforces verbal instructions
Modeling	Use of a live or videotaped model aids in client skill development by demonstrating a proper or desired behavior or technique
Feedback	Providing the client with immediate feedback improves client learning and skill development through evaluation of progress and performance
Negative consequences (punishment)	Use of adverse consequences deters the client from repeating a behavior, because negative feedback decreases the likelihood of repeating an undesired behavior This technique is most effective when used as an early intervention strategy in cases of undesired behavior
Positive consequences (reward)	Use of positive consequences, or rewards, strengthens behavior and encourages the repetition of a behavior Rewards include praise, special privileges, token systems, and material goods
Distraction	Use of other audiovisual stimuli, such as listening to music through headphones or watching a videotape, decreases uncooperative behavior by providing stimuli on which the client can focus her attention during dental hygiene care
Communication	Choosing words and phrasing that reflect empathy, respect, and warmth enhances client and provider interaction and builds trust
Hand signals	Allowing the fearful client to raise her hand as a sign to stop treatment promotes the client's feelings of safety and security
Touch	Use of a reassuring touch displays warmth and understanding toward the anxious client
Relaxation, hypnosis, sedation	Use of additional techniques that require counseling or drugs may be needed for clients who demonstrate extreme levels of anxiety or fear or uncooperative behavior

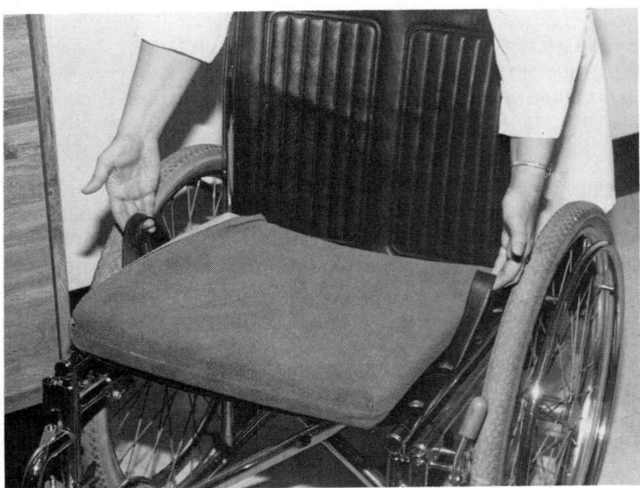

FIGURE 26–15
Handles and seat cushions are commonly used on wheelchairs to keep the client positioned correctly in the chair.

obtained. Parents must be cautioned not to apply any dentifrice or topical agents in this position because the child may aspirate more easily in a supine position. The disabled child who is more cooperative with oral hygiene care may be given ingestible toothpaste to use, a safe alternative for children with neuromuscular or behavioral problems.

To meet the client's human need for safety, proper positioning is critical because of the disabled client's increased risk of aspiration. It is essential to use good evacuation techniques throughout care with the aid of a dental assistant, especially in those cases when increased salivation is present (Fig. 26–16). Rubber dams should be used for dental sealant placement, amalgam recontouring, and placement of temporary restorations to further prevent the risk of aspiration of dental materials. Use of a mouth prop is very helpful for treating most disabled clients, especially for those clients with muscle weakness or muscle spasms. Use of a mouth prop may minimize fatigue for those clients with muscular disorders or involuntary muscular tremors. Clients who are seizure-prone or who experience involuntary spasms should always be treated with a mouth prop to prevent closure of the mandible onto the operator's fingers. The mouth prop should be attached to the napkin clips around the client's neck via a piece of dental floss or string so that in the event of an emergency, the mouth prop can be readily pulled from the mouth.

Most disabled clients can be treated successfully in the oral healthcare environment with few adaptations. The client is usually the best source of information for advice on how to approach positioning and movement. Ideally, all clients should be treated in the dental chair, but on occasion, a client in a wheelchair may be too sick or weak to transfer into the dental chair. Some clients who have catheters may be too risky to transfer for fear of dislodging the tubing during the process. Other clients are afraid of transferring out of the wheelchair and may refuse to do so, even if they have the physical capability. Extremely overweight or physically large clients may be difficult to transfer, and it may not be safe for the dental hygienist to attempt to move the client alone. Regardless of reason, the client in a wheelchair may be treated from the chair position if treatment

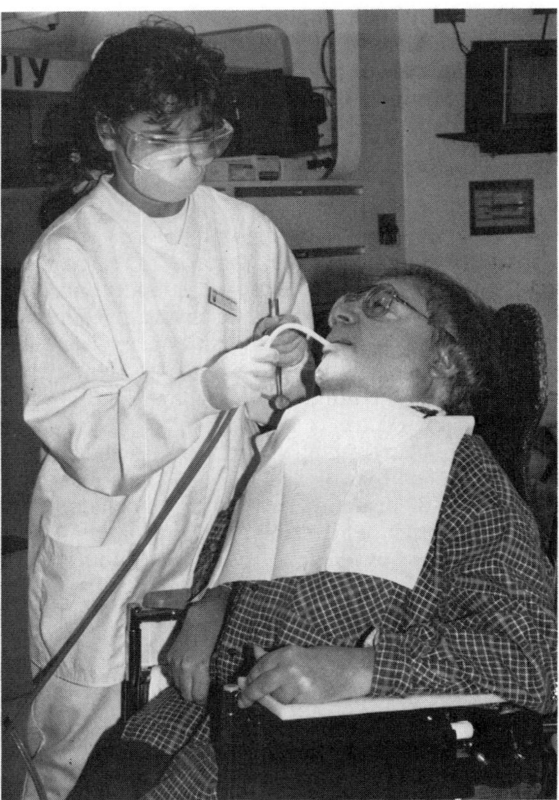

FIGURE 26–16
Good evacuation techniques are essential to prevent aspiration.

areas are wide enough for positioning of the client either alongside or behind the dental chair. The dental unit light can be adjusted for illumination, and most hoses for handpieces and suction can reach the working area.

Clients who remain in the wheelchair need additional head support during care, which can be obtained by using a portable headrest or by turning the client around in the wheelchair so that the head is leaning against the back of the dental chair's headrest.[29] The dental hygienist must be cautioned that treating multiple clients from this position during the day may cause personal physical strain, such as back, neck, and leg fatigue, and therefore, clients who cannot be transferred should be treated early in the day while the hygienist is well rested (Fig. 26–17). After providing client care from this compromised position, the hygienist should take a break for adequate rest and muscle stretching before treating another client. A list of client stabilization and supportive devices is found in Table 26–4.

WHEELCHAIR TRANSFER TECHNIQUES

Most disabled clients can be transferred safely and easily into the dental chair if proper techniques are used throughout the procedure. Various wheelchair **transfer techniques** are available for use depending upon the physical strength and abilities of both the client and practitioner. Prior to attempting a transfer, several steps must be taken to assess the client's ability to participate.[30]

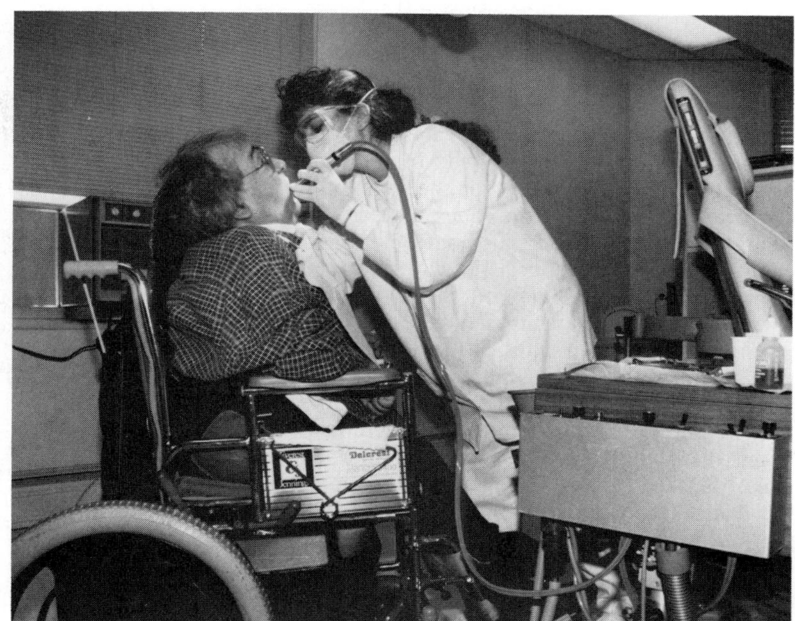

FIGURE 26–17
Treating clients who remain in their wheelchairs can cause considerable fatigue and muscle soreness for the hygienist.

Transferring from Wheelchair to Dental Chair

First, the client's health history must be carefully assessed to determine the client's current health status, the nature of the condition that dictates the use of a wheelchair, existing physical strength, risk of inducing muscle spasm, and areas of the body that could possibly become injured if moved incorrectly. In addition, the client should be questioned regarding the use of urinary appliances, such as catheters and collecting bags, that may become dislodged during transfer. A kinked catheter may result in inadequate drainage of the bladder, causing an accumulation of toxic waste, and thus trigger an emergency situation. It is important to ask the client about the use of urinary appliances so that proper care can be taken not to dislodge the appliance

TABLE 26–4
CLIENT POSITIONING AND STABILIZATION DEVICES

Item	Manufacturer	Contact
Mouthprops	Kent Dental	1-800-345-8202
Client assistive devices		Abet Medical
For home use:	Flaghouse	(Distributor)
Universal straps	Preston	2816 Limekiln Pike
Velcro straps	Sammons	Glenside, PA 19038
		215-576-7151
Wheelchair transfer boards	Therafin	
Seatbelts	Quickie	
	Thompson	
	P.R.C.	
	Canyon	
Restraints	Skillcare	
	Posey	
Portable dental chair Portable dental unit	ADEC	ADEC Equipment Company P.O. Box 111 Newberg, OR 97132 1-800-547-1883
Portable dental units (carry units/mobile carts)	Dentalaire	Dentalaire Products International 1820 S. Grand Avenue Santa Ana, CA 92705 714-540-9969
Portable dental unit (Transcare Portable Self-Contained Unit)		Healthco 2866 Banksville Road Philadelphia, PA 1-800-222-1708
Portable dental operatories Portable dental chairs and stools Portable dental x-ray equipment Portable dental units	M-Dec Corporation	Mobile Dental Equipment Corporation 16604 SE 17th Place Bellevue, WA 98008 1-800-321-6332

during the transfer. The client's physician should be consulted about specific medical concerns raised during the health history review prior to attempting any transfer movement.

Second, the client's physical ability to participate with the transfer should be assessed. Many clients who have undergone physical therapy for their condition may be accustomed to transfer techniques, especially if they have been taught to transfer at home by themselves. Some clients have the ability to assist with the transfer, although they may be unfamiliar with the actual procedural steps involved. Still other clients may perceive that they have the physical strength and skills needed to assist the dental hygienist with the transfer, when actually they do not possess these abilities. Misconceptions about abilities to transfer may be dangerous if the transfer is attempted without verifying whether the client's perceptions and abilities are realistic. Also, the client's willingness to transfer is essential for the dental hygienist to know; it is important to remember that during any transfer procedure there is a certain level of dependency upon the practitioner by the client, especially during lifting from the wheelchair. An uncooperative client who overestimates or underestimates his abilities or a client who resists transfer attempts poses significant management challenges for the hygienist, as well as increased risk for injury to both the client and the practitioner.

Third, the client's level of coordination and balance should be discussed to determine the need for assistance with the transfer process. Assistance may be required from another operator, or may be obtained with the use of a *transfer belt* or *transfer board.* Transfer belts are secured around the client's waist to provide a place to hold the client in the event that the person begins to slip or fall during the transfer process.[30] Transfer belts are especially useful with clients who have little to no upper body strength, such as quadriplegics. Transfer boards are used to assist the client with good upper body strength by helping him slide out of the wheelchair across the board and into the dental chair. The wheelchair must be positioned beside the dental chair, and the arms to both chairs must be removed to accommodate the board. One end of the board is placed underneath the client and the other end is laid across the dental chair. The client uses upper arm and body strength to pull the body across the board, while the board provides support from underneath the client's legs. Transfer boards also are useful with clients who are overweight or are otherwise too big for one person to safely move alone. Transfer belts may be used as an added precaution during a sliding transfer with a board.

In addition to client safety, the operator's safety should be ensured as well. Several safety precautions must be taken by the operator before attempting any transfer procedure. First, the operator should never attempt to transfer a client alone. Although the one-person transfer technique requires only one individual to maneuver the client, an additional person must always be available to provide assistance if needed. The presence of an additional person to help greatly reduces the risk of falling or injury to the client during a transfer. Second, the operator should never attempt alone to transfer a client who is very tall or heavy, especially those clients who have no upper body strength. These clients have a much greater chance of falling, because of their lack of coordination and balance, and they may injure both themselves and the operator. Third, all transfer movements performed by the operator should be done with the feet separated for good balance and with the knees bent to protect against back strain. Fourth, all lifting procedures should be performed with the legs while keeping the back straight and slightly bent forward at the waist to prevent muscular back injury to the operator. Finally, the operator should never attempt to twist the back while lifting the client out of the wheelchair and into the dental chair; twisting may cause severe muscular back strain and injury. Instead, the operator should move with small steps to position the client.[31]

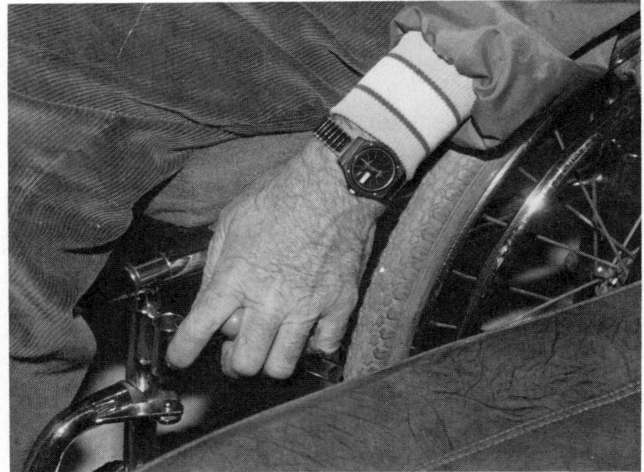

FIGURE 26-18
Prior to transfer, lock the wheels on the wheelchair.

Prior to beginning the transfer procedure, the client should be informed of the steps to be used during the process. The hygienist should take the time to explain the steps to reduce client anxiety and to answer questions. If the client is expected to assist with the transfer, he must be informed of how and when his assistance is needed. A simulation with the client is very helpful prior to performing the actual procedure, especially for those clients who have never been transferred previously. To prepare for

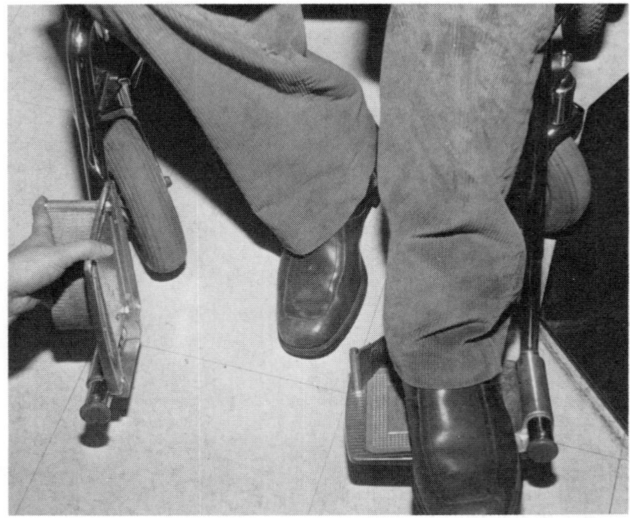

FIGURE 26-19
Footrests on the wheelchair should be folded back, so the client's feet can be correctly positioned for transfer.

transferring the client, the following procedures are performed:[31]

1. Position the wheelchair beside the dental chair. The wheelchair should be parallel with the dental chair, with the seats aligned, or with the seat of the dental chair slightly lower than the wheelchair in relation to the floor.
2. Position the wheelchair so that the wheels are facing forward. This position of the wheels helps to steady the chair and reduces the chance of tipping during the transfer.
3. Lock the wheels on the wheelchair (Fig. 26–18). For clients who use electronically operated wheelchairs, the appropriate adjustments should be made to secure the brakes on the chair, after which the motor should be turned off.
4. Remove the footrests from the chair. Footrests may also be folded back so that the client's feet do not become caught during the transfer process. The client's feet should be gently placed on the floor by the operator to prevent spasm and to position the feet for the appropriate transfer (Fig. 26–19).
5. Remove the arms of both the wheelchair and the dental chair. If the arm of the dental chair is not removable, it should be positioned as far back as possible so that it does not interfere with the transfer (Fig. 26–20).
6. Check the area for any sharp edges or cords that could cause injury during the transfer process.
7. Unfasten the client's safety belt. After the belt is removed, the operator must support the client to prevent falling.
8. Transfer any special padding used underneath the client to the dental chair. Gently rock the client forward while an assistant removes the padding from the wheelchair and places it onto the dental chair.

Some clients are able to transfer themselves into and out of the dental chair with little to no assistance. These transfer techniques are called "semi-dependent transfers," and the dental hygienist is used only to provide support and assistance on an "as needed" basis by the client. Each client has a different level of need; there are no strict guidelines to follow when assisting a client with these maneuvers. The most important concept for the hygienist to remember is to be readily available to ensure the safety of the client during the transfer process.

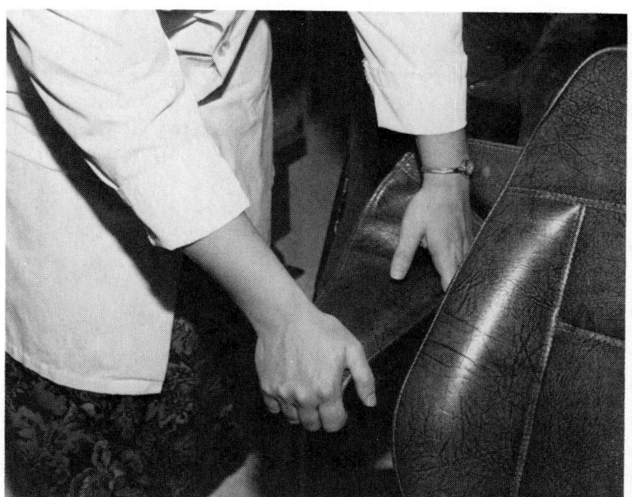

FIGURE 26–20
The arm of the dental chair should be positioned as far back as possible so it does not interfere with the transfer.

The two main transfer techniques used for dependent clients are the one-person and two-person transfer lifts. Each lift contains specific criteria to follow for client and operator safety. Prior to initiating either of these lifts, the hygienist should prepare the client for transfer according to the aforementioned criteria. The procedures used for the lifts are shown below.[30,31]

PROCEDURE 26–1

TRANSFERRING A CLIENT FROM WHEELCHAIR TO THE DENTAL CHAIR (ONE-PERSON LIFT)

Steps	Rationale
1. A transfer belt is securely positioned around the client's waist just below the ribcage.	Use of a transfer belt ensures client safety.
2. The operator inserts his hands underneath the client's thighs, and gently slides the client forward in the wheelchair seat so that the client's buttocks are positioned on the front portion of the seat.	This position brings the client's center of gravity closer to the operator, which facilitates the transfer.
3. The client's feet are then placed together and are held in place on either side by the operator's feet. The operator then closes his knees on the client's knees, thus supporting and stabilizing the client's legs, which allows the client to bear some of his own weight during the lift.	Supporting the client's legs helps prevent the client from falling forward onto the operator during the lift.
4. The client's arms are then placed over the shoulders of the operator, and the client is instructed to rest his head on the left shoulder of the operator.	This position allows the operator to see behind the client and to clearly view the dental chair.
5. The operator grasps the client around the waist and holds the transfer belt securely between both hands. If there is no transfer belt available, use an overlapping wrist grasp for greater stability.	Overlapping the arms to grasp the belt is recommended to provide added stability.

CONTINUED ON FOLLOWING PAGE

Steps	Rationale
6. The client is now positioned for the lift. The operator rocks gently backwards onto the heels and, using the leg muscles, lifts the client off the seat. The client is now resting against the operator.	
7. The operator pivots on the foot closest to the dental chair, and maneuvers the client over the seat of the dental chair. This should be done in a smooth motion.	
8. The client is lowered onto the dental chair by the operator by bending at the knees. The operator must not release the transfer belt around the client until the client is securely placed into the chair.	Bending at the knees reduces the risk of injury to the operator. Maintaining hold of the transfer belt ensures client safety.
9. The operator releases the right hand to lift the client's legs onto the chair while still holding the transfer belt with the left hand. The armrest of the dental chair is repositioned for the client's safety.	Repositioning the client establishes client stability and safety.

PROCEDURE 26–2

TRANSFERRING A CLIENT FROM A WHEELCHAIR TO THE DENTAL CHAIR (TWO-PERSON LIFT)

Steps	Rationale
1. The first operator stands behind the client, and reaches around the client's torso underneath the client's armpits. The operator crosses his arms in front of the client, and grasps the client's hands at the wrists with his opposite hands (right over left, left over right). The operator then slides his arms down so that his arms are positioned under the client's ribcage on the abdomen.	The stronger of the two operators is placed behind the client to support the majority of the client's weight.
2. The second operator is positioned on the right side of the wheelchair at the client's legs and feet (Fig. 26–21). Bending at the knees, the operator slides one arm underneath the client's thighs slightly above the knees, while the other arm is placed underneath the client's ankles to support the feet.	The second operator provides support for the client's lower extremities during transfer.

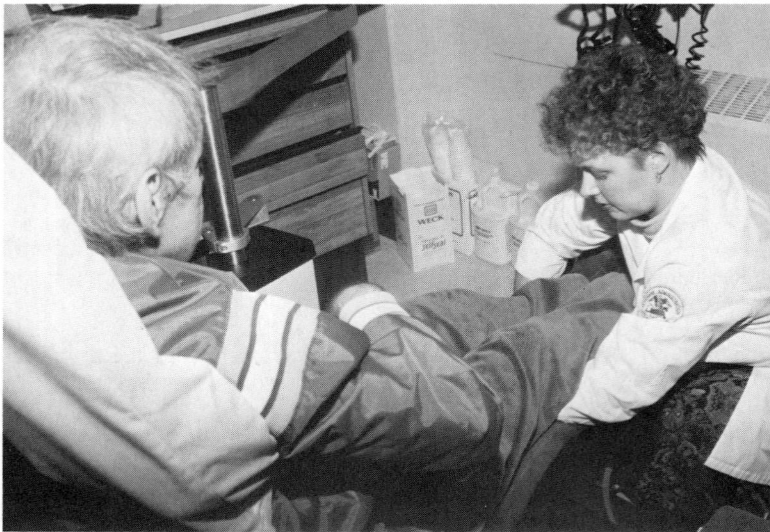

FIGURE 26–21
The second operator is positioned on the right side of the wheelchair at the client's legs and feet.

Steps	Rationale
3. The client is lifted simultaneously by both operators. The lift is done at a prearranged signal, such as at the end of a count ("1,2,3, lift"). One person should coordinate the lift, preferably the operator who is supporting the client's torso, the operator who is lifting the most weight.	Use of a prearranged signal eliminates the risk of loss of client support by one or both operators during the lift. Loss of client support places the client and the operators at risk to injury.
4. The client is lifted in one smooth motion and is placed in the dental chair.	
5. The operator holding the legs releases the grasp on the client, and repositions the client in the chair. The other operator does not release the client until the client is stabilized and the arm of the dental chair is replaced (Fig. 26–22).	Repositioning the client establishes client stability and safety.

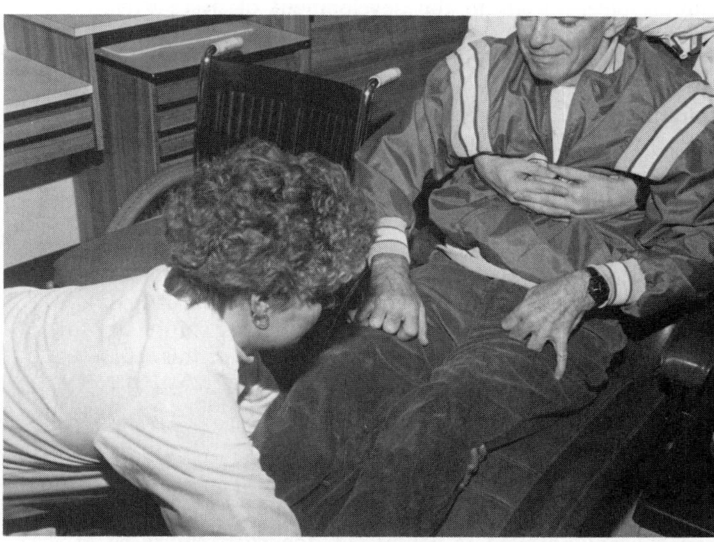

FIGURE 26–22
The first operator supports the client while the second operator positions and stabilizes the client after transfer.

After the client has been transferred, several steps must be taken to ensure that the client is stable and secure in this new position:[31]

1. Center the client in the chair, making certain that the client is balanced and comfortable.
2. Adjust pillows for support, and add additional supportive devices, such as belts or rolled towels for padding, if necessary.
3. Assess the risk for the development of pressure sores. Straighten clothing that may bind the client, especially around the legs and arms, and readjust any padding underneath areas that are in contact with the dental chair that may not normally support the client's weight.
4. Check the client's catheters or other urinary appliances to be certain that there is no urinary backflow. The appliances should be positioned so that there is a gravitational downflow of urine.
5. Recheck the position of the armrest on the dental chair. The armrest must be locked into place for adequate client safety.

Complications Involved in Wheelchair Transfer

There are several risks associated with wheelchair transfers with which the dental hygienist must be familiar.

Muscle Spasms

Movement of a client may stimulate muscle spasms, and the hygienist must be prepared to protect the client from injury if spasms occur. Continuous spasms may be reduced by gently massaging the affected area or simply by waiting until the muscle relaxes. Use of supportive pillows may reduce the incidence of spasms induced by movement. Anxiety can also contribute to spasms; therefore, the hygienist should talk to the client to reduce fear and to address any concerns prior to initiating the transfer.

Pressure Sores

Individuals who use wheelchairs are prone to developing pressure sores known as decubitus ulcers. Decubiti form in areas where there is blood pooling, such as on the buttocks and on the backs of the thighs. Decubiti can be extremely painful and easily become infected. The dental hygienist must question the disabled client during the health history review about the presence of decubiti. To prevent decubiti from occurring, clients must perform *weight shifts* every 20 minutes to relieve pressure from the skin. When clients are transferred into the dental chair, supportive devices and weight shifts must be incorporated into the client's appointment management plan. Changes in skin integrity must be monitored carefully and should be brought to the attention of the client's physician.

Bowel and Bladder Elimination Schedules

Clients who are transferred into the dental chair may need to be reminded of the time so that the client may adhere to his bowel and bladder elimination program. Adequate time must be allotted to transfer the client back into the wheelchair if the client needs to use the restroom during an appointment. The schedule of the client's program should be recorded in the health history document.

Autonomic Dysreflexia

The presence of any of these conditions poses significant risk for the development of **autonomic dysreflexia,** a severe condition that can be fatal if left untreated. The presence of noxious stimuli, such as urinary backflow or pain from decubitus ulcers, leads to the development of dysreflexia, manifested by a variety of symptoms in the client. The client may appear disoriented and flushed and may exhibit profuse sweating and goosebumps. The most characteristic manifestation of dysreflexia is an extremely elevated blood pressure, which ultimately results in stroke. The dental hygiene practitioner who is alerted to any of these clinical signs must stop work immediately, check the client's blood pressure, and begin to look for the cause of the reaction. Usually, treatment of the cause produces an immediate, favorable response, such as when a kinked catheter is straightened. Any suspicion of dysreflexia must be treated as a severe medical emergency, and assistance must be summoned immediately. Because of the nature of this risk, it is imperative that *no client who is transferred to the dental chair be left unattended.*

Transferring the Client Back to the Wheelchair

When the appointment is completed, the client must be transferred from the dental chair back into the wheelchair. The same procedures are conducted to move the client, with special attention given to replacing the padding and supports underneath the client before seating him in the wheelchair. The wheels of the chair must always be locked when transferring the client back into the wheelchair.

Transfer techniques require practice to perform safely and successfully. Routinely practicing these techniques, especially for those who conduct actual client transfers infrequently, helps to ensure competence in performing transfer procedures. The assistance of physical therapists in training and practice can be helpful to those hygienists who are unfamiliar with interacting with clients in wheelchairs. Transfer techniques, when used in daily practice, can enable hygienists to treat a variety of clients who may otherwise not receive necessary preventive oral healthcare services.

THE DENTAL HYGIENIST AS EDUCATOR, HEALTH PROMOTER, ADVOCATE, AND RESEARCHER

Educator

Aside from the role of clinician, the dental hygienist may serve in a variety of roles when interacting with clients with special needs. The underlying purpose that drives the process of dental hygiene care is educating those who present with special needs or who care for those with special needs, and to improve the process by applying current research findings to practice. The dental hygienist serves as **educator** throughout the clinical experience with the client and in teaching continued care with clients, families, and caregivers. Teaching begins at the initial client contact and is used while assessing the client's human needs related to dental hygiene care, designing and evaluating self-care programs, and monitoring client progress throughout the person's lifetime, as her needs change.

Education is also a critical factor that validates the dental hygienist's role as a member of the **interdisciplinary care** team who collaboratively treats clients with special needs. As a consultant, the dental hygienist may work closely with physicians, nurses, physical and occupational therapists, and dietitians in identifying needs, setting goals, and planning client health programs. The dental hygienist may work directly with any of these professionals in designing individualized programs for clients who present with unique and challenging management problems. Through in-service education, the dental hygienist can help other healthcare providers understand the importance of oral health status as it relates to client human needs. The dental hygienist can teach these professionals how to effectively screen for early signs of oral disease and encourage those providers to make referrals for early dental hygiene intervention and oral health promotion.

Families and caregivers of the client require educational oral health services to clarify information and to learn how to maximize their roles as healthcare providers for the client. The dental hygienist works closely with these individuals who play an important role in managing the activities of daily living either with or for the client. Teaching strategies used with families and caregivers frequently include demonstrations and repetition; therefore, the dental hygienist must allot an adequate amount of time to work with these individuals and to answer questions and address concerns. The dental hygienist who conveys a genuine concern for these caregivers will find that they are responsive and willing to receive information to better care for their dependents. Occasionally, the dental hygienist may encounter a caregiver who does not wish to be responsible for the daily oral healthcare practices of another person. When the dental hygienist experiences frustration in trying to convince a caregiver to participate, it is wise to address the issue with the individual and identify alternative solutions to avoid jeopardizing the client's health.

Health Promoter

As a health promoter, the hygienist serves the client through the development and implementation of preventive programs that not only focus on early detection and intervention but that also enable the client to achieve oral wellness. Dental hygienists can also promote wellness in these clients by encouraging health to continue through proper oral healthcare behaviors, by participating in educational programs such as health fairs and by volunteering for community service. All of these actions constitute **health promotion.**

Advocate

As an **advocate,** the dental hygienist supports disabled clients not only in the healthcare arena but also by promoting the rights of these clients as contributing members of society. Many disabled populations are underserved because of the high costs of healthcare and the numerous barriers to care. Opportunities abound for dental hygienists to work with these populations to improve their access to dental hygiene services. Participation on councils, local boards, and in area support groups helps other members of the community identify dental hygienists as leaders in **client advocacy.** Holding leadership positions in organizations, initiating community programs, and contributing to both the lay and professional communities through speaking engagements and publications generates action and effects change for citizens with special needs (see Resource List for Information Regarding Disabilities chart).

Researcher

Dental hygienists serve in **non-traditional care settings,** such as long-term care institutions, group homes, and via cooperation with home health agencies to reach those clients whose human needs often go unattended. The profession of dental hygiene assumes responsibility for teaching these clients to control oral disease, and leads in the provision of preventive oral healthcare by reaching out to the community, conducting research to improve knowledge and practice, and by utilizing every available resource to ensure access to quality dental hygiene services. Dental hygiene **researchers** continue to investigate new methods of oral hygiene care for clients with special needs and serve an important role in information transfer, ensuring that the latest valid research findings are applied in practice to improve client care.

SUMMARY

Table 26–5 provides a comprehensive list of medical conditions requiring special care from the dental hygienist and guidelines for the dental hygienist to follow.

RESOURCE LIST FOR INFORMATION REGARDING DISABILITIES

American Association of Public
Health Dentistry
10619 Jousting Lane
Richmond, Va 23235

American Bar Association
Commission on Legal Problems of the Elderly
1800 M Street, N.W.
Washington, D.C. 20036
202-331-2297

American Dental Association
Special Care in Dentistry
211 East Chicago Avenue, Room 1616
Chicago, IL 60611
800-621-8099

American Dental Hygienists' Association
444 North Michigan Avenue, Suite 3400
Chicago, IL 60611
312-440-8900

American Geriatrics Society, Inc.
770 Lexington Avenue, Suite 400
New York, NY 10021
212-308-1414

American Health Care Association
1200 15th Street, N.W.
Washington, D.C. 20005
202-833-2050

American Public Health Association
1015 15th Street, N.W.
Washington, D.C. 20005
202-789-5600

American Society for Geriatric Dentistry
211 East Chicago Avenue
Chicago, IL 60611

Association for Children with
Retarded Mental Development
162 Fifth Avenue, 11th Floor
New York, NY 10010

Association for Retarded Citizens (see local listing)

American Society on Aging
833 Market Street, Room 516
San Francisco, CA 94103
415-543-2617

Board of Education
Division of Special Populations
Presidential Building
415 12th Street, N.W.
Washington, D.C. 20004
202-724-3636

Department of Employment Services
Disability Compensation Program
1200 Upshur Street, N.W.
Washington, D.C. 20011
202-576-7090

Department of Health and Human Services
200 Independence Avenue, S.W.
Washington, D.C. 20024
Information: 202-475-0257
Administration on Developmental
Disabilities: 202-245-2890
Handicapped Employment Program: 202-245-6568

Easter Seals (see local listing)

Gerontologic Society of America
1275 K. Street, N.W.
Suite 350
Washington, D.C. 20005-4006

Gray Panthers
National Office
311 South Juniper Street
Philadelphia, PA 19107
202-545-6555

Health Security Action Council
1757 N Street, N.W.
Washington, D.C. 20036
202-223-9685

Legal Counsel for the Elderly
1331 H Street, N.W., Suite 1005
Washington, D.C. 20005
202-234-0970

CONTINUED ON FOLLOWING PAGE

RESOURCE LIST FOR INFORMATION REGARDING DISABILITIES *Continued*

Medicaid/Medicare Management Institute (MMMI)
6401 Security Boulevard
Baltimore, MD 21235
301-594-9526

Multiple Sclerosis Society (see local listing)

National Association for Home Care
519 C Street, N.E.
Washington, D.C. 20002
202-547-7424

National Association of Home Health Agencies
426 C Street, N.E., Suite 200
Washington, D.C. 20002
202-547-1717

National Association of Social Workers
7981 Eastern Avenue
Silver Spring, MD 20910
301-565-0333

National Geriatrics Society
212 W. Wisconsin Avenue, Third Floor
Milwaukee, WI 53203
414-272-4130

National Hospice Organization
1901 N. Fort Myer Drive #307
Arlington, VA 22209
703-243-5900

National Information Center for Children with Handicaps
7926 Jones Branch Drive
McLean, VA 22102
703-893-6061

National Organization on Disability
910 16th Street, N.W.
Washington, D.C. 20006
202-293-5960

National Rehabilitation Information Center
8455 Colesville Road
Silver Spring, MD 20910
301-588-9284

Office of Human Rights Handicap Coordinator
Frank D. Reeves Center
2000 14th Street, N.W.
Washington, D.C. 20009
202-939-8740

United Cerebral Palsy (see local listing)

United Way (see local listing)

Federal Government
Department of Health and Human Services

Administration on Aging
Office of Public Information
330 Independence Avenue, S.W.
Room 4247
Washington, D.C. 20201
202-245-0724

Federal Council on Aging
Room 4545 Cohen Building
330 Independence Avenue, S.W.
Washington, D.C. 20201
202-245-2451

Health Care Financing Administration (HCFA)
Office of Public Affairs
200 Independence Avenue, S.W.,
Room 435H
Washington, D.C. 20201
202-245-6113

National Center for Health Services Research (NCHSR)
3700 East-West Highway, Room 7-44
Hyattsville, MD 20782
301-436-8970

National Center for Health Statistics (NCHS)
Scientific and Technical Information Branch
3700 East-West Highway
Hyattsville, MD 20782
301-436-8500

National Institutes of Health (NIH)
Division of Public Information
9000 Rockville Pike
Building 1, Room 309
Bethesda, MD 20205
301-496-5787

Office of Disease Prevention and Health Promotion
330 C Street, N.W.
Washington, D.C. 20201
202-472-5660
Also operates National Information Clearinghouse:
800-336-4797

National Clearinghouse on Aging
Administration on Aging, DHHS
330 Independence Avenue, S.W.
Washington, D.C. 20201
202-245-0995

RESOURCE LIST FOR INFORMATION REGARDING DISABILITIES *Continued*

The Institutes

National Institute on Aging
9000 Rockville Pike
Building 1, Room 5C-36
Bethesda, MD 20205
301-496-9625

National Library of Medicine
301-496-6221

National Cancer Institute
301-496-5615

National Eye Institute
301-496-2234

National Institute of Allergy and Infectious Diseases
301-496-2263

National Institute of Arthritis, Diabetes, Digestive and Kidney Disease
301-496-5887

National Institute of Child Health and Human Development
301-496-3454

National Institute of Dental Research
301-496-3571

National Institute of Environmental Health Sciences
Research Triangle, NC 27709
919-541-3201

National Institute of General Medical Sciences
301-496-5231

National Institute of Neurological and Communicative Disorders and Stroke
301-496-3167

National Institute of Arthritis and Musculoskeletal and Skin Diseases
301-496-4000

National Institute on Deafness and Other Communication Disorders
301-496-4000

Other Government Agencies
Commission on Social Services

Mental Retardation and Developmental Disabilities Services Administration
202-673-7678

Rehabilitation Services Administration
202-727-3227

Hearing Impaired Services
202-727-0981

Services to Handicapped and Disabled
202-727-0955

Visually Impaired Services
202-727-0907

Disability Determination Division
202-727-8584

TABLE 26–5
SIGNIFICANT FACTORS RELATED TO THE DENTAL HYGIENE CARE OF INDIVIDUALS WITH SPECIAL NEEDS

Condition	Medical Manifestations	Barriers to Care	Associated Risk Factors	Care Considerations	Prevention/Education and Health Promotion Issues	Common Oral Manifestations
Mental retardation	Syndrome? Associated medical conditions/other disabilities Treatment regimens	Limited financial resources Degree of reliance on others Limited mental ability	Oral motor dysfunction General incoordination Cariogenic foods/reinforcers Self-abuse Resistant behavior	Gagging: radiographs, instrument placement, positioning Mental impairment: communication, cooperation, and stability in chair Limited finances: alternative care plans	"Tell-show-do" approach Simple language Frequent repetition and positive reinforcement Involve caretakers Frequent evaluation appointments Alternatives for food reinforcers	Thickness of the lips; irregular eruption patterns; tooth anomalies; oral habits such as clenching, bruxing, mouthbreathing, tongue thrusting; dental caries, gingivitis, and periodontal disease
Down syndrome	Heart defects? (antibiotic premedication) Decreased resistance to infection Frequent respiratory infections	Same as for mental retardation	Same as for mental retardation	Same as for mental retardation plus: Small oral area: oral access for procedures Hearing disorders: communication	Same as for mental retardation plus: Stress oral hygiene and periodontal maintenance	Same as for mental retardation plus: open mouth with protruding tongue; enlarged tonsils and adenoids; large, fissured tongue; microdontia and peg lateral incisors; class III malocclusion; posterior crossbite; flat facial profile
Autism	No major problems	Behavior Degree of reliance on others Communication Minimal language skills	Eating disorders or fetishes Resistant behavior	Dependence on "routines": procedure sequencing Lack of useful language: communication Learning disabilities/sensitivity to stimuli: communication distractions in the operatory	Combine verbal and nonverbal communication techniques and positive reinforcers Teach toothbrushing as a "motion" rather than a function Avoid metaphors and complex language structures	Neglected oral care; intraoral trauma due to self-injurious, aggressive behavior
Learning disabilities/minimal brain dysfunction	Medications and potential side effects	Depends on type of disability	Depends on disability Oral motor dysfunction General incoordination	Depends on disability Disorientation/hyperactivity; stability in chair, length of appointments, physical contact	Tap skill areas Use combination of teaching approaches Maintain attention through eye contact and physical contact Involve caregiver when necessary	No specific oral manifestations

Emotional/mental illness	Medications and potential side effects Psychological causes of reported symptoms/diseases, fears	Limited financial resources in some cases Emotional concerns, fears about oral healthcare Disturbed thought processes	Depends on nature of disturbance Inadequate diet or strange food practices Phobias relating to oral care Self-abuse Side effects of medications	Anxiety, fear, aggression: stability in chair, cooperation, communication	Reality orientation techniques Possible dietary counseling Involve caretakers Positive reinforcement and repetition Decrease phobias and self-abuse Fluoride supplements if xerostomia from medications	Intraoral trauma due to self-injurious, aggressive behavior; xerostomia due to medications may contribute to dental caries, decreased salivary buffering capacity, gingivitis, glossitis, stomatitis, acute parotitis, candidiasis, angular cheilitis
Depressive disorders	Greater-than-average sensitivity to medication Medications and potential side effects	Compliance failure Possible financial barriers Disturbed thought processes	Insomnia or hypersomnia Psychomotor agitation or retardation Loss of energy Decreased ability to think, make decisions, and concentrate Ideas of death and suicide Inadequate diet or strange food habits	Obtain informed consent Give checklists for specific instructions Variable pain response During oral hygiene avoid guilt-inducing language Modify time of appointments, duration of visits, and type of procedures, if needed	Encourage a regular awakening ritual Recommend three small meals a day with a snack in between Recommend fruit snacks and milk before bed to enhance sleep Encourage a regular exercise program Involve caregivers if necessary Saliva substitute and fluoride application if xerostomia is present	Same as for emotional/mental illness
Anxiety disorder	Greater-than-average sensitivity to medication Medications and potential side effects	Compliance failure Possible financial barriers Emotional concerns/fears of dental care Disturbed thought processes	Motor tension (jumpiness, jitters, tension headaches, etc.) Autonomic hyperactivity (heart pounding, clammy hands, dry mouth, etc.) Apprehensive expectation (anxiety, worry, etc.) Vigilance and scanning behavior (poor concentration, insomnia, easily distracted) Inadequate diet or strange food habits	Obtain informed consent Utilize relaxation techniques Explain all procedures and outcomes to avoid hyperventilation, tachycardia, and/or hypersensitivity to pain Investigate all medications prior to administration of anesthesia Possible use of nitrous oxide or a minor tranquilizer before treatment Consider possibility of alcohol or drug abuse by person prior to dental visit Modify time of appointments, duration of visits, and types of procedures, if needed	Recommend elimination of nicotine, caffeine, alcohol, salt, and sugar from diet Educate person about the interaction between fear and anxiety and physical manifestations of each Involve caregiver when necessary Saliva substitute and/or fluoride application if xerostomia is present	Xerostomia due to medications that may contribute to dental caries, decreased salivary buffering capacity, gingivitis, glossitis, stomatitis, acute parotitis, candidiasis, angular cheilitis

Table continued on following page

TABLE 26–5
SIGNIFICANT FACTORS RELATED TO THE DENTAL HYGIENE CARE OF INDIVIDUALS WITH SPECIAL NEEDS *Continued*

Condition	Medical Manifestations	Barriers to Care	Associated Risk Factors	Care Considerations	Prevention/Education and Health Promotion Issues	Common Oral Manifestations
Schizophrenia	Antipsychotic medications Parkinsonism Extrapyramidal signs and symptoms of medications: akathisia (change of body position frequently or rising and pacing the floor); dyskinesia (abnormal movement); nystagmus (oscillatory movement of the eyeballs); restlessness Cardiovascular signs and symptoms of medication effects: orthostatic hypotension; tachycardia; cholinergic effects	Compliance failure Possible financial barriers Emotional/concerns fears of dental care Disturbed thought processes	Delusions Auditory hallucinations Functional impairment Illogical thinking Incoherence Neglected oral hygiene Side effects of medications	Disturbed self-image—concentrate on aesthetic component Distrust and paranoia Extreme sensitivity to the feelings of others Continued contact with professionals managing disorder Perform procedures in an organized, straightforward manner Obtain informed consent Modify time of appointment, duration of visits, types of procedures performed, if needed	Encourage regular appointments and help from caregiver when needed Saliva substitute and fluoride application if xerostomia is present Recommend elimination of nicotine, caffeine, alcohol, salt, and sugar from diet	Same as for emotional/mental illness
Eating disorders	Symptoms: Anorexia— amenorrhea, abnormally functioning endocrine glands, hypothermia, lanugo hair, bradycardia, electrolyte imbalance, compulsive physical activity, dry/cracked skin, brittle nails, cardiac arrhythmias Bulimia— hypokalemia, electrolyte imbalances, urinary infections, renal damage, cardiomyopathy, peripheral myopathy, constipation, abdominal pain	Psychological status Denial of symptoms Guilt and shame Avoidance Intense fear of weight gain Relapse Expense of treatment Length of treatment Client compliance	Eating patterns Frequent vomiting Xerostomia Depression Life-threatening risk factors include conflict, life crises, major life changes, need for control, need for approval	Coordinated care: physicians, nutritionist, and psychologist Carious or eroded teeth: restoration Anxiety: psychosedation Pit and fissure sealants, if appropriate Study models to monitor progression of tooth structure loss	Saliva substitute or sugar-free gum for xerostomia Rinsing with sodium bicarbonate after vomiting rather than using toothbrushes Emphasize self-control of oral hygiene and oral disease Neutral pH sodium fluoride rinses or stannous fluoride gels used daily Stress good oral health in terms of appearance and body image Frequent brushing but not after vomiting Use of a mouth protector	Anorexia: dental caries Bulimia: enamel erosion, dental caries, salivary gland enlargement, oropharyngeal inflammation, xerostomia, dentinal hypersensitivity, raised appearance of restorations, smooth and dished-out appearance of lingual surfaces of teeth

	Amount of weight loss Presence and frequency of bulimia Medical and psychological interventions Eating patterns Binge-purge cycle Associated psychiatric disorders					
Alzheimer's disease	Multiple medical problems Medications Reduced bowel and bladder control Fatigue from abnormal sleep patterns	Behavior Finances may be limited by disability and medical problems Communication Wheelchair confinement Uncooperative Dependence on others	Oral motor dysfunction Depression or disorientation leading to oral neglect General motor dysfunction Deficit in cognitive and psychomotor skills Potential for injury	Fluctuating moods and disorientation: length of appointments, communication, cooperation Motor problems: oral access, radiographs, stability in chair Memory loss: data collection Establish oral wellness early in course of disease	Involve caretakers Involve client when most lucid and positive Simple instructions and frequent repetition Positive reinforcement Frequent maintenance care Prevent oral injuries	Poor oral hygiene, increased incidence of oral injuries and periodontal disease
Epileptic disorders	Medications and side effects Seizure information: Type and degree of control Specific manifestations Presence of aura Frequency General management History of status epilepticus	Transportation if cannot drive Disturbance in self-image	Side effects of medications Potential for orofacial trauma during seizures	Seizure activity: precipitating factors, care planning, appointment scheduling, stability in chair, communication Tissue overgrowth from phenytoin Prolonged bleeding time from valproic acid	Optimal oral hygiene and frequent maintenance visits to decrease gingival overgrowth from phenytoin First-aid instructions for oral trauma Positive reinforcement and self-image building	Gingival hyperplasia secondary to phenytoin, evidence of past oral injuries, e.g., scar tissue, fractured teeth
Visual impairment	Degree of impairment? Sensitivity to light Treated versus untreated conditions	Partial or total dependence on others Attitudes and stereotypes about disability and toward dog guides Limited income if not fully employed Locating dental providers Physical obstacles to oral healthcare	No specific factors	Sight impairment: appointment scheduling, explanation of procedures, clinician position, communication, positioning of light, mobility into clinic, data collection, noise level Dog guide: placement in comfortable place in office	Watch tone of voice Comment on any changes in procedures Describe everything graphically Demonstrate procedures on finger, etc. Precede actions with verbal descriptions Teach toothbrushing Use audio aids or physical models for teaching Involve caregiver when appropriate	Poor oral hygiene, gingivitis, periodontitis, dental caries

Table continued on following page

TABLE 26–5
SIGNIFICANT FACTORS RELATED TO THE DENTAL HYGIENE CARE OF INDIVIDUALS WITH SPECIAL NEEDS *Continued*

Condition	Medical Manifestations	Barriers to Care	Associated Risk Factors	Care Considerations	Prevention/Education and Health Promotion Issues	Common Oral Manifestations
Hearing impairment	Degree of impairment? Functioning of hearing aid	Partial or total dependence on others Limited income if not fully employed Locating dental providers Communication: sign language, lip reading, inaccurate pronunciation	No specific factors	Hearing impairment: appointment scheduling, explanation of procedures, clinician position, communication, data collection, noise interference, use of aid during appointment	Determine appropriate communication techniques Provide paper and pencil if desired Involve translator if needed Watch facial expressions Demonstrate when possible Make cards with frequently used phrases Use physical models for teaching Involve caregiver when appropriate	Poor oral hygiene, gingivitis, periodontitis, dental caries
Cleft lip or palate	Hearing impairment Upper respiratory tract infections Prosthetic appliances Medications	Fear of healthcare providers Self-image problems	Missing or malaligned teeth Oral motor dysfunction Feeding disorders	Cleft: clear communication, instrument positioning or fulcruming, suctioning and prevention of aspiration	Involve caretaker when appropriate Instruct in cleaning prosthetic aids Nutritional counseling if needed	Cleft lip: unilateral or bilateral fissure in the upper lip Cleft palate: unilateral or bilateral fissure in the palate
Cerebral palsy	Associated disorders Medications Other therapies Respiration impaired? Presence of primitive reflexes Degree of impairment	Communication Transportation if in wheelchair or cannot drive May have limited financial resources Dependence on others for care in many cases Mobility problems if in wheelchair Provider attitudes toward condition Self-image problems	Oral motor dysfunction General motor dysfunction Suboptimal fluoride intake possible Special diets	Fear: dental procedures, cooperation Primitive reflexes: client or clinician position, stability, instrument positioning or fulcruming, oral access, suctioning and amount of water used, protection of airway, radiographs Use of wheelchair: transfers to dental chair, mobility in office, office accessibility	Involve caretakers as appropriate Be patient with slowness of responses and progress Use combination of communication methods Assess needs for physical assistance or adaptive aids for home care Frequent evaluations Daily fluoride therapy Nutritional counseling if needed	Facial grimacing, abnormal oral muscle function, facial asymmetry, malocclusion, mouthbreathing, tongue thrusting, bruxism, poor oral hygiene, gingivitis, periodontitis, and dental caries

Bell's palsy	Therapies, especially prednisone Duration of condition Use of steroids Possible surgery to achieve facial symmetry	Self-image problems Language skills	Oral motor dysfunction	Lack of eye closure: protection of eyes (goggles) Oral motor dysfunction: protection of airway	Caution regarding effects of anesthesia Frequent rinsing or toothbrushing for food retention on affected side	Bilateral weakness or paralysis of facial muscles; drooping of one corner of mouth; excessive salivation and drooling
Myasthenia gravis	Medications History of radiation therapy or surgery History of myasthenic crises	Communication Client may hold chin to help during speaking	Oral motor dysfunction Myasthenia crisis may be precipitated by excitement, surgery, alcohol intake, infection, loss of sleep	Weakness increases during day: scheduling appointments Oral motor dysfunction/paralysis/impaired breathing, protection of airway, use of rubber dam, suctioning, chair position Weak voice: communication	Frequent evaluation to prevent infection Frequent rinsing or toothbrushing for food retention	Dysphagia, disturbed speech, expression, mastication, and swallowing
Systemic lupus erythematosus	Multiple organ systems affected Symptoms include fatigue, fever, cardiac lesions, kidney disease, neurological involvement, hematological disorders, butterfly rash, discord lupus, photosensitivity	Self-image problems and embarrassment due to facial rash	May affect blood vessels, brain, heart, kidneys, and white blood cells	Possible need for antibiotic premedication if cardiac valvular pathology is present Possible need for supplemental steroids in conjunction with stressful dental procedures Possible need for antibiotic therapy with surgical procedures; if immunosuppression is a problem consult with physician	Create a relaxing oral healthcare environment Client evaluation is essential after oral healthcare	Classic butterfly rash on cheeks and bridge of nose; oral ulceration, erythema, and keratosis that may involve the vermilion border, buccal mucosa or gingiva; fissuring of the tongue; temporomandibular joint involvement
Parkinson's disease	Medications and side effects Rigidity of larger joints Sensitivity to heat	Mobility to and in office Communication Embarrassment about condition	Oral motor dysfunction Side effects of drugs Possible inadequate diet	Tremors: stability, instrumentation, radiographs Sensitivity to heat: temperature of operatory Muscular pain and joint rigidity: chair position, appointment length Slurred speech: communication	Frequent evaluation Frequent rinsing and toothbrushing Adaptive equipment or assistance if needed Fluoride supplements Counseling about side effects of medications	Excessive salivation and drooling; difficulty in swallowing, tremors in lips, tongue, neck, and head

Table continued on following page

TABLE 26–5
SIGNIFICANT FACTORS RELATED TO THE DENTAL HYGIENE CARE OF INDIVIDUALS WITH SPECIAL NEEDS *Continued*

Condition	Medical Manifestations	Barriers to Care	Associated Risk Factors	Care Considerations	Prevention/Education and Health Promotion Issues	Common Oral Manifestations
Arthritis	Medications Degree of impairment Joints affected Joint replacement (premedication may be needed) Joint pain Heberden's nodes	Mobility to and in office Limited finances if disabled Weakness or fatigue decreases motivation to seek care	General motor impairment Drug-related complications such as prolonged bleeding, adrenal suppression, and bone marrow suppression	Joint pain: chair position, appointment length Antibiotic premedication for joint replacement Limited oral opening: positioning, instrumentation, radiographs Prolonged bleeding due to long-term aspirin therapy Client comfort Client may need supplemental steroids	Adaptive equipment or assistance if needed Counseling about side effects of medications Prevent sources of oral infection in clients with joint replacement for stressful dental hygiene procedures	Oral mucositis; increased oral infection related to antimetabolite drug therapy; increased bleeding due to antimetabolite, aspirin, and nonsteroidal antiinflammatory therapy
Multiple sclerosis	Medications and side effects Degree of facial pain Degree of impairment Sensitivity to heat	Mobility to and in office, especially if in wheelchair Depression or moodiness affects motivation Limited finances if on disability	Special diets Side effects of drugs Fine motor coordination problems Oral motor dysfunction Infection Fatigue and stress	Weakness and numbness: wheelchair transfer, stability, appointment length Oral motor dysfunction: protection of airway Mood changes: communication, acceptance of treatment, cooperation Sensitivity to heat: room temperature Periods of exacerbation/remission: appointment scheduling	Adaptive equipment or assistance may be needed More frequent rinsing and brushing Assistance in dietary counseling Supplemental fluoride More frequent evaluation to prevent infections	Facial pain, facial numbness occurs in some; abnormal facial muscle movements; facial myokymia
Muscular dystrophies	Medications Other therapies Type and degree of involvement Prognosis Check for obesity, scoliosis, or cardiopulmonary involvement	Depends on type Mobility to and in office, especially if in wheelchair Limited financial resources Weakness and possible decreased lifespan decreases motivation Locating accessible office facilities	Oral motor dysfunction General motor weakness and incoordination Dietary inadequacies Mouth breathing	Depends on type and degree of involvement Muscle weakness: stability in chair, wheelchair transfers, radiographs, instrumentation, appointment length Oral motor dysfunction: protection of airway, communication	Frequent evaluation More frequent brushing and rinsing Fluoride supplements Adaptive equipment or physical assistance for oral care	Facial muscle weakness, mouth breathing, poor oral hygiene

				Incoordination: restorative treatment planning, and possible emergency care Limited life span: care planning		
Spinal injuries	Depends on level of injury Medications Respiratory involvement Decubitus ulcers Incontinence/encopresis Contractures Heterotopic ossifications Body temperature regulation Potential for autonomic hyperreflexia Type of adaptive equipment	Mobility to and in office, especially if in wheelchair or on respirator Limited financial resources unless employed Psychosocial concerns/depression/substance abuse Locating accessible office facilities Poor self-image	Depends on level of injury Oral motor dysfunction Limited or total dependence on others Special diets	Psychological state: communication, cooperation Spasticity, tremors: stability Paralysis: mobility, wheelchair transfers, stability in chair, length of appointment Impaired respiration/oral motor dysfunction: chair position, use of rubber dam, protection of airway, instrumentation	Adaptive equipment or physical assistance needed Fluoride supplementation Consider psychological state Emphasize self-control and self-determination of oral health status	Dental caries, periodontal disease associated with poor oral hygiene
Spina bifida	Depends on type Similar to spinal injuries Shunt for hydrocephalus (antibiotic premedication) Seizure disorders	Depends on type and degree of impairment Similar to spinal injuries	Similar to spinal injuries, except oral motor dysfunction not apparent	Similar to spinal injuries, although psychological state not as poor Prophylactic antibiotic premedication required for clients with shunts	Learning disabilities influence oral health education methods Fluoride supplementation	No specific oral manifestations
Viral hepatitis	Type Degree of liver impairment Immunity versus active state versus carrier state Follow-up with physician if status unclear Good history Need for antigen or antibody test to verify carrier state	No known barriers	Potential for transmission of virus Potential for abnormal bleeding in cases of significant liver damage Potential for altered drug metabolism Carrier may be asymptomatic	No treatment if active state Avoid use of aerosol-producing equipment (e.g., air polisher, air/water syringe, ultrasonic scaler)	No specific concerns unless a chronic carrier Isolation of toothbrush from others if a carrier Counseling regarding transmission via saliva if type B or C Discuss blood testing to determine carrier state if unknown	May have bleeding tendency

Table continued on following page

TABLE 26–5
SIGNIFICANT FACTORS RELATED TO THE DENTAL HYGIENE CARE OF INDIVIDUALS WITH SPECIAL NEEDS *Continued*

Condition	Medical Manifestations	Barriers to Care	Associated Risk Factors	Care Considerations	Prevention/Education and Health Promotion Issues	Common Oral Manifestations
Acquired immunodeficiency syndrome (AIDS)	Systems involved Degree of impairment Consult with physician Kaposi's sarcoma Treatment regimens Predisposition to multiple opportunistic infections Immunosuppression	Finding dentist who will treat Stigmas associated with disease Decreased motivation/depression Limited finances if unemployed Fear of rejection	Oral infections Homosexual/bisexual behavior Intravenous drug abusers Transfusion recipients Hemophiliacs Unprotected sex Artificial insemination	Gingivitis should be treated to prevent necrotizing ulcerative periodontitis Oral infections: care planning, transmission potential Kaposi's sarcoma: care planning Psychological state: communication, motivation Referral to dentist for rapid treatment of odontogenic infection Prophylactic antibiotics should be considered	Dietary counseling and fluoride supplements while on special diet Palliative care for oral infections Increased attention to oral hygiene	Oral malignancies, i.e., Kaposi's sarcoma Oral opportunistic infections, i.e., *Candida,* histoplasmosis, herpes simplex, herpes zoster cytomegalovirus, hairy leukoplakia Multiple episodes of oral candidiasis Esophageal candidiasis Periodontitis
Sexually transmitted diseases (gonorrhea, syphilis, genital herpes)	Determine status: history of disease, active disease reported or observed, in high-risk group Treatment regimen and compliance Follow-up care Medication sensitivity Complications from long-standing untreated cases	Psychosocial stigma of diseases	Potential for disease transmission	Oral lesions: palliative care	Counseling regarding disease transmission concerns	See specific disease entities below
Syphilis	Primary stage: chancre at the site of inoculation Secondary stage: oral mucosal patches Latent stage: gumma, neurosyphilis, cardiovascular syphilis Treatment: penicillin G	Psychosocial stigma of disease	Potential for transmission Risk of congenital syphilis in the newborn Untreated person is infectious	Threat of transmission from oral lesions to the oral healthcare provider	Counseling regarding disease transmission concerns	Chancre, mucosal patches (ulcerations on the oral mucosa, tongue, palate, pharynx, lips), gumma, interstitial glossitis Condylomata lata

Gonorrhea	In males: severe dysuria, frequency of urination, urethral discharge, prostatitis, epididymitis In homosexuals: gonococcal proctitis and pharyngitis In females: vaginal discharge, dysuria, urinary frequency, vaginal bleeding, menstrual abnormalities, cystitis Treatment: procaine penicillin G or tetracycline	Identifying the presence of the disease	Carrier may be asymptomatic Potential for disease transmission	Possibility of transmission from oral lesions to the oral healthcare provider	Counseling regarding disease transmission concerns	Gonococcal arthritis of the temporomandibular joint; infrequent but can include pharyngitis, tonsillitis, stomatitis, ulceration, and formation of pseudomembranous coating
Tuberculosis	Strongly suggestive history Treatment regimen (compliance and effectiveness) Appropriate follow-up care Instances of reinfection Organ systems affected	Stigma of condition	Potential for disease transmission	Disease transmission: same as for hepatitis Avoid use of aerosol-producing equipment Palliative treatment of oral lesions	No specific recommendations except prevention of disease transmission	Oral ulceration, tuberculous involvement of cervical and submandibular lymph nodes (cervical lymphadenitis)
Cystic fibrosis	Degree of impairment, and prognosis Dietary changes Treatment regimens Chronic pulmonary disease Abnormal viscous secretions causing damage to major organs, such as the lungs, pancreas, and liver	Small stature may cause embarrassment Prognosis may decrease motivation Finances may be limited	Decreased resistance to infections Pulmonary complications compounded by problems of malabsorption and malnutrition Recurrent attacks of pneumonia, bronchiectasis	Mucous accumulations/impaired breathing: chair position, appointment scheduling and length, coughing, protection of airway, use of rubber dam Fear of medical situations: cooperation Susceptibility to infections: appointment scheduling Tetracycline staining: aesthetics, care planning	Fluoride supplements if dry mouth Frequent oral care due to mouth breathing Coordinate dietary suggestions with other professionals Saliva substitute due to decreased salivary output Recommend tartar control dentifrice	Enlargement of submandibular gland, increased calculus formation, xerostomia

Table continued on following page

TABLE 26–5
SIGNIFICANT FACTORS RELATED TO THE DENTAL HYGIENE CARE OF INDIVIDUALS WITH SPECIAL NEEDS *Continued*

Condition	Medical Manifestations	Barriers to Care	Associated Risk Factors	Care Considerations	Prevention/Education and Health Promotion Issues	Common Oral Manifestations
Bronchial asthma	Type and severity of asthma Frequency and severity of attacks Precipitating factors Treatment regimens History of hospitalizations or status asthmaticus Instruct patient to bring inhalers if used	Fear of medical and dental environments	No specific risk factors Factors may precipitate an acute asthmatic attack, e.g., stress, exposure to sulfites	Anxiety control: possible premedication or use of nitrous oxide Medications/precipitating factors: contraindications to prescribing or using certain drugs, appointment scheduling, medical emergency preparedness Have bronchodilator present Use of local anesthetic without epinephrine or levonordefrin	Model relaxed, stress-free environment No specific preventive requirements Avoid known precipitating factors Instruct client to bring bronchodilator Avoid use of aspirin Need for meticulous oral hygiene	Oropharyngeal candidiasis infection due to inhaled steroid treatment
Congenital heart disease	Type and if repaired Extent of limitations Medications Prognosis Need for antibiotic premedication Physician consultation	Financial constraints from medical bills Frequent illness Possibly debilitated state Overprotective attitude of parents	Decreased resistance to infections	Consultation with allergist Bleeding potential in some cases: care planning, need for laboratory tests, possible referral to specialist Heart condition: antibiotic premedication, stress management protocols, appointment length, chair position	Emphasize danger of intraoral infections in terms of aggravating heart condition Prevention of infective endocarditis Frequent maintenance care	Orofacial tissue may appear bluish if cyanosis is present or may appear ruddy if polycythemia is present; if thrombocytopenia is present, tissues may show small hemorrhages; oral infections if leukopenia is present
Rheumatic heart disease	Residual effects of rheumatic fever: heart murmurs, myocarditis, pericarditis, cardiomegaly, electrocardiographical changes, pericardial rub, congestive heart failure Physician consultation regarding need for antibiotic premedication	No specific barriers	Rheumatic fever	Heart defects: need for antibiotic premedication Consultation with cardiologist Complete as much oral healthcare as possible during 2 to 3 hours following the waiting period after the loading dose	Prevention of infective endocarditis Stress oral hygiene to prevent oral infections and self-induced bacteremias Frequent maintenance care	None

Rheumatic fever	Carditis, polyarthritis, chorea, erythema marginatum, subcutaneous nodules, arthralgia, fever, tachycardia, abdominal pain, generalized weakness, epistaxis	No specific barriers	Pharyngeal infection with group A streptococci	Heart defects: need for antibiotic premedication	Prompt treatment of pharyngeal infection Prevention of recurrence with antibiotic therapy	None
Cardiac arrhythmias	Symptoms Medications and side effects Presence of pacemaker and type	If pacemaker, avoidance of certain electrical equipment	No specific risk factors Clients who are cocaine users can develop arrhythmias from cocaine-epinephrine interactions	Pacemaker: avoidance of electromagnetic equipment Arrhythmias: stress management protocol, drug precautions, bleeding potential from medications	No specific preventive regimens Saliva substitute	Oral complications due to antiarrhythmic drugs: Procainamide: mucosal ulcerations and drug-induced lupus erythematosus Propranolol: mucosal ulcerations and petechiae Disopyramide: xerostomia Quinidine: mucosal ulcerations
Surgically corrected cardiovascular problems	Date of surgery Type of surgery Medications and side effects Foreign material used, e.g., Dacron Presence of artificial heart valves	No specific barriers	Potential for bleeding and infective endocarditis	Bleeding potential if on anticoagulant medications Dacron surgical correction and artificial heart valves: need for antibiotic premedication Coronary bypass graft surgery: need for antibiotic premedication up to 6 months postoperatively Consultation with cardiologist	No specific regimens	None
Hypertensive disease	Vital sign monitoring Physician consultation or referral Medications and side effects and other treatment regimens Cause: primary or secondary Predisposing or general risk factors Severity, symptoms Possibility of orthostatic hypotension	Anxiety about oral care	Side effects of medications Potential for stroke, myocardial infarction, and renal failure Potential for adverse drug interactions between vasoconstrictors and antihypertensive drugs	Identify cardiac problems that require modification of care plan Hypertension: stress management protocols, chair position, care planning, monitoring vital signs, appointment scheduling, contraindications to treatment	Counseling regarding reducing general risk factors Palliative care for oral infections from medications Fluoride supplements for xerostomia Create stress-free environment Prevent postural hypertension	Xerostomia associated with antihypertensive therapy; oral lesions associated with mercurial diuretic; orofacial paresthesia associated with acetazolamide Possible lichenoid reactions from thiazides, methyldopa, propranolol, and labetalol

Table continued on following page

TABLE 26–5
SIGNIFICANT FACTORS RELATED TO THE DENTAL HYGIENE CARE OF INDIVIDUALS WITH SPECIAL NEEDS *Continued*

Condition	Medical Manifestations	Barriers to Care	Associated Risk Factors	Care Considerations	Prevention/Education and Health Promotion Issues	Common Oral Manifestations
Hypertensive disease *Continued*				Medications: drug interactions, gag reflex, local anesthetics, bleeding potential Avoid sudden changes in chair positions Avoid procedures that can increase blood pressure Refer to physician if necessary		
Ischemic heart disease (coronary atherosclerotic heart disease)	Current health status Angina or myocardial infarction episodes Hospitalizations Medications and side effects Surgery or pacemakers	Possible debilitated state Medical and other expenses Anxiety about dental hygiene care If pacemaker, avoidance of electromagnetic equipment	Side effects of medications Susceptibility to infections if debilitated	Heart condition: same considerations as for hypertensive disease and preparation for medical emergency, contraindications for treatment if uncontrolled or recent attack (within 6 months) Avoid care within 6 months after infarction Medications: same as for hypertensive disease Short morning appointments Monitor vital signs Pacemaker: avoidance of electromagnetic equipment Verify use of vasoconstrictors Cardiologist consultation Treat only when condition is controlled	Palliative care for side effects of medications Counseling regarding decreasing general risk factors Special oral hygiene instructions if hospitalized or bedridden Frequent maintenance Create stress-free environment	Pain in the lower jaw brought on by physical activity; oral ulceration associated with allergic or toxic reactions to drug therapy; prolonged bleeding associated with dicumarol
Congestive heart failure	Same as for severe ischemic or hypertensive heart disease	Mobility	Pulmonary congestion and edema	Prone to nausea and vomiting during oral healthcare Keep client upright in chair	Frequent maintenance and evaluation Create stress-free environment	Oral infection, spontaneous gingival bleeding, ecchymoses and petechiae all related to polycythemia (thrombocytopenia, leukopenia, thrombosis)

Cerebrovascular accident (stroke)	Type of involvement, degree of limitation Seizures? Medications and side effects Other therapies	Communication Limited financial resources Accessibility if adaptive equipment or wheelchair is needed Partial or total dependence on others	Oral motor dysfunction Side effects of medications Impaired general motor coordination Dietary inadequacies Transient ischemic attack Previous stroke, hypertension, cardiac abnormalities, atherosclerosis, diabetes mellitus, elevated blood lipid	Memory impairment, communication, data collection Oral motor dysfunction/paralysis, instrumentation, jaw stability, radiographs, care planning Impaired emotional control: cooperation, communication Short morning appointments General paralysis: mobility, possible wheelchair transfers, stability in chair Minimize use of vasoconstrictors	Use combination of teaching approaches Reinforce and repeat instructions Monitor vital signs Frequent maintenance Fluoride supplementation Tobacco cessation intervention Adaptive aids or supervision for oral care Avoid sensory overload Reorient patient to situations Use one-step instructions	Prolonged bleeding related to drug therapy, e.g., anticoagulant and antiplatelet drugs
Sickle cell anemia	Precipitating factors for crises Symptoms and severity Associated conditions Transfusions? Laboratory tests needed?	Periods of pain Debilitated condition at times Fear of dental environment Limited financial resources because of medical bills Racial prejudice	Susceptibility to infections Low stress tolerance	Sickle cell crises: appointment scheduling, motivation, emergency care only Susceptibility to infections: periodontal maintenance, physician consultation for possible antibiotic premedication Reduce client stress Emphasis on preventive oral healthcare Consultation with physician Avoid medications that depress respiration	Dietary analysis/counseling Frequent maintenance care because of associated alveolar bone problems and need to control oral infection Involvement of others in care Create a stress-free oral healthcare environment Emphasis on optimal preventive oral health behaviors	Enamel hypoplasia, delayed eruption, pallor of the oral mucosa; decreased radiodensity of mandible and maxilla, increased size of marrow spaces, and loss of trabecular pattern
Leukemias	Type Treatment regimens, frequency, Presence of anemia, thrombocytopenia, and infection	Stages of acute disease versus remissions Fear of dental environment	Side effects of chemotherapy or radiation therapy Susceptibility to infections Oral hemorrhage	Bleeding potential: preappointment laboratory tests, appointment scheduling, physician consultation, surgical procedures Potential for oral and systemic infections: periodontal maintenance, antibiotic premedication Ideally, provide invasive care prior to chemotherapy or radiation therapy	Palliative care for oral lesions Frequent evaluation Fluoride program Involvement of others in care program Saliva substitutes Eliminate potential sources of oral infection Meticulous oral hygiene Daily antimicrobial mouthrinses	Gingival bleeding secondary to thrombocytopenia, oral infection, gingival hypertrophy Oral complications from chemotherapy include odontogenic infection, oral hemorrhage, oral mucositis (*Candida,* herpes simplex virus)

Table continued on following page

TABLE 26–5
SIGNIFICANT FACTORS RELATED TO THE DENTAL HYGIENE CARE OF INDIVIDUALS WITH SPECIAL NEEDS *Continued*

Condition	Medical Manifestations	Barriers to Care	Associated Risk Factors	Care Considerations	Prevention/Education and Health Promotion Issues	Common Oral Manifestations
Leukemias *Continued*				Acute versus remission stages: care planning, appointment scheduling Chemotherapy or radiation therapy: care planning Consultation with oncologist		
Hemophilias	Type and severity Frequency and location of bleeds Treatment regimens Joint replacements? Hepatitis? Seizures? Inhibitor status Laboratory tests needed?	Finding dentist who will treat Resources for emergency care	Potential for oral bleeds Hepatitis, cirrhosis or AIDS associated with frequent clotting factor replacement therapy	Bleeding potential: preappointment laboratory tests, surgery, physician consultation, factor replacement therapy, instrumentation, radiographs, use of rubber dam, suctioning, use of AMICAR Joint replacements: antibiotic premedication Hepatitis carrier: disease transmission procedures	Use of oral rinses and soft-bristled brush Counseling regarding first aid for oral trauma Frequent evaluation	Gingival bleeding, poor oral hygiene associated with fear of causing bleeding
Diabetic syndrome	Type and severity Insulin regimens Dietary regimen Complications Hypertension and other heart conditions Frequency of episodes of hypoglycemia or hyperglycemia	Finding dentist who will treat if chronic complications are present	Susceptibility to infections Decreased salivary flow in some Decreased resistance to periodontal disease Poor healing Susceptibility to oral *Candida* infection Complications associated with disturbances in vision and kidney function	Comprehensive health history Insulin/sugar balance: potential for medical emergency, appointment scheduling, stress management protocol Potential for infection: periodontal maintenance, possible antibiotic premedication, treatment planning Potential for delayed healing Associated conditions	Frequent maintenance visits Dietary analysis Fluoride program Need for bacterial plaque control Minimize stress Prevention of oral diseases Control of oral infections Adherence to preventive oral health behaviors Prevention of insulin shock or diabetic coma	Caries incidence in poorly controlled diabetes due to higher concentrations of glucose in saliva and decreased salivary flow, xerostomia Parotid gland enlargement, oral candidiasis, delayed healing and burning mouth syndrome, diabetic neuropathy in the oral region Periodontal disease may be accelerated

Thyroid disease	Type and etiology Symptoms and severity Medications Examples: Graves' disease (thyrotoxicosis) Can cause cardiac dysrhythmias, gastrointestinal problems	Swelling of tongue in hypothyroidism may cause difficulty in speech communication	Abnormal dental development Thyroid crisis is life-threatening	Sensitivity to drugs: care planning, postoperative instructions, preparation for medical emergency Mental retardation in some "Thyroid storm" or "thyroid crisis" precipitated by surgery, infection, trauma, or uncontrolled thyroid disease Heat or cold intolerance	Special hygiene instruction if mentally retarded Good oral hygiene to prevent infection Prevention of "thyroid crisis" Create a low-stress environment Encourage client to adhere to antithyroid medications No palpation of thyroid gland	Hypothyroidism: puffy lips and protruded tongue, underdeveloped mandible with wide appearance of the maxilla; spongy gingivae; delayed eruption; swelling of the tongue; difficulty in speech Hyperthyroidism: accelerated eruption rate of teeth Enlarged thyroid gland
Acromegaly	Excessive secretion of growth hormone in the adult Enlarged hands, coarse facial features Enlarging pituitary neoplasm may give rise to headaches and compression of optic nerve	Finding a dentist who will treat Visual disturbances may occur	Predisposition to diabetes mellitus, hypertension, cardiomyopathy, dysrhythmias Complex endocrine abnormalities may occur	May need corrective jaw surgery	Emphasis on controlling and preventing oral disease Education about the value of orthodontic treatment	Mandibular overgrowth that can lead to a class III malocclusion, enlarged tongue, flaring of the anterior teeth, further eruption of teeth with the development of hypercementoses, apposition of new bone in the alveolar ridges, marked thickening of bone
Pregnancy	Rise in progesterone levels Significant changes in the immune response Trimester side effects Nutritional status	Comfort of the pregnant woman Nausea and sensitivity to various odors Frequent sickness	Vulnerability of fetus during first trimester Development of pyogenic granulomas Increased incidence of gingivitis Possible dietary inadequacies	Safest period to provide routine care is second trimester Short appointments Allow client to change position and assume a semireclining position Fetal sensitivity: avoidance of drugs, radiographs, elective dental procedures Pressure of fetus on mother: chair position, orthostatic hypotension (turn on left side to alleviate)	Meticulous oral hygiene Education on the relationships among bacterial plaque, hormonal level, and periodontal disease Education on the relationship between caries process and gastric acids from vomiting Emphasis on controlling and preventing oral diseases Prevent super hypotensive syndrome Education on care of infant's oral cavity and baby bottle syndrome Prenatal counseling	Gingival enlargement, inflammation, and bleeding; pyogenic granuloma

Table continued on following page

TABLE 26–5
SIGNIFICANT FACTORS RELATED TO THE DENTAL HYGIENE CARE OF INDIVIDUALS WITH SPECIAL NEEDS *Continued*

Condition	Medical Manifestations	Barriers to Care	Associated Risk Factors	Care Considerations	Prevention/Education and Health Promotion Issues	Common Oral Manifestations
Pregnancy *Continued*					Good oral hygiene to decrease response to bacterial plaque Daily home fluoride therapy during episodes of vomiting Supplemental fluoride drops for nursing infant	
Chemical dependency	Types of drugs used Symptoms Treatment interventions Potential for drug interactions or overdose Emotional stability during appointment	Emotional state Denial of drug problem Demanding requests for use of nitrous oxide or pain medications Disoriented behavior	Neglect personal hygiene Potential for oral trauma Potential link (not documented) to oral cancer Potential drug interaction with local anesthetic	Coordinated care: professional team and family if in treatment program Use of drugs for procedure: restrict Strict guidelines for keeping appointments necessary	Frequent brushing and flossing Teach oral self-examinations Avoid mouth rinses containing alcohol Topical fluoride program	Oral trauma, xerostomia, mucosal lesions from irritants, dental caries and periodontal disease, extrinsic stains on teeth

Chronic alcoholism	Patient's perception of severity of problem Symptoms Treatment program Nutritional deficiencies Chronic complications Degree of liver impairment	Limited finances if not employed Potential for no-show appointments	Susceptibility to infection Nutritional deficiencies Nausea and vomiting Potential for oral trauma	Liver impairment and bleeding potential: preappointment laboratory testing, drug metabolism, instrumentation, treatment planning Inebriated states: emergency care, appointment scheduling, treatment planning, data collection Associated medical problems (see management for each problem)	Nutritional counseling Frequent evaluation Fluoride programs Frequent soft tissue evaluation for oral cancer Counseling regarding first aid for oral trauma Firm approach regarding need for good oral hygiene Instill responsibility for oral care Recommend saliva substitute	Parotid swelling, xerostomia, alcoholic breath, glossitis, leukoplakia, oropharyngeal cancer, dental caries and periodontal disease, oral trauma
Chronic renal failure	Symptoms and severity Hypertension Dialysis? Transplant? Special diets Need for antibiotic premedication	Finding dentist who will treat Debilitated condition at times Limited finances Fear of dental environment	Susceptibility to oral infection Dietary inadequacies	Hypertension and kidney failure: vital signs, drug interactions, drug metabolism Bleeding tendency: preappointment blood tests, instrumentation, physician consultation Arteriovenous shunt: antibiotic premedication Dialysis: appointment scheduling Transplants: premedication with steroids or antibiotics	Frequent evaluations because of increased calculus Emphasis on good oral hygiene to prevent infection Palliative care for oral lesions Dietary counseling Daily home fluoride therapy Tartar control toothpaste	Dental caries and periodontal disease related to oral neglect; oral ulcerations and stomatitis from medications; candidiasis, increased calculus formation, anemic mucosa, oral petechiae and hemorrhage, ground-glass appearance of alveolar bone on radiograph, halitosis and bad taste in mouth, enamel hypoplasia

Data from Entwistle, B. M. Dental hygiene care for individuals with special needs. In Darby, M. L. (ed.). Comprehensive Review of Dental Hygiene, 3rd ed. St. Louis: C. V. Mosby, 1994, pp. 588–596.

References

1. Goldenson, R. M. Dimensions in the field. In Goldenson, R. M., Dunham, J. R., and Dunham, C. S. (eds.). The Disability and Rehabilitation Handbook. New York: McGraw-Hill, 1978, pp. 3–11.
2. Dunham, C. S. Social-sexual relationships. In Goldenson, R. M., Dunham, J. R., and Dunham, C. S. (eds.). The Disability and Rehabilitation Handbook. New York: McGraw-Hill, 1978, pp. 12–20.
3. Mosher, J. Employment and job placement. In Goldenson, R. M., Dunham, J. R., and Dunham, C. S. (eds.). The Disability and Rehabilitation Handbook. New York: McGraw-Hill, 1978, pp. 71–85.
4. Shaffer, S., Margon, C., and Stiefel, D. J. Principles of rehabilitation (Project DECOD). Seattle: University of Washington School of Dentistry, 1985, pp. 1–29.
5. Kliment, S. A. Removing environmental barriers. In Goldenson, R. M., Dunham, J. R., and Dunham, C. S. (eds.). The Disability and Rehabilitation Handbook. New York: McGraw-Hill, 1978, pp. 110–119.
6. Uniform Federal Accessibility Standards, part II. Federal Register, 49(153):31528–31613, August, 1984.
7. Laurie, G. Housing and home services. In Goldenson, R. M., Dunham, J. R., and Dunham, C. S. (eds.). The Disability and Rehabilitation Handbook. New York: McGraw-Hill, 1978, pp. 101–109.
8. Lee, M., and Sonis, A. An instrument to assess dental students' attitudes toward the handicapped. Special Care Dentist 3(3):117, 1983.
9. Stoltenberg, J. L. and Walker, P. O. Student dental hygienists' and dental hygiene educators' attitudes toward the handicapped. Journal of Dental Hygiene 63(3):117, 1989.
10. Bishop, J. A study of dental hygienists' attitudes towards working with elderly patients. Dental Hygiene 53(3):125, 1979.
11. American Association of Dental Schools. Curricular Guidelines for Dental Hygiene Care for the Handicapped. Journal of Dental Education 48(5):266, 1984.
12. American Association of Dental Schools. Curriculum guidelines for dentistry for the person with a handicap. Journal of Dental Education 49(2):118, 1985.
13. Kimmelman, B. B. The need for and utility of dental service among people with severe disabilities. Special Care Dentist 9(1):10, 1989.
14. Dunham, J. R., and Dunham, C. S. Psychosocial aspects of disability. In Goldenson, R. M., Dunham, J. R., and Dunham, C. S. (eds.). The Disability and Rehabilitation Handbook. New York: McGraw-Hill, 1978, pp. 28–35.
15. Dunham, J. R., and Dunham, C. S. Psychosocial aspects of disability. In Goldenson, R. M., Dunham, J. R., and Dunham, C. S. (eds.). The Disability and Rehabilitation Handbook. New York: McGraw-Hill, 1978, pp. 28–35.
16. Guidelines for Reporting and Writing about People with Disabilities. Philadelphia: Center for Independent Living, 1984.
17. Vocational Rehabilitation Act of 1973, 503, 504, P.L. 93–112, 87 Stat 335, 793–794 U.S.C.S.
18. Barnes, G. P., Allen, E. H., et al. Dental treatment needs among hospitalized adult mental patients. Special Care Dentist 8(4):173, 1988.
19. Hiltbrunner, A. V. Argument against providing dental care for the severely cognitively impaired patient. Gerodontics 4(4):168, 1988.
20. Shuman, S. K. Ethics and the patient with dementia. Journal of the American Dental Association 119(6):747, 1989.
21. Walshe, T. Approach to patients with degenerative disorders of the nervous system. Gerodontics 4(4):156, 1988.
22. Venus, C. A. Interacting with patients who have communication disorders. Texas Dental Journal (107):11, 1990.
23. Blaine, H. L., and Nelson, E. P. A mouthstick for quadriplegic patients. Journal of Prosthetic Dentistry 29(3):317, 1973.
24. Hock, D. A. The use of the maxillary interocclusal splint as a mouthpiece for the mouthstick prosthesis. Journal of Prosthetic Dentistry 62(1):56, 1989.
25. O'Donnell, D., and Robinson, W. A simple self-retaining mouth appliance for physically disabled individuals. Quintessence International 19(1):63, 1988.
26. Smith, R. Mouthstick design for the client with spinal cord injury. American Journal of Occupational Therapy 43(4):251, 1988.
27. Polyzois, G. L. Custom mouth protectors: An aid for autistic children. Quintessence International 20(10):775, 1989.
28. Neil, S. M., and Saunders, M. J. The general dentist's role in swallowing and speech aid appliances. Texas Dental Journal 107(2):19, 1990.
29. McGhay, R. M. A simple headrest for patients confined to wheelchairs. Journal of Prosthetic Dentistry 44(3):347, 1980.
30. Felder, R. S., Gillette, V. M., and Leseberg, K. Wheelchair transfer techniques for the dental office. Special Care Dentist 8(6):256, 1988.
31. Schubert, M. M., Hale, J. M., Friedel, C. A., and Marvinney, S. L. Wheelchair transfers in the dental office (Project DECOD). Seattle: University of Washington School of Dentistry, 1989, pp. 1–27.

Suggested Readings

Birch, J. W. Mainstreaming: Educable mentally retarded children in regular classes. Reston, VA: Council for Exceptional Children, 1974.

Education for All Handicapped Children Act of 1975, P.L. 94–142, 20 U.S.C.S.

Ferguson, F. S., Berentsen, B. J., Marinelli, R. D., and Richardson, P. S. A predoctoral program in dental care for the developmentally disabled. Journal of Dental Education 54(9):576, 1990.

Hicks, J. S. Educational programs. In Goldenson, R. M., Dunham, J. R., and Dunham, C. S. (eds.). The Disability and Rehabilitation Handbook. New York: McGraw-Hill, 1978, pp. 53–66.

Mund, S. Vocational rehabilitation; employment; self-employment. In Goldenson, R. M., Dunham, J. R., and Dunham, C. S. (eds.). The Disability and Rehabilitation Handbook. New York: McGraw-Hill, 1978, pp. 67–87.

Niessen, L. C. New directions—constituencies and responsibilities. Journal of Public Health Dentistry 50(2):133, 1990.

Thornton, J. B., Al-Zahid, S., et al. Oral hygiene levels and periodontal disease prevalence among residents with mental retardation at various residential settings. Special Care Dentist 9(6):186, 1989.

U.S. Department of Health, Education, and Welfare. Vocational rehabilitative programs: Implementation provisions. Washington, DC, 1975.

27

Dental Hygiene Care for the Edentulous Individual

OBJECTIVES

Mastery of the content in this chapter will enable the reader to:

- Understand the demographics, etiology, and disease patterns associated with edentulous persons
- Appreciate the psychological factors involved in the loss of natural teeth, deficits in the client's wholesome body image, and loss of appreciation and respect
- Identify the types of dentures used in complete denture therapy
- Acknowledge the physiological changes in the oral environment of the edentulous client and their contribution to the client's human need for wholesome body image and a biologically sound dentition
- Explain the limitations associated with tooth loss
- Provide recommendations to ease adaptation to new dentures
- Discuss the implications of dental hygiene care for successful prosthodontic therapy
- Recognize the denture-induced oral lesions and oral manifestations of systemic disease that compromise the client's human need for integrity of skin and oral mucous membranes and freedom from pain and stress
- Educate the edentulous client about expectations, daily preventive denture and oral hygiene measures, the need for self-determination and responsibility, continued care and maintenance programs, and proper nutrition required to maintain oral health
- Assess deficits in the need for nutrition in the edentulous client and suggest guidelines for a nutritionally balanced diet
- Assess deficits in the edentulous client's need for wholesome body image; a biologically sound dentition; skin and oral mucous membrane integrity; conceptualization and problem solving; nutrition; safety; self-determination and responsibility; appreciation and respect; freedom from pain and stress; and value system
- Plan dental hygiene care for an edentulous client

INTRODUCTION

The word **edentulous,** derived from the Latin word *edentatus,* is defined as being without teeth or lacking teeth. Normally, individuals are not conscious of the many critical daily functions for which teeth are used: eating, speaking, facial expression, and appearance. However, once the teeth are lost, the person is quick to realize how eating becomes more difficult, speech is not as distinct, and facial tissues lose their support, which ultimately impair the person's appearance and other people's perceptions of the person. In addition to these obvious changes, the supporting alveolar bone progressively resorbs. The dental hygienist must be especially cognizant of the human need deficits that may arise in the client who is edentulous.

Although the percentage of edentulous persons tends to increase with age, it is not uncommon to find clients in their second through fifth decade of life who are denture wearers. Although maintaining the oral health of the edentulous individual entails the same basic elements of preventive and therapeutic care as those provided for clients who have a complete dentition, edentulous clients have specialized needs.

This chapter presents information on the demographics, etiology, and disease patterns associated with edentulous persons; psychological and physiological factors associated with edentulism; types of dentures; oral lesions induced by dentures; denture limitations; and recommended continued maintenance and nutritional strategies for persons who are edentulous. Throughout the chapter, implications for meeting human need deficits as a part of the dental hygiene process are discussed.

DEMOGRAPHICS

Changing patterns in oral disease and attitudes toward oral healthcare have decreased the number of completely edentulous individuals. The National Survey of Oral Health of United States Adults conducted by the National Institute of Dental Research and National Institutes of Health found a gradual yet significant decline in the number of edentulous persons.[1] However, given longer lifespans and the increasing size of the elderly segment of the population, current surveys indicate that the total number of edentulous individuals is between 20 and 25 million, suggesting that the provision of complete dentures is common in the oral healthcare environment.

The percentage of edentulous persons among U.S. populations increases dramatically with age.[1] The 1985 National Survey of Oral Health of U.S. Adults estimated 41% of the senior population to be completely edentulous, while only 2% had all their teeth.[2] Miller and colleagues also reported that only 13% of edentulous seniors had been to the dentist within the last 12 months, and 67% of them had not visited the dentist within the last 3 years.[1] This evidence suggests a critical role for the dental hygienist in encouraging regular maintenance care and recognizing oral changes that often go unnoticed by the client (see Chapter 30, Dental Hygiene Care for the Older Adult).

ETIOLOGY

Two major factors contribute to a person's edentulous status:

- Rampant caries
- Periodontal diseases

In general, the primary reason for tooth loss before age 35 years is dental caries, while periodontal diseases are responsible for tooth loss during the third through the fifth decade of life. Furthermore, the rate at which individuals lose their teeth is influenced by four primary elements:[3]

- Intraoral tissue quality and host resistance
- The economic and social status of the person
- The quality of oral hygiene performed at home
- The quality and frequency of professional oral healthcare

PSYCHOLOGICAL FACTORS RELATED TO EDENTULISM

In all phases of the dental hygiene process, the client's mental attitude and values can influence the success of care, and the edentulous person is no exception. The human need for a wholesome body image often is in deficit because of the complete loss of natural teeth, and this deficit may be exacerbated by the fear of aging, decreased sexuality, feelings of insecurity, fear of rejection, loss of self-esteem, and unrealistic expectations involving complete denture replacement. The dental hygienist should carefully assess the client who experiences wholesome body image deficits as a result of denture problems and difficulties in adaptation to the edentulous state. Care for these clients requires that the dental hygienist listen attentively; demonstrate caring, nonverbal behavior; provide information and reassurance; and reinforce positive attributes about the client's body image. These humanistic behaviors help meet the client's human need for appreciation and respect and nurture trust and self-acceptance by the client.

The dental hygienist should engage the client in an open dialogue to discuss oral problems and complaints. Such interaction between client and dental hygienist may reveal the underlying cause of the human need deficits. Careful documentation of the client's concerns also may assist the dentist in the dental diagnosis and selection of dental treatment procedures. Clients' mental attitudes are classified into four categories as described by House:[4]

- Philosophical
- Exacting
- [Dissatisfied]
- Indifferent

Although it is difficult to label a client's emotional state, Table 27–1 describes characteristics of each of the four categories of mental attitude discussed below.

TABLE 27–1
HOUSE'S PSYCHOLOGICAL ASPECTS OF THE EDENTULOUS CLIENT

Client Classification	Characteristics
Philosophical	Loss of natural dentition following satisfactory professional oral healthcare; accepts and adjusts to the edentulous state easily; calm, rational, understanding, and cooperative in regards to dental and dental hygiene needs; most favorable prognosis and pleasant to treat
Exacting	Possesses the same positive attributes as the philosophical client, but requires extreme care; compulsive, accurate and precise; very demanding; reluctant to accept advice; lack of confidence in the clinician; dental hygienist must be tolerant of and respond to demands of the client
[Dissatisfied]	Unfavorable adjustment to the complete denture; uncooperative, excitable, irritable, insistent, impatient and apprehensive; emotionally unstable; places impossible demands upon the dental hygienist; may require professional counseling
Indifferent	Blames the clinician for present dental condition; disinterested in dental treatment; apathetic; unwilling to follow instructions, but accedes reluctantly upon the advice of family; passively cooperative; poor prognosis until client becomes committed to dental and dental hygiene treatment

Data from House, M. M. Full Denture Techniques. Lecture, Study Club #1. Whittier, California, 1935. With permission from Renner, R. P. Complete Dentures: A Guide for Patient Treatment. New York: Masson Publishing USA, Inc, 1981, pp. 19–20.

Philosophical Attitude

The philosophical client who has developed confidence in the dental hygienist knows that the best care for a successful outcome is being rendered. Few, if any, modifications in providing care are necessary for the philosophical client. Previous satisfaction with professional oral healthcare permits the client to accept the judgment of oral healthcare professionals without question.

Exacting Attitude

Clients in the exacting classification previously had poor results with dental treatment, although they have tried to be cooperative. Human need deficits in conceptualization and problem solving, in addition to deficits in appreciation and respect, may arise. Throughout all phases of dental hygiene care, a kind and sympathetic attitude is crucial to successful outcomes for exacting clients. More time and effort is necessary to develop their confidence and help them to understand the details of their problems. A careful and thorough examination is necessary to engender the client's trust.

Dissatisfied Attitude

The dissatisfied/hysterical client is extremely critical of oral healthcare providers because of many previously failed attempts to obtain a denture made to his specifications. From the outset, the dental hygienist must be in firm control and influence the progression of care. Poor health often contributes to the irritable nature of the hysterical client, and thus a medical consultation is advisable prior to treatment. A rewarding outcome is possible with dissatisfied/hysterical clients if the dental hygienist can reverse their negative attitudes with patience and education.

Indifferent Attitude

Indifferent clients have little concern for oral health, and thus more time must be spent to meet their human needs for a wholesome body image, value system, and appreciation and respect. Although at times providing care for the indifferent client may be discouraging, persistence by the dental hygienist can have favorable outcomes. Initially, the dental hygienist should focus on the client's human need deficit for appreciation and respect by exhibiting both verbal and nonverbal behaviors of interest and praise. Attentive listening may assist the dental hygienist in identifying, and incorporating the client's value system into the process of care. Furthermore, acceptance, reassurance, and positive reinforcement during dental hygiene care may help develop the client's self-esteem and wholesome body image.

TYPES OF DENTURES

Transition from natural dentition to completely artificial dentition is a major life event that most individuals find difficult. This situation can cause client deficits in the human needs for a wholesome body image, freedom from stress, and nutrition. If these needs cannot be appropriately met, or if the client believes that these needs cannot be met, the success of complete denture therapy may be jeopardized.

Several types of dentures, ranging from partial to complete, are used by dentists to meet clients' needs for a sound dentition, for a wholesome body image, and for nutrition (Fig. 27–1). The **partial denture** is used to replace some, but not all, of the natural teeth. Partial dentures may be fixed or removable (see Fig. 27–1). A **fixed partial denture** is permanently attached to natural teeth and is also called a bridge. It cannot be removed by the client. The components of fixed partial dentures include:

- **The abutment:** the tooth or teeth used to anchor the prosthesis
- **The pontic:** the artificial tooth or teeth that occupy the edentulous space

The **removable partial denture** can be removed and replaced by the client. This type of partial denture may be supported by retainer clasps around the natural teeth, or it may be supported by a combination of natural teeth and oral tissue.

The **transitional partial denture** is used to restore edentulous areas until the remaining natural teeth are extracted. On occasion, this is advantageous for the individual for whom difficulty in adaptation or tolerance of complete dentures is anticipated.

The **overdenture,** often used by the dentist as a transitional denture, is placed over retained roots that have been reduced to levels just above the gingiva. Overdentures, however, also may be used as permanent dentures. The advantages of using overdentures compared with conventional complete dentures include decreased rate of alveolar resorption, improved proprioception, and additional dental support and retention. In addition, better preservation of alveolar ridge height results in greater facial contours, which is both cosmetically and psychologically valuable for the client.

Immediate dentures are constructed prior to extraction of remaining teeth and delivered on removal of the teeth to maintain normal mechanical and physiological functions of the orofacial components. In addition, the newly edentulous person can avoid potential social embarrassment from being without teeth.

Implant dentures are designed to fit over implant fixtures that are inserted partially or entirely into living bone. The increased stability and retention derived from this type of prosthetic appliance have renewed the hopes of the edentulous population for an acceptable alternative to natural teeth. Research efforts continue to define the clinical applications for the use of dental implants (see Chapter 28, Dental Hygiene Care for the Individual with Osseointegrated Dental Implants).

PHYSIOLOGICAL FACTORS IN TOOTH LOSS

Although complete dentures can restore many of the important oral functions lost when a person becomes edentulous, remodeling of the orofacial tissues is invariably encountered. The placement of dentures introduces unfamiliar forces compared with those of the natural dentition. Related changes in the oral environment are composed of residual ridge and alveolar bone resorption, oral mucous membrane remodeling, and loss of orofacial muscle tone. Although these factors are physiological in nature, they can contribute to disturbances in the client's human need for a

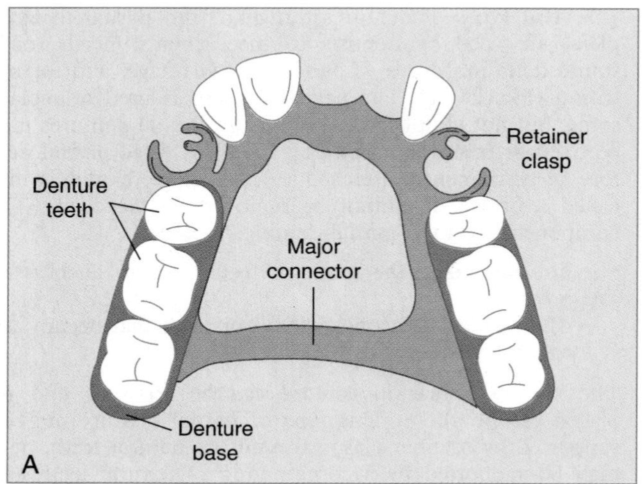

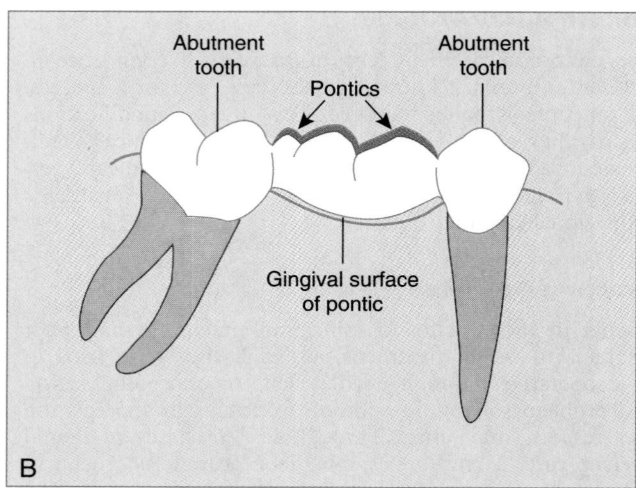

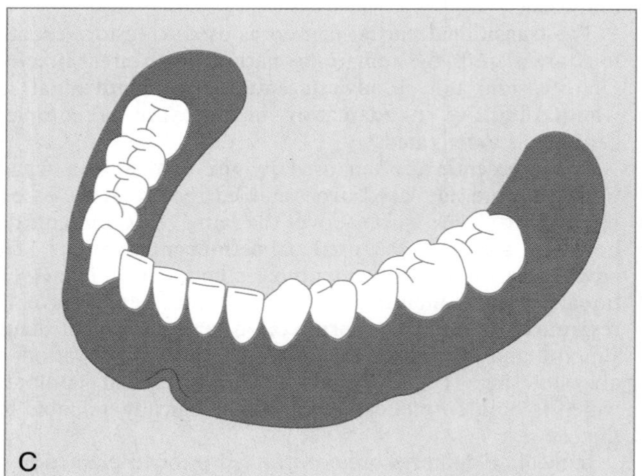

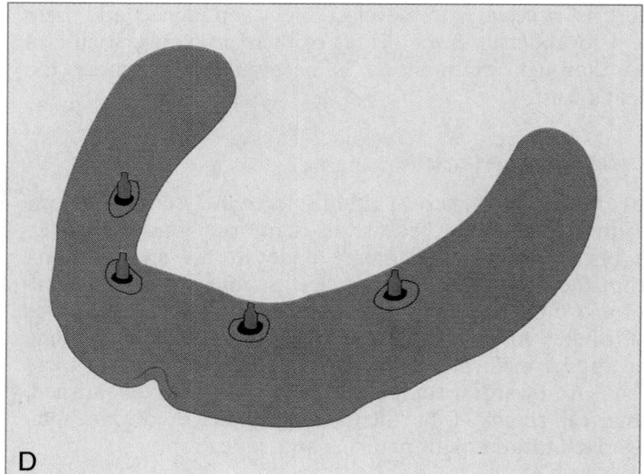

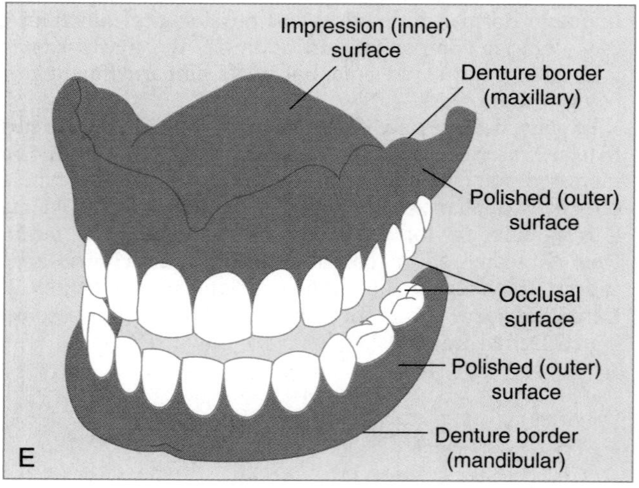

FIGURE 27–1
Types of dentures. *A*, Removable partial denture. *B*, Fixed partial denture. *C*, Overdenture. Mandibular complete denture. *D*, Implant denture. *E*, Complete denture.

wholesome body image. In addition, deficits may arise in the client's human need for skin and oral mucous membrane integrity, a biologically sound dentition, and freedom from pain and stress.

Bone Resorption

Following tooth extraction, major bony changes, such as residual alveolar ridge resorption, occur within the first year and continue throughout life. The correlation between degree of alveolar bone resorption and the duration of edentulousness is well documented.[5–9] Although the rate of resorption can vary enormously between individuals, it is generally accepted that well-fitting dentures tend to decrease the rate of resorption.[10] Furthermore, in addition to an improvement in oral mucosal health, reduced resorption is observed when dentures are removed at night.[9,11] Local factors, including trauma from dentures or opposing teeth on dentures, may affect the rate of resorption so that the dentures become ill-fitting. Some investigators believe that systemic factors, such as metabolic bone disease, postmenopausal osteoporosis, and a calcium-poor diet, also contribute to severe mandibular atrophy in edentulous individuals.[12]

Generally, older individuals resorb bone at faster rates than younger individuals because of anatomic, metabolic, functional, and prosthetic factors.[3] Often the problems that arise as a result of residual bone resorption are magnified as the person ages. For example, in some older adults, severe resorption of the mandibular alveolar ridge may expose the contents of the mandibular canal, and thus pressure from a prosthesis causes extreme discomfort. Additionally, compression of an exposed mental nerve at or near the crest of the alveolar ridge with only a thin layer of oral mucosa overlying it may cause pain and paresthesia of the lower lip and chin. If on assessment the dental hygienist finds a deficit in the client's need for a biologically sound dentition and freedom from pain and stress, immediate referral to the dentist would be indicated. Also, the dental hygienist should educate the client about the causes of bone resorption and suggest methods of minimizing the rate of resorption, including removal of the denture at night, regular evaluation to ensure well-fitting dentures, and a calcium-rich diet. Furthermore, it is imperative that edentulous clients understand the importance of annual professional oral healthcare for evaluation of the integrity of the tissues and oral mucosa and for adjusting, relining, or remaking the denture.

Some edentulous clients erroneously perceive that dentures last a lifetime without further modifications; however, in reality new dentures should be made at least every 4 to 8 years. Hence, client education during the process of care is a priority for the edentulous individual. To meet clients' human needs for conceptualization, problem solving, and safety, the dental hygienist may focus educational efforts toward:

- The importance of daily oral hygiene measures and continued care appointments
- The indications for use of denture adhesives
- The potential hazards of over-the-counter denture repair kits

For example, **denture adhesives** may stabilize and retain the denture by increasing the peripheral seal. However, individuals with well-fitting dentures should not need denture adhesives. For some anxious individuals, denture adhesives may provide security to allay the fear of social embarrassment from sudden dislodgement of the denture. Available in powder, paste, or film formulations, denture adhesives may aid client adaptation to new dentures, increase comfort in an anxious client, and reduce dislodgement of dentures in clients with severe alveolar ridge resorption.[13] Moreover, the client should be discouraged from attempting to adjust his own denture and refrain from using commercial products, such as denture cushions, denture relining, and repair kits. Besides jeopardizing the integrity of oral tissues, permanent destruction of the prosthesis may result.

Resorption of the alveolar ridges undoubtedly diminishes the stability and retention of the denture as the bony ridges continue to flatten with time. As a general rule, the bony changes observed in the mandibular arch differ significantly from those in the maxilla (Fig. 27–2). The mandibular arch resorbs in a downward and facial direction in the posterior region.[14] This progressive widening in the mandibular molar region occurs because the width of the inferior border of the mandible is greater than the overlying alveolar process. In the anterior segment of the mandibular arch, resorption initially occurs downward and lingually and then continues to move forward with time. In comparison, resorption from the maxilla proceeds in an upward and lingual direction both anteriorly and posteriorly. The resulting ridge relation of the mandible and the maxilla is a crossbite position so that the maxillary arch is confined within the mandibular boundaries, and the client appears prognathic. The rate of resorption is four times greater in the mandible than in the maxilla.[15]

On occasion, irregular patterns of alveolar ridge resorption can create numerous sharp spikes, especially in the mylohyoid ridge. A considerable amount of pain can develop as the mucous membrane covering becomes trapped between the hard denture base and the sharp bone.

Other bony contours resulting from either growth abnormalities or alveolar resorption may create undesirable consequences and should be surveyed while examining the client's edentulous mouth. **Exostoses,** benign bony outgrowths, frequently occur on the hard palate and lingual aspect of the mandibular alveolar ridge and are known as palatal and mandibular tori, respectively. Sometimes they are removed surgically prior to denture construction to prevent the possibility of irritation of the overlying oral mucosa by the tori. Similarly, large maxillary tuberosities potentially can provide an unsatisfactory fit of the prosthetic appliance.

Alveolar ridge contour can be classified into four types (Fig. 27–3).[10]

- Normal
- Flat or resorbed
- Narrow, sharp, or V-shaped
- Prominent bulbous or undercut

These bony configurations vary considerably among edentulous clients, especially in the mandible. With the exception of the normal ridge, each classification can present significant problems to the denture wearer if it is not addressed by the dentist. The dental hygienist must recognize the loss of retention, stability, and support of the dentures and call it to the attention of the dentist. Hence, collaboration between the dentist and the dental hygienist is necessary to restore the human need deficits of edentulous clients and provide quality care.

The soft tissues primarily associated with the denture appliance are the tongue, floor of the mouth, cheeks, lips, and the mucosa overlying the edentulous ridge. The oral mucosa is divided into three categories, all of which are composed of stratified squamous epithelium overlying connective tissue:

- Masticatory
- Lining
- Specialized mucosa

In general, the epithelium of the masticatory mucosa is keratinized, whereas the lining mucosa is not. In health, both the hard palate and the edentulous ridge consist of keratinized epithelium. Adjacent to the surface epithelium, connective tissues consisting of dense collagenous fibers that are contiguous with the lamina propria complete the mucous membrane covering of the bony ridge. Providing primary support and resiliency for the denture, the underlying connective tissue firmly attaches to the alveolar bone.

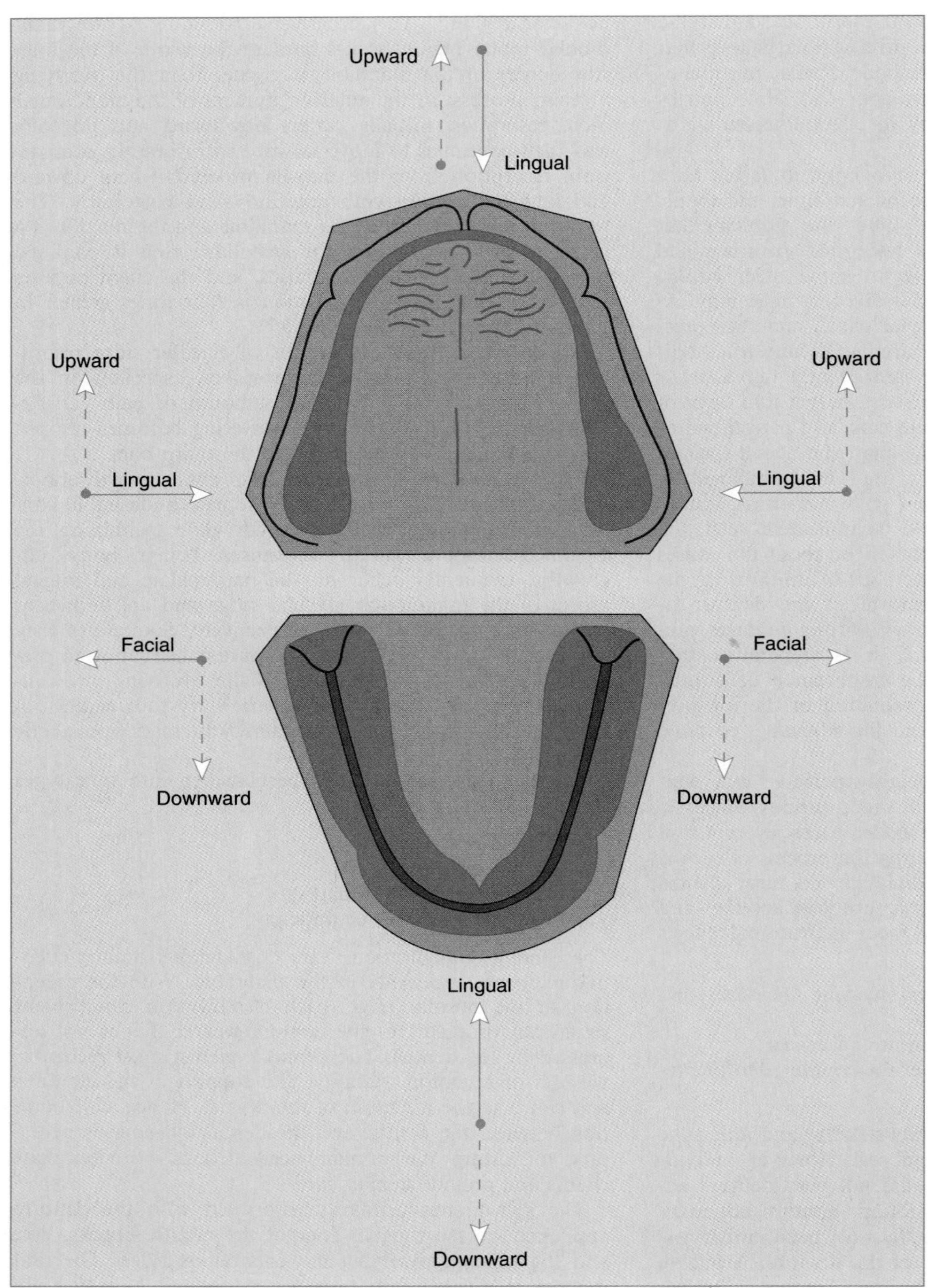

FIGURE 27–2
Directions of alveolar ridge resorption in the maxillary and mandibular arches.

In addition, the connective tissue layer contains the blood and nerve supply to the mucosa and may have glandular, fat, or muscle cells present.

Substantial variation of soft tissues exists between individuals primarily because of age and health status. Younger edentulous clients exhibit relatively thick denture-bearing mucosa, whereas older clients frequently have thin, tightly stretched, easily blanched tissues.[14] Clinical assessment factors include the color, mobility, and quality of the involved tissues. The simplest approach to soft tissue assessment is to examine the relationship of the denture with respect to the adjacent structures both visually and digitally.

Soft Tissue Changes

Understanding the soft tissue response to placement of dentures enables the dental hygienist to assess the client's skin and oral mucous membrane integrity. Both long-term wear of dentures and soft tissue changes related to aging can significantly impact the plan of care. Furthermore, trauma or injury to mucosal tissues may or may not be tolerated by the client. For example, a large majority of clients experience chronic mucosal irritation. Early recognition of this inflammatory or hyperplastic response may prevent further destruction of the underlying tissues. The

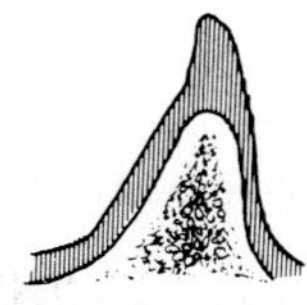
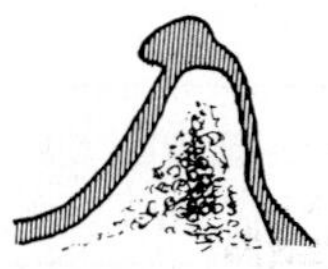

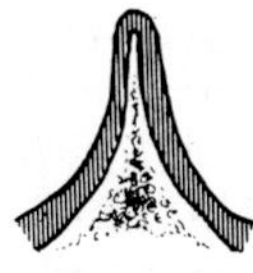
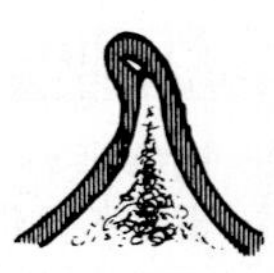

FIGURE 27–3
Effects of dentures on sharp, fibrous, and bony ridges. *A*, Sharp fibrous ridge. *B*, Sharp bony ridge. (With permission from Mack, A. Full Dentures. Dental Practitioner Handbook No. 13. Bristol: Butterworth-Heineman Limited, 1978, p. 21.)

PROCEDURE 27–1

CONTINUED DENTAL HYGIENE CARE AND MAINTENANCE FOR THE EDENTULOUS CLIENT

ASSESSMENT

Steps	Rationale
1. Update the client's health history to identify systemic disorders, current medications, and conditions that may affect the dental hygiene care plan and the client's ability to wear complete dentures	Often, the dental hygienist is the first to recognize systemic diseases with oral manifestations. The systemic health of the client can seriously affect oral health and the subsequent success of dentures
2. Review the personal history records of the client, and note details such as age, occupation, and culture	The client's personal details and priorities considerably influence the care plan. Age-related changes can directly impact the successful use of complete dentures. The client's occupation and culture may dictate his priorities of denture and oral hygiene care
3. Review the dental history of the client	The present oral health status may directly reflect a client's previous tendency toward developing oral disease, past dental and dental hygiene care efforts, personal oral hygiene care, and values toward care
4. Ask the client to explain in detail the denture problems experienced, and listen attentively to the complaints	This enables the dental hygienist to gain insight on the true nature of the denture problem as well as to learn about the client's personality and value system
5. Perform comprehensive assessment of facial structures and soft tissues	The assessment phase of the dental hygiene process must include an evaluation of the head and neck regions for early recognition of abnormalities that may signal human need deficits related to oral health and disease
6. Assess the temporomandibular joints (TMJ) and associated musculature as the client opens and closes the mouth and slides the jaw from side to side	TMJ disorders can develop following extended wear of ill-fitting dentures
7. Observe and record irregularities in the facial symmetry, level of the occlusal planes, amount of freeway space, and center line position of the dentures during conversation with the client	Functional difficulties may indicate improper fit of the prosthesis
8. Survey external soft tissues to evaluate contour and inflammation with special regard to labial structures	Adequate facial support by dentures is necessary to maintain normal facial appearance. In addition, angular cheilitis may indicate an intraoral *Candida* infection or other systemic disease
9. Assess the oral soft tissues for evidence of local or systemic diseases, and record color, texture, size, shape, presence or absence of pain, and condition of the overlying epithelium	Early recognition of disturbances in skin and mucous membrane integrity, such as inflammation, traumatic injury, and chemical irritations, that may indicate need for referral to dentist for further evaluation to prevent progression of the problem
10. Visually inspect the denture-bearing mucosa and palpate it	Determining the resilience of the overlying mucosa and submucosa assists in evaluating the denture fit and changes produced with increasing age
11. Assess the structure and form of the alveolar ridges	Presence of flabby tissue, uneven underlying bone, and bony spikes contributes to poor stability and retention of the denture

CONTINUED ON FOLLOWING PAGE

PROCEDURE 27–1

CONTINUED DENTAL HYGIENE CARE AND MAINTENANCE FOR THE EDENTULOUS CLIENT *Continued*

Steps	Rationale
12. Note changes in associated structures, including the tongue, floor of the mouth, and oropharynx	Careful assessment of these structures may reveal loose-fitting dentures, lack of wear of the prosthesis, chronic low-grade trauma, systemic conditions, or oral carcinoma
13. Assess the oral hygiene status of the client by surveying the oral cavity for chronic fungal infections and accumulation of bacterial plaque and food debris	Improper denture care, continuous wear of the denture at night, and decreased oral hygiene may potentiate infection and poor denture adaptation
14. Determine the retention of the denture by attempting to displace the prosthesis away from supporting tissues. The posterior border seal of the maxillary denture is checked by attempting to pull the anterior teeth forward	Retention is absolutely necessary for satisfactory physiological performance and appearance of the denture and for the client's ability to speak properly
15. Assess the fit of the dentures by first seating them and then attempting to move them in anteroposterior and lateral directions	A proper denture fit determines the overall success of the prosthesis and, in addition, prevents debilitating conditions such as excessive alveolar ridge resorption
16. Assess the stability of the denture with respect to denture position during normal oral functions	The stability of the denture is directly associated with retention and fit
17. Indicate any changes in occlusion and articulation	The client's freeway space and occlusal vertical dimension are important to appearance and comfort
DENTAL HYGIENE DIAGNOSIS	
18. Review the information collected during the assessment phase, including the health/dental history, extraoral/intraoral examination, denture evaluation, and client's chief complaint. Present all significant findings to the dentist of record	All information obtained during the assessment phase is organized for collaboration with the dentist so that a comprehensive care plan can be developed. The dental hygienist can highlight areas of concern for the dentist and greatly expedite dental care
19. Analyze both objective and subjective assessment data, and identify the human need deficits that are verifiable and that are amenable to dental hygiene care	Having a dental hygiene diagnosis ensures that dental hygiene care will be planned to meet the unique needs of the client
PLANNING	
20. Determine the goals of the dental hygiene care plan within the overall goals of the comprehensive dental treatment plan	Dental hygiene care is prioritized based on the client's human need deficits. The role of the dental hygienist is to provide preventive and preparatory services for the client prior to prosthodontic treatment by the dentist
21. Develop the proposed care plan with the client, and describe the importance of the dentist–dental hygienist–client relationship throughout all phases of prosthodontic treatment	Communication is extremely important to the successful care of the edentulous client. Client motivation and acceptance are enhanced if the client understands his responsibilities in the care plan
22. Establish, in conjunction with the client, goals that will be achieved as a result of dental hygiene care	Goals can be evaluated to ensure progress and measure the outcome of care
IMPLEMENTATION	
23. Review daily oral and denture hygiene care. Identify specific areas of neglect, and suggest methods for improvement of bacterial plaque control	Reinforcement of bacterial plaque control measures is vital to the maintenance of oral health in edentulous clients
24. Use disclosing solution to stain accumulations of bacterial plaque and calculus on the denture	This can be a motivational tool to demonstrate the need for improved denture hygiene practices
25. Counsel the client on the importance of proper nutrition. Emphasize the need for a diet high in protein, dairy products, and complex carbohydrates	Diet counseling can correct nutrient imbalances that compromise the integrity of oral tissues in edentulous clients
26. Fill a small plastic bag with cleansing solution, submerge the denture in it, and place the bag in an ultrasonic unit. If this method is unavailable, carefully scale the prosthesis	Ultrasonic cleaning is a safe and effective alternative to manual scaling for removing all calculus and extrinsic stain from the denture

Steps	Rationale
27. Lightly polish the denture with an extremely fine polishing agent (tin oxide) *on the external surfaces only,* and thoroughly rinse under warm water	Restoration of denture shine may inspire the client to maintain its cleanliness
EVALUATION	
28. Advise the client on the next continued care appointment and expectations as to the longevity of the denture from that visit	Reminding the client to maintain a regular recall schedule is essential to continued denture successes
29. Measure achievement of client goals	Measurement of goals prevents supervised neglect and erroneously dismissing a client who might still need dental hygiene care
30. Formulate an evaluation statement regarding the level of client goal attainment	This documents the client's level of goal attainment in the record

dental hygienist should carefully document any deficits in skin and mucous membrane integrity, inform both the client and the dentist of all deviations from normal, and recommend to the client procedures for daily care of the oral soft tissues to prevent further destruction.

The denture-bearing tissues react differently from individual to individual. For example, differences in the thickness of the mucosa in conjunction with varying degrees of keratinization can be expected in the mouth of the edentulous client. Some edentulous persons may develop a **denture-induced fibrous hyperplasia** as a result of fibrous tissue proliferation following alveolar bone resorption under an ill-fitting denture (Fig. 27–4). Although detection is sometimes difficult because of nearly normal color and texture, this flabby hyperplastic tissue is identified by palpating freely movable tissue over edentulous ridges or on the vestibular mucosa. If this tissue is observed, the client has a human need deficit in the area of skin and mucous membrane integrity related to an ill-fitting denture; therefore, the dental hygienist should refer the client to the dentist for evaluation and treatment. Depending on the severity of hypermobile tissue, dental treatment may involve a period of tissue rest, denture adjustment, and/or surgical excision to reduce the excess tissue. Keratinization of edentulous alveolar ridges may be completely absent, or it may progress to a hyperkeratinized state. This **focal (frictional) hyperkeratosis** is classified as a hyperkeratotic white lesion of the oral mucosa that should resolve with time on discontinuation of the underlying trauma.

FACTORS AFFECTING THE ORAL MUCOSA OF INDIVIDUALS WHO WEAR ORAL PROSTHESES

Factors such as age, systemic diseases affecting the oral environment, denture occlusion and fit, oral hygiene habits, and continuous wear of the prosthesis influence the condition of the mucosa covering the bony ridges. The following

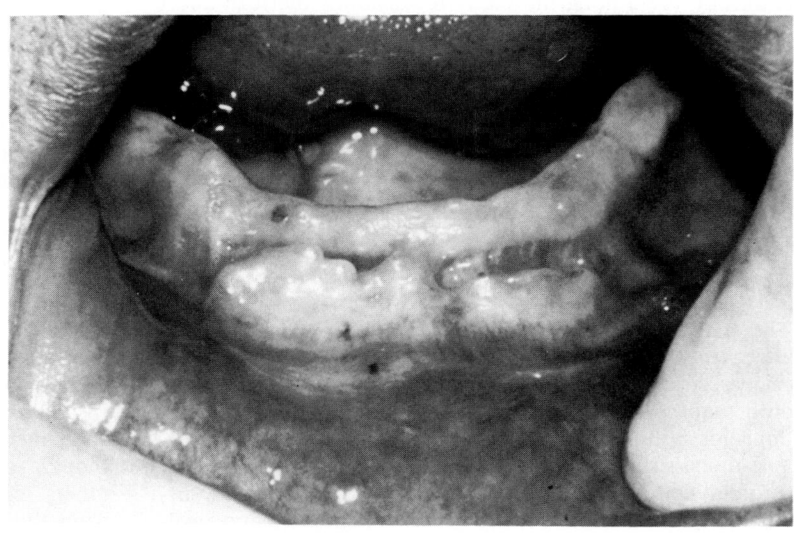

FIGURE 27–4
Denture-induced fibrous hyperplasia. (With permission from Regezi, J. A., and Sciubba, J. Oral Pathology: Clinical-Pathologic Correlations, 2nd ed. Philadelphia: W. B. Saunders, 1993, p. 204.)

discussion addresses these significant factors as they relate to the dental hygiene process within the human needs conceptual model.

Age

Deficits in body image may develop as normal and abnormal physical changes appear with increasing age. Cultural and societal attitudes and values may alter an aging person's self-concept, and thus the dental hygienist's acceptance and positive reinforcement of the client can improve the outcomes of care.

The effect of aging on the oral mucosa and skin characteristically results in atrophy of the tissue, with diminished elasticity and resiliency. Commonly, the denture-bearing tissues of the aged appear smooth and glazed. The thinning of the oral epithelium increases the vulnerability of the denture-bearing mucosa to stress, pressure, and disease. For example, the older adult may experience inflammation and ulceration of the thin, friable mucosa that is unable to withstand the masticatory stresses or relatively mild mechanical irritation. Often, older adult edentulous clients exhibit a decrease in thickness of the oral mucosa, but the extent varies, depending on the client's dental history, systemic health, medications, and nutritional status.

Systemic Diseases

Systemic health contributes to the oral health of an individual. Poor general health results in denture problems, such as friable denture-bearing mucosa. For example, a person with kidney dysfunction may have dehydrated mucosal tissues because of a water imbalance, and thus the mucosa becomes more vulnerable to trauma. Decreased tolerance to stress, impaired healing, emotional strain, and medications related to poor systemic health can adversely affect the oral soft tissues. Systemic conditions that may require modification of dental hygiene care include cardiovascular diseases, hypertension, allergies, psychological problems, and chronic diseases such as diabetes, anemia, and postmenopausal osteoporosis.

Medications taken for systemic diseases can affect a client's oral condition and must be documented and updated during each continued care visit. Hormones, digitalis, nitroglycerin, diazepam (Valium), and chlordiazepoxide (Librium) are among the many medications that can affect the oral environment of the edentulous client. Xerostomia, a common side effect of diuretic, antihypertensive, and antidepressive drugs, interferes with complete denture retention and stability as a result of a loss of mucosal lubrication.[16] Uncontrollable tongue and facial movements may develop with psychotropic medications. Drugs such as cortisone, thyroid hormone, and estrogen may perpetuate a chronic soreness of the mucosal tissues.[17]

Denture Occlusion and Fit

The state of the oral mucosa overlying the ridges directly affects the comfort of the denture. As might be expected, a thicker covering is more resilient and provides more padding than a thin mucosa. Unfortunately, dental interventions for minimizing the discomfort associated with a friable mucosa are limited, although soft lining materials such as tissue conditioners and resilient liners may alleviate discomfort for some individuals. **Tissue conditioners** and **resilient liners** are composed of soft, flexible elastomer polymers that are intended to treat chronic soreness and protect the supporting tissues from functional and parafunctional occlusal stresses. Specific indications for tissue conditioners as an adjunct to denture adjustment or fabrication of a new prosthesis include the following:

- Traumatized mucosa from ill-fitting dentures
- Bruxism
- Papillary hyperplasia
- Debilitating systemic diseases[18]

However, misuse of tissue conditioners can cause additional irritation to the denture-bearing mucosa. Important concepts to convey to clients about the use of commercially available tissue conditioners follow:

- Minimum thickness of 1 mm is necessary for tissue conditioners to be effective
- Proper powder-to-liquid ratios are required to obtain the correct consistency
- A soft diet is recommended for the first 8 hours after application to prevent loss of shape
- A soft toothbrush or cotton is used to cleanse the soft lining material under cold water
- Denture cleansers should not be used because they can alter the physical properties of the conditioner
- A new application of material every 3 or 4 days is critical for successful recovery of the tissues

Resilient liners are similar to tissue conditioners, but they have an increased longevity of 6 months to 5 years. Despite their increased length of use, it is important to note that resilient liners are only temporary solutions to chronic problems. The indications for the use of resilient liners include the following:

- Severe alveolar ridge resorption
- Clients with contraindications to surgery
- Bruxism
- Xerostomia
- Pain relief for oral structures that consistently become irritated

Oral Hygiene Habits

The state of an edentulous client's oral mucosa can reveal information about her daily home care. Accumulation of bacterial plaque, stain, and calculus on the denture and oral mucosa may lead to offensive odors and mucosal irritations, such as denture stomatitis, papillary hyperplasia, and chronic candidiasis. Recognition of any of these conditions mandates that the client be educated about the importance of preventive oral hygiene measures necessary to maintaining the health of the mucosal tissues.

Continuous Wear of Dentures

Clients should be instructed to remove the denture for an extended period each day, preferably at night. Because of the stresses of mastication exerted by dentures, the residual alveolar ridges and oral mucosa may become compromised. In addition, the potential for an inflammatory condition to arise increases if the tissues are not allowed to rest. Although some client's tissues tolerate the stresses better than others, clients should be advised to remove the denture from the mouth during each 24-hour period. While out of the mouth, the denture should be placed in a container filled with water to prevent drying and subsequent damage to the denture base material.

PROBLEMS ASSOCIATED WITH TOOTH LOSS

Although complete dentures can facilitate restoration of the edentulous person's human need for a biologically sound dentition and a wholesome body image, successful adaptation depends on the attitude and commitment of the individual. At the outset, the client must be informed of the limitations of complete dentures and their effectiveness as substitutes for natural dentition. Clients who receive complete dentures should be informed about the physical manifestations of bone resorption related to appearance, potential speech difficulties, and the effects of a denture on masticatory efficiency. The physiological changes of the edentulous person associated with aging are of special concern, since these changes are magnified in the older population. Understanding age-related changes allows the dental hygienist to recognize common denture problems experienced by older adults; address human need deficits in body image, appreciation and respect, freedom from pain and stress, and nutrition; and counsel these clients about daily oral health behaviors. If realistic expectations and goals for proper denture care are outlined early, the client can successfully adapt to the artificial dentition. Client education should emphasize the value of dentures in restoring function and health; instructions for use, care, and cleaning of the prosthesis; and the importance of regular professional evaluations.

Physical Appearance Related to Bone Resorption

Alveolar bone resorption can dramatically affect both the physical appearance and the wholesome body image of the edentulous individual. Modifications in appearance often are clearly visible following extensive alveolar bone resorption, such as loss of facial height, reduced lip support, and

PROCEDURE 27–2

DAILY ORAL AND DENTURE HYGIENE CARE

Equipment

Soft denture brush
Dilute sodium hypochlorite solution or commercial denture cleanser
Warm water
Denture cup
Basin
Towel
Soft nylon toothbrush

Steps	Rationale
1. Explain the importance of daily oral hygiene for both the dentures and the associated soft tissues	A routine home care regimen prolongs the useful life of the dentures, promotes healthy intraoral tissues, and promotes the general well-being of the client
2. Describe the potential consequences of oral and denture hygiene neglect	The client should be aware of halitosis, inflammation, trauma, or negative remodeling effects on the oral environment
3. Summarize the client's responsibilities in monitoring his oral function and health status	Clients taught to recognize early problems of denture fit, mastication, food impaction, chronic cheek biting, speech, and tissue inflammation may prevent further discomfort and destruction
4. Advise against the use of denture home repair kits or retention products, and encourage the client to return to the dentist for proper adjustments	Improper denture modification results in further damage to the oral tissues and the denture itself
5. Discourage the use of denture adhesives with a stable and retentive prosthesis. Under the supervision of the dentist, a small amount may be evenly applied over the inner impression surface that directly contacts the oral mucosa	Generally, the use of adhesives indicates the need for adjustment of the denture, rather than a need for adhesives
6. Remind the client to brush the denture following each meal and before retiring or, at the very least, to rinse it under running water	Bacterial plaque and food debris readily collect on the denture and may foster a variety of problems of the oral mucosa
7. Describe techniques for self-examination of the denture for proper fit, denture deposits, and abraded inner and outer surfaces	Accumulation of plaque, calculus, and heavy stain, and abraded surfaces should be removed by the dental hygienist for proper cleaning. Adjustment problems should be referred to the dentist to avoid further problems

CONTINUED ON FOLLOWING PAGE

PROCEDURE 27-2

DAILY ORAL AND DENTURE HYGIENE CARE *Continued*

Steps	Rationale
8. Inform the client that some commercially available denture powders and pastes are too abrasive for dentures and are not recommended for general use	The coarse abrasives present in some denture powders and pastes may cause a loss of shine, surface character, and fit of the prosthesis
9. Suggest regular use of fresh denture immersion cleansers daily or biweekly as needed. Recommend a dilute sodium hypochlorite solution as a cleanser: 1 teaspoon household bleach per 8 ounces of water. Soak for 5 to 10 minutes, and rinse thoroughly	Chemical cleansers bathe all denture surfaces, aid those clients who lack manual dexterity to care for the dentures, prevent accidental breakage of dentures, and can be easily used while the dentures are out of the mouth. Dilute hypochlorite solutions provide nontoxic, bactericidal, and fungicidal actions. Solutions should be changed daily
10. Advise removal of the denture when possible and at night while at rest	Continuous wearing of dentures inhibits the natural cleansing mechanisms of the tongue and saliva and increases bacterial plaque retention
11. Assemble supplies	Set up the necessary materials for proper cleaning technique. The client may prefer a soft nylon toothbrush, but must be reminded to access all areas without overexuberant brushing, which may damage the denture
12. Fill a basin with water, and line the bottom with a small towel	This prevents breakage of the denture should it be accidentally dropped
13. Gently remove the denture, and rinse away the saliva and loose debris	Prevents slippage of denture when grasping it to brush it
14. Firmly grasp the denture in the palm of one hand, and hold near the water-filled basin	A secure hold without excessive pressure is adequate, since undue stress may break the denture
15. Remove any denture adhesive material with a brush	All gross debris should be removed from the denture to permit cleaning of all areas
16. Demonstrate the use of a denture brush with a mild soap solution to remove accumulations on the inner impression and outer polished surfaces, and adapt the brush as necessary	All denture surfaces must be cleansed thoroughly. Areas difficult to access require special attention
17. Rinse the denture and brush under running water to completely remove all denture cleanser	Residual cleanser may cause irritation to the oral mucosa
18. Inspect the denture for any remaining bacterial plaque, food debris, or cleanser by visual and tactile examination	This ensures that all debris has been removed
19. Place prosthesis in a denture cup filled with room-temperature tap water or denture cleanser, and cover it	When left out to rest the tissues, dentures are placed in solution to prevent dehydration and distortion of the acrylic resin
20. On removal of the denture, rinse the mouth with warm water or a saline solution	Removal of large debris from the oral cavity is essential to maintaining a healthy oral environment
21. Débride the denture-bearing mucosa by using the client's tongue to sweep over the area	A superficial débridement of the edentulous areas can assist in the cleansing process
22. Use a soft toothbrush or soft cloth daily to clean the edentulous mucosa by employing long strokes in a posterior to anterior direction	Removal of food and oral epithelial debris is not a trivial matter in attempting to maintain sound supporting tissues for dentures
23. Using the thumb and index finger, massage the edentulous tissues daily by applying pressure and then releasing it continually along the ridge. Alternatively, mechanical stimulation with the side of the bristles of a multitufted soft toothbrush in a vibratory manner can provide similar results	This provides mechanical stimulation to increase the keratinization of the oral mucosa and circulation in these tissues and, ultimately, to increase the resistance to denture trauma

increased chin prominence (Fig. 27–5). The effects of physical alterations attributed to bone resorption include decreased denture stability, unbalanced occlusion, TMJ disorders, and a dissatisfaction with appearance. Additionally, an unsatisfactory jaw relationship evolves so that extensive resorption allows an original normal jaw relation to appear as a class II malocclusion. Usually a pleasing appearance is most critically judged by the clients themselves. However, the astute dental hygienist who compliments clients on their positive attributes and features can assist in building the self-esteem of the client.

Speech Disturbances

Speech patterns invariably are affected by loss of teeth and associated structures and the acquisition of oral prostheses. On placement of new oral appliances, transient speech difficulties in articulation and the degree of oral resonance are to be expected, but they should disappear.[19] To facilitate adaptation to speaking with an oral appliance, clients should be instructed to read aloud. If a speech disturbance persists longer than a few days, the denture may be ill-fitting and should be examined by a dentist. A speech deficit

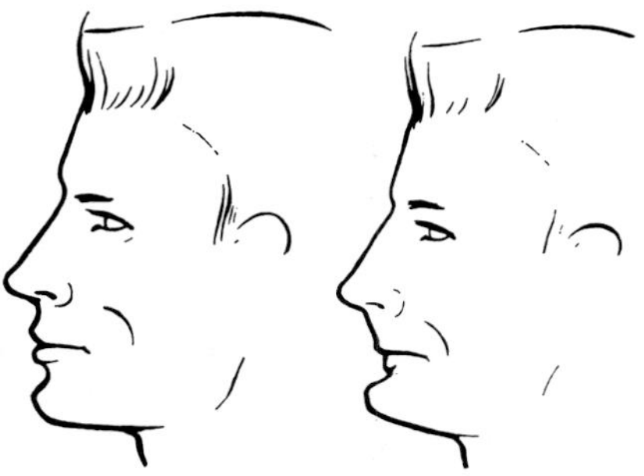

FIGURE 27-5
Physical modifications of the edentulous, including overclosure, decreased lip support, and increased chin prominence. (With permission from Mack, A. Full Dentures. Dental Practitioner Handbook No. 13. Bristol: Butterworth-Heineman Limited, 1978, p. 64.)

may also arise in conjunction with bone resorption, since a loosely fitting denture is difficult to control.

Masticatory Efficiency

Masticatory efficiency with complete dentures is estimated to be one-sixth that of individuals who have a natural dentition.[3] The two primary reasons for the marked reduction in masticatory abilities are:

- Loss of periodontal support and stability
- Loss of periodontal proprioception

The periodontal ligament support area is critical to the stability of a partial denture or full dentures confined to one arch only. Yet, in the edentulous person periodontal ligament support is one-fourth to one-half that which supports the natural dentition. Furthermore, proprioception is a major component in the body's reception and interpretation of sensation. Without this feedback of movement and position by the pressoreceptors in the periodontal ligaments, chewing ability precipitously declines.

Biting and chewing forces decrease 10-fold and 3-fold, respectively, in the person with complete dentures. Although the muscles of mastication are adequate, the mucous membrane covering the edentulous ridge cannot withstand the pressures exerted. This may be especially true for the elderly person with a thin, friable mucosa covering the bony ridges.

The edentulous person's ability to adapt to the foreign prosthesis greatly influences the eating pleasures, the eating proficiency, and the overall health of the individual. The quality and quantity of nutritional intake are not necessarily modified in the edentulous individual. Nonetheless, if the denture is ill-fitting, the nutritional status of the person may suffer. Hence, eating becomes a chore and less pleasurable. The dental hygienist can facilitate the client's human need for nutrition and the success of the denture therapy by assessing the client's nutritional status and providing dietary counseling to ensure that nutritionally rich foods, such as vegetables, meats, and fruits, are not ignored. The client will experience greater success with his new denture if he is taught to avoid repeated incision using anterior teeth, gum chewing, and eating sticky foods. The client should also be instructed to consume food in smaller pieces, lengthen chewing time, evenly distribute food to both the left and the right sides of the mouth while chewing. Practicing these behaviors is critical to masticatory efficiency and denture stability.

DENTURE-INDUCED ORAL LESIONS

Periodic maintenance appointments provide the dental hygienist with an excellent opportunity to identify soft tissue lesions related to dentures and to refer these clients to the dentist for evaluation and treatment.

Although several studies have demonstrated no correlation between cancer at specific sites and the wearing of dentures,[20-22] denture irritation may be considered a cocarcinogenic factor in some predisposed individuals.[23] Although it is highly unlikely that chronic irritation due to ill-fitting dentures will cause oral carcinoma, trauma induced by dentures and other mechanical irritations probably accelerate the progression of the disease.[24] For this reason, the dental hygienist should be especially attentive to its signs and symptoms, for example, ulceration/erosion, erythema, induration, fixation, chronicity, lymphadenopathy, and leukoplakia. (See Chapter 34 for a discussion on oral cancer.)

A wide spectrum of oral mucosal conditions in the denture wearer are associated with improper oral hygiene care, extended wear of the denture, or reaction to poor prosthesis fit. More specifically, denture-induced lesions are subdivided into four categories (Figs. 27-6 to 27-8):

- Reactive/traumatic
- Infectious
- Mixed reactive and infectious
- Systemic disease-related lesions

Each lesion is categorized according to its typical etiological factors and clinical features (Table 27-2). Generally, relining or remaking of the denture by the dentist and/or client education can eliminate the irritation.

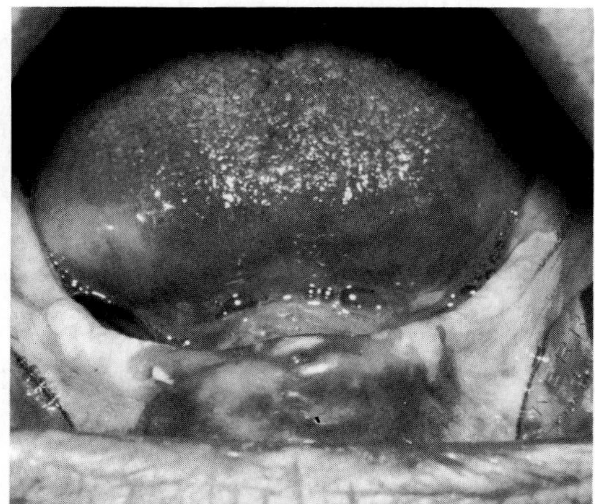

FIGURE 27-6
Reactive/traumatic lesion—focal (frictional) hyperkeratosis. (With permission from Regezi, J. A., and Sciubba, J. Oral Pathology: Clinical-Pathologic Correlations, 2nd ed. Philadelphia: W. B. Saunders, 1993, p. 99.)

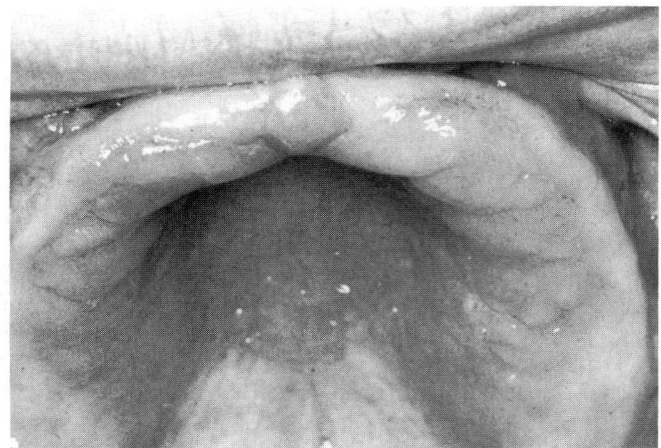

FIGURE 27–7
Infectious lesion—chronic candidiasis infection, palatal papillary type. (With permission from Regezi, J. A., and Sciubba, J. Oral Pathology: Clinical-Pathologic Correlations, 2nd ed. Philadelphia: W. B. Saunders, 1993, p. 124.)

Reactive/Traumatic Lesions

Reactive/traumatic lesions commonly are secondary to either acute or chronic injury. Lesions included in this category are ulcers, focal (frictional) hyperkeratosis, and denture-induced fibrous hyperplasia. An overexuberant repair response produces hyperplastic tissue that often is painless, but pain may develop if the fibrous lesion is traumatized or ulcerated. Surgical excision and removal of the irritating factor are effective methods of treating reactive lesions.

Infectious Lesions

Denture stomatitis, angular cheilitis, and **burning mouth syndrome** are infectious lesions typically associated with wearing dentures. The most common inflammation of the denture-bearing mucosa is denture stomatitis (Fig. 27–9). Despite the minimal pain associated with denture stomatitis, it is often referred to inappropriately as "denture sore mouth." With a predilection for females, the incidence varies between 20 and 40% of the edentulous population.[25] However, it can be observed in as many as 65% of the older adult population who wear complete maxillary dentures.[24]

Chronic Candidiasis

The majority of denture-related infections, including denture stomatitis, probably are due to a chronic *Candida* infection and can effectively be treated by a dentist using a topical antifungal agent, such as nystatin. Prescribed by the dentist for use at home, nystatin cream is applied to both the affected tissues and the dentures to eliminate the fungi. Topical antifungal agents should be used by the client for approximately 1 week following disappearance of clinical symptoms.

A chronic *Candida* infection is primarily responsible for the development of denture stomatitis,[26] although recent studies implicate bacteria as the etiological agent.[27,28] The predominant bacteria isolated were gram-positive *Streptococcus* species; however, *Lactobacillus, Bacteroides,* and *Actinomyces* species also were detected regularly. Other contributing factors include bacterial plaque accumulation on dentures; chronic, low-grade soft tissue trauma due to ill-fitting dentures; an unbalanced occlusal relationship; and continuous wearing of the denture at night. In some circumstances, systemic conditions such as diabetes, anemia, menopause, malnutrition, and malabsorption of nutrients in the digestive tract can predispose an individual to a candidal infection.

The oral manifestations of this infection appear on the palatal mucosa rather than on the mandibular alveolar mucosa. The clinical features demonstrate variations in surface texture ranging from a smooth, velvety appearance to a more nodular or hyperplastic form. With severe infections, surfaces may appear eroded, with small confluent vesicles. Characteristically, the bright-red color of the denture-supporting mucosa is confined within a well-defined denture border.

Angular Cheilitis

Angular cheilitis frequently appears in conjunction with the mucosal inflammation caused by the *Candida albicans* in-

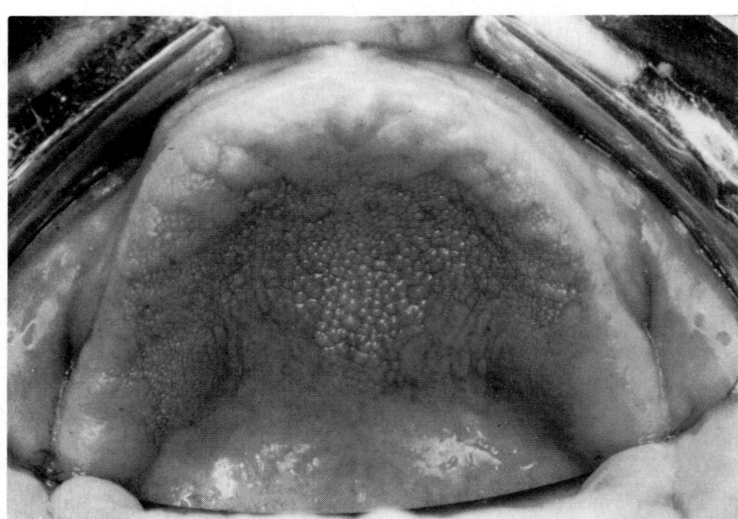

FIGURE 27–8
Mixed reactive and infectious lesions—papillary hyperplasia associated with candidiasis infection. (With permission from Regezi, J. A., and Sciubba, J. Oral Pathology: Clinical-Pathologic Correlations, 2nd ed. Philadelphia: W. B. Saunders, 1993, p. 177.)

TABLE 27–2
CHANGES IN THE ORAL TISSUES OF THE EDENTULOUS CLIENT SUGGESTING A DEFICIT IN HUMAN NEED FOR SKIN AND ORAL MUCOUS MEMBRANE INTEGRITY

Oral Manifestation	Due To	As Evidenced By
Reactive Lesions		
Acute ulcers	Ill-fitting denture Chemical agent irritation: denture adhesive denture cleanser self-medication	Yellow-white exudate Red halo Varying pain and tenderness
Chronic ulcers	Same as above	Yellow membrane Elevated margin Little or no pain
Focal (frictional) hyperkeratosis	Chronic rubbing or friction of denture	White patch Asymptomatic
Denture-induced fibrous hyperplasia (epulis fissurata, denture hyperplasia)	Ill-fitting denture	Folds of fibrous connective tissue Varying color Asymptomatic Typical on vestibular mucosa at denture flange contact
Infectious Lesions		
Denture stomatitis (denture sore mouth)	Chronic *Candida albicans* infection Poor oral hygiene care Continuous wear of dentures Ill-fitting denture Systemic factors: anemia, diabetes, immunosuppression, menopause Systemic antibiotics Chemical agent irritation: denture adhesive denture cleanser self-medication Denture base allergy	Generalized redness of mucosa Velvet-like appearance Pain and burning sensations Typical under maxillary denture
Angular cheilitis	Chronic *C. albicans* infection Pooling of saliva in commissural folds Riboflavin deficiency	Fissured at angles of mouth Eroded Encrusted Moderate pain
Burning mouth syndrome	Chronic *C. albicans* infection Ill-fitting denture Systemic factors: anemia, xerostomia, vitamin B deficiency	Intense pain and burning sensations Normal-appearing mucosa
Mixed Lesions		
Papillary Hyperplasia	Chronic *C. albicans* infection Chronic low-grade denture trauma	Multiple round-to-ovoid nodules—"cobblestone" appearance Generalized red mucosa background Rarely ulcerated Typical under maxillary denture
Systemic Conditions		
Paget's disease	Cause unknown May be metabolic abnormality	Initial bone resorption phase Enlargement of skull, maxilla, or mandible in bilateral and symmetrical manner Flattened palatal vault Pain in bones initially

fection (Fig. 27–10). The condition results from small amounts of saliva accumulating at the commissural angles, which promotes the colonization of yeast. Clinically, angular cheilitis appears as cracked, eroded, and encrusted surfaces at the commissural folds and may cause moderate pain. Often it is secondary to overclosure resulting from a reduction in the client's vertical dimension. A vitamin B (riboflavin) deficiency resulting from inadequate nutrition also can cause angular cheilitis. Dental treatment requires elimination of the trauma by correcting the denture and reduction of the *Candida* infection by prescribing antifungal drugs. Dental hygiene care to prevent the recurrence of this condition includes instructing the client in thorough daily cleansing of the infected denture using chemical immersion. A weak sodium hypochlorite solution is used to soak the denture overnight. This inexpensive, safe, and effective cleansing solution consists of the following:[29]

1 tablespoon (15 mL) sodium hypochlorite (household bleach)

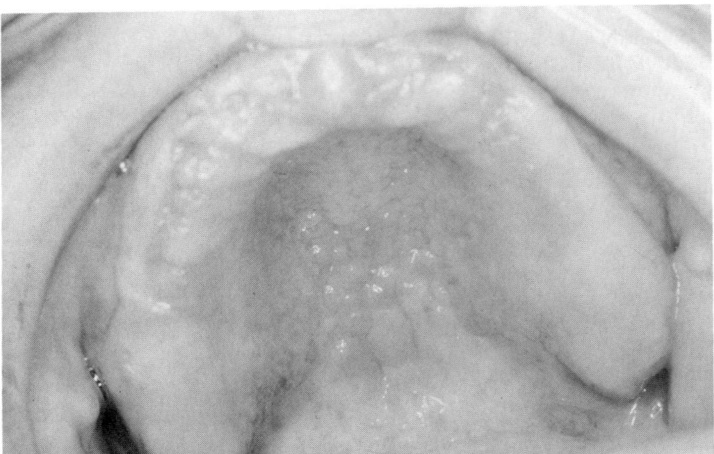

FIGURE 27–9
Denture stomatitis. (With permission from Regezi, J. A., and Sciubba, J. Oral Pathology: Clinical-Pathologic Correlations, 2nd ed. Philadelphia: W. B. Saunders, 1993, p. O-44.)

1 teaspoon (4 mL) Calgon detergent
4 ounces (114 mL) water

The denture must be rinsed thoroughly with water prior to reinsertion into the oral cavity.

Mixed Reactive and Infectious Lesions

Both trauma and infection are etiological factors contributing to mixed reactive and infectious lesions, such as **papillary hyperplasia.** A "cobblestone" appearance often describes the granular papillary projections that result from a hyperplastic tissue response. This condition can predispose or potentiate the growth of *Candida albicans* under the denture and further complicate the problem. Multiple dental therapies are used to resolve the lesions, including surgical excision, antifungal agents, soft tissue conditioners and liners, and strict oral hygiene measures.

Systemic Disease–Related Lesions

Oral manifestations of systemic disease may create additional problems for the edentulous client. **Paget's disease** is a chronic, nonmetabolic disease of bone characterized by a slowly progressive enlargement of the maxilla, mandible, and skull. Typically, edentulous clients with Paget's disease complain of newly acquired ill-fitting dentures as the alveolar ridges widen. The unknown etiology and slow progression of Paget's disease allow only for symptomatic treatment.

Xerostomia and the Edentulous Client

The many etiological factors of xerostomia and extreme difficulties experienced by the edentulous client warrant an understanding of its oral manifestations. The critical role of saliva in the maintenance of oral health is well established.[30,31]

Normal salivary flow is essential for denture retention and function. A thin film of saliva provides adhesive action as well as lubrication and cushioning effects. When the mucosa becomes dry, movement of the denture can easily cause frictional irritation of the denture-bearing mucosa. Other symptoms also may arise as a result of oral dryness, including altered taste perceptions, cracked lips, a fissured

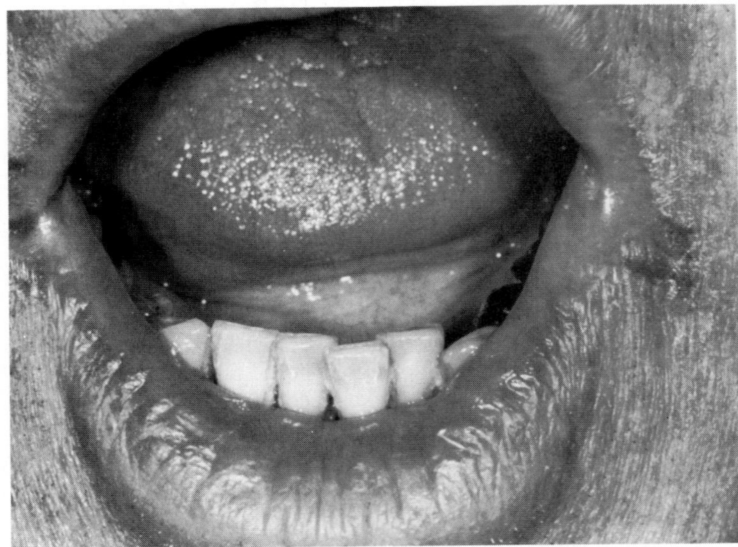

FIGURE 27–10
Angular cheilitis. (With permission from Regezi, J. A., and Sciubba, J. Oral Pathology: Clinical-Pathologic Correlations, 2nd ed. Philadelphia: W. B. Saunders, 1993, p. 123.)

tongue, and generalized "burning" of the oral cavity. Although the exact causative agent of xerostomia may be difficult to identify, the most common etiological factors are Sjögren's syndrome, emotional and anxiety states, anemia, negative fluid balance, polyuria states, selected nutritional and hormonal deficiencies, drugs or medications, acquired immunodeficiency syndrome, and therapeutic radiation.[24] Contrary to widespread belief, diminished salivary output is not directly associated with increased age; rather, other factors should be considered if xerostomia is observed in older adults.[32,33]

Dental hygiene care for the denture client with xerostomia can be challenging, since most remedies provide only temporary relief. The dental hygienist may recommend saliva substitutes and frequent mouth rinses, especially during meals, to keep the mouth lubricated and temporarily provide symptomatic relief. Recommendations for the management of soft tissue dryness include coating the tissue surface of dentures with petroleum lubricating jelly, silicone fluid, or denture adhesive material.

CONTINUED CARE AND MAINTENANCE PROGRAM

Education is the primary strategy for meeting client human need deficits in conceptualization and problem solving, and is the foundation of the preventive program for the edentulous client. From the outset of care, the edentulous person must be educated regarding expectations, oral hygiene practices, denture use and care, and periodic maintenance appointments. Successful prosthodontic therapy greatly depends on clients who achieve a sense of self-determination and responsibility regarding their oral health status. The dental hygienist encourages clients to set personal goals for maintenance of oral health and suggests behavior patterns and techniques that are compatible with the client's lifestyle, cultural customs, values, and physical capabilities. A dental hygiene care plan for an edentulous client is illustrated in the case study that follows.

The newly edentulous person commonly requires a denture adjustment within the first 6 months to 1 year. The useful life of complete dentures is estimated to range from 4 to 8 years. During this time, annual continued care visits are essential to denture longevity and to identify the need for denture duplication, rebasing, or replacement. However, some individuals with poor oral hygiene require biannual visits. Each continued care appointment should incorporate all aspects of the dental hygiene process, including assessment, diagnosis, planning, implementation, and evaluation as guided by any identified human need deficits related to oral health (see Procedure 27-1).

During assessment, the dental hygienist encourages the client to describe his complaints in his own words to help

DENTAL HYGIENE CARE PLAN: THE EDENTULOUS CLIENT

Jeremy Myers, age 67, was a new client at the University dental hygiene care center. Recently widowed, Mr. Myers lived alone in an apartment complex for retired individuals and relied solely on social security payments for living expenses. The client wore a complete maxillary denture and had the majority of his natural mandibular dentition remaining. Following a review of the client's health, dental, and dental hygiene history, the dental hygienist assessed the human need deficits experienced by the client that related to dental hygiene care. The client complained of a sore palate and "loose denture which hurts especially while eating." On intraoral examination, the dental hygienist noticed a generalized redness on the palatal mucosa. The denture was easily displaced when the retention of the prosthesis was evaluated. Furthermore, periodontal assessment of the natural dentition revealed periodontal probe depths of 4 to 5 mm, bleeding on probing, and moderate bacterial plaque and calculus throughout the mandible.

OBJECTIVE DATA

1. Denture with poor retention
2. Generalized red inflamed mucosa under maxillary denture
3. Moderate bacterial plaque and calculus on mandibular dentition

SUBJECTIVE DATA

1. Denture feels loose
2. Painful hard palate
3. Difficult to eat

Dental Hygiene Diagnosis	Due To or Related To	As Evidenced By	Goal/Expected Behavior
Deficit in the need for a biologically sound dentition	• Ill-fitting dentures • Poor oral hygiene	• Client's expression of difficulty in chewing • Denture with decreased retention on displacement • Presence of moderate plaque and calculus on mandibular teeth	• By 3/19 refer to dentist for denture adjustment • By 4/1 client shows improved oral hygiene • By 4/30 client able to eat efficiently

Continued on following page

DENTAL HYGIENE CARE PLAN: THE EDENTULOUS CLIENT *Continued*

DENTAL HYGIENE INTERVENTIONS

1. Refer client to dentist for relining or remaking of denture.
2. Educate the client about the importance of daily oral hygiene care for the denture, mucosal tissues, and remaining natural dentition.
   - Show the client the signs and symptoms associated with the denture irritation and periodontal disease
3. Teach the client about the periodontal disease process.
   - Compare healthy periodontal tissues to diseased sites in the client's own mouth to develop his awareness of his condition

EVALUATIVE STATEMENTS

1. April 1 goal met. Client's denture has proper fit and occlusion.
2. April 30 goal met. Mucosal irritation resolves, and client reports that he is able to eat.
3. April 1 goal met. Client exhibits a 3-point reduction in the plaque index.

Dental Hygiene Diagnosis	Due To or Related To	As Evidenced By	Goal/Expected Behavior
Deficit in the need for skin and mucous membrane integrity of the head and neck	• Deficit in knowledge about denture-induced lesions of the oral cavity • Deficit in knowledge about the periodontal disease process and bacterial plaque as an etiological agent	• Ill-fitting denture • Generalized pain and inflammation under maxillary denture • Poor oral hygiene • Probing depths of 4 to 5 mm • Moderate bacterial plaque and calculus	• By 3/19 refer to dentist for denture adjustment and treatment of mucosal inflammation • By 4/1 client shows improved oral hygiene • By 4/30 client will verbalize the value of periodic continued care visits and daily home care

DENTAL HYGIENE INTERVENTIONS

1. Refer client to dentist for relining or remaking of denture and therapeutic treatment of mucosal inflammation.
2. Educate the client about denture-induced lesions, and review prevention techniques.
   - Describe the potential consequences of oral and denture hygiene neglect
   - Demonstrate techniques for self-examination of the denture for proper fit, denture deposits, and abraded surfaces
   - Teach the client daily oral and denture hygiene care
   - Advise the client to return at least annually for professional continued care visits
3. Explain the process of periodontal disease to the client.
4. In collaboration with the dentist, scale and root-plane mandibular dentition after immediate denture problems are addressed.
5. After 1 month, evaluate periodontal tissues, edentulous mucosa, and personal oral and denture hygiene care.

EVALUATIVE STATEMENTS

1. April 1 goal met. Client achieves oral mucous membrane integrity following denture adjustment and therapeutic treatment for mucosal inflammation.
2. April 1 goal met. Probing depths improve to 3 to 4 mm, and no bleeding on probing is observed.
3. April 30 goal unmet. Client still questions the validity of oral care for a person with dentures.

Dental Hygiene Diagnosis	Due To or Related To	As Evidenced By	Goal/Expected Behavior
Deficit in the need for freedom from pain	• Chronic *C. albicans* infection • Poor daily oral hygiene • Ill-fitting dentures	• Client's expression of pain on hard palate and when eating • Clinical signs of chronic inflammation	• By 3/19 refer to dentist for immediate care • By 4/1 mucosal irritation resolves using antifungal therapy • By 4/30 client can eat comfortably

DENTAL HYGIENE CARE PLAN: THE EDENTULOUS CLIENT *Continued*

			• Verbalizes the need for daily oral hygiene

DENTAL HYGIENE INTERVENTIONS

1. Assess level of pain experienced by client by encouraging him to describe in detail his denture problem.
2. Refer client to the dentist for immediate care to adjust denture and treat mucosal inflammation.

EVALUATIVE STATEMENTS

1. April 30 goal met. Client reports no pain when eating.
2. April 1 goal met. Client exhibits no mucosal inflammation.
3. Goal partially met. Client shows improved oral hygiene care.

Dental Hygiene Diagnosis	Due To or Related To	As Evidenced By	Goal/Expected Behavior
Deficit in need for self-determination and responsibility	• Inadequate daily oral and denture hygiene care • Lack of knowledge about his role in maintenance of oral health • Unaware of methods of self-examination of denture and oral tissues	• Mucosal irritation • Ill-fitting denture for extended period • Poor oral hygiene • Unhealthy periodontal tissues	• By 3/19 client will verbalize importance of maintaining daily oral self-care • By 4/1 client accepts responsibility for oral wellness

DENTAL HYGIENE INTERVENTIONS

1. Assess the present oral health behaviors from data collected in the client's health, dental, personal, and social history and from direct observation of the oral cavity and denture.
2. Suggest to the client oral and denture hygiene behaviors necessary to obtain and maintain oral health.
3. In collaboration with the client, set goals related to dental hygiene care within the overall goals of the comprehensive treatment plan.
4. Motivate the client to develop self-determination and accept responsibility for oral health.
5. After 1 month, evaluate the denture occlusion and fit and client's acceptance of oral and denture hygiene care.

EVALUATIVE STATEMENTS

1. April 1 goal met. Client claims responsibility for his oral wellness.
2. April 1 goal met. Client is capable of maintaining oral health by daily self-care.

Dental Hygiene Diagnosis	Due To or Related To	As Evidenced By	Goal/Expected Behavior
Deficit in need for nutrition	• Lack of knowledge about need for nutrition to maintain tissue integrity • Limited financial resources • Skill deficit in food preparation	• Decreased tissue integrity • Moderate bacterial plaque	• By 3/19 client verbalizes the need to take active role in healthy nutrition for oral and general health • By 4/1 tissue integrity improves with proper nutrition and fluid intake

Continued on following page

DENTAL HYGIENE CARE PLAN: THE EDENTULOUS CLIENT *Continued*

DENTAL HYGIENE INTERVENTIONS

1. Assess deficits in nutrition and fluid intake.
2. Set nutritional goals with the client that include his lifestyle, financial resources, physical capabilities, living conditions, and cultural preferences.
3. Counsel client on nutritional guidelines for the edentulous older adult.
4. Evaluate client response to nutritional goals in 1 month.

EVALUATIVE STATEMENTS

1. April 1 goal met. Client shows normal healing patterns.
2. April 1 goal met. Client maintains structurally and functionally competent body parts.
3. April 1 goal met. Client's dietary assessment indicates intake of nutrient-rich foods necessary for health maintenance.

assess the nature of the problem. For example, sometimes a client with good muscular control of his denture may perceive an ill-fitting denture as satisfactory. In comparison, another individual reports a well-fitting denture to be loose when, in fact, occlusal interferences exist. All deficits in the client's need for a biologically sound dentition are assessed throughout the appointment and accurately documented in the client's record. As a cotherapist with the dentist, the dental hygienist is attentive to the individual human need deficits of the edentulous client and refers these concerns to the dentist.

Clients should be advised of the importance of daily care of both the dentures and the associated soft tissues (see Procedure 27–2). Both verbal and written instructions can reinforce the home care regimen, especially for the elderly individual. A simple reminder to rinse the dentures and mouth after each meal can help eliminate accumulation of food debris and bacterial plaque. Written instructions or other formal educational materials that include proper denture hygiene and cleansing of the oral tissues provide the client with specific recommendations for maintaining oral health. Pertinent information to teach the client includes:

- Types of chemical cleansing agents; frequency and duration of their application; and other instructions for their use
- Materials and techniques for mechanical cleaning of the prosthesis
- Cleansing and massage of the oral tissues
- Warnings of potentially harmful effects of improper denture care and neglect of oral hygiene
- Special instructions for cleaning of soft lining materials, if necessary

At continued care visits, the dental hygienist should assess the client's ability to perform meticulous oral hygiene care at home.

Commercial Denture Cleansers

Maintaining denture hygiene is essential both for aesthetic concerns and for prevention and treatment of oral infections in the client with dentures. Proper hygienic care can be confusing for the edentulous client because of the many commercially available products as well as home remedies. Commercially available denture cleansers can be divided into six groups:

- Abrasive powder or paste cleansers
- Chemical soak cleansers
- Acids
- Enzymes
- Antimicrobials
- Ultrasonic devices

Table 27–3 describes their mechanism of action, advantages, and disadvantages. When selecting a denture cleanser, the safety of the denture wearer and of the denture is a paramount concern. If abrasive powders and pastes are used improperly, they pose the highest risk of damage to the denture materials. Denture acrylic can become abraded, and this ultimately may lead to an altered fit if a hard bristle brush or extreme vigor is used when cleaning the prosthesis.

The relative efficacy of denture cleansers partially depends on the manual dexterity of the client. Brushing with abrasive powders and pastes is suitable for the client who is motivated and has the dexterity to clean thoroughly all surfaces. However, this denture cleansing method is the most difficult, especially for the physically challenged or older adult client. Chemical soak cleansers are effective alternatives to mechanical cleansing. Alkaline peroxide and hypochlorite solutions can be recommended for dentures with and without metal components, respectively. Hypochlorites are reported in the majority of clinical studies to be the most efficacious soaking method for dentures constructed with only acrylic materials. Caution must be taken to avoid completely the use of acid solutions and to limit the duration of use of hypochlorites to 15 minutes on any metal-containing prostheses.[34] If an offensive taste and odor linger following the hypochlorite soak, alkaline peroxide may be used subsequently. A comparative study of the antimicrobial capabilities of an abrasive paste and a chemical soak denture cleanser suggests that a denture cleanser soak in conjunction with brushing with an abrasive paste is necessary for complete denture hygiene.[35] Most important, the edentulous client must understand the reasons for denture hygiene maintenance and the potential risks and benefits provided by the variety of denture cleansers available today.

TABLE 27–3
DENTURE CLEANSING PRODUCTS

Product	Mechanism of Action	Advantages	Disadvantages
Chemical Soak Cleansers			
Alkaline hypochlorite	Dissolves mucins and organic substances of denture plaque matrix	1. Bactericidal 2. Fungicidal 3. Bleaches stains 4. May inhibit calculus formation	1. Corrodes metals 2. Odor and taste may be unacceptable 3. May bleach acrylic if used in high concentration or for prolonged periods
Alkaline peroxide	Mechanical cleansing effect by the release of oxygen (bubbling)	1. Some antibacterial effect 2. Removes stain	1. None
Abrasive Cleansers			
Powders and pastes	Mild abrasives such as calcium carbonate assist mechanical cleaning by brushing	1. Removes bacterial plaque 2. Removes extrinsic stain	1. Ineffective and harmful to denture materials if used improperly 2. Dentures may become ill-fitting if used improperly
Acids			
Hydrochloric acid with or without phosphoric acid	Dissolves the inorganic components of denture deposits	1. Removes calcium phosphate deposits 2. Removes stain 3. Effective at dilute concentrations (3–5%)	1. An in-office procedure only 2. Careful handling of acids required 3. Corrodes metal
Ultrasonic Devices	Conflicting evidence regarding effectiveness of ultrasonic action per se; chemical solution may provide cleansing action	1. Removes bacterial plaque 2. Enhances effectiveness of disinfectants	1. Commonly an in-office procedure 2. Uncertain efficacy of ultrasonic action
Antimicrobials			
Chlorhexidine gluconate 2% solution (not approved for use on dentures in United States)	Antimicrobial action by chemical agent	1. Antibacterial 2. Antifungal	1. Only temporary relief of denture stomatitis symptoms 2. Stains denture teeth
Enzymes	Enhances dissolution of protein components in denture plaque matrix when used in combination with chemical soak solutions	1. Removes bacterial plaque	1. None

Adapted from Abelson, D. C. Denture plaque and denture cleansers: Review of the literature. Gerodontics 1:202–226, 1985. ©1985 Munksgaard International Publishers, Ltd., Copenhagen, Denmark.

NUTRITION FOR THE PERSON WHO IS EDENTULOUS

Many of the lesions associated with denture wearing are a result of multiple factors, such as ill-fitting dentures, poor denture and oral hygiene care, and prolonged wearing of the prosthesis. However, a deficit in the client's human need for nutrition also contributes to denture-induced lesions. Nutritional deficiencies are seldom noticed and, therefore, infrequently corrected. For example, a client deficient in the B-complex vitamins may appear with oral symptoms of atrophic glossitis, angular cheilitis, or cracking, fissuring, or ulceration of the lips. These clinical signs may be interpreted as a chronic *Candida albicans* infection rather than a nutritional deficiency. Although difficult to identify, a disturbance in the client's need for nutrition can be detected by the dental hygienist who is cognizant of the changes related to nutritional deficiencies experienced by the denture wearer. Following nutritional assessment, the dental hygienist should inform the dentist of potential nutritional problems and recommend to the client dietary measures that may improve oral health.

Nutritional Factors

Key nutritional factors in the edentulous client include the causes and effects of:

- Negative water balance on oral structures
- Negative calcium balance on alveolar bone
- Nitrogen-protein balance on muscle weakness and tissue fragility of oral tissues[36]

Water is an essential nutrient for all body functions. Hence, evidence of tissue dehydration can be recognized throughout the body, especially in elderly individuals, as wrinkled skin, loss of muscle mass, decreased sweat and

TABLE 27-4
NUTRITIONAL GUIDELINES FOR MAINTENANCE OF ORAL HEALTH IN THE EDENTULOUS CLIENT

Nutritional Goal	Rationale
1. Eat a variety of foods.	1. A well balanced diet is essential to meet the client's human need for nutrition for repair and maintenance of structurally and functionally competent body parts. Eating a different food within each food group according to the food pyramid increases the likelihood of getting all the necessary nutrients.
2. Select foods high in complex carbohydrates: fruits, vegetables, whole-grain bread and cereals.	2. Often elevated in older adults, blood glucose levels rise less if complex carbohydrates are consumed rather than simple sugars. Also, fiber is a major component of these foods which promotes normal bowel function and may reduce serum cholesterol.
3. Protein-rich foods including lean meat, poultry, fish, dried peas, and beans are required daily.	3. Protein is required to maintain the strength and integrity of tissues especially when exposed to physiologic stresses.
4. Daily requirements for calcium intake are obtained primarily from dairy products, but some nondairy foods also contain substantial amounts of calcium. Milk, cheese, yogurt, ice cream, collard greens, broccoli, oysters, canned salmon, sardines, and tofu made with a calcium coagulant are excellent dietary sources of calcium.	4. Dietary calcium intake is critical to maintain bone mass. Alveolar bone has been shown to be an early site of calcium withdrawal if dietary calcium intake is low.
5. Consume vitamin C containing fruit juices and citrus fruit every day.	5. Vitamin C is essential for repair and healing of wounds and for absorption of other vitamins and minerals.
6. Limit intake of processed foods high in fat and sodium.	6. Increasing evidence has linked high fat intake to heart disease, certain cancers, and obesity. High sodium intake may cause hypertension.
7. Limit intake of bakery products high in fat and simple sugars.	7. Bakery products are often high in calories and/or low in nutrients.
8. Drink eight glasses of water daily.	8. Water is an essential nutrient for all body functions.

Adapted from Zarb, G. A., Bolender, C. L., Hickey, J. C., and Carlsson, G. E. Boucher's Prosthodontic Treatment for Edentulous Patients, 10th ed. St. Louis: C. V. Mosby, 1990, p. 112.

sebaceous gland secretions, dry eyes, xerostomia, and a smooth, atrophic tongue. The best dietary recommendation for dehydrated clients is to consume vegetable soup because both water and nutrients are more effectively retained in this form.

A negative calcium balance results in osteoporosis, which can precipitate rapid and extensive resorption of the alveolar ridges. Common in the aging person, a defect in calcium intake, absorption, or transport may be responsible for the bony changes. Low-fat milk and milk products are good dietary sources of calcium.

Depletion of protein most notably affects muscle mass but also may increase tissue fragility and cracking of the lips. A decrease in mass and strength of the muscles of mastication is especially evident in the older adult and can be monitored by placing the finger in the vestibule of the mouth and asking the client to clench his teeth. Edentulous clients should be encouraged to maintain a high-protein diet to facilitate maintenance of muscle mass. Recommendations for quality sources of protein include meat, fish, beans, tofu, and legumes.

Undoubtedly, the nutritional quality of food depends on the method of preparation. Variations in food preparation result from the client's physical capabilities, living conditions, and cultural preferences. Hence, dietary advice should include cooking instructions that maximize the nutrient value of the diet with consideration of individual circumstances and preferences. For example, meat and fish are most nutritious when broiled or boiled rather than fried. In addition to limiting fat intake, boiling foods breaks down complex proteins to more easily digestible components. On the other hand, fried protein-rich foods lose some nutritional value because the protein coagulates and becomes more difficult to digest.

Nutrition and the Older Adult Who is Edentulous

In general, the edentulous older adult's diet is of great concern to the dental hygienist. A deficiency of essential nutrients magnifies the tissue friability and diminished repair potential observed in geriatric clients. Many older adults live under circumstances that predispose them to poor nutritional habits, such as low incomes, inadequate kitchen facilities, loneliness, and poor physical health. A lack of knowledge and interest in proper nutrition also contributes to malnutrition in the older adult. Often the older adult's dietary intake is affected by wearing dentures, and deficiencies in protein, calcium, and B-complex vitamins may be present.[3] Normally these nutrients are essential in the maintenance and repair of oral tissues and bone. Many older adults have limited ability to digest and absorb food. This problem can be exacerbated by ill-fitting dentures, which may elicit chewing difficulties and diminish consumption of fibrous foods. Hence, digestion, absorption, and utilization of nutrients are impaired. The two most common dietary tendencies of the aged edentulous person are their:

- Preference for a soft diet high in carbohydrate and refined sugar
- Consumption of fewer protein-rich and high-fiber foods

For these reasons, the dental hygienist should routinely assess nutritional habits and suggest healthy food alternatives to promote weight control and a nutritionally balanced diet (Table 27–4). This can be effectively accomplished if simple, well-defined, concise guidelines are constructed so that no major changes in food habits and preferences are made. The client and the dental hygienist can set nutritional goals that reflect individual human need deficits, taking into account lifestyle, financial resources, and cultural preferences. With the edentulous client, nutritional deficits should always be considered when determining factors that contribute to a denture-related problem.

References

1. Miller, A. J., Brunelle, J. A., et al. Oral Health of United States Adults: The National Survey of Oral Health in U.S. Employed Adults and Seniors: 1985–1986, National Findings. Bethesda: National Institute of Dental Research, NIH Publication no. 87-2868, 1987.
2. Brunelle, J. A., Miller-Chisholm, A. J., and Löe, H. Oral Health of United States Adults: The National Survey of Oral Health in U.S. Employed Adults and Seniors: 1985–1986, Regional Findings. Bethesda: National Institute of Dental Research, NIH Publication no. 88-2869, 1988.
3. Renner, R. P. Complete Dentures: A Guide for Patient Treatment. New York: Masson Pub. USA, 1981.
4. House, M. M. Full Denture Techniques. Lecture, Study Club #1. Whittier, California: 1935.
5. Campbell, R. I. A comparative study of the resorption of alveolar ridges in denture wearers and non-denture wearers. Journal of the American Dental Association 60:143, 1960.
6. Carlsson, G. E., and Persson, G. Morphological changes of the mandible after extraction and wearing of dentures: A longitudinal, clinical, and x-ray cephalometric study covering five years. Odontologisk Revy 18:27, 1967.
7. Jozefowicz, W. The influence of wearing dentures on residual ridges: A comparative study. Journal of Prosthetic Dentistry 24:137, 1970.
8. Kelsey, C. C. Alveolar bone resorption under complete dentures. Journal of Prosthetic Dentistry 25:152, 1971.
9. Kalk, W., and de Baat, C. Some factors connected with alveolar bone resorption. Journal of Dentistry 17:162, 1989.
10. Mack, A. Full Dentures: The Treatment of the Edentulous Patient. Bristol: John Wright and Sons Ltd., 1978.
11. Tautin, F. S. Should dentures be worn continuously? Journal of Prosthetic Dentistry 39:372, 1978.
12. Devlin, H., and Ferguson, M. W. J. Alveolar ridge resorption and mandibular atrophy: A review of the role of local and systemic factors. British Dental Journal 170:101, 1991.
13. Karlsson, S., and Swartz, B. Effect of denture adhesive on mandibular denture dislodgement. Quintessence International 21:625, 1990.
14. Zarb, G. A., Bolender, C. L., et al. Boucher's Prosthodontic Treatment for Edentulous Patients, 10th ed. St. Louis: C. V. Mosby, 1990.
15. Tallgren, A., Lang, B. R., et al. Roentgen cephalometric analysis of ridge resorption and changes in jaw occlusal relationships in immediate complete denture wearers. Journal of Oral Rehabilitation 7:77, 1980.
16. De Franco, R. L., and Ortman, L. F. Diagnosis and treatment planning. In Winkler, S. (ed.). Essentials of Complete Denture Prosthodontics, 2nd ed. Littleton, MA: PSG Pub. Co., 1987, pp. 37–55.
17. Friedman, S. Diagnosis and treatment planning. Dental Clinics of North America 21:237, 1977.
18. Gonzales, J. B. Preventing and treating abused tissue. In Winkler, S. (ed.). Essentials of Complete Denture Prosthodontics, 2nd ed. Littleton, MA: PSG Pub. Co., 1987, pp. 81–87.
19. Basker, R. M., Davenport, J. C., and Tomlin, H. R. Prosthetic Treatment of the Edentulous Patient, 2nd ed. London: Macmillan Press, 1983.
20. Wynder, E. L., Bross, I. J., and Feldman, R. M. A study of the etiological factors in cancer of the mouth. Cancer 10:1300, 1957.
21. Browne, R. M., Camsey, M. C., et al. Etiological factors in oral squamous cell carcinoma. Community Dentistry and Oral Epidemiology 5:301, 1977.
22. Gorsky, M., and Silverman, S., Jr. Denture wearing and oral cancer. Journal of Prosthetic Dentistry 52:164, 1984.
23. Silverman, S., Jr., and Shillitoe, E. J. Etiology and predisposing factors. In Silverman, S., Jr. (ed.). Oral Cancer, 3rd ed. New York: The American Cancer Society, 1990.
24. Regezi, J. A., and Sciubba, J. J. Oral Pathology: Clinical-Pathologic Correlations. Philadelphia: W. B. Saunders, 1989.
25. Neill, D. J., and Nairn, R. I. Complete Denture Prosthetics, 3rd ed. London: Wright, 1990.
26. Davenport, J. C. The oral distribution of *Candida* in denture stomatitis. British Dental Journal 129:151, 1970.
27. Koopmans, A. S. F., Kippuw, N., and de Graaff, J. Bacterial involvement in denture-induced stomatitis. Journal of Dental Research 67:1246, 1988.
28. Verran, J. Preliminary studies on denture plaque microbiology and acidogenicity. Microbial Ecology in Health and Disease 1:51, 1988.
29. Ortman, L. F. Patient education and complete denture maintenance. In Winkler, S. (ed.). Essentials of Complete Denture Prosthodontics, 2nd ed. Littleton, MA: PSG Pub. Co., 1987, pp. 331–340.
30. Mandel, I. D., and Wotman, S. The salivary secretions in health and disease. Oral Science Reviews 8:25, 1976.
31. Baum, B. J. Salivary glands and saliva: Recent advances in understanding their functions and role in oral health. New Dentist 9:21, 1979.
32. Baum, B. J. Evaluation of stimulated parotid saliva flow rate in different age groups. Journal of Dental Research 60:1292, 1981.
33. Heft, M. W., and Baum, B. J. Unstimulated and stimulated parotid salivary flow rate in individuals of different ages. Journal of Dental Research 63:1182, 1984.
34. Abelson, D. C. Denture plaque and denture cleansers: Review of the literature. Gerodontics 1:202, 1985.
35. Dills, S. S., Olshan, A. M., et al. Comparison of the antimicrobial capability of an abrasive paste and chemical-soak denture cleansers. Journal of Prosthetic Dentistry 60:467, 1988.
36. Massler, M. Nutrition and the denture-bearing tissues. In Winkler, S. (ed.). Essentials of Complete Denture Prosthodontics, 2nd ed. Littleton, MA: PSG Pub. Co., 1987, pp. 15–21.

Suggested Readings

Baum, B. J. Evaluation of stimulated parotid saliva flow rate in different age groups. Journal of Dental Research 60:1292, 1981.

Ring, T. Healthcare reform: A national dilemma. Access 6:10, 1992.

28 Dental Hygiene Care for the Individual with Osseointegrated Dental Implants

OBJECTIVES

Mastery of the content in this chapter will enable the reader to:

- Define the key terms related to dental implants
- Define the basic components of a dental implant
- Define the various types of dental implants and explain the rationale for each
- List the materials for each type of implant
- List the criteria necessary for the success of osseointegration
- Discuss the general indications for use of dental implants
- Discuss the contraindications for dental implants
- Discuss the benefits of dental implants
- Discuss the potential complications associated with dental implants
- Describe periimplantitis and related dental hygiene interventions
- List the armamentarium for providing professional dental hygiene care for dental implant clients
- Describe the sterilization procedure for plastic scalers used with dental implants
- List the oral hygiene aids for dental implants and discuss the application of each in the oral hygiene care of clients with dental implants
- Discuss motivational strategies that can be used by the dental hygienist to encourage client adherence to a daily home care plan.
- Develop an oral hygiene care plan for a client based on the type of dental implant and the client's personal preferences and oral hygiene behaviors
- Describe the dental hygiene process of care for clients with dental implants

INTRODUCTION

Implant dentistry offers an alternative to clients who cannot function adequately (physically or psychosocially) with conventional dental prostheses, or who experience insufficient retention with conventional prosthetic appliances. For example, an edentulous client (Fig. 28–1) who has limited bony support for a denture (narrow or atrophic alveolar ridge) is a potential candidate for dental implants. Studies have shown that clients who wear dentures chew at only 25% of efficiency as compared to individuals with natural teeth. With implants, chewing efficiency rises to 96%.[1] In addition, implants can be beneficial to those who have lost a single tooth or just a few teeth, making it possible for clients to avoid wearing a removable partial appliance as well as a full denture. Implants provide a comfortable, functional, and attractive system and stable replacement of natural teeth for the right candidate.

"Natural tooth function" is the term used to describe the secure feeling of having a stable foundation upon which to bite, chew, and grind. Tooth loss attributed to periodontal diseases, dental caries, or trauma prevent many individuals from proceeding with natural tooth function. Although conventional restorative and prosthetic dental care assists clients in adapting to their lost dentition through fixed and removable dental prosthetic appliances, osseointegrated dental implants clearly provide some clients with a chance to regain their natural tooth function.[1]

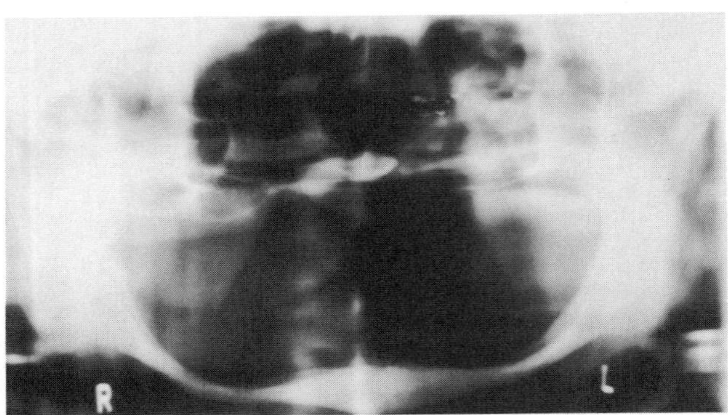

FIGURE 28-1
Radiograph of a very atrophic mandible. (Courtesy of A. K. Lakha.)

Personal and professional oral hygiene care is vital to the success of dental implants and provides an opportunity for collaboration between dentists and dental hygienists. The dentist and dental hygienist, each with certain roles and expertise, work as co-therapists with the client to achieve the common goal of providing natural tooth function for the client. The dentist evaluates clients and meets their reconstructive needs; the dental hygienist uses the dental hygiene process to identify human needs deficits related to the maintenance of the mucous membrane integrity of the periimplant tissues. Some human needs that are particularly relevant to the client who chooses dental implants include the need for:

- Wholesome body image
- Skin and mucous membrane integrity of the head and neck
- Nutrition
- Conceptualization and problem solving
- Appreciation and respect
- Self-determination and responsibility

This chapter describes the various types of osseointegrated dental implants, the implant process, and the principles associated with the dental hygiene process of care for clients with dental implants.

OSSEOINTEGRATED DENTAL IMPLANTS

An osseointegrated **dental implant** is a stable functional replacement for one or more missing teeth that consists of an anchor, an abutment, and a prosthetic tooth or appliance (Fig. 28-2). The anchor is a metal device that is inserted within the bone tissues of the mandibular or the maxillary arch. The metal is frequently coated with a synthetic material that acts as a biocompatible interface to enhance bone formation. **Titanium** is the preferred metal for an implant anchor because of its biocompatibility with bone tissues. Other metals consist of vitallium, cobalt alloys, ceramic, aluminum, and vanadium. After the implant anchor is inserted, healing requires approximately 4 to 6 months in the maxilla and 3 to 6 months in the mandible. During the healing period, the edentulous client uses a relined denture until the abutments are attached to the implant anchors.

The surgical insertion of the **abutments** involves exposing the underlying implant anchor and attaching the abutment to the implant anchors by a center screw. The abutment acts as a connection between the implant anchor and the prosthetic appliance. The gingival tissue around the abutment needs approximately 3 weeks to heal in the maxilla and 1 week in the mandible. Oral hygiene and bacterial plaque control must be reinforced at this time for proper healing. With poor oral hygiene and an increased amount of bacterial plaque present, the periimplant tissue may be susceptible to inflammation and infection **(periimplantitis).**

The prosthetic tooth or appliance is fabricated by the dentist or prosthodontist and is the final attachment. The prosthetic appliance can consist of a crown, a bridge, or a denture and is placed following the healing period of the abutment insertion, which takes a few weeks.

Although there are various types of implants, the three most common are subperiosteal, transosteal (transosseous), and endosteal (endosseous) implants (Table 28-1). The American Dental Association (ADA) considers the subperiosteal and endosteal implants to be the safest and most effective.[2]

Subperiosteal Implant

The **subperiosteal** implant (Fig. 28-3) consists of a titanium metal framework made by surgically separating the alveolar tissue and exposing the edentulous ridge and taking an impression of the ridge. The client is placed under general anesthesia. The alveolar tissue is sutured, a study model is made, and the laboratory technician casts a framework to the model of the bone. After the titanium framework has been fabricated from the impression of the jawbone, the gingival tissue is surgically reexposed and the framework is placed on top of the bone and under the periosteum. The gingival tissue heals over the framework. The implant does not osseointegrate to the bone, but affixes itself to the bone by a fibroosseous connective tissue. Posts connected to the metal framework protrude through the gingiva to hold a fixed or removable crown, bridge, or denture. Other examples of a subperiosteal implant are shown in Figures 28-4 through 28-6.

The subperiosteal implant is indicated when the width and depth of the alveolar bone are narrow or when the alveolar ridge is atrophic. Subperiosteal implants may fail because of a poorly designed prosthetic appliance or an infection that begins at an abutment site and travels throughout the implant framework.

Transosteal Implant

The **transosteal** implant (staple implant) also consists of a titanium metal framework and is placed by the dental specialist through the chin and into the mandible while the client is under general anesthesia. Because the design of the transosteal implant is strictly for placement in the mandible, it cannot be placed in the maxilla. The design of this framework, shown in Figures 28-7 and 28-8, differs from the subperiosteal framework in that the transosteal implant is placed through the lower portion of the jaw and the subperiosteal implant is placed on the alveolar ridge after the gingival tissue has been separated and exposed by flap surgery. Transosteal implants are most commonly placed when a client with a narrow mandible needs strength and

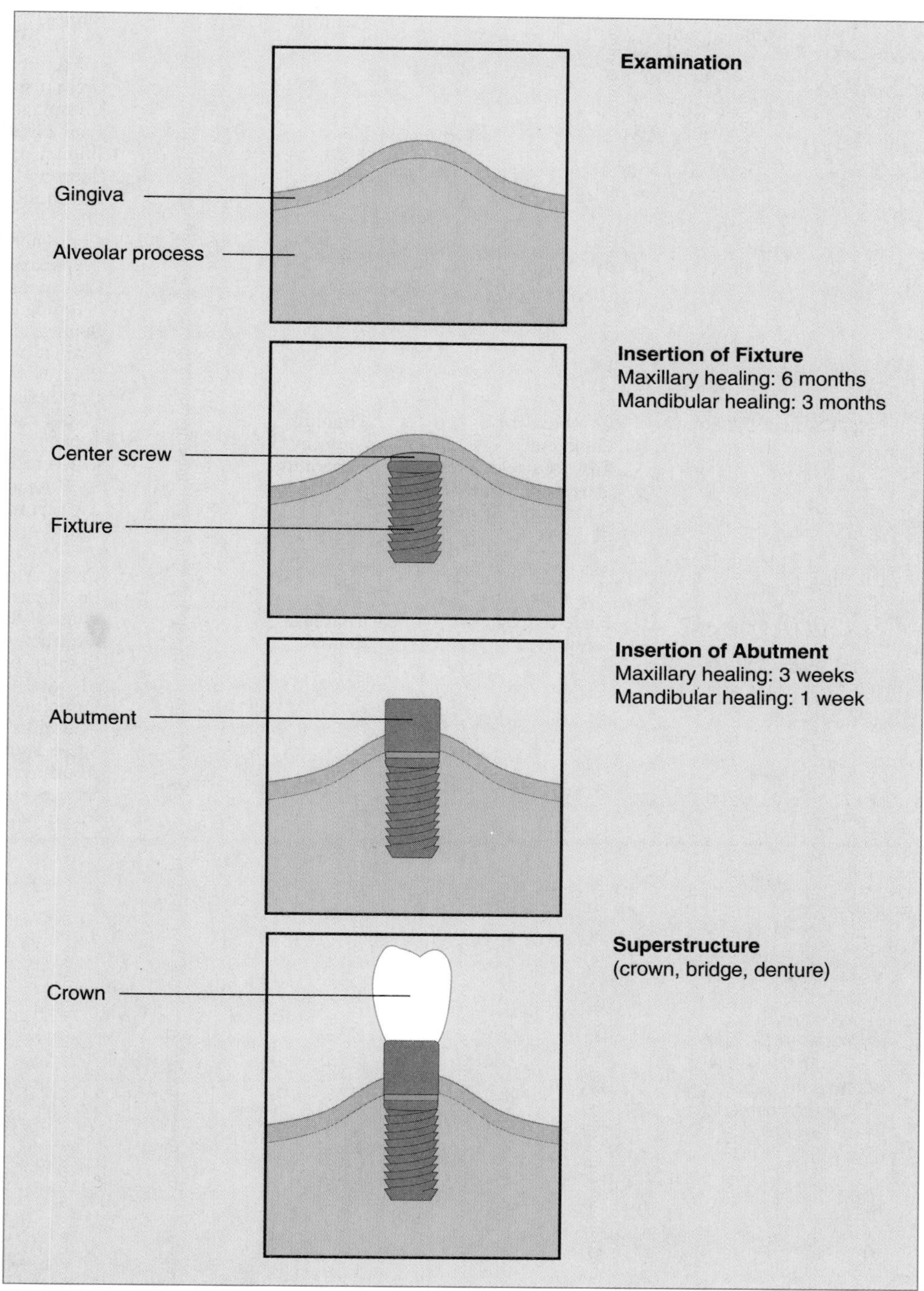

FIGURE 28–2
Sequence of treatment with osseointegrated dental implants.

TABLE 28–1
DENTAL IMPLANTS AND THEIR CHARACTERISTICS

Implant	Location	Types	Material	Description of the Implant Process
Subperiosteal (See Figs. 28–3 to 28–6)	"On top of the bone"	Mandibular Staple bone plate	Cobalt-chromium Molybdenum (Vitallium) Titanium	Surgical flap to expose bone Impression of bone taken Suture Cast metallic unit made from impression Second surgical flap to place implants Four posts into bone Framework in place Suture Prosthesis placed OR Computer tomography scan approximate casts Cast metallic unit from tomography Surgical flap made Framework in place Suture Prosthesis placed
Transosteal (transosseous) (See Figs. 28–7 to 28–9)	"Through the bone"	Complete arch Unilateral Cast framework rests over the bone of the mandible or maxilla	Titanium Aluminum Vanadium	Five- to seven-pin metal plate Fitted to the inferior border of mandible Two terminal pins protrude into oral cavity to hold overdenture Crossbar placed Prosthesis placed
Endosteal (endosseous) (See Figs. 28–10 to 28–14)	"Within the bone"	Blade-shaped Screw type	Titanium Ceramic	Surgical flap Drill hole in bone Body or fixture placed Mucosal tissue sutured Osseointegrate in 3–6 months Second surgical flap Abutment or neck placed Suture Prosthesis placed

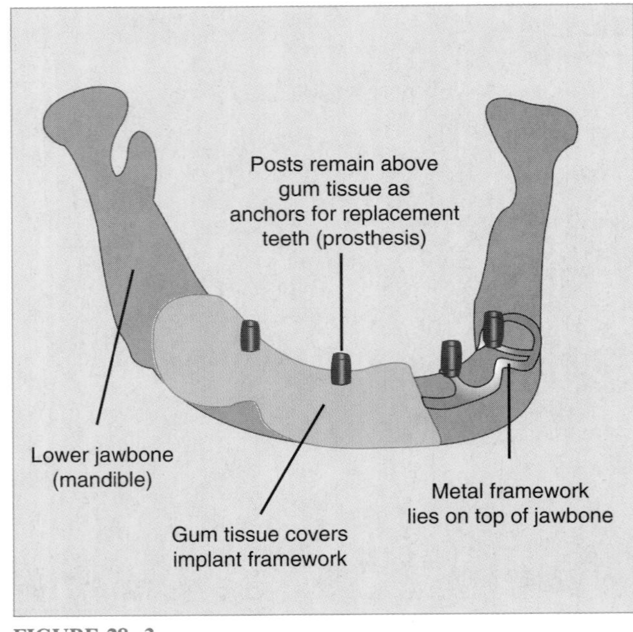

FIGURE 28–3
Subperiosteal implant.

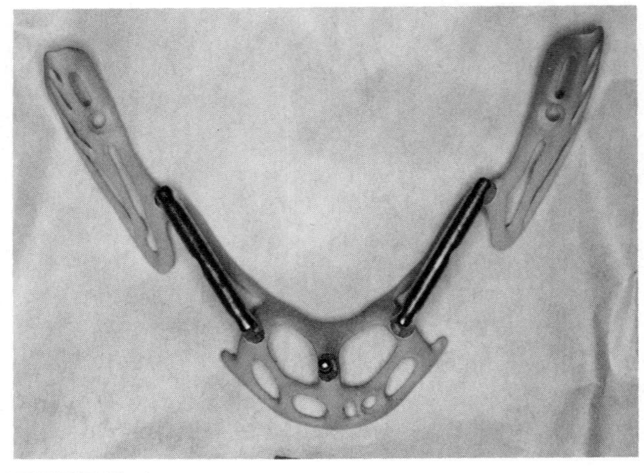

FIGURE 28–4
Calcitek subperiosteal implant. (Courtesy of M. A. Conover.)

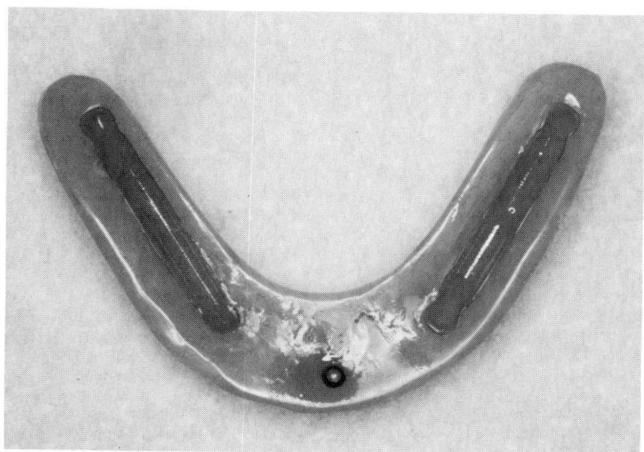

FIGURE 28-5
Overdenture used with a subperiosteal implant. (Courtesy of M. A. Conover.)

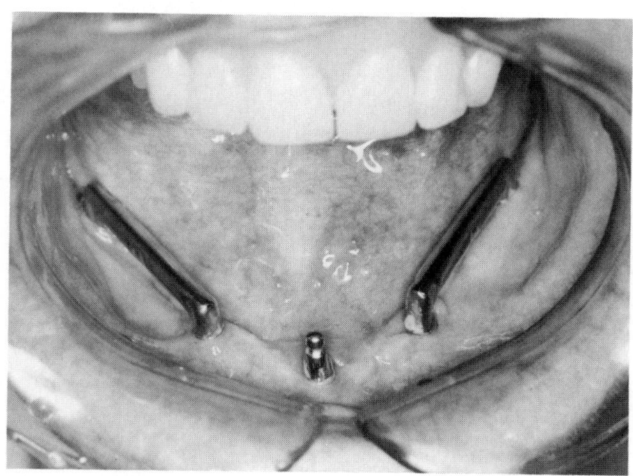

FIGURE 28-6
Client with the subperiosteal implant surgically placed. (Courtesy of M. A. Conover.)

support for chewing, biting, or grinding. A client who cannot tolerate conventional lower dentures because of severe bone resorption (Fig. 28-9) needs a transosteal implant. An extraoral 5-cm incision is made through the anterior portion of the mandible to place this implant; it should be noted that no other implant requires this incision. A high-speed drill is used to make holes through the mandible. The transosteal implant consists of a plate and five or seven parallel dowels. Once the holes are made, the implant is tapped and screwed into the mandible. The dowels that protrude through the mandible act as the abutments for the prosthetic appliance that sits on top of the transosteal implant. Compared to other surgical techniques, the surgical placement of the transosteal implant has an increased probability of infection, which can lead to implant failure. For this reason, transosteal implants are rarely used.

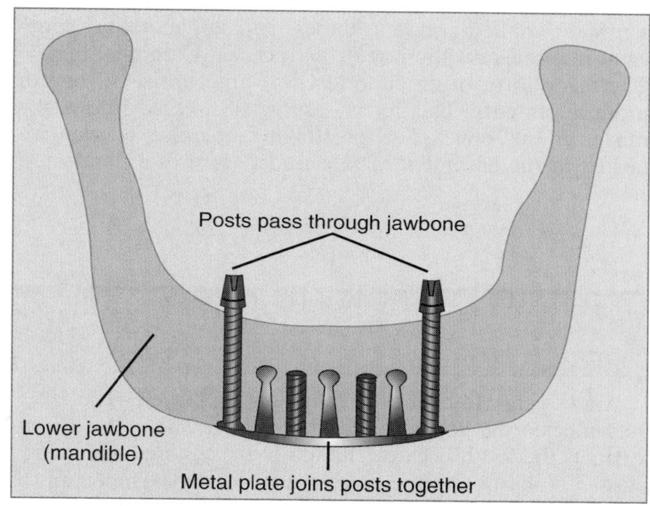

FIGURE 28-7
Transosteal implant.

Endosteal Implant

There are two forms of the **endosteal** implant:

- Blade form
- Cylinder form

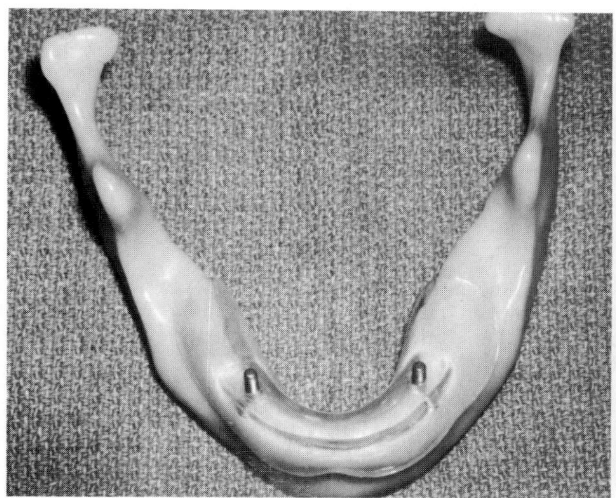

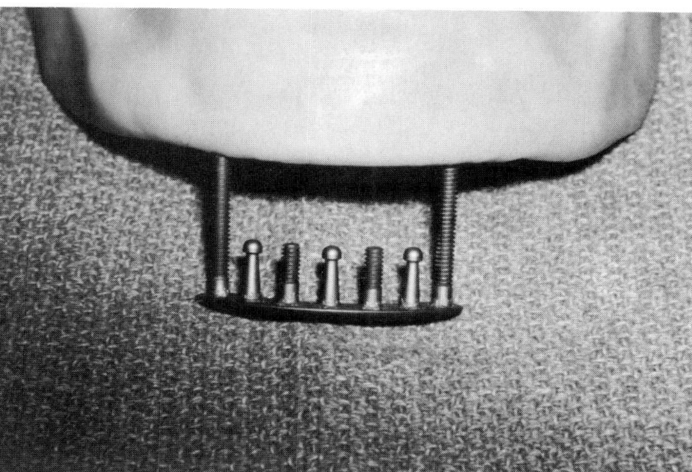

FIGURE 28-8
Hall transosteal implant with guided stent. (Courtesy of M. J. McDonald.)

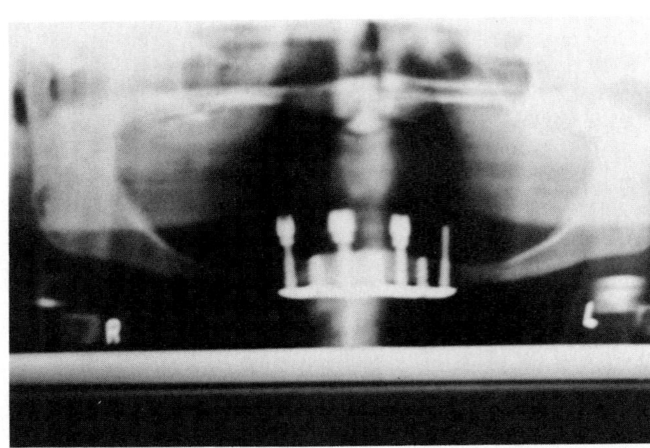

FIGURE 28-9
Radiographic example of transosteal implant surgically placed. (Courtesy of M. J. McDonald.)

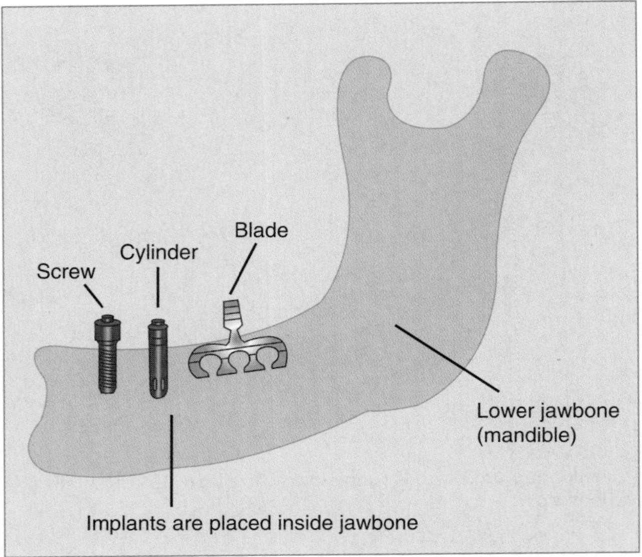

FIGURE 28-10
Endosteal implant.

The cylinder form of an endosteal implant consists of a screw, a small titanium cylinder, and an abutment surgically inserted into the bone[3] that acts as a "root system."[3] The blade form of an endosteal implant consists of one or more abutments. This form is surgically placed into a slot made in the bone. The prosthetic appliance is then attached to the abutment. The cylinder form of an endosteal implant is the most widely used implant. This type of implant has been very successful and has provided increased efficiency and improved aesthetic result. An example of an endosteal implant is shown in Figure 28-10.

CASE STUDY. A SINGLE IMPLANT WITH A FIXED PROSTHETIC TOOTH

An 18-year-old client has fallen on his bicycle. The fall has affected the upper left central incisor. The oral surgeon extracts the tooth because the tooth is diagnosed as having class 3 mobility and the gingival tissue has developed an infection with exudate. After the client's condition is assessed, dental treatment is planned for one implant in this area. The anchor is surgically inserted by the oral surgeon. The restorative dentist or prosthodontist fabricates a crown to match the natural tooth that the client lost, and the fixed prosthetic tooth is secured to the top of the single implant (Fig. 28-11). This type of implant can be removed only by the dentist.

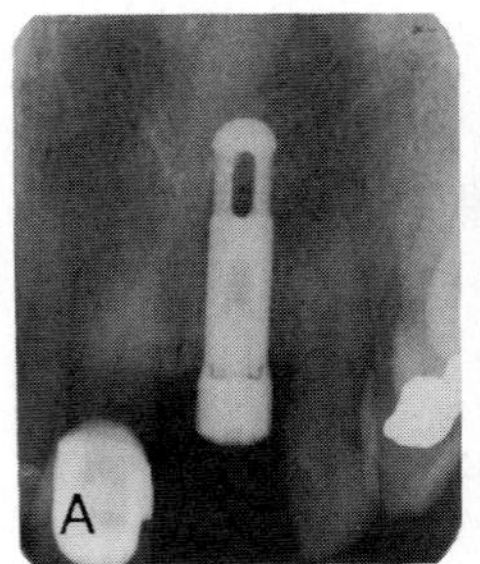

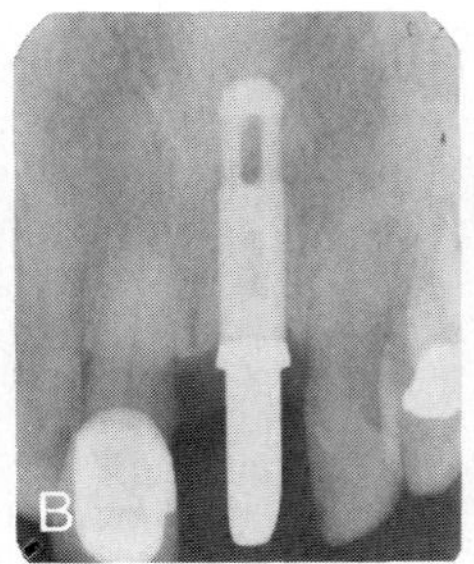

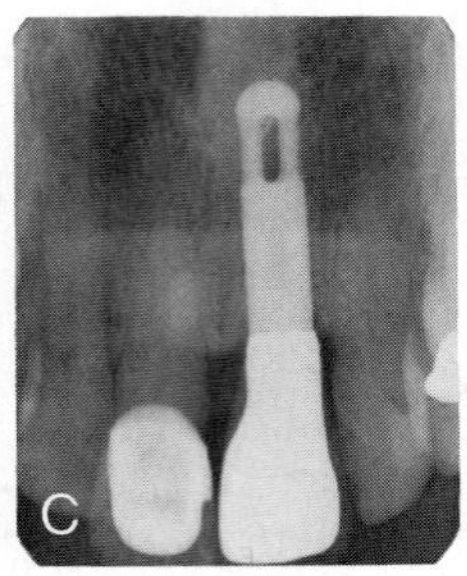

FIGURE 28-11
Radiographs of a single fixed dental implant. *A*, Dental implant placed with healing cap. *B*, Dental implant with abutment. *C*, Dental implant with fixed restorative crown. (Courtesy of K. Larsan.)

TABLE 28–2
MOBILITY INDEX FOR FREE-STANDING ENDOSTEAL IMPLANTS AND ATTACHED PROSTHESES

Use of two single-ended metal instruments to determine mobility
Rock the implant to test horizontal mobility
Test vertical mobility by applying pressure occlusally

Grade	Clinical Impression
0	No mobility
1	Slight buccolingual mobility, <0.5 mm
2	Slight buccolingual mobility, >0.5 mm but <1.0 mm
3	Mobility >0.5 mm in buccolingual and mesiodistal directions
4	Depressible, salivary percolation (bubbling around implant)

With permission from Koth, D., McKinney, R. V., Jr., and Steflik, D. Clinical Dentistry: Evaluation of the Implant-Gingival Tissue Interface. Hagerstown, MD: Harper & Row, 1984, p. 121.

CASE STUDY. A CLIP AND HADER-BAR IMPLANT WITH A REMOVABLE PROSTHETIC APPLIANCE OR DENTURE

A 70-year-old client has developed severe periodontal disease. Her facial contours have collapsed from extensive bone resorption. The general dentist and dental hygienist have discussed the diagnosis and care options with the client and have referred her to an oral surgeon for extraction of all remaining teeth. In consultation with the client, the general dentist and oral surgeon plan treatment to include a full removable upper denture and a lower endosteal implant system. The endosteal implant will consist of a two-implant system with a Hader-bar between the implants and a full lower removable denture with a clip to hold it in place (Fig. 28–12). With this dental implant approach, the client can readily remove the full lower denture. The client's ability to remove the prosthetic appliance promotes long-term success of the implant by allowing daily access to the bacterial plaque accumulation and debris. The maxillary removable prosthetic appliance adds rounded facial contours and alleviates deep furrows.

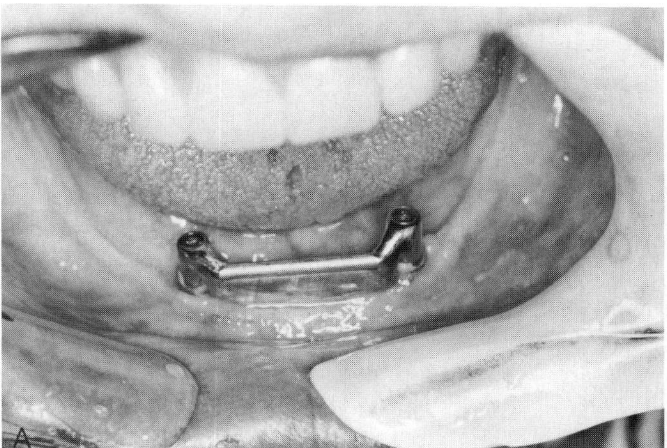

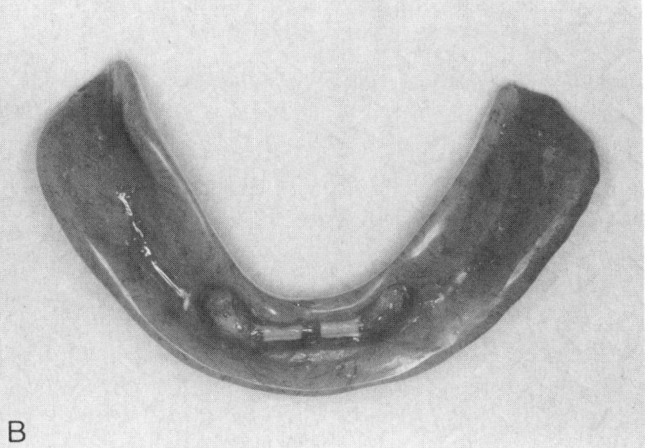

FIGURE 28–12
Crossbar endosteal implant and a clip-on type of overdenture. (Courtesy of M. A. Conover.)

CASE STUDY. A BALL, CROSSBAR, AND SOCKET IMPLANT WITH A REMOVABLE PROSTHETIC APPLIANCE

This cylinder form of implant system is similar in function to that of the clip and Hader-bar implant with a removable prosthetic appliance described above. The design, however, is different in that a ball is on the implant abutment and the socket is within the prosthetic appliance (Fig. 28–13).

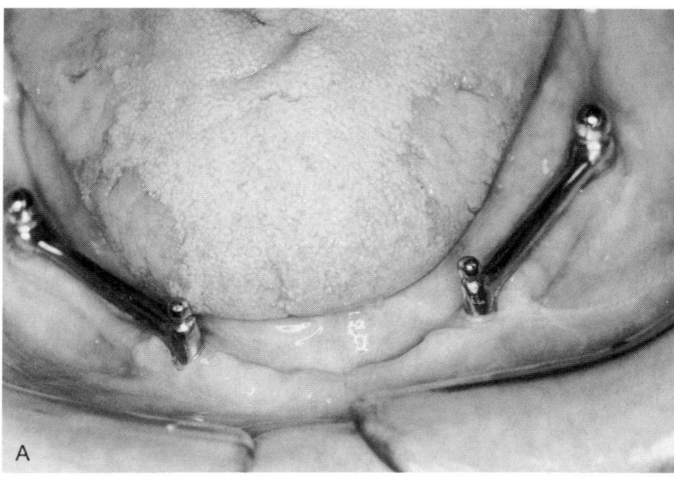

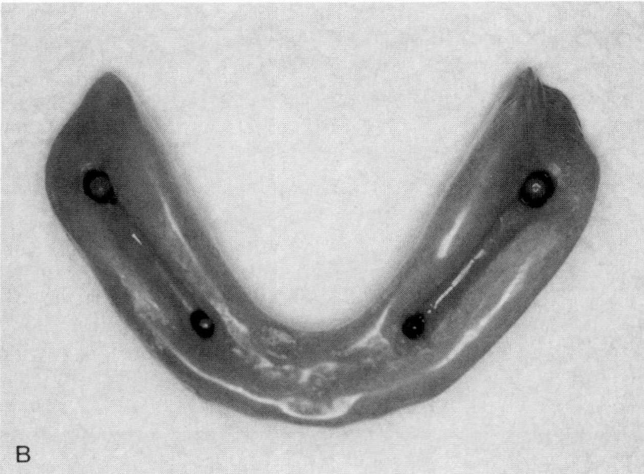

FIGURE 28–13
Ball and crossbar endosteal implant and the socket-type overdenture. (Courtesy of M. A. Conover.)

CASE STUDY. A TWO-IMPLANT SYSTEM COMBINED WITH A TWO-UNIT CROWN RESTORATION AND A CANTILEVER BRIDGE

A client developed a benign tumor within the lower right portion of the mandible. The oral surgeon extracted two molars, removed the tumor, and inserted synthetic bone in place of the tumor to promote bone growth. A few months later, two implants were placed in the mandibular right premolar area. The oral surgeon is hesitant to place another implant in the mandibular right molar region for fear of disturbing the inferior alveolar nerve. Therefore, a two-unit crown restoration with a cantilever bridge was fabricated (Fig. 28–14). A cantilever bridge allows for an occluding surface in the posterior area without having to place a third implant.

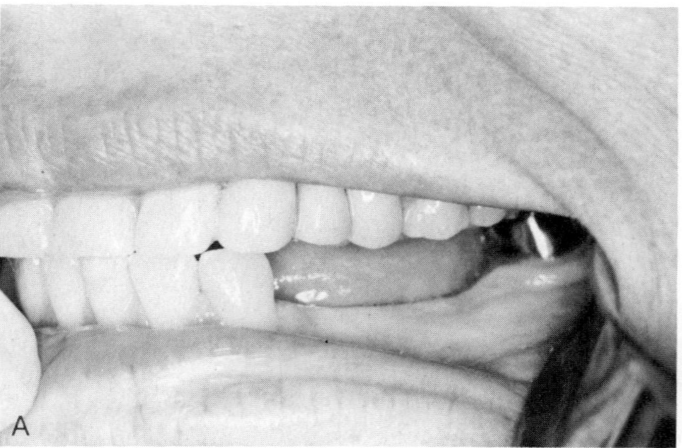

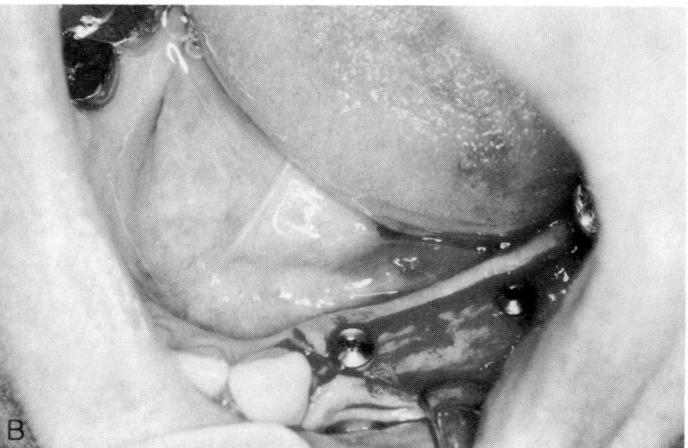

FIGURE 28–14
Partial edentulism and two endosteal implants surgically placed. (Courtesy of M. A. Conover.)

CASE STUDY. A BLADE IMPLANT SYSTEM

A 71-year-old client lost her right posterior molars and second premolar when she was in her early twenties. The bone has resorbed, leaving her with a knife-edged ridge that would not allow a cylinder form of implant. The oral surgeon places a blade form of implant and attaches a prosthetic bridge to the implant (Fig. 28–15).

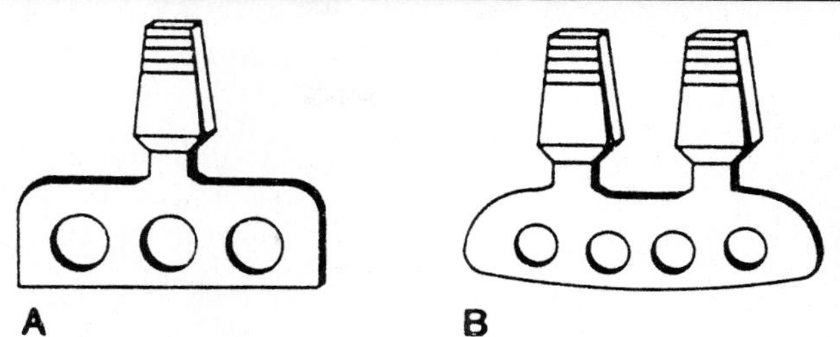

FIGURE 28–15
Blade implant. (With permission from Wilkins, E. M. Clinical Practice of the Dental Hygienist, 6th ed. Philadelphia: Lea & Febiger, 1989, p. 360.)

CASE STUDY. A FULL MAXILLARY AND MANDIBULAR FIXED PROSTHESIS

A 68-year-old client complains of an ill-fitting conventional denture that she cannot tolerate any longer. She has a strong desire for a fixed restorative implant system. The oral surgeon places a cylinder form of endosteal implant in the maxillary and mandibular arches. The fabricated prosthetic appliance **(overdenture)** is fixed to the endosteal implants. This implant system provides the client with the greatest comfort and stability. In addition, the psychological dilemma associated with removing the prosthetic appliance is eliminated. These appliances closely resemble the client's natural tooth function. However, the facial contours are difficult to reshape and rebuild. Fixed appliances also are limited to the amount of bulk and volume they can contain to reshape the facial contours ideally.

THE IMPLANT PROCESS

The implant process consists of a three-step surgical and restorative treatment plan.[3]

Step One: The First Surgical Procedure

At the first surgical appointment, the client is placed under general or local anesthesia. General anesthesia is commonly used with the placement of transosteal implants. In addition, a local anesthetic may be administered into the gingival tissue for hemostasis. A **surgical guide stent,** a clear resin device containing holes, is constructed (Fig. 28–16) to allow the oral surgeon to maintain the angulation and the axis for drilling the bone and for placement of the fixture. The dental implant anchor is placed into the drilled holes of the bone by the oral surgeon. After the surgical placement of the implants, the periosteum is sutured over the implant for a healing period. After surgery, the client experiences a sensation similar to that of having a tooth extracted.

A process called **osseointegration** (Fig. 28–17) is a biological phenomenon that occurs after surgery.[4] This process was discovered in the 1950s by a Swedish professor, Per-Ingvar Brånemark, M.D., Ph.D.[4] In osseointegration, the living bone cells directly fuse to a unique space-age metal, titanium or Vitallium, that exhibits excellent biocompatibility. The bone cells grow tightly around the metal anchor and firmly hold it in place (Fig. 28–18). The success of the dental implant is dependent on the osseointegration process, wherein the bone fuses to the implant.

Because the mandibular bone is less dense than the maxillary bone, the mandible does not require as long a healing or osseointegration period as does the maxilla. In general, dental implants placed in the mandibular bone heal and osseointegrate within 3 to 6 months, whereas the maxillary bone takes approximately 4 to 6 months to heal and osseointegrate. At the end of the first year, the osseointegration process should be stable.

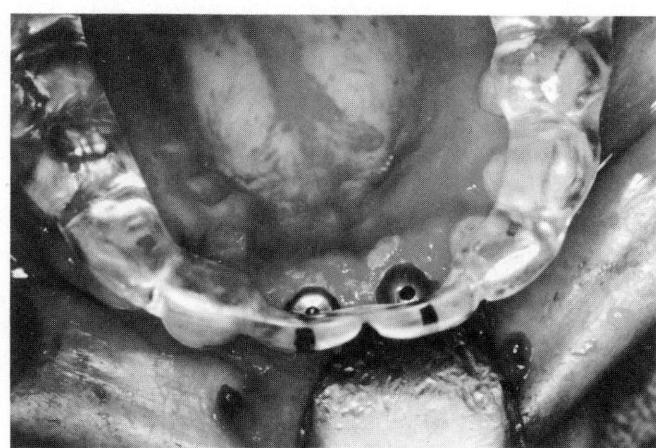

FIGURE 28–16
Surgical guide stent.

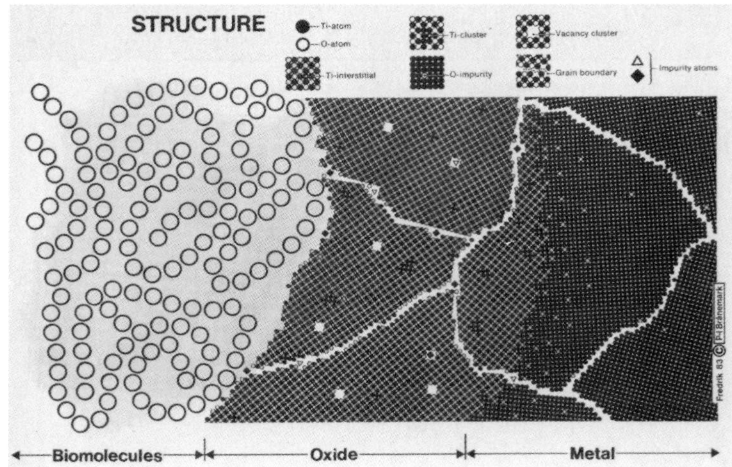

FIGURE 28–17
Diagram of bone cells directly attaching to a titanium metal. (Courtesy of Professor Per-Ingvar Brånemark, Institute for Applied Biotechnology, Gothenburg, Sweden.)

The success of osseointegration depends on the following factors:

- Quality and quantity of existing bone
- Strict asepsis during gentle surgical insertion
- Extreme precision in the dimensions and surface characteristics of the titanium anchorage units
- Adequate uninterrupted healing time of bone
- A sound **superstructure**
- A uniform "bite" once the bridgework is attached
- Daily oral hygiene care by the client (Fig. 28–19)
- Long-term clinical and radiographic follow-up (Fig. 28–20).

The Brånemark system is the only system with the acceptance of the ADA for the placement of dental implants. The ADA contends that: "The Brånemark system is acceptable for use in selected fully edentulous patients. Responsibility for proper selection of patients for adequate training and experience in the placement of the implant and for providing appropriate information for informed consent rests with the dentists." [2,4]

Step Two: The Second Surgical Procedure

After the implants have osseointegrated, as determined by radiographic appearance, a second surgery is performed. The implants are surgically uncovered at the second surgical appointment in order to place the abutments on top of the exposed implants. The implants are then surgically recovered by suturing the periosteum together with the abutments protruding through the periosteum. **Healing caps** (Fig. 28–21) are placed to allow the tissue to heal for oral hygiene access to the implant abutments and for the prosthodontist or restorative dentist to secure the prosthetic appliance in place. The healing caps are removed after 2 to 4 weeks.

Step Three: The Fabrication of Prosthetic Appliance or Restorative Crown

The third stage of the implant process begins with fabricating the prosthetic appliance. It may require several appointments to achieve a desirable fit. The prosthetic design

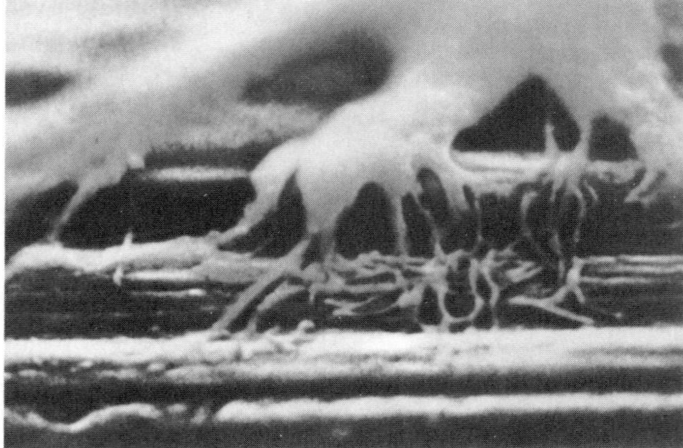

FIGURE 28–18
Bone cells fusing to a titanium implant, which is osseointegration. (Courtesy of Professor Per-Ingvar Brånemark, Institute for Applied Biotechnology, Gothenburg, Sweden.)

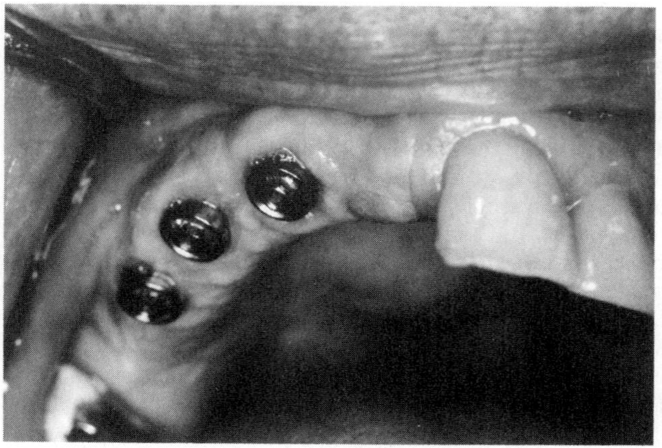

FIGURE 28–19
A result of a client who has healthy periimplant tissue and good oral hygiene compliance. (Courtesy of A. K. Lakha.)

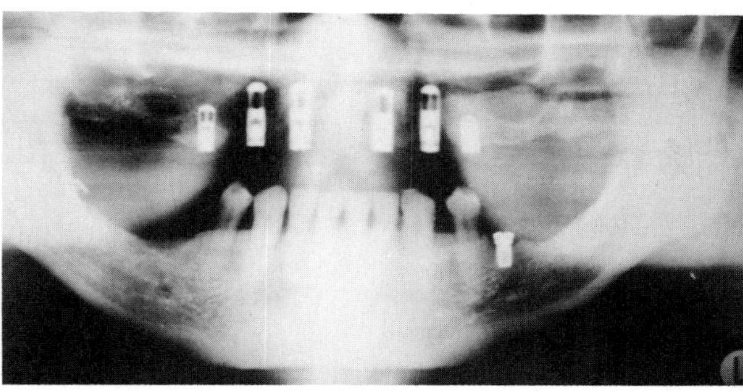
A

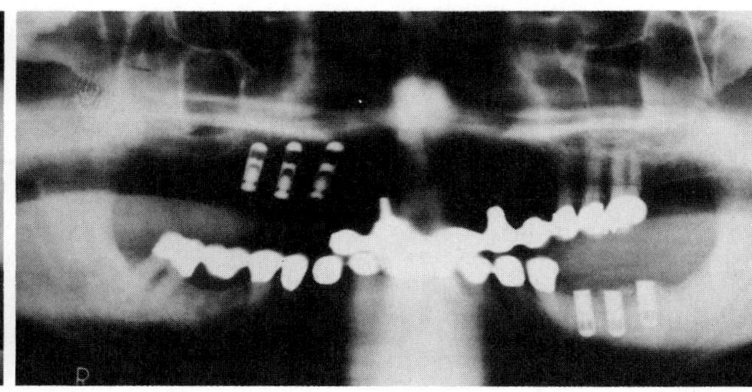
B

FIGURE 28–20
Radiographs of endosseous implants used for clinical follow-up. (Courtesy of A. K. Lakha.)

is an extremely important step. The decision to use a removable or fixed prosthetic appliance determines the exact fit of the occlusal plane and cuspal inclination. The design of the prosthetic appliance should ensure a wide interproximal space for access during daily bacterial plaque control. One to 2 weeks after the placement of the prosthetic appliance, oral hygiene education should be provided by the dental hygienist. Within a few months, the natural tooth function should be restored.

CANDIDATE SELECTION PROCESS

The dental hygienist's assessments assist the dentist in determining whether implants should be recommended for the client. A questioning system like the one below to assess systematically whether the client is a good candidate for dental implants has been shown to be beneficial.

- When you eat, do your dentures cause pain?
- Do your dentures fit adequately?
- Are your teeth mobile or displaced?
- Do you have any concerns about your dentures?
- Will you commit time to take care of your dental implants on a daily basis?
- Will you keep your appointments?
- Will you be able to wait 6 months for the final dental implant system?

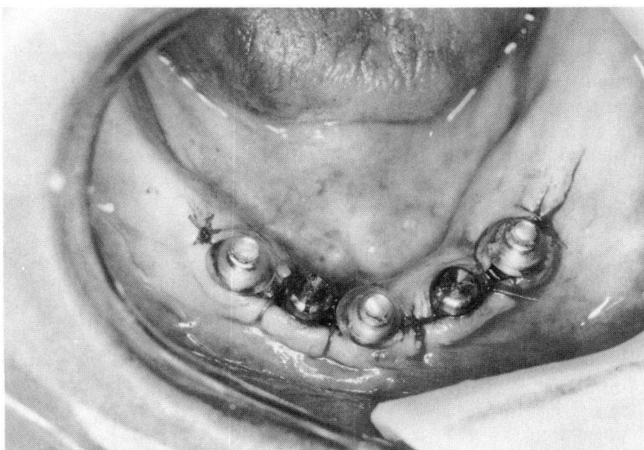

FIGURE 28–21
Endosseous implants with healing caps. (Courtesy of M. A. Conover.)

The oral healthcare team gathers information regarding pertinent health history, medications, allergies, chief complaints, missing teeth, current prosthetic appliances, radiographs, and diagnostic models. This information allows the dentist to determine which type of implant to use and a definitive care plan. Figure 28–22 depicts an oral surgery dental implant referral form used to summarize the pertinent information.

Table 28–3 lists indications and contraindications for dental implants that should be considered in identifying appropriate candidates for dental implantation. Indications and contraindications of dental implants should be discussed candidly with the client. The necessity for client compliance with oral hygiene recommendations should be emphasized and explained in detail. Many clients believe that the implant is a new tooth that will tolerate mistreatment better than a natural tooth. This myth must be dispelled, and the client must realize that the gingival tissue around the dental implant needs more mechanical oral hygiene care than the gingival tissue around a natural tooth. Many dental implant candidates have lost their natural teeth as a result of poor bacterial plaque control and periodontal disease. Therefore, these individuals may be more susceptible to failure of the dental implant. To determine a level of commitment to daily oral hygiene care, a dental hygienist should also evaluate the client's value system regarding oral health by asking questions about how he feels about his mouth and his oral health behaviors. A motivated client with a good level of manual dexterity is an important requirement in a candidate for dental implants because compliance with oral hygiene recommendations is critical to the health of the implant tissues. In fact, a willingness to perform daily bacterial plaque control is a criterion that separates a good implant candidate from a poor one.

If the client has one or more chronic contraindications, the oral health team may want to consider another mode of treatment. Once contraindications are resolved, the client can be reevaluated for implants.

BENEFITS AND RISKS

The benefits and risks should be thoroughly explained verbally and in writing to clients who show interest in dental implants. Table 28–4 summarizes these benefits and risks.

DENTAL IMPLANT REFERRAL FORM

Date: ______________________________

Client: ______________________________ Phone: ______________

Referring Doctor: ______________________________

Client's Chief Complaint:

- ☐ Difficulty in eating
- ☐ Functional difficulty
- ☐ Aesthetics
- ☐ Prosthetic discomfort
- ☐ Facial image
- ☐ Other ______________________________

Dental Treatment Plan:

Partially Edentulous

- ☐ Single tooth replacement
- ☐ Implant bridge to natural teeth
- ☐ Totally fixed implant bridge

Totally Edentulous

- ☐ Full arch fixed prosthesis
- ☐ Hader bar, clip removable prosthesis
- ☐ Ball and socket removable prosthesis

Alternative Treatment: ______________________________

Diagnostic Records:

- ☐ Periapical radiographs/full mouth series
- ☐ Panorex
- ☐ CT scan
- ☐ Tomograph
- ☐ Study models

FIGURE 28–22
Dental implant referral form.

TABLE 28–3
INDICATIONS AND CONTRAINDICATIONS FOR USING DENTAL IMPLANTS

Indications	Contraindications
Good general physical and mental health to facilitate client acceptance of the dental implant	Blood dyscrasias (prevent proper healing and clotting)
A commitment to a daily bacterial plaque control regimen to avoid periimplantitis	Certain cardiovascular diseases
Manual dexterity to ensure that bacterial plaque control procedures can be performed effectively on a daily basis	Chronic renal diseases
A sufficient quantity and quality of alveolar bone to retain the dental implant	Corticosteroidal use
Continuous cooperation and communication between client and oral healthcare team	Debilitating or uncontrollable disease or compromised healing conditions such as that resulting from radiation therapy
	Diabetic clients susceptible to gingival and periodontal disease
	Hypersensitivity of tissues to specific implant materials
	Metabolic diseases
	Psychiatric disorders
	Rheumatoid disease
	Inadequate client motivation
	Inability of client to maintain optimal daily hygiene care
	Local gingival infection
	Noncorrectable heavy grinding or bruxing problem
	Pregnant client
	Systemic infection
	Unattainable prosthetic reconstruction
	Unrealistic expectations of the client

TABLE 28–4
BENEFITS AND RISKS OF DENTAL IMPLANTS

Benefits	Risks
The improved ability to masticate and speak adequately	Failure to osseointegrate (See Fig. 28–20)
Enhanced client's self-confidence and esteem due to improved aesthetics and function	Improper client selection
Decreased amount of bone resorption	Improper control of immediate stress or load force
Decreased tissue ulceration and unnecessary pressure	Improper oral hygiene care (See Fig. 28–21)
Elimination of direct force on the gingival tissue and alveolar crest	Inadequate allowance of healing time and interface development
Increased retention of the prosthetic appliance	Inadequate control of manufacture quality
Preservation of the remaining bone structure	Inadequate implant or prosthetic design
	Periimplantitis (See Fig. 28–22)
	Surgical complications

Benefits

Dental implants allow clients to chew food properly, facilitating essential digestive processes. In addition, clients with dental implants report that they enjoy their food more; their speech is improved; and their comfort, appearance, self-confidence, and self-esteem are increased compared to their previous condition. Other benefits include decreased bone resorption, tissue ulceration, and pressure; elimination of direct force on the gingival tissue and alveolar crest; increased retention of the prosthetic appliance; and preservation of the remaining bone structure. Findings from studies of more than 4,000 implant placements show an overall success rate of 96% over a 20-year period. If clients show interest in dental implants, knowledge of the benefits associated with implant reconstruction can assist them in determining whether they want dental implants placed.

Risks

There are few risks involved with placing dental implants. However, an implant may fail because of a **dehiscence** (a hole in the buccal or labial plate of the alveolar process caused by placing an implant in an area of insufficient bone) or periimplantitis resulting from inadequate personal or professional oral hygiene care, or the inability of the body to accept the space-age metal of the implant. Dental implants might also fail because of failure to osseointegrate, improper client selection, improper control of immediate stress or **load** force exerted on the implant, inadequate allowance of healing time and interface development, inadequate control of manufacturing quality of the dental implant, inadequate prosthetic design, and surgical complications. The dental hygienist should explain potential risks to the client so that the client can make an informed decision about dental implants or other treatment options.

DOCUMENTATION AND INFORMED CONSENT

The dentist must inform the dental implant candidate of the treatment plan, the specific time requirements to complete the plan, the specific dental hygiene regimen required, and the benefits and risks of having dental implants. To educate the client regarding the lifestyle changes associated with dental implants, the dental hygienist makes use of study models, photographs, pamphlets, and radiographs as needed. After relevant information is received and understood by the client, an informed consent document should be signed and dated by the client and clinicians involved (Fig. 28–23). After the placement of the implants, the person should be given a card to keep in his wallet to identify

DENTAL IMPLANT CONSENT

Acknowledgement of Receipt of Information

State law requires that you be given certain information and that we obtain your consent prior to beginning any treatment. What you are being asked to sign is a confirmation that we have discussed the nature and purpose of the treatment, the known risks associated with the treatment, and the feasible treatment alternatives; that you have been given an opportunity to ask questions; that all your questions have been answered in a satisfactory manner. Please read this form carefully before signing it and ask about anything that you do not understand. We will be pleased to explain.

Consent for Dental Implant

I hereby authorize and direct the oral and maxillofacial surgeon whose name appears below with associates or assistants of his choice to perform surgery upon me (or upon the person identified below as the patient, for whom I am empowered to consent) to insert dental implant(s) in my upper and/or lower jaw.

Nature and Purpose of the Procedure

I understand incision(s) will be made inside my mouth for the purpose of placing one or more metal structures in my jaw(s) to serve as anchor(s) for a missing tooth or teeth or to stabilize a crown (cap), denture, or bridge. I acknowledge that the oral and maxillofacial surgeon whose name appears below has explained the procedure, including the number and location of the incisions to be made, in detail. I understand that the crown (cap), denture, or bridge will later be attached to this implant by a general dentist or prosthodontist and that the cost for that work is not included in the charge for this procedure. I also understand that this implant should last for many years, but that no guarantee that it will last for any specific period of time can be or has been given. I have been informed that the implant must remain covered under the gum tissue for at least three months before it can be used and that a second surgical procedure is required to uncover the top of the implant. Finally, I understand that this is a relatively new procedure. I have received literature, anesthesia information, pre and post surgical instructions and diet information and have read and understand the information.

FIGURE 28–23
Consent form for dental implant. (Courtesy of Richard Smith, D.D.S., UCSF Oral and Maxillofacial Surgery Clinic.) *(Figure continues on following page.)*

Alternatives to a Dental Implant

The alternatives to the use of a dental implant, including no treatment at all; construction of a new standard dental prosthesis; augmentation of the upper or lower jaw by means of a vestibuloplasty, skin and bone grafting, or with synthetic materials; and implantation of another type of device have been explained to me as have the advantages and disadvantages of each procedure and I choose to proceed with insertion of the dental implant.

Authorization of Ancillary Treatment

I also authorize and direct the oral and maxillofacial surgeon whose name appears below with associate or assistants of his choice to provide such additional services as he or they may deem reasonable and necessary, including, but not limited to, the administration of anesthetic agents; the performance of necessary laboratory, radiological (x-ray), and other diagnostic procedures; the administration of medications orally, by injection, by infusion, or by other medically accepted route of administration; and the removal of bone, tissue and fluids for diagnostic and therapeutic purposes and the retention or disposal of same in accordance with usual practices.

Authorization for Supplemental Treatment

If any unforeseen condition arises in the course of treatment which calls for the performance of procedures in addition to or different from that now contemplated and I am under general anesthesia or sedation, I further authorize and direct the oral and maxillofacial surgeon whose name appears below with associates or assistants of his choice to do whatever he deems necessary and advisable under the circumstances.

No Guarantee of Treatment Results

I understand that there is no way to accurately predict the bone healing capabilities of any particular patient following the placement of the implant and that complications do occur; and I confirm that I have been given no guarantee or assurance by the oral and maxillofacial surgeon whose name appears below, or by anyone else, as to the results that may be obtained from treatment.

Risks and Complications Associated with Dental Implants

I have been informed and understand there are risks and complications from surgery, drugs and/or anesthetics.

Surgical Complications

Surgical incisions performed outside the mouth leave a scar on the skin, and although a good cosmetic result is hoped for, it cannot be guaranteed. Other surgical complications include but are not limited to, infection, tissue discoloration (bruising), alteration in taste and/or numbness, tingling, increased sensitivity of the lips, tongue, chin, cheek or teeth which may last for an indefinite period and may be permanent. Also possible are injury to teeth if present, loss of bone, bone fractures, nasal or sinus penetration, chronic pain, bleeding and decreased ability to open the mouth. I have also been informed that any procedure which is performed outside the mouth will leave a scar on the skin, and that although a good cosmetic result is hoped for, it cannot be guaranteed.

I also understand that any of these treatment complications may necessitate additional medical, dental, or surgical treatment; may necessitate wiring of my teeth or jaws; and may require an additional period of recuperation at home or even in the hospital. Finally, I have been told that this treatment may not be successful, that problems may arise during the procedure which may prevent placement of the implant, and that rejection of this implant is possible which would necessitate its removal at any time after placement. Should this happen, I understand that it may be possible to insert another implant after a suitable healing period.

Drug and Anesthetic Complications

There may be irritation of, or damage to, the vein in which anesthetic medications are injected. I understand there are certain drugs and anesthetic risks, which could involve serious bodily injury, and are inherent in any procedure requiring their use.

Risks Associated with No Treatment

I understand that should I NOT have this implant procedure, one or more of the following *may* occur: faster dissolving of the jaw bone structure, increased difficulty wearing conventional dentures, increased loss of bony support of the face, lips and cheeks, increased difficulty chewing, pain and numbness, and fracture of a very thin jawbone.

Importance of Patient Compliance

I agree and understand that the degree of success of any dental treatment is directly related to my cooperation and that, if I fail to cooperate as requested and instructed, I may suffer temporary or permanent injury to my dental and general health and to the dental work performed by my dentist.

FIGURE 28–23
Continued

I understand that the success of dental implants depends to a great extent on my maintenance of meticulous oral hygiene throughout my mouth and especially around the implant posts where they come through the gum tissue.

I understand that smoking, alcohol, and improper dietary practices may affect bone and gum healing and may limit the success of the implant. I agree to follow home care and dietary instructions as prescribed.

I agree to return at regular intervals as specified by the doctor for inspection of my mouth and implant cleansings by the doctor or the hygienist and to have performed such dental services as may be needed to maintain my oral health. This will involve regular and long term follow-up care for the life of the implant.

I agree to report immediately any evidence of pain, swelling or inflammation around my implant(s) and arrange to attend the clinic if necessary. A reasonable fee will be charged for these visits commencing one year after placement of my implants(s).

I agree not to eat or drink anything for 6 hours prior to my surgery/anesthesia. Medications, drugs, anesthetics and precriptions may cause drowsiness and lack of awareness and coordination, which can be increased by the use of alcohol or other drugs. Thus, I have been advised not to operate any vehicle, automobile, hazardous devices, or work while taking such medications and/or drugs; or until fully recovered from their effects. I understand and agree not to operate any vehicle or hazardous device for at least twenty-four hours after my release from surgery or until further recovered from the effects of anesthetic medication and drugs that may have been given to me in the office or hospital for my care. I agree not to drive myself home after surgery and will have a responsible adult drive me or accompany me home after my discharge from surgery.

Contingencies

If, for any reason, it is deemed that the implant is not serving properly, it is agreed that one of the following options is acceptable to me:

1. The implant(s) will be removed at no extra charge (except where the services of an anesthetist or hospital are necessary). A more conventional denture can then be constructed, or
2. the case will be redone with similar or different type implants at a reduced fee.

Fees and Financial Arrangements

The fees and financial arrangements have been explained to me and are satisfactory.

Authorization of Use of Dental Records

I authorize photographs, x-rays, or other viewing of my care and treatment during its progress may be used for educational purposes and research.

I hereby state that I have read and that I understand this consent form, that I have been given an opportunity to ask any questions I might have had, that those questions have been answered in a satisfactory manner. I also understand that I am free to withdraw my consent to treatment at any time.

Date ____________________ Time ____________________

Signature of Patient ____________________

Signature of Relative or

Representative (where required) ____________________

Witness ____________________

I certify that the matters set forth above were explained to the patient, that the patient was given an opportunity to ask questions, that all questions asked were answered in a satisfactory manner, and that all the blanks in this form were filled in prior to signature by the patient. Where this form has been signed by the patient rather than his (her) representative, I certify that, in my judgment, the patient was competent to understand the matters discussed and to give his (her) consent to treatment.

Oral and Maxillofacial Surgeon ____________________

Courtesy of UCSF Oral and Maxillofacial Surgery Clinic, Richard Smith, D.D.S.

FIGURE 28-23
Continued

Dental Implant Wallet Card
Client: Dana Lowe
Implant Date of Placement: 12-27-94
Location of Implant: #27, 22, 6, 11
Implant Manufacturer: IMZ Interpore
Registration No.: 256943
Type of Implant: Internal Hex 3.25 cylinder

Location of your dental implant may not be determined by visual inspection. This information is important and should be kept with you in case of your relocation or your decision to see a new dentist.

A

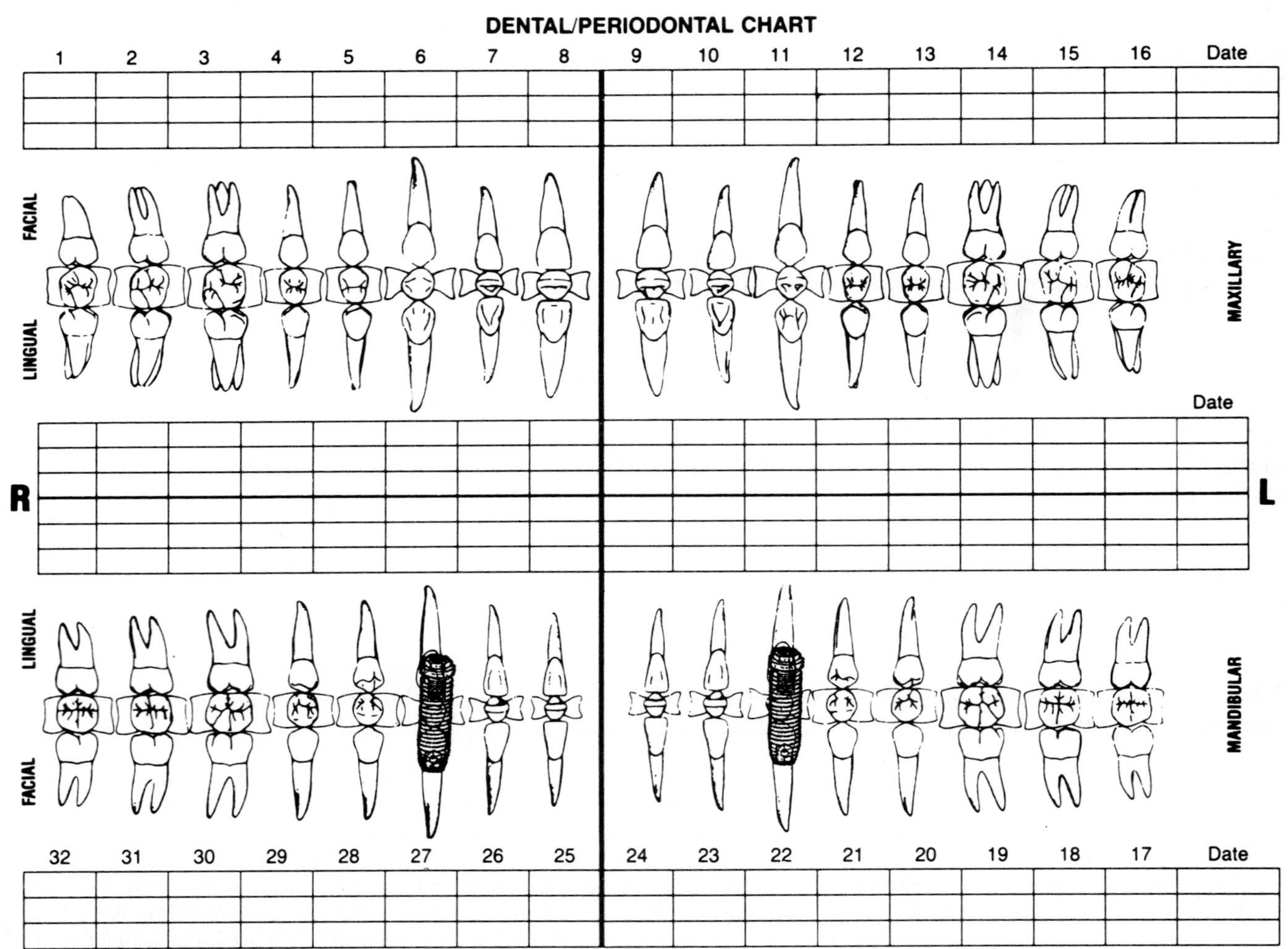

B

FIGURE 28–24
A, Dental implant wallet card. *B*, Dental implant stamp used to show location of dental implant for documentation in the client record.

NUMBER OF CHARTABLE ITEMS: ________

COMMENTS

PEDO

A B C D E F G H I J

R L

T S R Q P O N M L K

B

FIGURE 28–24
Continued

the locations, type of dental implant, and date the implant was placed (see Fig. 28–24*A*). A dental implant sticker or uniquely colored chart should be used in the client record to distinguish the dental implant client from other clients.

THE DENTAL HYGIENE PROCESS OF CARE FOR THE CLIENT WITH DENTAL IMPLANTS

Assessment

During the assessment phase of dental hygiene care, the practitioner must be able to identify and document signs and symptoms of oral problems and risk factors associated with the dental implant. Client data collected and analyzed include:

- Changes in the health history
- The location of implants using the implant stamp (Fig. 28–24B).
- The conditions of the oral mucosa
- Discomfort, pain, or infection related to the implant
- The color, texture, and overall condition of the gingival periimplant tissues, as measured by the:

  Attached periimplant tissue index (Table 28–5)
  Periimplant tissue bleeding index (Table 28–6)
  Periodontal probing depths
  Bleeding on probing
  Presence of exudate in sulci around abutments

TABLE 28–5
ATTACHED PERIIMPLANT TISSUE INDEX

Create tension by retracting lips laterally to form the mucoperiimplant tissue junction.
Use the probe to measure the external surface of the periimplant tissue and measure from the mucoperiimplant tissue line to the periimplant tissue margin to determine width

Grade	Clinical Impression
0	No keratinized epithelium
1	1 mm or less keratinized epithelium
2	2 mm or less than or equal to 2 mm and greater than 1 mm keratinized epithelium
3	Greater than 2 mm keratinized epithelium

With permission from Koth D., McKinney, R. V., Jr., and Steflik, D. Clinical Dentistry: Evaluation of the Implant-Gingival Tissue Interface. Hagerstown, MD: Harper & Row, 1984, p. 121.

TABLE 28–6
PERIIMPLANT TISSUE BLEEDING INDEX

Visual assessment and use of a plastic probe determines grade of periimplant tissue

Grade	Clinical Impression
0	No inflammation Periimplant tissue of normal color and stippling with no bleeding on probing
1	Mild inflammation Periimplant tissue with slight change in color and stippling with slight hyperemia, no bleeding upon probing
2	Moderate inflammation Periimplant tissue hyperemic with redness, edema, glazing, and loss of stippling, bleeding upon probing
3	Severe inflammation Periimplant tissue markedly red, edematous, ulcerated, and tendency toward spontaneous bleeding on finger pressure

With permission from Koth, D., McKinney, R. V., Jr., and Steflik, D. Clinical Dentistry: Evaluation of the Implant–Gingival Tissue Interface. Hagerstown, MD: Harper & Row, 1984, p. 117.

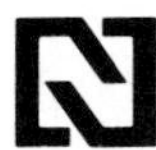

Brånemark System®
Maintenance Record

Patient Name ____________________

Chart # ____________ Referring Dr. ____________ Alternate Recalls Y / N

MEDICAL ALERT

MAINTENANCE INTERVAL

Months	Minutes
2	30
3	45
4	60
6	90

NEXT APPOINTMENT

1. ______
2. ______
3. ______
4. ______

CHARTING CODE (cc)*

B-Bleeding	M-Mobility
C-Calculus	N-Normal
D-Discharge/Suppuration	NK-Nonkeratinized
E-Edematous, Soft	P-Plaque
F-Fibrous Enlargement	R-Redness
K-Keratinized	S-Sensitivity

Special Considerations:

DATE ______
DDS√: Y / N FEE: ______

CHANGES
Medical History Y / N ______
Dental History Y / N ______
EO/IO Exam Y / N ______
Radiographs: (type)

PROCEDURES PERFORMED

Tissue Assessment Y / N
Prosthesis removed Y / N
Calculus removed Y / N
Coronal polish Y / N

HOME CARE INSTRUCTIONS

Recommended: ______

Uses: ______

Patient compliance: good / poor

Comments: ______

Signature: ______

PROBING DEPTHS (of natural teeth)

	1-8	1-7	1-6	1-5	1-4	1-3	1-2	1-1	2-1	2-2	2-3	2-4	2-5	2-6	2-7	2-8
Fa																
*cc																
Li																
*cc																

UPPER
Patient's right side upper jaw
Patient's left side upper jaw
1-1 2-1
Quadrant No 1
Quadrant No 2
1-8 2-8
4-8 3-8
Quadrant No 4
Quadrant No 3
4-1 3-1
Patient's right side lower jaw
Patient's left side lower jaw
LOWER

Designate Implant Abutment Site In Blue

	4-8	4-7	4-6	4-5	4-4	4-3	4-2	4-1	3-1	3-2	3-3	3-4	3-5	3-6	3-7	3-8
Li																
*cc																
Fa																
*cc																

FIGURE 28–25
Maintenance record. (Courtesy of Nobelpharma.)

- Amount of bacterial plaque and calculus formation as measured by disclosing solution and the plaque and calculus index (Table 28–7)
- Visualization of salivary percolation as a result of applying pressure to the crown of the implant and causing bubbles to form at the sulcus, indicating a breakdown of the biological seal
- Mobility of the bridgework as measured by the mobility index (see Table 28–2)
- Results of indicated microbiological monitoring tests
- Marginal bone height surrounding the fixture as indicated on radiographs
- Oral hygiene knowledge, beliefs, and habits

Figure 28–25 shows a sample assessment form used in establishing the client's baseline status that can be used in conjunction with the human needs assessment form found in Chapter 2.

Identification of deficits in the 11 human needs related to dental hygiene care enables the hygienist to plan and implement dental hygiene interventions and to collaborate with the dentists to prevent the possibility of implant failure and promote the likelihood of long-term success. Actual or potential problems associated with the dental implant should be documented on the appropriate form and called to the attention of the dentist.

Planning

Depending on the client's human need deficits identified during assessment, the dental hygienist, in conjunction with the client and the dentist, sets goals and develops a dental hygiene care plan. Oral health practices are influenced by client knowledge, beliefs, values, habits, lifestyles, and health needs. The dental hygienist must consider these factors when planning professional dental hygiene care and daily care for clients with dental implants.

A variety of appropriate personal oral physiotherapy aids and techniques are available for a client to use. For example, some clients may prefer to use an interdental brush rather than a gauze strip to clean the implant interproximally. Client preferences significantly affect the client's acceptance of oral health recommendations and should be incorporated into the dental hygienist's care plan. The dental hygienist must work collaboratively with the client to ensure that the proposed dental hygiene care plan is understood and accepted by the client.

If the client has a human need deficit in conceptualization and problem solving related to oral health and disease, adequate time must be allowed to explain the following concepts:

- The etiology and pathogenesis of periodontal disease and importance of bacterial plaque control in prevention of oral diseases and in maintenance of oral health
- Expectations of the client during the maintenance phase of care to sustain the health of the periimplant tissues and to prevent periodontal disease and dental caries in the existing natural dentition

TABLE 28–7
PLAQUE AND CALCULUS INDEX

Visual assessment and use of a plastic probe

Grade	Clinical Impression
0	No plaque in the periimplant tissue area The amount of plaque is determined by running a pointed plastic probe across the implant surface at the entrance of the periimplant crevice No calculus
1	A film of plaque can be removed but is not visible to the clinician; or supragingival calculus extending no more than 1 mm below the periimplant tissue margin and adjacent area of the implant The plaque may be recognized only by running a probe across the implant surface
2	Visible plaque within the periimplant crevice or on the implant and periimplant tissue margin and adjacent periimplant tissue surface; moderate accumulation of soft debris; or subgingival calculus extending more than 1 mm into the crevice or moderate amounts of supra- and subperiimplant calculus can be seen visually
3	Heavy accumulation of plaque within the crevice or on the implant surface and periimplant tissue margin and adjacent implant surface; an abundance of soft matter or heavy accumulation of supra- and subperiimplant calculus

With permission from Koth, D., McKinney, R. V., Jr., and Steflik, D. Clinical Dentistry: Evaluation of the Implant–Gingival Tissue Interface. Hagerstown, MD: Harper & Row, 1984, p. 121.

Implementation

The oral environment surrounding the dental implant consists of keratinized and nonkeratinized periimplant tissues. A biological seal is created and adapts to the titanium abutment. The microbial flora within the sulcus of a dental implant is composed of microbial flora similar to that found around a natural tooth. Bacterial plaque and dental calculus can accumulate around the abutment and the prosthetic appliance. Supragingival calculus is more common than subgingival calculus, is less tenacious than calculus around a natural tooth, and flakes off easily. The low surface energy of the titanium abutment and the attraction of proteins with low surface affinity account for this phenomenon. The metabolic end products of oral spirochetes may cause cytotoxicity to gingival tissues by producing and releasing proteolytic enzymes (that dissolve fibrin) and trypsin-like enzymes (that disrupt cell-to-cell adhesion). Periimplant inflammation (Fig. 28–26) can occur around

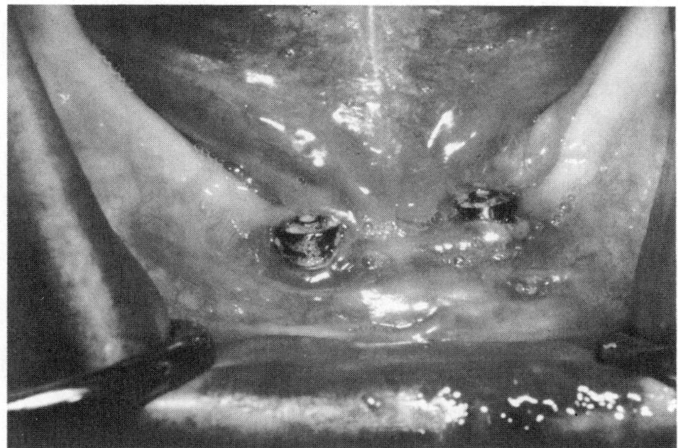

FIGURE 28–26
Example of poor oral hygiene care; note the increased amount of plaque. (Courtesy of A. K. Lakha.)

the implant abutment if plaque and calculus continue to accumulate. The marginal bone height for the implant decreases and may lead to failure or rejection of the implant. Failing endosseous dental implants may be associated with higher levels of subgingival spirochetes within the periimplant tissues. The client must perform effective daily oral hygiene home care and obtain continued professional dental hygiene care to maintain the success of the dental implant.[8]

In providing care for the client with dental implants, the main goal of the dental hygienist is to work with the client and dentist to maintain optimal gingival health and bony support of the dental implant. To accomplish this the dental hygienist instructs the client on appropriate home care aids to clean the implants daily (Table 28–8) and provides professional oral hygiene care in the oral healthcare setting at regular intervals.

Personal Oral Hygiene Care[6–9]

Daily rigorous personal oral hygiene care for the prevention of infection is critical to the health and success of the dental implant. Ongoing bacterial plaque control education should be customized based upon client preferences and

TABLE 28–8
HOME CARE AIDS FOR CLEANING DENTAL IMPLANTS

Oral Hygiene Aid	Type	Frequency	Location	Technique
Disclosing agent Intraoral mirror Pen light Face mirror	Solution, tablets Magnified	Two times per week in front of mirror under adequate light or as needed	Throughout oral cavity	Place solution on cotton swab or chew tablet Carefully paint solution on abutments Perform examination with intraoral mirror, facial mirror and pen light
Assortment of toothbrushes	Small-head soft bristles	Two to three times per day or as needed	Front and on top surfaces	General care to prosthetic appliance
End-tuft interspace toothbrush	Tapered or flat	Two to three times per day or as needed	Front and back surfaces	Carefully brush abutment cylinders Plastic handle placed under hot water can be customized by changing angulation Dipped in chlorhexidine
Rubber tip	Tapered	As needed	All surfaces	Use at gum line
Electric rotary toothbrush	Rotary	Two times per day or as needed	In between teeth, under prosthesis and around abutments	Low speed Dipped in chlorhexidine Sweeping motion
Dentifrice	Gel	Two times per day or as needed	All surfaces	Use on any oral hygiene aid
Proxabrush	Tapered or cylindrical (plastic-coated)	As needed	Between teeth	Use from front to back areas Between teeth Dipped in chlorhexidine
Superfloss	Fuzzy gauze	As needed	Around posts with limited spaced areas	Use on posts or underneath bridged areas
G-floss	Flat cotton	As needed	Around posts with limited spaced areas	
Implant flossing cord	Red—thick Green—thin	As needed	Around posts with limited spaced areas	Insert from front and thread through Slide back and forth
Cotton	Yarn 1-inch moist gauze	As needed	Under pontics or saddles	See-saw motion
Antimicrobial agents	0.12% chlorhexidine gluconate solution	Short-term use	Direct application to specific sites	Apply with cotton swab May use with any oral hygiene aid or oral irrigator
Wood	Porte polisher Wooden picks Stimudents	As needed	Any brand	Use to remove any increased amount of bacterial plaque and debris
Oral irrigators	Water-powered chemotherapeutic solution	As needed	Periimplant tissue	Use with caution; never at the implant junction Low water pressure Horizontally angled tip and flow Chemotherapeutic solution may be added

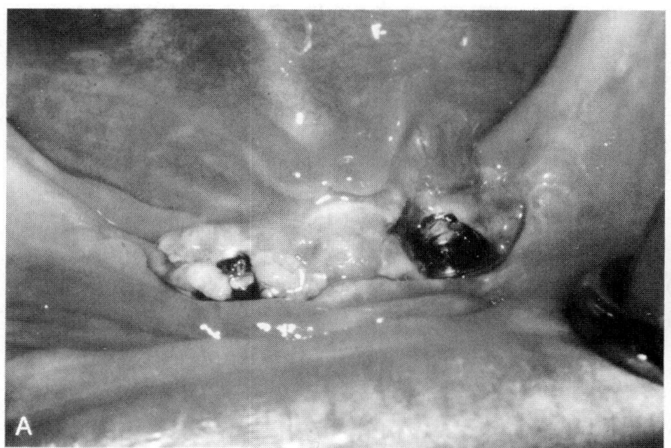

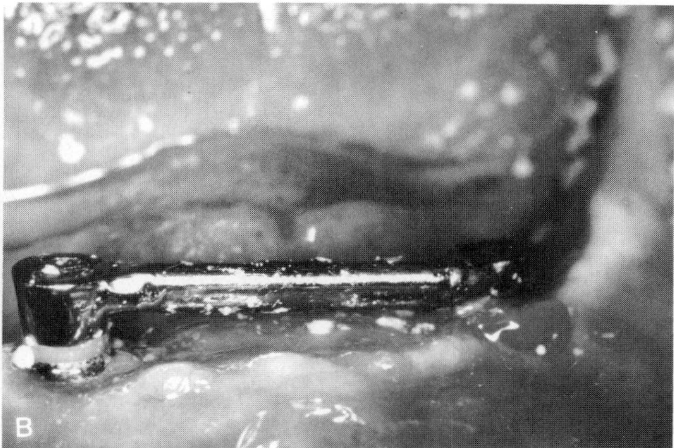

FIGURE 28–27
Periimplantitis, an infectious and soft tissue disease, around implant. (Courtesy of A. K. Lakha.)

with regard to abutment length and position; the prosthetic design and the ease of plaque removal between the appliance and gingival tissue; client motivation, compliance, and manual dexterity; and health of the periimplant tissue. Clients who have lost their teeth because of periodontal disease as a result on inadequate bacterial plaque control (neglect) need thorough education on the need for consistent oral hygiene care. The hygienist must impress upon these clients that their implants also are vulnerable to periodontal disease (periimplantitis) (Fig. 28–27).

Oral hygiene self-care techniques require meticulous attention and reinforcement by the dental hygienist. The dental hygienist should demonstrate use of the oral hygiene aids and provide written instructions and educational pamphlets. Adequate time during the appointment is necessary for the client to practice using each homecare aid while the dental hygienist is observing. Reinforcement, good communication, and understanding are necessary to increase the client's awareness of the importance of the recommended oral hygiene regimen, especially at each maintenance care appointment.

To prevent plaque-retentive scratches on the dental implants, clients should be instructed *never* to use a rigid toothbrush, safety pins, paper clips, or metal objects to self-clean the implants or abutments. The dental hygienist should monitor the oral tissues to ensure that the client is not causing trauma with an oral hygiene aid. Daily oral hygiene care may include a variety of excellent oral hygiene aids. As a dental implant client's oral condition changes, so do his dental hygiene needs. For example, if a client has an increased amount of hemorrhaging, the dental hygienist may need to reassess the client's condition and modify his home care to include a daily application of a chemotherapeutic agent such as 0.12% chlorhexidine gluconate, phenolic solutions, plant alkaloids, or a new implant cleaning strategy.

RECOMMENDED STRATEGIES FOR CLEANING DENTAL IMPLANTS

(see Chapter 16)[6–9]

Disclosants

Disclosing agents, for professional and home use, are applied to teeth and dental implants for bacterial plaque visualization. For example, the client may not see plaque on the lingual aspect of abutments or on the posterior portion of a bridge without the aid of a disclosant. These agents (tablets or solution) can be used initially on a regular basis and then used periodically as a monitoring strategy once good oral hygiene habits have been confirmed.

Intraoral Mirror and Penlight

A magnifying intraoral mirror and penlight should be used by the client in conjunction with the use of disclosants for an adequate visual examination of the localized bacterial plaque accumulation.

Assortment of Toothbrushes

Clients with dental implants should clean their implants, teeth, and gums two to three times daily with a toothbrush directed at a 45-degree angle toward the soft tissues. Because titanium is less rigid than a natural tooth, the surface of the abutment can be damaged with hard-bristled toothbrushes, which can lead to bacterial plaque accumulation. Also hard-bristled toothbrushes can lead to gingival or periimplant recession. Therefore, soft-bristled brushes are recommended. To prevent trauma to the delicate mucosa surrounding the abutment during toothbrushing, the soft bristled brush should have a small, compact head for reaching the facial, lingual, and occlusal surfaces. The toothbrush can be dipped into a 0.12% chlorhexidine gluconate solution to enhance plaque control. Clients also should invest adequate time brushing their prosthetic appliance.

Unituft Interspace Brushes—Tapered or Flat

The unique design of the unituft interspace brush allows the client to focus on one implant or tooth at a time (Fig. 28–28). The brush has soft-bristled nylon fibers that do not damage the periimplant tissue. The facial and lingual surfaces of dental implants can be reached with the unituft interspace brush with either the tapered or flat design. The plastic handle can be placed under hot water and bent to a position for greater access to hard-to-reach areas. The unituft toothbrush is recommended for use two to three times per day to remove bacterial plaque accumulation and to

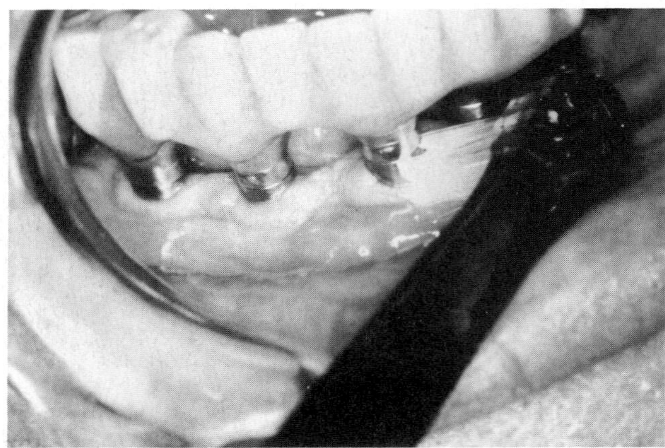

FIGURE 28-28
Application of an end-tuft toothbrush to an endosseous implant. (Courtesy of J. Kleinman.)

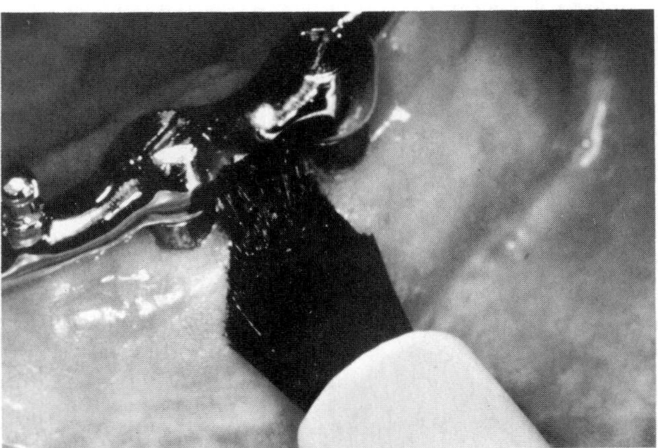

FIGURE 28-30
Application of Rotadent (ProDentec) electric rotary brush to an endosseous implant. (Courtesy of J. Kleinman.)

strengthen the periimplant and gingival tissue. The unituft brush can be dipped into a 0.12% chlorhexidine gluconate solution to enhance plaque control.

Motor-Powered Rotary Brushes

Rotary brushes should be prescribed for clients with limited dexterity to thoroughly clean around the abutments and interproximal areas under the prosthetic appliance (Figs. 28-29 and 28-30). Use of a low speed is indicated to prevent damage to the periimplant tissue. The brushes can be dipped into 0.12% chlorhexidine gluconate and used with a sweeping motion. The oscillating motion of the brush should follow the curvature of the dental implant along the gingiva. Electric rotary brushes are recommended for use one to two times per day.

Plastic Nylon-Coated Interdental Brush–Tapered or Cylindrical

Interproximal areas of dental implants can be reached with a cone-shaped or cylindrical interdental brush (Fig. 28-31). To avoid alteration of the abutment surface, nylon-coated wires are required rather than the conventional metal-wired brushes. Interdental brushes should be discarded when the nylon coating has worn down to the metal wire. The interdental brush can be used from the facial or lingual areas and interproximally. Interdental brushes are recommended for use at least one time per day. The interdental brush also may be used with 0.12% chlorhexidine gluconate.

Rubber Tip

The rubber tip may be used to remove debris accumulation from all surfaces including the gingival sulcus towards the coronal and abutment surface. The rubber tip also may stimulate and massage the periimplant tissue. Performance of this procedure is recommended once daily.

Dentifrice

Abrasive dentifrice can alter the abutment surface. Therefore, a gel or fine abrasive, anticalculus dentifrice such as Crest or Colgate antitartar formulas is indicated for use by clients with implants twice daily in conjunction with an oral hygiene aid.

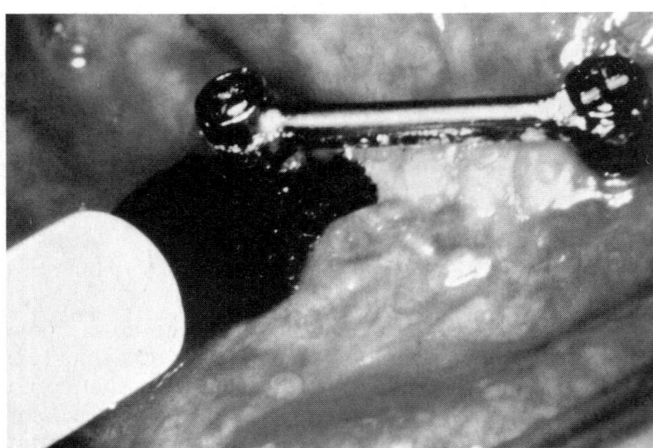

FIGURE 28-29
Application of a Rotadent (ProDentec) electric rotary long-tip brush to clean the crossbar of an endosseous implant. (Courtesy of J. Kleinman.)

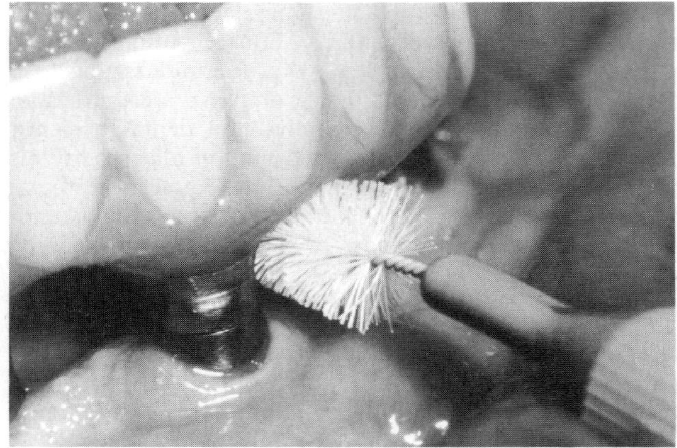

FIGURE 28-31
Application of a John O. Butler nylon-coated proxabrush to an endosseous implant. (Courtesy of J. Kleinman.)

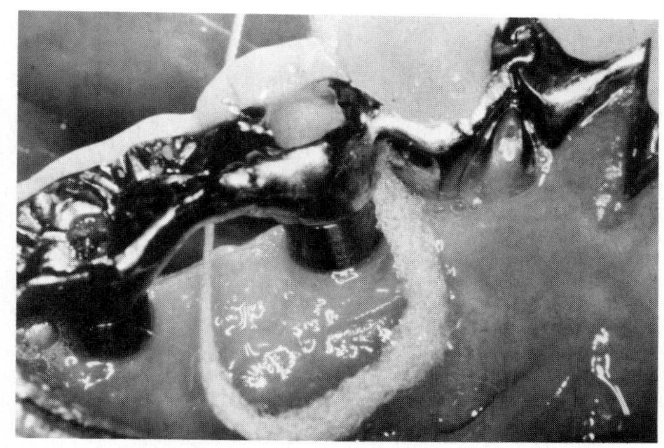

FIGURE 28–32
Application of Oral B Superfloss to an implant. (Courtesy of Oral B.)

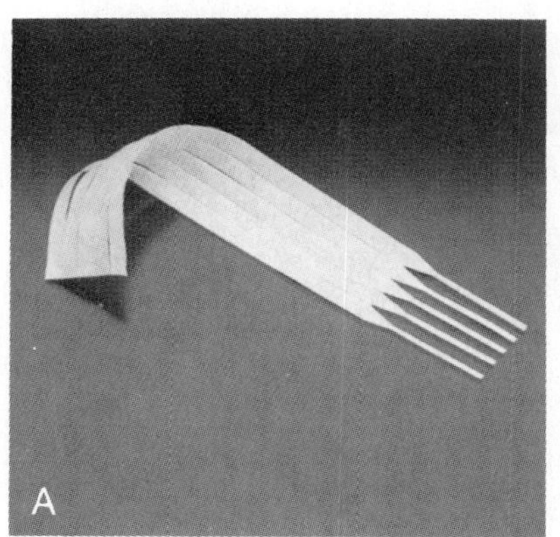

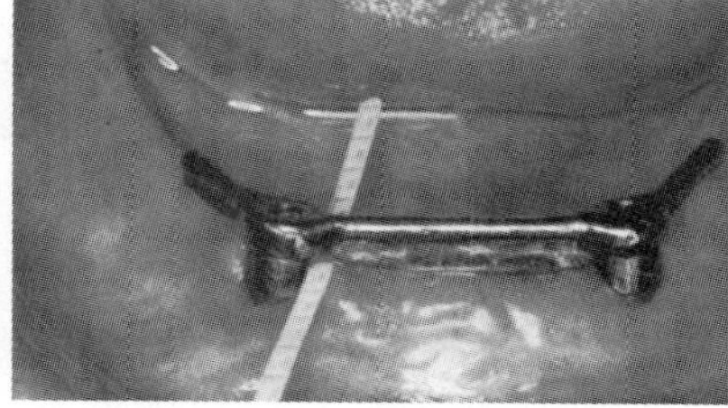

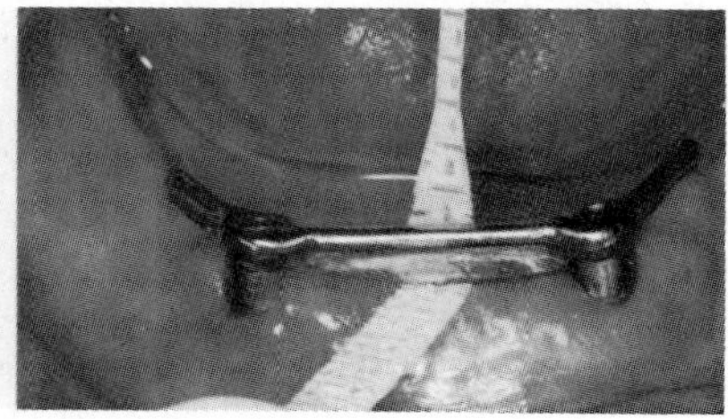

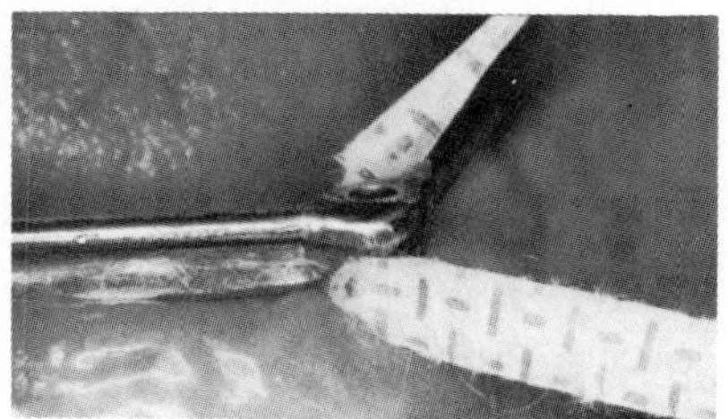

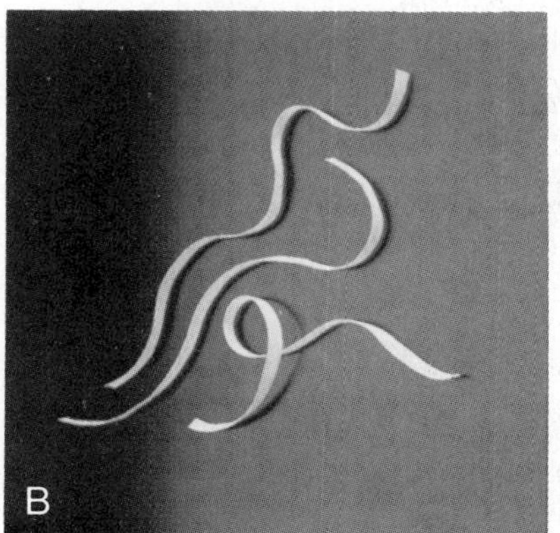

INSTRUCTIONS:

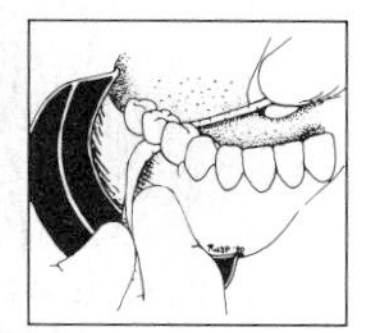

Use tapered, stiffened end to thread under fixed bridges where space allows.

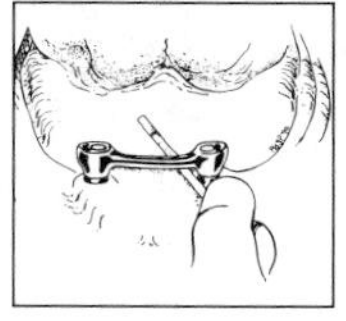

Tapered, stiffened end also allows ease in threading under connecting bars or implant overdenture prosthesis.

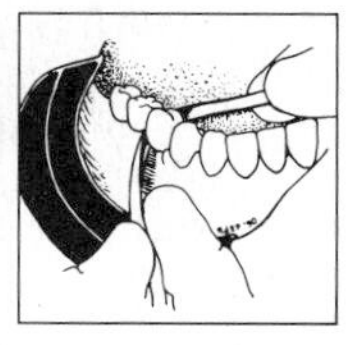

Wrap in a "C" shape around the abutment tooth, then use a back and forth polishing motion.

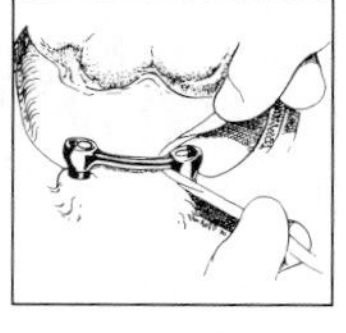

Floss may be wrapped in a "C" shape around natural tooth or implant coping and a back and forth polishing motion applied for optimal plaque removal.

D

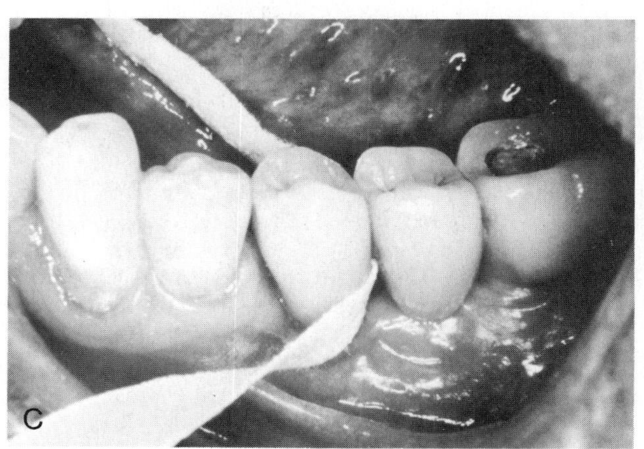

FIGURE 28–33
A, Tapered G-Floss. *B*, G-Floss. *C*, Application of G-Floss to an implant. *D*, Instructions on how to use G-Floss. (Courtesy of 3i-Implant Innovations.)

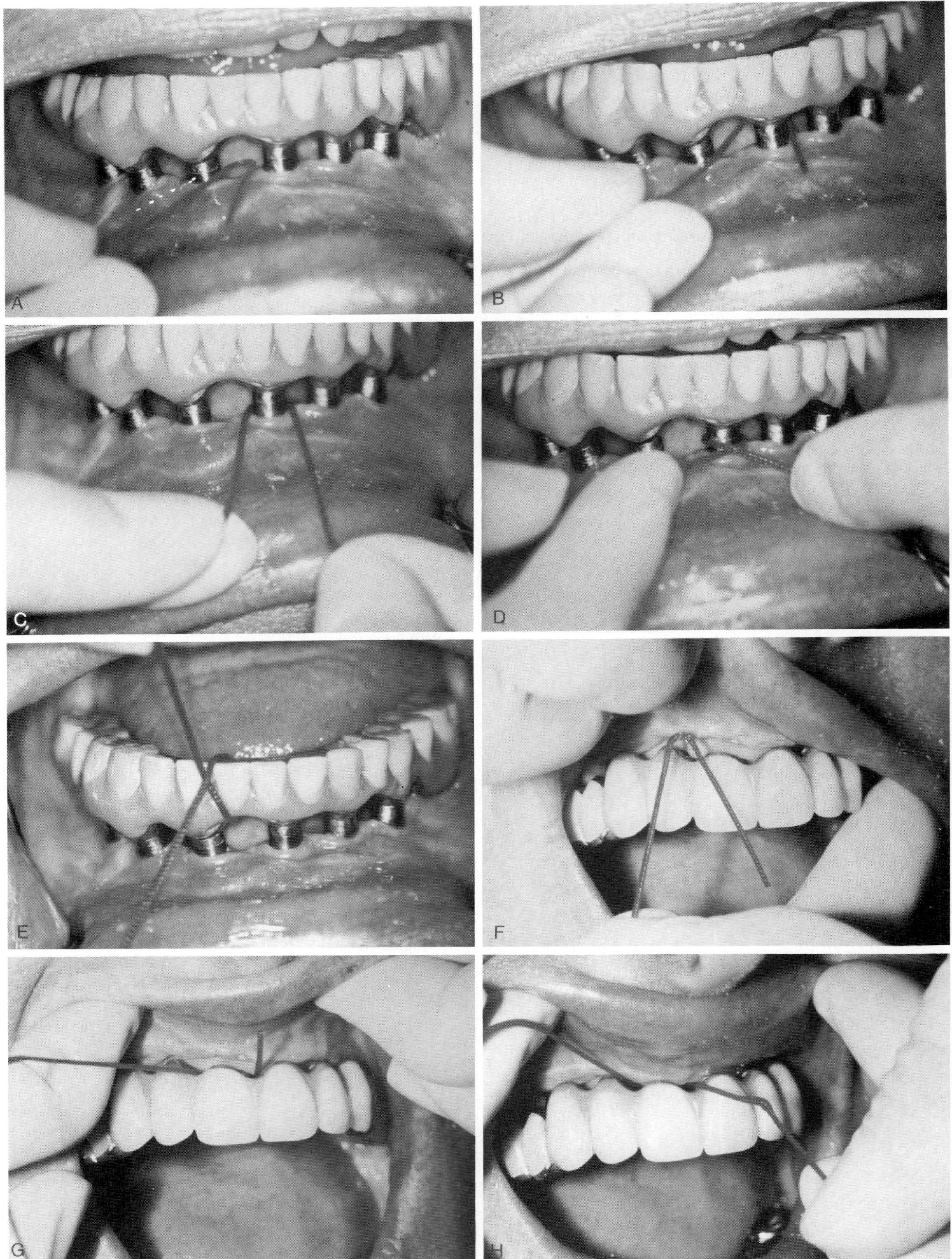

FIGURE 28–34
Systematic demonstration of how to use the John O. Butler Postcare Implant Flossing Cord. (Courtesy of J. Kleinman.)

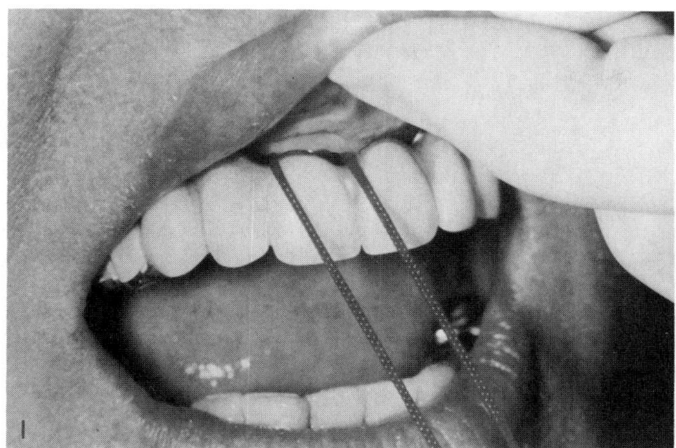

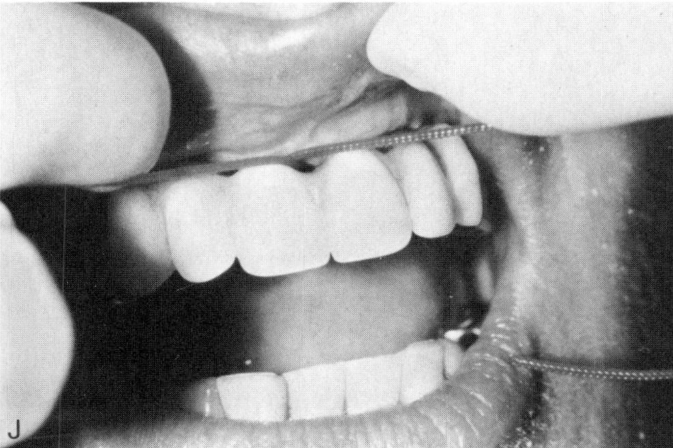

FIGURE 28–34
Continued

Dental Floss and Dental Tape

If abutments are spaced close to each other, dental floss or tape should be used to clean their proximal surface at least once a day (Figs. 28–32 to 28–34). Once the floss is placed around the implant, it can be crisscrossed and pulled in a shoeshining motion to clean the abutment. Floss or tape can be used in conjunction with a floss threader to allow easy access through the embrasure or limited areas. Other aids, such as shoelaces, ribbon, yarn, and gauze, may also be used.

Oral Irrigation

An oral irrigator may be indicated for use in limited access areas where there is evidence of soft tissue inflammation surrounding the abutment cylinder. The flow rate of the unit should be set at the lowest force. Solutions used in the oral irrigator may include water and a phenolic mouth rinse, a plant alkaloid mouth rinse, or a 0.12% chlorhexidine gluconate mouth rinse.

Antimicrobial Agent

For approximately 5 to 7 days after the abutment connection surgery, use of a capful of the antimicrobial 0.12% chlorhexidine gluconate solution as a 30-second rinse is recommended twice daily to help gingival sulcus healing. A cotton swab, soft toothbrush, unituft interspace brush, motor-powered rotary brush, or interdental brush may be used for the direct application of an agent to a specific site. However, use of chlorhexidine gluconate as a rinse for more than a month may cause staining of natural teeth or the prosthetic appliance. This antimicrobial solution is prescribed by the dentist and can be continued as recommended.

PROFESSIONAL DENTAL HYGIENE CARE

Comprehensive dental hygiene care for clients with dental implants requires a program of personal and professional

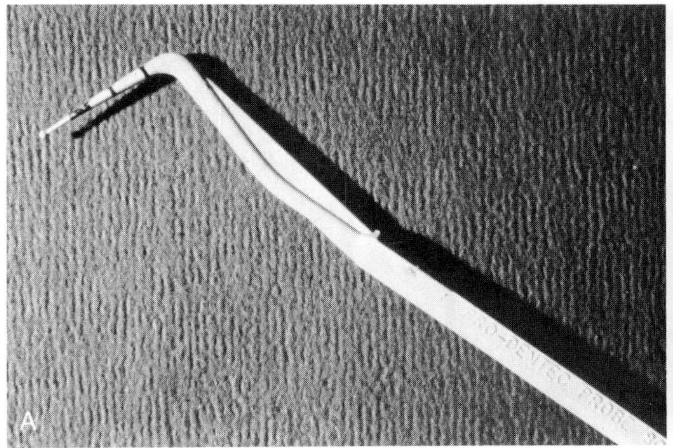

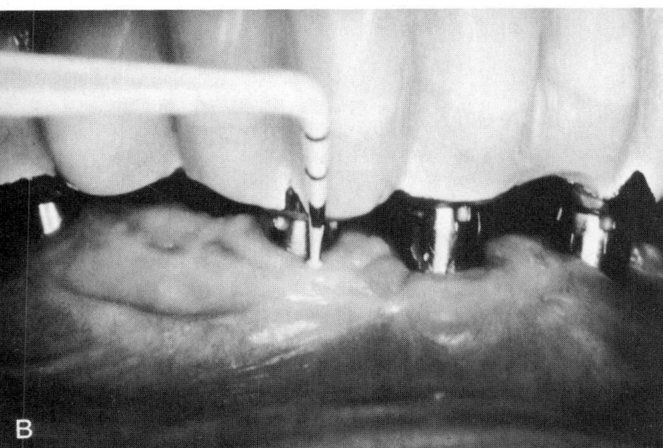

FIGURE 28–35
Plastic, flexible probe (ProDentec) to measure sulcus; it does not alter the abutment surface. (Courtesy of J. Kleinman.)

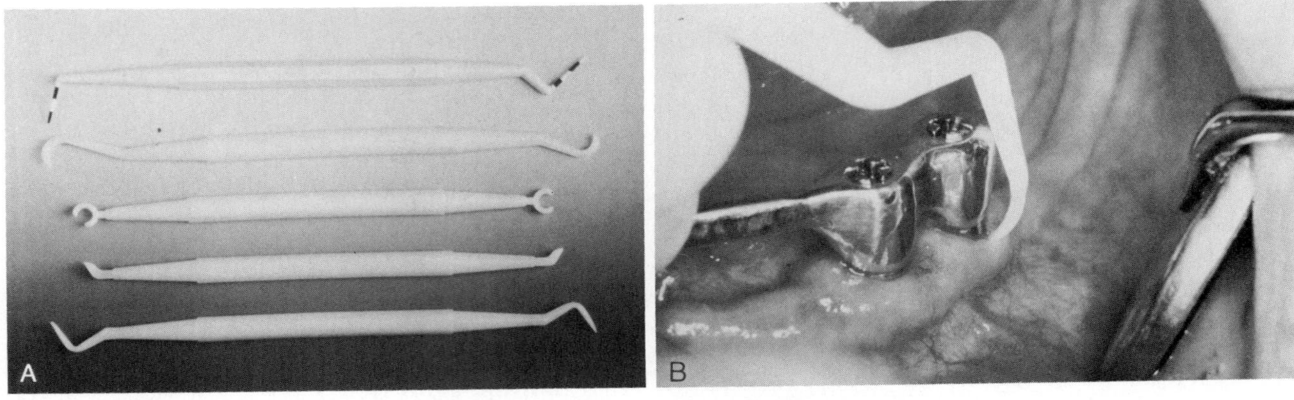

FIGURE 28–36
A, A set of Brevet plastic scalers. *B*, Plastic scaler adaptation to buccal area of implant abutment. (*B* courtesy of 3i-Implant Innovations.)

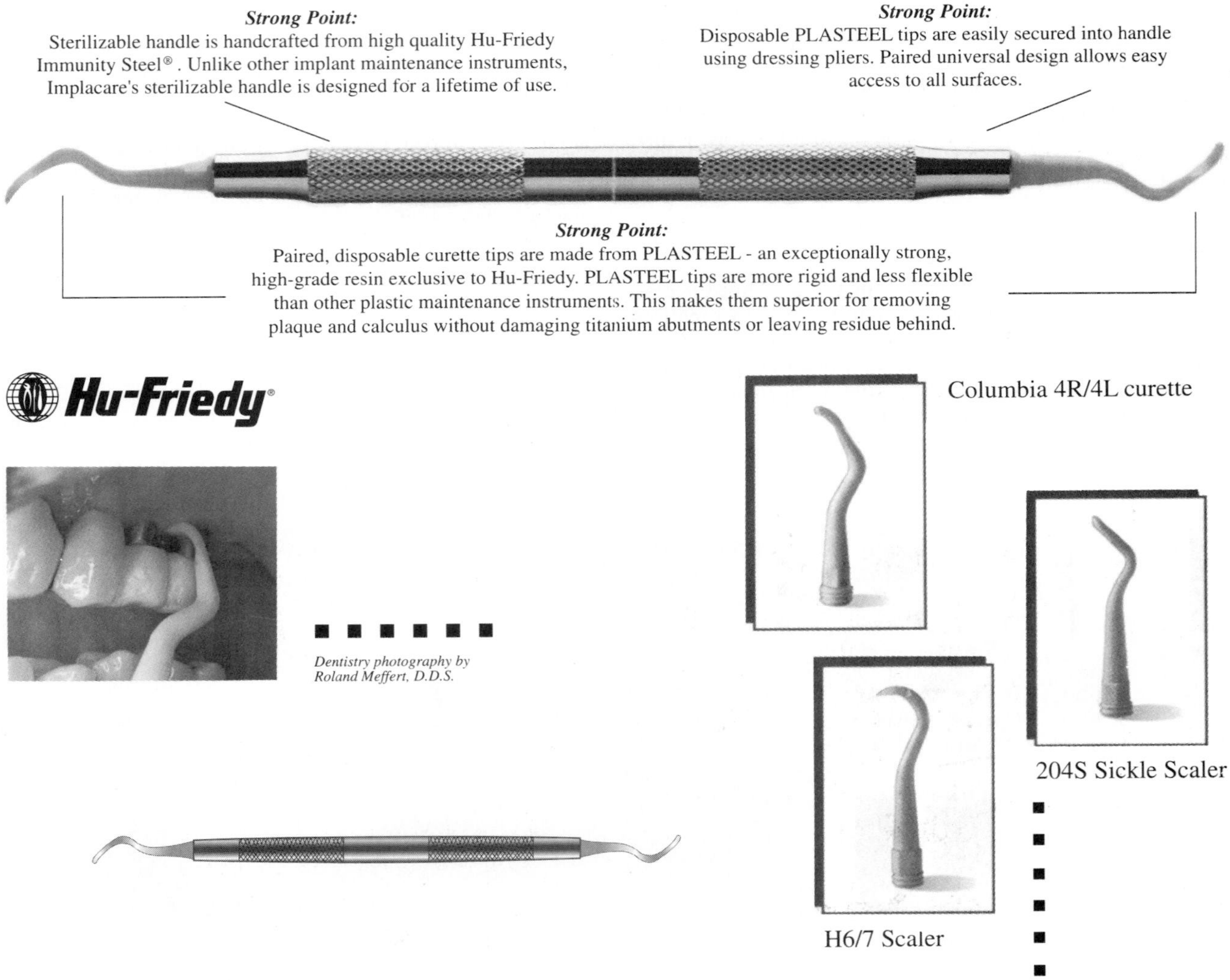

Strong Point:
Sterilizable handle is handcrafted from high quality Hu-Friedy Immunity Steel®. Unlike other implant maintenance instruments, Implacare's sterilizable handle is designed for a lifetime of use.

Strong Point:
Disposable PLASTEEL tips are easily secured into handle using dressing pliers. Paired universal design allows easy access to all surfaces.

Strong Point:
Paired, disposable curette tips are made from PLASTEEL - an exceptionally strong, high-grade resin exclusive to Hu-Friedy. PLASTEEL tips are more rigid and less flexible than other plastic maintenance instruments. This makes them superior for removing plaque and calculus without damaging titanium abutments or leaving residue behind.

Hu-Friedy®

Dentistry photography by Roland Meffert, D.D.S.

Columbia 4R/4L curette

204S Sickle Scaler

H6/7 Scaler

FIGURE 28–37
Hu-Friedy developed the Implacare Maintenance Instrument with disposable Plasteel tips that screw into the handle. (Courtesy of Hu-Friedy. Dentistry photography by Roland Meffert, D.D.S.)

oral hygiene care for the client based on identified human need deficits related to oral health status.

The clinical armamentaria needed to provide professional dental hygiene implant care includes the following:

- An antimicrobial solution such as 0.12% chlorhexidine gluconate
- A plastic disposable syringe or gingival irrigation unit
- A plastic periodontal probe (Fig. 28–35)
- A set of plastic Teflon-coated scalers (Figs. 28–36 through 28–38)
- A set of gold-tipped Gracey scalers such as an 11–12 or a 13–14 (Fig. 28–39)
- A set of graphite scalers (Fig. 28–40)
- A wood-tipped porte polisher
- A sonic scaler with a disposable polysulfon plastic tip (Fig. 28–41)
- A strip of 2 × 2-inch gauze
- Thick (red) and thin (green) implant floss
- A small portion of gel dentifrice or tin oxide
- A rubber cup and pointed polisher
- A soft, multitufted toothbrush with a compact head

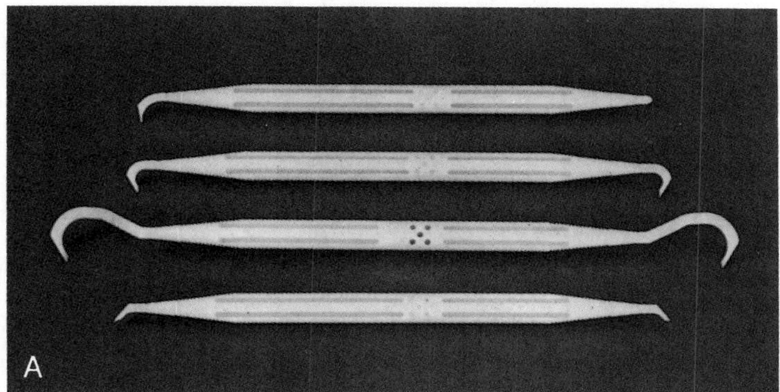

The Universal Scaler DIA 238, the Lingual Scaler DIA 239, the Posterior Scaler DIA 267, and the Buccal Scaler DIA 240 (from top to bottom).

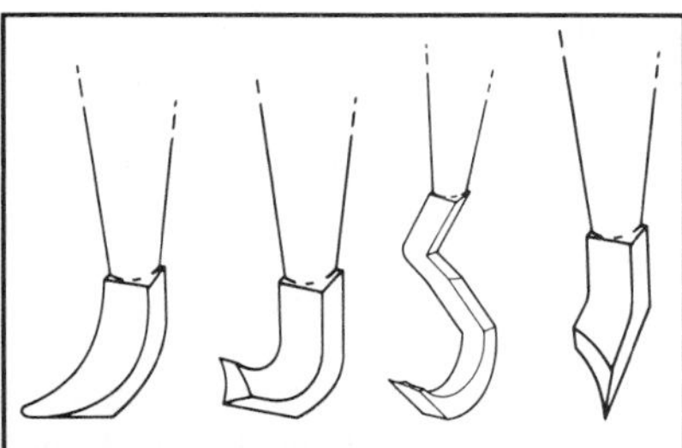

The edge of (from left to right) the universal, lingual, posterior, and buccal scaler.

B

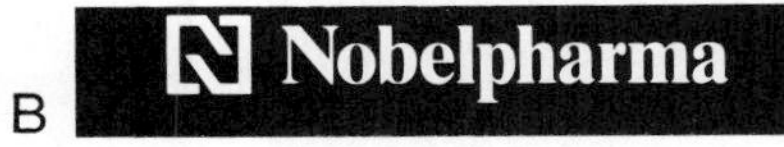

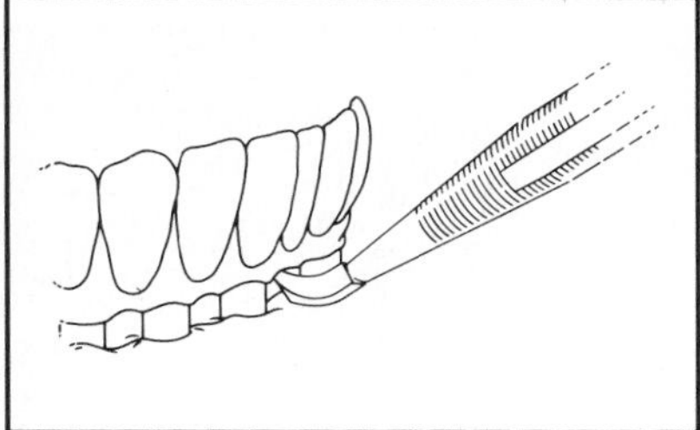

The universal scaler is used for cleaning the apical portion of the framework.

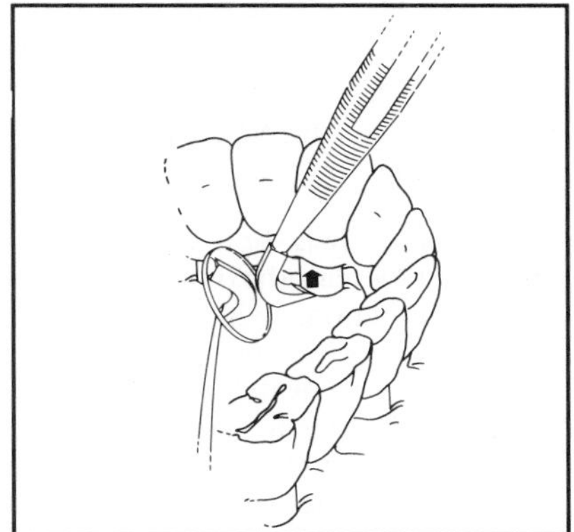

To clean the lingual side of the abutment, the lingual scaler is moved apicoronally and the work is done via a mirror.

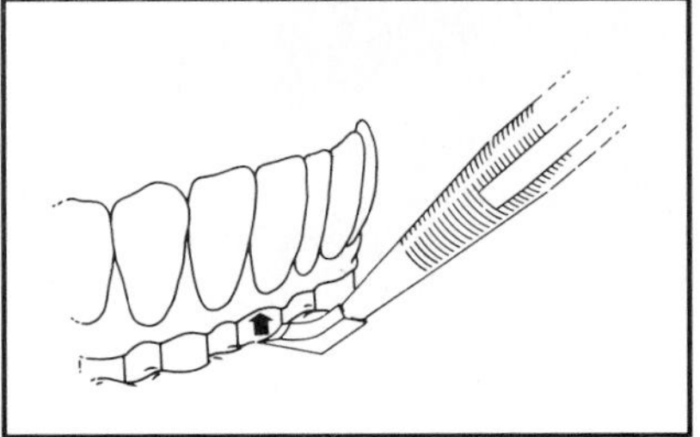

C *The edge of the buccal scaler is designed to fit the buccal surface of the abutment. The instrument is moved apicoronally.*

FIGURE 28–38
A to *C*, Nobelpharma's design of four plastic scalers. (Courtesy of Nobelpharma.)

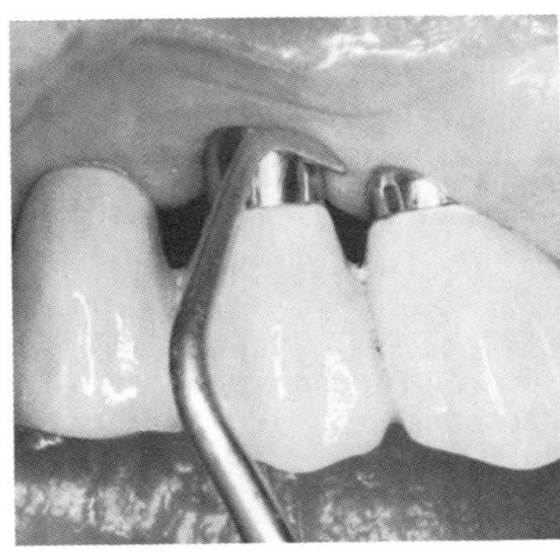

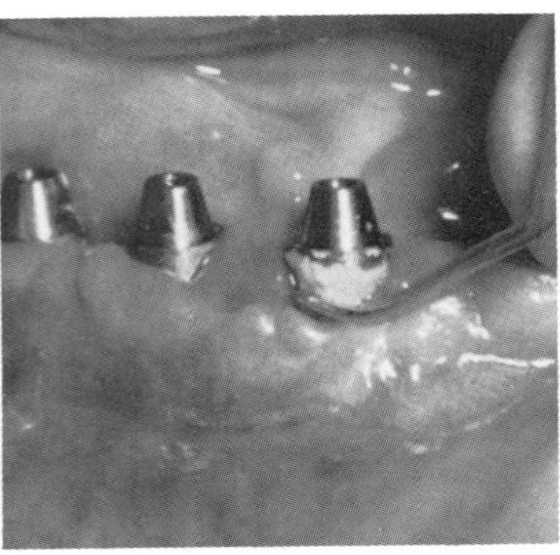

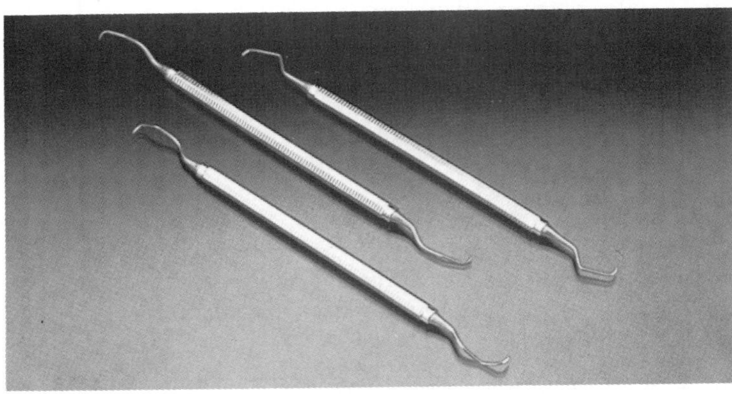

FIGURE 28–39
Application of gold-tipped scalers to an implant. (Courtesy of 3i-Implant Innovations.)

design and other appropriate auxiliary tools for self-care instruction

Periimplant tissue irrigation with an antimicrobial solution such as 0.12% chlorhexidine gluconate is performed prior to instrumentation. Irrigation reduces the pathogenicity of bacterial colonies and reduces the risk of a local infection. Therefore, irrigation should be implemented by the dental hygienist prior to the use of a scaling instrument. A plastic disposable syringe or a powered oral irrigation unit may be used to accomplish this irrigation procedure because both techniques allow access to the periimplant sulcus and deliver the antimicrobial solution to the periimplant sulcus easily and effectively. Chlorhexidine gluconate 0.12% is an excellent antimicrobial agent to use for periimplant tissue irrigation. If staining of the natural teeth or prosthesis is a problem, the antimicrobial solution may be applied locally with a cotton applicator rather than rinsing. A phenolic solution is acceptable if a client cannot tolerate the stain or taste of the antimicrobial solution.

Periodontal probing around the periimplant tissue has been a controversial issue among clinicians and researchers. Current consensus is that probing should not be used as a routine procedure on dental implant clients.[6,8] The possibility of disturbing the **biological seal** that attaches the healthy periimplant tissue to the titanium abutment can cause a local infection within the unattached sulci and can lead to implant failure. Probing should be used with caution to

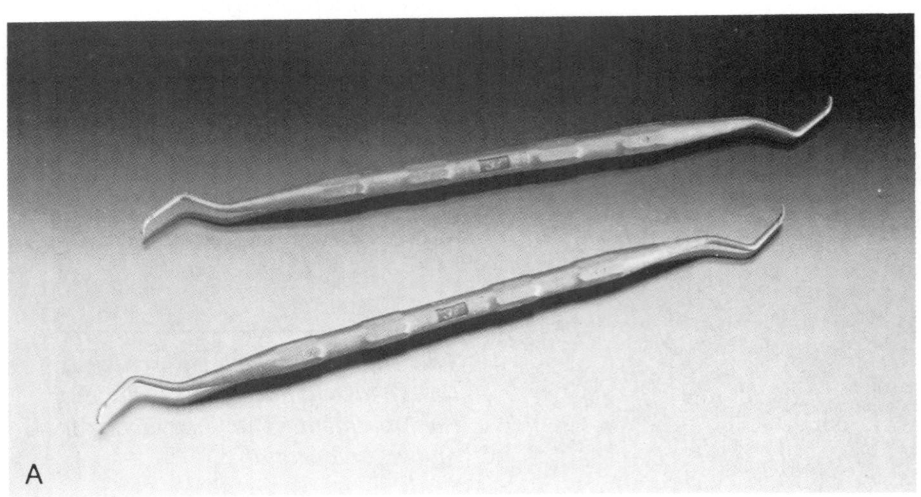

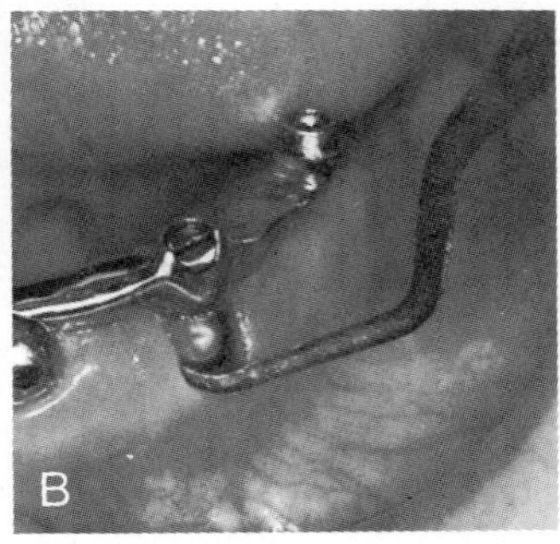

FIGURE 28–40
A, Graphite scalers. *B*, Application of graphite scaler to the dental implant.

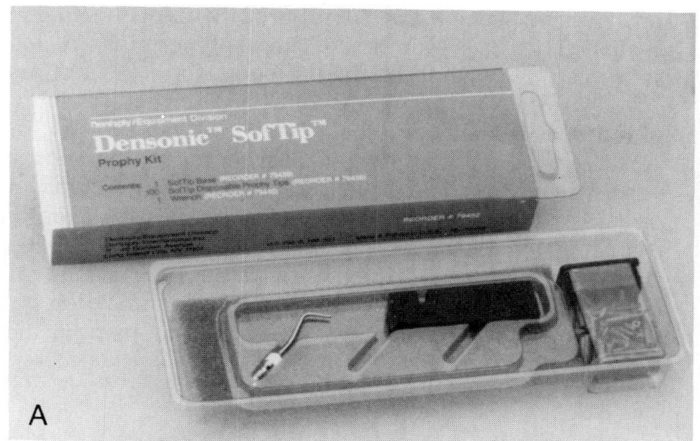

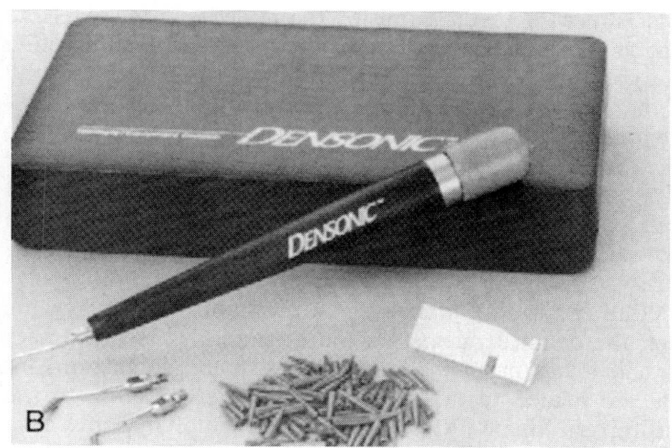

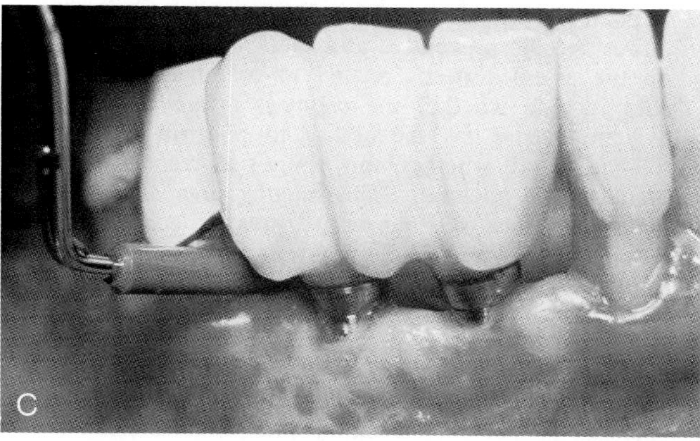

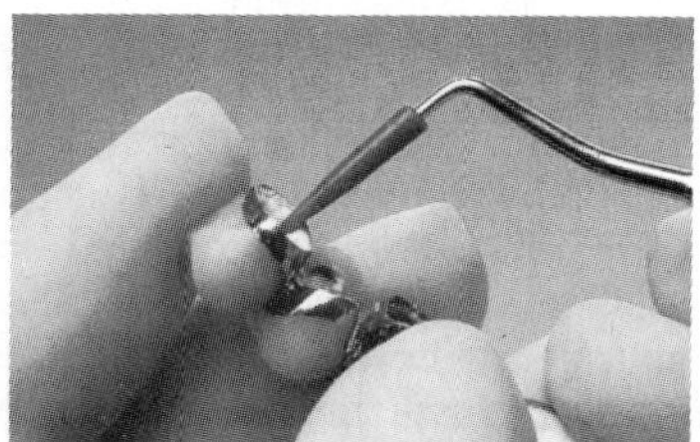

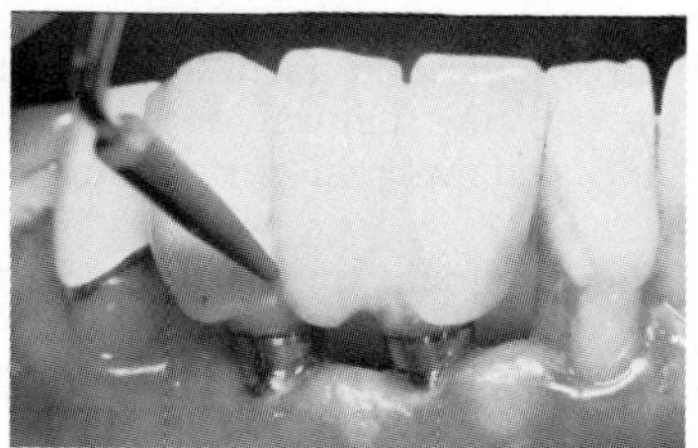

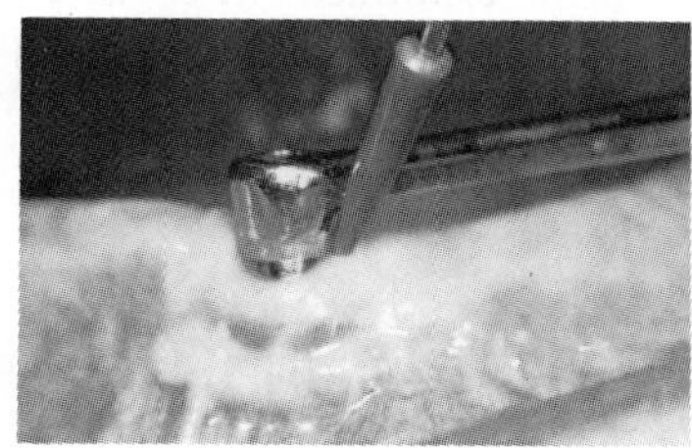

FIGURE 28–41
A, The Densonic SofTip Kit. *B*, A disposable polysulfon plastic Densonic SofTip used on the end of a Star Titan S or SW Scaler does not alter or harm the surface of a titanium implant. *C*, Application of the Densonic SofTip to the dental implant. (Courtesy of Dentsply.)

determine depth of severe marginal bone loss or periimplant problems. If probing is necessary, a plastic disposable probe should be used.

Screw retention should be assessed at each maintenance care visit. A loose screw can cause mobility of the bridge and dental implant.

The dental hygienist may select several types of instruments to remove adherent bacterial plaque and dental calculus. However, instrument rigidity and design, prosthetic appliance design, location of bacterial plaque, and calculus tenacity should be carefully assessed before instrumentation. Because the surface of the titanium abutment can be easily abraded by metal scalers, sonic instruments, and abrasive agents, the following methods and materials are contraindicated for use on dental implants: metal scalers, metal tip inserts of sonic and ultrasonic instruments, air polishing devices, and rubber cup polishing with flour of pumice or abrasive paste.[6] However, a polysulfon disposable tip may be used with a sonic scaler to remove tenacious calculus deposits.

Plastic, Teflon-coated, graphite wood-tipped, and gold-tipped Gracey instruments have been developed for use in scaling dental implants. The plastic and Teflon-coated instruments are designed to prevent abrasion to the titanium implants. The wood-tipped instrument or porte polisher is designed to prevent scratches on the implant surface. Half of a round, pointed toothpick inserted through the end of an interdental brush handle is considered a very safe and effective scaler for use around dental implants. However, wood-tipped instruments should be used only once and then thrown away to prevent splintering and damage to the periimplant tissue. The gold-tipped Gracey instruments are fabricated from a special gold alloy that is softer than titanium and, therefore, does not roughen the surface of the abutments or cause retention of acquired deposits. Gold-tipped Gracey scalers should not be sharpened because the gold is then removed, exposing the underlying metal. (Note that some clinicians and researchers believe that graphite and gold-tipped scalers may change the surface topography of the implant and should be avoided.) Polishing is recommended with a gel dentifrice or tin oxide in a rubber cup or rubber point. Buffing the abutments "shoeshine style" with longs gauze strips or floss is very effective for bacterial plaque removal. An ordinary cotton shoestring can help to remove bacterial plaque underneath the prosthetic appliance.

While providing professional mechanical oral hygiene care, the dental hygienist should continually assess whether the client has problems associated with the dental implant that are related to oral hygiene or to the condition of the periimplant tissue. At this time, the dental hygienist also has an excellent opportunity to offer emotional support and to educate clients about oral health practices. By incorporating recommended dental hygiene interventions for dental implants into the routine continued care appointment, the dental hygienist can efficiently meet the oral hygiene needs of dental implant clients. For example, depending on the client's assessed needs, the dental hygienist can monitor the condition of the periimplant tissue; remove acquired deposits from natural teeth and implants; discuss the related oral hygiene needs; provide specific oral hygiene instructions customized to an individual client's needs; reinforce bacterial plaque control education; evaluate the client's acceptance of and ability to perform recommended oral hygiene regimens; encourage client compliance with implant examinations; take necessary radiographs; and facilitate prevention of dental caries in the existing natural dentition by applying fluoride therapy and sealants and performing nutritional counseling.

Clients with dental implants should maintain a 3- to 4-month (or as needed) continued care schedule (Table 28–9) for professional dental hygiene care. Once a year, the fixed prosthetic appliance should be removed by the dentist and the stability of the implant examined. The bacterial plaque and dental calculus accumulated on the appliance also should be removed using the same procedure as with conventional dentures.

Evaluation

The client's oral health status should be continually evaluated throughout dental hygiene care to monitor goal attainment, coordinate dental and dental hygiene care plans, and enhance client compliance with recommended personal oral hygiene care. Screw retention of the implant should be evaluated at each continued care appointment. A loose screw can cause mobility of the dental implant and associated prosthesis, that is, the bridge. The client should be monitored annually by the dentist or oral surgeon who placed the implant. Every 18 to 24 months, the removable superstructures should be disassembled for evaluation and cleaning. Radiographs of the implant should be taken and evaluated by the dentist every 6 to 12 months. A client should contact the dentist if there is an increased amount of swelling, a fever, or sensitivity in the mandible or sinus area that is not resolved with prescription pain medications.[10]

TABLE 28–9
CONTINUING CARE SCHEDULE FOR CLIENTS WITH DENTAL IMPLANTS

Once implant is placed	Oral hygiene education and instruction
Radiographic evaluation of bone and periodontal structures	Every 3 months for first year and annually, thereafter, unless necessary
Continuing care appointment	Every 3 months for first year and thereafter, evaluate for 4-month continuing care appointments
Removal of prosthesis or implant parts	Annually, during continuing care appointment
Any signs of infection	Return to general dentist in 10–14 days, or refer to specialist

Note: Be sure to commit client to the next continuing care appointment before your appointment ends.

CONCLUSION

Dental hygiene care is vital to the long-term success of implants. Optimal dental implant health for the client requires specific preventive and therapeutic procedures based on the assessed needs related to oral health status. Such data include whether the client is aware of specific oral hygiene needs, has the ability to perform recommended self-care, and whether the client's current oral hygiene practices are adequate. The sulcular area around the implant or insert is the primary area of concern. Implant mobility and signs of inflammation and exudate around the implant sulcus should be recognized, documented, and called to the attention of the client and dentist. Using metal instruments or metal ultrasonic instruments to scale implants is not recommended. Metal instruments may cause scratches and irregularities on the implant, leading to bacterial plaque accumulation and inflammation. If metal instruments are used, they should be made of metals of equal or more pliability than titanium. Stainless steel is harder than titanium and may scratch the titanium implants more readily. Plastic, gold-tipped, Teflon-coated, graphite, or wooden instruments may be used for scaling. Dental hygiene care plans should be individualized according to the client's human needs related to oral health.

References

1. Adell, R., Lekholm, U., Rockler, B., Branemark, P. I. A 15 year study of osseointegrated implants in the treatment of the edentulous jaw. International Journal of Oral Surgery 10:387, 1981.
2. American Dental Association Council on Dental Materials, Instruments, and Equipment. Journal of the American Dental Association 113(12):949, 1986.
3. Smith, R., Koumjian, J. Understanding Dental Implants—Comfort and Confidence Again. Daly City, Krames Communication, 1988.
4. Brånemark, P. I. Osseointegration and its experimental background. Journal of Prosthetic Dentistry 50:399, 1983.
5. Nobelpharma. Clinical guidelines for hygiene maintenance of patients treated with the Branemark system. Chicago: Nobelpharma Co., 1988.
6. Meffert, R. M. The importance of periodontal maintenance for the dental implant. Journal of Practical Hygiene 1(1):27, 1992.
7. Ogren, E. M. The hygienist's role in successful implant treatment. Journal of Practical Hygiene 1(3):29, 1992.
8. Daniels, A. The importance of accurate charting for maintaining dental implants. Journal of Practical Hygiene 2(5):9, 1993.
9. Minichetti, J. C., and Coplanis, N. Consideration in the maintenance of the dental implant patient. Journal of Practical Hygiene 2(5):15, 1993.
10. Meffert, R. M. How to treat ailing and failing implants. Implant Dentistry 1(1):25, 1992.

29 Dental Hygiene Care for the Individual with Cardiovascular Disease

OBJECTIVES

Mastery of the content in this chapter will enable the reader to:

- Define the key terms used
- Discuss cardiovascular disease risk factors
- Identify the general signs and symptoms of cardiovascular disease, specifically those of rheumatic heart disease, bacterial endocarditis, valvular heart defects, cardiac arrhythmias, hypertension, coronary heart disease, congestive heart failure, and congenital heart disease
- Describe the psychological responses related to cardiovascular disease
- Describe the care of clients with cardiovascular disease, specifically rheumatic heart disease, valvular heart defects, hypertension, coronary heart disease, and congestive heart failure
- Discuss the oral complications associated with cardiovascular disease
- Complete an assessment of a client with cardiovascular disease
- Determine a dental hygiene diagnosis related to the individual with cardiovascular disease
- Develop a dental hygiene care plan for clients with cardiovascular disease
- Determine the need for emergency medical care in a client with cardiovascular disease, specifically, coronary heart disease
- Select alternative dental hygiene care procedures for the individual with cardiovascular disease
- Identify alternative dietary choices that meet the client's nutritional needs for cardiovascular and oral health

INTRODUCTION

National statistics indicate that one of five persons has some form of cardiovascular disease and more than 1 million people die of it annually.[1] Therefore, the probability of treating a medically compromised client with cardiovascular disease in dental hygiene practice is high.

The major structures of the heart and their basic functions are found in Figure 29–1. A review of the normal cardiovascular structure and physiology establishes the baseline for a discussion of pathological conditions.

Diseases of the heart consist of many types. Symptoms vary; in some cases the disease may become debilitating, whereas in others it may go unrecognized. The role of the dental hygienist is to understand the condition and take the necessary precautions to ensure successful dental hygiene care as directed by the human needs of the client.

Interdisciplinary approaches towards healthcare are the norm. Many cardiovascular diseases are considered multifaceted and present treatment risks. When treating the individual with cardiovascular disease, the dental hygienist's role as clinician, educator, client advocate, manager and coordinator of oral healthcare, and researcher become apparent. The dental hygienist also has an opportunity to promote optimal health in clients with no apparent cardiovascular disease via such services as blood pressure screening, nutritional counseling, and tobacco cessation programs.

This chapter provides information on the various forms of cardiovascular disease. The person with cardiovascular disease (or with the potential for cardiovascular disease as evidenced by the risk factors) may have human need deficits, the fulfillment of which can be facilitated through dental hygiene care. These deficits may relate to the human need for a wholesome body image; freedom from pain and

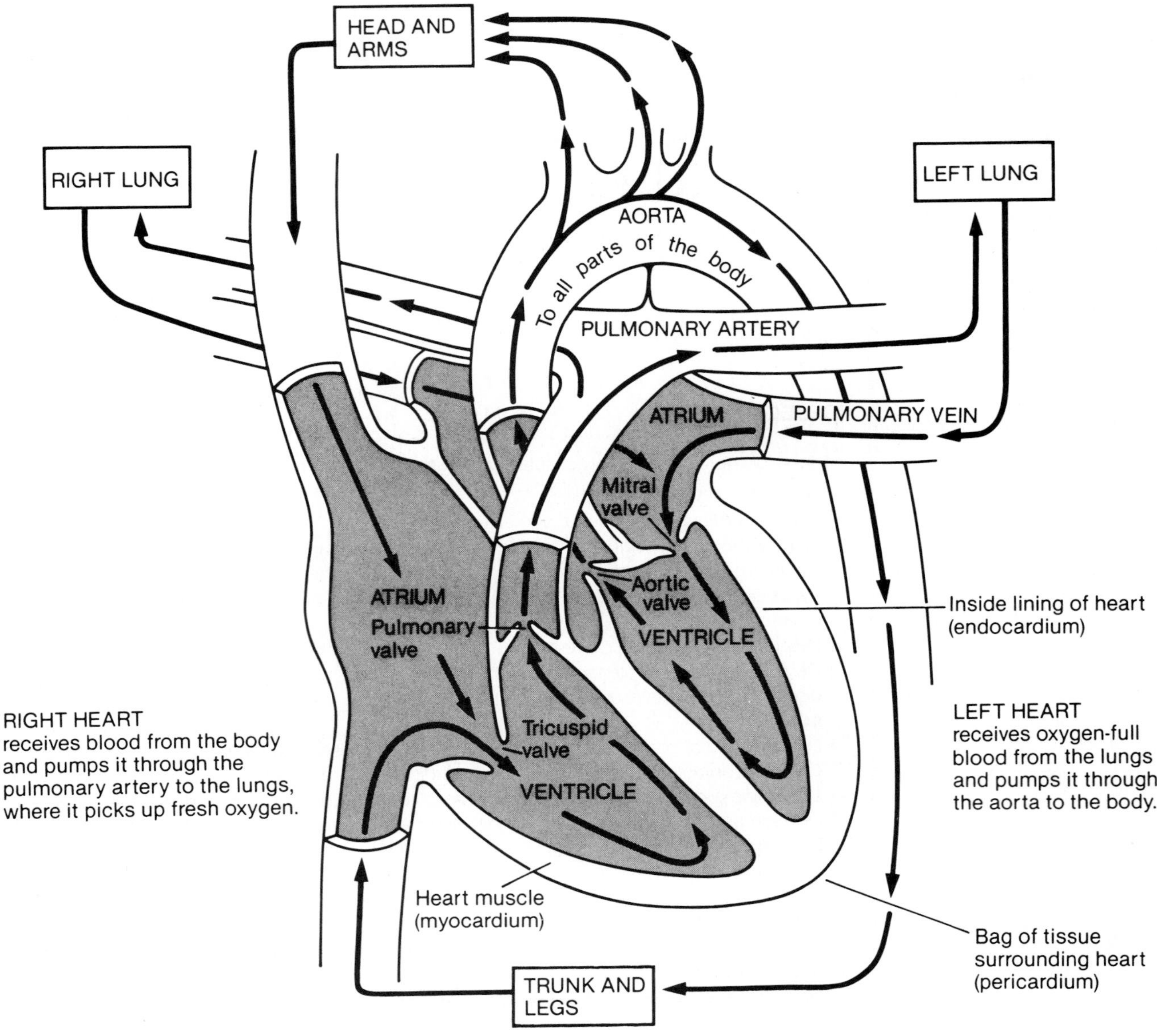

FIGURE 29–1
Diagram of the heart. (Reproduced with permission from Kinn, M. E., Woods, M. A., and Derge, E. F. The Medical Assistant: Administrative and Clinical, 7th ed. Philadelphia: W. B. Saunders, 1993, p. 548.)

stress; skin and mucous membrane integrity of the head and neck; nutrition; safety; biologically sound dentition; self-determination and responsibility; and values system. The relationship of these human needs to dental hygiene care for the client with cardiovascular disease is discussed throughout the chapter.

CARDIOVASCULAR DISEASE

Cardiovascular disease (CVD) is defined as an alteration of the heart and/or blood vessels that impairs function. World health statistics indicate that cardiovascular disease is responsible for 48% of deaths in developed countries.[1]

Although the prevalence rate is high, research has demonstrated that CVD is preventable.[2,3] The following characteristics or risk factors are associated with poor cardiovascular health:

- Family history of cardiovascular disease
- Increased age
- Gender
- Diabetes mellitus
- High cholesterol, sodium, and dietary fat intake
- Tobacco use
- Obesity
- Sedentary lifestyle
- Stressful lifestyle

Primary prevention and health promotion are methods of improving health status and reducing the risk of developing cardiovascular disease (Table 29–1).

Prevention of adult cardiovascular disease in childhood

TABLE 29–1
RISK FACTORS FOR CORONARY HEART DISEASE

Personal Factors	
Age (nonmodifiable)	Pathological changes within the coronary arteries, which are severe enough to cause symptoms, appear predominantly in persons over age 40 years
Sex (nonmodifiable)	Men are four times as likely to suffer from coronary heart disease as are women up to age 40 years
Genetic predisposition (nonmodifiable)	Family members who have suffered from cardiovascular disease
Personality traits (modifiable)	Hard-driving, competitive individuals who worry excessively about deadlines and who consistently overwork
Professional stresses (modifiable)	Occupations that impose tremendous responsibility, e.g., doctors, executives
Disease Patterns	
Hypertension (modifiable)	Individuals with a sustained blood pressure of 160/95 or higher double their risk of suffering a myocardial infarction
Obesity (modifiable)	Weight 30% or more above that considered standard for an individual of a certain height and build
Lipid abnormalities (modifiable)	Serum cholesterol of over 200 mg/100 mL or a fasting triglyceride of more than 250 mg/100 mL
Diabetes mellitus (modifiable)	Fasting blood sugar of more than 120 mg/dL, or a routine blood sugar of 180 mg/dL
Adverse Environmental Problems	
Cigarette smoking (modifiable)	Smoking two packs of cigarettes per day causes the risk of coronary heart disease to increase four-fold
Sedentary occupation and life style (modifiable)	Lack of exercise tends to promote mental depression and obesity
High-caloric, high-fat diet (modifiable)	Overeating and consuming fatty-rich foods promote obesity, lipid abnormalities, and diabetes

and youth is advocated by the American Academy of Pediatrics.[4] Early intervention to change risk-related behavioral patterns may decrease the prevalence of heart disease in the population.

Rheumatic Heart Disease

Rheumatic heart disease refers to the cardiac manifestations of rheumatic fever. Approximately, 2 to 3% of persons who have suffered a beta-hemolytic streptococcal infection develop rheumatic fever.[5] **Rheumatic fever** is an acute or chronic systemic inflammatory process characterized by attacks of fever, polyarthritis, and **carditis.** The latter may eventually result in permanent valvular heart damage.

The most destructive effect of rheumatic fever is carditis, which is found in up to 50% of individuals exhibiting signs and symptoms of rheumatic fever.[5] Carditis may affect the **endocardium, myocardium, pericardium,** or heart valves. Valvular damage is responsible for the familiar heart murmur associated with rheumatic fever or rheumatic heart disease. The heart murmur is defined as an irregularity of the auditory heart beat caused by a turbulent flow of blood through a valve that has failed to close. The valves most commonly affected are the mitral valve and the aortic valve. The damaged valves are susceptible to infection that may lead to bacterial endocarditis. Severe rheumatic carditis may cause difficulty in breathing, elevation of the diastolic blood pressure, and increasing signs of heart failure.

The significance of rheumatic fever to the professional dental hygienist is related directly to the provision of dental hygiene care. Dental hygiene care involves the manipulation of soft tissue, which in itself can introduce microorganisms into the bloodstream, causing infective endocarditis in a client with a history of rheumatic fever. Specifically, the American Heart Association recommends that antibiotics be delivered prior to dental and dental hygiene care to prevent bacterial endocarditis. The risk of infection increases if such a precaution is not taken prior to dental or dental hygiene care. As a licensed professional, the dental hygienist is responsible for the well-being of the client during dental hygiene care.

Bacterial Endocarditis

Bacterial endocarditis is an infection of the endocardium, heart valves, or cardiac prosthesis resulting from bacterial invasion. It is characterized by the formation of vegetative growths of *Staphylococcus aureus, Staphylococcus epidermidis, Streptococcus viridans,* and, the most prevalent, alpha-hemolytic streptococci on the heart valves or endocardial lining.[6] Although staphylococci and streptococci are found in most cases, yeast, fungi, and viruses have also been identified. If left untreated, endocarditis is usually fatal, but with proper antibiotic treatment, 70% of patients recover.[7]

There are two types of bacterial endocarditis: acute bacterial endocarditis (ABE) and subacute bacterial endocarditis (SBE). ABE and SBE differ in their method of onset.

Acute bacterial endocarditis is a severe infection with a rapid course of action. It is usually caused by highly pathogenic microorganisms, such as *S. aureus* and *S. epidermidis* capable of producing widespread disease.[6]

Subacute bacterial endocarditis is a slow-moving infection with nonspecific clinical features. Clients usually exhibit a continuous low-grade fever, marked weakness, fatigue, weight loss, and joint pain. Dental and dental hygiene procedures that involve the manipulation of soft tissue may be responsible for the development of SBE. Bacterial endocarditis, subacute or acute, is treated with a course of antibiotic therapy.

In general, bacterial endocarditis is caused by the formation of a **bacteremia** (the presence of microorganisms in the bloodstream). During dental and dental hygiene therapy a transient bacteremia is produced. Tissue trauma from instrumentation coupled with the state of dental and periodontal diseases determine the severity of the infection.

As bacterial endocarditis progresses, the circulating microorganisms attach to the damaged heart valves or other susceptible areas and proliferate to produce colonies. The result of this invasion includes cardiac failure from continued valvular damage and embolization (vessel obstruction) because of fragmentation of the colonized microorganisms.

High-risk clients include those who present with rheumatic heart disease, valvular heart defects, prosthetic heart valves, cardiac pacemakers, and previous episodes of bacterial endocarditis. To meet the human needs of these people for safety, preventive antibiotic therapy is required, as recommended by the American Heart Association and the American Dental Association Council on Dental Therapeutics prior to procedures that produce bacteremias (see Chapter 10, Tables 10–3 to 10–4).

Four essential steps the dental hygienist must take to control infection and prevent bacterial endocarditis are listed below.

1. Identify high-risk individuals by accurately reviewing the health history and questioning the client during assessment.
2. Ensure that preventive antibiotic coverage is administered 1 hour before dental or dental hygiene procedures that produce bacteremias, so optimal blood levels are established.
3. Prevent unnecessary trauma during intraoral procedures, to reduce the severity of the bacteremia.
4. Help the client maintain a high level of oral health through education and skill development to reduce the number of microorganisms in the mouth and the presence of disease.

Valvular Heart Defects

Valvular heart defects are commonly associated with rheumatic fever but also may be caused by congenital abnormalities or may develop after bacterial endocarditis.[8] The three main valves of the heart are the mitral valve, the aortic valve, and the tricuspid valve (see Fig. 29–1). A valve can produce cardiovascular damage if it is malfunctioning. Valvular malfunction can occur by **stenosis,** an incomplete opening of the valve, or **regurgitation,** a backflow of blood through the valve because of incomplete closure.

When malfunction occurs by either stenosis or regurgitation, the left ventricle hypertrophies to compensate for the increased amount of blood. This, in turn, causes the left atrium to hypertrophy, leading to pulmonary congestion and right ventricular failures. The client ultimately develops congestive heart failure if the condition is left untreated.

Corrective surgery is the method of treatment for all valvular heart defects. Most of the valves can be repaired; however, prosthetic valves are available if necessary. During assessment, if the client reports the presence of a prosthetic heart valve or a valvular heart defect, prophylactic antibiotic premedication is needed before dental hygiene care is done. Consultation with the client's physician is recommended to validate the client's current health status.

Mitral Valve Prolapse

Mitral valve prolapse, also known as Barlow syndrome, is one of the most frequently occurring valvular heart defects.[9] When the left ventricle pumps blood to the aorta, the mitral valve flops backward (prolapses) into the left atrium, resulting in a valvular condition termed mitral valve prolapse (MVP). Other names for MVP are "floppy mitral valve syndrome" and the "click murmur syndrome," referring to the sound the valve makes when it flops backward (Fig. 29–2). Although complications are rare with MVP, some do occur. Therefore, the client is always placed on antibiotic premedication for dental hygiene therapy as a precaution (see Chapter 10, Table 10–3).

An **echocardiogram** is the test most often used to determine the presence of MVP. Ultrasound (sound waves) is used to evaluate the heart size, as well as chamber and valve function, during an echocardiogram. The procedure takes approximately 1 hour and produces pictures of the heart with the use of a scanner (transducer).

Clients with MVP may complain of palpitations, chest pain, nervousness, shortness of breath, and dizziness. Treatment is not always necessary and is aimed at alleviating symptoms. Medications are given to control chest pain, slow the heart rate, reduce palpitations, and/or lower anxiety. During client assessment, medications are always recorded on the health history form and reviewed via the *Physician's Desk Reference* to verify action, indications, and contraindications.

Cardiac Arrhythmias

Cardiac arrhythmias are dysfunctions of the **heart rate** and **rhythm.** The dysfunction arises from disturbances in nerve impulse formation or nerve impulse conduction and is categorized according to the part of the heart in which it originates. Common arrhythmias include bradycardia, tachycardia, atrial fibrillation, premature ventricular contractions (PVCs), ventricular fibrillation, and heart block.

Arrhythmias may develop in both normal and diseased hearts. In healthy hearts the arrhythmia may be associated with physical and emotional stresses (e.g., exercise, emotional shock). These arrhythmias usually subside in direct response to stimulus reduction. Diseased hearts develop arrhythmias directly associated with the cardiovascular disease present, most commonly rheumatic heart disease, arteriosclerotic heart disease, and coronary artery heart disease.[8] In some cases, a cardiac arrhythmia may develop in response to drug toxicities and electrolyte imbalances.

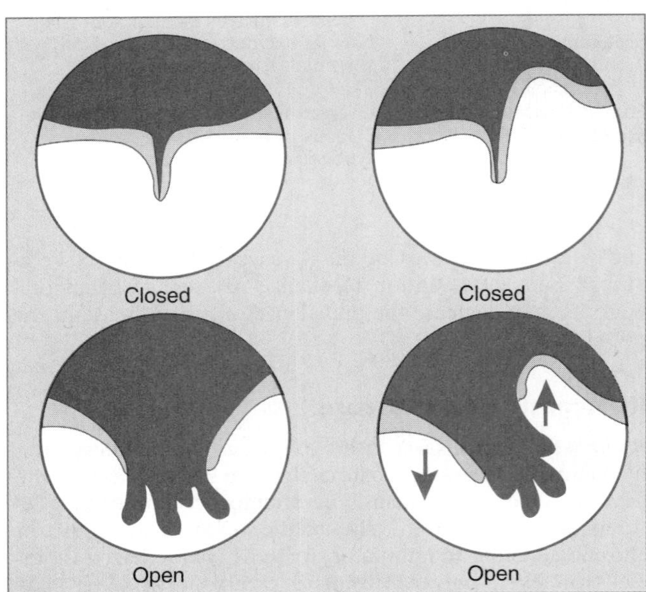

FIGURE 29–2
Diagram of a normal and a prolapsed mitral valve. (Courtesy of Mid-Island Hospital, Bethpage, NY.)

Bradycardia

Bradycardia is defined as slowness of the heart beat, as evidenced by slowing of the pulse rate to less than 60 beats per minute. Naturally this occurs during sleeping; however, increased bradycardia can lead to fainting and convulsions. If during dental hygiene care a client presents with an episode of bradycardia following a normal pulse rate of 80 beats per minute, emergency medical treatment is necessary. This individual may be encountering the initial symptoms of an acute **myocardial infarction** (heart attack). To meet the client's human need for safety, emergency medical treatment would include discontinuance of the dental hygiene appointment, administration of oxygen, and activation of the emergency medical system (EMS).

Tachycardia

Increased heart beat is termed **tachycardia.** This arrhythmia is associated with an abnormally high heart rate, usually above 150 beats per minute. Tachycardia can increase the individual's chance of developing angina pectoris, acute heart failure, pulmonary edema, and myocardial infarction if not controlled.[8] These diseases are related directly to the amount of work the heart is doing and its decreased cardiac output. Treatment consists of antiarrhythmic drug therapy to control tachycardia and reduce the potential of recurrence.

Atrial Fibrillation

An irregularity in ventricular beats, **atrial fibrillation** is the result of inconsistent impulses through the atrioventricular (AV) node transmitted to the ventricles at irregular intervals. During client assessment, the pulse rate may appear consistent with periods of irregular beats. Medical treatment intervention is focused on the causative factors, not on the condition itself. Congestive heart failure, mitral valve stenosis, and hyperthyroidism may be linked to atrial fibrillation.

Premature ventricular contractions (PVCs) are easily identified as pauses in an otherwise normal heart rhythm. The pause develops from an abnormal focus of the ventricle, allowing the ventricle to be at a refractory (resting) period when the impulse for contraction arrives. The feeling of the heart skipping a beat is PVC. PVCs increase with age and are associated with fatigue, emotional stress, and excessive use of coffee and tobacco.

In dental hygiene practice, recognition of PVCs may have some significance in the client with cardiovascular disease. If five or more PVCs are detected during a 60-second pulse examination, medical consultation is strongly recommended. Individuals who are distressed and who have five or more detectable PVCs per minute may be undergoing an acute myocardial infarction or ventricular fibrillation.[10] To meet the client's human need for safety, terminate dental hygiene procedure, place the client on oxygen, and activate the EMS.

Ventricular Fibrillation

Ventricular fibrillation is one of the most lethal arrhythmias. Immediate medical attention is necessary or cardiac arrest will result. This arrhythmia is characterized as an advanced stage of ventricular tachycardia with rapid impulse formation and irregular impulse transmission. The heart rate is rapid, disordered, and contains no rhythm. The immediate medical treatment for ventricular fibrillation is precordial shock, or use of electric current to halt the arrhythmia. The electric current depolarizes the entire myocardium at the time of shock, allowing the cardiac impulses to gain control of the heart rate and rhythm. This should reestablish cardiac regulation. Following precordial shock the person is placed on drug therapy to maintain regulation of the cardiac rate and rhythm.

Heart Block

Heart block is an arrhythmia caused by the blocking of impulses from the atria to the ventricles at the AV node. There are three forms of heart block: first degree, second degree, and third degree. Each form is dangerous; however, third-degree heart block presents the greatest danger, that of **cardiac arrest.**

First-degree heart block is usually associated with coronary artery disease or digitalis drug therapy. The individual with first-degree heart block usually is asymptomatic with a normal heart rate and rhythm. In second-degree heart block, the atrial and ventricular rates are disordered. Impulses from the AV node are fully blocked in irregular patterns. Third-degree heart block is the blocking of all impulses from the atria at the AV node resulting in atrial and ventricular dissociation. The ventricles begin beating in response to their pacemaker cells, producing an independent heart beat from the atrium.

All cardiac arrhythmias are medically diagnosed using an electrocardiogram (ECG) and/or a Holter monitoring system. The ECG is a graphic tracing of the heart's electrical activity. It can determine the heart rate, rhythm, and size. Each arrhythmia is associated with a specific graphic pattern indicating a definitive medical diagnosis.

Cardiac Pacemaker

The **cardiac pacemaker** is an electronic stimulator used to send electrical currents to the myocardium to control or maintain the heart rate. The pacemaker may be designed to control one or both of the heart chambers.

There are two types of pacemakers: temporary and permanent. The temporary pacemaker is used in emergency situations to correct ventricular standstill or arrhythmias that are not responding to other forms of treatment. The permanent pacemaker is inserted into the body and electrodes are transvenously placed in the endocardium and used for 5 to 10 years before battery replacement is necessary.[7] The two general methods of cardiac pacing for the permanent pacemaker are fixed-rate pacing and demand or standby pacing.

Fixed-rate pacing is based on a preset or fixed impulse. Pacemakers operating on a demand or standby pacing system operate only when needed to stimulate ventricular contraction. These systems contain mechanisms that sense when the client has an independent heart beat and stimulates the heart only when the rate deviates from normal. This type of pacing system is most commonly used and is replacing the fixed-rate pacing system because of its increased sensitivity to the body's natural metabolic requirements.[7]

Although the pacemaker helps sustain life in those individuals who without its use would die, technical problems still interfere with its operation (e.g., infection development at the site where the pacemaker is inserted, periodic battery replacement, and dislodgment of the endocardial electrode leads).

Cardiac pacemakers are sensitive to electromagnetic interferences that may alter or cease their function. In dental hygiene practice, devices that apply an electric current directly to the client are most likely to cause interference. These devices include ultrasonic scaling systems, electrode-sensitizing equipment, and pulp testers. To meet the person's human need for safety, client care is modified with respect to these devices because the use of such equipment is contraindicated. Additional protection of the pacemaker can be accomplished by placing a lead apron on the client. The lead apron helps interrupt interferences that may be created by other electronic dental equipment, such as the air polisher, slow- or high-speed handpiece, and electronic periodontal probe.

The physician of record should be contacted to verify clients' needs for prophylactic antibiotic premedication before dental hygiene care. Premedication is usually recommended for the first 6 months following the implantation of the pacemaker.

If the cardiac pacemaker fails or malfunctions during the dental hygiene appointment, the client may experience difficulty breathing, dizziness, a change in the pulse rate, swelling of the legs, ankles, arms, and wrists, and/or chest pain. When this situation arises the following procedures are necessary to meet the client's human need for safety:

1. Turn off all sources of interference.
2. Activate the EMS.
3. Be prepared to administer **cardiopulmonary resuscitation (CPR).**

Hypertensive Cardiovascular Disease

Hypertension is not considered a disease but rather a physical finding or symptom. Hypertension is defined by the American Heart Association as a persistent elevation of the systolic and diastolic blood pressures above 140 mm Hg and 90 mm Hg, respectively.[11] A sustained elevation of the blood pressure affects the heart and leads to hypertensive heart disease resulting in heart failure, myocardial infarction, cerebrovascular accident (stroke), and kidney failure. Therefore, hypertension may be a predisposing factor for vascular diseases or the result of a pathologic condition.

Hypertension affects 60 million people in the United States. However, one-half of the hypertensive population is thought to be undiagnosed. Many diagnosed cases of hypertension are not treated or the treatment is inadequate, leaving the client in an uncontrolled state and his human need for safety in deficit.

Blood pressure evaluation is accomplished by use of a **sphygmomanometer.** This device measures the force of blood through the arteries (systolic pressure) and the force of blood through the arteries when the heart is resting (diastolic pressure). Routine blood pressure evaluations can identify individuals with hypertensive heart disease and should be a component of the dental hygiene assessment. Early identification of these clients minimizes the occurrence of medical emergencies, helps meet the client's human need or safety, and proves life saving for individuals who are unaware of their condition.

There are two major types of hypertension: primary and secondary. Primary hypertension, also known as essential idiopathic hypertension, with etiology unknown, is the most common type, constituting 90% of all cases.[8] It is characterized by a gradual onset or an abrupt onset of short duration. Secondary hypertension is found in 10% of cases and is the result of an existing disease such as those of the cardiovascular system, renal system, adrenal glands, or neurologic system.[8]

Predisposing factors of hypertension include family history, race, stress, obesity, a high dietary intake of saturated fats or sodium, use of tobacco or oral contraceptives, fast-paced lifestyle, and age. With respect to race, it is estimated that 25% of the African-American population has some form of hypertension as opposed to the American whites, who have 11%.[2]

Because hypertension usually follows a chronic course, the client may be asymptomatic. Some of the early clinical signs and symptoms are occipital headaches, vision changes, ringing ears, dizziness, and weakness of the hands and feet. As the condition persists, advanced signs and symptoms can be observed. These include hemorrhages, enlargement of the left ventricle, congestive heart failure, angina pectoris, and renal failure. The dental hygienist should refer clients for medical diagnosis if the client is suspected of having a hypertensive disorder.

Treatment

Treatment of hypertension is based on lifestyle changes and antihypertensive drug therapy. The goal is to reduce and maintain the diastolic pressure level at 90 mm Hg or lower. Some clients need only to watch their dietary consumption of sodium and saturated fats, whereas others must reduce their daily stress level and alter their lifestyle. When a client needs drug therapy, periodic monitoring is essential. Some drugs may stabilize the condition temporarily and then an elevation can occur, indicating an alternative drug selection is needed. Trial and error periods determine the correct drug of choice.

The drugs used for hypertension can be grouped into three categories: diuretics, sympatholytic agents, and vasodilators. Diuretics are used to promote renal excretion of water and sodium ions. The most commonly prescribed diuretic is furosemide (Lasix). Sympatholytic agents modify the sympathetic nerve activity. Some of these drugs include propranolol (Inderal), reserpine (Serpasil), and catapres (Clonidine). The last category of antihypertension drugs is the vasodilator group. These act to increase blood vessel size and facilitate blood flow. Commonly prescribed vasodilators are diazoxide (Hyperstat) and prazosin (Minipress). Although drug therapy is necessary in some cases, side effects do exist and may vary according to dosage. Clients receiving hypertensive drug therapy may experience some or all of the following: fatigue, gastrointestinal disturbances, nausea, diarrhea, cramps, xerostomia, hypotension with dizziness, and depression.

Dental hygiene considerations are related to meeting the client's human need for safety through early identification of hypertension. The anxiety and stress associated with dental and dental hygiene care may raise the client's blood pressure to dangerous levels that may result in a cerebrovascular accident or myocardial infarction. Therefore, to meet the client's human need for freedom from stress, it is important to monitor blood pressure during the assessment phase of the dental hygiene process and consider the measurements in the plan of care. The following four situations have been formulated based on initial blood pressure measurement and family history information. Each situation demonstrates the appropriate dental hygiene care modification necessary to meet a specific human need.

CASE STUDY. NO HISTORY OF HYPERTENSION, ELEVATED BLOOD PRESSURE

During the assessment phase of the dental hygiene appointment, the client reports no history of a hypertensive disorder and no symptoms of hypertension, however, a clinical blood pressure reading of 160/100 mm Hg was obtained. One dental hygiene diagnosis may be a human needs deficit in safety due to a potential for heart attack or stroke as evidenced by an elevated blood pressure of 160/100 mm Hg. The dental hygiene care plan for this individual may include repeated blood pressure measurements during the assessment phase, approximately 10 minutes apart. If, after repeated measurements, the diastolic pressure is still above 100 mm Hg, the appointment should be limited to assessment and planning; no treatment should be implemented. The client must be referred to the physician of record for medical consultation and diagnosis. After medical evaluations have been completed, if the client is classified as nonhypertensive, it can be inferred that anxiety concerning dental hygiene care was the reason for the elevated blood pressure. Blood pressure must be monitored at each appointment thereafter and strategies implemented to meet the client's human need for freedom from stress.

CASE STUDY. CLIENT UNDER TREATMENT FOR HYPERTENSION

During the assessment phase of dental hygiene care, the client indicates that he is hypertensive and under the care of a physician. The client may have a deficit in the human need for freedom from stress and pain, or safety. To meet these human needs, the dental hygiene care plan may include the administration of nitrous oxide-oxygen analgesic to reduce client anxiety.

CASE STUDY. CLIENT NONCOMPLIANT WITH HYPERTENSION TREATMENT

The client indicates that she is hypertensive and has discontinued her medical treatment program. She also indicates that she takes her medication irregularly based on her symptoms. This client has uncontrolled hypertension and has an unmet human need for safety. The dental hygiene process of care for this client is stopped after assessment until her hypertension is stabilized. The client should be referred back to her physician for further medical evaluation and treatment.

Although the dental hygiene care for this client is postponed, the remaining appointment time can be used for facilitating the client's human need for safety via educational strategies directed toward the importance of controlling hypertension and the possible effects if it is left uncontrolled.

CASE STUDY. CLIENT WITH HYPERTENSION AND ACUTE SYMPTOMS

During the assessment phase the client demonstrates hypertension with diastolic readings above 110 mm Hg and symptoms (e.g., headache, dizziness, restlessness, decreased level of consciousness, blurred vision, palpatations) indicative of hypertensive disease. To meet the client's human need for safety, this client should be directed to his physician for immediate medical consultation and evaluation. Dental hygiene treatment should be delayed until the hypertensive disorder is under control.

Because hypertension can be related to anxiety and stress, the dental hygienist must determine if the client has a human need for stress control and, if affirmative, manage the client and environment to reduce the apprehension associated with therapy. Some stress control strategies may include encouraging the client to express fears and concerns; encouraging client participation in goal setting and care plan development, explaining all procedures completely, obtaining informed consent, demonstrating humanistic behaviors, and discussing the client's apprehensions directly.

Coronary Heart Disease

Coronary heart disease, also known as "coronary artery disease" and "ischemic heart disease," is the result of insufficient blood flow from the coronary arteries into the heart or myocardium. The disorders associated with this condition are arteriosclerotic heart disease, angina pectoris, coronary insufficiency, and myocardial infarction. Signs and symptoms generally include chest pain; or discomfort in the jaw, neck, throat, interscapular area, and left arm. Other signs and symptoms are related to the associated disorder.

The prevalence of coronary heart disease is extremely high, affecting over 4 million people in the United States. The occurrence of this disease is influenced by the age, sex, race, diet, lifestyle, and environment of the individual.

Age is considered a factor associated with coronary heart disease after age 40 years. Pathologic changes in the arteries are noticeable with age, usually producing symptoms of disease.

Gender is a predisposing factor in coronary heart disease. For example, men are four times as likely to suffer from the disease as are women up to age 40 years. However, after age 40 years the prevalence of coronary heart disease among women and men is the same. It is important to note that women younger than 40 years are at an increased risk of developing coronary heart disease if they are taking oral contraceptives.

Statistics indicate that race also may be a factor associated with the development of coronary heart disease. White men and nonwhite women are at a higher risk for developing the disease than nonwhite men and white women. Researchers are still trying to determine which genetic factors are involved.

Epidemiologic evidence has demonstrated that populations consuming a low-cholesterol, low-fat diet have little coronary heart disease, whereas populations whose diet consists of foods rich in cholesterol and saturated fat have a very high rate of coronary heart disease.

Social and economical environments can contribute to an individual's chance of developing the disease. The disease is seven times more prevalent in North America than South America and urban populations are at a higher risk than rural dwellers.[7] Cigarette smoking and stressful job situations can also increase an individual's chance of developing the disease at an early age.

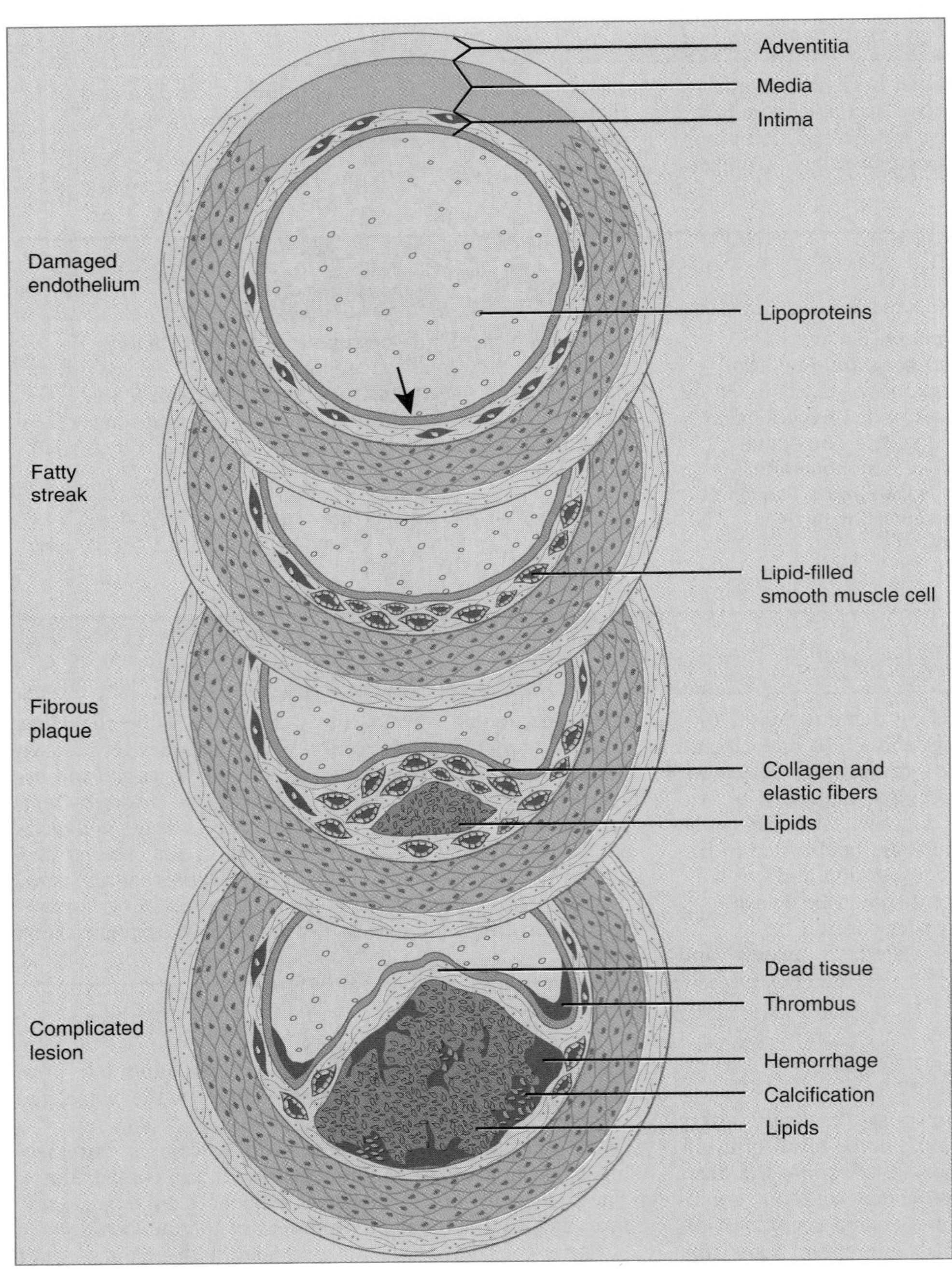

FIGURE 29–3
Types of atherosclerotic lesions. (With permission from Debakey, M., and Grotto, A. The Living Heart. New York: David McKay Publishing Co., 1977.)

The major cause of coronary heart disease is atherosclerosis, a narrowing of the lumen of the coronary arteries thereby reducing the volume of blood flow. The narrowing of the lumen is accomplished by the deposition of fibrofatty substances containing several types of lipids and cholesterol. The deposits thicken with time and eventually close the vessel (Fig. 29–3). Other causes of coronary heart disease are congenital abnormalities of the arteries, changes in the arteries because of infection, vascular changes from autoimmune disorders, and coronary embolism (blood clot).

Atherosclerosis

Atherosclerosis usually develops in high-flow, high-pressure arteries and has been linked to many risk factors. Elevated levels of blood lipids (the result of an increased dietary intake of cholesterol and saturated fat), hypertension, obesity, smoking, stress, diabetes, family history, and insufficient exercise are the most common risk factors.

Prevention of Atherosclerosis Seven behaviors are associated with the prevention of coronary heart disease: regular check-ups, a prudent diet, regular exercise, avoidance of stress, avoidance of tobacco, controlling high blood pressure, and knowledge of the warning signs of a heart attack. If these behaviors are practiced consistently they can reduce the risk of heart disease.

A reduction of saturated fat and cholesterol in the diet has been recommended by the American Heart Association and has gained public attention. Many people are making food choices based on this recommendation. Major food companies are introducing foods that are low in cholesterol and saturated fats, and restaurants are expanding their menu options for diet-conscious patrons.

Food choices to control dental diseases and improve oral health are part of comprehensive dental hygiene care. Factors associated with coronary heart disease must be taken into consideration when providing nutritional dental counseling to a client. In facilitating the client's human need for nutrition, the dental hygienist should be able to recognize the importance of dietary choices related to coronary heart disease and incorporate that knowledge in the nutritional education session. Table 29–2 lists food choices and avoidances for the client at risk for coronary heart disease. This table can be used as a nutritional counseling resource with individuals who have coronary heart disease.

The three basic manifestations of coronary heart disease are angina pectoris, myocardial infarction, and sudden death.

Angina Pectoris

Angina pectoris is the direct result of inadequate oxygen flow to the myocardium. The individual with angina feels a burning, squeezing, or crushing tightness in the chest that radiates to the left arm, neck, and shoulder blade. The person typically clenches his fist over his chest or rubs his left arm when describing the pain. These sudden attacks of angina pectoris usually follow physical exertion, emotional excitement, or exposure to cold.

Medical treatment for angina pectoris is aimed at two goals: (1) to reduce myocardial oxygen demand, and (2) to increase oxygen supply. The method of therapy consists primarily of physical rest to decrease oxygen demand and the administration of nitrates, such as nitroglycerin, to provide more oxygen.

Nitroglycerin (glyceryl trinitrate) is categorized as a vasodilator. It increases blood flow (oxygen supply) by expanding the arteries. Administration can be sublingual for immediate absorption or by nitroglycerin pads and patches for time-released medication absorbed by the skin and incorporated into the bloodstream. Obstructive lesions that do not respond to drug therapy may need surgery.

To meet the client's human need for safety and freedom from stress, dental hygiene considerations associated with angina pectoris include identification of the client's condition and frequency of angina attacks. Clients who report frequent episodes of pain should be referred to their physi-

TABLE 29–2
ALTERNATIVE FOOD CHOICES BASED ON THE CHOLESTEROL–SATURATED FAT INDEX (CSI) FOR CLIENTS AT RISK FOR CORONARY HEART DISEASE

		Choices/Alternatives (scale 1–4) 1 = Best choice, 4 = worst choice			
Food Item	**Avoidances**	**1**	**2**	**3**	**4**
Meats		Fish	Poultry	Lean beef	Fatty beef
Fish		White fish Snapper Perch, sole	Salmon	Shellfish	
Poultry		Chicken (no skin)	Turkey (no skin)		
Beef Pork		10% fat ground sirloin	15% fat ground round	20% fat ground chuck	30% fat ground beef Pork
Lamb		Flank steak		Pot roast	Lamb steaks, chops Roasts
Eggs		Egg whites	Egg substitutes	Whole egg	
Fats	Coconut oil, Palm oil Cocoa butter	Vegetable oil	Soft margarine	Soft shortening	Butter
Cheeses		Pot cheese Low-fat cottage cheese	Cottage cheese	Part-skim mozzarella	Cheese spreads
Frozen desserts	Ice cream	Water ices Sorbets	Sherbert Frozen yogurt	Ice milk	Ice cream 10%

cian of record. Dental hygiene appointments should be short in duration and preferably scheduled for the morning. The atmosphere should be friendly and conducive to relaxation. If the client becomes fatigued or develops significant changes in pulse rate or rhythm during the appointment, termination of the appointment is suggested.

Dental Hygiene Care for the Client With Angina Pectoris

Prior to initiating dental hygiene care for a client with a history of angina pectoris, the client's supply of nitroglycerin should be placed within reach of the dental hygienist. The potency of nitroglycerin is lost after 6 months outside of a sealed container; consequently, fresh supplies should be available in the oral healthcare environment. If an emergency develops, dental treatment should be stopped and the client placed in an upright position. The client should be reassured and given nitroglycerin sublingually. The EMS should be called if the client continues to experience pain after the administration of nitroglycerin. Vital signs must be monitored and the results recorded on the client's record.

Myocardial Infarction

Myocardial infarction, the second manifestation of coronary heart disease and one of the leading causes of death in the United States,[8] is defined as a reduction of blood flow through one of the coronary arteries, resulting in an infarct. An infarct is an area of tissue that undergoes necrosis because of the elimination of blood flow. A myocardial infarction is commonly known as a heart attack.

The predisposing factors associated with myocardial infarction are similar to those found in atherosclerosis because the major etiology is arterial blockage. Some myocardial infarctions result in death, whereas others produce cardiac complications. Sudden death from myocardial infarctions usually occurs before hospitalization and within 1 hour of the onset of symptoms and may be the result of ventricular fibrillation.

Symptoms associated with a myocardial infarction are similar to those experienced by an individual with angina pectoris; however, the pain usually persists for 12 or more hours and begins as a feeling of indigestion. Other clinical manifestations include a feeling of fatigue, nausea, vomiting, and shortness of breath.

Treatment A combination of therapies to reduce cardiac workloads and increase cardiac output is the currently suggested treatment. Cardiac workload reduction therapies include bed rest, morphine for pain reduction and sedation, and oxygen if necessary. To increase cardiac output, therapy associated with the control and reduction of cardiac arrhythmias is recommended. Medical treatment includes antiarrhythmic drugs and possibly a cardiac pacemaker. Nitroglycerin is indicated to relieve chest pain and increase the cardiac output by intensifying the blood flow and redistributing blood to the affected myocardial tissue.

Dental Hygiene Care for the Client With Myocardial Infarction

Dental hygiene therapy is complicated if the client is on anticoagulant drug therapy to reduce the possibility of another heart attack. Anticoagulants increase bleeding time and may have to be stopped several days prior to dental hygiene or surgical treatment that involves tissue manipulation. Some cardiologists believe that it is more dangerous to take the individual off the anticoagulant than it is to keep the individual on the drug and provide care; therefore, confirmation from the client's cardiologist is recommended to meet the client's human needs for safety. Other changes associated with dental or dental hygiene care include consultation with the attending physician to verify the client's condition and to discuss client management associated with the prescribed dental hygiene care. Arranging for appointments in the morning and for shorter-than-usual intervals should be undertaken to reduce stress and anxiety, thereby facilitating the client's human need for freedom from stress.

Emergency situations that arise in the oral healthcare setting resulting in a myocardial infarction should be managed by an emergency medical team. Oral health professionals are responsible for monitoring vital signs, administration of nitroglycerin, and the performance of CPR if the client undergoes cardiac arrest. CPR certification should be maintained by all oral health professionals.

The last manifestation of coronary heart disease is sudden death. Sudden death occurs during the first 24 to 48 hours after the onset of symptoms. The majority of sudden cardiovascular deaths are caused by ventricular fibrillation. For example, ventricular fibrillation results in ventricular standstill (cardiac arrest) if insufficient blood is pumped into the coronary arteries to supply the myocardium with oxygen. Biologic death results when oxygen delivery to the brain is inadequate for 4 to 6 minutes. Therefore, CPR must be administered to maintain enough blood oxygen to sustain life. Transportation to the hospital for emergency medical care is necessary.

Congestive Heart Failure

Congestive heart failure is defined as a syndrome characterized by myocardial dysfunction that leads to diminished cardiac output or abnormal circulatory congestion. The weakened heart develops compensatory mechanisms to continue to function. These mechanisms include tachycardia, ventricular dilation, and enlargement of the heart muscle.

The causative factors associated with congestive heart failure are arteriosclerotic heart disease, hypertensive cardiovascular disease, valvular heart disease, pericarditis, circulatory overload, and coronary heart disease. Each of these factors contributes to the gradual failure of the heart by one of the following mechanisms reducing the inflow of blood to the heart, increasing the inflow to the heart, obstructing the outflow of blood from the heart, or damaging the heart muscle itself.

Congestive heart failure can occur as two independent failures, termed left-sided and right-sided heart failure. However, because the heart functions as a closed unit, both pumps need to be functioning properly or the efficiency of the heart is diminished.

Medical treatment of congestive heart failure is directly related to the removal of the cause. Usually the corrective therapy associated with the underlying disease eliminates the presence of congestive heart failure. Some cases require additional methods of rehabilitation such as dietary control, reduced physical activity, and drug therapy. Drugs most frequently used for the control of congestive heart failure are diuretics and digitalis. Diuretics are used to reduce the retention of salt and water; digitalis is used to strengthen myocardial contractility.

Dental Hygiene Care for the Client With Congestive Heart Failure

Dental hygiene care usually is not altered for the client with congestive heart failure if the individual has a monitored condition. However, some precautions should be taken. Clients taking digitalis are prone to develop nausea and vomiting during dental procedures.[12] Therefore, procedures that may promote gagging should be performed with extra care. In addition, the dental hygienist should be aware of any underlying heart conditions that are responsible for the congestive heart failure. These conditions must be evaluated and appropriate precautions taken.

The major adjustment in the dental hygiene care plan for a client with left-sided congestive heart failure is related to client-operator positioning. Because the client has difficulty breathing in a supine position, and to meet the client's human need for safety and freedom from pain and stress, the correct position is upright inclined. Therefore, operator positioning must be changed to compensate for the client's repositioning. The dental hygienist must remember that although the client-operator positioning has been altered, the principles of instrumentation must be maintained.

If an emergency arises with a client who has congestive heart failure, medical assistance should be obtained. The client is usually conscious and demonstrating difficulty breathing. The mode of treatment is to position the person upright to facilitate breathing, administer oxygen if necessary, and monitor vital signs.

Congenital Heart Disease

Congenital heart disease affects approximately 1% of live births and constitutes 3% of all cases of heart disease after infancy.[12] There are many types of congenital heart malformations. Those most commonly observed are the ventricular septal defect, the atrial septal defect, and the patent ductus arteriosus.

The etiology of congenital heart disease is generally unknown; however, genetic and environmental factors have been attributed to poor intrauterine development. Genetic conditions are related to heredity and are apparent in some situations. The environmental factors are based on the health of the mother. Rubella (German measles) and drug addiction have produced delayed fetal development and growth retardation associated with the cardiovascular structure.

Ventricular Septal Defects

Ventricular septal defects are responsible for up to 30% of all congenital heart defects and are described as a **shunt** (opening) in the septum between the ventricles.[5] The opening allows the oxygenated blood from the left ventricle to flow into the right ventricle, as shown in Figure 29–4. Small defects that close spontaneously or are correctable by surgery have a good prognosis. Larger defects that are left untreated or are irreparable usually result in death from secondary cardiovascular complications. The ventricular septal defect can be detected by a characteristic heart murmur audible at birth.

Clinical manifestations of ventricular septal defects vary with the size of the defect, infant age, and the effect of the deviated blood passage on the cardiovascular structure. Large ventricular septal defects cause hypertrophy of the ventricles, resulting in congestive heart failure.

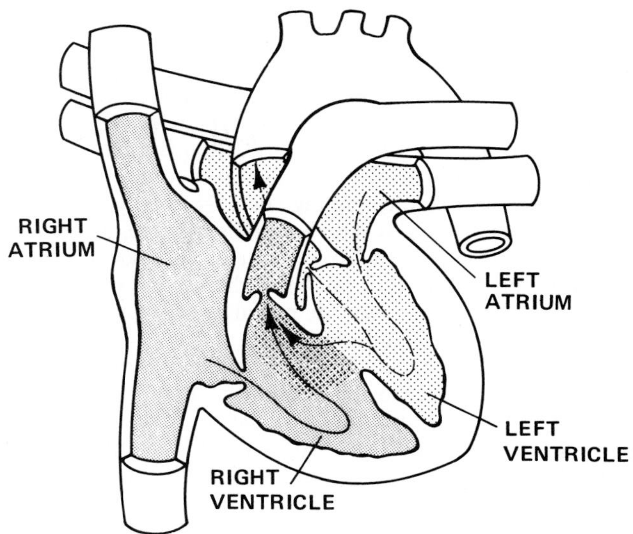

FIGURE 29–4
Ventricular septal defect. (With permission from Bleck, E., and Nagel, D. Physically Handicapped Children: A Medical Atlas for Teachers, 2nd ed. Needham Heights, MA: Allyn & Bacon, 1982.)

Atrial Septal Defect

The atrial septal defect, described as a shunt (opening) between the left and right atria, is responsible for approximately 10% of congenital heart defects. The blood volume overload eventually causes the right atrium to enlarge and the right ventricle to dilate (Fig. 29–5).

Clinical manifestations related to atrial septal defects are few. The client usually is asymptomatic and the defect goes undetected. However, in adults, clinical symptoms become more pronounced. The client is easily fatigued and becomes short of breath after mild exertion. Treatment includes cardiovascular repair surgery, observance of developing atrial arrhythmias, and monitoring of vital signs.

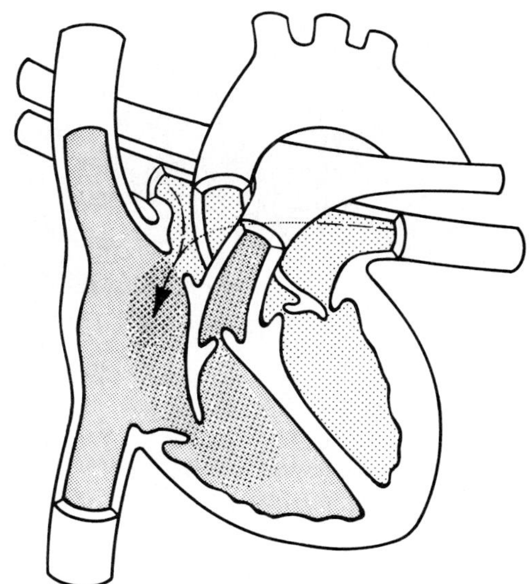

FIGURE 29–5
Atrial septal defect. (With permission from Bleck, E., and Nagel, D. Physically Handicapped Children: A Medical Atlas for Teachers, 2nd ed. Needham Heights, MA: Allyn & Bacon, 1982.)

Patent Ductus Arteriosus

The congenital heart defect termed "patent ductus arteriosus" affects twice as many females as males and is the most common congenital heart defect found in adults.[5] During development, the fetal heart contains a blood vessel called the "ductus arteriosus." This vessel connects the pulmonary artery to the descending aorta. Normally, following birth the vessel closes. If the vessel fails to close, a congenital heart defect is formed. Failure to close is associated with premature births and thus failure of the vessel's contracture necessary for closure. Patent ductus arteriosus also has been linked to the rubella syndrome.

The shunting of blood in a patent ductus arteriosus defect is from the aorta to the pulmonary artery (Fig. 29–6). This type of blood flow results in the recirculation of oxygenated blood through the lungs. Thus, the left atrium and ventricle have an increased workload from increased pulmonary blood return, which can result in congestive heart failure. If left untreated, severe obstructive pulmonary vascular disease may develop.

Clinical manifestations of patent ductus arteriosus include respiratory distress, susceptibility to respiratory tract infections, and slow motor development. Treatment consists of surgical correction and the elimination of symptoms associated with secondary complications.

Tetralogy of Fallot

Tetralogy of Fallot is a rare and complex congenital heart defect. It is generally associated with cyanosis. The defect is composed of four congenital abnormalities: ventricular septal defect, pulmonary stenosis, right ventricular hypertrophy, and malposition of the aorta.[5] The blood shunts right to left through the ventricular septal defect, permitting unoxygenated blood to mix with oxygenated blood, resulting in cyanosis. Treatment of this defect includes measures to relieve cyanosis, and palliative and corrective surgery.

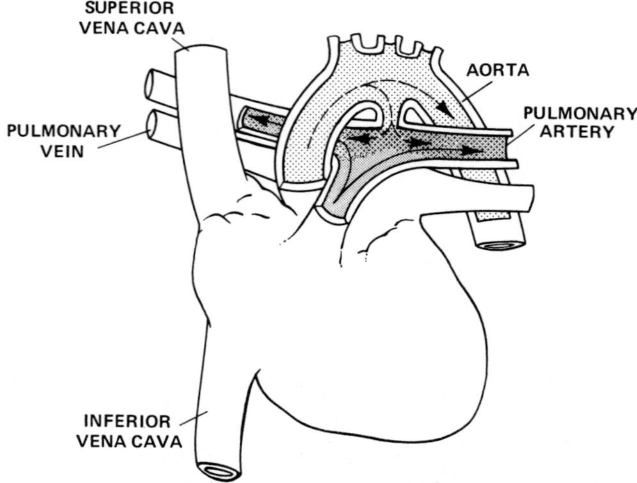

FIGURE 29–6
Patent ductus arteriosus defect. (With permission from Bleck, E., and Nagel, D. Physically Handicapped Children: A Medical Atlas for Teachers, 2nd ed. Needham Heights, MA: Allyn & Bacon, 1982.)

Dental Hygiene Care for the Client With Congenital Heart Disease

Because many of the clients with congenital heart defects are susceptible to bacterial endocarditis, the primary concern of the dental hygienist is prevention of this life-threatening condition. Even those clients who have had surgery to correct congenital defects are susceptible during the healing phase. Prophylactic antibiotic coverage suggested for the client with congenital heart disease is the same as for the client with rheumatic heart disease (see Chapter 10, Table 10–3). Secondary concerns are focused toward the management of cardiovascular complications such as congestive heart failure and cardiac arrhythmias resulting from the congenital defect.

Dental hygiene care for the client with congenital heart disease includes medical consultation to confirm drug usage and the current medical status, prophylactic antibiotic coverage to prevent bacterial endocarditis, and assessment of symptoms secondary to the disease that may indicate treatment alteration.

CARDIOVASCULAR SURGERY

Cardiovascular surgery has revolutionized medical treatment for the individual with certain cardiovascular diseases. It is now possible to perform heart transplants, repair congenital heart lesions, and replace diseased heart valves. Procedures used to surgically treat heart disease can be classified into two categories: open and closed.

Open heart surgery is necessary for those procedures that are complex and need direct visualization of the heart while being performed. Examples are heart transplants, heart valve replacements, and coronary bypass surgery. This type of surgery is always performed with the use of a heart-lung machine. The machine completely controls cardiopulmonary function, enabling surgeons to operate for long periods of time without interfering with the individual's metabolic needs.

Coronary Bypass Surgery

Coronary bypass surgery is a common procedure used to replace closed arteries. The American Heart Association estimated that 332,000 bypass operations were conducted in 1987. The procedure is performed by removing a part of the leg vein or chest artery and then grafting it onto the coronary artery, thereby creating a new passageway for the blood. This type of surgery can be done for more than one artery at a time and is named accordingly (double bypass, triple bypass). The benefits of coronary bypass surgery include relief from angina, increased tolerance to exercise, improved quality of life, and extended life span.[13] A person who has had a bypass operation has no contraindications to dental hygiene therapy.

Valvular defect repair or replacement also is performed frequently. Prosthetic cardiac valves for valve replacement have been available for 25 years and outcome after surgery has steadily improved.[13] However, clients with artificial heart valves are especially susceptible to infections. Individuals who have artificial heart valves must be premedicated with an antibiotic prior to dental hygiene care.

Heart Transplantation

Heart transplantation is a viable option for individuals with end-stage heart disease in which no other therapeutic intervention is considered effective. One hundred twenty hospitals in the United States perform cardiac transplantation; however, the dilemma associated with this therapeutic approach is finding donors. The waiting period has doubled from 7 days in 1985 to 2 weeks in 1986 and is increasing annually.[14]

Future goals and implications of heart transplantation include the development of a safe, reliable, permanent, totally implantable artificial heart device. Ideally, the device should allow a recipient to carry out normal activities. The development of such a device may increase availability of this lifesaving procedure for those eligible recipients who at this time await donors.

Dental Hygiene Care for the Client Who Has Had a Heart Transplant

A major concern of the heart transplant patient is infection and transplant rejection. Prior to performing dental hygiene care, consultation with the client's cardiologist is recommended to determine if additional premedication is indicated. Most transplant patients are put on long-term preventive antibiotic therapy to control systemic bacteremias and reduce the possibility of transplant rejection. If possible, dental and dental hygiene care should be performed prior to cardiac surgery to eliminate the presence of active oral infection and to control dental diseases over the remaining life span. Such an approach not only meets the client's human need for skin and mucous membrane integrity but also empowers the individual with responsibility over his oral health status. The client's feeling of self-determination over oral health is particularly important at a time when control over cardiac health is impossible.

Closed Heart Surgery

Closed heart surgery is usually associated with **cardiac catheterization.** The most common closed heart surgery is termed **angioplasty.** The procedure involves the use of a catheter (a long, slender tube) with a tiny balloon at the end that is inserted into the coronary artery. Specifically, the balloon is inserted in places where the artery narrows, inflated to flatten fatty deposits, and deflated to allow the increased blood flow to compress and redistribute the atherosclerotic lesion. This procedure is recommended for those individuals who have a small atherosclerotic lesion constricting blood flow. If the lesion cannot be corrected by the angioplasty procedure, bypass surgery may be necessary.

Dental Hygiene Care for the Client Who Has Had Closed Heart Surgery

No contraindications are associated with dental or dental hygiene treatment unless the individual is taking anticoagulant medication. As in all cardiac-associated situations, consultation with the client's cardiologist is recommended.

ORAL MANIFESTATIONS OF CARDIOVASCULAR MEDICATIONS

Some medications used in cardiovascular disease therapy have a profound effect on the oral cavity and may cause a disturbance in the client's human need for skin and mucous membrane integrity, a biologically sound dentition, and/or safety. These medications typically include those that treat hypertension (diuretics), heart transplant stabilization (immunosuppressants), and coronary heart disease (anticoagulants). Individuals taking these medications should seek regular dental hygiene care to compensate for their increased vulnerability to dental and periodontal diseases.

Most medications used for the treatment of hypertension have the side effect of xerostomia. This condition can increase the individual's risk of developing dental caries and periodontal disease by reducing the amount of salivary flow and may lead to dental hygiene diagnosis of defects in the human needs for sound dentition and for skin and mucous membrane integrity of the head and neck, respectively. In addition, those individuals who have exposed root surfaces are extremely susceptible to root surface caries. Self-administered fluoride therapy and the use of saliva substitutes should be incorporated into the individual's home care regimen.

Immunosuppresants used for the stabilization of heart transplants increase the individual's risk of developing periodontal disease or may exaggerate a preexisting condition, leading to a dental hygiene diagnoses of a deficit in skin and mucous membrane integrity. Another dental hygiene diagnosis to consider is a deficit in the human need for safety because immunosuppressants place the individual at risk for developing opportunistic infections of the oral cavity such as candidiasis, herpes simplex, herpes zoster, and acute necrotizing ulcerative gingivitis (ANUG). In addition to regular professional dental hygiene care, these individuals should be instructed to use antimicrobial mouth rinses as part of their home care regimen to reduce the threat of disease.

Blood thinners (anticoagulants) are used in the therapy for coronary heart disease. Persons with a history of heart attack or cerebrovascular accident usually are placed on this type of medication to increase blood flow. The side effects are prolonged bleeding and spontaneous oral bleeding in the presence of infection. These individuals must maintain a healthy periodontium to reduce the possibility of periodontal disease. Professional oral hygiene care and preventive home care practices that appeal to the client's human needs for self-determination, safety, and value of oral health provide a framework within which optimal oral wellness can be maintained.

DENTAL HYGIENE PROCESS OF CARE

The individual who is identified as having a cardiovascular disease, symptom, or defect is a special needs client. This type of client is considered at high risk, one whose life may be threatened by daily activities. High-risk clients have a human need for safety because they increase the possibility of having emergency situations in the oral healthcare setting. These high-risk patients also may increase the chance of lawsuits arising from the application of certain treatment procedures.

Managing the client with cardiovascular disease begins with applying the dental hygiene process of care within a human needs framework.

Assessment

When assessing the individual with a potential cardiovascular disease the current medical status becomes important. The dental hygienist must verify the type of cardiovascular disease present to provide safe and effective care. Because many individuals do not know they are affected, the assessment process becomes a challenge. Vital signs play an important role in determining cases of hypertension, cardiac arrhythmias, and congestive heart disorders. Health histories reveal behaviors such as difficulty breathing upon mild exertion and use of extra pillows to sleep, which may be indicative of an underlying cardiovascular disease.

When clinical data suggest a potential cardiac problem, the dental hygienist, as a client advocate, should request that the individual consult with a physician for further evaluation. Clinical findings that suggest a potential cardiovascular problem always should be shared with the client to alleviate any unnecessary fears and to encourage adherence with the dental hygienist's recommendation to seek medical consultation. Direct client-practitioner communication may put the individual at ease and demonstrate concern from the health professional. All dental and dental hygiene procedures should be postponed until a definitive medical diagnosis is obtained.

If the disease is known and reported on the health history, the dental hygienist must verify the current status with the physician of record prior to initiating dental hygiene care. Determining the current status of a cardiovascular disease includes its onset, treatment, and degree of severity. Verification can be conducted by consulting the individual's physician and/or questioning the client.

In addition to identifying the disease, the dental hygienist must determine the type of medical care the client is undergoing (drug therapy, surgical intervention, cardiac pacemaker implantation, etc.). As previously discussed, certain cardiovascular therapies influence the planning and implementation of dental hygiene care. The *Physician's Desk Reference* and *Merck Manual* should be available in the healthcare setting to assist the dental hygienist in determining treatment precautions.

After assessing the client's state of health, the dental hygienist must analyze these findings and make a dental hygiene diagnosis that identifies the actual or potential human need deficit related to oral health and disease.

There are several key human needs of the individual with cardiovascular disease that can be identified during the health history and dental history interview and intra- and extraoral examination. These include the human need for a wholesome body image, freedom from pain and stress, nutrition, safety, and value system. Other human needs also may be apparent. Each person should be assessed as an individual to identify human needs and to gather information necessary to motivate the client toward oral health.

A disturbance in the individual's body image may occur as a result of having to live with cardiovascular disease. The potential for optimal oral health, a direct benefit of dental hygiene care, can facilitate one's perception of body image.

Freedom from pain and stress associated with cardiovascular disease includes both physical and emotional stressors. The client generally has systemic pain from the cardiovascular disease and emotional distress from the treatment methods and life-threatening implications of the disease.

The assessment of physical pain is based on objective and subjective data. The most common physical pain of the individual with cardiovascular disease identified during the assessment phase is chest pain accompanied by difficulty breathing. If the client complains of physical pain that cannot be alleviated, referral to the physician is recommended. If the pain is associated with dental hygiene procedures, alterations in the care plan are necessary to meet the client's need for freedom from pain.

Treatment of cardiovascular disease may cause emotional stress to the client. Cardiovascular surgery, dietary restrictions, and side effects of drug therapy contribute to emotional distress because they alter the individual's lifestyle. The oral healthcare environment can augment the **anxiety** in an individual who is already having difficulty adapting to stress. Stress control strategies must be implemented consciously as a therapeutic dental hygiene intervention if the client's human need for freedom from stress is to be met.

Dietary restrictions may have a negative emotional effect on the individual with cardiovascular disease. Foods are closely related to lifestyle, habits, financial status, overall feelings of well-being, and cultural background. Some individuals experience difficulty adjusting to special dietary requirements. Many people enjoy mealtime and the social interaction and relaxation that it brings. When dietary behaviors are restricted or controlled, the individual may become depressed. The healthcare professional should recognize the actual or potential alteration in the human need for nutrition created in the client with cardiovascular disease. Interacting with the client to find food substitutions that are appealing and that support oral and cardiovascular health is a helpful strategy.

Safety is a human need related to dental hygiene care and the individual with cardiovascular disease. It is a fact that oral procedures cause the potential for infection, stress, anxiety, and fear. If the client's safety is not ensured, the potential for a life-threatening medical emergency is increased.

The client with cardiovascular disease is at risk in stressful situations, especially those who have angina pectoris, hypertension, previous myocardial infarctions, and congestive heart failure. The assessment of this human need is accomplished by monitoring the client's reactions to dental hygiene procedures and assessing past responses in responses in oral healthcare situations. Muscular tenseness, excessive perspiration, and verbal cues are indications of a potential emergency and mean that the client's need for safety is not being met.

Individuals with cardiovascular disease may have an oral health values deficit and may place dental hygiene care low on their priority list. Understandably, these individuals typically are more concerned with their life-threatening medical condition than with preventing oral diseases. However, an accurate assessment of the client's personal beliefs, behaviors, and values can identify motivators (needs) that can lead to a commitment to therapeutic goals and priorities (Fig. 29–7).

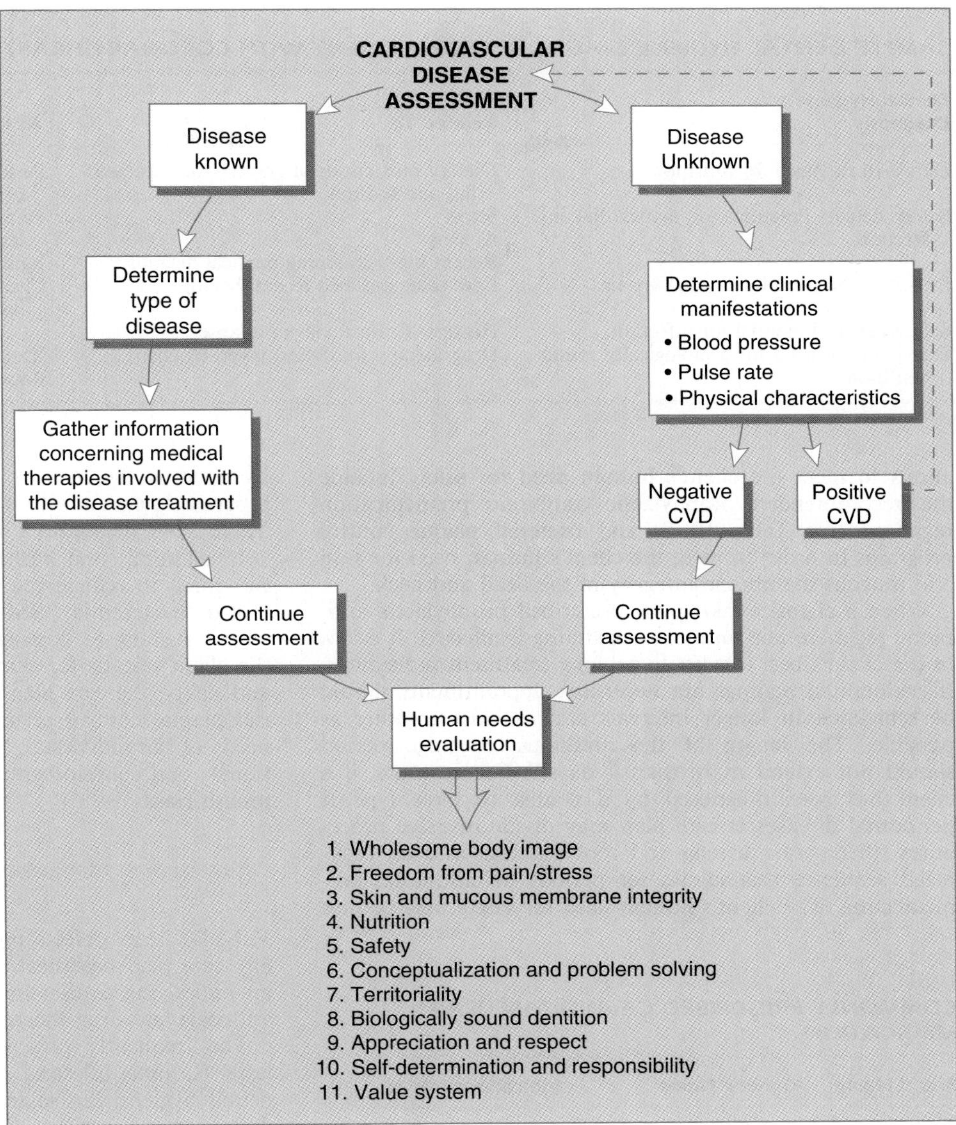

FIGURE 29-7
Dental hygiene assessment flow chart for the individual with a potential for cardiovascular disease.

Dental Hygiene Diagnosis

Dental hygiene diagnoses identify human need deficits based on information known about the client to direct dental hygiene care in a holistic and humanistic fashion. After the dental hygiene diagnoses are verified, the dental hygiene care plan can be developed with the client. As changes occur in the client's human needs as evidenced by his physical and psychological condition, the dental hygiene diagnoses change, and consequently the care plan is revised.

Diseases of the cardiovascular system give rise to several human needs related to the condition and its treatment that can be addressed through professional dental hygiene care. Table 29-3 illustrates sample dental hygiene diagnoses for a client with coronary heart disease.

The dental hygiene care plan formulated for the client with cardiovascular disease is complex, and many factors influence the care plan development. Care planning is one way to prevent unnecessary emergencies and ensure that the unique client human need deficits are the focus of the therapeutic interventions.

When developing a dental hygiene care plan for the client, special attention should be given to drug therapies to ensure that no contraindications are present and that oral cavity side effects are identified. Table 29-4 lists the most commonly prescribed drugs for the treatment of cardiovascular disease.

In addition to drug therapies, the client's cardiovascular disease characteristics and the human need deficits they precipitate should be evaluated for their potential to influence dental hygiene interventions. Tables 29-5 and 29-6 list dental hygiene care precautions related to clients with various cardiovascular diseases. These tables can be used when developing the dental hygiene care plan for the client with a cardiovascular disease.

Care Planning for Clients With Rheumatic Heart Disease

The client with rheumatic heart disease is susceptible to bacterial endocarditis as a result of dental hygiene procedures that cause a transient bacteremia. Care plan consider-

TABLE 29–3
SAMPLE DENTAL HYGIENE DIAGNOSES FOR A CLIENT WITH CORONARY HEART DISEASE

Dental Hygiene Diagnosis	Related To	As Evidenced By
Deficit in the need for nutrition	Dietary restrictions of cholesterol, saturated fat, and sodium	Periods of depression and frustration concerning dietary habits
Safety deficit: Potential for myocardial infarction	Stress Anxiety Recent life-threatening medical diagnosis	Pain in chest, jaw, neck, throat, interscapular area, and left arm Agitation
Deficit in the need for a value system	Low value ascribed to oral health	Client reports a lack of interest in performing daily oral hygiene care
Safety deficit: Potential for infection	History of mitral valve prolapse	
Deficit in the need for a biologically sound dentition	Drug therapy (diuretics) taken by client	Xerostomia Root caries

ations to meet the client's human need for safety include the recommended prophylactic antibiotic premedication regimens (see Table 10–3) and bacterial plaque control programs in order to meet the client's human need for skin and mucous membrane integrity of the head and neck.

When a client is taking the prescribed prophylactic antibiotic regimen, appointment scheduling is affected. It is not in the client's best interest to prolong treatment procedures. If periodontal scalings are necessary, appointments should be scheduled in longer intervals and as close together as possible. The length of the antibiotic coverage period should not extend more than 7 days.[15] For example, if a client has been diagnosed by a dentist to have type II peridontal diseases, a care plan may divide invasive procedures (therapeutic scaling and root planing) into an organized sequence that allows for periods off antibiotic premedication. The client's human need for safety may be met by dividing the invasive treatment appointments into two separate intervals with a lag time separating each interval. Table 29–7 illustrates a sample dental hygiene care plan.

In addition, oral health stability must be maintained by the client to reduce the possibility of developing a self-inflicted bacteremia. Self-inflicted bacteremias can occur when brushing or flossing in a diseased condition. To meet the client's needs for skin and mucous membrane integrity and safety, the care plan should include an extensive bacterial plaque control program designed to meet the unique needs of the individual. Such a program may include additional oral physiotherapy aids and daily antimicrobial mouth rinses.

TABLE 29–4
COMMONLY PRESCRIBED CARDIOVASCULAR MEDICATION

Brand Name	Generic Name	Indications for Use
Glycosides		
Lanoxin	Digoxin	Congestive heart failure Atrial fibrillation
Diuretics		
Dyazide Maxide Lasix	Triamterene Hydrochlorothiazide Furosemide	Congestive heart failure and hypertension
Beta Blockers		
Tenormin Inderal Lopressor	Atenolol Propranolol Metoprolol	Hypertension and angina
Calcium Channel Blockers		
Cardizem Procardia Calan	Diltiazem Nifedipine Verapamil	Hypertension and angina
ACE (Angiotensin Converting Enzyme) Inhibitors		
Capoten Vasotec	Captopril Enalapril	Hypertension

Care Planning for Clients With Valvular Heart Defects

Valvular heart defects present in the client do not require any care plan modifications unless they are associated with an underlying cardiovascular condition or are treated with anticoagulant drug therapy.

The frequently prescribed anticoagulants heparin, warfarin (Coumadin), and indanedione derivatives affect the dental hygiene care plan if scaling or root planing procedures are indicated or if the gingivae have a tendency to bleed spontaneously.

When the client is taking anticoagulant therapy, the client's physician should be consulted to determine if a reduction should be made in the dosage of anticoagulant medication or if it is safer for the client to maintain the prescribed dosage. The reduction in medication dosage should increase the normal prothrombin time by 2 seconds. The normal prothrombin time varies between 10 and 16 seconds; the optimal prothrombin time for dental hygiene therapy should be between 20 and 32 seconds on the day of the scheduled procedure.[16]

When damaged heart valves are replaced by prosthetic valves, the area is considered susceptible to bacterial endocarditis and the client has a deficit in the human need for safety related to dental hygiene care. Care plan modifications should follow the standard prophylactic antibiotic regimen listed in Table 10–3 (see Chapter 10).

Care Planning for Clients With Hypertensive Disorders

Dental hygiene care for the hypertensive individual is planned according to the actual or potential human need deficit of the client. If the individual's hypertension is un-

TABLE 29–5

QUICK REFERENCE TO THE SIGNS, SYMPTOMS, AND TREATMENT OF INDIVIDUALS WITH CARDIOVASCULAR DISEASES

Disease	Signs and Symptoms	Medical and Surgical Treatment
Rheumatic heart disease	Carditis, polyarthritis, chorea, erythema marginatum, subcutaneous nodules, fever	Bed rest and medications associated with manifestations
Bacterial endocarditis	Initial high fever, cardiac decompensation, heart murmur	Antibiotic therapy
Valvular heart defects	Fatigue, shortness of breath, and pulmonary edema If left untreated congestive heart failure will develop	Valvular repair of replacement with a prosthetic heart valve
Mitral valve prolapse	Palpitation, chest pain, nervousness, shortness of breath, dizziness	Treatment is not always necessary and is aimed at alleviating symptoms
Cardiac arrhythmias	Bradycardia: pulse rate less than 60 beats/minute Tachycardia: pulse rate above 150 beats/minute	Antiarrhythmic drug therapy or cardiac pacemaker
Hypertension	Headache, fatigue, diminished exercise tolerance, shortness of breath	Antihypertension drug therapy and dietary control of sodium
Coronary "ischemic" heart disease	Angina pectoris, discomfort in jaw, neck, throat, interscapular area, left arm	Bed rest and administration of nitroglycerin
Congestive heart failure	Fatigue, weakness, dyspnea, cough, anorexia	Treatment is directed at the underlying etiology
Congenital heart disease	Dependent on type of defect	Surgery to correct defect

TABLE 29–6

QUICK REFERENCE TO DENTAL HYGIENE CARE IMPLICATIONS FOR INDIVIDUALS WITH CARDIOVASCULAR DISEASE

Disease	Implications for Dental Hygiene Care	Dental Hygiene Care Precautions
Rheumatic heart disease	When carditis is present the client is susceptible to bacterial endocarditis and requires antibiotic premedication prior to invasive dental hygiene therapy Special attention should be given to home care practices because self-inflicted bacteremias may occur when oral disease is present	Careful manipulation of soft tissues during instrumentation to reduce the presence of a transient bacteremia
Bacterial endocarditis	Client susceptible to reinfection in the presence of a transient bacteremia Prophylactic antibiotic premedication is indicated for invasive dental hygiene procedures	Invasive dental hygiene procedures should include careful manipulation of soft tissue
Valvular heart defects	Bacterial endocarditis may occur following dental hygiene procedures that cause transient bacteremias Clients receiving anticoagulant medication may have a prolonged bleeding time	If anticoagulant medication is being used and scaling procedures are planned, the dosage of anticoagulant medication should be discussed with the client's cardiologist
Mitral valve prolapse	Prophylactic antibiotic premedication given as a precaution	Careful manipulation of soft tissue during invasive dental hygiene procedures.
Cardiac arrhythmias	Electrical interferences can cause pacemaker malfunction	Usage of dental hygiene equipment that interferes with pacemaker function is contraindicated
Hypertension	Stress and anxiety associated with dental hygiene treatment may increase blood pressure	If blood pressure is uncontrolled, dental hygiene care is contraindicated Implement stress and anxiety-reducing strategies; create atmosphere conducive to relaxation
Coronary "ischemic" heart disease	Stress and anxiety associated with dental hygiene treatment may precipitate an angina attack	Nitroglycerin should be available during dental hygiene treatment Implement stress- and anxiety-reducing strategies; create atmosphere conducive to relaxation
Congestive heart failure	None if patient is under appropriate medical care	Client should be treated in upright position to decrease fluid collection in the lungs

TABLE 29-7
SAMPLE DENTAL HYGIENE CARE PLAN FOR A CLIENT TAKING PROPHYLACTIC ANTIBIOTIC PREMEDICATION

Dental Hygiene Diagnosis	Goal	Expected Outcomes	Dental Hygiene Interventions
Safety deficit: Potential for developing a resistance to prescribed antibiotic if taken for more than 7 days at a time Deficit in the skin and mucous membrane integrity of the head and neck	Complete invasive dental hygiene treatment so that the antibiotic coverage period does not extend past 7 days Reduce gingival bleeding by 9/92 Reduce periodontal probing depths by 9/92	Complete chart of periodontal probing depths Dentition and periodontium free from soft and hard deposits Root surfaces smooth and free from diseased cementum Bleeding index score reduced by 50% Periodontal probing depths reduced by at least 1 mm	Schedule treatment into five appointments Week 1, appointments one and two, probe entire mouth, scale and root plane maxilla; bacterial plaque control with toothbrush and floss Week 2, host response time, no treatment Week 3, appointments four and five, evaluate tissue state of maxilla; scale and root plane mandible; bacterial plaque control continued Week 4, host response period, no treatment One month after treatment, evaluate outcome

controlled, treatment procedures are postponed until regulation of the disorder is achieved. If the client is being treated with antihypertensive agents and clinical blood pressure evaluations are within normal limits, dental hygiene care can continue to meet other human needs related to oral health and disease.

The care plan considerations for the individual with controlled hypertension include meeting the human need for freedom from pain and stress through stress and anxiety reduction strategies and local anesthetic drug modification to reduce the potential for medical emergencies. Stress and anxiety reduction is accomplished by planning short appointments, preferably in the morning when the client is well rested and better prepared to handle a stressful situation. Another way to reduce the stress and anxiety associated with dental hygiene care is to provide nitrous oxide-oxygen analgesia for the client if he has no contraindication to this drug (see Chapter 23). Finally, gaining the client's respect and confidence by demonstrating support and concern should be incorporated into every client-dental hygienist interaction.

Drug considerations for the use of local anesthetics in clients with hypertensive heart disease are based on the avoidance of vasopressors, which are used in local anesthetics to constrict blood vessels. Blood vessel constriction concentrates the anesthetic in the desired area and prevents its dissipation.

A side affect of vasopressors is an elevation in blood pressure. In the normal person, a slight elevation in blood pressure does not cause damage. However, hypertensive individuals are at increased risk of cerebrovascular accident, myocardial infarction, and congestive heart failure.

Care Planning for the Client With Coronary Heart Disease

The client who is identified as having coronary heart disease is susceptible to angina pectoris and myocardial infarctions. Both of these conditions influence the dental hygiene process of care. The client with angina pectoris should be treated in a stress-free environment to meet the client's human need for safety and freedom from pain and stress. This individual should be scheduled for short morning appointments in an attempt to control the environment, and it is appropriate to offer nitrous oxide-oxygen analgesia to reduce stress if no contraindications to the drug exist (see Chapter 23. If the client develops chest pain during the appointment, administration of nitroglycerin sublingually is recommended. Dental hygiene care may continue based on individual circumstances.

Myocardial infarction does not indicate a change in care plan procedures unless it has occurred within 6 months of the appointment. Dental hygiene therapy should be postponed until the individual is 6 months or more postinfarction with no complications. The client's medical status should be confirmed with the cardiologist of record during the assessment phase of care.

The drugs used to treat or control myocardial infarctions (anticoagulants, digitalis, and antihypertensive agents) can necessitate care plan alterations. Anticoagulant drugs were already discussed; the same concerns and considerations should be taken whenever these drugs are used. Digitalis is a drug used to increase the contractility of the heart. The improvement in force makes the heart more efficient as a pump, increasing its volume in relation to cardiac output. This type of drug, botanical in origin, is classified as a glycoside. The most commonly prescribed digitalis drug is digoxin (Lanoxin).

Oral health professionals can detect early signs of digitalis toxicity in clients. Clinical signs include anorexia, nausea, vomiting, increased salivation, and lower facial pain resembling the type associated with trigeminal neuralgia.[17] If digitalis toxicity is not detected early, cardiac irregularities can develop. These irregularities include arrhythmias that can progress to ventricular fibrillation and sudden death.

Antihypertensive agents used to control myocardial infarctions are similar to those used to control hypertension. These agents do not influence care plan procedures unless the underlying condition is not controlled.

In addition, clients with coronary heart disease may experience periods of fear, depression, and disturbances in body image, associated with a change in lifestyle (e.g., dietary restrictions, exercise, and maintaining low stress). The dental hygienist needs to be aware of the client's psychological condition influencing human needs to motivate a change in oral health.

Care Planning for Clients With Cardiac Pacemakers

Individuals wearing cardiac pacemakers may be susceptible to bacterial endocarditis, and the pacemaker function can be affected by electrical interference in the oral healthcare setting. Care plans should denote a standard prophylactic antibiotic regimen when necessary to prevent bacterial endocarditis. Care plans also should incorporate nonelectrical procedure alternatives to reduce the possibility of functional interference (e.g., hand instrumentation, tooth desensitization with a nonelectronic apparatus, and pulp testing performed by tooth percussion). These interventions facilitate fulfillment of the client's human need for safety.

Care plan development for the individual with a cardiac pacemaker also can be affected by the drugs used to treat the client's underlying medical condition—anticoagulants and antihypertensive agents. The monitoring and assessment of drug therapy provide the dental hygienist with the information necessary to modify treatment.

Care Planning for Clients With Congenital Heart Disease

The individual with congenital heart disease does not require extensive alterations in the dental hygiene process of care. These conditions are treated with standard prophylactic antibiotic regimens similar to those required by individuals with rheumatic heart disease or artificial heart valves. If the individual develops congestive heart failure, then care plan considerations should follow those outlined in the next section.

Care Planning for Clients With Congestive Heart Failure

Individuals who are closely monitored by a physician do not require a change in conventional dental hygiene procedures. However, the client with uncontrolled symptoms does present a problem in the dental hygiene care environment. These individuals should be treated in an upright position to decrease collection of fluid in the lungs. The drugs used by physicians to treat heart failure function include those that increase heart efficiency and decrease edema. The drugs of choice are digitalis and some diuretics.

Factors associated with the cause of congestive heart failure should be considered in the dental hygiene care plan. Care plan alterations are based on the causative factors (hypertension, valvular heart disease, congenital heart disease, and myocardial infarction) in association with the individual's current medical status.

Care Planning for Clients After Cardiovascular Surgery

Currently, no set procedures are available relating to dental hygiene care and the individual who has had cardiovascular surgery. When in doubt, consult with the cardiologist. However, it is important to note that prosthetic valvular heart replacements and those cardiac surgeries that make the client susceptible to infection require prophylactic antibiotic premedication.

The complications from dental hygiene care observed in clients who have had cardiovascular surgery are associated with the drug therapy used rather than the surgery itself. Most postsurgical clients are placed on medication to increase healing, suppress immune response, reduce infection, and/or decrease clot formation. Careful evaluation of drug contraindications and reactions is necessary.

Implementation

Implementation of dental hygiene care for the client with cardiovascular disease takes into consideration the possibility of a medical emergency occurring. The most life-threatening emergency situation is cardiac arrest. The basic responsibilities of the dental hygienist are to

- Contact the EMS
- Monitor vital signs and state of consciousness
- Administer oxygen
- Provide basic life support (CPR)

One of the key aspects of emergency care is the dental hygienist's composure and attitude toward the client. Remaining calm in an emergency requires understanding the cause of the problem and course of treatment to be undertaken.

Other medical emergencies associated with cardiovascular disease are attacks of angina pectoris and myocardial infarctions. Below is a list of basic steps to take in the event of an emergency.

- Make certain the client is comfortable, loosen restricting garments, position the client so the head is slightly elevated
- Angina pectoris—immediately administer nitroglycerin sublingually and 100% oxygen with a face mask or nasal cannula
- Monitor vital signs
- Myocardial infarction—transfer client to an emergency facility as soon as possible
- Be prepared to administer CPR if necessary
- Stay with the client until he or she is transferred to the care of a physician

Legal Issues

In addition to the implementation of the care plan procedures and the avoidance of medical emergencies, the client with cardiovascular disease could pose a potential malpractice threat if treatment procedures are not performed correctly. The following legal doctrines underscore the legal issues that confront the healthcare professional as a result of a medical emergency.[10]

Doctrine 1—The original "incident" may submit the practitioner to liability for causing additional harm (even death) resulting from later negligent care and treatment addressed to the original injury.

Doctrine 2—The original "incident" may submit the practitioner to liability for causing additional harm (even death) resulting from later care and treatment (not negligent).

Doctrine 3—The original "incident" may submit the practitioner to liability for causing additional harm

TABLE 29–8
SAMPLE EVALUATION OF DENTAL HYGIENE INTERVENTIONS

Goals	Evaluative Measures	Expected Outcomes
Complete invasive dental hygiene therapy so that antibiotic coverage period is not extended beyond 7 days	Review treatment appointment scheduling for appropriate time intervals	Dentition and periodontium free from soft and hard deposits Root surfaces free from diseased cementum
By 9/92, reduce gingival bleeding By 9/92, reduce periodontal probing depths	Document client's periodontal condition for treatment results using periodontal probing depths and a gingival bleeding index	Periodontal probing depths reduced by at least 1 mm Minimal to no gingival bleeding

(even death) resulting from later care and treatment, when an inherent risk, like infection, is the aftermath.

If a client with cardiovascular disease develops chest pain in the oral healthcare setting and begins to feel anxious, the provider should

1. Stop dental hygiene care.
2. Alert the dentist.
3. Together with the dentist manage the immediate emergency situation.

If dental hygiene care is continued and the client undergoes a myocardial infarction, liability charges may be brought against the practitioner according to the first doctrine.

Health history documentation and update is the basis of client assessment. If dental hygiene care is performed on a client who was not appropriately interviewed about his health history and that status is documented on an acceptable health history form, the oral health professional could be held responsible for any damage resulting from care, as stated in the second doctrine.

An example of the third doctrine concerns prophylactic antibiotic premedication for the prevention of bacterial endocarditis. If a client reports on the health history that he has a cardiac condition that requires an antibiotic premedication regimen and he is not premedicated, then the oral health professional is liable for the risk of infection and complication thereof following treatment. Medical emergency situations must be prevented and properly managed or malpractice issues could arise.

Evaluation

Oral healthcare professionals use the evaluation process to measure the current health status of the client in light of the established client goals. By reviewing the assessment data, dental hygiene diagnoses, care plan, and intervention used, one can determine where weaknesses occurred and modify the process of care if necessary. Table 29–8 illustrates an evaluation of dental hygiene interventions for the care plan devised in Table 29–7.

References

1. World Health Organization. World Health Statistics: Annual Report. Washington, DC: WHO, 1990.
2. Conner, W., and Bristow, D. Coronary Heart Disease. Philadelphia: J. B. Lippincott, 1985.
3. Downey, A., Cresanta, J., et al. Cardiovascular health promotion in children: "Heart smart" and the changing role of physicians. American Journal of Preventive Medicine 5(5):279, 1989.
4. Kimm, S., Gergen, P., et al. Dietary patterns of U.S. children: Implications for disease prevention. Preventive Medicine 5(5):279, 1989.
5. Hamilton, H. (ed.). Diseases: Causes and Diagnosis. Springfield, PA: Intermed Communications, 1982, pp. 1083, 1091, 1102.
6. Bisno, A., Dismukes, W., et al. Antimicrobial Treatment of Infective Endocarditis due to Viridans Streptococci, Enterococci, and Staphylococci. Journal of the American Medical Association 261(3):1471, 1989.
7. Luckmann, J., and Sorensen, K. C. Medical-Surgical Nursing: A Psychological Approach, 2nd ed. Philadelphia: W. B. Saunders, 1980, p 87.
8. Rose, L., and Kaye, D. (eds.). Internal Medicine for Dentistry, 2nd ed. St. Louis: C. V. Mosby, 1990, pp. 452, 464, 478, 479.
9. Jeresaty, R. Mitral Valve Prolapse. New York: Raven Press, 1979, p. 2.
10. McCarthy, F. Essentials of Safe Dentistry for the Medically Compromised Patient, 2nd ed. Philadelphia: W. B. Saunders, 1980.
11. Gifford, R. Office evaluation of hypertension. Circulation 79(3):721, 1989.
12. Little, J., and Falace, D. Dental Management of the Medically Compromised Patient. St. Louis: C. V. Mosby, 1980, p. 69.
13. Callaghan, J., and Wartak, J. Open Heart Surgery; Theory and Practice. New York: Praeger, 1986, pp. 46, 53.
14. Baumgartner, W., Retiz, A., and Achuff, S. Heart and Heart-lung Transplantation. Philadelphia, W. B. Saunders, 1990, p. 86.
15. Danjani, A., Bisno, A., et al. Prevention of bacterial endocarditis: Recommendations by the American Heart Association. Journal of the American Medical Association 264(22):2919, 1990.
16. Kutscher, A., Goldber M., et al. (ed.). Pharmacology for the Dental Hygienist, 2nd ed. Philadelphia: Lea & Febiger, 1982, p. 146.
17. Holroyd, S., Wynn, R., et al. Clinical Pharmacology in Dental Practice. St. Louis: C. V. Mosby, 1988, p. 274.

Suggested Readings

American Dental Association. Patients with Cardiovascular Disease. American Dental Association; Council on Community Health, Hospital, Institutional and Medical Affairs. Chicago: ADA Publishers, Sept., 1989.

Baltch, J. Bacteremia following dental cleaning in patients with and without penicillin. American Heart Journal 104:1335, 1982.

Byrne, D., and Rosenman R. (eds.). Anxiety and the Heart. New York: Hemisphere Publishing, 1990.

Garfunkez, A., Massot, S., and Galili, B. Oral treatment needs for patients requiring heart surgery. Special Care Dentist 167:7, 1987.

Gordon, R., and Kammel, W. Premature mortality from coronary heart disease: The Framingham study. Journal of the American Medical Association 215(12):1617, 1971.

Hollinger, J., and Moore, E. Cardiovascular considerations in general dentistry. Dental Survey 54(10):16, 1978.

Newkirk, C. The hypertensive dental patient: Detection and treatment. Dental Hygiene 51(5):205, 1977.

Sullivan, B. The cardiac patient; Chemoprophylaxis considerations. Dental Hygiene 60(10):462, 1986.

Tzukert, A., Leviner, E., and Sela, M. Prevention of infective endocarditis not by antibiotics alone. Oral Surgery Oral Medicine and Oral Pathology 62(4):385, 1986.

30

Dental Hygiene Care for the Older Adult

OBJECTIVES

Mastery of the content in this chapter will enable the learner to:

- Define the key terms used
- Discuss the dominant sociopsychological and biological theories of aging
- Describe the significant demographic characteristics of the population over age 64
- Identify the major socioeconomic attributes of the older population including family, educational, and economic factors
- Describe normal age-related changes of the cardiovascular, pulmonary, musculoskeletal, neurosensory, gastrointestinal, genitourinary, and integumentary systems
- Describe prevalent chronic diseases associated with aging and discuss the implications for dental hygiene care
- Identify oral changes commonly found in the older adult
- Discuss oral changes that occur as a result of diseases or medications
- Explain potential alterations in the dental hygiene process of care that need to be considered when treating an older adult
- Address the special human needs related to oral health and disease of homebound and institutionalized older adults
- Consider the impact of the changing oral health status of older adults on the dental hygiene profession
- List some dental hygiene diagnoses related to the older adult

INTRODUCTION

The terms "geriatrics" and "gerontology" are often used synonymously, although there is a difference in their implications. **Geriatrics** is the branch of medicine concerned with the illnesses of old age and their treatment. **Gerontology** is the scientific study of the factors affecting the normal aging process and the effects of aging. In a true sense these terms are not interchangeable. A **gerontologist** is an individual who investigates numerous factors that affect the aging person and the aging process.

A lifetime of unique experiences has rendered older adults a heterogeneous group. Life at any given moment is the result of physiological capabilities, environmental variables, psychosocial factors, and a sense of one's own skills and alternatives. Therefore, the human needs of each older adult must be assessed individually, without prior assumptions based on preconceived stereotypes or myths.

Gerontologists have divided study of the older population into several categories based on age:

- **Young-old** (65–74 years)
- **Middle-old** (75–84 years)
- **Old-old** (85-plus years)

Some sociologists have classified those between the ages of 55 and 64 years as the **"new-old"** and those over 95 years as the **"very old."** Whatever terms are used, two important facts exist. First, characterizations of age should be based on ability, not chronological age; and second, the majority of older adults perform at a high level of independent function. The preponderance of older adults with functional limitations and compromised health are over the age of 75 years.

When considering the aging process within the context of human need theory, the importance of distinguishing between chronological and functional age becomes paramount. **Chronological age** refers to age as measured by calendar time since birth, whereas **functional age** is based on performance capacities. Although a calendar may signify a particular age, functional ability should be the standard that differentiates a person's capability to maintain activity.

SOCIAL ASPECTS OF AGING

No single theory can explain why and how people age. Rather, an intermingling of sociopsychological, environmental, physiological, and lifestyle factors contributes to

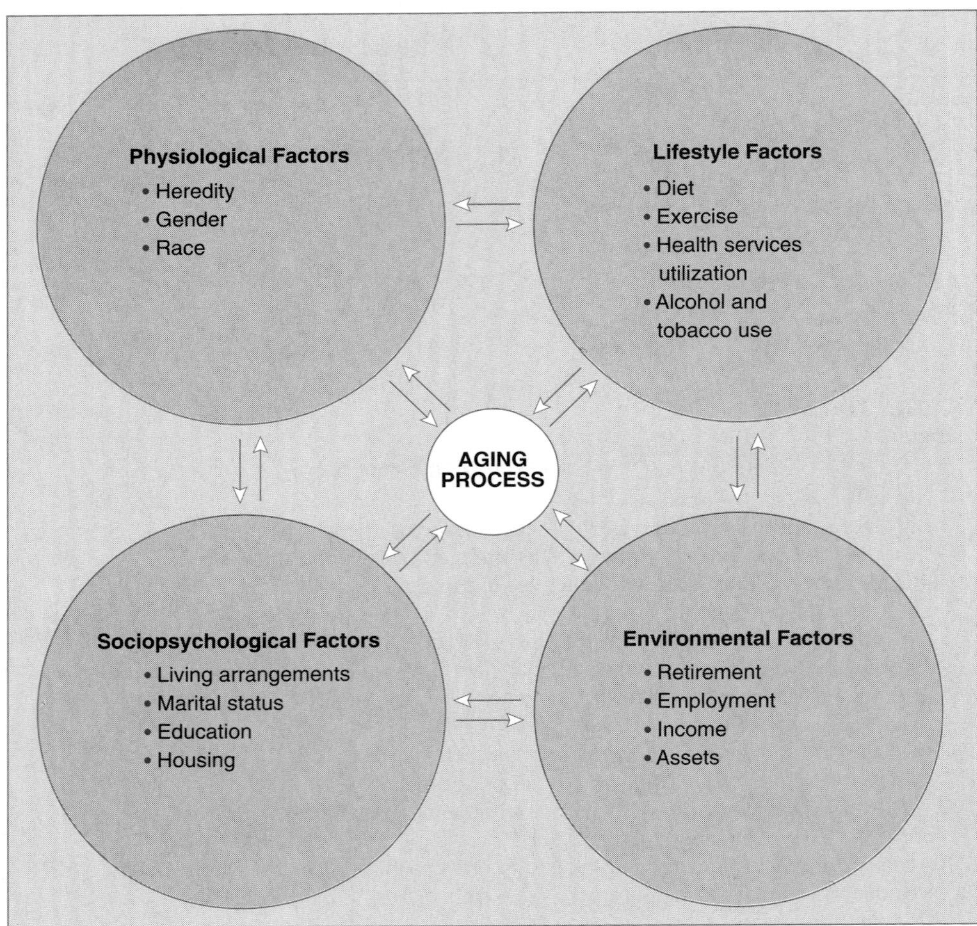

FIGURE 30–1
A conceptualization of factors influencing the aging process. (Modified from Esberger, K. K., and Hughes, S. T. Nursing Care of the Aged. Norwalk, CT: Appleton & Lange, 1989, p. 22; reprinted with permission.)

the aging process, either in accelerating or in retarding its progress, and produces a different course for each individual. Aging is a progressive yet fluid process, with each factor affecting the other. Figure 30–1 proposes a conceptualization of the major categories of contributing factors interacting with the others and affecting the aging process.

Understanding the theories of aging, those that have validity and those that contribute to stereotypes, enables the dental hygienist to facilitate human need fulfillment in the older adult through the dental hygiene process of care.

Social science researchers looking at aging focus on numerous factors affecting the lives of older persons. One theory cannot and should not be used to explain everything about the aging process. The importance of the interdisciplinary focus becomes paramount when trying to study the aging process. No one area—social, psychological, environmental, or biological—can predict how individuals age and adapt. Therefore, dental hygienists must be aware of the dynamic processes that influence each older client. The resources listed in this chapter should be helpful to the hygienist in understanding issues dealing with the aging process.

Social Theories of Aging

Disengagement Theory

The **disengagement theory** represents the first major hypothetical system designed to consider development of the latter stages of normal aging. The premise of this theory is that when a person reaches old age, he begins to withdraw from society and sever social ties, and that society in turn withdraws from the individual.[1] Proponents of this theory claim that disengagement is inevitable and mutually satisfying for both the individual and the society. For example, with retirement the older person is freed from normative control over his behavior and thus becomes the sole judge of what is appropriate for him. The older person's withdrawal from the workplace allows society to place younger workers into the workforce, thus creating an equilibrium and a continuation of the social system. In reality, however, how disengagement benefits the older adult is difficult to determine. How does the older adult benefit from withdrawal from social situations? Also, it may be argued that disengagement disrupts society because of loss of experienced workers in the workforce. Again, many economists argue a societal need for absolute manpower for many jobs that have normally been occupied by younger cohorts. Critics of this theory claim that people do not naturally disengage; withdrawal is a manifestation of depression needing psychological intervention.[2] Table 30–1 presents the dental hygiene implications using the human need theory for the social theories.

Activity Theory

A theory that assumes an opposite view is the **activity theory.** This theory states that a positive relationship exists

RESOURCES FOR THE AGING

Addiction Research Foundation
33 Russell Street
Toronto, Ontario, Canada, M5S
Publication: Substance Abuse Among the Elderly

Alzheimer's Disease and Related Disorders Association
(800)621-0379

American Association of Retired Persons
1909 K Street, N.W.
Washington, D.C. 20049

American Heart Association, National Center
7320 Greenbille Ave.
Dallas, TX 75231
Publication: An Older Person's Guide to Cardiovascular Health

American Foundation for the Blind
15 W. 16th Street
New York, NY 10011
Publication: About Aging and Blindness

American Health Care Association
1200 15th Street, N.W.
Washington, D.C. 20005
Publication: Thinking About a Nursing Home?

Arthritis Information Clearing House
P.O. Box 9782
Arlington, VA 22209

Center for Health Promotion and Education
Centers for Disease Control
1600 Clifton Road, N.E.
Atlanta, GA 30333

National Institute on Aging
National Institutes of Health
Building 31, Room 5C-36
9000 Rockville Pike
Bethesda, MD 20205

National Diabetes Information Clearinghouse
Box NDIC
Bethesda, MD 20205
Publication: Diabetes and Aging

National Institute of Neurological and Communicative Disorders and Stroke
Building 31, Room 8A-06
9000 Rockville Pike
Bethesda, MD 20205

The American Parkinson Disease Association
166 John Street
New York, NY 10038

between individuals' level of participation in social activities and their life satisfaction. Therefore, the theory proposes that continuation of a moderately active lifestyle will maintain a sense of well-being. Lost roles (worker, mother, spouse, etc.) must be replaced with other roles. For example, through retirement, an individual may lose a particular social structure, but by replacing it with new relationships and interests, life satisfaction remains the same. Testing of this theory shows, however, that the type of activity is more important than frequency; informal interactions and social activities with friends have a greater positive effect on life satisfaction than frequency of endeavors.[3,4]

TABLE 30–1
SOCIAL THEORIES OF AGING

Theory	Hypothesis	Limitation	Dental Hygiene Implication
Disengagement theory (Developed in late 1950s)	Aging individuals and society gradually withdraw from each other for mutual benefit	Theory undermined by the recognition that each individual has a different aging process, and the process often damages the aged and society	Understand how one's withdrawal from society can affect one's self-concept and motivate behavior Facilitate human needs for self-determination, responsibility, and a wholesome body image
Activity theory (Developed in late 1960s)	Aging individuals should be expected to maintain norms of middle-aged: employment, activity, replacement of lost relationships	Age-related physical, mental, and socioeconomic losses may present barriers to maintaining activity	Encourage client to seek other support systems to share/continue activities Discuss appropriate bacterial plaque control instruction and self-examinations
Continuity theory (Developed in late 1960s)	Aging depends on a person's psychological make-up and habitual methods of coping	Ability to continue in valued social roles depends upon an individual's social resources and the opportunities afforded by the social system	Foster behavior patterns to maintain oral wellness Facilitate human needs for freedom from stress, self-determination, and responsibility

Table continued on following page

TABLE 30–1
SOCIAL THEORIES OF AGING *Continued*

Theory	Hypothesis	Limitation	Dental Hygiene Implication
Age stratification theory (Developed in early 1970s)	Attempts to formulate a whole life conception of aging Old age is a process of becoming socialized to new or revised role definitions reflecting a fluid relationship among people, their social contexts, and their opportunities	Change is dependent on an intertwined series of feedback loop and revolving around the size of the population, the roles available, and the differences in the timing of individuals and social needs	Recognize the values and beliefs associated with oral health and disease within a defined-age stratum Facilitate human needs for value system, conceptualization, and problem solving
Social environment theory (Developed in late 1970s)	Depicts aging as a negotiated sequence depending on resources held by the trading partners	Adjustment is contingent on maintaining supportive environments and individual resources for manipulating unfavorable situations	Recognize the impact of individual resources on the procurement of therapeutic services Facilitate human needs for self-determination and problem solving
Political-economic theory (Developed early 1980s)	Aging is influenced by the relationship between the distribution of power and the form of economic organization	Lack of empirical evidence to support claims	Serve as client advocate Facilitate human needs for appreciation, respect, and self-determination

Continuity Theory

The **continuity theory** speculates that habits, preferences, associations, and coping abilities are part of an individual's personality, and they are continued throughout life. Therefore, coping strategies acquired throughout life remain fairly constant for older adults during their daily lives. Unlike the activity theory, the continuity theory does not assume that lost roles need to be replaced. Social roles may be discontinued at the beginning of old age but an individual's need for an identity, self-esteem, and social contact continues. It is important to keep in mind that not everyone has an equal opportunity to continue in valued social roles.

Social Environmental Theory

The **social environmental theory** emphasizes the functional status surrounding the daily lives of the older adult. Values and beliefs generated in particular situations exert an undeniable degree of control over individuals in that they constitute the cultural backdrop in which the older adult tests adaptability and personal worth. Adaptation and self-fulfillment are both active and reactive, negotiated by people in their effort to master a situation while extracting from it what they need to retain a positive self-image. Three basic premises are implicit in nearly all social environmental models:

- An emphasis on normative expectations derived from particular contexts
- Attention to individual capacities for interaction
- A focus on the subjectively evaluated correspondence between ability and that which is expected in a particular situation

Older adults are much more likely to feel a sense of well-being if all three components are reasonably consonant. However, adjustment is based on maintaining supportive environments and individual resources.[5]

DEMOGRAPHIC ASPECTS OF THE AGED

Number and Proportion of Older Adults

The older population group of the United States has grown steadily since the turn of the century when fewer than one in 10 Americans were 55 years and older and one in 25 was 65 years and older. Currently, the proportion aged 55-plus years constitutes approximately 21% of the population, whereas those 65 years and over comprise over 12% of the population. This represents a substantial expansion since 1900 when the older population, those over 65 years, was 4%. These changes, both total number and proportion, represent significant increases since 1900.

Life span is the maximal length of life potentially possible of a species–the age beyond which no one can expect to live. For humans, this number is approximately 110 to 120 years. **Life expectancy** is the average number of years lived by any group of individuals born in the same period, and is computed at birth. For example, individuals born in 1990 (varies depending on culture, gender, and race) can expect to live approximately 75.4 years, whereas individuals born at the turn of the century had life expectancies of 47 years. Several fundamental processes account for the increase in life expectancy. Fertility rates have declined significantly since the baby boom era (1945 to 1960), and mortality has declined, especially infant and childhood mortality. Medical progress coupled with technological advances have further prolonged the lives of those who would have died. Therefore, increases in longevity are not so much because of increases in life span but because more people are surviving young life, fertility rates have decreased, and medical technology has improved.

The number of people who reach age 65 years in a given year depends heavily on the number of births 65 years earlier. The baby boom generation is expected to create a "gerontology" boom in approximately the year 2020 with one in five Americans being over the age of 64 years. After

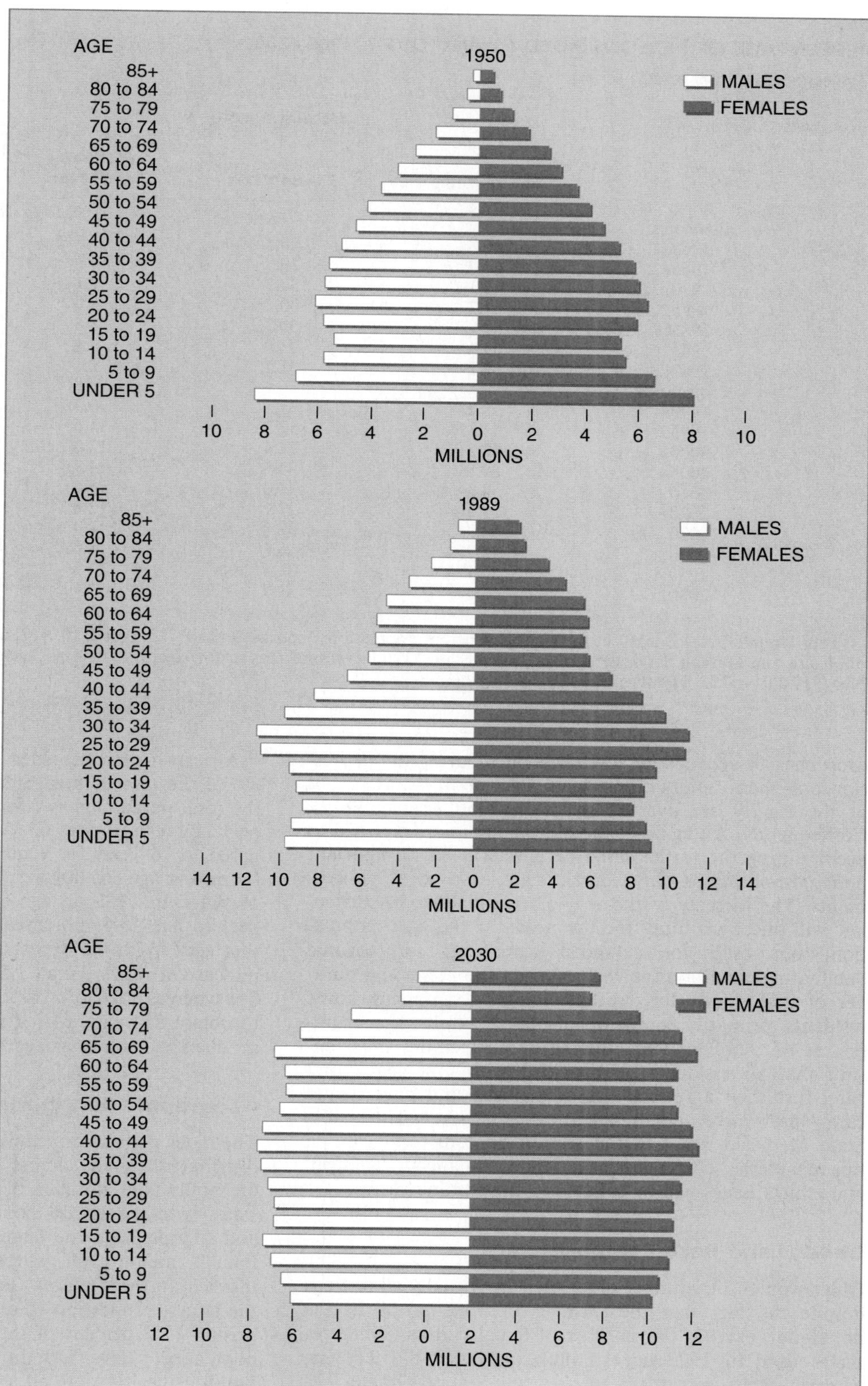

FIGURE 30–2
U.S. population pyramids, by age and gender: 1950, 1989, and 2030. (From U.S. Bureau of the Census. Estimates of the population of the United States, by single years of age, color and sex: 1900 to 1959. Current Population Reports, Series P-25, No. 311, 1965; U.S. Bureau of the Census. Projections of the population of the United States, by age, sex, and race: 1988 to 2080. Current Population Reports, Series P-25, No. 1018, 1989; U.S. Bureau of the Census. U.S. population estimates, by age, sex, race and Hispanic origin: 1989. Current Population Reports, Series P-25, No. 1057, 1990.)

the year 2020, the gerontological age group will increase at a slower rate because of the decrease in the size of the birth groups during the 1960s. Figure 30–2 demonstrates a change from a pyramid-shaped society (1950) to a more equal-shaped society (2030).

Not only has the older population of the United States grown in size and proportion in the total population during this century, but it also has become more aged. Currently, 9.6% of those in the 65-plus group are 85 years and older. This percentage should grow steadily to 15.5% by 2010,

TABLE 30–2
PERCENTAGE OF PERSONS AGED 65 AND OVER: 1960–2080
(Projection data from middle series)

Year	Percent aged—			Median Age of 65 and Over Population
	65–74 Years	75–84 Years	85 Years and Over	
Estimates:				
1960.........	66.3	28.1	5.6	71.9
1965.........	64.4	29.7	5.9	72.3
1970.........	62.1	30.7	7.1	72.6
1975.........	61.3	30.7	8.0	72.5
1980.........	60.9	30.3	8.8	72.8
1985.........	59.6	31.0	9.4	73.0
1987.........	59.2	31.2	9.6	73.1
Projections:				
1990.........	58.2	31.5	10.3	73.3
1995.........	56.1	32.3	11.6	73.8
2000.........	52.3	34.4	13.3	74.5
2005.........	50.8	34.5	14.7	74.2
2010.........	53.4	31.0	15.5	74.2
2020.........	59.5	27.7	12.8	73.0
2030.........	54.9	32.8	12.4	74.0
2040.........	45.2	36.8	18.0	76.1
2050.........	46.1	31.6	22.3	76.1
2080.........	44.6	31.7	23.7	76.4

From United States Bureau of the Census. Current Population Reports, Series P–25, Nos. 519, 917, and 1022. United States Department of Health and Human Services. Health United States, 1990. National Center for Health Statistics, Centers for Disease Control, DHHS Pub. No. (PHS) 91–1232, Hyattsville, MD, 1991.

drop back to account for low birth rates during the depression era, then rapidly climb again to a point where 22.3% of the elderly are over 85 years in 2050 (Table 30–2). Consequently, the aging of the older population expected to occur during the forthcoming decades will have important policy implications for federal, state, and local governments. The increase of the very-old population, in particular, will affect planning for the needs of the aged population, not only for extended care, but for chronic debilitating conditions as well. Already the increasing number of frail elderly has created changes for nursing home residents, primarily composed of old-old adults. For example, as of October 1990, nursing home facilities must ensure that all residents be provided with emergency oral care, furnished a referral list of dentists, and have dental care—preventive and therapeutic—as promulgated by the State Medicaid Act (see the section on long-term care in this chapter).[6] Understandably, many financial, political, and ethical issues will be debated in the coming years.

Gender and Race Composition

Older women outnumber older men in virtually all settings despite the fact that the number of male births in the population exceeds the number of female births. White females born in 1990 have a life expectancy of 79 years, whereas white males' life expectancy approximates 72 years. Table 30–3 shows projected life expectancy at birth and the percentage of differences between race and gender. The reasons for females' longer life expectancy are multiple. Although genetic variations contribute to the difference, social influences, regional differences, healthcare utilization, and other factors compound the situation.

African-American older adults comprise approximately 8% of the total United States population, although 12% of the total population is African-American.[7] In 1988, life expectancy at birth was 69 years for African-Americans compared to 76 years for whites. Differences in life expectancy by race at age 65, however, are smaller in terms of number of years. In 1985, at age 65, African-Americans could expect to live 15.5 more years, 1.3 years less than whites at that age.[8] With life expectancy after 65 years continuing to increase, a white female has a 33% chance of living to age 85, whereas 28% of African-American females can expect to obtain 85 years. Males, regardless of race, have a one in six chance of reaching age 85 years.[9]

Geographic Distribution and Mobility

The older population, similar to the total population, is not distributed equally across the United States (Fig. 30–3). Generally, the number of older adults is greatest in the states with the largest populations. California, New York, and Florida have the largest older populations, with more than 2 million each, whereas Alaska, Wyoming, and Vermont have the smallest number of aged adults. Florida has the largest proportion of residents aged 65-plus years, comprising 17.7 percent of the total population. As the older population grows both in number and age, demands for housing, health, and protective services will increase, particularly in heavily proportioned states.

Not only are the older adults distributed unequally across the states, but within cities and in rural areas predictable patterns of residence can be observed. Whereas the 1970 census found that most older people resided in metropolitan areas, the 1980s have shown a shift to the suburbs.

TABLE 30–3

LIFE EXPECTANCY AT BIRTH AND AGE 65, BY RACE AND GENDER: 1900–1987*

	All Races			White			Black		
Year	Both Sexes	Men	Women	Both Sexes	Men	Women	Both Sexes	Men	Women
At birth:									
1900[1,2]	47.3	46.3	48.3	47.6	46.6	48.7	33.0[3]	32.5[3]	33.5[3]
1950[2]	68.2	65.6	71.1	69.1	66.5	72.2	60.7	58.9	62.7
1960[2]	69.7	66.6	73.1	70.6	67.4	74.1	63.2	60.7	65.9
1970	70.9	67.1	74.8	71.7	68.0	75.6	64.1	60.0	68.3
1980	73.7	70.0	77.4	74.4	70.7	78.1	68.1	63.8	72.5
1987	75.0	71.5	78.4	75.6	72.2	78.9	69.4	65.2	73.6
At age 65:									
1900–02[1,2]	11.9	11.5	12.2	—	11.5	12.2	—	10.4[3]	11.4[3]
1950[2]	13.9	12.8	15.0	—	12.8	15.1	13.9	12.9	14.9
1960[2]	14.3	12.8	15.8	14.4	12.9	15.9	13.9	12.7	15.1
1970	15.2	13.1	17.0	15.2	13.1	17.1	14.2	12.5	15.7
1980	16.4	14.1	18.3	16.5	14.2	18.4	15.1	13.0	16.8
1987	16.9	14.8	18.7	17.0	14.9	18.8	15.4	13.5	17.1

* 1900 to 1980 data: National Center for Health Statistics. Health, United States, 1988. DHHS Pub. No. (PHS) 89-1232, Washington, D.C.: Department of Health and Human Services, 1989.
1987 data: National Center for Health Statistics. Life Tables. Vital Statistics of the United States, 1987, Vol. II, Section 6, 1990.

[1] 10 states and the District of Columbia.

[2] Includes deaths of nonresidents of the United States.

[3] Figure is for the nonwhite population.

Older persons are found in disproportionately high numbers in suburbs that were established before World War II. These older suburbs also have lower average resident income levels, more rental housing, lower home values, and higher population densities. Although some older persons have moved out to the suburbs as older adults, others have grown old in place; they moved to the suburbs in midlife, raised their families, and remained after their children had grown and left. Currently, only about one-third of all older people live in what is considered inner-city neighborhoods. The exception is the minority aged, with more than one-half of older African-Americans living in central cities.

Other parts of the country, the Sunbelt states, also are experiencing an aging of their population because of the migration of older persons during early retirement years. Older adults are following a general migration pattern oc-

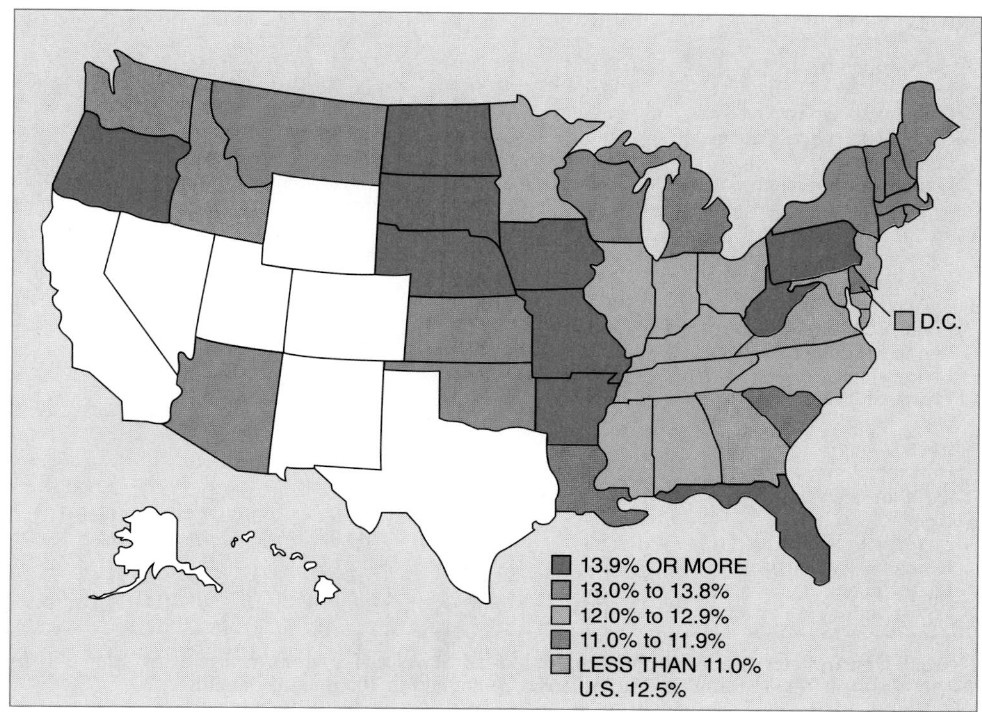

FIGURE 30–3
Persons aged 65+ years as a percentage of total population: 1989. (From U.S. Bureau of the Census. State population and household estimates: 1989. Current Population Reports, Series P-25, No. 1058, 1990.)

curring throughout the country. Older persons who move to another state are relatively affluent, are well educated, and are frequently accompanied by their spouses. Many have existing ties to the new area, such as family, friends, or property. Recently there is evidence of a new trend called **countermigration,** in which a small number of older adults who moved to another state at retirement move back home or to a state where family members live.

SOCIAL AND ECONOMIC ASPECTS OF THE AGED

Marital Status and Living Arrangements

Marital status and living arrangements of older persons vary tremendously by gender. Most men, for example, spend their later years married and in family settings, whereas most older women spend their later years as widows outside of family settings. Several reasons account for this discrepancy: women have a longer life expectancy and tend to outlive their husbands, men often marry women who are younger than themselves, and men who lose a spouse through divorce or death are more likely to remarry than are women in similar situations. Older widowed men have remarriage rates over eight times higher than those of women.[10]

Two-thirds of older, noninstitutionalized people live in a family setting. As with marital status, however, these statistics vary considerably by gender, and the differences grow larger with advancing age. For example, nearly four of every five men 75 years and older live with their spouses or other family members, compared to less than one-half of women in this age group (Table 30–4). In addition, the proportion of persons 85 years and over living alone climbed from 39% in 1980 to 47% in 1990.[10]

More than 70% of older adults live in their own homes compared to approximately 60% of the nonaged population. Homes owned by older adults generally are older and in greater need of maintenance than housing of younger

TABLE 30–4
LIVING ARRANGEMENTS OF NONINSTITUTIONALIZED OLDER PEOPLE BY AGE, GENDER, RACE, AND HISPANIC ORIGIN: 1989

	65+		65 to 74		75 to 84		85+	
Living Arrangement	**Men**	**Women**	**Men**	**Women**	**Men**	**Women**	**Men**	**Women**
All Races								
Total (thousands)	12,078	16,944	7,880	9,867	3,506	5,669	693	1,408
Percent	100.0	100.0	100.0	100.0	100.0	100.0	100.0	100.0
Living with spouse	74.3	40.1	78.4	51.4	70.4	28.1	48.2	9.1
Living with other relatives	7.7	16.9	6.4	13.5	8.7	19.1	17.3	32.6
Living alone	15.9	40.9	13.3	33.5	18.4	50.5	32.6	54.0
Living with nonrelatives	2.1	2.0	2.0	1.5	2.5	2.3	1.7	4.3
White								
Total (thousands)	10,798	15,204	7,050	8,767	3,136	5,174	612	1,263
Percent	100.0	100.0	100.0	100.0	100.0	100.0	100.0	100.0
Living with spouse	76.3	41.2	80.6	53.3	72.3	28.7	47.9	8.8
Living with other relatives	6.6	15.4	5.3	11.8	7.7	17.5	16.8	31.1
Living alone	15.3	41.4	12.5	33.5	17.9	51.5	33.7	55.5
Living with nonrelatives	1.8	2.0	1.7	1.4	2.0	2.3	1.6	4.6
Black								
Total (thousands)	981	1,455	619	913	300	416	62	126
Percent	100.0	100.0	100.0	100.0	100.0	100.0	100.0	100.0
Living with spouse	56.1	27.9	58.6	33.4	51.0	20.7	(B)**	11.9
Living with other relatives	15.6	29.7	15.0	26.4	17.0	32.2	(B)	45.2
Living alone	23.9	39.8	22.8	37.7	24.7	43.5	(B)	42.9
Living with nonrelatives	4.6	2.6	3.7	2.5	7.3	3.6	(B)	0.0
Hispanic Origin*								
Total (thousands)	447	557	301	350	120	176	26	31
Percent	100.0	100.0	100.0	100.0	100.0	100.0	100.0	100.0
Living with spouse	65.5	37.7	69.8	47.4	62.5	23.3	(B)	(B)
Living with other relatives	15.2	35.5	12.6	30.0	18.3	43.2	(B)	(B)
Living alone	17.4	25.7	15.0	21.1	19.2	33.5	(B)	(B)
Living with nonrelatives	1.8	1.4	2.7	1.4	0.0	0.6	(B)	(B)

From United States Bureau of the Census. Marital Status and Living Arrangements: March 1989. Current Population Reports, Series P–20, No. 445, 1990 (percentage distributions may not add to 100 due to rounding).

* People of Hispanic origin may be of any race.

** (B) Base less than 75,000.

homeowners. Although age of housing is not necessarily an index of physical condition, it does bear a relationship to size and ease of maintenance. Many older persons live in homes that are too large for current family size and need. Many older adults with physical disabilities have limited resources to adapt older, larger homes to their physical needs.[11]

Education

Older adults are less likely to have graduated from high school than the entire population 25 years and older. Approximately 55% of individuals of 65-plus years were high school graduates as compared with 77% of the 25-plus population during 1989.[7]

As presented in Table 30–5, no significant differences in educational attainment exist by gender. However, large differences are noted between older whites and older nonwhites. In 1989, a majority (58%) of older whites had completed 12 or more years of school, whereas among middle-old nonwhites, about one-third had completed high school.[12] Differences by age group in educational attainment, unlike those in health status or income, are almost entirely the result of the **cohort effect.** That is, educational attainment is primarily a function of the prevailing attitudes and educational opportunities for a group at a point in time. The older population of today received the bulk of its formal education early in this century when educational opportunities were more limited than in recent decades, and when the economic structure of the country put less emphasis on structured learning. Although educational attainment of the older population is below that of the younger population, the difference is expected to decrease with subsequent cohorts of older adults.

Economic Status and Workforce Participation

Older adults, as a group, have a lower economic status than other adults in the United States. This difference primarily results from changes in status (retirement, marital status) often associated with aging. In retirement, older persons lose earnings and become reliant instead upon Social Security benefits, supplemented with pensions and the assets (for some older adults) they have accumulated over their lifetimes. With limited potential to improve their income through work, older persons become economically vulnerable to circumstances over which they have no control: the loss of a spouse, changes in sources of income, deterioration of their health and self-sufficiency, and inflation.

Many older adults have the economic benefits and resources that enable them to meet their needs for food and shelter in retirement quite comfortably. However, the economic status of the aged is far more varied than that of any other age group. Although some older persons have substantial resources, others have virtually none. Comparisons

TABLE 30–5
SELECTED MEASURES OF EDUCATIONAL ATTAINMENT BY AGE GROUP, GENDER, RACE, AND HISPANIC ORIGIN (NONINSTITUTIONALIZED): 1989

Measure of Educational Attainment and Age	Sex			Race and Hispanic Origin*								
				White			Black			Hispanic Origin*		
	Total	Men	Women	Total	Men	Women	Total	Men	Women	Total	Men	Women
Median years of school completed:												
25+	12.7	12.8	12.6	12.7	12.8	12.7	12.4	12.4	12.4	12.0	12.0	12.0
60 to 64	12.4	12.5	12.4	12.5	12.5	12.4	10.7	10.6	10.7	9.3	9.6	8.9
65+	12.1	12.1	12.2	12.2	12.2	12.2	8.5	8.1	8.7	8.0	8.1	8.0
65 to 69	12.3	12.3	12.3	12.4	12.4	12.4	9.5	9.1	9.8	8.4	8.5	8.3
70 to 74	12.2	12.2	12.2	12.3	12.3	12.3	8.4	8.2	8.6	8.0	8.1	7.9
75+	10.9	10.5	11.3	11.6	11.1	11.9	7.8	7.0	8.2	7.1	7.0	7.1
Percent with a high school education:												
25+	77	77	77	78	79	78	65	64	65	51	51	51
60 to 64	66	65	67	69	68	71	39	43	37	34	37	31
65+	55	54	56	58	57	59	25	22	26	28	26	29
65 to 69	63	61	65	67	65	68	31	28	33	33	31	35
70 to 74	57	56	58	60	59	62	21	20	22	25	21	29
75+	46	44	48	49	47	50	21	18	23	23	21	24
Percent with four or more years of college:												
25+	21	25	18	22	25	19	12	12	12	10	11	9
60 to 64	14	19	10	15	21	10	5	7	4	6	5	7
65+	11	14	9	12	15	10	5	4	5	6	7	5
65 to 69	13	16	10	13	17	10	5	3	6	9	9	9
70 to 74	11	13	9	11	13	10	3	3	3	3	3	3
75+	10	12	9	11	13	9	6	4	6	4	7	3

From United States Government. Aging America: Trends and Projections, 1991 Edition. U.S. Department of Health and Human Services, Washington, D.C.: U.S. Senate Special Committee on Aging, DHHS Pub. No. 91–28001, 1991.
* People of Hispanic origin may be of any race.

of average statistics conceal the fact that an unusually high proportion of older adults have incomes and other economic resources below or just barely above the poverty level.

Poverty rates vary greatly by gender, race, and marital status. For example, in 1990 7.8% of aged men were living below the poverty level, compared with 14% of aged women. The low incomes of older women are largely associated with a pattern of lifelong economic dependency on men and with marital status changes that occur in old age. The oldest women are the poorest, with one in five living below the poverty level. For whites, 9.6% of the aged were poor, as compared with 30.8% of African-Americans and 20.6% of Hispanics.[13]

Historically, minority populations (racial, gender, cultural minorities) have had fewer opportunities for profitable employment. African-American and Hispanic aged people have substantially lower incomes than their white counterparts. The median income of African-American and Hispanic males of 65-plus years is about two-thirds that of white males. The poverty rates are much higher among minority aged than among white aged. Older African-American women are especially poor, with nearly 64% of black females living in poverty (Fig. 30–4).[13]

Older adults depend more heavily on Social Security benefits for their income than they do on any other source. In 1990, 38% of all income received by aged adults came from the government in the form of Social Security payments.[14] Income from assets is the second most important income source for older adults. Earnings from paid employment are a particularly important source of income to the young-old, but this source declines in importance with age.

The occupational structure of the labor force has undergone changes with a decreasing emphasis on agricultural and blue collar jobs and an increasing emphasis on white collar and service occupations. In 1989, nearly two-thirds of workers 65 years and older were in professional and service occupations. The shift from physically demanding jobs to those in which skills or knowledge are the important prerequisite may increase the potential of older workers to remain in the labor force longer.

PHYSIOLOGICAL ASPECTS OF AGING

Senescence is the term that describes the normal physiologic process of growing old. Goldman indicates four characteristics of physiologic aging: it is universal, progressive, detrimental, and intrinsic.[15] The fact that everyone, given time, eventually experiences physical changes in all of the body systems makes aging universal. Physical changes that occur are normal for all people but take place at various rates and depend on accompanying circumstances (environmental, psychosocial, lifestyle factors, and biological) in an individual's life. Typically, normal age changes have been studied in collaboration with pathological or disease conditions, leading to the misconception that age changes indicate illness or disease. Research continues to uncover evidence that many changes thought to be directly related to the aging process are actually a result of disease or lifestyle influences. For example, a decrease in salivary production was thought to be a normal aging feature. Within the last decade, however, research has shown that no decrease in salivary production occurs in healthy older adults; diminished salivary flow is, instead, a byproduct of medications or disease.

The process of aging occurs at different rates among individuals and in different systems within the same individual. Pathological changes may develop simultaneously; therefore, it is important to distinguish, when possible, between that which is physiologically age-related change and that which is the result of disease. The difference is important because of the need to recognize disease patterns and relate their significance to oral health changes observed during assessment.

Biological Theories of Aging

Most theorists agree that a unifying theory does not yet exist that explains the mechanics and causes underlying the biological phenomenon of aging. Basically, biological theories can be divided into molecular and nonmolecular theories. Each hypothesis provides a clue to the aging process, but many unanswered questions remain. The following is a description of the predominant biological theories.

Molecular Theories

The **cell theory** has been the topic of frequent scientific investigation in examining the aging phenomena. The cell has three specific components that have contributed to the basic framework of other biological theories. The three cell components include cells that reproduce, cells that do not reproduce, and intercellular substances and materials.[16]

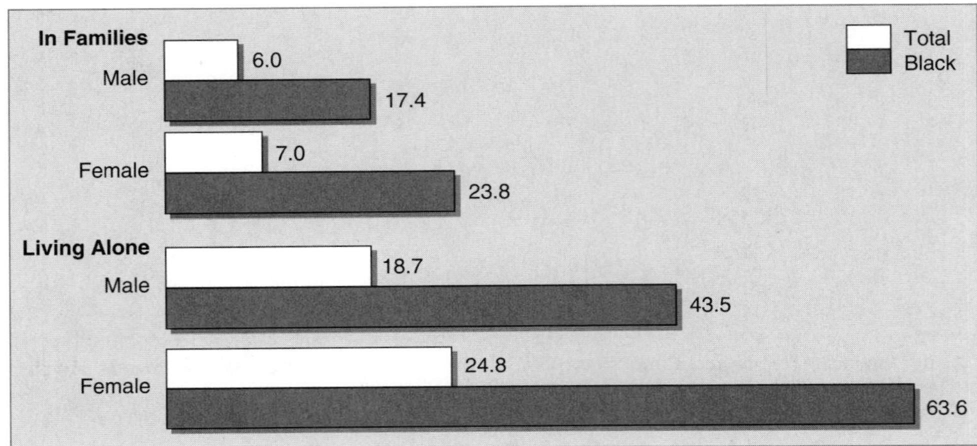

FIGURE 30–4
Persons aged 65 years and over with income below the poverty level (in percentage). (From Grad, S. Income of the population 65 or over, 1988. Pub. No. 13-11871, Washington, DC: U.S. Social Security Administration, U.S. Department of Health and Human Services. Health United States, 1990. National Center for Health Statistics, Centers for Disease Control, DHHS Pub. No. (PHS)91-1232, Hyattsville, MD, 1991.)

The theory based on cells that reproduce proposes that during reproduction some of the new cells are nonfunctioning or less effective than the other cells that were replaced. As the aging process progresses and there is an accumulation of inefficient and nonfunctioning cells, the organism's functional ability becomes apparent. For example, the skin is an organism wherein cells are continuously being replaced. With age, the skin takes on visible changes such as wrinkling, roughness, and dryness. The theory related to cells that do not reproduce suggests that with age the cells progressively wear out or are destroyed. For example, the central nervous system (comprised of cells that do not reproduce) gradually develops an accumulation of nonfunctioning cells. Subsequently, the system becomes less efficient and unable to handle the usual work load.

The **somatic mutation theory** suggests that when cells are exposed to radiation or chemicals an alteration of deoxyribonucleic acid (DNA) occurs, thus increasing the incidence of chromosomal abnormalities. These mutations are a time-dependent accumulation of chromosome abnormalities that become apparent in later life. Ultimately a decrease in cellular function and organ efficiency results. For example, somatic cells that are nondividing, such as brain and muscle cells, have a limited lifespan and are not replaced when injured or dead.[17]

The **error theory** postulates that cells may become inoperative because of copying errors in repeated divisions. For a message to be transmitted to the cell, DNA depends on the ribonucleic acid (RNA) stored in the nucleus. Changes in the structure of RNA may result in progressive modifications in copying so that newer cells are incapable of recognizing essential components of themselves. This nonrecognition forces the body's immune system to work against itself. For example, cancer is the result of abnormal cells produced within the body.[18]

The premise of the **programmed theory** is that the lifespan of an organism is programmed within the genes of the organism. The program sets the rate and time that an individual proceeds through the lifespan and dies. For example, the graying of hair, wrinkling of skin, and beginning of menopause are intrinsically correlated with time. These changes are considered normal aging alterations that are not pathological.[19]

Nonmolecular Theories

The **immunologic/autoimmune theory** proposes that with age the immune system undergoes involuntary changes after puberty. The result is twofold. First, the body's production of antibodies necessary to fight off infections declines. Second, as normal immune patterns change in one direction, autoimmune responses change in the opposite direction. Cells normal to the body are misidentified as foreign matter and are attacked by the body's own immune system.[5]

The **crosslinkage theory** (also referred to as the collagen or connective tissue theory) suggests that chemical reactions create strong bonds between molecular structures that are normally separate. As the body ages, there is an increase in the number of crosslinks in extracellular components, which results in fibers becoming more rigid.[17] For example, a lack of elasticity in the walls of the circulatory system signifies the probable onset of atherosclerosis and high blood pressure. Because collagen makes up about 30% of body protein, alterations in the fibers can produce significant changes in the older adult's functioning, thus the human need for self-determination may be compromised.

The **free radical theory** postulates that free radicals contain unpaired ions that exist momentarily and are highly reactive chemically with other substances, such as unsaturated fats. The molecular structure of free radicals differs from that of ordinary molecules in that they possess an extra electric charge (free electron). This charge instigates a one-time, irreversible, and energy-wasteful reaction that damages or alters the original structure or function of the cell membrane. Although body cells possess the capacity to eliminate unwanted waste and materials, neutralize byproducts, and repair damage, free radical accumulation is thought to be faster than the repair process of the organism.[17]

In summary, the fundamental mechanisms of the aging process are becoming less obscure but remain extremely variable among human beings. A search for a universal factor or factors is complicated by the fact that signs of aging do not appear in all individuals at the same chronological age. Knowledge of the various biological theories of aging is helpful in understanding physiological manifestations and some mental changes that may affect the older client with whom the dental hygienist works.

Health Status and Self-Assessment

Health assessment of older persons includes a functional appraisal in addition to a health history. A functional assessment consists of evaluating the fundamental tasks and demands of daily life. The items generally agreed on as comprising a functional assessment are divided into **activities of daily living** (ADLs) and **instrumental activities of daily living** (IADLs). ADLs are those abilities that are fundamental to independent living, such as bathing, dressing, toileting, transferring from bed or chair, feeding, and continence. More complex daily activities, such as using the telephone, preparing meals, and managing money, are examples of IADLs.

The majority of older adults have one or more chronic conditions, but most older adults view their health positively. Results from the 1989 Health Interview Survey demonstrate that approximately 71% of noninstitutionalized older adults describe their general health as excellent, very good, or good, compared with others their age.[20] Less than 30% report that their health is fair or poor. Little difference exists in perception of health between males and females. Income, however, appears to play a significant role in perception of health. Nearly 26% of older people with incomes over $35,000 described their health as excellent compared to others their age, whereas only about 10% of those with incomes less than $10,000 reported excellent health.[21] Income is directly related to the ability to receive healthcare services, which functions as a factor in overall health.

The pattern of illness and disease has changed over the past century. Acute conditions were predominant during the early 1900s, whereas chronic conditions present more prevalent health problems for older adults today. The leading chronic conditions for older adults are arthritis, hypertensive disease, hearing impairments, and heart conditions. Figure 30–5 presents common chronic conditions of persons aged 65 years and older. Dental hygienists can facilitate the fulfillment of the human needs for safety and self-determination by recognizing age-related and pathology-induced physical changes.

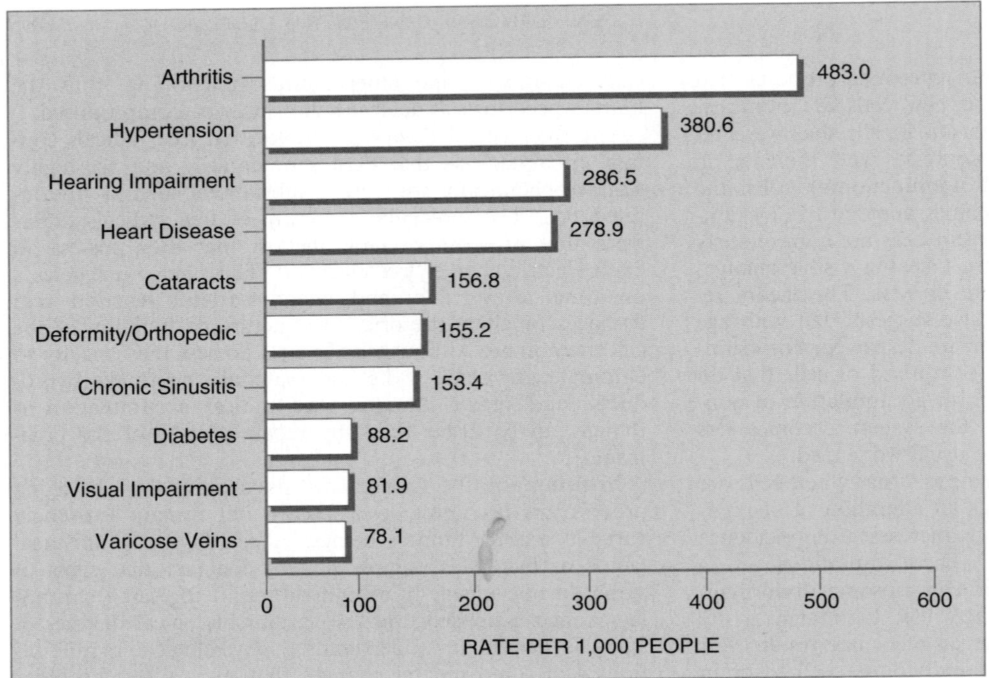

FIGURE 30–5
Common chronic conditions of persons aged 65 and over (noninstitutionalized). (From National Center for Health Statistics. Current Estimates from the National Health Interview Survey, 1989. Vital and Health Statistics Series 10, No. 176, 1990.)

The plurality of young-old and middle-old persons are relatively healthy and often are not limited in activity despite having chronic conditions. Health and mobility do decline generally, however, with advancing age. By the eighth and ninth decades of life, the chances of having limited activity and needing health and social services increase significantly.

Health Promotion and Aging

The majority of health conditions and diseases are the result of cumulative lifestyle habits and environmental factors. Diet, activity level, alcohol abuse, and tobacco usage all play a significant part in the development or exacerbation of disease(s).

On the positive side, research indicates that older adults, on average, take better care of their health than does the general population. Individuals of 65-plus years are less likely than younger adults to drink alcohol, be overweight, smoke, or report that stress has adversely affected their health (Table 30–6). The lower rates of drinking alcohol and smoking can be attributed to the tendency toward discontinuing these habits in older age, whether done spontaneously or in response to a medical condition or advice, and to the higher mortality rates of those who were drinkers or smokers at younger ages.

Older adults, however, are less likely to engage in regular physical exercise. Inactivity poses serious health hazards to both young and old. Lack of exercise can lead to coronary artery disease, hypertension, obesity, tension, chronic fatigue, premature aging, poor musculature, osteoporosis, and inadequate flexibility. Many older adults, and younger adults also, believe that aged individuals are too old to begin or participate in a fitness program. However, research

TABLE 30–6
PERSONAL HEALTH HABITS OF OLDER ADULTS

Characteristic (%)	Sleeps 6 Hours or Less	Never Eats Breakfast	Smokes Every Day[1]	Less Physically Active Than Contemporaries	Had 5 or More Drinks On Any One Day[2]	Current Smoker	30% or More Above Desirable Weight[3]
All people 18+[4]	22.0	24.3	39.0	16.4	37.5	30.1	13.0
Age							
18 to 29 years old	19.8	30.4	42.2	17.1	54.4	31.9	7.5
30 to 44 years old	24.3	30.1	41.4	18.3	39.0	34.5	13.6
45 to 64 years old	22.7	21.4	37.9	15.3	24.6	31.6	18.1
65 + years	20.4	7.5	30.7	13.5	12.2	16.0	13.2
65 to 74 years old	19.7	9.0	32.4	15.8	NA	19.7	14.9
75+ years	21.5	5.1	27.8	9.8	NA	10.0	10.3

[1] Percentage of current smokers.
[2] Percentage of drinkers who had five or more drinks on any one day in the past year.
[3] Based on 1960 Metropolitan Life Insurance Company standards. Data are self-reported.
[4] Excludes people whose health practices are unknown.
United States Government. Aging America: Trends and Projections, 1991 Edition. U.S. Department of Health and Human Services, Washington, D.C.: U.S. Senate Special Committee on Aging, DHHS Pub. No. 91–28001, 1991.

indicates that even those with chronic conditions can benefit from an appropriately designed fitness program.[22,23]

Dental Hygienist's Role in Health Promotion

The dental hygienist as an educator and health promoter can provide appropriate wellness information and reinforce positive lifestyle habits of older clients, thus facilitating the human need for self-determination, and a wholesome body image. For example, some beneficial health activities may include:

- Begin or maintain a physical activity program
- Consume a nutritious diet low in fermentable carbohydrates, sugars, and fats
- Limit exposure to ultraviolet light
- Avoid exposure to pollutants such as alcohol, tobacco, noise, and polluted air and water
- Prevent infections and diseases; identify and treat them early if they do occur
- Practice appropriate oral hygiene behaviors
- Manage stress effectively
- Remain mentally active and alert

Age-Related Physiological Changes

Age-related and pathology-induced changes in the human body occur at differing chronological ages. Table 30–7 displays physiological changes usually found in older adults; however, the occurrence and degree of difference vary from individual to individual. Several body systems are presented with the accompanying dental hygiene care modifications.

TABLE 30–7
PHYSIOLOGICAL CHANGES THAT MIGHT BE PRESENT IN OLDER ADULTS

Cardiovascular Changes	
Cardiac output	Heart loses elasticity; therefore, decreased heart contractility in response to increased demands
Arterial circulation	Decreased vessel compliance with increased peripheral resistance to blood flow resulting from general or localized arteriosclerosis
Venous circulation	Does not exhibit change with aging in the absence of disease
Blood pressure	Significant increase in the systolic, slight increase in the diastolic, increase in peripheral resistance and pulse pressure
Heart	Dislocation of the apex because of kyphoscoliosis; therefore, diagnostic significance of location is lost
Murmurs	Diastolic murmurs in over half older adults; the most common at the base of the heart because of sclerotic changes on the aortic valves
Peripheral pulses	Easily palpated because of increased arterial wall narrowing and loss of connective tissue; feeling of tortuous and rigid vessels
	Possibility that pedal pulses may be weaker as a result of arteriosclerotic changes; colder lower extremities, especially at night; possibility of cold feet and hands with mottled color
Heart rate	No changes with age at normal rest
Respiratory Changes	
Pulmonary blood flow and diffusion	Decreased blood flow to the pulmonary circulation; decreased diffusion
Anatomic structure	Increased anterior-posterior diameter
Respiratory accessory muscles	Degeneration and decreased strength; increased rigidity of chest wall
	Muscle atrophy of pharynx and larynx
Internal pulmonic structure	Decreased pulmonary elasticity creates senile emphysema
	Shorter breaths taken with decreased maximum breathing capacity, vital capacity, residual volume, and functional capacity
	Airway resistance increases; less ventilation at the base of the lung and more at the apex
Musculoskeletal Changes	
Muscle strength and function	Decrease with loss of muscle mass; bony prominences normal in older adults, since muscle mass decreased
Bone structure	Demineralization, more porous
	Shortening of the trunk as a result of intervertebral space narrowing
Joints	Become less mobile; tightening and fixation occur
	Activity may maintain function longer
	Normal posture changes; some kyphosis
	Range of motion limited
Anatomic size and height	Total decrease in size as loss of body protein and body water occurs in proportion to decrease in basal metabolic rate
	Increased body fat; diminished in arms and legs, increased in trunk
	Decreased height from 2.5 to 10 cm from young adulthood
Nervous System Changes	
Response to stimuli	All voluntary or automatic reflexes slower
	Decreased ability to respond to multiple stimuli
Sleep patterns	Stage IV sleep reduced in comparison to younger adulthood; increased frequency of spontaneous awakening
	Stay in bed longer but get less sleep; insomnia a problem, which should be evaluated

Table continued on following page

TABLE 30–7
PHYSIOLOGICAL CHANGES THAT MIGHT BE PRESENT IN OLDER ADULTS *Continued*

Nervous System Changes	
Reflexes	Deep tendon reflexes responsive in the healthy older adults
Ambulation	Kinesthetic sense less efficient; may demonstrate an extrapyramidal Parkinson-like gait
	Basal ganglions of the nervous system influenced by the vascular changes and decreased oxygen supply
Voice	Decreased range, duration, and intensity of voice, may become higher pitched and monotonous
Sensory Changes	
Vision	
Peripheral vision	Decreases
Lens accommodation	Decreases, requires corrective lenses
Ciliary body	Atrophy in accommodation of lens focus
Iris	Development of arcus senilis
Choroid	Atrophy around disk
Lens	May develop opacity, cataract formation; more light necessary to see
Color	Fades or disappears
Macula	Degenerates
Conjunctiva	Thins and looks yellow
Tearing	Decreases; increased irritation and infection
Pupil	May differ in size
Cornea	Presence of arcus senilis
Retina	Observable vascular changes
Stimuli threshold	Increased threshold for light touch and pain
	Ischemic paresthesias common in the extremities
Hearing	Less perceptible high-frequency tones; hence greatly impaired language understanding; promotes confusion and seems to create increased rigidity in thought processes
Gustatory	Decreased acuity as taste buds atrophy; may increase the amount of seasoning on food
Gastrointestinal Changes	
Mastication	Impaired because of partial or total loss of teeth, malocclusive bite, and ill-fitting dentures
Swallowing and carbohydrate digestion	Swallowing more difficult as salivary secretions diminish
Esophagus	Decreased esophageal peristalsis
	Increased incidence of hiatus hernia with accompanying gaseous distention
Digestive enzymes	Decreased production of hydrochloric acid, pepsin, and pancreatic enzymes
Fat absorption	Delayed, affecting the absorption rate of fat-soluble vitamins A, D, E, and K
Intestinal peristalsis	Reduced gastrointestinal motility
	Constipation because of decreased motility and roughage
Genitourinary and Reproductive Changes	
Renal blood flow	Because of decreased cardiac output, reduced filtration rate and renal efficiency; possibility of subsequent loss of protein from kidneys
Urination	In men, possibility of increased frequency as a result of prostatic enlargement
	In women, decreased perineal muscle tone; therefore, urgency and stress incontinence
	Increased nocturia for both men and women
	Possibility that polyuria may be diabetes related
	Decreased volume of urine may relate to decrease in intake but evaluation needed
Incontinence	Increased occurrence with age, specifically in those with dementia
Integumentary Changes	
Texture	Skin loses elasticity; wrinkles, folding, sagging, dryness
Color	Spotty pigmentation in areas exposed to sun; face paler, even in the absence of anemia
Temperature	Extremities cooler; decreased perspiration
Fat distribution	Less on extremities; more on trunk
Hair color	Dull gray, white, yellow, or yellow-green
Hair distribution	Thins on scalp, axilla, pubic area, upper and lower extremities; decreased facial hair in men; women may develop chin and upper lip hair
Nails	Decreased growth rate; ridges form on nails

Reprinted with permission from Elbersole, P., and Hess, P. Toward Healthy Aging: Human Needs and Nursing Response, 3rd ed. St. Louis: Mosby–Yearbook, 1990.

Cardiovascular Changes

Some physiological changes that occur in the cardiovascular system are the result of aging of the body and are independent of pathological processes. These physiological changes affect the efficiency with which the cardiovascular system functions and alter the function of the whole body. Because the cardiovascular system is the link to providing the oxygen and nutrients needed by tissues for metabolic requirements, changes in it affect the entire body.

The most common change in the older person's heart is within the myocardium—the thick layer of muscle. Muscle fibers decrease and some are replaced by fibrous tissue; consequently, oxygen is used less efficiently. Research indicates that stiffening of heart muscle fibers is not permanent but is partially modifiable with physical conditioning.[24] Generally, heart size remains about the same throughout the lifespan if no change occurs in an individual's activity level or disease is not present. With age, the heart valves stiffen and become thicker as the collagen degenerates and fatty deposits accumulate. Cardiac output is decreased with aging, although the decrease can be retarded, to some degree, by physical conditioning.

Decreased elasticity of arteries is responsible for various vascular changes that affect blood flow to body organs such as the heart, liver, and kidneys. Circulation in the coronary arteries diminishes by approximately 35% after the sixth decade, and increased resistance to peripheral blood flow occurs at a rate of about 1% per year.[25] With normal aging, some atherosclerosis is normal, but it can be exacerbated to a pathological state by a diet high in saturated fat. However, under nonstressful conditions, the older person's cardiovascular system can adapt to its functional ability if the system is not greatly damaged.

Cardiovascular Disorders

Cardiovascular disease accounts for more than 50% of all deaths among the aged, and is the primary cause of hospital admissions of older adults. The majority of individuals over 65 years have cardiovascular disease, most commonly in the form of coronary heart disease or hypertension. The prevalence of cardiovascular disease varies widely by gender and race. For example, men are more likely than women to experience hypertension and heart attacks (myocardial infarction). Estrogen appears to reduce females' susceptibility to most cardiovascular diseases until menopause. After menopause, however, heart disease for females equals that of males in the absence of estrogen replacement therapy.

The oral complications and care plan modifications depend on the type and severity of cardiovascular disease and the physical condition of the older adult. Because stress and anxiety related to dental hygiene care may increase blood pressure, resulting in myocardial infarction or cerebrovascular accident, precautions should be taken to meet the older adult's human needs for safety and freedom from stress (Table 30–8).

As with other body systems, cardiovascular changes that

TABLE 30–8
ALTERATIONS IN THE DENTAL HYGIENE CARE OF OLDER ADULTS WITH CARDIOVASCULAR DISEASE

Atherosclerotic Disease

Potential Risk Relating to Dental Hygiene Care	Prevention of Medical Complication
1. Stress and anxiety related to oral healthcare visit may precipitate angina attack in the oral healthcare setting 2. Myocardial infarction may occur when older adult is in the oral healthcare setting 3. Sudden death caused by disruption of cardiac rhythm or cardiac arrest without acute myocardial infarction may occur in the oral healthcare setting Dental Hygiene Care Plan Modifications 1. Older adults with stable form of angina Any routine oral healthcare 2. Older adults with unstable form of angina Only care needed to deal with or prevent oral pain or infection or both Oral Complications Usually none; however, on rare occasions older adults may have lower jaw pain of cardiac origin (referred pain); history of what initiates the pain and how it is relieved should provide clue to its cardiac origin	1. Detection of older adult with history of angina pectoris 2. Referral of older adult thought to have untreated angina based on health history for medical evaluation and treatment 3. Older adult under medical treatment for angina—during oral healthcare visit every attempt should be made to reduce stress a. Concern and warm approach by oral healthcare professionals b. Make older adult feel free to talk about fears c. Morning appointments d. Short appointments e. Premedication—diazepam (Valium), 5 to 10 mg; prophylactic nitroglycerin, one tablet preoperatively f. Nitrous oxide-oxygen analgesia g. Effective local anesthetic—epinephrine 1:100,000 can and should be used; aspirate; inject slowly 4. Reinforce importance of risk factors that can be influenced by older adults 5. If older adult develops chest pain during hygiene care, stop procedure and give older adult nitroglycerin tablet sublingually a. If pain continues longer than 2 or 3 minutes, monitor vital signs and give up to two nitroglycerin tablets one at a time during the next 15 minutes; if pain persists and older adult's condition is stable, transport older adult to hospital emergency room; call for medical aid and be prepared to render cardiopulmonary resuscitation b. If older adult has stable type of angina and pain is relieved within 2 or 3 minutes with nitroglycerin, dental hygiene care may be continued or terminated depending on circumstances

Table continued on following page

TABLE 30–8
ALTERATIONS IN THE DENTAL HYGIENE CARE OF OLDER ADULTS WITH CARDIOVASCULAR DISEASE *Continued*

Atherosclerotic Disease

Potential Risk Relating to Dental Hygiene Care	Prevention of Medical Complication
	c. Older adult with unstable angina whose pain is relieved with nitroglycerin within 2 to 3 minutes should have appointment terminated and physician informed of what happened 6. Terminate appointment if older adult becomes fatigued or develops change in pulse rate or rhythm 7. Avoid use of vasopressors except for epinephrine 1 : 100,000 in local anesthetic a. Do not use vasopressors to control local bleeding b. Do not use gingival packing material that contains vasopressor

Congestive Heart Failure

Potential Risk Relating to Dental Hygiene Care	Prevention of Medical Complications
1. Sudden death resulting from cardiac arrest or arrhythmia 2. Myocardial infarction 3. Cerebrovascular accident 4. Infection 5. Bacterial endocarditis if heart failure is caused by rheumatic heart disease, congenital heart disease, etc. 6. Shortness of breath 7. Drug side effects a. Orthostatic hypotension (diuretics, vasodilators) b. Arrhythmias (digoxin, overdosage) c. Nausea, vomiting (digoxin, vasodilators) d. Palpitations (vasodilators)	1. No routine oral healthcare until under good medical management 2. Older adults under good medical management Cause of heart failure and any other complications must be considered in the dental hygiene care plan a. Hypertension b. Valvular disease (rheumatic heart disease) c. Congenital heart disease d. Myocardial infarction e. Renal failure f. Thyrotoxicosis g. Chronic obstructive lung disease 3. Antibiotics to prevent postoperative infection 4. Older adult should be in upright position during care to decrease collection of fluid in lung 5. Bleeding time and prothrombin time should be obtained before any surgical procedures; if abnormal, consult with primary care physician 6. Terminate appointment if older adult becomes fatigued, etc. 7. Drug considerations a. Digitalis—older adult more prone to nausea and vomiting b. Anticoagulants—dosage should be reduced so that prothrombin time is 2½ times normal value or less (takes 3 to 4 days) c. Antidysrhythmic drugs d. Antihypertensive agents e. Use of vasoconstrictors

Dental Hygiene Care Plan Modifications	Oral Complications
1. Cause of heart failure, presence of complications, and older adult's current status must be considered 2. In some older adults, only urgent dental needs should be taken care of (by conservative methods) 3. In older adults under good medical management with no complications Any indicated dental hygiene care	1. Infection 2. Bleeding 3. Petechiae 4. Ecchymoses 5. Drug-related a. Xerostomia b. Lichenoid mucosal lesions

Hypertensive Disease

Potential Risk Relating to Dental Hygiene Care	Prevention of Medical Complications
1. Stress and anxiety related to oral healthcare visit may cause increase in blood pressure; in older adult with already elevated blood pressure as a result of hypertensive disease, myocardial infarction or cerebrovascular accident may be precipitated 2. If blood pressure is significantly elevated, excessive bleeding may occur following surgical or scaling procedures 3. Older adults being treated with antihypertensive agents may	1. Detection and referral of older adults with marked elevation of blood pressure and those with moderate prolonged elevation of blood pressure for medical evaluation and treatment 2. Older adults being treated with antihypertensive agents a. Reduce stress and anxiety of oral healthcare visit by premedication, short appointments, morning appointments, and concerned atmosphere by oral healthcare professionals;

TABLE 30–8

ALTERATIONS IN DENTAL HYGIENE CARE OF OLDER ADULTS WITH RESPIRATORY DISEASE
Continued

Hypertensive Disease

Potential Risk Relating to Dental Hygiene Care	Prevention of Medical Complications
become nauseated and vomit, may become hypotensive, or may develop postural hypotension 4. Excessive use of vasopressors will cause significant elevation of blood pressure, which in these older adults may be very dangerous 5. Many antihypertensive agents will potentiate sedative action of barbiturates 6. Sedative medication used in older adults taking certain antihypertensive agents may bring about hypotensive episode(s)	let older adult talk about fears and concerns related to oral healthcare visit; nitrous oxide-oxygen analgesia can be used, but hypoxia must be avoided b. If older adult becomes stressed, terminate appointment c. Avoid orthostatic hypotension by changing chair positions slowly and supporting client when he gets out of chair d. Avoid stimulating gag reflex—nausea e. Avoid excessive use of vasopressors 3. Drug considerations a. Use of local anesthetics with small concentration of vasopressor (epinephrine 1:100,000) and not more than three cartridges; aspirate before injection and inject slowly b. Do not use vasopressors to control local bleeding c. Do not use gingival packing material that contains vasopressor d. Reduce dosage of barbiturates and other sedatives whose actions are enhanced by many antihypertensive agents e. Epinephrine should not be used in any form in older adult being treated with antihypertensive agent pargyline (Eutonyl) or any other monoamine oxidase inhibitor

Dental Hygiene Care Plan Modifications	Oral Complications
1. In uncontrolled hypertension No routine oral healthcare 2. In older adults under good medical management with no complications such as renal failure or congestive heart failure Any indicated dental hygiene care	1. Excessive bleeding in client with uncontrolled hypertension following scaling procedures 2. Xerostomia in older adults overtreated with diuretic agents 3. Mercurial diuretics may cause oral ulceration or stomatitis as an allergic reaction to drug 4. Acetazolamide may cause facial paresthesia

Myocardial Infarction

Potential Risk Relating to Dental Hygiene Care	Prevention of Medical Complications
1. Cardiac arrest 2. Myocardial infarction 3. Angina pectoris 4. Congestive heart failure 5. Bleeding tendency secondary to anticoagulant 6. Infective endocarditis complicating implanted pacemaker 7. Electrical interference with pacemaker	1. No routine oral healthcare until at least 6 months after infarction because of increased risk of new infarction and arrhythmias 2. Consultation with older adult's physician before starting routine oral healthcare to confirm older adult's current status and need for antibiotic prophylaxis for older adults with transvenous pacemakers 3. Morning appointments 4. Short appointments 5. Termination of appointment if older adult becomes fatigued or short of breath, develops change in pulse rate or rhythm, or develops chest pain—inform older adult's physician 6. Use of local anesthetic with epinephrine 1:100,000 (no more than three cartridges); aspirate before injecting; inject slowly 7. Premedication before appointment to reduce stress associated with oral healthcare visit—diazepam, 5 to 10 mg 8. Anticoagulant medication—if surgery or scaling procedures are planned, physician should be contacted and dosage of anticoagulant reduced so that prothrombin time will be twice normal or less—will take 3 to 4 days; check to see if desired result was obtained day of procedure by having another prothrombin time done 9. Digitalis—older adult more prone to nausea and vomiting; avoid stimulating gag reflex 10. Antisialagogues—atropine, methantheline may cause tachycardia; check with older adult's physician before using 11. Antiarrhythmic agents—quinidine, procainamide—nausea and vomiting may occur; hypotension may occur; oral ulceration may indicate agranulocytosis 12. Antihypertensive agents 13. Avoidance of use of instruments such as ultrasonic scaler with older adults who have pacemaker

Table continued on following page

TABLE 30–8
ALTERATIONS IN THE DENTAL HYGIENE CARE OF OLDER ADULTS WITH CARDIOVASCULAR DISEASE *Continued*

Dental Hygiene Care Plan Modifications	Oral Complications
1. Older adults 6 months or more after infarction with no complication Any routine oral healthcare 2. If complications such as congestive heart failure are present Dental hygiene care should be limited to immediate needs only	Usually none except those related to drugs used to treat older adult's medical problem

Data from Little, J. W., and Falace, D. A. Dental Management of the Medically Compromised Patient, 4th ed. St. Louis: Mosby–Yearbook, 1993; pp. 6–14, 48, 49, 175–196.

normally accompany aging occur at different rates in every individual. The rate of the aging process of the cardiovascular system is dependent on an individual's lifestyle, environment, and heredity. Ebersole and Hess label normal changes as intrinsic, whereas factors within the control of the individual are called extrinsic.[17] Extrinsic cardiovascular risk factors that can be eliminated or modified by the individual are presented in Chapter 29.[17] Dental hygienists can be of vital service as both educators and role models. The dental hygienist must advocate a "heart healthy" lifestyle with clients through health education and promotion activities, therefore meeting multiple human needs, for example, wholesome body image, freedom from pain and stress, nutrition, self-determination, and responsibility.

Respiratory Changes

Alterations in the respiratory system and pulmonary performance occur gradually, allowing the older adult to continue to breathe effortlessly in the absence of pathological states. Confronted with a little exertion or stress, however, dyspnea and other symptoms can appear.

The efficiency of the respiratory system declines with age, as evidenced by decreased elasticity of the muscles of the chest and increased rigidity of internal lung stuctures. The ultimate result is less efficiency in emptying of lungs and a reduction in the diffusion of oxygen. Coupled with cellular and humoral immunity decline, older adults are rendered susceptible to respiratory infections and other diseases.

Pulmonary Disorders

Pulmonary diseases are a significant cause of death and disability in older adults. Moreover, many respiratory diseases are linked directly to or are exacerbated by lifestyle practices, chiefly smoking. Chronic obstructive pulmonary diseases (chronic bronchitis and emphysema) are caused primarily by inhalation of smoke, and to a lesser degree by air pollution. Older adults are susceptible to several life-threatening respiratory diseases including asthma, pneumonia, and influenza. In addition, the older individual is more likely to have inactive tuberculosis than any other age group.

Dental hygiene care for persons with respiratory disease includes modifications in positioning (upright posture) in the dental chair so that breathing is not impeded. Clients with asthma who utilize an inhaler should bring it to their appointment. In addition, a low-stress environment (whenever the oral healthcare setting is the least active) can reduce the probability of an asthmatic attack. In individuals with active tuberculosis, treatment is best provided in a hospital setting with appropriate isolation, sterilization, mask, gloves, gown, and special ventilation systems. Because of the special precautions, treatment is usually limited to emergency care only (Table 30–9).[26]

Musculoskeletal Changes

Musculoskeletal changes associated with the aging process affect the posture, function, and gait, and may take on a

TABLE 30–9
ALTERATIONS IN DENTAL HYGIENE CARE OF OLDER ADULTS WITH RESPIRATORY DISEASE

Asthma

Potential Risk Relating to Dental Hygiene Care	Prevention of Medical Complications
Precipitation of asthmatic attack	1. Identification of asthmatic older adult by health history 2. Determination of character of asthma a. Type (allergic or nonallergic) b. Precipitating factors c. Age at onset d. Frequency and severity of attacks e. How usually managed f. Medications being taken g. Necessity for past emergency care 3. Avoidance of known precipitating factors

TABLE 30–9
ALTERATIONS IN DENTAL HYGIENE CARE OF OLDER ADULTS WITH RESPIRATORY DISEASE
Continued

Asthma

Potential Risk Relating to Dental Hygiene Care	Prevention of Medical Complications
	4. Consultation with physician for severe, active asthma 5. Drug considerations a. Regularly taken medications b. Recent corticosteroid use may require supplementation c. If inhaler is used, older adult should bring it to appointment d. Anxious older adult (nitrous oxide-oxygen analgesia or diazepam) should be premedicated. e. Avoid (if possible) (1) Antihistamines (2) Anticholinergics (3) Narcotics (4) Aspirin (5) Nonsteroidal antiinflammatory drugs (6) Penicillin 6. Provision of stress-free environment
Dental Hygiene Care Plan Modifications	**Oral Complications**
Avoidance of the air polishing device	None

Tuberculosis

Potential Risk Relating to Dental Hygiene Care	Prevention of Medical Complications
1. Tuberculosis may be contracted by dental hygienist from actively infectious older adult 2. Older adults can be infected by oral healthcare professionals who are actively infectious	1. In older adults with active tuberculosis a. Consultation with physician before dental hygiene care b. Care limited to emergency care only c. Care in hospital setting with proper isolation, sterilization, mask, gloves, gown, ventilation d. When older adult produces consistently negative sputum and remains in chemotherapy Care provided same as normal patient 2. In older adults with past history of tuberculosis a. Approach with caution; obtain good history of disease and its treatment (treatment of at least 6 to 18 months' duration); appropriate review of systems is mandatory b. Should give history of periodic chest x-ray films and examination to rule out reactivation c. Consult with physician and postpone care if: (1) Questionable history of proper care (2) Lack of appropriate medical supervision since recovery (3) Signs or symptoms of relapse d. If present status "free of active disease" Care provided same as normal older adult 3. In older adults with recent conversion to positive skin test (PPD) a. Should have been evaluated by physician to rule out active disease b. May be receiving isoniazid (INH) for 1 year prophylactically c. Care provided same as normal patient 4. In older adults with signs or symptoms of tuberculosis a. Referral to physician and postpone treatment b. If treatment necessary, care provided as in category 1
Dental Hygiene Care Plan Modifications	**Oral Complications**
None required	1. Oral ulceration, tongue most common 2. Tuberculosis involvement of cervical and submandibular lymph nodes

Modified from Little, J. W., and Falace, D. A. Dental Management of the Medically Compromised Patient, 4th ed. St. Louis: Mosby–Yearbook, 1993, pp. 48–53; used with permission.

variety of appearances. There is a general flexion and forward projection of the head and neck. The back becomes humped, the hips, wrist, and knees slightly flexed, the muscles of the arms and legs flabby and weak, and the overall height reduced. Movement and gait become slower and appear clumsy, and the older adults appears less than agile.

With aging, the skeletal system undergoes a reduction in the skeletal mass. Vertebral disks become thin, causing a shortening of the torso. Posture and structural changes occur primarily because of calcium loss from bone and as a result of atrophy of cartilage and muscle. The loss of muscle mass can be attributed to a decrease in the number and size of muscle fibers. Fibrous tissue replaces muscle tissue when muscle regeneration no longer occurs, resulting in a decrease in the power of the muscle. Movement, motor power, and locomotion are complex physiological functions that have interrelationships with the circulatory and nervous systems. Changes in these systems directly affect physical activity and muscle reflex capabilities.[27] The loss of bone mass coupled with changes in muscle fibers affect bone strength, placing the older client at greater risk for fractures. Fractures, in turn, can lead to decreased mobilization, which contributes to further bone mass loss. Immobilization is a primary factor associated with institutionalization of older adults (see the section on long-term care later in this chapter).

Ligaments, tendons, and joints become hardened, more rigid, and less flexible, predisposing these structures to tears. Worn cartilage around joints combined with a diminished lubricating fluid in the joints can lead to slow, painful movement.

Musculoskeletal System Disorders

Arthritis is a major source of discomfort and disability for many older adults, accounting for serious limitations in activity. The term "arthritis" is a generic term that literally means inflammation of a joint. There are more than 100 different kinds of arthritis, but the most common among the aged are **osteoarthritis** and **rheumatoid arthritis.**

Osteoarthritis, the most common joint disease, is usually encountered in persons older than 50 years. The disease is a defect of articular cartilage, characterized by the gradual loss of cushioning. As cartilage is lost, the resultant exposure of rough underlying bone ends can cause pain and joint stiffness. Bone growths or spurs may appear, producing joint enlargement. As the condition continues, low-grade inflammation of the synovial membrane develops. Thus, inflammation is a secondary effect rather than the initial lesion of osteoarthritis. Weight-bearing joints including the spine, knees, and hips are commonly affected sites, whereas the wrist and knuckles are not. Surgical intervention may be necessary to relieve pain and correct joint deformity.

Rheumatoid arthritis is a chronic, systemic disease affecting connective tissue throughout the body. The hands and feet are most commonly affected in addition to the knee, hip, ankle, and shoulder. Symptoms of rheumatoid arthritis include malaise, fatigue, fever, anemia, and nodules that develop on soft tissues.

Joint diseases are seldom identified as causes of death, but they can interfere significantly with one's body image, self-determination and freedom from pain. Rheumatoid arthritis can greatly affect the older person's ability to perform ADLs such as preventive oral healthcare. Modifications in oral hygiene aids such as enlarged handles or extension devices and automated mouth cleaning devices may be necessary for individuals to meet their needs for a biologically sound dentition and skin and mucous membrane integrity of the oral cavity.

The older client frequently needs the dental hygienist to facilitate human need fulfillment for safety. For example, the older adult who has undergone joint replacement may need to be premedicated to prevent bacteremia from occurring; clients using aspirin or nonsteroidal antiinflammatory drugs must be monitored for increased bleeding; and antibiotic premedication may be indicated for some individuals prior to treatment (Table 30–10) (see Chapter 10 for antibiotic premedication).

Osteoporosis is a condition involving demineralization of the bone and a decrease in bone mass caused by excessive leaching of calcium from the bone matrix. Generally, bone is constantly being broken down and rebuilt at the same rate. However, in osteoporosis, the rate of breakdown exceeds the buildup rate, causing a net loss of bone mass. These changes significantly reduce bone strength, making bones, especially those in the back, hip, and forearm more susceptible to fractures. Osteoporosis can result in diminished height, stooped posture (dowager's hump), and chronic pain, and it is the major cause of skeletal fractures in postmenopausal women and all older persons.

The disease is four times more prevalent in women than men. Females are more prone to the disease because they have less bone mass initially and because changes during menopause lower calcium and estrogen levels. Loss of bone mass begins in the fourth decade, but it is seldom diagnosed until after a fracture occurs. Over their lifetimes, women lose 25 to 30%, whereas men lose 12% of their bone mass because of osteoporosis.[28]

Several intrinsic factors have been identified as increasing the risk of osteoporosis, including gender, race, heredity, and body frame. Although these factors cannot be altered, lifestyle practices can influence the integrity of bone and the bone thinning process (Table 30–11).

The National Research Council of the National Academy of Science has established a daily maintenance dose of calcium that prevents the body from drawing on its mineral stores in bone. For the older woman, 1,000 to 1,200 mg of calcium is recommended and 1,500 mg if the woman is not taking estrogen therapy.[17] Approximately four glasses of nonfat or low fat milk provide 1,200 mg of calcium. For individuals who are lactose intolerant, many green vegetables, sardines, and nuts can serve as sources of calcium. Calcium is best absorbed from dairy products and food, however dietary supplements (calcium carbonate tablets) can be consumed. Calcium carbonate supplements are absorbed best when taken with meals. Older adults who have a family history of kidney stones should seek a physician's advice before using calcium supplements.

There are several screening techniques that detect the degree of bone loss. However, the tests cannot predict who will suffer from fractures and who will not. The procedure is costly, imprecise, and unreliable and many experts do not recommend it to screen women without symptoms. Because the common treatment for osteoporosis is estrogen supplementation, a women not wanting to take estrogens should not undergo the test. Research indicates that estrogen as replacement therapy is not only beneficial in preventing osteoporosis, but also is effective in reducing the risk of cardiovascular diseases. Osteoporosis screening is not helpful for women 10 years after menopause because even if osteoporosis is noted, estrogen treatment has been shown to be ineffective if started that late.[29–31]

TABLE 30–10
ALTERATIONS IN DENTAL HYGIENE CARE OF OLDER ADULTS WITH JOINT DISEASE

	Potential Risk Relating to Dental Hygiene Care	Prevention of Medical Complications	Dental Hygiene Plan Modifications	Oral Complications
Osteoarthritis	Joint pain, stiffness, and loss of mobility Bleeding tendency from aspirin or nonsteroidal antiinflammatory drugs	Short appointments Ensure physical comfort a. Position changes b. Comfortable chair position c. Physical supports Pretreatment bleeding time if taking large dosage of aspirin or nonsteroidal antiinflammatory drugs	Dictated by severity of disability; if severe, extensive care not indicated; encourage and facilitate oral health-promoting behaviors	Temporomandibular joint involvement
Rheumatoid arthritis	Joint pain and immobility Bleeding tendencies secondary to aspirin and nonsteroidal antiinflammatory drugs Bone marrow suppression from gold salts or penicillamine resulting in anemia, agranulocytosis, or thrombocytopenia Adrenal suppression secondary to steroids	Short appointments ensure physical comfort a. Position changes b. Comfortable chair position c. Physical supports Management of drug complications a. Aspirin/nonsteroidal antiinflammatory drugs —obtain pretreatment bleeding time b. Gold salts/penicillamine Obtain complete blood count with differential bleeding time c. Corticosteroids—discuss need for supplements with physician	Dictated by severity of disability and temporomandibular joint involvement; if severe, extensive care not indicated; temporomandibular joint surgery may be helpful; encourage oral health-promoting behaviors	Temporomandibular joint ankylosis Stomatitis secondary to gold salts
Joint prosthesis	Deep infection around joint prosthesis secondary to bacteremia from oral manipulation is thought to be possible problem	Obtain good health history, including medications and surgery Consult with physician, present care plan, and ask for suggestions regarding need for prophylactic premedication Must minimize effects of bacteremia for all oral procedures by using antibiotic premedication; same drugs and dosage schedule can be used as for prevention of bacterial endocarditis in older adults with rheumatic heart disease; orthopedic surgeon often will have personal preference concerning drug	None	May need antibiotic prophylaxis before all oral health care Older adults with acute oral infection must be treated aggressively by local and systemic means; cases have been reported in which acute oral infection has resulted in infection around prosthesis

Data from Little, J. W., and Falace, D. A. Dental Management of the Medically Compromised Patient, 4th ed. St. Louis: Mosby–Yearbook, 1993, pp. 46, 58, 59, 72, 73.

Dental hygienists should advocate adequate calcium intake for all clients to facilitate the human need for safety and a biologically sound body and dentition in later life. Maximum bone deposition occurs by the mid-30s. Consequently, after age 35, calcium products and calcium supplements can, at best, maintain bone quantity and quality.

Neurosensory Changes

As aging occurs, both structural and functional neurological changes become evident. Structural changes includes loss of neurons, loss of total brain weight, and development of neurofibrillary tangles. Functional changes include a decrease in synaptic transmission between neuronal cells and a longer reaction time in the neuromuscular and autonomic nervous systems. In addition to a decreased amount of synaptic transmission, the neurons are slower in sending these transmissions. The **electroencephalogram** (EEG) is a measure of brain wave activity. EEG tracings of the older person show delayed activity compared to EEG results in a younger person.

TABLE 30–11
INTRINSIC AND EXTRINSIC FACTORS ASSOCIATED WITH OSTEOPOROSIS

Intrinsic	Extrinsic
Female gender	Inadequate weight-bearing exercise
White race	Inadequate calcium intake
Small-boned body frame	Use of alcohol and tobacco products
Northern European ethnicity	Chronic medication usage
Slender	Corticosteroids
	Isoniazid
	Tetracycline
	Aluminum-containing antacids
	Diseases
	Hyperparathyroidism
	Kidney disease
	Rheumatoid arthritis
	Diabetes mellitus
	Chronic obstructive pulmonary disease

Cognitive Function

The distinction betweeen normal and abnormal brain changes in the aging process has been studied intensively during the past 40 years. Early studies encouraged the stereotype of the older adult as being forgetful and incapable of learning. More recent studies of the aging brain show that there is no serious cognitive decline in the absence of disease, trauma, or stress.[17] Furthermore, results show that intellectual decline is not an outcome of aging alone but is caused by many conditions such as poor nutrition or hormonal changes.[32] An older adult usually takes longer to learn the same information as a younger adult, but given sufficient time, the end result is similar. Investigations of memory indicate that more time is needed for recall of information; however, differences are found between short- and long-term recall. Short-term memory appears to decline after age 65 years. Alternatively, older adults seem to have a very large capacity for long-term memory. Usually, long-term information is highly organized by time and place or meaningful relations. For example, an older adult may be able to describe an event that occurred in childhood in exacting detail but may not remember the activities of the previous day. Some researchers speculate that much of the short-term information may be perceived as meaningless, thus not stored.[5] Other investigations suggest that alterations in memory are probably more the result of social and health factors than of irreversible effects of age.[33,34] It is important to note that the majority of intellectual testing of older adults has been through cross-sectional research design rather than longitudinal investigations. Consequently, the same group or cohort of older adults was not evaluated over the time needed to provide reliable data regarding changes in that group. Rather, older adults were compared to younger adults, which may not account for differences such as level of education, sensory changes, and motivation between the groups.

Changes in cognitive functioning and sensory changes affect the older adult's likelihood of understanding, performing, and adhering to a preventive oral hygiene program. Dental hygienists must be cognizant of these alterations, whether age-related or pathologically induced, to facilitate human need fulfillment in the older adult through dental hygiene care.

Sensory Changes

Sensory modalities are in a constant state of transition and compensations are increasingly required over the course of the lifespan. Eventually, a reduced efficiency of all of the sensory organs occurs, requiring adaptation by the older adult so that he feels competent and satisfied in the later years. Frequently, the older adult with impaired vision or hearing may be unfairly labeled as stubborn, eccentric, or senile. Dental hygienists need to be aware of sensory changes in older adults in order to adapt their oral hygiene instruction when appropriate. For example, an older adult with diminished eyesight may not be able to read the instructions for a prescribed procedure and, therefore, does not implement the suggested method. The following is a discussion of changes in vision, hearing, taste, smell, and touch with related oral hygiene implications.

Several physical and chemical changes occur in the eye as an individual ages. The eye becomes less accommodating because the lens becomes more rigid and does not change shape as easily to see objects at close range and at a distance. **Presbyopia** is the term for this degenerative change. The lens becomes more opaque and yellows with age. Compounded by a reduced pupil size, the older adult may have difficulty discerning certain color intensities, especially the cool colors. Blue, green, and violet are filtered out and may be difficult to differentiate. Warm colors, including red, yellow, and orange, are generally more easily seen, which makes it advisable to mark objects such as steps, handrails, and operatory equipment with colors that stand out. More light is needed for the older person to see the same objects that a younger person visualizes, and glare presents a significant problem. Finally, the cells in and around the eye lose water and shrink. Pockets of skin, or bags, appear around the eyes and can interfere with vision if the lids sag far enough over the eyes. The lacrimal glands, which keep the eye moist, produce less fluid, leading to the drying of the eye and increased irritation.

Visual Disorders Three disorders, **cataracts, glaucoma,** and **age-related macular degeneration** (AMD), represent the most common visual problems of the older adult. Each can be responsible for serious loss of vision.

Cataracts are the most common disability of the aged eye. If an individual lives long enough, she will develop cataracts to some degree. A cataract involves an opacity of the normally transparent lens. As the lens loses its transparency, there is interference with the passage of light. Risk factors include female gender, smoking, malnutrition, exposure to sunlight and ultraviolet radiation, and advanced age. Treatment consists of surgical removal of the opaque lens. Surgery is indicated when vision loss interferes with the performance of activities. Eyeglasses, contact lenses, or intraocular lens implants are used to compensate for the loss of the lens. Research currently is being conducted to determine the relationship between vitamins (vitamins C and E) and nutrients (zinc) on delaying the development of cataracts.[35]

Glaucoma, a condition in which intraocular pressure increases, is the second most common visual problem in the aged and the primary cause of blindness among African-American older adults. Glaucoma occurs from an obstruction in the normal escape route of the nutrient fluid within the chambers of the eye. When this flow is obstructed, intraocular pressure builds because the production of fluid occurs faster than it can be eliminated. Eventually, pressure is transferred to the optic nerve, leading to irreparable damage. If left untreated, glaucoma leads to blindness. Risk factors include advanced age, diabetes, family history, race, hypertension, and myopia (nearsightedness). Treatment consists of medication to keep the pupil constricted and decrease fluid production. Surgery may be required to provide new channels for fluid elimination. Dental hygienists should be aware of the symptoms of glaucoma, which include complaints of eyes feeling tired, headaches, halos around light, and blurred vision. The symptoms seem to be more evident early in the morning, and one or both eyes may be affected. Clients describing these symptoms should be referred to their primary care physician.

Age-related macular degeneration (AMD) occurs because of deterioration in the membrane between the retina and underlying blood vessels. Damage occurs to the macula, the key focusing area of the retina. As a result, there is a decline in central visual acuity, which makes it difficult to perform tasks such as driving or reading. The etiology of AMD is not well understood but appears to be most strongly associated with age. Genetic factors, smoking, serum cholesterol, and light iris color also seem to play a role. Treatment, with varying success, involves use of lasers to seal off or destroy the abnormal blood vessels. In addition, closed circuit television and magnifying glasses can assist individuals affected with AMD.

The reduced ability to focus the eye and the presence of cataracts may make it difficult for the older adult to navigate, especially in unfamiliar surroundings such as the oral healthcare setting. Also, decreased kinesthetic sensitivity in the elderly person results in postural instability. Providing written directions and educational materials in large print greatly assists the visually impaired person and meets the human need for self-determination and responsibility.

Hearing Disorders Impaired hearing is common among older persons, with 30% of females and more than one-half of males over 65 years exhibiting significant hearing loss.[36] **Presbycusis** is defined as the progressive loss of hearing as a result of the aging process. There are two major types of hearing loss that may occur in the older adult: conductive and sensorineural. *Conductive hearing loss* is an interruption in the transmission of sound waves caused by damage to the auditory nerve or a buildup of ear wax. *Sensorineural deafness* is related to a disorder of the inner ear; a loss of nerve cells in the eighth cranial nerve results in a loss of hearing high frequency sounds. Presbycusis and noise-induced loss are coexistent in many instances.

The ability to hear is a major means of communication. Hearing loss is not only frustrating to the older adult, but also it may threaten an individual's safety and self-esteem. Dental hygienists should look for signs of hearing loss such as anger, confusion, withdrawal, inappropriate responses, and lack of response. Compensation for hearing loss includes the dental hygienist speaking slowly, distinctly, and in a low voice tone. Individuals should be addressed face to face with the face mask removed when possible. Gestures also may be used to enhance and clarify conversation. Shouting or speaking in high-pitched tones and using simplistic language should be avoided. Individuals who have hearing loss because of conduction deficits may use a hearing aid or an assisted listening device to compensate for the loss.

Changes in Taste As a person ages, modest changes in the sensation of taste occur as a result of diminished number and functional ability of the taste buds. Up to 60 years, the ability to perceive sweet, sour, bitter, and salt does not appear to change. During the sixth decade of life, some gradual erosion of the ability to taste salt is apparent but not significant. Although an individual may lose taste on part of the tongue (from trauma or viruses), other parts of the tongue overcompensate for at least part of the loss.[37] The inability to distinguish various tastes or flavors is often caused by other factors such as diminished sense of smell.

Loss of Olfaction Loss of olfaction (smell) with age is not well understood. Age-related degenerative changes in the olfactory bulb or damage of the nerves that service the olfactory bulb may be responsible for impaired olfactory function.[38] The receptors in the olfactory bulb that perceive smell tend to atrophy in the aging process and the individual is unable to smell odors as distinctly as do younger adults. Diminished smell results in a decline in taste perception. As a result, affected older adults may have a diminished appetite with the potential for malnutrition. Whether observed deficits in olfactory acuity have functional significance for the quality of life among older adults is unclear. Undoubtedly, more research is warranted in this area.

Loss of Kinesthetic Ability Touch, or **kinesthetic sensitivity,** refers to the ability to discriminate temperatures, perceive spatial relationships, and discern pain. With advanced age, older adults lose their kinesthetic ability, leaving them vulnerable to accidental falls and postural instability. Understandably, the dental hygienist wants to promote the human need for safety for the older adult. Attention should be devoted to securing loose rugs, and furniture and equipment placement. Additionally, a decrease in tactile sensations can affect fine motor discrimination for hand-to-eye coordination. Coupled with arthritic complications, some older adults may have difficulty manipulating oral hygiene devices.

Neurosensory Disorders

Three disabling, prominent neurological disorders in older adults are **cerebrovascular accidents** (CVA), **dementia,** and **Parkinson's disease.**

Cerebrovascular Accident A CVA or stroke is caused by a thrombus (usual cause in older adults) or a hemorrhage that results in a cerebral infarct. CVA is the most common neurological cause of problems related to coordination and mobility. Strokes rank third as the most common fatal affliction in the later half of life. Survivors of strokes often experience temporary or permanent paralysis and may require adaptive aides or assistance in performing oral hygiene care. As with other medically compromised persons, medications consumed may lead to specific dental hygiene diagnoses that require alterations in dental hygiene treatment and referral (Table 30–12). Prevention of strokes includes smoking cessation, hypertension control, aspirin therapy, and removal of symptomatic blockages.

Dementia Also called organic brain syndrome, dementia is a progressive brain impairment that interferes with normal intellectual functioning. Classic symptoms include significant losses of at least three of the following: cognition, memory, language, recognition, visual and spatial skills, and personality. All behaviors may not be present at all times and they may vary in intensity. Those with mild organic brain syndrome cannot abstract and assimilate new information. In severe cases the individual loses self-care skills and becomes incontinent. Dementia is classified as either reversible or irreversible.

The incidence of dementia increases with age, afflicting 5% of those 65 to 75 years and over 20% of those 85-plus years old. Some degree of dementia is present in over one-

TABLE 30–12
ALTERATIONS IN DENTAL HYGIENE CARE OF INDIVIDUALS AFTER A STROKE

Potential Risk Relating to Dental Hygiene Care	Prevention of Medical Complications	Dental Hygiene Care Plan Modifications	Oral Complications
Dental hygiene care could precipitate stroke Bleeding secondary to drug therapy	Identification of stroke-prone older adult from health history (hypertension, smoking, transient ischemic attacks) Reduce older adult's risk factors for stroke For past history of stroke a. For current transient ischemic attacks (TIAs)—no elective care b. Drug considerations —aspirin/dipyridamole (Persantine), obtain pretreatment bleeding time —Coumadin drugs, obtain prothrombin time under 35 seconds c. Short morning appointments d. Monitor blood pressure e. Avoid use of vasoconstrictor, or at least use sparingly f. No epinephrine in retraction cord	Dependent on physical impairment Modified oral hygiene aids may be needed	None

Modified from Little, J. W., and Falace, D. A. Dental Management of the Medically Compromised Patient, 4th ed. St. Louis: Mosby–Yearbook, 1993, pp. 58, 59.

half the nursing home residents. It is estimated that 45 to 50 billion dollars are spent each year in maintaining those with organic brain syndrome.[39]

Historically, dementia was believed to be an acceleration of the normal aging process caused by arteriosclerosis of the arteries that supply the brain with oxygen. Researchers now find that dementia can be caused by a number of factors: brain tumors, fever, trauma, environmental toxins, chronic lung disease, alcoholism, drug abuse, and stroke. The majority of dementias are irreversible and result in progressive, permanent mental impairment.[39]

Alzheimer's Disease (AD) This disease is irreversible and is the most common form of dementia. It is characterized by the accumulation of neurofibrillary tangles and senile plaques within the cerebral cortex. The etiology is unknown, although there are indications that AD is familial. The prevalence of the disease is low among the young-old and middle-old; it is prevalent (20%) among those of 85 years and older. AD is a primary factor affecting the institutionalization of older adults in the later stages of the disease.

Individuals with AD progress through three stages lasting from 2 to 15 years or longer (Table 30–13). Providing oral healthcare for AD clients can be difficult in the later stages of the disease because of their inability to tolerate dental and dental hygiene care. To meet the client's human need for freedom from stress and for respect, the recommended course of action is to complete dental and dental hygiene care in the early phase of the illness when client cooperation is achievable.

Approximately one-third of individuals with AD have seizure disorders requiring phenytoin. Consequently, gingival hyperplasia is a common oral finding in the presence of poor oral hygiene. Other medications, anticholinergics, may induce salivary gland dysfunction resulting in xerostomia

TABLE 30–13
STAGES OF ALZHEIMER'S DISEASE

Stage 1—Mild Impairment (2 to 4 Years)
Memory loss (predominant symptom) Forgetfulness Spatial disorientation Inability to perform complex routine activities Errors in judgment Neglect of appearance Inability to find objects Denial of deficits
Stage 2—Moderate Impairment (2 to 10 Years)
Increasing memory loss Flat affect Wandering Sudden mood change Repetitive movements Constant motion Unclear speech Restlessness at night Sensory deficits Intensified personality deficits
Stage 3—Severe Impairment (1 to 3 Years)
Confinement to bed or chair Unresponsiveness Rigidity Incontinence Seizures Delusions High risk of infections

and lead to the dental hygiene diagnosis of a deficit in the human need for skin and mucous membrane integrity of the head and neck.

The dental hygiene care plan should begin with a thorough health history including all medications consumed. Depending on the stage of the disease, assistance in obtaining an accurate history may need to be obtained from the caregiver or physician. The oral examination is similar for all clients, but a mouth prop may be useful during the examination and treatment. The dental hygiene care plan must be realistic for the client's medical and physical condition and oral health condition. Also, the oral hygiene care plan must delineate the role of the caregiver in the maintenance of daily oral hygiene care. Aggressive prevention with frequent maintenance care appointments (every 2 to 3 months) averts the need for extensive treatment at a time when the client is unable to cooperate for the dental and dental hygiene care.[40]

As the disease progresses, the individual with AD has difficulties with verbal abilities and with understanding the meaning of what is said. Frequently, their behavior becomes the primary means of communication with others. Similarly, as verbal abilities deteriorate, AD clients become more sensitive to nonverbal behavior of their caregivers. Dental hygienists should look directly at AD clients when speaking and establish eye contact to focus their attention. Verbal and nonverbal messages need to match because individuals with AD are inclined to respond to the nonverbal message. For example, the meaning of "relax" is not understood if said in a tense tone of voice. Verbal communication should consist of exact, positive words or simple sentences delivered in a slow, calm, low voice.[41]

Daily oral hygiene for individuals with AD usually rests with the primary caregiver. In order to meet their human need for skin and mucous membrane integrity of the head and neck and for a biologically sound dentition, home care for dentate clients should include toothbrushing with a fluoridated toothpaste. Because flossing can be difficult, an interdental brush is recommended for interdental cleaning. Fluoride rinses are contraindicated because AD clients have difficulty understanding that the substance should not be swallowed, but daily caregiver-applied fluorides (toothbrush-applied gels) may be indicated as an adjunctive therapy. Saliva substitutes are useful for clients with xerostomia.

The second most common type of dementia is multiinfarct dementia. Small strokes occur within the brain, which causes an insufficiency of blood to some areas and consequent death of the brain tissue. Appearance is sudden, with symptoms of dizziness, headaches, and decreased energy in addition to the classic dementia symptoms. The course of this type of dementia is erratic. Initially, individuals may recover lost function, but as more small strokes occur, the chance of recovery decreases. This type of dementia is associated with hypertension.

Parkinson's Disease This is a chronic, progressive disorder caused by pathological changes in the basal ganglia of the cerebrum, resulting in a deficiency of dopamine. It is characterized by muscle rigidity, involuntary tremors, loss of postural stability, and slowness of spontaneous movement; there is no impairment in intellectual function (see Chapter 26).

Individuals with Parkinson's disease demonstrate excess salivation and drooling. The facial expression is motionless with diminished eye blinking. Tremors in lips and tongue are common, and many individuals have difficulty in swallowing. Adaptive aids and enlarged toothbrush and floss handles should be provided for these clients to facilitate self-care and hence self-determination whenever possible.

Other Disorders

Several other multifactorial conditions are prevalent among the aged that affect the practice of dental hygiene. The following are some additional diseases that may alter dental hygiene care of older adults.

Anemia

Anemia is a common blood disorder among older adults. The two types of anemia seen most frequently are iron-deficiency anemia and pernicious anemia. Iron-deficiency is the most frequent form of anemia, seen more often in females. Chronic aspirin intake, often noted in clients with arthritis, can be a contributing factor leading to blood loss. Pernicious anemia, a progressive disease, is caused by vitamin B_{12} and folic acid deficiency in older adults. Anemia due to inadequate iron intake can make the tongue appear red, smooth, and painful. Pernicious anemia results in a beefy red tongue. Other oral tissues are usually pale or yellowish in color. A person with severe forms of anemia may not be able to tolerate dentures or toothbrushing because of discomfort. This condition has obvious implications for human need fulfillment in the areas of nutrition, freedom from pain, skin and mucous membrane integrity, and a biologically sound dentition.

Diabetes Mellitus

Diabetes mellitus among older adults is the seventh most frequent overall cause of death (see Chapter 31 for a description of the disease). Current estimates suggest that approximately 9% of all older persons in the United States suffer from diabetes. Older women appear slightly more susceptible than older men. At all ages, African-Americans are affected more often than whites.

Oral complications in individuals with uncontrolled diabetes are related to excessive loss of fluids **(xerostomia),** increased susceptibility to infection, and delayed healing times. Often a high prevalence of periodontal disease, angular cheilitis, and mucosal changes are found among clients with uncontrolled diabetes. Dental hygiene care depends on the diagnosed human needs of the client that can be met with dental hygiene care, and the severity of the disease (Table 30–14). For example, some common dental hygiene diagnoses associated with the diabetes might include deficits or disturbances in the following human needs: freedom from stress, skin and mucous membrane integrity of the head and neck, nutrition, and safety. Uncontrolled or unstable diabetes usually indicates the need for antibiotic premedication to reduce the possibility of infection and meet the client's human need for safety. Appointments should be scheduled midmorning following the client's breakfast if possible, therefore meeting the human need for safety and freedom from stress.

Alcoholism

Alcohol has been identified as an important causative factor for many chronic diseases. One of the most significant effects of alcohol abuse is liver damage that impairs other organ systems. Liver damage may appear as alcoholic hepatitis or cirrhosis, a chronic inflammatory disease of the liver.

TABLE 30–14
ALTERATIONS IN DENTAL HYGIENE CARE OF OLDER ADULTS WITH DIABETES

Potential Risk Relating to Dental Hygiene Care	Prevention of Medical Complications
In uncontrolled diabetes a. Infection b. Poor wound healing In older adult treated with insulin—insulin reaction In older adult with diabetes, early onset of complications relating to cardiovascular system, eyes, kidney, and nervous system; angina, myocardial infarction, cerebrovascular accident, renal failure, peripheral neuropathy, blindness, hypertension, congestive heart failure	Detection by a. Health history b. Clinical findings c. Screening blood sugar Referral for medical diagnosis and treatment Older adult receiving insulin—prevent insulin reaction a. Advise older adult to eat normal meals before appointments b. Schedule appointments in morning or midmorning c. Advise older adult to inform you of any symptoms of insulin reaction when they first occur d. Have sugar in some form to give in case of insulin reaction Older adults with diabetes being treated with insulin who develop oral infection may require increase in insulin dosage; consult with physician in addition to local and systemic aggressive management of infection Drug considerations a. Insulin—insulin reaction b. Hypoglycemic agents—on rare occasions aplastic anemia, etc. c. In severe diabetics avoid general anesthesia
Dental Hygiene Care Plan Modifications	**Oral Complications**
In well-controlled diabetes, no alteration of dental hygiene care plan is indicated unless complications of diabetes present such as Hypertension Congestive heart failure Myocardial infarction Angina Renal failure	Accelerated periodontal disease Periodontal abscesses Oral ulcerations Numbness, burning, or pain in oral tissues

Modified from Little, J. W., and Falace, D. A. Dental Management of the Medically Compromised Patient, 4th ed. St. Louis: Mosby–Yearbook, 1993, pp. 18, 19; reprinted with permission.

Alcohol affects the cardiovascular system (cardiomyopathy) and nervous system (organic brain syndrome). Also, alcohol has been identified as a contributing factor in malnutrition leading to general poor health and anemia. Persons who abuse alcohol are likely to suffer accidents, falls, and serious injury compromising their human need for safety.

Oral manifestations commonly observed in alcoholics include increased bleeding tendencies and bruises, and poor oral hygiene may be evident because of overall neglect (Table 30–15). In this situation, dental hygiene interventions would be planned to meet the client's human need for nutrition, freedom from stress, and skin and mucous membrane integrity of the head and neck.

ORAL CONDITIONS IN THE AGED

As with other physiological alterations, the distinction between age-related oral changes and those disease-induced is not always clear or conclusive. Disease, consequences of disease, and use of medications often manifest oral changes and pathology independent of the aging process. Many oral conditions are a result of lifetime oral hygiene and preventive practices.

In this century, perhaps the most significant change in older adults' oral status is the decline in edentulousness. Data show that although 55% of the 65- to 74-year-olds were edentulous in 1957 and 1958, the proportion had decreased to approximately 40% in 1985 and 1986.[42] Changes in treatment philosophies (restore rather than extract), improved treatment modalities, and advances in prevention have played a significant role in reducing tooth loss among older adults, especially the young-old. It is expected that the rate of edentulousness will probably continue to decline for future cohorts of older adults.

Age-Related Oral Changes

Dentition

With age, teeth undergo several changes including alterations in the enamel, cementum, dentin, and pulp. Enamel becomes darker in color because of lifetime consumption of stain-producing foods and drink and the formation of secondary dentin. The enamel surface develops numerous cracks (acquired lamellae) and obtains a translucent appearance. The enamel surface has calcium and phosphate constantly dissolved and redeposited during the active phases of caries. During the active phases of caries dissolution, the surface appears clinically dull with slight exploration revealing a chalky surface. Arrested dental caries in older adults often appear as a brownish-black discoloration because of lifelong uptake of dyes in enamel lamellae.[43]

Occlusal fissures frequently appear darkly stained in older adults partly as a result of previous active dental caries that have changed into an inactive stage. Occlusal attrition often smoothes the occlusal area, which reduces microbial accumulation in the fissure. These fissures may appear slightly sticky on probing, but they may not need

TABLE 30–15
ALTERATIONS IN DENTAL HYGIENE CARE OF OLDER ADULTS WITH CIRRHOSIS OF THE LIVER CAUSED BY ALCOHOLISM

Potential Risk Relating to Dental Hygiene Care	Prevention of Medical Complications
Bleeding tendencies Impaired ability to metabolize certain drugs	Detection of alcoholic older adult a. Health history by older adult b. Clinical examination c. Repeated detection of odor on breath d. Information from friends or relatives Consultation with physician to verify current status Laboratory screening a. Complete blood count b. Bleeding time c. Thrombin time d. Prothrombin time Minimize drugs metabolized by liver
Dental Hygiene Care Plan Modifications	**Oral Complications**
Because oral neglect is commonly seen in alcoholics, older adults should demonstrate interest in and ability to care for dentition before any significant dental hygiene care	Neglect Bleeding Ecchymoses Petechiae Glossitis Angular cheilosis Impaired healing Parotid enlargement

Modified from Little, J. W., and Falace, D. A. Dental Management of the Medically Compromised Patient, 4th ed. St. Louis: Mosby-Yearbook, 1993, pp. 52–54. reprinted with permission.

restoring. Therefore, vigorous exploring must be avoided in order not to damage mechanically the porous part of the fissure enamel thus compromising the individual's human need for a biologically sound dentition.

Cementum undergoes compositional changes, including an increased fluoride and magnesium content. Abrasion of the crowns of teeth is compensated for by deposition of cementum at the apical end and bifurcated areas of the roots. This secondary cementum is normally deposited slowly and continuously throughout life.

Two independent changes are found within the dentin:

- Secondary dentin formation
- Obturation of dentinal tubules (dentin sclerosis)

As a result, the vitality of the dentin is greatly decreased, and aged dentin may become entirely insensitive and impermeable.

The pulp undergoes the same changes that occur in similar tissues elsewhere in the body; pulpal blood supply decreases, the number of cells decrease, and the amount of fibers increase in aged adults. Because pulp calcifications increase with advancing age, the size of the pulp chamber is reduced. Pulp calcifications appear to form in both erupted and unerupted teeth.[44]

Both coronal and root caries are active in the older adult population. Dental caries were once considered childhood phenomena, but research suggests that older adults are more likely to develop new coronal dental caries at a greater rate than school-aged children.[45]

Root caries are most prevalent among older populations because of gingival recession, exposed root surfaces, and tooth longevity. Coronal caries may occur on sound root surfaces or as recurrent decay (Fig. 30–6). Research demonstrates that approximately 60 to 70% of older adults with teeth develop root caries.[42] Mandibular molar and premolar teeth are most frequently involved. The best predictors of root caries include coronal caries, calculus, plaque, and the use of medications with xerostomic effects.[46,47] Root caries can develop rapidly in the absence of adequate oral hygiene, and in the presence of xerostomia, suboptimal periodontal health, and ingestion of fermentable carbohydrates. Dental caries have implications for human need fulfillment in the areas of freedom from pain and a biologically sound dentition. A suggested protocol for dental caries control is reviewed in Table 30–16.

Attrition is common along the incisal and occlusal surfaces as a result of a lifetime of wear, habits, and dietary factors. Severe attrition can result in visible dentin (Fig. 30–7). Many of today's older adults utilized a stiff tooth-

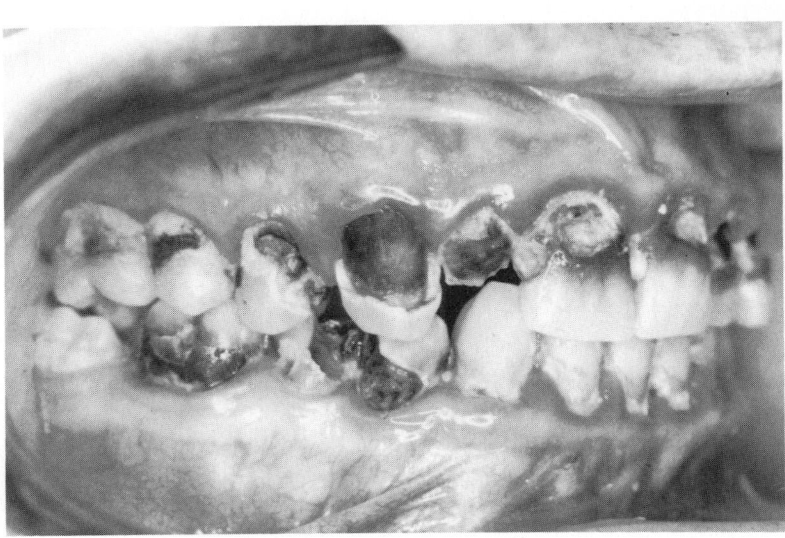

FIGURE 30–6
Rampant root caries. (With permission from Regezi, J. A., and Sciubba, J. J. Oral Pathology: Clinical-Pathologic Correlations, 2nd ed. Philadelphia, W. B. Saunders, 1993, p. 523.)

TABLE 30–16
PROTOCOLS FOR DENTAL CARIES CONTROL

Caries Free	Caries Risk	Carious Lesion/Rampant
Soft tissue management Remove overhanging restorations Reduce root surface sensitivity Plaque removal daily: "A-1" oral hygiene Fluorides: for caries prevention Fluoride in drinking water Dentifrice: Sodium fluoride (NaF) (with 3 brushings) Overdenture used for fluoride tray daily Regular reevaluation Oral health status: teeth, gingiva Health status	Soft tissue management Remove overhanging restorations Reduce root surface sensitivity Plaque removal daily: "A-1" oral hygiene Fluorides: for remineralization, for caries prevention Fluoride in drinking water Dentifrice: NaF (with 3 brushings) Daily rinse (0.05% neutral NaF) Professional NaF topical application at maintenance appointments Overdenture used for fluoride tray daily Saliva substitute with fluoride for xerostomia Increased frequency of reevaluation Oral health status Health status Increased emphasis on counseling for noncariogenic diet	Soft tissue management Appointments for restoration of carious lesions Remove overhanging restorations Reduce root surface sensitivity Plaque removal daily: "A-1" oral hygiene Fluorides: for remineralization Fluoride in drinking water Dentifrice: NaF (with 3 brushings) Daily rinse (0.05% neutral NaF) Weekly rinse (0.20% NaF) Professional NaF topical application at maintenance appointments Overdenture used for fluoride tray daily Saliva substitute with fluoride for xerostomia Increased frequency of reevaluation Oral health status Health status Diet control: eliminate cariogenic foods

Modified from Wilkins, E. M. Root caries: The problem and the protocol. Dental Hygienist News 4(1):6–7, 1991; reprinted with permission.

brush and abrasive paste in the past. Consequently, **abrasion** of the teeth, especially in the cervical area and on root surfaces, may be evident (Fig. 30–8). Abrasion, although common among older adults, is the result of a physiochemical process rather than a result of aging. Although modern dentifrices are not sufficiently abrasive to severely damage intact enamel, they can cause remarkable wear of cementum and dentin if the toothbrush is used in a horizontal rather than vertical direction. Dental hygienists can assist individuals in maintaining a biologically sound dentition and freedom from pain through appropriate oral hygiene educational instructions.

Periodontium

Advanced stages of periodontal disease are typically manifested in people of 45 years and older; age is often erroneously associated with causing the disease. Research indicates that the affect of age on the progression of periodontitis is considered negligible when good oral hygiene is maintained.[48]

The level of periodontal health in middle age can be used as a predictor of periodontal disease in later life. Data suggest that the prevalence and severity of periodontal disease will likely decrease within a few decades as the present

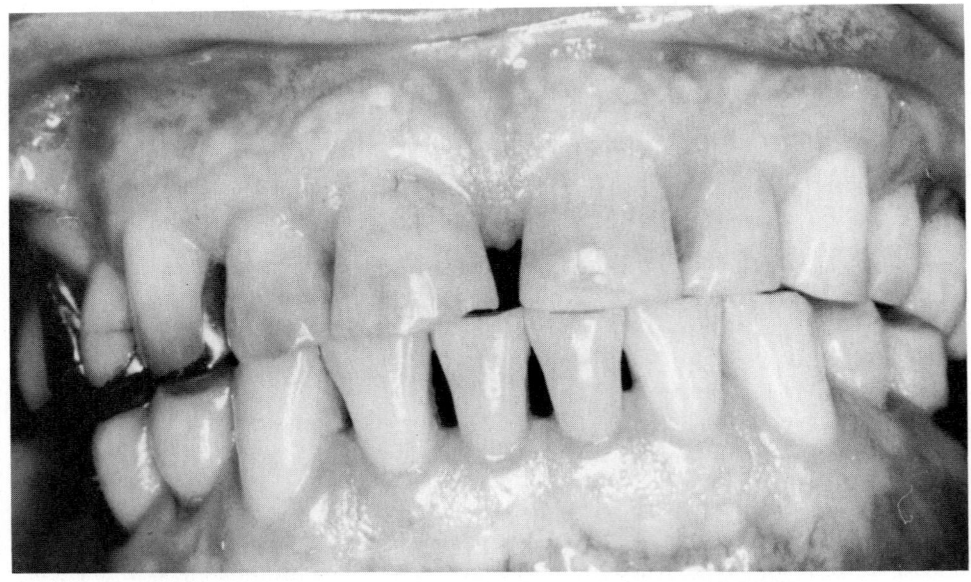

FIGURE 30–7
Attrition of adult dentition. (With permission from Ibsen, O. A. C., and Phelan, J. A. Oral Pathology for the Dental Hygienist. Philadelphia: W. B. Saunders, 1992, p. 81.)

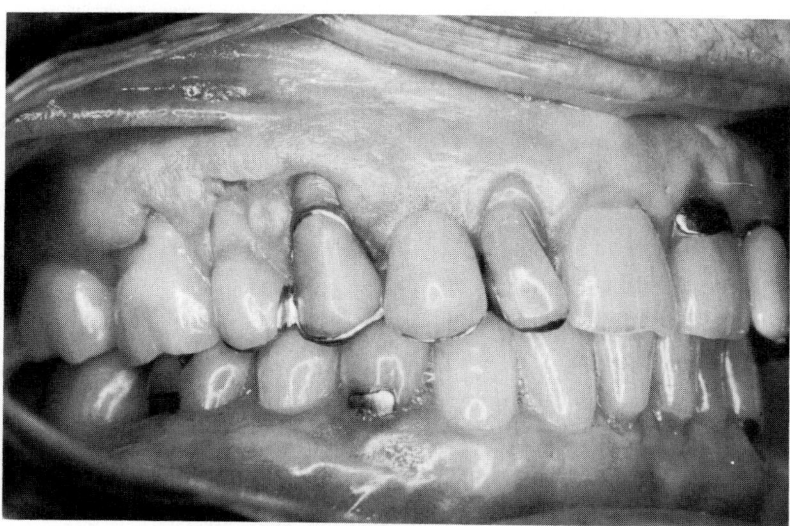

FIGURE 30–8
Toothbrush abrasion of cervical zone of maxillary teeth. (With permission from Regezi, J. A., and Sciubba, J. J. Oral Pathology: Clinical-Pathologic Correlations, 2nd ed. Philadelphia: W. B. Saunders, 1993, p. 501.)

younger age groups, with better oral hygiene and less gingival disease, move into their 60s and 70s.[49] For many of today's older adults, however, periodontal treatment needs still exist. The National Institute of Dental Research (NIDR) survey of adult oral health revealed that 34% of those over 65 years had at least one site with significant periodontal destruction, attachment loss of 6 mm or greater, compared with approximately 8% of the 18- to 64-year-old group.[50] Other studies found similar results with the majority of older adults exhibiting moderate levels of periodontitis (attachment levels of 4 to 6 mm) that can be controlled and treated. Older adults do not appear to present significant increases in gingival bleeding with ascending age but have more calculus compared to younger adults. Recession is frequently evidenced, predisposing the older adult to root caries and abrasion.

Age-Related Changes in the Periodontium

Alveolar Bone

The most significant tissue consideration in determining the relationship between age and periodontal disease is the quality of alveolar bone. There is an increase in bone porosity and diminution of cortical width with aging, but this increased porosity has been found to be unrelated to the presence of teeth and does not lead to crestal resorption. Research shows that crestal bone loss with aging is minimal in healthy persons, although evidence suggests that bone resorption activities do diminish with age.[51]

Soft Tissue Changes

Gingival epithelium reportedly shows no significant morphological changes with age, although there is evidence of a thinning of the epithelium, diminished keratinization, and increased cellular density.[51]

A reduction in cellular elements and an increase in fibrous intercellular substance have been noted in gingival connective tissue. A reduced number of nerves in the gingiva and increased evidence of nerve degeneration with increasing age have been found, along with arteriosclerotic changes in gingival vessels. An increase in gingival width seen with aging has been attributed to growth of the alveolar process, along with eruptive movements of the teeth and supporting tissue, suggesting a compensatory response of the dentogingival unit to age-related changes.[51]

Periodontal Ligament

Alteration in periodontal ligament cellular function, increases in calcification, and arteriosclerosis are seen with advancing age. Research suggests that periodontal arteriosclerosis may exacerbate pathological changes in animal studies, but the effect in humans is unclear.[51]

Bacterial Plaque

Limited studies with conflicting results have compared the composition of plaque at differing ages. Studies have shown, however, a greater plaque accumulation in older age groups, suggesting that factors affecting plaque accumulation in clients (gingival recession, reduced salivary flow) may be related.[52]

Numerous morphological, biochemical, and metabolic changes can be observed in the periodontium with aging, but the overall significance of these factors as they affect susceptibility and progression of periodontal disease is unclear. It appears, however, that in the absence of disease, the clinical changes in the periodontal structures attributable to aging alone are therapeutically insignificant.

Periodontal disease can be treated and periodontal health maintained successfully in the aged. Professional care, adequate oral hygiene, and frequent periodontal maintenance therapy increase the likelihood of maintaining periodontal health among older adults. Dental hygienists are the primary oral healthcare providers prepared to assist older adults in meeting the multiple human needs of wholesome body image, freedom from pain, mucous membrane integrity, and a sound dentition.

Oral Mucosa and Lips

The degree of change in the oral mucosa due to aging versus the consequence of disease is unclear. Some mucosal alterations are a result of systemic factors (for example,

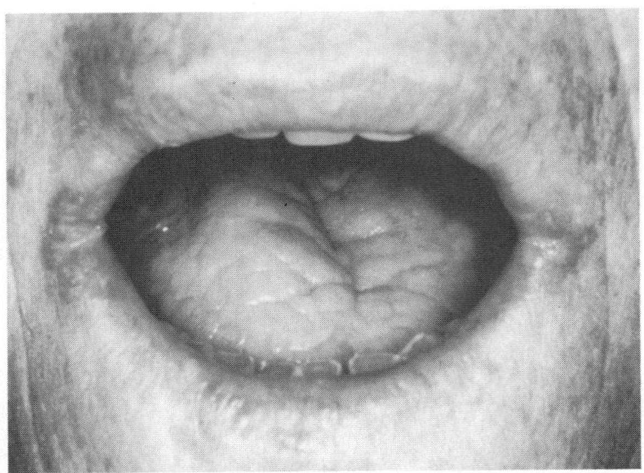

FIGURE 30-9
Angular cheilitis in a patient with pernicious anemia. (With permission from Ibsen, O. A. C., and Phelan, J. A. Oral Pathology for the Dental Hygienist. Philadelphia: W. B. Saunders, 1992, p. 428.)

xerostomia) and are not related to aging, per se. Systemic disease and medication use cause some older adults to have changes in their oral mucosa, including atrophy of epithelium and connective tissues with a decrease in vascularity. Clinically, the oral mucosa appears dry, smooth, and thin. In the absence of disease, however, the oral mucosal status of older adults is comparable to that of younger adults, suggesting that aging alone does not lead to changes in the appearance of oral mucosa.[53] Fungal infections (candidiasis), however, may result from utilization of broad-spectrum antibiotics, such as amoxicillin, and xerostomia-causing medications.

Lips may appear dry and drawn as a result of dehydration and loss of elasticity within the tissues. **Angular cheilitis,** commonly evidenced among the aged, clinically appears as fissuring at the angles of the mouth, with cracks, erythema, and ulcerations (Fig. 30-9). Moistness from drooling, deficiency of vitamin B_2 (riboflavin), and infection by *Candida albicans* are the etiologic factors associated with the disease. Dental hygienists can meet multiple human needs including skin and mucous membrane integrity, nutrition, and wholesome body image.

Ill-fitting dentures or poor denture hygiene can result in mucosal irritation, including **denture stomatitis, papillary hyperplasia,** and **denture-induced fibrous hyperplasia.** Denture stomatitis appears as a localized or diffuse red inflamed area that is sometimes ulcerated (Fig. 30-10). Papillary hyperplasia is characterized by closely arranged pebble-shaped, red, edematous projections on the palatal vault (Fig. 30-11). The signs of denture-induced fibrous hyperplasia include single or multiple elongated folds near the border of a ill-fitting denture (Fig. 30-12). The human need for mucous membrane integrity necessitates that the dental hygienist provide palliative treatment and refer the individual to the dentist for further evaluation.

Hard Tissues

Osteoporosis, primarily, and resorption, to a lesser degree, effect decreases in bone mass and increases in porosity. Also, a reduction in metabolism and reduced healing capacities can influence the quality of bone. The human need fulfillment for a biologically sound dentition may be compromised as a result.

Alveolar bone quality can affect significantly the older adult's ability to wear oral prosthetics. Difficulty in mastication can occur as a result, leading to a deficit in the person's human need for nutrition.

Tori and exostoses do not require treatment unless they interfere with placement of prosthesis or are chronically

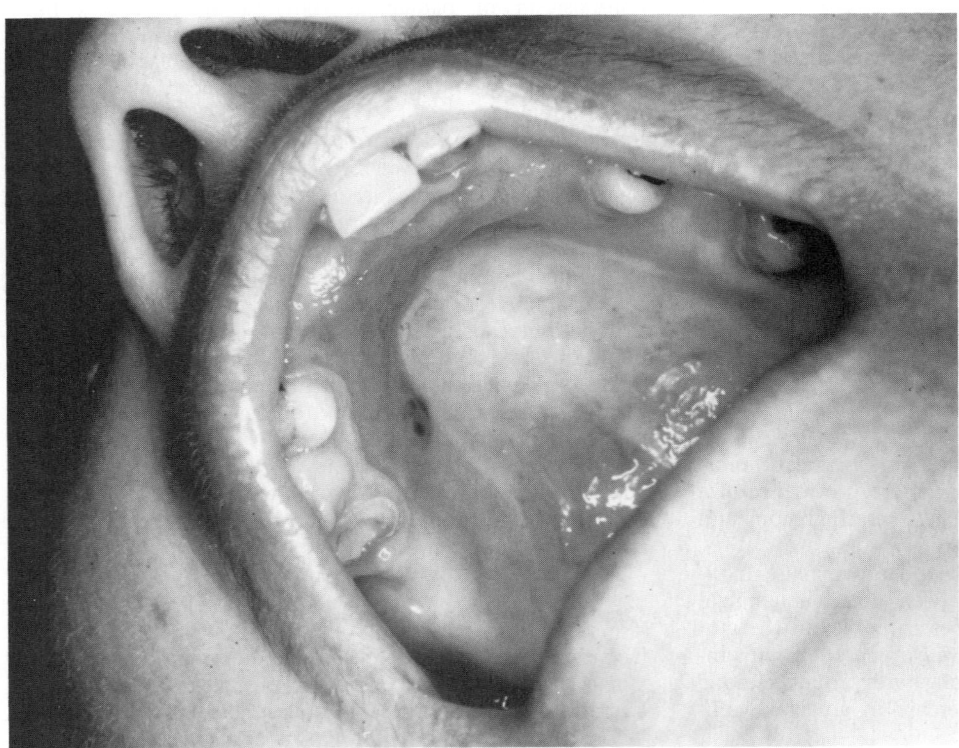

FIGURE 30-10
Denture stomatitis. (With permission from Ibsen, O. A. C., and Phelan, J. A. Oral Pathology for the Dental Hygienist. Philadelphia: W. B. Saunders, 1992, p. 195.)

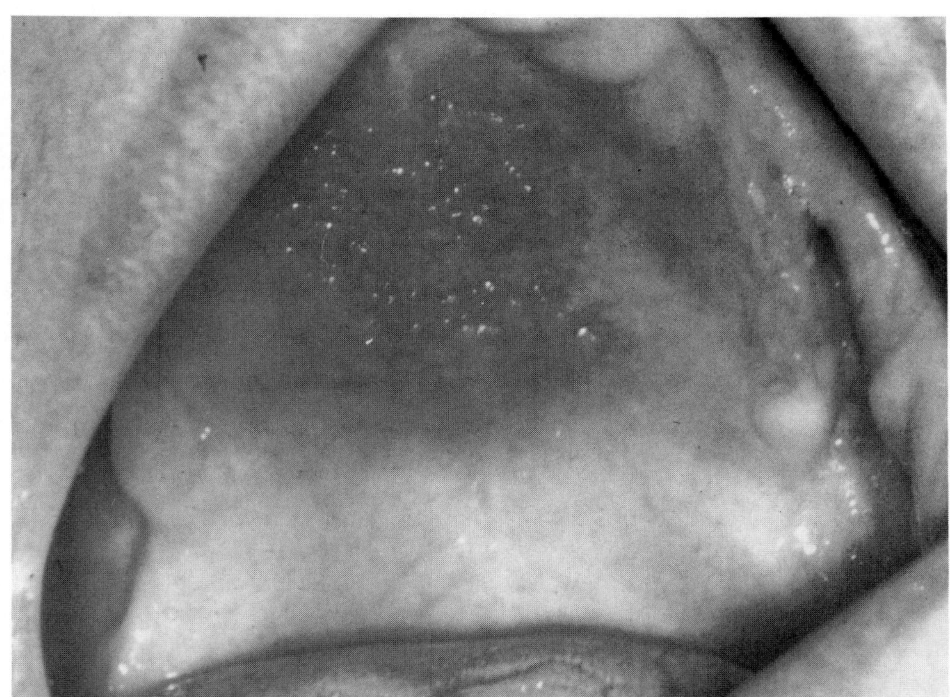

FIGURE 30-11
Papillary hyperplasia. (Courtesy of Dr. Edward Zegarelli.)

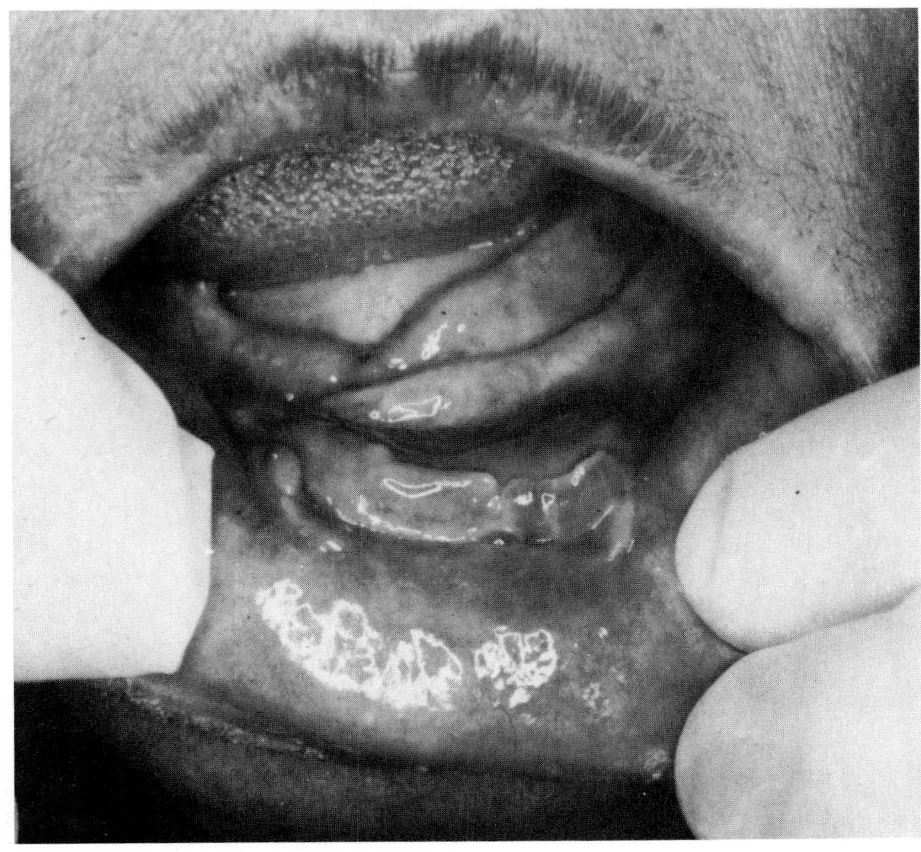

FIGURE 30-12
Denture-induced fibrous hyperplasia. (With permission from Ibsen, O. A. C., and Phelan, J. A. Oral Pathology for the Dental Hygienist. Philadelphia: W. B. Saunders, 1992, p. 111.)

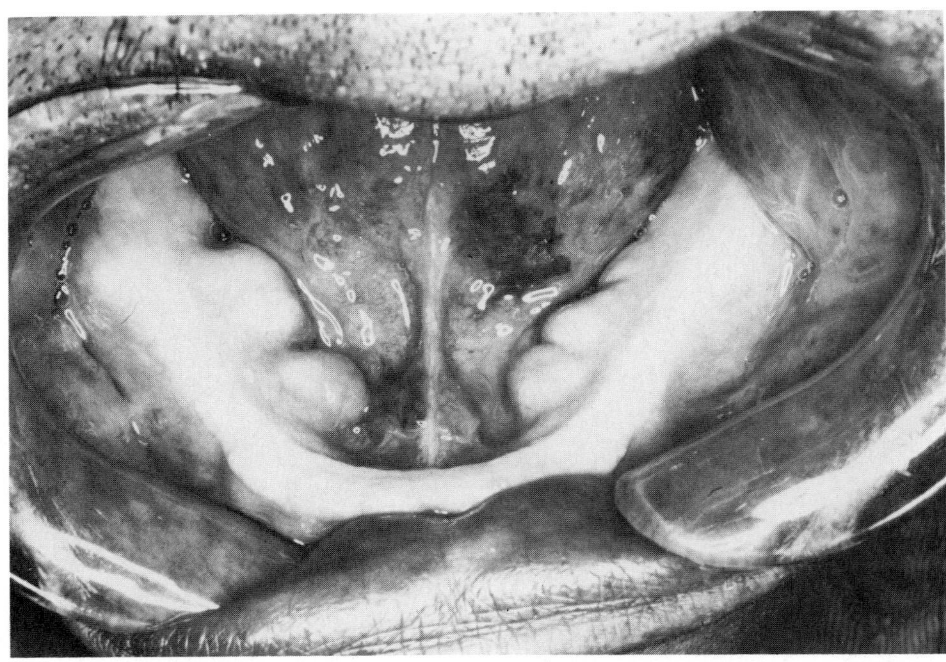

FIGURE 30-13
Mandibular tori. (With permission from Ibsen, O. A. C., and Phelan, J. A. Oral Pathology for the Dental Hygienist. Philadelphia: W. B. Saunders, 1992, p. 340.)

irritated. Approximately 25% of the adult population have these bone growths (Fig. 30-13).

Tongue

Changes in the tongue may include a decrease in the number and sensitivity of papillae. Combined with a decline in the sense of smell, some foods have less appeal, and nutritional needs may not be met. In addition, the tongue often increases in size in edentulous mouths or as a result of disease (for example, pernicious anemia).

Sublingual varicosities are customary findings among the aged; however, they are not problematic. Clinically, they appear as deep red or bluish-black dilated vessels on either side of the midline on the ventral surface of the tongue (Fig. 30-14).

Because of nutritional factors, older adults frequently have anemia as a result of iron deficiencies. Atrophic glossitis is a symptom of this condition, and the tongue appears smooth, shiny, and denuded. Often individuals complain of a burning sensation. The dental hygienist can assist the individual to maintain freedom from pain by recommending an oral lubricant to reduce discomfort and by providing dietary counseling.

Salivary Glands

Research has shown fairly well that reductions in salivary flow are not a result of the normal aging process. Decreases

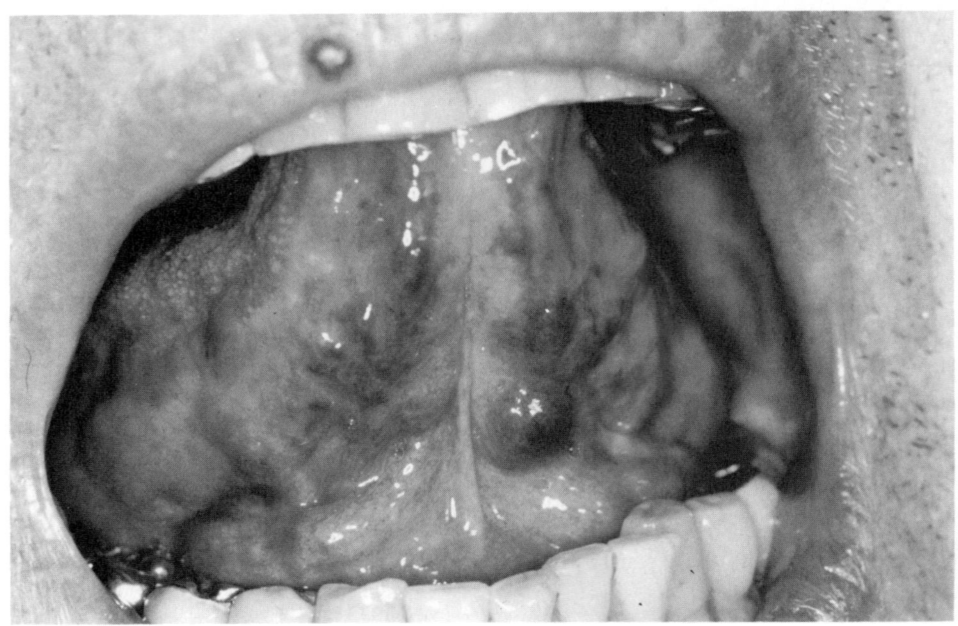

FIGURE 30-14
Sublingual varicosities. (Courtesy of Dr. David Zegarelli.)

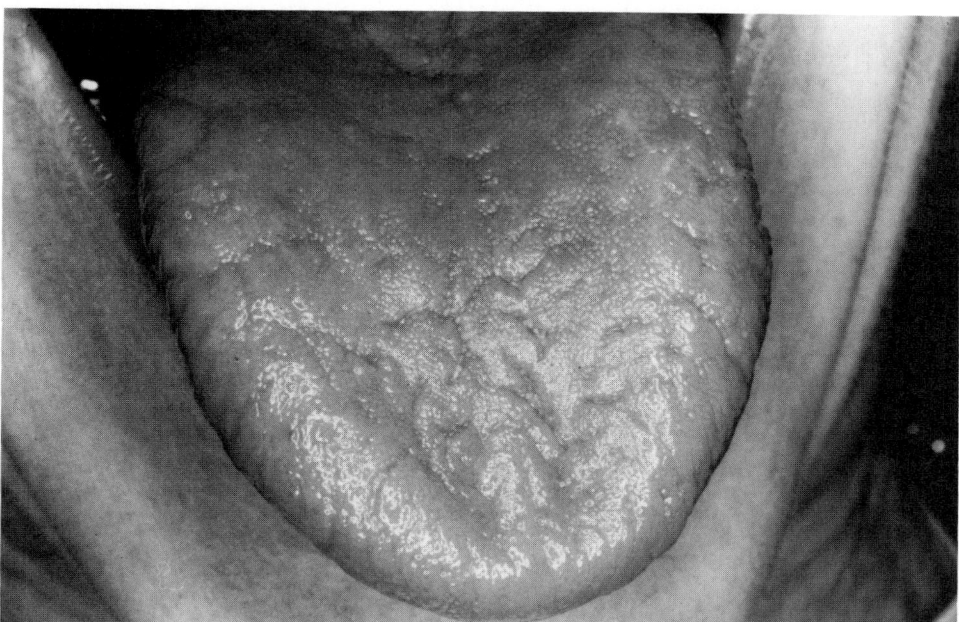

FIGURE 30-15
Sjögren's syndrome with severe xerostomia. (With permission from Ibsen, O. A. C., and Phelan, J. A. Oral Pathology for the Dental Hygienist. Philadelphia: W. B. Saunders, 1992, p. 170.)

in salivary flow are usually attributed to systemic disease, radiation therapy, tumors, or medications that cause temporary or permanent xerostomia.

Signs and symptoms of salivary reduction should be carefully evaluated to determine the cause. In the absence of medications, underlying diseases and the possibility of salivary gland tumors should be investigated.

Sjögren's Syndrome

Sjögren's syndrome is an autoimmune disorder of the salivary glands occurring most frequently in postmenopausal women. Approximately 60% of people with this disorder are older than 50 years.

Clinically, the oral mucosa is extremely dry and saliva is ropy. Initially the tongue shows marked atrophy of the papillae, and later the surface becomes smooth and lobulated (Fig. 30-15).

To meet the need for mucous membrane integrity, persons with Sjögren's syndrome should be instructed to use saliva substitutes. For dentate individuals, fluoride therapies (rinses or daily gels) may be recommended to help meet the need for a sound dentition.

Drug-Induced Oral Changes

Approximately one-fourth of all prescription and over-the-counter drugs are used by older adults. **Polypharmacy** is a term to describe treatment with multiple drugs. Polypharmacy stems from multichronicity, the prescribing methods of physicians, and the beliefs and practices of the older adult toward illness and treatment. On average, most older adults take more than three therapeutic agents and the institutionalized elderly use between five and seven drugs concomitantly.

Several physiological changes of aging that influence drug therapy have been identified. These changes include alterations in the kidney and liver function that inhibit the metabolism and excretion of drugs; intestinal blood flow is reduced and the solubility and ionization of drugs is altered; and the aging brain experiences a loss of neurons and changes in neurotransmitters affecting the administration of central nervous system-acting drugs and neuronal blockers. All of these changes influence the effects of drugs and can exacerbate adverse reactions.[54]

Medications most frequently used by older adults include analgesics, diuretics, oral hypoglycemics, antihypertensives, antidepressants, and sedatives. Table 30-17 lists many drugs consumed by older adults. Multiple medical problems, along with multiple drug use, can lead to a high rate of adverse drug reactions. Many drugs produce oral changes in the mouth because of side effects or as a consequence of the drug (Table 30-18). Dental hygienists play an important role in identifying medication usage and potential side effects in meeting the human need for safety.

Xerostomia

Xerostomia is a common side effect of many drugs. Currently more than 300 medications have been identified as causing xerostomia (Table 30-19).

Saliva lubricates the oral mucosa, assisting speech and swallowing, and facilitates the retention of oral appliances. Diminished salivary flow can alter taste, contribute to plaque formation and dental caries, and cause the oral mucosa to appear dry and inflamed. For edentulous persons, denture retention and comfort may become difficult. If xerostomia is severe, a medical consultation is necessary to determine the probable cause. Some drugs cause xerostomia to a lesser degree than others and may be substituted.

Older adults with chronic medical conditions should be asked to bring their medications to their appointment for identification. Possible side effects need to be determined prior to dental hygiene care.

Individuals with xerostomia may find nonprescription saliva substitutes helpful, especially at meal time and for assisting in denture retention. Some contain fluoride, which can prevent dental caries in dentate individuals.

TABLE 30–17
COMMON DRUGS TAKEN BY OLDER ADULTS

Classification	Generic Name	Brand Name	Indications	Adverse Reactions
Analgesics	Aspirin	Bayer Empirin	Mild-moderate pain, fever, inflammation, arthritis, post-extraction pain, thromboses	G.I. upset, prolonged bleeding time, rash, tinnitus
	Ibuprofen	Advil Motrin	Same	G.I. upset, prolonged bleeding time, drowsiness, blurred vision, tinnitus, rash, edema, alopecia
Sedatives Benzodiazepines	Diazepam Alprazolam Oxazepam	Valium Xanax Serax	Anxiety, tension, muscle relaxant, antiemesis	Drowsiness, dizziness, nausea, transient hypotension, abdominal discomfort, xerostomia, ataxia, confusion
Antidepressants Tricyclic antidepressant	Nortriptyline	Aventyl	Depression	Xerostomia, orthostatic hypotension, blurred vision, tachycardia, drowsiness, epinephrine potentiation
	Imipramine Amitriptyline	Tofranil Elavil		
Cardiovascular Glycosides	Digoxin	Lanoxin	Congestive heart failure, arrhythmias	G.I. upset, trigeminal neuralgia, visual disturbances, arrhythymias, epinephrine potentiation
Antiarrhythmic	Quinidine	Cin-Quin Quinora	Arrhythmias	G.I. upset, lightheadedness, pallor, fever, headache, vertigo, hypotension, rash, tinnitus, thrombocytopenia
Beta blocker	Propranolol	Inderal	Hypertension, headaches, hyperthyroid, arrhythmias	Bradycardia, bronchospasm, tension, xerostomia, fatigue, G.I. upset
Nitrates Nitrites	Nitroglycerin	Nitrostat	Angina	Fainting, hypotension, severe headaches
Diuretics	Triamterene Triamterene HCZ	Dyrenium Dyazide	Hypertension, edema	Orthostatic hypotension, dizziness, xerostomia, electrolyte imbalance
Neuronal blockers	Reserpine	Serpasil	Hypertension	Stuffy nose, xerostomia, orthostatic hypotension, depression, hypotension, bradycardia, nervousness, drowsiness, weight gain, G.I. upset
CNS-acting drug	Methyldopa Clonidine	Aldomet Catapres	Hypertension, edema	Anemia, sedation, edema, weight gain, stuffy nose, orthostatic hypotension, xerostomia, lichenoid eruptions, bradycardia
Anticoagulants	Warfarin	Coumadin Panwarfin	Pulmonary embolism, thrombophlebitis	Hemorrhage, diarrhea, nausea, dermatitis, mouth ulcers, fever

Reprinted with permission from Swapp, K. M. Drugs and the geriatric patient: A dental hygiene perspective. Journal of Dental Hygiene 64(7):326–331, 1990. Copyright 1990 by the American Dental Hygienists' Association.

Drug-Induced Hyperplasia

Persons taking anticonvulsants such as phenytoin may exhibit gingival hyperplasia as a side effect (Fig. 30–16). Adequate plaque control, particularly if started before the administration of phenytoin, may reduce the magnitude of gingival overgrowth. Also, clients with prescribed antiangina drugs (nifedipine) may exhibit hyperplasia.

Candidiasis

Conditions that promote *C. albicans* overgrowth are prolonged antibiotic therapy or depression of defense mechanisms by immunosuppressants. Candidiasis is characterized by a thick, white coating on the tongue or oral mucosa. Persons with candidiasis may have difficulty maintaining their oral hygiene or wearing dentures as a result of pain, thus compromising their human need for freedom from pain.

DENTAL HYGIENE PROCESS OF CARE

Care planning and implementation are determined by the dental hygiene diagnosis, type, and severity of chronic conditions and the cognitive abilities of the older adult. Attitude of the client, level of self-care, expectations, and financial ability all play a significant role as well. Table 30–20 is a presentation of dental hygiene diagnoses related to the older adult.

Because the elderly have a lower stress tolerance and tire more easily than a younger person, short appointments in the morning are recommended. A written note of date and time of each appointment should be provided.

Assessment and Dental Hygiene Diagnoses

Assessment of overall physical factors begins in the reception area. It is important to observe gait and balance because some elderly may require assistance to the treatment area. An arm should be extended for clients who appear unsteady or have severe visual impairments. The dental chair should be positioned at the level of the knees or higher if the person has difficulty bending the knees, therefore facilitating the human need for safety. Also, the arm of the chair should be placed back as far as possible. If the client uses a wheelchair, transfer to the dental chair is necessary. The client should be asked if assistance is needed or which method of wheelchair transfer is preferred.

TABLE 30–18
DRUG-INDUCED ORAL CHANGES

Condition	Description	Class	Generic/Brand Names
Xerostomia	Dry, smooth, shiny oral mucosa	Diuretics	Triamterene HCZ/Dyazide
		Antihistamines	Diphenhydramine/ Benadryl
		Antidepressants	Imipramine/Tofranil
		Antihypertensives	Reserpine/Serpasil
		Antiarrhythmics	Atropine sulfate/Atropine
		Anti-Parkinsonism	Benztropine/Bensylate
Trigeminal neuralgia	Sharp, stabbing pain, aching of teeth and of lower jaw	Beta blockers	Propranolol/Inderal
		Tricyclic antidepressants	Nortriptyline HCl/Aventyl
		Cardiac glycosides	Digoxin/Lanoxin
Glossitis, stomatitis	Lesions on tongue, small multiple ulcers	Anticoagulants	Warfarin/Coumadin
		Salicylates	Aspirin/Bayer
		Barbiturates	Pentobarbital/Nembutal
Erythema multiforme	Vesicles or bullae, fever, impaired physical condition	Antituberculars	Rifampin/Rifadin
		Anticonvulsants	Phenytoin/Dilantin
		Antibiotics	Tetracycline/Vibramycin
		Antianxiety	Meprobamate/Meditran
		Antibacterial	Clindamycin/Cleocin
Lichenoid eruptions	White striations, erythematous patches, erosions, or ulcerations	CNS-drugs	Methyldopa/Aldomet
		Diuretics	Furosemide/Lasix
		Antiarrhythmics	Quinidine/Cin-Quin
Oral candidiasis	(Thrush) multiple white patches	Antibiotics	Tetracycline/Vibramycin
		Corticosteroids	Prednisone/Orasone
		Antifungal	Griseofulvin/Fulvicin-U/F
Hairy tongue	Elongation of filliform papillae	Corticosteroids	Prednisone/Deltazone
		Antibiotics	Tetracycline
		Antifungal	Griseofulvin/Fulvicin-U/F
Gingival hyperplasia	Overgrowth of papilla and marginal gingiva	Anticonvulsant	Phenytoin/Dilantin

Reprinted with permission from Swapp, K. M. Drugs and the geriatric patient: A dental hygiene perspective. Journal of Dental Hygiene 64(7):326–331, 1990. Copyright 1990 by the American Dental Hygienists' Association.

TABLE 30–19
DRUGS CAPABLE OF CAUSING XEROSTOMIA

Classification	Example
Anticholinergics	atropine, scopolamine, propantheline
Antihypertensives	guanethidine (Ismelin), clonidine (Catapres)
Antihistamines	diphenhydramine (Benadryl), chlorpheniramine (Chlor-Trimeton)
Antipsychotics	chlorpromazine (Thorazine), promazine (Sparine), thioridazine (Mellaril)
Anoretics	amphetamines, diethylpropion
Narcotics	meperidine (Demerol), morphine
Anticonvulsants	carbamazepine (Tegretol), lithium carbonate (Lithane)
Antiparkinsonian	benztropine (Cogentin), trihexyphenidyl (Artane)
Antineoplastics	busulfan (Myleran), procarbazine HCl
Antispasmodics	dicyclomine hydrochloride (Bentyl)
Sympathomimetics	ephedrine
Antidepressants	tricyclic (doxepin, amitriptyline), MAO inhibitors (isocarboxazid, phenelzine)
Antianxiety agents	meprobamate (Miltown), benzodiazepines (Valium, Librium, Serax, Ativan), hydroxyzine (Atarax)
Muscle relaxants	orphenadrine (Norflex), cyclobenzaprine (Flexeril)
Diuretics	hydrochlorothiazide (Hydrodiuril)
Antiemetics	metoclopramide (Reglan)

Reprinted with permission from Felder, R. S., Millar, S. B., and Henry, R. H. Oral manifestations of drug therapy. Special Care in Dentistry 8:119–124, 1988. Copyright © 1988. Reprinted by permission of ADA Publishing Co., Inc.

Vision impairments may necessitate assisting the elderly adult in completing the health history. Ideally, a health history in large print allows visually impaired clients to complete the form themselves. The person should be addressed in a low pitch with the face mask removed. Shouting is not only unnecessary but ineffective. Background noises such as music should be eliminated if possible. Individuals with hearing aids should be requested to keep them on while reviewing the client history or discussing oral hygiene methods; however, the volume should be reduced when using a rotary handpiece. Older adults accompanied by others should be addressed directly, not the family member or caregiver. By speaking directly to the elderly client, infantilization is not promoted, therefore meeting the human needs for appreciation and respect and self-determination.

The health history should include the client's personal, medical, and dental background. Personal history, for example, may show that clients are widowed (may live alone, may have reduced income), which could affect their ability to receive dental care. The health history should include previous and past medical conditions. Both prescription and over-the-counter medications currently being used must be reviewed for oral implications. A current *Physicians' Desk Reference (PDR)* is indispensable for medications that are unfamiliar or not prescribed as the common drug of choice. Some individuals suffering from more than one disease may experience adverse effects from multiple drug use. The practitioner must consult with the client's physician if there is doubt regarding treatment. Evaluation of vital signs, including respiration, pulse, blood pressure, and temperature (if indicated), should be performed and recorded. In addition to completing a thorough health his-

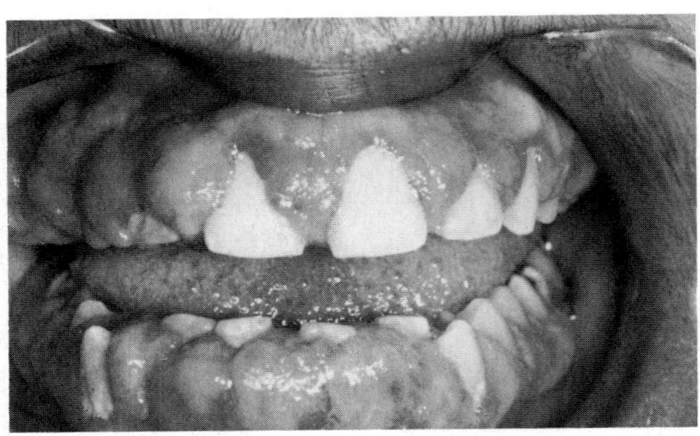

FIGURE 30–16
Gingival hyperplasia. (Courtesy of Dr. Edward Zegarelli.)

tory, the practitioner should be patient and listen to information that the client shares.

The extraoral examination can reveal abnormalities in the skin of the face and neck, lymph nodes, salivary glands, and underlying muscles. The mandible should be examined for movement, and the temporomandibular joint should be palpated for crepitation, tenderness, or limitations in movement. A client with arthritis may not be able to open his mouth fully.

A client's breath can indicate periodontal disease, systemic disease, or alcohol abuse. Lips must be evaluated for signs of angular cheilitis, muscle inelasticity, and lesions. A thorough intraoral examination is necessary to determine if any abnormal lesions are present. A complete dental charting and periodontal assessment must be part of every dental history to provide documentation for reevaluation. The quantity and quality of saliva must be assessed to ascertain if saliva substitutes should be recommended.

Radiographs and other diagnostic aids such as study models should be used as indicated and appropriate. Referral for biopsy may be indicated for suspicious lesions.

Oral hygiene status including bacterial plaque distribution, calculus, and stains must be assessed. Assessment of the client's ability to perform oral hygiene practices is essential. The older person's home care practices should be modified rather than attempts made to change completely the habits of 50-plus years. Compensation for physical changes such as arthritis and impaired vision may affect their ability to carry out oral hygiene recommendations, therefore compromising the human need for wholesome body image.

If the client's vision and dexterity permits, individuals should be instructed to perform self-assessments of their plaque control methods and oral soft tissue examination. Periodic evaluation of their bacterial plaque control measures can be accomplished by using disclosing solution or gingival and plaque indices. Individuals should be advised to conduct an oral self-examination monthly to look for lesions that are painless and do not heal within 2 weeks.

Planning

Dental hygiene care planning for older adults is often more complex than that for younger persons because the vast majority have at least one chronic condition. Also, normal

TABLE 30–20
SAMPLE DENTAL HYGIENE DIAGNOSES RELATED TO THE OLDER ADULT

Dental Hygiene Diagnoses	Related To	As Evidenced By
Deficit in the need for self-determination and responsibility	Lack of skill Impaired manual dexterity Impaired mental ability	Inadequate oral health behaviors Plaque, calculus, gingival bleeding Inability to hold or adapt dental floss Inability to hold toothbrush
Value system deficit	Low value ascribed to oral health	Reports no interest in keeping mouth and dental prostheses plaque free Lack of interest in seeking regular dental hygiene and dental care
Deficit in the need for safety: potential for infection	History of joint replacement therapy Diabetes Cancer Radiation and chemotherapy-induced mucositis and xerostomia	Did not take premedication prior to appointment Uncontrolled bleeding Mucositis
Deficit in the need for conceptualization and problem solving	Knowledge deficit Impaired mental ability	Expresses confusion about the need for bacterial plaque control Evidence of bacterial plaque and gingival bleeding
Deficit in the need for a biologically sound dentition	Ill-fitting dentures Poor oral hygiene	Mucositis Angular cheilosis Loss of weight Root caries
Deficit in the need for freedom from stress	Limited capacity to manage stress	Agitation, verbal expression of fear and anxiety Unable to concentrate Allows others to answer questions
Deficit in the need for nutrition	Ill-fitting dentures Alcohol abuse High sugar intake Lack of resources Lack of social network	Reports of ill-fitting dentures that interfere with eating Substandard body weight History of heavy alcohol consumption Rampant caries Report of oral pain

aging alterations may create a compromised oral situation. Treatment modalities need to be developed based on individual considerations between the client, dental hygienist, dentist, and at times the physician and physical and occupational therapists.

A person's attitude towards oral health affects care planning and outcomes. Many older adults view oral problems as an inevitable part of aging. Also, research suggests that older people perceive a lower need for dental care than that which is actually required.[55–57] Therefore, some older adults do not use dental services as frequently as recommended or do so only when dental emergencies occur.

Implementation

During instrumentation, as little trauma as possible should occur to the gingiva because of reduction in healing capabilities. Loss of elasticity of lips and oral mucosa may make retraction uncomfortable.

Persons with a history of periodontal disease need periodic scaling and root planing. Depending on the periodontal classification, scaling should be completed by quadrants to allow for short appointment times. Routinely, premedicated individuals should have as much care as possible at one time; however, the person's medical condition may compromise lengthy appointments.

Exposed root surfaces are susceptible to dental caries, and a topical fluoride should be administered to help meet the need for a biologically sound dentition. The role of bacterial plaque and diet in relation to dental caries formation needs to be stressed. A desensitization treatment and dentifrice also may be recommended to help ensure freedom from pain if root surfaces are sensitive.

At the completion of the appointment, the chair back should be straightened slowly. The client should be allowed to sit up for a short time before dismissal. The dental hygienist should pay close attention to see if the client needs assistance out of the chair. Postoperative instructions should be reviewed and a written copy provided as indicated.

Evaluation

Clients need to be reevaluated to assess care results and modifications if necessary. If possible, maintenance appointments should be frequent—every 3 or 4 months if realistic.

Fluoride Therapies

Home use of topical fluoride products has been advocated for individuals with signs of primary or secondary dental caries. In addition to using fluoride dentifrice, clients can use a daily nonprescription fluoride rinse. Clients who have undergone head and neck radiation therapy, who suffer from severe xerostomia, or who have rampant caries may need to have a daily gel prescribed by the dentist.

Saliva Substitutes

Saliva substitutes are recommended for individuals with xerostomia. Saliva substitute is a preparation with physical and chemical properties similar to those of real saliva. A suitable substitute should coat the mucosa and teeth to keep them moist, reduce enamel solubility, and reduce the accumulation of plaque. Saliva substitutes can be used without limit on the frequency of use. The substitute is usually sprayed into the mouth and distributed through the mouth with the tongue. Several over-the-counter products are available, with some containing fluoride. The flavored varieties are usually more acceptable than the flavorless.

COMMUNITY HEALTH SERVICES

Institutionalized elderly comprise approximately 5% of the elderly population. Homebound, semidependent elderly account for another 5 to 6%. The numbers may be small, but these groups of elderly have the greatest oral needs and most difficulty reaching dental services.

The functionally dependent are more likely to be edentulous and may not have used dental services for more than 8 years. Furthermore, research suggests that over 80% have dental needs with nearly 40% requiring immediate attention. Among dentate individuals, three-fourths need scaling and prophylaxis. Root caries are another common problem with this population. Oral hygiene status is consistently found to be deplorable.[58–60]

Several factors can be identified that have created this neglect. First, people who are in a **long-term care facility** (LTCF) or are homebound may not be able to care for themselves. They may have numerous complicated and interrelated problems, and dental care may not be a priority. In addition, dental professionals have not been active in providing services because of their own attitudes toward treating the frail elderly, low financial return, and state practice acts that limit dental hygienists' ability to work unsupervised in LTCFs or with the homebound.

The homebound elderly have additional problems to overcome. Some suffer from malnutrition, withdraw socially, or perceive that their speech is adversely affected. These factors can elicit low self-esteem leading to depression. Problems of not eating and withdrawal can be exacerbated as a result.

Provision of routine dental services is not included under **Medicare** (federal) benefits; Medicaid (state) dental benefits and eligibility vary by state, however, preventive dental care for elderly is usually not a priority. Given the high dental needs of homebound or institutionalized elderly, systems to provide care need to be established and advocated.

Traditional Dental Office

For individuals not bedridden, the traditional dental office may be the most appropriate site to provide care. This is the ideal setting because all equipment and materials are readily available. Many of the elderly do not have a means of transportation to the dental office. Consequently, they cannot reach professional oral healthcare without the availability of a special transportation service. However, because of the time and expense involved, dental offices may be reluctant to contract out for this type of program. Usually a van must be available with a staff member to accompany the client. Several factors need to be taken into account when treating a frail, elderly person.[61]

Appointment time—Short morning appointments should be scheduled. Most elderly are physically strongest in the morning. However, because many cannot sit for long periods, 2 hours should be the limit, including transportation time.

Accessibility into the dental office—Parking lots, ramps,

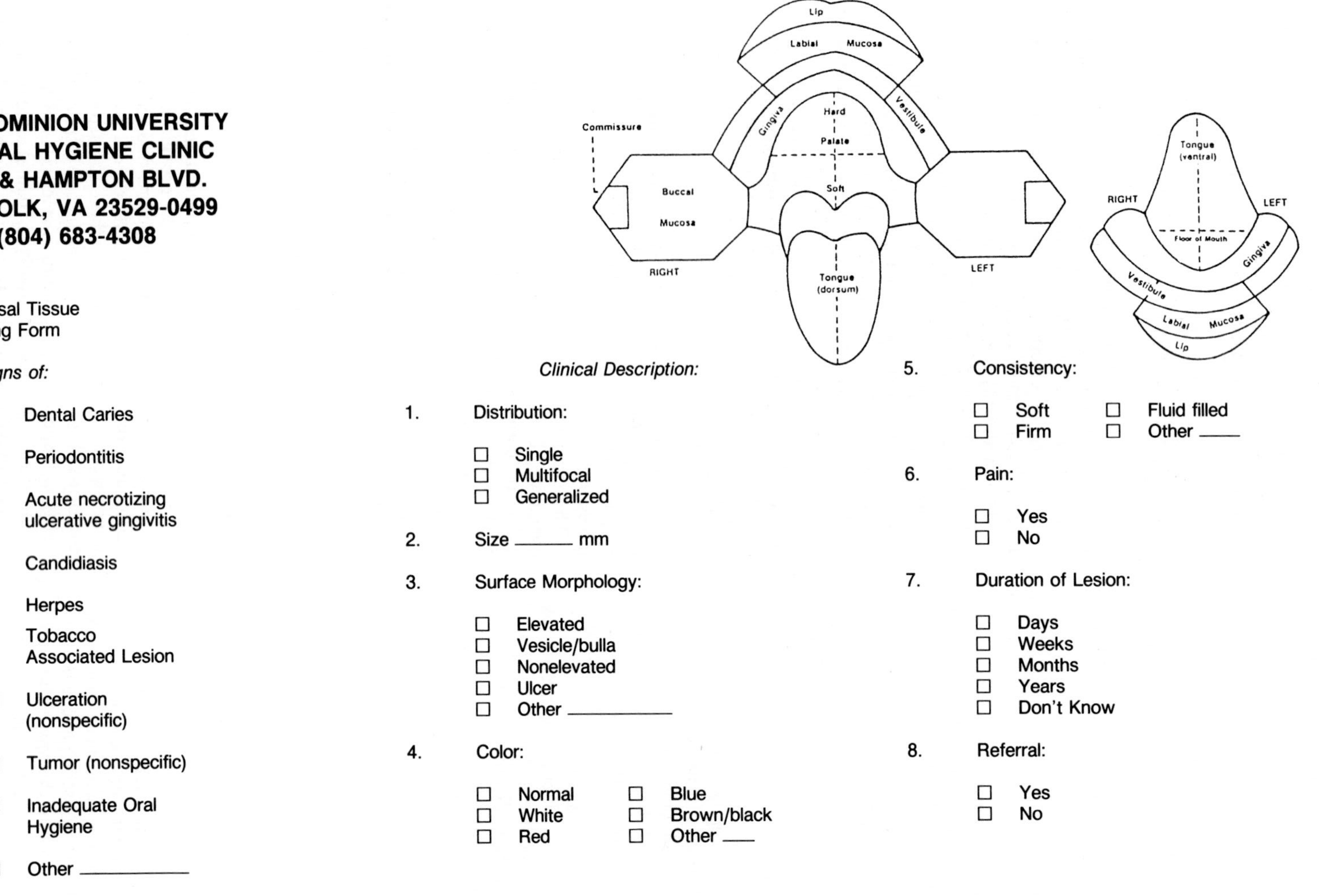

OLD DOMINION UNIVERSITY
DENTAL HYGIENE CLINIC
47th & HAMPTON BLVD.
NORFOLK, VA 23529-0499
(804) 683-4308

Oral/Mucosal Tissue
Screening Form

Clinical Signs of:

- ☐ Dental Caries
- ☐ Periodontitis
- ☐ Acute necrotizing ulcerative gingivitis
- ☐ Candidiasis
- ☐ Herpes
- ☐ Tobacco Associated Lesion
- ☐ Ulceration (nonspecific)
- ☐ Tumor (nonspecific)
- ☐ Inadequate Oral Hygiene
- ☐ Other ________

Clinical Description:

1. Distribution:
   - ☐ Single
   - ☐ Multifocal
   - ☐ Generalized
2. Size ______ mm
3. Surface Morphology:
   - ☐ Elevated
   - ☐ Vesicle/bulla
   - ☐ Nonelevated
   - ☐ Ulcer
   - ☐ Other ________
4. Color:
   - ☐ Normal
   - ☐ White
   - ☐ Red
   - ☐ Blue
   - ☐ Brown/black
   - ☐ Other ___
5. Consistency:
   - ☐ Soft
   - ☐ Firm
   - ☐ Fluid filled
   - ☐ Other ___
6. Pain:
   - ☐ Yes
   - ☐ No
7. Duration of Lesion:
   - ☐ Days
   - ☐ Weeks
   - ☐ Months
   - ☐ Years
   - ☐ Don't Know
8. Referral:
   - ☐ Yes
   - ☐ No

I understand that this was *not* a thorough oral examination and that I need to see a licensed dentist for a dental diagnosis and possible treatment.

____
Signature of Client   Date

____
Signature of Examiner   Date

FIGURE 30–17
Oral assessment referral form. (Modified from U.S. Department of Health and Human Services. Oral Health Surveys of the National Institute of Dental Research. Washington, DC: Public Health Service, National Institutes of Health, Publication no. 91–2870, Jan. 1991, p. 95.)

and doorways must accommodate wheelchairs. Legally, the Americans with Disabilities Act of 1993 mandates access to all public facilities.

Communication with facility—Most facilities require that services provided and instructions be in writing.

Legal considerations—The elderly client may not be capable of providing informed voluntary consent. Therefore, the practitioner will need to have written permission from the individual's physician, family, or facility.

Multiple health conditions and drug therapies—Many elderly individuals have a multitude of chronic health conditions. Consultation with the physician may be necessary.

On-Site Dental Programs

Providing care in the facility or home has several advantages over the traditional dental office:

- Frail elderly do not withstand favorably the disruption of being transported
- Incontinent or catheterized individuals are best treated at their place of residence
- It is less disruptive to the facility
- A familiar environment reduces anxiety

Some LTCFs have dental operatories set up within the facility. In others where it is not practical to establish an operatory, mobile equipment can be used. Mobile equipment and vans can be used for homebound persons as well.

Role of the Dental Hygienist

Dental hygienists serve in an important capacity with the institutionalized and homebound elderly:

- Providing clinical dental hygiene care
- Providing in-service education programs for staff
- Marking dentures for identification
- Giving fluoride applications
- Developing individual care plans
- Modifying oral hygiene aids (see Fig. 30–17 for a sample client assessment form that can be used with homebound, hospitalized, or long-term care residents)

Nursing staff and aides are important intermediaries for dental professionals. Staff should be encouraged to refer elderly individuals to the dental office or consulting dentist if they detect unusual signs, such as swelling or discoloration, or if they hear a verbal complaint. Although they may refer clients for a normal anatomic landmark, the staff member should be complimented for being attentive and caring.

For homebound individuals, establishment of a prevention program using visiting nurses or home healthcare workers is needed when family members are not available. Some states have developed dental programs that use mobile vans with both professionals and students providing services for homebound elderly. Dental hygienists can collaborate with local agencies, dental and dental hygiene associations, and dental hygiene educational institutions to develop oral screening, referral, and preventive programs for homebound elderly.

References

1. Cumming, E., and Henry, W. E. Growing Old: The Process of Disengagement. New York: Basic Books, 1961, pp. 27–30.
2. Kart, C. S., Metress, E. K., and Metress, S. P. Aging, Health and Society. Boston: Jones and Barlett Publishers, 1988.
3. Lemon, B. W., et al. An explanation of the activity theory of aging activity types and life expectation among inmovers to a retirement community. Journal of Gerontology 27(4):511, 1972.
4. Longino, C. F., and Kart, C. S. Explicating activity theory: a formal replication. Journal of Gerontology 37(6):713, 1982.
5. Hendricks, J., and Hendricks, C. D. Aging in Mass Society: Myths and Realities, 3rd ed. Boston: Little, Brown, 1986.
6. Federal Registrar, Vol. 54, No. 21. Washington, DC: Government Printing Office, February 2, 1989.
7. U.S. Bureau of the Census. Projections of the population of the United States, by age, sex and race: 1988-2080. Current population Reports, P-25, No. 1018. Washington, DC: U.S. Government Printing Office, 1989.
8. National Center for Health Statistics. Advance report on final marriage statistics, 1984. Monthly Vital Statistics Report. Vol. 36, Supplement (2), June 1987.
9. U.S. Bureau of the Census. Statistical Abstract of the United States, 1985, 105th ed. Washington, DC: U.S. Government Printing Office, 1985.
10. U.S. Bureau of the Census. Marital status and living arrangements: March, 1990. Current Population Reports, P-20, No. 450. Washington, DC: U.S. Government Printing Office, 1991.
11. U.S. Bureau of the Census. Demographic and socioeconomic aspects of aging in the United States. Current Population Reports, P-23, No. 138. Washington, DC: U.S. Government Printing Office, 1984.
12. U.S. Bureau of the Census. Population profile of the United States, 1989. Current Population Reports. Special Studies Series P-23, No. 159. Washington, DC: U.S. Government Printing Office, 1989.
13. U.S. Bureau of the Census. Money income and poverty status in the United States, 1989. Current Population Reports, P60, No. 168. Washington, DC: U.S. Government Printing Office, 1990.
14. Grad, S. Income of the population 65 or over, 1988. Pub. No. 13-11871. Washington, DC: U.S. Social Security Administration, 1990.
15. Goldman, R. Decline in organic function with age. In Rossman, R. L. (ed.). Clinical Geriatrics, 2nd ed. Philadelphia: J. B. Lippincott, 1979, pp. 113–116.
16. Busse, E. W. Biologic and sociologic changes affecting adaption in mid and late life. Annals of Internal Medicine 15(7):115, 1971.
17. Ebersole, P., and Hess, P. Toward Healthy Aging: Human Needs and Nursing Response, 3rd ed. St. Louis: C. V. Mosby, 1990.
18. Orgel, L. F. The maintenance of the accuracy of protein synthesis and its relevance to aging. Proceedings of the National Academy of Science, 67:1476, 1970.
19. Wilson, D. L. The programmed theory of aging. In Rockstein, M. (ed.). Theoretical Aspects of Aging. New York: Academic Press, 1974.
20. Current estimates from the National Health Interview Survey, 1989. Vital and Health Statistics, Series 10, No. 176, 1990.
21. Aging America, 1991.
22. Johnson, B. E., Crommer, M. E., et al. Wellness center. Journal of Gerontologic Nursing 12:37, 1986.
23. Neville, K. Promoting health for seniors. Geriatric Nursing 9:14, 1988.
24. Special Committee on Aging. U.S. Department of Health and Human Services, Public Health Service, NIH Pub. No. 81-2328. Washington, DC: National Institute on Aging, 1981.
25. Cunningham, W. R., and Brookbank, J. W. Gerontology: The Psychology, Biology, and Sociology of Aging. New York: Harper & Row, 1988, pp. 87–88.
26. Little, J. W., and Falace, D. A. Dental Management of the Medically Compromised Patient, 3rd ed. St. Louis: C. V. Mosby, 1988.
27. Esberger, R. N., and Hughes, S. T. Nursing Care of the Aged. Norwalk, CT: Appleton & Lange, 1989.
28. Lindsay, R. The aging skeleton. In Haug (ed.). Physical and Mental Health of Aged Women. New York: Springer, 1985, pp. 131–133.
29. Benett, J. Postmenopausal women: Reasons for selection of

estrogen replacement therapy. Proceedings of the NIH Conference: Aging: The Quality of Life. Washington, DC: February 1992.

30. Grundy, S. M. Nutrition, aging, and disease: The metabolic crossroads. Proceedings of the NIH Conference: Aging: The Quality of Life. Washington, DC: February 1992.
31. Shulman, L. Osteoporosis, osteoarthrosis, and other musculoskeletal disorders in the elderly. Proceedings of the NIH Conference: Aging: The Quality of Life. Washington, DC: February 1992.
32. Jarvik, L. "Aging of the brain: How can we prevent it?" Journal of Gerontology 28(6):396, 1988.
33. Perlmutter, M., and Hall, E. Adult Development and Aging. New York: John Wiley & Sons, 1985, pp. 98–100.
34. Botwinick, J. Aging and Behavior. New York: Springer, 1984, pp. 62–63.
35. Sperdute, C. Visual changes and aging. Proceedings of the NIH Conference: Aging: The Quality of Life. Washington, DC: Feb. 1992.
36. Jerger, J. Changes in the auditory system. Proceedings of the NIH Conference: Aging: The Quality of Life. Washington, DC: February 1992.
37. Baum, B. Changes in the oral cavity. Proceedings of the NIH Conference: Aging: The Quality of Life. Washington, DC: February 1992.
38. Bartoshik, L. Changes in taste and smell. Proceedings of the NIH Conference: Aging: The Quality of Life. Washington, DC: February 1992.
39. Plum, F. The Brain: Lighthouse of the aging years. Proceedings of the NIH Conference: Aging: The Quality of Life. Washington, DC: February 1992.
40. Niessen, L. C., and Jones, J. A. Alzheimer's disease: A guide for dental professionals. Special Care in Dentistry 6(1):6, Jan.–Feb. 1986.
41. Harper, M. S. Management and Care of the Elderly. Newbury Park, CA: Sage Publications, 1991.
42. U.S. Department of Health and Human Services. Oral Health of United States Adults. The National Survey of Oral Health in U.S. Employed Adults and Senior: 1985–1986. National Institute of Dental Research. NIH Publication No. 87-2969, 1987.
43. Fejerskow, O., and Nyvad, B. Pathology and treatment of dental caries in the aging individual, 1986. In Holm-Pedersen, P., and Loe, H. Geriatric Dentistry: A Textbook of Oral Gerontology. Copenhagen: Munksgaard, 1986.
44. Thomas, B. O. Gerodontology: The study of changes in oral tissues associated with aging. Gerodontology 8(4):119, 1989.
45. Hand, J. S., Hunt, R. J., and Beck, J. D. Incidence of coronal and root caries in an older adult population. Journal of Public Health Dentistry 48(1):14, 1988.
46. Kitamura, M., Kiyak, H. A., and Mulligan, K. Predictors of root caries in the elderly. Community Dental Oral Epidemiology 14:34, 1986.
47. DePaola, P. F., Soparker, P. M., and Tavares, M. The clinical profiles of individuals with and without root surface caries. Gerodontology, 8(1):9, 1989.
48. Abdellatif, H. M., and Burt, B. A. An epidemiological investigation into the relative importance of age and oral hygiene status as determinants of periodontitis. Journal of Dental Research 66:13, 1987.
49. Johnson, B. D. Aging or disease? Periodontal changes and treatment consideration in the older dental patient.
50. National Institute for Dental Research (NIDR). Oral Health of U.S. adults: 1985–1986. Publication No. 86-2868, Washington, DC: U.S. Government Printing Office, 1987.
51. Johnson, B. D. Aging or disease periodontal changes and treatment considerations in the older adult patient. Gerodontology 8(4):109–118, 1989.
52. Holm-Peterson, P., Folke, L. E. A., and Gawronski, T. H. Composition and metabolic activity of dental plaque from healthy young and elderly individuals. Journal of Dental Research 59:771, 1980.
53. Wolff, A., Ship, J. A., Tylenda, C. A., Fox, P. A., and Baum, B. J. Oral mucosal appearance is unchanged in health, different aged persons. Oral Surgery Oral Medicine Oral Pathology 71:569, 1991.
54. Swapp, K. M. Drugs and the geriatric patient: A dental hygiene perspective. Journal of Dental Hygiene, 64:326, 1990.
55. Holtzman, J. M., Berkey, D. B., and Mann, J. Predicting utilization of dental services by the aged. Journal of Public Health Dentistry 50(3):164, 1988.
56. Kiyak, H. A. Psychosocial factors in dental needs of the elderly. Special Care Dentistry 1(1):22, 1981.
57. Strayer, M.S., Branch, L. G., Jones, J. A., and Adelson, R. Predictors of the use of dental services by older veterans. Special Care Dentistry 8(5):209, 1988.
58. Beck, J. D., and Hunt, R. J. Oral health status in the United States: Problems of special patients. Journal of Dental Education 49(6):407, 1985.
59. Berkey, D. B., Berg, R. G., Ettinger, R. L., and Meskin, L. H. Research review of oral health status and service among institutionalized older adults in the United States and Canada. Special Care Dentistry 11(4):131, 1991.
60. MacEntee, M. I., Wyatt, C. C. L., and McBride, B. C. Longitudinal study of caries and cariogenic bacteria in an elderly disabled population. Community Dental Oral Epidemiology 18:149, 1990.
61. Ettinger, R. E., Rafal, S., and Potter, D. E. Dental care programs for chronically ill homebound patients, for residents of nursing homes, and for patients in geriatric hospitals, 1986. In Holm-Pedersen, P., and Loe, H. (eds.). Geriatric Dentistry: A Textbook of Oral Gerontology. Copenhagen: Munksgaard, 1986.

Suggested Readings

Felder, R. S., Millar, S. B., and Henry, R. H. Oral manifestations of drug therapy. Special Care Dentistry 8:119, 1988.

Havinhurst, R. J. A social psychological perspective on aging. The Gerontologist 8(2):67, 1968.

Riley, M. W., Johnson, M., and Foner, A. Aging and Society, Vol. 3: A Sociology of Age Stratification. New York: Russell Sage Foundation, 1972.

31 Dental Hygiene Care for the Individual with Diabetes

OBJECTIVES

Mastery of the content in this chapter will enable the reader to:

- Describe the difference between type I, insulin-dependent diabetes mellitus (IDDM), and type II, non–insulin-dependent diabetes mellitus (NIDDM)
- List the symptoms of diabetes
- Describe the chronic complications of diabetes mellitus
- State the medications prescribed for the individual with diabetes
- Identify the appropriate prophylactic antibiotic prescribed for the diabetic client
- Recognize a diabetic emergency and take appropriate action for management
- Appreciate the lifestyle adjustments made by the individual with diabetes to control the disease
- Understand the control of the diabetic condition through control of oral infections
- Develop client-centered dental hygiene care plans for the individual with diabetes
- Recognize oral complications of diabetes mellitus:
  Salivary and oral changes
  Periodontal changes
  Infection and wound healing
  Tongue changes
  Opportunistic changes
- Apply the dental hygiene process of care to the individual with diabetes
- Apply the principles of oral health instruction to the individual experiencing the psychological aspects of the diabetic condition
- Recognize or suspect the diabetic condition when oral tissues fail to respond to traditional treatment

INTRODUCTION

Diabetes mellitus is one of the most widespread diseases in the United States, affecting an estimated 14 million people. Half of these are unknown or undiagnosed cases. Every year, 700,000 more Americans are diagnosed with diabetes. Diabetes ranks seventh among leading causes of death in the United States. Individuals with diabetes face not only a shortened lifespan but also the probability of developing acute and chronic health complications.

Diabetes mellitus is a group of disorders commonly characterized by:

- Relative or absolute lack of insulin or improperly functioning insulin
- An impairment in the body's ability to metabolize carbohydrates, fats, and protein, and as a result
- Abnormalities in the structure and function of blood vessels **(microangiopathy)** and nerves **(neuropathy)**

The result of the diabetic condition is **hyperglycemia,** a condition of abnormally increased blood **glucose.**

CLASSIFICATION OF DIABETES AND OTHER CATEGORIES OF GLUCOSE INTOLERANCE

In understanding diabetes, it is essential to separate the disease into three major clinical types:

Type I—insulin-dependent diabetes mellitus
Type II—non–insulin-dependent diabetes mellitus
Other types—including diabetes mellitus associated with certain conditions and syndromes (Table 31–1).

All categories are described below. A comparison of the characteristics of type I and type II disease is presented in Table 31–2.

TABLE 31-1
CLASSIFICATION OF DIABETES MELLITUS AND OTHER CATEGORIES OF GLUCOSE INTOLERANCE

Clinical Classes
Diabetes Mellitus
Type I: Insulin-dependent diabetes mellitus
Type II: Non-insulin-dependent diabetes mellitus
Nonobese
Obese
Other: Other types of diabetes associated with certain conditions or syndromes: pancreatic disease, hormonal conditions, chemical- or drug-induced disease, genetic symptoms, insulin-receptor abnormalities, and others[a]
Impaired Glucose Tolerance
Nonobese
Obese
Impaired glucose tolerance associated with certain conditions or syndromes: pancreatic disease, hormonal conditions, chemical- or drug-induced diabetes, genetic symptoms, and insulin-receptor abnormalities
Gestational Diabetes mellitus
Statistical Risk Classes
Previous abnormality of glucose tolerance[b]
Potential abnormality of glucose tolerance

[a] The subcategory "Other" includes diabetes associated with malnourished populations, comparable to the subclass "Malnutrition-Related Diabetes Mellitus" included in the World Health Organization classification.
[b] Normal glucose tolerance but increased risk of developing diabetes.
Reprinted with permission from National Diabetes Data Group: Classification and diagnosis of diabetes mellitus and other categories of glucose intolerance. Diabetes 28(12):1042–1043, 1979. Copyright © 1979 by American Diabetes Association, Inc.

Type I—Insulin-Dependent Diabetes Mellitus

Type I diabetes mellitus (IDDM), which involves about 15% of the diabetic population, usually occurs in children and young adults but can strike at any age. A severe deficiency of insulin is characteristic in this type, and treatment requires regular lifelong administration of insulin by injection to prevent ketosis and sustain health.

An abrupt onset of symptoms characterizes this disease, although present evidence suggests a preceding period of slowly developing autoimmune damage to the pancreatic B cells.[1] Genetic predisposition related to the presence of certain human leukocyte antigens (HLAs) that influence immune activity directed against islet cells appears to be essential for type I diabetes to develop, but alone it is not the cause.[2] Environmental factors, particularly certain viral agents such as coxsackievirus, mumps, and congenital rubella, are postulated to play an etiological role in predisposed individuals.[3] Type I diabetes presents more commonly in winter than in summer, also suggesting environmental factors (i.e., viral infection). Figures 31–1 and 31–2 show current theories on the development of type I diabetes mellitus.

Results of twin studies suggest a genetic difference in type I and type II diabetes, a concept further supported by

TABLE 31-2
CHARACTERISTICS OF TYPE I AND TYPE II DIABETES MELLITUS

Factor	Type I	Type II
Age at onset	Usually in young, but may occur at any age	Usually in persons older than 40 years of age, but may occur at any age
Type of onset	Usually abrupt	Insidious
Genetic susceptibility	HLA-related DR3, DR4, and others	Frequent genetic background; not HLA-related
Environmental factors	Virus, toxins, autoimmune stimulation	Obesity, nutrition
Islet-cell antibody	Present at outset	Not observed
Endogenous insulin	Minimal or absent	Stimulated response is (1) adequate but delayed secretion, or (2) reduced but not absent
Nutritional status	Thin, catabolic state	Obese, or may be normal
Symptoms	Thirst, polyuria, polyphagia, fatigue	Frequently none, or mild
Ketosis	Prone: at onset or during insulin deficiency	Resistant, except during infection or stress
Control of diabetes	Often difficult with wide glucose fluctuation	Variable; helped by dietary adherence
Dietary management	Essential	Essential; may suffice for glycemic control
Insulin	Required for all	Required for 20 to 30%
Sulfonylurea	Not efficacious	Efficacious
Vascular and neurological complications	Seen in majority after 5 or more years of diabetes	Frequent

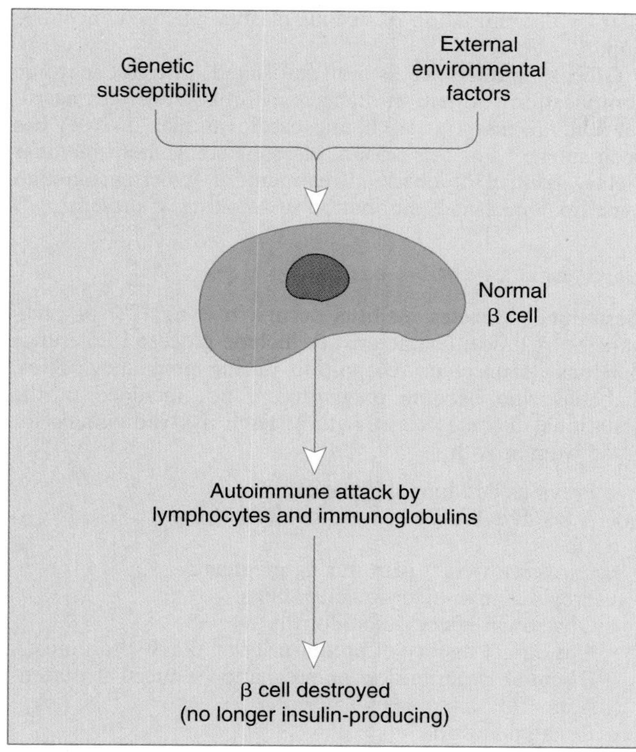

FIGURE 31-1
Current view of the pathogenesis of type I diabetes mellitus. (Redrawn from Galloway, J. A., Potvin, J. H., and Shuman, C. R. [eds.]. Diabetes Mellitus, 9th ed. Indianapolis: Lilley Research Laboratories, 1988.)

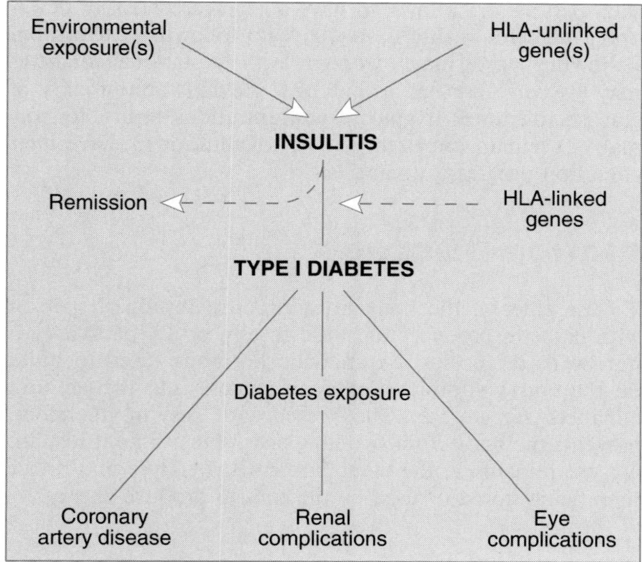

FIGURE 31-2
"Insulitis" is recognized pathologically as lymphocytic infiltration of pancreatic islets. Schematic diagram of the natural history of type I diabetes mellitus and its complications. (Redrawn with permission from Krolewski, A. S., Warram, J. H., et al. Epidemiologic approach to the etiology of type I diabetes mellitus and its complications. The New England Journal of Medicine 317:1390, 1987. Reprinted with permission from *The New England Journal of Medicine.*)

HLA and family studies. More than 95% of individuals with type I diabetes possess certain HLAs, compared with only 40% of type II and nondiabetic individuals.[4] A predisposition to type I diabetes, rather than the disease itself, seems to be inherited because approximately 50% of nondiabetic individuals have HLA DR3 or DR4, yet only about 0.1% of that population develop type I diabetes.

Type II — Non-Insulin-Dependent Diabetes Mellitus

Type II diabetes mellitus (NIDDM) is recognized as a heterogeneous disorder with abnormalities in insulin secretion, reduced sensitivity to insulin, and excessive hepatic glucose production.[5] Figure 31-3 summarizes the metabolic abnormalities that contribute to hyperglycemia in type II diabetes. People with type II diabetes constitute approximately 80 to 85% of the diabetic population. Type II diabetes usually occurs in individuals older than 40 years of age. Symptoms may be gradual, and weight loss is uncommon. Persons with type II diabetes often respond to weight reduction, dietary management, exercise, and oral hypoglycemic agents (sulfonylurea medications). Persons with type II diabetes may require insulin therapy to achieve good control or during illness, which is an important distinction between insulin-dependent and insulin-treated individuals.

Type II diabetes is recognized as having a strong genetic basis, as evidenced by studies of twins and familial transmission. Type II diabetic twins are 91% **concordant** (both twins have the disease).[6] If nongenetic or environmental factors were important, **discordance** (only one twin is affected) in twins would be common. It is commonly believed that obesity is a cause of type II diabetes; however, the lighter weight twin most often develops diabetes first,[4] and an estimated 10 to 40% of individuals with type II diabetes are not obese.[7] Obesity may worsen glucose intolerance but is not a cause.

Type II diabetes is predominantly inherited; however, it has no association with HLA or B cell destruction. Insulin is present in the circulation, and in **nonobese type II diabetes** the insulin response after a meal is preserved, al-

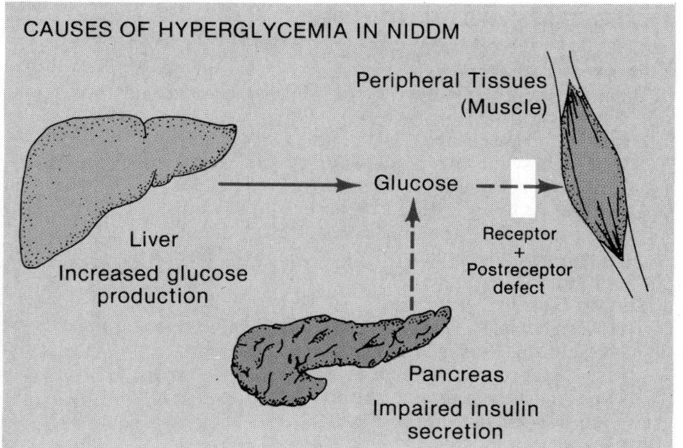

FIGURE 31-3
Causes of hyperglycemia in type II diabetes. (Redrawn with permission from Olefsky, J. M. Diabetes mellitus. In Wyngaarden, J. B., Smith, L. H., and Bennett, J. C. (eds.). Cecil's Textbook of Medicine, 19th ed. Philadelphia: W. B. Saunders, 1992, p. 1295.)

though peak concentration is delayed, causing hyperglycemia. Early type II diabetes does not result from insulin deficiency but from sluggish responsiveness in insulin secretion and resistance to its action. The defect that causes type II diabetes remains unidentified.

Other Types of Diabetes Mellitus

The subclass "other types" is heterogeneous and includes specific disorders in which the etiological relationship is known, such as diabetes as a result of pancreatic disease, endocrine disease, chemical agents, or drugs. In other disorders, such as genetic syndromes associated with glucose intolerance, an etiological relationship is suspected. Rare and highly specific causes of diabetes and insulin resistance include defects in insulin receptors located on the cell membrane, or conditions such as lupus erythematosus in which insulin-receptor antibodies may develop. In addition to the presence of the specific condition or syndrome, diabetes mellitus also is present. To place an individual in the subclass "other types," two diagnostic determinations must be observed:

- The presence of type I or II diabetes and
- The presence of the associated condition or syndrome

A partial listing of disorders that constitute this subclass of diabetes is shown in Table 31–3.

Impaired Glucose Tolerance

The designation **impaired glucose tolerance** applies to individuals whose plasma glucose concentrations lie between normal values and values diagnostic of diabetes. Impaired glucose tolerance may progress to NIDDM or IDDM diabetes over time, but the majority of glucose concentrations remain the same or improve to normal plasma glucose concentrations. Impaired glucose tolerance can be determined only by results of an oral glucose tolerance test consisting of a standard glucose challenge followed 2 hours later by determination of venous plasma glucose concentration.

Glucose intolerance is not associated with the chronic complications evident in diabetes mellitus; however, **macrovascular disease** (i.e., ischemic cardiovascular disease) has been shown.[8] For this reason, disease management includes dietary control of obesity, treatment of hypertension and hyperlipidemia, and elimination of smoking, if present.

TABLE 31–3
OTHER TYPES OF DIABETES MELLITUS: DISORDERS AND SYNDROMES*

Pancreatic Disease
Pancreatitis, carcinoma, cystic fibrosis, hemochromatosis, pancreatectomy
Hyperendocrinopathy
Cushing's syndrome, pheochromocytoma, glucagonoma, aldosteronoma, acromegaly
Chemical- or Drug-Induced Disease
Glucocorticoids, most thiazide diuretics, phenytoin, oral contraceptives, phenothiazines, tricyclic antidepressants, clonidine, lithium
Certain Genetic Syndromes
Hyperlipidemia, Turner's syndrome, myotonic dystrophy, leprechaunism, Prader-Willi syndrome
Insulin-Receptor Abnormalities
Type A—altered receptor response
Type B—receptor antibodies
Other Types
Diabetes associated with malnourished populations

* For additional examples of secondary forms of diabetes, see West (1978), and the National Diabetes Data Group (1979), in reference list and suggested readings list.

Gestational Diabetes Mellitus

Gestational diabetes mellitus occurs in 3 to 12% of pregnancies.[9] Clinical characteristics include glucose intolerance that has its onset or recognition during pregnancy. Thus, diabetics who become pregnant are not included in the gestational diabetes classification. High-risk individuals include women with:

- Previous gestational diabetes
- A positive family history for diabetes
- Obesity
- Excessive weight gain during pregnancy
- Previous high-birth-weight infants
- Obstetrical history of stillbirths
- Obstetrical history of prematurity or polyhydramnios
- Essential hypertension or pregnancy-induced hypertension
- Renal glucosuria[7]

The normal pregnancy state affects both fetal and maternal metabolism and, even in the nondiabetic individual, exerts a diabetogenic effect. Gestational diabetes generally reverts following birth because the condition is a consequence of the normal antiinsulin effects of pregnancy hormones and the diversion of natural glucose to the child.

If unrecognized or untreated, gestational diabetes increases the risk of perinatal complications. Furthermore, such persons are known to have an increased risk of developing diabetes within 5 to 10 years following parturition. Following parturition, women with gestational diabetes may (1) be reclassified as having a previous abnormality of glucose tolerance, if glucose concentrations return to normal, (2) remain impaired glucose tolerant, or (3) have their condition progress to diabetes.

PATHOPHYSIOLOGY

To use glucose, the body must produce **insulin.** A person with diabetes produces too little insulin or a type that cannot be used. Insulin, an anabolic hormone (used to build up the body), stimulates entry of glucose into the cell and enhances fat storage. The presence of insulin, therefore, prevents the body from breaking down fat. Without insulin, glucose remains in the blood stream (hyperglycemia) rather than being stored or used by the cells to produce energy.

INSULIN DEPRIVATION

The net effect of insulin deficiency is that blood glucose concentration rises (hyperglycemia). Without insulin, the glucose derived from a meal cannot be utilized or stored. When the blood glucose level rises above 150 mg/dL, the kidney tubules become incapable of resorption. Glucose appears in the urine (glucosuria), taking with it a large

TABLE 31–4
SIGNS AND SYMPTOMS OF KETOACIDOSIS

Common Cardinal Symptoms	Other Symptoms
"Fruity" acetone breath	Recurrence of bedwetting
Frequent urination	Repeated skin infections
Excessive thirst	Malaise
Unusual hunger	Drowsiness
Weight loss	Headache
Weakness	Marked irritability
Nausea	
Dry skin and mucous membranes	
Flushed facial appearance	
Abdominal tenderness	
Rapid, deep breathing	
Depressed sensory perception	

amount of fluid, raising the volume of urine (polyuria) and, therefore, necessitating frequent urination. Dehydration follows, leading to excessive thirst (polydypsia).

Ketoacidosis may follow hyperglycemia (see Table 31–4 for signs and symptoms) when blood glucose levels rise to above 400 mg/dL. Impaired carbohydrate metabolism, which the body interprets as energy starvation, necessitates use of fats and proteins to satisfy energy requirements. Ketoacids and ketone bodies (acetone) are produced as a result of catabolism (lipolysis) of fatty acids. Ketones accumulate in the tissues, are excreted in the urine (ketouria), and circulate in the blood (ketonemia), causing a drop in the pH of the blood and leading to diabetic coma.

CLINICAL SIGNS AND SYMPTOMS OF DIABETES

In type I diabetes, the predominant problem seems to be impaired insulin action, whereas in type II diabetes the predominant problem seems to be a resistance to insulin action. A considerable overlap exists, however, in clinical features of the two forms of diabetes. The deficiency of insulin action leads to derangements of the intermediary metabolism of carbohydrates, protein, and lipids. In clinical practice, the suspicion of diabetes is gleaned from history and physical findings (Table 31–5). The symptoms listed below are indications of probable diabetes mellitus:

- Fatigue
- Thirst
- Polyuria
- Weight loss
- Recurrent infection

A family history of diabetes, obesity, unfavorable obstetrical experiences (see section on gestational diabetes), premature atherosclerosis, and neuropathic disorders also are indications of probable diabetes mellitus.

CHRONIC COMPLICATIONS

In addition to an impairment of insulin production, people with both types of diabetes mellitus show a tendency for severe, multisystem, long-term complications, including microvascular and macrovascular disease. Diabetic retinopathy, nephropathy, neuropathy, and aggravated atherosclerosis mar the ultimate prospects for health and for long lifespan for many individuals with diabetes mellitus[10] (Table 31–6). Elevated plasma glucose values have been most closely associated with development of micro- and macrovascular disease.

All complications affect clients with both type I and type II diabetes, although clinical manifestations and consequences differ greatly. Generally, kidney and eye diseases predominate in type I disease (persons diagnosed early in life) and atherosclerotic disease predominates in type II disease (those diagnosed later), and neuropathy occurs in both.

DIABETIC EMERGENCIES

An individual may have uncontrolled diabetes, increasing the likelihood of an emergency situation:

- Comas
  - Hypoglycemia
  - Ketoacidotic hyperglycemia
  - Nonketotic hyperosmolar hyperglycemia
  - Lactic acidosis
  - Uremia
  - Nondiabetic coma
- Infection
- Myocardial infarction
- Stroke
- Emergency surgery

The occurrence of stupor or coma in diabetes may be due to several causes. The diabetic condition may be un-

TABLE 31–5
KNOW THE WARNING SIGNS OF DIABETES

Insulin-dependent diabetes is characterized by the sudden appearance of:
Constant urination
Excessive thirst
Extreme hunger
Dramatic weight loss
Irritability
Obvious weakness and fatigue
Nausea and vomiting
These symptoms appear suddenly. Any of these signals can mean diabetes.

Non–insulin-dependent diabetes symptoms may develop slowly.
Any of the insulin-dependent symptoms and/or:
Recurring or hard-to-heal skin, gum, or bladder infections
Fatigue
Blurred vision
Tingling or numbness in hands or feet
Itching
Any one of these signals can mean diabetes. Contact your doctor and ask for a test for diabetes.

TABLE 31–6
COMPLICATIONS OF DIABETES MELLITUS

Affected Area	Complications
Eyes	Retinopathy Cataracts Glaucoma
Kidneys	Glomerulonephritis Nephrosclerosis Pyelonephritis
Mouth	Gingivitis Dental caries Periodontitis
Reproductive system	Stillbirths Miscarriages High-birth-weight babies Congenital defects Neonatal deaths
Skin	Xanthoma diabeticorum Pruritus Furunculosis Limited joint mobility
Vascular system	Arteriosclerosis Microangiopathy Large-vessel disease Myocardial infarction
Peripheral nerves	Earliest recognized complication Somatic neuropathy Autonomic neuropathy

diagnosed, or the person with type I disease may not have followed the required insulin regimen. Stress, infection, or increased level of activity may contribute to the onset of an emergency situation.

Hypoglycemia

Hypoglycemia, the most common metabolic emergency in persons with type I diabetes, is a condition resulting from an excess of insulin and a deficiency of glucose. Severe episodes occur in one of five individuals each year. Minor episodes occur every 2 weeks on average in each insulin-treated person. In clients with type II disease treated with sulfonylurea agents, hypoglycemia is more common than generally recognized and may be severe, especially in older persons treated with longer acting agents.[11]

Hypoglycemia has been defined as a blood glucose concentration below 50 mg/dL (80 to 120 mg/dL is normal). Signs and symptoms of hypoglycemia result from a lack of glucose in the brain and compensation by the nervous system for this lack of glucose (Table 31–7). The main causes of hypoglycemia in persons with type I disease are shown in Table 31–8.

Individuals with diabetes can manage mild hypoglycemia themselves by ingesting glucose, sweet drinks, or milk. Between 10 and 20 g of glucose (about the amount in an 8-ounce glass of 2% fat milk, a 4-ounce glass of orange juice, three pieces of hard candy, or eight Lifesavers candies) are generally adequate, although many persons take considerably more because they fear prolonged hypoglycemia. More severe hypoglycemia also can be treated by oral ingestion of carbohydrate, but friends or relatives may have to administer it. If the person is unconscious, treatment requires intravenous dextrose solution or an intramuscular injection of 0.5 to 1.0 mg glucagon, followed on awakening by oral complex carbohydrate with a protein source (i.e., small meat or cheese sandwich or cottage cheese and fruit).

TABLE 31–7
SIGNS AND SYMPTOMS OF HYPOGLYCEMIA

Lack of Glucose to the Brain (Neuroglucopenia)	Nervous System Compensations (Adrenergic Discharge)
Confusion	Anxiety
Blurred vision	Sweating
Paresthesia—tingling in arms and legs	Pallor
Fatigue	Tachycardia
Stupor	Palpitations
Convulsions	Hunger
Unconsciousness (coma)	Restlessness
Irritability	Excitability
Impaired concentration	Trembling
Headache	Headache
Somnolence (sleepiness or drowsiness)	Nausea
Psychiatric disorders—stupor	Dizziness
Transient sensory or motor defects—weakness, slurred speech	

Hyperglycemic Ketoacidotic Coma

Although the percentage of all diabetes deaths caused by hyperglycemia ketoacidotic coma (diabetic coma) has decreased dramatically, from more than 60% in preinsulin days to 1% at present, it is still considerable, especially in younger individuals.[12] Prevention is the best treatment; however, emergency treatment requires hospitalization to correct fluid and electrolyte imbalances (Table 31–9).

Coma resulting from absolute insulin deficiency is found in persons with acute-onset type I diabetes in whom diagnosis was unknown or delayed and in individuals with known diabetes who discontinued or decreased their insulin dose for some reason. Coma resulting from relative insulin deficiency[12] may be caused by infection or other stress states in which there is an increase in secretion of antiinsulin hormones (i.e., glucagon, cortisol, and catecholamines) (Table 31–10). The situation is often compounded by a person's not eating and, therefore, mistakenly decreasing

TABLE 31–8
CAUSES OF HYPOGLYCEMIA IN INSULIN-DEPENDENT (TYPE I) DIABETES MELLITUS

Type	Cause
Insulin	Inappropriate insulin regimens Day-to-day variability in absorption Insulin antibodies Inappropriate site rotation Factitious hypoglycemia Renal failure
Food	Delayed intake Decreased intake
Exercise	Increased energy requirements Increased insulin absorption
Other	Impaired counterregulation Liver disease Hypoendocrine states Alcohol Potentiating drugs "Hypoglycemic unawareness" (absence of signs and symptoms, long-standing diabetes, autonomic neuropathy)

TABLE 31–9
HYPOGLYCEMIA COMPARED WITH HYPERGLYCEMIA

Signs and Symptoms	Hypoglycemia	Hyperglycemia
Onset	Rapid (minutes)	Slow (days/weeks)
Thirst	Absent	Increased
Nausea and vomiting	Absent	Frequent
Vision	Double	Dim
Respirations	Normal	Difficulty—hyperventilation
Skin	Moist, pale	Hot, dry, flushed
Tremors	Frequent	Absent
Blood pressure	Normal	Hypotension

his insulin dose. Infection is the most common precipitating factor and is present in more than 50% of all persons with diabetic ketoacidotic coma.[13]

A series of biochemical events explains the basis of severe ketoacidosis, and signs and symptoms are presented in Table 31–11. Clear guidelines on maintaining control should be provided to the diabetic client with intercurrent infection to clear the infection early. These guidelines are listed below.

- Increase self-monitoring of blood glucose (or urine glucose if blood-monitoring equipment is not available) to four times daily (fasting, before lunch, before evening injection, bedtime)
- Test for urine ketones twice daily
- If not eating normally, replace carbohydrate content of meals and snacks with sugar-containing drinks or milk; ensure adequate fluid intake (2 to 3 L/day)
- If two preceding blood tests show glucose level greater than 200 mg/dL (11.1 mmol/L), increase the next insulin dose by 4 units (2 short-acting, 2 intermediate)
  If, in addition, the ketone test is positive, increase by 6 units (2 short-acting, 4 intermediate)
  Continue this with each injection*
- If vomiting supervenes or blood glucose is greater than 300 mg/dL plus positive ketones for more than 24 hours, call for urgent medical advice

*Alternatively, the total daily dose can be given as four equal divided doses of short-acting regular insulin with carbohydrate taken after each injection. This allows flexibility for increasing insulin, but is necessary only for seriously uncontrolled diabetes with infections.

TABLE 31–10
CAUSES OF HYPERGLYCEMIA KETOACIDOTIC COMA

Absolute Insulin Deficiency
Newly presenting type I diabetes with B-cell depletion
Incorrect insulin dosage (omitted or decreased)

Relative Insulin Deficiency
Stress states
- Infection
- Myocardial infarction
- Trauma
- Cerebrovascular accident

Drugs and endocrine disorders
- Steroids
- Adrenergic agonists
- Hyperthyroidism
- Pheochromocytoma
- Thiazide diuretics

Treatment of diabetic ketoacidosis requires hospitalization to restore the disturbed metabolic fluid and electrolyte state to normal. Fluid (salt and water) rehydration, insulin, potassium, broad-spectrum antibiotic therapy, and treatment of precipitating factors are the main elements of diabetic coma treatment.

DISEASE MANAGEMENT

Diet Therapy

Diet remains "the hallmark of diabetes therapy" despite therapeutic advances in insulin formulations, delivery systems, and oral medications.[14] Diabetic diets are designed to provide appropriate quantities of food at regular intervals, supply daily caloric requirements to aid in achieving or maintaining desirable body weight, and reduce fat intake to correct an unfavorable lipid profile conducive to atherosclerosis.

In type II diabetes, reduction in hyperglycemia is corre-

TABLE 31–11
PRESENTING FEATURES OF SEVERE DIABETIC KETOACIDOSIS

Feature	Possible Cause
Symptoms	
Thirst	
Polyuria	Hyperglycemia, osmotic diuresis
Fatigue	Dehydration, protein loss
Weight loss	Dehydration, protein loss, catabolism
Anorexia	(?)*
Nausea, vomiting	Ketones (?), gastric stasis, ileus
Abdominal pain	Gastric stasis (?), ileus, electrolyte deficiency (?)
Muscle cramps	Potassium deficiency (?)
Signs	
Hyperventilation	Acidemia
Dehydration	Osmotic diuresis, vomiting
Tachycardia	Dehydration
Hypotension	Dehydration, acidemia
Warm, dry skin	Acidemia (peripheral vasodilatation)
Hypothermia	
Impaired consciousness or coma	Hyperosmolality
Ketotic breath	Hyperketonemia (acetone)
Blood Chemistry	
High blood glucose }	
High blood ketone bodies }	Insulin deficiency
(glycosuria, ketonuria) }	
Low arterial blood pH	Ketone bodies
Low arterial pCO_2	Metabolic acidosis
Normal or low arterial pO_2	Pulmonary arteriovenous shunting (?)
Low plasma bicarbonate	Metabolic acidosis
Low plasma sodium	Hyperglycemia
Variable plasma potassium	Loss through diuresis, acidemia, dehydration
Leukocytosis	Raised ketone bodies

* (?) Indicates speculated cause or unknown cause.

Reprinted from Alberti, K., and Phil, D. Diabetic emergencies. In Galloway, J. A., Potrin, J. H., and Shuman, C. R. (eds.). Diabetes Mellitus, 9th ed. Indianapolis: Lilley Research Laboratories, 1988.

lated with weight loss. In type I diabetes, nutritional strategies primarily involve monitoring the percentage of carbohydrate (55 to 60% of total calories) to protein (12 to 20% of total calories) intake. Meal planning for diabetics is based on the food exchange lists system of the American Diabetes Association. If dietary management alone fails to achieve desirable glycemic control in type II diabetes, treatment with insulin or a sulfonylurea hypoglycemic agent is considered by the physician.

Two of the most important clinical advances in the management of diabetes mellitus have been the introduction of home self-monitoring of blood glucose with small automated devices and use of glycosylated hemoglobin (HbA_{1c}) laboratory tests by the physician to determine if long-term (3-month) glycemic control has been attained.

Insulin Therapy

The person with type I diabetes has essentially no pancreatic insulin, is unresponsive to oral sulfonylurea hypoglycemic agents, and is ketosis-prone and therefore dependent on lifelong administration of insulin by subcutaneous injection. There are three types of insulin, categorized by time of action:

- Rapid-acting
- Intermediate
- Long-acting

Table 31–12 illustrates insulin types that may be used alone or in combination. Dosages, frequency, and times of administration are dependent on several factors:[15]

- Prescribed treatment program
- Lifestyle
- Exercise
- Food intake
- Dietary habits
- Certain medications
- Trauma
- Infection
- Physical stress
- Emotional stress
- Pregnancy
- Hyperthyroidism
- Hyperpituitarism[15]

Various factors influence insulin treatment regimens.

- Client's ability to detect and counterregulate hypoglycemia
- Client's capacity to comply with diet, exercise, self-monitoring of blood glucose, and insulin regimen guidelines
- Client's educational level, lifestyle, and home support system
- Client's endogenous insulin secretory status, including type of diabetes (type I or type II)
- Client's age and weight (including degree of ponderosity and growth status)
- Concurrent medical conditions, including pregnancy
- Client's pharmacodynamic response to or ability to use specific types of insulin or insulin prescriptions
- Availability of competent professional supervision

TABLE 31–12
TYPES OF INSULIN PREPARATIONS

Type	Onset of Action	Peak Effect (hr)	Duration (hr)
Rapid			
Regular or crystalline	15 min	2–3	5–7
Semi lente	30 min	3–6	12–16
Intermediate			
NPH	3 hr	6–10	18–24
Globin zinc	3 hr	8–12	18–24
Lente	3 hr	8–12	18–24
Prolonged			
Protamine zinc (PZI)	3½ hr	14–20	30–36
Ultra lente	3½ hr	16–18	36

THE DENTAL HYGIENE PROCESS OF CARE

Well-controlled diabetes occurs when the client's blood glucose is within the normal range as a result of a careful balance of medication, diet, and exercise. Clients with well-controlled diabetes can be treated safely, provided that the person's daily routine is not affected. Diabetics with well-controlled disease have a reduced incidence of dental caries.

Infections of any type can cause a profound disturbance of glycemic control, potentially leading to ketoacidosis and diabetic coma. When infection is present, counterregulatory hormone secretion increases (specifically, that of cortisol and glucagon), leading to hyperglycemia and increased ketogenesis. Infection is the most common precipitating factor for severe ketoacidosis. In the client with poorly controlled diabetes, phagocytic function is impaired and resistance to infection decreased.[16] Prevention of oral diseases and infections is critical to the diabetic control of the client, and poor diabetic control may aggravate the oral disease status.

Some key unmet human needs related to the dental hygiene care of the individual with diabetes may include:

- Wholesome body image
- Skin and mucous membrane integrity
- Nutrition
- Conceptualization and problem solving
- Self-determination and responsibility
- Freedom from stress

For example, emotional stress induced by an oral healthcare appointment causes the release of epinephrine, which mobilizes glucose from glycogen stored in the liver. Stress, therefore, can contribute to a hyperglycemic condition becoming ketoacidotic. Periods of waiting and treatment time should be minimized to meet the client's human need for freedom from stress.

Diabetes in people on intensive regimens of multiple insulin injections and daily self-monitoring of blood glucose may abruptly become uncontrolled as a result of an active periodontal infection. When unrecognized, the periodontal infection may cause the human needs for skin and mucous membrane integrity and safety to become compromised. In addition, Table 31–13 reflects some unmet human needs and their effect on outcomes of self-monitoring of blood glucose.

TABLE 31–13
SOME UNMET HUMAN NEEDS IN INDIVIDUALS WITH DIABETES AND THE EFFECT ON OUTCOMES OF SELF-MONITORING OF BLOOD GLUCOSE

Unmet Human Need	Client's Feeling	Example: Client's Behavioral Response
1. Wholesome body image	I want to be 100% okay.	Seeking perfection; therefore, records results as 100% okay.
2. Appreciation and respect	I want you to be pleased, proud.	Seeking approval; therefore, I give you information that makes you pleased, proud.
3. Self-determination	I want to be in charge.	Seeking independence; therefore, I give you records that show what I want you to see.
4. Freedom from pain/stress	I don't want you to punish me.	Avoiding punishment; therefore, I give you records so that you think I don't deserve punishment.
	I don't want you to question or accuse me.	Avoiding confrontation and criticism; therefore, I give you records that encourage you to leave me alone.
	I don't want to hear if I'm good or bad.	Avoiding judgment; therefore, I give you records that you won't have to comment about.
	I don't want to pay attention to diabetes and feel sad.	Avoiding depressions; therefore, I won't test so that I won't have to face sadness.
	I don't have diabetes.	Expressing denial; therefore, I need not test.
	I hate diabetes, or I hate how you make me deal with diabetes.	Expressing resentment or anger; therefore, I won't do what you ask me to do.
	I cheated.	Expressing guilt; therefore, "I'll hide it."

Reprinted and adapted with permission from Skyler J. S., and Reeves M. L. Intensive treatment of type I diabetes mellitus. In Olefsky, J. M., and Sherwin, R. S. (eds.). Diabetes Mellitus: Management and Complications. New York: Churchill Livingstone, 1985, pp. 31–79.

Client Assessment

The most important factor in assessing a client is a thorough health history.[17] Using an "investigative" approach, the dental hygienist questions the client regarding the signs and symptoms of ketoacidosis (see Table 31–5) to determine an undiagnosed diabetic condition. High-risk characteristics for developing diabetes include:

- Age over 40 years
- Diabetic family members
- Obesity
- Females who have had high-birth-weight babies (i.e., 10 or more pounds)

Diabetes-prone individuals are those who have:

- A history of hypertension
- Cardiovascular disease
- Arteriosclerosis
- Gout
- Pancreatitis
- Cholecystitis
- Hyperlipidemic states

Among the aging, classic symptoms do not usually become manifest. Rather, clinical findings are those related to chronic complications of the disease, such as vascular disorders or neuropathic syndromes.

If the person is a known diabetic, the client and health history interview should address:

- The date of onset of diabetes
- Type of diabetes
- Regularity of appointments with a physician
- Methods for controlling diabetes (medication, diet, and exercise)
- Date of last insulin reaction
- Method of testing diabetic control (blood or urine)
- Results of testing (trends and day of appointment)
- Medication schedule and dosages
- Complications from diabetes such as diabetic retinopathy or kidney disorders

Oral assessment may reveal a variety of oral conditions common in poorly controlled diabetes (Table 31–14). Common oral findings include:

- Cheilosis
- Xerostomia
- Glossodynia
- Enlarged salivary glands
- Increased glucose in saliva
- Fungal infections such as candidiasis (thrush)

Uncontrolled diabetes means an increased incidence of dental caries as a result of dehydration, resulting in reduced saliva secretion. Increased glucose content of saliva also may contribute to caries activity. Other oral complications associated with diabetes may affect nutrition by causing the person to select foods that are easy to chew but are nutritionally inadequate.

Diabetic individuals are considered to be predisposed to destructive periodontitis; however, in well-controlled diabetes, individuals do not necessarily have greater frequency of gingivitis or periodontitis than nondiabetic individuals.[18–20] Several factors may contribute to the diminished resistance to infection of people with diabetes. Elevated glucose levels in oral fluids as well as microvascular changes (i.e., thickening of the basement membrane of capillaries) in the gingival tissues contribute to these complications.[21] Impaired leukocyte functions of chemotaxis, phagocytosis, and bactericidal activity can reduce resistance to periodontal infection during periods of poor diabetes control.[22–24]

Poorly controlled diabetes may, therefore, contribute to periodontal disease. Concurrently, periodontal problems can complicate or worsen the diabetic condition.

TABLE 31–14
ORAL COMPLICATIONS OF DIABETES MELLITUS

Clinical Signs and Symptoms	Pathophysiology
Salivary and oral changes	
Xerostomia	Increased fluid loss
Bilateral, asymptomatic parotid gland swelling with increased salivary viscosity	Increased fatty acid deposition Increased salivary glucose levels Compensatory hypertrophy due to a decrease in saliva production
Increased dental caries, especially in the cervical region	Secondary to xerostomia
Unexplained odontalgia and percussion sensitivity (acute pulpitis)	Pulpal arteritis from microangiopathies
Lingual erosion of anterior teeth[a]	Complications of anorexia nervosa and bulimia
Periodontal changes	
Periodontal diseases[b]	Degenerative vascular changes
Tooth mobility	Microangiopathies
Rapidly progressive pocket formation	Local factors
Gingival bleeding	
Yellow, soft, rapidly forming calculus	Local factors Decreased granulocytosis
Subgingival polyps	Etiology unknown
Infection and wound healing	
Slow wound healing (including periapical lesions after endodontics) and increased susceptibility to infection	Hyperglycemia reduces phagocytic activity Ketoacidosis may delay chemotaxis of granulocytes Vascular changes lead to decreased blood flow Abnormal collagen production
Oral ulcers refractory to therapy, especially in association with a prosthesis	Microangiopathies Neuropathies
Increased incidence and prolonged healing of dry socket	Degenerative vascular changes Postextraction infection
Tongue changes	
Glossodynia	Neuropathic complications Xerostomia Candidiasis
Flabby tongue and indented lateral borders	Neuropathies leading to decreased muscle tone
Median rhomboid glossitis (glossal central papillary atrophy)	*Candida albicans*
Other changes	
Opportunistic infections: *Candida albicans* and Mucormycosis	Repeated use of antibiotics Compromised immune system
Acetone or diabetic breath (seen when the person is close to a diabetic coma)	Ketoacidotic state
Increased incidence of lichen planus (as high as 30%)	Diabetes mellitus, hypertension, and lichen planus have been called the Grinspan syndrome[c]

[a] Although not a complication of diabetes per se, this pattern is seen when the person wants to maintain the weight-loss aspect of diabetes while ignoring or tolerating the hyperglycemic side effects. The client may not be taking his or her proper insulin doses and may not be truthful when asked about this.

[b] This disease is seen in up to 40% of diabetic patients. Adequate periodontal therapy may result in decreased insulin requirements.

[c] This syndrome has been the subject of controversy (Smith, M. J. A. Oral lichen planus and diabetes mellitus: A possible association. Journal of Oral Medicine 32(4):110, 1977).

Adapted and reprinted with permission from The Compendium of Continuing Education in Dentistry. From Skoczylas, L. J., Terezhalmy, G. T., Langlais, R. P., and Glass, B. J. Dental management of the diabetic patient. Compend Contin Educ Dent 9:394, 1988.

Planning

A comprehensive dental hygiene care plan focuses on the client's human need deficits and allows the clinician to manage the risks of potential diabetic emergencies, thereby meeting the client's overriding human need for safety. Appointments should be brief to minimize anxiety and stress and avoid interference with medication and meal or snack schedule. Morning appointments are best because most people with diabetes are under best control at this period of the day. An hour to an hour and a half after breakfast is best for appointments to avoid the peak action time of medication. Regular (fast-acting) insulin, often taken in the morning or at each meal, peaks within 2 to 3 hours following the injection. Oral hypoglycemic agents do not cause peaks as does injected insulin.

Therapeutic scaling and root planing are contraindicated for people in the uncontrolled diabetic condition. Clients should be treated in consultation and referred to the physician of record for systemic evaluation. Dental hygiene care should not begin until the diabetic condition is controlled.

When planning care for the client with diabetes, the dental hygienist also must consider interventions such as:

- Nutritional and dietary analysis
- Fluoride therapy
- Salivary replacement therapy
- Antimicrobial subgingival irrigation of periodontal pockets
- Collaboration with the physician and certified diabetes educator

TABLE 31–15
ALTERATIONS IN DENTAL HYGIENE CARE OF OLDER ADULTS WITH DIABETES

Potential Risk Relating to Dental Hygiene Care	Prevention of Medical Complications
1. In uncontrolled diabetic older adult a. Infection b. Poor wound healing 2. In older adult treated with insulin a. Insulin reaction 3. In diabetic older adult a. Early onset of complications relating to cardiovascular system, eyes, kidney, and nervous system, angina, myocardial infarction, cerebrovascular accident, renal failure, peripheral neuropathy, blindness, hypertension, congestive heart failure	1. Detection by a. Health history b. Clinical findings c. Screening blood sugar 2. Referral for medical diagnosis 3. Older adult receiving insulin—prevent insulin reaction a. Advise older adult to eat normal meals before appointments b. Schedule appointments in morning or midmorning c. Advise older adult to inform you of any symptoms of insulin reaction when they first occur d. Have sugar in some form to give in case of insulin reaction 4. Older adults with diabetes being treated with insulin who develop oral infection may require increase in insulin dosage—consult with physician in addition to local and systemic aggressive management of infection 5. Drug considerations a. Insulin—insulin reaction b. Hypoglycemic agents—on rare occasions aplastic anemia, etc. c. In severe diabetics avoid general anesthesia
Dental Hygiene Care Plan Modifications	**Oral Complications**
In well-controlled diabetic older adult No alteration of dental hygiene care plan is indicated unless complications of diabetes present, such as 1. Hypertension 2. Congestive heart failure 3. Myocardial infarction 4. Angina 5. Renal failure	1. Accelerated periodontal disease 2. Periodontal abscesses 3. Oral ulcerations and opportunistic infections 4. Numbness, burning, or pain in oral tissues 5. Xerostomia 6. Glossodynia 7. Prolonged healing

Data from Little, J. W., and Falace, D. A. Dental Management of the Medically Compromised Patient, 4th ed. St. Louis: C. V. Mosby, 1993; reprinted with permission. (Prepared by Pamela P. Brangan, BSDH, MPH, MS.)

A sample dental hygiene care plan is presented later in the chapter. Other management concerns are shown in Table 31–15.

Implementation

Oral Health Instruction

Prevention of oral infections through personal oral hygiene care is critical in the maintenance of diabetic control. Individuals with diabetes require frequent oral assessments and continued dental hygiene care to ensure adequate healing and prevention of infection. Oral health instruction should:

- Stress meticulous oral home care
- Relate the greater risk of infection and increased healing times to the need for good oral hygiene
- Teach the client to use daily subgingival irrigation for target delivery of antimicrobial agent to reduce potentially pathogenic microorganisms
- Inform clients about the maintenance of the dentition for chewing good foods, because diet and nutrition are essential in the control of diabetes
- Emphasize that individuals with diabetes may not tolerate dentures well because of oral conditions

Therapeutic Scaling and Root Planing

Destructive periodontitis found in diabetes may not respond well to subgingival scaling, débridement, and bacterial plaque control. However, the removal of all hard and soft deposits and toxic elements from crowns and root surfaces of teeth is critical in the prevention of periodontal infection in people with diabetes. Unnecessary tissue manipulation and trauma should be avoided to promote healing and minimize the risk of postoperative infection.

Well-controlled diabetes with no evidence of infection does not require antibiotic coverage.[25,26] In fact, antibiotic use in diabetic patients may lead to oral or systemic fungal infections. If an infection is present, preoperatively or postoperatively, antibiotic therapy is mandatory. Prophylactic antibiotic therapy prior to periodontal instrumentation should be considered following consultation with the client's physician. The dental hygienist must consider that diabetic microangiopathy causes blindness and kidney disease. Therefore, if a client exhibits eye disorders, he also may suffer from kidney disease. Antibiotics that are excreted renally may be retained in the body of the diabetic client with kidney disease, causing toxic effects. Erythromycin is excreted renally, and penicillin is preferred with diabetic clients, provided that there is no history of allergies. When administering local anesthetics, minimal use of vasoconstrictors is required because epinephrine is capable of raising blood glucose.

Evaluation

The evaluative phase of the dental hygiene process of care is paramount for the client with diabetes. The periodontal

DENTAL HYGIENE CARE PLAN: THE CLIENT WITH DIABETES

Dental Hygiene Diagnosis	Goal/Expected Behavior
Deficit in the need for conceptualizaton and problem solving	• By 12/1, client verbalizes the role of bacterial plaque in causing periodontal disease • By 12/1, client verbalizes the role of oral infection in glycemic control
Deficit in the need for self-determination and responsibility	• By 1/1, client controls hyperglycemia through elimination of periodontal disease

DENTAL HYGIENE INTERVENTIONS

1. Present "bleeding gums" as an indicator of a bacterial infection.
2. Demonstrate bacterial plaque control measures.
3. Demonstrate value of oral antimicrobial agents for control of inflammation and techniques for application.
4. Scale, root plane, and irrigate with antimicrobial agent.
5. Monitor oral health behavior through frequent evaluation.
6. Provide appropriate follow-up evaluation of tissue response.

EVALUATIVE STATEMENTS

1. Client explains the interrelationships of diabetic control and periodontal/gingival infection.
2. Client's personal oral health behavior is congruent with maintenance of glycemic control.
3. Client practices oral self-care techniques to enhance glycemic control.

Dental Hygiene Diagnosis	Goal/Expected Behavior
Deficit in the need for nutrition (undernutrition and increased frequency of carbohydrate consumption)	• By 2/1, client verbalizes the need for adequate nutrition • By 2/1, client participates in dietary counseling.

DENTAL HYGIENE INTERVENTIONS

1. Relate nutritional needs in terms of both diabetes control and integrity of the periodontium.
2. Relate the frequency of meals and snacks to need for bacterial plaque control.
3. Relate the importance of healthy dentition and periodontium to optimal diet consumption.
4. Design bacterial plaque control measures consistent with frequency of carbohydrate consumption.
5. Referral to certified diabetes educator for design of a dietary prescription and meal planning.

EVALUATIVE STATEMENTS

1. Client reports normal blood glucose levels.
2. Client indicates compliance with individual dietary prescription and meal plan.

tissues of the client with well-controlled diabetes respond well to nonsurgical periodontal therapy. Delayed healing, however, may indicate hyperglycemia, which decreases the normal healing properties of leukocyte phagocytosis, chemotaxis, and adherence properties.[27] Collaboration with the physician should follow periodontal instrumentation when healing is delayed. Outcomes of dental hygiene care contribute significantly to the long-term systemic health of the diabetic client.

Additional Considerations

The oral health educator/promoter may find a very receptive and interested co-therapist in the certified diabetes educator (CDE) or health education consultant. Many hospitals interested in marketing through community service are developing diabetes centers. The dental hygienist can provide these centers with expertise in oral disease prevention education and oral health screenings and referrals to reduce the threat infection poses to the individual with diabetes.

References

1. Gorsuch A. N., et al. The natural history of type I (insulin-dependent) diabetes mellitus: Evidence for a long pre-diabetic period. Lancet 2:1363, 1981.
2. Irvine, W. J., and Teviol, O. (eds.). Immunology of Diabetes Mellitus. Edinburgh, Scientific Publications, 1979.
3. Craighead, J. E. Viral diabetes mellitus in man and experimental animals. In Skyler, J. S., and Cahill, G. F. (eds.). Dia-

betes Mellitus. New York: York Medical Books, 1981, pp. 23–30.
4. Pyke, D. A. Diabetes and heredity. In Galloway, J. A., Potvin, J. H., and Shuman, C. R. (eds.). Diabetes Mellitus, 9th ed. Indianapolis: Lilley Research Laboratories, 1988, pp. 16–25.
5. Pfeiffer, E. F., and Galloway, J. A. Type II diabetes mellitus and oral hypoglycemic agents. In Galloway, J. A., Potvin, J. H., and Shuman, C. R. (eds.). Diabetes Mellitus, 9th ed. Indianapolis: Lilley Research Laboratories, 1988, pp. 140–157.
6. Barnett, A. H., Eff, C., et al. Diabetes in identical twins: A study of 200 pairs. Diabetologia 20:87, 1981.
7. National Diabetes Data Group (NDDG). Classification and diagnosis of diabetes mellitus and other categories of glucose intolerance. Diabetes 28(12):1039, 1979.
8. Keen, H. Chronic complications of diabetes mellitus. In Galloway, J. A., Potvin, J. H., and Shuman, C. R. (eds.). Diabetes Mellitus, 9th ed. Indianapolis: Lilley Research Laboratories, 1988, pp. 16–25.
9. Gabbe, S. G. Diabetes mellitus: Obstetrical management. In Davidson, J. K. (ed.). Clinical Diabetes Mellitus: A Problem-Oriented Approach. New York: Thieme, 1986, pp. 485–495.
10. DCCT Research Group. The effect of intensive treatment of diabetes on the development and progression of long-term complications in insulin-dependent diabetes mellitus. The New England Journal of Medicine 329:977, 1993.
11. Alberti, K. G., and Phil, B. M. Diabetic emergencies. In Galloway, J. A., Potvin, J. H., and Shuman, C. R. (eds.). Diabetes Mellitus, 9th ed. Indianapolis: Lilley Research Laboratories, 1988, pp. 253–275.
12. Schade, D. S., Eaton, R. P., et al. Diabetic Coma: Ketoacidotic and Hyperosmolar. Albuquerque: University of New Mexico Press, 1981, p. 250.
13. Hockaday, T. D. R., and Alberti, K. G. Diabetic coma. Clinical Endocrinology 1:751, 1972.
14. Galloway, J. A., Potvin, J. H., and Shuman, C. R. (eds.). Diabetes Mellitus, 9th ed. Indianapolis: Lilley Research Laboratories, 1988, p. 86.
15. Rothwell, B. R., and Richard, E. L. Diabetes mellitus: Medical and dental considerations. Special Care in Dentistry 4(2):58, 1984.
16. Wheat, L. J. Infection and diabetes mellitus. Diabetes Care 3:187, 1980.
17. Campbell, P. R., Shuman, D., and Bauman, D. B. ADHA graduate student/faculty research project: Health history. Journal of Dental Hygiene 67:378, 1993.
18. Ervasti, T., Knuuttila, M., et al. Relation between control of diabetes and gingival bleeding. Journal of Periodontology 56(3):154, 1985.
19. Harrison, R., and Bowen, W. Periodontal health, dental caries, and metabolic control in insulin-dependent diabetic children and adolescents. Pediatric Dentistry 9(4):283, 1987.
20. Tervonen, T., and Knuuttila, M. Relation of diabetes control to periodontal pocketing and alveolar bone level. Oral Surgery Oral Medicine Oral Pathology 61(4):346, 1986.
21. Saadoun, A. P. Diabetes and periodontal disease: A review and update. Periodontal Abstracts 28:116, 1980.
22. Leeper, S. H., Kalkwarf, K. L., and Strom, E. A. Oral status of "controlled" adolescent type I diabetes. Journal of Oral Medicine 40(3):127, 1985.
23. McMullen, J. A., Van Dyke, T. E., et al. Neutrophil chemotaxis in individuals with advanced periodontal disease and a genetic predisposition to diabetes mellitus. Journal of Periodontology 52(4):167, 1981.
24. Manouchehr-Pour, M., Spagnuolo, P. J., et al. Comparison of neutrophil chemotactic response in diabetic patients with mild and severe periodontal disease. Journal of Periodontology 52(8):410, 1981.
25. Foster, D. W., and McGarry, J. D. The metabolic derangements and treatment of diabetic ketoacidosis. The New England Journal of Medicine 309(3):159, 1983.
26. Cooper, G., and Platt, R. *Staphylococcus aureus* bacteremia in diabetic patients. American Journal of Medicine 73(5):658, 1982.
27. Nolen, C. M., and Beatyttn Bagdade, J. O. Further characteristics of the impaired bacterial function of granulocytes in patients with poorly controlled diabetes. Diabetes 27:880, 1978.

Suggested Readings

Basker, R. M., et al. Patients with burning mouths: A clinical investigation of causative factors, including the climacteric and diabetes. British Dental Journal 145(1):9, 1978.

Bressler, R., and Galloway, J. A. Insulin treatment of diabetes mellitus. Medical Clinics of North America 55:861, 1971.

Bressler, R., and Galloway, J. A. Insulin treatment of diabetes mellitus. Medical Clinics of North America 62:663, 1978.

Diabetes and Oral Health. Journal of the American Dental Association 115:741, 1987.

Eisenbarth, G. S. Autoimmune beta cell insufficiency—diabetes mellitus type I. Triangle 23:111, 1984.

Farman, A. G. Cellular changes and *Candida* in diabetic outpatients having glossal papillary atrophy. Journal of the Dental Association of South Africa 33(8):425, 1978.

Galloway, J. A. Chemistry and clinical use of insulin. In Galloway, J. A., Potvin, J. H., and Shuman, C. R. (eds.). Diabetes Mellitus, 9th ed. Indianapolis: Lilley Research Laboratories, 1988, pp. 117–118.

Galloway, J. A., and deShazo, R. D. The clinical use of insulin and the complications of insulin therapy. In Ellenberg, M., and Rifkin, H. (eds.). Diabetes Mellitus: Theory and Practice, 3rd ed. New Hyde Park, NY: Medical Examination Publishing, 1983, pp. 519–538.

Greenstein, G. Effects of subgingival irrigation on periodontal status. Journal of Periodontology 58:827, 1987.

Grupper, C., and Avril, J. Lichen erosif buccal, diabete et hypertension (syndrome de Grinspan). Bulletin de la Societe de Dermatologie et de Syphiligraphie 72(5):721, 1965.

Krolewski, A. S., Warram, J. H., Rand, L. I., and Kahn, C. R. Epidemiologic approach to the etiology of type I diabetes mellitus and its complications. The New England Journal of Medicine 317(22):1390, 1987.

McKinney, R. V., and Singh, B. B. Oral manifestations not well recognized as early signs of diabetes mellitus. Journal of the Georgia Dental Association 47(4):19,

Motegi, K., Nakano, Y., et al. Clinical studies on diabetes mellitus and diseases of the oral region. Bulletin of the Tokyo Medical and Dental University 22(3):243, 1975.

Reiner, A. Oral implications of diabetes. Annals of Dentistry 36(2):46, 1977.

Roland, J. M., and Bhanji, S. Anorexia nervosa occurring in patients with diabetes mellitus. Postgraduate Medical Journal 58(680):354, 1982.

Russotto, S. B. Asymptomatic parotid gland enlargement in diabetes mellitus. Oral Surgery 56(6):594, 1981.

Ryan, D. E., and Bronstein, S. L. Dentistry and the diabetic patient. Dental Clinics of North America 26(1):105, 1982.

Santiago, J. V. Alternate routes of and methods of insulin delivery. In Galloway, J. A., Potvin, J. H., and Shuman, C. R. (eds.). Diabetes Mellitus, 9th ed. Indianapolis: Lilley Research Laboratories, 1988, p. 183.

Shuman, C. R. Diabetes mellitus: Definition, classification, and diagnosis. In Galloway, J. A., Potvin, J. H., and Shuman, C. R. (eds.). Diabetes Mellitus, 9th ed. Indianapolis: Lilley Research Laboratories, 1988, p. 183.

Skyler, J. S., and Reeves, M. L. Intensive treatment of type I diabetes mellitus. In Olefsky, J. M., and Sherwin, R. S. (eds.). Diabetes Mellitus: Management and Complications. New York: Churchill Livingstone, 1985, pp. 31–79.

Smith, M. J. A. Oral lichen planus and diabetes mellitus: A possible association. Journal of Oral Medicine 32(4):110, 1977.

Stege, P., Visco-Dangler, L., et al. Anorexia nervosa: A review including oral and dental manifestations. Journal of the American Dental Association 104(5):648, 1982.

Szmukler, G. I., and Russell, G. F. M. Diabetes mellitus, anorexia nervosa, and bulimia. British Journal of Psychiatry 142(1):305, 1983.

West, K. M. (ed.). Epidemiology of Diabetes and Its Vascular Lesions. New York: Elsevier-North Holland, 1978.

32 Dental Hygiene Care for the Individual with Mental Retardation

OBJECTIVES

Mastery of the content in this chapter will enable the reader to:

- Define the key terms used
- Discuss the etiologies of mental retardation, autism, and Down syndrome
- Describe the behavioral and physical characteristics of the client with mental retardation, autism, and Down syndrome
- Discuss the dental hygiene process of care used for a client with mental retardation, autism, and Down syndrome
- Identify the factors to consider when planning educational interventions for a client with mental retardation, autism, and Down syndrome
- Outline an oral health instructional unit designed to overcome communication barriers inherent in the client with autism
- Describe medical conditions that may accompany Down syndrome and their effect on dental hygiene care
- Identify the importance of a comprehensive assessment that should be used for the Down syndrome client
- Recognize the specific dental and oral manifestations seen in the client with Down syndrome

INTRODUCTION

Mental retardation is defined as "a significantly subaverage intellectual functioning accompanied by significant deficits or impairments in adaptive functioning and manifests during the developmental period before 18 years of age."[1] Mentally retarded persons usually have an intellectual quotient (IQ) below 70 and have impairments in communicative, social, and daily living skills.

Because dental hygienists have a prominent role in providing preventive oral care for persons with mental disabilities, it is important that dental hygienists be aware of the various types of mental disability so that they can facilitate human need fulfillment in this special population.

ETIOLOGY

The etiologies of mental retardation typically are grouped into three categories: prenatal, at birth, and postnatal causes.

Research reveals that approximately 90% of mental retardation is of prenatal origin.[2] Several prenatal causes of mental retardation include phenylketonuria, congenital hypothyroidism, and chromosomal abnormalities. Phenylketonuria is a metabolic disorder wherein the infant does not inherit the enzyme necessary to digest the amino acid phenylalanine. If recognized early, dietary alterations can be made to minimize mental retardation. Congenital hypothyroidism is a defect in endocrine functioning that can result in mental retardation. Cretinism, which is associated with hypothyroidism, is the result of partial or complete absence of the thyroid gland.[1,2] Down syndrome is a type of retardation that results from a chromosomal abnormality.

Other prenatal conditions that can cause mental retardation are congenital rubella, congenital syphilis, congenital toxoplasmosis, and fetal alcohol syndrome. Immunization for rubella has decreased the number of babies born with mental retardation from congenital rubella syndrome. The rubella syndrome also can cause cataracts, cardiac anomalies, microcephaly, and deafness.

Congenital syphilis is the transfer of syphilis from mother to fetus. Other dental signs of congenital syphilis are Hutchinsonian incisors, mulberry molars, and microdontia.

Neonatal congenital toxoplasmosis is the infection of the fetus across the placenta with the protozoa *Toxoplasma gondii,* which is carried in raw meat and fecal material. Major hazards may not be apparent in the mother (symptoms can be evident only as a cold) but fetal impact may be dramatic. For example, 85% of surviving newborns may be mentally retarded and may have other complications such as blindness or convulsions.

Fetal alcohol syndrome, caused by the consumption of alcohol during pregnancy, has been shown to cause abnormal development and growth in children. Symptoms shown by children may include slow growth before and after birth, a small head, facial irregularities (narrow eye slits, sunken nasal bridges), defective heart and other organs, malformed arms and legs, genital abnormalities, and mental retardation. Behavioral problems also are evident, such as hyperactivity, extreme nervousness, and a poor attention span. The amount of alcohol intake that results in fetal alcohol syndrome has not been determined.

Injury at birth is not a frequent cause of mental retardation. If mental retardation does occur at birth it is usually a result of a difficult labor and delivery that causes anoxia (lack of oxygen) to the infant.

Postnatal causes of mental retardation are classified in three groups: acute illness, traumatic events, and progressive disorders. Encephalitis, measles, meningitis, and other illnesses accompanied by a high fever may cause mental retardation. Accidents that lead to a fractured skull, concussion, or unconsciousness also may cause mental retardation. Progressive disorders are defined as disorders that increase in extent or severity, and these disorders may be accompanied by mental retardation. For example, a child with cerebral palsy who has a motor disability also may have an intellectual defect resulting in mental retardation.[1,2]

LEVELS OF MENTAL RETARDATION

Dental hygiene professionals must determine the level of retardation, make an accurate assessment of the client's abilities, and plan oral health interventions that take these abilities into account. The level of retardation also is important to assess in determining if the client is capable of giving informed consent for dental hygiene care.

Levels of mental retardation are categorized as mild, moderate, severe, and profound. Persons with **mild retardation** have an IQ of approximately 50 to 70. These clients are designated as educable mentally retarded and are able to learn some academic skills. Persons with mild retardation can learn simple skills in detail, but their attention spans and memories are short. Mild retardation is sometimes not evident until a child enters school and demonstrates a poor learning ability. For clients with mild retardation, dental hygiene professionals should explain and demonstrate oral hygiene instructions and teach activities instead of concepts. Clients with mental retardation require public recognition, praise, and reward for progress.

Moderate mental retardation is classified by an IQ of approximately 35 to 49. Persons with moderate mental retardation can learn self-care, social adjustment, and economic usefulness, but very few academic skills. The client's functional abilities are limited and learning is slower. Poor hand and finger coordination may be evident; therefore, clients should be taught only the fundamental skills by employing the show-and-tell method. Every successful step performed during therapy and oral hygiene instruction should be rewarded with both tangible and verbal praise. Oral hygiene instructions should be reviewed at each appointment because of the short memory and attention span of clients with moderate retardation. The primary caregiver should be encouraged to supervise the client's daily oral hygiene regimen to ensure that optimal home care is practiced.

Severe retardation is seen in persons with an IQ of approximately 20 to 34. This level of retardation allows the person to acquire some oral care skills with supervision. These clients learn by habit training, which consists of repeating procedures and movements continuously so that the client can grasp the procedures. It is important to include the caregiver in teaching oral hygiene instructions to clients with severe mental retardation. Depending on the environment, all successfully performed skills should be rewarded by the dental hygienist or the caregiver. See Table 32–1 for suggested awards.

Profound retardation is characterized by an IQ below 20. These clients are incapable of total self-care, social skills, or economic usefulness and require continued supervision and care from the primary caregiver. Many clients with profound retardation remain withdrawn and usually have an inability to interact with others. The caregiver is responsible for the client's oral hygiene care; therefore, the dental hygiene professional should educate the caregiver to meet the daily oral hygiene needs of the person with profound mental retardation.[1,2,3]

GENERAL CHARACTERISTICS OF PERSONS WITH MENTAL RETARDATION

A range of characteristics accompany mental retardation, many of which are consistent with the specific type of mental retardation. Astute oral healthcare professionals avoid the overgeneralization of mentally retarded individuals and instead take into account the specific and individual needs of each person.

TABLE 32–1
REWARDS THAT CAN BE USED TO REINFORCE POSITIVE BEHAVIOR FOR CLIENTS WITH MENTAL RETARDATION

Social rewards	Attention, smiles, hugs, praise and other signs of approval and affection
Activity rewards	Any activity a person enjoys—watching television, playing a game, going to a party
Material rewards	An item that a person can use, play with, wear, or consume—toys, money, food, clothing

Adapted from Stiefel, D. J., and Stull, D. E. Motivation, compliance, and preventive behavior. In Ingersoll, B. D. (ed.). Behavioral Aspects in Dentistry. New York: Appleton-Century-Crofts, 1982, pp. 100–101.

Health

Persons with mental retardation usually have less physical stamina than persons in the general population. Furthermore, they manifest delayed physical development and usually have speech and physical defects. Mental retardation also is accompanied by poor motor coordination, vision, and hearing. It is not uncommon to see persons with mental retardation who are overweight or underweight as a result of environmental factors such as poor parental or poor institutional care, or from genetic and metabolic factors such as phenylketonuria. Also, persons with mental retardation may have poor dental and oral health as a result of malnutrition, limited self-care capabilities, and the presence of economic barriers to care. As part of assessing the client's human needs for nutrition and a biologically sound dentition, the dental hygienist must consider the client's diet, possible chewing or swallowing difficulties, and the possibility of dietary restrictions.

Mental and Motor Abilities

Mentally retarded persons usually have a short memory span and an inability to concentrate. These persons may have limited speech. A lack of adaptive, associative, or organizing skills also is seen. Persons with mental retardation usually have an inability to see differences or likenesses between objects. Success is usually found from concrete rather than abstract experiences. These persons usually are more adept in manual skills than academic skills. Depending on the severity of the retardation, some clients may be able to render their own oral hygiene care.

Social and Emotional Abilities

Persons with mental retardation are viewed as "followers" rather than the "leaders," that is, they tend to imitate others. Mentally retarded persons frequently show behavioral problems to gain attention or release emotion. Some maladaptive behaviors may be destructive, including aggressiveness directed toward others, property destruction, and self-injurious behavior. These persons have an awareness of not belonging and become discouraged easily. Criticism is not taken positively and there is an inability to learn through experience.

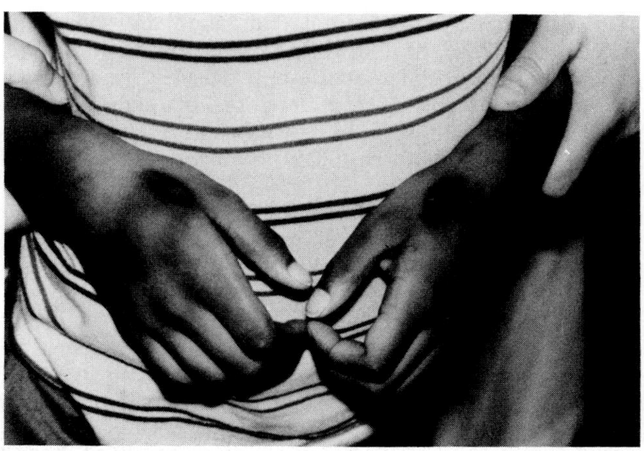

FIGURE 32–1
Physical outcome of self-injurious behavior in a child with mental retardation. (Courtesy of Dr. F. T. McIver, Department of Pediatric Dentistry, University of North Carolina School of Dentistry.)

Oral Manifestations

Oral manifestations observed in mentally retarded clients often coincide with a specific type of syndrome.

A client may bite the lips or the lining of the mouth as a type of self-injurious behavior. Figure 32–1 shows an autistic child who has bitten his hands as a type of self-injurious behavior. Persons with mental retardation also have been known to hit themselves in the mouth to gain attention or release emotion.[4] Griffin and colleagues offer nine strategies for managing self-injurious behavior: (1) differential reinforcement of another behavior; (2) positive reinforcement; (3) ignoring unwanted behavior; (4) positive reinforcement of wanted behavior; (5) psychoactive medication; (6) restraint; (7) counseling; (8) application of consequences after behavior; and (9) overcorrection.[5] These are fully explained in Table 32–2.

TABLE 32–2
NINE STRATEGIES FOR MANAGING SELF-INJURIOUS BEHAVIOR IN DENTAL HYGIENE CLIENTS WITH SPECIAL NEEDS

Strategy	Defined	Examples
Differential reinforcement	Reinforcement of any behavior other than the self-injurious behavior	Draw interest away from injurious behavior
Positive reinforcement	Used in order for a person to repeat a desired behavior	Praise—"you really did well"; "good job"
Ignoring unwanted behavior	Refusing to take notice of behavior	Consciously ignoring a negative behavior
Positive reinforcement of wanted behavior	Reinforcement when the wanted behavior is directly addressed	"You really brushed those back teeth well"
Psychoactive medication	Medication that alters one's psychological state	Neuroleptics, antidepressants, psychostimulants
Restraint	Confinement of a person physically	Papoose board, Velcro straps
Counseling	Professional guidance of a person using psychological methods	Offer support, positive reinforcement, and trust
Application of consequences after behavior	Punishment after the unwanted behavior to reinforce the idea that the behavior was unacceptable	Time out, not allowing a reward after treatment
Overcorrection	When an unwanted behavior is done and it is corrected by requiring duties above and beyond the specific behavior	Joe colors on the wall, he should clean more of the wall than where he colored

Lips of clients with mental retardation are sometimes larger than those of the general population, and tooth anomalies such as microdontia and delayed eruption patterns are usually present from developmental abnormalities. Wear of the tooth surfaces from bruxism has been observed, which seems to be linked to anxiety and emotional distress.

The consequences of bruxism can include dental attrition, functional problems such as temporomandibular joint disorders, and eventually sensitivity and pain. Wear is usually seen in the incisors and canines and increases with age. By the age of 30 to 49 years, wear becomes so significant that restorative measures may be needed. Bruxism may be the result of a lack of personal contact and also has been viewed as a type of self-stimulation.[6] Increased wear of teeth also may be the result of psychopharmacological therapy that causes xerostomia and oral dyskinesia.[7] Before treatment can be given for these problems, a complete assessment must be made to reveal the origin of the behavior and its chronicity.

Periodontal disease prevalence has been documented in mentally retarded individuals. The prevalence of periodontal diseases is attributed to lack of professional care, lack of funds to support care, increased susceptibility of the client, and poor oral hygiene. Mentally retarded persons usually depend on someone else to facilitate their access to oral healthcare, and a lay person's assessment for the oral healthcare need is likely to differ from that of a dentist or dental hygienist.

INSTRUCTIONAL INTERVENTION FOR MENTALLY RETARDED CLIENTS

Most (89%) mentally retarded persons seen in the oral healthcare environment are mildly retarded. A smaller percentage (6%) is moderately retarded, and 4.5% is severely or profoundly retarded.[3] When teaching oral hygiene skills, the oral healthcare professional should teach based on the client's mental age, not chronological age. A client's mental age can be determined by the following formula, where CA represents chronological age and MA represents mental age.

$$MA = CA \times IQ \div 100:$$

Estimation of MA = :

Mildly retarded	2/3 × CA
Moderate	1/2 × CA
Severe	1/3 × CA
Profound less than	1/4 × CA

As with any client, the key to managing a mentally retarded client is a humanistic approach coupled with a comprehensive care plan designed according to the individual's assessed abilities and human need deficits related to dental hygiene care. Once this is accomplished, oral healthcare professionals should begin instructions with familiar activities, praise small accomplishments, and use a gentle but firm demeanor. Extra instructional time may be required for conveying new information. If problems occur (e.g., crying, frustration) the dental hygienist must be prepared to repeat an earlier achievement level to meet the client's need for freedom from stress. Effective communication with the mentally retarded client leads to a trusting relationship, which in turn allows the oral healthcare experience to be successful for both the client and oral healthcare provider.[3] Several approaches that can be used to form this trusting relationship are presented in the Strategies for Establishing a Trusting Relationship with Clients who are Mentally Challenged chart.

When providing care to clients with mental retardation, using the dental hygiene process can increase the likelihood that the visit will be successful. While conducting the client assessment, the dental hygienist must also collect data about the daily self-care status of the client (e.g., toilet training, oral hygiene habits, developmental level, eating habits). The client's primary caregiver may be able to suggest behavior guidance to increase the likelihood of a pleasant experience for both the client and the oral healthcare professional. Several critical factors to consider during the dental hygiene process include the client's diet and ability to chew, oral hygiene potential, client interests, parent's and caregiver's interests and values, client's and parent's or caregiver's level of cooperation, and cost of care.

MANAGEMENT OF THE CLIENT WITH DOWN SYNDROME

Down syndrome is the most common and frequently observed chromosomal abnormality in the human race. This syndrome, first observed by Langdon Down (1866) in a group of mentally handicapped individuals, occurs in all socioeconomic levels, geographic regions, ethnic groups, and cultures. The occurrence of babies born with Down syndrome is 1 in 800 live births, but because 75% of Down syndrome fetuses spontaneously abort, this does not repre-

STRATEGIES FOR ESTABLISHING A TRUSTING RELATIONSHIP WITH CLIENTS WHO ARE MENTALLY CHALLENGED

- At the first appointment, help the client become familiar with the surroundings
- Schedule time for the oral healthcare team to meet the client; try to alleviate any anxieties by getting to know the client and by the client getting to know the team
- The first appointment should be short and nonthreatening
- Explanations should be given slowly with one instruction given at a time
- Use the tell-show-do technique when teaching oral hygiene instructions; teach one technique at each appointment to avoid overwhelming the client
- Make sure the client understands the instructions by having the client demonstrate how to perform the procedure (i.e., brushing or flossing)
- Reward the client often for positive behavior[3]
  Rewards might include: verbal positive reinforcement such as "good job," tangible reinforcement such as a toy or special outing arranged by the caregiver, public recognition such as a certificate that can be displayed in the client's home or work setting
- If the client can read, provide handouts, designed at the appropriate level of reading comprehension, that can be taken home

Modified from Stiefel, D. J., and Stull, D. E. Motivation, compliance, and preventive behavior. In Ingersoll, B. D. (ed.). Behavioral Aspects in Dentistry. New York: Appleton-Century-Crofts, 1982, p. 171.

sent a true occurrence rate of Down syndrome.[8] When considering the birth rate of 1 in 800 and the estimation of approximately 4 million births in the United States in 1990, about 5,000 newborns with Down syndrome would be expected. Because of the prevalence of Down syndrome, dental hygienists are likely to provide care for clients with this condition. Therefore, dental hygienists must be prepared theoretically and clinically to meet the needs of persons with Down syndrome.

Genetics as Etiology

Down syndrome is a chromosome abnormality that affects chromosome number 21 and results in a defined set of physical characteristics and mental retardation. Three manifestations of chromosomal abnormality can occur; these include trisomy 21, translocation, or mosaicism. The majority (95%) of people with Down syndrome have the effects of trisomy 21. **Trisomy 21** is a failure of a pair of number 21 chromosomes to segregate (nondisjunction) during the formation of either an egg or sperm prior to conception.[9] Trisomy 21 is not inherited and has no known etiology. The incidence is correlated with increased maternal age. For example, mothers under 30 years of age have a one in 1,000 chance of giving birth to an infant with Down syndrome; those 35 years of age have a one in 400 chance; and for those 40 years of age, the chances increase to one in 100.[10] **Translocation** is hereditary and occurs when a piece of chromosome in pair 21 breaks off and attaches to another chromosome, usually chromosome 14, 21, or 22. Translocation occurs in approximately 4 to 5% of those children with Down syndrome. The third type of chromosomal anomaly associated with Down syndrome is **mosaicism.** Mosaicism occurs in only 1% of children with Down syndrome. Mosaicism is a result of an error in one of the first cell divisions shortly after conception. Regardless of the type of chromosomal anomaly, the presence of three number 21 chromosomes are responsible for the specific physical characteristics and mental deficiencies seen in persons with Down syndrome.[11]

Physical and Mental Characteristics

Approximately 50 different physical characteristics have been observed in infants with Down syndrome; however, not every infant with Down syndrome manifests all 50 characteristics. Only the most common characteristics are discussed in this chapter.

The skull of a child with Down syndrome usually appears small and is shortened in diameter anterior to posterior (from forehead to the crown). A hypoplasia of midfacial bones also is apparent. Strelling pointed out that the eyes, nose, and mouth are small and grouped closely together at the center of the face.[12] The eyes present with prominent epicanthal folds, which are folds of skin extending from the root of the nose to the median end of the eyebrow.[12] The iris of the eye is speckled with marks called Brushfield spots. The nose is reduced in size, nostrils are upturned, and there is a depression of the nasal bridge. Deviations in the nasal septum also are common. Because of the flat nasal bridge and the underdevelopment of the midfacial region, the face of a Down syndrome person appears flat.[11,13] This flat facial profile is the most frequently observed characteristic of Down syndrome.[14]

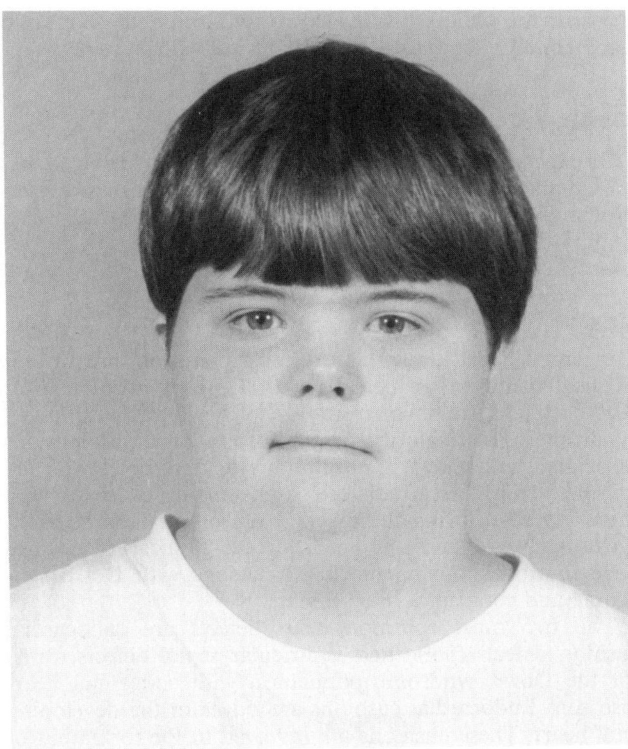

FIGURE 32–2
Facial profile of a Down syndrome client. (Courtesy of Dr. F. T. McIver, Department of Pediatric Dentistry, University of North Carolina School of Dentistry.)

Figure 32–2 depicts the facial features of a Down syndrome client. The ears of a person with Down syndrome may appear small and abnormal in structure. In most cases the ears have a lack of distinct contour, which results in a round or square appearance; the hands may appear short and broad with nails that are hyperconvex (Fig. 32–3).[15] Persons with Down syndrome tend to be short and overweight.

Down syndrome persons usually present with an IQ between 25 and 50.[16] Despite the limitations of their IQ, the

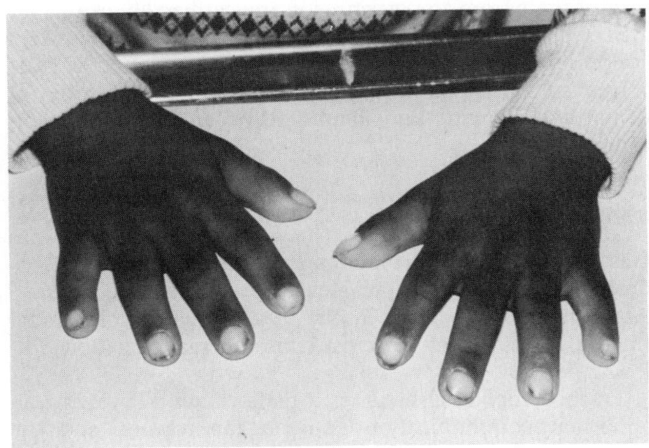

FIGURE 32–3
Hands of a Down syndrome client. (Courtesy of Dr. F. T. McIver, Department of Pediatric Dentistry, University of North Carolina School of Dentistry.)

majority of children with Down syndrome develop into happy and in some cases self-reliant individuals.

Medical Considerations

Life expectancy for persons with Down syndrome is approximately 35 to 40 years of age.[17] Lives of Down syndrome persons can be lengthened by quality healthcare and healthy lifestyle behaviors.

Congenital Heart Disease

Congenital heart disease is the most common and serious medical condition in persons with Down syndrome. Cardiac problems are observed in 40% of newborns with Down syndrome. The majority of cardiovascular malformations associated with Down syndrome are acutely or chronically life-threatening. Heart disease is the major cause of high mortality rate during the first 2 years of the infant's life.[18] Fortunately, advances in medical and surgical procedures have improved the prognosis for persons with Down syndrome and congenital heart disease.

The two most common heart defects are endocardial cushion defects (36%) and ventricular septal defects (33%) for the Down syndrome population with congenital heart disease.[19] Endocardial cushions are ridges in the developing fetal heart. These cushions are involved in the formation of the septum that separates the right and left ventricles, formation of the septum that separates the right and left atria, and the formation of the two valves between the atria and ventricles. Symptoms of these heart defects are severe heart failure, frequent pneumonia, and poor growth. Also frequently seen in Down syndrome is pulmonary artery hypertension. This is characterized by constriction of the blood vessels in the lungs, which causes back pressure and overload on the right ventricle. Pulmonary artery hypertension is often a consequence of the increased flow to the lungs caused by the heart defects.[18]

Many other cardiac abnormalities are observed in Down syndrome. Multiple abnormalities exist in approximately 30% of persons with Down syndrome.[11] Medical care depends on the severity of the symptoms. When providing oral healthcare to a person with Down syndrome, the dental hygiene professional must obtain a detailed health history of the person to determine if any cardiac abnormalities are present. Antibiotic premedication is prescribed when congenital heart defects are present because defective heart valves are susceptible to bacterial endocarditis as a result of dental hygiene care (see Chapter 10 on antibiotic premedication).

Gastrointestinal Disorders

Gastrointestinal malformations are observed in Down syndrome with an overall prevalence of approximately 12%.[20] Abnormalities can occur in any area of the gastrointestinal tract: a discussion of the most common malformations follows.

Tracheoesophageal fistula is a malformation involving an abnormal communication between the trachea and the esophagus. This anomaly causes ingested substances to be aspirated into the lungs. Treatment is surgical in all cases. Pyloric stenosis is characterized by a constriction of the outlet of the stomach that prevents food from passing from the stomach to the small intestine. Symptoms seen in infants include projectile vomiting and extreme hunger. The symptoms usually appear at 1 to 2 months, and medical diagnosis can be made by observing clinical symptoms and confirmed by analysis of radiographs.

Duodenal atresia is a malformation wherein the duodenum is obstructed. An annular pancreas leads to duodenal obstruction as a result of the pancreas surrounding the duodenum and constricting the lumen. These abnormalities are present at birth and symptoms are seen at feeding. Although the cardinal sign of duodenal atresia is bilious vomiting, medical diagnosis is made by analysis of an abdominal radiograph. Imperforate anus is the absence of an anal opening and is diagnosed at the time of birth. Hirschsprung's disease is the absence of the nerve cells in the rectum and colon that stimulate intestinal motility. The major sign is severe constipation with soft stools.[11]

Orthopedic Concerns

Orthopedic problems are usually a result of low muscle tone. Atlantoaxial subluxation, a cervical spine instability characterized by an abnormal increase in mobility within the joint between the first two cervical vertebrae in the neck, occurs in 10 to 20% of persons with Down syndrome.[21] Most children have no symptoms of atlantoaxial subluxation; but if symptoms are present (i.e., neck pain, change in gait, extremity weakness, spasticity, and limited neck movement) they are related to spinal cord compression.

Scoliosis (curvature of the spine) is frequently detected in Down syndrome but is usually mild.[11] Persons with Down syndrome usually have excessive external rotation and abduction of the hip. As a result of these hip anomalies, a wide-angled gait and widespread legs when sitting are evident.[13]

Other Disorders

Thyroid disorders are common in persons with Down syndrome. In older persons with Down syndrome, as many as 50% have thyroid disorders, with hypothyroidism being the most common.[22] The classic symptoms of hypothyroidism include delayed growth, short stature, obesity, lethargy, and dry skin.

Hearing impairments occur in 75% of persons with Down syndrome.[23] Hearing loss is usually mild to moderate and is often caused by persistent fluid in the middle ear. Ear infections also are common in Down syndrome. Cataracts occur in 30 to 60% of persons with Down syndrome; however, most cataracts do not affect vision or require surgery.[24]

Seizure activity is seen in infants and young children with Down syndrome at the same occurrence rate as in the general population. However, at age 20 to 30 grand mal seizures are seen more frequently in persons with Down syndrome. Oral healthcare professionals should be aware of gingival changes caused by medications taken to control seizure activity. Phenytoin (Dilantin) is a drug often prescribed to control epileptic seizures; it often causes gingival hyperplasia in varying degrees of severity. Figure 32–4 shows moderate gingival changes, and Figure 32–5 shows severe gingival changes from phenytoin therapy.

Alzheimer's disease has been linked to Down syndrome. Anatomical changes of Alzheimer's disease appear to be almost universal in adults with Down syndrome over the age of 35 years.[25] Despite the anatomical changes of Alzheimer's disease seen in adults with Down syndrome, most do not show signs of Alzheimer's disease.

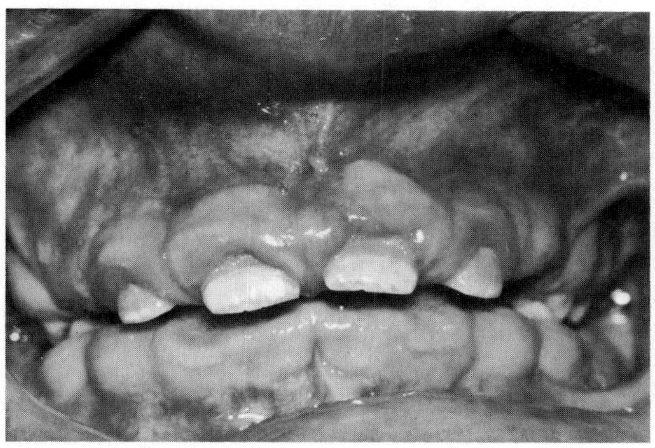

FIGURE 32–4
Moderate gingival changes associated with Dilantin (phenytoin) therapy for seizure control in a client with Down syndrome. (Courtesy of Dr. F. T. McIver, Department of Pediatric Dentistry, University of North Carolina School of Dentistry.)

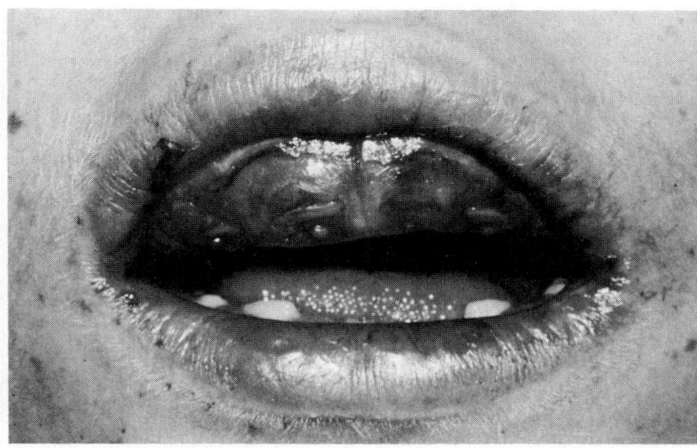

FIGURE 32–5
Severe gingival changes associated with Dilantin therapy for seizure control in a client with Down syndrome. (Courtesy of Dr. F. T. McIver, Department of Pediatric Dentistry, University of North Carolina School of Dentistry.)

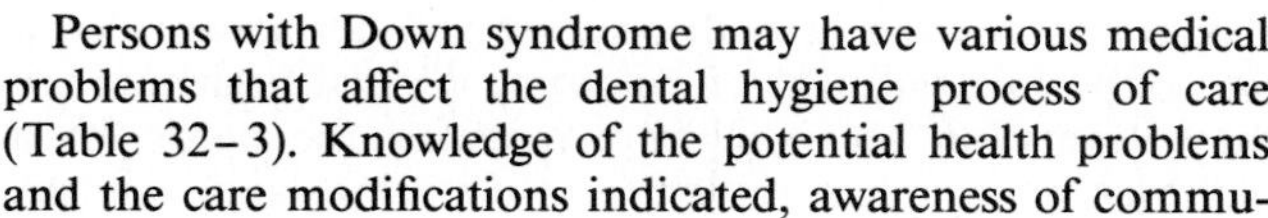

Persons with Down syndrome may have various medical problems that affect the dental hygiene process of care (Table 32–3). Knowledge of the potential health problems and the care modifications indicated, awareness of community services and resources, presence of good client and family rapport, and use of a collaborative approach in meeting the client's healthcare needs are required to achieve oral health and wellness. A knowledge of organiza-

TABLE 32–3
MEDICAL CONSIDERATIONS FOR CLIENTS WITH DOWN SYNDROME

Concern	Clinical Expression	When Seen	Prevalence	Management
Congenital heart disease	Endocardial cushion defect Septal defects Tetralogy of Fallot	Newborn or first six weeks	40%	EKG, chest x ray, pediatric cardiology consultation, echocardiogram, surgical repair
Hypotonia	Reduced muscle tone Increased range of joint mvt. Motor function problems	Throughout life Improvement with maturity	100%	Guidance by physical therapy early intervention program
Delayed growth	Typically at or near the third percentile of general population	Throughout life	100%	Early nutritional support, appropriate expectations, use DS growth charts, check heart/thyroid
Developmental delays	Some global delay, degree varies Specific processing problems Specific expressive language delay	First year, monitor Throughout life	100%	Early intervention Special education Language therapy
Hearing problems	Serous otitis media Small ear canals Conductive impairment	Check by 6 months Review annually	50–70%	Audiology, tympanometry ENT consultation Myringotomy tubes if needed
Ocular problems	Refractive errors Strabismus Cataracts	Eye exam in early months Regular follow-up	50% 35% 15%	Ophthalmologic consultation and appropriate treatment
Cervical spine problem	Atlantoaxial instability Skeletal cervical anomalies Possible spinal cord compression	X ray by 3 years	10%± 1–2%±	Orthopedic, neurology, neurosurgery ?Restriction of high-risk activity Surgical stabilization if symptomatic
Thyroid disease	Hypothyroidism (rarely hyper-) Decreased growth, activity	Some congenital, most 2nd decade + check age 1, repeat	?15%+	Replacement therapy (medication)
Obesity	Excessive weight gain	Esp. 2–3 yrs, 12–13 yrs and in adult life	Common	Caloric restriction Activity/exercise Watch thyroid function
Seizure disorder	Primarily generalized (grand mal) Also, myoclonic, hypsarrhythmia	Any time	5–10%	Neurology consultation, EEG Medication
Emotional problems	Inappropriate behavior, depression	Mid/late childhood, adulthood	Common	Mental health assistance, family counseling
Premature senescence	Behavior changes; functional losses	>5th decade	Increase with age	Specialized support, neurology

Also, variable occurrence of: congenital gastrointestinal anomalies, Hirschsprung's disease, leukemia, hepatitis B carrier state, keratoconus, dry skin, hip dysplasia, diabetes, mitral valve prolapse

Adapted with author's permission from Crocker AC. The spectrum of medical care for developmental disabilities. In Crocker A. C., Rubin I. L. (eds.). Developmental Disabilities—Delivery of Medical Care for Children and Adults. Philadelphia: Lea & Febiger, 1989, p. 10.

NATIONAL ORGANIZATIONS FOR CLIENTS WITH SPECIAL NEEDS

National Down Syndrome Congress
1800 Dempster
Park Ridge, IL 60068-1146
312-823-7500

National Association for Retarded Citizens
2501 Avenue J
P.O. Box 6109
Arlington, TX 76006
1-800-433-5255

National Association for Down Syndrome
P.O. Box 4542
Oak Brook, IL 60521
312-325-9112

tions in the community aids the oral healthcare professional in meeting client needs beyond the scope of dental hygiene (see National Organizations for Clients with Special Needs chart). These organizations may not be in the immediate location of clients, but they may be able to supply knowledge of the closest organization for referral and support. The yellow or blue pages of the telephone directory under Social Services, Disabilities, or Mental Retardation can supply local assistance.

Oral Manifestations

Persons with Down syndrome exhibit specific dental and oral characteristics. A Down syndrome person often may be seen with the mouth open and the tongue protruding. It has been thought that there is an increase in the size of the tongue; however, Jensen, Cleal, and Yips indicated that the tongue seems enlarged as a result of an underdeveloped maxilla, a narrow palate with broadened alveolar ridges, and enlarged tonsils and adenoids, all of which produce a small oral cavity.[26] Fissuring of the tongue and enlargement of the vallate papillae are observed in 37 to 60% of persons with Down syndrome.[9] Typically, a person with Down syndrome has an underdeveloped maxilla accompanied by prognathism of the mandible.[27]

The teeth are commonly found to be small (microdontia) in persons with Down syndrome. Teeth in the maxillary arch are generally more affected in size than the teeth in the mandibular arch.[28] Garn and colleagues reported that the maxillary second molars, lateral incisors, and canines were reduced in size, with the most posterior teeth reduced to the greatest extent.[29] Abnormalities in tooth morphology also are seen in Down syndrome persons. Cohen and colleagues discovered that morphological abnormalities appear more frequently in the maxillary arch than in the mandibular arch.[30] The most frequently affected permanent teeth in the maxillary arch were the second molars (52%), lateral incisors (42%), canines (41%), first molars (40%), and central incisors (35%). In the mandibular arch the first and second premolars were most frequently affected (63% and 48%). Tetracycline staining may be evident as a result of the significant number of infections requiring antibiotic medication in children with Down syndrome during their first few years of life.[31]

Congenitally missing teeth occur in persons with Down syndrome at a much higher rate than that in the general population. Barkla reported that of 122 individuals with Down syndrome, 12% had one or more congenitally missing primary teeth.[32] The most frequently missing permanent teeth in Down syndrome persons are the lateral incisors. Within each quadrant it is common to find the most posterior tooth to be missing more than the most anterior tooth. Malocclusion also is seen frequently, with mandibular overjet and posterior crossbite occurring in virtually all persons with Down syndrome.[33] Figure 32–6 depicts a Down syndrome person with severe overjet and other maloccluding teeth. Correction of maloccluding teeth is usually not indicated. If crossbites are corrected, an earlier tissue breakdown may occur as a result of the underdeveloped maxilla and its relation to basal bone. Lingual movement of mandibular teeth is not indicated because of the tendency of persons with Down syndrome to have large protruding tongues. Other reasons contraindicating orthodontic treatment include: susceptibility to periodontal disease, poor oral hygiene skills, and questionable tolerance to orthodontic appliances.[27] Also, it has been observed that tooth eruption is delayed in both primary and permanent dentition of persons with Down syndrome. Dental hygienists use the information obtained from assessing the needs for a biologically sound dentition and for skin and mucous membrane integrity when planning care and oral hygiene instructions.

Individuals with Down syndrome have a high incidence of **periodontal disease.** Shaw and Saxby compared the type of periodontal disease seen in clients with Down syndrome to that seen in juvenile periodontitis.[34] These researchers concluded that clinical similarities in periodontal involvement are apparent, and it is probable that juvenile periodontitis and the type of periodontal disease seen in clients with Down syndrome are both functions of immunodeficiencies rather than poor oral hygiene alone. Periodontal disease has been reported to begin as early as age 5 years, and by adulthood nearly all Down syndrome persons are affected.[35]

Figure 32–7 depicts a Down syndrome client with marginal gingivitis and enamel hypoplasia. Figure 32–8 shows

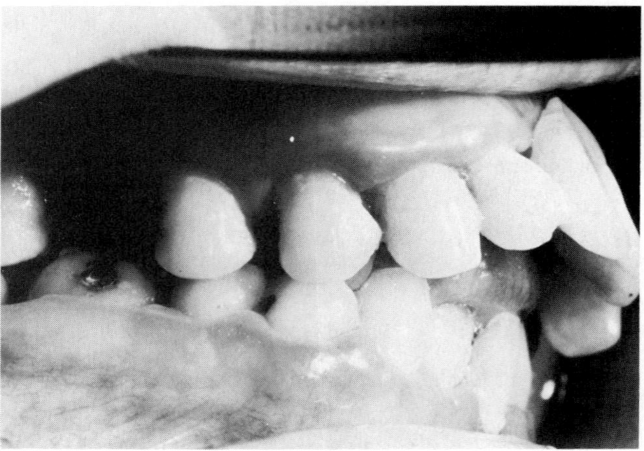

FIGURE 32–6
Malocclusion in a Down syndrome client. (Courtesy of Dr. F. T. McIver, Department of Pediatric Dentistry, University of North Carolina School of Dentistry.)

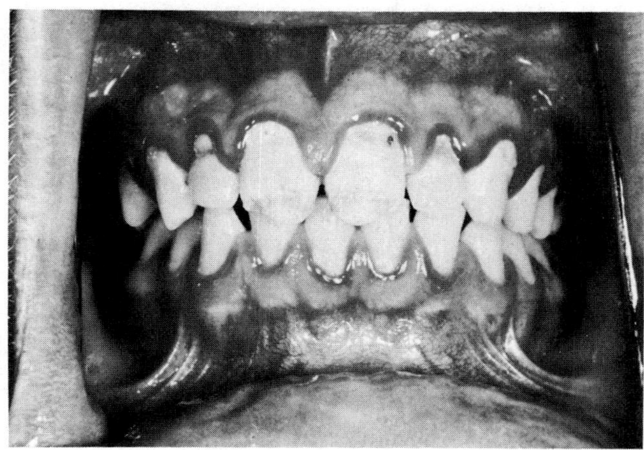

FIGURE 32–7
Marginal gingivitis and enamel hypoplasia in an individual with Down syndrome. (Courtesy of Dr. F. T. McIver, Department of Pediatric Dentistry, University of North Carolina School of Dentistry.)

more severe periodontal problems in a Down syndrome client. Periodontal disease is more frequently seen in individuals living in institutions as compared to individuals living in the community. This finding may be the result of the lack of education given to the healthcare providers in these institutions, diet, and inadequate daily preventive oral health behavior. In Down syndrome individuals living in the community, the level of oral hygiene practiced and the extra care given by their caregivers may be sufficient to slow down the disease process.[36]

If oral healthcare professionals can incorporate effective oral hygiene care as a part of the client's daily routine, gingival and periodontal conditions may be prevented or controlled. Maintaining a high level of oral hygiene is very difficult for persons with Down syndrome; therefore, oral healthcare professionals must educate caregivers and stress the importance of close supervision during oral hygiene procedures and diet habits that promote oral health and wellness.

Tooth loss occurs in about 50% of individuals with Down syndrome, which may be attributed to the high prevalence of periodontal disease in this population.[33] Other oral manifestations of Down syndrome may include hypoplastic enamel, shortened roots, and a low caries rate.[27] Therefore, it is imperative that persons with Down syndrome employ appropriate oral disease control strategies, follow good dietary habits, receive restorative care, and receive pit and fissure sealants and fluoride therapy. Dental hygienists can provide in-service education sessions on the oral health needs of the Down syndrome persons to healthcare providers and caregivers, and can promote policies and practice that lead to optimal wellness in this population.

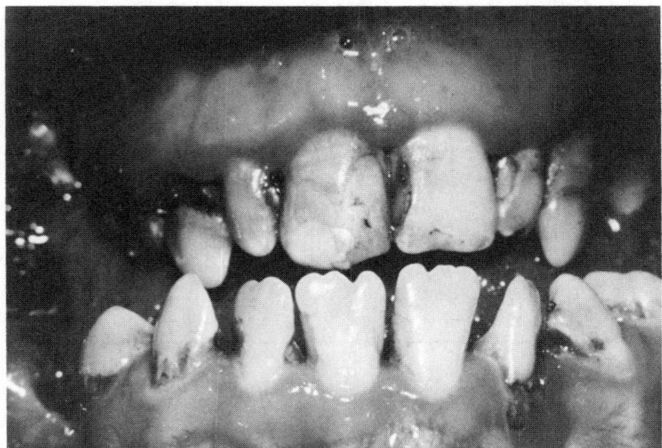

FIGURE 32–8
Severe periodontal disease in a Down syndrome client. (Courtesy of Dr. F. T. McIver, Department of Pediatric Dentistry, University of North Carolina School of Dentistry.)

The dental hygiene professional must ensure that oral hygiene instructions are presented to the client and a family member or primary caregiver in a clear and concise manner. Persons capable of performing their own oral hygiene procedures should be encouraged to do so. Electric or powered toothbrushes may enable persons with minimal motor control to perform their own oral hygiene care, thereby facilitating the human need for self-determination. If persons can perform their own preventive oral behaviors, they own the task and are likely to perform the behavior regularly. There is evidence that persons with Down syndrome learn better from visual teaching than auditory teaching; therefore, teaching and learning interventions should be augmented with visual materials such as pictures, models, and diagrams.[37]

Persons with Down syndrome are content and affectionate individuals, but they can become aggressive if confused or disoriented. Although speech patterns are retarded, the majority of adults speak intelligently with a husky quality of voice. The key point to remember is that the client does not comprehend the need for care or that it is beneficial. It is important to assess the mental level of the client via the formula discussed at the beginning of the chapter, or by behavioral patterns, responses during conversation, and questioning the caregiver. Everything related to care should be introduced slowly, explained, and shown if possible. Humanistic behavior should be used to calm the client's fears. Some Down syndrome clients with higher IQs (mild and slightly moderate retarded) can become involved and appreciate the attention given to them during the dental hygiene visit. If these clients are unmanageable it is usually because they are frightened, have had a previous traumatic dental experience, or their mental limitations do not allow them to comprehend the procedure. Preoperative medications and general anesthesia can be prescribed and administered if necessary. When care requires use of a general anesthetic agent, a thorough health history review is imperative and all possible needs should be met while the person is anesthetized.[27] A sample dental hygiene care plan for the client with Down syndrome follows.

DENTAL HYGIENE CARE FOR THE CLIENT WITH AUTISM

Autism is a developmental disorder and disability characterized by a persistent aloneness. This condition was brought to the attention of the public by the 1989 Academy award–winning movie, *Rain Man.* Other names have been used to describe autism, including Kanner's syndrome, early infantile autism, primary autism, infantile or childhood autism, and childhood psychosis. Individuals with autism relate poorly to people and would rather spend

DENTAL HYGIENE CARE PLAN: CLIENT WITH DOWN SYNDROME

Dental Hygiene Diagnosis	Goal/Expected Behavior	Dental Hygiene Interventions	Evaluative Statements
Deficit in the need for a wholesome body image	• By 9/1, client will be satisfied with the physical appearance of her teeth and related oral structures	• Provide education to client and caregiver about personal oral hygiene practice that will improve the look and health of the mouth	• Client verbalizes that she likes the way her teeth and gums look
Deficit in the need for integrity of the skin and mucous membranes of the head and neck	• By 10/5, client will have healthy gingival tissues	• Perform scaling/root planing • Provide oral hygiene instruction and continued evaluation of progress	• No evidence of inflammation or bleeding on probing
Deficit in the need for a biologically sound dentition	• By 11/20, client will have a reduced plaque index • Client will have reduced caries activity	• Provide oral hygiene instruction • Apply topical fluoride and sealants	• Lower plaque index scores by next visit • No evidence of caries activity
Deficit in the need for nutrition	• By 9/25, client will prepare routine meals that include the four basic food groups	• Provide nutritional counseling to client and primary caregiver	• Client ingests healthier foods that promote healthy teeth and gingiva
Deficit in the need for safety	• Ensure safety and protection at each visit	• Take thorough health history • Follow protocols for infection control; use antibiotic premedication • Introduce procedures slowly and in language on the client's level • Convey a humanistic and interested attitude	• Client looks forward to and enjoys dental hygiene visits • No untoward effects on the client as the result of dental hygiene care
Deficit in the need for conceptualization and problem solving	• By 10/4, client will recognize the importance of monitoring bacterial plaque accumulation in her own mouth	• Assess client's mental level and oral health knowledge • Provide client with disclosing solution and/or tablets and oral hygiene instruction • Demonstrate use of mouth mirror	• Client participates in daily self-evaluation of oral hygiene care, using disclosing tablets, hand mirror, and a mouth mirror
Deficit in the need for appreciation and respect	• By 11/1, client should feel good about her oral hygiene • By 11/1, client will achieve increased social acceptance related to oral hygiene and fresh breath	• Understand and accept client's feelings, emotions, and attitudes • Incorporate empathy, support, and rewards for client	• Client reports that she feels more accepted by others because of her clean mouth and fresh breath
Deficit in the need for self-determination and responsibility	• By 10/5, client will assume responsibility for and perform oral hygiene care regularly	• Allow client to perform her own oral hygiene care when possible • Teach caregiver to supervise home dental hygiene care	• Client accurately demonstrates oral hygiene procedures
Deficit in the need for a value system	• By 10/15, client will comprehend the need for dental hygiene treatment	• Exhibit positive attitude toward client's needs • Explain why good oral health is important	• Client verbalizes that dental hygiene care is beneficial to her oral health

quality time with objects. Many autistic persons have been inaccurately referred to as feebleminded or schizophrenic. For most dental hygienists, the provision of care for an autistic person is likely because statistics indicate that autism is more common than blindness and nearly as common as deafness.[38]

In 1943, Leo Kanner first described a condition in children that he called autism. Kanner characterized an autistic child by the inability to relate in an ordinary manner to people and situations from the beginning of life. Children with autism are sometimes described as "self-sufficient"; "living life in a shell"; "happiest when alone"; "acting as if people were not there"; and "giving the impression of silent wisdom." From the beginning, the child desires an extreme autistic aloneness that ignores, disregards, and shuts out anything that comes from outside of the child. The child has an all-powerful need for being left undisturbed. Everything and anything that changes his external environment is looked on as an intrusion. The above features are seen from the very beginning of life. The first characteristic sign of autism is the lack of posture on being picked up and the failure to adjust the body to that of the person holding the child. Autism is classified as a life-long disorder. Many children with autism come from highly intelligent families.

Communication

Autistic children are usually devoid of speech or have abnormal language. Their "language" consists mainly of naming nouns and adjectives that identify objects, and indicating colors and numbers that represent nothing specific. This type of "language" is referred to as excellent "rote memory." Language becomes a valueless or grossly distorted memory exercise with no use for the purpose of communication. In other words, autistic children meaninglessly parrot what they hear (echolalia). When sentences are formed, they are mostly parrot-like repetitions of word combinations that have been heard. For the autistic child, words become inflexible and cannot be used with any other reference but the original acquired meaning. Autistic children repeat and use personal pronouns just as they are heard. For example, if an autistic child desires milk, he may say, "Are you ready for your milk?" Children with autism slowly learn to speak of themselves in the first person and of the person addressed as second person; this occurs around the age of 6 years.[39] Also, it is noted that children with autism avoid eye-to-eye contact, facial expressions, and any other form of nonverbal communication.[1]

Behavior

The behavior of an autistic child is controlled by the obsessiveness for sameness that no one can disrupt but the child. Living monotonously repetitious lives makes them feel secure.

Food is the first intrusion that an autistic infant has to face. Babies with autism may find eating difficult, which may result in vomiting.[39] Their unsuccessful struggle against the intrusion of food leads to a limited selection of food choices.[1] If food selection includes regular sucrose intake, dental caries may be a major concern.

Despair and confusion can be caused by minor changes in routine, everyday tasks, and furniture arrangement. Autistic children also react to loud noises and moving objects with horror. The noise or motion of an object or person is not feared by the child, but rather the disturbance may threaten the child's aloneness.[39] Another characteristic of autism is stereotypical body movements such as rocking, spinning, sniffing, handclapping, and swaying.[1]

Physical Characteristics

Persons with autism are usually normal physically, although autism may occur along with other conditions such as metabolic disturbances (i.e., phenylketonuria, Tay-Sachs disease), Down syndrome, and epilepsy. Some acquire skill in fine muscle coordination, whereas others have a clumsy gait or poor gross motor performance.

Interpersonal Relationships

Children with autism are more interested in objects than people because objects rarely change in appearance or position. The sameness of objects does not threaten the child, allowing the child to have undisturbed power and control. Autistic children are not afraid of people but of the objects they acquire. For example, an autistic child is scared of a pin pricking his body, not the person doing the pricking. Dental hygienists should try to alleviate a fear of dental instruments by explaining each procedure and the use of each instrument to the client.

The children are not interested in surrounding conversation. When addressed, autistic children respond quickly to "get it over with" so they can continue their activity, or they may not respond at all. Family members derive the same response as a casual acquaintance. Similarly, autistic children are very interested in pictures of people but not in people themselves. The pictures of people cannot disturb their environment.

Progress

By the age of 5 or 6 years, language becomes more communicative because the autistic child has experienced a number of patterns. Food is accepted, noises and motions tolerated, and panic tantrums subside. The children also experience increased contact with people, especially people who satisfy their needs, answer their questions, and help them do things (such as reading). By the age of 6 or 8 years, autistic children play alongside other children (parallel play) but never with a group. They also acquire reading skills quickly at this age.[39] As autistic children grow older several changes begin to occur. They are still in their world of aloneness and sameness but emerge from solitude to varying degrees. Some people are accepted into their life, because they finally compromise and gradually extend feelers into a world to which they have been total strangers. Other behaviors exhibited by autistic persons at various age periods are shown in Table 32–4.

Etiology and Treatment

The etiology of autism is unknown. Several theories exist, including psychogenic, genetic, biochemical deficits, and neurophysiological theories. No single theory has been completely accepted.

The care of clients with autism is consistent with the theory held by the healthcare provider. Types of treatment include psychotherapy, body stimulation, sensory awareness, psychoeducational intervention, group therapy, communication therapy, special education, medications, and behavioral therapy.[40,41]

Dental Hygiene Process

The dental hygienist who is prepared and willing to provide care for the autistic client across the life span makes oral healthcare a positive experience. Although the human needs related to dental hygiene care vary with each person, two common dental hygiene diagnoses may include a deficit in the human need for self-determination, as evidenced by poor dental hygiene habits, and a deficit in the human need for freedom from stress, as evidenced by lack of client cooperation.[42] Also, an understanding of the range of oral manifestations related to the human need for a biologically

TABLE 32–4
POSSIBLE BEHAVIORS EXHIBITED BY AUTISTIC PERSONS

Age Period	Response to Environment	Social/Play Skills	Language‡ Communication Skills	Feeding/Eating	Motor Development
Infancy	"Good": The infant is quiet and placid, seldom cries, and is fascinated by lights. or "Irritable": The infant screams and may quiet only with vigorous rocking or car rides. Fights washing, dressing, and feedings. Stiff, hard to cuddle. Body rocks, head bangs.	Unresponsive to parents' presence. Poor response to social games. Little eye contact. No reaching or pointing. No interest in baby toys. May enjoy roughhousing.	Ignores speech. Ignores loud sounds. Is fascinated with soft sounds. Has decreased verbalizations.	Poor sucking. Refusal to eat lumpy foods. Does not cry when hungry.	On schedule or uneven. May bypass a motor stage, such as creeping.
Toddler	Self-stimulating behaviors—rocking, head banging. Sleep patterns irregular. Resists changes in routine. Disturbances in response to stimuli: • Is fascinated with some sounds. • Uses touch, taste, and smell to extremes. • Ignores objects of usual childhood interest. Zeros in on details. • Uses peripheral vision. • Recognizes parents by outline rather than by features. • Does not respond to painful stimuli.	Inappropriate use of an attachment to objects. Stereotypic, repetitive play. May be extremely passive. May be destructive, aggressive, and self-injurious. Difficult to manage. Frequent tantrums.	Unresponsive to voice, tone, or name. Echolalia-delayed or immediate. Screams. Leads adult by the arm. Responds to simple commands.	Likes pureed foods. Will eat only a limited variety of foods. Does not recognize foods in other forms, such as a banana without the peel.	Prolonged cruiser. Tiptoe walks. May be normal. May be hyperactive.
Preschool	Toddler responses continue.	Aloof and expressionless. Delayed toilet training. More affectionate. Socially embarrassing behaviors. Tantrums continue. Stereotypic, repetitive play continues. Passivity may continue.	Echolalia may develop. Meaningful speech is produced with effort—poor pronunciation and voice control. Unable to understand most speech. Can understand short, concrete sentences. Confusion with pronouns, similar sounding words, and word order. Uses and understands limited gestures.	Food jags.	May be normal. May jump, spin, flap arms/hands. May be graceful or clumsy. Fine motor ability may differ from gross. Difficulty with copying movements. May walk with elbows bent, hands together, and wrists dropped. May be earthbound. Hyperactivity may continue.
School Years	Behaviors (tantrums) decrease. Sleep irregularities may continue. Continues to have disturbances in response to stimuli.	Increased affection. Increased social skills. May help with simple household chores.	Language skills may increase. Same problems as preschooler may continue.	Food jags continue. May begin trying new foods.	Increased motor skills. Unusual walk. Earthbound behavior continues. Splinter skills may develop. May pace, jump, spin.
Adulthood	Same as school years	Increased affection Increased social skills.	Language skills continue to increase.	Diet broadens. Food jags continue.	Motor skills continue to increase. Earthbound behavior continues. Relatively self-sufficient.

Reprinted with permission of Jannetti Publications, Inc., publisher, from Zoltak, B. B. Autism: Recognition and management. Pediatric Nursing 12(2):90–94, 1986, based on data from Autism Society of America. How They Grow: A Handbook for Parents of Young Children with Autism. Washington, DC: 1984; Paluszny, M. Autism, A Practical Guide for Parents and Professionals. Syracuse, NY: Syracuse University Press, 1979; and Wing, L. Children Apart: Autistic Children and their Families. Washington, DC: National Society for Autistic Children, 1974.

sound dentition and for mucous membrane integrity of the head and neck is critical. Oral care may have been neglected as a result of language difficulties, anxiety, and lack of social contact.[43] Psychotropic medications may be used as adjuncts to other treatments, causing decreased salivation.[44] Persons with autism also may have epilepsy requiring oral medication such as phenytoin (Dilantin) which produces gingival enlargement, especially when the individual has poor bacterial plaque control.[45,46]

Often, individuals with autism have deficits in their need for nutrition because of such behavior as fixation to a diet, preference for soft or sweet foods that require little chewing, and lack of tongue coordination. Autistic people are known to pouch their food (hold in their mouth, for example in their cheeks) instead of swallowing. Therefore, these persons may have poor dietary habits and poor oral hygiene.[47,48] All of the aforementioned should be assessed and taken into consideration while planning dental hygiene care for the individual.

The first priority when providing care for an autistic client is to form a trusting relationship. This can be accomplished by slowly introducing the assessment to allow the person with autism to become familiar and comfortable with the oral healthcare environment. With children, the procedure can be demonstrated on the parent first with the child watching. Parents also can be used to issue instructions or commands to the autistic child. The majority of parents are supportive and like to share in their children's care and accomplishments.[49]

During communication with autistic clients, firmness should be used, with frequent verbal approval for appropriate responses.[50] Problems may be influenced by unclear commands or poor sentence structure. The oral healthcare team should define everything that the autistic client finds confusing. A positive approach from the beginning helps to ensure a successful oral health outcome.[40]

Many methods have been used to care for persons with autism, including hospitalization, sedation and tranquilizing, and behavior modification. **Behavior modification** seems to be the preferred method because it uses positive reinforcers to get the desired response. Drash's eight steps in behavior modification for the dental client with autism are shown in the box above.

Many autistic persons can be successfully treated when the oral healthcare team is aware of and uses appropriate communication strategies. Following are sample dental hygiene diagnoses for the client with mental retardation and a sample dental hygiene care plan.

STEPS IN BEHAVIORAL MODIFICATION FOR THE INDIVIDUAL WITH AUTISM

1. Use extensive positive social reinforcement to put the client at ease.
2. Use a very simple reward system and explain the system to the client. For example, the client could be given a toy if good behavior is exhibited throughout the appointment. If the client is an adult, a trip to his/her favorite restaurant may be appropriate. The reward should be suited to the individual client.
3. Give constant positive social reinforcement throughout each appointment.
4. Following each desired behavior, provide verbal praise immediately and precisely.
5. Give instructions in a reassuring manner with each desired behavior.
6. Make sure the points always entitle the person to a prize at the end.
7. Do not discuss dental treatment needed during dental hygiene care.
8. Conclude each session with excessive praise.

Data from Drash, P. W. Behavior modification: New tools for use in pediatric dentistry with the handicapped child. Dental Clinics of North America 18:617, 1974; reprinted with permission.

DENTAL HYGIENE DIAGNOSES FOR THE CLIENT WITH MENTAL RETARDATION

Dental Hygiene Diagnoses	Related To	As Evidenced By
Deficit in the need for self-determination and responsibility	• Lack of skill • Impaired mental ability • Impaired muscular coordination	• Inadequate oral health behavior • Presence of bacterial plaque • Presence of gingival bleeding
Deficit in the need for value system	• Low value placed on oral health	• Reports no previous regular dental or dental hygiene care • Fails to report for scheduled appointments • Reports that "false teeth" would be fine
Deficit in the need for conceptualization and problem solving	• Knowledge deficit regarding the periodontal disease process and the caries process	• Inability to verbalize that bacterial plaque causes gum bleeding and tooth decay
Deficit in the need for a biologically sound dentition	• Inadequate care by primary caregiver • Inadequate self-care • Lack of resources • Dilantin therapy	• Active carious lesions • Report of oral pain • Missing teeth

Table continues on following page

DENTAL HYGIENE DIAGNOSES FOR THE CLIENT WITH MENTAL RETARDATION *Continued*

Dental Hygiene Diagnoses	Related To	As Evidenced By
Deficit in the need for skin and mucous membrane integrity	• Inadequate care by primary caregiver • Inadequate self-care • Lack of resources • Dilantin therapy	• Presence of gingival bleeding • Periodontal attachment loss of 4–7 mm, generalized • Hyperplastic gingival tissue overgrowth • Primary caregiver reports that client is on public assistance
Deficit in the need for nutrition	• Knowledge deficit • Lack of resources • Uncontrolled oral pain	• Reports poor nutrition intake • Reports oral pain that interferes with eating • Experiences concern about meeting all living expenses • Reports eating junk foods frequently
Deficit in the need for wholesome body image	• Inadequate self-care • Inadequate care from primary caregiver • Inadequate professional dental care	• Client does not like how his mouth looks • Presence of extrinsic stain on teeth • Halitosis • Primary caregiver reports that people do not like to come close to the client because of his halitosis

DENTAL HYGIENE CARE PLAN: CLIENT WITH MENTAL RETARDATION

Dental Hygiene Diagnosis	Goal/Expected Behavior	Dental Hygiene Interventions	Evaluative Statements
Deficit in the need for self-determination and responsibility	• By 1/15, client will participate in his daily oral healthcare	• Provide education to client and caregiver on toothbrushing and dental flossing	• Client can independently perform oral hygiene with minimal supervision
Deficit in the need for skin and mucous membrane integrity	• By 1/25, client will have healthy gingival tissues	• Provide scaling and/or root planing and oral irrigation with antimicrobial agent	• Client has no evidence of inflammation or bleeding on probing
Deficit in the need for a biologically sound dentition	• By 2/20, client will have a reduced caries index score	• Provide oral hygiene instruction and continued evaluation of progress • Apply topical fluoride and sealants	• Client has lower caries index score by next appointment
Deficit in the need for nutrition	• By 5/2, client will prepare meals that include the four basic food groups	• Provide nutritional counseling to client and primary caregiver	• Client regularly eats foods that promote healthy teeth and gingiva as well as general health
Deficit in the need for a value system	• By 4/9, client will demonstrate a commitment to having a healthy mouth	• Introduce procedures slowly and in language on the client's level • Convey a friendly and interested attitude • Provide rewards for oral health and healthy behavior • Make each appointment fun	• Client looks forward to and enjoys dental hygiene visits • Client verbalizes that his teeth and gums are important to him

DENTAL HYGIENE CARE PLAN: CLIENT WITH MENTAL RETARDATION *Continued*

Dental Hygiene Diagnosis	Goal/Expected Behavior	Dental Hygiene Interventions	Evaluative Statements
Deficit in the need for conceptualization and problem solving	• By 4/20, client will understand the relationship between bacterial plaque on the teeth and periodontal disease	• Assess client's mental level and oral health knowledge • Provide instruction on the role of bacterial plaque in causing oral disease • Provide instruction on the use of disclosing solution and/or tablets	• Client participates in daily self-evaluation of oral hygiene care using disclosing tablets • Client verbalizes the role of bacterial plaque in causing periodontal disease
Deficit in the need for a wholesome body image	• By 5/11, client should feel good about how he looks after good oral hygiene	• Understand and accept client's feelings, emotions, and attitudes • Incorporate empathy and support for client	• Client verbalizes that he likes the way his healthy teeth and gingiva look • Client feels more accepted by others because of his clean mouth and fresh breath
Deficit in the need for self-determination and responsibility	• By 5/11, client will feel an "owning" of the tasks and perform the behavior regularly	• Client performs his own oral hygiene care when possible	• Client demonstrates good oral hygiene procedures with minimal direction and supervision

References

1. American Psychiatric Association. Diagnostic and Statistical Manual of Mental Disorders, 3rd ed. rev. Washington, DC: American Psychiatric Association, 1987, pp. 41–42.
2. Blodgett, H. E. Mentally Retarded Children: What Parents and Others Should Know. Minneapolis: University of Minnesota Press, 1971, pp. 9, 15–22.
3. Ingersoll, B. D. Behavioral Aspects in Dentistry. New York: Appleton-Century-Crofts, 1982, pp. 170–171.
4. Dura, J. R., Torsell, A. E., et al. Special oral concerns in people with severe and profound mental retardation. Special Care in Dentistry 8(6):265, 1988.
5. Griffin, J. C., Williams, D. E., et al. Self-injurious behavior: A state-wide prevalence survey of the extent and circumstances. Applied Research in Mental Retardation 7:105, 1986.
6. Oilo, G., Hatle, G., et al. Wear of teeth in a mentally retarded population. Journal of Oral Rehabilitation 17(2):173, 1990.
7. Rydgren, K. O. Side-effects of odontological interest of psychopharmacotherapy. Swedish Dental Journal 69:85, 1976.
8. Wegman, M. Annual summary of vital statistics. Pediatrics 86:835, 1990.
9. Cooley, W. Common syndromes and management issues for primary care physicians. Clinical Pediatrics 30(4):233, 1991.
10. de La Cruz, F. F., and Muller, J. Z. Facts about Down syndrome. Children Today 12(6):2, 1983.
11. Tingey, C. Down Syndrome: A Resource Handbook. Boston: College-Hill, 1988, pp. 5–8, 11–14, 34–39.
12. Strelling, M. K. Diagnosis of Down's syndrome at birth. British Medical Journal 2:1386, 1976.
13. Caselli, M. A., Cohen-Sobel, E., et al. Biochemical management of children and adolescents with Down syndrome. Journal of the American Podiatric Medicine Association 81(3):119, 1991.
14. Hall, B. Mongolism in Newborns: A Clinical and Cytogenetic Study. London: Berlingska Boktrychkeriet, 1964, pp. 478–481.
15. Erlick, N. E., Engel, E. D., and Davis, R. H. Dermatoglyphics: A diagnostic tool for chromosomal abnormalities in podiatric medicine. Journal of the American Podiatry Association 71:409, 1981.
16. Thompson, J. S., and Thompson, M. W. Genetics in Medicine. Philadelphia: W. B. Saunders, 1986, p. 119.
17. Thase, M. E. Longevity and mortality in Down syndrome. Journal of Mental Deficiency 26:177, 1982.
18. Spicer, R. L. Cardiovascular disease in Down syndrome. Pediatric Clinics of North America 31(6):1331, 1984.
19. Rowe, R. D., and Uchida, I. A. Cardiac malformation in mongolism: A prospective study of 184 mongoloid children. American Journal of Medicine 31:726, 1961.
20. Scola, P. S. Genitourinary system. In Pueschel, S. M., and Pynders, J. E. (eds.). Down Syndrome: Advances in Biomedicine and the Behavioral Sciences. Cambridge: Ware Press, 1982, p. 207.
21. Antony, R. M. Atlantoaxial instability: Why the sudden concern? Adapted Physical Activity Quarterly 3:320, 1986.
22. Pueschel, S. M., Tingey, C., et al. New perspectives on Down syndrome. Baltimore: Brookes, 1987, pp. 123–124.
23. Schultz, M. C., and Pueschel, S. M. Audiological assessments. In Pueschel, S. M. (ed.). The Young Child with Down syndrome. New York: Human Science Press, 1984, p. 340.
24. Pueschel, S. M. Clinical aspects of Down syndrome from infancy to adulthood. American Journal of Medical Genetics 7[Suppl.]:52, 1990.
25. Wisniewski, K. E., Wisniewski, H. M., and Wen, G. Y. Occurrence of neuropathological changes and dementia of Alzheimer's disease in Down's syndrome. Annals of Neurology 17:278, 1985.
26. Jensen, G. M., Cleal, J. F., and Yips, A. S. G. Dentoalveolar morphology and developmental changes in Down syndrome (trisomy 21). American Journal of Orthodontics 64:607, 1973.
27. Brown, R. H. Dental treatment of the mongoloid child. Journal of Dentistry for Children 32:73, 1965.
28. Cohen, M. M., and Winer, R. A. Dental and facial characteristics in Down's syndrome (mongolism). Journal of Dental Research 44(2[Suppl]):197, 1965.
29. Garn, S. M., Cohen, M. M., et al. Relative magnitudes of crown size reduction and body size reduction in 47-trisomy G. Journal of Dental Research 50:513, 1971.
30. Cohen, M. M., Blitzer, F. J., et al. Abnormalities of the permanent dentition in trisomy G. Journal of Dental Research 49:1386, 1970.
31. Gullikson, J. S. Oral findings in children with Down syndrome. Journal of Dentistry of Children 40(4):293, 1973.
32. Barkla, D. H. Congenital absence and fusion in the deciduous

dentition in mongols. Journal of Mental Deficiency Research 7:102, 1963.

33. Pueschel, S. M., and Scola, F. H. Atlantoaxial instability in individuals with Down syndrome: Epidemiologic, radiographic, and clinical studies. Pediatrics 80:555, 1987.
34. Shaw, L., and Saxby, M. S. Periodontal destruction in Down's syndrome and in juvenile periodontitis: How close is the similarity? Journal of Periodontology 57(11):709, 1986.
35. Saxen, L., and Aula, S. Periodontal bone loss in patients with Down's syndrome: A follow-up study. Journal of Periodontology 53:158, 1982.
36. Swallow, J. N. Dental disease in children with Down's syndrome. Journal of Mental Deficiency Research 8:102, 1964.
37. Elliott, D., Weeks, D. J., and Elliott, C. L. Cerebral specialization in individuals with Down syndrome. American Journal of Retardation 92:263, 1987.
38. Rutter, M. Medical aspects of the education of psychotic children. In Weston, P. (ed.). Some Approaches to Teaching Autistic Children: A Collection of Papers. London: Pergamon Press, 1965.
39. Kanner, L. Autistic disturbances of affective contact. Nervous Child 2(3):217, 1943.
40. Burkhart, N. Understanding and managing the autistic child in the dental office. Dental Hygiene 58(2):60, 1984.
41. Entwistle, B. Dental hygiene care for individuals with special needs. In Darby, M. L., 3rd, (ed.). Comprehensive Review of Dental Hygiene. St Louis: Mosby–Year Book, 1994.
42. Shapira, J., Mann, J., et al. Oral health status and dental needs of an autistic population of children and young adults. Special Care in Dentistry 9:38, 1989.
43. Wilkins, E. M. Clinical Practice of the Dental Hygienist. Philadelphia: Lea & Febiger, 1989, pp. 647–653.
44. Palmai, G. Patterns of salivary flow in depressive illness and during treatment. British Journal of Psychiatry 113:1297, 1967.
45. Stewart, R. E., Barber, T. K., et al. (eds.). Pediatric Dentistry: Scientific Foundations and Clinical Practice. St. Louis: C. V. Mosby, 1981, p. 841.
46. Hassell, T. M. Epilepsy and the Oral Manifestations of Phenytoin Therapy. Basel, Switzerland: Karger, 1981, p. 121.
47. Kopel, H. M. The autistic child in dental practice. Journal of Dentistry for Children 44:302, 1977.
48. Nowak, A. J. Dentistry for the Handicapped Patient. St. Louis: C. V. Mosby, 1976, p. 108.
49. Zoltak, B. B. Autism: Recognition and management. Pediatric Nursing 12(2):90, 1986.
50. Kamen, S., and Skier, J. Dental management of the autistic child. Special Care in Dentistry 5(1):20, 1985.

33 Dental Hygiene Care for the Individual With HIV Infection

OBJECTIVES

Mastery of the content of this chapter will enable the reader to:

- Define the key terms
- Describe the growing acquired immunodeficiency syndrome (AIDS) epidemic
- Describe the action of the human immunodeficiency virus (HIV)
- Explain the systemic manifestations of HIV infection
- Identify the oral manifestations of HIV infection
- Discuss dental hygiene care for HIV-positive clients within the context of a human needs framework

THE INTRODUCTION OF AIDS TO HUMANITY

Acquired immunodeficiency syndrome (AIDS) is an immunosuppressive disease characterized by specific suppression in the immune response and associated with a wide variety of opportunistic infections. Over 1 million Americans are living with human immunodeficiency virus (HIV) recognized to cause AIDS, and more than 179,000 individuals are diagnosed with AIDS.[1] Although many die daily, more become infected and start a journey that, thus far, leads to premature death.

The first documented cases of AIDS in the United States were reported in June 1981 by the Centers for Disease Control. These cases involved five young, previously healthy homosexual males with a rare and aggressive pneumonia usually associated only with severe immunodeficiency. Subsequently, multiple cases of oral **Kaposi's sarcoma** were identified in the homosexual population. Previously Kaposi's sarcoma was found only in elderly men of Mediterranean heritage, and then only on the legs. Retrospective analysis of several deaths in the United States and abroad in the 1970s were suspicious of AIDS. In fact, frozen serum samples from these cases revealed the presence of HIV antibodies. AIDS cases also were reported in Haiti and several countries in Africa in the early 1980s. In 1982 the first AIDS cases were identified in people with hemophilia.[2]

Although the disease was first recognized among homosexual men, from the early days it has also been observed in the heterosexual population, especially in Africa. There, the epidemic of AIDS is particularly severe, affecting between 2 and 12% of the population in central African countries,[2] where more than 7 million people are infected.[3]

In 1983 the human immunodeficiency virus was isolated and recognized as a retrovirus that infects T lymphocytes and other cells. It was first named lymphadenopathy-associated virus (LAV) by French scientists, and human T-lymphotrophic virus type III (HTLV-III) concurrently by American scientists. It has also been called AIDS-associated retrovirus (ARV). In 1986 the International Committee on Taxonomy of Viruses agreed to call the AIDS virus human immunodeficiency virus (HIV). In 1985 a second virus, HIV-2, was isolated. Found primarily in western Africa, it is similar to the simian AIDS virus.[2]

EPIDEMIOLOGY OF HIV INFECTION

HIV infection and AIDS are now widespread in the United States. Currently, 1 to 1.5 million Americans are infected with HIV. More than 160,000 have died, and estimates are that 40,000 to 60,000 new cases in the United States will be diagnosed per year. By the end of 1993, it is estimated that there will be 390,000 to 400,000 cases of AIDS in the United States. The World Health Organization estimates that 10 million people in the world are HIV-positive, and that by the year 2000, there will be 15 to 20 million cases of HIV infection. Although first thought to be a disease related to the gay lifestyle, then associated with contaminated needle use, the disease is spreading into all sectors of society. It occurs in all racial and ethnic groups regardless of sexual orientation, can be contracted at any age, and appears to be on the increase in women and in the 13- to 24-year-old population.[4]

Healthcare workers, too, are at risk for exposure to HIV infection. Of all the AIDS cases reported to the Centers for Disease Control and Prevention as of December 1992, 4.8% of 184,163 AIDS cases were healthcare workers. Thirty-two individuals became HIV-positive after documented occupational exposure, seven more have developed AIDS. In addition, 69 other healthcare workers who were not in known risk categories for AIDS possibly acquired HIV through occupational exposure, but seroconversion after exposure was not documented. All other healthcare workers had other risk factors associated with subsequent HIV infection.[5]

UNDERSTANDING HIV INFECTION

The HIV epidemic in the United States and the world is a catastrophe of extraordinary proportion. HIV affects millions worldwide, knows no gender, socioeconomic, or ethnic boundaries, and is nearly 100% fatal: all dental hygienists will treat and probably already have treated HIV-infected individuals. Therefore, a basic understanding of how the immune system is altered by the HIV virus, and how the course of the disease progresses, is essential for the dental hygienist.

The Immune Response in HIV Infection

The immune response is an extremely complex reaction in the body that is still imperfectly understood despite years of intense study and research. HIV infection causes a deficiency in the immune system, thus the name acquired immunodeficiency syndrome—AIDS.

The three major cell types involved in the acquired immune response to HIV are **T lymphocytes, B lymphocytes,** and **macrophages.** T lymphocytes have many functions and titles. Accordingly, the most significant in understanding the mechanism of HIV infection is the T-helper cell, especially the one bearing the CD4 protein molecule on its surface. The depletion and reduced function of CD4-bearing T-helper lymphocytes is probably the major feature of HIV infection. In general terms, T-helper lymphocytes respond to an antigen (in this case, HIV) by modulating the immune response; they activate other T lymphocytes to proliferate, produce cytokines such as interleukins, or become cytotoxic. T-helper lymphocytes also regulate the B lymphocyte response.

B lymphocytes are lymphocytes that have differentiated postnatally in the bone marrow. These cells can be activated to differentiate into antibody-producing plasma cells. In HIV infection, there are three types of antibodies or immunoglobulins formed: antibodies specific to the viral protein, autoantibodies (antibodies to self, formed against host HIV-infected cells), and nonspecific hyperglobulinemia (increased antibody or immunoglobulin in serum). The antibodies produced against HIV are nonprotecting, as are the autoantibodies and hyperglobulinemia.

The macrophage is the predominant cell that initiates the immune reaction to antigens by engulfing and processing the antigen, then presenting it to the T-helper lymphocyte and other cells. It has been suggested that the macrophage is the major reservoir of HIV and may contribute to **immune dysfunction** by improper functioning.[6]

Another type of T lymphocyte, one with cytotoxic and suppressor activity, bears the CD8 molecule on its surface. This cell mediates most of the antigen-specific cytotoxicity (for example, killing cells perceived as foreign, such as virus-infected ones). In addition, these CD8-bearing T cells also can suppress immune responses by other lymphocytes by the release of factors that regulate function. In summary, HIV infection results in a poorly regulated immune response from the improper interaction of many cells involved in the immune response.

Natural History of AIDS Infection

Advances have been made toward elucidating the life cycle of HIV in the human body and understanding the sequence of events that leads from infection, through latency, to AIDS and eventual death.

HIV belongs to the group of **retroviruses** in which the genetic material is in the form of ribonucleic acid (RNA). Associated with the RNA core are the reverse transcriptase enzymes, which convert the viral RNA into deoxyribonucleic acid (DNA), a process that is the "reverse" of the usual process of DNA being transcribed into RNA.

Once inside the host, the HIV seeks out a target cell, such as the CD4-bearing T-helper lymphocyte because the CD4 surface molecule functions as a receptor for the virus. HIV binds to the CD4 molecule, enters the cell, and becomes uncoated. The viral RNA is transcribed by means of the enzyme reverse transcriptase into linear DNA. This linear double-stranded DNA becomes circular, passes from the cytoplasm into the nucleus, where it incorporates itself into host chromosomal DNA. Here the integrated piece of viral genome can remain latent for the lifetime of the host cell. Alternatively, it can synthesize new viral RNA, which in turn forms the viral protein. This viral complex of protein and associated RNA buds through the cell membrane and acquires a glycoprotein envelope and, thus, becomes a mature HIV virus. These new particles may be released at the cell surface or may spread by direct cell-to-cell transmission with no significant virus being released into the body fluid.

The integrated HIV DNA may remain latent or may cause effects on the target cell. The virus may kill the target cell or may cause the infected cells to combine with others to form functionally ineffective giant cells. Although other cells are infected, the predominant cell killed or inactivated is the CD4-bearing T-helper lymphocyte. This loss in T-helper cell numbers causes a reduction or loss of ability to mount a normal immune response, rendering the HIV-infected individual susceptible to infection from a large variety of bacteria, fungi, and other viruses.

HIV involves also the central nervous system, probably affecting the glial cells by a mechanism not completely understood. This effect may explain the neurological defects seen at any stage in HIV infection, ranging from memory deficit to frank dementia.

Certain cells of the large bowel also may be infected with HIV, possibly resulting in the persistent diarrhea associated with the infection. This particular avenue of infection may explain the extreme wasting seen in persons with AIDS that has resulted in the disease being called the "slim disease."

Persons infected with HIV do form antibodies to the

virus, but the antibodies do not appear to be effective in neutralizing the infection. Individuals with positive antibody titers in the blood, termed *seropositive,* also can have HIV simultaneously cultured from the blood. When HIV antigen appears in the blood after antibody formation (not the initial infection period) the period of latency of infection is likely over, and the disease begins to progress toward AIDS. In fact, HIV antigen presence in the blood is considered predictive of disease progression.[2] The list below summarizes the major immunologic features of HIV infection.

- CD4-presenting T-helper cells are the primary cells infected
- HIV infection both depletes and reduces function of T-helper cells
- B lymphocytes are activated, producing nonprotecting antibodies
- Protective immune response becomes less effective
- The body is susceptible to infection

Primary Infection

HIV virus is transmitted by three known routes: sexual contact, blood, and mother to unborn child. Not everyone who is exposed to HIV becomes infected, and it remains to be elucidated through research what percentage becomes ill and why others are resistant.

Although primary clinical symptoms occur (Table 33–1),[7] they can resemble those of other viral diseases and tend to resolve after a few weeks. HIV infection is screened through laboratory findings of antibody to HIV in the blood and confirmed by direct detection of viral antigen, using the western blot test. After initial infection, the ensuing latent period may last for years. Greenspan reported the incubation times for five cohorts of AIDS patients progressing from HIV infection to AIDS. The period of latency was up to 9.8 years.[2]

When primary infection does occur, it is characterized by a variety of clinical, serological, and immunological signs and symptoms. Clinical signs are of most significance to dental hygienists.

Opportunistic Infection

Opportunistic infections are common in HIV-infected individuals as a result of their compromised immune responses. There are many infections associated with AIDS ranging from persistent "jock itch" to severe candidiasis of the mouth and pharynx and severe pneumonias. Table 33–2 lists some of the infections commonly observed in persons with AIDS.[2] These infections are just a sample of the severe infectious diseases, difficult to control and life-threatening, of persons with AIDS.

TABLE 33–1
CLINICAL SIGNS OBSERVED IN INDIVIDUALS WITH PRIMARY HIV INFECTION

General	Fever, pharyngitis, lymphadenopathy, headache, joint pain, muscular pain, malaise, weight loss, nausea, diarrhea
Dermatologic	Red maculopapular rash, mucocutaneous ulceration

TABLE 33–2
SOME DISEASES OBSERVED IN INDIVIDUALS WITH HIV INFECTION

Disease	Characteristics
Candidiasis	Located in the esophagus
Cytomegalovirus	Retinitis resulting in loss of vision
Kaposi's sarcoma	In persons under 60 years
Lymphoid interstitial pneumonia or pulmonary lymphoid hyperplasia	Affecting a child 13 years of age or younger
Mycobacterial disease	Disseminated to two or more sites including lungs, skin, cervical, or hilar lymph nodes
Pneumonia	Caused by *Pneumocystis carinii*
Toxoplasmosis	Affecting the brain of a person older than 1 month of age

ORAL LESIONS ASSOCIATED WITH AIDS

Considerable investigation has been conducted on the oral lesions associated with HIV infection because most HIV-infected individuals experience them at some time. Eighty percent of HIV-infected persons followed in Europe showed signs of oral lesions.[8] A number of lesions are commonly found in persons with AIDS; others are less common. The significance of recognizing HIV-associated oral lesions is that they are often among the first signs manifested by the HIV-positive individual as the immune deficiency progresses into AIDS. In addition, atypical periodontal lesions are associated with HIV infection. Recognition and understanding of these lesions and their treatment considerations are essential for contemporary dental hygiene practice.

Common Lesions

Lymphadenopathy

Cervical lymphadenopathy is commonly identified in HIV-positive persons. It is almost always present at initial HIV infection and often found at later stages of the disease.

Candidiasis

A variety of *Candida albicans* infections may be seen in HIV infection. The most common types are pseudomembranous candidiasis (Fig. 33–1; see color section), the erythematous or atrophic candidiasis, and angular cheilitis (Fig. 33–2; see color section). **Pseudomembranous candidiasis** is often referred to as **thrush.** The lesions are soft, white plaques on the oral tissues that, when wiped away, leave red and bleeding patches of mucosa. Atrophic *Candida* infection presents as smooth red patches on the tongue, palate, or mucosa (**erythematous** or **atrophic** *Candida* infection). These lesions are more easily missed than white patches. **Angular cheilitis** presents as redness, cracks, or fissures at the corners of the mouth. Medical treatment of *Candida* infection is by use of a variety of topical or sys-

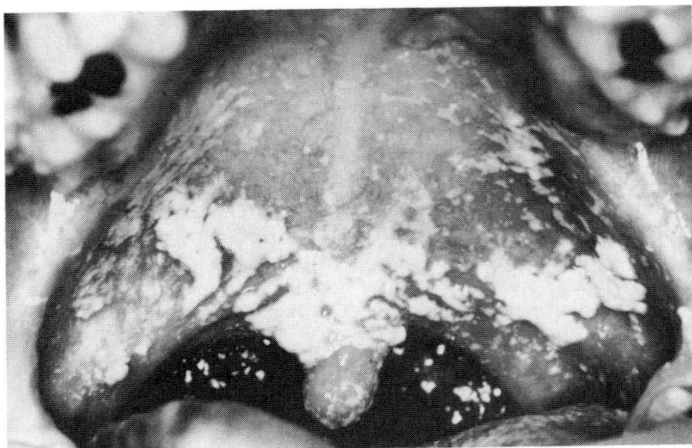

FIGURE 33-1
Pseudomembranous candidiasis in an individual with AIDS manifested as white plaques on the palate. (Courtesy of James R. Winkler, D.D.S., Switzerland.)

temic antifungal drugs.[9] Nystatin, amphotericin B, or clotrimazole are commonly used topical medicines, and ketoconazole and fluconazole are systemic drugs used to control *Candida* infections.[10]

Herpes Simplex Virus

Recurrent herpes simplex virus infections occur in the HIV-infected population and are more severe and persistent than in the non-HIV population. Herpetic infection has the typical appearance of recurrent herpes but can have severe consequences for HIV-infected persons. The pain associated with herpes lesions can significantly restrict the HIV-positive individual's intake of food, thus compounding weight loss and poor nutrition.[12]

Hairy Leukoplakia

In **hairy leukoplakia,** thick, white lesions are usually seen on the lateral borders of the tongue. The lesions can present with long, finger-like projections, thus the name hairy leukoplakia. Epstein-Barr virus is associated with this lesion. Hairy leukoplakia has been reported most often in HIV-infected individuals, but some reports suggest that other persons with severe immunosuppression may display hairy leukoplakia (Fig. 33-3; see color section). Hairy leukoplakia may be an opportunistic disease and may be a predictor of poor prognosis for individuals infected with HIV.[9]

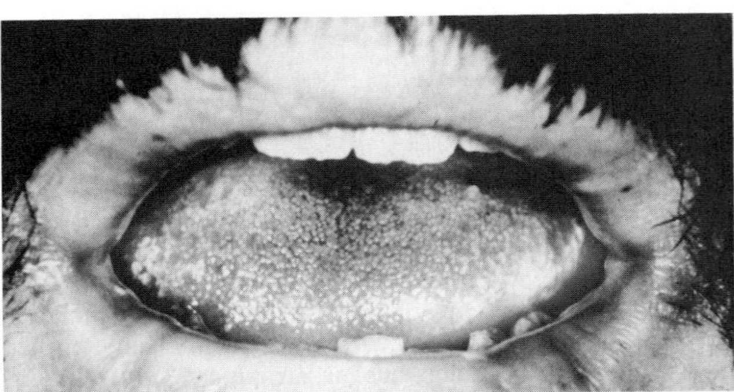

FIGURE 33-2
Angular cheilitis in a person with AIDS seen as cracked sores at the right corner of his mouth. (Courtesy of James R. Winkler, D.D.S., Switzerland.)

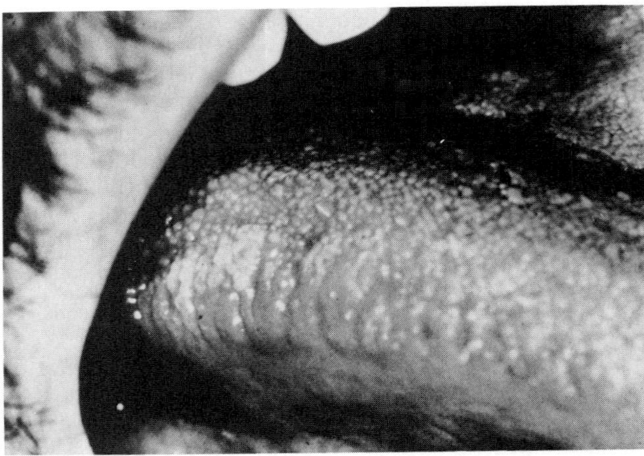

FIGURE 33-3
Hairy leukoplakia in an individual with AIDS located on the right lateral border of the tongue. (Courtesy of James R. Winkler, D.D.S., Switzerland.)

Kaposi's Sarcoma

Kaposi's sarcoma is a malignant endothelial cell neoplasm rarely seen in individuals under the age of 60 except in the HIV-infected populations. The lesions appear on the skin or in the mouth as reddish or purplish nodules that may be flat or raised. A single lesion or multiple lesions may be present (Fig. 33-4; see color section). It has been reported that 50% of those with Kaposi's have oral lesions and that about 10% have only oral lesions.[10]

Lesions of the Periodontium

Specific gingival and periodontal diseases are seen in HIV-positive individuals. These are termed **linear gingival erythema, necrotizing (ulcerative) gingivitis, necrotizing (ulcerative) periodontitis,** and, in extremely severe cases, **necrotizing stomatitis.** Successful dental hygiene care of individuals with these oral diseases depends on understanding

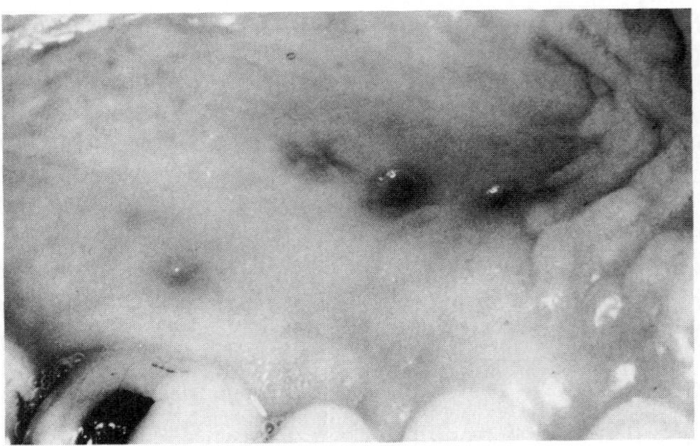

FIGURE 33-4
Oral Kaposi's sarcoma lesions on the palate of an individual with AIDS. (Courtesy of James R. Winkler, D.D.S., Switzerland.)

the unique features of the disease process in HIV-infected individuals. In addition, Kaposi's sarcoma lesions associated with the dentition are of particular concern to the dental hygienist in caring for HIV-infected persons.

Gingival Diseases

HIV-associated gingival diseases appear as an atypical gingivitis characterized by extreme redness in the gingiva. They can present as a fiery red border to the gingiva, either localized or generalized, termed linear gingival erythema; or a fiery red edematous gingivitis not limited to the attached gingiva, now called necrotizing (ulcerative) gingivitis. The extreme redness can extend right into the alveolar mucosa, which also may be bright red, and red petechia-like patches on the gingiva also may be observed. *Candida albicans* may play an etiological role in these diseases. They are not very responsive to simple mechanical removal of bacterial plaque and calculus. Additional chemotherapeutic agents are required to control the pathogens that cause the infection. It is now thought that gingival lesions may well be the precursor to necrotizing ulcerative periodontitis.[13]

Treatment of HIV-associated gingival diseases consists of aggressive removal of local irritants: bacterial plaque control, scaling, and root planing. The use of local anesthetics also may be necessary for the client's comfort. Thorough root instrumentation is followed by irrigation with a povidone-iodine solution such as a 10% oral suspension of Betadine for some pain relief and an antimicrobial effect. The iodine solution is applied as a low-pressure intrasulcular lavage using a disposable syringe and blunt needle. Treatment should be performed as expeditiously as possible with iodine lavage used at each appointment. Allergy to iodine should be ruled out during the assessment phase and prior to its use as an irrigant. Saline is an acceptable alternative if the client has an iodine allergy. Chlorhexidine is contraindicated for intrasulcular lavage in individuals with HIV-associated diseases because the alcohol and flavoring agents may cause irritation.[14]

Postoperative recommendations should include conventional mechanical bacterial plaque control and twice-daily use of chlorhexidine as a mouth rinse. Sometimes a course of antibiotics such as metronidazole is needed to control the disease process.[14]

Management of HIV-associated gingival diseases is critical because they can be an early sign of HIV infection and, without proper aggressive therapy, they may progress to more severe periodontal involvement (Fig. 33–5; see color section).

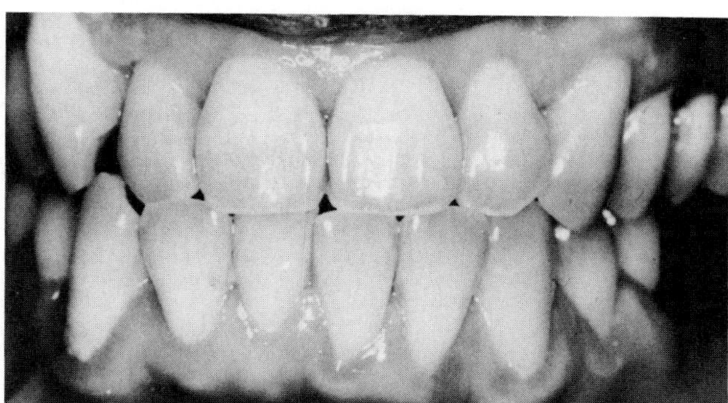

FIGURE 33–5
Necrotizing ulcerative gingivitis associated with HIV infection prior to care: The gingival margin shows color change to bright red that may extend onto the alveolar mucosa. (Courtesy of James R. Winkler, D.D.S., Switzerland.)

Periodontal Lesions

In general, HIV-associated periodontal lesions resemble necrotizing ulcerative gingivitis (NUG) superimposed on sites of rapidly progressing periodontitis. This disease is characterized by edema and erythema of marginal and attached gingiva, necrosis of the tissues, pain in the bone surrounding the area, spontaneous bleeding, and extremely rapid disease progression. The disease may be localized or generalized and may lead to tooth loss in a matter of days or weeks. Most persons presenting with acute necrotizing ulcerative periodontitis relate symptoms of severe pain in the bone, nocturnal bleeding, and clots in the mouth.[13] The disease is characterized by severe attachment loss but not necessarily deep pocketing, probably as a result of the necrotic effects of infection on the gingiva. In addition, the amount of bacterial plaque present may not correlate with the extreme tissue destruction observed. Extreme cases in which lesions extend onto oral tissues beyond the periodontium are termed necrotizing stomatitis.

The oral flora associated with necrotizing ulcerative periodontitis is similar to the flora associated with periodontal disease in non–HIV-infected persons. The subgingival bacterial plaque has been shown to harbor high proportions of the same periodontal pathogens found in non–HIV-infected persons with periodontal lesions. A notable difference is that subgingival yeasts have been identified in 62% of adult HIV-infected persons with periodontal disease, compared with 16.8% of non–HIV-infected people with periodontal disease.[15] Although the precise mechanisms of destruction in HIV infection are not understood, it is likely that the presence of increased amounts of *Candida,* xerostomia, and altered lymphocyte action create the extremely destructive periodontal disease process sometimes seen.[9,10]

Treatment of necrotizing ulcerative periodontitis consists of the same aggressive removal of local irritants as performed when treating the gingival condition. In addition, periodontal surgery may be required to remove necrosed tissues, including bone. Local irrigation of the gingiva and affected tissues with iodine solution (e.g., Betadine, a 10% oral suspension of povidone-iodine or saline solution in the case of iodine sensitivity) is necessary following root instrumentation at each appointment. Disposable syringes with blunt needles are required to adequately irrigate the affected tissues. Persons treated for necrotizing ulcerative periodontitis require close monitoring and evaluation. Postoperative care requires good mechanical bacterial plaque control, twice-daily chlorhexidine rinses for chemical bacterial plaque control, and antibiotics such as metronidazole to control the oral flora (Fig. 33–6; see color section).[10]

Kaposi's Sarcoma

Oral Kaposi's sarcoma lesions often appear on the gingiva associated with the teeth. In these cases the tumors may be significantly enlarged by the presence of bacterial plaque and calculus.[16] Dental hygienists and dentists are sometimes hesitant to treat the gingival condition for fear of harming the Kaposi's lesions or causing significant bleeding. However, in some cases tumor reduction can be enhanced by nonsurgical periodontal care.

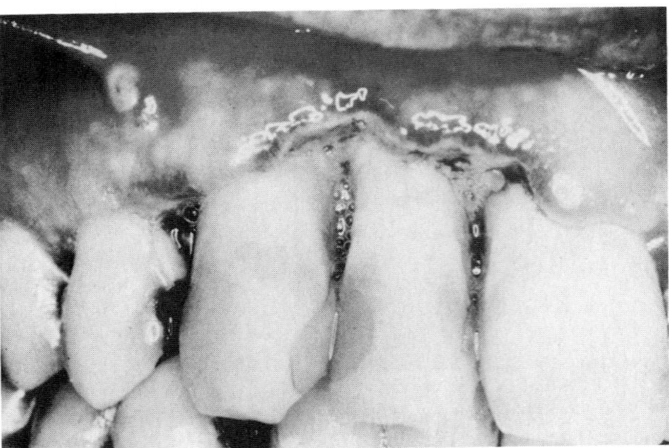

FIGURE 33-6
Necrotizing ulcerative periodontitis in an individual with AIDS showing color change, necrosis, and sloughing of the periodontal tissues. (Courtesy of James R. Winkler, D.D.S., Switzerland.)

Kaposi's lesions on the gingiva associated with the teeth require excision or other tumor reduction therapy just like Kaposi's sarcomas located away from the teeth. The Kaposi's lesions tend to diminish in size and are managed successfully through excision, radiation treatment, or antitumor drug therapy. Treatment appears to be more successful when thorough scaling, root planing, and oral hygiene procedures also are carried out. The dental hygienist must not avoid treating the teeth and gingiva because of the presence of closely associated, often large and red to purple lesions (Fig. 33-7; see color section). Thorough bacterial plaque removal and scaling and root planing are essential to maximizing the effects of tumor therapy.[16]

Dental Hygiene Care of Periodontal Conditions

Thorough dental hygiene care is required in the treatment of all HIV-infected individuals. Knowledge of periodontal conditions associated with HIV infection permit regular assessment and evaluation of HIV-infected clients and provision of adequate care.

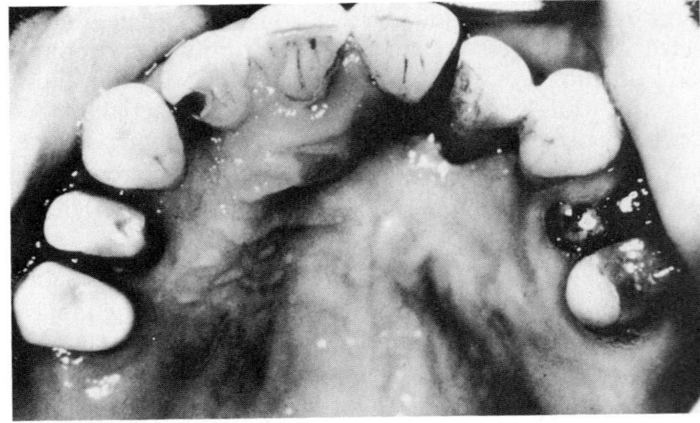

FIGURE 33-7
Kaposi's sarcoma associated with the teeth before treatment; dark lesions are present around the teeth and on the palate. (Courtesy of James R. Winkler, D.D.S., Switzerland.)

The dental hygienist must assess the special needs of every HIV-infected client and plan, implement, and evaluate the dental hygiene care. The care plan must include education of the client, therapeutic scaling and root planing, irrigation of the sulcus areas, provision of posttreatment instructions, and evaluation. In the case of recognized gingival and periodontal diseases and the myriad oral lesions such as those of Kaposi's sarcoma, care must be in collaboration with the dentist and physician. Sometimes, as in the case of severe necrotizing ulcerative periodontitis or necrotizing stomatitis, the need for surgical treatment is so urgent that periodontal surgical intervention may be done at the same appointment as the dental hygiene care.

Table 33-3 summarizes the recommendations for dental and dental hygiene care of common HIV-associated oral conditions. HIV-positive clients can be provided with a rinse of 0.12% chlorhexidine prior to treatment to reduce the number of organisms in the mouth during the provision of care. However, this has not been proved to have value in prevention of disease transmission. Whenever chlorhexidine is used, clients must be informed of possible side effects, including staining of the teeth, discoloration of the oral mucosa, and altered taste sensation.

Less Common Lesions

A variety of infections, neoplasms, and other oral lesions have been described in HIV-infected persons. Although rare, they should be recognized and treated to make HIV-infected individuals more comfortable. The dental hygienist plays a role in performing oral examinations and informing clients of the presence of lesions so treatment may be encouraged.

Less common disease entities may be seen at any time during the course of HIV infection. Treatment is provided by medical and dental experts and is evolving as new drugs become available and experience with the disease of AIDS grows. This summary is based on the work of Scully and associates.[10,11]

Pharyngitis—Sore throat often accompanied by fever is seen in individuals with HIV infection. Pharyngitis should be treated by the client's physician.

Human papillomavirus—Infection with this virus results in benign wart-like projections on the oral epithelium. Cryosurgery, laser therapy, or excisional surgery may be used by dentists to control the lesions.

Cytomegalovirus—Infection with this virus can result in chronic oral ulcers. They may respond to antiviral medication recommended by the client's dentist or physician.

Tuberculosis—Tuberculosis is most commonly associated with HIV-infected drug abusers in Africa. Cervical lymphadenopathy and oral ulcers may be present and should be evaluated by the client's dentist or physician.

Cellulitis—Cellulitis, a spreading inflammation of cellular or connective tissue, may result from oral infections. Vigorous treatment with various antibiotics has been recommended.

Lymphoma and other neoplasms—Oral lymphomas of the non-Hodgkin's type are recognized in HIV-infected individuals. They are usually rapidly growing masses around the face or neck, and they may be associated with Epstein-Barr virus. Lymphomas are usually man-

TABLE 33–3
GUIDELINES FOR DENTAL AND DENTAL HYGIENE CARE OF HIV-ASSOCIATED ORAL CONDITIONS

Necrotizing (Ulcerative) Gingivitis	Necrotizing (Ulcerative) Periodontitis	Dentition-Associated Kaposi's Sarcoma
Possible need for antibiotic premedication	Possible need for antibiotic premedication	Possible need for antibiotic premedication
Consultation with the person's physician	Consultation with the person's physician	Consultation with the person's physician
Oral hygiene instruction	Oral hygiene instruction	Oral hygiene instruction
Repeated blood tests prior to invasive procedures	Possible blood tests prior to invasive procedures	Possible blood tests prior to invasive procedures
Therapeutic scaling and root planing	Therapeutic scaling and root planing	Therapeutic scaling and root planing
10% povidone-iodine subgingival irrigation	10% povidone-iodine subgingival irrigation	10% povidone-iodine subgingival irrigation
Possible antifungal and antibiotic medication	Possible antifungal and antibiotic medication	Possible antifungal and antibiotic medication
Chlorhexidine rinse regimen twice daily	Possible periodontal surgery	Surgery or other antitumor therapy
Follow-up evaluation and retreat as needed	Chlorhexidine rinse regimen twice daily	Chlorhexidine rinse regimen twice daily
2- to 4-month continued care intervals when controlled	Follow-up evaluation and retreat as needed	Follow-up evaluation and retreat as needed
	2- to 4-month continued care intervals when controlled	2- to 4-month continued care intervals when controlled
Fluoride therapy	Fluoride therapy	Fluoride therapy
Nutritional counseling	Nutritional counseling	Nutritional counseling

aged medically with radiation therapy. Squamous cell carcinoma has been reported in a few HIV-infected individuals, but a significantly increased risk has not been identified.

Aphthous ulcer—Persistent and recurrent aphthous ulcers have been identified. Topical or systemic corticosteroids recommended by the dentist or physician are used to treat them.

Gangrenous stomatitis—This condition has been described in several HIV-infected persons. The lesions are resistant to treatment, but systemic antimicrobials and steroids prescribed by the client's physician and dentist may help.

Oral purpura—Petechiae, ecchymoses, and spontaneous bleeding have been reported in HIV-infected individuals.

Salivary gland disease—Xerostomia and salivary gland enlargement have been reported in HIV-infected persons. Conventional management of xerostomia by the client's dentist or physician using saliva substitutes and water is often sufficient to relieve symptoms.

Neuropathies—Cases of facial pain and sensory loss resembling Bell's palsy have been reported.

Oral hyperpigmentation—Brown or black oral pigmentation has been reported and may be related to drug therapy.

Exfoliative cheilitis—This condition has been reported in up to 9% of HIV-infected individuals.

Cat scratch disease—Oral vascular lesions similar to Kaposi's lesions have been related to cat scratch disease.

IMPORTANCE OF RECOGNITION

Some of the earliest lesions to appear indicating HIV infection are present in and around the oral cavity; therefore, recognition of signs of oral diseases related to HIV infection is a paramount responsibility for dental hygienists.

Recognition of these lesions and early referral of clients for further medical and dental evaluation and supportive care can have enormous positive consequences for the individual involved and for helping stem the AIDS epidemic. The earlier HIV infection is detected, the earlier individuals can be assessed, treated, and monitored. Zidovudine (2′-azido-3′-deoxythymidine [AZT]) is the most prescribed medication in the treatment of HIV infection. The drug inhibits reverse transcriptase enzymes, interfering with the replication of the virus.[16] AZT antiviral therapy has been shown to prolong the latency period of infection and help infected persons lead normal lives for longer periods.[2] Also, HIV-infected individuals, if identified early, can get counseling to improve the quality of life, protect loved ones, and refrain from infecting others.

CONSIDERATIONS IN TREATMENT OF HIV-INFECTED PERSONS

Centers for Disease Control and Prevention (CDCP) Definition of AIDS and HIV Infection

Differentiation between HIV-positive status and the diagnosis of AIDS was until recently defined by a complex system considering the occurrence of one or more opportunistic infections present in people with immunosuppression. As of January 1, 1993, the Centers for Disease Control and Prevention (CDCP) in Atlanta revised the classification system for AIDS to permit a more accurate assessment of the number of cases in the United States, therefore permitting a more accurate reporting of cases and a better understanding of the effect of AIDS on the healthcare system. The revised CDCP AIDS definition includes all HIV-infected persons with less than 200/mm^3 CD4 T-lymphocytes or a CD4 T-lymphocyte percentage in total lymphocytes of less than 14%.[17] In addition, the diagnosis of AIDS is reported for the clinical conditions listed in Table 33–4, regardless of CD4 count. The new definition includes three conditions

TABLE 33–4
CDCP-DESIGNATED AIDS-ASSOCIATED CONDITIONS

Candidiasis	Of the bronchi, trachea, or lungs
Candidiasis	Esophageal
Coccidioidomycosis	Disseminated or extrapulmonary
Cryptococcosis	Extrapulmonary
Cryptosporidiosis	Chronic intestinal (>1 month duration)
Cytomegalovirus disease	Other than liver, spleen, or nodes
Cytomegalovirus retinitis	With loss of vision
HIV encephalopathy	
Herpes simplex	Chronic ulcer(s) (>1 month duration), or bronchitis, pneumonitis, or esophagitis
Histoplasmosis	Disseminated or extrapulmonary
Isosporiasis	Chronic intestinal (>1 month duration)
Kaposi's sarcoma	
Lymphoma	Burkitt's lymphoma
Lymphoma	Immunoblastic
Lymphoma	Primary in the brain
Mycobacterium avium complex or *M. kansasii*	Disseminated or extrapulmonary
Mycobacterium tuberculosis	Disseminated or extrapulmonary
Mycobacterium	Other species or unidentified species disseminated or extrapulmonary
Pneumocystis carinii	Pneumonia
Leukoencephalopathy	Progressive multifocal
Salmonella septicemia	Recurrent
Toxoplasmosis	Of brain
Wasting syndrome	As a result of HIV
Pulmonary tuberculosis	Lungs
Recurrent pneumonia	Lungs
Invasive cervical cancer	Females only

not previously considered in diagnosis: pulmonary tuberculosis, recurrent pneumonia, and invasive cervical cancer. The revised surveillance system acknowledges the association between life-threatening illnesses and the number of CD4 lymphocytes present in the blood in addition to AIDS-associated infections. It now reflects the use of CD4 counts as integral parts of the medical management of this infection, and to determine initiation of treatment. For example, antiretroviral therapy, the use of AZT, is commonly begun when CD4 counts fall to 500/mm^3, and prophylactic inhalation therapy (pentamidine) to prevent *Pneumocystis carinii* is recommended because the disease is associated with CD4 counts below 200/mm^3.

This simplified and expanded AIDS surveillance definition is expected to have a significant impact on dramatically increasing the number of reportable AIDS cases. Of the one million HIV-infected individuals in the United States, more than 150,000 are expected to have CD4 counts below 200/mm^3 and no associated illness that previously would have made their cases reportable as AIDS. A sharp increase in the national tabulation of AIDS is anticipated. In addition, more women are expected to be reported as having AIDS because some of the opportunistic infections that plague them, such as recurrent and persistent vaginal candidiasis, were not included in the earlier definition of AIDS.

AIDS and the Practice of Dental Hygiene

Increased knowledge of the continuum of immunodeficiency that is HIV infection on the one end and death from AIDS on the other has heightened public awareness and concern for the epidemic. Clearly, the time for feeling safely removed from this disease, whether professionally or personally, is past.

AIDS has served as a potent reminder that infectious diseases have not been conquered and that epidemics are not yet things of the past.

Dental hygienists have a legal and ethical responsibility to treat HIV-infected individuals just as they care for other persons presenting for care.[18] The likelihood of contracting the HIV virus from an infected person, although hard to quantify, is low. Based on glove puncture rates and rates of hepatitis B seroconversions among surgeons, it has been reported that the rate of HIV seroconversion falls somewhere between 1 in 4,500 and 1 in 130,000 cases.[19] Although this rate is clearly below 1%, fear of treating HIV-positive individuals is not uncommon.

HIV-infected people are often young individuals who have suddenly had their sense of safety and well-being shattered. They are struggling to live with HIV and striving to have a healthy lifestyle to help control the disease. HIV-infected individuals are most often eager, cooperative, and appreciative clients who are happy to comply with recommendations for professional care. However, the HIV-infected client may initially be reluctant or fearful of the clinician's response to knowledge of his or her HIV infection. The client may have been shunned by others and fear the same when visiting the dental hygienist. One effective means to initiate a professional relationship and restore a sense of safety to both client and dental hygienist is to shake hands upon introduction. The courtesy of this polite touch infuses the professional care with confidence and defuses unwarranted fear and alienation.

All healthcare workers, including dental hygienists, must use adequate sterilization and barrier infection control procedures (see Chapters 7, 8, 9).

Education and interaction with clients is a critical element of dental hygiene care in this age of HIV infection, no less important than infection control. It has been reported that 30% of the population has thought about contracting AIDS in the dental office.[20] This information was published prior to the galvanic announcement that the first person known to have contracted AIDS from a healthcare worker contracted that HIV infection from her dentist. In fact, that dentist is reported to have transmitted the HIV infection to at least six patients and has sparked a spirited debate about the merits of mandatory HIV testing (and notification of clients treated) for healthcare workers.[21]

That debate is not yet resolved. However, suggestions for better communication with the population of clients presenting for care have been made. A number of strategies can help inform and diffuse to clients an atmosphere of knowledge, appreciation, and understanding of the realities of protecting people through universal infection control protocol. These steps, elucidated by Bender,[22] suggest that practitioners:

1. Have literature available for clients. A toll-free AIDS hotline has been established by the government for samples of free literature: 1-800-342-2437.
2. Have specific questions on the health and dental history form: e.g., Have you tested positive for HIV? Is your knowledge of HIV High? Average? Low?
3. Question clients regarding responses to questions to stimulate dialogue.
4. Assess the client's psychological resources such as family and personal coping mechanisms if HIV infection is suspected.
5. Assess your personal response to HIV so that care for infected persons can be provided out of concern, not fear.
6. Have referral sources available, including those for members of the oral health team if emotional support is necessary.

Dental hygienists are committed to oral disease prevention and the promotion of wellness. Application of the human needs framework to the dental hygiene process of care facilitates this commitment to prevention and wellness.

APPLICATION OF THE DENTAL HYGIENE PROCESS OF CARE FOR THE HIV-INFECTED CLIENT AND THE CLIENT WITH AIDS

Assessment

During the assessment phase of dental hygiene care, the dental hygienist must be particularly sensitive to observing conditions identified in the literature as indicative of HIV infection. For example, while validating the health history and during the interview, the client might report high-risk sexual behavior, intravenous drug use, or blood transfusion in the early 1980s prior to adequate screening of the blood supply. Medications that an HIV-positive person might be taking include zidovudine (Etrovir or AZT) or a newer, less common medication used to delay the onset of AIDS, didanosine (DDI). The client may also report recent hospital stays for conditions associated with HIV status, as listed in Table 33–4.

Extraoral assessment may reveal purplish-red nodules on the skin indicative of Kaposi's sarcoma. Intraorally, some conditions may include spontaneous gingival bleeding, severe marginal and papillary gingival redness, evidence of candidiasis, petechiae, hairy leukoplakia, or Kaposi's sarcoma lesions.

In order to provide the best care possible and to meet the client's human need for safety, the dentist or dental hygienist should consult with the client's physician. The oral healthcare team may want to obtain from the physician results of the HIV-positive individual's most recent blood tests. Clients' platelet count, prothrombin time, and partial prothrombin time are sometimes used to predict excessive postoperative bleeding.

Dental Hygiene Diagnosis

Several of the 11 human needs identified in the model by Walsh and Darby[23] are relevant to dental hygiene care for the individual infected with HIV. For example, the HIV-infected person may be dissatisfied with the appearance of the gingiva or embarrassed by extraoral Kaposi's sarcoma lesions indicating a deficit in the human need for a wholesome body image. There may be considerable anxiety about disclosing the HIV status to the oral healthcare provider, suggesting a deficit in the area of freedom from stress. Presence of HIV-associated gingival and periodontal diseases demonstrates a deficit in skin and mucous membrane integrity of the head and neck. Possible nutritional deficits, perhaps compounded with diarrhea, may mean difficulty in sustaining periodontal healing and maintenance. Health history may reveal a drug sensitivity to iodine that requires the substitution of saline solution for oral irrigation after therapeutic scaling and root planing to meet the human need for safety.

Planning

Planning of dental hygiene care must be integrated with the overall dental treatment plan. Meeting the client's human need for freedom from pain and stress and human need for safety should be priorities in the plan of care. Additional medication for oral candidiasis or other conditions may be needed during the course of care and thus consultation with the client's physician and dentist is a must.

Because the gingiva of an HIV-positive individual may be tender and bleed easily, it is common for the HIV-infected person to avoid conscientious daily oral hygiene. Client deficits in the human need for conceptualization and problem solving, self-determination and responsibility may be important areas for the dental hygienist to address. The dental hygienist needs to plan to evaluate the client's knowledge of bacterial plaque and oral disease processes, as well as the person's dexterity level, prior to selecting strategies that lead the client to *optimal* oral health status. Human need deficits in skin and mucous membrane integrity and nutrition also should be addressed in the plan of care. In addition to oral hygiene instructions, scaling, and root planing, the dental hygienist may plan to recommend an over-the-counter mouth rinse or a chlorhexidine mouth rinse to assist in the control of supragingival bacterial plaque and gingivitis. The dental hygienist may be required to provide nutritional counseling aimed at encouraging sufficient nutrients to support healing and oral maintenance. The client also may be consulting or may need to consult a nutritionist, and thus the dental hygienist also may be sharing responsibility with this member of the healthcare team.

Implementation

Once formulated, the plan of care is implemented according to the goals and priorities established by the client and oral healthcare team. The dental hygienist might prefer to perform therapeutic scaling and root planing procedures by hand; ultrasonic instrumentation generates extensive aerosols.

Evaluation

After comprehensive dental hygiene care has been completed, the dental hygienist should evaluate the client to ensure that the goals outlined in the plan of care have been achieved. Evaluation should take place at frequent intervals (2 to 4 months) to provide opportunities to assess continually the client's oral health, daily oral hygiene practices, and nutrition. Continued dental hygiene care and evaluation at short intervals may be necessary to assist the client to promote oral health and control oral conditions associated with HIV infection. At the evaluation phase of the dental hygiene process, other human need deficits may be identified that require further planning and care. Therefore, the process of care cycle repeats itself.

References

1. Centers for Disease Control and Prevention. HIV/AIDS Surveillance Report, June, 1991.
2. Greenspan, D., Greenspan, J. S., Schiot, M., and Pindborg, J. AIDS and the Mouth. Chicago: Mosby–Year Book, 1990.
3. WHO predicts 10-fold rise in AIDS cases. The Nation's Health. Washington, DC: American Public Health Association newspaper, April 1992.
4. AIDS The Second Decade. US News and World Report 100(23):21, 1991.
5. Centers for Disease Control and Prevention. Facts about HIV/AIDS and Health Care Workers. Atlanta, GA: December 1992.
6. Crowe, S., and Mills, J. Infections of the immune system. In Stites, D. P., and Terr, A. (eds.). Basic and Clinical Immunology, 7th ed. Norwalk, CT: Appleton & Lange, 1991, p. 698.
7. Tindall, B., and Cooper, D. Primary HIV infection: Host responses and intervention strategies. AIDS 5(1):1, 1991.
8. Van der Waal, I., Schulten, A. J. M., and Pindborg, J. J. Oral manifestations of AIDS: An overview. International Dental Journal 41:3, 1991.
9. Greenspan, J. S., Greenspan, D., and Winkler, J. R. Diagnosis and management of the oral manifestations of HIV infection and AIDS. Infectious Disease Clinics of North America 2(2):373, 1988.
10. Scully, C., Laskaris, G., et al. Oral manifestations of HIV infection and their management. I. More common lesions. Oral Surgery Oral Medicine and Oral Pathology 71(2):158, 1991.
11. Scully, C., Laskaris, G., et al. Oral manifestations of HIV infection and their management. II. Less common lesions. Oral Surgery Oral Medicine and Oral Pathology 71(2):167, 1991.
12. Greenspan, D., and Greenspan, J. S. Oral mucosal manifestations of AIDS. Dermatologic Clinics 5(4):733, 1987.
13. Winkler, J. R., and Murray, P. A. Periodontal disease. California Dental Association Journal 15(1):20, 1987.
14. Winkler, J. R., Murray, P. A., Grassi M., and Hammerle, C. Diagnosis and management of HIV-associated periodontal lesions. Journal of the American Dental Association (Suppl.) Nov. 1989, p. 25-S.
15. Zambon, J. J., Reynolds, H. S., and Genco, R. J. Studies of the subgingival microflora in patients with acquired immunodeficiency syndrome. Journal of Periodontology 61(11):699, 1990.
16. Shiboski, C. H., and Winkler, J. R. Gingival Kaposi's sarcoma and periodontitis. Oral Surgery, Oral Medicine, Oral Pathology 76(1):49, 1993.
17. Centers for Disease Control and Prevention. 1993 revised classification system for HIV infection and expanded surveillance case definition for AIDS among adolescents and adults. Morbidity and Mortality Weekly Report 41(RR-17):1, 1992.
18. Tolle-Watts, S. L., and Shuman, D. AIDS education in dental hygiene programs in the United States and Canada. Journal of Dental Hygiene 65(3):124, 1991.
19. Kohn, M. Contagious symbols: The inflated fear of AIDS among health care professionals. AIDS and Public Policy Journal 5(3):107, 1990.
20. Gerbert, B., Maguire, B. T., and Spitzer, S. Patients' attitudes toward dentistry and AIDS. Journal of the American Dental Association (Suppl.) Nov. 1990.
21. King, L., and Lyons, S. HIV-infected practitioners: Hygienists speak out. Access 5(3):21, 1991.
22. Bender, P. Educating and interacting with your patients. Journal of the American Dental Association (Suppl.) Nov. 1989, p. 22-S.
23. Walsh, M. M., and Darby, M. Application of the human needs conceptual model of dental hygiene to the role of a clinician; Part II. Journal of Dental Hygiene 67(6):335, 1993.

Suggested Readings

DeVore, L. R. Dental and dental hygiene treatment of an HIV+ individual. Case Studies in Oral Disease 1(1):1, 1993.

Palmer, C. AIDS and dentistry: The governmental view. Journal of the American Dental Association (Suppl.) Nov. 1989, p. 3-S.

Tindall, B., and Cooper, D. Primary HIV infection: Host responses and intervention strategies. AIDS 5(1):1991.

34 Dental Hygiene Care for the Individual with Cancer

OBJECTIVES

Mastery of the content in this chapter will enable the reader to:

- Define the key terms used
- Discuss cancer risk factors
- Identify the general signs and symptoms of cancer
- Describe the psychological responses related to cancer
- Describe the treatment of oral squamous cell carcinoma and its complications
- Discuss the oral complications of different types of cancer therapies
- List dental hygiene diagnoses associated with individuals who have cancer
- Develop a dental hygiene care plan for clients with cancer
- List appropriate dental hygiene interventions for a client with cancer
- Develop evaluation criteria for the client with cancer

INTRODUCTION

The National Institutes of Health formally recognizes the critical role that dentists and dental hygienists play in early detection of abnormal tissue changes in the overall care of the individual with cancer.[1]

Cancer is not a single disease, but a broad classification of more than 100 types (Fig. 34–1). The common element in **cancer** is the abnormal and unrestricted growth of cells that can invade and destroy surrounding normal body tissues, sometimes spreading to other parts of the body. The difference between a malignant and a benign neoplasm is that a benign tumor is usually circumscribed and encapsulated, usually grows slowly, and is composed of cells that resemble the tissue from which it arises. A **malignant** neoplasm or cancer not only infiltrates locally but also has the potential to *metastasize* or spread to distant sites. The cells are usually atypical or dysplastic and may not resemble the parent tissue.

The branch of medicine that studies and treats cancer is called **"oncology,"** and the physician specialist is an **"oncologist."** When cancers are left untreated, they result in significant morbidity and death. In the United States, only heart disease caused more deaths in adults. Cancer kills more children between the ages of 3 to 14 years than any other disease.[2]

RISK AND PROTECTIVE FACTORS FOR CANCER

Carcinogenic, or cancer-causing influences may be both environmental and genetic. The National Cancer Institute implicates tobacco as the single major cause of preventable cancer deaths. Other environmental carcinogenic agents are alcohol, chemicals, radiation, sunlight, hormones, and asbestos. There is evidence that certain viruses are linked to the development of cancers, especially cancers of the liver, nasopharynx, cervix, and lymphatic system. The American Cancer Society and The National Cancer Institute promote certain lifestyles and diets that may decrease the risk of cancer (Fig. 34–2). Dental hygienists can use this information to promote overall health awareness and concern for the individual.

SIGNS AND SYMPTOMS OF CANCER

In early stages, most cancers exhibit no symptoms. Depending on the type of cancer, the most common presenting signs are:

- Change in bowel or bladder habits
- A sore that does not heal

Leading Sites of Cancer Incidence and Death—1993 Estimates

Cancer Incidence by Site and Sex*

Male	Female
Prostate 165,000	Breast 182,000
Lung 100,000	Colon & Rectum 75,000
Colon & Rectum 77,000	Lung 70,000
Bladder 39,000	Uterus 44,500
Lymphoma 28,500	Lymphoma 22,400
Oral 20,300	Ovary 22,000
Melanoma of the Skin 17,000	Melanoma of the Skin 15,000
Kidney 16,800	Pancreas 14,200
Leukemia 16,700	Bladder 13,300
Stomach 14,800	Leukemia 12,600
Pancreas 13,500	Kidney 10,400
Larynx 10,000	Oral 9,500
All Sites 600,000	All Sites 570,000

Cancer Deaths by Site and Sex

Male	Female
Lung 93,000	Lung 56,000
Prostate 35,000	Breast 46,000
Colon & Rectum 28,800	Colon & Rectum 28,200
Pancreas 12,000	Ovary 13,300
Lymphoma 11,500	Pancreas 13,000
Leukemia 10,100	Lymphoma 10,500
Stomach 8,200	Uterus 10,100
Esophagus 7,600	Leukemia 8,500
Liver 6,800	Liver 5,800
Brain 6,600	Brain 5,500
Kidney 6,500	Stomach 5,400
Bladder 6,500	Multiple Myeloma 4,600
All Sites 277,000	All Sites 249,000

*Excluding basal and squamous cell skin cancer and carcinoma in situ.

Source: American Cancer Society, *Cancer Facts & Figures—1993.*

FIGURE 34–1
American Cancer Society incidence and deaths by site and sex, 1993 estimates. (With permission from American Cancer Society, Cancer Facts and Figures 1993.)

- Unusual bleeding or discharge
- Thickening or lump in breast or elsewhere
- Indigestion or difficulty in swallowing
- Obvious change in a wart or mole
- Nagging cough or hoarseness

(From the American Cancer Society)

Pain is not often a symptom in early stages of cancer. A person who has one of the seven common signs of cancer for longer than 2 weeks should see a doctor promptly.

PSYCHOSOCIAL AND DEVELOPMENTAL RESPONSES RELATED TO A CANCER DIAGNOSIS

A medical diagnosis of cancer immediately presents a major disruption of life and threat of loss: loss of life from the disease, and loss of control, self-esteem, and function from the treatment of the disease. The acute emotional reaction is one of turmoil, shock, and disbelief. Concerns about trauma to the family, loss of work, and drain on finances cause additional anxiety.

The individual with cancer enters a grieving process with manifestations not unlike those of a person undergoing bereavement: grieving for loss of one's own life and lifestyle. Common psychological manifestations of cancer include anxiety, depression, and hopelessness.[3] Kubler-Ross described the stages associated with a potentially fatal disease as denial, anger, bargaining, depression, and acceptance.[4] These do not follow a systematic progression but may surface repeatedly at any time. They are considered normal but may be considered pathological when they result in unrealistic perceptions, extreme and uncharacteristic behaviors, progression to suicidal tendencies, or inappropriate delay in or resistance to treatment.

Some of these stages are an important part of the person's coping mechanism. Denial can initially serve to save and protect psychological integrity.[5] Anger often is a signal that the individual desires to fight for his life and is at-

WHAT ARE THE PROTECTIVE FACTORS?

Eat more cabbage-family vegetables. Important studies show these vegetables (also known as cruciferous) appear to protect you against colorectal, stomach and respiratory cancers. They include broccoli, cauliflower, brussels sprouts, all cabbages and kale.

Add more high-fiber foods. A high-fiber diet may protect you against colon cancer. Fiber occurs in whole grains, fruits and vegetables including peaches, strawberries, potatoes, spinach, tomatoes, wheat and bran cereals, rice, popcorn, whole-wheat bread.

Choose foods with Vitamin A. It may help protect you against cancers of the esophagus, larynx and lung. Fresh foods with beta-carotene like carrots, peaches, apricots, squash and broccoli are the best source, not vitamin pills.

Do the same for Vitamin C. This vitamin may help protect you against cancers of the esophagus and stomach. You'll find it naturally in lots of fresh fruits and vegetables like grapefruit, cantaloupe, oranges, strawberries, red and green peppers, broccoli, tomatoes.

Add weight control. Obesity is linked to cancers of the uterus, gallbladder, breast and colon. Exercise and lower calorie intake help you avoid gaining a lot of weight. Walking is ideal exercise for most people, and primes you for other sports. Check with your physician before strenuous activity, or a special diet.

WHAT ARE THE RISK FACTORS?

Trim fat from your diet. A high-fat diet increases your risk of breast, colon and prostate cancer. Fat-loaded calories mean a weight gain for you, especially if you don't exercise. Cut overall fat intake by eating lean meat, fish, skinned poultry, low-fat dairy products. Avoid pastry, candies.

Subtract salt-cured, smoked, nitrite-cured foods. Cancers of the esophagus and stomach are common in countries where these foods are eaten in large quantities. Choose bacon, ham, hot dogs or salt-cured fish only occasionally, if you like them a lot.

Stop cigarette smoking. Smoking is the biggest cancer risk factor of all—the main cause of lung cancer and 30% of *all* cancers. Smoking at home means more respiratory and allergic ailments for kids. Pregnant women who smoke harm their babies. Chewing tobaccos are harmful, too, as risks for mouth and throat cancers. Pick a quit day now and call us (American Cancer Society) for help.

Go easy on alcohol. If you drink a lot, your risk of liver cancer increases. Smoking *and* drinking alcohol greatly increases risk of cancers of the mouth, throat, larynx and esophagus. If you do drink alcohol, be moderate in your intake.

Respect the sun's rays. Too much sun causes skin cancer and other damage to your skin. Protect yourself with sunscreen—at least #15, wear long sleeves and a hat, especially during midday hours—11 a.m. to 3 p.m. Don't use indoor sunlamps, tanning parlors or pills. If you see changes in a mole or a sore that does not heal, see your physician.

FIGURE 34–2
Life and dietary styles to reduce cancer risks. (Redrawn with permission from American Cancer Society, Cancer Facts and Figures 1993.)

tempting to regain the control that was lost with the initial diagnosis. These reactions must be respected by the health-care professional and allowed to surface and to be expressed at appropriate levels.

Persons in all stages of the life cycle experience the aforementioned stages, but different age groups may have varied reactions. Older adults sometimes are resigned to a life-threatening diagnosis and may resist treatment. Some enter a significant depression because of the fear that they will become a physical and financial burden on their loved ones. Adult men may resent their loss of control and of their role as caretaker and provider. This may be the first time in their adult lives when someone else assumes care of their needs, which produces guilt and loneliness. Younger persons may express more anger and resentment than older people and may feel threatened by loss of career, sexuality, and family. Children have varied responses according to their age. Children younger than 5 years of age fear abandonment or separation. From ages 6 to 10, the greatest fear is that of bodily harm; children in this age group have some awareness of death. The greatest fear for children older than 10 years of age is that of death. Coupled with this fear may be difficult communication with adults.[6]

ORAL SQUAMOUS CELL CARCINOMA AND OTHER CANCERS OF THE ORAL CAVITY

Approximately 9 of every 10 oral malignancies are **oral squamous cell carcinoma.** Most occur in persons older than 40 years of age, but all persons should have a routine oral cancer screening, especially those in high-risk categories.

The prevalence in men is more than twice as high as in women. This ratio, however, has been narrowing, with probable cause being the increase in smoking by women.

The use of all tobacco products (cigarettes, smokeless/spit tobacco, cigars, and pipes) and alcohol is associated with an increased risk for oral squamous cell carcinoma. This risk is higher with increased product use. Individuals who use tobacco and drink alcohol heavily are at 10 times greater risk for developing oral cancer than persons who do not smoke or drink. The high prevalence of squamous cell carcinoma in countries such as India, where there is common use of betel nuts, slaked lime, and spices, demonstrates the impact of other environmental, cultural, and social factors. The role of diet and viruses, especially the human papillomavirus and the herpes simplex virus, is currently being investigated. At the present time, there are no conclusive studies that demonstrate a correlation between denture trauma or other chronic irritation and the development of oral cancers.

The American Cancer Society's *Facts and Figures* reports that in 1993, the overall 5-year survival rate for all stages of squamous cell cancer of the oral cavity was approximately 52%. There were approximately 9,000 deaths from oral cancer, and another 3,750 persons with laryngeal cancer died. Prognosis is highly variable and dependent on the stage and location of the disease when first diagnosed. National Cancer Institute data collected between the years 1973 to 1984 demonstrated that persons with a small localized oral squamous cell cancer had a 72% 5-year survival rate, compared with only 34% for a late stage oral cancer.[7] The public often does not comprehend the serious nature of oral cancers, perhaps because it associates disease in the mouth with dental care that is not life-threatening.

The most common presenting signs of squamous cell carcinomas of the oral cavity, pharynx, and larynx are:

- Swelling, lump, growth, or area of induration or hardness anywhere in or about the mouth or neck, which is usually painless
- **Erythroplakia** patch (velvety, deep red)
- **Leukoplakia** patch (white or red/white patch)
- Any sore (ulcer, irritation) that does not heal after 2 weeks
- Repeated bleeding from the mouth or throat
- Difficulty in swallowing or persistent hoarseness

Histologic studies demonstrate that 90% of red or combined red and white mucosal lesions and only 20% of white lesions in high-risk areas are dysplastic or carcinomatous.[8] Red or combined red and white lesions therefore should be considered to be more dangerous than white lesions and should be evaluated carefully.

The most common intraoral sites for squamous cell cancer are the lateral borders and ventral surfaces of the tongue, floor of the mouth, and the oropharynx. Any of the signs and symptoms that persist for longer than 2 weeks after removal of potentially irritating factors and/or application of therapeutic measures must be considered a cancer until proven benign by biopsy and microscopic evaluation.

Histologically, squamous cell carcinoma is assessed by the pathologist according to the similarity of appearance of the cancer cells to the cells from which it was derived. Cells that appear like the parent cells are classified as "well-differentiated" or "moderately differentiated." If they do not resemble the original cells, they are classified "undifferentiated" or "anaplastic." The less differentiated cells generally indicate a more aggressive cancer.

Other cancers less frequently found in the oral cavity include adenocarcinomas of salivary gland origin, lymphomas, melanoma, and bone and soft tissue sarcomas. Cancers that begin in other parts of the body may metastasize to or exhibit manifestations in the oral cavity. The most common metastases are from tumors in the lung, breast, colon, and kidney. Manifestations of leukemia, lymphomas, and multiple myeloma may also be present within the oral cavity.

PREVENTION OF ORAL SQUAMOUS CELL CARCINOMA

The dental hygienist has an opportunity to educate people, especially those in high-risk categories, about the early signs and symptoms of oral cancer and self-evaluation skills. Teaching aids and pamphlets are available free of charge from local units or state divisions of the American Cancer Society or the National Cancer Institute (1-800-4-CANCER). Dental hygienists also may participate in community health fairs or public education seminars through local hospitals or health clinics. Educational posters and pamphlets describing oral cancer and self-examimation procedures can help the public become aware of the dangers of oral cancer. These interventions can help clients fulfill their human needs for conceptualization, problem solving, self-determination, and responsibility.

Mashberg and Silverman advocate the use of toluidine blue dye to detect malignant lesions.[7,9] Studies indicate that carcinomas and carcinoma-in-situ stain dark blue with a topical application. The dye acts as an evaluation tool in addition to the clinician's subjective impression. There is a 2 to 6.7% false negative rate, but this is less than the percentage with subjective clinical judgment alone. *The dye is not diagnostic, and a suspicious lesion must be biopsied to confirm malignancy.* If a lesion does not stain positive, the person should have potential irritants removed and *then be instructed to return in 10 to 14 days for additional evaluation.* If the lesion is in a high-risk area and does not resolve within this time period, a biopsy with histological confirmation should be done (see Chapter 11).

Another prevention strategy that dental hygienists can implement is tobacco education and cessation programs. As stated earlier, tobacco is considered the number one carcinogen in the United States. Tobacco not only is responsible for an increased incidence of oral cancer but also is implicated in cancers of the larynx, esophagus, lung, pancreas, uterus, cervix, and bladder. From the years 1976 to 1987, the percentage of adult smokers in the population dropped from 37% to 29%.[2] Unfortunately, there has been an increased use of smokeless tobacco products, especially among adolescents and young men. In several studies, users of smokeless tobacco say that they thought the product was safe because it was not burned and there were no warning labels on it. It is known, however, that "dipping snuff" or using other smokeless tobacco products exposes the body to levels of nicotine equal to or above those of cigarettes. These products also have high levels of carcinogens, heavy metals, and other toxic agents.[10] Tobacco companies are now required to put warning labels on all smokeless tobacco products.

There are several tobacco cessation programs available to dental professionals for use in their office. One that is free of charge and is well researched is available through the American Cancer Society and the National Institutes of

Health in Bethesda, MD. Part A of this program provides information about getting office personnel ready to provide tobacco intervention services by organizing

- The office team
- A tobacco-free office environment
- Records, codes, and procedures
- Client literature

Part B of this program provides information on how to use the "Four A's":

- ASK clients about tobacco
- ADVISE clients who want to stop
- ASSIST clients in stopping
- ARRANGE for follow-up services

Community and school programs are especially beneficial for educating children about the dangers of smokeless tobacco. Children in the fourth through sixth grades are especially vulnerable to beginning a tobacco habit because they are starting team sports and they like to emulate professional athletes who are often seen on television with a cheek pouch of tobacco. Children and teenagers are often not concerned about a cancer that may take several years to develop, but they may consider an immediate threat to their appearance (wholesome body image) with risk of foul breath, gingival recession, tooth decay, and tooth loss. Coaches of children and teenagers also need to learn about the nicotine addiction associated with smokeless tobacco so that they do not promote a habit that will lead to a lifelong tobacco addition.

People who drink heavily often deny they have an alcohol problem, but sometimes a cancer diagnosis provides a significant threat, and they ask for assistance in quitting their alcohol habit. The National Council on Alcoholism has an office in most large cities and acts as a resource for alcohol programs. Alcoholics Anonymous is another excellent program with chapters worldwide.

CANCER TREATMENT

The choice of cancer treatment is dependent on the type and stage of cancer. It may include surgery, chemotherapy, radiation, hormones, and/or immunotherapy. Some cancers respond to a single mode of treatment, whereas others require multimodality treatment strategies. The goal of cancer treatment is to totally remove or destroy the malignant cells from the body. Unfortunately, treatments available today are not able to target only the cancer cells, and normal healthy cells must sometimes be destroyed during the treatments. This may result in significant psychological stress and physical morbidity or death.

The goals of multidisciplinary care are to cure the disease and prevent and palliate the side effects of therapy. Ideally, a care plan is developed at a conference or tumor board attended by members of the oncology team. The care plan includes not only the initial therapy protocol but also the management of the side effects of the treatment and a plan for reconstruction and rehabilitation. Oral health professionals should encourage their involvement in care planning. The dental hygiene process within a human needs conceptual framework is used to assist in management of the oral complications associated with cancer therapy and prevent some of the systemic problems that may occur.

TREATMENT OF ORAL CANCERS

Choice of treatment for oral cancer is dependent on the stage of disease at the time of diagnosis. A small lesion of less than 1 cm may require only surgery or radiation therapy. Larger cancers, especially those that have spread to the lymph nodes in the neck, require surgery and radiation therapy. Chemotherapy is not a curative treatment for oral squamous cell cancer, but it may be used as an adjunct prior to surgery or radiation therapy to reduce the size of the tumor, or as a palliative treatment for recurrent and advanced tumors.

Surgical Treatment and Associated Complications

Surgery is chosen as primary treatment when oral cancer is not sensitive to radiation therapy; when lymph nodes, salivary glands, or bone are involved; or when there is a recurrence of tumor in an area that has already received a therapeutic dose of radiation. The disadvantage of surgery is the sacrifice of important functional oral structures.

Acute physical complications after head and neck surgery may include infection; airway obstruction; fistula formation; necrosis in the surgical site; impairment of swallowing, hearing, vision, smell, and speech; and compromised nutritional status. Long-term complications include speech impairment, malnutrition from the inability to swallow foods, drooling, malocclusion, temporomandibular disorders, facial deformity, and chronic pain in the shoulder muscles.

There may be significant psychosocial problems associated with surgery of the head and neck because the results of the cancer and its treatment are often visible and humiliating and can be psychologically devastating.[11] Physical impairments cannot be completely disguised by clothing, prostheses, or cosmetics. In today's society self-image is often equated with bodily image. As a result, some individuals experience depression, withdrawal and social death, anger, and/or stigmatization.[12] Some who are heavy smokers and drinkers experience guilt because of the association of these habits to oral cancer.[13] Preventing oral disease, promoting oral health through dental hygiene care, and assisting with tobacco and alcohol cessation can facilitate the person's human need for a wholesome body image and self-determination.

Surgical procedures for cancers of the head and neck may result in long-term disability. These problems may be short-term if reconstructive surgery and rehabilitation are possible. A retrospective study of 477 individuals treated for oral cancers at Memorial Sloan-Kettering Cancer Center in New York City demonstrated that 76% were able to return to a normal lifestyle within a year after treatment. Those interviewed attributed this finding to the excellent treatment, "tender loving care," and support they received from the oncology rehabilitation team.[11] The human needs approach to dental hygiene care articulates well with the oncology rehabilitation team approach that has proved successful.

Radiation Therapy and Associated Complications

Therapeutic radiation employs the use of ionizing radiation in the form of external beams of x-rays or gamma rays or external beams of electrons, or internally implanted sources of gamma rays.

TABLE 34–1
POTENTIAL COMPLICATIONS OF RADIATION THERAPY TO THE ORAL CAVITY AND SALIVARY GLANDS

Acute	Chronic
Xerostomia	Xerostomia
Mucositis	Rampant dental caries
Infection	Telangiectasia, friable mucosa
Taste alteration	Infection
Dysphagia	Muscle fibrosis and trismus
Impaired nutrition	Decreased vascularization
	Soft tissue necrosis
	Osteoradionecrosis
	Dentofacial malformations
	Impaired nutrition

Radiation therapy may be used by itself for the treatment of oral squamous cell carcinoma when the lesion is small and superficial and when a surgical procedure would result in significant functional or cosmetic morbidity. It is often used in combination with surgery, either postoperatively to eliminate residual disease or preoperatively to reduce the size of the tumor. Surgeons generally prefer to operate prior to a therapeutic dose of radiation because of delayed wound healing of irradiated tissue. Radiation therapy also may be used in the treatment of other cancers of the head and neck, including lymphomas and salivary gland tumors.

Radiation damage to normal cells may be acute and may resolve after completion of the therapy. Other normal cells may not have the capacity to repair themselves, resulting in long-term complications. After the first week of radiation, the client begins to experience some of the acute side effects whereas other complications may not become evident until after completion of radiation therapy (Table 34–1). At this time, the person's human needs for nutrition and integrity of the skin and mucous membranes become paramount in dental hygiene care.

Alteration of Taste

When the oral cavity is within the field of radiation, the client begins to experience an alteration of taste (dysgeusia) following the first few treatments. After the first 3 weeks of radiation clients may complain of complete taste loss, affecting the human need for nutrition. Eating ceases to be a pleasurable activity and clients must force themselves to eat only to maintain nutritional status. Taste acuity usually returns a few months following the completion of radiation therapy.

Salivary Gland Dysfunction

Exposure of the salivary glands to radiation is unavoidable when treating tumors of the oral cavity and neck because they are in close proximity to the lymphatic system and cannot be shielded. Ionizing radiation induces fibrosis and atrophy of the salivary gland tissue, especially the serous acinar cells. This results in diminished salivary flow and thickened sticky secretions. Salivary gland dysfunction is highly dependent on the individual and the dose and field of radiation. A dry mouth **(xerostomia)** can result in speech dysfunction, extreme discomfort, and difficulty with eating. Clients often complain bitterly about the complications associated with xerostomia.

Currently, it is not known if the radiation effects on salivary glands during childhood are permanent. There is some evidence from empirical data indicating that prepubertal children do not suffer significant irreversible salivary gland damage from high doses of radiation.[14]

Mucositis

After the first week of radiation, the client begins to experience the effects of damage to the oral and pharyngeal mucosal cells. The mucosa first becomes edematous and inflamed. Later the tissue becomes thinned, pseudomembranes form, and the tissue becomes denuded; producing severe pain, unpleasant odors, nutritional deficiency from inability to eat, and difficulty in talking **(mucositis).** Lack of saliva increases the risk of ulceration and bleeding. Following completion of all radiation treatments, gradual resolution of the mucositis can be expected although the epithelium undergoes permanent fibrosis and the tissue may be thin, fragile, and may show evidence of telangiectasia (a vascular lesion of dilated small blood vessels).

Infection

The human need for safety associated with the potential for oral infection is a common need observed in persons undergoing radiation therapy. Secondary infections of the oral mucosa are common and may intensify the mucosal irritation. The fungal organism *Candida albicans* is most often implicated, but any organism may be responsible for infection when the tissues are severely compromised from xerostomia, mucositis, altered nutrition, and inadequate oral hygiene.

To meet the individual's human need for safety, early detection and treatment of an oral infection is imperative to prevent exacerbation of mucositis that may require interruption of cancer therapy. *Optimal oral hygiene* and *absence of dental-related sources of infection* have been shown to reduce oral and systemic infection during therapy.[15]

"Radiation Caries"

Rampant demineralization of the tooth structure usually begins within the first year following radiation therapy unless intensive oral hygiene and preventive measures are instituted. Figure 34–3 shows the typical pattern of this demineralization process. The destruction results from decreased salivary flow, changes in the chemical composition of the saliva, and a more acidic dental plaque.[16–19] The altered quantity and quality of the saliva prevent the natural remineralization of the tooth structure with calcium and phosphate. With dry and friable tissues, these clients may change to a soft, high carbohydrate diet, adding to the risk of caries development. Studies have not demonstrated a significant negative effect of direct radiation on the tooth structure.

Altered Tooth and Jaw Development

The latent effects of therapeutic radiation therapy to children with cancers of the oral cavity and associated structures vary with radiation dose and field, and stage of growth and development. Radiation has the potential to

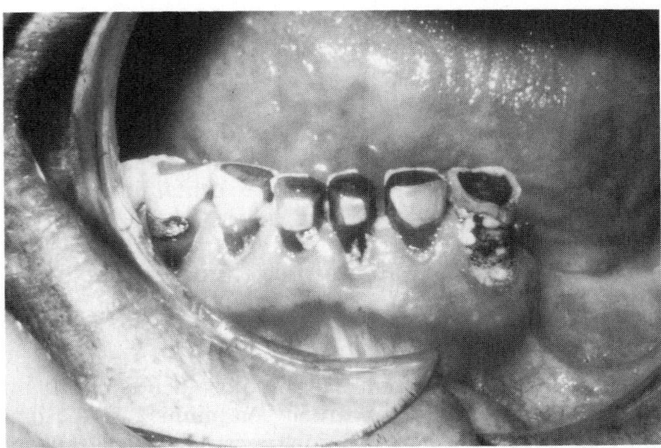

FIGURE 34-3
Radiation caries.

alter or arrest craniofacial growth and tooth development. Older children who receive minimal doses may experience only slightly altered root development, whereas younger children treated at an age when their jaws and teeth are under development may experience gross malformation of the dentition and may suffer significant skeletal deformities.[20]

Trismus

Limited jaw opening may result from tumor involvement of muscles or from fibrosis of the muscles or temporomandibular joint ligaments after a high dose of radiation. Children may actually experience hypoplastic development of the muscles. Trismus usually occurs within 6 months after therapy and remains a lifelong problem. It can result in significant discomfort and can interfere with eating, talking, and posttreatment examination.

Soft Tissue Necrosis and Osteoradionecrosis

Radiation therapy may irreversibly injure the vascularity of soft tissue and bone. Therefore, bone and soft tissue within a radiation field become hypovascular, hypocellular, and hypoxic.[21] Thus, the bone and/or soft tissue may not have the capacity to heal after a surgical procedure or trauma, such as from a prosthetic appliance. **Osteoradionecrosis** is defined as exposed bone that does not respond to treatment over a 6-month period of time. There is a higher risk of radionecrosis as the dose of radiation and the volume of irradiated bone and tissue increase. Nonhealing soft tissue or bone may become secondarily infected and the client may eventually experience intolerable pain and jaw fracture. The mandible appears to be more susceptible than the maxilla because of its limited blood supply. Clients who are at the greatest risk are those who have surgery or trauma to tissue and bone after radiation, or clients who have dental infection in close approximation to bone compromised by radiation. Prevention of osteoradionecrosis by preradiation therapy dental evaluation and treatment is mandatory. Following radiation, the teeth and periodontium must be professionally managed at intervals to ensure *excellent oral hygiene, early intervention, and minimal disease.* The dental hygienist is an extremely important member of the professional team to manage this potential problem, meeting the person's human need for safety.

Surgical and Prosthetic Rehabilitation of the Person with Head and Neck Cancer

Planning for rehabilitation of the person with head and neck cancer begins at the time of medical diagnosis. When a surgical resection creates facial defects and oral dysfunction, the client must be assured that there is a plan to restore at least partial function and improve cosmetic appearance. The oral and maxillofacial surgeon, the maxillofacial prosthodontist, the general dentist, and the dental hygienist all may play a role in the initial care planning. The dental hygienist's sensitivity to the person's human need for a wholesome body image, appreciation, and respect is most important at this time.

Maxillary defects result in unintelligible speech because of nasal voice quality, difficulty in eating, thickened nasal and sinus secretions, and facial disfigurement. Optimal management begins at the time of surgery when the prosthodontist may place a surgical obturator to help correct these problems. Approximately 3 to 4 months after surgery, if no complications arise, a permanent prosthesis is fabricated. This usually allows the most effective restoration for the client because speech, swallowing, mastication, and facial contour all can effectively be restored with a prosthesis instead of reconstructed with plastic surgery.

Mandibular defects are often created during surgery for oral cancers. If mandibular stabilization is not accomplished, the defect results in deviation of the mandible and loss of interocclusal relationship. This can be prevented by intermaxillary fixation or stabilization of the mandible with an external fixation appliance placed at the time of surgery and maintained during the healing process (Fig. 34-4). Sometimes immediate reconstruction is possible with alloplastic implant or surgical flaps. After several months of healing and no evidence of recurrent tumor, the mandible may be reconstructed. One method involves attaching a titanium tray to the mandible stubs. The tray is packed with iliac crest cancellous bone, which over time generates a new jaw.

Following extensive intraoral surgery, the client may need a surgical procedure to release the tongue from the floor of the mouth, a skin graft, and vestibuloplasty to create a vestibule for saliva pooling and to allow for extension of denture flanges. These procedures also aid in speech, mastication, and swallowing.

Following radiation therapy to the oral cavity, clients who are partially or fully edentulous require conservative

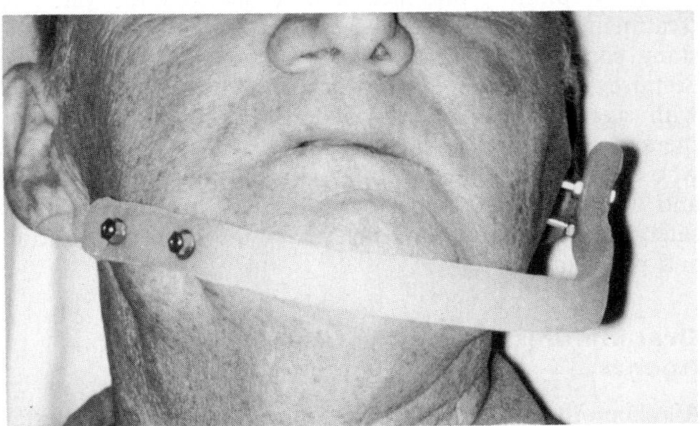

FIGURE 34-4
External fixation after surgical hemimandibulectomy.

prosthetic management because of permanent radiation manifestations. The thinned and friable tissue, scarring and fibrosis from surgery, and lack of lubrication and protective qualities of the saliva make denture placement difficult and place the client at risk for soft tissue breakdown and osteoradionecrosis. Some clients are never able to wear dentures. Detailed education, close professional supervision, and client acceptance of recommendations are necessary for successful prosthetic rehabilitation.

Chemotherapy and Associated Complications

Chemotherapeutic drugs have been used for the treatment of cancer for more than 40 years. In the 1960s, combinations of chemotherapeutic agents resulted in significant improvement in cure rates for some cancers. Other cancers are not cured by chemotherapy alone, but the drugs are used in combination with surgery and/or radiation to destroy cancer cells that may have spread systemically. Sometimes chemotherapy is used by itself for a period of time to control a tumor that cannot be eradicated.

Chemotherapy alone is not a curative treatment for oral squamous cell carcinoma, but it is sometimes used adjuvantly with surgery and radiation, or may be used to palliate advanced tumors. Prior to surgery, it may be given to reduce the size of very large tumors. Drugs given for oral cancer may result in **myelosuppression** and mucositis. Currently all chemotherapy protocols for oral squamous cell carcinoma are under investigation, with improvement in long-term survival rates still to be assessed. Chemotherapy for malignancies outside the head and neck may result in oral complications.

The most common overall complication of chemotherapy is infection as a result of myelosuppression. Local infection may lead to sepsis and death.[22] Other complications of chemotherapy include electrolyte imbalances, bleeding and hemorrhage, and acute toxicity from the drugs, including nausea and vomiting, photosensitivity, central nervous system dysfunction, alopecia (hair loss), and poor nutritional status.

Chemotherapy is not only physically demanding but also stress-producing. The human need for a wholesome body image is often compromised because the physical effects of the drugs destroy a person's self-image. These persons need the support of their caregivers. They should be encouraged to focus on positive attributes and benefits of the short-term therapy. Some individuals who experience no debilitating symptoms from their cancer question the value of treatments that make them feel so ill. Others express constant concern about the effectiveness of the treatments. Some experience an overall feeling of being "off-balance" with significant mood swings. Persons undergoing cancer therapy need support from family, friends, and caregivers who are good listeners, who allow a full range of emotions, and who encourage hope to address the human needs for safety and freedom from stress and for conceptualization and problem-solving.

Oral Manifestations of Chemotherapeutic Agents

All chemotherapy protocols do not result in oral manifestations but many have either a direct or indirect effect on the mouth. Some chemotherapeutic agents may directly destroy normal cells, resulting in nausea, vomiting, neurotoxicity, and/or mucosal ulcerations. Sonis and colleagues reported that approximately 40% of persons treated for *non–head and neck malignancies* experienced oral complications.[23] In 1988, these investigators reported that oral problems related to myelosuppression may be significantly and favorably affected through aggressive preventive dental intervention. They also reported that younger patients had a higher frequency of oral problems than did older patients, possibly because of differences in mucosal cell turnover rates.

Mucositis

The direct cytotoxic action of chemotherapeutic agents on the oral mucosa results in atrophy or thinning of the oral mucosa, erythema, and ulceration. Because the oral mucosa regenerates approximately every 10 days, mucosal changes usually begin within 7 to 10 days following the administration of stomatotoxic drugs. Ulcerations usually appear individually but may progress to diffuse and confluent lesions, especially on the nonkeratinized mucosal surfaces of the mouth. The lesions are often very painful, causing difficulty in eating and talking. Lesions usually last until the bone marrow begins to recover. The person's human need for freedom from pain as a result of the severity of mucositis may be favorably affected by dental hygiene interventions that create a clean and well-hydrated oral environment, good nutritional status, and control of secondary infection.

Infection

Suppression of the bone marrow by chemotherapeutic drugs results in neutropenia, or a reduction in the neutrophils that are responsible for combating infection.

Oral mucosal infections occurring during periods of immunosuppression are commonly caused by normal oral flora such as Streptococcus and Staphylococcus bacteria and Candida fungi and herpes simplex virus, but any organism may be responsible. Chronic and subclinical dental infections of periodontal, periapical and/or pulpal origin may be exacerbated when the patient is in an immunosuppressed condition. Clinical signs of inflammation (redness, pain, swelling, heat) may be reduced or absent during periods of neutropenia, making it difficult to assess the mouth for infection.

Oral infections can result in significant morbidity for the client undergoing chemotherapy. Oral infections not only intensify mucositis, but with a breach in the oral mucosa, dental and mucosal infections may lead to septicemia and death in clients with profound **immunosuppression.** Recently major cancer centers have reported an increased incidence of alpha-streptococcal sepsis with life-threatening shock syndrome in individuals treated intensely with chemotherapy.[24] Alpha-streptococcal invasion of the normal oropharyngeal flora is implicated as the source of these septic episodes. Therefore, the person undergoing chemotherapy that results in the suppression of bone marrow has a human need for safety associated with true infection or a potential for infection.

Bleeding or Hemorrhage

Myelosuppression from chemotherapy may result in **thrombocytopenia** and reduction of other clotting factors. Clients with platelet counts under $50,000/mm^3$ may experience oral bleeding during invasive dental procedures. The occurrence of spontaneous gingival bleeding increases with a platelet count below 20,000/mm^3.[25] When there is a disruption of the mucosal integrity and/or periodontal disease, clients are at greater risk of bleeding. This fact emphasizes the need for early intervention, soft tissue management, and periodontal maintenance care.

Salivary Gland Dysfunction

Some clients complain of a dry mouth, thickened secretions, or excessive drooling during chemotherapy. Studies are inconclusive as to the drugs' affects on salivary glands. Persons who complain about dysfunction need palliation from saliva substitutes and adequate hydration to prevent further exacerbation of other oral complications.

Dental Caries

Rampant tooth decay is not directly caused by the toxicity of chemotherapeutic drugs. However, clients with a chronically dry mouth, or persons who increase their intake of high carbohydrate foods because of eating problems, may experience an increase in caries development. Depending on severity of this problem, various preventive regimens may be prescribed.

Children who are chronically ill may be given nighttime bottle feedings and/or diets high in sugar. During periods of stress, parents and caregivers may allow an unbalanced diet to avoid additional stress from confrontation. Counseling primary caregivers about cariogenic foods and behaviors is important to meet the person's human need for a sound biological dentition.

Neurotoxicity

Some chemotherapeutic agents derived from plant alkaloids (such as vincristine) may cause severe, deep, and often bilateral odontogenic-like pain. When no dental pathology can be found, the drug may be implicated. The pain subsides within a few days after administration of the drug.

Altered Tooth Development

Studies have shown that some chemotherapy drugs given before the age of 10 years, and especially before the age of 5 years may alter root development.[23a]

Bone Marrow Transplantation and Complications

Bone marrow transplantation (BMT) is a therapeutic procedure used to treat a variety of hematologic diseases including aplastic anemia, leukemias, lymphomas, neuroblastoma, and immunodeficiency diseases. It is also being used at some cancer centers to treat some solid tumors.

Bone marrow transplantation begins with the donation of normal bone marrow. Multiple aspirations of marrow are drawn from the donor's iliac crests under sterile conditions and anesthesia. The individual with cancer then goes through a "conditioning phase" when they are given superlethal doses of chemotherapy and sometimes total body irradiation (TBI). The goal is to destroy all of the malignant cells and suppress the immune system to permit engraftment of the normal bone marrow. After the client has been conditioned, the marrow is intravenously infused into their blood. The marrow stem cells travel to the marrow cavities and, if engraftment takes place, the cells begin to reproduce within 2 to 4 weeks.

A significant problem that exists for clients who undergo an **allogeneic bone marrow transplant** is **graft-versus-host disease** (GVHD). This results from an immunological reaction wherein the donor marrow cells react against the host tissue antigens. If this occurs within the first 100 days after transplant it is called acute GVHD and is characterized by dermatitis, enteritis, and hepatitis. If it occurs after the first 100 days, it is termed chronic GVHD with manifestations similar to those of autoimmune disorders. These may include skin diseases, keratoconjunctivitis, oral mucositis, xerostomia, esophageal and vaginal strictures, pulmonary insufficiency, intestinal problems, and chronic liver disease. Both forms of GVHD can result in fatal infections. To prevent GVHD, various types of immunosuppressive therapy are used.

The other major problem after transplant is decreased immunological function, making the transplanted individual susceptible to opportunistic infections. After the first year, most recover their immune function unless they have developed chronic GVHD.

Oral Manifestations of Bone Marrow Transplantation

During the first 30 days of transplantation, the client experiences cytotoxic and immunosuppressive oral manifestations from the chemoradiotherapy conditioning. These may include severe mucositis, ulceration, hemorrhage, infection, and xerostomia. Infections during the first 30 days intensify the mucositis and ulcerations, opening a portal of entry for organisms into the blood.

During the next several months, the client's acute manifestations begin to resolve unless he develops GVHD. Common complaints with GVHD are xerostomia and mucositis. Also, there may be evidence of lichen planus–like or lupus–like lesions, sometimes becoming erosive. Generalized atrophy of the mucosa and changes consistent with scleroderma may be seen. Viral infections, including herpes simplex virus and fungal infections are common.

After the first 100 days after transplant, persons with no evidence of GVHD usually do not have any oral complaints other than varying degrees of xerostomia. Those persons with persistent xerostomia may develop rapid demineralization of the tooth structure and oral infections.

Patients who are scheduled for bone marrow transplantation should undergo a thorough oral and dental evaluation and necessary treatment prior to transplant. All potential sources of infection and irritation should be treated because chronic, nonsymptomatic oral infections may become acute during immunosuppression and/or GVHD and may lead to sepsis and even death. The role of the dental hygienist in controlling oral infections is clearly established.

DENTAL HYGIENE PROCESS OF CARE FOR THE INDIVIDUAL WITH CANCER

The dental hygienist, as a member of the oncology team, has the opportunity to prevent and/or ameliorate many of the oral and systemic complications associated with cancer

RESOURCES FOR HOSPITAL INSERVICE PROGRAMS

University of Missouri–Kansas City School of Dentistry
An instructional series with 80 slides, accompanying manual and professional education booklet entitled "Oral Management of the Cancer Patient" is available for rent or purchase. Call 816-235-2064 or write: Instructional Resource Librarian, Dental Library, UMKC School of Dentistry, 650 East 25th Street, Kansas City, MO 64108-2795.

American Cancer Society
Local units or state divisions provide both public and professional posters and pamphlets on various cancer-related topics.

Moi-Stir Products, Kingswood Laboratories
Supplier of hospital oral care products (swabs and saliva substitute). Provide some educational materials and samples of products. Call 317-846-7452 or write: Kingswood Laboratories, Inc., 1119 3rd Avenue, SW, PO Box 567, Carmel, IN 46032

Sage Medical Products
Supplier of hospital oral care kits and products. Will provide samples. Call 1-800-323-2220 or write Sage Medical Products, 680 Industrial Drive, Cary, IL 60013

treatment by designing a dental hygiene care plan that promotes a clean and healthy oral cavity. (See Resources for Hospital Inservice Programs chart.)

Prior to the initial dental hygiene care appointment, consultation must be sought with other oncology team members involved in the care of the person with cancer. Open and continuous communication with physicians and nurses reduces the risk of providing care that compromises the client's condition. (See the Information Sought Through Consultation with Oncology Team Prior to Dental Hygiene Care chart).

Assessment

A client scheduled for surgery to the oral cavity requires an expedient assessment to identify sources of infection (human need for safety) that may delay postoperative healing.

The pretherapy assessment is most critical for a client scheduled for radiation therapy to the oral cavity and/or salivary glands. Once the mandible and maxilla have been irradiated, the client is at lifelong risk for the development of osteoradionecrosis. Because this risk is potentiated by trauma to the bone from surgery or prosthesis irritation, all infections, irritations, bone pathology, and teeth that cannot be maintained for the client's lifetime should be identified for removal. This includes not only teeth with gross caries and refractory periodontal disease, but also teeth that potentially may not be maintained because of the client's lack of personal motivation, physical or mental ability, and/or financial resources.

A client with a clean and healthy mouth will experience fewer oral complications and systemic infections during chemotherapy; therefore, to meet the client's human needs for skin and mucous membrane integrity and safety, a client scheduled for chemotherapy must be assessed to identify potential sources of irritation that may potentiate mucositis or sources of intraoral infection that may spread through the bloodstream and result in sepsis and possibly death. Assessment of a potential BMT recipient should identify sources of irritation and infection or any oral problem that may arise within the first year following the transplant when the client is in an immunosuppressed condition. Clients with potential GVHD are at an increased risk for oral and systemic infections, as well as xerostomia and rampant tooth decay.

Client Interview

The client interview provides critical information that influences future oral hygiene care and dental treatment. Social support of the person with cancer is an important part of the treatment process. Therefore, those closest to the individual should be involved in the client interview and education whenever possible. In order to meet the individual's need for appreciation and respect, clients who have had a laryngectomy or those with a surgical speech defect should be provided a pad of paper and pencil to assist in answering questions. If they use a communicative assistive device (e.g., an electro-larynx) the dental hygienist should encourage its use. It is difficult to understand a client who

INFORMATION SOUGHT THROUGH CONSULTATION WITH ONCOLOGY TEAM PRIOR TO DENTAL HYGIENE CARE

All Oncology Clients
Medical diagnosis of cancer
Stage of disease
Proposed cancer treatment plan and date of initiation
Other medically-compromising conditions that affect dental treatment or wound healing
Infection risk
Nutritional status
Significant psychosocial issues
Current hematological status including clotting factors and absolute neutrophil count

Additional Information for Clients Receiving Chemotherapy
Proposed protocol schedule
Potential oral and systemic complications
Presence of indwelling central venous catheter

Additional Information for Clients Receiving Radiation to the Oral Cavity and Salivary Glands
Specific field of radiation
Total dose of radiation (cGy or rad)

Additional Information for Clients Undergoing Head and Neck Surgery
Extent of surgical resection

Additional Information for Clients Undergoing Bone Marrow Transplant (BMT)
Type of BMT
Proposed use of total body irradiation
Presence of indwelling central venous catheter
Previous oral complications associated with cancer therapy

is just beginning to use the device, but time and patience increase the client's self-confidence, thus promoting mutual trust and respect.

It is important for the dental hygienist to verify what clients understand about their cancer diagnosis and medical treatment prior to discussing the dental hygiene component of care. This facilitates the person's human need for conceptualization and problem solving. Physicians employ different strategies for telling clients about their disease. Most doctors feel it is their ethical and legal responsibility to disclose fully the consequences of a cancer diagnosis and complications associated with treatment. Some doctors, however, tell the client only what they seem to be able to comprehend at the time of initial diagnosis, and have not completed the educational process when the person is referred for dental consultation. Even when a physician offers a full explanation to the person and the family, *emotional factors often prevent a clear understanding and comprehension of all information.* Ethically, it is inappropriate to give a judgmental opinion about the client's care plan. It is appropriate and important, however, to offer empathy and listen to the client's fears. Taking time to listen to the client's perceptions decreases client and family stress, promotes consistency, encourages cooperation among members of the oncology team, and assists the dental hygienist in assessing the client's human needs that shape the dental hygiene process of care.

The client's dental history is reviewed, including frequency of care, dental experiences that were unpleasant or painful, and current attitude and knowledge about the teeth and mouth and oral self-care habits. This information assists the dental hygienist in assessing the client's image of the teeth and mouth and the value placed on oral health. This is the time also to assess the client's fear of dental procedures so that deficits in the human need for freedom from pain and stress can be met. A client who has had a recent surgical procedure to the head and neck may be in the process of acceptance of the facial deformity and functional alterations. Encouragement to talk about these issues aids the client in moving towards acceptance of the new body image. The interview also reveals the client's socioeconomic status, and cultural and ethnic influences that may affect perceptions of cancer, health beliefs, coping strategies, social support system, dietary habits, and ability to adhere to the supportive care.

Other important information includes environmental factors such as history of childhood development in an area with fluoridated water and exposure to carcinogens. History of tobacco use and alcohol intake is important information to seek from the client with oral squamous cell carcinoma. Amount, duration of use, and attempts to quit should be documented. The dental hygienist should ask the client if he understands the association of tobacco and alcohol to oral cancer, and if he has a desire to quit these habits. Information about oral habits such as mouth breathing, clenching, and bruxing is documented and followed with clinical evaluation.

Important psychosocial information related to human needs includes the client's self-concept, coping resources, and body image, and the family or "significant other's" perception of the client. One of the most common psychological responses to cancer is depression. Signs of depression include a loss of interest in daily activities, lack of motivation, loss of energy and appetite, insomnia or hypersomnia, feelings of worthlessness, diminished ability to think, psychomotor agitation, and suicidal thoughts. Some clients appear to accept their diagnosis but are actually repressing their fears and anxiety, which can lead to depression.

Most chemotherapeutic agents do not have any direct psychological effects, but a few may cause confusion, depression, delirium, lethargy, and fatigue. In the assessment process, if the dental hygienist is concerned about the psychological state of the client, consultation with the members of the oncology team about various human need deficits is always appropriate to clarify the cause of the problems.

Assessment of Health History and Dietary Habits

A review of the client's health history should include past and present illness and allergies. Preexisting illness and allergies may influence the dental hygiene process of care. It is also important to document the history of the cancer symptoms and first diagnosis. This information provides insight into the client's perception of self-acceptance, values, and coping strategies. A recurrence of a previously treated cancer also influences the client's hope for successful medical treatment, the perception of prognosis, and the values about preventive care.

Dietary habits and daily food intake should be discussed to assess the individual's human need for nutrition. Of special importance is assessment of sugar intake because often the sequelae of cancer therapy are decreased or altered salivary flow and oral dysfunction and pain, significantly increasing the risk for dental caries.

Assessment of Current Oral and Dental Status

When possible, a complete extra- and intraoral assessment should be accomplished prior to initiation of cancer therapy by the dentist and dental hygienist team. Objective data from a radiographical and clinical assessment reveal the current oral and dental status, as well as the client's previous oral healthcare, and indicate the client's personal motivation and adherence to oral hygiene self-care measures. Standardized assessment indices for bacterial plaque, calculus, gingival bleeding, periodontal disease, and dental caries should be used. The oral tissues should be inspected for color, texture, evidence of edema, interruption of or alteration in mucosal integrity, operculums, bleeding, and lesions. It should be noted whether the oral secretions are scanty, absent, ropy, or excessive.

To assess the need for a biologically sound dentition, the teeth should be inspected for enamel or dentinal defects, fractured restorations and overhangs, mobility, pain, disturbance in eruption, and occlusion. Function and fit of prostheses should be checked. Children scheduled for radiation therapy and bone marrow transplantation should have their tooth development and exfoliation pattern documented. Orthodontic appliances should be noted. A full head and neck examination, including lymph nodes in the neck and the temporomandibular joint, should be accomplished. Bone pathology detected on radiographs should be noted.

Dental hygiene diagnoses identify problems to direct dental hygiene care prior to initiation of cancer therapy, during therapy, and after the client has completed all proposed therapy but continues to experience chronic and per-

TABLE 34–2
SAMPLE DENTAL HYGIENE DIAGNOSES PRIOR TO CANCER THERAPY FOR ORAL SQUAMOUS CELL CARCINOMA TREATED WITH SURGERY, RADIATION, AND CHEMOTHERAPY

Dental Hygiene Diagnoses	Related To	As Evidenced By
Deficit in the need for self-determination and responsibility	• Lack of skill • Impaired physical oral function • Impaired mental ability	• Inadequate oral health behaviors • Bacterial plaque, calculus, gingival bleeding • Teeth with suspicious lesions • Periodontal attachment loss of 5 to 7 mm
Deficit in the need for value system	• Low value ascribed to oral health	• Reports no previous regular dental hygiene care, education, or interest
Deficit in the need for conceptualization and problem solving	• First experience with cancer treatment • Impaired mental ability • Knowledge deficit regarding oral manifestations of cancer therapies	• Reports no previous exposure to cancer • Minimal preparation by other health professionals
Deficit in the need for nutrition	• Weight less than body requirement • Knowledge deficit • Lack of resources • Alcohol abuse • Emotional distress	• Reports poor nutritional intake • History of heavy alcohol consumption • Report of oral pain • Body weight more than 10% below standard • Inflamed and fissured tongue • Uncontrolled oral pain • Gingival bleeding
Deficit in the need for safety: potential for infection	• Inadequate self-care • Inadequate nutrition • Impending surgery • Impending immunosuppression from to chemotherapy • Impending radiation- and chemotherapy-induced mucositis and xerostomia	
Deficit in the need for a wholesome body image	• Feelings of lack of control • Impending cancer therapy with mutilating side effects • Tongue mass	• Spouse reports dissatisfaction with teeth and halitosis • Speech dysfunction • No interest in care of teeth and oral tissues • Concern expressed about impending cancer surgery
Potential deficit in the need for a biologically sound dentition	• Knowledge deficit • Inadequate self-care • Impending radiation to salivary glands	

manent side effects. The preliminary pretherapy dental hygiene diagnoses, derived from baseline data, results in care consistent with the client's human needs. As therapy progresses and the client moves through various physical changes and psychosocial stages related to the cancer, the dental hygiene diagnoses change and the care plan is continually revised.

Initially, when clients are faced with a life-threatening cancer diagnosis, they are unable to conceptualize the importance of care beyond their most basic physiological and survival needs. As these needs appear to be no longer at imminent risk, the client often begins to accept the diagnosis and may be capable of participating in supportive care. A client in the dental office with a previous positive attitude about the teeth and oral hygiene may reveal totally different values during times of stress. It cannot be assumed that this client will continue the previous level of personal oral hygiene care. On the other hand, it should not be assumed that persons with a seemingly overwhelming cancer diagnosis do not have the ability to participate in successful rehabilitation. At appropriate times, a clear understanding of the oral problems associated with cancer therapy must be effectually communicated and trust established by mutual participation in the development of oral health goals. Tables 34–2, 34–3, and 34–4 illustrate sample dental hygiene diagnoses prior to, during, and after cancer therapy.

Planning

The client undergoing cancer therapy or one in **end-stage disease** requires a care plan directed toward meeting actual or potential needs associated with the oral and systemic complications of cancer therapies. The dental hygiene care

TABLE 34–3
SAMPLE DENTAL HYGIENE DIAGNOSES DURING CANCER THERAPY

Dental Hygiene Diagnoses	Related To	As Evidenced By
Deficit in the need for safety: potential for oral and systemic infection	• Immunosuppression • Presence of indwelling venous catheter • Xerostomia • Mucositis • Partial knowledge deficit • Inadequate nutrition • Stress from cancer therapy	
Deficit in the need for self-determination and responsibility: potential to optimize oral health	• Client demonstrates acceptance of cancer • Client asks questions about side effects and preventive measures • Demonstrates interest in treatment plan • Beginning to participate in decision making	
Deficit in the need for safety: potential for oral injury	• Mucositis • Immunosuppression • Parasthesia from surgery • Improper use of oral topical anesthetic	
Deficit in the need for a wholesome body image	• Oral and speech dysfunction • Alopecia (hair loss) • Facial deformity	• Dysfunction of tongue from surgical resection • Effects of chemotherapy resulting in hair loss • External fixation and facial scars • Makes self-derogatory remarks
Deficit in the need for conceptualization and problem solving	• Stress from cancer therapy • Knowledge deficit • Partial self-care deficit	• Repeats questions regarding self-care • Expresses confusion about treatment plan • Evidence of bacterial plaque and gingival bleeding
Deficit in the need for skin and mucous membrane integrity of the head and neck	• Cytotoxic effects of cancer therapy • Partial self-care deficit	• Inflammation • Edema • Ulceration • Bacterial plaque • Thick oral secretions
Deficit in the need for nutrition	• Side effects of cancer • Stress • Less than body requirement	• Mucositis • Xerostomia • Taste loss • Dysphagia • Nausea • Anxiety • Weight more than 10% below standard

plan for the client with cancer is based on one or more of the possible goals listed in Table 34–5 and Table 34–6.

Implementation

Clients referred by a physician for dental care in conjunction with cancer therapy should present a referral letter or form bearing the physician's signature. Dental professionals participating on oncology teams may provide oncologists with printed referral forms that include important information about the medical status of the client, the specific cancer therapy, and necessary precautions (Fig. 34–5). A documented and physician-signed referral permits submission of the bill for dental and dental hygiene services to the patient's medical insurance company. Most medical insurance policies do not cover dental-related treatment, but because the dental care is requested as part of the overall management for the client with cancer, a request can be made for a special review of the claim by the insurance company's arbitration board to determine if some or all of the bill may be reimbursed as a medical expense. A letter to the insurance company requesting a special review with an explanation of the rationale for dental care provides the best opportunity for reimbursement of expenses. As a change agent and consumer advocate, the dental hygienist has the opportunity to educate healthcare consumers, third-party reimbursers, and government institutions about the

TABLE 34–4
SAMPLE DENTAL HYGIENE DIAGNOSES AFTER CANCER THERAPY

Dental Hygiene Diagnoses	Related To	As Evidenced By
Deficit in the need for a wholesome body image	• Surgical disfigurement • Oral dysfunction • Fear of unknown • Emotional instability	• Unable to verbalize fears • Withdrawn • Anxious • Psychomotor agitation • Makes self-derogatory remarks
Deficit in the need for nutrition	• Oral dysfunction • Less than body requirements	• Edentulous • Pain in temporomandibular joint • Body weight more than 10% below standard
Deficit in the need for a biologically sound dentition	• Radiation therapy–induced xerostomia • Partial self-care deficit	• Signs of dental caries on cervical ⅓ and incisal edges of teeth. • Pain with oral hygiene measures • Difficult mastication
Deficit in the need for safety	• Previous exposure to therapeutic radiation	• Verbalizes fear of radiographs
Deficit in the need for self-determination and responsibility	• Denial • Mental ability • Deficit in self-care	• Reports no longer using fluoride trays • Presence of bacterial plaque

importance and benefits of dental and dental hygiene interventions in the care of medically compromised patients.

It is important to remember that dental hygienists are responsible for clearly communicating with other oncology team members regarding procedures their state practice acts legally allow them to perform. Most medical professionals have limited knowledge of dental hygiene care and may request the hygienist to perform functions that are outside legal and regulatory guidelines. The dental hygienist can assist the client in obtaining necessary dental care with a referral to the appropriate professional.

Prior to Cancer Therapy

Referral to a Dentist Conditions found by the dental hygienist that require diagnosis by a dentist should be referred immediately to a dentist for evaluation and treatment. Clients scheduled for surgery need to have all potential sources of infection and irritation eliminated. Those clients to receive radiation therapy to the oral cavity and salivary glands need oral surgical procedures accomplished 14 to 21 days prior to initiation of therapy. Fabrication of new dental prostheses is delayed until several months after radiation therapy ends when all acute side effects of radiation have resolved. Restorative needs should be cared for prior to the onset of painful mucositis. Before chemotherapy begins, clients should have all surgical procedures done at least 7 days prior to periods of immunosuppression, all sources of infection and irritation removed, and all projected dental needs met.

Psychosocial Issues The initial client appointment is an important time when trust and assurance are established. In order to meet the client's human need for appreciation and respect and freedom from pain, the client must feel acceptance in a nonjudgmental environment and sense that his self-esteem will be preserved. The client is a "person living with cancer" not a "cancer case." Additional time is necessary to allow the client to express his feelings. All feelings should be acknowledged and anger should not be mitigated too quickly. To meet the person's need for self-determination and responsibility, the client should be encouraged to participate in care planning, which provides an opportunity to regain some of the control over his life which was lost to the cancer. Eye contact is important to help eliminate feelings of isolation and stress, especially for clients who have suffered surgical facial deformity and who have disturbances in body image. It may help clients to be reminded that the treatment is aimed at the disease, not their personhood. Clients who seem to be immobilized by human need deficits of a psychosocial nature may require a referral to a social worker or psychologist on the oncology team.

Education Adequate time must be allotted for the education session because the stress related to a cancer diagnosis can easily impede the normal learning process. The nursing literature adequately documents the importance of pretherapy education for the reduction of stress and anxiety and the level of side effects.[26,27] It is important to engage in the teaching process with full regard for the client's psycho-

TABLE 34–5
POSSIBLE GOALS FOR MEETING THE HUMAN NEEDS OF INDIVIDUALS WITH CANCER

Goals	Human Needs Met by Achievement of Goals
Reduce client's anxiety and knowledge deficit related to dental and dental hygiene care, cancer therapy, and associated needs	Freedom from pain Conceptualization and problem solving Safety
Achieve a positive client attitude about the importance of oral hygiene during and after cancer therapy	Self-determination and responsibility Value system
Provide optimal professional dental hygiene care Reduce the risk of oral and systemic infection, oral trauma, and malnutrition	Integrity of oral mucous membrane Nutrition Biologically sound dentition Safety
Palliation of painful tissues	Freedom from pain
Achieve appropriate oral hygiene measures in cooperation with the client to encourage acceptance and responsibility for oral hygiene self-care Promote preventive measures against cancer	Self-determination and problem solving Safety

TABLE 34–6
SAMPLE DENTAL HYGIENE CARE PLAN PRIOR TO CANCER THERAPY

Dental Hygiene Diagnosis	Goal/Expected Behavior	Dental Hygiene Interventions	Evaluative Statements
Deficit in the need for self-determination and responsibility	By 9/31, client will participate in design and practice of oral self-care skills	Explain risks of poor oral hygiene during cancer therapy Demonstrate plaque control measures In cooperation with client, design self-care procedures with regard for impaired function Provide written instructions or printed educational materials	Client exhibits good plaque control habits Client exhibits no evidence of plaque or debris on index Client exhibits no evidence of oral bleeding on probing

Oncology Dental Support Clinic
University of Missouri-Kansas City
School of Dentistry
650 E. 25th, Kansas City, MO 64108

______________________________ is referred for an oral/dental evaluation and treatment.

This adjunctive medical care is essential so that the patient may complete cancer therapy.

________________________ ____________
Physician's Signature Date

Diagnosis: ______________________________

Proposed therapy: ______________________________

If therapy includes radiation to the salivary glands or oral cavity, please indicate field of therapy:

If therapy is myelosuppressive, please give current:

absolute granulocyte count ____________________

platelet count ____________________

Does the patient have a central venous catheter?

______ (yes) ______ (no)

Does the patient need antibiotics prior to dental treatment?

______ (yes) ______ (no)

Additional important medical information:

To schedule an appointment, contact the Special Patient Care Clinic at 235-2160 or the Oncology Dental Support Clinic Coordinator, Ms. Gerry Barker (RDH, MA), at 235-2300.

APPOINTMENT DATE: ____________ **TIME:** ____________

FIGURE 34–5
Dental oncology referral form. (Redrawn and modified by permission of the University of Missouri-Kansas City School of Dentistry.)

logical human need status. Clients in a state of denial are not able to comprehend the importance of preventive oral healthcare until they begin to accept their cancer and therapy plan. Others, stressed by the financial burden of medical treatments, may not place priority on dental and dental hygiene treatment when compared to their impending lifesaving cancer therapy. Those who are depressed and see their prognosis as grave do not value the importance of long-term dental hygiene care until they begin to see cause for hope.

In view of the constraints placed on the client by all of the medical diagnostic tests necessary before cancer therapy and the amount of new information related to cancer treatment, the dental hygienist must utilize the most effective teaching strategies possible. Whether teaching adults with cancer or the parents of a child with cancer, the teaching process can be strengthened by using adult education theory.[28] All material presented should address a problem that clients perceive is important to them, and clients should be allowed to express themselves and make as many of the decisions regarding their self-care as possible. This strategy meets clients' human need for self-determination and responsibility. It is also important to include family members or friends in the education process because they may be more capable of comprehending the information and asking appropriate questions. Whenever possible it is important to give the client either handwritten instructions or printed materials specific to immediate needs to reinforce the verbal communication.

Education of children may be aided by booklets and videos. Many of these are available about oral healthcare in general, and most children's hospitals have audiovisual departments that produce videos for client education. Some cancer centers now teach children about their disease and its treatment with child-sized puppets with medical apparatus similar to that used during cancer therapy. If available, these puppets can be used for teaching mouth care by including a toothbrush and other oral care products in the puppet's "backpack."

Information about the oral manifestations of the cancer therapy may not have been provided by the physician and nurse; therefore, it is important to ask clients what they understand and then provide additional information that is concise and in an easy-to-understand language. (See the Oral Oncology Research and Cancer Resources chart.) A brief overview of the potential problems is appropriate with assurance that additional information will be given as the therapy progresses.

Oral Hygiene Instruction and Self-Care Assistance with oral hygiene self-care is important prior to initiation of cancer therapy to establish good hygiene before the oral tissues are compromised (see Table 34–7). Use of a disclosing agent aids in instruction and helps the client identify areas that need closer attention in self-care procedures. This also provides an opportunity for the dental hygienist to explain the composition of bacterial plaque and the risk of oral and systemic infections during cancer therapy. Assessment of the client's self-care technique should be accomplished if possible, and the person should be assisted in establishing plaque removal techniques that will be useful prior to and during therapy. If a client is scheduled for therapy that will significantly compromise the oral tissues, initial teaching should be given regarding alternate methods for cleansing the mouth. These methods are then elaborated upon during therapy. Clients also should be warned that because many hospital-supplied toothbrushes are inexpensive and made with unpolished hard bristles, they should take a new extra-soft nylon bristled toothbrush when admitted as hospital inpatients. These dental hygiene strategies facilitate clients' human needs for self-determination and responsibility, and conceptualization and problem solving.

ORAL ONCOLOGY RESEARCH AND CANCER RESOURCES

Oral Oncology
NIDR, National Institute of Dental Research
PO Box 54793
Washington, DC 20032

Cancer Resources
Cancer Information Service (CIS)
1-800-4-CANCER

National, Public, Professional, and Patient Resources
American Cancer Society
1599 Clifton Road, NE
Atlanta, GA 30329
404-320-3333

Leukemia Society of America, Inc.
733 Third Avenue
New York, NY 10017
212-573-8484

American Association of Cancer Education (professional education)
Educational Research and Development
University of Alabama at Birmingham
401 CHSD University Street
Birmingham, AL 35294

Oncology Nursing Society
1016 Greentree Road
Pittsburgh, PA 15220-3125

National Hospice Organization
1901 North Moore Street
Suite 901
Arlington, VA 22209
703-243-5900

Smoking and Alcohol Cessation Counseling Clients usually are told by other members on the oncology team that they should quit using tobacco products and limit excessive alcohol intake during cancer therapy. Reinforcement by the dental hygienist is important. As mentioned earlier in this chapter, there are programs available through the National Cancer Institute and American Cancer Society to aid the dental hygienist in helping clients quit a tobacco habit. Referral to a professional program or support group may be necessary and desired by the client. This strategy serves to meet the client's human need for safety and freedom from stress.

Nutritional Counseling The nutritional status of clients affects their overall response to cancer therapy, as well as their psychological well-being. The nutritionist on the oncology team assumes primary responsibility for monitoring the nutritional status of the client and counseling him on diet selection. The dental hygienist has the responsibility for consulting with the nutritionist and educating the client about diet selection and dietary habits to promote a clean and healthy oral environment and reduce caries development. Before cancer therapy begins, the dental hygienist

TABLE 34–7

ORAL HYGIENE PRODUCTS USED DURING CANCER THERAPY (see CHAPTER 16)

Product	Description	Indication/Rationale/Use	Precautions
Toothbrushes	Several available with extra or super-soft bristles. Some with storage covers. Child-size may be helpful for clients with limited opening. Some available with suctioning capability	Plaque removal after meals when not severely compromised from surgery, chemotherapy, or bone marrow transplantation. Tongue must be brushed, especially in clients on soft or liquid diets	Beware of inexpensive hospital-supplied hard, unpolished bristled toothbrushes. Benefit vs risk of brushing may need to be assessed in clients with severely compromised condition
Floss	Unwaxed or waxed	Important for plaque removal at least 1 time/day	Assess client's dexterity. Assist if necessary. Discontinue only when client is at high risk of bleeding and bacteremia
Dentifrices	Commercial without strong flavoring agents. Paste made from baking soda and water is an alternative	Aid in plaque removal	Strong flavoring agents may intensify mucositis. Fully rinse baking soda residue from oral cavity
Foam or sponge-sticks Large cotton-tipped applicators	Alternative to toothbrushes. Available from medical supply. Some impregnated with cleansing agents	Use to cleanse oral cavity during periods of severe neutropenia when toothbrushing precipitates bleeding. May also be used to apply topical medications	Does not adequately remove plaque. Do not soak in solution; sponge top may fall off stick and client can aspirate. May abrade friable tissue Do not use lemon-glycerine swabs. They are acidic and drying to the tissues
Gauze	Alternative to toothbrush. Use 2 × 2 or 4 × 4 squares	Use to cleanse oral cavity during periods of severe neutropenia when toothbrushing precipitates bleeding. Moisten in water, saline 0.9% (1 tsp NaCl to 16 oz H_2O), or baking soda solution. Wrap around finger and cleanse teeth, tongue and tissues	Does not adequately remove plaque
Baking soda/saline rinse	Mucolytic cleansing solution: ½ tsp baking soda ¼ tsp salt 16 oz water	An alkaline soothing rinse used to cleanse mouth every 2 to 4 hours for clients with mucositis, xerostomia, thick secretions, or after emesis. May be used in irrigation bag to assist in rinsing painful mouth. Rinse with plain water after use	High sodium content. Instruct client not to swallow solution. Not to be used by clients on sodium restricted diet
Isotonic sodium chloride solution (0.9% aqueous)	1 tsp salt 16 oz water	Soothing and cleansing rinse for clients with mucositis. Same concentration as cellular fluids	High sodium content, as above
Hydrogen peroxide 3% diluted with water	Dilute H_2O_2 with 5 parts water or saline solution	To loosen hardened debris in inaccessible area. Treatment of acute oral infection	Should not be used for over 3 days, or in clients with recent oral surgery. May disrupt new granulation tissue. Acidity may be irritating. Continued use may change normal oral flora and result in hairy tongue
Carbamide peroxide 10%	Place several drops on infected area, expectorate after 1 minute	For cleansing area of acute periodontal infection	May be irritating to tissue. Avoid excessive use. Discontinue if infection does not resolve
Chlorhexidine gluconate 0.12%	Bactericidal mouth rinse	Prophylactic or therapeutic mouth rinse to reduce dental plaque and oral microbes. Rinse for 30 seconds with 1 capful b.i.d.	Product available in United States is prepared with alcohol; may be irritating and drying. May cause staining; removable with dental prophylaxis. May alter taste perception
Commercial mouthwashes	Dilute heavily with water	May serve as mouth freshener.	Most commercial mouthwashes have a high concentration of alcohol or phenol which is very drying and irritating to tissues unless diluted heavily with water. Flavoring agents may intensify mucositis

should assess the client's human need for nutrition. From this information, the dental hygienist determines the client's understanding of the relationship of a well-balanced diet to dental caries, periodontal disease, and infection. When the client is ready psychologically to assimilate preventive behaviors, the client and the dental hygienist should choose foods that are desirable to the client but are low in sugar and oral retention qualities. The client should understand that it is often difficult during therapy to eat a well-balanced diet containing foods that promote oral health, but the pretherapy teaching aids the client in setting goals and in food selection.

Dental Hygiene Instrumentation The dental hygienist performs a variety of dental hygiene interventions, as well as other procedures the dentist delegates, such as removal of overhangs and polishing of restorations. A clean and well-hydrated oral environment and control of periodontal disease reduces the risk of oral infection and bacteremia.

Fluoride Therapy When the client is scheduled for radiation therapy to the salivary glands or total body irradiation for BMT, custom fluoride gel trays are fabricated for daily application of either 0.4% stannous fluoride gel or 1% neutral pH sodium fluoride gel to prevent rampant dental caries. The dental hygienist may be responsible for taking impressions for study models to fabricate the custom trays (Fig. 34–6). These may be sent to a dental laboratory or the trays may be made in the dental clinic using a vacuum unit. The fluoride trays are made from a soft-vinyl mouthguard material. They should be adapted to extend slightly above the cervical line of the teeth, with full coverage of all teeth. The tray edges *must* be absolutely smooth and nonirritating to the client's oral tissues to prevent soft tissue breakdown. The client begins use of the fluoride trays at the initiation of therapy. Clients are instructed to first brush and floss their teeth and then place a thin ribbon of fluoride gel in each of the trays. They place the trays on their teeth and leave them in place for 5 to 10 minutes. Upon removal, they rinse the trays well with water, but do not rinse their mouth or eat anything for 30 minutes. This must be done once each day. It is important to let the client decide upon a time of day when cooperation with the routine is most likely. Many clients feel it is easiest to use the trays when they are bathing or showering. In this way, the procedure is incorporated into a regular daily routine.

During Cancer Therapy

Once therapy has been initiated it is important to continue to support the client, but the dental hygienist must understand that most cancer therapy is physically and psychologically demanding. Unrealistic scheduling of appointments must be avoided. Frequent phone calls to the client or family member emphasize the importance of regular oral hygiene self-care and help in determining when it is appropriate to schedule the client for dental hygiene care and further education.

With each appointment, the dental hygienist should repeat the oral assessment, update the health history, and assess the client's human needs to determine his level of disease acceptance and readiness for new interventions. It must be remembered that anger and bargaining may be signs of acceptance of the diagnosis and an attempt to regain control of his life. These times offer the dental hygienist an opportunity to direct the client's interest to positive involvement in oral self-care and dietary planning. An attempt should be made to incorporate the client as much as possible into decisions about the dental hygiene care plan and self-care. Education during care should be centered on the immediate real and impending complications of therapy.

Clients Undergoing Chemotherapy When scheduling a client undergoing chemotherapy for an appointment it is imperative to consult the oncologist regarding the status of the client's blood counts and clotting factors (See the Blood Count Guidelines for Dental Treatment During Chemotherapy chart). As previously mentioned, many chemotherapeutic agents suppress the bone marrow, resulting in immunosuppression and bleeding problems. A dental procedure could initiate uncontrolled bleeding or result in a bacteremia causing sepsis and death. The final decision regarding the safest time to schedule oral health care appointments is made by the oncologist. If necessary, the

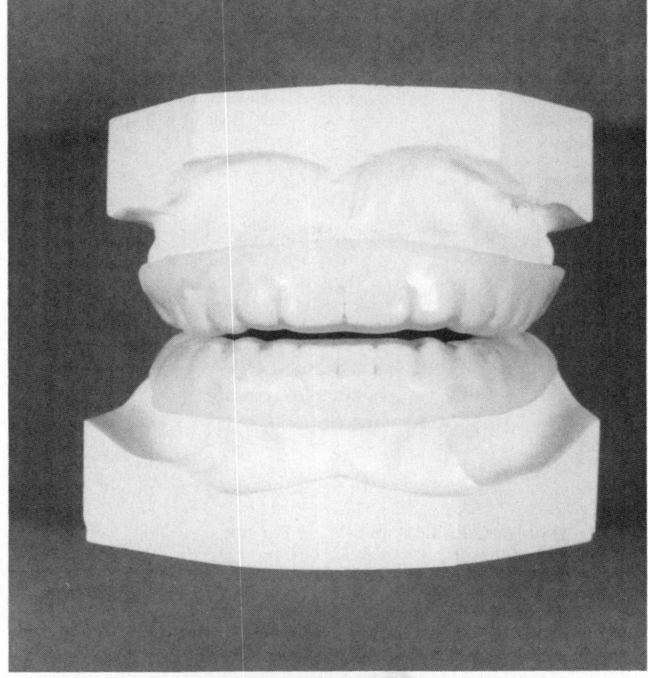

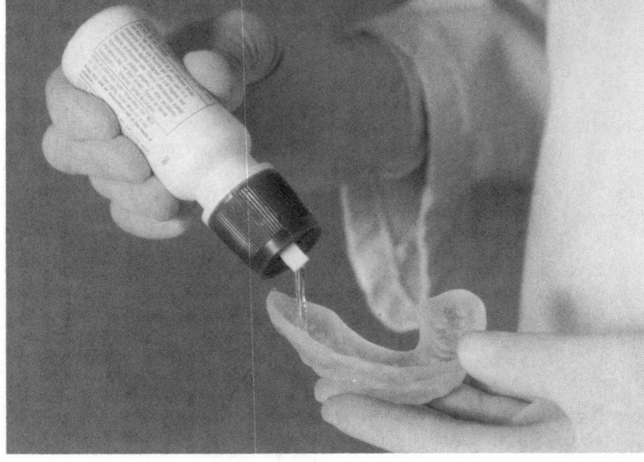

FIGURE 34–6
Custom fluoride trays.

BLOOD COUNT GUIDELINES FOR DENTAL/ DENTAL HYGIENE CARE DURING CHEMOTHERAPY*

- Absolute neutrophil (granulocyte) count more than 1,000/mm^3
- Adequate clotting factors
- Platelet count more than 50,000/mm^3

* Consultation with oncologist is imperative

oncologist may recommend antibiotic prophylaxis prior to dental and dental hygiene care.

Another reason for antibiotic prophylaxis prior to dental treatment exists when the client has an indwelling central venous catheter for delivery of chemotherapy (Fig. 34–7). Some individuals begin chemotherapy without a central venous catheter but have one placed later during therapy. Therefore, in order to meet the client's human need for safety, each time a client is seen it is necessary to ask if he currently has one in place. As previously stated, the catheter may become contaminated from bacteria or fungi, or bacterial endocarditis may occur after a dental or dental hygiene procedure. Jaspers and Little described the risk of endocarditis as intermediate.[29] Currently no data are available to indicate which prophylactic antibiotic regimen should be used in this patient population prior to dental procedures. Spuller recommends the current American Heart Association endocarditis prophylaxis special regimen because of the prevalence of catheter sepsis and endocarditis.[30] (See Chapter 10 for antibiotic premedication.) Again, the oncologist should be consulted, and ultimately it is her decision as to what antibiotics are necessary.

When the client has immunosuppression and/or is experiencing mucositis and oral ulcerations (deficits in the human need for skin and mucous membrane integrity) it is important to offer suggestions to aid in keeping the mouth clean and well hydrated. The risk of oral and systemic infection increases when bacterial plaque is not consistently and mechanically removed. It may be difficult for the client to practice routine care when the mouth is inflamed and ulcerated. The pain from mucositis can be so extreme that it is impossible to brush the teeth and even difficult to swish water in the mouth.

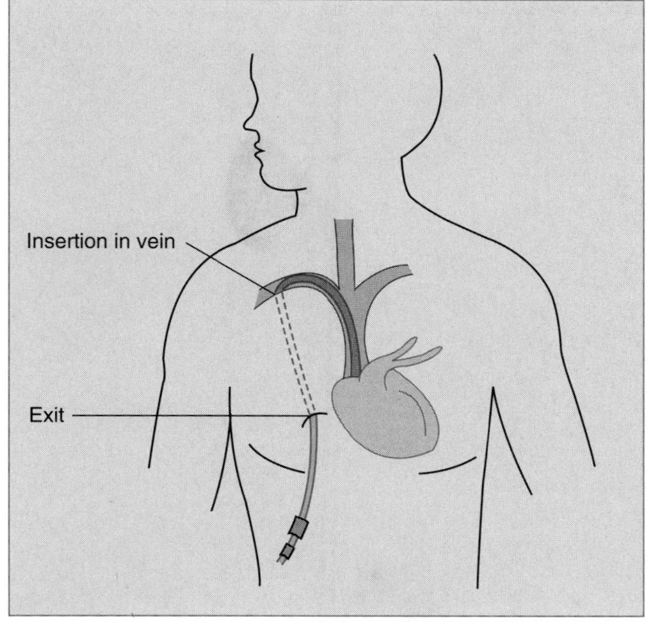

FIGURE 34–7
Placement of an indwelling central venous catheter.

Some cancer centers have clients discontinue toothbrushing and flossing when they have severe myelosuppression. This practice is controversial, however, because careful toothbrushing and flossing decrease bacterial plaque and local infection and therefore reduce the risk of potentially life-threatening systemic infection.[31] Oral hygiene procedures must be tailored to the individual's skill and condition but must not cause mucosal trauma. Toothbrushes are available that are super-soft and nonabrasive. Sponge sticks and large moist cotton-tipped applicators are supplied for oral care to hospitals through medical supply companies. These devices and moistened gauze are not as effective in bacterial plaque control. A suction toothbrush is available commercially, or one can be made by drilling a hole in the back of the head of a toothbrush and attaching suction tubing. Figure 34–8 illustrates several oral hygiene aids for medically compromised individuals. When nondisposable products are used, they must be rinsed well and kept dry. Rinsing in an antimicrobial solution may be advisable. Disposable products should never be reused. Regardless of the means for mechanical plaque removal, the client should be encouraged to rinse frequently with sodium bicarbonate or saline water rinses. This soothes and hydrates the inflamed tissues, aids in bacterial plaque removal, and neutralizes pH if the client is vomiting. A useful method for irrigating the mouth during episodes of painful mucositis is shown in Figure 34–9. The disposable enema or irrigation bag is hung over a sink and filled with a solution of 1 tsp of baking soda, ½ tsp of salt, and 32 oz of water. The solution is directed throughout the mouth with the hose and is allowed to flow out into the sink to avoid swallowing.

Use of mouth rinses that contain alcohol or phenol are contraindicated because they are drying and irritating. Chlorhexidine gluconate mouth rinse has been shown in some studies to be beneficial in reducing oral infections and severity of mucositis during cancer therapy.[32] These rinses, when prepared with alcohol, should be evaluated for their antimicrobial benefit versus the irritating effect of the alcohol (Table 34–7). High pressure water irrigating devices are not recommended during periods of immunosuppression and thrombocytopenia because of the risk of bacteremia and bleeding. When the client's condition is not compromised he should be scheduled for regular preventive oral healthcare. (Table 34–8 shows a sample dental hygiene care plan during cancer therapy.)

Clients with mucositis and ulceration sometimes require topical anesthetics and coating agents in addition to the soothing bland rinses (See the Topical Anesthetics and Coating Agents for Palliation of Mucositis During Cancer Therapy chart). To meet the human need for safety, all clients, especially children and their parents, should be cautioned that the agents may anesthetize the soft palate and epiglottis, potentially causing aspiration of food. Excessive use may potentiate mucositis. Some clients require systemic analgesics and sometimes even narcotics to control the pain of mucositis.

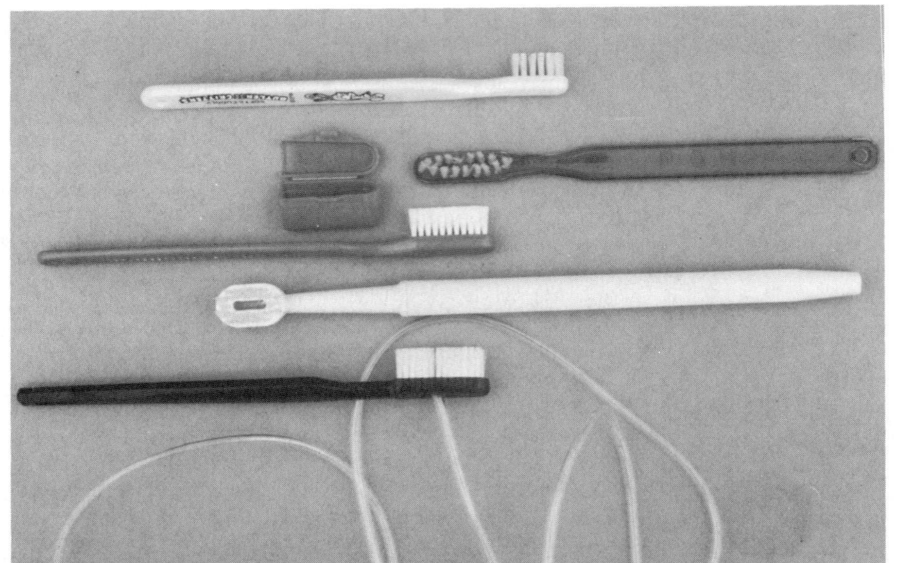

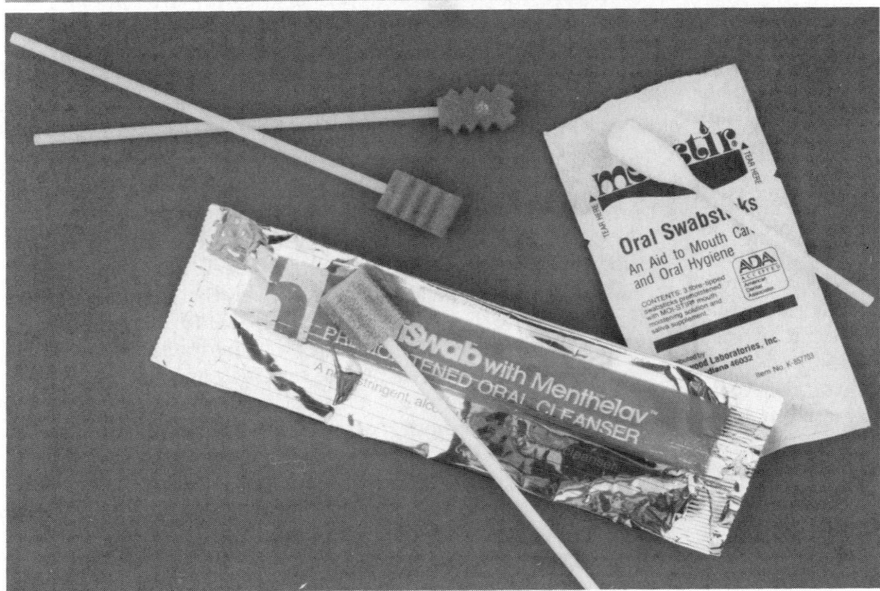

FIGURE 34–8
Oral hygiene aids for medically-compromised individuals.

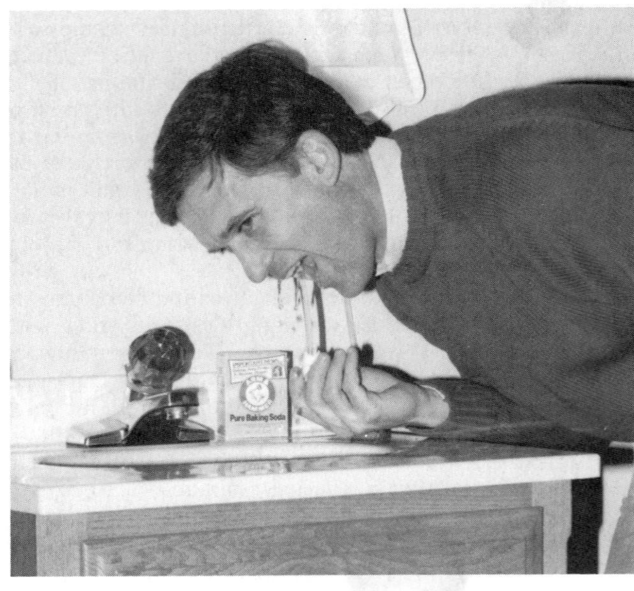

FIGURE 34–9
Irrigation of mouth during episodes of painful mucositis.

TABLE 34–8
SAMPLE DENTAL HYGIENE CARE PLAN DURING CANCER THERAPY

Dental Hygiene Diagnosis	Goal/Expected Behavior	Dental Hygiene Interventions	Evaluative Statements
Deficit in the need for safety: potential for oral infection	By 3/15, client will have mucosal tissues that are within normal limits for therapy protocol without evidence of infection	Request that physician order for culture of suspicious lesions Listen to client's concerns about cancer therapy Reassure client Refer client to dietitian for nutritional counseling Teach client about risk of oral infection leading to sepsis, and self-care inspection and preventive measures Refer client to dentist for dental diagnosis	Teeth and oral tissue free from soft and hard deposits and exudate Oral tissue remains intact without evidence of excessive bleeding Client reports alterations in oral tissues Client understands relationship of oral health and decreased infections Client lists measures to prevent oral infection Client complies with dental and nutritional referrals

Potential bleeding problems associated with chemotherapy can be avoided by careful assessment of the client's clotting factors and bleeding times and consultation with the oncologist. Generally, a platelet count of at least 50,000/mm^3 is recommended prior to invasive dental or dental hygiene procedures.[33] If a dental or dental hygiene procedure is absolutely necessary during periods of thrombocytopenia, platelet support therapy may be given by the oncologist. Adequate bleeding times are dependent upon the extent of the oral procedure. The client should also be warned that trauma from improper toothbrushing or a poorly fitting dental prosthesis may initiate bleeding when platelets are low.

TOPICAL ANESTHETICS AND COATING AGENTS FOR PALLIATION OF MUCOSITIS DURING CANCER THERAPY

Prescribed by Physician or Dentist

Topical Anesthetic		Coating Agent
Diphenhydramine hydrochloride (parenteral form without alcohol)	mixed with	Kaopectate[a] Maalox[b] Alternagel[c] Carafate suspension[d]

Lidocaine viscous, 2%
Dyclonine hydrochloride

Over-the-counter Products

Benylin Cough Syrup[e]/Kaopectate[a] or other coating agent mixed 1:1
Benzocaine in Orabase[f] (for isolated ulcers)
Oratect Gel[g] (for isolated ulcers)

Warning

- Excessive use of topical anesthetics and coating agents may potentiate mucositis
- Topical anesthetics may decrease gag reflex, resulting in aspiration of food
- Mixtures should not be swallowed
- Excellent oral hygiene must be maintained when using coating agents; many contain high concentration of sugar

[a] Upjohn Co., Kalamazoo, MI
[b] Rorer Consumer, Fort Washington, PA
[c] Stuart Pharmaceuticals, Wilmington, DE
[d] Marion Laboratories, Kansas City, MO
[e] Parke-Davis, Div. of Warner Lambert, Morris Plains, NJ
[f] Colgate-Hoyt, Norwood, MA
[g] MGI PHARMA, Inc., Minneapolis, MN

All persons on chemotherapy do not experience xerostomia or ropy saliva, but when they do they should be offered palliative measures to help manage this debilitating and uncomfortable side effect. Commercial saliva substitutes are available as over-the-counter products. They have the advantage over plain water because they contain carboxymethylcellulose, a lubricating viscous agent, and they have the minerals and electrolytes found in normal saliva. Some have fluoride to help prevent dental caries. However, they do not contain the protective proteins and mucoproteins found in saliva. They usually offer the client longer lasting relief than plain water, but some clients do not feel the cost is justified for the limited relief. Some clients make their own lubricating solution by adding ½ tsp of glycerine to 8 oz of water. The glycerine adds a lubricating ingredient to the water. Additional suggestions for a dry mouth include: rinsing frequently with baking soda or saline, letting ice chips melt in the mouth, or sucking on sugarless popsicles. Some stimulation of the salivary glands may be possible with sugarless gum or candies. Rooms should be humidified with cool-mist humidifiers. Tobacco, alcohol, and alcohol-containing products should be strongly discouraged because of their drying effects. The lips should be lubricated with a water-based lubricant or lanolin. Pure petrolatum provides only an occlusive agent and does not moisturize the perioral tissues. (See the Suggestions for Xerostomia chart.)

Clients with dentures should be evaluated frequently and encouraged to call the dental office whenever necessary to seek early intervention for an oral complication or dental-related sources of pain, irritation, or dental trauma. Oral tissues may change significantly during chemotherapy from edema, inflammation, ulceration, and/or weight loss. Clients should understand that when denture irritation occurs, the prosthesis should be removed from the mouth to avoid further trauma. Persons with oral infections may reinfect their mouths with poorly cleansed dentures. It is

SUGGESTIONS FOR XEROSTOMIA

Saliva Substitutes

Commercial saliva substitutes offer limited duration of relief from xerostomia

Xero-lube	Scherer Laboratories, Dallas, TX
Salivart	Westport Pharmaceuticals, Westport, CT
Moi-Stir	Kingswood Laboratories, Carmel, IN
Mouth-Kote	Parnell Pharmaceuticals, Foster City, CA
Oral Balance	Laclede Research Labs, Gardena, CA

Moisture Replacement

High-moisture foods (gelatins, melons, ices, sugar-free popsicles, and ice chips)
Air humidifier
Frequent baking soda and saline rinses

Saliva Stimulants

Sugar-free candies (citrus-flavored)
Sugar-free chewing gum

Lip Care

Moisten lips with water-based lubricant; then coat with lanolin or lip balm with wax base or petrolatum

Avoid

Tobacco products
Alcohol
Highly seasoned foods
Commercial mouthwash containing alcohol or phenol

important for the client to clean and disinfect the dentures daily and keep them out of the mouth while sleeping. Denture soaking solutions must be changed daily and the soaking container cleansed and rinsed thoroughly.

Clients Undergoing Radiation Therapy to the Oral Cavity and Salivary Glands

The client undergoing radiation therapy to the oral cavity and salivary glands begins to experience some of the side effects after the first week of therapy. If all nonsurgical dental or dental hygiene procedures have not been accomplished prior to initiation of radiation, they should be done within the first 2 weeks of therapy before the onset of mucositis. Throughout therapy, it is important to support the client with suggestions to palliate the acute symptoms of radiation therapy and provide oral hygiene care that will assist in keeping the mouth clean.

A clean, well-hydrated mouth during radiation therapy reduces the severity of mucosal ulceration and risk of oral infection. Once the client begins to experience mucositis, it is necessary to modify oral hygiene procedures to be nonirritating and atraumatic but adequate to remove bacterial plaque and thickened saliva. (See the Oral Hygiene Measures During Radiation Therapy chart.) Toothbrushes should be extra soft and may be further softened in hot water. Use of commercial toothpastes with strong flavoring agents may have to be temporarily discontinued and replaced with a paste made of baking soda and water. If toothbrushing becomes impossible because of painful tissues, the teeth, gingiva, and tongue may be swabbed with gauze moistened in warm water. Frequent mouth rinses of baking soda and/or saline water should be suggested. Use of an irrigation bag, as described under the section on chemotherapy, is helpful when the mouth is too sore to swish the mouth rinse. Dental flossing should be continued as long as possible and resumed as soon as the mucositis resolves. All commercial mouthwashes with alcohol or phenol should be avoided because of their drying and irritating effects. Although half-strength peroxide and water solutions are sometimes used in hospitals to remove encrusted secretions or for acute infections, they are not recommended for long-term use because they are acidic and may alter the normal oral flora. Some dental oncology units at major cancer centers use a 10% carbamide peroxide preparation for short-term control of acute periodontal infections.

Clients with dentures should be instructed to leave the dentures out of their mouths as often as possible. If the field of radiation encompasses all of the oral tissues, it may be impossible for the client to wear dentures because of significant oral tissue changes from edema and inflammation. The client should keep the dentures as clean as possible and should store them in a soaking solution that is changed daily to avoid microbial contamination. These clients often eat a soft or liquid diet and the tongue becomes coated and infected. Therefore, they should understand also the importance of keeping the mouth well cleansed and the tongue brushed.

These clients begin to experience a change in their saliva after the first week of radiation. They first complain of a thickened and ropy saliva, and as the treatments progress their mouths become dryer. One long-term study of 42 persons who had undergone cancericidal doses of radiation therapy to all of the major salivary glands at M. D. Anderson Hospital in Houston reported a 67% decrease in saliva after 1 week of radiation, a 76% loss after 6 weeks, and a 95% loss 3 years after completion of radiation.[34] Clients who undergo radiation therapy to the neck involving the submandibular and sublingual salivary glands with only partial inclusion of the parotid glands complain mostly of a thick ropy saliva. These clients benefit greatly from the baking soda and saline water rinses. A baking soda solution is mucolytic, which aids in cleansing and refreshing the mouth. Suggestions for xerostomia are in the box at the top of this page. Studies have demonstrated the effectiveness of a pharmaceutical sialogogue, pilocarpine, for stimulation of residual salivary gland tissue.[35,36]

ORAL HYGIENE MEASURES DURING RADIATION THERAPY

Recommend	Avoid
Extra-soft bristled toothbrush, or if necessary moist gauze wrapped around finger, or sponge or cotton-tipped applicator	Unpolished hard-bristled toothbrush
Bland toothpaste or paste made with baking soda and water	Mouthwash with alcohol or phenol
Dental flossing without injury	Peroxide rinses
Baking soda, salt water rinses (irrigation bag for delivery)	Cleansing agents with irritating flavoring agents

All clients receiving cancericidal doses of radiation therapy to any of the salivary glands must have custom fluoride trays made for daily application of a fluoride gel to aid in prevention of rampant tooth demineralization. There may be a period of time during therapy when severe mucositis prevents fluoride application. During this time, the client is encouraged to increase oral rinses and hydration of tissues and resume the daily fluoride gel application as soon as the mucositis resolves.

When the tongue is in the field of radiation the client experiences a partial or full taste loss. This is an acute effect, and usually the taste sense returns after healing from the total radiation. Although taste loss may not appear to be a significant side effect, it is one that makes radiation therapy almost intolerable. Eating becomes a chore, clients complain that all food tastes like mush or straw, and their human need for nutrition suffers. The clients are helped by having someone listen to their complaints. They should be assured that taste dysfunction is a normal side effect of radiation but they should be encouraged to continue eating. Referral for nutritional counseling may be necessary to avoid weight loss and medical complications.

Usually by the third week of radiation the client begins to experience mucosal inflammation and pain, and as the treatments progress small ulcerations enlarge to a confluent and pseudomembraneous mucositis. Severe mucositis sometimes requires a short interruption of therapy to allow regeneration of normal cells. Topical anesthetics and coating agents give temporary relief but often the need for freedom from pain requires systemic analgesics. The same agents used for chemotherapy-induced mucositis may be recommended. Highly seasoned foods and strong flavoring agents found in dentifrices may not be tolerated.

The client receiving radiation therapy to the muscles of mastication should be placed on an exercise program to prevent fibrosis of the muscles and trismus. The jaw should be exercised three times a day by opening and closing the mouth, 20 times, as wide as possible without causing pain.

During radiation therapy, care of the perioral tissues should be directed by the radiation oncologist. Some lip lubricants can potentiate the effects of the radiation and cause significant radiation dermatitis. Physicians order their preferred product for skin care during therapy.

Clients Undergoing Bone Marrow Transplantation

Once the client has entered the BMT center, he is not allowed to leave the unit until the bone marrow has engrafted and his blood counts have returned to a normal range. Therefore, all dental treatment must be accomplished prior to the transplant. A dental hygienist working in a hospital setting with a BMT unit may assist with daily oral assessment and oral hygiene procedures. Oral care regimens vary among transplant centers, but generally oral care is given every 2 to 4 hours. Protocols range from simple saline rinses and antimicrobial rinses to aggressive oral débridement.

Nutritional Counseling During Cancer Therapy

The side effects of cancer therapy often result in high risk for dental caries. The client may be placed on a soft and bland diet or liquid high carbohydrate diet because of recent oral surgery and/or mucositis from therapy. They may also be encouraged to eat small frequent meals and snacks to increase their caloric intake and counteract nausea and vomiting. Additional complications arise from a dry mouth or thickened saliva, taste dysfunction, inability to practice good oral hygiene because of an oral surgical procedure, and/or a lack of interest in eating because of depression and stress. When severely malnourished, the client may be placed on parenteral nutrition, completely eliminating the mechanical oral cleansing action of foods.

Diets of children during cancer therapy are often a problem because there are so many times when the child is too sick to eat that parents allow them to eat anything they want when they are feeling well. Regular meals, especially in a pediatric hospital setting, are difficult to achieve.

In working with the nutritionist, the dental hygienist should continue to emphasize the importance of a well-balanced diet for prevention of infection and promotion of healing after the insult of therapy. In turn, the nutritionist can assist the client in planning meals low in sugar when possible. The suggestion may also be made to add cheeses to the diet when eating sugar-containing foods to reduce cariogenicity.

When possible, the dental hygienist should alert other oncology team members about the high concentration of sugar in some medications, especially antifungal suspensions. Alternatives may be suggested, such as sugar-free troches or suppositories.

Clients with a painful mouth may be helped by suggesting one of the topical anesthetic or coating agents prior to eating mentioned in the box on page 973. Also, the client with oral ulcerations or a dry mouth may find it helpful to eat foods high in moisture or they may thin their food with liquids and take frequent sips of water while eating. Irritating hot, spicy, or acidic foods should be avoided. All meals and snacks should be followed by oral hygiene measures and adequate hydration of the tissues.

A client who has had an oral surgical resection should be encouraged to use a spoon to place small bites of food on the unaffected side and as far back as possible. Forks should be avoided until incisions heal. It may be necessary for clients to feed themselves liquids with a large syringe.

The Client Following Cancer Therapy

Following any kind of cancer therapy, the dental hygienist continues to have an important role in the care of the client. With each appointment or contact with the client the dental hygienist must reassess the client's human needs related to oral health and disease. Even when clients have been reassured that their cancer has successfully responded to therapy, they continue to experience stress, anxiety, and concern about possible recurrence of the cancer. Some need to continue to adapt to an altered body image resulting from the long-term side effects of the therapy. Some clients continue to be dependent on the caregivers and need to reestablish their independence and regain their self-confidence. Occasionally individuals treated for cancer want to place everything associated with the cancer therapy behind them and ignore critical preventive long-term self-care procedures. Continued education and frequent contact and support are essential. The dental hygienist should tailor the client's oral self-care to the individual's status and human needs, and place as much responsibility on the client as possible.

The Client After Head and Neck Surgery

The person who has surgery for oral cancer often requires a long postoperative hospital course. A dental hygienist working in a hospital can offer to provide nursing inservice sessions on oral assessment and oral hygiene care during cancer therapy. Eilers and colleagues published an excellent article on developing a nursing inservice program.[37] Additional resources are shown in the box on page 968. Acting as a liaison between the surgical and dental teams, the dental hygienist can facilitate ongoing prosthodontic and oral surgery consultations. The dental hygienist also may work with the client teaching insertion, removal, and cleansing of a surgical prosthesis or stent. The oral tissues need frequent assessment for irritation and comfort. The oral cavity and all remaining teeth must be maintained in optimal condition with frequent gentle cleansing and hydration. This is usually accomplished with irrigation bag or bulb syringe saline rinses and gentle débridement with large cotton-tipped applicators, sponge swabs, or gauze. Care must be taken when cleansing and suctioning not to disrupt new granulation tissue.

The Client After Radiation Therapy to the Oral Cavity and Salivary Glands

The care of the client after radiation therapy to the oral cavity and salivary glands requires lifelong frequent dental and dental hygiene maintenance care. Because damage from cancericidal dose radiation therapy to the salivary glands and jaw bones is permanent, clients are at permanent risk for development of rampant "radiation caries" or demineralization of the tooth structure and osteoradionecrosis. Continued care appointments are scheduled at intervals to ensure excellent oral hygiene, maintenance of sound tooth structure, and avoidance of soft tissue irritation. The use of the custom fluoride trays with fluoride gel must continue on a daily basis for the rest of the client's life.

With each appointment the dental hygienist should assess the client's nutritional status and dietary intake. Adjustments should be made to return to a normal and noncariogenic diet as the acute side effects of radiation therapy resolve. Referral for nutritional counseling may be necessary (Table 34–9).

A thorough head and neck assessment for oral cancer and function of the muscles of mastication, temporomandibular joint, and prosthetic appliances should be done at each appointment. Deficits in the needs for integrity of the skin and mucous membrane of the head and neck and for biologically sound dentition require immediate referral to the dentist. Dental disease in an area of irradiated bone is managed as conservatively and as atraumatically as possible and sometimes is accompanied with antibiotic prophylaxis. If trismus occurs, treatment consists of introducing tongue blades between the teeth for several minutes each day, gradually increasing the number until adequate opening is achieved. This may be painful and requires patience and perseverance. Dental treatment of osteoradionecrosis is conservative but generally requires conservative surgical removal of necrotic tissue, antibiotics to prevent infection, and, ideally, hyperbaric oxygen therapy to stimulate vascularization and new bone growth. When conservative measures fail, surgical resection is usually indicated.

The Client After Chemotherapy

Once a client has completed the required rounds of chemotherapy, most of the oral manifestations completely resolve. With full recovery of the bone marrow, all problems associated with acute cytotoxicity, immunosuppression, and thrombocytopenia should disappear. Some clients, after long and intensive chemotherapy, take months to recover fully and experience chronic oral infections such as candidiasis and herpetic infections. Continual assistance with oral hygiene is required to prevent unnecessary infections. Assessment of clients' nutritional intake is important to determine if they have resumed a noncariogenic and normal diet.

The Client After Bone Marrow Transplantation

After clients are released from a transplant unit they may have residual effects of the conditioning phase of treatment and may remain susceptible to infections for several months because of immunosuppressive therapy. Some continue to experience xerostomia which predisposes them to an altered oral flora and infections, trauma, and rampant dental caries. Clients with graft-versus-host-disease experience additional complications of a thinned and friable mucosa and mucosal lesions.

The dental hygienist must assist the client in establishing consistent and effective oral hygiene methods that do not create additional trauma and irritation. Bland rinses, gentle but thorough and consistent cleansing of the teeth and tissues, and saliva substitutes are important.

TABLE 34–9
SAMPLE DENTAL HYGIENE CARE PLAN AFTER CANCER THERAPY

Dental Hygiene Diagnosis	Goal/Expected Behavior	Dental Hygiene Interventions	Evaluative Statements
Deficit in the need for nutrition	By 12/6, client will be able to masticate food without pain By 12/6, client will consume adequate food to maintain weight	Refer client to a prosthodontist for rehabilitation Make nutritional referral; consult with nutritionist about cariogenic food to avoid Encourage self-feeding and food selection Reinforce nutritionist's recommendations	Client reports daily intake consistent with recommendations Client's weight within 10% of standard body weight

PROCEDURE 34–1

PERFORMING ORAL HYGIENE CARE FOR NONAMBULATORY CLIENTS

Equipment

Protective gloves, face mask, protective eyewear
Towel
Extra-soft toothbrush with suction (adapted toothbrush or suction equipment)
Dental floss and holder
Bite block
Cleansing agent: ingestible toothpaste, baking soda, and/or denture cleanser
Pitcher of water and cup or bulb syringe or irrigation bag filled with water and hung on an intravenous pole
Water-based lubricant
Emesis basin

Steps	Rationale
1. Position bed to comfortable height	Facilitates access and acceptable body mechanics for the dental hygienist
2. Don face mask and protective eyewear; wash and glove hands	Maintains universal infection control protocol
3. Position client; sitting, or on side	Facilitates drainage and prevents aspiration of debris and fluids
4. Place towel under client's head	Maintains position and comfort of the client
5. Place emesis basin at chin	Facilitates drainage of saliva and debris from the client's mouth
6. Assemble suction equipment	Suction equipment prevents aspiration of saliva and debris
7. Position bite block between teeth if necessary	Aids client in keeping the mouth open
8. Apply lubricant to lips	Prevents trauma to dry lips
9. Assess oral cavity	Enables dental hygienist to identify needs and plan appropriate care
10. Cleanse teeth, tongue, and mucosal tissues with appropriate technique and aids (dependent upon client's condition)	Provides both palliative and therapeutic oral care; a clean, well-hydrated oral environment reduces the risk of oral infection and bacteremia
11. Suction, rinse with clear water, repeat suction (catch return flow in basin)	Facilitates removal of oral debris and client comfort
12. Apply lubricant to lips	Prevents trauma to dry lips
13. If client has dentures, brush dentures over towel-lined sink and soak in clean soaking solution, rinse well; either put back in client's mouth or store in clean water; instruct client to leave dentures out of mouth while sleeping	Provides palliative, cosmetic, and therapeutic care to the edentulous client; prevents damage to dentures; promotes client comfort; prevents oral infection
14. Saliva substitute may be palliative	Increases client comfort
15. Excessive drooling may require a gentle suction device	Facilitates removal of oral debris and client comfort

Deficits in the needs for integrity of the skin and mucous membrane of the head and neck and for a biologically sound dentition should be immediately referred for dental evaluation and treatment. Dental procedures deemed necessary are done only after consultation with the oncologist to assess the client's immune status and need for antibiotic prophylaxis or platelet support. Elective dental procedures are delayed until the client has full hematological function, sometimes up to a year or longer after treatment. Rampant dental caries from xerostomia are prevented with daily application of fluoride gel in custom fluoride trays.

The Client with End-Stage Disease

Oral and dental care is sometimes ignored during this stage of life, but a mouth free of discomfort and bad odors is extremely important. The mouth becomes the center of existence during terminal disease because it maintains nutritional status and is used to communicate needs and emotions to loved ones. A mouth free of bad odors helps to maintain self-esteem and aids in social communication, preventing some of the loneliness experienced during the terminal stage. All care must be designed to provide quality of life and the best care *for the client's needs.* Care that enhances the person's dignity and facilitates personal comfort, normal eating, and social communication is of critical importance.

The dental hygienist should provide education about the importance of oral hygiene for the client, family, hospice volunteers, and other caregivers. Many people do not realize how important the mouth becomes to the dying individual. Simple explanations and procedures reduce the stress related to this time period. This is also a wonderful way for family members to assist in the care of their loved one because it aids so much in their overall comfort. This may be especially true for parents of dying children. Many medical procedures must be done by nurses or physicians, but oral care procedures are simple and provide an opportunity for the parent to participate with tender care.

The dental hygienist can help the client and other caregivers to design oral hygiene procedures that effectively remove plaque but are nonirritating and provide adequate tissue hydration. All highly-flavored dentifrices and mouthwashes should be avoided. A small amount of pleasant-flavored mouthwash may be added to water to refresh the client's mouth. Saliva substitutes may be important for the client with xerostomia. Baking soda and saline solutions aid in cleansing thickened secretions from the mouth.

Procedures may need to be designed for bed-ridden clients. (See Procedure 34–1.) The client should be rolled on the side or placed in a sitting position to prevent aspiration. If necessary, a bite block should be placed between the teeth on one side which later can be placed on the other side to aid in cleansing each area of the mouth. The lips may be lubricated with a water-based lubricant. Petrolatum-based products should be avoided because aspiration of nonwater-soluble agents can result in pneumonia. The teeth, tongue, and buccal mucosa are cleansed either with dental floss and an extra-soft toothbrush or gauze dampened in warm water or a moistened sponge stick. An ingestible toothpaste is available commercially. A bulb syringe and small basin may be helpful for delivering and collecting the rinses and water.

Clients with dentures should be encouraged to wear their dentures as long as they fit well and do not irritate the tissues. They must be kept immaculately clean and kept out of the mouth while the client is sleeping. Clients with ill-fitting dentures should be referred to a dentist for care.

Clients with xerostomia may need daily application of fluoride gel to prevent rampant tooth decay. Even though death is anticipated, avoidance of potential dental problems that could result in oral discomfort or infection should be prevented with referral for dental evaluation and treatment. Clients with excessive drooling may need a gentle suction device. Medications may be ordered by the physician to help reduce salivary flow.

Evaluation

The needs of clients with cancer vary tremendously, depending on stage of disease, treatment, and psychological status. Dental hygiene interventions play an important role in reducing the risks of the disease and its treatment, and in meeting clients' human needs to promote quality of life. These interventions are evaluated repeatedly by the clients' responses as they move through the various phases of treatment and psychological adjustments to their disease (Table 34–10).

PSYCHOSOCIAL SUPPORT FOR THE PROFESSIONAL

Working with the client with cancer may be very rewarding but also may be stressful and difficult. Medical and oral health professionals who treat clients with terminal disease must be able to accept death as part of life and acknowledge their own mortality. The fact that some persons are going to die because all therapy is not curative must be accepted by the oncology team. This may be difficult for dental hygienists because of their strong association with

TABLE 34–10
SAMPLE EVALUATION OF DENTAL HYGIENE INTERVENTIONS

Goals	Evaluative Measures	Evaluative Statement
By 5/1, client participates in design/practice of oral self-care	Apply disclosing agent to teeth Inspect the oral cavity and teeth for evidence of bacterial plaque, gingival inflammation Utilize standardized measurements and indices Observe the client's self-care skills Observe the client demonstrate self-care routine correctly Listen as the client verbalizes oral health knowledge	Goal met. Teeth and oral tissues free of bacterial plaque Goal met. No evidence of gingival inflammation or bleeding Goal partially met. Improvement in oral hygiene standardized measurement scores
By 5/15, client's mucous membrane is of normal color and texture; integrity intact, without debris, bacterial plaque, or bleeding	Inspect oral tissues for presence of inflammation, bleeding, debris, and/or exudate Inspect integrity of mucosal tissues Palpate tissues for tenderness Observe client's verbal and nonverbal response	Goal met. Teeth and oral tissues free of soft and hard deposits, exudates Goal met. Oral tissue intact without evidence of inflammation or bleeding
By 6/20, client is able to adequately masticate food without pain, consume adequate food to maintain weight, and report daily diet without high cariogenic foods	Weigh client Inspect and discuss daily diet	Goal not met. Client weight not within 10% of standard body weight Goal not met. Client reports daily diet intake inconsistent with recommendations

preventive medicine. Another difficult task may be dealing with their own vulnerability to cancer.

Professionals must maintain a balance between the needs of their clients and their personal needs. Maintaining open communication with other oncology team members about personal frustrations, feelings of guilt for not being able to help a client, and personal sadness and grief for the loss of a client help to abate overwhelming feelings and depression. A well-balanced life of work and recreation also is important.

The positive aspects of working in oncology come from the association with individuals who are acutely aware of their priorities in life and must focus on living one day at a time. So many of these clients share their personal strengths with their caregivers. By being open and receptive, one can learn many important lessons from them. Another benefit comes from being able to provide care that offers immediate and significant improvement in the quality of life. When clients understand the importance of good oral hygiene during therapy and when palliative measures give comfort and reduce stress, they are openly and intensely appreciative. Keeping these aspects in mind compensates for negative feelings and provides a professional environment that is stimulating, challenging, and very gratifying.

References

1. National Institutes of Health. Consensus development conference on oral complications of cancer therapies: Diagnosis, prevention, and treatment. Journal of the American Dental Association 119:179, 1989.
2. American Cancer Society. Cancer Facts and Figures—1993. Atlanta, GA: 1993.
3. Groenwald, S. L., Grogge, M. H., et al. Cancer Nursing Principles and Practice, 2nd ed. Boston: Jones and Bartlett, 1990, pp. 347–357.
4. Kubler-Ross, E. On Death and Dying. New York: Macmillan, 1969, pp. 38–137.
5. Hinton, J. The cancer ward. Advances in Psychosomatic Medicine 10:78, 1980.
6. Spinetta, J. J., Deasy-Spinetta, P., et al. Emotional Aspects of Childhood Leukemia, A Handbook for Parents. New York: Leukemia Society of America, 1986.
7. Silverman, S. Oral Cancer, 3rd ed. Atlanta: American Cancer Society, 1990.
8. Shafer, W. G., and Waldron, C. A. Erythroplakia of the oral cavity. Cancer 36:1021, 1975.
9. Mashberg, A., and Samit, A. M. Early detection, diagnosis, and management of oral and oropharyngeal cancer. CA 39(2):67, 1989.
10. American Cancer Society. Smokeless Tobacco, A Medical Perspective. Atlanta, GA: 1987.
11. Argerakis, G. P. Psychosocial considerations of the post-treatment of head and neck cancer patients. Dental Clinics of North America 34(2):285, 1990.
12. Bernstein, N. R. Emotional Care of the Facially Burned and Disfigured. Boston: Little, Brown, 1976, pp. 23–39.
13. Thawley, S. E., and Panje, W. R. Comprehensive Management of Head and Neck Tumors. Philadelphia: W. B. Saunders, 1987, pp. 69–78.
14. Berkowitz, R. J., Ferretti, G. A., and Berg, J. H. Dental management of children with cancer. Pediatric Annals 17(11):715, 1988.
15. Peterson, D. E. Pretreatment strategies for infection prevention in chemotherapy patients. In NCI Monograph No. 9. U.S. Public Health Service. Washington, DC: U.S. Government Printing Office, 1990, pp. 61–72.
16. Brown, L. R., Driezen, S., et al. Effect of radiation-induced xerostomia on human oral microflora. Journal of Dental Research 54:740, 1975.
17. Driezen, S., Brown, L. R., et al. Radiation-induced xerostomia in cancer patients. Cancer 38:273, 1976.
18. Makkonen, T. A., Tenovuo, J., et al. Changes in protein composition of whole saliva during radiotherapy in patients with oral and oropharyngeal cancer. Oral Surgery Oral Medicine Oral Pathology 62:270, 1986.
19. Shannon, I. L., Starcke, E. N., and Wescott, W. B. Effect of radiotherapy on whole saliva. Journal of Dental Research 56:639, 1977.
20. Sanders, J. E. Implications of cancer therapy to the head and neck on growth and development and other delayed effects. In NCI Monograph No. 9. U.S. Public Health Service. Washington, DC: U.S. Government Printing Office, 1990, pp. 163–168.
21. Marx, R. E., and Johnson, R. P. Studies on the radiobiology of osteoradionecrosis and their clinical significance. Oral Surgery Oral Medicine Oral Pathology 62:270, 1986.
22. Cancer Manual. Boston: American Cancer Society, Massachusetts Division, 1990.
23. Sonis, S. T., Sonis, A. L., and Lieberman, A. Oral complications in patients receiving treatment for non-head and neck malignancies. Journal of the American Dental Association 97:468, 1978.

23a. Rosenberg, S. W., Kolodney, H., Wong, G. Y., and Murphy, M. L. Altered root development in long-term survivors of pediatric acute lymphoblastic leukemia. Cancer 59:1640, 1987.

24. Wingard, J. R. Infectious and noninfectious systemic complications. In NCI Monograph No. 9. U.S. Public Health Service. Washington, DC: U.S. Government Printing Office, 1990, pp. 21–28.
25. Lockhart, P. B. Dental management of patients receiving chemotherapy. In Peterson, D. E., and Sonis, S. T. (eds.). Oral Complications of Cancer Chemotherapy. Boston: Martinus Nijhoff, 1983, pp. 113–149.
26. Rainey, L. C. Effects of preparatory patient education for radiation oncology patients. Cancer 58(5):1179, 1986.
27. Villejo, L., Flynn, V., and Klucharick, S. Strategies for cancer patient education: Overcoming barriers. Cancer Bulletin 40(6):365, 1988.
28. Padberg, R. M., and Padberg, L. F. Strengthening the effectiveness of patient education: Applying principles of adult education. Oncology Nursing Forum 17(1):65, 1990.
29. Jaspers, M., and Little, J. Infective endocarditis: A review and update. Oral Surgery Oral Medicine Oral Pathology 57:606, 1984.
30. Spuller, R. L. The central indwelling venous catheter in the pediatric patient: Dental treatment considerations. Special Care in Dentistry 8(2):74, 1988.
31. Peterson, D. E. Bacterial infections: Periodontal and dental disease. In Peterson, D. E., and Sonis, S. T. (eds.). Oral Complications of Cancer Chemotherapy. Boston: Martinus and Nijhoff, 1983, pp. 79–91.
32. Ferretti, G. A., Brown, A. T., et al. Oral antimicrobial agents—chlorhexidine. In NCI Monograph No. 9. U.S. Public Health Service. Washington, DC: U.S. Government Printing Office, 1990, pp. 51–56.
33. Wright, W. E., Haller, J. M., et al. An oral disease prevention program for patients receiving radiation therapy and chemotherapy. Journal of the American Dental Association 110:43, 1985.
34. Driezen, S., Daly, T. E., and Drane, J. B. Oral complications of cancer radiotherapy. Postgraduate Medicine 61:85, 1977.
35. Greenspan, D. Management of salivary dysfunction. In NCI Monograph No. 9. U.S. Public Health Service. Washington, DC: U.S. Government Printing Office, 1990, pp. 159–162.
36. Johnson, J. T., Ferretti, G. A., et al. Oral pilocarpine for post-irradiation xerostomia in patients with head and neck cancer. The New England Journal of Medicine 329:390, 1993.
37. Eilers, J., Berger, A. N., and Peterson, M. C. Development, testing and application of the oral assessment guide. Oncology Nursing Forum 15(3):325, 1988.
38. Rosenberg, S. W., Kolodney, H., et al. Altered dental root development in long-term survivors of pediatric acute lymphoblastic leukemia. Cancer 59(5):1179, 1986.

39. Sonis, A. L., Tarbell, N., et al. Dentofacial development in long-term survivors of acute lymphoblastic leukemia. Cancer 66:2645, 1990.

Suggested Readings

Bodey, G. P., Buckly, M., and Sathe, Y. S. Quantitative relationships between circulating leukocytes and infection in patients with acute leukemia. Annals of Internal Medicine 64:328, 1966.

Dahlof, G., Barr, M., et al. Disturbances in dental development after total body irradiation in bone marrow transplant recipients. Oral Surgery Oral Medicine Oral Pathology 65:41, 1988.

Guggenheimer, J., Verbin, R. S., et al. Factors delaying the diagnosis of oral and oropharyngeal carcinomas. Cancer 64:932, 1989.

Little, J. W., and Falace, D. A. Dental Management of the Medically Compromised Patient, 4th ed. St. Louis: Mosby–Year Book, 1994, pp. 460–482.

Schimpff, S. C. Hahn, D. M., and Brouillet, M. D. Infection prevention in acute leukemia: Comparison of basic infection prevention techniques with standard room reverse isolation or with reverse isolation and added air filtration. Leukemia Research 2:231, 1978.

Schnaper, N., and Kellner, T. K. Psychosocial effect of cancer on the patient and family. In Peterson, D. E., Elias, E. G., and Sonis, S. T. (eds.). Head and Neck Management of the Cancer Patient. Boston: Martinus Nijhoff, 1986, pp. 503–508.

Sonis, S. T., and Kunz, A. Impact of improved dental services for non-head and neck malignancies. Journal of the American Dental Association 65:19, 1988.

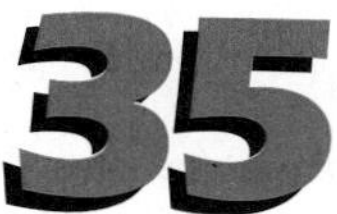

Dental Hygiene Care for Individuals with Eating Disorders

OBJECTIVES

Mastery of the content in this chapter will enable the reader to:

- Define the key terms used
- Differentiate between anorexia and bulimia nervosa as eating disorder syndromes using the DSM-III-R criteria for diagnosis
- Discuss psychological and physical characteristics of the anorexic and bulimic client
- Describe systemic complications that can arise as sequelae to anorexic and bulimic behaviors
- Identify oral characteristics of the bulimic, anorexic, and bulimorexic client
- Identify the components of a comprehensive assessment that should be used for clients with eating disorders
- Outline dental hygiene diagnoses and interventions to be considered for each oral manifestation associated with these eating disorders
- Identify community resources that can serve as a referral source for psychological treatment of the client with eating disorders
- Describe a technique for confronting and referring a newly identified anorexic or bulimic client for psychological therapy
- Outline an appropriate plan for education and oral management for bulimic and anorexic clients during the psychological treatment phase
- Identify treatment modalities for both reversible and irreversible oral manifestations of bulimia and/or anorexia
- Value the role of oral health professionals in identification and referral of clients with eating disorders
- Develop a personal and professional ethics system related to understanding the issues of professional responsibility and liability in referring clients for psychological therapy

EATING DISORDERS

Eating disorders are a topic of interest and concern to health professionals in many disciplines. Aberrant eating may be manifested in a variety of forms. The American Psychiatric Association recognizes five distinct diagnoses of eating disorders:

- Anorexia nervosa
- Bulimia nervosa
- Atypical eating disorder
- Pica
- Rumination[1]

Pica and rumination are aberrant eating disorders restricted to infancy and childhood. Atypical eating disorders may include the nonspecific categories such as obesity and compulsive overeating, although the extent of psychopathology associated with these conditions varies widely. Because little information exists regarding the effect of these disorders on oral health, they are not discussed further in this chapter. However, data obtained from various sources indicate that the prevalence of anorexia nervosa, bulimia nervosa, and bulimorexia (the vacillation between anorexic and bulimic behavior) has steadily increased over the past two decades. It is generally believed that Western society's preoccupation with body image and thinness has resulted in an increased prevalence of these disorders. Although increased awareness by our society of these problems gives the impression that these are new and unusual disorders, evidence from historical references and detailed case histories in the medical literature indicates that both anorexia and bulimia were well documented as early as the mid-18th century.

Clients suffering from these disorders present a unique challenge to oral health professionals. Behaviors associated with eating disorders result in significant physical and oral sequelae and, over time, increased mortality rates. A comprehensive understanding of the psychosocial, physical, and oral dimensions of these disorders is critical for the dental hygienist. Eating disorders are complex, and successful care requires the coordinated effort of various health professionals: individual and family therapy by specially trained psychologists; psychiatrists and social workers (psychological, family, and social components); medical support by physicians and nurses with experience in eating disorders (medical component); education and reorientation of eating and exercise habits from nutritionists and exercise therapists (dietary and recreational components); and support and treatment of oral manifestations of the illnesses by the oral health team (oral health component) (Fig. 35–1).

Persons with eating disorders are likely to seek oral healthcare because of concern with the changing appearance of teeth or complaints of oral discomfort. As a result, it is likely that the dental hygienist could be the first health professional to identify oral and physical manifestations characteristic of these disorders in clients. Individuals with eating disorders are reluctant to acknowledge the gravity of their obsession with food and weight, and protect carefully the secret of their obsessive, compulsive behavior. The dental hygienist then becomes essential in the initial recognition and referral of the client to the medical and psychological treatment system, as well as integral to the support of the oral environment.

Anorexia Nervosa

Anorexia nervosa, the least common of the eating disorders, has a high profile in society because of publicity related to many public figures who have either died from self-starvation or have made public their diagnosis. The term "anorexia" is a misnomer and may lead to confusion. Anorexia literally means "loss of appetite," whereas the client suffering from anorexia suppresses and denies sensation of hunger.

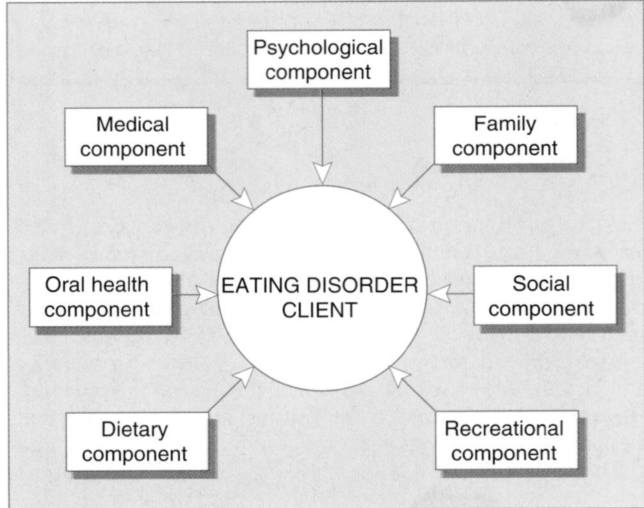

FIGURE 35–1
A multidisciplinary approach to providing care to individuals with eating disorders.

Diagnosis of this obsessive/compulsive disorder is based on criteria established in the *Diagnostic and Statistical Manual for Mental Disorders* (see DSM-III-R Criteria for Medical Diagnosis of Anorexia and Bulimia Nervosas chart). Features typical of anorexia include a failure to maintain normal body weight, an intense fear of gaining weight even though underweight, a distorted body image, and amenorrhea for at least three consecutive menstrual cycles. The stereotypical image of the extremely emaciated person may or may not be accurate in clients with anorexia. Body weight more than 15% below normal for the person's age and height does not ensure an emaciated appearance. In fact, some clients may appear "fashionably" thin. Clients with anorexia use rigorous physical exercise as an expression of their fear of weight gain. Because of their severely distorted body image, anorexic clients frequently complain of feeling or looking fat when they are obviously thin or underweight. Diagnostically, the distortion of body image represents the critical difference between individuals with anorexia and individuals with a quest for thinness. Anorexia nervosa is suspected in a client when no other physical illnesses are present to account for these physical and mental changes.

DSM-III-R CRITERIA FOR MEDICAL DIAGNOSIS OF ANOREXIA AND BULIMIA NERVOSAS

Anorexia Nervosa

- Refusal to maintain body weight over a minimal normal weight for age and height (e.g., weight loss leading to maintenance of body weight 15% below that expected; or failure to make expected weight gain during period of growth, leading to body weight 15% below that expected)
- Intense fear of gaining weight or becoming fat, even though underweight
- Disturbance in the way in which one's body weight, size, or shape is experienced (e.g., the person claims to "feel fat" even when emaciated, believes that one area of the body is "too fat" even when obviously underweight)
- In females, absence of at least three consecutive menstrual cycles when otherwise expected to occur (primary or secondary amenorrhea). (A woman is considered to have amenorrhea if her periods occur only following hormone (e.g., estrogen) administration

Bulimia Nervosa

- Recurrent episodes of binge eating (rapid consumption of a large amount of food in a discrete period of time)
- A feeling of lack of control over eating behavior during eating binges
- The person regularly engages in self-induced vomiting, use of laxatives or diuretics, strict dieting or fasting, or vigorous exercise in order to prevent weight gain
- A minimal average of two binge eating episodes a week for a least 3 months
- Persistent overconcern with body shape and weight

The onset of anorexia commonly begins in early adolescence (approximately 11 to 14 years old). The condition may go through a period of remission only to reemerge in late adolescence or early adulthood. Prevalence rates have been estimated from 0.5 to 1% in white females of school age.[2,3] Accurate determination of these rates is difficult because reluctance to admit that a problem exists is typical for individuals with anorexia. Incomplete prevalence rates are available for women in other racial or ethnic groups; however, several studies have indicated that Asian, African-American, Hispanic and American Indian adolescent females are also at risk for eating disorders.[4–6] It has been estimated that 5 to 10% of anorexic clients are men.[7–9] Limited data are available on the cultural, ethnic, or racial groups of anorexic men.

Bulimia Nervosa

Bulimia nervosa is more common than anorexia, with prevalence rates estimated at 8 to 20% of college-age women.[10,11] As with anorexia nervosa, precise prevalence rates are difficult to compile because of the secretive behavior associated with the disorders. The difference between anorexia and bulimia nervosa is in the manifestations of the conditions. Diagnostic criteria for bulimia include recurrent episodes of binge eating followed by self-induced vomiting, use of laxatives or diuretics, excessive exercise, a feeling of lack of control over the behavior, and a consistent concern with body image and weight.

Bulimia literally means "ox hunger" and accurately describes this abnormal craving for food. Bulimics may gorge with large quantities of food (up to 25 times the normal daily intake) then eliminate the consumed food by vomiting or using laxatives. Binge foods typically are high in carbohydrate content and low in food value. Binge eating episodes are most often followed by vomiting. Sixty to 80% of bulimics vomit repeatedly as the primary method of ridding themselves of the engorged food.[12]

Compared to anorexia, the onset of bulimia begins later in adolescence or early adulthood (ages 17 to 25 years) and is more likely to be associated with a perception of adolescent obesity. Like anorexia, the vast majority of bulimics are women, with only 5% reported as males.[13]

The frequency of binge eating differs among bulimics. Approximately 66% succeed in controlling binge eating for several days then succumb to overeating weekly or biweekly, whereas 10% overeat daily, especially during the evening.[14]

Anorexia and bulimia can occur concomitantly, with clients alternating between self-starvation and binge-purge behaviors. It has been estimated that approximately 47% of individuals with a history of anorexia nervosa adopt bulimic behaviors within 1.5 years after the appearance of anorexia.[15] Individuals who originally develop bulimia have been known to develop anorexia later in the course of the illness. The diagnosis of **"bulimorexia"** is used when these disorders occur concomitantly.[16] No distinct diagnostic criteria have been developed for bulimorexia, but characteristics of preoccupation with food and body weight are typical.

Etiology of Anorexia and Bulimia

Current theories regarding the etiology of anorexia and bulimia suggest a complex interrelationship between both developmental and genetic components. Information in this area is limited, but evidence from studies on twins suggests the possibility that a genetic element may exist that predisposes an individual to develop an eating disorder. Studies examining the prevalence rates of anorexia and bulimia in identical versus fraternal twins have shown a higher concordance rate of these disorders in the identical twin groups.[17,18] Whether this genetic predisposition is related to depression, neurochemical abnormalities, or affective instability is still unknown.

The developmental components of both disorders are more completely understood. Developmentally, anorexia and bulimia are similar in that the individual fails to progress normally through appropriate developmental stages during childhood and adolescence. This developmental disturbance frequently results from disturbed parent-child relationships.[19] Classic family dynamics of the anorexic client include parental overprotection, rigidity, lack of conflict resolution, alcoholism, and/or use of the child to diffuse parental conflict. In contrast, family histories of bulimics show a classic profile of highly dependent and enmeshed family relations that are aggressive, full of conflict, and without "normal" boundaries. Clients with both anorexia and bulimia may report family histories of alcoholism, emotional or sexual abuse, or parental abandonment (either perceived or real) during childhood.

Effects of Eating Disorders

The effects of anorexia and bulimia on the general well-being of an individual are significant. Unlike many illnesses that have solely physiological etiologies, the psychological profile combined with physiological sequelae can result in complex physical manifestations that must be understood by professional dental hygiene practitioners.

Psychosocial Dimension

The chart following shows contrasts between anorexia and bulimia with regard to the psychosocial dimension. Examples are common but may not relate to all eating disorder clients in all circumstances.

In the individual with anorexia, distortion of body image and obsession with food restriction results in self-starvation behavior accompanied by compulsive exercise. Control over hunger and body represents an inappropriate psychological coping mechanism. Clients with anorexia use this control of food and perfectionistic behavior to feel more competent and in control of life. Although the symptomatic behaviors may appear to be the problem, it is the denial of family conflict and resulting depression that are the true problems.

In bulimia, low self-esteem and subsequent feelings of inadequacy are reinforced in the guilt and embarrassment associated with binge and purge behavior. Ironically, the behavior itself becomes self-reinforcing, because achievement and maintenance of low weight are perceived by people with bulimia as bringing increased attractiveness and more friends.

Bulimic clients do not experience distortion of body image or rigidity of thought characteristic of anorexia. In fact, the individual suffering from bulimia can think abstractly and may superficially appear quite successful in the management of life. Affective expression may appear gregarious to the casual observer; however, underlying the facade is an obvious flattened affect resulting from the associated anxiety, guilt, and dysphoria.

PSYCHOSOCIAL CONTRAST BETWEEN ANOREXIA AND BULIMIA NERVOSA

Anorexia Nervosa

- Shy and socially introverted
- Extreme self-control; rigid compliance with high standards
- Marked feelings of unworthiness and inadequacy; shallow social relationships
- Constricted expression of feelings
- Intelligence unimpaired, but thinking is concrete

Bulimia Nervosa

- Gregarious; may be socially introverted at times
- Alternates between self-control and impulsivity (e.g., drug/alcohol abuse)
- Unstable sense of worth and personal effectiveness; dependent relationships
- Affect labile or characterized by anxiety or guilt
- Intelligence unimpaired; thought can be abstract

Adapted from French, R. N., and Baker, E. L. Anorexia nervosa and bulimia. Indiana Medicine 77(4):241–245, 1984.

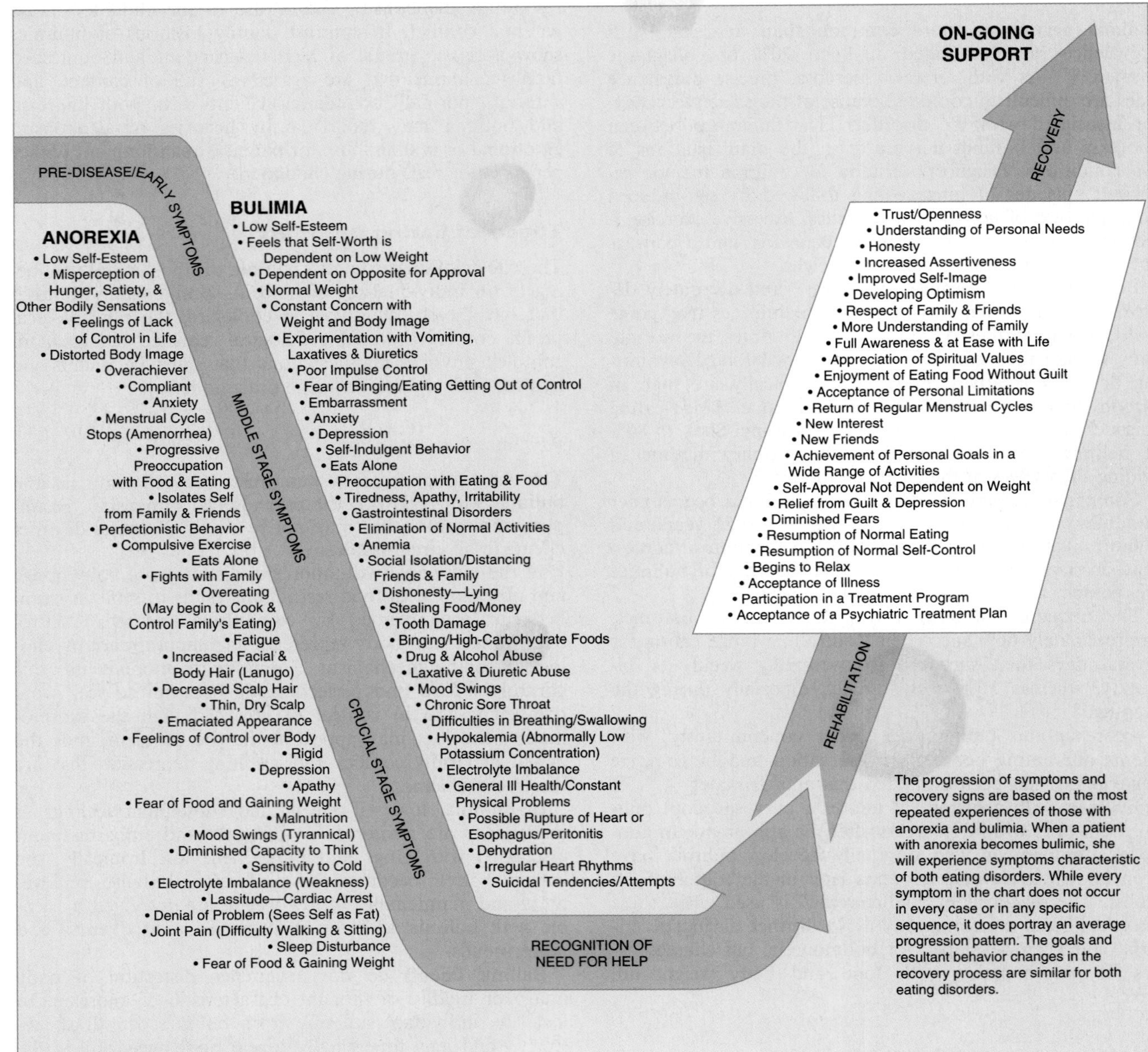

FIGURE 35–2
Anorexia nervosa–bulimia: a multidimensional profile. (Courtesy of CompCare, Eating Disorders Program, 16305 Swingle Ridge Drive, Suite 100, Chesterfield, MO 63017.)

Impaired psychological development and concomitant distortion of attitudes in the client with eating disorders provide the foundation for continued dysfunction and progression of the disorder. Anorexic clients rarely seek professional assistance on their own and may resist recommendation and offers of help from family members and friends. In contrast, the bulimic client is more likely to seek professional intervention because of frustration with recurrent binge and purge behaviors and obsession with food.

Awareness of the psychodynamics of eating disorders and distortion of attitudes is critical for the dental hygiene practitioner who treats both diagnosed and undiagnosed clients with anorexia and bulimia nervosa.

Physiological Responses

Many body systems are at risk for disruption as a result of the behaviors associated with an eating disorder. These physiological findings for clients with anorexia and bulimia are summarized in Figure 35-2.

In anorexia, restricted food intake and resulting undernutrition impair overall functioning and health of an individual. The most common physiological effect of anorexic behavior is hormonal deficiency.[20,21] In females, prolonged decrease in estrogen along with decreased body fat contributes to amenorrhea and decreased bone density (osteoporosis). In males, decreased testosterone levels may result in impotence and decreased libido. Other endocrine disturbances result in altered metabolism and abnormal temperature regulation which are demonstrated by findings of bradycardia, hypotension, dry skin, and lower-than-normal body temperature in anorexia.[20]

Cardiovascular, gastrointestinal, renal, and hematologic systems may be compromised in clients with anorexia.[22] Vital statistics in the anorexic client may reveal low pulse rates and hypotension. Decreased blood pressure and cardiac output result in thinning of the left ventricle and decreased heart chamber size over time. Other cardiac abnormalities may include arrhythmias and heart murmurs. These abnormalities are thought to result from long-standing electrolyte imbalances and decreased cardiac function.

Gastrointestinal changes result from decreased food intake and dehydration. These may include decreased intestinal motility and gastric emptying with resulting constipation and abdominal pain.[22] It is unlikely that anorexic clients would complain of these symptoms, but a comprehensive health history taken during client assessment may identify these gastrointestinal disturbances.

Kidney dysfunction may result from dehydration, electrolyte imbalance, and reduced glomerular filtration rate. As a result, anorexic clients may be predisposed to an increased incidence of kidney stones, increased blood urea nitrogen, and peripheral edema upon refeeding.

Hematological changes in anorexia are usually mild and without serious clinical consequences. These changes may include anemia, thrombocytopenia, and leukopenia.[22] Clients may appear pale or may report chronic fatigue during the health history interview.

The repeated binge and purge behavior in the bulimic client may result in dangerous complications, which when left untreated can become life-threatening. Excessive vomiting, and diuretic and laxative abuse lead to dehydration and electrolyte imbalance. Loss of potassium is a particular threat because the resulting hypokalemia and metabolic alkalosis may result in cardiac or renal failure.[23] Six to 10% of individuals afflicted with untreated bulimia for more than 10 years have cardiac arrests.[24]

Although probably ineffective in preventing caloric absorption, many bulimics may abuse laxatives as an attempt to prevent weight gain. When laxative use ceases, chronic constipation and rebound edema may occur.

Use of syrup of ipecac to induce vomiting following binge periods is particularly dangerous. Ipecac syrup contains emetine, which can destroy fibers of the heart muscle. Chronic ingestion and absorption of ipecac can lead to fatal myocardial dysfunction. In addition, repeated binging and vomiting can cause gastric dilatation, esophagitis, esophageal tears, or rupture.[22]

Fasting, vomiting, and purging may cause protein malnutrition and weight loss, resulting in endocrine disturbances similar to those found in the anorexic client.[20] Menstrual dysfunction or irregularities occur in 50 to 60% of women afflicted with bulimia. Although this is not a diagnostic criteria of bulimia, the frequency of occurrence of amenorrhea in this population is significant.

During the dental hygiene process, assessment of vital signs, health and dental history, and general observations assist the dental hygienist in recognizing the physiological changes associated with the client with eating disorders.

Lanugo, a fine downy hair usually found on the lower half of the face and upper extremities, may be present in anorexia. Dry skin and hair, as well as decreased scalp hair, are predictable findings as the eating disorder progresses. Hypothermia and increased sensitivity to cold may be evident when anorexic clients wear inappropriately warm clothing when environmental temperatures are moderate. These physical characteristics are associated with the latter stages of the disorder.

In bulimia and bulimorexia, presence of a callus on the knuckle(s) can occur from repeated self-induced vomiting. It has been estimated that 8 to 29% of this population may exhibit this type of callous.[25] Commissure lesions, dry cracked lips, and intraoral trauma may be evident; both have been found to be common findings in the bulimic individual. Figure 35-2 summarizes the progressive development of physical, psychological, and physiological symptoms and signs associated with anorexia and bulimia.

Oral and Perioral Findings

Oral manifestations of eating disorders, particularly bulimia and bulimorexia, are the most frequent and obvious disturbances identified in these populations (Table 35-1). Dental hygiene clients may exhibit one or more of these manifestations, but few individuals exhibit all.

Dental Erosion **Perimylolysis** or dental erosion, is the most common dental finding in the vomiting eating disorder client.[25-27] However, this erosion is not usually detected until the vomiting has persisted for 2 years.[28] Chemical erosion on the lingual, occlusal, incisal, or facial surfaces of the teeth occurs when the enamel is decalcified and softened by gastric acids. Subsequent mechanical erosion then occurs when the tongue or toothbrush moves against the teeth.

Early perimylolysis is difficult for practitioners to identify because tooth loss usually is subtle. Figure 35-3 shows erosive changes that are the first to be detected in the client with frequent vomiting behavior. Slight pitting is evident on the incisal surfaces of the anterior teeth and a cupping appearance may be present on the cusps of the posterior

TABLE 35-1
EFFECT OF EATING DISORDERS ON THE ORAL AND PERIORAL TISSUES

Anorexia Nervosa	Bulimia and Bulimorexia
Parotid enlargement	Parotid enlargement
Diminished taste acuity	Diminished taste acuity
Dehydration (diuretic abuse)	Commissure lesions
	Dry, chapped lips
	Xerostomia
Enamel erosion	Perimylolysis
Self-induced trauma	Self-induced trauma
Cheek/lip chewing	Palatal abrasion
	Palatal hematoma
	Ulcerations
	Cheek/lip chewing
Increase in dental caries	Increase in dental caries
	Knuckle callus

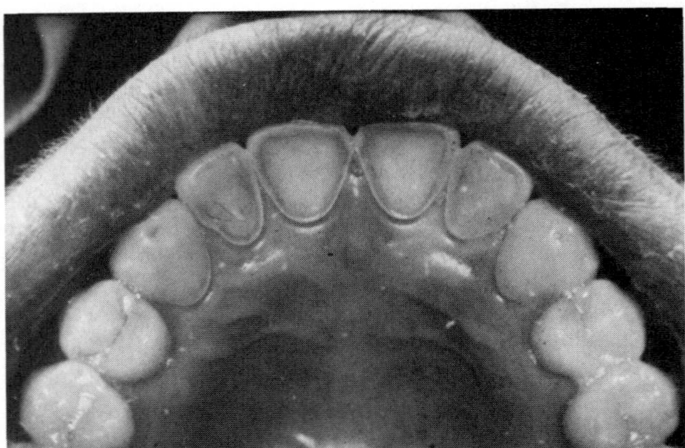

FIGURE 35-4
Extensive periomylolysis characterized by loss of lingual, occlusal, and incisal enamel.

teeth. This dished-out appearance should be differentiated from the typical flattened appearance that occurs from abrasion. As perimylolysis progresses, the teeth exhibit a loss of normal anatomical features, such as developmental grooves and pits, and they develop a mat-like surface with rounded margins. This may become so extensive that a complete loss of enamel is evident (Fig. 35-4). Loss of lingual and incisal enamel on anterior teeth weakens the tooth structure, making them more susceptible to chipping. Teeth of clients with eating disorders may appear translucent and moth-eaten anteriorly, with an open bite (Fig. 35-5). Loss of enamel around amalgam restorations results in a raised-island appearance of the amalgam. Teeth without restorations show a significant loss of occlusal contours (Fig. 35-6).

Xerostomia and Dental Caries **Xerostomia** and dry chapped lips may occur if the client is dehydrated from vomiting or diuretic or laxative abuse (Fig. 35-7). In addition, decreased salivary flow can predispose the client to an increased dental caries rate. Not all studies support the theory that individuals with eating disorders have an increased prevalence of dental caries, but it has been hypothesized that high carbohydrate intake, changes in oral pH, and/or decreased saliva quantity and/or quality may result in a higher caries rate.[27,29-31]

Intraoral and Extraoral Findings Other intraoral findings may include the presence of traumatic lesions such as ulcerations or hematomas on the hard and soft palates, cheek and lip bites, and commissure lesions resembling angular cheilitis.[25] It is thought that the commissure lesions occur when oral tissues are dehydrated and vomiting is frequent. Figure 35-8 shows a bulimic client with pronounced commissure lesions.

Extraorally, **parotid enlargement** has been observed in both anorexia and bulimia. This enlargement has been termed "nutritional mumps" and is noninflammatory in nature.[32-34] Biopsy specimens of enlarged parotid glands in eating disorder clients show increased fatty infiltration and fibrosis *without* chronic inflammatory cell infiltrate.

Although not obvious from the intraoral examination, diminished taste acuity has been reported by clients with eating disorders.[35] This alteration in taste sensation is thought to be a result of malnutrition, specifically trace metal deficiency, or hormonal abnormalities. Changes in hormonal levels have been shown to decrease sensations of taste and smell.

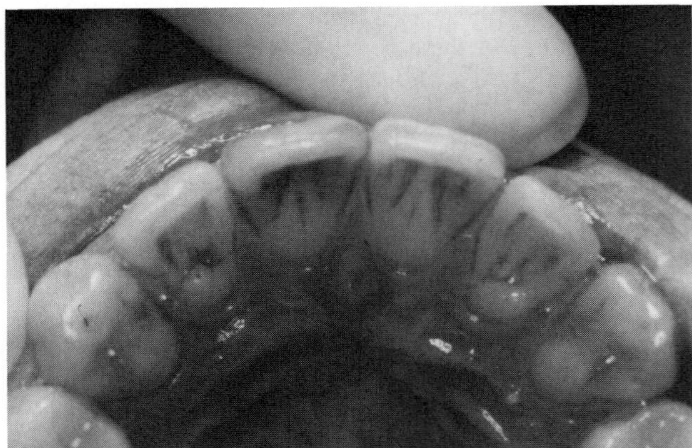

FIGURE 35-3
Early erosive cupping on cusps resulting from perimylolysis. (Courtesy of Dr. Connie Drisko, University of Missouri-Kansas City, School of Dentistry.)

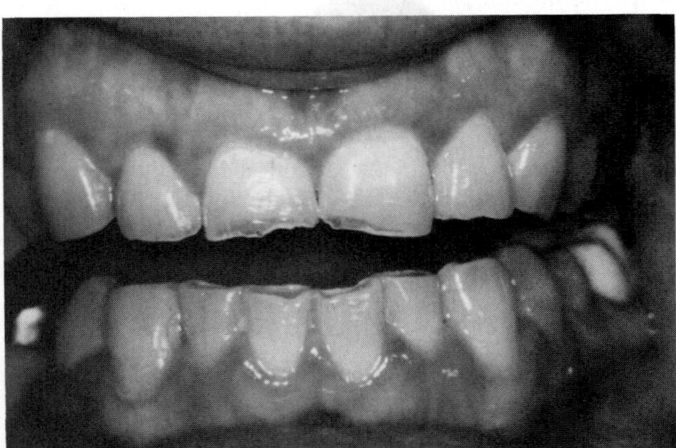

FIGURE 35-5
Moth-eaten appearance of anterior teeth resulting from loss of lingual enamel walls and subsequent weakening and chipping of incisal edges.

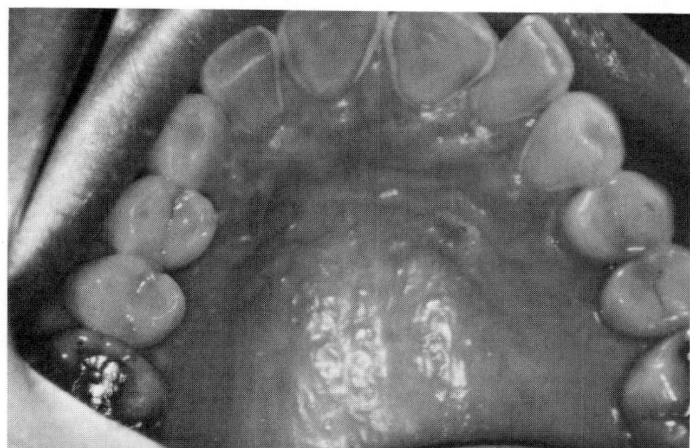

FIGURE 35-6
Loss of normal occlusal contours from perimylolysis.

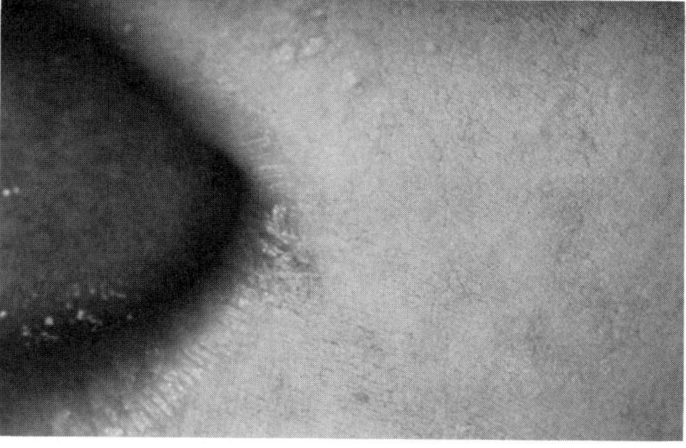

FIGURE 35-8
Presence of commissure lesions in the bulimic client. (Courtesy of Dr. Connie Drisko, University of Missouri-Kansas City, School of Dentistry.)

HUMAN NEEDS OF THE CLIENT WITH EATING DISORDERS

The complex nature of eating disorders generally results in an individual in whom many of the basic human needs are not met. As evidenced by the diagnostic criteria for both anorexia and bulimia, these clients have strong unmet needs for a wholesome body image and for appreciation and respect. In anorexia and bulimia, an altered body image coupled with low self-esteem make the aforementioned human needs primary issues in dental hygiene care. The dental hygiene diagnosis of a wholesome body image deficit as it relates to oral and perioral changes in the person with aberrant eating behaviors is important for the clinician to identify. This need is often the primary motivating factor for the client to seek oral health services and is usually preeminent of all other human needs in the client's mind.

Freedom from pain and stress is often another human need in deficit for persons with eating disorders. The professional dental hygienist should be sensitive to the wide variation of perceived oral discomfort that the client may experience. For clients with perimylolysis or high caries rate, a dental hygiene diagnosis of a deficit in the human need for a biologically sound dentition may be applicable. For the client with decreased salivary flow, a diagnosis of a deficit in the need for skin and mucous membrane integrity of the head and neck associated with xerostomia also may be appropriate. Clients are likely to have more than one unmet human need.

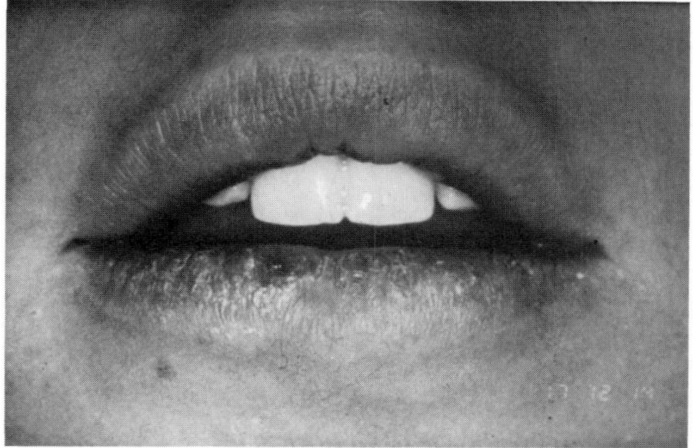

FIGURE 35-7
Perioral evidence of dehydration. Note evidence of dry, cracked lips. (Courtesy of Dr. Connie Drisko, University of Missouri-Kansas City, School of Dentistry.)

Other human need deficits commonly present in the eating disorder client are related to the needs for nutrition, self-determination and responsibility, and safety. A clear understanding of the multifaceted components of anorexia and bulimia are necessary for professionals to assess and provide appropriate dental hygiene care.

DENTAL HYGIENE PROCESS OF CARE FOR CLIENTS WITH EATING DISORDERS

A **multidisciplinary approach** to care of the client with an eating disorder based on a human needs conceptual framework may increase the success rate of psychological treatment of the disorder. Such an approach focuses on human need deficits that can be fulfilled through professional dental hygiene care. The role of the dental hygienist and the oral healthcare team varies according to the circumstances surrounding the client's status.

For individuals with an eating disorder who have not been medically diagnosed, the dental hygienist as a client advocate may be the health professional who identifies the need for referral to the psychological and medical support system. A working knowledge of organizations and individuals within the region or state who specialize in caring for individuals with eating disorders allows the dental hygienist to guide the client for appropriate therapy. This knowledge can be obtained by contacting mental health organizations or eating disorder treatment facilities within the community. These organizations may not be in the immediate geographic locale, but they are generally knowledgeable about available support throughout the region. Some national organizations that can serve as a starting point are displayed in the National Organizations chart.

Creation of a liaison or a formal referral protocol with eating disorder treatment centers or with individuals who

NATIONAL ORGANIZATIONS

American Anorexia/Bulimia Association, Inc. (AABA)
420 East 76th Street
New York, NY 10021
212-734-1114

Anorexia Nervosa and Associated Disorders, Inc. (ANAD)
P.O. Box 271
Highland Park, IL 60035
708-432-8000, ext. 3307, or 708-831-3438

Anorexia Nervosa and Related Eating Disorders, Inc. (ANRED)
P.O. Box 5102
Eugene, OR 97405
503-344-1144

Bulimia, Anorexia Self-Help, Inc. (BASH)
6125 Clayton Avenue, Suite 215
P.O. Box 39903
St. Louis, MO 63139
314-567-4080 or 1-800-227-4785

National Anoretic Aid Society, Inc. (NAAS)
1925 East Dublin Granville Road
Columbus, OH 43229
614-436-1112

specialize in these disorders is necessary. Frequently, mental health professionals treating eating disorder clients need oral healthcare professionals to whom they can refer clients who are experiencing oral problems. A liaison between the oral health team and psychological and medical team will open the door for mutual referrals and collaboration.

Assessment

Assessment of all dental hygiene clients involves collection of data on the client's comprehensive health history, intra- and extraoral status, physical status, and oral status. In addition, intraoral photographs and study models are helpful in establishing baseline data to be used for subsequent evaluation of enamel erosion and soft tissue abnormalities. When the clinician observes deviations from normal in client assessment data that suggest an eating disorder, follow-up questioning to provide additional information is necessary. A comprehensive assessment that includes appropriate questioning to validate findings and rule out all other explanations for the findings is of the utmost importance. Information presented in the chart Possible Etiologies for Oral Findings may be helpful to determine other possible reasons for findings that appear to be indicative of an eating disorder.

For example, although the presence of commissure lesions and/or dry chapped lips on a dental hygiene client may indicate a finding typical of an eating disorder, these findings also may be present following other illnesses, such as influenza, that cause dehydration and/or undernutrition. Usually, clients who have been ill and have dehydration sequelae willingly convey this information upon questioning.

In addition, although dental erosion is the most common oral finding in bulimia and bulimorexia, it has also been associated with vomiting as a result of gastric disturbances (such as hiatal hernia, duodenal or peptic ulcers, previous pregnancies, and chemotherapy), high citric acid fruit juice intake, habitual eating or sucking on chewable vitamin C tablets or sweet-and-sour type candies, Antabuse therapy for alcoholism, medications containing hydrochloric acid, and exposure to industrial acids. Moreover, intraoral trauma may result from an accident, or may be evidence of self-mutilation indicative of psychological problems other than eating disorders. Clients with xerostomia from medications, such as antidepressants or antihypertensives, may use sucrose-containing mints or gum to relieve dryness associated with decreased salivary flow. Commonly, these clients experience an increase in dental caries rate that can easily be identified by examining the health history and questioning the client. For example, asking "Have there been any dietary changes that have increased your exposure to sugar or sugar containing foods?" or "Can you tell me a little about your snacking habits?" provide an opportunity to discuss eating habits in a nonthreatening manner. Follow-up questions related to frequency or patterns of snacking or sugar consumption provide additional information while allowing the dental hygienist to observe the client's demeanor regarding discussion of food.

During assessment of a client with a suspected eating disorder, it is imperative that the dental hygienist gather specific information in a professional, nonjudgmental manner. Concluding the presence of an eating disorder without

POSSIBLE ETIOLOGIES FOR ORAL FINDINGS COMMONLY ASSOCIATED WITH CLIENTS WHO HAVE EATING DISORDERS

Perimylolysis and Erosion: Differential Diagnosis

- Gastric or physical disturbances with associated vomiting (e.g., previous pregnancies, chemotherapy, hiatal hernia, duodenal or peptic ulcers)
- High citric acid fruit or fruit juice intake
- Antabuse therapy (and associated vomiting) for alcoholism
- Habitual eating or sucking on vitamin C tablets or sweet-and-sour type candies
- Medications containing hydrochloric acid
- Exposure to industrial acids

Parotid Enlargement Differential Diagnosis

- Salivary neoplasms
- Inflammatory diseases (e.g., mumps, infectious mononucleosis, tuberculosis, sarcoidosis, histoplasmosis)
- Metabolic disturbances (e.g., malnutrition, alcoholic cirrhosis, diabetes mellitus)
- Autoimmune diseases such as Sjögren's syndrome
- Parotid duct obstruction
- (AIDS) Acquired immunodeficiency syndrome

Xerostomia

- Medications (e.g., antihypertensives, antidepressants, antipsychotics, antihistamines
- Systemic diseases (e.g., diabetes, Sjögren's syndrome)
- Dehydration from recent flu-like illnesses or high fever)

Commissure Lesions

- Loss of vertical dimension or overclosure
- Vitamin B deficiency

Name: ________ Age: _____ Marital Status: ________
Occupation: ______________________

I. HISTORICAL INFORMATION
 A. Type of Disorder: ____________
 B. History of Disorder:
  1. Age at onset: ____________
  2. Current status: Length of disorder: ________
   Active: ________ Inactive: ________
  3. Frequency of episodes: ____________
  4. Periods of abstinence: ____________
  5. Precipitating factors: ____________
 C. Significant Sociocultural/Familial History
II. PAST MEDICAL/ORAL HEALTHCARE FOR DISORDER
 A. Medical Treatment:
 B. Psychological/Psychiatric Counseling:
 C. Oral Health History:
  1. Recognition/counseling:
  2. Preventive measures:
  3. Restorative therapy:
  4. Frequency of examination/treatment appointments:
III. CURRENT STATUS
 A. General Health: ___ Most Recent Physical Exam: ___
 B. Under Active Medical/Psychological Therapy:
 C. Medications (dosages): ____________
 ____
 D. Under Control (Length of Time): ____________
 E. Assessment Findings:
  1. Extraoral
   a. Arms, hands, fingers: ____________
   b. Face, cheeks, lips, commissures: ________
   ____
  2. Intraoral
   a. Pharynx:
   b. Palate:
   c. Tongue:
   d. Buccal mucosa:
   e. Gingiva:
   f. Maxillary teeth:
   g. Mandibular teeth:
   h. Dentinal hypersensitivity:
   i. Salivary glands:
   j. Salivary flow:
IV. CARE OPTIONS
 A. Medical/Psychological Referral:
 B. Eating Disorder Treatment Center Referral:
 C. Support Group Referral:
 D. Dental Hygiene Care/Dental Treatment:
  1. Palliative:
  2. Preventive:
  3. Emergency:
  4. Definitive:
V. ADDITIONAL COMMENTS

FIGURE 35–9
Assessment instrument for the individual previously diagnosed with an eating disorder.

adequate assessment is to be avoided at all costs. To conclude prematurely that a client has an eating disorder puts the client and clinician in an unnecessary and uncomfortable position.

Assessment of the client who reports a known history of bulimia, anorexia, or bulimorexia involves several important components. In the client with a diagnosed eating disorder, historical information regarding the eating disorder, past medical and dental care, and current status of the oral environment and treatment interventions is necessary to provide appropriate care for the client. This evaluation should provide a clear depiction of the extent of the eating disorder as it relates to associated behaviors, current status regarding psychotherapy and/or supportive care, and current physical and oral findings (see Assessment of the Client with a Suspected and Previously Diagnosed Eating Disorder chart). Figure 35–9 shows an additional data collecting instrument that can be used for this purpose.

Dental Hygiene Diagnosis

Dental hygiene diagnosis should be accomplished by the identification deficits in the 11 human needs related to dental hygiene care based on all data collected during the client assessment phase; data is needed to determine the need for client referral into the medical or psychological healthcare system. *Actual diagnosis of the eating disorder is not a function of members of the oral health team because this can be determined only by a thorough psychological evaluation.*

ASSESSMENT OF THE CLIENT WITH A SUSPECTED AND PREVIOUSLY DIAGNOSED EATING DISORDER

Health History Component	Assessment Technique
■ Physical appearance and gait Skin, build, weight, hair, pallor	Observation
■ Vital signs: Blood pressure Heart rate Body temp (optional)	Objective measurement
■ Systemic diseases: Current and past status	Interview
■ Systems review	Interview

Continued on next page

ASSESSMENT OF THE CLIENT WITH A SUSPECTED AND PREVIOUSLY DIAGNOSED EATING DISORDER *Continued*

Health History Component	Assessment Technique
■ Medications: Drug name Dosage Duration of medication Reason for medication	Interview
■ Exercise or physical activity: Frequency and duration Type of activity	Interview
■ Oral home care habits	Interview
■ Dietary habits or restrictions	Interview
Extraoral assessment	
■ Salivary and lymph glands	Palpation
■ Temporomandibular joint	Palpation and auscultation
■ Skin Color Moisture Facial hair (lanugo) Lesions	Observation
■ Perioral structures Commissure lesions Lip integrity Trauma	Observation
Intraoral assessment	
■ Soft tissue assessment Condition of mucous membranes Unexplained trauma (especially palatal)	Observation and palpation
■ Assessment of signs of caries and oral hygiene	Radiographic and manual examination
■ Periodontal assessment	Observation and measurement of probing depths and attachment level
■ Tooth wear Presence or absence Location Appearance (cupped or moth eaten versus abraded)	Observation, study models

A client usually manifests several human need deficits arising directly or indirectly from the eating disorder. Many oral manifestations result from alterations in physiological functioning that are direct sequelae to behaviors associated with anorexia and/or bulimia. For example, repeated binge eating of carbohydrates followed by vomiting and laxative abuse may result in increased dental caries activity ensuing from frequent sucrose intake, lowered oral pH, and eventual systemic dehydration with subsequent xerostomia. Dental hygiene diagnoses relating to this complex interrelationship of variables include identifying deficits in the human needs for a biologically sound dentition, in nutrition, freedom from pain, and wholesome body image.

In addition to the obvious dental hygiene diagnoses relating to the integrity of the skin and mucous membrane and a biologically sound dentition, other dental hygiene diagnoses deserve particular discussion. Deficits in the client's human needs for territoriality, appreciation and respect, and self-determination and responsibility are diagnoses that, if not met, compromise the success of all future dental hygiene care. The psychological dynamics of the eating disorders are tightly intertwined with the client's human need for wholesome body image, sense of privacy (territoriality), and personal respect and self-determination. Consequently, any additional threat to these human needs, such as a breach in confidentiality or respect for the client's well-protected psychological domain, is perceived negatively by the client and hinders the ability of the oral healthcare team to be effective in the client's overall healthcare.

The dental hygiene diagnosis of a human need deficit in self-determination and responsibility varies depending on the type of eating disorder identified. For example, in the anorexic client, self-control is a human need that motivates the individual to action. Consequently, the client will likely exhibit greater adherence to ideal oral health behaviors if she understands the concept of personal control over oral health and disease. In contrast, lack of self-control and self-determination characterizes the bulimic client. Therefore, it is likely that the client inadequately monitors her behaviors necessary to enhance oral health. A sample of a dental hygiene diagnosis for eating disorders follows.

DENTAL HYGIENE DIAGNOSES FOR CLIENTS WITH EATING DISORDERS BASED ON THE HUMAN NEED CONCEPTUAL MODEL OF DENTAL HYGIENE

Dental Hygiene Diagnosis	Due or Related To	As Evidenced By
Deficit in the need for a wholesome body image	• Self-induced vomiting • Dietary habits High citric acid intake Excessive diet soda intake Carbohydrate binging • Bruxing habits • Work hypertrophy from binge and purge behavior	Client expression of dissatisfaction with: • Tooth discoloration • Loss of tooth structure • Appearance of an open bite • Visible dental caries • Parotid gland enlargement
Deficit in the need for freedom from pain and stress	• Frequent vomiting • Diminished saliva flow rate • Limited capacity to manage stress • Diuretic/laxative abuse • Fear of being "found out" • Potential changes in salivary components • Lack of willingness to communicate fully • Denial of or providing false explanations for oral manifestations • Avoidance of dental hygiene care and frequent appointment cancellation	• Exposed dentin from enamel erosion • Dental caries activity • Xerostomia/dehydrated oral tissues • Oral discomfort • Dentinal hypersensitivity • Low self-esteem and feelings of inadequacy • Introversion and feelings of social isolation • Depression • Guilt and embarrassment
Deficit in the need for integrity of the skin and mucous membranes	• Laxative, diuretic and vomiting abuse • Use of fingers and other objects to cause vomiting • Depression	• Dehydration of oral environment • Self-induced trauma during purging • Self-abusive behavior
Deficit in the need for nutrition: undernutrition or poor quality of food intake	• High carbohydrate, low nutrient diet • Self-starvation • Anemia • Alteration in body metabolism • Decreased cardiac function	• Increased dental caries rate • Dry skin/hair • Enlarged parotid glands • Bradycardia/low blood pressure/low body temperature • Thin or pale appearance • Fatigue
Deficit in the need for appreciation and respect	• Low or endangered esteem • Need for acceptance by others • Feelings of guilt	• Verbalization of fears • Hesitancy to discuss problems openly • Withdrawal from clinician
Deficit in the need for territoriality: Potential for violation of client's psychological domain Potential for compromise of client's confidentiality and privacy	• Guilt or anxiety over behavior • Rigidity of thought process • Inability to trust others • Potential for violation of client's psychological space • Potential for angering client	• Lack of willingness to acknowledge obvious oral manifestations • Lack of willingness to participate in goal planning • Fabrication of poor excuses to explain observed oral and perioral findings
Deficit in the need for self-determination and respectability Potential to sacrifice oral wellness Potential for self-destructive behavior	• Unstable sense of self • Feelings of unworthiness • Anxiety	• Lack of "ownership" of problems • Impaired self-care • Evidence of self-inflicted oral trauma

Planning

The planning phase for the client suspected of having an eating disorder should include:

- Referral of the client into the medical and psychological therapy systems
- Establishment of a liaison or formal referral protocol with the psychological treatment team
- Support of the client's human needs during and following psychological treatment

Planning for the client with a previously diagnosed eating disorder includes the last two phases. Members of the oral health team must recognize their limitations in treating clients with these disorders. Oral and dental treatment, either palliative or definitive, may be necessary, but the primary role of the oral health team in the client with a suspected eating disorder is to offer the client **psychological referral** to meet her human need for safety. Establishment of a caring, nonjudgmental environment based on mutual trust is necessary to achieve a successful referral. Attention to the client's need for freedom from pain through palliative oral care initially is recommended if the client is experiencing discomfort.

Involving the client in setting mutual goals should be a primary consideration. Setting goals that are:

- Specific
- Based on the dental hygiene diagnoses
- Measurable by both client and professional

are crucial to the planning process. Sample dental hygiene care plans for the bulimic and anorectic client follow.

DENTAL HYGIENE CARE PLAN: THE CLIENT WITH BULIMIA

Dental Hygiene Diagnosis	Goal	Dental Hygiene Interventions	Evaluative Statement
Deficit in the need for freedom from pain and stress	By 12/3, client will have normal oral function with no discomfort By 11/1, client communicates openly with dental hygienist and participates in management of oral conditions	Fabricate mouthguard for dental coverage during vomiting episodes and/or fluoride application	Client complies with recommended treatment for ameliorating dental/oral discomfort
	Dental caries activity will be decreased for at least 1 year	Recommend daily use of neutral sodium fluoride gel/ rinse and/or desensitizing dentifrice Demonstrate bacterial plaque control measures Explain risks of vomiting to hard oral tissues—increased sensitivity	No evidence of progressive enamel/dentin loss (perimylolysis) No evidence of caries activity after 1 year
		Refer to DDS for palliative/ definitive coverage of exposed dentin Provide client with verbal and nonverbal reinforcement demonstrating acceptance of client's illness	Client reports changes in bulimic behavior that affects oral conditions Client does not actively seek dental hygiene/dental services
	By 10/3, client will use mouthguard during vomiting episodes		Goal partially met—client uses mouthguard during some vomiting episodes
Deficit in the need for self-determination and responsibility	Client participates in treatment of bulimia by attending all medical/ psychological and dental treatment appointments for 1 year By 10/2, client participates in management of oral conditions by utilizing oral self-care skills By 10/5, client will self-monitor plaque	Refer client for psychological intervention Involve client in design of self-care skills that coordinate with concomitant psychological therapy Liaison with other healthcare providers to coordinate multidisciplinary care Provide appropriate evaluation and feedback	Client complies with referral to mental health specialist/ eating disorder treatment facility Client demonstrates successful use of self-care skills No evidence of bacterial plaque or gingivitis No evidence of oral trauma from self-care

DENTAL HYGIENE CARE PLAN: THE CLIENT WITH BULIMIA
Continued

Dental Hygiene Diagnosis	Goal	Dental Hygiene Interventions	Evaluative Statement
	By 11/20, client will self-monitor gingival bleeding	Use media and instructional aids to support skill development in bacterial plaque removal	
Deficit in the need for a wholesome body image	Client participates in active psychological treatment for 6 months By 7/20, client will accept dental hygiene/dental interventions as a coordinated effort towards comprehensive treatment By 8/15, client will verbalize that her mouth looks and feels better	Referral to and continued liaison with medical/psychological team Refer to dentist for aesthetic/definitive dental treatment intervention Provide education regarding client's expressed dissatisfaction with oral condition	Client indicates that she has been going for psychological treatment Client expresses acceptance of oral conditions after treatment Client has realistic expectations for alterations in appearance of oral conditions from dental treatment Client states that her mouth looks and feels better

Planning care for clients with perimylolysis should be aimed at eliminating pain, maintaining existing tooth structure, and preventing further erosion. To this end, planning may include one or more of the following: self-applied daily fluoride therapy, mouthguard fabrication to provide coverage for teeth during vomiting episodes, client education, and/or desensitization of dentinal hypersensitivity with either prescribed or over-the-counter agents. Clients exhibiting xerostomia as a result of dehydration may benefit from a saliva substitute and client education with respect to the influence of xerostomia on the oral hard and soft tissues.

Implementation

Once the dental hygiene assessment and diagnosis have been completed, consultation between the dentist and dental hygienist affords both healthcare providers an opportunity to view the data collaboratively. At the initial decision-making junction, it should be determined, based upon psychosocial and ethnocultural factors, whether the dental hygienist or dentist is the best person to confront the client with the objective findings and suspicion of an eating disorder **(professional confrontation).** As a general rule, the dental hygienist is the oral health professional most likely to be successful in a confrontation because she does not represent an "authority figure" in the mind of the client as might the dentist. However, it is important to note that female clients may be more receptive to a confrontation by a female clinician whereas males may be more receptive to a male clinician.[31] No matter who conducts the initial confrontation, a matter-of-fact, nonjudgmental approach must be maintained. Many clinicians are initially uncomfortable with the prospect of confronting a client with a suspected eating disorder and may inadvertently communicate this discomfort nonverbally to the client. To prevent this, the inexperienced dental hygienist would benefit from role playing to practice these types of a confrontational situations prior to an actual experience. Using desensitizing and follow-up questions, such as those found in the Guidelines for Confronting and Referring a Person with a Suspected Eating Disorder chart provide the professional with the opening to apprise the client that these changes are commonly associated with eating disorders.

The actual confrontation should occur in a confidential setting and should be accomplished using desensitizing questions followed by more specific questions. If dental erosion is the most obvious oral finding, asking questions that eliminate other possibilities for erosion permits the clinician to gain valuable information while desensitizing the client to the more direct interview to follow. The confrontational interview should be conducted by asking direct questions while maintaining eye contact. Of interest, the client's body language frequently provides clues as to whether the suspicion of an eating disorder is accurate. Although some clients openly admit a problem with an eating disorder, many have become quite accomplished at denial and maintain that posture throughout much of that and subsequent appointments. Most clients with eating disorders, however, experience discomfort at being confronted with objective information they have attempted to hide. This may pose a threat to their need for psychological territoriality. The dental hygienist should be aware of nonverbal cues, such as loss of eye contact by the client or dropping of the head with a look of "shame." These clues are usually an indication that the clinician is on the right track with the questions even though the client may verbally respond negatively.

Individuals with eating disorders commonly react to the initial confrontation with various emotions. Two common responses are

- Denial accompanied by tears
- Outright anger

It is important that the dental hygienist maintain a professional demeanor during emotional outbursts and afford re-

GUIDELINES FOR CONFRONTING AND REFERRING A PERSON WITH A SUSPECTED EATING DISORDER

Confrontation

Setting:
Use of a private setting meets the client's human need for respect by assuring client confidentiality.

Approach:
Be firm, formal, objective and concerned. Keep in mind that eating disorder behavior is a symptom of low self-esteem, depression, and long-standing emotional problems.

Present and review findings observed. Explain lack of other possible etiologies as evidenced by responses to differential diagnoses questions.

Ask if client engages in behaviors associated with the disorder (e.g., "Do you vomit after eating sometimes?", "Do you restrict the amount of food that you usually eat?")

Inquire "Have you ever heard of bulimia/anorexia?"

Reassure that eating disorders are not uncommon without conveying to the client that he/she is not a unique and special individual.

Referral

Refer the Individual:
To meet the client's human need for conceptualization and problem solving, give specific information on resources for professional evaluation and offer support.

Encourage the client to contact resource personnel for evaluation.

To meet the client's human need for self-determination and responsibility, explain that it is the client's choice to seek assistance.

Contact the Professional Person to Whom You Are Referring the Client:
Inform counselor or therapist of referral.

Discuss symptoms and signs of concern.

Discuss areas of difficulty with confrontation and referral and appropriateness of referral.

Follow-up and Support:
To meet the client's need for valuing health and wellness, communicate satisfaction when evaluation or therapy has occurred.

Recognize that seemingly small accomplishments may be major to the recovering client.

Expect that the client will have periods of recurrence of eating disorder behaviors.

Support recovery, not the illnesses.

Do's and Don'ts:
Do be prepared. Anticipate resistance and defensiveness.

Don't confront with inadequate preparation and evidence.

Do focus on observed signs and symptoms and concern for health. Don't diagnose a medical, psychological or dental problem.

Do convey concern—but in a firm, formal manner.

Do explain that help is available.

Do explain that the client must decide on his/her own whether to seek assistance

Don't be misled by sympathy evoking tactics or be manipulated by resistance and defensiveness. Stay focused on observed findings and concern for individual.

Don't generalize or insinuate. Be specific.

Don't moralize or make value judgments. Maintain a professional demeanor.

inforcement to the client that the oral, physical, and/or health history findings are typical of an eating disorder and have no other etiological explanation, if in fact that is the case. Many clients are relieved at being discovered and are receptive to suggestions for referral to an eating disorder specialist. *Suggesting* that the client make an appointment with an identified eating disorder specialist or treatment center for an evaluation is a less threatening approach than making a definitive statement that the client has an eating disorder. Many clients are receptive to having the dental hygienist initiate a consultation appointment for them at an eating disorder treatment center. Others prefer to take the referral information with them to initiate the consultation appointment on their own. Either way, it is important that the client assume personal responsibility for attending a consultation appointment. It can be suggested that the client bring a trusted friend or relative along on the evaluation appointment if she feels awkward seeking help on her own. Following the confrontation appointment, the dental hygienist should adequately document the discussion that was held and the decisions regarding referral for evaluation in the client's permanent dental record so that subsequent evaluation and monitoring can be achieved.

Clients may initially deny that they have an eating disorder yet over time may become comfortable enough with the dental hygienist to be receptive to intervention. Persistence on the part of the oral health team when no other explanations can be identified for the findings is crucial because eating disorders can be life-threatening. Ethically, failure to refer a client who has obvious signs of an eating disorder for subsequent psychological evaluation is neglecting one's professional responsibility as a healthcare provider.

Establishment of the Dental/Medical/Psychological Team Liaison

Once a client with a suspected eating disorder has been confronted and referred for psychological counseling, a liaison between the oral health team and psychological/medical team can be established. Phases 2 (establishing a liaison) and 3 (management of the oral environment) of the implementation process are identical for recently confronted clients as well as those who present to the oral healthcare setting with a positive history of bulimia, anorexia, or bulimorexia.

Success of oral healthcare is largely determined by the client's ability to control behaviors associated with the eat-

CONSENT FORM

I hereby give consent for my dentist and dental hygienist to contact all healthcare providers and therapists involved in the treatment of my eating disorder. I understand that coordination of care among these health professionals is in my best interests. In addition, I understand that all consultation and discussion among these individuals will be held in strict confidence.

Client Signature Date

Witness Date

FIGURE 35-10
Sample client consent form.

ing disorder. For this reason, open dialogue among all health providers prevents segmented care planning and permits an integrated approach to client care. Many bulimic and bulimorexic clients with extensive erosion require significant dental reconstruction. Lack of coordination between healthcare providers may mean dental failure if the reconstruction is completed before the client has made adequate progress in her psychological therapy and control of vomiting behaviors. Use of a signed release form allows oral health professionals to contact and collaborate with the psychological and medical healthcare providers and is recommended when caring for a client with an eating disorder. A sample release form is shown in Figure 35-10.

Professional liaison between the oral healthcare team and the psychological support team permits the oral health team to have a better understanding of the client's specific psychological problems and increases the success rate of all therapeutic interventions. Often, there are important issues that the client is confronting in psychological therapy. These issues may influence the timing and ultimate success of definitive oral care. Without dialogue between the oral health team and mental health team, oral health professionals may make care decisions that fail to address the human needs of the client. If clients are aware that all health providers are working together for their total good, then they are less likely to claim that "all is well" in order to have short-term desires met. It is not uncommon for clients with eating disorders to attempt to manipulate healthcare providers during the course of therapy. Dental hygienists and dentists must maintain a collaborative interdisciplinary approach to healthcare for maximal success with the client with eating disorders.

Management and Support of Oral Tissues

Implementation of individualized education and preventive strategies to support a healthy oral environment is a primary focus of this phase of the dental hygiene process. To meet the client's human need for conceptualization and problem solving, oral health education assists the client in understanding the effect of eating disorder behaviors on oral health and provides self-care strategies to ameliorate or control the associated problems. When providing client education, health-promoting behaviors and management of oral problems as they relate to body image, self-determination, and nutrition should be emphasized. Potential health hazards, such as cardiac irregularities, endocrine disturbances, renal dysfunction, electrolyte imbalance, and predictable negative sequelae such as death should be deemphasized because this approach can result in alienation of the client.

Oral health education strategies for the eating disorder client are provided in the Oral Health Education and Promotion chart. These strategies may not be relevant for all clients, but an overview of general concepts should be included in each educational program.

Etiology of Oral Manifestations Associated with the Disorder An overview of the etiology of identified problems is necessary prior to individualized oral hygiene instructions. For example, clients with significant perimylolysis as a result of repeated vomiting need to understand that the low pH of stomach contents causes chemical demineralization of tooth enamel. If toothbrushing follows vomiting episodes, mechanical abrasion of the presoftened tooth surfaces is likely. The etiology of all oral manifestations should be adequately explained to clients.

Effect of Eating Disorder Behaviors on the Oral Environment Client education also includes an overview of systemic physiological changes typical of the specific eating disorder as it relates to changes in the oral environment. For example, dehydration commonly is associated with bulimia, anorexia, and bulimarexia, especially when vomiting or drugs such as diuretics or laxatives are used to control weight gain. Systemic dehydration results in decreased salivary flow, which in turn decreases the host's resistance to dental caries activity.

Self-starvation and decreased body fat alters endocrine function, which in turn has the potential of causing osteo-

ORAL HEALTH EDUCATION AND PROMOTION FOR THE EATING DISORDER CLIENT

Oral Health Education Programs Should Include

Etiology of the observed oral characteristics associated with the eating disorder behaviors

Effect of eating disorder behaviors on the oral environment and dental structures

- Current status
- Potential progression of problems

Effect of dietary habits on dental and oral health

- Frequency of eating
- Types of foods and drinks consumed

Individualized oral hygiene instruction

Oral Health Promotion Should Include

Specific management and control of oral/dental manifestations of the disorder

- Amelioration of existing problems
- Prevention of progression of other characteristics
- Management of oral discomfort associated with dentinal hypersensitivity

Recommendation for daily, at-home use of a neutral sodium fluoride rinse or gel

Recommendation of sodium bicarbonate or magnesium hydroxide rinses, or saliva substitute, as necessary

Construction of an oral mouthguard for protection during vomiting episodes porosis early in life. It has not been determined to what degree early osteoporosis affects periodontal bone support later in life, but it is important that anorexic and bulimarexic clients be cognizant of potential changes in bone density as they relate to overall health.

Clients with parotid gland enlargement may express concern about the unaesthetic appearance of the enlargement. Knowledge that the enlargement usually decreases once the eating disorder behaviors are brought under control provides the client with additional motivation for following through with psychotherapy.

Effect of Diet on Oral Health Individuals with eating disorders commonly have unusual eating habits that potentially alter normal oral health. For example, foods containing simple carbohydrates such as cookies, cake, and other sweets are common binge foods for the bulimic. Counseling on the effect of repeated binge eating, frequent sucrose intake and/or extreme intake of dietary carbonated drinks should be shared with the client if applicable. Dietary habits in anorexia frequently include excessive intake of diet soda beverages in place of food. Continual consumption of low pH diet soda beverages in the presence of diminished salivary flow may result in dental erosion and accompanying dentinal hypersensitivity. By adequately assessing eating habits, the dental hygienist can provide appropriate education individualized to the client's needs.

Oral Hygiene Instruction and Self-care Oral hygiene instruction for eating disorders includes techniques for bacterial plaque removal that are directed at preventing periodontal diseases and dental caries. In addition, oral hygiene instruction encompasses self-care measures that promote health and prevent further destruction of hard and soft oral tissues. These strategies are aimed at meeting the client's human needs for integrity of skin and mucous membrane in the head and neck and for a biologically sound dentition.

Normal brushing should be encouraged for all clients, but clients with bulimia and bulimorexia should be discouraged from toothbrushing after vomiting. It is believed that immediately brushing teeth following exposure to the acidic vomitus may increase loss of tooth structure. Use of sodium bicarbonate (1 tsp in 8 oz of water) or magnesium hydroxide (milk of magnesia) rinses following vomiting episodes cleanses the mouth of vomitus while neutralizing the acidic environment of the oral cavity.

For clients with evidence of dental erosion and/or dentinal hypersensitivity, use of a home fluoride treatment should be given top priority. Daily use of 1.1% neutral sodium fluoride gel, administered either by a custom-fabricated tray or brushing, or a 0.2% sodium fluoride mouth rinse provides maximal protection while strengthening enamel to prevent additional erosion. Use of a stannous fluoride gel for home application is contraindicated because these agents have a low pH that may increase sensitivity and the potential for additional erosion. Clients can be advised that the custom-fabricated fluoride trays can also be used without the fluoride to protect teeth during periods of out-of-control binge and purge episodes. Use of desensitizing fluoridated dentifrices may provide additional benefit for clients with exposed dentin from erosion.

Recommendations for saliva substitutes are appropriate if the client reports discomfort from xerostomia. Many clients currently under psychological or psychiatric treatment for eating disorders are medicated with prescription antidepressants. Xerostomia resulting from these medications combined with systemic dehydration can create a situation that the dental hygienist needs to address during client education. For individuals who find saliva substitutes unpleasant, frequent water rinsing or sipping or sucking on crushed ice chips can be recommended.

Dental Hygiene Instrumentation During instrumentation (scaling, root planing, and removal of extrinsic stain), concern should be taken by the dental hygienist to provide thorough care while protecting sensitive hard and soft tissues. Maintaining a moist, clean environment by frequent rinsing of the oral cavity during instrumentation meets the client's need for freedom from pain and skin and mucous membrane integrity, especially if the individual suffers from xerostomia. Selective polishing or use of a low abrasive polishing agent should be considered when clients have had extensive enamel erosion resulting in dentin exposure. Many polishing pastes are excessively abrasive to dentin (e.g., pumice and/or medium- or coarse-grade agents) and can result in additional deficits in the human need for a biologically sound dentition (e.g., loss of tooth structure and increased dentinal hypersensitivity). Selective polishing is recommended if the individual does not have extrinsic stains or if the dental hypersensitivity impedes client comfort during stain removal.

Implementation of the dental hygiene process of care and necessary palliative treatment of discomfort (e.g., use of desensitization treatments) may be timed prior to and during psychological treatment. Additional restorative and prosthetic dental care, when required, should be coordinated with the psychological and medical teams once the client is receiving treatment.

Evaluation

Evaluation of dental hygiene care for the client with an eating disorder is composed of two parts:

- An objective evaluation based on mutual goals previously established by the dental hygienist and client
- A subjective report by the client

Objective Evaluation

For an objective evaluation, comparison at baseline and subsequent appointments of data collected on human needs deficits that relate to plaque accumulation, periodontal status, dental caries, enamel erosion, dentinal hypersensitivity and oral tissue health is critical. Many changes that occur over time are subtle and defy detection unless an accurate comparison can be made of the client's previous status. This is especially true in cases where perimylolysis is a significant finding. Clients who are under psychological treatment, but are not under control of the binge and purge behavior, may lead the oral health team to believe that the dental erosion has ceased. Objective comparison of pre- and posttreatment oral photographs and study models can verify or negate the subjective report by the client.

Subjective Evaluation

The subjective evaluation can provide additional information that the dental hygienist can use for future care planning. Using the worksheet for these clients guides the dental hygienist in obtaining subjective information on the dynamics of eating disorder behaviors and provides the client with the opportunity to be a participant in the evaluation process. Preservation of a caring, professional environment assures the client that confidentiality is maintained while oral health needs are met humanistically. The oral health team must be aware during evaluation of the client that successful treatment of anorexia, bulimia, and bulimarexia takes intensive therapy followed by many years of aftercare. It is common for clients who have successfully controlled eating disorder behaviors for several weeks or months to revert periodically to previous behaviors, especially when stressful life events occur. Awareness and verbal acknowledgment of this by the dental hygienist during evaluation permit clients to share honestly areas of progress as well as areas of distress. This information can then be used in conjunction with the objective data and reports from other attending health professionals to guide subsequent care.

On occasion, objective and subjective evaluations conflict. For instance, a client with previously documented dental erosion may report that binge and purge episodes have been under control for 6 months and that she is no longer in need of psychological treatment. However, comparison of current dental status to intraoral photographs and diagnostic models obtained 1 year previously may indicate that the erosion has been progressive and that a significant amount of tooth loss has occurred since that time. Discussing these discrepancies with the client and expressing concern about the reported cessation of aftercare therapy is crucial. Frequently the oral health team becomes instrumental in encouraging the client to seek additional psychotherapy when it is apparent that previous therapy has been unsuccessful. In this situation, it may even become necessary for the oral health team to refuse definitive dental treatment unless the client is in therapy and coordination between psychologist and oral health professionals can occur.

Continual evaluation of the client's oral health status, as well as status of psychological therapy, is one of the most critical functions of the dental hygienist when managing an individual who suffers from anorexia, bulimia, or bulimarexia. At several points during the dental hygiene process of care, the clinician may need to reassess the client's condition, revise care goals, plan alternative strategies, implement these strategies, and reevaluate the outcome. The dynamic nature of the dental hygiene process of care for clients with an eating disorder creates a challenge for the professional dental hygienist.

References

1. American Psychiatric Association. Diagnostic and Statistical Manual of Mental Disorders, 3rd ed. rev. Washington, DC: American Psychiatric Association, 1987.
2. French, R. N., and Baker, E. L. Anorexia nervosa and bulimia. Indiana Medicine 77:241, 1984.
3. Crisp, A. H., Palmer, R. I., and Kalucy, R. C. How common is anorexia nervosa? A prevalence study. British Journal of Psychiatry 128:549, 1976.
4. Mumford, D. B., and Whitehouse, A. M. Increased prevalence of bulimia nervosa among Asian schoolgirls. British Medical Journal 297:718, 1988.
5. Snow, J., and Harris, M. Disordered eating in south-western Pueblo Indians and Hispanics. Journal of Adolescence 12(3):329, 1989.
6. Robinson, P., and Andersen, A. Anorexia nervosa in American blacks. Journal of Psychosomatic Research 19(2):183, 1985.
7. Andersen, A. E. Anorexia nervosa and bulimia in adolescent males. Pediatric Annals 13:901, 1984.
8. Crisp, A. H., and Toms, D. A. Primary anorexia nervosa or weight phobia in males: Report on thirteen cases. British Medical Journal 1:334, 1972.
9. Hall, A., Delahunt, J. W., and Ellis P. M. Anorexia nervosa in the male: Clinical features and follow-up of nine patients. Psychiatric Review 19:315, 1985.
10. Drewnowski, A., Hopkins, S., and Kessler, R. The prevalence of bulimia nervosa in the U.S. college student population. American Journal of Public Health 78(10):1322, 1988.
11. Pyle, R., Mitchell, J., et al. The incidence of bulimia in freshmen college students. International Journal of Eating Disorders 2(3):75, 1983.
12. Wolcott, R. B., Yager, G., and Gordon, G. Dental sequelae to the binge-purge syndrome (bulimia): Report of cases. Journal of the American Dental Association 109:723, 1984.
13. Lucas, A. R. Bulimia and vomiting syndrome. Contemporary Nutrition 6:1, 1981.
14. Russell, G. Bulimia nervosa: An ominous variant of anorexia nervosa. Psychosomatic Medicine 9:429, 1979.
15. Garfinkle, P. E., Moldofsky, M. D., and Gardner, D. M. The heterogeneity of anorexia nervosa: Bulimia as a distinct subgroup. Archives of General Psychiatry 37:1036, 1980.
16. Boskind-Lodahl, D. Cinderella's step-sisters: A feminist's perspective on anorexia nervosa and bulimia. Signs: Journal of Women in Culture and Society 2:342, 356, 1976.
17. Holland, A. J., Sicotte, N., and Treasure J. Anorexia nervosa: Evidence for a genetic basis. Journal of Psychosomatic Research 32(6):561, 1988.
18. Hsu, L. K., Chesler, B. E., and Santhouse, R. Bulimia nervosa in eleven sets of twins: A clinical report. International Journal of Eating Disorders 9(3):275, 1990.
19. Hudson, J. I., Pope, H. G., et al. Family history study of anorexia nervosa and bulimia. British Journal of Psychiatry 142:133, 1983.
20. Newman, M. M., and Halmi, K. A. The endocrinology of anorexia nervosa and bulimia nervosa. Neurologic Clinics 6(1):195, 1988.
21. Beaumont, P. Anorexia and bulimia nervosa: The dieting disorders. BASH (Bulimia and Anorexia Self-Help newsletter) 7(11):265, 1988.
22. Herzog, D., and Copeland, P. Eating disorders. New England Journal of Medicine 313:295, 1985.
23. Koh, E., Ohishi, S., et al. Clinical evaluation of hypokalemia in anorexia nervosa. Japanese Journal of Medicine 28(6):692, 1989.
24. Casper, E. C., Eckert, E. D., et al. Bulimia: Its incidence and clinical importance in patients with anorexia nervosa. Archives of General Psychiatry 37:1030, 1980.
25. Drisko, C., Drisko, R., et al. Oral health status of anorexics and bulimics: A case control study (abstr.). Journal of Dental Research 68(Spec. issue):285, 1989.
26. Roberts, M. W., and Li, S. H. Oral findings in anorexia nervosa and bulimia nervosa. Journal of the American Dental Association 115:407, 1987.
27. Milosevic, A., and Slade, P. D. Orodental status of anorexics and bulimics. British Dental Journal 167:66, 1989.
28. Simmons, M. S., Greydon, S. K., and Salmen, C. W. Dentist's role in diagnosis of bulimia via screening for erosion (abstr.). Journal of Dental Research 64(Spec. issue):186, 1986.
29. Hellstrom, L. Oral complications in anorexia nervosa. Scandinavian Journal of Dental Research 85:71, 1977.
30. Hurst, P. S., Lacey, J. H., and Crisp, A. H. Teeth, vomiting, and diet: A study of the dental characteristics of seventeen anorexia nervosa patients. Postgraduate Medical Journal 53:298, 1977.
31. Altshuler, B. D., Dechow, P. C., et al. An investigation of the oral pathologies occurring in bulimia nervosa. International Journal of Eating Disorders 9(2):191, 1990.
32. Levin, P. A., Falko, J. M., Dixon, K., et al. Benign parotid enlargement in bulimia. Annals of Internal Medicine 93:827, 1980.
33. Burke, R. C. Bulimia and parotid enlargement: Case report and treatment. Journal of Otolaryngology 15(1):49, 1985.

34. Brady, J. P. Parotid enlargement in bulimia. Journal of Family Practice 20:496, 1985.
35. Jirik-Babb, P., and Katz, J. Impairment of taste perception in anorexia and bulimia. International Journal of Eating Disorders 7(3):353, 1988.

Suggested Readings

Cowan, R. D., Sabates, C. R., et al. Integrating dental and medical care for the chronic bulimia nervosa patient: Report of case. Quintessence International 22(7):553, 1991.

Drisko, C., Gross, K., et al. Prevalence of factitious injuries in eating disorder patients (abstr.). Journal of Dental Research 68(Spec. issue):367, 1989.

Kassett, J. A., Gwirtsman, H. E., et al. Patterns of onset of bulimic symptoms in anorexia nervosa. American Journal of Psychiatry 145(10):1287, 1988.

Pope, H. G., Hudson, J. I., and Jonas, J. M. Bulimia in men: A series of fifteen cases. Journal of Nervous and Mental Disease 174(2):117, 1986.

VII LEADERSHIP AND MANAGEMENT

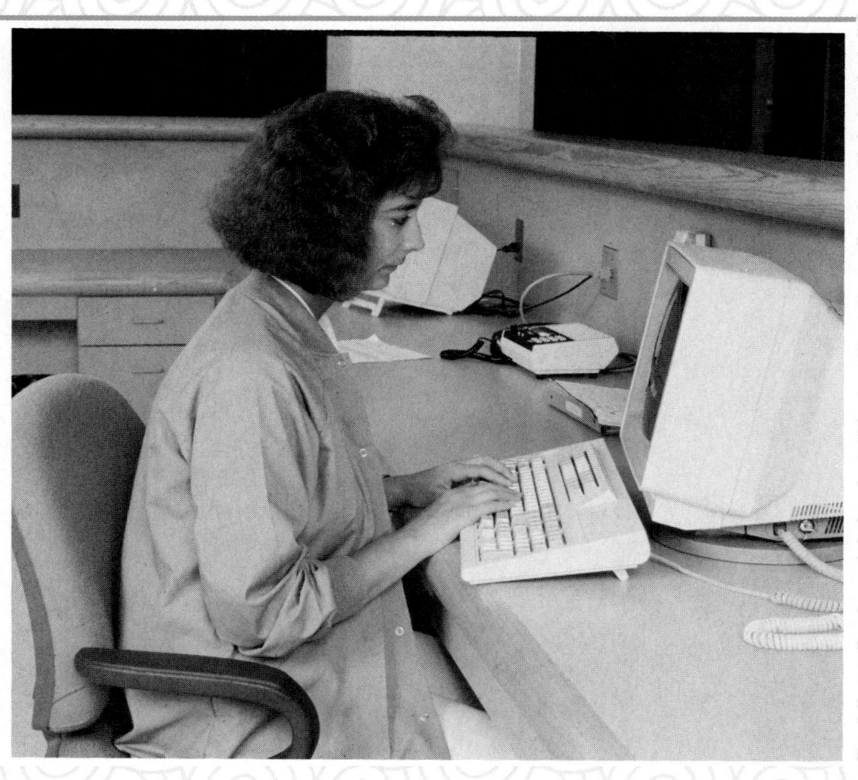

36 Dental Hygiene Management and Leadership

OBJECTIVES

Mastery of the content of this chapter will enable the reader to:

- Define the key terms used
- Differentiate between leadership and management
- Explain why leadership skills are important to the dental hygienist
- Describe the four classic styles of leadership: authoritarian, democratic, laissez-faire, and situational
- Explain how the dental hygienist uses the leadership process to benefit the client, the oral health team, society, and the dental hygiene profession
- Explain how leadership and management skills can be used to effect change
- Describe the dental hygienist's role as a change agent

INTRODUCTION

Dental hygienists spend a large portion of their professional careers in organizations such as private practices, academic institutions, public schools, public health departments, and acute care or long-term care facilities. Within an organization, a dental hygienist might serve in the roles of subordinate, manager, or both. The purpose of this chapter is to guide the dental hygienist in developing effective management and leadership skills that can be used by the dental hygiene clinician, manager, change agent, consumer advocate, educator, or researcher.

Successful organizations have effective leaders. To meet the demand for effective leaders in dental hygiene, dental hygienists must learn and develop leadership skills early in their careers, apply leadership theory in various dental hygiene roles, on a daily basis, and in a wide variety of situations and circumstances. The dental hygienist must understand basic management and leadership theory, principles of management, and strategies for achieving organizational goals through people. This information, if applied, can be helpful to the professional dental hygienist striving for success in both employment and volunteer settings.

When a dental hygienist becomes involved in an organization as an employee or volunteer, her first goal is to become a successful subordinate. The concept of "the successful subordinate" should not be underestimated. Before one advances in any organization, one must be recognized as a valued member. In any organizational hierarchy, an employee is always subordinate to another person within the organization. Even the president is subordinate to the board of directors. In the private practice setting, the dental hygienist might be subordinate to the office manager, who is then subordinate to the dentist who owns the practice; in a professional association, the committee members are subordinate to the committee chairperson.

Several elements are critical to being an effective subordinate:

- Knowing the organization, its philosophy, its mission, and its goals
- Understanding the jobs of those one works with, including the job of the official leader
- Understanding one's job in relation to the jobs of other employees in the organization
- Understanding human needs and viewing human needs as motivational factors that influence behavior[1]

What Is a Manager?

A **manager** is a person who accomplishes goals and objectives through other people. The dental hygienist may be employed as a manager in situations as diverse as a client's oral health, a research project, a healthcare setting, a dental public health department or project, a dental hygiene program, a government program, or some aspect of a professional association or corporation. A dental hygienist, in a managerial role, needs to:

- Establish short- and long-range goals
- Participate in strategic planning
- Formulate policies and procedures
- Coordinate human, material, and financial resources
- Motivate and evaluate workers
- Solve problems
- Make decisions
- Resolve conflicts
- Effect change

These activities might take place in dental or dental hygiene practice settings, institutions of public and higher education, public health agencies, or business and industry. The functions of a manager and those of a leader frequently overlap. Although managers' positions differ among settings and organizations, several functions are common to all managers.[2]

"Managers work with and through other people." In this capacity, managers work with people internal and external to the organization and as such serve as channels of communication. Managers use motivational strategies to encourage peak performance of the work group and to maintain enthusiasm and job satisfaction.[2]

"Managers are responsible and accountable." As such, managers are responsible for tasks completed by others as well as themselves. For example, the achievements and failures of subordinates are a direct reflection on managerial effectiveness. The stress level of managers is great because of their responsibility for the work of those who they indirectly control.[2]

"Managers balance competing goals and set priorities." In any organization, a manager is faced with having to achieve numerous objectives, with limited human and material resources. This challenge is most evident during a time of economic recession when organizations are downsizing. The manager must be able to set short- and long-range goals, establish priorities that are congruent with the mission of the organization, assign workloads and resources necessary for goal attainment, and disseminate information. Human and organizational needs and demands are in constant competition for limited resources, making the job of the manager particularly difficult. The manager applies human need theory to understand and satisfy the needs of the workers and the organization.[2]

"Managers must think analytically and conceptually." They must be able to dissect a problem systematically, see its components, generate alternative solutions, and then evaluate the impact of the various approaches. At all times, the manager must have a vision of where the plans are taking the organization, and the implications of her actions and inactions. Often, the manager must make decisions under condition of extreme ambiguity.[2]

"Managers are mediators." Conflict is a normal, not abnormal, occurrence in organizations. Managers must devote regular attention to resolving disputes that are likely to occur between co-workers. Dedication to this managerial role and skills in conflict management and negotiation augment the effectiveness of the manager.[2]

"Managers are politicians." Managers must build professional relationships with people in and external to the organization in an attempt to promote organizational goals. This involves communication, interpersonal skills, the process of change, persuasion, motivating, networking, and team building. Managers must "play politics" to build support through IOUs, alliances, and coalitions.[3] Such networks of mutual obligation with others in the organization provide the political base necessary to win support for new plans, decisions, and ideas and muster cooperation for their implementation and evaluation.[2]

"Managers are diplomats." Managers represent the perspectives of their subordinates and their organization at meetings and conferences and as such serve as official spokespersons and ambassadors. Managers must embody the philosophy and image of the organization of which they are a part.[2]

"Managers make difficult decisions." Problems are a usual occurrence within the realm of the manager. The manager's problems are augmented because the problems encountered by subordinates are the problems of the manager. Typical problems that challenge the manager's decision-making ability include budgetary problems, personnel problems, political problems, and resource allocation.[2]

THE MANAGEMENT PROCESS

Management can be described as a series of parts that make up a process. Five main activities comprise the **management process:**

- Planning
- Organizing
- Leading
- Motivating
- Controlling

Emphatically, the functions presented in the model do not necessarily occur in a sequence (Fig. 36–1); rather, various combinations of these functions may occur simultaneously as the manager pursues the objectives of the organization. Furthermore, these functions are influenced by factors such as the manager's scope of authority, the personality of the organization, and resource limitations. The model is presented as a useful beginning approach to viewing the functions of the manager and is not meant to be a definitive replication of the real world.

Planning

Planning is the beginning and most fundamental component of the management process. Planning is second nature to most dental hygiene professionals who typically use planning in the dental hygiene process of care and in applying the scientific method. Planning is proactive and requires initiative on the part of the dental hygienist. Organizational needs differ from client human needs, and managers must integrate both organizational and human needs and prepare in advance to meet them. Planning is essential for setting the course or direction of the members of the organization. The manager uses plans to establish objectives and develop strategies or programs for achieving these objectives. Plans may be short-term, that is, established to outline directives for the day or week; or may be long-term, requiring implementation over a 1- to 5-year period.

Through planning, the manager in collaboration with subordinates decides what to do, when to do it, how it should be done, and who should do it.[4] Some of the areas

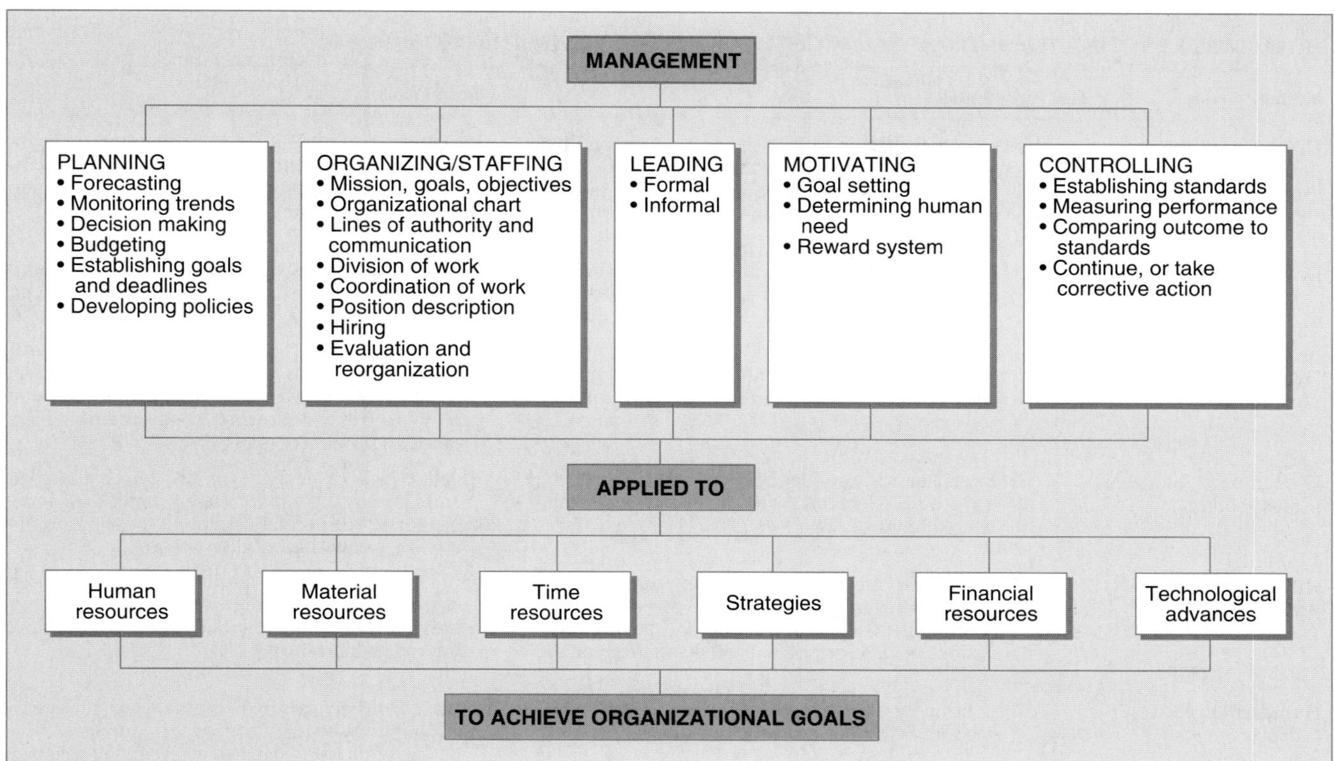

FIGURE 36-1
The management process.

that need to be spelled out during the planning process include goals, objectives, standards, schedules, methods, budgets, staffing, policies, procedures, and rules. The planning process has several benefits for the manager and organization. Good planning helps minimize the risk of uncertainty, ensures the best possible use of all resources, focuses attention on achieving organizational goals, defines the criteria of measurement for evaluating goal attainment, establishes a work schedule, and clarifies needs for human and material resources. Lyles[5] offered several suggestions for improving the planning process:

- Ensure proper input; the manager should make every effort to obtain contributions from anyone who is willing to make them
- Make sure that goals set are realistic; although goals should encourage growth, they should not be so unrealistic so as to frustrate the workers
- Plans should be specific and measurable; specific plans are more easily understood and communicated and implemented than general plans
- Actively communicate the plan; plans must be understood fully to be carried out successfully
- Be flexible; even the best plans must be modified for unforeseen reasons

Organizing and Staffing

The organizing function involves the creative grouping of human and material resources so that the established plans can be carried out. The manager must design the most effective grouping of people, resources, and responsibilities to achieve the organization's objectives. The best conceived plans will fall short if the manager cannot organize resources or obtain the resources necessary to make goal attainment a reality. Some of the elements of the manager's organizing function include:

- The organizational chart
- Division and coordination of work
- Position descriptions, rules, and policies and procedures

These elements create an operational structure that facilitates the flow of information, the span of management, and goal attainment. The organizing structure of the organization should evolve from demands of the organization and should be revamped when they no longer fulfill organizational needs.

Once the organizational structure is in place, the right people must be recruited and hired to make the organization work. The managerial responsibility known as staffing ensures that the organization has the human resources to achieve its goals. The staffing function includes planning personnel needs; recruitment; selection, hiring, and firing; personnel orientation, training, and development; and position reassignment.

Leading

Leading refers to the manager's role influencing people to work toward the achievement of the organization's goals. Through effective **leadership,** the manager influences the performance of employees. Models and theories on leading behaviors suggest that various leadership styles may be appropriate at some time, depending on the situation.

Motivating

Motivating is a managerial function that enables the manager to influence the employees she manages. Motivating

TABLE 36–1
HUMAN NEEDS THAT THE INDIVIDUAL MIGHT SEEK TO FULFILL IN THE WORKPLACE

Human Need	Definition	Descriptors
Human need for acceptance of self and others, by others	A receptive attitude toward self and others, and by others, which recognizes the value or worth of the person without implying approval of particular human behaviors and without implying affection	Recognition of abilities and limitations; recognition of virtues and faults; feeling of contentment and satisfaction with one's self; experiences positive regard from others
Human need for activity	A behavior or action requiring an expenditure of energy by the person with volition and intent	Muscular action/organic functioning; a changed relationship between person and environment; organized response toward a specific result; purposeful use of memory
Human need for appreciation	The act of taking critical notice of and giving a determination of the quality, the value of the person	Understanding and enjoyment; consideration; courtesy; thoughtfulness; response to another person's behavior; caring; cognizant of importance and uniqueness of person
Human need for autonomy, choice	Maintenance of ego-identity when making decisions and selections with independence from external control	Relative lack of dependence on others; the right and the power to rule oneself; emotional independence; purposeful selection; conscious deliberation; knowledge of alternatives
Human need for belonging	Being a part of, having a secure position in a group, as a family, of significant others, a community, a social/cultural group and having possessions, goods, or personal effects that are one's own	One's place within the family, an occupation, an organization a bonding with; membership, affinity; connectedness; close caring relationship; interrelatedness
Human need for confidence	The belief in the sureness, reliability of self and one's ability, other persons, and things	Trust; certitude; assured expectation of experiences based on past similar or comparable experiences; having faith in oneself; self-reliance; consistency
Human need for challenge	An act of striving to accomplish a goal through the expenditure of special effort or dedication	Response to a call for a cause action-oriented; make demands upon the imagination; take issue with; focused energy; thought provoking; stimulate
Human need for conceptualization and problem solving	The ability to grasp ideas and abstractions, to reason, to make sound judgments about one's life and circumstances, to resolve situational uncertainties, answer perplexing questions requiring solutions and resolution	Acquisition and use of knowledge; decision making; induction; deduction; generalization; ordering of data; intellectual discrimination of facts and opinions; hypothesizing; critical thinking; understanding cues and responding
Human need for humor	The perception, the frame of mind to enjoy and express a sense of the clever, the funny, the comical	Amusement; light-heartedness and wit; recognition of the incongruencies and peculiarities in a situation; looking on the "bright side"; laughter; comedy; mood elevating
Human need to love and be loved	The experience of human energy given and/or received freely and honestly in the form of warm personal attachment and strong affection directly to self, God, parents and kin, spouse, children, significant others, friends and neighbors, the community of human beings; and reciprocated in kind	Devotion; passion; charity; compatibility; adoration; affinity; erotic love; attraction; to hold dear; affectionate concern; friendship
Human need for personal recognition	The experience of acknowledgement of achievement, worth, service, or merit, to be regarded favorably with admiration and approval by others	Reward; public honor; homage; reverence; high regard, approbation; to be looked up to; privileged position; favorable impression; experience of success
Human need for self-determination and responsibility	The exercise of personal restraint, firmness of purpose and accountability for one's behavior and actions as a result of interaction between the person's internal powers of thought and emotions and the external forces in the physical and social environment	Regulation of one's self; doing what one ought to do; deciding for oneself; accountability
Human need for self-fulfillment, to be, to become	The act of realizing one's ambition, desires, purpose in life through one's own efforts as knowing and understanding oneself and the environment in which the person finds oneself, then achieving one's potential and culminating in the fullest state of being for the person	Self-understanding; goal-fulfillment; time-honored self-achievement; futuristic striving; personhood; striving for meaning; Creator's purpose for human beings; satisfaction; self-actualization
Human need for structure, law, and limits	A state of conduct in accordance with stated and learned principles that are sanctioned by one's	Protection, stability; authority; obedience; preservation of self and others

TABLE 36–1
HUMAN NEEDS THAT THE INDIVIDUAL MIGHT SEEK TO FULFILL IN THE WORKPLACE *Continued*

Human Need	Definition	Descriptors
	conscience, natural law, God, and are within the boundaries of the rules, customs, and practices of one's family, community, and culture providing a stable organized environment in which to live	
Human need for tenderness	The state of being treated with consideration, gentleness, concern by others and reciprocation of this to others	A gentle word; protective of vulnerable others; sensitivity to feelings of others; compassionate; caring; cherishing
Human need for value system	An internalized designation of the importance of or worth of people, institutions, things, activities, and experiences in one's life	Intrinsic desirability; judgment; set of beliefs, norms, and goals; intrinsic worth

Data from Yura, H., and Walsh, M. The Nursing Process, 5th ed. Norwalk, CT: Appleton & Lange, 1988.

employees is based on concepts inherent in human need theory. As human beings, individuals have numerous human needs that they seek to fulfill in the workplace (Table 36–1). When human needs are unsatisfied, individuals pursue goals that may satisfy their unmet human needs. The astute manager attempts to identify unfulfilled needs in her employees and assigns workloads and responsibilities that lead to human need fulfillment.

Within the conceptual framework of human need theory, the employee's attempt to satisfy her human needs is termed **motivation.** If the manager assumes that the employee is motivated by unmet human needs, then the unsatisfied need is a motivator. Some human needs can never be completely satisfied. For example, as we satisfy self-esteem, autonomy, self-respect, and recognition, our need for them becomes greater. Various needs are of greater and lesser importance to us throughout the life cycle, with personal growth needs becoming more important as they are satisfied. Within the sphere of the manager, motivation may include the defined human needs as well as opportunities for advancement, promotion, greater responsibility, status, growth, interesting work, and financial gain (see Managerial Strategies to Motivate Employees Using Human Needs Framework chart). The motivating function can be a powerful tool if the manager takes the time to understand employees' needs, and then is able to match an employee's motivation to satisfy a human need with a responsibility that needs to be carried out to achieve an organizational goal. An employee's motivation is influenced by factors that directly affect her human need fulfillment.

Poor performance may be the result of factors internal or external to the subordinate. Internal subordinate factors include lack of effort, lack of ability, lack of expertise, emotional or personal problems, burnout, and stress. External factors are problems beyond the subordinate's control such as inadequate material or human resources, lack of information, and financial limitations. When poor performance is recognized, the manager must try to change the situation by first determining the cause of the poor performance and then attempting to work with the subordinate to control or eliminate the causative factors and meet the employee's needs. Solutions may include modifying the responsibilities, time off to resolve a personal problem, arranging for staff development or continuing education, securing more resources, reorganizing to improve resource allocation and utilization, providing more information, or setting clearer performance goals and deadlines. When these strategies are ineffective, the manager may need to monitor the subordinate more closely to identify new incentives or inducements that may improve performance. Warnings, reprimands, and punishments may also be effective. Strategies for rewards and punishment are shown in Table 36–2. To be most effective, rewards and punishments should be linked to the factors that best motivate the subordinate, such as the subordinate's human need.

MANAGERIAL STRATEGIES TO MOTIVATE EMPLOYEES USING A HUMAN NEEDS FRAMEWORK

Managerial Strategies	Motivators Involved Based on Human Need
Removing some controls while retaining accountability	Self-determination and responsibility
Increasing the accountability of individuals for their own work	Self-determination and responsibility
Giving a person a complete natural unit of work (module, division, areas, and so on)	Autonomy
Granting additional authority to an employee in his activity; job freedom	Self-determination and responsibility
Making periodic reports directly available to the worker rather than to the supervisor	Appreciation and respect
Introducing new and more difficult tasks not previously handled	Challenge, conceptualization and problem solving
Assigning individuals specific or specialized tasks, enabling them to become experts	Challenge, conceptualization and problem solving

Modified from Scanlan, B. K. Principles of Management and Organizational Behavior. New York: John Wiley & Sons, 1973. Reprinted by permission of Burt K. Scanlan.

TABLE 36–2
REWARDS AND INCENTIVES USED BY DENTAL HYGIENE MANAGERS

Intrinsic Rewards	Extrinsic Rewards
Responsibility	Salary recommendations
Recognition (public/private)	Promotions
Information	Workloads
Esteem	Discretionary funds
Endorsements	Resource allocation
Autonomy	Job opportunities
Growth	Staff support
Mentorship	Committee assignments
Achievement	Relief from assignments
Advancement	Leaves of absence
Challenge	Schedule
Belonging	Fringe benefits
Respect	

Note: Punishment is withholding any of these rewards.

Controlling

Good planning, strong organization, and effective leadership have little chance for success unless there exists an adequate system of control.[6] *Control* is the process used by managers to assure that activities are carried out as planned. Through the control process, the manager measures progress toward goal attainment and takes corrective action as necessary. The controlling function of management ensures that the human and material resources within the organization actually move the organization toward the stated goals. The manager controls by:

- Establishing performance standards
- Measuring current performance against established standards
- Initiating change to correct performance that fails to meet standards

In designing a management control system, the manager must determine critical elements to be monitored, the standards and measurements to be used, the frequency of measurement, and the direction the results will take. The control process is applied to employee performance, budget and finance, services provided, and products generated.

MANAGEMENT THEORY

Management theory helps dental hygienists to predict the effect of their roles as managers. Without management theory, managers would be using hunches rather than a body of knowledge to guide actions. Each school of management offers a different conceptual model for defining and solving managerial problems and each offers valuable insights to dental hygienists exercising managerial roles. Table 36–3 summarizes some of the major theories of management.

One management approach of particular note is interactive management. Interactive management theory purports that successful leaders are those who can adapt their behaviors to meet the needs of other people. "Interactive management is a relationship building process that focuses on dealing with people as individuals in order to build trust, openness, and honesty in the manager-employee relationship, thereby improving productivity in the organizational setup."[7] To accomplish this the manager identifies and adjusts effectively to behavioral style differences to manage employees as unique individuals.

In the behavior style model, *assertiveness* is defined as the degree of control an individual tries to exert over others and the situation based on the amount of forcefulness one uses to express his thoughts and feelings to other people. Assertive behavior is divided into high and low assertiveness. Table 36–4 lists adjectives to describe each of the assertive styles. Responsiveness, the other major dimension

TABLE 36–3
MAJOR THEORIES OF MANAGEMENT

Theory/Theorists	Major Propositions	Contributions	Limitations	Application to Dental Hygiene
CLASSICAL APPROACH: Scientific Management Theory Robert Owen (1771–1858) Frederick W. Taylor (1856–1915) Henry L. Gantt (1861–1919) Frank B. Gilbreth (1868–1924) Lillian M. Gilbreth (1878–1972)	• Improving the conditions of the workers will lead to increased productivity and profits • Publishing worker productivity information leads to increased worker productivity, pride, and competition • Division of labor enhances efficiency and productivity • The best method for performing a task should be determined scientifically • Workers should be assigned responsibility according to who is best suited for the job • Workers should be scientifically educated and developed • Cooperation between labor and management should be cultivated	• Concept of the assembly line. • Concepts of time and motion • Concept of work design • Concept that tools can be made to increase efficiency • Beginning of the application of scientific principles to management	• Overlooked the social needs of workers • Overlooked the issue of job satisfaction • Did not achieve complete efficiency and harmony in the workplace	• May cause burnout • Economic gains are not the only thing that matters; people want to feel important and want a voice on issues that matter to them

TABLE 36–3
MAJOR THEORIES OF MANAGEMENT *Continued*

Theory/Theorists	Major Propositions	Contributions	Limitations	Application to Dental Hygiene
	• Management's aim is to help workers reach their full potential as human beings • Decreasing unnecessary motion decreases fatigue and increases productivity • A team of people, each responsible for a single task, can outproduce an equal number of people who are each responsible for all the tasks • Workers are rational, and as such are interested only in higher wages			
Classical Organizational Theory Henri Fayol (1841–1925)	• Management is not a talent but a learned skill • Business operations can be divided into six activities: technical, commercial, financial, security, accounting, and managerial • Defines management as planning, organizing, commanding, coordinating, and controlling • Developed Fayol's 14 Principles of Management[6a]	• Formal managerial training in schools • Management principles can be applied to all types of group activity • Certain principles underly effective managerial behavior	• Too general for today's complex organizations • More appropriate for the conditions found in the past • Less applicable to today's more educated worker • Did not achieve complete efficiency and harmony in the workplace	• Individuals can learn to be effective managers • Dental hygiene managers can continue to improve their managerial skills
BEHAVIORAL APPROACH: Human Relations Chester I. Barnard (1886–1961) Hugo Munsterberg (1863–1916) Elton Mayo (1880–1949)	• People join formal organizations to achieve things they could not achieve alone[6b] • Organizational effectiveness occurs when the organization's goals and the aims and needs of the workers are kept in balance[6b] • Good human relations stimulates worker productivity; poor human relations decreases worker morale and efficiency[6c] • For good human relations, managers must understand what motivates employees • Being singled out for special attention causes people to increase their work efforts[6c] • Social environment of the workers influences productivity[6c]	• Integrated principles from sociology and psychology with management theory • Discovery of the Hawthorne effect • Concept of the "social man" who is more motivated by social needs than by management control • True concern for workers increases productivity • Focused on manager's style and management training • Concepts of group processes and group rewards	• Does not completely describe workers in the workplace • Improving job satisfaction and work conditions does not dramatically improve productivity	• Humanistic theory applied by the dental hygiene manager can improve job satisfaction and work group cohesiveness
Behavioral Science	• A person is motivated to satisfy a hierarchy of needs: physical, safety, social, recognition, self-actualization • Each person is unique; a manager must try to influence workers according to their individual needs	• Concept of the self-actualizing man • Concepts of motivation, group behavior, interpersonal relations in the workplace and the importance of work	• Does not fully explain what motivates people • Often viewed as too complex to apply in the real world • Conflicting views of various behavioral scientists inhibit managers from applying behavioral theory	• Human need theory can be used by the dental hygiene manager to motivate people by helping them to fulfill their human needs and the needs of the organization simultaneously

Table continues on following page

TABLE 36–3
MAJOR THEORIES OF MANAGEMENT *Continued*

Theory/Theorists	Major Propositions	Contributions	Limitations	Application to Dental Hygiene
QUANTITATIVE APPROACH: Operations Research Management Science	• Problem solving can be accomplished best by bringing together experts who work together (operations research team) • Team of specialists use management science techniques to solve a problem and formulate a rational basis for decision making	• Management science techniques of mixed team specialists, mathematical modeling, computer modeling • Can be applied to budgeting and cash flow management, scheduling, and inventory control • Greatest application is to the managerial functions of planning and controlling	• Not readily applicable to human relations, organizing, staffing, and leading	• Quantitative techniques can be applied to solve some complex problems in dental hygiene including the economic value of dental hygiene services
SYSTEMS APPROACH:	• The organization is a unified, purposeful system composed of interrelated parts • Activity in one part of an organization affects the activities of every other part[6d,6e] • Management decisions are made only after their impact on other parts of the organizations is studied • Parts that make up the whole organization are referred to as subsystems • The entire organization is greater than the sum of its parts (synergy) • Open systems interact with their environment; closed systems do not • The system boundary (flexible ⟶ inflexible) separates the system • Resources flow into the system from the environment, undergo transformation, and exit the system as outputs, goods/services) • Feedback is information used to assess the system	• Concepts of subsystems, synergy, open and closed systems, system boundary, flow, feedback • Enables managers to maintain a balance between needs of the parts of the organization and the needs of the entire organization		• Enables dental hygienists to view and study their roles in the broader context of the entire work-unit, organization, or healthcare system
CONTINGENCY APPROACH:	• The manager must identify which technique will result in the attainment of goals given a particular situation, under a particular circumstance, and at a particular time • Builds upon systems theory by focusing on the *nature* of the relationships between the parts of an organization	• Recognizes that one approach will not be effective in all situations • Emphasizes flexibility in the application of management principles • Emphasizes that the complexity of the situation must be thoroughly considered in making managerial decisions • Some view the contingency approach as a leading branch of management today	• Not yet considered a true theory by some; does not address all aspects of systems theory	• Dental hygiene managers must thoroughly analyze the situation and their own behaviors to result in an effective management style

TABLE 36–3
MAJOR THEORIES OF MANAGEMENT *Continued*

Theory/Theorists	Major Propositions	Contributions	Limitations	Application to Dental Hygiene
INTERACTIVE MANAGEMENT APPROACH:	• The manager must identify behavioral style differences in employees and adjust her behavior accordingly • Management is a relationship building process that focuses on employees as individuals • Focuses on dealing with people as individuals in order to build trust in the manager-employee relationship	• Recognizes that successful leaders are those who can adapt their behaviors to meet the needs of other people • Recognizes that all employees are unique • Provides tangible suggestions for managing different behavioral styles	• Often difficult to subordinate one's behavioral style to that of another	• Dental hygiene managers must identify behavioral styles in co-workers and must be able to meet behavioral style needs to develop a climate of mutual trust

of behavioral style, is defined as the readiness with which one expresses emotions and develops relationships. Responsive behavior also is divided into high and low dimensions. Table 36–5 list descriptors for each type of responsive behaviors.

Figure 36–2 presents the two assertiveness extremes on a horizontal axis and the two responsiveness extremes on the vertical axis. Responsiveness and assertiveness levels vary across individuals. Any person may be high on both, low on both, high on one and low on the other, or somewhere in between on one or both scales. When the two scales are combined (Fig. 36–3), they form four quadrants that divide assertive and responsive behavior into four behavioral styles. One's behavior style describes the way that individual tends to interact with others in social and work situations naturally.

Knowledge of the four behavioral styles helps a manager understand why persons behave as they do, and this understanding allows more effective interaction with them to build productive relationships. Figure 36–4 lists characteristics of each behavioral style and Figure 36–5 lists behaviors related to each style.

Behavioral flexibility refers to the ability to change and adopt one's style to different interpersonal situations in order to make another feel more at ease. Behavioral flexibility is integral in the concept of interactive management. Table 36–6 presents strategies for implementing behavioral flexibility in interaction with each of the four behavioral styles to build productive relationships.

Each behavioral style has its own characteristic manner of reacting to stress in unproductive behavior. The Expressive attacks, the Driver dictates, the Analytical withdraws, and the Amiable submits. To avoid unproductive behavior in others, one must be able to meet their behavioral style needs. When one meets another's behavioral style needs, a climate of mutual trust begins to develop. According to interactive management, if a manager is able to identify differences in people, then she can treat them the way they want to be treated (the platinum rule—do unto others as they would have you do unto them). Following the platinum rule then leads to less tension along with higher levels of trust and credibility.

LEADERSHIP THEORY

Leadership is the ability to influence, motivate, or direct others toward the achievement of predetermined goals.

TABLE 36–4
ASSERTIVENESS DESCRIPTIONS

Low Assertiveness	High Assertiveness
Quiet	Verbose
Mild opinions	Strong opinions
Avoids risks	Takes risks
Meditative decisions	Swift decisions
Pleasing first impression	Powerful first impression
Shy	Active
Reserved	Confident
Supportive	Confronting
Easygoing	Impatient
Slow actions	Fast actions
Listens	Talks

From Hunsaker, P. L., and Alessandra, A. J. The Art of Managing People. New York: Simon and Schuster, 1986. Copyright © 1986 by Phillip L. Hunsaker and Anthony J. Alessandra. Reprinted by permission of Simon & Schuster, Inc.

TABLE 36–5
RESPONSIVENESS DESCRIPTIONS

Low Responsiveness	High Responsiveness
Aloof	Personable
Formal and proper	Relaxed and warm
Fact oriented	Opinion oriented
Guarded	Open
Controlled	Dramatic
Disciplined	Flexible
Task oriented	Relationship oriented
Hides personal feelings	Shares personal feelings
Thinking oriented	Feeling oriented

From Hunsaker, P. L., and Alessandra, A. J. The Art of Managing People. New York: Simon and Schuster, 1986. Copyright © 1986 by Phillip L. Hunsaker and Anthony J. Alessandra. Reprinted by permission of Simon & Schuster, Inc.

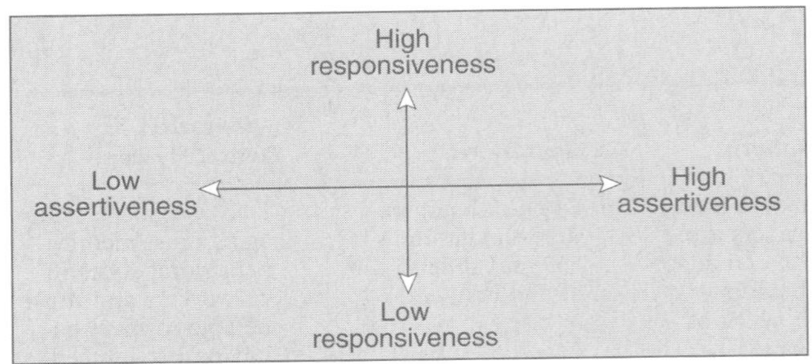

FIGURE 36-2
Assertiveness and responsiveness scales related to behavioral styles. (Redrawn by permission of Simon & Schuster, Inc. from Hunsaker, P. L., and Alessandra, A. J. The Art of Managing People. New York: Simon & Schuster, 1986. Copyright © 1986 by Phillip L. Hunsaker and Anthony J. Alessandra.)

Leaders take existing information and translate it into new and better ways of doing something. The leader may influence an individual, a client, a group, or an organization.

- "Leadership is based on an understanding of the way an organization could and should work (not how it does).
- Leadership uses deliberation and collective action, not unilateral action.
- Leadership involves all interested parties; it is concerned about who is in the conversation.
- Leadership is concerned with vision, not status quo.
- Leadership concerns problem-solving and problem-definition.
- Leadership is exercised by groups, individuals, or nations."[8]

Leadership may be formal or informal. A formal leader is one who leads via her legitimately superior position *(positional power)* within a group or organization. An informal leader holds a subordinate position within a group but influences others via her *personal power.* Dental hygienists who exercise leadership can bring about desired changes in clients' oral health patterns and behaviors, the employment setting, healthcare policy, community oral health practices, the healthcare system, and the dental hygiene profession in general. Therefore, leadership is an important process to master.

Effective leaders are sensitive to the human needs and roles of subordinates and peers, know managerial techniques and when to apply them, have a strong desire to effect change and a commitment to work with people to achieve goals. According to Bennis,[9] organizations with effective leaders empower the workforce with four evident themes:

- People feel significant; everyone feels that he or she makes a difference to the success of the organization, . . . people feel that what they do has meaning and significance
- Learning and competence matter, leaders value learning and mastery, and it clear that there is no failure, only mistakes that give us feedback and tell us what to do next
- People are part of a community, where there is leadership, there is a team, a family, a unity. Even people who do not especially like each other feel the sense of community
- Work is exciting; where there are leaders, work is stimulating, challenging, fascinating, and fun. Leaders articulate and embody the ideals toward which the organization strives.[9]

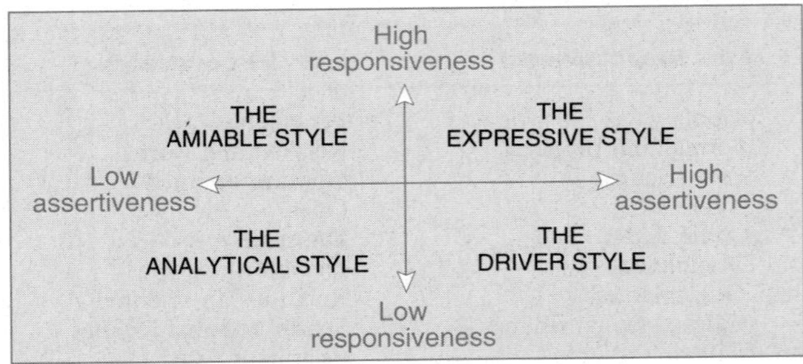

FIGURE 36-3
Four behavioral styles. (Redrawn by permission of Simon & Schuster, Inc. from Hunsaker, P. L., and Alessandra, A. J. The Art of Managing People. New York: Simon & Schuster, 1986. Copyright © 1986 by Phillip L. Hunsaker and Anthony J. Alessandra.)

Leadership Style

Autocratic, democratic, and laissez-faire styles of leadership are most frequently encountered in organizations. It is generally believed that one **leadership style** is not superior to another. Rather, each leadership style can be effective under certain conditions or in certain situations. Dental hygienists should develop their leadership skills in the style context with which they are most comfortable and should learn which situational variables are most compatible with the various leadership styles. Variables that make each leadership situation unique include the dental hygienist's personality, the characteristics of the group, the climate of the organization, and the nature of the tasks to be completed.

Authoritarian Leadership

In **authoritarian leadership,** the leader exerts close control over people. The leader's behaviors can be characterized as task-oriented, controlling, and directive with little autonomy given to the subordinates. The authoritarian leader perceives herself as the expert (authority) and solicits little input from the subordinates. Decision making, problem solving, planning, and evaluating all remain within the purview of the authoritarian leader, without delegation or consideration of the subordinates' needs, ideas, or beliefs. The authoritarian leader motivates through external rewards, such as pay, benefits, working conditions, promotions.

Many dental hygienists have worked under autocratic leadership. This approach has been used in some private practice settings and educational institutions where the employer or program director uses a "top-down" management style with little regard for self-determination on the part of the employee. Authoritarian leaders are described as highly task oriented with little regard for employee relations. This type of manager may believe that power and control must remain with the "boss" in order for the organization to be effective, that employees are not capable of significant decision making, or that she loses power, prestige, and respect if employees are given a greater voice in the operation of the organization.

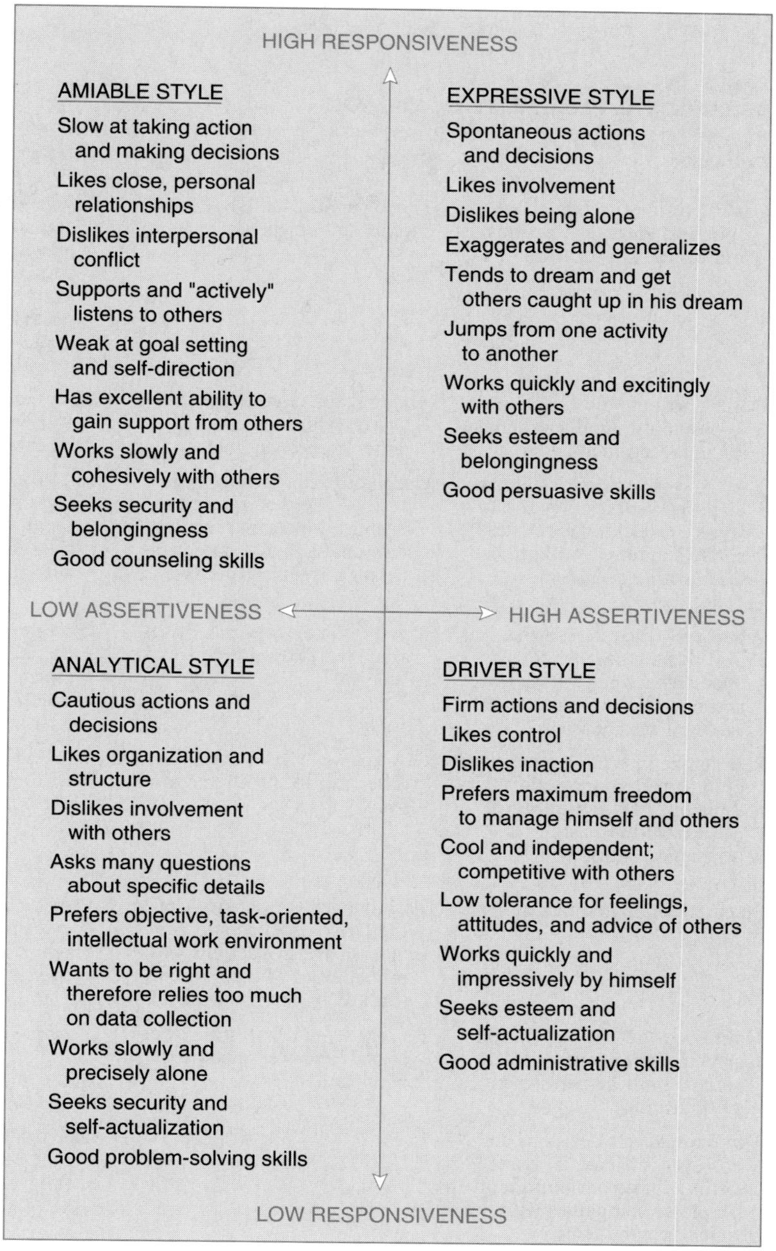

HIGH RESPONSIVENESS

AMIABLE STYLE

- Slow at taking action and making decisions
- Likes close, personal relationships
- Dislikes interpersonal conflict
- Supports and "actively" listens to others
- Weak at goal setting and self-direction
- Has excellent ability to gain support from others
- Works slowly and cohesively with others
- Seeks security and belongingness
- Good counseling skills

EXPRESSIVE STYLE

- Spontaneous actions and decisions
- Likes involvement
- Dislikes being alone
- Exaggerates and generalizes
- Tends to dream and get others caught up in his dream
- Jumps from one activity to another
- Works quickly and excitingly with others
- Seeks esteem and belongingness
- Good persuasive skills

LOW ASSERTIVENESS ↔ HIGH ASSERTIVENESS

ANALYTICAL STYLE

- Cautious actions and decisions
- Likes organization and structure
- Dislikes involvement with others
- Asks many questions about specific details
- Prefers objective, task-oriented, intellectual work environment
- Wants to be right and therefore relies too much on data collection
- Works slowly and precisely alone
- Seeks security and self-actualization
- Good problem-solving skills

DRIVER STYLE

- Firm actions and decisions
- Likes control
- Dislikes inaction
- Prefers maximum freedom to manage himself and others
- Cool and independent; competitive with others
- Low tolerance for feelings, attitudes, and advice of others
- Works quickly and impressively by himself
- Seeks esteem and self-actualization
- Good administrative skills

LOW RESPONSIVENESS

FIGURE 36–4
Predominant characteristics of each behavioral style. (Redrawn by permission of Simon & Schuster, Inc. from Hunsaker, P. L., and Alessandra, A. J. The Art of Managing People. New York: Simon & Schuster, 1986. Copyright © 1986 by Phillip L. Hunsaker and Anthony J. Alessandra.)

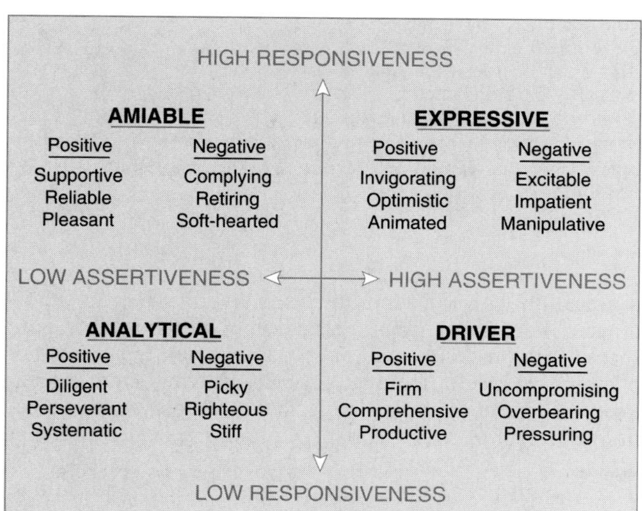

FIGURE 36–5
Positive-negative description of each behavior style. (Redrawn by permission of Simon & Schuster, Inc. from Hunsaker, P. L., and Alessandra, A. J. The Art of Managing People. New York: Simon & Schuster, 1986. Copyright © 1986 by Phillip L. Hunsaker and Anthony J. Alessandra.)

TABLE 36–6
BEHAVIORAL FLEXIBILITY GUIDELINES

Expressives	Drivers	Analyticals	Amiables
Get Expressives to talk about opinions, ideas, and dreams, and try to support them	Try to support the Driver's goals and objectives	Try to support the Analytical's organized, thoughtful approach. Any contributions you can make toward her objectives should be demonstrated through actions rather than words (send literature, brochures, charts, etc.)	Try to support the Amiable's feelings
Don't hurry the discussion. Try to develop mutually stimulating ideas together	Ask questions that allow the Driver to discover things rather than being told	Be systematic, exact, organized, and prepared with the Analytical	Project that you are interested in him as a person
The Expressive does not like to lose arguments, so try not to argue. Instead, explore alternative solutions you both can share with enthusiasm	Keep your relationship businesslike. Do not attempt to establish a personal relationship unless that is one of the Driver's specific objectives	List advantages and disadvantages of any plan you propose, and have viable alternatives for dealing effectively with the disadvantages	Take time to effectively get the Amiable to spell out personal objectives. Make sure you get him to differentiate what he wants from what he thinks you want to hear
When you reach agreement, iron out the specific details concerning what, when, who, and how. Be sure you both agree on the specifics	If you disagree with the Driver, argue the facts, not personal feelings	Give the Analytical time to verify your words and actions (because she *will* take the time)	When you disagree with the Amiable, do not debate facts and logic. Discuss personal opinions and feelings
Summarize in writing what you both agreed upon, even though it may not appear necessary (don't ask permission—just do it)	Give recognition to the Driver's ideas, not to the Driver personally	The Analytical likes things in writing, so follow up your personal contacts with a letter	If you and the Amiable quickly establish an objective and come to a fast decision, explore potential areas for future misunderstanding or dissatisfaction
Be entertaining and fast moving	To influence the decisions of the Driver, you should provide alternative actions with probabilities of their success (backed by facts, if available)	Provide solid, tangible, factual evidence (not someone's opinion) that what you say is true and accurate	Be agreeable with the Amiable by casually moving along in an informal, slow manner
Make sure you both are in full agreement concerning when actions must be performed (specification)	Be precise, efficient, time disciplined, and well organized with the Driver	Do not rush the decision-making process	Show the Amiable that you are "actively" listening and you are "open" in your discussion
The Expressive's decisions are positively affected if you use testimonials from important people or companies with which he can identify		An Analytical likes guarantees that her actions cannot backfire	The Amiable likes guarantees that actions will involve a minimum of risk. Offer personal assurances of support. However, do not overstate your guarantees, or you will lose his trust
		Avoid gimmicks that you believe might help you in getting a fast decision (the Analytical will think something is wrong with your plan)	

From Hunsaker, P. L., and Alessandra, A. J. The Art of Managing People. New York: Simon and Schuster, 1986.

Democratic Leadership

The **democratic leader** believes in the strengths inherent in people. Such a leader assumes that people like work and welcome opportunities that expand their responsibilities, competence, and skills. The democratic leader *does not* view himself as an authority, but rather assumes that a wealth of knowledge rests within the work group. This leader's behaviors can be characterized by frequent communication with the subordinates, active listening to subordinates' needs and ideas, delegation of responsibility, and shared responsibility with subordinates in key areas of planning, decision making, problem solving, and evaluation. The democratic leader facilitates employee participation, development, and equality among the leader and subordinates. The democratic leader may be described as having a high regard for both goal attainment and human relations. Such a leader motivates by using external as well as internal factors such as self-esteem, public recognition, job satisfaction, and respect to fulfill subordinates' human needs.

A dental hygienist who serves as the educational leader in oral healthcare setting may effectively use the democratic style of leadership to plan for office staff development. Rather than independently deciding on the courses staff members should take, the dental hygienist, in the leader role, calls a staff meeting so that the group may identify their own educational weaknesses and areas of interest. Together, the group also considers the needs of the setting and then reviews the educational opportunities that would improve individual knowledge and skill as well as overall organizational effectiveness. The dental hygienist develops the final plan with clear contributions from the group. The democratic style of leadership has been used effectively.

Laissez-faire Leadership

Laissez-faire or "hands-off" leadership refers to the person who avoids assuming leadership behaviors. With this type of leader, planning, decision making, and problem solving is ignored in hopes that problems will go away. The laissez-faire leader is characterized as being low on task orientation and low on human relations. Laissez-faire leadership can be good or bad depending on the strengths of the subordinates. If the subordinates are strong, they can assume the role of the leader and become totally self-directed. However, if the work group is weak, chaos can prevail and organizational effectiveness can suffer. For example, a laissez-faire leadership style may be observed in an organization when one employee is overtly lax in following established policies and procedures. Although this dental hygienist frequently abuses office privileges, making more work for her colleagues, the office manager merely ignores the behavior rather than solving the problem.

LEADERSHIP AND MANAGEMENT

Dental hygienists need effective leadership and management skills to help families, community groups, and society achieve oral health and wellness goals. The dental hygiene profession also needs effective dental hygiene leaders who can influence the direction of the profession and implement positive change. A dental hygienist in a leadership or managerial role uses specific skills to:

- Influence individual or group goals, commitment, motivation, and behavior
- Identify strategies and resources for goal attainment
- Influence the climate of the group or organization

The terms *manager* and *leader* are used interchangeably in this section because ideally a manager is a good leader and vice versa.

Leadership is the ability of an individual to influence people toward goal attainment. Comparing this definition to the earlier definition of management, it is clear that effective leaders and managers both have much in common, and it is possible to be a leader and a manager, a leader and a subordinate, and a manager and a subordinate at the same time.

Research and theory development on leadership suggest some answers about how leaders are developed; however, as of yet there is no grand theory of leadership. As in all complex, multifactored phenomena, great variability exists in the way leadership is conceptualized, observed, exercised, and measured.

Trait Theory of Leadership

Prior to 1949, most studies of leadership focused on the personality traits that distinguished leaders from nonleaders. Trait theorists believed that people born with certain attributes were most likely to evolve into leaders. In other words, leaders were born and not made. As researchers tested the trait theory, findings revealed that the theory was incorrect. Traits were inconsistently found across all leaders and more than 100 traits were identified as essential to effective leadership. Years of study have failed to identify one personality trait or set of qualities that can be used to identify effective leaders.[10,11]

Given that the majority of dental hygiene managers are women, it is interesting to note that men and women have dramatically different leadership traits. According to Rosener men tend to lead by command and control, that is they given an order, explain the reward for a job well done, and keep their knowledge and power to themselves.[12] Female managers generally lead by sharing power and information, interacting positively with subordinates, encouraging participation, and matching subordinates' personal goals with institutional goals. Rosener believes that this female leadership model is especially appropriate for the corporate climate of the 1990s where international and cultural influences, the increase in women and minorities in the workplace, and rapidly changing technology require accurate decisions on complex and competing issues. Women's tendency to share knowledge, power, and responsibility might be what is needed next.

Behavioral Theory of Leadership

The behavioral approach to leadership attempts to identify aspects of leader and manager behavior associated with effective leadership by examining the behavioral differences between effective and ineffective leaders (Fig. 36–6).

Effective managers maintain a mental agenda of objectives and strategies and an ever-expanding network of allies capable of implementation. The approach of focusing on what leaders *did* (behaviors) rather than what leaders *were* (traits) marked a new direction in understanding leadership. Unlike traits that one is born with, behaviors can be learned, and therefore leadership training could be accomplished.

Situational Theory of Leadership

Current perspectives on leadership theory suggest that unique **situational leadership** factors determine leader effectiveness, such as the tasks to be accomplished, the educational and skill level of the subordinates and leader, the organizational environment, the leader's personality and past experience (Fig. 36–7). This belief is based on studies showing that effective leadership is related not to a particular set of traits, but rather on how well the leader's traits match the characteristics of the situation.[13] Researchers who have tried to determine the *situational variables* that cause one leadership style to be more effective than another have found key variables to be important.[2] These variables should be analyzed by the dental hygienist facing managerial responsibilities.

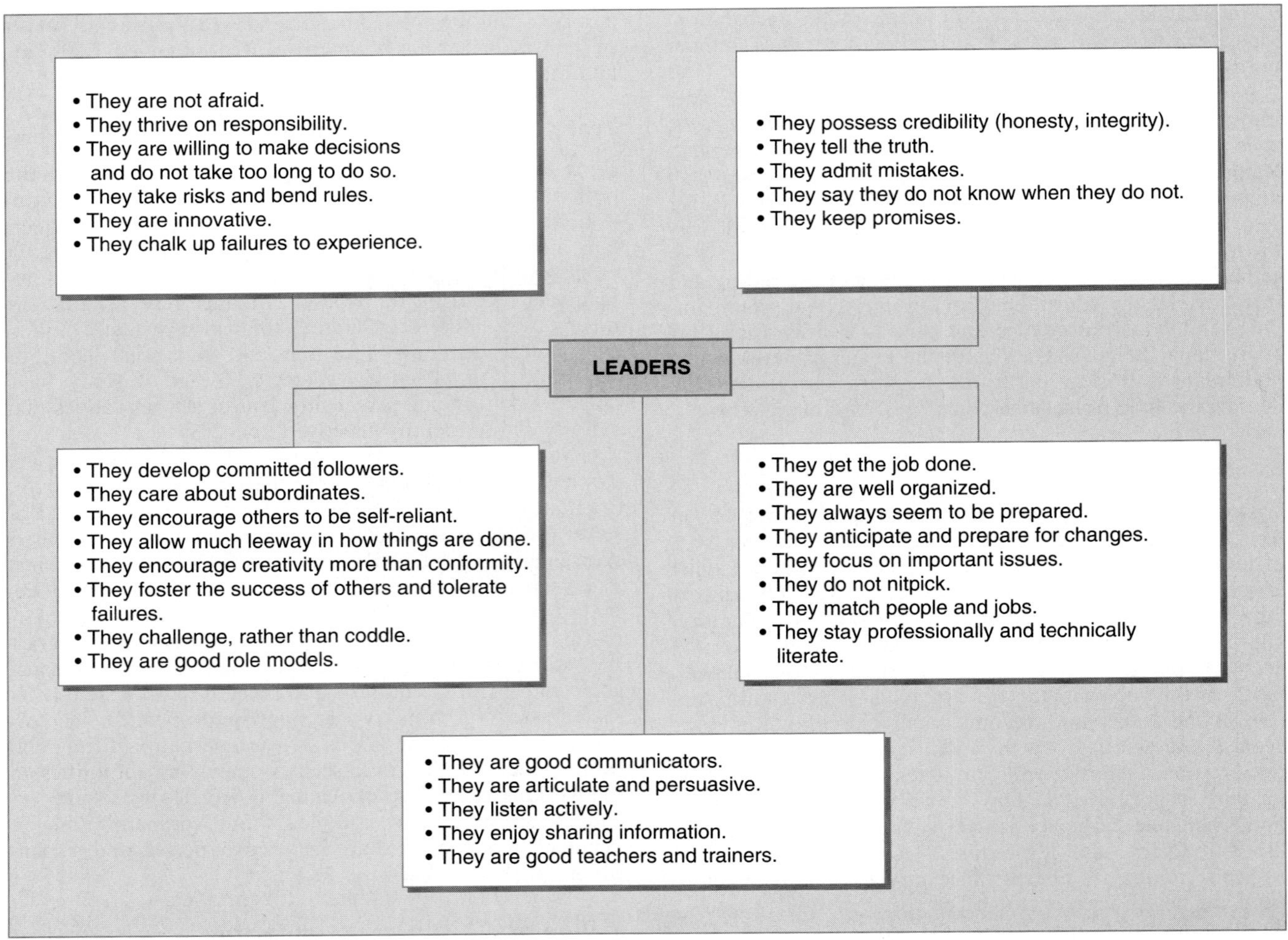

FIGURE 36–6
Behavioral characteristics of effective leaders. (Adapted and redrawn from Umiker, W. Management Skills for the New Health Care Supervisor. Gaithersburg, MD: Aspen, 1988, pp. 98–99. With permission of Aspen Publishers, Inc. © 1988.)

Leader's Personality, Past Experiences, and Expectations

Managers develop a leadership style that is most natural for their personality, beliefs, attitudes, expectations, and past experiences. For example, if the manager believes that subordinates are lazy and dislike work, the manager may adopt a more authoritative style of leadership. A manager who trusts his employees and who believes that job satisfaction comes from autonomy, self-respect, and recognition from others may be more employee-oriented.

Expectations and Behavior of Superiors

Higher level managers serve as role models for lower level managers. Qualities that are valued by the high-level manager (for example authority, human relations, peace-keeping, productivity) may cause the lower level manager to adopt those types of behaviors, too! Fleishman[22] found that new behaviors learned by supervisors tended to be abandoned if they were not consistent with their immediate supervisor's leadership style. Moreover, role expectations from supervisors, colleagues, and subordinates influence leader behavior to meet those expectations.

Subordinates' Characteristics, Expectations, and Behavior

Subordinates who are affected by the manager are important in determining the manager's leadership style. Highly educated and trained subordinates respond best to a manager who gives them autonomy, whereas lesser trained employees need more direction from an authoritative manager.

Subordinates who have had past experience with an authoritative manager may be uncomfortable with a democratic manager who asks for employee participation in decision making. The astute manager gives strong consideration to subordinates' characteristics, past experiences, and reactions in order to develop a leadership style that meets the demands of the situation.

Task Requirements

The nature of the task carried out by subordinates affects the type of leadership style the manager should use. Task-oriented leadership may be more effective for subordinates who work in isolation or whose job requires precise procedures. A people-centered leadership style is more appropri-

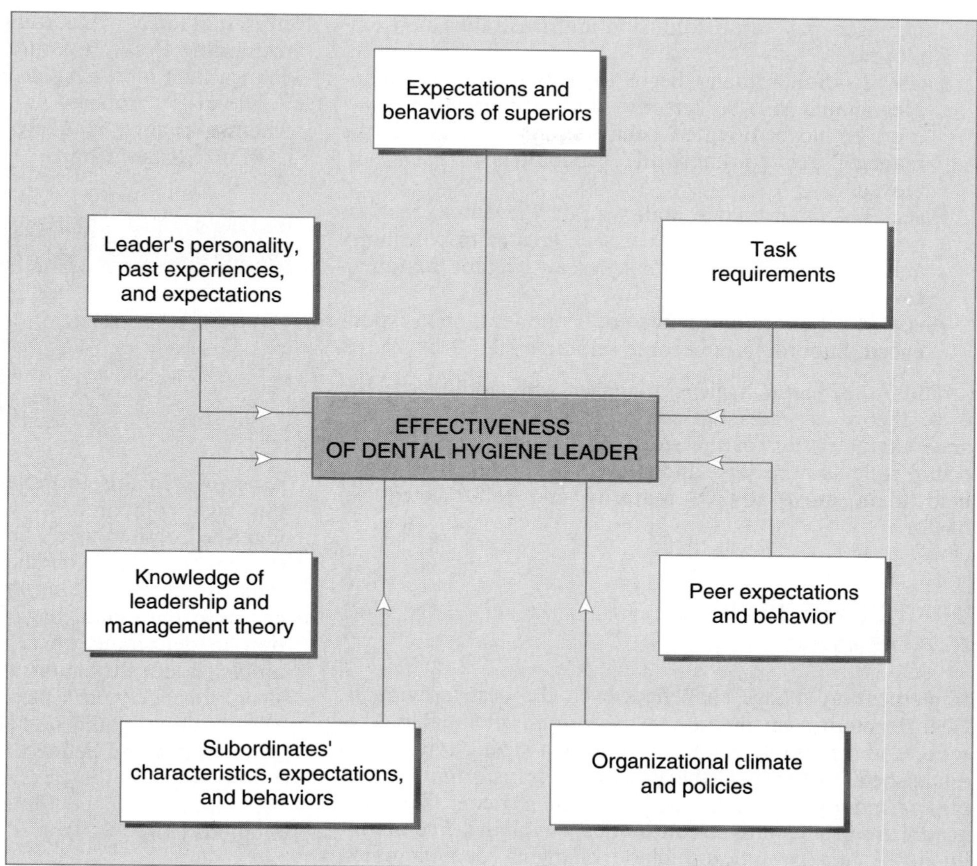

FIGURE 36–7
Factors influencing leader effectiveness in dental hygiene. (Modified from James A. F. Stoner/R. Edward Freeman, Management, 5e, © 1992, p. 481. Reprinted by permission of Prentice Hall, Englewood Cliffs, New Jersey.)

ate when the subordinate's job allows for creativity, autonomy, and collaboration among workers.

Organizational Climate and Policies

The personality of the organization influences the behaviors and expectations of the manager and subordinates. Organizations that enforce strict policies and procedures designed to meet organizational goals at all costs encourage leadership behavior that demands accountability, close supervision, and control over subordinates.

Peer Expectations and Behavior

Managers in collegial relationships with other managers in the organization exert peer pressure that influences the others' leadership style. Subordinates may complain that the expectations in their department differ from those in another department. Criticisms such as "You're too soft on your employees" may pressure some managers to alter their leadership style to meet the expectations of their peer managers. Managerial effectiveness depends in part on how well the manager recognizes the influence of these key variables, overcomes constraints and role conflicts, and pursues opportunities that arise.

The Life Cycle Theory of Leadership

The life cycle theory of leadership, developed by Hersey and Blanchard, predicts that the most effective style of leadership varies with the maturity of the subordinates.[14] In this context, maturity is defined as the subordinate's desire for achievement, willingness to accept responsibility, and task-related ability and experience. The model of the life cycle theory, shown in Figure 36–8, suggests a dynamic, four-phase relationship between a manager and subordinates:

Phase 1—Subordinates first enter the organization. Individuals new to an organization require a directive (task-oriented) style of management; a nondirective

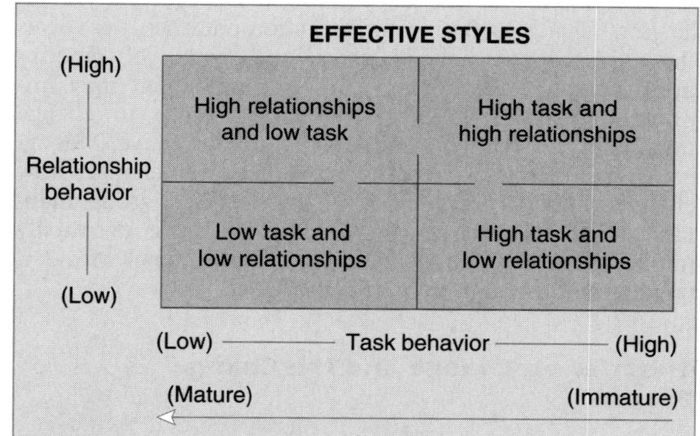

FIGURE 36–8
Life cycle theory of leadership. (Redrawn with permission from Stoner, J. A. F. Management, 2nd ed. Englewood Cliffs, NJ: Prentice Hall, 1982, p. 487; and adapted from Paul Hersey/Kenneth H. Blanchard, Management of Organizational Behavior: Utilizing Human Resources, 3e, © 1977, p. 165. For updated information on situational leadership, contact the Center for Leadership Studies, Escondido, CA.)

manager may cause confusion and frustrate a new employee.

Phase 2—Subordinates begin to learn their jobs. Manager should still be directive and task oriented; however, employee-oriented behaviors can increase as the manager gets to know the capabilities of each employee.

Phase 3—Subordinates' ability and achievement motivation increase and employees seek greater responsibility and autonomy. Manager's style can become nondirective.

Phase 4—Subordinates become confident and experienced. Subordinates become self-directed.

Thus, the dental hygiene manager who applies the life cycle theory of leadership constantly assesses the performance characteristics of the subordinates, modifies her leadership style as necessary, and supports staff development to help them move toward maturity and self-directed behavior.

EFFECTING CHANGE THROUGH LEADERSHIP

Implementing change challenges even the best individuals. Change requires an investment of human and material resources and is implemented only after a strong rationale is established. "**Change** is the process of transforming, altering, or modifying something."[15] Dental hygiene, like other healthcare professions, is continuously evolving. Factors influencing this evolution include changing demographics, cultural diversity, changing status of women in society, consumerism, rising cost of healthcare, ever-expanding knowledge and technology, special needs of subgroups, threats from other professional groups, and economic uncertainties.

"**Planned change** is a purposeful, systematic effort to alter or bring about change through the intervention of a change agent."[15] "The **change agent** is the individual who is responsible for taking a leadership role in managing the process of change."[2] Although the manager serves as a change agent, this role can also be assumed by various individuals within a work group. An outside change agent may be necessary if the entity to be changed is particularly challenging. Change within an organization commonly involves the need for new policies, procedures, goals, job descriptions, personnel, technology, and programs that may improve organizational effectiveness. Resistance to change must be overcome if the manager is to be effective. Managers must be able to recognize the need for change, how change can best be implemented, and facilitate group adaptation to the change made. Because change is eventually implemented through people, people must be involved if the change process is to be effective.

Theories on Change and the Change Process

Kurt Lewin's force-field theory explains that behavior is the result of an equilibrium between *driving* and *restraining forces*.[16] When most of us desire to see a change implemented, our natural tendency is to push. However, the equally natural tendency of those being pushed is to push back. In other words, driving forces activate their own restraining forces. According to Lewin's theory, decreasing restraining forces is a more effective way of implementing change than increasing driving forces.

Theorists proposed a simple formula to determine whether change is likely to be successful, wherein $C = (ABD) > X$ (see Chart).

C = (ABD) > X

C = Change
A = Level of dissatisfaction with the status quo
B = Clearly identified desired state
D = Practical first steps toward the desired state
X = Cost of the change[17]

As shown in this formula, the cost of the change may be too high compared with the level of dissatisfaction, the identified desired state, and the steps needed to implement the change. If so, resistance to change will outweigh the intent to change. Using this formula as a model for change can help the dental hygiene manager to analyze the situation to determine where intervention is needed. "For example, if dissatisfaction with the current state of affairs is strong on everyone's part, but there is no concrete notion of how things could be better, then the ideal state needs to be identified and defined."[2,17]

The steps of the *change process* are similar to those of the dental hygiene process and other problem-solving methods (Fig. 36–9):

Assessment

- Recognize when a change is needed.
- Collect data to verify the problem to be solved through change, and identify the desired state that will result from the change.

Diagnosis

- Label the problem that has created a need for change.

Planning

- Generate alternative solutions/approaches to the problem for which change is needed. Analyze the alternative approaches in terms of advantages, disadvantages, consequences of each, resources needed, cost, level of support. Decide upon a course of action from the alternatives analyzed.
- Design a plan for change: state objectives, outline methods, develop timetable, involve people, assign responsibilities, assign resources, and monitor stability.

Implementation

- Implement the plan for change.
- Monitor for unforeseen problems.

Evaluation

- Determine if the desired outcome and stated objectives have been achieved as a result of the implemented change.
- If necessary, reassess the situation and modify the plan for change.
- Stabilize the change by directing human and material resources to make the change permanent. Provide incentives and reward commitments to change. Rewards

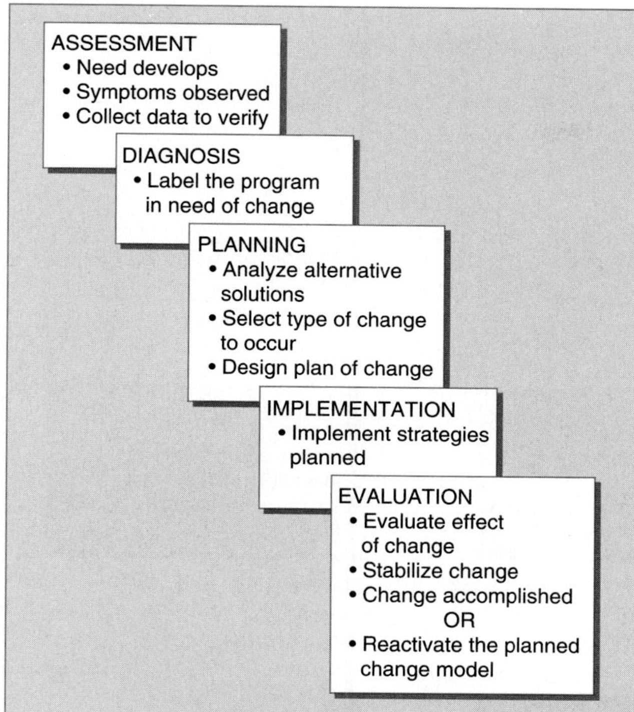

ASSESSMENT
• Need develops
• Symptoms observed
• Collect data to verify
DIAGNOSIS
• Label the program in need of change
PLANNING
• Analyze alternative solutions
• Select type of change to occur
• Design plan of change
IMPLEMENTATION
• Implement strategies planned
EVALUATION
• Evaluate effect of change
• Stabilize change
• Change accomplished
OR
• Reactivate the planned change model

FIGURE 36–9
A planned change model based on the dental hygiene process.

and incentives should meet the human needs of the people involved.

MANAGING RESISTANCE TO CHANGE

There are several sources of resistance to change.[18–20]

Uncertainty about the causes and effects of change. People are creatures of habit. They like tradition and routine because of the degree of predictability that it brings to the workplace. People may resist change because they fear the unknown.

Threat to self. People may feel that the change affects them personally, such as loss of self-esteem, power, prestige, more or less work and responsibility, change in peer relationships, or loss of other benefits. For example, a dental hygienist in a private practice setting might feel threatened when a fellow dental hygienist is asked to plan and implement a new marketing program for the practice. Another dental hygiene educator may resist the department's plan to expand its dependence on computer technology because she views the change as making her responsibilities more complex.

Lack of understanding. People who do not understand the reasons for the change or how the change can help them and the organization may resist change. Some dental hygienists may resist the trend toward higher levels of professional education or the need for dental hygiene research because they do not understand that society can be best served through these professional advancements.

Overcoming Resistance to Change

Dental hygienists, in managerial and leadership roles, need strategies for overcoming resistance to change. Resistance may be subtle or overt, passive or aggressive. Effectively managing resistance to change requires strength, knowledge, perceptions, knowledge of group dynamics and the characteristics of the work group, and a leadership style that is appropriate for the situation. Other reasons for resistance to change are displayed in Table 36–7.

The dental hygienist, as a change agent, benefits from using the following strategies proposed by Koller and Schlesinger:[18]

Education and communication. Always inform people about the planned change and completely explain the necessity of it. Use individual, one-on-one discussion, group meetings, formal presentations, and elaborate media campaigns if necessary.

Participation and involvement. Involve potential resistors in the process of change. Research confirms that resistant to change can be reduced or eliminated by having those involved participate in the plan of change.[19,21] Provide regular opportunity for open communication and feedback.

Facilitate and support. People in the transition of change may feel overlooked, rejected, unimportant, or inadequate. The manager must be sensitive to the human needs of the workers by communicating support and understanding. Other activities might include staff training and development, rewards (choice of schedule, public recognition, new title, bonuses, time off), and emotional support.

Negotiation and agreement. This technique seeks to achieve compromise agreements with the resistors of change. Perhaps a benefit desired by the resistor could be offered in return for support of the change. For example, if the constituent dental hygiene association was interested in gaining support of the nurses' association on a legislative issue, they may negotiate and agree to publicly support nursing on a future issue of concern to nurses in the state.

Manipulation and co-optation. People can be manipulated to support change by selectively releasing or

TABLE 36–7
REASONS FOR RESISTANCE TO CHANGE

External	Internal
Disagreements about benefits of change	Threat to self
Information not channeled appropriately	Lack of understanding
Poor planning	Limited tolerance for change
Lack of administrative support	Fear of increased responsibility
Lack of facilities	Change may be seen as punishment
Undefined goals and objectives	Concerns about future competence
	Lack of knowledge
	Lack of motivation

Data from Byrd, G. from Bassett, L. C., and Metzger, N. Achieving Excellence—A Prescription for Health Care Managers. Maryland: Aspen Publishers, 1986, p. 93; Potter, P. A., and Perry, G. A. Fundamentals of Nursing: Concepts, Processes, and Practice, 2nd ed. St. Louis: C. V. Mosby Co., 1993, p. 824; and Taylor, C., Lillis, C., and LeMone, P. Fundamentals of Nursing, 2nd ed. Philadelphia: J. B. Lippincott, 1993, pp. 372–373.

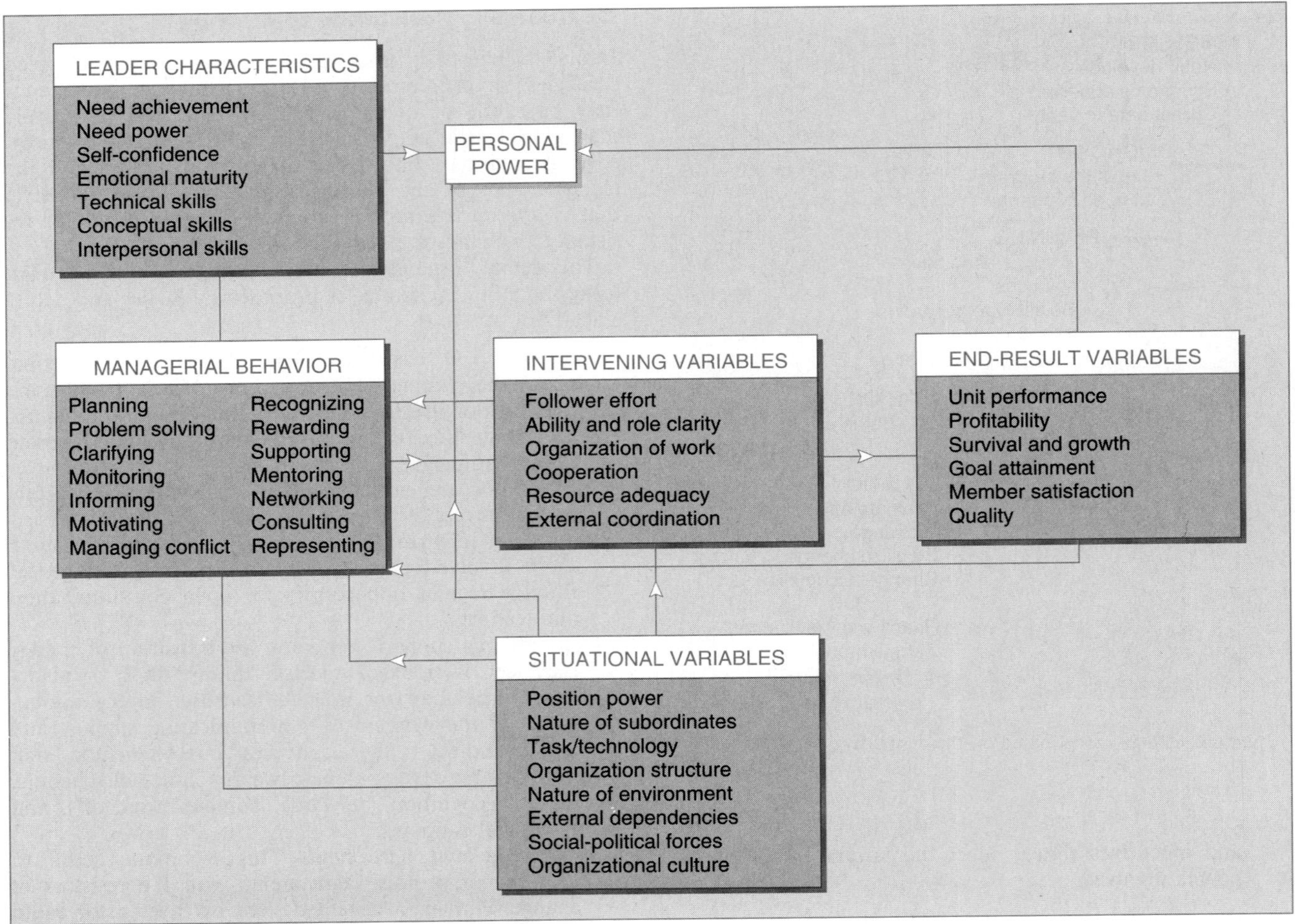

FIGURE 36–10
An integrating conceptual framework. (Redrawn with permission from Yuki, G. Managerial leadership: A review of theory and research. Journal of Management 15[2]:274, 1989.)

withholding information. A key person can be strongly encouraged (co-opted) to support a change by providing the person with special benefits if the change is not resisted. The ethics of these tactics must be questioned.

Explicit and implicit coercion. This strategy requires the manager to force people to support a change by exercising punishments such as lack of promotion, loss of job, salary decrease, or job transfer. This method can create poor relations between the manager and subordinates.

External change agent. When a manager predicts resistance to change, an expert external to the organization can be brought in to make recommendations for change. As in any change process, the external change agent should involve the participants who will be effected by the change. This approach is observed readily when consultants are hired to solve specific problems in school, institution, department, business, or private practice.

CURRENT STATUS OF LEADERSHIP THEORY

Currently, different sets of variables from past theories appear to be converging into a new meaningful configuration. The model shown in Figure 36–10 incorporates elements of most of the major leadership theories into a unique conceptual framework that encompasses the major variables relevant to leadership effectiveness. As research continues, this conceptual framework may be transformed into a grand theory capable of explaining and predicting effective leadership. For now, the framework provides a blueprint that identifies variables significant to the leadership process. Dental hygiene managers should consider these variables for developing an effective leadership style.

A dental hygiene leader invests time in studying the situational variables of the organization (characteristics of the subordinates, the organizational climate), the nature of the tasks to be accomplished, her own predominant leadership style, and the leadership style that has the greatest likelihood of success given the unique circumstances of the situation. Assumptions about subordinates (people like or dislike work, people must be coerced to work, people must be highly directed or given little direction to achieve organizational goals, people seek responsibility and autonomy, or people like to be closely supervised) have a significant influence on the leadership style adopted by the manager. The effective dental hygiene manager must be able to empower subordinates with a sense of ownership, mutual trust, and opportunity for participatory decision making. Within the human needs framework, the leader must rec-

SELF-STUDY QUESTIONS FOR MANAGERS

- Where do I get my information, and how? Can I make greater use of my contacts? Can other people do some of my scanning? In what areas is my knowledge weakest, and how can I get others to provide me with the information I need? Do I have sufficiently powerful mental models of those things I must understand within the organization and in its environment?
- What information do I disseminate? How important is that information to my subordinates? Do I keep too much information to myself because disseminating it is time consuming or inconvenient? How can I get more information to others so they can make better decisions?
- Do I tend to act before information is in? Or do I wait so long for all the information that opportunities pass me by?
- What pace of change am I asking my organization to tolerate? Is this change balanced so that our operations are neither excessively static nor overly disrupted? Have we sufficiently analyzed the impact of this change on the future of our organization?
- Am I sufficiently well-informed to pass judgment on subordinates' proposals? Can I leave final authorization for more of the proposals with subordinates? Do we have problems of coordination because subordinates already make too many decisions independently?
- What is my vision for this organization? Are these plans primarily in my own mind in loose form? Should I make them explicit to guide the decisions of others better? Or do I need flexibility to change them at will?
- How do my subordinates react to my management style? Am I sufficiently sensitive to the powerful influence of my actions? Do I fully understand their reactions to my actions? Do I find an appropriate balance between encouragement and pressure? Do I stifle their initiative?
- What kind of external relationships do I maintain, and how? Do I spend too much of my time maintaining them? Are there certain people whom I should get to know better?
- Is there any system to my time scheduling, or am I just reacting to the pressures of the moment? Do I find the appropriate mix of activities or concentrate on one particular function or problem just because I find it interesting? Am I more efficient with particular kinds of work, at special times of the day or week? Does my schedule reflect this? Can someone else schedule my time (besides my secretary)?
- Do I overwork? What effect does my work load have on my efficiency? Should I force myself to take breaks or to reduce the pace of my activity?
- Am I too superficial in what I do? Can I really shift moods as quickly and frequently as my work requires? Should I decrease the amount of fragmentation and interruption in my work?
- Do I spend too much time on current, tangible activities? Am I a slave to the action and excitement of my work, so that I am no longer able to concentrate on issues? Do key problems receive the attention they deserve? Should I spend more time reading and probing deeply into certain issues? Could I be more reflective? Should I be?
- Do I use the different media appropriately? Do I know how to make the most of written communication? Do I rely excessively on face-to-face communication, thereby putting all but a few of my subordinates at an information disadvantage? Do I schedule enough of my meetings on a regular basis? Do I spend enough time observing activities firsthand, or am I detached from the heart of my organization's activities.
- How do I blend my personal rights and duties? Do my obligations consume all my time? How can I free myself from obligations to ensure that I am taking this organization where I want it to go? How can I turn my obligations to my advantage?

Reprinted by permission of *Harvard Business Review*. An exhibit from "The manager's job: Folklore and fact." by H. Mintzberg, March-April 1990, p. 174.

ognize human needs of the individuals in the work group and use managerial strategies that facilitate human need fulfillment. The Self-Study Questions for Managers chart can help dental hygienists assess their managerial skills and analyze their situations to understand their managerial and leadership behaviors.

References

1. Gabaro, J. L., and Kotter, J. P. Managing your boss. Harvard Business Review 58(1):92, 1980.
2. Stoner, J. A. F. Management, 2nd ed. Englewood Cliffs, NJ: Prentice-Hall, 1982.
3. Kanter, R. M. Power failure in management circuits. Harvard Business Review 57(4):65, 1979.
4. Steiner, G. A. Strategic Planning: What Every Manager Must Know. New York: Free Press, 1979.
5. Lyles, M. A., and Mitroff, I. I. Organizational problem formulation: An empirical study. Administrative Science Quarterly 25(1):102, 1980.
6. Strong, E. P., and Smith, R. D. Management Control Models. New York: Holt, Rinehart, 1968, pp. 1–2.

6a. Fayol, H. Industrial and General Armamentarium (trans.). Geneva: International Management Institute, 1930.

6b. Barnard, C. I. The Functions of the Executive. Cambridge, MA: Harvard University Press, 1938.

6c. Mayo, E. The Human Problems of an Industrial Civilization. New York: Macmillan, 1953.

6d. von Bertalanffy, L., Hempel, C. G., Bass, R. E., and Jonas, H. General system theory: A new approach to unity of science. Human Biology 23(4):302, 1951.

6e. Boulding, K. E. General systems theory—the skeleton of science. Management Science 2(3):197, 1956.

7. Hunsaker, P. L., and Alessandra, A. J. The Art of Managing People. New York: Simon & Schuster, 1986.
8. Morse, S. W. Leadership for an uncertain century. National Forum, The Phi Kappa Phi Journal 71(1):2, 1991.
9. Bennis, W. Learning some basic truisms about leadership. Phi Kappa Phi Journal 71(1):12, 1991.
10. Yukl, G. A. Leadership in Organizations. Englewood Cliffs, NJ: Prentice-Hall, 1981, p. 90.
11. Jennings, E. E. The anatomy of leadership. Management Personnel Quarterly 1(1):1, 1961.
12. Rosener, J. B. The female leadership model. Harvard Business Review 68(6):1, 1990.

13. Cartwright, D., and Zander, A. (eds.). Group Dynamics, 3rd ed. New York: Harper & Row, 1968.
14. Hersey, P., and Blanchard, K. H. Management of Organizational Behavior, 3rd ed. Englewood Cliffs, NJ: Prentice-Hall, 1977.
15. Taylor, C., Lillis, C., and LeMone, P. Fundamentals of Nursing, 2nd ed. Philadelphia: J. B. Lippincott, 1993.
16. Lewin, K. Field Theory in Social Science: Selected Theoretical Papers. New York: Harper, 1951.
17. Beckhard, R., and Harris, R. T. Organizational Transitions: Managing Complex Change. Reading, MA: Addison-Wesley, 1977, pp 25–27.
18. Kotter, J. P., and Schlesinger, L. A. Choosing strategies for change. Harvard Business Review 57(2):106, 1979.
19. Lawrence, P. R. How to deal with resistance to change. Harvard Business Review 47(1), 1969.
20. Kaufman, H. The Limits of Organizational Change. Tuscaloosa: University of Alabama Press, 1971.
21. Coch, L., and French, J. R. P., Jr. Overcoming resistance to change. Human Relations 1(4):512, 1948.
22. Fleishman, E. A. Leadership climate, human relations training, and supervisory behavior. Personnel Psychology 6(2):205, 1953.

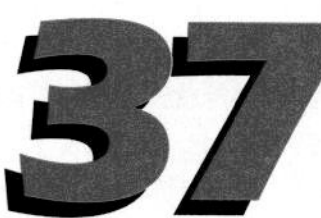

Practice Management and Professional Development

OBJECTIVES

Mastery of the content in this chapter will enable the reader to:

- Develop a mission statement and goals for the dental hygiene component of a dental practice
- Describe the behavior necessary for successful client management
- List and define the elements necessary for a complete case presentation
- Explain the importance of client noncompliance and the legal implications
- Outline the three types of appointment book management systems
- Discuss economic considerations for a profitable practice, including production, collection, and office overhead
- Develop a marketing plan for a dental practice, including strategies for increased client satisfaction and methods of evaluation of the project
- Explain the contributions of the dental hygienist to the dental practice
- Define the terms of dental hygiene employment and give examples of how they can be combined to fully describe the nature of an employment arrangement
- Compare and contrast the methods of remuneration, including elements of risk and security and range in value for each
- Create an employment compensation package, including method of compensation and fringe benefits, with total annual income value
- Design an employment contract, including elements of setting, job description, compensation, terms of employment, performance evaluation, and termination procedures
- Evaluate job performance, including expectations and techniques necessary for changing performance
- Write an employment resume and cover letter
- Outline a sample job interview, including sample questions for the dental office representative and possible questions the candidate may receive with appropriate responses
- Describe job search strategies, including a list of job sources and a prioritized list of job selection criteria
- Explain why stress and burn-out are common among dental hygienists and list stress management techniques
- Describe employment alternatives to clinical dental hygiene
- Develop a plan for personal financial management, including an annual budget, adequate insurance coverage, investment goals, and a retirement plan
- List the special tax deductions allowable to dental hygienists and the documentation necessary to support them

INTRODUCTION

Management and leadership skills are essential for dental hygienists to participate in the practice management and administration of the dental or dental hygiene practice. Participation in management adds a dimension of administrative responsibilities to the daily routine and affords professional growth opportunities. A basic understanding of business management contributes to the efficiency of the employment setting, increases the dental hygienist's position as a valued team member, and enhances job satisfaction.

DEFINITION OF PRACTICE MANAGEMENT

Practice management can be defined as the organization, administration, and direction of the professional practice in a style that facilitates quality client care, efficient use of time and personnel, reduced stress to staff members and clients, enhanced professional and personal satisfaction for staff, and financial profitability.

The development of a *mission statement* is a basic tool for the successful management of dental or dental hygiene practices. The mission statement is supported by specific goals that describe what is to be done within the practice. Objectives describing how each goal is to be accomplished are defined by measurable components. All members of the staff participate in the development of the mission and goals statements, agreeing by consensus on the final statements. It is this set of guidelines that is used to direct all management activities of the practice.

ELEMENTS OF PRACTICE MANAGEMENT

The **team concept** within the dental or dental hygiene practice comprises the interaction and interdependence of the entire office staff to promote the unity and efficiency of the group. The oral health team is composed of the client, dentists, dental hygienists, dental assistants, office manager, receptionists, dental laboratory technicians, and bookkeepers. With the knowledge of the mission statement and goals for the practice, each member of the staff accepts responsibility to strive toward the accomplishment of these guidelines.

Personnel Management

The interpersonal team elements include daily communications and regular staff meetings. Staff meetings provide an opportunity to review organizational goals, evaluate progress, share information, air grievances, and solve problems together to find agreed-upon solutions. Interpersonal team building creates quality human relations between all office personnel, clients, and members of the professional community. The organizational team elements include manuals that delineate **office policies and procedures** that are applicable to all members of the organization. These manuals systematize the practice and clearly familiarize personnel with responsibilites for which they are accountable.

Team building is the synergistic process of developing group goals with motivation and commitment. The dental hygienist contributes to the strength of the team by:

- Sharing information
- Participating in the formulation of goals and objectives
- Activating, evaluating, and revising plans
- Encouraging the participation of all staff members in these processes

Client Management

Successful client management is dependent on the belief that the client is the most important person in the oral healthcare environment. Each individual has physical, psychological, spiritual, and emotional human needs that are influenced by previous experiences, level of intelligence, and socioethnocultural factors.[1] See Chapter 5, Behavioral Foundations for the Dental Hygiene Process, and Chapter 6, Cultural Diversity and the Dental Hygiene Process, for communication strategies used for successful client management.

Policies for Clients

Policies are established for clients to provide consistency and guidance for expectations. This document may begin with a statement of the setting's philosophy, such as the intention to provide quality oral healthcare and the team members' desire for client satisfaction. It also delineates policies such as arriving promptly for scheduled appointments, timely notice expected if an appointment needs to be changed or cancelled, financial responsibility and arrangements, third-party coverage, and responsibility for minor or dependent relatives. Other issues may be outlined regarding medical precautions and the need for oral radiographs and collaboration with other dental and health professionals when necessary. These policies should be presented to clients in writing during the first visit to the office setting. Once the content is understood, the client signs and dates the statement of office policies.

Reference to these policies may be made during correspondence with the client, which may be sent when management problems occur such as failed appointments or failure to meet financial obligations. Written correspondence to the client about the dental or dental hygiene diagnosis and care plan is generally completed by the office manager; however, there are other times when the dental hygienist may be responsible or may wish to communicate with clients in writing. For example, a follow-up letter may be useful as a review of important points made during an appointment or as a reinforcement to encourage use of new skills or development of new oral health behaviors. There may be need for a note to remind the client to schedule a regular or an overdue appointment. Furthermore, the dental hygienist may wish to send a note of personal congratulations, well wishes, sympathy, or thanks. All such types of correspondence help to establish the dental hygienist as a unique professional within the team and promote perception of a caring attitude.

Case Presentations

A **case presentation** is defined as the process of explaining assessment findings to the client along with options and recommendations for therapy to reach agreement on a care plan. The dental hygienist may be responsible for case presentations to clients within a general dental or dental hygiene practice. In some cases, the dentist may perform the data collection, dental diagnosis, and recommended care plan for both restorative and periodontal care, and then assign the dental hygienist the responsibility of making the case presentation to the client. To meet the client's human needs for safety, freedom from stress, and conceptualization and problem solving, it is important that the discussion be held in a manner that is informative and nonthreatening to the client, using terminology that the individual can easily understand. The client's dental chart, periodontal maintenance record, radiographs, intraoral photographs, and study models may be useful visual aids during the process. The elements of a complete case presentation are presented in Table 37-1. (See Chapter 15: The Dental Hygiene Care Plan.)

Client Motivation

An effective case presentation is the key to client acceptance of care and motivation. In this case, the dental hygienist wants to motivate the client to proceed with the recommended dental hygiene intervention to meet the client's human needs that can be fulfilled through dental hygiene care. Motivated clients assimilate new information more rapidly than unmotivated clients.

Client motivation is best achieved when the information presented satisfies human needs and coincides with the client's own culture, beliefs, attitudes, and values. Strategies that can be used by the dental hygienist to motivate the client include:

- Making the information relevant and meaningful
- Relating information by building on the client's existing knowledge, experience, attitudes, and feelings
- Using success or rewards to promote learning, rather than criticism or punishment
- Planning reinforcement in the learning process, including repetition and recalling previous successes (see Chapter 5, Behavioral Foundations for the Dental Hygiene Process)

TABLE 37-1

ELEMENTS OF A COMPLETE CASE PRESENTATION TO A DENTAL OR DENTAL HYGIENE CLIENT

Information
Data collected and clinical assessment are shared with the client using visual aids such as radiographs or a periodontal maintenance record, when appropriate.
Education
An explanation of the significance of the assessment findings is given to the client, including short- and long-range possibilities and consequences of the conditions present. At this time, the practitioner should ask questions and initiate discussion that bring the client into the conversation so a determination can be made of the client's level of understanding and client priorities, and interest in pursuing care. Media and other instructional strategies should supplement client education.
Options
A list of alternative methods of care is given to the client, including benefits, time involved, risk of doing the treatment, risk of not doing the treatment, and cost for each.
Choice
A selection for care is made by the client based on his understanding of the information presented, priorities, desire for treatment, and perceived needs.
Agreement
The client and professional concur on a course to follow, including sequencing of care and assignment of responsibilities. The dental hygienist, as an advocate, supports the informed decision made by the client. A written summary of the case presentation may be composed by the dental hygienist and mailed to the client following this appointment.

Adapted from Dental Risk Management Foundation. Dental Risk Management—A Practical Guide. San Francisco, 1988.

Client Nonadherence

Nonadherence, or **noncompliance,** is a lack of client cooperation with recommended oral healthcare. It is significant because it can result in compromised care, unsatisfactory care outcomes, and litigation.[2] In the event of a lawsuit, the judicial decision, outcome, or amount of settlement may be altered based on negligence of the practitioner if nonadherence was ignored. There are several examples of nonadherence that may occur during dental hygiene care:

- Routinely tardy arrival for scheduled appointments or necessity for an early departure from the appointment
- Repeated postponement or cancellations
- Failure to appear for scheduled appointments
- Unwillingness to have necessary diagnostic tests, such as radiographs
- Unwillingness to accept recommended specific procedures or the care plan
- Unwillingness to accept referrals to specialists
- Failure to use medications as prescribed
- Failure to follow the recommended oral hygiene regimen

The management of client nonadherence begins with recognizing it when it happens. The following list describes the process of documenting client nonadherence to prescribed care.

1. Record recommended care
2. Describe all instructions that have not been followed
3. Describe the specific behavior of the client
4. Record in quotations verbalization of nonadherence by the client
5. Note any discussion of the consequences of not following recommendations or instructions that occur between office personnel and the client

Clients whose uncooperative behavior impedes professional care may be legally discontinued from the practice by following precise legal protocols. Practitioners are advised to be familiar with these protocols to avoid litigation associated with client abandonment. (See Chapter 39, Ethical and Legal Decision Making in Dental Hygiene.)

Records Management

Written client records are the most valuable permanent document of past dental or dental hygiene care and provide the "written memory" of the events and conversations that transpired during each appointment. Maintaining accurate records **(records management)** enhances smooth office operations as well as other functions. Client records serve a variety of purposes including a sourced for organizing data collected, an evaluation tool to aid in dental and dental hygiene diagnosis and care planning, protection of the client regarding general health and discovery of oral diseases, a communication tool for client education and behavior modification, a guideline for performing consistent care, a proof to third-party insurers to justify necessary treatment, a demonstration of accountability for responsible care, and legal protection to present documentary evidence for defense if necessary. Written records include the dental and periodontal charts; health history; records of examinations, diagnosis, and care delivered; informed consent and informed refusal forms; and copies of prescriptions. Nonwritten records consist of photographs, radiographs, models, and cephalometric tracings.

Table 37–2 compares elements of notes documenting care. All notes are to be thorough, accurate, and legible, with facts separated from opinion. Writing should be done in a timely manner, either during the appointment or immediately after the completion of care. It is likely that some information is forgotten and therefore left out of the client record if all chart entries are made at the end of the day. Records should be kept indefinitely, even if the client transfers to another oral healthcare setting.

Time Management—Scheduling of Clients

Effective time management is essential to the success of the practice. The appointment book is the mechanism for controlling time by allotted increments to scheduled appointments, lunch breaks and staff meetings, and days off for personal time, holidays, vacations, and professional conferences. A variety of appointment book management systems are used for client scheduling:

Unlimited future booking—This allows appointments to be scheduled as far in advance as is necessary to accommodate all clients. This requires careful advance planning by the dental hygienist for time away from the practice.

Restricted appointment booking—This limits scheduling to a specified time period, such as 1 to 3 months. Clients who are not prescheduled during this time are added to a call list and telephoned when appointments become available. This system requires less advance planning for taking time off.

Telephone contact file—This is a waiting list of clients in need of appointments who are available on short notice to fill changed appointments and cancellations. All dental and dental hygiene practices should maintain such a list. Below is a list of appropriate clients for the telephone contact file.

- Clients new to the practice
- Clients needing multiple appointments
- Clients who cancel existing appointments
- Clients who need appointments within a specified time frame, such as prior to a vacation, home from college for a limited time only, terminating insurance benefits, and coordination with other dental care
- Clients with an existing scheduled appointment who wish to receive care sooner than scheduled
- Clients known to have flexible schedules who are able to make appointments on short notice

The information for the telephone contact file includes:

- The client's name
- Daytime telephone number with notation of work or home phone
- Type of appointment needed and time required
- Special requests or needs during the appointment such as antibiotic premedication or local anesthesia
- Preferred day or time of appointment and date of existing scheduled appointment

If a client is telephoned to fill an available time and cannot accept the appointment, the client declination should be recorded in the file. Examples of this approach are presented in Figure 37–1.

Time allotments are designed for each client depending on the care needed. Generally 45 minutes to 1 hour is the time delineated for dental hygiene care with additional time scheduled for new clients or clients with periodontal conditions, special needs, or management challenges.

Entries in the appointment book should include:

- Pencil led entries, including the client's name and daytime telephone number

TABLE 37–2
DOCUMENTING ORAL HEALTHCARE

Minimum Documentation	Complete Treatment Notes
Date	Date
	Clinical observations
Significant findings	Significant findings
	Summary of discussions regarding conditions present
	Options for care
	Decisions made by client
Services rendered	Services rendered
	Instructions presented to client
	Items dispensed to client
	Recommendations for future care
Initials of practitioner	Initials of practitioner
Fee	Fee

June Johnson 516-223-4657—work 4 Quad Root Planing—1 hour each Q Local Anesthesia M/W/F before 10 A.M.
Susie Thomas 516-756-2188—home Child Prophy and Fluoride—1/2 hour Any day after 3 P.M. *Called 11/21/95: client declined appointment*
Tim Scott 712-299-0506—work Perio Maintenance—1 hour Has 12/5 appointment Tuesdays, anytime *11/20/95 = NO*

FIGURE 37–1
Examples of client information included in a telephone contact file.

- The service to be given or type of appointment planned
- The length of appointment time in units and any special instructions such as need for premedication
- Local anesthesia or client concerns

An example of appointment scheduling is shown in Figure 37–2.

Periodontal Maintenance Systems

Continued care periodontal health systems (recall systems) are designed to organize and maintain periodontal assessments and preventive or maintenance care on a regular schedule according to individual client needs. In some practices, the dental hygienist is responsible for developing and managing the periodontal maintenance system. Such a system ensures that a maximal number of clients receive care within a given dental or dental hygiene practice. Advance scheduling may be done to set a definite future appointment with a reminder postcard and telephone call to the client shortly before the reserved date. Monthly reminder cards may be sent to notify clients without appointments that it is time to return for the periodontal maintenance (Fig. 37–3). This system shares responsibility with the client, who is encouraged to make the appointment, while the office manager may retain a cross-reference file for follow-up. Many practices telephone clients to remind them of the scheduled visit as a protection from forgotten and missed appointments. Usually a combination of all continued care systems is available within the office with implementation based on client preference.

References are necessary to keep track of clients in various types of scheduling. A triplicate appointment card may be used with one copy given to the client, a second copy filed in the chart, and the third serving as a postcard reminder to be mailed prior to the appointment (Fig. 37–4). A *tickler file* may be used to collect monthly groupings of cards for clients needing appointments (Fig. 37–5). Each card contains a record of previous appointments, current needs, and ways to best contact and schedule the client. An alphabetical file may be used to list client's name, previous

Monday, March 15	
8	John Jacobs
15	Perio maintenance
30	BWX
45	W: 525-5258
9	Susan Woods
15	1 Quad root plane
30	Local anesthesia
45	W: 828-2143
10	Matt Lewis
15	Perio maintenance
30	W: 526-1122
45	
11	Dorothy Walker
15	New client
30	Exam, FMX
45	Hygiene therapy
12	H: 444-6989
15	↓
30	
45	Lunch
1	
15	
30	Jennifer Thomas
45	Perio recall
2	W: 828-6446
15	Bessie Sicular
30	Perio maintenance
45	H: 527-2895
3	Bobby O'Brien
15	Pedo oral Px
30	Tami O'Brien
45	Pedo oral Px
4	Mom: 526-3832
15	Joseph Camp
30	1 Quad root plane
45	Local anesthesia
5	W: 444-7172
15	

FIGURE 37–2
Sample schedule from appointment book.

Dear ____________________:	STAMP
It is time to schedule an appointment for your _______ month examination and periodontal maintenance therapy.	
Your last visit was: _____________. Please call to set a date and time!	Client Name Street Address City, State, Zip
__________ *Signed* ___________ Registered Dental Hygienist for Harold F. Greenburg, D.D.S. 618-525-5255	

FIGURE 37–3
Client reminder card.

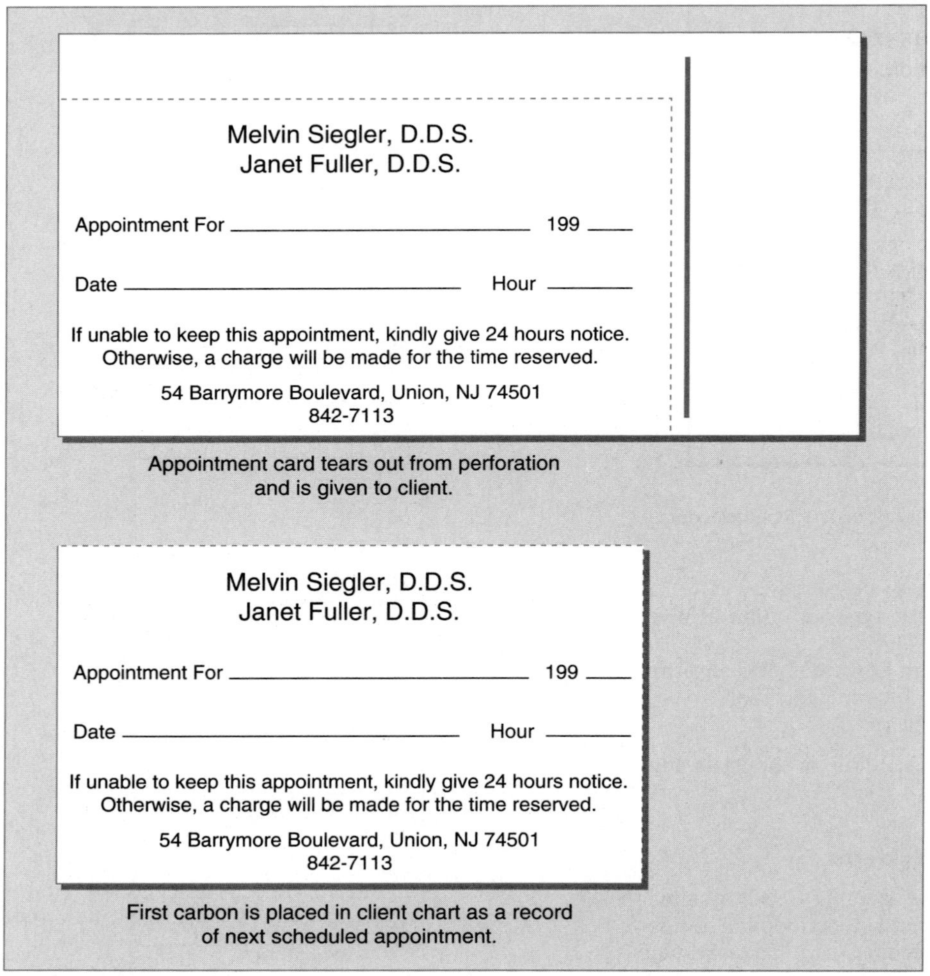

Melvin Siegler, D.D.S.
Janet Fuller, D.D.S.

Appointment For ______________________ 199 ___

Date ______________________ Hour ______

If unable to keep this appointment, kindly give 24 hours notice.
Otherwise, a charge will be made for the time reserved.

54 Barrymore Boulevard, Union, NJ 74501
842-7113

Appointment card tears out from perforation and is given to client.

Melvin Siegler, D.D.S.
Janet Fuller, D.D.S.

Appointment For ______________________ 199 ___

Date ______________________ Hour ______

If unable to keep this appointment, kindly give 24 hours notice.
Otherwise, a charge will be made for the time reserved.

54 Barrymore Boulevard, Union, NJ 74501
842-7113

First carbon is placed in client chart as a record of next scheduled appointment.

FIGURE 37–4
Triplicate appointment card.

appointment date, services rendered, plus needed care. Cross-references may be designed to combine any number of these techniques.

Reclamation is a process of periodic purging of all files to identify clients whose care is incomplete, who have missed appointments, or who have been absent from the practice and are in need of care. Once identified, clients may be telephoned or notified by mail of the date of the last appointment and need for prompt oral healthcare. The dental hygienist may be responsible for managing the chart reviews as part of quality assurance measures to determine which clients are overdue for appointments and need to be contacted.

Economic Considerations

The financial considerations of a practice include a determination of the office income and expenditure (e.g., productivity, overhead expenses, collections, and profit). Expenses include:

- Rent, lease, and utility expenditures
- Equipment purchase and maintenance
- Lease-hold improvements
- Supplies
- Employee salaries and fringe benefits
- Accounting expenses
- Insurance payments for policies the employer carries for the building or personnel

The *office overhead,* based on these expenses, is a determination of the dollar amount it costs per hour to run the office; the *office production* is the total fees billed for services performed. *Collection* is the amount of money that is actually paid to the office from clients and dental insurance companies.

Financial arrangements must be confirmed with each client in advance of performing oral healthcare. The office policy statement presented to new clients should summarize the financial arrangement options and responsibilities. The dental hygienist may be the person who discusses financial issues with the client, especially for extensive dental hygiene care. To encourage prompt fee collections, some practices offer a small discount to clients who make payments in full at the time services are rendered. If the office requires a *down payment* prior to extensive treatment or carries a balance for 60 to 90 days, the client needs to be informed of these policies. Special long-term financial arrangements may also be offered to some clients.

Dental insurance enhances the ability of many clients

Melvin Siegler, D.D.S.
Janet Fuller, D.D.S.

Appointment For ______________________ 199 ______

Date ______________________ Hour ______

If unable to keep this appointment, kindly give 24 hours notice.
Otherwise, a charge will be made for the time reserved.

54 Barrymore Boulevard, Union, NJ 74501
842-7113

Second carbon is a postcard, filed by the month and then mailed as a reminder two weeks prior to appointment.

FIGURE 37–4
Continued

who otherwise might not have been able to afford oral healthcare. However, many misunderstandings arise about oral healthcare financing when clients do not fully comprehend how insurance coverage is determined or the limits of their benefits. Oral health insurance coverage varies from company to company and also from policy to policy within the same company. It is important to explain to clients that they are responsible personally for the fees incurred. Even with the help of the office staff in completing and submitting insurance claims, it is the client's responsibility to investigate and understand his individual insurance coverage.

Realizing a profit in dentistry and dental hygiene is enhanced with a well-managed practice, involving the elements of personnel, clients, records, appointment scheduling, and foresight and wisdom in economic considerations. Although it is presently illegal for a dental hygienist to own and operate a *dental* practice, it is legal for a dental hygienist to own and operate a dental hygiene practice in the state of Colorado; therefore, it is essential for the hygienist to understand the economic aspects of the business of oral healthcare. With this knowledge, the hygienist can optimize the managerial role, fully contribute in the area of practice management, and enjoy the rewards of a financially successful practice.

Office Facility Management

Dental hygiene care rooms and equipment must be carefully cleaned and maintained to reach the maximal lifespan of these costly items. Written guidelines are useful to direct personnel in the care of all such items. Such guidelines include:

- Information on special cleansing and lubricating agents
- People to contact for necessary repairs
- Intervals for cleaning and oiling
- Assignment of the person responsible for equipment resources management

A material resources inventory file for dental hygiene services and oral hygiene products dispensed to clients is best maintained on a manual or computer-managed inventory control system (Fig. 37–6).

Adequate stock should be kept on hand, but an excess accumulation of items should be avoided to prevent shelf life and storage problems. An inventory control system consists of:

- A list of supplies and materials used
- The manufacturer or distributor
- Cost of the item
- Quantity and frequency of ordering

Maintaining the date of each order and the date received establishes a predictable pattern of shipping time for future orders. It is most efficient for one person to be responsible for materials resources management, such as ordering the supplies for the office and inventory control. However, it is often the dental hygienist who controls the inventory for oral hygiene products.

JUNE
Steven Armstrong 516-223-4576—work
Last = 2/4/95
4-month perio maintenance—1 hour
T/Th afternoons

JUNE
Janice and Johnny Tenny 516-221-7588—mom
Last = 12/10/95
6-month prophy w/ fluoride—1/2 hour each
must be scheduled together
M/T/W after 3:30 P.M.

FIGURE 37-5
Tickler appointment cards.

MARKETING DENTISTRY AND DENTAL HYGIENE

Marketing is a structured, organized approach to selecting and servicing markets, and a researched approach to informing the public of a service.[3,4] Marketing includes:

- Formulating and managing a program
- Selecting a specific group toward which efforts are directed (target marketing)
- The target market's needs and desires
- The market mix, commonly known as the four Ps of marketing (product/service, pricing, place, and promotion)

Marketing is regarded as a business practice and social institution because it is a means of satisfying certain needs of people.[3] A *marketing plan* for the dental or dental hygiene practice involves the planning and management of services that benefit clients at a profit to the practice.[5] The purpose of marketing dentistry and dental hygiene is to obtain and maintain the needed share of the client population market to keep the practice productive as desired, and to inform society of the benefits of the practice. The profits from a productive practice include both financial gain and personal satisfaction for the staff members.

Date Ordered	Product Name	Quantity & Cost	Supplier & Phone	Date Rec'd

FIGURE 37-6
Format for a material resources inventory file.

The marketing plan should include the four Ps of marketing:

- Product/service
- Price
- Place
- Promotion

Product/service might include philosophy and objective of the practice, services provided, and quality of care. Price considers cost and oral healthcare financing mechanisms. Place encompasses the entire location and environment of the practice. Promotion includes strategies that communicate with target markets or external public groups.

The personnel involved in marketing relations are numerous. A manager is needed to coordinate the marketing plan, delegate responsibilities to staff members, monitor the marketing budget, establish an overall time schedule, and evaluate the effectiveness of the marketing plan. Effective practice marketing is cost-effective if the client pool is increased. Within the oral healthcare setting, the dentists, dental hygienists, dental assistants, receptionists, office managers, and dental laboratory technicians must be familiar with the plan and incorporate its elements into daily practice. The business consultants employed by the practice—bookkeeper, accountant, and attorney—contribute ideas and communicate the credits of the practice to their community contacts. Other healthcare professionals—physicians, allied healthcare providers, product suppliers, and prominent community and business members—are similarly involved with the knowledge of the practice's reputation and can refer to the practice. The best participants in the marketing plan for dentistry and dental hygiene are the clients. Satisfied clients who believe that their needs have been met by quality oral health services, at a reasonable fee, in a caring environment recommend the practice to friends, relatives, and business associates.

Practice Promotion

Practice promotion occurs when all staff members project the desired professional image and gain public exposure on behalf of the practice (see Marketing Strategies for Practice Promotion chart). Client satisfaction does more for practice promotion than any other strategy for marketing.

Client Satisfaction

To appeal to a broad-based population, the office must offer a spectrum of oral services including preventive, therapeutic, maintenance, restorative, cosmetic, counseling, and reconstruction services or the practice should develop a professional network to ensure clients ready access to oral health services that might be needed. Quality care is the key to obtaining **client satisfaction.** Clients recognize dentists and dental hygienists sensitive to human needs who maintain technical expertise and who are respectful of staff whose skills also are apparent and fully utilized. The oral health team sets a pattern committed to consistent dependable care, with an attitude of caring and gentleness. Personalized attention, respecting each client as an individual, listening carefully, thoroughly discussing reported symptoms, and being responsive all are methods that help develop special relationships appreciated by the client. As a consumer advocate, the dental hygienist stays abreast of

MARKETING STRATEGIES FOR PRACTICE PROMOTION

- Writing articles for the local newspaper on oral disease prevention, dental service updates, dental emergency care, and evaluation of over-the-counter oral health products
- Inviting a local newspaper reporter to the practice to write a feature article
- Participating in broadcast media programming, local radio and television, with special interest information, talk shows, and community service announcements
- Participating in civic, religious, and fraternal group activities where the practice professionals meet many new people
- Using business contacts within the community client population
- Sponsoring community projects or athletic team sports
- Participating in community cultural and recreational events
- Becoming a public speaker
- Teaching health information and cardiopulmonary resuscitation workshops to consumers and other professionals
- Becoming a student, attending local classes and workshops
- Meeting and cooperating with neighboring health professionals, providing business cards and referral slips
- Volunteering professional services and demonstrations
- Performing oral health screenings in schools, health fairs, career days, community and athletic programs, civic groups and special events
- Actively participating in the professional association
- Participating creatively in the community
- Having an open house to welcome neighbors to meet the dental office staff members
- Buying advertising space or time within the telephone book, local newspaper, radio, and other community media
- Using direct mail methods, sending oral health education materials, practice brochures, or a newsletter to the client population or the local community at large

consumer trends and educates clients about oral healthcare changes as new services become available. When explaining care plans, alternatives are offered, including explanations of all options and costs of each, with clear recommendations given. All current treatment modalities are offered to clients, or referrals are made to specialists who offer such treatments. Clients need to understand the difference between what is necessary treatment and what is ideal. The client's informed decision is then fully supported. (See Elements of a Dental or Dental Hygiene Practice that Enhance Client Satisfaction chart.)

Written and telephone communications further enhance client satisfaction with the dental or dental hygiene practice. A practice brochure can be developed and distributed to describe the philosophy of care, introduce the staff, describe services offered, list office hours plus emergency arrangements, and note special features about the practice. Written outlines of assessed needs and sequencing of appointments help the client to review and recall verbal case presentations. Sending the client copies of letters to or from other health professionals concerning needed or ongoing care informs the client of the shared interest in his oral health. Mailing clients brief personalized notes of thanks, congratulations, well wishes for recovery, and sympathy communicates appreciation and caring. Telephone contacts with clients should be maintained on a positive, satisfactory note. The dental hygienist can use follow-up telephone calls after lengthy or complex treatments to check on comfort and healing or to reassure anxious clients. Such strategies address clients' human needs for appreciation and respect and for freedom from pain and stress associated with oral disease and care.

Client satisfaction leads to staff member satisfaction. The dentist and dental hygienist can recognize one another and all staff members by expressing appreciation for daily cooperation and team spirit, offering congratulations for jobs done well, noting client loyalty, and recognizing referrals

ELEMENTS OF A DENTAL OR DENTAL HYGIENE PRACTICE THAT ENHANCE CLIENT SATISFACTION

- Offer extended business hours such as early morning, evening, and weekend appointments
- Appeal to all age ranges, from children to senior citizens
- Involve client in understanding dental disease processes, with encouragement to take responsibility for his own oral health maintenance, making decisions about care, setting goals, and committing to long-term oral health maintenance
- Provide an effective "continued care" system for oral health maintenance with repeated instructions on prevention and periodically checking techniques, individualizing instructions according to client's needs
- Have waiting time based on an efficiently managed practice, with realistic scheduling of time for appointments and advising clients of anticipated length of appointments
- Promote positive psychological attitudes by all staff members, creating an upbeat atmosphere
- Establish warm, respectful interpersonal relations between office personnel and clients
- Create a pleasant, comfortable, attractive office decor maintained in constant cleanliness
- Provide "give away" items during office visits such as oral hygiene aids, health education brochures, toys and balloons for children, or flowers to clients for special occasions
- Charge fair and reasonable fees
- Offer a variety of financial arrangements
- Process dental insurance forms expediently
- Maintain rapport with specialty practices to facilitate referrals, coordination of treatment, and close follow-through regarding clients who are referred to other professionals for special care
- Arrange appointments quickly when need requires expediency
- Always immediately accommodate emergency clients

TABLE 37–3
MARKETING EFFECTIVENESS EVALUATION

Quantitative Elements	Qualitative Elements
Internal	
1. Maintain a count of clients treated during each month to demonstrate evidence of practice growth a. Returning clients seeking maintenance care and examinations b. Active restorative, cosmetic, and reconstructive appointments c. New clients and how each was referred 2. Perform a quarterly or annual comparison of gross revenues with production and collection 3. Complete a complex financial analysis 4. Calculate productivity per month, week, day, and hour	1. All staff members list their activities for practice promotion. 2. Interview staff members for evaluative comments regarding current marketing programs. 3. Staff members offer suggestions for future marketing strategies.
External	
1. Compare financial reports with others published in the area 2. Meet with local practices and make comparisons of all numbers	1. Interview clients with questionnaire regarding oral needs, desires, satisfaction with the practice, and services offered 2. Ask clients for suggestions regarding improving the practice and their recommendations for change 3. Survey community professional sources for additional information that assists in evaluating marketing effectiveness; ask about further services that might increase referrals

received from staff members' marketing efforts. Verbal "thank yous" and small tokens of appreciation promote continued success. Table 37–3 presents methods of evaluating marketing effectiveness.

INTEGRAL CONTRIBUTIONS OF THE DENTAL HYGIENIST

The dental hygienist benefits the dental practice beyond tangible clinical skills and services. These nontangible benefits or "integral" contributions make the hygienist indispensable to the oral healthcare team.[6] Generally recognized as an "oral disease prevention specialist," the dental hygienist is known for expertise in educating clients in the knowledge and techniques necessary to care for their own oral health. Further, dental hygiene strategies encourage clients to become responsible for the maintenance of their own oral health, thereby fulfilling the client's human need for self-determination and responsibility. By performing the multiple roles of clinician, researcher, consumer advocate, change agent, educator and oral health promoter, and manager, the hygienist facilitates release time for the dentist, thereby allowing the dentist's time for restorative and surgical services.

The dental hygienist is a professional associate of the dentist in a collaborative relationship, communicating together about clinical findings and care options. Respect and recognition of one another's level of competence promote reciprocal sharing of professional ideas and assignment of responsibility. By participating together in case evaluations and care planning, maximal use is made of the dental hygienist's knowledge, skills, and experience. The establishment of a cooperative, diplomatic atmosphere allows for constructive evaluation and criticism that enhance learning and professional growth.

The dental hygienist markets dental and dental hygiene care, reporting oral needs to clients or projecting services that may be needed in the future. The dental hygienist is a practice builder, interacting with clients as a professional relations specialist, interpreter to facilitate communications with the dentist, confidant, practice ambassador, and friend. Public relations are promoted when the hygienist speaks highly and enthusiastically about the value of oral health.

Dental hygienists participate in office staff meetings in both a "team player" role and a leadership role. All personnel attend staff meetings to share information, generate ideas and solve problems together. In addition, the hygienist is responsible for the evaluation of dental hygiene care in the management of the dental hygiene portion of the practice. The role is therefore expanded to include practice analysis and revision recommendations plus implementing changes as needed to create an improved situation. The dental hygienist also may contribute to the management of the practice in general and in cooperation with the existing organizational hierarchy. The professional dental hygienist exerts leadership to ensure that these **integral contributions** positively affect the overall success of the practice.

EMPLOYMENT

Employment Arrangements

The employer-employee relationship, wherein the dental hygienist works as an employee within the practice structure, is the most common arrangement for dental hygiene employment. In this arrangement, all financial concerns of operating the practice are the responsibility of the employer. The employer pays the employee on an hourly wage, salary, or commission basis, withholding federal, state, and Social Security taxes from the employee's paycheck. **Employment arrangements** may be any of the following: the dental hygienist's employer may be a dentist; dental hygienist; an independent management firm; a health maintenance organization; or a national, state, county, or private agency employing individuals for dental offices or other employment settings. Financial arrangements between the dentist and dental hygienist are solely the concern of those two individuals and are separate from and not controlled by any dental practice act.

In some states a dental hygienist may work as an *independent contractor.* The actual requirements for establishing an independent contractor status are set by the Internal Revenue Service (IRS), which explains the contractual arrangement between the dentist and self-employed dental hygienist. In this situation, the dental hygienist provides services to the clients of the dentist while adhering to the state dental practice act. An independent contractor dental hygienist may hire employees and function as an employer. The financial arrangements for operating the dental hygiene portion of the practice are contracted between the dentist and dental hygienist. No taxes are withheld by the dentist from the hygienist's paycheck; instead the hygienist pays self-employment (Social Security) tax and files estimated income tax payments. It is illegal for a dentist-employer to arbitrarily assign the status of independent contractor to a dental hygienist-employee.

Independent dental hygiene practice, legal only in Colorado, allows the direct delivery of care to clients by dental hygienists in a separate dental hygiene facility without the supervision of a dentist. The dental hygienist assumes all financial responsibility for the practice, is self-employed, and functions as an employer to the employees of the facility. Professional collaboration occurs with general and specialty dental practices, as well as with other health providers to assure clients access to various services that might be needed.

Terms of Employment

Various **terms of employment** that may apply to dental hygiene depending on the practice setting and arrangements made with the employer are explained in the Terms of Employment chart. These terms may be integrated to fully describe the nature of the employment agreement.

Employment Rights

Dental hygiene employment falls under the Non-discrimination Act, Title VII of the Civil Rights Act of 1964. The law establishes equal employment opportunity for all during the hiring process and throughout the course of employment. Further, it requires fairness and impartiality with regard to race, color, religious belief, gender, national origin, and age. The Pregnancy Discrimination Act of 1979 also applies to dental hygiene employment. It prohibits discrimination on the basis of pregnancy, childbirth, or related medical conditions. This law protects women from being fired or refused a job or promotion because of pregnancy. Furthermore, it provides that following maternity leave, the job will be returned with no loss in seniority or fringe benefits.

Minimal standards for working conditions are set by each state and include guidelines pertaining to hours and days of work, minimum wage and reports for pay, employee records, uniforms and equipment, meal periods and eating area, rest periods and rest facilities, and environmental temperature. The Occupational Safety and Health Standards Board (OSHA) sets minimum federal requirements for industrial safety.

Compensation

The methods of remuneration for dental hygiene employment are varied and determined by agreement between the employee and employer. It is the initial task and responsibility of the dental hygienist to establish the best possible financial arrangements with the employer. With continuous employment in one oral healthcare setting, it is later the task and challenge of the dental hygienist to negotiate for improved financial arrangements (see Methods of Compensation chart).

TERMS OF EMPLOYMENT

Permanent
The employee service with the employer is relatively secure and of unlimited duration

Temporary
The employee service is known to be of limited duration

Probationary
A service trial period, usually 1 to 3 months, for employee and employer to work together, then evaluate one another. During this period the employee may resign or be dismissed immediately for any reason

Full Time
The employee works solely in one office, or for one employer in multiple offices, the customary number of hours that the facility functions. Normally, 30 to 40 hours per week constitutes full-time employment

Part Time
The employee works less than full, customary hours of the facility's operation, usually less than 30 hours per week

Job Sharing
Two or more people share one full-time job by the day, week, month, or year. The time can be split in any fashion agreeable to the job sharers and the employer. The salary and benefits are divided proportionally with the time worked

Regular Hours
Work time that coincides with normal office hours

Staggered Hours
Established, consistent working hours that fit the life schedule of the employee. These hours vary from the routine office hours but are stable daily for the employee

Flex Time
Work time that changes daily, with the employee arriving and leaving whenever she or he chooses or depending on the daily workload.

Fringe Benefits

Fringe benefits are services paid by the employer in addition to regular wages. Fringe benefits are desirable because of the tax advantage of their being received directly from the employer rather than buying them with after-tax paycheck dollars. Legally required benefits that must be offered by the employer are Social Security, including old age benefits, survivor's benefits in the case of death of the employee, disability benefits for some medically caused total disabilities, and hospital insurance after age 65 (Medicare); workers' compensation, which protects the employee from medical expenses and loss of income in the event of injury on the job or job-related disability (disability insurance is required in some states to provide benefits for nonoccupational accidents or illnesses); and unemployment insurance, which provides benefits to individuals involuntarily unemployed.

Optional fringe benefits or "perks" fall into the categories of paid absences, insurance benefits, and professional ex-

METHODS OF COMPENSATION

Fixed Salary
A guaranteed fixed wage for hourly, daily, weekly, or monthly employment

Salary Plus Commission
A base salary is paid, plus an additional percentage of fees charged for dental hygiene services

Commission with Guaranteed Minimum Salary
A percentage of fees charged for dental hygiene services is paid with an assured minimum wage per day regardless of daily gross production

Commission
Earnings are based on a percentage of fees charged for dental hygiene services (Note: it is illegal for an employer to pay a commission to an employee based on fees collected)

Independent Contractor
The dental hygienist sets and collects all fees and pays overhead costs with the profit fluctuation based upon production, collection, and expenses

Overtime
Usually for hourly wage earners only, time-and-a-half is paid for all hours in excess of the contracted hours per week

Compensatory Time Off ("Comp Time")
Hours or days off given for excess time worked beyond the established work week; used in place of overtime pay

Profit-Sharing Bonus
A work incentive awarded to employees after profit goals are achieved for a specified period; may be calculated monthly, quarterly, or annually

Fringe Benefits
Paid services in addition to regular wages. Some benefits are required by law and some are optional services offered by the employer or requested by the dental hygienist. Fringe benefits paid for by the employer are tax deductible to the employer

penses (see Optional Fringe Benefits chart). Benefits may be paid for directly by the employer or there may be reimbursement for expenses to the employee.

Employment Contracts

The **employment contract,** or letter of agreement, is a written contract describing the terms of employment agreed on by the dental hygienist–employee and the dentist-employer. It functions to clarify the specific details of employment issues for both parties and in so doing establishes a stable working relationship between the two. Although it provides psychological security for both parties, it may or may not be legally binding. In some cases, the employer provides a letter of agreement prior to beginning employment. In other cases, the employment setting functions on a less formal basis, and it becomes the responsibility of the dental hygienist–employee to draw up an employment contract for the employer to sign. Many dental hygienist–employees work without an employment contract and do not experi-

OPTIONAL FRINGE BENEFITS

Paid Absences

Sick Leave
Salary paid during occasional short-term illnesses; usually sick leave benefits are allowed to accumulate if not used, or unused days are paid at the end of the year as a bonus

Holidays
Salary paid for usual, nationally observed holidays

Vacation
Salary paid for vacation time off, the amount of which varies according to the length of service with the employer. Vacation pay may be cumulative; for part-time employees, vacation days are prorated (divided proportionally with the work schedule)

Educational Leave
Salary paid for time off to attend educational programs that are work-related

Professional Activities
Salary paid for time off to attend professional meetings that are work- or career-related

Emergency Personal Leave
Paid time off for unexpected events such as a family illness, death, or funeral; jury duty, legal depositions, or court appearances; or extreme weather conditions.

Maternity Leave
Time off, usually without pay, but with the guarantee of job protection on return from leave; reasonable time limits usually apply

Extended Leave
Usually leave without pay for a few weeks to several months for the purpose of travel, family, or personal needs. The position is held during the absence with an agreed-upon time of return

Sabbatical, Developmental, or Research Leave
Usually leave without pay or reduced pay for a few weeks to several months for the purpose of education or research. The position is held during the absence with an agreed-upon time of return

Insurance Benefits
Health insurance
Dental insurance
Vision insurance
Liability (malpractice) insurance
Long-term permanent disability insurance
Life insurance
Pension plans
(See also sections on professional insurances and retirement)

Professional Expenses
Professional license renewal
Uniform allowance
Professional education assistance
Professional activities
Professional journals or texts
Transportation expenses
Expense account
Child care
Professional services
Staff functions

COMPONENTS OF AN EMPLOYMENT CONTRACT

Terms of Agreement
- Names of employee and employer
- Job title
- Date the contract takes effect
- Date the contract expires
- Option of contract renewal

Settings and Terms of Employment
- Address(es) of the employment
- Name(s) of supervising dentist(s)
- Agreement of both parties to adhere to the rules and regulations of the state dental practice act
- Statement of equipment, supplies, and instruments to be provided by the employer
- Work arrangement of days of work and workload by hours and scheduling of appointments

Job Description
- Specific services to be performed
- Other work responsibilities
- Opportunities for growth and promotion

Compensation
- Method of remuneration
- Starting wage
- Payroll schedule
- Increases in pay, including dates of review and basis for review
- Fringe benefits, listed individually with requirements for qualification, vesting increments, and accrual techniques
- Overtime compensation agreement
- Payment for time not worked such as holidays, vacation, sick leave, etc.

Probationary Period
- Terms and date of probation
- Agreement for mutual evaluation
- Employment termination options for each party

Performance Evaluation
- Dates for review
- Method of evaluation
- Criteria for performance success

Termination Procedures
- Advance notice required
- Statement of cause
- Employee replacement procedures

Signatures
- Employee and date signed
- Employer and date signed
- Witness(es) optional

ence problems; however, to avoid misunderstanding, written clarification of points of discussion is very helpful. Several components may be included in the employment contract (see Components of an Employment Contract chart). A sample contract is displayed in Figure 37–7.

Job Performance

The job performance of the dental hygienist is determined by a combination of the individual's own professional style and the completeness of the job description, plus procedure and policy manuals provided by the employment setting. The office procedure manual delineates responsibility and describes routines. A specific job description for the position of dental hygienist clearly defines all aspects of performance, outlines expectations, and serves as a guideline for performance review.

Standard of care describes the level of clinical performance required for the position of dental hygienist in that

---

Beginning June 1, 1995: Nancy Sutton, R.D.H., B.S., shall work as employee of Jack Joplin, D.D.S., as employer.

Ms. Sutton shall work as a Registered Dental Hygienist with Expanded Duties.

She shall work Mondays, Wednesdays, and Fridays from 8:00 A.M. until 5:30 P.M. The work schedule will be established by client need, determined by the dentist and dental hygienist, with appointment lengths of 30 minutes minimum for pedodontic clients and 45 minutes minimum for adult clients. A lunch break of 1 hour will be allowed daily.

Policy and procedures of the office, as outlined in the office manuals, will be followed by the employee. A complete job description is contained therein.

The starting salary will be $200 per day. After a 3-month probationary period, a performance evaluation will be completed by both the employee and the employer. At that time, the parties will evaluate their work compatibility to convert to permanent employment or to select a date for job termination. With permanent employment, the parties will establish a benefits package to equal $1,000 per year. A merit-based salary increase will occur every 6 months for the first year, and annually every year thereafter.

The employee will use the office space, equipment, and supplies provided by the employer. Special instrument and equipment needs will be considered on request by the employee. All uniforms will be purchased and maintained at the expense of the employer.

Additions to this agreement will be put in writing as they are developed.

I have read this contract and agree with the contents.

______________________	______________________
Nancy Sutton, R.D.H., B.S.	Jack Joplin, D.D.S.
Date __________	Date __________

FIGURE 37–7
Employment contract.

setting, practice philosophy and goals, and other special qualifications that maintain consistency among staff members. The policy manual applies to all personnel and is designed to outline the practice principles and how they are to be implemented. The success of the practice is dependent on staff members adhering to these standards. Client and personnel satisfaction is enhanced by following the contents of the office policy. Beyond a description of the personnel involvement in the team approach to delivering dental care, specific standards for quality assurance and education are outlined. Personnel policies, employment regulations, and work arrangements are included. Guidelines of professional ethics and conduct further assure quality client care with an ability to minimize liability. Office safety and emergency protocols prevent confusion and provide guidance for unified actions if unexpected situations occur. Finally, service to the community as an overall theme with specific contributions is described in the policy manual.

Job expectations are established when both the dental hygienist–employee and employer write the job description together and discuss and agree on level of performance and results. Specifically, this includes a listing of the basic responsibilities, standards of performance, importance of the functions, skills necessary to perform the job, and goals and limits for achieving the expectations. Beyond the area of job description, success in any setting is dependent on working with other people. Job satisfaction for the dental hygienist comes from human needs that are fulfilled in the employment setting (see Chapter 36, Leadership and Management). As one gains competence, responsibility, recognition and respect, and a sense of belonging, job satisfaction follows.

Performance Evaluation

The **performance evaluation** is a communication tool based on an agreed-upon performance plan. It is a valuable tool because it provides a progress report for the employee, it recognizes and supports desired behavior, develops strengths, pinpoints weaknesses, and gives specific direction for change. The performance evaluation may assist in determining a salary increase or can be used as a legal supporting document for employee dismissal.

A job evaluation is always performed at the completion of the probationary period if the employee is new, then once or twice a year for the duration of employment. In addition to the written document, daily verbal feedback as an evaluation *process,* rather than an event, facilitates successful employee performance.

Completing the performance evaluation requires that both the dental hygienist–employee and employer prepare the evaluation, then meet together to share, compare, and discuss the results (see Elements of the Performance Evaluation and Formats Used for Employee Performance Review charts).

The content of the performance evaluation addresses all areas of the job description such as:

- Participation with the practice and staff as a team member
- Knowledge of the dental hygiene field
- Clinical competence
- Interpersonal skills
- Dependability to the office and work schedule
- Responsibility for the treatment area and material resources
- Work habits
- Initiative, management, leadership, and problem-solving skills.

A sample performance evaluation is shown in Figure 37–8.

ELEMENTS OF THE PERFORMANCE EVALUATION

- Measure progress toward the goal of task and behavior performances
- Compare actual results with the agreed-on plan, citing specific incidents
- Praise accomplishments when performance meets or exceeds stated standards
- When differences occur, determine the cause, then consider alternatives to facilitate reaching desired outcomes
- If corrective action is indicated, state the specific plan with measurable results, and gain agreement of both parties
- Modify performance standards if indicated and agreed on by both parties
- Enhance communications between the employer and the employee, giving an opportunity for "coaching" to achieve performance goals, rather than merely "judging" performance

Improving Job Performance

The three elements required for changing job performance are planning, evaluation, and incorporation. Planning is begun by identifying the specific performance discrepancies, listing desired standard of performance in comparison with the present level of performance, analyzing the discrepancy, and defining what needs to be done differently. The employee and employer reach mutual agreement on the desired change, being certain that each party is clear about the details of the plan.

FORMATS USED FOR EMPLOYEE PERFORMANCE REVIEW

Management by Objective
Lists objectives together with a time frame using specific measurable criteria

Standard Office Procedure
Describes how well each responsibility is performed, according to the written job description

Critical Incidents
Descriptive file of events, both positive and negative, pertaining to job performance

Multiple Appraisers
A team of staff members participates in the performance assessments, and a compiled evaluation is presented to the employee

Employee Name: ______________________ Date: __________

Registered Dental Hygienist

Evaluation completed by: ______________________

	EXCELLENT	ACCEPTABLE	NEEDS IMPROVEMENT
PROFESSIONAL BEHAVIOR:			
1. Attitude	____	____	____
2. Cooperation	____	____	____
3. Responsibility	____	____	____
4. Initiative	____	____	____
5. Communications	____	____	____
6. Contributions to Office	____	____	____
CLIENT MANAGEMENT:			
1. Information & Instruction	____	____	____
2. Assistance in Decision Making	____	____	____
3. Respectful	____	____	____
4. Contribution to Comfort	____	____	____
5. Client Acceptance	____	____	____
RISK MANAGEMENT:			
1. Infection Control	____	____	____
2. Protect Self/Client from Injury	____	____	____
PROCESS OF CARE:			
1. Systematic Approach	____	____	____
2. Performs All Necessary Care	____	____	____
3. Care Procedures (List specific concerns)			
______________________			
______________________			
______________________			
______________________			
______________________			
4. Documentation Skills	____	____	____
5. Evaluation Skills	____	____	____
6. Modification of Care	____	____	____
7. Coordination with Other Care	____	____	____

CHANGES/GROWTH SINCE LAST EVALUATION:

____

____

____

GOALS FOR CHANGE/GROWTH:

____

____

____

FIGURE 37–8
Employee performance evaluation.

Illustration continued on following page

COMMENTS:

____

____

____

SIGNED:

_____________________________________ Date: ________
Supervisor

_____________________________________ Date: ________
Employee

FIGURE 37–8
Continued

The evaluation phase requires immediate feedback and reinforcement of the new, desired actions. Progress is monitored, with reinforcement given often at first and gradually tapering down. The guidelines for change are steadily reviewed and followed. It is important that specific acknowledgment be made when the desired changes are achieved.

Job Termination

Job termination may occur through dismissal by the employer or resignation by the employee. In the event of dismissal, the dental hygienist should make all attempts to understand clearly the grounds, asking for the true, complete picture, with clarification of any vague statements. Employees should be aware that it is the work performance that is unacceptable, and not the person. The employee should clarify the severance arrangements, including the date of termination, severance pay, and benefits accrued and due to the employee. Termination requires behaving professionally and with dignity, while allowing an opportunity to acknowledge feelings and mourn the loss of the job. Following a job dismissal, the terminated job must be put in perspective to re-enter the job market. This is a time for the dental hygienist to inventory career goals, update a resume, begin the interviewing process with specific ideas of new job requirements to achieve professional satisfaction, and then move confidently to the next career stage.

When the dental hygienist decides to resign from a job, notice of intentions is to be given to the employer as soon as possible, prior to telling any of the office co-workers. The notification process involves a clear statement of grounds for resigning or a statement of time for career change or advancement. Clarification is made of the severance arrangements, including the date of termination, benefits accrued and due, and whether there is an intention to find and/or train a successor. Departing employees should tie up loose ends and depart with dignity, behaving in a professional manner.

SEEKING EMPLOYMENT

Writing a Resume

The *resume* is a brief, written summary that highlights achievements and enhances the introduction of the dental hygienist to create a professional first impression. The resume is like an advertisement, intended to stimulate the reader to want to learn more. It presents an inventory of professional qualifications, assets, and goals that can generate a job interview or eliminate a purposeless interview and leaves a visible reminder of the applicant to the potential employer following an interview. The resume types are defined as *blanket,* which is a general resume for all jobs in the relevant field, and *specific,* which is designed with one particular job in mind. The resume styles can be either *descriptive* in the traditional sense of listing education, experience, and qualifications in reverse chronological order, or *functional,* which states effective accomplishments that support a specific job position and reflect ability in individual skills areas (see Components of a Quality Resume chart).

Honesty and accuracy are the most important elements of resume writing; be certain all contents are correct. Prospective employees should use concise phrases with descriptive terminology, demonstrate confidence and professional interest, emphasize individual qualities and avoid listing general responsibilities, be credible, and avoid exaggeration. The resume format is brief; one page is preferred, although two pages are acceptable; typed, typeset, and word-processed presentations are acceptable. Overall, the resume must appear polished, neat, and accurate, with correct spelling and grammar; and organized with bold functional headings to introduce each category. Spaces and wide margins are used for easy readability. An original or high quality photocopy on medium-weight, white or ivory-colored paper looks most professional. Carbon copy resumes are unacceptable. Sample resumes appear in Figures 37–9 and 37–10.

Preparing a Cover Letter

The cover letter introduces the applicant and the resume and may highlight the most important qualifications of the dental hygienist. A comment on how the applicant learned about the job availability is contained in the cover letter, plus a demonstration of interest in the practice. Statements that demonstrate an understanding of the employer's needs and how the applicant's skills specifically match this job demonstrate a clear interest in the position and appeal to the employer's pride in his practice. The cover letter format is brief and simple, in one to two paragraphs, and should not repeat the content of the resume. It should be an original page, individually typed and not photocopied. The cover letter is to be neat, accurate, typed letter-perfect on bond paper with correct spelling and grammar, and addressed to the person of authority, using the person's name

COMPONENTS OF A QUALITY RESUME

Personal Identification
- Name
- Address
- Telephone

Job Objective
Statement of the exact job being sought, giving resume focus
- Brief philosophic statement
- Professional goals

Career Summary
Creating a sense of the applicant and what has been accomplished professionally
- Skills
- Strengths
- Assets

Academic History
Schooling applicable to the job objective
- College/university
- Date of graduation
- Degree(s) received
- Honors and awards
- Dental hygiene licensure
- Special certificates

Professional Employment Experience
Summarize any responsibilities not generally encompassed by the normal dental hygiene job description and note any special awards received. New licentiates can list special skills/interests from school, jobs in related fields, or academic honors and awards
- Private practice
- Teaching
- Administrative
- Research
- Government agencies

Professional Data
(Optional)
- Professional affiliations
- Community and professional services
- Publications
- Presentations given
- Continuing education courses attended
- Professional projects

References
(Optional) If included, be certain reference sources are notified and willing to speak highly of applicant
- "Available upon request" or
- List two sources

Personal Information
Unnecessary and should be eliminated including gender, age, race or color, religion, marital status, children, health conditions, height, weight, interests or hobbies

---

Cindy Browne, R.D.H., B.S. 415-882-3434
1661 "M" Street
San Francisco, CA 94112

JOB OBJECTIVE

Registered dental hygienist seeking employment with additional responsibilities in local anesthesia, soft tissue management, and nitrous oxide–oxygen analgesia.

LICENSURE & EDUCATION

California Registered Dental Hygienist License DH 38991
B.S. in Dental Hygiene—June 1994
University of California at San Francisco
School of Dentistry

WORK EXPERIENCE

1990 to 1995—Summers
Dental Assistant in various dental offices in San Francisco.
Employed as a "temporary" for an employment agency.

REFERENCES

Jennifer Jones, R.D.H., M.S., Director
Dental Hygiene Program at UCSF
Telephone: 415-444-1234

Additional references available on request from former employers.

PRIMARY AIMS

I wish to contribute my skills and knowledge to a prevention-oriented dental practice. My goal is to become part of an office team whose members are mutually supportive and positive in their approach to client care.

FIGURE 37–9
Sample of a "new graduate" resume.

and title (Fig. 37–11). The cover letter is signed and the resume is enclosed.

Interviews

The purpose of an interview is to provide a mutual opportunity for reciprocal information exchange and to evaluate for congruent job objectives.[7] The interviewer appraises the candidate's resume, work qualifications, professional philosophy, and behavior. The candidate appraises the interviewer and the employment situation with regard to job description and responsibility, practice philosophy, staff members as potential co-workers, office environment, working conditions, and opportunity for job satisfaction, professional growth, challenge, and responsibility.

Susan Jensen, R.D.H., M.S. 415-525-5566
11 California Way
San Francisco, CA 92110

LICENSURE & EDUCATION

California Registered Dental Hygienist License DH3322
Certification in Expanded Functions: Local Anesthesia, Soft Tissue Curettage, and Nitrous Oxide–Oxygen Analgesia
M.A. Education, San Francisco State University: 1975
B.S. Dental Hygiene, University of Southern California: 1970

EMPLOYMENT

Dental Hygienist in General Dental Practice 1985 to Present
Rodney Mann, D.D.S., San Francisco

Dental Hygienist in Periodontal Practice 1970 to 1985
Robert Hanson, D.D.S., San Francisco

TEACHING

Instructor of Dental Hygiene 1975 to Present
Diablo Valley College

COMMUNITY

Community Oral Health Projects 1970 to 1994

REFERENCES available on request.

CAREER GOALS

I would like to build on my skills and interests in health education and communications within a people- and prevention-oriented dental practice. My professional satisfaction comes from contributing thorough periodontal assessment and quality periodontal therapy services of lasting value.

FIGURE 37-10
Sample resume of a veteran hygienist.

Interview styles may follow a specific structured pattern of formatted questions or may be loosely structured and broad, allowing for interaction between the interviewer and the candidate. A combination-type interview is most common. In rare cases there may be a *group* interview, when several candidates are grouped together at one time with the expectation by the interviewer that one candidate will emerge superior to the others. Or there may be a *board* interview, in which there is one candidate meeting with several interviewers. In this case, each interviewer asks questions.

A screening process precedes scheduling an interview. The initial evaluation identifies potentially acceptable positions for the dental hygienist–applicant and eliminates those employment settings that are unacceptable. The screening may be done via the telephone and may include a series of basic questions about the position. The dental hygienist–applicant pays close attention to the office "tone" during these conversations. An interview appointment is scheduled if the office passes the initial screening. Applicants should confirm the date, time, and location of the interview and obtain directions to the office. An expected, agreed-upon length of time is established for the appointment and the interviewer is determined. In some cases the potential employer is not the person who conducts the preliminary interview, rather, the senior dental hygienist or the office manager may process the bulk of applicants before the dentist meets "the finalists."

Preparation for the interview requires self-knowledge for the dental hygienist–applicant. The dental hygienist must

1234 Main Street 415-321-4455
San Francisco, CA 94110

October 15, 1995

John Joplin, D.D.S.
444 No. University Avenue
San Francisco, CA 94115

Dear Dr. Joplin,

Dental hygiene care is the foundation of a sound dental practice. Persons maintained on a continued care basis will enjoy a healthy periodontium and dentition as well as keep your practice viable and growing.

As a registered dental hygienist skilled in periodontal care and effective communications, I would like to contribute to the increasing success of your practice. My emphasis is on client assessment and treatment sequencing with certification in local anesthesia and nitrous oxide–oxygen analgesia.

I would enjoy meeting with you to hear your views about dental hygiene care within your dental practice. My resume is enclosed for your review. You will see by the workshops I have attended that I have a strong interest in periodontics and practice enhancement.

I shall be calling next week to set a meeting date.

Sincerely,

Nancy Smith, R.D.H., B.S.

FIGURE 37–11
Cover letter.

define personal standards and qualifications (e.g., skill strengths and weaknesses, employment expectations and desires, professional philosophy, and short- and long-term career goals). The position should be studied and selected if it meets these standards. Learning the characteristics of the practice, the dentist and the staff members, and the client population are important. Speaking with current or former employees, college alumni, or other dentists and professionals in the area is beneficial. The object is to find out as much as possible about the philosophy and work environment of the practice before appearing for the interview, then tailor a job-interview style to match personal strengths to the needs of the practice. Some applicants practice by role-playing a mock interview by writing out possible questions asked of candidates and presenting answers out loud. Some write out questions for the interviewer about the practice and the available position. A colleague may critique the rehearsal.

The preliminary interview is an opportunity to establish rapport between the interviewer and the candidate. The candidate presents qualifications as represented on the resume and shares the professional philosophy. Strengths of education and experience are stressed, demonstrating the candidate's potential as an employee. New licentiates can address lack of experience with "eagerness to learn" attitudes.

The interviewer presents the position represented by the job description, the dental hygienist's responsibilities, nature of participation with the practice team, and opportunity for professional growth. The practice philosophy and description of the office atmosphere and work environment also are presented. Two questions commonly asked of the candidate during the preliminary interview are:

"What are your professional goals?"
"Why should we hire you?"

Preparation is necessary to be able to answer each with three or four specific responses that demonstrate how the candidate can benefit the practice. There may be an initial discussion of compensation presented at this interview. Compatibility is established by linking the candidate's skills and strengths with the job description and needs of the practice. Plans may be discussed to accommodate for weaknesses in the match. Both parties may work from written notes or a list of important questions. The preliminary interview is concluded with a summary of the findings, a statement of incompatibility from either party, an invitation to return for a follow-up interview, or possibly a job offer.

The second interview, or selection interview, provides an opportunity for both the candidate and the office staff members to have a second look at each other. A thorough discussion of the details of the job should include the job description and office policies and procedures, work schedule, compensation package of starting wage and benefits, and the frequency of raises.

Techniques for Successful Job Interviews

The following recommendations may enhance the success of employment interviews:

- Know and believe in yourself. Memorize your professional goals and accomplishments. Keep spirits high and do not get discouraged. Heed personal intuition during interviews and when making the job selection decision
- Be prompt. Do not arrive late to the interview, nor more than 15 minutes early. If you know you are going to be late, telephone the office prior to the appointed time with an apology and appropriate explanation plus an estimated time of arrival
- Wear attire that makes a professional impression
- Dress as though you represent the organization with which you are interviewing
- Greet the practice receptionist or secretary with friendliness and respect; this is the first impression made
- Present a personal style that is friendly, self-assured, and sincere. Convey interest and eagerness to learn about the practice. The first 1 to 2 minutes are critical to candidate selection: quickly establish comfort and rapport to set the tone for the rest of the interview
- Address the interviewer by name, especially when greeting and upon leaving the appointment; wait for the interviewer to begin the questioning first and follow the interviewer's lead. Listen carefully to each question and answer the actual question asked, responding with direct, thoughtful, concise answers. Ask for clarification if a question is not clearly understood; if there is an unanswerable question, say so; do not fake it. Be articulate and answer with details to establish a memorable impression; give examples of proven

ability and professionalism, but try not to repeat what is on the resume. Establish credibility and trust; above all, be honest and do not misrepresent yourself

- Avoid offering information about your personal life, which is irrelevant to the position. Listen carefully for any problems, difficulties, negatives, or disappointments subtly exposed by the interviewer. Be diplomatic and tactful; avoid complaining or negatively judging past experiences, jobs, employers, colleagues, schools or teachers; do not exaggerate past work performance; and focus on professional, not personal, statements
- Interview the interviewer on a parity basis. Be proactive with prepared comments about practice philosophy and professional goals. Ask specific, intelligent questions that will provide the information needed to determine if this is the position sought. Failing to ask questions is a common error made by job candidates; questions demonstrate an interest in the job. Always ask, "What qualifications are you looking for in the dental hygienist who fills this position?" If the response indicates this is a mismatch, the candidate can say so and cut the interview short; if desirable, the candidate can stress matching qualities. It is reasonable to ask about the work style of the practice such as daily pace, whether they generally stay on schedule, level of dental hygienist responsibility, and frequency of collaboration between staff members; as well as longevity of current or previous employees and reasons for employee departure from the practice
- Nonverbal communications and body language send the message of self-confidence. Shake hands firmly upon introductions, display a dental hygiene smile, maintain good posture, be seated only at the invitation of the interviewer, retain a calm body position and use eye contact throughout the interview
- Be cautious to contain nervous habits, e.g., do not fidget, smoke, or chew gum
- Demonstrate that the primary reason for the interview is to gain information about the position, and resist the temptation to ask about money. Although there may be brief mention of the wage or salary range during the interview, any salary negotiations should occur after a job offer is received
- Depart from the interview with a smile, a handshake, and a clear idea of the employer's notification schedule. Thank-you notes are optional, generally having little effect on enhancing a job offer because almost all interview decisions are made the day of the interview. The contents of the note may reiterate interest in the position and summarize why the practice should be interested in the candidate. In the event of a second interview, the first thank-you note can win friends in the job setting and communicate gratitude

Job Search Strategies

Preparation for the job search begins by clarifying career goals. A careful assessment can prevent a poor employment match and, later, job dissatisfaction. One should imagine the ideal job situation, with elements that motivate and gratify, then seek or create one that closely fits this image.

Applicants should investigate the job market, studying local trends in career opportunities, job descriptions, work loads, and the possibility of job sharing, compensation packages, job turnovers, and layoffs (see Sources for Locating Dental Hygiene Employment chart). Be aware of the full value of the dental hygienist to the dental practice. Send a resume promptly so as to be among the first seen. Do not underrate personal abilities and do not undercut a wage.

SOURCES FOR LOCATING DENTAL HYGIENE EMPLOYMENT

- Friends, colleagues, and other professional contacts using the word-of-mouth approach **(networking)**
- Verbal or printed announcements at meetings and conferences
- Dental hygiene association employment placement services
- Dental society employment placement services
- Private healthcare providers' employment placement agencies
- Public or county health departments
- Dental hygiene school employment opportunities bulletin boards
- Dental hygiene and dental association newsletters and journals, section on employment vacancies
- Employment opportunity bulletin boards in large office buildings
- Professional people in the geographic vicinity where work is sought; people mentioned in association newsletters, association leaders, authors, speakers, and educators
- Local dental association membership directories, alumni association membership directories, telephone books with local dental office listings
- Dental supply houses or supply salespersons
- Newspaper classified advertisements

Job Selection Considerations

When considering which job to select, the dental hygienist compares career needs and desires with what is being offered by the potential employer. There are many factors to take into account[8]:

- Overall practice ambiance and atmosphere
- Practice philosophy, goals, and values
- Personal harmony felt with the office atmosphere and staff members
- Interactions with clients (e.g., "professionally distant" or "personal and caring")
- Practice standards and quality of care provided
- General job description including the specific responsibilities of the job and the scope of dental hygiene care provided
- General work conditions such as workload, scheduling, pace, hours, equipment, supplies, and instruments
- Overall role of the dental hygienist within the practice including level of respect and responsibilities
- Compensation package consisting of salary, fringe benefits, opportunity for bonuses, and schedule for remuneration increases
- Concern with feelings of belonging to the practice "team"

- Opportunity for professional growth and personal satisfaction
- Job security with an assured client load plus established record of employee longevity
- Practice open to innovation or content to maintain the status quo
- Location of employment setting, commuting and parking situation
- Practice well-established or new and growing, stable or restructuring and in transition, large or small staff

The right choice for job selection should satisfy the greatest number of professional desires and needs possible. Applicants should choose the employment setting that offers the most. Feeling excited about starting a new job is a good beginning.

CAREER DEVELOPMENT

Planning a career is defined as following a course related to some noteworthy activity or pursuit that forms the total of one's lifework in a chosen field. An *occupation* is defined as a regular or principal business or line of work, while a *job* is defined as a position of employment to gain a livelihood. A *career* is differentiated by offering a wide range of activities within one field. The elements of a career in dental hygiene include:

- Continuing education to expand knowledge and skills in the field
- Maturation of professional skills
- Making responsible contributions for directing the success of client care or other work objectives and creating a positive work environment
- Participation in the growth of the profession through research, education, politics, organizational leadership, and/or public awareness
- Gaining personal gratification through these various involvements

The goals of career development are to select short-term objectives that support long-range goals for professional achievement and growth. A written record of career goals is used to continually guide direction and contribute to commitment. Goals are revised for growth, advancement, or change, as needed.

Presentation of the Professional Image

The dental hygienist's professional image is consistently projected through affect, or overall behavior of self-confidence and caring about the health and well-being of others. Presenting a self-confident appearance and positive body language conveys a professional image. The dental hygienist may be represented by business cards or business stationery. The cards and stationery can be used for exchange at job interviews; dental professional meetings, conferences, and educational programs; and nondental professional associations, agencies, and professional contacts. Furthermore, cards, stationery, and personalized memo pads can be used during professional correspondence and practice promotion.

The design of these items incorporates the dental hygienist's name and professional degrees, title, and other identifying information. Home or office address and telephone number may be used. The quality of paper and design should project a professional image. The dental hygienist may need more than one card design to represent different affiliations and activities.

Starting a New Job

Presentation of a professional image is the first step of starting a new job. The dental hygienist quickly establishes, then maintains the "professional personality" in both client care and intraoffice interactions. Initial employment includes investigating to learn about the new position and other staff members' job responsibilities. This behavior gains respect and builds a loyalty base from both clients and co-workers. Newcomers learn from mistakes and seek help when assistance is needed; they are flexible to learn from the new job and persistent to develop excellence. They ease through the work day knowing what is expected and that expectations are being met, with assurance of the feeling of being respected and appreciated by clients, dentist, and co-workers and having a sense of job security develop over the years within a given practice. New licentiates need to allow time to establish a solid track record and develop clinical skills in communications, management, and leadership.

Stress and Burn-out Among Dental Hygienists

Stress is the strain or tension from compulsive pressures, usually resulting in a diminished capacity for resistance. **Burn-out** is the combination of physical, emotional, and behavioral changes in an individual as a response to high-intensity or long-duration stress, when one's adaptive capabilities are exceeded (see Sources of Stress and Burn-out in a Dental Hygiene Career chart).

Various strategies can be employed to reduce stress and burn-out, beginning with an identification of the reasons causing the feelings. Some people analyze feelings to achieve self-awareness of the internal issues. Others evalu-

SOURCES OF STRESS AND BURN-OUT IN A DENTAL HYGIENE CAREER

- The **"giving" role** of healthcare providers is emotionally draining, with little "received" in return
- Working in an **"intimate zone"** of the human body
- The **intense interpersonal relations** with clients and staff members
- Dental hygiene **job tasks** that are **repetitive** and monotonous
- **Lack of intellectual stimulation**
- **Lack of feeling appreciated** which leads to reduced self-esteem
- **Feelings of being taken for granted** that lead to reduced self-worth
- **Sensing a lack of accomplishment** of personal and/or professional goals
- Generalized **lack of change**

With permission from Dreyer R. Is burnout inevitable? Career Directions for Dental Hygienists 10(11):1, 1983.

ate the environment and work situation to make external changes, then reprioritize goals or reevaluate methods used to accomplish reconfirmed goals. A conscious attempt should be made to incorporate changes that reduce stress by delegating responsibilities, being creative, and trying something new. People should modify behavior to enjoy life by taking classes, learning new skills, maintaining physical fitness, enjoying recreation, trying techniques for body and mind relaxation, and adopting new behaviors.

Networks for Professional Enhancement

Professional connections can be accomplished by **"networking,"** or sharing and extending professional contacts to establish friendships and business relationships. The functions of networks are to exchange knowledge and information and to develop a professional and morale support system for achievement of professional goals. These groups can keep members informed of professional developments and job opportunities and assist in making job changes. The members may be professional colleagues, college classmates and faculty, or friends and relatives.

Employment Alternatives to Private Practice Dental Hygiene

Most dental hygiene employment opportunities are in the private practice sector; however, employment alternatives might include positions in:

- Dental hygiene and dental schools
- Public schools
- Community oral health projects
- Consulting in practice management and teaching in continuing education
- Private enterprise
- Acute and chronic care facilities, nursing and convalescent homes, residential care facilities, homes for the elderly, and hospices
- Oral health products industry
- Insurance industry
- Government service in the armed forces, Veteran's Administration, Public Health Service, Indian Health Service, or state agencies.
- Health professionals placement agency
- Scientific research and theory development
- Professional and public organizations
- Professional media development
- Dental hygiene practice in foreign countries

PROFESSIONAL AND PERSONAL FINANCIAL MANAGEMENT

Management of finances is a lifetime endeavor and involves a combination of factors. Compensation is paramount at the beginning of the career, and sound financial planning should begin immediately. Knowledge of annual tax deductions and liabilities guides spending and an eye to the future for retirement planning encourages a savings program.

Compensation Considerations

Financial security must be attained by the dental hygienist throughout the career. Initially, wages and fringe benefits are to be evaluated for coverage of living expenses, paid time off, insurance coverage, and savings. The compensation package must cover these needs for monthly bills and annual financial objectives. It is essential that the dental hygienist also consider long-term economic needs. **Financial planning** is the process of setting financial goals for the future by taking intentional steps to achieve financial security.

Steps to Financial Planning

Financial planning begins with an evaluation of the present financial situation by computing net worth, which is the difference between assets (amount owned) and liabilities (amount owed). This calculation includes real property, life insurance, stocks, bonds, retirement accounts, household and personal property, and bank accounts. Net worth is determined on an annual basis to check progress in reaching financial goals; then a review and update of the plan are done.

Set goals for the future, stating specific objectives for short-term accomplishments and long-range goals. Plan to spread investments over the years. In determining the long-range goals, include the desired income at retirement. List other objectives, including income now and in 5 years, then 10 years, etc. Specify investments such as residential property, securities, retirement accounts, education of children, travel, and others for personal needs and desires.

Plan a budget as an effective money management tool. Use the outline of both short- and long-term goals to develop the budget. Anticipate basic needs and expenses and allocate funds for these. Analyze spending habits, control impulse buying, and live within the income limits. Do plan some fun and recreation as well as consideration for emergency expenses. Determine how to compensate for unexpected bills. Regularly monitor actual expenses as compared with the budget to evaluate whether the budget is realistic. Keep records for a complete and accurate accounting. The records help determine if the planning is appropriate as well as assisting with taxes, expense accounts, and forecasting the financial future.

The dental hygienist needs to establish an individual credit rating. This facilitates getting loans, a mortgage, or other credit. It also allows for independent financial functioning. Once credit is established, use it effectively. Major purchases may be spread over a long period and paid off with a reasonable finance charge. Avoid unnecessary debts, finance charges, and penalties for late payments.

One should pay oneself first, with interest, dividends, and appreciation. Begin with small guaranteed accounts and investments that make the money work for you. Select interest-bearing checking accounts, savings accounts, money market accounts, mutual funds, bonds, certificates of deposit, and United States Treasury bills. In addition, establish a reserve fund for emergencies that does not disturb the other accounts.

Purchasing a home is the most important initial major investment, usually the largest single investment of a lifetime. Providing a home eliminates paying rent to someone else, offers safety and security, provides financial leverage as collateral, gains appreciation, and offers tax advantages. Diversify other investments to spread the risks, obtain the highest possible return, and gain income-producing securities.

The dental hygienist needs to protect personal income with disability insurance, as a safeguard for earning power (see the section on disability insurance). Immediately upon initial employment, the dental hygienist needs to begin a retirement fund that will receive contributions throughout all the working years (see the section on retirement planning).

Investment Goals

The goals for investments are varied and should be considered prior to selecting each investment. Choose investments for as many of the following purposes as possible. To:

- Produce income
- Provide a tax advantage
- Hedge inflation
- Show capital growth and appreciate in value
- Furnish safety and security
- Have liquidity conversion potential
- Maintain them management-free or with minimal expense

Professional assistance for financial planning is recommended. A carefully planned strategy to achieve financial goals is best done with the expertise of specialists who can help with laws, regulations, taxes, intricacies, and refinements. These specialists include bankers, real estate brokers, stockbrokers, insurance brokers, investment advisors, accountants, and attorneys.

The types of investments are numerous. For each, one must consider how much risk one is willing and able to assume, considering both short- and long-term investments plus evaluating income needs now and in the future. The tangible investments (hard assets) include real estate; gold, silver, coins, and gems; plus antiques, art, stamps, and rare books. The intangible investments (paper with a guarantee, securities, or liquid assets) include banks, savings and loans offering interest-bearing checking accounts, savings accounts, money market accounts, and certificates of deposit; government securities such as Treasury bills, notes and bonds, savings bonds, federal agency lending programs, short-term tax-exempt notes, and municipal bonds for estates, counties, and municipalities; and investment firms with money market funds, stocks, corporate bonds, mutual funds, tax-deferred annuities, commodities and financial futures, limited partnerships, tax shelters, trust deeds, and foreign currency.

Estate Planning

Estate planning is defined as providing for intentional disposition of possessions and assets on one's death to organize family resources and provide for the family's future. Estate planning requires careful financial planning and management during one's lifetime. It intentionally creates, defines, and retains assets of the estate, provides for disability, and plans and provides for retirement. A well-planned estate can spread family income and ensure prudent money management during one's lifetime. Estate planning is valuable in establishing trusts to reduce administrative and management costs and protect assets, as well as minimize or avoid taxes imposed on estates and inheritances. Finally, the estate plan guarantees that the financially secure property will be disposed of as one desires.

Professional Insurances

Liability. The dental hygienist may purchase insurance policies to protect professional and personal assets. *Liability (malpractice) insurance* is a plan that protects the insured against liability arising out of professional service (see the section on fringe benefits). It is recommended that a dental hygienist carry a personal malpractice policy, even if the employer carries similar insurance that extends coverage to all employees. Dental hygienists should note that the employer's policy is in effect to represent the dental hygienist only if the dentist is also named in a lawsuit. If the employer and dental hygienist are both named and later the dentist is dropped from the suit, the liability insurance may no longer apply for the hygienist (see Chapter 39, Ethical and Legal Decision Making in Dental Hygiene). Furthermore, all insurance policies have limits of liability. If the limits to protect the dentist are met, and no financial coverage is left to protect the hygienist, the dental hygienist alone is responsible for covering all court costs, attorney fees, and injury expenses. Finally, when carrying one's own policy, the dental hygienist has the right to select an attorney, rather than be forced to accept an attorney assigned by the employer's policy. Hygienists should be familiar with all the terms of any policy purchased.

Disability Insurance. Disability insurance or workers' compensation is defined in the section on fringe benefits. When selecting a disability policy, the dental hygienist must first determine the minimal monthly expenses that must be paid by the insurance policy, should she become disabled, because this insurance coverage provides a percentage of the basic wage. After investigating other sources of income during disability, such as a state disability insurance paid on all employees, a minimum monthly total is determined to assist in policy selection. Some policies pay an additional benefit during the time of hospitalization. Partial benefits may be available if the insured is able to return to work on a limited basis. The benefit period may be a specified number of years, the length of the disability, until the insured can be retrained in a new job, until regular retirement benefits begin, or for a lifetime. The premium price is determined by the amount paid by the policy if disability occurs and the length of "elimination" or waiting period before the policy begins to make payments to the insured. Hygienists should read the policies carefully because the term "disability" may be defined in a variety of ways.

Life Insurance. Life insurance is classified as term or whole life insurance. Term insurance, covering a specific temporary time period, or whole life insurance, a long-term investment policy that builds on cash value and may pay dividends or provide borrowing equity, may be selected. It is recommended that the dental hygienist seek professional guidance in selecting a life insurance policy.

Taxes

Taxes are the largest single item in the personal budget. Therefore, it is important to receive all tax breaks available. The "tax bracket" is the combined federal and state percentage of taxes paid on the total dollars earned. In the United States tax system, it is advantageous to maximize tax deductions so as to reduce tax liabilities, thereby creating the lowest tax bracket possible. The tax bracket helps to determine the best types of investments.

Professional Tax Deductions

In addition to the tax savings available to all taxpayers, professionals are entitled to special tax adjustments, deductions, and credits if these expenses are employment-related.

The IRS requires that the individual maintain a calendar of professional activities that are tax deductible, with an explanation of each event, including the date, activity, relationship to the job, the sponsor, location, cost, and transportation required. The expense record includes proof of all costs, such as receipts, cancelled checks, or credit card vouchers. Federal records should be maintained for at least 3 years after filing, and copies of the federal and state income tax returns are to be kept forever. Professional expenses are deducted only to the extent that the professional is not reimbursed and can establish the right to deduct them.

Professional expenses that are tax deductible to dental hygienists include travel and transportation costs related to professional activities, professional education, uniforms, and miscellaneous professional expenses. Activities with related travel and transportation deductions may be office staff meetings, conferences and meetings of professional organizations, speaking engagements performed by the dental hygienist as a community service, educational programs, study group meetings, seeking employment, and commuting between two jobs on 1 day.

Travel Expenses. Travel expenses are the ordinary and necessary expenses incurred while away from home (overnight) for the purpose of a professional or job-related activity. Travel expenses are deducted as "Employee Business Expenses" on IRS Form 2106, as an adjustment to income. Travel expenses include fares for airplanes, trains, and buses; meals and lodging; automobile expenses, and related necessary expenses such as telephone calls and laundry. Transportation expenses are the actual cost of transportation to professional activities while not away from home (not overnight). They are allowed only as itemized deductions on Schedule A of IRS Form 1040. Basic commuting between home and job and back home again is not allowed as a transportation expense. These items include actual automobile expenses, bus and cab fares, plus bridge tolls and parking fees. There are two methods of computation for travel and transportation expenses. One is by the "mileage rate system" in which the IRS states a specific amount allowed for each mile driven. Instructions and the amount allowed for any given year appear on Form 2106. The other is the "actual expenses method," which requires the computation of the ratio of professional mileage to total mileage driven for the year. It represents the actual operating costs such as gasoline, oil, repairs, maintenance, licenses, insurance, depreciation or lease payments, and loan interest. Both options require keeping an odometer diary at the beginning and end of each trip. Nonprofessional travel portions are to be excluded from the total mileage. There are special rules for travel outside the United States. Refer to IRS guidelines for details and qualifying regulations.

Educational Expenses. Professional education expenses may be deducted as ordinary and necessary if they meet the express requirements of the employer or the law for retaining professional status and/or licensure. Because many states require a minimum number of hours of continuing education annually as a prerequisite to license renewal, this deduction is easy for the dental hygienist to apply. Professional education expenses may also be deducted to maintain or improve skills required in performing the responsibilities of the present profession, including education that leads to a degree. This allows a tax deduction for a dental hygienist with an associate degree to return to college to earn a baccalaureate degree. Furthermore, if new educational requirements are placed on the profession, all necessary education expenses to meet these stipulations are deductible. Expenses for training in a new profession may not be deducted. Specific costs that are deductible include tuition, fees for correspondence courses, books, supplies, travel, and transportation expenses. Proof of attendance may be required in the event of a tax audit.

Uniform Expenses. Professional uniforms are defined as work clothes that are specifically required as a condition of employment and are not suitable for general or everyday wear. They must be recognizable as "uniforms." The purchase and maintenance costs are deductible including laundering, dry cleaning, repairs, and alterations. Uniform items for dental hygienists are dresses; pants and tops; laboratory coats and jackets; clinic shoes; caps; white or support hosiery; protective clothing such as protective eyewear, masks, and gloves; plus name tags and professional pins.

Miscellaneous Expenses. Other miscellaneous professional expenses include dues to professional organizations; employment-seeking expenses such as agency fees, resume typing and printing, telephone calls, postage, travel and transportation expenses; liability (malpractice) insurance premiums; instruments, professional equipment and supplies; medical examinations that are required by the employer; subscriptions to professional and trade journals; professional legal expenses; professional license renewal; and postage, local and long-distance telephone calls for professional reasons.

Child and dependent care expenses are allowed for children or disabled dependents while one is at work or seeking employment. For specific qualifications and regulations, see IRS Form 2441 titled "Credit for Child and Dependent Care Expenses." Certain retirement account contributions may be deducted as an adjustment to income, before the adjusted gross income is determined. All interest earned on these accounts is not taxed during working years. Refer to IRS guidelines for details of which accounts qualify and see the section in this chapter on retirement planning.

Tax Audits

Tax returns are reviewed by IRS agents and IRS computers for errors and omissions, deductions that are beyond the normal range relative to a given profession, and other variables. A letter of notification is sent to the taxpayer indicating specific categories for audit. The examination may be done through the mail, as a correspondence audit, or in the office of the IRS. The burden of proof of all allowable deductions is on the taxpayer. All related records are presented to the auditor for consideration and evaluation as legitimate deductions. Although all auditors rely on the same reference sources, each examiner may interpret the law differently. The auditors have equal responsibility to both the taxpayer and the government. Although they primarily investigate to increase collections, they also identify overpayments.

Following the review of data presented, if additional taxes are due from the taxpayer, the auditor will calculate a revised bill, including interest. Repetitive audits for the same items are not allowed for 2 years following a clear audit. If an audit finds additional tax liability, the audit can be repeated on that item until the audit is clear. A taxpayer can be audited every year for different categories. Do not eliminate legitimate deductions to avoid an audit. By collecting documentation and completing a diary, taxpayers have all proof necessary to satisfy an auditor.

Retirement Planning

Retirement planning is best begun at the beginning of the dental hygienist's career, so that a definite program is in place and funds have been invested over the years to adequately provide for retirement. Focus on goals that include lifestyle, home location, and living conditions. Consider activities, travel, recreation, hobbies, and business involvement. Attempt to project living costs, factoring in cost of living increases, and the income required to accommodate the retirement plans, allowing for possible illness or disability. Resources for income during retirement include Social Security payments, retirement funds, whole life insurance policies, and other planned investments. A formal plan, reviewed periodically, is helpful.

There are many types of tax deferred retirement accounts. It is best to consult a professional advisor for assistance in selecting a plan that meets the investor's specific needs. In a tax deferred program, taxes on amounts deposited and interest earned are deferred until withdrawal. These accounts reduce the annual adjusted gross income, thereby reducing the income tax debt. If the dental hygienist's employer has a corporate, Simplified Employee Pension Plan (SEP), or Keogh retirement program and the employee qualifies to be included in the plan by job title and hours of employment, the hygienist needs to study the requirements and contributions schedule for such a plan. Become familiar with the guidelines on vesting; allowance of additional contributions by the employee, beyond the contributions of the employer; and termination procedures, if the employee leaves the office. In such cases, the dental hygienist may take his portion of the fund (amount vested) and "roll it over" into an individual retirement arrangement (IRA) without paying tax consequences.

The IRA is allowable for anyone with earned income who is not included in another pension plan provided by an employer. There is also an exclusion if the employee's spouse is covered by a tax deferred retirement plan. If neither spouse is covered by an employer's pension plan, each spouse may have a separate IRA, even if one spouse does not earn an income. The mechanisms for these arrangements include savings accounts, mutual funds, retirement bonds, retirement annuities, and trust accounts. The IRS outlines all the rules and regulations for qualifying for an IRA, including maximum contribution allowable, dates for contributions, termination, and withdrawal. Changes occur periodically, and it is recommended that the taxpayer review details each year.

Wills

A *will* is a written, legal arrangement for distribution of assets when death occurs. The dental hygienist needs a legal will regardless of age, marital status, or dependents, to direct disposal of belongings. A will provides for financial and guardian care of minor children or disabled dependents, covers payments of debts of the decedent, and can lessen delay in distributing the estate.

The contents of a will identify beneficiaries, identify all aspects of financial affairs, divide the assets; a codicil can direct distribution of special items. Wills are best prepared in consultation with an attorney to ensure validity and protect the overall interests of the individual. Although a person may write a will without legal assistance, laws for each state vary about the validity of handwritten wills. Consult the rules for your state if you choose to write a will without the guidance of an attorney.

Probate is the legal process alerting the community of the death, then attending to the financial distribution of the estate. An executor, assigned to carry out the provisions of a will, directs the financial concerns of the estate following death (e.g., gathers and preserves the property, collects all income due, pays bills and taxes, provides recordkeeping to the court, then identifies and distributes all remaining assets as stated in the will).

A *living trust* is a legal document similar to a will, but with some advantages. There is no probate with a living trust, all court proceedings and delays are eliminated, privacy is maintained because a living trust is not a public document, and estate taxes can be reduced or eliminated. Property and assets are held in the name of the trust, rather than an individual, and the trust is controlled by the individual establishing it or another individual as assigned. Professional asset management can be performed by a trustee. A trust is individually tailored to the needs and desires of the person or couple for whom it is created. It can be designed to contain all provisions with a means to handle almost every contingency that may arise during a lifetime, including illness and disability. It is flexible and can be changed or cancelled at any time. Consult an attorney knowledgeable in living trusts for more information.

References

1. Saxton, D. F., Nuzent, P., and Pelikam P., et al. Mosby's Comprehensive Review of Nursing, 14th ed. St. Louis: C. V. Mosby, 1993, p. 11.
2. The Dentists' Insurance Company: Patient non-compliance. TDIC Newsletter 3:3, 1982.
3. Nielsen, C. Marketing the dental hygiene program. Journal of Dental Hygiene 63(7):322, 1989.
4. Keim, W., and Keim, M. Marketing the Program. San Francisco: Jossey-Bass, 1981.
5. Milone, C. L., Blair, W. C., and Littlefield, J. E. Marketing for the Dental Hygiene Practice. Philadelphia: W. B. Saunders, 1982, p. 18.
6. Lampner, J. Effective Career Management for Hygienists. Los Altos, CA: Lange Medical Publications, 1977, p. 15.
7. Medley, H. A. Sweaty Palms: The Neglected Art of Being Interviewed. Belmont, CA: Wadsworth, 1978, p. 108.
8. Woodall, I. R. Legal, Ethical, and Management Aspects of the Dental Care System, 2nd ed. St. Louis: C. V. Mosby, 1983, pp. 106–113.

Suggested Readings

American Dental Hygienists' Association. Current employment conditions for practice. Annual Report 1979–1980.

Blanchard, K., and Johnson, S. The One Minute Manager. New York: William Morrow and Company, 1982.

Darby, M. L. (ed). Mosby's Comprehensive Review of Dental Hygiene, 3rd ed. St. Louis: C. V. Mosby, 1994.

Dental Risk Management Foundation. Dental Risk Management —A Practical Guide. San Francisco, 1988, pp 652–690.

Dreyer, R. Is burnout inevitable? Career Directions in Dental Hygiene 10(11):1, 1983.

Lyles, R. I., and Joiner, C. Supervision in Health Care Organization. New York: John Wiley & Sons, 1986.

Scanlon, B. K. Principles of Management and Organizational Behavior. New York: John Wiley & Sons, 1973.

38 Computer Applications in Dental Hygiene

OBJECTIVES

Mastery of the content in this chapter will enable the reader to:

- Define key terms used
- Discuss how computer functioning is critical to the dental hygienist in the roles of clinician, change agent, consumer advocate, researcher, educator and health promoter, and administrator and manager
- Discuss general computer components and their functions
- Describe the basis for computer selection in a dental hygiene environment
- Describe some current computer applications in clinical dental hygiene practice
- Discuss the legal and ethical issues of computer usage in dental hygiene practice

INTRODUCTION

Computer technology and knowledge are commonplace, and a basic understanding of the principles of computer functioning and possible applications is essential for the contemporary dental hygienist. This chapter focuses on the advantages and disadvantages of automation and introduces basic components and functioning of the computer, particularly the microcomputer. Just as the dental hygiene profession has its own language, the world of computers also has a unique dialect, and thus common terminology is introduced and explained.

Quite simply a **computer** is a machine that stores, organizes, and communicates information given to it by an operator to save time and effort. Microcomputers are available in countless settings such as businesses, schools, and households, and the microcomputer industry has rapidly expanded. Computers have become less expensive and more accessible to the general population. For this reason, a "demystification" has occurred regarding the computer and its operation. Myriad resources exist in the form of training manuals, books, magazines, and courses devoted to learning to use a computer. Computer technology exists to perform a substantial portion of the tasks involved in office management.

With decreased costs of equipment and easy-to-use applications, automation can save considerable time and costs in professional practice. Because the dental hygiene process of care involves the collection, analysis, and evaluation of information to restore or maintain the oral health of clients, computer automation can contribute significantly to this process.[1] For these reasons, dental hygienists need a clear vision of what they want computers to accomplish in their particular settings and how they will use the information computers generate.

OVERVIEW OF COMPUTER SYSTEMS

Computers traditionally have been classified as **mainframes, minicomputers,** or **microcomputers** generally corresponding to large, medium, and small machines, respectively. In the past, these distinctions also were based on the speed or power of the computer's **central processing unit (CPU).** Today, however, these distinctions are less relevant because the most powerful microcomputers compete with minicomputers and minicomputers compete with mainframes. A more useful differentiation might be between personal computers (microcomputers) dedicated to personal use and computers in centrally administered, multiuser systems (mainframes and minicomputers). Even this contrast is not always appropriate because microcomputers can be configured as multiuser systems.[2]

The term "computer" usually denotes that part of the machine that actually computes. The rest of the computer system serves as the interface between the user (or operator) and the computer. Thus, the computer may be considered the "brains" of the computer system.[3] Commonly, the equipment or machinery of the computer system is referred to as the **"hardware,"** whereas the instructions or programs for different applications, such as word processing capabilities or games, are referred to as the **"software."** The computer pictured in Figure 38–1 is a typical representation of a microcomputer. The basic components include a **video-**

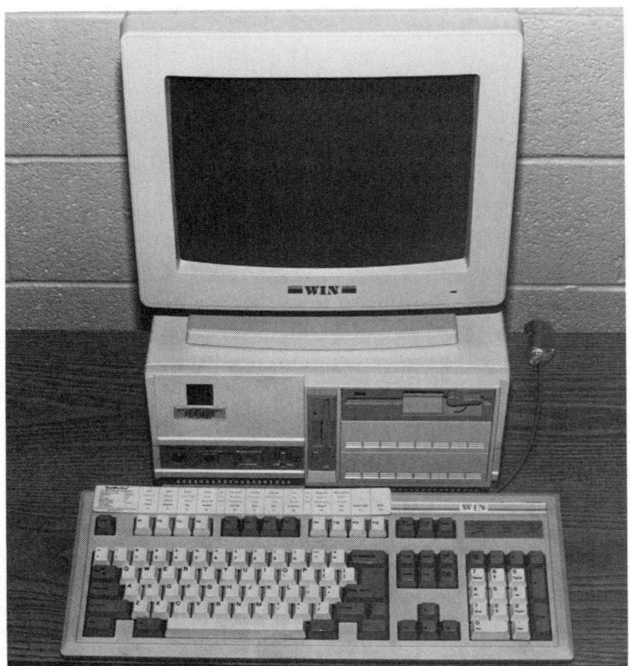

FIGURE 38-1
A typical personal computer system.

display (or **monitor**), a **system unit,** and a **keyboard** (with keys much like a typewriter); a power source also is necessary for functioning. Depending on the model and make of a computer, the system may appear slightly different from one unit to the next.

If one examined the inside of the system unit, an abundance of electronics could be observed; this is called the **electronic logic.** Vast quantities of electronic logic are created as microscopic circuits on small pieces of silicone element no larger than a dime, and are referred to as **"chips"** (Fig. 38-2).[3] The system unit contains essential operating elements as follows:

CPU—The central processing unit (or brains of the unit) consists of the **microprocessor,** clock, program counter, and control and interrupt circuits to allow external devices, such as the keyboard, to transfer messages to the CPU. The CPU is responsible for all data processing performed by the machine.

I/O—The input/output (I/O) is organized by "ports" or small groups of I/O lines that allow reading and writing capacities between the CPU and the logic portion of the I/O.

Memory—There are two types: ROM (read only memory) and RAM (random access memory). This electronic memory is how the computer remembers information and may be an internal component of the machine or housed externally.

A simplified model of computer system functioning is displayed in Figure 38-3.

A computer operates by responding to two types of electrical signals—on or off. This operation might be correlated to a light bulb in which the light source may be on or off, thus regulating illumination. All functioning of the computer is represented by a series of on and off signals, each of which is referred to as a BInary digiT, or **bit;** a sequence of 8 bits is called a **byte.** Each character (upper and lower case letters, numerical digits, punctuation symbols, and special characters) is represented by its own special code within a byte by a number between 1 and 128. One type of code is called the American Standard Code for Information Interchange (ASCII); which is a standard code used by microcomputers and peripheral devices.[4]

For the computer to operate, the CPU must manage the data for a specific task and the instructions needed to process that data (or programs). The CPU includes some of the instructions to manage tasks within the main memory, which is also called primary storage. Secondary storage is another component of the computer system and usually is in the form of magnetic disks. Secondary storage permits the storage of more data than the CPU's main memory can allow.[5]

Memory in the computer is designated by two types: random access memory and read only memory. **Random access memory (RAM)** is temporary storage of information and is reusable (see Common Terms Describing Random Access Memory chart). A good analogy of RAM is a blackboard and chalk in which the RAM can be used over and over again after it is wiped clean. In fact, once the power is removed, contents of RAM are lost. The RAM stores the programs and data loaded during a work session; RAM is the primary central storage for the computer.

Read only memory (ROM), as the name implies, cannot be used to store information entered by the user. Contents of the ROM are fixed and are not lost when power is

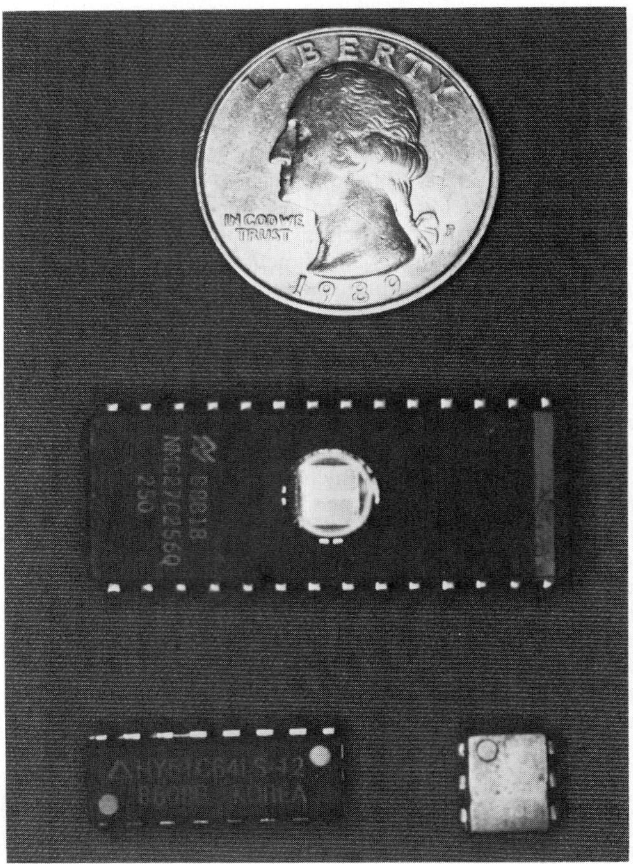

FIGURE 38-2
Computer chips.

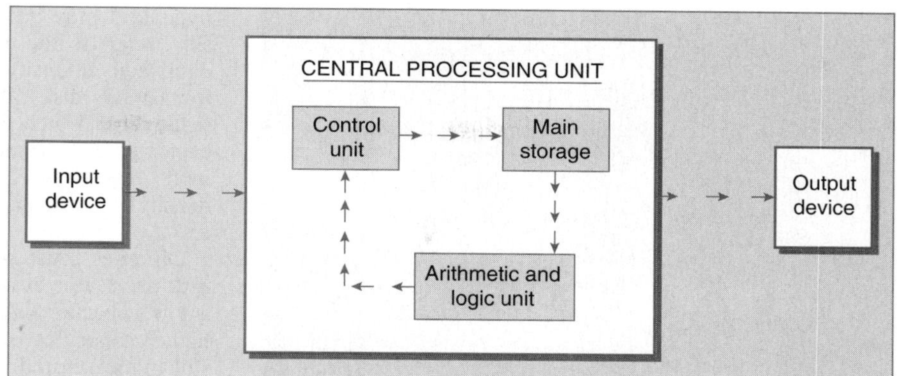

FIGURE 38–3
A simplified model of computer functioning.

removed. The ROM stores important information the computer needs to perform all of its functions and executes the built-in programs. Many terms are used to describe RAM included with a system, and an understanding of these terms is essential to knowing what programs and software can be operated on the selected system. The factors represented by these terms are important because they determine the speed of the CPU in performing operations and may be critical to the user when selecting a computer for a specific purpose.

Inside the computer, information travels from chip to chip on a set of circuits called a **data bus.** In 8-bit systems, for example, all 8 bits of information can travel concurrently and in parallel. If more than 8 bits of data are required, it is necessary to wait until the bus is available before another byte can travel. In 16- and 32-bit-wide systems, the data can be transferred simultaneously; this translates to an increase in operating speed. Figure 38–4 illustrates a 16-bit memory device. The clock within the CPU produces regular, periodic voltage pulses that initiate and synchronize all CPU actions.[4] The clock frequency (or machine time) is measured in megahertz (MHz), millions of cycles per second, and can range from 1 to 16 MHz. Essentially, the faster the cycle time, the more rapid the processing time of the computer. Figure 38–5 displays the computer circuitry known as the board.

As computer technology has advanced so too has the speed of microprocessors. Early machines were equipped with 8088 microprocessors that were capable of transmitting information from 4 to 10 MHz. The 80286 was introduced with the IBM-PC AT model and was capable of 8 to 16 MHz. With the newer microprocessors, 80386, the data path was extended to 32 bits and the machine processes information four times faster than the original 8088 machines. The relatively new appearance of a 80486 microprocessor is setting innovative standards in speed and data transfer.

Different terms may be observed in the computer literature regarding CPUs that may be confusing when consumers are shopping for a computer. The term "PC-compatible" means that the computer uses the 8088 CPU and is compatible with hardware and software manufactured for the IBM PC. The term "AT-compatible" means that the CPU has a 80286 microprocessor and is compatible with 286 machines. Finally, "computerese" may be used in labeling microprocessors, and one may see "286," "386," or "486," which means that the computer runs on the 80286, 80386, or 80486 microprocessors, respectively.

Disk Drives

The computer requires some mechanism by which to store and save the information entered into it, otherwise it would function like a typewriter. The **disk drive** is the storage mechanism and is of two types:

- Flexible (or **floppy**) disk drive
- Fixed (or **hard**) disk drive.

All software is packaged on disks, and thus most machines have at least one floppy disk drive. Computer manufacturers frequently provide a choice of adding a second drive so that there is less inserting and removing of disks.

A hard disk drive operates with a higher speed and capacity than a floppy disk drive. The hard disk customarily is fixed inside the computer, but it may be housed in an external drive case. External hard disks are available for adding storage to an existing computer system. Unlike the floppy disk counterpart, a hard disk cannot be removed from its casing. Hard disks are available with different

COMMON TERMS DESCRIBING RANDOM ACCESS MEMORY

Term	Example	Definition
Bit	Bit	Taken from the term "binary digit," a bit is the smallest unit of data measurement; a bit is an electrical representation that is either 0 or 1
Byte	Byte	The equivalent of 8 bits or one character
Kilobyte	640K	1,024 bytes of information; 640K is read as "640 thousand bytes"
Megabyte	4M	One million bytes of information; 1M is read as "one megabyte" or "one meg," for short

Adapted from Murray, K. Introduction to Personal Computers. Carmel, IN: QUE Corp., 1990.

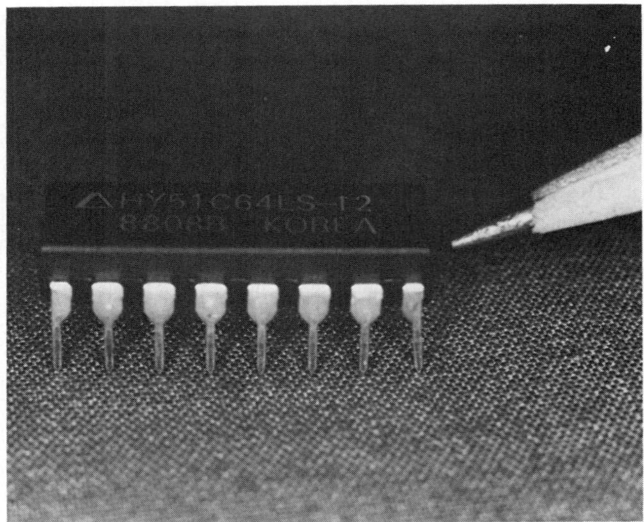

FIGURE 38–4
A 16-bit memory device.

amounts of storage from 20 megabytes (M) to as high as 160M. When selecting a hard disk, a good rule of thumb is to purchase as much storage space as is affordable.

Floppy Diskettes

Figures 38–6 and 38–7 depict two types of removable or **floppy diskettes** used in microcomputers. Although both classes of diskettes are termed "floppy disks," the 3.5-inch diskette has a plastic casing and is more rigid and less vulnerable to mishaps in handling than the 5.25-inch diskette and is sometimes called a "rigid" diskette. More commonly, however, the diskettes are referred to by their respective sizes, either 5.25-inch or 3.5-inch.

Diskette size is predicated on the size and type of the disk drive accompanying the machine. Both sizes of floppy disks hold a limited amount of information (referred to as "disk capacity") which is measured in kilobytes or megabytes and may be of high or low density. The term "density" refers to the manner in which the disk is able to store data; high intensity disks can store more information than low density disks in the same amount of space. Of the two sizes, the 3.5-inch diskette is the newer version and has the capacity to store more bytes of information than the 5.25-inch diskette—720K (low density) and 1.4M (high density)—compared to 360k and 1.2M in the 5.25-inch disk.

Diskettes must be purchased to be compatible with the disk drive. For example, a high capacity disk drive can use a low capacity diskette, but not vice versa. In spite of the higher capacities of 3.5-inch disks, commercial software is still manufactured using the 5.25-inch version, and popular programs are offered in both sizes. However, most hardware can be customized to contain either size of disk drive. When purchasing disk drives, selecting one of each drive offers the most flexibility in software utilization.

A diskette stores information via electrical impulses sent to it from the disk drive. Because disks are magnetized, they are sensitive to magnetic source fields and should be handled with care. Diskettes also are sensitive to radiation and for that reason should be stored away from radiation sources such as x-ray tube heads. Protecting diskettes from contamination with liquids such as disinfectant solutions is another precaution. These concerns are particularly important when diskettes are used in a client care area. Avoiding sensitization from magnetic disturbances such as laboratory bench engines and contamination from plaster dust also are concerns when computers are located in laboratory areas (see Guidelines for Handling Diskettes chart).

Input Devices

Communication in a computer system usually is conducted to or from the microcomputer using a keyboard, mouse system, display monitor, printer, and other **input/output** devices. Microcomputers generally are configured to accommodate several ways for the operator to send information to the computer and for the computer to send information back to the user. For example, most micro-

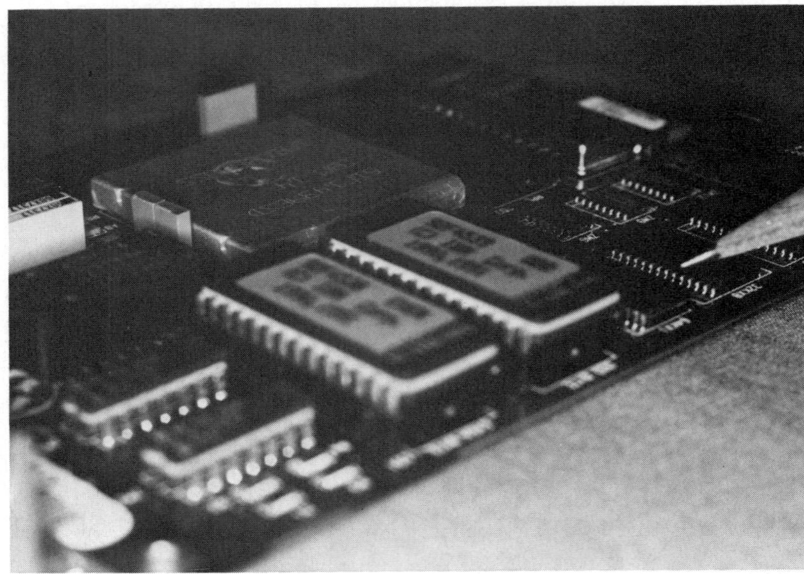

FIGURE 38–5
Computer board.

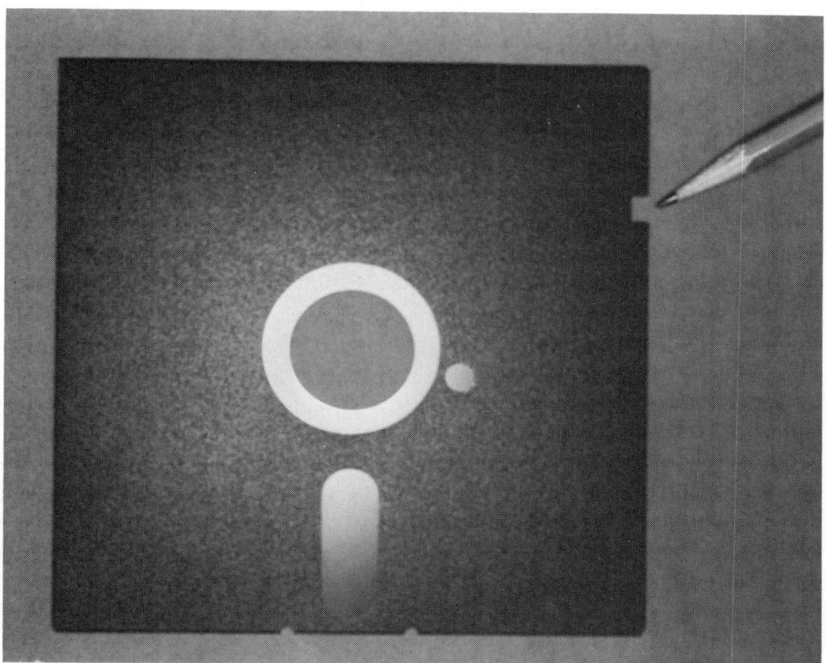

FIGURE 38-6
A 5.25-inch floppy diskette.

computers are designed to use both a printer and a monitor for output.

Keyboard

A computer **keyboard** resembles a typewriter keyboard and is available in two types—standard and expanded. The expanded keyboard is equipped with a numerical keypad to the right of the board in addition to the standard numerical keys (Figure 38-8). An expanded keyboard is useful when data to be entered in the computer consist primarily of numbers. Keyboards are sensitive components of the computer and should be kept free of dust and dirt. Eating or drinking near a keyboard is not recommended to avoid unintentional contamination of the keyboard. A useful accessory to a keyboard is a keyboard cover that can protect the keyboard when not in use. When used in client care areas, employing a clear, flexible keyboard cover is advisable to protect the keyboard during use and to allow disinfection between clients.

Mouse System

A **mouse** system offers an alternative mechanism by which to enter information in the computer; often this includes moving objects on-screen. A small hand-held device that is

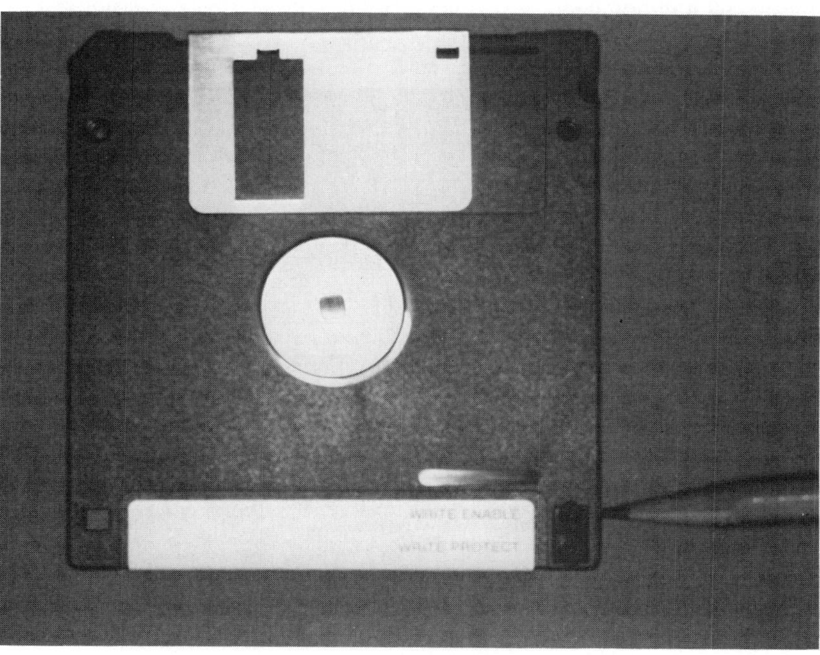

FIGURE 38-7
A 3.5-inch floppy diskette.

GUIDELINES FOR HANDLING DISKETTES

- Never write on a floppy diskette with a ballpoint pen or a pencil; use a felt-tip pen or marker to write on a diskette label
- Do not eat, drink, or smoke around a computer and exposed diskettes
- Take care not to bend a diskette; use a rigid case for storing or transporting
- Do not get a diskette wet
- Do not expose diskettes to extreme heat or cold—never leave a diskette in a car
- Avoid laying diskettes on magnetized surfaces, such as the CPU, keyboard, or a telephone
- Check the contents of new diskettes with virus-detecting software before using them for the first time
- Avoid placing or storing diskettes near radiation sources such as a microwave oven or an x-ray unit
- Store diskettes in a dust-free environment when not in use

rolled along the desktop surface, the mouse is most often used with graphics programs to select and move objects on the monitor screen. The mouse acts as a pointing device by controlling the position of the "cursor" or position indicator on the screen. Once the cursor is placed on the option or command located on the screen, a button on the mouse is tapped with a finger (or "clicked") to initialize the command, and the mouse is moved to indicate where the object or text is to be created on the screen. The area on the screen that displays the options or choices is called the **menu.** Communication to the computer occurs through pressure-sensitive electrodes inside the mouse housing. A useful accessory to a mouse is a mouse pad that allows the mouse to move smoothly and serves as an accurate tracking surface. It also protects the mouse from dust on a desktop. Figure 38–9 shows the tracking device on the mouse and a mouse pad.

Optical Character Recognition

Optical character recognition (OCR) equipment (called "scanners" for short) is another computer input device. This equipment can scan a printed page and then communicate the information to the computer without the operator having to manually type the material. These devices can offer a real time savings to businesses that need to enter preprinted documents into the computer. A drawback to OCRs is that they have yet to be perfected and often they are sensitive to poor quality paper, dirt, or smudges, thereby altering exact copying of the original document.[6]

Monitor

Selecting a good quality **monitor** is quite important, particularly if the computer is to be used for long periods of time. Like other aspects of the computer, a variety of features is available. The largest differences between monitors are the screen colors, whether color or monochrome, and the **resolution** or crispness of the image. Poor screen resolution can cause eye strain if the monitor is viewed for long periods of time, and thus the ability of the monitor to present crisp, well-formed characters is a critical factor in selection.

Monochrome monitors present in amber, green, or white. These monitors may be sufficient for most applications, but the ability to use colors is an option of many software packages and may add interest to the work task. In some cases the ability to use color is useful in displaying different text options and for graphics purposes. For example, in a word processing package an underlined word may appear in green and a boldfaced word in orange.

A very important aspect of monitor selection is to be certain that the monitor, software, and **display adapter** all operate together. The display adapter is actually a board that inserts into the computer machinery and to which the monitor connects. The board serves as an intermediary between the CPU and the monitor for creating the visual display. Fortunately, many software applications function with a variety of display configurations. Graphics software requires a graphics display adapter and a monitor that can

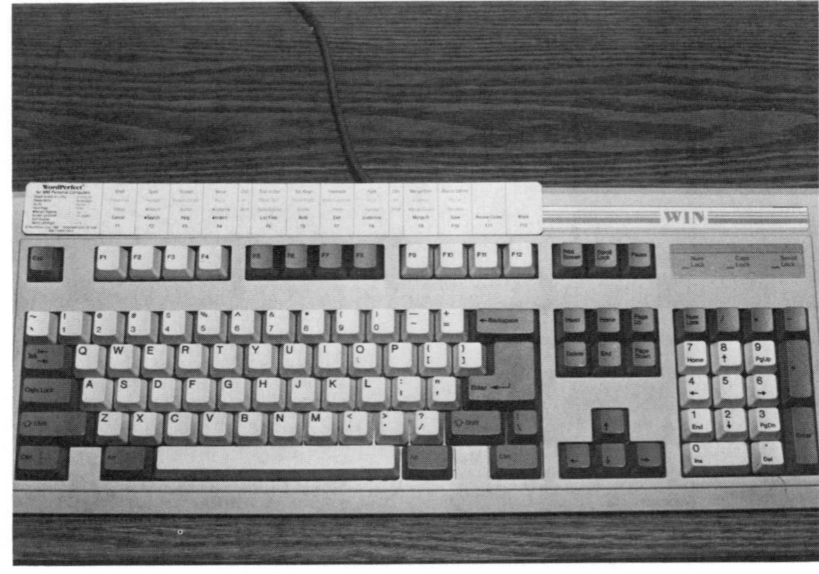

FIGURE 38–8
Expanded keyboard.

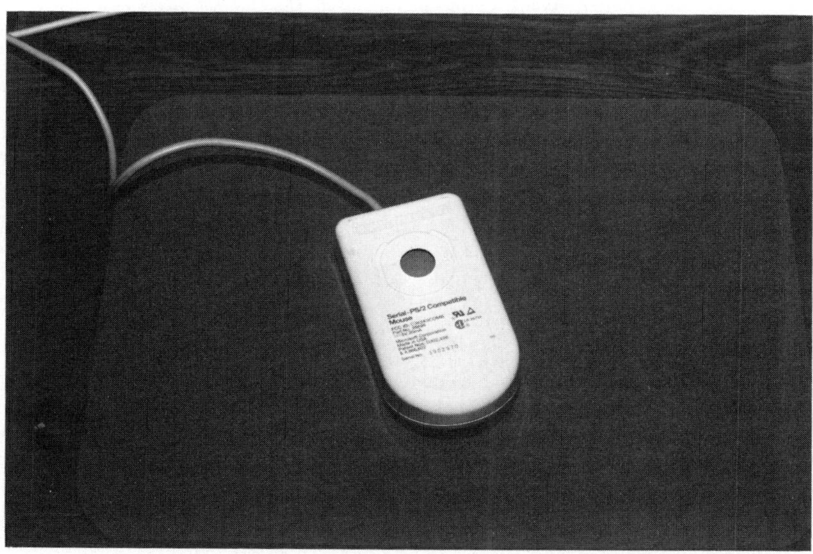

FIGURE 38–9
Mouse tracking ball and mouse pad.

support graphics. If graphics are an important feature of the computer system, selection of the display adapter is crucial.

To understand the display adapter, one must be familiar with the concept of a **pixel.** A pixel is merely a pinpoint of light on the monitor, and each image on the screen is composed of thousands of pixels. The more pixels that the screen can display, the higher the screen's resolution.[6] A variety of display adapters is available: monochrome display adapter (MDA), color graphics adapter (CGA), enhanced graphics adapter (EGA), video graphics array (VGA), and the Hercules monochrome graphics card. Each of these offers different pixel display capabilities and thus different resolution potential. Text and graphics resolution is best using a VGA or a Hercules graphics board, and most major software supports these display adapters.

Output Devices

Printers

Printers offer some of the greatest variety of features in a computer system, and the basis for their selection should be predicated on the intended use. The most common varieties of printers are the impact printer (**daisy wheel** and **dot-matrix printers**) and the **laser printer.** Differences between these types of printers relate to their mechanisms for creating a printed document, speed of operation, and image quality. Furthermore, some printers offer more variety in font size, graphics abilities, and page formatting. All printers allow the user to produce a paper copy often referred to as a **hard copy.** This is in contrast to information viewed on the computer monitor, which is called **soft copy.**

Impact Printers Impact printers consist of daisy wheel and dot-matrix printers and are so called because their mechanism for printing is much like a typewriter in that they use a print head that strikes a ribbon. These types of printers dominated the market until 1984 and the introduction of the laser printer. Impact printers can accomplish some printing tasks that lasers cannot, such as printing multipart forms, and they are relatively inexpensive. These are some of the reasons that impact printers continue to be popular despite the availability of faster and better image-producing laser printers. An explanation of how each of the printers operates is important to understanding their differences.

The simplest type of printer is the daisy wheel which comprises a print wheel containing all of the available characters. When printing, the wheel spins until the desired character is in position and then a hammer strikes the wheel, forcing the character to strike the ribbon and imprint on the paper. A drawback to the daisy wheel printer is that printing is limited to the characters that fit on the print wheel. Another drawback is the noise of the printer created during impact of the print wheel. Hearing a typewriter printing at a constant speed might provide an idea of how a daisy wheel printer sounds.[7]

A term associated with printers is **letter quality,** meaning that the final product should resemble the same quality as that of a typewriter. Because daisy wheel printers use an impact mechanism, the text produced is letter quality. This characteristic, however, also can constitute a downfall in that printer ribbons can wear out, print wheels can break, and letters can become misaligned. Although daisy wheel printers produce a final product faster than a typist can, other types of printers are faster. Depending on the task to be performed, the quality of print may still be acceptable with an impact printer even though speed may be lacking. For example, printing rough drafts of papers or research notes may be acceptable using a daisy wheel printer.

Dot-matrix printers are a bit more complicated in that the print head contains small pins—usually nine or 24 (Figure 38–10). The pins strike the ribbon in the pattern required to form a character. Dot-matrix printers also are capable of printing graphics and different typefaces (styles) and sizes of characters when used in conjunction with applicable software packages.

Laser Printer With a laser printer, a laser source exposes a photosensitive drum in a dot pattern that forms the image. Negatively charged toner then clings to the positively charged areas of the drum. As paper enters the printer it also is given a strong positive charge that causes the toner to be transferred to the paper. Finally, the toner is bonded to the paper using heat and pressure.[8] Figure 38–11 illustrates a typical laser printer. Laser printers create nearly flawless text and have the capacity for high-quality graphics, typeface and size (font) selection, and

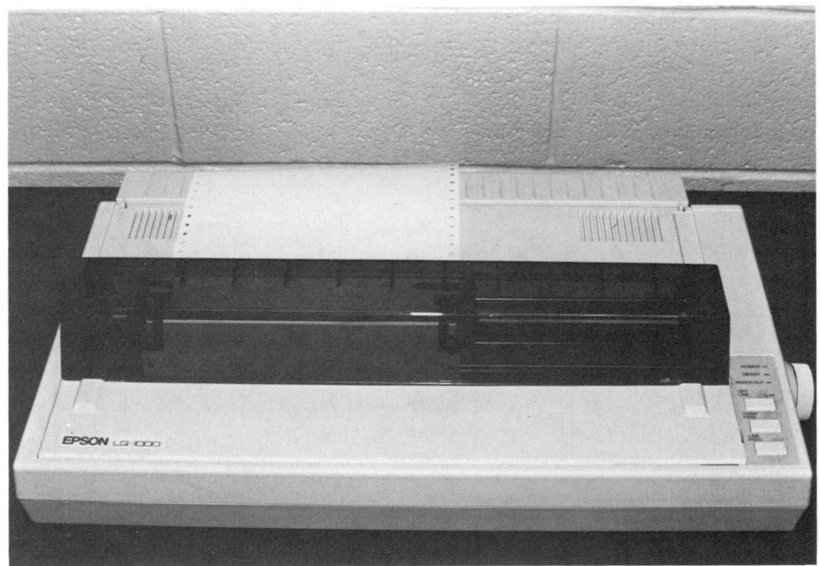

FIGURE 38–10
Dot-matrix printer.

quiet operation. Figure 38–12 provides examples of print from each of the three types of printers discussed, and Figure 38–13 illustrates examples of different typefaces printed using a laser printer. The drawback to laser printers is that they are more expensive to purchase and operate than impact printers; however, if a crisp, clean-looking business document is important to the image of the dental hygiene setting, a laser printer should be considered for purchase.

Modem

Like the mouse system, the **modem** is a computer accessory and serves as a means for communication between computers. A compression of the term "modulator demodulator," the modem receives information from the user's computer and transforms it into electrical pulses that are then transmitted through a telephone line. The receiving modem on the remote computer receives the pulses and transforms (or demodulates) them into a pattern that can be understood by the computer. The modem may be internal or external to the computer. Generally, external modems are more expensive than internal modems because of the additional parts such as the housing and cables. Communications software also is necessary for communication to take place and must be used by both the transmitting and receiving computers.[7]

Operating Features

The **operating system** is the program that controls basic functioning of the computer system and provides a mechanism for working with disks and files as well as running software applications. Operating systems vary among computers, and purchased software applications must be able to function using the system that is present in the microcom-

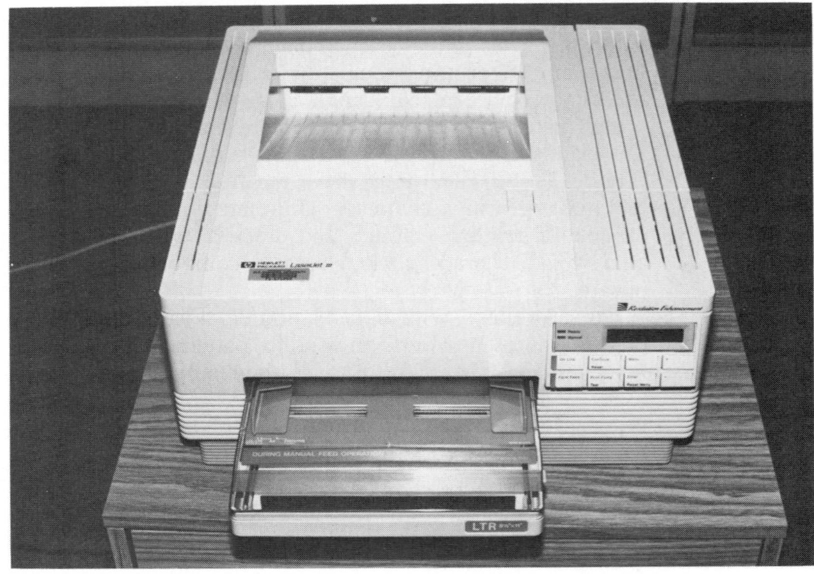

FIGURE 38–11
Laser printer.

This is a sample of daisy wheel print from an NEC 3510. This is a sample of daisy wheel print from an NEC 3510. This is a sample of daisy wheel print from an NEC 3510. This is a sample of daisy wheel print from an NEC 3510. This is a sample of daisy wheel print from an NEC 3510. This is a sample of daisy wheel print from an NEC 3510. This is a sample of daisy wheel print from an NEC 3510.

This is sample print from a 24 pin dot-matrix printer. This is sample print from a 24 pin dot-matrix printer. This is sample print from a 24 pin dot-matrix printer. This is sample print from a 24 pin dot-matrix printer. This is sample print from a 24 pin dot-matrix printer. This is sample print from a 24 pin dot-matrix printer.

This is a sample of laser print. This is a sample of laser print. This is a sample of laser print. This is a sample of laser print. This is a sample of laser print. This is a sample of laser print. This is a sample of laser print. This is a sample of laser print. This is a sample of laser print. This is a sample of laser print.

FIGURE 38–12
Sample of daisy wheel, dot-matrix, and laser print.

This is an example of CG 8-point Italics

This is an example of Courier 10cpi Bold

This is an example of Univers 12-point bold italics

This is an example of Univers 14-point

This is an example of Univers 50-point

FIGURE 38–13
Examples of different typefaces.

puter. Some functions of the operating system perform without the user's knowledge, but some functions are accessible, for example, those to manage files. Some application packages are started from the operating system level, although the system may be rearranged to begin certain programs upon starting the computer. For example, rather than beginning with operating system commands, the computer may be programmed to load a calendar application package so that the day's schedule may appear first when turning on the computer. Commercial software usually is designed to begin immediately with the application and the user is not required to enter operating system commands.

Line-Oriented Operating System

DOS is an example of a **line-oriented operating system** in which a specialized language is needed to communicate with the computer. For example, the following statement is a common DOS command that may be used:

Copy A:*.* C:

The purpose of this statement is to copy all files (*.*) from a floppy disk drive (the A: disk) onto the hard disk (C: drive). When using DOS commands, the statements must be typed precisely using the proper spaces and punctuation dictated by DOS syntax. Learning this special language may be a challenge to the novice computer user, but once experience with a few common commands is gained, it is relatively easy to communicate needs.[9] Other common operating systems include CP/M, UNIX, XENIX, and OS/2.

Graphic User Interface

The other major category of operating system is the **GUI,** or **graphic user interface.** Rather than relying on a special language, this system employs resources that are more recognizable to the average individual. A GUI system uses small pictures or symbols referred to as **icons,** to which the computer user can point and click to activate by using a mouse. Shaded colorings of the icons on the monitor indicate if a system is turned on or off.

The concept of a **window** is another operating feature in conjunction with GUIs that should be understood by new computer users. Windows are a category of operating environment rather than an operating system. Windows allow users to function with several applications at one time. A window is depicted as a boxed-in area of a computer screen that is controlled by a specific application program. Windows are common in GUIs for moving among programs and are switched on by using the mouse. The Macintosh computer is probably the best known of the graphic user interface systems although several programs, such as WordPerfect for Windows, for use with IBM-PCs and compatibles have been introduced with GUI capabilities.[10–12]

Programs

Programs are comprised of instructions to the computer written in a language that the computer can understand and then execute; these instructions are in the form of a computer language or **programming language.** Each language has a mechanism, such as a translator, that transposes the program into the machine language of the computer. Several hundred languages are available; however, there are a few commonly used languages such as BASIC, PASCAL, COBOL, and FORTRAN (Table 38–1).

TABLE 38–1
COMMON COMPUTER PROGRAMMING LANGUAGES

Language	Usage
BASIC	Acronym for Beginners All-Purpose Symbolic Instruction Code; first high-level language for programming on microcomputers; used in a variety of applications from business to computer science
COBOL	Derived from Common Business Oriented Language; used primarily in business applications
FORTRAN	Stands for FORmula TRANslation; standard language for science and engineering used for programming mathematical formulas
PASCAL	Combines features of BASIC and FORTRAN; used on microcomputers and within business, science, and engineering

The process of writing a program is called "coding," and each language has its own rules for syntax and logic—syntax being the correct use of the language, such as the placement of commas, periods, spaces, and so on. The process of testing a program for errors in syntax and logic is termed "debugging."[13] Most software programs for the microcomputer are "user-friendly" in that the operator does not need to know a computer language to operate the software program; however, an avid user may want to design some individually useful applications using a simple BASIC program.

STANDARD SOFTWARE APPLICATIONS

There are numerous application packages that form the standard for most computer operations. The goal of this discussion is to present an introduction to these applications, including word processing, desktop publishing, spreadsheets, data base management, graphics, and communications (Table 38–2). The variety of manufacturers and capabilities of different software packages is far beyond this general discussion; therefore, a few major types are presented for examples. Manufacturers are continually updating their products and the dental hygiene computer manager/administrator and user should investigate options fully before purchasing.

Word Processing

Word processing software allows the manipulation of text in a manner not possible by typewriters. Some advantages of word processing applications are listed below:

- Provides easy entry of text and editing features
- Stores text for reuse
- Allows on-screen formatting to control tabs, margins, columns, and special features such as superscript
- Facilitates accurate document generation by including features such as spelling and grammar checkers as well as a thesaurus

TABLE 38-2
TYPES OF SOFTWARE APPLICATIONS

Type of Software	Description
Word processing	Manipulates text; allows for on-screen editing or formatting; some packages offer sophisticated functions such as different sizes of print as well as a thesaurus and grammar checkers
Spreadsheets	Automates accounting functions; uses concept of rows and columns similar to an accountant's pad; allows for data entry and calculations
Data management	Manages data via entry, storage, sorting, and retrieving information; predicated on the concept of records and fields; reports can be generated in a variety of forms from the same data set
Graphics	Creates visual images from simple drawings to sophisticated models, prepared artwork, photographic-like images
Desktop publishing	Integrates text and graphics to produce professional-looking documents
Integrated software	Software with combined applications such as word processing, data management, spreadsheets, and graphics
Communications	Software used with a modem to allow one computer to communicate with another
Educational	Designed for instructional purposes with a wide variety of programs available ranging from learning tax law to reading skills
Recreational	Wide variety of games and entertainment; games for fun, relaxation or skill testing; can range from racing cars to chess

- Augments a professional image (e.g., allows a variety of letter sizes and typesetting features)

Text may be revised, moved, or copied on-screen. Once the final format is achieved, the text can be printed, resulting in a polished document that has been created with fewer paper drafts than is possible on an ordinary typewriter. Many word processing packages also include options to check spelling and grammar and provide a thesaurus. These mechanisms enhance writing style and ease, particularly for individuals who are not proficient writers. Furthermore, studies suggest that writing accomplished on a computer tends to be better writing than that which is done with paper and pencil.[14-16] These results suggest that dental hygiene educators may want to implement the use of word processing for student writing assignments.

Desktop Publishing

When a computer user has the need to develop documents that are of typeset quality, **desktop publishing** software should be investigated. This software has the capability to create professional looking work that is suitable for newsletters, manuscripts, fliers, pamphlets, research questionnaires, and other documents in which a bold, professional appearance is desirable. Figure 38-14 gives an example of a document combining text with graphics created using WordPerfect 5.1.

A desktop publishing feature that allows the user to produce quality art in documents is **clip art.** This graphics ability entails importing professional images without having to be an artist. Many kinds of images are available from dozens of companies and can include borders, animals, cartoons, holiday themes, people, symbols, signs, and even common dental images. The scope of availability of clip art is almost limitless; if a particular piece of artwork is required, it is likely that someone has published it. Figure 38-15 is a sample of the clip art packaged by LifeArt in the Dental Collection.

Graphics

Graphics program software is an application that allows the user to create artwork on the screen. The categories of graphics software are paint programs, draw programs, presentation graphics programs, and computer-aided design programs (or CAD). Paint programs are relatively easy to use by employing a choice of tools, colors, and patterns to paint the screen. Draw programs can generate sophisticated graphics, but are more complicated to learn than a paint program.

Presentation graphics allow the user to create charts and materials used in presentations and can replace the use of overhead transparencies when graphics are displayed with a color video monitor instead. Computer-assisted design programs (CAD) build from draw programs, but add greater dimension. Figures can be rotated and modified in three dimensions; this capability gives the illusion of animation. Harvard Graphics is a popular CAD program and is used frequently in business. Figure 38-16 was created using Harvard Graphics. Uses of graphics programs by dental hygienists may include artwork for journal publications or professional presentations, logos for newsletters and special letterhead, and charts and graphs to illustrate technical information.

Spreadsheets

Spreadsheets are the electronic equivalent of an accountant's pad and pencil. Automated functions of the program allow formulas to be performed, thus eliminating the need for a calculator or adding machine. The advantage to a spreadsheet program is that data are reusable and can be modified or reworked as much as needed.[7] Other benefits of using spreadsheet programs follow:

- Column and row format is easy to understand
- Formulas for calculations are saved
- Columns, rows, and formulas can be moved
- Various formats are possible for financial reporting
- Graphs can be created from data in the spreadsheet

Rows and columns are available in the spreadsheet and the number of these depends on the particular software program (Fig. 38-17). The intersection of each row and column is a cell into which data and formulas are entered for calculating, sorting, and formatting. Spreadsheet programs can be useful in a number of activities in which a dental hygienist might be involved:

- Bookkeeping tasks
- Financial tasks
- Accounts receivable and payable
- Research proposal budgets
- For dental hygiene educators to record and compute students' grades.

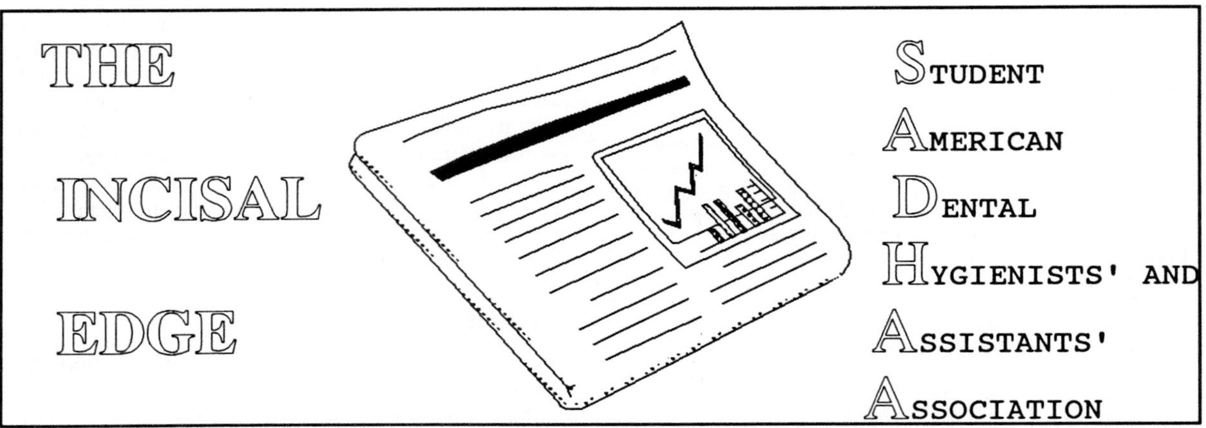

VOLUME I ISSUE I FALL 1991
NEWSLETTER EDITOR: RHONDA SOUTHERS

1991–92
SADHAA OFFICERS

President .... Meg Richardson
Vice President .... Sherri Smith
Treasurer .... Lauren Ryan
Secretary & Editor .... Rhonda Southers
Historians .... Denise Barbara & Fred Ochave
Faculty Advisor .... Michele Darby

PRESIDENT'S MESSAGE

We have a very talented and diverse body of students, staff, and faculty within the School of Dental Hygiene and Dental Assisting. Together we can really make a mark for ourselves on campus and within the community and oral health professions.

Although there is a good response from members to serve on committees, several could use additional support. Please consider serving on a committee. At our first SADHAA meeting you will be asked about your preference.

Welcome to another year with SADHAA, and to the new members a warm welcome to you! This year is going to be very exciting and a little different from previous years.

The emphasis will be on unity and involvement of all students and faculty in each of our academic programs. Dental Assistants, Sophomores, Juniors, Seniors, Degree Completion, Graduate Students, and Faculty: Plan to work together to achieve our common goals. Let's Get Involved!!

FIGURE 38–14
Sample document created using a desktop publishing package.

Data Management

Everyone manages data in some form or another, whether it is making a shopping list or managing a client's continued care (recall) file. Depending on the amount and frequency of data management, an individual may increase efficiency and productivity by using data base management (DBM) programs (or **data base programs**). A data base (DB) is simply the collection of information and can include payroll, inventories, bibliographies, notes, and other types of information. Data management software offers a means by which to enter, organize, and update information. A variety of features are available in different software programs to manage a data base; depending on specific needs, the user may select a simple or intricate system. A simple program may allow the user to create a mailing list and print labels from a client data base, whereas an elaborate program might be more desirable for large data sources in which sorting and programming are required. Like spreadsheet software, one advantage to data base management software is that data are reusable. Once entered, the data can be sorted or rearranged to create different reports and perform other functions without reentering the original information.

A manager who works with information about people, places, or products may benefit from the use of a data management program.[7] Client lists, inventories, and name and address information are just some examples of appropriate tasks that are easily handled by data management programs. A long-standing standard in commercial data base management software is the dBase IV program manufactured by the Ashton-Tate Corporation. This program can perform many data management functions and is relatively easy to employ even by novice users. Figure 38–18 is a simulation of a screen displaying a data base program.

Communications

Computers are rapidly becoming a communication standard. Their applications include electronic mail, telecommunications, and access to public information services. Communication among computers can be as simple as using a modem with a microcomputer and appropriate software to converse with a computer across town or communication within an elaborate network of computers that are able to access the same software packages. A number of common terms regarding computer communication are identified below and are essential to learn before embarking on computer information transfer.

Baud—The amount of information transmitted per second; for example, a 1200-baud modem is capable of

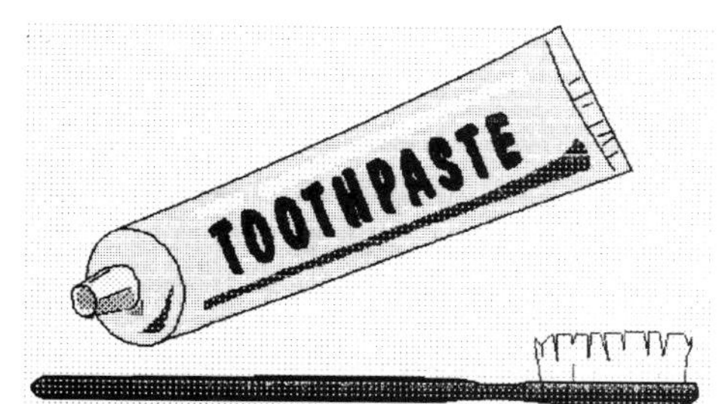

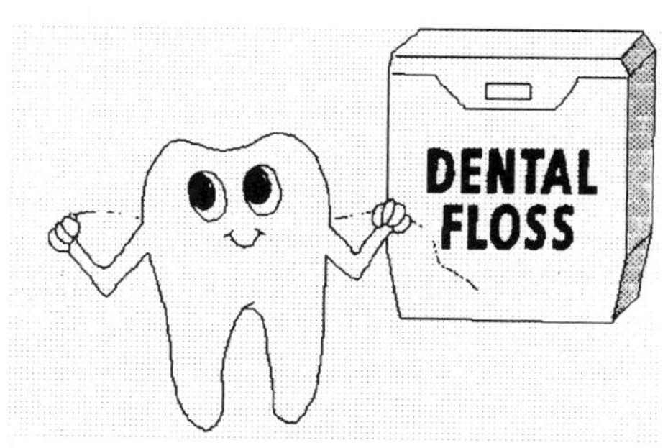

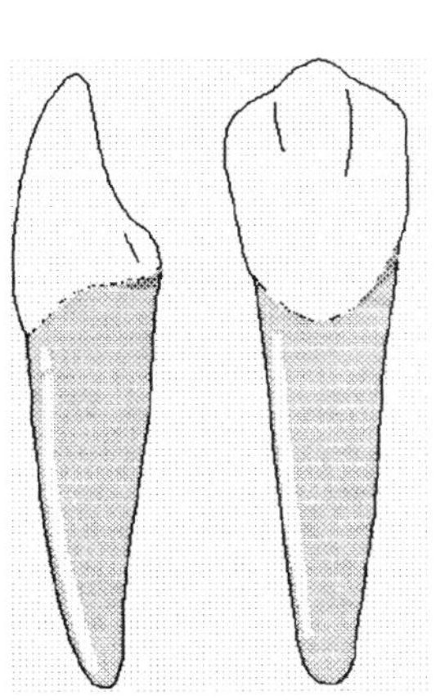

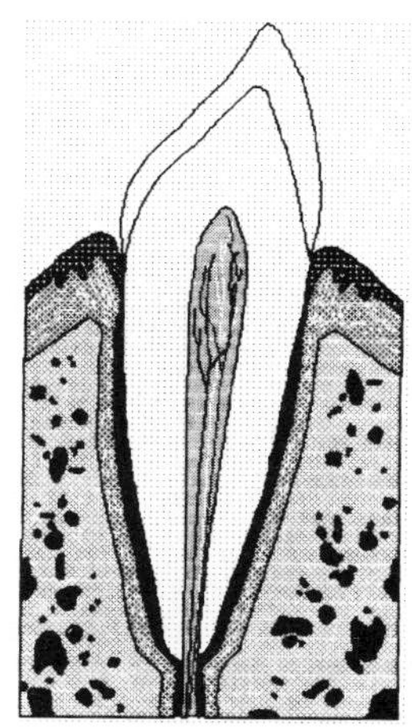

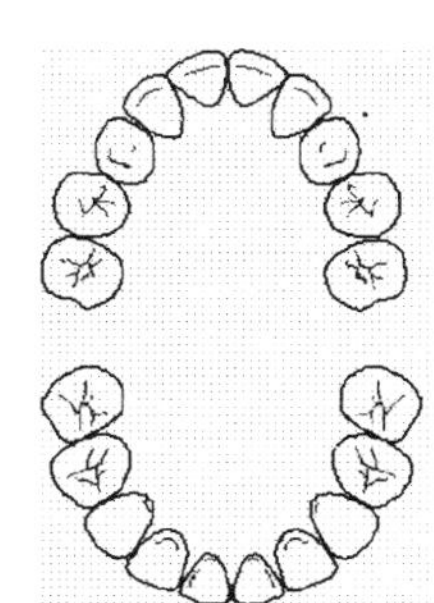

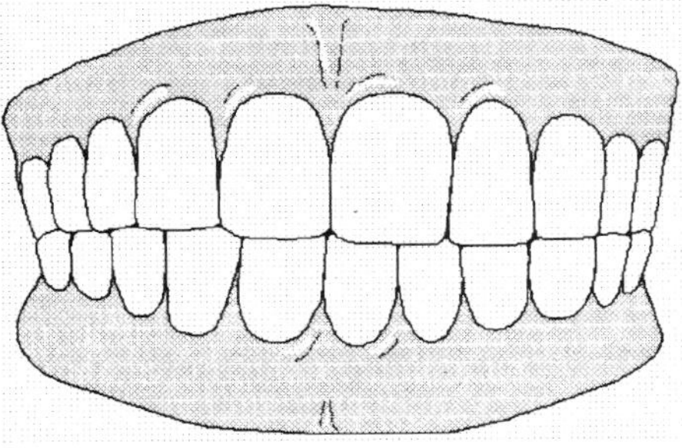

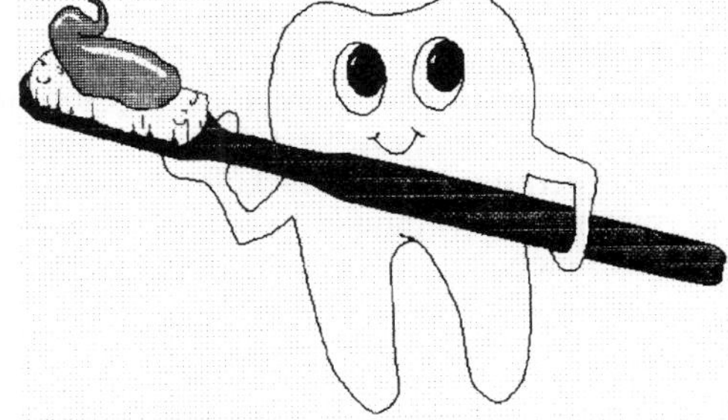

FIGURE 38–15
Sample clip art from LifeArt Dental Collection. (Courtesy of Techpool Studios.)

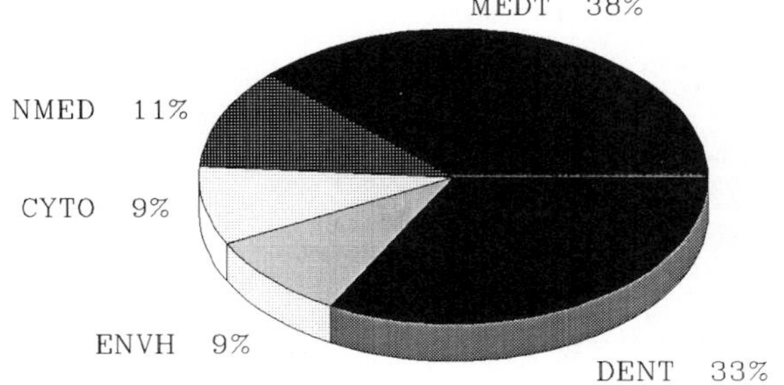

FIGURE 38–16
Chart created with Harvard Graphics 3.0.

```
D7: [W12]                                                                READY

          A           B           C           D        E         F         G         H
1
2                                 Budget Sheet - Research Proposal
3
4
5
6               Costs                     Year 1          Year 2            Total
7
8               PI                     $11,200.00      $11,200.00        $22,400.00
9               Co-PI                   $6,000.00       $6,000.00        $12,000.00
10              Fringe Benefits           $800.00         $800.00         $1,600.00
11              Travel                  $2,000.00       $2,000.00         $4,000.00
12              Special Equipment       $5,000.00           $0.00         $5,000.00
13              Other Direct Costs      $5,200.00       $2,000.00         $7,200.00
14
15              Total Costs:           $30,200.00      $22,000.00        $52,200.00
16
17
18
19
20
07-Oct-92   01:44 PM
```

FIGURE 38-17
Sample printout of a spreadsheet program.

sending and receiving 1,200 bits of information per second (bps)

Bulletin Board—A computer service accessed by using a modem; computer users may post notices or exchange information

Downloading—The process of transferring information from one computer system to another (for example, transferring lengthy files from a mainframe to the user's microcomputer to read at a later date)

Electronic mail—Means of communication similar to an answering machine except that it is performed using computer technology; messages can be received or left for other computer users on the electronic mail system

Uploading—Process of using a modem connection to transfer information from the user's computer to another computer (for example, uploading raw data from a microcomputer to a mainframe for statistical analysis)

Computer Networks

Computer **networks** involve the sharing of resources and information and, thereby, eliminate the need for departmental systems and mainframe computers as primary resources, thus reducing the cost of operations.[9] Multiple computers in a business can be connected by cable and can use the same network server microcomputer that physically houses the software applications; this eliminates the need for purchasing multiple copies of the same software packages. Networks also allow the sharing of peripheral devices, such as a laser printer. A **local area network** or **LAN** is a small group of microcomputers connected via cable over a

Continued Care Appointment Schedule
DATABASE

Last Name: Smith
First Name: Tom
Address: 123 Main Street
City: Anytown
State: VA
Zip Code: 23456
Recall Period: 6 months
Next Recall Date: 01/05/93
Days Available: M (T) W (R) F
Times Available: (800) 900 1000 1100
1300 1400 1500 1600

FIGURE 38-18
Sample screen of a simple database program.

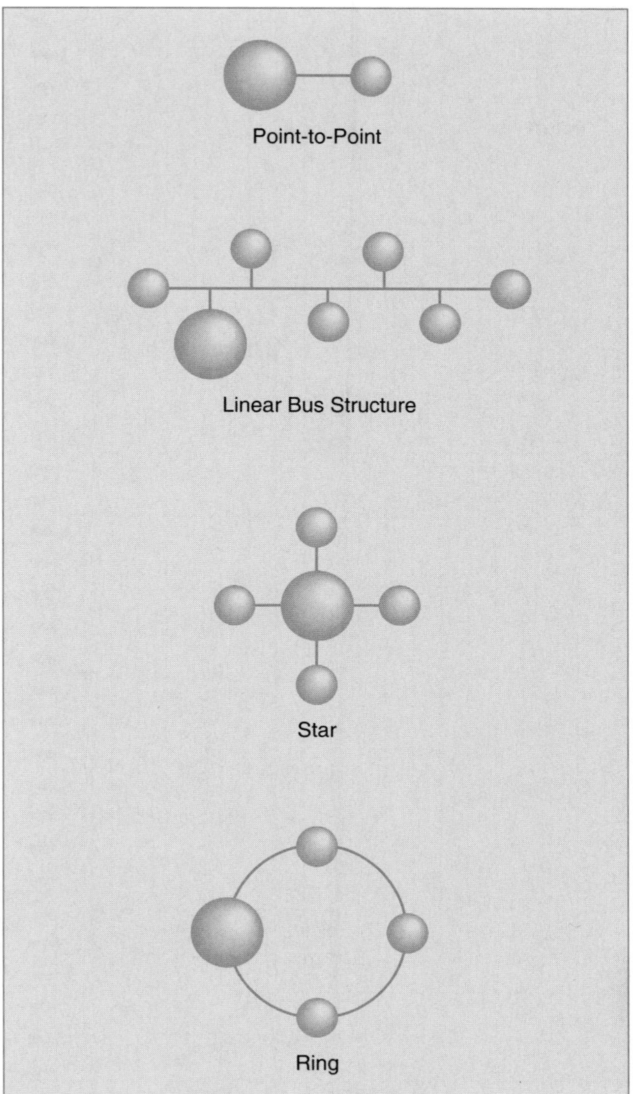

FIGURE 38–19
Typical network configurations. (*Note:* Larger circle represents the network server, while the smaller circle represents the workstation.)

short distance. A typical application for a LAN is within a department or in a student computer laboratory. The shape of the network cabling system varies and is of special interest to the dental hygiene administrator because of the practical considerations of installation. Figure 38–19 illustrates some typical network configurations. The connection of multiple LANs is a supernetwork or **WAN, wide area network.** Local and wide area networks exist because of the expansive use of microcomputers and the development of data transmission standards.[9]

Teleconferencing

Teleconferencing, or telecommunications, which encompasses communicating using a computer and transmitting information through telephone lines, is a growing avenue for communication. The advantage of this form of communication is that individuals can exchange information without having to convene at one site and yet communicate just as frequently and easily as they can at conventional meetings. All that is needed to participate is a microcomputer, a telephone line, and a modem. Users reach telephone numbers through a local access telephone number so that long distance charges are not necessary. TELENET is the name for General Telephone and Electric's computer communications network.[17]

An advantage of teleconferencing is that participants do not have to wait their turn and are not interrupted by others using the system. A printed transcript of the discussions is produced easily. The program keeps track of each participant individually and includes participants' names and the date and time of each response. There are many potential uses for teleconferencing such as submitting journal articles for review, editing, and publishing on-screen. The time lag between submission and publication is reduced significantly compared to conventional methods. Within the specialty of public health, teleconferencing is already a vital means of information exchange between departments located across the country.[17,18] Within dental hygiene education, teleconferencing could possess a similar role for conducting meetings and reviewing journal article submissions.

Electronic Mail

Electronic mail can be defined as the delivery of messages from a sender to a receiver by electronic means and is often termed "E-mail." Electronic mail can include FAXs (acronym for facsimiles), which employ some type of printer or communication device using word processing software packages for uses such as sending an interoffice memo.

Information Services

Information services, also known as **bulletin board services (BBS),** are electronic communication services that operate on large mainframe computers and can house a variety of topics. Regardless of the type of computer used, a modem can link the user to local bulletin board services that share user group information or trade computer games, and even can perform financial functions such as electronic check writing. Two popular commercial information services are CompuServe and Prodigy in which information access includes news, weather, sports, travel, games, shopping, and financial information, to name a few.[7]

Integrated Software

Integrated software, an appropriate description of this application, is a program that combines several programs into one. Some application programs that may be present in an integrated software package include word processing, a spreadsheet, data management, graphics, and communications. Integrated software is useful to managers who perform a multitude of tasks, but who desire one package to handle these functions. An example of an integrated application is when a client list is entered via a data management portion of the software, and then a spreadsheet program performs accounting of fees charged to and payments made by the clients on the data base. With integrated software, the clients' names do not have to be entered a second time for the spreadsheet program. Furthermore, if the user wants to send each of these clients a business letter, the

Trans-Optic® by NCS EP-46309:321 A22' ? Printed in U.S.A.

STUDENT NUMBER

0–9 (nine columns)

COURSE

0 1 2 3 4 5 6 7 8 9

TODAY'S DATE

JAN FEB MAR APR MAY JUN JUL AUG SEP OCT NOV DEC

DAY | YEAR

APPT NO

PATIENT NUMBER

0–9 (nine columns)

PT BIRTHDAY

JAN FEB MAR APR MAY JUN JUL AUG SEP OCT NOV DEC

YEAR

SEX M F

CLINIC ACTIVITY

CLINIC AST

COMP SERV

INST NO

PATIENT CLASS

CAL	PER	STA	DEN
1	1	1	D
2	2	2	M
3	3	3	P
4	4	4	E
5	5		
	6		

TIME-IN HR (8 9 10 11 12 1 2 3 4 5) MIN

TIME-OUT HR (8 9 10 11 12 1 2 3 4 5) MIN

STATUS COMP INC

OLD DOMINION UNIVERSITY

PATIENT NAME:

STUDENT NAME: PRINT LAST NAME FIRST MI

INSTRUCTOR SIGNATURE:

SCHOOL OF DENTAL HYGIENE AND DENTAL ASSISTING
NORFOLK, VIRGINIA 23529

ASSESSMENT

U M N MEDICAL/DENTAL HISTORY
U M N ORAL EXAMINATION
U M N DENTAL CHARTING
U M N PERIODONTAL CHARTING & ASSESSMENT
U M N REASSESSMENT

PLANNING

U M N TREATMENT PLANNING
U M N OHI PLANNING

IMPLEMENTATION

U M N ORAL HEALTH INSTRUCTION
U M N SCALING/ROOT PLANING
U M N EXTRINSIC STAIN REMOVAL

RADIOGRAPHS

U M N ASSESS OF PATIENT NEED
U M N TECHNIQUE
U M N INTERPRETATION/UTILIZATION
FMX EXO OCC PAN
PA 1 2 3 4 5 6 7 8 9 10 11 12
BW 1 2 3 4 5 6 7 8 9 10 11 12

COMPREHENSIVE SERVICES

AMALGAM I 1 2 3 4 5 6 7 8 9 10 11 12
POLISHING II 1 2 3 4 5 6 7 8 9 10 11 12
V 1 2 3 4 5 6 7 8 9 10 11 12
SEALANTS 1 2 3 4 5 6 7 8 9 10 11 12

AIR/POWDER ABRASIVE
TOPICAL ANESTHESIA
CARIES ACTIVITY TEST
ULTRASONIC SCALING
DESENSITIZATION
FLUORIDE TREATMENT
IMPRESSIONS
INTRAORAL PHOTOGRAPHS
MOUTH GUARD
NUTRITIONAL COUNSELING
PEER REVIEW
PERIODONTAL PACK
PHASE MICROSCOPE
PROSTHETIC CLEANING
PULP VITALITY TEST
RUBBER DAM APPLICATION
STUDY MODEL
SUBGINGIVAL IRRIGATION

EVALUATION/MANAGEMENT

U M N EVAL. OF D.H. TREATMENT
U M N CLINIC ASSISTANT
U M N DECISION MAKING
U M N PREV. DISEASE TRANS.
U M N TIME MANAGEMENT

TECHNIQUE EVALUATION

GENERAL

Y N Seeks assistance when needed.
Y N Uses approp. precautions to prev. dis. trans.
Y N Completes record.
Y N Uses appropriate symbols/terminology.
Y N Explains purpose & findings to patient.
Y N Records all findings & procedures legibly in ink.
Y N Uses proper patient/operator/equipment positions.
Y N Uses adequate direct & indirect lighting.

HEALTH HISTORY

Y N Elaborates on positive responses.
Y N Id. conditions which contraindicate/modify treatment.
Y N Records all required information or medications.
Y N Updates records each appointment.

ORAL EXAMINATION/CHARTING

Y N Records deviations/variations. | Y N Perio. Assess.
Y N Extraoral. | Y N Perio. Charting.
Y N Soft tissue. | Y N Dental Charting.
Y N Calculus. | Y N Occlusion.

PLANNING

Y N Establishes & implements comprehensive plan.
Y N Establishes logical sequence of treatment.
Y N Discusses plan with instructor & patient.
Y N Makes alterations in plan when indicated.

INSTRUMENTATION

Y N Uses sharp instrument.
Y N Avoids tissue trauma.
Y N Makes definitive decisions.
Y N Uses correct scaling technique.
Y N Uses correct exploring technique.
Y N Selects appropriate armamentaria.
Y N Uses appropriate grasp & fulcrum.
Y N Establishes logical sequence.

EXTRINSIC STAIN REMOVAL

Y N Adapts rubber cup & brush to surface.
Y N Uses proper speed and pressure.
Y N Selects appropriate polishing agent.
Y N Uses dental floss.

SPECIAL CONSIDERATIONS

Y Excessive hemorrhage.
Y Sensitive gagging response.
Y Tenacious calculus.
Y Sensitive tooth surface.
Y Malposed/missing teeth.
Y Special patient management.

FIGURE 38–20
Customized clinical grade sheet. (Courtesy of Old Dominion University, School of Dental Hygiene and Dental Assisting, Norfolk, Virginia.)

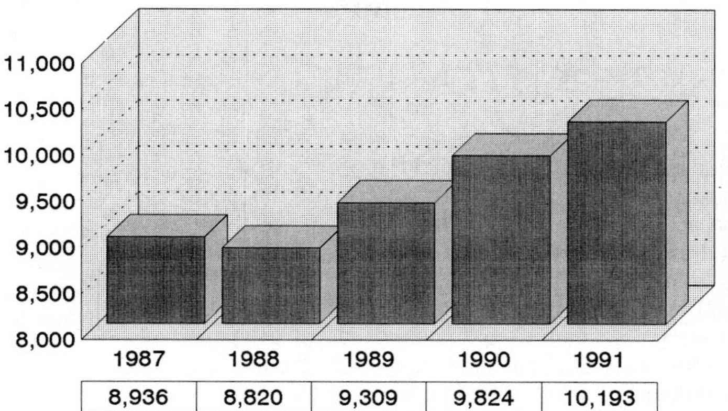

FIGURE 38–21
Computer-generated graph from statistical data. (From 1991 Annual Report: Council on Dental Education, American Dental Association.)

program can insert the names and addresses in the document and generate mailing labels, saving the user considerable time. Another advantage to integrated software is that the cost is less than that if the same types of application packages were purchased separately. In addition, the computer user does not have to learn three or more different programs because the integrated software employs similar menus and options throughout the package. PFS: First Choice, distributed by Software Publishing Corporation, is a popular integrated software package for the PC. Microsoft Works (Microsoft Corporation), initially developed for the Macintosh computer, now has a version for the PC and is another popular integrated software package.

Custom Software

Computer software that is written by a programmer for a specialized task is custom software. Obviously, one would not want to pursue significant programming work and the associated costs to develop a word processing package when standard applications are available for purchase. However, there may be specialized applications required in large businesses for which a software program is needed and the resources for achieving this are not readily available. For example, at Old Dominion University, the School of Dental Hygiene and Dental Assisting had custom software developed by on-campus programmers for its students' clinical performance system (Fig. 38–20). An advantage to custom software is that it precisely performs its intended function; the disadvantage is that the purchaser is dependent on the programmer for quality of the custom program, and rewriting of the software, in the event of its loss, is costly.[9]

Research Applications

Statistical software packages for computing are a category unto themselves; however, they may be of interest to the dental hygiene researcher and educator and therefore are worthy of discussion. Computers have a long-standing history in statistical applications; however, statistical packages for microcomputers are a relatively new application and are becoming more sophisticated over time. "Microcomputers can be a cornerstone in improved research productivity because of the tasks they allow us to perform faster, better, and more efficiently."[2] Providing independence from central computing facilities, microcomputers allow dental hygiene researchers easier access to their data and statistical packages for computation. The researcher is not competing with other users to use the mainframe, thus providing better time management.

Commercial software packages are available that use statistical methods already familiar to the dental hygiene researcher, such as Statistical Package for the Social Sciences (SPSS) and Statistical Analyses System (SAS); therefore, the user does not have to learn a new program for statistical testing, and data can be entered using a word processing software package. Dental hygiene students and novice researchers may find microcomputer statistical software packages easier to use and less intimidating than mainframe applications when first attempting statistical analyses. Furthermore, there are software packages that can create pie charts and three-dimensional graphs from statistical outcomes for use in publications and presentations. These statistical graphics are usually termed "business graphics" to distinguish them from animation and engineering graphics (Fig. 38–21). At present, most PC software packages for statistical analysis have limitations that may be a drawback for some researchers, such as the use of small data sets and limited variable names. It is expected that soon these problems will be overcome with the evolution in computer technology.

Access to library data bases for electronic literature searches is a significant avenue for developing a thorough literature review and can be obtained through a personal computer. Access to this medium may be through an on-line communication system or the use of CD-ROMs (compact discs–read only memory). The large data bases of interest to dental hygienists include the Cumulative Index to Nursing and Allied Health Literature (CINAHL), National Library of Medicine data base (NLM), Psychological Abstracts (PsycINFO), and the Educational Resources Information Center (ERIC) data bases.

A burdensome task in research report writing is bibliographic and citation management. Even careful writers may omit citations, thinking they will return to the task after a sentence or paragraph is drafted. Many word processing packages offer options for automatically handling footnotes or creating reference lists and bibliographies. This makes citation preparation in a final document much easier as well as avoiding interference during the writing of the text.[2]

SELECTION OF A COMPUTER SYSTEM

The first step in the decision-making process should be the evaluation of the setting and definition of the needs that can be addressed by a computer system. Once these issues are addressed, investigation of systems, operating arrangements, and personnel training can follow. The implementation of computers into most settings can replace paper and pencil operations as well as handle much of the paperwork storage for materials that previously were filed.[19] However, the usefulness of computers is only as good as the original organizational system; in other words, the computer can deal only with the information provided to it, thus records must be in order before converting. Often automation magnifies problems that existed in a poorly managed business practice.[20]

The dental hygiene manager must have clear definitions of the need for automation and which tasks the computer will perform. For example, the size and frequency of the tasks to be completed and the potential future growth of the business are significant considerations when selecting computer hardware and software. Writing out specific objectives for that which the computer is to accomplish is a good idea, and objectives that are designed in measurable terms can help to demonstrate improved performance levels.

Before selecting a system for purchase, the individual evaluating computer hardware and software choices should learn about the products on the market. Some sources of information include enrolling in computer courses, talking to vendors and reading their literature, participating in seminars sponsored by vendors, talking to other users, using demonstration diskettes, and reading popular magazines on computers. Merely examining a system at a major convention may provide some basis for comparison, but time constraints and the pressure of other observers may not furnish the best demonstration. Reviewing systems of interest and talking with vendors back home are highly recommended.

Computer hardware and software costs continue to decrease, but a computer purchase is still a major business investment and systems should be evaluated for performance as well as price. An inexpensive system may not offer all that was expected once it is implemented, so it is important to select the system that best meets the needs of the work setting.[21] Some criteria that can be used for hardware selection are listed below:

- Determine whether desired software applications will operate on the computer system of interest
- Determine whether a single user or multiple users will operate the equipment because different systems are indicated
- Determine how much main memory (RAM) is required to operate the application software
- Determine how much hard disk storage is required to store and load programs and files
- Calculate future growth and consider the amount of required memory and storage
- Determine data output requirements and the type of printer needed
- Determine data communication requirements and whether a modem is needed
- Determine whether a mouse is required to operate the software of interest
- Evaluate the reliability of the system
- Determine how much to spend on the system

Finding reliable vendors is probably the most significant factor when selecting a computer. Ongoing support and efficient service can mean the difference in successful operation and the least disturbance of daily operations when the need for repairs or consultation arises. Contractual arrangements and responsibilities of the dealer are extremely important issues and are often overlooked during computer purchase. Some issues that should be examined include:

- Warranty information
- Annual maintenance fees
- Responsibility of the dealer for repair, training, and consultation
- The experience of repair personnel

Purchasing a computer system from a reliable vendor who has been in business for some time rather than a mail order house probably offers the best service over time.[22]

Preparing the office environment needs some consideration in view of space allocation for hardware placement as well as the storage of software and other supplies. Work tables and chairs specifically designed for use with computers are not essential, but ones fashioned for ergonomic efficiency may be considered for the health and comfort of an employee who uses the computer for long periods of time.

Once the environment is readied and equipment is installed, employees need to receive training on the use of the hardware and software applications. This may be difficult at first if employees have little or no experience with computers. It is important to expect mistakes and to be patient. With adequate training and experience, the skill, speed, and accuracy of employees using the computer should increase.

INTEGRATING COMPUTERS INTO PRACTICE

Integrating computers into the oral healthcare setting can be a frustrating task if not approached in a diligent and organized manner. An implementation approach that can make this transition smoother includes some commonsense considerations: staff participation, timing, and utilization approaches. As mentioned previously, the first task is to organize existing paper records in the office; if they are well-organized, less time is spent in general organization. It is important to remember that automating the business takes considerable time, particularly if it is a large office.[23]

Involving staff is a significant consideration in the ease of automation as well as successful integration of computers into practice. Much of the work of implementation is the responsibility of the staff, and thus securing their cooperation is very important. Also, their attitudes towards computers and office automation can govern the success or failure of the endeavor. Enlisting their participation from the very beginning of the project is vital. Organizational meetings as well as staff demonstration workshops are suggested in the early stages of decision making. Also, having the staff provide recommendations regarding the organization of office records prior to computerization is helpful because they are the individuals who encounter them on a daily basis. Identifying the roles and responsibilities of staff persons once computers are installed is an important issue that may help alleviate fears regarding their future employment. Often, individuals believe that the computer can replace them in the office. Updating the office manual is a good avenue for addressing staff responsibilities before the equipment is installed in the office.[24]

The normal business schedule should not be severely affected during computer implementation. Having a plan for all stages and a time schedule for implementation is extremely important. All data are not entered in 1 day and because it is important that data entry be accurate, adhering to a plan is essential. Entering data can be a tedious endeavor. Making this step an educational exercise for the staff is recommended to alleviate boredom as well as to serve as an audit mechanism.[23]

Training of the staff is important to obtain the full benefit from the system. Sessions should be planned at intervals rather than crammed into a single day. It is easier to absorb smaller portions of information over a period of time rather than several days of intensive training. There should be specified time periods for training rather than snatches of time between other tasks; this also helps to stress the importance of learning how to use the system accurately and reduces employee anxiety during the change process.[24]

Ideally, the computer should be used in some manner from the very first day of installation, whether for word processing or for entering accounts. However, not all aspects of the system should be expected to be operational from the beginning; for example, in the clinical practice setting it is important to begin entering active client accounts, allowing the system to be functional in a progressive fashion. It may be useful to experiment with the system at first and gain confidence before entering actual data. A common procedure is to run a parallel system initially; this means to use the old and the new system simultaneously for a limited time period to check the accuracy of the new system. Generally, a month is enough time to observe if the new system is working properly, after which the old system should be discontinued.[24] It is important to suppress the urge to make the system operational too quickly; a computer can be likened to a new employee, in which case it takes some time to observe full efficiency and production.[23] Staff members need time to adjust to a new system of office procedures, but once this has occurred, efficient and effective utilization of the computer system should evolve.

INFORMATION MANAGEMENT SYSTEMS IN DENTAL HYGIENE SETTINGS

A plethora of commercial software is available dealing with dental business management functions; selecting the package most useful to a specific environment should be dependent on the size of the organization, the scope and nature of the functions to be automated, and business growth estimates. Currently, in the oral healthcare environment, the most widely used computerized management systems include client billing and insurance form processing.

Using a computerized management system for billing generally encompasses entering the practice fee schedule and preparing a bill based on services rendered to the client. Statements that are produced are legible and professional in appearance and readily available at the end of an appointment. Computer usage for billing also maximizes collection of accounts, thus minimizing time spent on billing.[25] Computerized management of employee records for payroll and tax purposes is another common application in business settings. Commercial packages specifically designed for this purpose are based on spreadsheet concepts previously discussed and are readily available.

As with billing, insurance forms are easily processed by computer. Data can be entered during the client visit and claim forms generated immediately. The client can be informed about insurance coverage during the office visit and questions can be answered without delay. Other functions for which the computer can be employed include:

- Posting payments directly to bank accounts
- Check writing
- General accounting functions such as accounts receivable and office expenses
- Payroll

Again, the computer serves as an effective management tool in reducing costs and increasing office productivity.

Appointment scheduling for clients in the clinical practice setting and other business settings, where meetings need to be arranged or employees scheduled, can be done easily through an appointment book or calendar program. Search functions in the program can identify available times based on certain criteria established by the operator. Appointment book programs can be used to manage large amounts of data along specified parameters established by the operator, for example, scheduling dental hygiene students for community oral health rotations or making faculty and student clinical assignments. Continued care (recall) appointments for clients also can be managed easily through an appointment program with search functions.

Marketing is probably one of the most significant areas in which computers can be used to enhance an organization. In the dental hygiene practice environment, computer records can be used to determine referral sources and then efforts can be directed toward stimulating clients from those sources. Dental hygiene schools need to evaluate their client pools to ensure optimal learning experiences for their students, and computer analysis is an ideal way to accomplish this task.[26] Internal marketing also can be a primary role for the dental hygienist in creating newsletters, policy and procedures manuals, infection control documentation, and in recognizing special events, such as birthdays.[25]

The University of California at Davis has begun mailing floppy disks containing recruitment material to potential students. An image of a dormitory room appears on the screen and the user can point to the items in the room using a mouse to obtain information on specific topics. For instance, clicking on the sports pennant provides information on athletics, and clicking on the checkbook furnishes details on fees. It is believed that the disks have a far greater impact than a brochure on prospective students.[27]

Computerized Client Records

Paper records are the primary vehicle for recording client care information, and whereas recent years have seen a trend towards computerization of components of the record, paper records are still the norm for most healthcare settings. As technology improves and the demand for healthcare information increases, it is likely that computerization of a standard client record will ensue.[28–30]

Automated records have been identified as a means to improve healthcare in three ways:

- Provide personnel with better data access and higher quality data, support decision-making and quality assurance activities, and provide clinical reminders to assist in client care
- Capture clinical information to enhance research programs
- Increase efficiency by reducing costs and improving staff productivity[31]

The necessity for automation of client records continues to escalate as demands for information throughout the health sector increase and as healthcare providers and clients become more accustomed to computers in everyday life.

CLINICAL PRACTICE APPLICATIONS

Computerized applications for client care are available in all aspects of the dental hygiene process. Some approaches are still in the experimental stages, but others have become common practices and are valuable tools to enhance dental hygiene practice.

Computer systems for diagnosis and treatment of oral disease presently are used rarely in the dental field, and many systems described in the literature still are experimental or in early generation stages.[32] These "expert" systems, or "intelligent" data bases, are more specialized than standard data base management systems in that they provide additional information. For example, in a data base file on oral lesions, the file could be queried about all possible disease manifestations that display a particular oral lesion; the expert system would suggest further tests, explain why those tests are warranted, and provide a specific dental diagnosis. Expert systems are products of a field of artificial intelligence that seeks to employ information in more useful ways than simple problem solving. They have been used for the medical diagnosis of infectious disease, interpretation of pulmonary tests, and initial screening of clients at medical centers.[33] Within the dental field, Wagner and Schneider describe their work in this area and propose that to be functional, decision support systems should include modules on health and dental history data; graphic presentation of the oral status including the dentition, periodontal tissues, and radiographs; images accompanied by text on diseases; differential diagnosis; therapeutic approaches including cost estimations; diagnosis and treatment of orofacial masticatory system; and client recall.[34]

The use of data bases for obtaining information on clients' medications and drug interactions is a comprehensive and time-saving approach to decision making and documentation. For instance, the Micromedix Company has established medical information data bases that identify and provide ingredients of more than one-half million commercial, pharmaceutical, and biological substances. Indexes for substances of concern in poison control, drug information retrieval, and for emergency and acute care settings are available through Micromedex data bases.[35] Access to computerized data bases such as this provides a mass of information to a practitioner, educator, researcher, or student that otherwise may take valuable time and effort to obtain.

Software programs that can reference numerous oral conditions of interest to dental hygienists are available. These programs offer electronic references to common diseases of the oral cavity and systemic diseases with dental significance. Menus by which diseases are referenced make these software applications easy to use. These programs can be used in educational programs, libraries, dental practices, and as client educational information. This is only one example of a software application that can be used by the dental hygienist.

Visualization of structures within the oral cavity is probably one of the best developed computer applications in clinical practice. Used in conjunction with a videocamera system, the computer can capture an intraoral image and simulate alterations, all the while projecting these on a video monitor. Computer **video imaging systems** can augment client education and practice marketing regarding cosmetic dentistry and smile enhancement.[36] The computer image furnishes an immediate picture of the dentition prior to actual dentistry being performed. Images show how the teeth and smile will appear after shading, shaping, or repositioning with bleaching, porcelain veneers, or other tooth-colored restorations. Use of this technology can reduce uncertainty for the client about the results of cosmetic dental

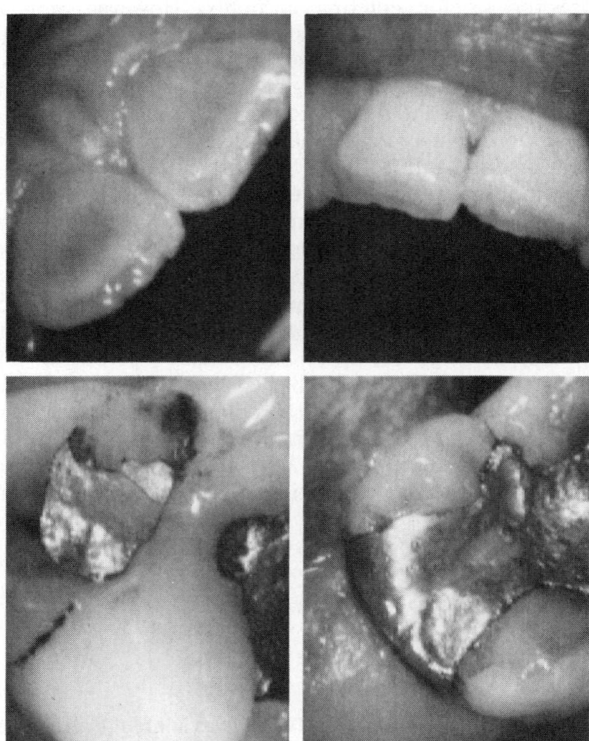

FIGURE 38–22
Computer video imaging output. (Courtesy of Dr. Gregory A. Schrumpf, Virginia Beach, Virginia.)

XYZ Dental Group, Ltd.
Dr. John Doe, DDS

PERIODONTAL CHART

Name: Newman, Paul Prov: Dr. Philip McKenzie	Pat#: NEWMPA	SSN: 127-21-6697 Date: 02-24-1992
Provider's Signature		Date
Notes: This is an actual printout from ** Chart-It ** For more information, please contact: SINGER Professional Services, Inc. 8401-K Mayland Drive Richmond, VA 23294 (804) 747-5289		

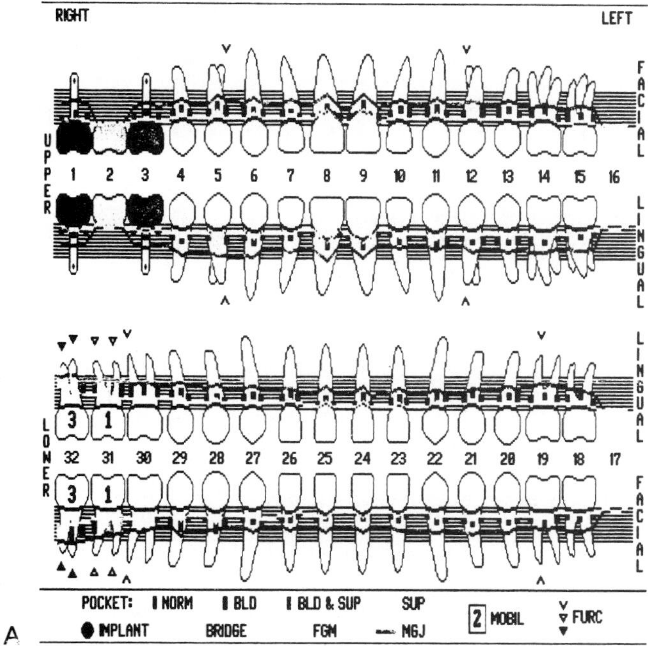

A

FIGURE 38-23
A, Computerized dental chart (CHART-IT). (Courtesy of Singer Professional Services, Inc. Copyright 1991, Singer Professional Services, Inc.) *B*, Sample of INTERPROBE printout. (Copyright 1989 Bausch & Lomb, Oral Care Division, Inc.)

procedures and can be a dynamic marketing tool. On-screen changes allow clients to view the changes they desire and practitioners to recommend possible treatment options.[32,37] In dental hygiene care, video imaging can be employed to show clients inflamed gingival tissues or lesions in the oral cavity (Fig. 38-22). When used in conjunction with tissue management programs, clients can evaluate along with the therapist changes in tissue health.

Examination of the periodontium involves the recording of more data than any other aspect of oral assessment and, therefore, is ideally suited to computer utilization.[38] Various computerized periodontal probing devices and charting mechanisms currently are available on the market. One example is Chart-It (Singer Professional Services Company), an automated charting system in which information can be entered using an electronic probe, light pen, or mouse. Each client's information is stored on a disk. Chart-It printouts include periodontal, restorative, and comparative data, statistical reports, and notes (Fig. 38-23*A;* see color section of this volume).

Interprobe, by Bausch and Lomb, is a periodontal examination and charting system that employs its own computer control unit, memory cards (disks), handpiece, dot-matrix printer, report forms, and disposable probes (see Fig. 38-23*B*). As a diagnostic tool, the Interprobe is used to measure pocket depths and document attachment loss, gingival recession, bleeding sites, suppuration, mobility, and furcation involvement. A single operator can use the device and enter data via a foot control. The probe handpiece is shaped like a traditional probe and uses disposable tips. The handpiece houses an optical encoder that measures the pocket depth and communicates this information to the control unit via the foot switch.[39] Measurements are instantaneous and data can be printed upon completion of the examination.

Oral health education can be provided using computerized educational packages. These self-paced programs can be used in the reception area to provide clients with educational information while they wait or can be employed during the visit as part of the oral healthcare program. Clients with access to computers at home or work may be provided with floppy disks to check out and use as supplemental or follow-up education.

Computer software is available to provide a complete

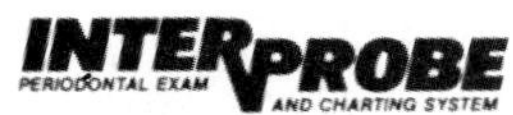

BAUSCH AND LOMB
5243 ROYAL WOODS PARKWAY
TUCKER GA 30084

PATIENT ANDERSON WM
SOCIAL SECURITY
EXAMINED BY
DATE 10/31/89

		1	2	3	4	5	6	7	8	9	10	11	12	13	14	15	16
MOBILITY		0	0	0	0	0	0+	0+	0	0	0	0	0	0	0	0	0
FURCATION	MESIAL					0							0				
	MIDDLE	0	0	0											0	0	0
	DISTAL					1							0				
POCKET	MESIAL	B 2.5	2.0	2.0	S 3.5	B 4.5	3.0	1.5	1.0	0.5	B 0.5	1.5	1.5	S 2.0	1.0	1.5	B 2.0
	MIDDLE	B 2.0	S 2.5	2.0	3.0	4.0	B 2.5	1.5	1.5	1.0	B 1.5	2.0	1.5	2.5	1.0	1.5	B 2.5
	DISTAL	2.0	2.0	2.5	B 3.0	4.0	2.0	1.5	1.5	1.0	1.0	2.0	2.0	2.0	2.0	1.0	S 2.0
RECESSION	MESIAL	B- 0.5	- 1.0	0.0	S- 2.0	B- 1.5	0.0	0.0	- 1.0	- 1.5	B- 0.5	0.0	- 0.5	S- 1.5	0.0	0.0	B- 1.5
	MIDDLE	B- 1.0	S- 1.0	0.0	- 1.5	- 1.5	B 0.0	0.0	- 1.0	- 1.0	B- 0.5	0.0	0.0	- 1.0	0.0	0.0	B- 1.0
	DISTAL	- 1.0	- 1.0	0.0	B- 1.5	- 1.0	0.0	0.0	- 1.0	- 1.0	- 1.0	0.0	0.0	- 1.0	0.0	0.0	S- 1.0
FACIAL	CEJ																
		1	2	3	4	5	6	7	8	9	10	11	12	13	14	15	16
LINGUAL	CEJ																
POCKET	MESIAL	B 2.5	2.0	2.5	* 3.5	B 4.5	* 3.0	1.5	1.0	0.5	B 1.0	1.5	1.5	S 2.0	1.5	1.5	B 2.5
	MIDDLE	B 2.0	* 2.5	2.5	3.0	4.0	3.5	1.5	1.5	1.0	1.5	2.0	B 2.0	2.5	1.5	1.5	2.5
	DISTAL	2.0	2.5	2.0	B 3.0	4.0	3.5	1.5	1.5	1.0	1.5	2.0	1.5	2.0	2.0	1.0	S 2.0
RECESSION	MESIAL	B- 1.0	- 1.5	0.0	*- 1.5	B- 1.5	*- 0.5	- 0.5	- 1.0	- 1.5	B- 0.5	0.0	- 0.5	S- 1.5	0.0	0.0	B- 1.5
	MIDDLE	B- 1.0	*- 1.0	0.0	- 1.5	- 1.5	- 0.5	0.0	- 1.0	- 1.0	- 0.5	0.0	B- 0.5	- 1.0	0.0	0.0	- 1.0
	DISTAL	- 1.0	- 1.0	0.0	B- 1.5	- 1.0	- 0.5	0.0	- 1.0	- 1.0	- 1.0	0.0	- 0.5	- 1.0	0.0	0.0	S- 1.5
FURCATION	MESIAL	0	0	0		0							0		0	0	0
	DISTAL	0	0	0		0							0		0	0	1

ANNOTATION CODE: B = BLOOD S = SUPPURATION * = BOTH

		32	31	30	29	28	27	26	25	24	23	22	21	20	19	18	17
MOBILITY		1+	0	0	0	0	1	0+	0+	0	0+	0	0	0	1	1+	1
FURCATION	MIDDLE	3	0	0											0	1	2
POCKET	MESIAL	5.0	3.5	2.5	2.5	1.5	2.0	2.5	1.5	1.0	2.0	2.5	S 2.0	3.0	4.0	4.5	5.5
	MIDDLE	6.0	3.5	B 3.0	3.5	2.0	2.0	2.5	1.5	1.0	2.0	2.5	2.0	3.5	4.5	B 4.0	4.5
	DISTAL	6.0	B 4.5	2.5	3.5	1.5	2.0	1.5	B 1.5	1.5	2.5	- 1.5	1.5	3.5	4.5	4.0	* 5.0
RECESSION	MESIAL	- 0.5	- 1.5	- 1.0	- 1.0	- 0.5	- 0.5	- 1.0	0.0	- 0.5	- 0.5	- 1.0	S- 0.5	- 1.5	- 1.0	- 1.5	- 1.5
	MIDDLE	- 1.0	- 1.0	B- 1.0	- 1.0	- 0.5	- 0.5	- 1.0	0.0	- 0.5	- 0.5	- 1.0	- 1.0	- 1.5	- 1.0	B- 1.5	- 1.5
	DISTAL	- 1.0	B- 0.5	- 1.0	- 1.0	- 0.5	- 0.5	- 1.0	B 0.0	0.0	- 0.5	- 1.0	- 1.0	- 1.0	- 1.5	- 1.5	*- 2.0
FACIAL	CEJ																
		32	31	30	29	28	27	26	25	24	23	22	21	20	19	18	17
LINGUAL	CEJ																
POCKET	MESIAL	* 6.5	2.5	3.0	B 2.5	1.5	2.0	3.0	3.0	2.5	1.5	2.0	1.5	* 3.0	B 4.0	4.0	* 5.0
	MIDDLE	6.5	3.0	S 3.0	3.0	1.5	2.0	3.0	S 2.5	2.5	2.0	* 2.5	2.0	* 3.5	3.0	3.5	B 6.0
	DISTAL	* 7.0	B 2.5	3.5	2.5	* 1.5	2.0	3.0	3.0	3.0	2.0	2.5	2.0	2.5	3.5	3.5	S 6.5
RECESSION	MESIAL	*- 1.0	- 1.0	- 1.0	B- 0.5	0.0	0.0	2.0	2.0	1.0	- 0.5	- 1.0	- 1.0	*- 1.0	B- 1.5	- 1.0	*- 1.0
	MIDDLE	- 1.5	- 1.0	S- 1.0	- 0.5	0.0	0.0	2.0	S 2.0	1.0	- 0.5	*- 1.0	- 1.0	*- 1.0	- 1.0	- 1.0	B- 1.0
	DISTAL	*- 1.0	B- 1.0	- 1.0	- 0.5	* 0.0	0.0	2.0	2.0	1.0	- 0.5	- 1.5	- 0.5	- 1.0	- 1.0	- 1.0	S- 1.0
FURCATION	MIDDLE	2	0	0											0	0	1

B

IP-414-119

FIGURE 38–23
Continued

dietary analysis upon entering a client's personal food intake. Output may include the client's nutritional intake or recommended dietary amounts based on age, sex, height, and weight. Using these types of data may be particularly helpful in counseling clients on special diets.

Computer applications in clinical dental hygiene practice continue to evolve. The dental hygiene practitioner and manager should keep abreast of new developments. Implementation of computer applications in all facets of practice can enhance dental hygiene diagnosis, documentation, care, education, and evaluation of client care.

LEGAL AND ETHICAL PERSPECTIVES

Although selecting the appropriate computer to purchase is of utmost importance, many buyers fail to become familiar with legal aspects of computer purchase. Purchasers need to have a clear understanding of the warranty accompanying the equipment and also aspects of coverage by maintenance contracts.

Software purchase and use also has legal implications that are covered primarily by copyright and license laws. Buyers should be familiar with these aspects prior to purchase so that expectations of the software use will meet their needs. Also, they can avoid the unintentional infringement of manufacturers' legal rights.

A final area of legal and ethical concerns in computer use deals with physical security. This issue encompasses both the protection of confidential information stored in the computer and use of equipment by authorized personnel as well as the physical securing of equipment against theft and environmental disasters. Protecting software data and programs from malicious destruction by computer viruses is another physical security concern. These issues are of utmost importance to the dental hygienist concerned with risk management.

Rights in Purchase — Contract and Warranties

The bulk of law dealing with computer acquisition encompasses purchase agreements.[40] Contracts for the purchase of computers and software applications are governed by the same fundamentals of contract law for commercial purchases.[41] And while there is no such thing as a perfect contract, there are some items that are essential in a contract to purchase hardware. The hardware should be identified by name and stock number including the common marketplace name, such as Macintosh, Commodore, TRS-80 Model III, and so forth. Manufacturers' specifications of the equipment should be appended as a numbered item to the contract if not included in the contract itself. The price of the equipment and whether warranties are priced separately are other considerations. If software are included or built into the hardware, it also should be addressed in the contract. Delivery terms should be set forth if the equipment is to be shipped — the vendor should retain the risk of loss until delivery to the purchaser. Terms and length of warranty should be specified as well as whether the vendor will provide a rent-free unit on loan in the event that equipment needing adjustment must be sent to a repair facility. The vendor or manufacturer should be able to indicate that the equipment has been registered with the Federal Communications Commission and that it meets codes and standards established under local, state, and federal regulations. If training is part of the agreement, this should be specified in writing. The contract should indicate the technical level of documentation manuals (repair instructions) and the expertise needed to understand them — these guides should be understandable by the average noncomputer expert. In the event of injury from the equipment, the manufacturer should bear the cost of damages and litigation.[41]

Some manufacturers offer the opportunity to purchase a maintenance contract, which is an extension of the warranty. This means that for an additional payment, the purchaser is entitled, for a specified time period, to repairs and replacements of defective parts. In most cases, the standard 90-day warranty is enough time to determine if the equipment functions properly. Also, if the computer model is known to be very dependable, the cost of an extended warranty might be reason enough to decline purchase of a maintenance contract. If, however, time for repair of malfunctioning equipment would cause significant business loss, a maintenance contract that ensures fast service may be a wise investment.[40]

Intellectual Property

Computer programs are recognized as literary works, and thus as intellectual property they are protected under copyright laws. For computer programs, the copyright law works much like that for books; limited copying of a book for personal purposes usually is not a violation of copyright law. For example, copying a chapter of a book to study in more depth at home is permissible. Making a backup copy of a copyrighted software program might be permissible by the manufacturer, if so specified in the agreement; however, making duplicates of copyrighted software programs to share with others is prohibited by law. Exceptions to this rule are the duplication of original disks to provide copies for use by the original purchasing agent. For example, software designed for teaching purposes may specify that a set number of copies can be made by the school for use in the case of multiple machines. In the case of software covered by a licensing agreement, sometimes making backup copies is prohibited and extra fees may be required to obtain a backup copy from the publisher. Copying software programs is a relatively easy and inexpensive task. Commonly, avid microcomputer users copy and share software programs (such as games) among themselves. Although the designer or manufacturer of a software program may not go to the expense to prosecute users making illicit copies, it is the responsibility of the individual user to maintain ethical standards and avoid violating copyright laws and thus possibly incurring expensive damage claims and legal costs.

Security Issues and Risk Management

Computer security issues include both physical security against environmental hazards as well as operational threats to security of hardware, software, and data files. Physical security includes protecting equipment and software against environmental hazards and natural disasters such as fires, floods, and the prevention of and recovery from loss. For example, placing equipment under water sprinkler systems, near major water lines, radiation sources, air conditioners, heating vents, laboratory plaster bins and other sources of dust is not advisable.[42] Temperature and humidity control is another important consideration in the physical placement of equipment in an environment. Creating backup copies of important files and software and storing these in another location are important precautions against loss of significant or costly data.

The protection of information processing operations also is a tenable concern in computer security and has created new problems for society.[43] Potential situations in which employees use company computers for their own means or when disgruntled employees or criminals sabotage files are legitimate concerns that should be addressed in computer security policies and procedures. Advances in computer technology permit vast quantities of data to be accumulated, analyzed, and stored. Within the healthcare industry, this has seriously compounded existing controversies regarding confidentiality of medical records. The violation of confidentiality is much easier in an efficient automated system.[44] Dental hygienists should be cognizant of these issues as significant progress in the computerization of clients' records ensues. Some general security measures for standalone systems are delineated below[45]:

- Lock all terminals when not in use
- Restrict access by unauthorized personnel
- Assign individual passwords for system access
- Never store or post passwords near the terminal
- Turn terminals off when not in use or when left temporarily
- Limit the number of users who have access to report-generator systems

In a partially integrated system where a user has access to information but does not enter data, there is little security risk and the same procedures recommended for a standalone unit are adequate. However, in a fully integrated system, for example where quality assurance files and client information are stored along with other applications, and live transfer of data is possible, security measures need to be more stringent. Security considerations need to include the location of terminals, security clearance for users, password protection on hard and removable disks, and strictly adhered to procedures for access and use.[45]

Passwords are a means to provide computer access to appropriate users and prohibit unauthorized users from accessing information. Passwords should be chosen carefully and should not include initials, social security numbers, or birth dates. They also should be unrelated to the application, particularly its name.[41] Passwords should not be exchanged or borrowed; they should not be posted or filed near the computer terminal.

Computer Viruses and How to Prevent Them

Understanding computer viruses is a complex task, but in simple terms a **virus** is any program that can cause harm to a computer.[46] The term "virus" was coined by the media, but it has evolved to an acronym meaning, *V*ital *I*nformation *R*esources *U*nder *S*iege. Comparable to human cold transmission, a virus can be obtained through contact with an infected program, ultimately causing the computer to malfunction. The extent of destruction from the virus depends on the strain of virus; a virus can take on many different forms, but most use the same mechanisms to spread.[9] Implementing a few routine operating procedures into common practice can prevent viruses or at least avoid costly destruction.

A virus is a program that infects existing programs; it may add strings of instructions to a program being run and may even multiply itself causing programs to become so large so as to exhaust disk space and significantly increase

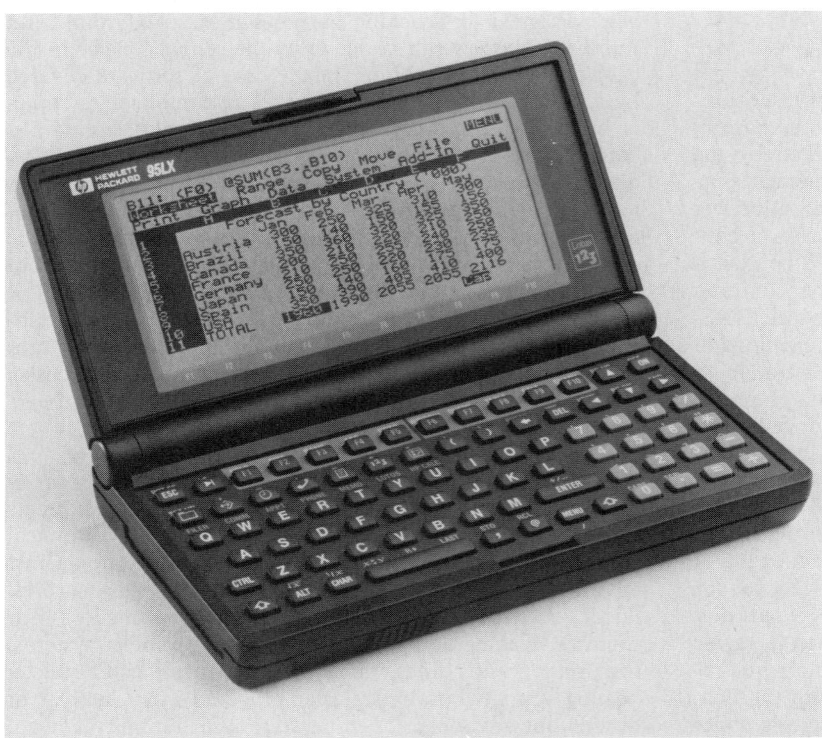

FIGURE 38–24
Hewlett-Packard 95LX Palmtop Computer. (Photo courtesy of Hewlett-Packard Co.)

processing time. Eventually, the program may be so large that it cannot be loaded on the PC and therefore renders the program inoperable.

A virus originates from an infected program, so any time an "outside" program is run on the microcomputer, there is risk of exposure. The source by which a virus enters the computer is an infected diskette. Exposure occurs when a diskette is used in a computer that has an infected program and then is transferred to another computer through use of the now-infected diskette. A technical repair person who unknowingly runs an infected diskette is an example of how a computer virus is transmitted among computers. Other common avenues of virus infection include co-workers who share a new program or game from their diskette or a work diskette shared among users operating different computers. A number of precautions can be followed to reduce the possibility of virus infection:

- Avoid using programs whose origin is unknown
- Do not allow others to run their programs on your computer
- Limit transporting diskettes between PCs, for example, between home and work
- Beware of programs **downloaded** from bulletin boards or use BBSs where software is checked before it is posted
- Make routine antivirus checks of all files
- Be able to recognize the signs of a virus and be alert to these signs
- Know how long it takes programs to load and recognize when they are taking longer than usual
- Remain cognizant of the size of files and recognize when they are larger than expected

A final defense strategy is to back up copies of essential work so that in the event of a virus important information is not lost.

To detect and remove a virus before it can cause damage, software antivirus programs have been developed to "vaccinate" the software. These programs scan the RAM and hard and floppy disks for viruses and identify their location, allowing the user to delete infected files or disk sectors or the virus program code.[47] Development and enforcement of security procedures is an essential objective for the professional administrator and manager; security procedures should be established as standard protocol in the work environment.[48]

NEW DEVELOPMENTS

Hardware and software innovations are evolving at a rapid pace. It is difficult to keep informed of all the new developments. A few "cutting-edge" technologies in input devices that are presently available and used in selected settings include:

- Voice recognition and voice activated computers
- Light pens
- Touch screens

These mechanisms for computer communication and input are particularly useful for novice computer users, children, and individuals with disabilities and assist in making computer use available to a wider population.

Laptop computers are small enough to transport; they weigh from 9 to 12 pounds. Capabilities for laptops can rival those of powerful desktop systems. They are designed for individuals who cannot leave the office behind. Laptops can be carried in cars, airplanes, cruise ships, and just about anywhere else. Batteries allow the operator freedom from an AC outlet and rechargers are available for the system. A laptop computer may appear to be like an inexpensive toy, but the price can be equivalent to that of a full desktop system.[7]

A newer development in microcomputer technology is the computerized **notebook** which is smaller than the laptop computer and comparable in size to a standard-sized notebook and weighs between 4 and 8 pounds. These computers offer a variety of options including 486 microprocessors, built-in hard disks, and spreadsheet and wordprocessing software. Even smaller than the notebook computer is the palmtop computer, which is about the size of a checkbook. The Hewlett-Packard 95LX palmtop PC is a 10-ounce computer with 512K of RAM. It includes Lotus 1-2-3, a personal information manager, a communications package, a file manager, and a financial calculator (Fig. 38–24).[49] Uses for notebook and palmtop computers in the dental hygiene field are endless. The user can enter client data in a clinical practice setting, dental hygiene student evaluations in a clinical or community oral health setting, or observations made during research investigations. The user can enter client data in a clinical practice setting, dental hygiene student evaluations in a clinical or community oral health setting, or observations made during research investigations. The information gathered and stored in the notebook computer then can be electronically transferred to other programs such as word processing for printing.[9] Potential applications for this new technology have yet to be investigated fully, but the advantages are readily apparent.

Within the realm of information transfer, a new application is electronic journals. The American Association for the Advancement of Science in a joint venture with Online Computer Library Center (OCLC) is publishing *The Online Journal of Current Clinical Trials,* which contains results of research on new and established medical treatments for diseases. The initial issue, published in July 1992, is believed to be the first peer-reviewed electronic publication containing graphs, charts, and illustrations. Computerization affords the ability to provide information to subscribers faster than paper publication and eliminates the time for printing and mailing. The journal initially is available to subscribers with IBM-compatible machines and with a 386 (or more powerful) chip. Also required for use are a software program called "Microsoft Windows 3.0," a mouse, a modem (9600 bps), and 4 megabytes of RAM. Technology for Apple Macintosh access to the *Online Journal* will be available in the future.[51] With wider usage of computers among the general population and the increased demand for rapid communication, electronic journals and teleconferencing likely will become commonplace for information transfer in the future.

References

1. Carpenter, C. R. Computer use in nursing management. Journal of Nursing Administration 13:17, 1983.
2. Madron, T. W., Tate, C. N., and Brookshire, R. G. Using Microcomputers in Research. Beverly Hills: Sage Publications, 1985.
3. Osborne, A. An Introduction to Microcomputers, vol. 1. Berkeley, CA: Osborne/McGraw-Hill, 1980.

4. Blum, B. I. Understanding computer basics, M.D. Computing. Computers in Medical Practice 1(1):59, 1984.
5. Schultheis, R., and Sumner, M. Management Information Systems. Homewood, IL: IRWIN, 1989, pp. 109–116.
6. Dayton, D. Computer Solutions for Business. Redmond, WA: Microsoft Press, 1987.
7. Murray, K. Introduction to Personal Computers, 2nd ed. Carmel, IN: Que, 1991.
8. WordPerfect Publishing Corp. Laser printer buyer's guide. WordPerfect The Magazine, October, 35, 1990.
9. Christensen, W. W., and Stearns, E. I. Microcomputers in Health Care Management. Rockville, MD: Aspen, 1990.
10. Nelson, E. Making the move: Is windows right for you? WordPerfect the Magazine, November, 41, 1991.
11. Skousen, P. B., ed. WordPerfect 5.1 for windows — a sneak preview. WordPerfect Report 4(4):1, 1990.
12. Biehl, A. WordPerfect does windows. WordPerfect the Magazine, November, 26, 1990.
13. Cassel, D., and Jackson, M. Introduction to Computers and Information Processing. Reston, VA: Reston, 1981, p. 261.
14. Halio, M. P. Student writing: Can the machine maim the message? Academic Computing 4(4):16, 1990.
15. Johnson, J. The Computer Revolution in Teaching. Accent on Improving College Teaching and Learning. National Center for Research to Improve Postsecondary Teaching and Learning. Ann Arbor, MI: University of Michigan, 1989.
16. Kirsch, M., Ribaudo, M., and Wiener, H. Computers and College Writing: Selected College Profiles. New York: National Project on Computers and College Writing, 1990.
17. Eklund, S. A. Is it time for CONFER, a computer-based conference for dental public health? Journal of Public Health Dentistry 78(4):45, 1988.
18. Weintraub, J. A., and Eklund, S. A. Development of a computer-based communication network for a dental specialty group. Journal of Dental Education 52(9):525, 1988.
19. Beckett, J. M. Computer utilization. Dental Economics 76(9):53, 1986.
20. Council on Dental Practice. Computer technology in dental practice. Journal of the American Dental Association 101:938, 1980.
21. Farr, D., and Farr C. Take another look at computers. Dental Economics 78(4):45, 1988.
22. Gerber, I. A. A guide to the purchase of dental computer hardware. New York State Dental Journal 54(9):52, 1988.
23. Bennett, W. J. A method of computer system implementation, Journal of the Virginia Dental Association 62(2):10, 1985.
24. Ehrlich, A. Computers: The Key to Improved Dental Practice Management. Champagne, IL: Colwell Systems, 1985.
25. Forrest, J. L., Williams, C., and Gurenlian, J. R. Improved communication through computer technology. Dental Hygiene 60(12):558, 1986.
26. Wooten, R. K. A computer-based approach to analyzing a patient pool. Journal of Dental Education 45(6):349, 1981.
27. Wilson, D. L. Floppy disks used to recruit students. The Chronicle of Higher Education 38(22):A22, 1992.
28. Dick, R. S., and Steen, E. B. (eds). The Computer-based Patient Record: An Essential Technology for Health Care. Institute of Medicine (U.S.) Committee on Improving the Patient Record. Washington, D.C.: National Academy Press, 1991.
29. Neiburger, E. J., and Diehl, M. C. The past and future of the electronic dental record from the practitioners' view. Journal of Dental Education 55(4):268, 1991.
30. Monteith, B. D. The electronic patient record and second generation clinical databases: Problems of standards and nomenclature. Journal of Dental Education 55(4):246, 1991.
31. GAO (General Accounting Office). Medical ADP Systems: Automated Medical Records Hold Promise to Improve Patient Care. Washington, D.C.: GAO, 1991.
32. Nathanson, D. Dental imaging by computer: A look at the future. Journal of American Dental Association 122:45, 1991.
33. Schrodt, P. A. Microcomputer Methods for Social Scientists. Beverly Hills, CA: Sage Publications, 1984.
34. Wagner, I., and Schneider, W. Computer-based decision support in dentistry. Journal of Dental Education 55(4):263, 1991.
35. Micromedix, Inc. Micromedic Information Systems. Denver, CO: 1992.
36. Golub-Evans, J. Imaging helps induce balky patients, colleagues to accept best treatment. Dentist, March:1, 1990.
37. Dzierzak, J. Computer imaging: Its practical application. Journal of the American Dental Association 122:41, 1991.
38. Duguid, R., and Cowley, G. C. Use of a computer to plot and compare periodontal pocket charts. Community Dentistry and Oral Epidemiology 10:320, 1982.
39. Bausch and Lomb Oral Care Division. Interprobe Periodontal Exam and Charting System. Tucker, GA, 1989.
40. Hagelshaw, R. L. The Computer Users's Legal Guide. Radnor, PA: Chilton, 1985.
41. Wolk, S. R., and Luddy, W. J., Jr. Legal Aspects of Computer Use. Englewood Cliffs, NJ: Prentice-Hall, 1986.
42. Romano, C. A. Privacy, confidentiality, and security of computerized systems. Computers in Nursing 5(3):99, 1987.
43. Forester, T. Computers and behavior. Phi Kappa Phi Journal, Summer, 18, 1991.
44. Hiller, M. D., and Beyda, V. Computers, medical records, and the right to privacy. Journal of Health Politics, Policy and Law 6(3):463, 1991.
45. Walsh, M., and Cortez, R. Quality assurance system must balance functionality with data security. Computers in Nursing 9(1):27, 1991.
46. Kane, P. Avoiding the virus crisis. WordPerfect the Magazine, February, 66, 1991.
47. Diehl, S., Wszola, S., Kliwere, B., and Stevens, L. Virus protection: Strong medicine for a fast cure. Byte 16(8):226, 1991.
48. Buss, M. D. J., and Salerno, L. M. Common sense and computer security. Harvard Business Review 82(2):112, 1984.
49. Dickinson, J. Put an XT in your pocket! PC Computing 4(5):101, 1991.
50. Wilson, D. L. New electronic journal to focus on research on medical treatments. The Chronicle of Higher Education 38(6):A27, 1991.
51. Online Journal of Current Clinical Trials (brochure), 1333 H Street, NW, Washington, D.C., 20005, 1992.

Suggested Readings

American Dental Association, Council on Dental Practice. Practice Management in the News. Chicago: American Dental Association, 1985.

Christianson, W. W., and Stearns, E. I. Microcomputers in Health Care Management. Rockville, MD: Aspen Publications, 1990.

Consumer Guide: Computer Buying Guide. Lincolnwood, IL: Publications International, 1991.

Enockson, P. G. A guide for selecting computers and software for small businesses. Reston, VA: Reston Publishing Co., Inc., 1983.

Jamsa, K. Welcome to Personal Computers. New York: Management Information Source, 1992.

Jay, A. T. Using computers and actually liking it. Dental Management 30(10):30, 1990.

Lyons, S. Attention practitioners: The data bank has its eye on you. Access 4(7):11, 1990.

McKeown, P. G. Living with Computers, 2nd ed. Orlando: Harcourt Brace Jovanovich, 1988.

Schmitz, H. H. Managing Health Care Information Resources. Rockville, MD: Aspen Publications, 1987.

39 Ethical and Legal Decision Making in Dental Hygiene

OBJECTIVES

Mastery of the content in this chapter will enable the reader to:

- Define the key terms used
- Describe key ethical principles and philosophies affecting healthcare
- Identify the issues emphasized in a code of ethics for dental hygienists
- Develop an awareness of ethical dilemmas encountered in the practice of dental hygiene
- Recognize a theoretical framework to assist in ethical decision making
- Describe the legal concepts and theories that apply to dental hygiene practice
- Develop an awareness of the legal concepts affecting the dental hygienist-client and dental hygienist-dentist relationship
- Recognize methods to reduce risks within the practice of dental hygiene
- Identify legal issues relevant to the various roles of the dental hygienist

ETHICS

Foundations of Ethical Decision Making

Personal Values and Professional Ethics

Ethics is a branch of philosophy that deals with thinking about morality, moral problems, and moral judgments. Some argue that ethics are individual, influenced by personal, cultural, religious, and familial experiences. Nash suggests that ethics is a concern for everyone as it forces the question of what one should do and why.[1]

A discussion of ethics from the perspective of a profession such as dental hygiene relates to what is professionally right or conforming to professional standards of conduct. This definition reflects the traditional view of a profession as a group that determines its own professional standards of ethics, writes its own code of ethics, and disciplines its own members. This traditional view is undergoing change to include a broader perspective that argues professional ethics are not merely what practitioners regard as custom but, rather, what the profession and society agree are appropriate rules of conduct. For example, codes of ethics point out that healthcare providers should not discuss a client's medical condition, disease, or illness with anyone without the individual's authorization.[2] Another example found within the American Dental Association (ADA) Code of Ethics is a statement that the dentist should inform the client of proposed care and allow the person to become involved in treatment decisions. The addition of society as a player in the development of ethical rules of conduct suggests a factor that is important in a discussion of ethical decision making.

A code of ethics, whether personal, professional or a combination, must recognize three relationships affected by ethical behaviors. The relationships include:

- The professional and the client
- The professional and the professional
- The professional and society

Thus, ethics in the practice of dental hygiene focuses on the moral duties and obligations of the professional to clients, colleagues, and society. The broader commitment to society is not always specifically reflected in codes of ethics. However, the influence of society in evaluating professional groups and their ethical conduct is increasingly evident. For example, articles in the lay press advocate that healthcare professionals reveal their positive human immunodeficiency virus (HIV) status to clients.

Historically, the health professions were viewed as groups that followed codes of ethics carefully and monitored the activities of their members. However, recurring charges of malpractice, impropriety, fraud, and the scrutiny of various public and private agencies have projected the health professions, including dentistry and dental hygiene, into the arena of public concern and criticism. Consumers, aware of inappropriate or perceived unethical behaviors, are contacting dental and dental hygiene professional organizations and peer review groups to express their concerns. Professional conferences and publications now address issues such as ethics, ethical decision making, quality assurance, and related issues.

There is a distinction between *legal obligations* and *ethical obligations.* Rules of conduct, promulgated by state or federal statutes, are by their nature obligatory customs or practices of a community (legal obligation). A dental hygienist must follow certain legal obligations or must face the consequences. For example, a hygienist is obligated by both federal and state statutes not to discriminate against specific classes of individuals or sexually harass another person. Such behaviors may result in legal action against the dental hygienist. The consequences for violating statutory laws may include fines or prison sentences, depending on the severity of the violation.

Rules of conduct promulgated by private groups, such as the American or Canadian Dental Hygienists' Association, serve as guidelines for conduct or ethical obligations. A professional who violates an ethical code or principle may frustrate a client or lose the respect of professional colleagues. However, there *may or may not* be legal consequence to an ethical violation. For example, the dental hygienist who refuses to provide care to individuals on Medicaid is violating the ethical standard that suggests dental hygienists should not discriminate. However, there are no legal consequences.

Accountability and Responsibility

A dental hygienist is accountable for the client care provided. **Accountability** refers to ability to answer for one's actions. Dental hygienists provide client care and should realize that they are accountable for their actions on many levels. Dental hygienists must answer to themselves, their clients, the profession, the employer or employing agency, and society (see How to Maintain Professional Accountability chart).

Professional accountability has the following purposes:

- To evaluate new professional practices and reassess existing ones
- To maintain standards of care
- To facilitate personal reflection, ethical thought, and personal growth on the part of health professionals
- To provide a basis for ethical decision making

Dental hygienists must be accountable for dental hygiene care and not rely on, or allow, members of other disciplines to assume that responsibility. Accountability for dental hygiene care contributes to the quality of care provided as well as to client satisfaction.

HOW TO MAINTAIN PROFESSIONAL ACCOUNTABILITY

Self
- Report any conduct or conditions that endanger clients
- Stay informed and practice current dental hygiene theory
- Make judgments and evaluate based on facts

Client
- Provide clients with thorough and accurate information about care
- Conduct dental hygiene care in a manner that ensures client safety and well-being
- Encourage communication within a professional client-provider relationship

Profession
- Maintain ethical standards in practice
- Encourage professional colleagues to follow the same ethical standards
- Report colleagues' unethical behavior to appropriate peer review entities

Employment Situation
- Follow appropriate policy and procedures

Society
- Maintain ethical conduct in care of all clients in all settings

Major Ethical Perspectives

Ethics has been addressed by philosophers, scientists, educators, and ethicists for centuries. A cursory review suggests three major ethical perspectives (see Major Ethical Perspectives chart).

John Stuart Mill, a nineteenth century English philosopher and economist, called his perspective utilitarian ethics. Propositions inherent in utilitarian ethics suggest that the rightness or wrongness of actions and practices is determined solely by the consequences produced for the general well-being of all the parties concerned. What makes an action right or wrong is the good or evil produced by the act, not the act itself. For example, consider the dental hygienist trying to decide whether to provide care to a client with a poor periodontal prognosis. The utilitarian would base a decision on what actions would bring about the greatest benefit for the most people. Therefore, that dental hygienist would be concerned about the consequences of wasting time and effort on a case that appears hopeless, when one could be providing caring to others who would have a better prognosis. Another example is the community-based dental hygienist who acquires funds to improve the oral health status of the target population. Although there are clients who need restorative and prosthetic care, the utilitarian would decide based on doing the most good for the larger population. Thus, a fluoride mouthrinse program may be selected to utilize the funds available.

MAJOR ETHICAL PERSPECTIVES

Utilitarian Ethics (John Stuart Mill)
- Greatest good for greatest number
- The end justifies the means
- Emphasis is on consequences to determine rightness or wrongness of actions and promises

Deontological Ethics (Immanuel Kant)
- A binding duty or obligation
- Means separate from the end
- Emphasis upon the morality of the act rather than on the consequences

Virtue Ethics (Aristotle/Plato)
- Based on character traits
- Virtue is moral
- Emphasis upon excellence of character

Immanuel Kant, eighteenth century German philosopher, advocated deontological ethics. Deontologists argue that an action is right when it conforms to the relevant principles of duty. This philosophy indicates that it is immoral to deceive, coerce, or fail to consult with others merely in order to promote one's own goals. Promises must be kept and debts must be paid because such actions are one's duty, not because of the consequences of such actions.

Again, consider the client with severe periodontal disease. The deontologist would consider duty as the primary consideration in deciding whether to accept the case. The decision is based on a sense of duty, not the consequences. Deontologists also believe that performance of acts in the past creates obligations in the present. If one has entered into a contract, one is bound, independent of the consequences, to the terms of that contract.

Aristotle and Plato, Greek philosophers of the fourth century B.C., advocated virtue ethics. Ancient traditions viewed virtuous traits such as benevolence as the primary function of morality. Within this context, the dental hygienist's decision to care for the client with severe periodontal disease is determined by a perception of whether treating the individual is consistent with an accepted model of a virtuous person, someone who is compassionate and conscientious, for example. One would decide affirmatively if it promoted progress toward excellence of character.

Fundamental Ethical Principles in Healthcare

Each individual seeking dental hygiene care presents a unique array of qualities, values, beliefs, and perceptions about professional care and the healthcare provider. The dental hygienist also possesses specific values, beliefs, and perceptions. The ethical principles that underlie healthcare are presented below:

- Autonomy
- Beneficence
- Nonmaleficence
- Justice
- Veracity

Autonomy is based on the principle of respect for persons. Individuals have a right to self-determination, that is, freedom to make their own judgments based on their own evaluations. Recognizing the autonomy of a client occurs when the individual involves the client in decision making regarding care, obtains informed consent, and maintains client confidentiality. Autonomy means the caregiver respects clients and provides them with enough information to make judgments about their care.

Beneficence may be considered as the provision of benefit, preventing evil or harm, removing evil or harm, or promoting good. Based on this principle, a healthcare professional is responsible for contributing to the health and welfare of others. William Frontera, a noted ethicist, explains that four elements are included in the beneficence principle:

- One ought not to inflict harm
- One ought to prevent harm
- One ought to remove harm
- One ought to do or promote good

Examples of dental hygiene actions following the principle include taking only necessary radiographs and not overexposing the client to radiation, and maintaining equipment to prevent client injury, such as replacing worn instruments so that instrument tips do not break off into a client's mouth.

Nonmaleficence is summarized by the phrase "above all, do no harm." A dental hygienist seeks to never harm a client. An example of potential harm is when a dental hygienist learns about a new, somewhat controversial homecare regimen for periodontal disease. The dental hygienist decides to recommend the regimen, although she has no personal experience with the method or the possible outcomes from its use. Her actions may be viewed as having the potential to inflict harm and are in opposition to the principle of nonmaleficence.

Justice relies on fairness and equality. A person is treated justly when given what he or she is due, owed, deserves, or can legitimately claim. All clients receiving dental hygiene care should be treated equally. A dental hygienist who provides substandard care to persons in a nursing home, because they are institutionalized, is not treating all clients equally.

A final principle to consider is **veracity,** or truth telling. This is critical to meaningful communication and, thus, to relationships between individuals. Dental hygienists are obligated to be truthful in interactions with clients and professional associates. For example, a dental hygienist fails to tell a client that during a sealant application procedure to tooth 19, the primary tooth anterior to 19 fractured. The dental hygienist is not demonstrating honesty in the hygienist-client relationship.

Codes of Ethics

The American Dental Hygienists' Association (ADHA) Code of Ethics describes the principles of ethical conduct for dental hygiene practice. The principles emphasize the obligations of the dental hygienist to provide oral healthcare using professional knowledge, judgment, and skill; maintain competence; respect clients; educate the public, and participate in organized dental hygiene. Codes of ethics serve as a component of the self-policing responsibility of a profession.

In 1985, the ADHA adopted "Standards of Applied Dental Hygiene Practice" to assist in guiding dental hygienists in providing clinical care (see Chapter 3, Table 3–1). The Standards serve as a framework for decision making as well as contributing to a philosophy of maintaining competence. The Canadian Dental Hygienists' Association and the National Dental Hygienists' Association also have a Code of Ethics.

Ethical Problems in Dental Hygiene

It is frequently difficult to separate ethical, moral, and legal issues in the many professional dilemmas faced by dental hygienists. In this section, examples of ethical dilemmas in different career situations are presented followed by a decision-making framework that may be useful in solving ethical dilemmas.

Private Practice

Dental hygienists are challenged constantly by unethical situations. A study of members of the ADHA identified three commonly encountered ethical dilemmas in dental hygiene practice[3]:

- Observation of behavior in conflict with standard infection control procedures
- Failure to refer clients to a specialist
- Nondiagnosis of dental disease

Examples are the colleague who uses a cold disinfectant rather than properly sterilizing instruments; the staff person who recycles disposable items, such as saliva ejectors or rubber cups; the new dental assistant who is unfamiliar with standard barrier techniques. Similar situations are ubiquitous.

Failure to refer to a periodontist occurs in dental hygiene care situations. For example, the dental hygienist responsible for client assessment observes deteriorating periodontal status in the client. The dental hygienist is employed by a general dentist who prefers not to refer. However, the dental hygienist recognizes that the skill level of the dental hygienist and dental staff cannot meet the periodontal needs of the client. The failure to refer, depending on the facts, may constitute dental malpractice. From the ethical perspective, the principle to provide oral healthcare using professional knowledge, judgment, and ability must be considered. The dental hygienist is ethically obligated to provide optimal oral healthcare. However, the dental hygienist in some states cannot legally refer. The dental hygienist must consider the alternatives for solving the dilemma. Alternatives may include working to change office policy, informing clients of their need to seek care in another office, or seeking another position. Each solution carries with it consequences such as angering the employer-dentist, frightening the client, performing an activity outside the scope of dental hygiene practice, or losing a valued position. An easy solution is difficult to find.

Consider the scenario when the dental hygienist-dentist team fails to detect dental disease. Perhaps thorough clinical evaluation of a client does not occur during a client visit. The dental hygienist has the skills to assess the client and collect and record data, but is not given an adequate amount of time to fulfill those responsibilities. A cursory dental caries examination is conducted by the dentist, but other oral diseases and disorders such as periodontal disease, cancer, malocclusion, or temporomandibular joint dysfunction are ignored. The ethical violation includes failure to provide optimal oral healthcare, compromising the public's confidence in members of the dental health profession and failing to educate about the range of oral healthcare practices that can be used. The failure to thoroughly assess the client also may be an example of dental malpractice.

In these aforementioned situations, the dentist-employer, dental hygiene and dental assisting staff, and clients are placed in a compromised situation both ethically and legally. If the dental hygienist chooses to address the poor quality of the client assessment, the consequences can be far-reaching. Job security, working relationships, and personnel evaluations may be jeopardized. The dental hygienist may be viewed as a "troublemaker." If the dental hygienist chooses not to address the client assessment protocol, there is the personal frustration of practicing unethically. Also, failing to comprehensively evaluate the client could result in failure to identify a disease state and possibly charges of malpractice.

Public Health

Dental hygienists employed in the public health arena are presented frequently with ethical problems because decisions must be made concerning allocating limited resources and maximizing benefits. Perhaps a public health dental hygienist wishes to implement a dental sealant program for elementary school children. Funding is limited and, thus all students are not able to participate in the program. How are the recipients selected? Should children receiving the benefits of water fluoridation also have the benefit of a dental sealant program? Or should those children without access to water fluoridation or other fluoride therapies participate in the sealant program? With knowledge that sealants are useful in preventing occlusal caries, children without the benefit of fluoridation are at a higher risk for developing smooth-surfaces dental caries. Does socioeconomic status play a role in access to dental services? In this situation, the ethical principles of providing optimal oral healthcare using sound professional judgment to meet the oral health needs of the public should guide the decision making. The dental hygienist may choose to maximize the preventive potential by using the funding to develop a sealant program in the fluoridated community. The outcome may be potentially reduced incidence of caries in the children living in the fluoridated community. In addition, another outcome may be that the children at risk for caries without access to fluoride or dental sealants continue to be at risk for caries.

In another situation, a dental hygienist is employed by the state department of public health. The responsibilities of the position include monitoring quality and quantity of oral health services provided by different public health clinics throughout the state. State law does not allow dental hygienists to practice unless there is a dentist on the premises. The dental hygienist responsible for assisting local dental clinics is aware that although dental hygienists are providing dental hygiene care in settings where a dentist is not always present, quality care is being provided to individuals with oral health needs. A legal and ethical dilemma exists. Should the dental hygienist at the local clinics continue care? Is it fair to discontinue services to particular groups because a local clinic cannot afford to employ a dentist full-time? To whom is the dental hygienist ethically responsible—the citizens of the state, the profession, or the state board? From a legal perspective, the dental hygienist is practicing outside the provisions of the law. The ethical principles advocating providing care and preventing dental disease can be used to argue that, ethically, the dental hygienist is meeting the obligation. However, ethical codes also strongly encourage dental hygienists to recognize and uphold the laws and regulations governing the profession. Thus, this truly becomes a difficult dilemma. Unethical and illegal behavior cannot be tolerated. The dental hygienist coordinating the clinics should seek to remedy the situation legislatively or through creative strategies such as staffing alternatives and affiliation agreements with local dentist providers or clinics.

Administration

Administrators, whether in educational or business-based institutions, face ethical dilemmas. Perhaps, for example, students in a dental hygiene program are assigned to provide dental hygiene care at an urban, hospital-based dental clinic. The clients treated at the dental clinic are high-risk candidates for acquired immunodeficiency syndrome (AIDS). The dental hygiene program director is aware that there is always the possibility of a puncture wound occurring, with the result that a dental hygiene student is injured by a contaminated instrument. Does the director choose not to have any students assigned to the clinic? Should students and their families be informed of the risk? The situation may create a dilemma in some settings. However, using the principle that all individuals should be treated without discrimination, as well as the knowledge that the students are practicing using the appropriate standard of care, all students should be assigned.

An administrator also must deal with ethical problems among colleagues. The administrator is asked to evaluate the faculty for merit raises. Not all faculty members contribute equally to their responsibilities. One tenured faculty member fulfills the minimum amount of responsibilities. However, if that faculty person's raise is not comparable to others, she will contribute even less and may accuse the administrator of discrimination. Some less productive faculty members may decide to quit, leaving the remaining faculty with the burden of heavier workloads, especially because the college is experiencing a hiring freeze. Does the administrator recognize all the faculty members as equally meritorious? Is there an obligation to report weaker faculty contributions to the administration? What obligation exists to the most productive faculty members?

The administrator must identify the specific problem and, with the questions previously raised, consider the alternatives. A solution may be to suggest a merit raise for the weak faculty person, then structure that faculty member's obligations to improve her productivity. The consequences include other faculty members' lowered morale when all faculty members receive merit raises, although not all are justified.

Research

Dental hygienists conduct research in a wide range of problem areas. Informal research occurs in the private practice setting when a dental hygienist surveys clients' attitudes, evaluates their acceptance of products and procedures, or compiles salary survey data. Dental hygienists also are involved in research activities conducted at educational institutions or in association with the manufacturing of oral- or health-related products.

Perhaps a dental hygienist is conducting research with a colleague to evaluate the effectiveness of a chemotherapeutic agent on selective pathogenic and nonpathogenic microorganisms. Funding for the research is being provided by the manufacturer. The dental hygienist discovers that, although the research design appears to be valid, the colleague is allowing personal bias to influence observations and interpretations. Both researchers are aware that if the research establishes the chemotherapeutic agent as effective, the pharmaceutical company who produces the agent will provide more generous funding in the future. Should the dental hygienist confront the colleague? Should the dental hygienist maintain the standard that has been set, and ignore the activities of the co-worker? Knowing that research is replicated, should the dental hygienist ignore what has occurred and assume that follow-up research will reveal the flaws of the current research?

Other examples of ethical problems in the research arena include:

- Individuals who steal another's idea or concept
- Individuals who take credit for a colleague's success in research
- Manipulation of data
- Intentional bias in sampling and failure to report research that does not support or confirm a hypothesis

Dental Hygienist–Dentist–Client Relationships

One of the most difficult and common problems is the situation in which the dental hygienist and dentist do not agree on the type of oral healthcare required for a client. A dental hygienist observes signs of soft tissue changes during the client's assessment. The dental hygienist suggests to the dentist that the lesion be biopsied. The dentist disagrees. The dental hygienist feels a responsibility to the client that conflicts with that of the dentist. Does the dental hygienist express concern to the client? Should the dental hygienist identify another dentist in the office to evaluate the client? Should the dental hygienist allow the dentist's decision to stand? Should the dental hygienist suggest that the client obtain a second opinion? The dental hygienist should consider all the alternatives and choose one that satisfies ethical principles. If the dental hygienist seeks another dentist in the office to evaluate the client, the dental hygienist may be satisfied with a second opinion. The consequences can include an unhappy dentist and frightened client. However, if a biopsy does occur, the personal and professional satisfaction gained by the dental hygienist and effects of the biopsy on the client's health outweigh the other consequences. However, dilemmas between the dental hygienist and dentist are not always easily solved.

Dental hygienists are employed in situations where they work under the policies and procedures outlined by the dentist-employer(s). When policies and procedures dictate that the dental hygienist is allowed 45 minutes for all dental hygiene care, notwithstanding evaluating the periodontal status of the client, that care must be completed in one appointment, or that everyone gets a "routine oral prophylaxis," the dental hygienist is being forced to provide substandard care. The dental hygienist is aware that the quality of care provided is poor. Should the dental hygienist work within the policies, ignoring the quality-of-care dilemma? Does the dental hygienist terminate the position? It may be difficult to leave a position because of location, salary, and benefits. Does the dental hygienist inform the client that care is limited, or recommend referral for a second opinion? Or does the dental hygienist attempt to provide optimal care and work more diligently?

A conflict also can arise when a client refuses specific treatment, decides to ignore a referral, or refuses to discontinue an unhealthy practice. What obligations, from an ethical standpoint, does the dental hygienist have to the client and the employer?

A client makes a decision based on information. Some ethical dilemmas created by client actions, or failure to act, could be eliminated if the client were given an appropriate amount of information. Overly brief appointments and ill-informed or uncommunicative staff do not adequately educate clients. Client education and service should remain a priority and guide office practice and policies.

Dental Hygienist–Dental Hygienist Relationships

Most dental hygienists set high standards for themselves and their colleagues. It is difficult to work in an environment in which the quality of care of a dental hygiene colleague is below the acceptable standard. For example, the dental hygienist colleague may be compromising client care by not thoroughly assessing the client, or may be performing services that are illegal or beyond the scope of dental hygiene care. Situations that may affect the client's care create an immediate dilemma. Does one report the activity to the employer, regulatory boards, or the ethics board of the professional association? Does one attempt to educate or update the colleague? Or does one ignore the situation, assuming it is the employer's responsibility?

In situations like these, talking with the dental hygienist in question may be the best alternative. The dental hygienist may be unaware of the quality-of-care issues or illegal activities. Confronting individuals while offering solutions to the problem is a good first step toward resolution.

Employer–Employee Relationships

In a dental or dental hygiene practice or other work environment, various professional, personal, and business relationships co-exist. A dental hygienist may enjoy a personal and professional relationship with an employer. However, there is concurrently a business relationship based on the employer-employee status. As an employee, one may be asked to function in a role or roles that create ethical problems. Perhaps a dental hygienist suspects that an employer is sexually harassing an employee. A dental hygienist observes that insurance fraud is occurring during billing procedures; or, the dental hygienist observes that a colleague has a substance abuse problem. One may immediately determine that the dental hygienist has an obligation to act on the situations observed. Is it the dental hygienist's responsibility to act or is it the employer's? Should the dental hygienist be concerned about the ethical and legal issues? Does one address the issue with the offending practitioner? And what if, after the problem is addressed, no change occurs? It is especially exasperating when one recognizes that the dental hygienist is expected to practice within the ADHA Code of Ethics, but is not in control of the work environment.

One of the ethical principles suggested in the ADHA Code of Ethics is to support organized dental hygiene. A significant number of dental hygienists are not members of their professional association. Are the dental hygienists who are not members of the association aware of the Code of Ethics? Is it the ethical obligation of a dental hygienist who is a member to encourage nonmembers to join the professional association? As a member of a professional association, a dental hygienist has access to scientific literature, continuing education courses, and other resources. Should these items be shared with nonmember dental hygiene colleagues? Each question raises multiple ethical dilemmas. The Code of Ethics encourages a teamwork philosophy. Educating nonmember dental hygienists about the association or sharing new knowledge or skill expertise supports the teamwork philosophy. One must also recognize that some colleagues may not be interested in upgrading the professional or educational aspect of their lives.

A Framework for Resolving Ethical Problems

Two approaches are presented to facilitate ethical decision making by dental hygienists. The first is based on the ethical reasoning model suggested by Gairola and Skaff and the second is based on the model suggested by Pollack and Marinelli for informed decision making.[4,5]

Process for Ethical Decision Making

The ethical reasoning process is based on a systematic approach to decision making. The following is a modification of the model suggested by Gairola and Skaff:[4]

1. Define the problem or conflict
2. Identify the ethical issues
3. Gather relevant information
4. Identify the alternatives
5. Establish an ethical position
6. Justify and defend the alternative
7. Act on the ethical choice

Adapted and reprinted from Gairola, G., and Skaff, K. O. Ethical reasoning in dental hygiene. Journal of Dental Hygiene 57(2):16, 1983. Copyrighted (1983) by the American Dental Hygienists' Association.

Define the Problem or Conflict. The problem may be defined by personal criteria, such as one's feelings, sense of professionalism, or moral code. The problem also may be defined by ethical or legal standards or a combination of ethical and legal principles. In some instances, the conflict arises because of a difference in philosophy, management style, or professional priorities. It is advisable to define precisely the problem or conflict to address the dilemma. It is vague to state, for example, that a conflict has arisen because of different educational backgrounds. It is more precise to identify the conflict as lack of consistency in referring for biopsy or client assessment techniques.

Identify the Ethical Issues What are the issues of the situation? Is there one major issue that can be defined? An ethical dilemma occurs when acting on one responsibility or duty results in not fulfilling another responsibility or duty. For example, when a conflict between the dental hygienist's suggestion to refer to a specialist versus the dentist's refusal to support the suggestion, the dilemma occurs between a professional obligation to follow the dentist's diagnosis versus the dental hygienist's obligation to assess the client's needs and provide quality care. From the client's point of view, the referral may satisfy the client's need for a specialist's evaluation and possible treatment. However, if the dental hygienist's recommendation is incorrect or based on some misconceptions, the second opinion creates an additional expense in time and money for the client, resulting in conflict within the employment setting and a frustrated client.

Gather Relevant Information When faced with an ethical dilemma, the dental hygienist must gather all relevant information, for example, personal data such as family status, age, lifestyle, habits, medical and dental facts, and the professional and personal values involved. Subjective and objective information are included to evaluate the science-based and human-based elements. As part of information gathering, one may want to reevaluate a client, investigate a diagnosis, or obtain a third opinion. If the dilemma is focused on an office protocol or policy, the dental hygienist may want to contact other oral healthcare providers, a lawyer, or a professional association representative to obtain information about standard practices. In any situation, data gathering requires further action on the part of the individual seeking to solve an ethical dilemma.

Identify the Alternatives What are the ethical alternatives? To answer the question, the dental hygienist should make an exhaustive list of the possible courses of action. For example, in one situation alternatives may include resigning from a position, confronting an employer, or calling the client on the telephone to express a concern or suggest a course of action. Each alternative may carry serious personal, financial, and professional implications.

In most situations, the list of alternatives should take into consideration all the parties involved—the client, dentist, dental hygienist, and co-workers. When listing the alternatives, some questions to consider include:

- Obligation(s) to the client (legal and ethical)
- Obligation(s) to others involved (client's family, employer, colleagues)
- Personal beliefs and values
- The client's legal rights, responsibilities, values, and interests
- Alternatives that protect the client's best interests
- Alternatives that protect the professional's best interests
- Alternatives that do the least amount of harm
- Practical constraints
- Professional judgment

Establish an Ethical Position Once alternatives are delineated, the dental hygienist must make a choice. In selecting the course of action, one may weigh which action promotes the best balance between the negative and positive aspects of the situation. Or one may evaluate the alternatives and choose the least negative alternative. In selecting the ethical position, one must keep in mind the consequences. For example, a dental hygienist chooses, in order to balance her recommendations versus the dentist's decisions not to refer a lesion for biopsy, to reschedule the client in 2 weeks and reevaluate the lesion. The consequences may include a harmonious working relationship, an opportunity to further study the possible pathology and keep open the opportunity that in 2 weeks, a more informed assessment can be conducted by both the dental hygienist and dentist. The conflict may be internal, within the work environment, or with the parties involved, such as the dentist-employer. However, if one is resolved that the ethical choice is the correct one, identifying the consequences assists the decision maker in anticipating and preparing for implementing or acting on the choice.

Justify and Defend the Alternative Once the consequences of a choice have been evaluated, and prior to acting on the choice, one should review the decision. What are the supporting ethical principles? What might be a strong argument against the position? Identifying an argument, aside from an ethical position, that supports the decision is helpful. Evaluation at this stage assists the decision maker prior to implementing or acting on the choice. Individuals need to evaluate their decisions. It may be that the consequences are so negative that another alternative or compromise might need to be considered.

Scenario

A recent dental hygiene graduate takes a position in an office with a staff consisting of two dentists, two dental hygienists, and three dental assistants. The dental hygienist works late one evening a week with the dentist. The dentist has been practicing for about 10 years. The dental hygienist notices that after dinner, and throughout the evening, the dentist steps into the laboratory and drinks from a bottle in a paper bag which he hides in the laboratory. He then gargles with mouthwash and returns to client care. His care of clients does not appear compromised. He treats clients and staff with respect; he completes care as planned and manages the office. He meets all the requests of the dental hygienist and the evening office hours run smoothly. However, the dental hygienist notes that this behavior is repeated week after week. The dental hygienist questions the staff about the drinking. The staff indicates that they find him a great dentist, the office environment is a good one, and they really like the job. They imply that they hope that the dental hygienist will ignore the situation so that everything will remain the same. Using the framework for ethical decision making, how would the dental hygienist use the model to assist in evaluating the decision?

Define the Problem The problem can be defined using a number of criteria. The dental hygienist may find it personally offensive that a person is drinking on the job and providing client care. The dental hygienist may feel that the quality of care provided by the dentist is compromised by the drinking, thus violating the ethical mandate of providing the most comprehensive care available. There may be legal issues such as negligent behavior on the part of the dentist. There are also interpersonal issues of the rest of the staff ignoring the situation and pressuring the dental hygienist to do the same. The problem is the dentist drinking and providing client care and compromising that client care as well as staff interaction.

Identify the Ethical Issue One must look specifically to the situation. One is responsible for protecting clients' well-being. A dental hygienist must also prioritize her responsibilities to the client against the wishes of the staff to ignore the situation. Working with someone in an alcoholic state may affect client care, decision making, and evaluation by the dentist. In the light of client care, the issue seems to be one of good versus bad. That is, it is good to report the dentist in order to protect the client; it is bad to allow the drinking to continue.

Gather Relevant Information The dental hygienist needs to seek more information. Are other staff members noticing the same behavior? How long has the pattern existed? Does the drinking occur throughout the whole day? Have there been any untoward incidents (accidents or emergencies) identified with the dentist's care or client management? Is the dentist participating in any alcoholic rehabilitation? Is there a crisis in the dentist's personal or professional life? The dental hygienist may want to document her observations and those of others, if appropriate.

In addition, the dental hygienist may want to investigate the types of services available to professionals with a substance abuse problem, for example, a program where a dentist with a substance abuse problem can obtain professional help. Perhaps a protocol is in place within the state dental society to work with the dentist to overcome his problem and maintain his professional status, or Alcoholics Anonymous may have information about programs that can be used. The dental hygienist may also want to research alcoholism and the characteristics of an alcoholic to assist in confirming behaviors, actions, or language indicating that a problem exists.

Identify the Alternatives The hygienist should make an exhaustive list of the possible alternatives. In this situation, they may include the following:

- Discussing observations with the dentist involved
- Discussing and confirming observations with fellow staff members
- Confronting a single staff member to get additional support
- Discussing the observations with others
- Ignoring the situation
- Contacting appropriate agencies, such as the dental association or state board
- Quitting the employment situation
- Refusing to work with the dentist
- Contacting the local dental hygiene or dental component for guidelines or advice
- Talking to peers to get ideas or solutions

In addition, there may be ethical alternatives that guide the decision-making process. For example, the dental hygienist is required by the ethical code to follow the rules and regulations governing the practice of dental hygiene. Thus, if a mandate exists requiring the dental hygienist to report situations when client care may be compromised, the alternative of choice is clearly delineated. In most ethical situations, the ethical codes are useful to help generate a list of alternatives for consideration. Some alternatives are more dramatic than others, but depending on the situation, they must be considered.

Establish an Ethical Position As part of the decision-making process, the consequences to the alternative suggestion must be considered. In this example, the dental hygienist chooses to confront the dentist and offer information about counseling services available to persons with a drinking problem.

Justify and Defend the Alternative In making the choice, one needs to consider the decision in light of supporting ethical principles. In this case, the principles include client care, professional behavior, and the well-being of the client. One may also consider a strong argument against the position, such as the dentist's possible denial, or a consequence such as the dentist terminating the dental hygienist's employment rather than admitting a substance abuse problem. The evaluation of the alternative is an ongoing part of the process. It is most likely that as each alternative is identified, the advantages and disadvantages are mentally reviewed by the dental hygienist. The mental exercise of justifying and defending assists the dental hygienist in the decision-making process and helps generate additional alternatives. The dental hygienist goes through a process of "what if" and finishes the sentence.

Act on the Ethical Choice The most difficult part of the process is acting on the choice. In the best scenario, the dentist welcomes the identification of a problem and seeks counseling to overcome it. The worst scenario may be denial and an effort on the part of the dentist to dismiss the dental hygienist. However, the guiding principles of nonmaleficence, professionalism, quality client care, and concern for fellow employees should strengthen the dental hygienist, whatever the consequences.

The dental hygienist may never feel totally comfortable with a final decision or choice. However, the suggested process encourages a decision maker to evaluate multiple options and to act based on acquired information. Feedback following any decision is useful in future problem solving and contributes to professional growth and development.

Informed Decision Making

The informed decision-making approach for resolving a dilemma supports the concept that dental hygienists, because of the frequent dilemmas encountered in job situations, owe it to themselves to make certain that decisions are informed.[5] In informed decision making, one initially identifies the dilemma and choices or solutions to resolve the dilemma. For each choice, the decision maker needs to identify the following:

- Risks
- Benefits
- Alternatives
- Expected outcomes

The informed decision-making model encourages use of the legal framework found in informed consent and helps focus the moral, legal, and ethical aspects of a problem or dilemma. In identifying risks, for example, one needs to consider the legal and ethical codes that may be violated. A dental hygienist needs to consider the risks to the client, practitioner, and practice. The benefits are also evaluated from both the practitioner's and client's perspective. Alternatives to the choice are considered to develop a resource pool if the initial choice proves unfavorable. Expected outcomes of a particular choice also must be considered. Will an ethical code be violated? Can the dental hygienist be accused of an illegal activity? Will employment status be jeopardized? Are further risks or benefits possible?

Informed decision making may provide an abbreviated method for ethical decision making that some find useful. Looking at choices, in light of legal and ethical codes and risks and benefits, raises the consciousness of the dental hygienist to the influencing factors in today's society. The principles may be utilized unconsciously by the practitioner in day-to-day activities. A dental hygienist must be comfortable with the process used and ultimately comfortable with the resolution of the problem, both personally and professionally.

JURISPRUDENCE

The ADA reports that one out of 10 dentists is sued. In light of escalating levels of litigation, dental hygienists must understand the legal issues surrounding the delivery of oral healthcare. Knowledge of the legal principles that affect the practice of dental hygiene is one step toward developing a personal and professional risk management philosophy.

Oral Health Professionals: At Risk

Clients have become more sophisticated and are interested in quality healthcare that is accessible and reasonably

ARE YOU CONTRIBUTING TO POTENTIAL MALPRACTICE SITUATIONS OR ILLEGAL DENTAL HYGIENE PRACTICE?

- I have never gone out of my way to report violators of the dental practice act. I assume the state board monitors that
- I sometimes treat clients with severe periodontal disease for years rather than refer them
- If I am running late on my schedule, I may not update a client's health history
- There is probably a procedure or two that a dental assistant performs in my office, that is not allowed under state law
- Prior to treating a client, I rarely explain the reason for the procedure or the risks involved because it takes too much time
- If a client insists, we do not always premedicate individuals who should be
- If I do not like a client, I may eliminate the name from my continued care list

If you checked any of these statements, you or your clients are at risk

priced. Thus, an individual who is dissatisfied with oral healthcare frequently looks to the legal system for assistance.

The list of malpractice suits filed against dental professionals has consistently grown longer (see Are You Contributing to Potential Malpractice Situations or Illegal Dental Hygiene Practice chart). Malpractice litigation of interest to dental hygienists includes:

- Failure to treat problems related to temporomandibular joint syndrome
- Failure to diagnose, refer, or treat periodontal disease
- Failure to obtain informed consent
- Failure to identify and protect a person with a medically compromising condition, such as a heart murmur
- Failure to maintain infection control
- Failure to maintain proper records
- Incorrect history taking

Oral health professionals are governed by a variety of rules and regulations and legal interpretations (Fig. 39–1), such as statutory laws enacted by legislators; administrative laws promulgated by regulatory boards; and common law or case law determined by judicial decisions in court cases. Each governing body, to varying degrees, affects the practice of dental hygiene. The professional is presumed to be aware of all the rules and regulations influencing dental hygiene practice and cannot claim ignorance of the law. Each level of regulation also outlines sanctions for violations, and a health practitioner who violates a particular rule may be adjudicated under multiple governing bodies. For example, a dental hygienist who administers nitrous oxide-oxygen analgesia in a state that restricts dental hygiene to traditional practice has violated the rules and regulations outlined by the state regulatory board and may, based on a review of the board, have her dental hygiene license revoked or suspended. In addition, the individual may be charged with a civil violation, such as negligence, or a criminal violation, such as administering drugs without a license, depending on state and local statutes, resulting in court action or fines.

A dental hygienist must be aware of the rules and regulations governing the practice of dental hygiene in the jurisdiction where licensing is maintained.

Introduction to Legal Concepts

The law is divided into civil and criminal categories. Although these categories are separate, one can be accused of both a civil and criminal violation simultaneously. **Civil law** includes offenses for violating private or contractual rights or, in simpler terms, a crime against a person. **Criminal law** is that law established for preventing harm against society and describes a criminal act as well as the appropriate punishment.

The two categories of law require distinctly different **levels of proof** to determine innocence or guilt. For a criminal act, the level of proof required is that *beyond a reasonable doubt.* In order to meet the level of proof, a jury or judge must be absolutely convinced that the criminal act occurred to establish guilt. If one is not absolutely convinced, an individual may be found innocent. A civil action requires a less strict level of proof. The level of proof required is a *preponderance of the evidence.* This level requires that the jury or judge, based on the evidence presented, must be 51% certain that someone is guilty or innocent. For example, a dental hygienist committed an error during client care. If the jury or judge is 51% sure that error caused a harm to the client, the dental hygienist may be found guilty of a civil action. The requirement of a preponderance of evidence to prove guilt or innocence is weaker than a requirement of proof beyond a reasonable doubt. Professional malpractice suits filed against oral health professionals are usually in the civil arena, thus the level of proof required is the preponderance of evidence. Understanding the level of proof required for civil lawsuits assists in explaining how dental hygienists or dentists are found guilty or innocent when charges are filed against them. In a criminal lawsuit, the individual found guilty is punished based on society's rules and regulations. Fines, prison terms, or other punishments are based on the specific criminal violation. In a civil lawsuit, a violation against a person has purported to have occurred. The remedy that person seeks is to be "whole" because some type of "damage" has occurred, and the manner in which one is made "whole" is to receive monetary damages.

The parties in a lawsuit include the plaintiff(s) and the defendant(s). In a legal dispute, the plaintiff is the person who brings the action or files the suit, the defendant is the person defending himself or denying the action charged.

Contract Principles and Relationships

Most malpractice lawsuits are civil in nature. A common concept of liability used in dental malpractice lawsuits is breach of contract, that is, failure to perform a promise. When one thinks of a contract violation, business transac-

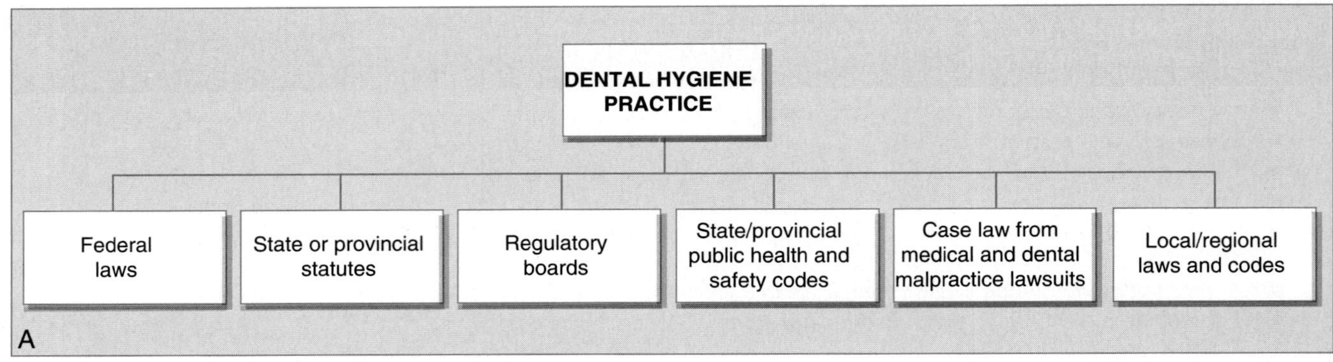

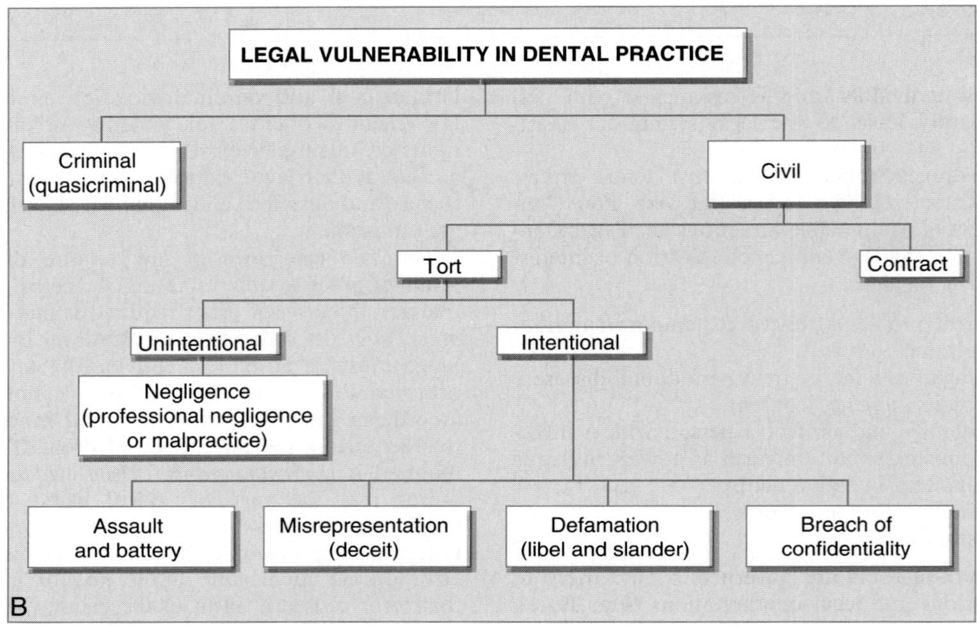

FIGURE 39–1
A, Diagram of governing bodies affecting the practice of dental hygiene. *B*, Diagram of legal vulnerability in dental practice. (*B*, Redrawn from Pollack, B. Risk Management Manual. Ft. Lauderdale, FL: National Society of Dental Practitioners, 1986, p. 12.)

tions come to mind, rather than oral healthcare. Applications of the breach of contract concept was originally limited to business transactions. However, society has become more consumer oriented, and the courts now recognize the dentist-client relationship as a contract. A legal definition states that a **contract** is an agreement between two or more consenting and competent parties to do or not to do a legal act for which there is sufficient consideration. Consideration is an exchange of something of value between two people, such as money.[6] The contractual relationship between the oral health practitioner and the client is one of two types. The first type is an implied contract. An implied contractual relationship can begin in a number of situations including the performance of a professional act, such as taking radiographs or expressing a professional opinion. There is no written document of agreement in an **implied contract,** however, the contractual relationship exists. The second type, an **express contract,** is one in which the terms are expressed and includes either a verbal or written agreement.

The contract, whether written or oral, may outline specific conditions or obligations that must be satisfied by the client or oral healthcare provider, such as fees, method of payment, or type of services to be provided. In addition, based on the contractual relationship, certain warranties or duties are required by both parties. The word "duty" in legal vernacular means obligatory conduct or service, or conducting yourself in a particular manner. Professionals in the legal system evaluate medical malpractice case law to determine the contractual rights and duties shared between the health practitioner and client based on the contractual relationship. Based on that contractual relationship, in accepting the client for care, the oral healthcare provider warrants to:[7]

- Be properly licensed and registered and meet all other legal requirements to engage in the practice of dentistry or dental hygiene
- Use reasonable care in providing services as measured against acceptable standards set by other practitioners with similar training
- Use methods acceptable to a respectable minority of similar practitioners
- Not use experimental procedures
- Complete care within a reasonable time

- Never abandon the client by abruptly stopping oral healthcare
- Obtain informed consent prior to examination or treatment
- Arrange care for the client during a temporary absence
- Ensure that care is available in emergency situations
- Make appropriate referrals and request necessary consultations
- Maintain **confidentiality** of information
- Maintain a level of knowledge in keeping with current advances in the profession
- Keep clients informed of their treatment progress and health status
- Inform the client of untoward occurrences
- Never exceed the scope of practice authorized by the license; never permit any person acting under another's direction to engage in unlawful acts
- Keep accurate records of the care provided to the client
- Comply with all laws regulating the practice of dentistry and dental hygiene
- Practice in a manner consistent with the code of ethics of the profession
- Charge a reasonable fee for services based on community standards
- Not attempt a procedure for which the practitioner is unqualified

Modified from Pollack, B. R. Dentist's Risk Management Guide. National Society of Dental Practitioners, 1990.

The duties or warranties listed are enforceable, although not written or stated in any document given to the client. A dental hygienist who uses an experimental periodontal therapy regimen rather than accepted procedures may be violating a contractual responsibility to use only standard procedures. A dental hygienist who casually discussed confidential information obtained from a client during the health history interview is violating a contractual obligation as well as committing a breach of confidentiality. A dental hygienist practicing outdated techniques is also violating a duty to remain current.

The client also has contractual duties based on the relationship including cooperating in care, paying fees, and keeping appointments. Private practitioners are frequently faced with clients who do not pay fees. Collection procedures may result based on the client's failure to meet the contractual obligation. Failing to cooperate in care, such as missed appointments or refusal to take premedication, does not necessarily result in a lawsuit filed by the dentist. Rather than a lawsuit, the dentist or dental hygienist may choose to dismiss the client from the practice.

If a breach of the contract occurs, the client can use the contract concept to remedy the situation and obtain damages. Perhaps a client discovers that a dental assistant, not a dental hygienist, is providing a level of care, root planing and scaling, that only a licensed dental hygienist is allowed to perform. The client was not harmed by the assistant. However, the dentist warranted, based on the contractual relationship between the dentist and client, that employees within the office were properly licensed and that the staff would never exceed the scope of practice authorized by a license, nor would the dentist ever allow someone to exceed that scope of practice. In this simple example, three violations have occurred and a breach of contract exists. At the same time, if the client has not met specific obligations, such as keeping an appointment, that client has breached that portion of the contract. The oral health professional would most likely not seek damages, but the failure of the client to meet his responsibilities may be reason to end the practitioner-client relationship.

Terminating the Practitioner-Client Relationship

Terminating the practitioner-client relationship frequently occurs in a dental or dental hygiene practice; however, the practitioner must be cautioned never to abandon the client. **Abandonment** is defined as a relinquishment of all connection with the client. The relationship between the oral health professional and client may end without charges of abandonment if:

- Both parties agree to end it
- The death of the client or oral health practitioner occurs
- The client ends the relationship by act or statement
- The client is cured
- The practitioner unilaterally decides to terminate care

If the practitioner seeks to end the relationship, specific steps are necessary. The client should receive written notification of termination and the reasons (e.g., lack of payment for services rendered or nonadherence to recommended care). The letter also should state that the individual will remain a client of the practice for a certain length of time, the date services will be terminated, and that, if necessary, emergency care will be provided for a designated time period. The letter also must suggest that the client seek another dental care provider and state that copies of the client's records will be forwarded to the new provider. The termination letter should be sent by certified or registered mail with return receipt requested (Fig. 39–2). The termination process is done carefully to assure continuity of care and diminish the possibility of charges of abandonment. A copy of the notification letter and returned receipt should be kept in the client's file.

Avoiding charges of abandonment becomes an issue in dental hygiene care when clients of record do not respond to a continued care notice. Although office procedures may not require that an individual receive notification that he is no longer a client of record, actions such as the written notification should be taken.

Another example of a situation that may require termination of the oral health professional-client relationship is when the client refuses necessary oral radiographs or premedication for the prevention of bacterial endocarditis. Rather than jeopardize the quality of care provided, the dental hygienist may suggest that the client be dismissed as a client of record from the practice. Again, the issue of abandonment becomes important. Written notification of termination is necessary to protect the dental hygienist and the employer.

Related Responsibilities

In addition to those warranties or duties outlined as part of the practitioner-client relationship, other related duties exist. A practitioner has the right to choose individuals to treat, that is, there is no duty to treat everyone seeking care. The law states that a practitioner may refuse to treat

September 3, 1994

Mr. Daniel Powers
12214 Harvard Road
Point Park, MI 48000

Dear Mr. Powers:

Our records indicate that you have failed to respond to six notices for periodontal maintenance care, sent over the two-year period from 1992 to 1994, requesting that you make an appointment for an examination and oral maintenance. Your lack of response to both mail and telephone messages suggests that you do not agree with our preventive philosophy. Thus, effective October 3, 1994, your relationship with this office is terminated. You will remain a patient in the practice for the next 30 days. Emergency treatment only will be provided during that 30-day period. I strongly suggest that you identify another oral healthcare provider. I shall be happy to forward a copy of your records once that practitioner is identified.

Mary L. Mesial, RDH, BS, PC

FIGURE 39–2
Letter of protection, terminating dental hygienist–client relationship.

an individual for any reason except race, creed, color, national origin, or certain condition, such as a handicap.

For example, a practice specializing in prosthodontic care may refuse to accept children as clients. As long as there is not a discriminatory reason such as ethnic origin, not accepting children as clients is legal. However, an office that fails to schedule individuals with Hispanic-sounding surnames, is discriminating based on national origin.

Dental hygienists should obtain information about the rules and regulations governing the care of clients within their state to avoid charges of discrimination. Different jurisdictions (states, commonwealths, provinces) have defined special groups that fall within certain statutory definitions relating to civil rights and discrimination. For example, in some states, persons with specific medically compromising conditions, such as HIV-infected persons, are protected by statutes related to the rights of the handicapped.

One can refuse to treat a client of record and not necessarily violate a contract obligation. A practitioner *should refuse* to treat a client if the practitioner does not have the skills or level of competence to provide the appropriate standard of care. The practitioner without the necessary skills is expected to refer the client to the appropriate oral health provider. Lawsuits have resulted from practitioners attempting to provide care that is beyond the practitioner's level of competence. Perhaps a dental hygienist evaluates the client's periodontal health and, although referral is indicated by the condition presented, the dentist chooses to provide treatment. If a certain skill level is required to provide the appropriate treatment (e.g., root planing and periodontal surgery) and those skills are not found within the personnel of that practice, the practitioner has failed to meet the obligation to refer. The referral is not viewed as a discriminatory practice, but rather is the appropriate action under contract principles.

Tort Principles

The legal basis most commonly used by clients to file suit against healthcare providers is the *negligence principle.* Negligence falls within the category of law known as torts. A **tort** is an interference with another's right to enjoy their person, property, or privacy.[6] The two categories of torts are intentional and unintentional. Intentional torts, as indicated by the title, are committed with intent on the part of the person. Intentional torts include battery, assault, false imprisonment, mental distress, breach of confidentiality, interference with property (e.g., trespass to land) and misrepresentation or deceit. Professional liability insurance frequently covers only the unintentional tort of negligence.

Intentional Torts

Intentional torts require that the person accused of the tort intended the harm that occurred. An intentional tort is a serious offense. It is difficult to discuss all the intentional torts in detail, however a few that are of interest to dental hygienists are highlighted.

An **assault** occurs when one intends to cause apprehension in someone, without touching them. An example of an assault may be threatening someone with a raised hand. A practitioner that threatens to harm someone, or causes fear, may be guilty of assault, such as in the example, "If you do not sit still, I am going to stick you with the needle."

A **battery** is a harmful or offensive contact with someone —touching someone without their permission. Examples in dental hygiene can include restraining a child without parental permission, placing dental sealants on teeth when consent was not obtained, or giving a fluoride treatment without the client's consent. In such cases, the person bringing the charges (plaintiff) argues that the contact was offensive, and the dental hygienist (defendant) could be charged with both assault and battery. Assault and battery are considered intentional torts and professional liability insurance may not provide coverage for charges filed under these categories. The dental hygienist should be cautious in all interactions with clients and obtain informed consent to prevent charges of assault and battery. (Informed consent is discussed later in the section.)

Deceit or misrepresentation can occur in the provision of oral healthcare. A failure to inform a client that an instrument tip has broken and is lodged in the sulcus is an example of deceit. A practitioner must always keep the client informed of his oral healthcare status and not misrepresent personnel or services rendered. If a dental hygienist is ill and is substituted by a dental assistant, there is an intent to misrepresent the dental assistant as a dental hygienist, and the employer is guilty of an intentional tort.

Another tort that could be classified as intentional is **breach of confidentiality.** A dental hygienist who violates the confidential relationship between the dental hygienist and client is committing a tort. For example, discussing a specific client's health history over lunch is inappropriate and a violation of confidentiality between the practitioner and client.

Unintentional Torts — Negligence

Unintentional torts, as indicated by their name, are *not* intended by the person accused of committing the tort. "Negligence" and "dental malpractice" are frequently used synonymously. It is important to become familiar with the more accurate terminology because understanding the more precise term and the criteria associated with the term may prevent negligent acts from occurring. **Negligence** is a failure of one owing a duty to another to do what a reasonable and prudent person would ordinarily have done under the circumstances. The characteristics of negligence are listed below.

- A duty or standard exists (e.g., health history taking; assessing blood pressure levels; assessing periodontal health, recording oral health status, referral)
- A breach or failure to exercise requisite care (e.g., failing to assess the patient, treat the patient; meet the standard of care for the practice of dental hygiene; incorrect use of anesthesia)
- A harm results (e.g., medical emergency; periodontal status declines; paresthesia)
- The harm is directly caused by the breach of duty

In the legal system, the plaintiff's responsibility is to prove that the defendant was negligent. The plaintiff must prove, by a preponderance of the evidence, all the elements listed above. For example, a dental hygienist is placing dental sealants on a child's teeth. The treatment area is a typical environment with the operator's supplies on the dental bracket tray. The supplies include a receptacle with acid etch material. The dental hygienist is etching the teeth while holding the acid etch–filled receptable. The child suddenly moves, the acid etch spills on the child, and a chemical burn occurs on the side of the child's face and neck. Has negligent behavior occurred? One would need to evaluate the elements of negligence to answer the question. The dental hygienist did not intend to burn the child; however, a duty existed to be cautious and careful while applying the acid etch. For the most part, the dental hygienist was practicing cautiously. However, the evidence may indicate that keeping the acid etch away from the child is recommended to avoid spilling. The dental hygienist failed to use certain precautionary measures (reasonably prudent man rule) and a harm resulted. The harm was proximately caused by the dental hygienist's actions, and thus the hygienist is found negligent by a judge or a jury. Again, the jury or judge would have to be only 51% sure that the dental hygienist's actions caused the harm. They may recognize that the child's actions influenced what occurred, but may still find the dental hygienist negligent.

Another example of negligent behavior could occur if a dental hygienist leaves infection control chemicals (like those used to clean out suction units) in a cup on a counter. If, when the dental hygienist is away from the treatment room, a client mistakes the liquid for water or mouthwash and drinks it, harm occurs although there was no intent to harm the client.

Standard of Care

An important aspect of a discussion of negligence is the standard of care. **Standard of care** is the degree of care a reasonably prudent person would exercise under the same or similar circumstances. The standard of care is not defined by the courts, but rather is determined by members of the profession. In negligence actions, in order to prove the standard of care and determine if the defendant is guilty or innocent, expert witnesses are called to testify. (Whether a lawyer may seek information from a professional association, such as ADHA's Standards of Practice, professional literature, or a nationally recognized group, such as the Centers for Disease Control and Prevention, as a source of acceptable standards.)

An expert witness is a member of the defendant's professional group with a similar background (e.g., in a periodontal malpractice lawsuit, a dental hygienist working in a periodontal practice). Lawyers for both the plaintiff and defendant may call into court expert witnesses that best satisfy their arguments. Thus, the dental hygienist, who may be defending specific actions, may identify an expert witness to support the standard of care demonstrated by that dental hygienist's practices. The plaintiff, on the other hand, has an expert witness testify that the dental hygienist did not meet the acceptable standard of care. The decision of guilt or innocence is left to the jurors and judge. Jurors, it should be noted, are primarily composed of non-healthcare providers. And, as indicated earlier, the level of proof required in civil actions is a preponderance of the evidence. After listening to the testimony of both the expert witnesses, the jurors must decide whether the plaintiff was or was not negligent. The dental hygienist is expected to meet the standard of care for the profession. Thus, if there is a failure to meet that standard, as determined by the jurors or a judge, the dental hygienist may be found negligent. For example, a dental hygienist fails to monitor and record a client's blood pressure prior to care. The client suffers a cardiac arrest during treatment related to high blood pressure. The standard of care for dental hygiene as outlined in the profession's standards of practice includes the skill of taking and recording the blood pressure as part of client assessment. This skill is and has been taught in dental hygiene educational programs for many years. The dental hygienist failed to meet the acceptable standard.

The failure to meet the standard of care can include either an act of omission, that is, not doing something, or an act of commission, performing an act inappropriately. Omitting a procedure or step because one is unaware that it is the current standard is not an acceptable excuse in a court of law. The changing dental hygiene practice environment requires a state-of-the-art knowledge base and competent skill level on the part of dental hygienists. Dental hygienists are obligated not only to seek continuing education but also to practice the concepts and techniques currently accepted.

If the standard of care for the local community is such that certain practices are occurring and the dental hygienist is not performing those tasks, the dental hygienist is negligent. At the same time, although the practice may not be one that is recognized by the local community, a national standard of care, in certain situations, must be considered and followed. The national versus the local standard conflict is apparent in examples concerning infection control or barrier techniques. Currently, the standard of care recommended by the Centers for Disease Control and Prevention and the ADA is for health professionals to use universal precautions for infection control during all dental procedures. However, dental practitioners in a local community may not follow the recommendations. Thus, a dental hygienist not utilizing the appropriate techniques is practicing, and perhaps meeting, a local standard, but not a national standard. If a negligent act occurs as a result of failing to use proper infection control procedures, the national standard may be the one that the dental hygienist is expected to meet.

Dental hygienists are licensed professionals and are expected to meet the appropriate standard of care. Although the dentist is ultimately responsible for the actions of the dental hygienist, the dental hygienist still may be found negligent in a court of law if a required duty is not met. The dental hygienist who provides care to a medically challenged person without the necessary antibiotic premedication or fails to treat a periodontally involved client with the appropriate services may be negligent. Typically, dental practitioners may be found negligent when harm is caused to the client as a result of failure to stay current. It is very difficult for any dental professional to accept a verdict of guilty of negligence because, as was noted earlier, there is no intent on the professional's part to practice inadequate dental hygiene care. However, members of the legal system attempt to evaluate the facts objectively; they evaluate the actions of the oral health practitioners and then assess the impact of those actions on the client. If harm occurs, practitioners of the legal system decide who is at fault and award damages, if appropriate.

Informed Consent

Another legal argument that falls within the negligence theory used by individuals in lawsuits brought against oral healthcare practitioners is lack of informed consent. **Informed consent** is a person's agreement to allow something to happen based on full disclosure of facts required to make an intelligent decision; **consent** is the individual's right to self-determination. As part of the consent process, clients must be informed of the material risks involved in care.

A material risk, as it is prescribed, is one that a "reasonable person" would consider in determining whether to proceed with the proposed treatment. Various court decisions have determined that the client has the final say in his care, must be of sound mind when giving consent, and the consent must be *informed* to be valid.[6]

To achieve informed consent in practice, clients must be told in a language that they understand:

- The nature and need for the procedure
- The benefits of the procedure
- The material risks in performing the procedure
- The prognosis if the procedure is performed or not performed
- The alternatives to the recommended procedure

In lawsuits that focus on the issue of informed consent, clients claim a lack of understanding of the risks involved in care, or that alternatives to treatment were not presented.

Consent can be documented using a standardized form that allows portions to be completed on a case-by-case basis (Fig. 39–3). Clients should sign the consent form. If care is modified or additional invasive procedures performed, consent should be obtained again.

Dental hygienists, depending on the jurisdiction, administer local anesthetics and nitrous oxide-oxygen analgesics, apply dental sealants, place restorative materials, and provide nonsurgical periodontal therapy that includes root planing and scaling. These and other procedures should be adequately explained to the recipient of care. Dental hygiene care includes some risks, as in the case of root planing using a local anesthetic which may result in a hematoma, parasthesia, and/or dentinal hypersensitivity. In addition to a separate form documenting consent, the fact that informed consent for such procedures was obtained should also be documented in the client record, in case the consent form is lost.

Documentation of refusal of care also is recommended. For example, the client may choose to refuse periodontal surgery and choose instead nonsurgical periodontal therapy followed by periodontal maintenance care every 3 months. The refusal and alternative should be clearly noted in the client's dental record. Moreover, specific explanations about the limitations of the alternative should be clearly outlined (Fig. 39–4).

In all documentation, one can develop a concise yet comprehensive manner of recordkeeping. It is suggested that office policy is developed so that informed consent is obtained in a consistent manner with all clients.

Informed consent can be a frightening experience for some clients. The dental hygienist must recognize that communication with the client is important, using the assumption that the information presented may assist the reasonable person to make an informed decision about care.

Dental hygienists must take the time to obtain informed consent and also allow the client an opportunity to ask questions. This opportunity to ask and have questions answered also must be documented in the client's record. Informed consent should be obtained for all surgical and invasive procedures as well as fluoride therapy, radiographs, and similar services.

Informed Refusal Against Dental Advice

A new risk of lawsuit, according to Pollack, occurs when the client refuses to follow the advice of the treating dentist

1. I consent to the recommended procedure or treatment ______________________________ to be completed by Dr. ____________.
2. The procedure(s) or treatment(s) have been described to me.
3. I have been informed of the purpose of the procedure or treatment.
4. I have been informed of the alternatives to the procedure or treatment.
5. I understand that the following risk(s) may result from the procedure or treatment: ______________________________.
6. I understand that the following risk(s) may occur if the procedure or treatment is not completed: ______________________________.
7. I do—do not—consent to the administration of anesthetic.
   a. I understand that the following risks are involved in administering anesthesia: ______________________________.
   b. The following alternatives to anesthesia were described: ______________________________.

All my questions have been satisfactorily answered.

Signature: ______________________________ Date

Representative: ______________________________ Date

Signature of Witness: ______________________________ Date

FIGURE 39–3
Consent form.

or dental hygienist.[7] A basic rule to follow when a client refuses advice is to inform the client of possible consequences. The rules follow those of obtaining informed consent to care. They include that the client be told in understandable language:

- The recommendation
- The reasons for the recommendation
- Risks to client's oral and general health

There must be discussion about the refusal and the effects as well as an opportunity to discuss the recommendation. An **informed refusal** form should be developed that includes the recommendation, a list of the consequences of refusal, a place for the date, signatures of the dentist, client, and a witness. A copy should be given to the client.

Statute of Limitations

The **statute of limitations** is the length of time an aggrieved person has to enter lawsuits against another for an alleged injury.[6] A statute of limitations places a time limit on a contract or tort action. Once the time period has ended, the lawsuit cannot be filed. For example, the statute of limitations for a contract action may be 3 years and a tort action 6 years. In some states, the statute of limitations starts either at the time an injury occurs or at the time the plaintiff discovers the injury. This ability to sue when an injury is discovered expands the length of time that someone can file a lawsuit. Perhaps a client is diagnosed with severe periodontal diseases 5 years after ending a client-provider relationship. The client still may be allowed to file a lawsuit. The risk constantly exists for a lawsuit to be filed. It is imperative that practitioners be aware of the statute of limitations and the rules governing this area within their state to assist in planning for recordkeeping and record storage.

Legal Concepts and the Dental Hygienist-Client Relationship

Dental hygiene practice focuses on the clients' comprehensive care. The dental hygienist must provide care within the scope of practice as defined by the State/Provincial Dental or Dental Hygiene Practice Act. Based on the legal principles previously discussed, the dental hygienist also must

Date	Progress Notes
8-1-94	Care plan suggests periodontal surgery. Explained justification for surgery, risks, and alternative of three-month maintenance care, with reevaluation of need for surgery; client opted for three-month maintenance care. Client states that she understands three-month regimen must be strictly followed. Explained limitations of maintenance care versus surgery. Client asked questions about procedures at maintenance appointment.
	I, Mary Gorski, refuse periodontal surgery as recommended by M. Mesial. I opt to cooperate in a three-month maintenance care appointment program for a nine-month period. The risks, benefits, and reasons for both treatment alternatives have been adequately explained, and my questions answered.

FIGURE 39–4
Progress notes.

fulfill legal duties and meet the standard of care in assessing, planning, implementing, and evaluating client care.

Confidentiality

The dental hygienist-client relationship raises additional areas of concern that extend the legal duties and obligations outlined. A client's care is confidential. Client data collected is confidential. To release confidential information without the permission of the client is an invasion of privacy. Examples of invasion of privacy include releasing client information to an unauthorized person, such as an employer, or discussing a client's health history outside the scope of treatment. Both violate the confidentiality between the healthcare provider and the client.

A person can waive confidentiality through words or actions. For example, an individual who is referred to a specialist waives confidentiality. The referring practitioner is expected to inform the specialist of the client's status. Or confidentiality can be waived by action of law, such as a requirement to report specific communicable diseases or the suspicion of child abuse to a state or provincial agency. A client's waiver of confidentiality should be documented in a progress note or separate form entitled Waiver of Confidentiality (Fig. 39–5).

Defamation

A communication that injures an individual's reputation may be libel **(written defamation)** or slander **(verbal defamation).** To be libelous or slanderous, the defamatory comment must not be true. However, if an individual's reputation is not harmed by the defamatory comment, there is no libel or slander. In certain defamation cases, malice (intent to inflict an injury) must be shown. If a lawsuit is filed, the plaintiff must show actual damages to property, business, trade, profession, occupation, or feeling. Thus, an informal comment to one person about an "incompetent dentist" by a recently fired dental hygienist would not be considered slander. The dentist's reputation was not harmed and those listening would consider the source and not necessarily believe the comment. Repeated comments by a dental hygienist in a periodontal practice stating that one periodontist is more skilled than another may result in a lawsuit, if the comments harm the dentist's reputation or influence clients' return to the practice.

I, ____________________, hereby grant permission
(Print Name)

to ______________________________
(Print Name of Doctor or Hospital)

to release information related to my health history, status, and care, and copies of my health record, radiographs, and any test results to:

____

at ______________________________

______________________________.

Signature: ______________________________
Date
(If a Minor, Parent or Guardian Must Sign)

FIGURE 39–5
Request for release of health information.

Legal Concepts and the Dental Hygienist-Dentist Relationship

Laws affect the dental hygienist-dentist relationship on multiple levels.

Discrimination in Employment

Federal and state regulations exist to govern the employer-employee relationship. In seeking employment, an individual is protected against unlawful discriminatory practices. Federal and state labor laws exist to protect both employers and employees. A federal statute, Title VII of the Civil Rights Act of 1969, prohibits **discrimination** based on race, color, religion, sex, or national origin as it relates to hiring, firing, terms, conditions, or privileges of employment. Sex discrimination includes discrimination based on pregnancy, childbirth, and related medical conditions such as gynecological or gender-related problems. Title VII applies to employers with 15 or more employees. However, human rights acts enacted in almost all states outlaw the same type of discriminatory activity and may affect employers with as few as one employee. State laws may also expand the types of discrimination banned (e.g., discrimination based on marital status, physical handicap, or sexual orientation). The Age Discrimination in Employment Act (ADEA) affects employers with 20 or more employees. The act states that discrimination on the basis of age between 40 and 70 is not allowed.

The Equal Employment Opportunity Commission (EEOC) deals with discrimination on any of the federally prohibited grounds. In some instances, the EEOC assists by investigating or advising on appropriate agencies to contact. There are strict guidelines dealing with timeliness of the complaint, such as a requirement to bring a complaint within 180 days. If the EEOC is unable to obtain a solution, an individual may have the right to file a lawsuit.

Dental hygienists who believe they have been discriminated against in the employment setting should contact their state civil rights agency.

Pregnancy and Employment Status

Because a significant percentage of dental hygienists are female, discrimination based on pregnancy is an important issue for dental hygienists. Federal law prohibits an employer from terminating or refusing to hire or promote a woman because she is pregnant. The EEOC is the agency that administers Title VII provisions. Guidelines distributed by the EEOC state that disabilities caused or contributed to by pregnancy or childbirth must be treated like any other disability. Mandatory leave arbitrarily set at a specific time for pregnant women without regard to their ability to work is also prohibited. Dental hygienists, in order to be informed and assist their employers, should obtain information from a local department of human rights if a maternity leave is anticipated.

Employer-Employee Relationships

Seeking employment is a common occurrence. The core of an employment application can include:

- Identification of the applicant (e.g., name, address, telephone number)
- Applicant's interests (jobs, salary levels)
- Summary of applicant's background including education, work history, and skills

A dental hygienist should be aware of both the rights and obligations of the potential employer and job candidate. Specific questions that are classified as unlawful preemployment inquiries are listed below:

- Applicant's maiden name
- Birthplace of applicant
- Age or date of birth (may ask if 18 years or older)
- Religious denomination or affiliation
- Complexion or skin color
- Photograph required
- Height, weight
- Marital status or children
- Arrests
- National origin
- Society or club memberships

One need not provide the information that falls within the unlawful category. Individual states also may have legislation that regulates employment. An excellent resource is a state department of civil rights or related agencies.

Unlike some employer-employee relationships, the dental hygienist rarely has a written contract for employment purposes. Traditionally, responsibilities of employment, financial arrangements, benefits, and length of employment are verbally agreed upon. The lack of a written agreement may leave the dental hygienist in a precarious situation. A written contract assists the dental hygienist and employer in clearly defining the relationship that exists. The contract is written documentation that clearly outlines the rights and responsibilities of the parties involved. Frequently, dentist-employers are not used to a written agreement between the dentist and the dental hygienist. A dental hygienist-employee needs to assist an employer so that a complete and fair contract is drafted. Categories that may be addressed are listed below. (The ADHA provides a sample employment contract to its members.)

- Position title and responsibilities
- Schedule days and hours of the week
- Remuneration
  - Amount
  - Pay period schedule
  - Benefits to be deducted
  - Manner remuneration will be calculated—commission, hourly, daily
- Schedules of review/evaluation
  - Influence on remuneration
  - Method of evaluation: formal/informal
- Fringe benefits
- Notification requirements for contract severance
- Specific expectations

In most jurisdictions, the dental hygienist works as an employee with the dentist. The law views this as a basic employer-employee relationship. In this type of relationship, there is direct control and supervision of the employee by the employer. The doctrine governing the relationship is **respondeat superior,** Latin for "let the superior/master answer." Based on the traditional structure of most state dental practice acts, the dentist-employer answers for the actions of the dental hygienist. It is important to note that the dental hygienist, as a licensed professional, is legally accountable and can be sued. However, because

IRS GUIDEPOSTS FOR INDEPENDENT CONTRACTORS

- Instructions—when, where, and how work is performed
- Training—requiring the worker to work with experienced employees, corresponding with the worker, requiring the worker to attend meetings or use other methods
- Integration—of the worker's services into business operations
- Services rendered personally—if services must be rendered personally, it is presumed the persons for whom services are performed are interested in methods used
- Hiring, supervising, and paying assistants—if the persons for whom services are performed hire assistants, that generally shows control; the reverse is also true
- Continuing relationship
- Set hours of work
- Full-time standard—if the worker performs full-time and restricts the employee from performing other work
- Doing work on the employer's premises—suggests control over the worker, especially if the work could be done elsewhere
- Order of sequence set—if the worker must follow a sequence set out by the entity for whom he is performing the services, this would indicate employer-employee relationship
- Oral or written reports—written reports indicate control
- Payment by hour, week, month—indicates employer-employee relationship; payment by job indicates independent contractor relationship
- Payment of business and/or travel expenses—if the person for whom services are performed pays for travel expenses, this generally indicates employer-employee relationship
- Furnishing of tools or material—by person for whom work is performed indicates employer-employee relationship
- Significant investment—lack of investment in facilities indicates employer-employee relationship
- Realization of profit or loss—by worker would indicate independent contractor; but the worker who cannot is generally considered an employee
- Working for more than one firm—if the worker performs work for more than one firm–unrelated–that generally indicates the worker is an independent contractor
- Making service available to the general public—on a regular basis indicates an independent contractor
- Right to discharge—indicates employer-employee relationship
- Right to terminate—by the employee without incurring liability, indicates employer-employee relationship

of the doctrine of respondeat superior, dentists are also named in lawsuits filed against dental hygienists. Including the dentist as one of the parties of a lawsuit is a reflection of the "deep pocket" theory. That is, the monetary damages sought can be increased because of the larger malpractice insurance coverage of the dentist-employer.

Another business relationship with the employer-dentist that may exist for the dental hygienist is that of an **independent contractor.** As an independent contractor, the dental hygienist is under contract to fulfill certain responsibilities, but has little guidance by the contracting party. The Internal Revenue Service has specific requirements to distinguish whether a person is an independent contractor or employee as it relates to federal taxes (see IRS Guideposts for Independent Contractors chart). The criteria include 20 different points to consider in determining the status of a worker. The key in reviewing the points is the control by the respective parties in the relationship and the substance of the relationship over form.

The independent contractor, in a sense, is self-employed. With the increased freedom of independent contracting, there is also an increased liability and total responsibility for income and social security taxes. An individual interested in an independent contracting agreement should investigate the area within the jurisdiction and seek legal advice.

Sexual Harassment

Over 10 years ago, the EEOC established sexual harassment as unlawful. Federal guidelines classify sexual harassment as a form of sexual discrimination. **Sexual harassment** is defined as sexual discrimination because it forces a female or male to work under adverse employment conditions. The EEOC defines sexual harassment as:

> Unwelcome sexual advances, requests for sexual favors and other verbal or physical conduct of a sexual nature when submission to such conduct is made either explicitly or implicitly a term or condition of an individual's employment; submission to or rejection of such conduct by an individual is used as the basis for employment decisions affecting the individual; or such conduct has the purpose or effect of unreasonably interfering with an individual's work performance or creating an intimidating, hostile or offensive working environment. (Fed. Reg., 1980)

Two types of sexual harassment occur. The first involves a superior-subordinate relationship in which the offender has control over the working conditions of the victim. Examples of sexual harassment include demands for sexual favors in exchange for better working conditions or reviews, raises, or promotions. A second form of sexual harassment is environmental. Examples may include unwelcome, demeaning verbal or physical conduct of a sexual nature creating a hostile, intimidating, or offensive work environment. The environment may interfere with the ability of the harassed employee to do the job; however, there is no tangible employment loss evident. Supervisors, co-workers, or nonemployees may be involved. Environmental sexual harassment is difficult to identify or control.[8]

Sexual harassment does occur in the dental practice environment. A dental hygienist reported that every time she asked for a dentist "to check" a client following a dental hygiene appointment, the dentist asked the dental hygienist to perform a sexual act. The dental hygienist became flustered and embarrassed and did not want to work alone with the dentist. Although the request for sexual favors was not related to salary or employee evaluation, it easily could have developed into that type of situation. The dentist's actions constitute sexual harassment. A second example may be a client who makes inappropriate remarks or gestures of a sexual nature. Clients, who are considered nonemployees, influence the environment in which a dental hygienist is employed. A dental hygienist should report the behavior of the client to the employer. The employer is obligated to make the working environment nonthreatening.

The EEOC requires that sexual harassment not occur in the workplace. An employer is required to maintain a professional, businesslike relationship among employees and prevent or stop all situations considered harassment. If an individual has been the victim of sexual harassment, immediate action is necessary. One should never be passive. An employee's response to either physical or verbal harassment must be prompt, serious, specific, and assertive. If faced with sexual harassment, one should:[9]

- Speak to the offender immediately indicating that the actions of the offender have created an uncomfortable environment
- Indicate to the offender that the statements or actions are absolutely improper
- Keep accurate notes of what was said, done, date, time, places, and witnesses, if any
- Talk to co-workers; determine whether there have been similar experiences shared by others
- If a refusal may affect the job, report the incident to a co-owner of the practice or appropriate supervisory personnel

Data from Gervasi, R. Sexual harassment and the politics of power. Dental Assistant 53:30, 1984.

If the situation is not remedied, several options exist. In practice settings that employ 15 or more employees, the district office of the EEOC is contacted. If there are fewer than 15 employees, there may be assistance available from a state agency such as the State Department of Civil Rights. Although hiring a lawyer may not be necessary, legal representation is helpful to guide the victim and represent the victim if the case progresses. The district EEOC office should be contacted as a source of information.

Termination of Employment

Based on the nature of dental hygiene employment, dental hygienists may have their employment terminated for little or no reason, defined as "at will." The small business atmosphere of dental practice allows the "at will termination" by either party to exist. However, certain states have developed legal remedies for those individuals wrongfully terminated. This area of the law is constantly evolving and changing. Some jurisdictions, for example, have laws that allow employers to terminate employees for good cause, that is, someone can lose his position with or without a reason or justification. A dental hygienist should be familiar with the state's policy on termination. Various states have developed criteria that must be met to prove either appropriate or inappropriate employer behavior. The termination process can also be outlined in a contract (e.g., termination requiring 2-week written notice). Based on the "at will" termination process, notice of termination is a courtesy but not a requirement to end employment.

Risk Management

A **risk management** program for an oral healthcare setting is recommended to assist dental staff to identify the following:[10]

- Potential risks
- Risk measurement
- Risk handling and treatment

The dental risk management consultant performs a comprehensive evaluation to determine areas of high risk within the dental practice setting. Much of the risk management materials focus on healthcare facilities such as hospitals. However, the principles apply to the oral healthcare environment. Kraus suggests potential exposure areas as:[11]

- Liability associated with professional performances of the staff
- General liability exposures for injuries to clients, guests, visitors, and others
- Property and casualty exposures associated with the office, building, and equipment
- Exposure to defamation actions among staff, office managers, and other personnel
- Exposure to financial losses in the business office through embezzlement and theft
- Exposure to contracts, warranties, and similar actions associated with the purchase and use of goods and services
- Fraud and abuse exposure associated with federal and state third-party reimbursement programs
- Exposure to losses associated with staff hiring, promotions, and termination practices

Data modified from Kraus, G. P. Health Care Risk Management. Owings Mills, Maryland: Rynd Communications, 1986.

Boyce adopts the list proposed by Kraus and adds the following checklist:[10]

- Is the health/dental history updated at every appointment?
- Does the staff fully document crucial data or conversations (e.g., "4-4-94 Generalized advanced periodontal disease with 7–9 mm pockets. Client has been advised of the condition, but refused recommended treatment. J. Schade-Boyce, RDH")?
- Does the office have a medical emergency procedure and has the procedure been rehearsed?
- Are the staff cardiopulmonary resuscitation (CPR) and first aid qualified?
- Is there a medical emergency kit available and are the drugs in it kept current?
- Is the staff practicing the latest infection control procedures according to Occupational Safety and Health Administration (OSHA) guidelines?
- Is the staff familiar with the uses of major equipment in the office (e.g., automatic processor, panoramic radiology, low- and high-speed handpieces, intravenous equipment, and autoclaves)?
- Are broken toys or sharp objects removed promptly from the reception area?
- Are the sidewalks, parking lots, or driveways clear of any debris (e.g., nails, glass, or ice)?
- Are the handicapped ramps operable?

Boyce's checklist provides a valuable introduction to concepts about risk management. Dental hygienists must consider risk management an integral part of their practice philosophy to protect themselves, their clients, and their colleagues.

Common themes appear in the risk management literature and workshops. The concepts consistently include: recordkeeping, informed consent, and staff credentials. These areas and other risk management issues are discussed to provide a framework for risk management.

Communication

Dental hygienists have long recognized the importance of good communication and its contribution to successful client management and care. Communication is important as a risk management tool. Communication is important on three levels:

- Dental hygienist-client
- Dental hygienist-employer
- Dental hygienist-colleagues

Dental Hygienist-Client Open communication between the dental hygienist and client minimizes misunderstandings, reducing the likelihood of lawsuits, and allowing for the direct and timely resolution of problems. A dental hygienist who spends 45 to 60 minutes in a one-on-one relationship with a client can reduce the potential of negligent actions. The one-on-one relationship with clients gives the dental hygienist an opportunity to explain the care that will occur and answer client questions.

Dental hygienists, through communication, can recognize problems early on and work to resolve them before they escalate. A client who senses a professional interest and expertise on the part of the dental hygienist may not be as prone to file a lawsuit if a procedure is unsuccessful. The client is knowledgeable that the dental hygienist conducted herself in the best manner possible and provided a reasonable level of care.

Dental Hygienist-Employer The dental hygienist can play a key role educating employers about the potential liabilities for dental hygienists and the preventive steps that can be applied to practice. Establishing standards for office protocol can be coordinated by the dental hygienist in conjunction with the employer. Maintaining a resource library that includes updated literature, textbooks and other related material, such as a current copy of the rules and regulations outlining the rights and responsibilities of licensed office staff, provides a quick resource if questions arise. Risk management for all staff members in any work environment contributes to long-term success. If a risk management philosophy is practiced and reinforced by the employees and the employer, legal risks are reduced for the entire staff.

Dental Hygienist-Colleagues The best resources for the development of a risk management philosophy are the personnel within the employment setting. Dental hygienists who are employed in the same setting can identify areas of vulnerability and solutions to reduce vulnerability. Consistent criteria for recordkeeping and referral can be developed; current scientific literature to support particular treatment modalities can be shared; office protocols and handbooks can be developed. Each activity contributes to improved practice habits. It is suggested that the dental hygienists employed in similar settings meet for a risk management day. The purpose of the meeting is to identify areas of potential risk and develop mechanisms to reduce that risk. Suggested activities are to:

- Brainstorm to identify risks in the practice of dental hygiene; these can include treatment techniques, client management, recordkeeping, communication, and preventive practices
- Have each dental hygienist review the plan of care for a client; write down the key steps followed by the dental hygienist
- Sample client records and review recordkeeping styles, abbreviations, charting records, informed consent, and other written aspects of care
- Discuss additional risky practices that have become apparent
- Develop a consensus that focuses on reducing risky behaviors and can be comfortably incorporated by all on a consistent basis; areas to consider include procedures for client care, charting techniques, abbreviations, referral guidelines, periodontal and other preventive therapies
- Develop a dental hygiene office manual, which can be a separate manual or incorporated as a component of a larger manual. The dental hygiene portion can focus on the dental hygiene staff, client assessment, treatment and evaluation, insurance information, risk management suggestions, recordkeeping protocol, standardized periodontal assessment and charting guidelines, and premedication information. Once consensus occurs, chapters can be delegated and written. The manual serves as a guidebook for what and whom. The office manual assists current employees and future employees. The manual is also helpful to other office staff and dentists
- Propose a similar risk management workshop for the dentists and assistants on staff

Dental Record

As outlined earlier, the **dental record** is important in risk management and can be a provider's best defense or worst enemy in a malpractice action. The dental record provides the following:

- Complete record of both the health and dental status at the time of the initial examination
- Comprehensive and chronological documentation of treatment provided
- Potential legal document on the client's behalf (e.g., use in corpse identification or insurance claims or fraud)
- Legal document for the defense of litigious claims against a dental practitioner
- Records as required in some states as part of the laws regulating professional practice
- Tool for quality assessment and assurance
- Communication mechanism among health professionals involved in the client's care

The practice of recordkeeping characterized by one-line notations, no signatures or date, and limited treatment entries are no longer acceptable. Excuses that documentation is time-consuming, contributes to a lengthy chart, or is not necessary are risk management liabilities. Documentation begins with initial client contact and continues throughout the relationship between the provider and the client, including reasons for terminating the relationship, if that occurs.

Identification Via Client Data

Client identification data are standard information such as name, address, telephone number, emergency contact person, legal guardian, physician of record, and insurance-related information. Practices have grown larger, client numbers have increased, and client populations reflect multicultural backgrounds. Inaccurate client data make it difficult to identify a record that may be critical in a lawsuit. A poorly kept record reflects on the oral healthcare provider. There may be an assumption that sloppy records reflect sloppy care.

Information about a client may change frequently so periodic updating should be routine. Updated material should be dated. A client's photograph, as part of the record, has been recommended for identification purposes.

Health and Dental History

There are significant variations in the forms used for health and dental history taking. Initial data collected serves as baseline information about the client. All health and dental history information should be pursued and answered. If an item on the history form is not appropriate, it should be indicated "NA" (not applicable). If the condition is normal, a notation such as "WNL" (within normal limits) is appropriate. Every question should be asked and some notation recorded.

Pollack reports that malpractice actions have occurred because of faulty history taking.[7] Errors commonly associated with the health history process include:

- Failure to discover potential drug incompatibility
- Failure to learn of drug allergy or potential drug allergy
- Failure to discover a medical condition that may result in serious injury to the client because of dental treatment, bleeding and healing problems

He also notes that errors associated with oral health problems include:[7]

- Failure to determine that a client presented with a history of temporomandibular joint dysfunction
- Failure to discover that a client exhibited a reaction to a local anesthetic
- Failure to discover problems associated with periodontal disease

Modified from Pollack, B. R. Dentist's Risk Management Guide. Ft. Lauderdale, FL: National Society of Dental Practitioners, 1990.

One needs to document the individuals involved in each step of the history-taking process. For example, the individuals identified should include names of those who completed the health history with the client, who reviewed the history with the client (if not the dentist or dental hygienist), and dates and signatures for each step.

Assessment data should be recorded in a consistent manner. A comprehensive initial charting of assessment data assists in evaluating the client's progress throughout care. For example, a client initially presents to the office with moderate periodontitis. If the condition does not improve, the practitioner has a record of the condition from the moment care began. Thus, the dentist or dental hygienist cannot be accused of contributing to the client's condition.

Treatment Information

Records of the care provided should be characterized by conciseness, accuracy, clarity, and comprehensiveness. Chart entries should include:

- Nature of the care provided
- Area where care is provided
- Type and dosage of anesthetic and/or analgesia used
- Details about conditions presented, gingival health, oral hygiene status, specific areas of change
- Language that is specific (e.g., a notation such as "some deep pockets in the posterior" provides little definitive information)
- Details of conditions during treatment such as hematomas, excessive bleeding
- Specific recommendations for postoperative instructions
- Medication prescribed or administered and dosages
- Client education conducted
- Continued care or maintenance schedule

All procedures, such as radiographs or dental sealant application, must be documented. Each client has one dental hygienist and remembers each visit. Each dental hygienist has a large clientele and needs to record information that may be required in future litigation. Cancellations, late arrivals, change of appointments, and conversations with front desk personnel should be documented. The record is a vital document and should be treated as such.

The record should reflect objective information; subjective information should be included only if it affects client care, for example, writing "Client was very apprehensive and asked many questions during the procedure," rather than "Client was a bother and questioned everything." A record must be maintained in a professional manner. It is advisable not to comment on client or guardian personalities or characteristics, such as "Mom is very protective."

The record can assist in the defense against a charge of breach of contract, negligence, or lack of informed consent. The lawyer for the plaintiff who reviews a thorough, complete record may determine that there is no reason to pursue a lawsuit. The record may clearly indicate that the practitioner has met all obligations and caused no harm. An incomplete or inaccurate record under close scrutiny provides multiple opportunities for the plaintiff's lawyer to prove inadequate or negligent care.

In managing client records, Pollack suggests the following:[7]

- Entries should be legible, written in black ink or ballpoint pen
- When there is more than one person making entries, entries should be signed or initialed
- When errors occur, they should not be blocked out so that they cannot be read. Instead, a single line should be drawn through the entry, and a note made above it stating "error in entry, see correction below." The correction should be dated at the time it is made
- Financial information should not be kept on the treatment record
- Entries should be uniformly spaced on the form. There should be no unusual or irregular blank spaces
- On health information forms, there should be no blank spaces in the answers to health questions. If the question is inappropriate, a single line is drawn through the question, or "not applicable" (NA) recorded in the box. If the response is normal, a "within normal limits" (WNL) notation is made
- All cancellations, late arrivals, and change of appointments are recorded
- Consents are documented including all risks and alternative treatments presented to the client, remarks made by the client
- The client is informed of any adverse occurrences or untoward events that take place during the course of care; a note on the record that the client was informed is necessary
- All requests for consultations and responses are recorded
- All conversations held with other health practitioners relating to the care of the client are documented
- All client records should be retained for at least the period of the statute of limitations equal to that of contract actions. In most jurisdictions it is 6 years. In the case of minors, it is until the person reaches the age of 24 years. Check for special laws in your local jurisdiction. If at all possible, *keep records forever*
- No subjective evaluations, such as an opinion about the client's mental health should be recorded on the treatment record unless the writer is qualified and licensed to make such evaluations
- Confidentiality of information contained on the record should be guarded
- The original record should not be surrendered to anyone, except by order of a court
- A record should never be altered once there is some indication that legal action is contemplated by the patient
- Heirs are instructed that they must retain the records of clients and comply with any written request for a copy

Modified from Pollack, B. R. Dentist's Risk Management Guide. Ft. Lauderdale, FL: National Society of Dental Practitioners, 1990.

Legal Issues Relevant to the Various Roles of the Dental Hygienist

Legal theories, such as contract and tort principles, are applicable to the roles of dental hygienists as practitioners, educators, administrators, consumer advocates, change agents, and researchers. The following discussion highlights specific areas of concern for individual roles.

Dependent Practitioner

Under the theory of respondeat superior, the dentist is ultimately responsible for the actions of the staff. In reviewing dental malpractice cases, the dentist is frequently named as the defendant in a dental malpractice lawsuit. However, members of the legal system recognize that a dental hygienist is a licensed professional responsible for client care as well as for the effects of professional actions and decisions.

The status of a dependent practitioner may be somewhat misleading. An individual is dependent as a result of the licensing and regulation laws of the state. However, the individual is not dependent on the employer to assume legal responsibility for one's action. The dependent practitioner is providing client care. Based on the educational background and licensed status, the dental hygienist has professional obligations and legal duties that must be fulfilled. Failure to fulfill specific legal duties may result in charges of negligence (malpractice). Each phase of client care has with it inherent responsibilities.

Knowledge of legal theories is useful in planning and providing client care. A dental hygienist may be charged with negligence if a breach of a duty occurs and harm results. One can omit a service resulting in negligence, such as assessing a client's blood pressure. A practitioner can also commit a negligent act, such as harming a client with an instrument or using hand-over-mouth technique practices to discourage inappropriate behavior in children. In any situation, the duty or standard of care expected is evaluated. A conflict arises when the dental hygienist cannot provide care at an acceptable standard. For example, an individual presents with a periodontal condition that requires four 1-hour appointments to adequately root plane and scale, followed by an appointment for reevaluation. The care planning philosophy of the dentist is to allow two appointments. The dental hygienist may fail to adequately treat the client in two appointments and may contribute to a declining periodontal status. The issue of the standard of care for the dental hygienist is addressed during the lawsuit. Thus, the dental hygienist is liable for professional actions taken.

Independent Practitioner

A subset of roles exists in independent dental hygiene practitioner status (e.g., care provider, business owner, and employer). As an independent practitioner, a hygienist is responsible for all the legal principles that influence client care, including negligence, referral, abandonment, and informed consent. An independent practitioner also is an employer and is responsible for knowledge of labor and employment laws, discrimination issues, tax principles, and related business obligations. Assessing and minimizing risks contributes to long-term success in practice.

An independent practitioner is advised to seek legal and business assistance for some of the following items. Contracts and other related agreements are necessary to a business owner and must be drafted, negotiated, and signed. Employer-employee relationships and office protocols must be developed and guidelines established. An independent practitioner is the owner of a business, and functioning as such requires managerial skills outside the realm of client care (e.g., building and equipment maintenance, material and human resources management, and strategic planning). State and federal laws affect many aspects of the business including hiring, firing, and evaluating personnel. Other laws affect the physical plant, such as incorporating barrier-free access or equipment selection and maintenance, as in OSHA guidelines.

The financial commitment to the practice is a significant one. Thus, protecting personal assets, as well as keeping personal and professional expenses separate, must be managed carefully. Separate accounts are advisable for ease of bookkeeping. In addition, separation of personal and professional assets is important so that personal assets cannot be taken if the business is affected by either financial or legal problems. An independent practitioner is responsible for policies and procedures used, quality of care provided, documentation, and the actions of employees. Given the litigious environment affecting dentistry and dental hygiene, in some instances, the independent practitioner is carefully and constantly scrutinized by those seeking to find errors or illegal activities. Thus, personally and professionally, the independent practitioner should be well versed in all the legal issues that can affect the dental hygienist. A clear understanding of the laws governing dental hygiene practice is imperative.

Independent Contractor

The independent contractor has an added dimension to dental hygiene practice. The legal principles take on broader implications. The independent contractor must recognize the contractual responsibilities inherent in both the business and professional relationships. The dental hygienist is contracting to provide services. Both parties in the relationship, the dental hygienist and the contracting party, have specific rights and responsibilities. For example, the dental hygienist assumes that the contracting party will pay a salary, and provide certain facilities and support staff. Failure to fulfill specific obligations of a contract is a breach or breaking of the contract. Dental hygienists should seek legal counsel prior to any commitment as an independent contractor. Issues such as labor laws, income tax and social security taxes, as well as liability issues are additional and important considerations. The independent contractor and practitioner must also remain cognizant of the legal issues affecting client care such as negligence, informed consent, referral, abandonment, and recordkeeping.

The dental hygienist, as an independent contractor, must view practice with a strong risk management philosophy. One must view the other party in the contract relationship—the dentist or dental practice—critically. A dental hygienist need not be put at risk because of the poor quality of care provided by someone else. Thus, during the interview process, prior to establishing a relationship, the dental hygienist should evaluate the employer in terms of potentially negligent activities, referral philosophies, infection control, and recordkeeping, to name a few. A working relationship that is based on a mutually agreed upon understanding that minimizes risks is important and protects both parties. Reviewing client records to observe how client care is managed may assist a dental hygienist in deciding whether to contract with a specific care provider.

Dissolution of the contract relationship after a preliminary period of time should be addressed as part of the initial negotiations. Rights and responsibilities of all parties should be clearly outlined so that the working relationship is defined. At the same time, the reasons and methods for ending the relationship also must be reviewed and agreed upon, such as reasons to dissolve and notice requirements.

Independent contracting requires careful scrutiny of tax laws and definitions of the independent contracting status. Legal counsel is suggested and should be contacted prior to committing to any relationship.

Educator

The roles of an educator include, and may not be limited to, mentor, manager, counselor, teacher, clinical supervisor, administrator, oral hygiene care provider, scholar, and researcher. The legal principles discussed can be applied to all levels of responsibility.

An educator has contact both with colleagues and students. Confidentiality, an obligation not to violate confidences shared, is one aspect of the relationships developed in an educational setting. In today's society, issues that must remain confidential have become more difficult to define. Educators are grappling with issues such as the student who confides a high-risk lifestyle for contracting AIDS, or a colleague who has had a positive HIV test. Institutions of higher education are developing policies to address such situations, but state and local laws may also address topics such as the students' rights and health issues. Discrimination may also be an issue in the educator-student or educator-colleague relationship. Educators must be certain that decisions affecting admission, hiring, clinical assignments, workload, promotion, and evaluation are not influenced by actions that are considered discriminatory. Informal comments previously made about an individual or group of individuals may resurface if allegations of discrimination occur. Clearly outlined policies for personnel hiring and management and student admission and continuance may assist in decreasing potentially discriminatory practices.

The educator who serves as a clinical instructor must recognize that the legal principles affecting client care apply to clinical education. Informed consent, standard of care, confidentiality, referral policies, and contract and tort duties must be purposefully applied. Clinical faculty members ultimately are liable for a student's actions. Thus, client interactions and care should be carefully monitored. Client information written by a student and co-signed by a faculty member should be read critically to assure accuracy and completeness. Student-faculty interactions in a clinical setting must be free of bias or potentially discriminatory practices. Similar issues apply to the educator who also may provide clinical care as part of an in-house faculty practice. Policies to prevent charges of abandonment must be developed and implemented. Careful documentation of client care, referral, and dismissal with standardized language may serve as a guideline for the faculty and assure consistency within the institution.

An educator may be involved in personnel supervision of clerical and clinical staff. Employee rights such as contractual responsibilities, employee evaluation, and dismissals involve legal issues. Again, the educator must consider written documentation, discriminatory practices, civil rights issues, and issues within the area of labor law and employer-employee relationships.

The educator also works with administrators. Issues such as the educator's contractual rights, civil rights, and related topics should be understood, and if an issue arises, legal counsel may be sought. Failure on the part of an institution to recognize specific rights may lead to a legal solution. Promotion and tenure, salary issues, and job descriptions and responsibilities have a legal component. Educators, like students and practitioners, must apply legal principles to control the risks involved when fulfilling the many roles within the profession of dental hygiene.

Educators also may be involved in research. The legal issues relevant to the role of a researcher are addressed later in this section.

Administrator/Manager

The administrator/manager works with individuals both on a colleague level and in an employer-employee relationship. The administrator/manager is involved, in many instances, in hiring, evaluating, and possibly dismissing colleagues or employees. Knowledge of federal and state laws affecting civil rights and sexual harassment, and the protection of those rights, is important policy to know and follow. Administrators must recognize that specific questions cannot be asked as part of an employment interview. Evaluation of an employee should be completed carefully and documented. In some instances, dismissal of an employee can occur only after a series of evaluations, warnings, and in some instances, counseling, is completed.

An administrator/manager has a responsibility to guide and educate. Again, colleagues who make discriminatory remarks, exhibit sexual misconduct, or conduct themselves inappropriately reflect on the administrator's ability to manage effectively.

Contracts are a common part of an administrator/manager's life. A contract, the agreement between two consenting parties, reflects certain rights and responsibilities. All parties involved require a clear understanding of the rights and responsibilities delineated in the contract. Failure to understand the contract may lead to charges of a breach of contract based on the failure to fulfill a responsibility. For example, if a breach of contract occurs, there may be financial ramifications. If an employee is inappropriately dismissed without due process of the law, the court may require that the employer be responsible for fulfilling the salary terms of the contract. Thus, although the employee is gone, the employer is still obligated under law to pay salary and benefits.

The administrator/manager may be responsible for assuring the safety of an employee from the tortious acts of another, for example, a responsibility to protect an employee from a client or student who may commit an assault or battery. In addition, a responsibility exists to prevent negligence in maintenance of the physical plant such as faulty steps, icy or wet entrances, or other dangerous situations.

The administrator/manager may be responsible for following federal or state mandates in areas such as employment or safety. OSHA regulations are an example of laws that must be followed. Adherence to laws, rules, and regulations within the workplace may be the responsibility of the manager.

Just as in clinical situations, documentation is important. Labor laws and related legal concepts may dictate what documentation is important and also appropriate. Employees have access to their employment files and, thus, one must be objective and thorough in documenting events and personal interactions.

State and federal laws, as well as the legal principles used to enforce them, seek to protect the rights of involved individuals. Administrator/managers must be cognizant of the critical nature of their role in controlling legal risks. Failure to follow established principles, using poor documentation, or misusing authority can lead to litigation. At the same time, an employee who abuses his position or the legal theories established to protect individual rights is creating a situation that can only result in someone calling into question the employee's intent or abilities to fulfill the job description.

Consumer Advocate

The advocate for consumer rights should be aware of legislation on legal issues, civil rights, healthcare, labor issues in employment of the handicapped, geriatrics, and issues regarding children and adolescents. The amount of information generated in both federal and state legislation is significant in both quantity and quality. The changing nature of the rules and regulations for specific groups, healthcare delivery and civil rights, to name a few, requires a herculean effort to remain updated. Consumer advocates should be selective in their efforts, focusing on areas that best meet personal needs and the needs of the population group(s) for which they advocate. Understanding the political system, how laws are enacted, and lobbying techniques assist the advocate to keep updated by pursuing information and getting on mailing lists to remain updated. Working with professional groups with similar interests also is a valuable resource for information or a need to react to a situation, such as a letter-writing campaign.

The issue of contracts and inherent rights and responsibilities can be applied in many situations. Did a group promising to provide services breach its contract? Did an agency violate the terms of its contract? Tort principles also apply. Was an individual negligent in his responsibilities? Was informed consent obtained? Is there a duty to an individual or group of individuals based on an interpretation of the law? Can one argue that some have misrepresented themselves or an issue? In most instances, a lawyer can assist in defining the legal principles that apply. The Code of Ethics for lawyers suggests that they perform some legal work *pro bono,* for free. Thus, an individual working as a consumer advocate may find legal assistance from someone willing to work *pro bono* and obtain valuable advice and guidance from the legal perspective.

Researcher

A dental hygienist in the role of a researcher should be familiar with issues such as confidentiality, informed consent, recordkeeping, and abandonment. Research protocols frequently address such issues, but a researcher must be careful not to overstep bounds that have been determined by institutional and federal guidelines. A researcher may be working with staff or research assistants who should also be educated to understand the basic legal concepts mentioned. Legal issues not addressed in this chapter, such as product liability, fund management, and tax issues, for instance, must also be considered by researchers.

CONCLUSIONS

The practice of dental hygiene involves decision making based on an understanding of the ethical and legal obligations influencing the professional. A dental hygienist must be aware of the impact of both ethics and law in clinical practice as well as alternative career choices. The Code of Ethics guiding the professional serves as a framework for decision making, but also assists the professional in meeting the needs of clients and colleagues. The legal system protects both the client and the dental hygienist. A dental hygienist may be an employer or employee and must be aware of the federal and state regulations and statutes impacting those roles. Risk management principles lay the foundation for a philosophy of protection of everyone's interests, while seeking to assure quality care or services.

References

1. Nash, D. A. Ethics . . . and the quest for excellence in the profession. Journal of Dental Education 49:198, 1985.
2. Gorlin, R. A. Codes of professional responsibility. Washington, DC: BNA, 1990, p. 207.
3. Gaston, M. A., Brown, D. M., and Waring, M. B. Survey of ethical issues in dental hygiene. Journal of Dental Hygiene 64:217, 1990.
4. Gairola, G., and Skaff, K. O. Ethical reasoning in dental hygiene. Dental Hygiene 57:16, 1983.
5. Pollack, B. R., and Marinelli, R. O. Ethical, moral and legal dilemmas in dentistry: The process of informed decision making. Journal of Law and Ethics in Dentistry 1:27, 1988.
6. Black, H. C. Black's Law Dictionary, 6th ed. St. Paul, MN: West, 1979.
7. Pollack, B. R. Dentist's Risk Management Guide. National Society of Dental Practitioners, 1990.
8. Waring, M. B., and Horn, M. L. Sexual harassment prevention and legal aspects. Dental Hygiene 61:206, 1987.
9. Gervasi, R. Sexual harassment and the politics of power. Dental Assistant 53:30, 1984.
10. Boyce, J. Risk management: An introduction for the dental practice. Dental Hygiene 58:504, 1984.
11. Kraus, G. P. Health care risk management. Owings Mills, Maryland: Rynd Communications, 1986.

Suggested Readings

Kohlberg, L. The Philosophy of Moral Development: Moral Stages and the Ideal of Justice. San Francisco: Harper & Row, 1981.
Weinstein, B. D. Dental Ethics. Philadelphia: Lea & Febiger, 1993.

40 Quality Assurance in Dental Hygiene

OBJECTIVES

Mastery of the content in this chapter will enable the reader to:

- Describe the evolution of quality assurance practices in oral healthcare
- Discuss why public agencies, third parties, and employers have an incentive to evaluate the quality of healthcare
- Define Professional Standards Review Organization
- Differentiate among quality assurance, quality assessment, and quality assurance mechanisms
- Describe the quality assurance cycle in terms of assessment, feedback to providers, corrective action, reporting on corrective action, and reporting to a responsible party
- Describe quality assessment in terms of the assessment of structure, process and outcome, evaluation, and correction
- Discuss the following quality assurance mechanisms: client surveys; client complaints; on-site evaluations; treatment record audits; clinical examinations; utilization review and peer review; formal educational requirements; accreditation standards; the accreditation process; national, state, and regional board examinations for licensure; and mandatory continuing education and retesting to maintain licensure
- Discuss the concept of standards and criteria as applied to quality assurance
- Recognize the suitability of the dental hygienist as a quality assurance manager
- Advocate quality assurance activities in the oral healthcare environment
- View the field of quality assurance as a viable career direction for the dental hygienist

INTRODUCTION

Quality assurance is "the assessment or measurement of, or judgement about, the quality of care and the implementation of any necessary changes to either maintain or improve the quality of care rendered."[1] Quality assurance includes "those activities designed to maintain or improve a standard of excellence in dental care."[2] The purpose of this chapter is to discuss quality assurance mechanisms as well as career opportunities for dental hygienists in this rapidly growing area.

HISTORY OF QUALITY ASSURANCE

Historically, physicians and dentists practiced autonomously and commanded an almost reverential respect from society. The earliest practitioners of the healing arts learned their skills by apprenticeship. As "professions" began to develop, standardization evolved in the form of textbooks, formal educational curricula, and professional licensure. These activities constituted the first attempts at quality assurance, and were designed to ensure the public a minimal level of competence in the practitioners of the healing arts.

Further developments in the field of quality assurance were limited until the advent of Medicare and Medicaid legislation in 1966. Suddenly the federal government found itself financing a large healthcare burden, with a considerable amount of fraudulent claims and unnecessary treatment. In response, **Professional Standards Review Organizations (PSROs)** were established in 1972 as mechanisms to monitor the quality, types, and frequency of services physicians were providing in hospitals. In 1974, PSROs were amended to include review of dental services. The staggering increases in medical costs, coupled with the increasing involvement of third-party payors, greatly contributed to quality assurance activities. PSROs continue to function today.

QUALITY ASSURANCE IN DENTISTRY

Initially, the PSROs did not include dental services. For a time, dentistry continued to practice autonomously and was relatively unaffected by the quality assurance fervor that the medical community experienced. Two factors were primarily responsible for a change in this situation. The first of these is a change in the way oral healthcare is financed. For example, traditional fee-for-service care is declining, whereas the number of health maintenance organizations, preferred provider organizations, exclusive provider organizations, and prepaid dental plans is increasing. A much greater focus on quality assurance has been driven by managed care programs and the organizations that purchase such plans. Employers and employees may be uncertain about selecting a dental practice from a list of unknown practitioners. Therefore, assurances of quality must be given and maintained. In addition, because the nature of some of these types of plans may lead to under-treatment of clients, third parties turn to quality assurance activities to monitor both quality and quantity of services.

The second reason for the increased interest in dental quality assurance is heightened consumer knowledge and demand for optimal care. Product manufacturers, mass media, and public school–based health education programs are reaching more people than ever before. Americans are purchasing more elective, expensive dental procedures, such as cosmetic dentistry and dental implants, than they did in the past. In return, consumers expect a high level of quality and accountability for services.[3,4]

The American Dental Association has maintained that "hygienist training is not sufficient to insure quality care without the supervision of a dentist."[5,6] Astute observers of the legal process would attest, however, that the dental hygienist is legally responsible for the care she renders and that malpractice suits can be brought individually against the hygienist in addition to the dentist.[3] Therefore, the dental hygiene profession actively promotes quality oral healthcare practices within its ranks via quality assurance mechanisms.

Formal dental hygiene educational settings provide ideal environments to observe quality assurance activities. Indeed, the dental hygiene student may find a discussion of quality assurance to be unnecessary "overkill." This response is understandable considering the scrutiny with which students and their clients are observed and evaluated. Within the academic setting, the dental hygiene process of care regarding quality assurance approaches the ideal. Consider, for example, the details of client assessment, the way the dental hygiene care plan is developed and client goals are formulated, and the methods by which comprehensive interventions are implemented and outcomes of care are evaluated. Both process and product criteria and standards exist to assure quality care.

Imagine the dental hygienist who has been in practice for 10 years, perhaps without the benefit of continuing education. Imagine further that the practice has inappropriate instruments and equipment, no protocol for universal precautions to ensure infection control, inadequate lengths of appointment times, and a lack of standards of practice against which contemporary dental hygiene students are evaluated. Although a recent study indicated that most clinical dental hygienists feel they provide quality services to their clients, lack of time allotted to dental hygiene appointments and other "dentist-related factors" were cited as having an adverse impact on the quality of treatment.[7] Practice outside of the academic setting can be less than ideal, although the care may be well within the standards for the community. In addition, the isolation of most dental hygienists in private practice settings increases the likelihood that, over time, the quality of care may decline. Therefore, all dental hygienists should understand and participate in quality assurance activities. These activities include several components that occur in a continuous cycle, known as the **quality assurance cycle.**

The Quality Assurance Cycle

Quality assurance has several key components (Fig. 40–1). These components operate in a cyclical fashion similar to that of the dental hygiene process of care (see Chapter 3). The first phase is quality assessment, during which quality is measured in some way. Once this assessment has been made, an evaluative phase occurs in which the gathered data are analyzed and the outcomes are reported to the appropriate parties. Finally, quality is confirmed or corrective action takes place. At this point the cycle is repeated, starting again with another assessment. Each component of this cycle is discussed in greater detail.

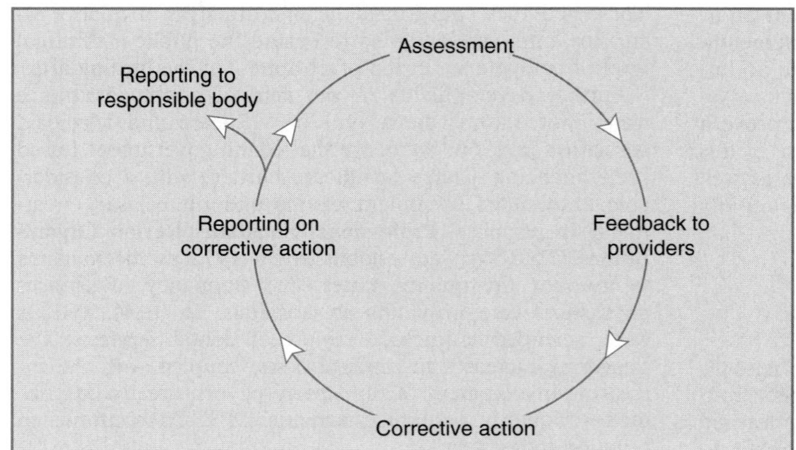

FIGURE 40–1
The quality assurance cycle. (Adapted and redrawn with permission from Jerge C. R., and Orlowski, R. M. Quality assurance and the dental record. Dental Clinics of North America 29:483, 1985.)

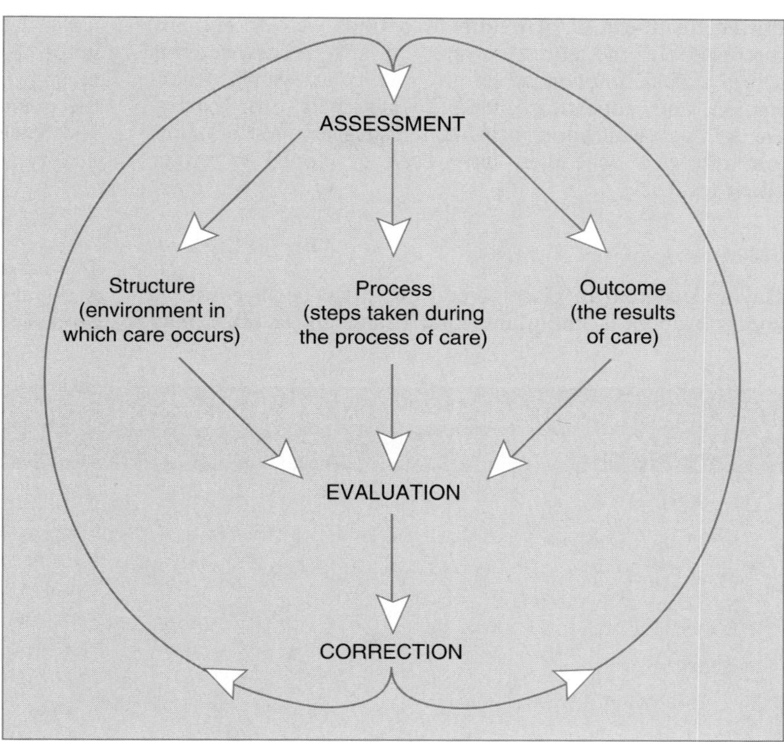

FIGURE 40–2
The quality assurance process.

Quality assessment measures the quality of care. It can be subjective or objective. Donabedian has divided client care into three areas that can be assessed[8]:—structure, process, and outcome (Fig. 40–2).

Structure refers to the setting in which client care occurs and includes such things as the condition of equipment and the integrity of materials. Infection control used within the oral health setting could be considered within the realm of structure.

Process refers to the steps taken during client care. Many dental hygiene programs evaluate students with process evaluations or task component analyses. "Formative evaluation" is another term for the evaluation of process. These evaluation methods proceed under the assumption that if all the proper decisions and steps were made and followed correctly during care, the result is quality of care. Making an assessment of the process of care also includes assessing the "art of care," that is, the quality of the client-provider interaction. The establishment of a positive client-provider relationship is an important aspect of care that should not be underestimated. It is often ultimately responsible for how well a person adheres to recommendations regarding the maintenance of personal health and may be an influencing factor for a client initiating a legal suit against a practitioner.

Assessing **outcome,** often referred to as "summative evaluation," is simply examining the results of care. Having a dental hygiene instructor evaluate a client's oral health status after a student has performed therapeutic scaling and root planing is an example of outcome assessment. With this type of assessment only the end product is assessed, not the means by which it was obtained. To use the previous example, if the instructor deems that all subgingival calculus and necrotic cementum were removed, it is immaterial which instruments and techniques (right or wrong) were used to achieve that outcome.

Quality Assurance Mechanisms

Quality assurance mechanisms exist by which structure, process, and outcome of client care can be assessed. Most quality assurance programs use a variety of tools in an attempt to assess all three components because no single component can give a clear picture of the quality of care provided. Rather, a combination of assessment mechanisms, based on the focus of the organization, is usually selected. Some of these tools are useful to the private practitioner wishing to monitor their own practice; others are relevant only to a large insurance corporation. Cost is another factor to consider when selecting appropriate quality assessment mechanisms. Not only does quality assurance require a personal commitment, it also requires a financial one. For the dental hygiene practitioner interested in self-evaluation, cost can generally be reduced by participating in the educational offerings of local professional societies and by employing quality assurance mechanisms on a small self-help scale. An explanation of some of the more commonly used quality assessment mechanisms follows.

Client Surveys

An often debated subject in the field of quality assurance is whether a client can accurately assess the quality of oral healthcare. Most clients cannot judge the quality of a particular service. However, seeking client opinion on the care they have received is an important way to assess the art of care. Client surveys measure client satisfaction, which is an essential component of quality of care. Also, questionnaires can elicit information regarding the process of care. Client questionnaires are an inexpensive way to assess quality and should be considered when designing a quality assurance program. For example, a client can report if the providers were wearing appropriate barrier protection at all times during treatment, or if treatment options were thoroughly discussed. In the purest sense of quality assurance, this serves a dual function of gaining quality assessment information and educating clients to do their own quality checks. Data collection instruments, such as questionnaires and interview schedules, have been developed to gather client feedback.[9]

Client Complaints

Having a system in place to address initial client concerns and grievances is important. Oral healthcare facilities may use a dental hygienist in the position of client care coordinator to facilitate individuals' care and manage client concerns.[10] From simple misunderstandings to questions about the quality of treatment, the dental hygienist as client advocate can stimulate the provision of improved access to quality oral healthcare.

On-Site Evaluations

The actual on-site visitation of an oral healthcare setting is a popular mechanism used by insurance companies and professional organizations to assess structure. Many ap-

AREAS ADDRESSED DURING AN ON-SITE QUALITY ASSURANCE EVALUATION OF AN ORAL HEALTHCARE SETTING

General Characteristics
- Is the setting geographically accessible to the clients?
- Does the practice have adequate office hours?
- Is the building in satisfactory condition?
- Is there handicapped access?

Reception Area
- Is there adequate seating?
- Is it clean and neat?
- Is it safe? Is there more than one exit? Are exits well marked? Is a fire extinguisher or sprinkler system available?
- Is a lavatory available that is clean and neat?

Business Area
- Is there adequate privacy?
- Is it clean and neat?
- Are all professional credentials displayed and current?
- Is there a copy of the state practice act on file?
- Is the office computerized?

Appointments
- Is there an adequate number of phone lines?
- Are emergencies handled promptly?
- Is there provision for handling after-hours calls?
- Is there a continued care (recall) system?
- Is the appointment book clean and neat?
- Is the wait for an appointment less than 2 weeks?

Medical Emergencies
- Is the staff currently certified in cardiopulmonary resuscitation?
- Is portable oxygen available?
- Is there a medical emergency kit?
- Is the kit complete, updated, and readily available?
- Is the staff trained and practiced for emergencies?

Radiology
- Is equipment modern and safe?
- Are film badge dosimeters worn by staff?
- Are lead aprons and collars used routinely?
- Are protective barriers adequate?
- Are radiographs developed properly?
- Are radiographic procedures carried out within the framework of OSHA regulations for infection control?

Infection Control
- Are fluid-resistant gowns, gloves, masks, and safety glasses worn during client care?
- Are safety glasses given to the clients?
- Is the method of disinfection appropriate?
- Is heat sterilization used?
- Is sterilization verified by appropriate measures?
- Are instruments stored properly?
- Is the office in compliance with OSHA regulations for infection control?
- Is the office in compliance with medical waste management laws of the state?

Treatment Areas
- Is there an acceptable mercury disposal system?
- Is equipment modern and in operable condition?
- Are treatment areas carpeted?
- Are the number and size of the treatment rooms adequate?
- Are treatment rooms clean with no unnecessary items?

Laboratory
- Is there a laboratory in the setting?
- Is it clean and neat with no cross-contamination?
- Does the laboratory work meet acceptable standards?
- Are prescriptions thorough and accurate?
- Is the laboratory in compliance with OSHA regulations?

Staff
- Is the staff professional in appearance and demeanor?
- Is the staff offered continuing education programs?
- Has the staff had the Heptavax or Recombivax immunization?
- Is the staff properly credentialed for their responsibilities?
- Is the staff aware of standard office policies and procedures?

proaches exist for on-site evaluation, but most use a comprehensive checklist to assess the important features of the oral healthcare environment, including an infection control protocol; medical emergency preparedness; credentials of the staff; documentation of client care; condition of equipment and materials; neatness and cleanliness of the environment; radiation, mercury, and nitrous oxide—oxygen safety; quality of laboratory work; and office policies including availability of routine and emergency appointments (see Areas Addressed During an On-Site Quality Evaluation of an Oral Healthcare Setting chart). Figure 40–3 shows a sample checklist of areas that may be addressed in an on-site evaluation. In addition, some on-site evaluations include direct observation of client care. The total assessment may take several hours to several days to conduct.

Treatment Record Audits

Client records review is a valid and frequently employed form of quality assessment.[11–16] By studying client records, examiners can assess the initial oral health status of the person, correctness of diagnosis and treatment decisions, and the outcomes of care (see Areas Addressed on a Treatment Record Review chart).

Clinical Examinations

Less commonly employed because of expense and malpractice considerations, direct examination of clients is an accurate but time-consuming way of assessing quality of care. To a limited extent, this type of direct peer review may

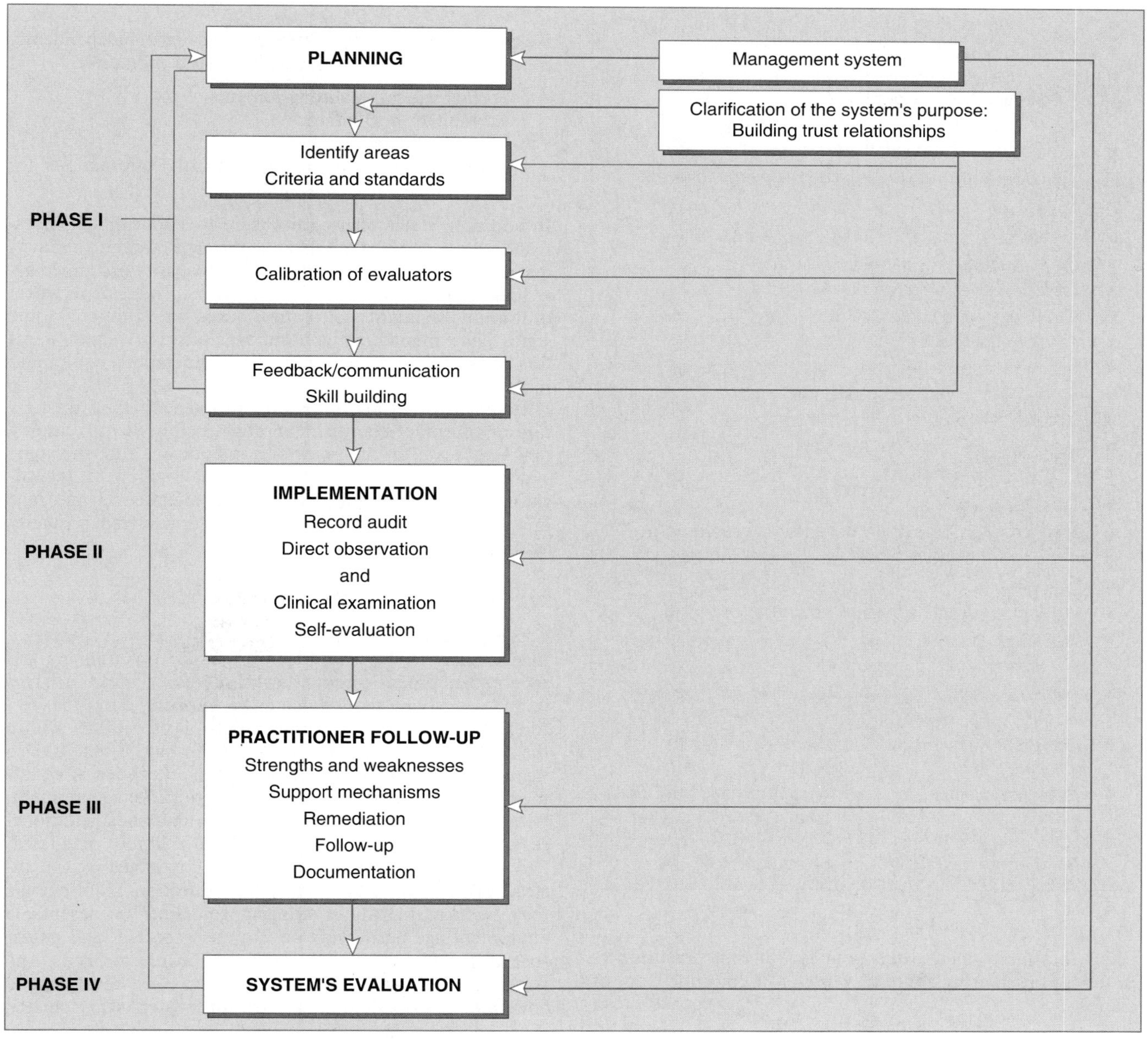

FIGURE 40–3
Quality assurance model for dental hygiene. (Adapted and redrawn with permission from Marcin, J., and Forrest, J. L. Quality assurance: A model for dental hygiene. Dental Hygiene 56(4):16, 1982. Copyrighted [1982] by the American Dental Hygienists' Association.)

AREAS ADDRESSED ON A TREATMENT RECORD REVIEW

Health History

- Is a comprehensive history present?
- Is it periodically updated and signed?
- Are medical alerts noted?
- Are medical consults sought and documented when needed?

Client Evaluation

- Are extraoral examinations performed and documented?
- Are intraoral examinations performed and documented?
- Are oral cancer examinations performed and documented?
- Is blood pressure taken when indicated?
- Is hard tissue charting present?
- Is periodontal charting present?
- Have the client's home care habits been evaluated?
- Based on the client's status as presented, were evaluation methods appropriate and complete?
- Are radiographs appropriate and diagnostic?
- Based on the record, do diagnoses appear complete?

Care Planning

- Have the client's problems been identified?
- Did the client receive a written care plan?
- Were alternatives presented to the client?
- Were services properly prioritized?
- Was informed consent obtained prior to care?
- Does the plan adhere to an appropriate sequence?
- Was the client's chief complaint addressed?
- Was care carried out in a timely manner?
- Did the care plan include a preventive program?
- Was the care plan appropriate for the client?

Services Rendered

- Do the progress notes reflect an orderly progression?
- Are the progress notes complete, signed, and dated?
- Was there any evidence of adverse outcome?
- Were any unexpected outcomes handled expeditiously?
- Are all entries in ink?
- Are materials and prescriptions documented?
- Are referrals sought when necessary and documented?
- Was the client's response to care documented?
- Based on the information, were selected materials appropriate?
- Was there an adequate preventive effort made, including a continued care (recall) schedule for the client?
- Do the radiographs indicate any treatment needs that are not addressed or were poorly addressed?

occur informally in a group practice wherein practitioners routinely observe each others' work on a common pool of clients.

Utilization Review

This quality assessment mechanism includes the examination of the types and number of oral health services given, as well as the patterns of care provided. It compares the practice patterns of a practitioner to those of all practitioners in a given area. Utilization review is practiced by insurance company examiners who can monitor claims and pretreatment estimates and is designed to assess the frequency and appropriateness of care.

Peer Review Committees

A peer review committee consists of a group of professionals with the same training who are asked to evaluate the performance of one of their colleagues. The review committee may be formal (such as a state board of dentistry) or informal (such as a study club), and it may respond specifically to complaints or as an ongoing mechanism to encourage quality practice.

External Mechanisms

Several quality assurance mechanisms exist independently of individually designed quality assurance programs:

- Formal educational requirements
- Accreditation standards
- The accreditation process
- National, state, and regional board examinations for licensure

In addition, states offering licensure by endorsement investigate the quality of applicants through written affidavits instead of clinical examination. These quality assurance activities serve to ensure that entering professionals meet minimum standards of competence. In addition, some states have mandatory continuing education requirements for license renewal and periodic radiographic equipment inspection.

State boards of dentistry are charged with the investigation of consumer complaints brought before them regarding oral healthcare. In the event of a malpractice suit, the court system may serve a quality assurance function by investigating the incident and punishing the offender. Hence, in a final sense, the court system may be considered a quality assurance mechanism.

Credentialing

Credentialing, like other external quality assurance mechanisms, refers to the assurance of qualified practitioners and reliable equipment through licensure and certification. This includes verifying that clinicians are properly educated, certified, and licensed to perform certain procedures within the scope of the jurisdiction's dental practice act. It also includes the proper certification and maintenance of equipment such as radiographic and sterilization equipment. Often the quality assurance program demands additional requirements of practitioners over those legally mandated. For example, credentialing may be conducted yearly instead of semiannually, continuing education requirements may be increased, more stringent guidelines on acceptable equipment age and condition may be expected, and dental specialists may be required to be board certified. The American Dental Hygienists' Association is developing a comprehensive credentialing program for dental hygienists.

Additional Mechanisms

Currently, several new quality assurance mechanisms are under investigation by state regulatory boards, insurance companies, and other organizations. These include requiring mandatory continuing education, levying fines for inadequate services, retesting to maintain licensure, requiring participating offices to be in compliance with an organization's quality assurance program, and negotiating lower malpractice insurance rates for those who participate in a quality assurance program.

The combination of quality assurance mechanisms used varies depending on the organization conducting the assessments (Table 40–1). Staffing, geography, finances, and legal authority of the organization are factors that influence which methods of quality assurance are employed. An individual practitioner interested in self-improvement selects very different mechanisms, for example, than a national insurance company.

Conducting Quality Assessments

Standards and Criteria

Three additional factors are necessary for quality assessment tools to be used successfully. The first is that **standards and criteria** be agreed upon to conduct assessments. There is some disagreement in the literature between the terms "standard" and "criteria." Here, *"standards"* are taken to mean the level of care expected to be accomplished by the provider of that care. *"Criteria"* are the specific factors that must be present in order to produce a high standard of oral healthcare *as judged by the authors of the criteria.* Therefore, what constitutes a "standard of care" in a local court system may fall short of the criteria in a quality assurance program looking at the same care provided in the academic setting. In the same manner, different quality assurance programs may have differing standards and criteria that reflect the programs' purpose and philosophy. Following is an example of a standard and its associated criteria.

Suppose that the clinical policy manual of an oral healthcare setting stated that all clients receive the necessary radiographs to ensure comprehensive diagnosis, treatment, and evaluation. This statement is their standard for quality assessment for radiographic surveys. Further criteria are needed, however, to arrive at a decision on whether a client received the correct prescription for radiographs.

TABLE 40–1
SUMMARY OF QUALITY ASSURANCE MECHANISMS

Mechanism	Membership	Type of Quality Addressed	Methods	Problems
System of professional education	• Faculty	• Theoretical and clinical knowledge, skills, judgments • Overall performance • Process, product, structure	• Direct supervision of work • Regular testing of process and product • Curricular guidelines • Standards of accreditation	• Variations in curricula • Inconsistent requirements • Inconsistent criteria • Graduation yields an assumption of competence
State boards (and Dental Hygiene Committees of the Board)	• Dentists, hygienists, lawyers, consumers appointed by governor	• Theoretical and clinical competence at the time of graduation • Product	• Written and practical examination for licensure • Direct observation	• Inadequate representation of true practice (invalid examination) • Once licensed, no provision for reexamination
		• Continuing competence	• Systems of reciprocity • Relicensure • Licensure by endorsement	• Criteria vary • Criteria vary; for a fee one can continue to have a license
		• Sample of one's performance	• Reprimands, suspension of licensure, or revoking of license for violation of State Practice Act	• Punitive, does nothing to correct the practitioner's lack of knowledge, skill, or judgment • Board generally focuses on criminal behavior, not quality of care
PSRO (Professional Standards Review Organization)	• Physicians and/or osteopaths	• Need for care • Conformance to professional standards • Appropriate level of care • Product	• Review of records by one's peers for quality and necessity of treatment	• Closed shop in that it is controlled by physicians and findings cannot be shared with public • Limited to medical care that is funded by Medicaid and Medicare • Evidence is not always apparent in the record • Extensive use of radiographs

Table continued on following page

TABLE 40–1
SUMMARY OF QUALITY ASSURANCE MECHANISMS *Continued*

Mechanism	Membership	Type of Quality Addressed	Methods	Problems
Group practice	• Dentists within the group • Dental hygienists within the group	• Overall performance • Product	• Direct observation • Review of records • Comparison of the individual's treatment, related statistics with the group norm, e.g., number of root planing procedures versus average number of root planing procedures of the group	• Evidence is not always apparent in the record • Extensive use of radiographs • Willingness to evaluate peers?
Third-party program Capitation programs Also, see indemnity plan (follows)	• Dentists who accept third-party reimbursement	• Quality of care rendered to clients sponsored by third-party payors • Product • Access to care • Satisfaction of patients as to cost control	• Review of records • Claims processing • Spot checks (posttreatment evaluation) • Systems developed to monitor and handle patient grievances • Systems for appropriate referrals to specialists	• Limited to third-party programs • Evidence is not always apparent in the record • Extensive use of radiographs • Number of claims from one dentist may be too limited a sample
Peer review committee Patient relations committee Arbitration committee	• Dentists from a component • Dental hygienists from a component	• Considers questions regarding the quality and appropriateness of care • Appropriateness of fees	• Records review • Interview with client involved • Interview with dentist involved • Direct client examination (posttreatment evaluation)	• Closed shop in that it is controlled by the dentists and findings are not shared with the public • Review is done ex post facto, initiated by client complaints • No punitive powers • Evidence is not always apparent in the record • Extensive use of radiographs
Continuing education	• Anyone who choses to participate	• Theoretical and clinical knowledge, skills, and judgment • Overall performance • Product, process	• Mandatory attendance • Self-evaluation • Continuing education registry • Direct observation	• Little control over courses offered • Accessibility to courses • No incentive to correct or improve • Voluntary in most states • Recordkeeping • Attendance does not yield competence
Standards of Practice (ADHA Commission for Assurance of Competence)	• All members of the professional association	• Overall performance	• Self-evaluation • Appeals to one's sense of ethics	• Voluntary • No incentive to correct or improve
Client feedback		• Client attitudes • Overall impression of care rendered • Overall impression of environment	• Questionnaire • Personal interview	• Do clients know quality when they see it?
Self-evaluation	• Dentist/hygienist who provides the service participates in the evaluation	• Technical quality of dental and dental hygiene care provided • Appropriateness of care	• Self-evaluation	• Voluntary • No incentive to correct or improve • No other performance to determine weaknesses

TABLE 40–1
SUMMARY OF QUALITY ASSURANCE MECHANISMS *Continued*

Mechanism	Membership	Type of Quality Addressed	Methods	Problems
Indemnity plan (goes along with third-party payment)		• Types of preparation for services provided by offices • Aberrant practices • Cost control • Appropriateness of care plans	• Pretreatment review of treatment plans • Develop practice profiles • Audits	• Does not advise dentist of treatment that may be needed for previously undiagnosed conditions
Purchasers of dental plans	• Employers • Union trust funds • Governmental agencies for government subsidy programs	• Adequacy performed by third-party payor • Cost of care • Quality of care	• Evaluate, validate, and judge quality assurance system	
ADA—American Dental Association	• Staff of the Office of Quality Assurance	• Quality of dental healthcare in general • Cost effectiveness • Access to care • Current healthcare environment	• Research • Scientific publications and programs • Accreditation of education programs • Testing for licensure • Peer review • Programs on dental therapeutic materials and equipment • Legislative activity • Demonstration projects • Information campaigns	• Slow implementation of programs • Individual dentists in community resist quality assurance

Such criteria might include:

- Clients over age 6 years who have had no previous radiographs shall receive a panograph and two bitewing radiographs
- Clients who have had no dental caries experience or periodontal disease within the previous year shall receive two bitewing radiographs every 2 years
- Risks and benefits of radiographic procedures are explained to all clients prior to exposure of films; those clients electing not to receive recommended radiographic surveys are required to sign an informed refusal form.

These aforementioned criteria are examples of possible criteria and there are many others that could be added. Currently, no universally or nationally agreed upon criteria exist for dental procedures. The Centers for Disease Control and Prevention along with Occupational Safety and Health Administration (OSHA) have, however, established criteria for universal precautions in infection control (see Chapters 7 to 9). As may be surmised from the preceding example, it is difficult to write inclusive criteria because there are always mitigating circumstances that arise and call for a different decision than the criteria set forth.

Several experts in the field of quality assurance have offered some standards and criteria that practitioners may find helpful.[1,17–19] Specific areas addressing the preventive and periodontal components of oral healthcare are of particular interest to the dental hygienist. For example, outlining a decision tree for recommending multiple fluoride therapy or the inclusion of smoking cessation and nutritional counseling in a practice may be of specific interest in dental hygiene quality assurance efforts.[1,18]

With specific regard to dental hygienists, an author at the University of California, Los Angeles (UCLA) wrote a set of practice assessment standards that state in part:

> The UCLA evaluators rate staffing as not acceptable if there are no hygienists . . . The basis for this criterion is that we have found that group practices, even small ones, almost always do not offer the same level of preventive services when there is no hygienist. Prophylaxes are performed in a few minutes by the dentist and, when subsequent radiographs are available, obvious calculus is seen to remain. Documentation of the status of the periodontium and of oral hygiene instruction is usually poor. Further, periodontal charting, even when disease is present, is not as thorough and deep scaling and root planing appear to be more record entries than a reality. This is not to say that hygienists always perform well, just that there is a clear superiority in the general dental groups we have observed.*[20]

The second factor important in conducting quality assessments is the rating scale used. Is the rater called upon to evaluate something as excellent, satisfactory, conditional, or unsatisfactory? If so, what must exist, or fail to exist, to merit each choice? Or is the rater simply asked to check a

* From Schoen, M. A quality assessment system: The search for validity. Journal of Dental Education 53:658, 1989.

list of items as present or absent, leaving the value judgments to another party? Still again, the rater may be called upon to answer open-ended questions about a practice, a client record, or an incident. Whatever grading scale is used must be understood clearly by those using it.

In designing criteria, standards, and a rating scale, planners can write either to the ideal or to an accepted minimal standard. Depending on which is chosen, the conceptualization of quality care is different and therefore is evaluated differently. If a minimal standard is used, it is expected that all practitioners meet or exceed the criteria to provide quality care. In contrast, if the criteria speak to a mythical ideal, a practitioner who "scores less" may still be rendering quality care. For example, suppose as part of a dental hygiene study club a dental hygienist was evaluating a colleague's practice to determine that colleague's standard of instrumentation and extrinsic stain and plaque removal. One assessment criterion states that "during an eight appointment day, *no* bacterial plaque will be visible on any client at dismissal." In conducting the evaluation, the dental hygienist may find bacterial plaque remaining on a total of three teeth during that day. Does this finding constitute poor quality care on the part of the dental hygienist being evaluated? If it were understood that the criterion reflected the ideal, the dental hygienist in question may score very well in this area.

In contrast, suppose a dental hygienist was conducting client surveys in a group practice. This practice's standard of care states that all clients are educated to care for their oral health on a daily basis to the best of their individual abilities. One criterion states that oral hygiene instructions will be provided by the dental hygienists on at least 70% of their clients' appointments. In response to the survey, clients reported receiving home care instructions only 40% of the time. Here, the criteria reflect a minimal standard that all the dental hygienists in the practice are expected to meet or exceed. Based on these findings, evaluators may conclude that this is an area where quality is lacking and needs to be corrected.

The third factor involved in successful quality assessment is the need for calibration among raters. This may not be crucial for a group dental practice interested primarily in self-assessment; however, it is vital if dental hygienists in a local professional association, for example, are conducting quality assessments in each other's oral healthcare settings. There is a critical need for all raters to understand the standards, criteria, and rating scales. For large organizations with raters in multiple geographic locations wherein interrater reliability cannot be easily achieved, it is preferable for the raters to simply assess the presence or absence of criteria; the value judgments are added at a central location by a few professionals whose judgments are calibrated.

Evaluation

Once an assessment has been made, an **evaluation** must take place. In most instances, evaluation is an end result; in quality assurance, evaluation is a middle step. Quality assessment data, once collected, are analyzed to determine whether the quality of care is at an optimal level or deficient in some area. The different types of quality assessments discussed earlier can be considered individually or in concert. A group practice may elect to look only at client surveys and later only at client record reviews. Larger organizations generally pool several types of assessment data to arrive at a more comprehensive evaluation.

To evaluate the data, it is often helpful to tabulate or summarize the data in some manner, and then compare the results to the preestablished criteria and standards. Practices that fail to conform to the standards are targeted for corrective action. Practices that meet or exceed the standards ideally should be rewarded; this is an area in quality assurance where greater emphasis should be placed. Most healthcare professionals are internally motivated by high professional ideals, and indeed most enter such professions to "help others." The stressful and often isolated environment in which oral healthcare is rendered, however, can lead to instances when quality of care is chronically lacking. A reward system need not be extravagant or expensive. The most common example of a reward system is in the academic setting where students are compensated for high performance through good grades, scholarships, honors, awards, and other mechanisms. It is hoped that satisfied clients and increased client referrals serve as a "reward" for quality service in the private sector; however, this cannot always be directly correlated to effort on the part of oral healthcare practitioners. Some other examples of positive reinforcers in a quality assurance program include: an afternoon off for employees, public recognition in a newsletter, specially funded continuing education courses, and financial bonuses.

Corrective Action

One final step, **correction,** remains to complete the quality assurance cycle. If the quality of care has been judged to be inadequate, corrective action must be taken to bring care back in line with the expected standard. Examples of corrective actions may include having a student complete remedial work, a mandate of continuing education from a state regulatory board, or refusal to allow a dental practice to participate on a preferred provider panel until deficiencies are corrected. Depending on the authority of the body conducting the assessment and evaluation, corrective actions also may include denial of a submitted care plan, fines, community service, or revocation of licensure. If, on the other hand, the quality of the care has been judged to be of a high standard, the cycle continues and assessment activities recommence.

If deficiencies are identified, a remedial system must be in place. The most common type of remediation is continuing education that is specific to the problem encountered. Although it has been suggested that continuing education can lead to an improvement in the quality of care, there is a lack of research studies to quantify this improvement.[21] Continuing education is particularly appropriate for the individual practitioner who is in need of improving specific skills or learning new ones. The staff meeting also can be used as a correction mechanism if the deficiency is small. In the earlier example where oral hygiene instructions were neglected by the dental hygienists, the quality assurance assessment outcomes are raised at a staff meeting and discussed to allow the group to solve the problem. Perhaps the appointments are only 30 minutes long, not allowing time for home care instructions. Perhaps the healthcare setting does not purchase media or oral hygiene aids, making client education unduly difficult. It is the goal of the staff meeting to develop a solution to the problem here, for example, to obtain a commitment from the dental hygienists to make client education a priority and thereby improve the quality of dental hygiene care in the setting.

Ideally, a reassessment is done at a later date to determine whether the corrective measures were successful.

A QUALITY ASSURANCE MODEL FOR DENTAL HYGIENE

Dental hygiene needs quality assurance programs at both local and national levels to meet clients' human needs for safety and to earn consumer trust. Research shows that many dental hygienists frequently encounter ethical dilemmas in their practices, which can affect the quality of care provided.[22] Despite academic preparation in ethics, practicing dental hygienists are often unable to resolve the ethical dilemmas they encounter. A quality assurance program provides a vehicle for problem solving within the practice environment.

When students are in a formal dental hygiene education program, the quality of their client care is "assured" by the licensed faculty under whom they practice. The setting is a teaching environment that practices skill assessment, evaluation, and correction. These conditions may vary in the private sector. With the complexity of contemporary clients (medical, ethnocultural, and psychosocial) as well as current concerns over infection control practices and oral disease prevalence, it is imperative that appropriate quality assurance mechanisms for dental hygiene care be designed to enable dental hygienists to consistently assure quality care and control the risk of litigation.

Even under the conditions of direct supervision, the dental hygienist treats clients with some degree of autonomy. That is to say, the dentist does not review each step in the dental hygiene process of care prior to permitting the dental hygienist to continue. In states with practice acts that allow general supervision and independent practice, the dental hygienist may give dental hygiene care in the absence of a dentist. Therefore, peer review programs that assure the quality of dental hygiene care to the consumer should be implemented. Such programs enable dental hygiene practitioners to assume responsibility for evaluating quality of care.

In 1982 a simple, cost-effective quality assurance program for dental hygiene was proposed (Fig. 40–3).[23] It was designed to be conducted at the private practice level by peer groups composed of a variety of practitioners and combined a number of quality assessment mechanisms, including record audits, direct observation, clinical examination, and self-evaluation. In this manner, costs in conducting the program were reduced.

QUALITY ASSURANCE AS A CAREER

Because of their preventive and education-oriented backgrounds and roles as client advocates, dental hygienists are ideal for promoting quality assurance within the oral healthcare environment. Employment opportunities exist for dental hygienists interested in pursuing a career in quality assurance. Employment may include coordinating client care at a dental school, supervising the infection control protocol at a hospital, traveling across the country evaluating dental practices for an insurance company, or managing the quality assurance program for a third-party insurer. An increase in the number of these positions is likely to occur as the demand for cost control and advanced technology escalate. A career in quality assurance can be professionally stimulating and economically rewarding and bears consideration as a career option for dental hygienists.

References

1. American Dental Association. Office of Quality Assurance. Guidelines for the Development of a Quality Assurance Audit System for Hospital Dental Programs, 1983.
2. Quality assurance: Five experts examine the issue. Journal of the American Dental Association 105:606, 1982.
3. Macdonald, G. A selected review of lawsuits brought against dentists: Their relevance to dental hygiene. Dental Hygiene 60:358,1986.
4. Galante, M. A. Dental flaws: Malpractice suits against dentists on the rise. National Law Journal 6:24, 1984.
5. Federal Trade Commission. Commission statement upon closing the dental hygienist portion of its investigation of dental industry practices. File 772, 3020, 1980.
6. American Dental Association. Comprehensive Policy Statement on Dental Auxiliaries. Chicago: ADA, 1986.
7. Boyer, E. Clinical dental hygienists' perceptions of quality dental hygiene care. Journal of Dental Hygiene 66:216, 1992.
8. Donabedian, A. A Guide to Medical Care Administration, vol. II. New York: New York Public Health Service Contract PH 108-66-153, The American Public Health Association, 1969.
9. Johnson, J. D., Scheetz, J. P., et al. Development and validation of a consumer quality assessment instrument for dentistry. Journal of Dental Education 54:644, 1990.
10. Miller, S. S., and DePaola, L. G. The concurrent patient care program: An introduction to the cotherapist approach to dental care. Journal of the Baltimore College of Dental Surgery 35(1):1, 1981.
11. Klyop, J. The dental profession's commitment to quality assurance. Dental Clinics of North America 29:521, 1985.
12. Vehkalahti, M., Rytömaa, I., and Helminen, S. Assessment of quality of public oral health care on the basis of patient records. Community Dentistry and Oral Epidemiology 20:102, 1992.
13. Marcus, M., Koch, A., and Gershen, J. A record review model for assessing dental practices. California Dental Association 7(10):51, 1979.
14. American Dental Association. The Dental Patient Record: Structure and Function Guidelines. Chicago: The Association, 1987.
15. Friedman, J. PSRO's in dentistry. American Journal of Public Health 65:1298, 1975.
16. Jago, J. Issues in assurance of quality dental care. Journal of the American Dental Association 89:854, 1974.
17. Morris, A. J., Bentley, J. M., Vito, A. A., and Bomba, M. R. Assessment of a private dental practice: Report of a study. Journal of the American Dental Association 117:153, 1988.
18. Schoen, M., Freed, J., Gershen, J. A., and Marcus, M. Appendix: Guidelines for criteria and standards of an acceptable quality general dental practice (special emphasis on group practice). Journal of Dental Education 53:662, 1989.
19. Aetna Life Insurance Company. Quality Assurance Program Manual: Aetna's Preferred Dental Plans, 1990.
20. Schoen, M. A quality assessment system: The search for validity. J Dent Educ 53:658, 1989.
21. Watkins, F. The Role of Continuing Education in Quality Assurance. National Round Table on Dental Quality Assurance, Summary of Proceedings, 1983.
22. Gaston, M. A., Brown, D. M., and Waring, M. B. Survey of ethical issues in dental hygiene. Journal of Dental Hygiene 64:217, 1990.
23. Marcin, J., and Forrest, J. L. Quality assurance: A model for dental hygiene. Dental Hygiene 56:16, 1982.

41 Research and Theory Development in Dental Hygiene

OBJECTIVES

Mastery of the content in this chapter will enable the reader to:

- Define the key terms used
- Compare and contrast various ways for acquiring knowledge
- Compare the methods for developing new knowledge in dental hygiene
- Describe how the scientific method is used in dental hygiene research
- Compare the research process to the dental hygiene process of care
- Identify why dental hygiene researchers and scholars are necessary
- Define scientific misconduct in research and provide examples
- Identify ethical issues in research
- Describe informed consent as it relates to research
- Describe the need for research in practice
- Describe strategies for enhancing research in practice and overcoming barriers
- Define a clinical dental hygiene problem
- Define theory and its characteristics
- Describe the progression of theory development
- Distinguish between research and theory and conceptual models and theory
- Describe how theory advances knowledge and practice
- Identify efforts of the American Dental Hygienists' Association to enhance dental hygiene research

INTRODUCTION

Research and theory are crucial for professional status. All professions are characterized by, among other things, the existence of a **body of knowledge.** This means that the knowledge base of the profession is well defined and well organized, is peculiar or specific to that discipline, and distinguishes it from other disciplines. This includes the concepts, propositions, and theories that provide the foundation for the practice of the discipline and give the practice its unique character. Practice based on research is necessary for the practitioner to make sound judgments and to deliver the most effective care possible.

Much has been written about how research provides the scientific basis underlying practice and makes the practitioner more certain about the outcomes of care. But practice, it is argued, is something more than the application of theoretical knowledge. For example, Donaldson and Crowley stated that "clinical practice is always to some extent empirical, pragmatic, intuitive, and artistic."[1] However, Dickoff, James, and Wiedenbach[2] have asserted that "theory is born in practice, is refined in research, and must and can return to practice." This latter statement reflects the interdependence among theory, practice, and research (Fig. 41–1).

For dental hygiene, research enables the profession to provide oral health services to the public that are efficacious; in other words, research helps ensure and validate that the care provided works and is not provided because of ritual, tradition, intuition, or personal preference.

In the oral healthcare environment, the dental hygienist as clinician and educator is a key disseminator of research findings. As such, the dental hygienist must be a critical consumer of research findings to make decisions about the relevance of the findings to current practice and client care. The practitioner must be able to evaluate research findings and then modify dental hygiene care to reflect current knowledge. Results of research also are conveyed to clients

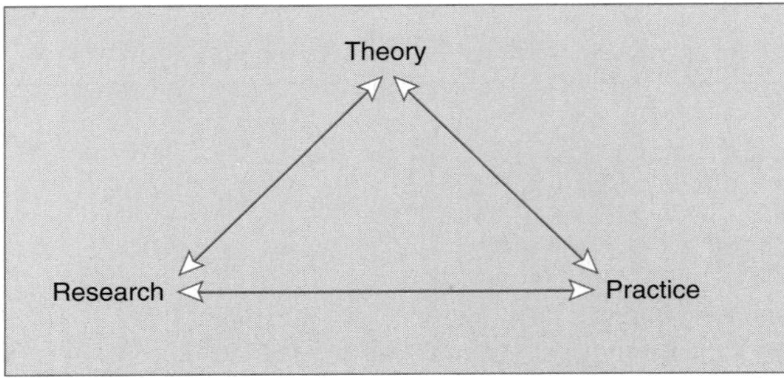

FIGURE 41-1
Reciprocal relationship among theory, research, and practice.

who query the dental hygienist about the effectiveness of over-the-counter healthcare products. The dental hygienist should recommend new products, aids, and equipment to clients and colleagues based on data obtained through research. Dental hygiene care is more likely to be "state of the art" when the practitioner has a research perspective.

This chapter provides an overview of the research issues relevant to the emerging profession of dental hygiene and strategies for enhancing research effectiveness.

ACQUIRING KNOWLEDGE

There are several **methods of acquiring knowledge:**

- Through tradition
- From experts
- Through experience
- By trial and error
- Through the scientific method

Tradition

Tradition is one of the oldest ways in which humans have passed on knowledge from one generation to the next. Learning to hunt or gather food for survival, modes of dress for significant occasions like a coronation, and religious practices and family or ethnic customs helps ensure that subsequent generations learn the necessary rules and roles to keep the practices alive. For many years in dental hygiene, as in nursing and other health professions, wearing a white uniform and cap was the traditional and accepted form of dress. Today a pinning ceremony in dental hygiene reflects a tradition of acknowledging that the student has completed the program. Although tradition is an efficient way of passing on knowledge one should guard against allowing it to become so ingrained that other more efficient and appropriate ways of doing things are overlooked.

Acquiring Knowledge From Experts

Another way of acquiring knowledge is from experts. It is common practice in our society to seek expert advice from attorneys, physicians, counselors, teachers, insurance agents, or accountants. Dental hygiene students usually seek the advice of their faculty or dental hygiene practitioners in the field. These individuals represent authority figures, and their views, although not without fault, are often accepted as absolute.

Learning Through Experience

Learning through experience is another way of knowing. "Without this process, a person would have to relearn a procedure every time it was performed. Practice leads to the development of routines that help build skills."[3] For example, a dental hygiene student learns to complete a periodontal assessment by first watching the instructor, then practicing the procedure on a classmate, then beginning to perform the procedure on a client. In learning to do this, the student begins to organize the process so that it is done completely and accurately and practices the procedure many times so that it is done quickly and confidently. The problem with this way of acquiring knowledge is that the procedure can be completed incorrectly or in an inefficient way so that learning becomes rote and new or better ways are overlooked.

Trial and Error

Trial and error can be observed from watching children play, adults tinker with gadgets around the house, or a dental hygiene student try a variety of oral physiotherapy aides with a client to determine which is effective. Although this method contributes to honing problem-solving skills in many instances, it is unsystematic and haphazard. In circumstances that involve a person's safety or health, trial and error is not the method of choice.

Scientific Method

The most objective means of acquiring knowledge is through the scientific method. The **scientific method** is characterized by "systematic, orderly procedures that, while not infallible, seek to limit the possibility for error and minimize the likelihood that any bias or opinion by the researcher might influence the results of research and thus the knowledge gained" (see Scientific Method chart).[3]

SCIENTIFIC METHOD

Problem Formulation
Identification and statement of a problem in need of solution or question in need of an answer

Hypothesis Formulation
Formulation of a solution or answer to the question that is observable, measurable, and consistent with what is already known in the field

Data Collection
Collection of facts that can be used to solve the problem, answer the question, or test the hypothesis

Analysis/Interpretation
Analysis and interpretation of the meaning of the data collected

Conclusions
Formulation of conclusions regarding the original research problem, question, or hypothesis

From Darby, M. L., and Bowen, D. M. Research Methods for Oral Health Professionals. St. Louis: C. V. Mosby, 1980, p. 2.

DENTAL HYGIENE AND THE SCIENTIFIC METHOD

Dental hygiene, like other sciences, is a synthesis of facts, ideas, concepts, and philosophies—a unique entity.[4] The current trend is for dental hygiene to use the scientific method as the most appropriate approach for acquiring knowledge and for developing its own body of knowledge. Although it is unlikely that dental hygiene will abandon conceptual models and theories from other disciplines, particularly in the social and biological sciences, it is crucial that dental hygiene continues to develop a knowledge base that is unique to dental hygiene.

The scientific method allows dental hygienists to define what they do and whether the care they give is effective because it is the most systematic, objective, and orderly approach to knowledge acquisition. For example, dental hygienists have acknowledged that communication and education are fundamental to fulfilling their responsibilities as preventive oral health specialists. Through the scientific method, research questions might address:

What types of communication are effective?
Does the type of communication vary depending on the cultural beliefs of a particular group or individual?
Which educational strategies are needed to address the needs of diverse groups and individuals?
Which educational strategies are most likely to motivate an individual, given cultural differences?
Which specific educational interventions are effective for diverse cultural groups?
Which educational interventions are more likely to promote oral health and prevent disease?

As a case in point, it has been found in the cultural beliefs of certain Southeast Asian groups that disease is not perceived to exist in the absence of pain or bleeding.

How does the dental hygienist modify clinical care and educational strategies for an individual in this group who has high blood pressure or periodontal disease when both pain and bleeding are absent?
How will client acceptance of preventive and therapeutic regimens be achieved?
What levels of anxiety are needed by the client to encourage compliant behaviors?
How do concepts of self-help and prevention apply to different ethnic groups?
Which existing behavioral models can be adapted and tested in dental hygiene practice?
Do the models vary based on factors such as ethnicity, race, age, or gender?
How do a particular ethnic group's needs fit into the paradigm for dental hygiene science?

One way of addressing some of the questions is to seek out authorities or experts in healthcare who have worked with a particular population and understand the group's culture. But a member of another healthcare profession who is an expert in Southeast Asian culture is not able to plan or implement the most appropriate dental hygiene intervention. Another way of addressing the problem is for the dental hygienist to rely on past experience or the trial and error approach and try different educational interventions. If the intervention is not successful, another approach may be attempted until a measure of success is achieved. Even if an intervention is successful with one individual or group, the success of this intervention with other individuals or groups is still questionable. Thus, research using the scientific method is critical to ensure that the problem is approached objectively, thoroughly, and systematically, and that practitioner bias and extraneous variables are controlled.

DEFINITIONS OF SCIENTIFIC AND DENTAL HYGIENE RESEARCH

All systematic inquiry designed for the purpose of advancing knowledge is called **research.**[5] Kerlinger, who provided what has become one of the most widely held definitions, stated that "Scientific research is the systematic, controlled, empirical, and critical investigation of hypothetical **propositions** about the presumed relations among natural **phenomena**" (emphasis added).[6] What this definition means is that when researchers use systematic, controlled methods for studying a problem, they can be more confident that the observations are accurate and not influenced by **bias** or belief or opinion of the investigator. The observations made during the study are **controlled,** which means that errors are regulated or limited, and alternative explanations are systematically ruled out. To be **empirical,** the evidence collected in the study must come from objective findings. By replicating the study, other investigators can examine the evidence and make the same observations. The results are open to review and critique by other researchers. To frame the design of the study, the researcher develops a set of statements, called **hypotheses,** that predict what is expected before the study begins. Finally, investigators study the relationship between or among certain characteristics or events. The relationship could be **correlational,** which means that one attribute changes as another changes but is not caused by another attribute or factor. For example, there is a greater incidence of tooth loss in the population over the age of 55 years. Yet just growing older is not the cause of tooth loss. Other factors contribute to tooth loss, such as dental caries, periodontal disease, and accidents. The relationship could be **cause and effect,** wherein the presence of one variable causes changes to occur in another variable. For example, sucrose has been shown to cause dental caries in laboratory animals.

Researchers study many types of relationships including how factors or characteristics cause other things to happen. Yet one should use caution in reviewing published research studies and avoid inappropriately interpreting results in terms of cause and effect relationships. Often investigators study how changes in characteristics are related to each other without determining why or how these changes occurred.

Dental hygiene research develops knowledge about oral health behaviors and the promotion of oral health over the lifespan. Even with this broad definition, dental hygiene research is in its infancy. Although the extent of research in dental hygiene contributing to the development of a body of knowledge unique to dental hygiene is limited, dental hygiene research uses various methods to study dental hygiene problems. One method, the **experiment,** uses highly controlled conditions with one group, the **control group** or comparison group, not receiving the treatment. For example, an experimental design was used to assess the effectiveness of toothbrushing, flossing, and subgingival irrigation with and without a chemotherapeutic agent in persons with moderate periodontal disease. The **experimental group** was required to brush, floss, and use subgingival irrigation with the chemotherapeutic agent whereas the control or comparison group brushed, flossed, and used subgingival irrigation without the chemotherapeutic agent. With another method, an **ethnographic study,** the researcher examines the role of the dental hygienist and the client during the oral health educational process. With this method, commonly used in anthropology and psychology, the researcher records and documents the verbal communication and the nonverbal behaviors of both the practitioner and the client during the educational process. This is in direct contrast to a **descriptive study** of a large number of dental hygienists' health promotion behaviors in which practitioners are surveyed and respond through a questionnaire regarding the frequency, amount of time, and mechanisms used in oral health education with clients. Of importance is that the actual problem being investigated is one of the factors that determines which research method is appropriate.

Research is divided into two main categories:

- Basic
- Applied

Both types can be used in developing knowledge about dental hygiene phenomena. **Basic research** is the systematic application of the scientific method leading to the establishment of new knowledge and theory. It is research for the sake of knowledge and without direct regard to application. For example, immunologists and cellular biologists have conducted in-vitro research to identify the virus that causes acquired immunodeficiency syndrome (AIDS). Other researchers, working independently and in tandem, continue to investigate at the cellular level how the virus reproduces and mutates, and they examine mechanisms that trigger the host to respond to the AIDS virus. Researchers conducting basic research usually share the results of their findings with other researchers who in turn apply the theories and research results from cellular biology, immunology, microbiology, and biochemistry to treatments that can directly benefit the client. Basic research tends to provide a theoretical foundation for applied research.

Applied research "adapts the theories developed through basic research to a practical situation or to the resolution of an existing problem. The basis for applied research is the desire to know or understand so that more effective and efficient techniques and approaches can be discovered and used."[7] For example, in the case of AIDS, researchers use the findings from basic research and apply what is known about the AIDS virus to disease transmission. This knowledge can be further applied by developing standard protocols for infection control and preventive behaviors. Research findings can be used in treatment—an example is the drug zidovudine (AZT; Retrovir)—and for research in developing a vaccine to prevent transmission of the AIDS virus.

THE RESEARCH PROCESS

The research process consists of phases or steps that can be compared to those of the dental hygiene process. Both are problem-solving processes used by dental hygienists (Table 41–1).

The **research process** is used to develop and test knowledge that can build concepts and theories and that can add to what is already known. Research findings can be applied to other situations as well. Dental hygienists may need to know why a particular problem occurs or what is the best way to deliver care for a diverse group of individuals experiencing a similar oral health problem.

TABLE 41–1
COMPARISON OF PHASES IN THE DENTAL HYGIENE PROCESS AND THE RESEARCH PROCESS

Phases in Dental Hygiene Process	Phases in Research Process*
Assessment	• Identify the research problem • Review the literature • Define concepts and variables • Estimate the success potential of the research
Dental hygiene diagnosis	• Define and formulate the specific research problem • State the hypothesis
Planning	• Continually review the literature • Select the research approach • Determine ethical implications • Identify the population and sample • Select the data-gathering methods and techniques • Identify assumptions and limitations • Select the data-gathering instrument • Design the data-gathering plan • Design the data analysis plan
Implementation	• Conduct pilot studies • Implement the research plan • Collect data
Evaluation	• Analyze and interpret data • Prepare the research report • Communicate findings

*Adapted from Darby, M., and Bowen, D. Research Methods for Oral Health Professionals. St. Louis: C. V. Mosby, 1980.

DENTAL HYGIENE RESEARCHERS AND SCHOLARS

The four points presented in the Directions for Dental Hygiene Research from the American Dental Hygienists' Association chart reflect the importance of developing a cadre of dental hygiene researchers and scholars who have the educational background, credentials, experience, and opportunity to advance the profession of dental hygiene by developing and expanding a body of knowledge unique to dental hygiene that has as its ultimate goal the improvement of the public's oral health. Although most dental hygiene research should be undertaken by dental hygienists who are trained to conduct scientific investigations, generally at the master's and doctoral level, opportunities exist for all dental hygienists to contribute to knowledge development. For instance, a practitioner can be a member of a research team who is trained to gather data on a group of clients receiving a specific dental hygiene care regimen. A dental hygiene student can participate as a subject in a study or in the data collection phase of an ongoing study by one of the student's faculty members.

Research and scholarship are equally important for the development of dental hygiene knowledge, but research and scholarship are not synonymous. Scholarship is not just

DIRECTION FOR DENTAL HYGIENE RESEARCH FROM THE AMERICAN DENTAL HYGIENISTS' ASSOCIATION

- Strengthen alliances among dental hygiene practitioners in the public, private, and educational sectors to facilitate the integration of dental hygiene research and services into appropriate levels of healthcare and to provide a more unified approach in the delivery and evaluation of dental hygiene care
- Focus research priorities on development of theory, assessment of the effectiveness of methods and technologies used in dental hygiene practice, and development of an epidemiological data base for making decisions on disease prevention and health promotion methods and priorities
- Promote and support master's degree programs in dental hygiene education to provide the faculty resources and research required to further develop the scientific basis for dental hygiene practice
- Promote and support education of dental hygienists at the doctoral level in social, biomedical, and behavioral sciences to develop scholars who are capable of formulating and conducting research that is based on existing theoretical constructs and has the potential for developing dental hygiene theory

Adapted from Steering Committee for the Workshops on the Future of Dental Hygiene Practice and Education. Prospectus for Dental Hygiene. Chicago: American Dental Hygienists' Association, 1988.

research or publication. Although a scholar may conduct research, a scholar is recognized in a discipline as an expert in a particular area. A scholar takes a leadership role in the field by developing a body of work through teaching, research, and theory development; presenting the work to a group of peers for critique; and expanding the field through reflective thought, application of concepts, and the creation of new knowledge.

Michels has argued that:

> Research and scholarship are not merely activities; they are a way of life and a way of thinking about life. Research and scholarship are founded on skepticism, distrust of authority, constructive criticism, clarity of thinking, trust in evidence, and recognition that knowledge is tentative, conditional, and probabilistic. Research and scholarship require . . . a way of thinking about the world and things in it that provokes the drive to search for the truth and the drive to share publicly not only the truth but the methods for searching for it. The drive to search for the truth, the drive to share the truth, and the methods of the search are relentless, uncompromising, and discomforting.*

The profession of dental hygiene not only needs researchers, it needs scholars as well. Research, a component of scholarship, advances the body of knowledge but is basically an activity. Scholars include research as part of their work, but scholars have career goals devoted to thinking broadly about advancing their discipline. Scholars apply theories and new ideas to their work daily and continually challenge established belief and tradition. Scholars are able to bring in perspectives from other disciplines, to view society broadly, and to analyze their discipline in relation to society. Dental hygiene needs scholars because it needs individuals who can think, who are exceptional teachers, who can solve problems, who are at ease with working with concepts, and who can develop theory.

ETHICAL ISSUES IN RESEARCH

Instances of misconduct in research in the past few years have necessitated a heightened concern within the research community as to its ability to detect and respond to scientific misconduct. **Scientific misconduct** is defined as fabrication, falsification, plagiarism, or other serious deviations from accepted practice in carrying out or reporting results from research. As the National Academy of Sciences has noted, error caused by the inherent limits on scientific theories can be discovered only through the gradual advancement of science, but error made by humans also occurs in science. Scientists are not infallible, and they do not have limitless working time or access to unlimited resources. Even the most responsible scientist can make an honest mistake. Mistakes made while trying to do one's best are tolerated in science; mistakes made through negligent work are not. Haste, carelessness, and inattention to detail not only damage the work of the particular investigator but damage the work of others as well.

Of all the violations of the ethos of science, fraud is the most serious. Fraud is the intent to deceive. Fraudulent behavior can include selecting only those data that support a hypothesis and concealing the rest, changing the findings to meet expectations, or fabricating the results. These behaviors are intentionally misleading and deceptive. Because science is a cumulative enterprise in which investigators test and build on the work of their predecessors, fraudulent observations and hypotheses tend eventually to be uncovered.[9]

Rights of Human Subjects

To develop new knowledge or test existing knowledge, research may involve the use of human subjects in procedures wherein the outcome is unknown. Researchers are obligated to inform all persons involved of the risks.

Informed consent in research is a formal process. Investigators develop a specific, comprehensive informed consent document for presentation to research subjects. Before beginning a research study, the protocol with the informed consent document must be submitted to an institutional review board for its review, modification, and approval. All of the elements of consent must be incorporated into the consent form (see Basic Elements of Informed Consent in Research chart).

The voluntary nature of the subject's participation in research is explicit among the elements of informed consent. Thus, alternative procedures that are of advantage to the client must be discussed. The right of clients to refuse to participate without penalty or loss of benefits to which they would otherwise be entitled must be made clear.

Institutional review boards work diligently to present the

* From Michels, E. Commentary: Enhancing the scholarly base: The role of faculty in enhancing scholarship. Journal of Allied Health 18(2):129–142, 1989.

BASIC ELEMENTS OF INFORMED CONSENT IN RESEARCH

- Statement that the study involves research along with an explanation of the purpose of and duration of participation
- A description of reasonably foreseeable risks
- A description of benefits
- A discussion of alternative procedures
- A statement describing the extent to which confidentiality of records identifying the subjects will be maintained
- For research involving more than minimal risk, an explanation as to whether compensation or treatments are available if injury occurs
- An explanation of whom to contact for answers to questions
- A statement that participation is voluntary and that the subject may discontinue participation at any time

risks and benefits of the potential research activity in terms that are most easily understood by the lay individual. To facilitate this, all institutional review boards are required to have at least one lay individual as a member. The board regularly confronts the dilemma of over- versus underinforming research subjects. Detailed descriptions of all potential adverse reactions may frighten individuals from participation. Underinforming may be equally dangerous to the subjects by not fairly or completely presenting the risks.

Federal regulations require that a consent document be informative and be presented to the subject in writing and worded in an understandable way (Fig. 41–2). In practice, the legal system requires that a professional not only disclose what is to be done but also ensure that the client understands this information. Investigators who are uncertain about the subject's comprehension should ask questions and provide an opportunity for the subject to ask questions.

STRATEGIES FOR INCREASING USE OF RESEARCH IN PRACTICE

Professional Conferences and Funding

The commitment of the American Dental Hygienists' Association (ADHA) and the Canadian Dental Hygienists' Association (CDHA) to research over the past decade has been exemplified through their financial support for research studies, national conferences and workshops on research, and the development of publications that disseminate research findings and address the development of research skills (Table 41–2). The associations have made a commitment to sponsoring research programs that have resulted in advancing the understanding of dental hygiene practice and have established a baseline for building dental hygiene theory through a strategic research plan.

As dental hygiene's professional honor society, Sigma Phi Alpha has taken a leadership role in advancing dental hygiene scholarship by funding scholarly programs at national meetings focused on developing dental hygiene's body of knowledge. To foster research in dental hygiene education, the honor society also has garnered support from dental products companies to award scholarships to graduate students.

Dental Hygiene Education

Bridging research and practice is accomplished through formal dental hygiene education. Dental hygiene programs include research in the curriculum and teach the value of research in practice. Emphasis is placed on lifelong learning and the role of continuing education as a valid mechanism for educating practitioners about the use of research principles in daily practice.

Periodically, collaborative programs are developed that bring researchers and dental hygiene practitioners together to increase awareness of new research and to identify areas of clinical practice in need of research. These collaborative programs serve as a way to transfer new knowledge to the practicing dental hygienist who then serves as the catalyst for applying the new knowledge in the oral healthcare environment. Such programs are used to develop guidelines to assist the practitioner in reviewing the literature and commercial product information, incorporating new findings in practice, recommending products to clients, and evaluating the outcomes of new interventions.

Research Publications

"The central function of journals is to provide current information related to practice, trends, and issues affecting a discipline."[10] Additional publications strictly devoted to dental hygiene research need to be developed to augment the dissemination of research information to practitioners and facilitate communication among researchers.

IDENTIFYING CLINICAL DENTAL HYGIENE PROBLEMS

A **clinical dental hygiene problem** is defined as a discrepancy between the way things are and the way they ought to be, or between what one knows and what one needs to know to eliminate the problem.[11] In other words, given current dental hygiene actions for a particular target group's oral health problems, how might care be improved or enhanced so that the results are better? Given what is currently known about dental hygiene care, what additional data are needed to plan actions for clients with a particular oral health problem?

Years of clinical practice experience are not essential for a dental hygienist to identify a clinical dental hygiene problem. Often the novice is more open than the experienced practitioner to the possibility that a procedure can be done differently than the expected routine. The dental hygienist needs to determine whether the problem is frequently occurring with a particular group of individuals, whether it can be consistently and accurately measured, and whether there is an alternative that could affect dental hygiene care.

Dental hygiene practitioners are primarily responsible for providing care or managing interventions that promote health/oral health and prevent oral disease. Globally, the practitioner may ask what interventions effectively promote health and prevent disease and under what conditions. Are certain interventions more effective in specific healthcare environments, with certain ethnic groups and certain age

Project Title: *Clinical Effectiveness of Hydrogen Peroxide–Sodium Bicarbonate Paste on Human Periodontitis Treated With and Without Scaling and Root Planing*

Investigator: (*Insert name*)

Date: (*Insert date*)

You are invited to participate in a study to investigate two home care methods. We hope to learn if there is any significant value obtained from brushing with a hydrogen peroxide–sodium bicarbonate paste to reduce periodontal disease compared to brushing with a fluoridated toothpaste. You were selected as a possible participant because you have a periodontal condition and do not have any medical complications that would affect participation.

Your participation will require that you follow the prescribed home care instructions accurately. You will be asked to brush your teeth with fluoridated toothpaste on one side of the mouth and use a hydrogen peroxide–sodium bicarbonate paste on the other side. The first treatment will include scaling your upper and lower teeth. We would like to examine the effect of cleaning your teeth combined with the home care regimen. You might experience some irritation to your gums if you should mix too much hydrogen peroxide with the sodium bicarbonate. You will be carefully instructed to avoid this irritation. We cannot and do not guarantee or promise that you will receive any benefits from this study. You may benefit from dental care procedures and education in the form of improved oral health.

I understand that the study will involve five appointments at the *(insert name of site)* over a two-month period. The first appointment will be two and one-half hours; each of the subsequent appointments will be 30 minutes. At the final appointment, the dental hygiene clinician will finish cleaning my teeth.

I have completed a health history and verify that all questions have been answered truthfully and to the best of my knowledge.

The investigation and the nature of my participation have been described to me in this form, and I understand the explanation. I understand that I am one of 30 individuals participating in this research project.

I understand that I may withdraw from the study at any time, and my decision will not prejudice further relations with *(insert name of site).*

I have been afforded an opportunity to ask questions concerning the purpose of this project, and all such questions have been answered to my satisfaction. I understand that should I have additional questions in the future about this project or the manner in which it is conducted, I may contact *(insert name of principal investigator)* at *(insert telephone number)* or *(insert name of co-investigator)* at *(insert telephone number).*

I understand that the results of this study may be published or presented orally, but I will not be identified individually.

I understand that participation in the study is strictly voluntary and no monetary compensation will be given.

I acknowledge that I was informed about any possible risks to my health and well-being that may be associated with my participation in this research. I understand that no medical or psychological assistance will be made available to me by either *(insert name of institution)* or any member of the research team as a result of any physical or emotional harm I may experience as a result of this research project. In the event I sustain physical injury as a result of participation in this investigation, if I am eligible for medical care, all necessary and appropriate care will be provided by *(insert name of site)* only. If I am not eligible for medical care, humanitarian emergency care will nevertheless be provided by *(insert name of site)* only.

I acknowledge that I have been advised of how I may obtain a copy of the results of this research project and that upon my making such a request, a copy will be provided without charge.

I understand that the information sought may mean better dental hygiene care for the public in the future.

I have been informed that I have the right to contact the *(insert name of institution)* Institutional Review Board for the Protection of Human Subjects or the *(insert name of site)* Subcommittee on Human Studies, Research and Development Committee should I wish to express any opinions regarding the conduct of this study. I further understand that all or a portion of the records concerning this study may be viewed by the *(insert name of appropriate federal agency).*

You are making a decision whether or not to participate. Your signature indicates that you have decided to participate, having read the information provided above.

________________________ __________
Signature of Volunteer Date

________________________ __________
Signature of Investigator Date

________________________ __________
Witnessed by Date

FIGURE 41–2
Consent to participate in research form. (From Lyne, S. M. Clinical Effectiveness of Hydrogen Peroxide–Sodium Bicarbonate Paste on Human Periodontitis Treated With and Without Scaling and Root Planing. Unpublished thesis. Old Dominion University, Norfolk, VA, 1984.)

TABLE 41-2
INITIATIVES IN THE DEVELOPMENT OF DENTAL HYGIENE RESEARCH 1970-1994

1970, 1973	• American Dental Hygienists' Association Policy on Research developed
1977	• Committee on Research established by American Dental Hygienists' Association House of Delegates
1977-79	• Committee on Research-sponsored workshops on research methods and scientific analysis
1978-79	• Dental hygiene program directors surveyed to determine attitudes toward research and level of research training in A.S., B.S., and M.S. programs
1979	• Research Grant Award Fund by American Dental Hygienists' Association Foundation established • Editorials on importance of research and articles on research methodology published in *Dental Hygiene*
1980	• Committee on Research merged to form Council on Educational Services and Research • Council on Educational Services and Research formulated three priority areas for funding of the Research Grant Award: quality of patient care, effectiveness of continuing education, dental hygiene practice
1980	• Research Initiative Task Force appointed and formalized a definition of research, mission of the Research Initiative, and 10 long-range goals
1982	• National survey of dental hygiene researchers conducted • First research forum held in conjunction with ADHA Annual Session. Eighteen papers were presented in education, community health, radiology, fluoridation, and behavioral and clinical research • Canadian Conference on Dental Hygiene Research held, sponsored by the University of Manitoba School of Dental Hygiene and Working Group on the Practice of Dental Hygiene, Department of National Health and Welfare
1984	• First American Dental Hygienists' Association-sponsored national conference on dental hygiene research held in Denver, Colorado (cosponsored with University of Colorado's Department of Dental Hygiene)
1987	• Second American Dental Hygienists' Association-sponsored national conference on dental hygiene research held in Iowa City, Iowa (cosponsored with University of Iowa's Department of Dental Hygiene)
1987	• Council on Research established as an independent American Dental Hygienists' Association Council (separated from Council on Educational Services and Research) • Research focus areas developed and disseminated
1989	• American Dental Hygienists' Association Institute for Oral Health provided funding for comprehensive literature reviews
1990	• "Building Alliances Through Dental Hygiene Research," special session held in conjunction with American Dental Hygienists' Association Annual Session in San Antonio, Texas
1993	• North American Conference on Dental Hygiene Research sponsored by the Canadian Dental Hygienists' Association in Niagara Falls, Canada
1994	• Third American Dental Hygienists' Association-sponsored research conference in Minneapolis, Minnesota
1994	• National Center for Dental Hygiene Research established at Thomas Jefferson University in Philadelphia, Pennsylvania

groups, and do they differ based on gender? With the prevalence of carpel tunnel syndrome (CTS) in the practitioner population, can the dental hygienist devise a new instrument, adapt existing instruments, or develop new principles of body mechanics to reduce the risk of CTS? By reading the dental hygiene literature and making observations in practice, practitioners can begin to identify dental hygiene problems that are relevant and meaningful for them and can ultimately make a difference to the oral health of society.

DEFINING THEORY

Without theory, research is little more than method applied systematically. A **theory** is a statement about the relationship of specifically defined concepts that describes, explains, or predicts some phenomenon and, in professional disciplines, prescribes action.[2,6,12] Theories generally are developed within a research tradition, that is, they are based on a particular view of reality and method of inquiry.[13] For example, Herzberg's motivation and hygiene theory is a statement about the relationship between factors that make people satisfied in their jobs and job performance and attitudes. This is an example of a management theory that prescribes action in relation to reward systems and job design. Numerous theories in psychology are used to conceptualize, describe, explain, and predict human behavior in a variety of contexts (e.g., Freudian theory, field theory, gestalt theory, and Skinnerian theory) (see Basic Characteristics of Theories chart).

Theories may be descriptive, explanatory, or predictive in nature, as each type described in Table 41-3.[4]

Disciplines are characterized as having a theoretical body of knowledge. As Darby has noted, whether dental hygiene emerges as a mature discipline depends on the direction its theory building will take.[4] Various types of theories need to be developed in dental hygiene. For example, grand theory takes an all-encompassing view of dental hygiene, a world view that attempts to explain and define dental hygiene—what it is, what it does, why it is important, and how it differs from other health professions. A grand theory of dental hygiene is derived not from observing what dental hygiene is (empirical phenomena), but rather from a philosophical position on what dental hygiene should be to be most effective. As such, a grand theory contains a significant value component that influences the acceptance and utility of the theory.[14] In contrast, midlevel theory has as its major goal the improvement of the practice of dental hygiene such as the most effective strategies for educating clients, managing anxiety, using a particular instrument, or developing self-care behaviors in clients. Most research on dental hygiene phenomena develops midlevel theory. Microtheories, also called partial theories, are summary statements of isolated observations of limited phenomena. Observations or case studies made by dental hygienists frequently yield information that enables the professional to develop components of a theory. These partial theories can evolve into midlevel theories with additional study.[4]

Theory Development

To more clearly understand what theory is, it is helpful to examine how theory evolves through the framework shown in Figure 41-3.[15] All theories begin with **facts** that we

TABLE 41–3
RELATIONSHIP BETWEEN TYPES OF THEORY AND RESEARCH

Types of Theory	Purpose of the Theory	Generated By	Examples in Dental Hygiene
Descriptive theory	Describes or classifies specific characteristics of individuals, groups, situations, or events by summarizing the commonalities found in discrete observations	Descriptive research	Osborn, J. B., Newell, K. J., Rudney, J. D., and Stoltenberg, J. L. Musculoskeletal pain among Minnesota dental hygienists. *Journal of Dental Hygiene* 64:132, 1990.
Explanatory theory	Specifies relations among the dimensions or characteristics of individuals, groups, situations, or events	Correlational research	Shannon, S. A. Variables that predict success on the National Board Dental Hygiene Examination. *Journal of Dental Hygiene* 63:73, 1989.
Predictive theory	Specifies the precise relationships between the dimensions or characteristics of a phenomenon or differences between groups	Experimental research	Lavigne, C. K., Nauman, R. K., Munley, M. M., and Suzuki, J. B. In vitro evaluation of air-powder polishing as an adjunct to ultrasonic scaling on periodontally involved root surfaces. *Journal of Dental Hygiene* 62:504, 1988.

Adapted from Fawcett, J. Analysis and Evaluation of Conceptual Models of Nursing, 2nd ed. Philadelphia: F. A. Davis, 1989, p. 21.

observe, directly or indirectly, quantify, and report. For example, fossils are found in rocks of a certain age, sterilization kills bacteria and viruses, water freezes at 32°F. However, facts alone provide limited information.

A **concept** expresses an abstraction formed by generalization from facts. For example, leadership, as a concept, is an abstraction formed from the observation of certain behaviors of individuals in positions of authority or influence. Also, prevention is a concept formed from the observation of an individual's behaviors that reduce the risk of injury or disease.

A **construct** is a concept with the added meaning of having been invented consciously and deliberately for a special scientific purpose. It is a concept that has been defined more specifically in that it can be observed and measured. For instance, intelligence is a concept, an abstraction from the observation of presumably intelligent and nonintelligent behaviors. As a scientific construct, intelligence means both more and less than it may mean as a concept. It means that scientists consciously and systematically use it in two ways. First, it is presented in theoretical schemes and is related in various ways to other constructs. Second, intelligence is so defined and specified that it can be observed and measured, such as through various intelligence tests. Definitions of concepts and constructs use other concepts or conceptual expressions in lieu of the expression being defined.[6]

Variables are observable and are symbols to which numerals or values are assigned. For example, in a previous example using prevention, components describing preventive behaviors can be given a numerical value that designates a strong or weak level of compliance on a component, such as "brushes or flosses regularly."

A **hypothesis** is a question, a conjectural statement, of the relationship between two or more variables. Collecting facts or identifying constructs is insufficient. If variables are selected that bear no relationship, the research is sterile, no matter how meticulous the subsequent observations and inferences.[16] The researcher must link variables together in some relationship. Knowing that a certain chemotherapeu-

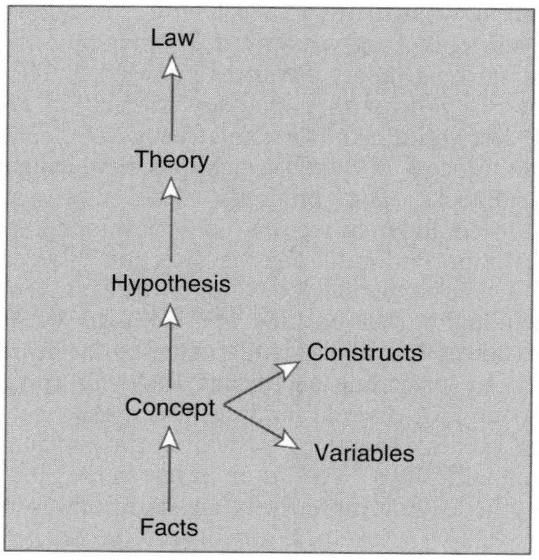

Law
Theory
Hypothesis
Constructs
Concept
Variables
Facts

FIGURE 41–3
Progression of theory development. (Adapted and redrawn from Owens, R. G. Organizational Behavior in Schools. Copyright 1970. Reprinted with permission of Allyn & Bacon.)

THE BASIC CHARACTERISTICS OF THEORIES

- Theories can interrelate concepts in such a way as to create a different way of looking at a particular phenomenon
- Theories must be logical in nature
- Theories are the basis for hypotheses that can be tested
- Theories contribute to and assist in increasing the general body of knowledge within the discipline through the research implemented to validate them
- Theories can be used by the practitioner to guide and improve their practice
- Theories must be consistent with other validated theories, laws, and principles

Adapted from The Nursing Theories Conference Group, Julia B. George, Chairperson. Nursing Theories: The Base for Professional Nursing Practice. Englewood Cliffs, NJ: Prentice-Hall, 1980, pp. 5–7.

tic agent alters bacterial plaque is useful if a relationship has been established with the control of oral disease.

The researcher links variables together with a hypothesis that states an expected relationship. That is, under one set of circumstances, certain facts should hold true. Hypotheses must be statements about the relationship between variables, and they must carry clear implications for testing the stated relations. A research study does not test variables, it tests relations between variables. For example, in a study of health promotion behaviors of dental hygiene practitioners, one hypothesis states there is a significant difference in health promotion behaviors between practitioners who have control over their clients' appointments and those who do not. This is stated to test the relationship between the variables related to behaviors and practice autonomy.

A **theory** is a set of interrelated constructs, concepts, ideas, definitions, and propositions that presents a systematic view of phenomena by specifying relations among variables with the purpose of explaining and predicting. A theory is the systematic relating of a set of general hypotheses. Theory can give rise to more hypotheses that can be tested and that will further strengthen or cast doubt on the theory. Some of the more widely recognized theories include the theory of relativity, the theory of evolution, and Maslow's theory of human need. Using a previous example, prevention is a concept but there are numerous theories about prevention in the social sciences, with anthropology, psychology, and sociology developing different perspectives and different methods to test their theories.

With repeated hypothesizing and testing over time, a theory can lead to empirical **law.** Once all possible relations have been tested and borne out, theory becomes law, such as the law of gravity.

Theory is Not. . . .

To better understand what theory is, it is often helpful to understand what theory is *not.* A theory is not something that is unproven or some sort of idle speculation ("I have a theory that sea water will cure the common cold"). A theory is not a philosophy or something that deals with values or what ought to be ("I have a theory that if everyone lived according to the Golden Rule there would be no war"). Theory is not merely a respectable term meaning impractical. How many times has someone stated "that's a great theory, but it isn't the way things work in practice"? If a theory does not work in practice, there is a problem with the theory. Theory is not a personal notion of how to get a job done. "I have a theory that if we do it this way. . . "[15]

Distinction Between Theory and Research

Research and theory are not synonymous, but they are mutually dependent. Michels has contrasted the difference between theory and research as follows:

> Without theory, research is little more than method and documentation applied systematically. Theory may be as simple as an hypothesis, as elegant as a mathematical model, or as elaborate and complex as a book-length theory of human learning, but theory is abstract in the sense that it consists of ideas and concepts that are connected together and to evidence by logical rules. Theory is not an act, but theorizing is. Theory is not merely rationale. . . Theory differs from rationale in that it both explains and predicts, and it is testable or falsifiable. Theory is the "so what" of research. Research without theory does not contribute to knowledge.*

Further, the contributions between theory and research are not all in one direction. Theory stimulates research and enhances the meaning of its findings; empirical research serves to test existing theories and to provide a basis for the development of new ones.

Research is a process of asking questions in a certain way or discovering better questions to ask. Theory explains phenomena by specifying which variables are related to other variables, thus enabling the researcher to predict the relationship from one variable to another. Theory can help us organize our knowledge into a systematic, orderly body. By establishing the limits of our knowledge, theory can assist the researcher in formulating problems for the study of unknown areas. In fact, the test of a good theory is how much research it generates.[6,17]

Distinction Between Theory and Conceptual Models

Theories, like conceptual models (see Chapter 1), are comprised of concepts and propositions; however, theories are much more specific than conceptual models (Table 41–4).[4] Conceptual models are valuable because they provide the organization for thinking, observing, and interpreting.[18] For example, if practitioners want to ensure that their practice is oriented toward health promotion, the practitioner needs to define health promotion, identify characteristics that could be observed and measured to know if the clients were implementing health promotion behaviors, and place these observations and measurements in a larger framework. However, conceptual models evolve not only from empirical observations and intuitive insights, but also from creatively combining ideas from other fields (see Major Focus of Seven Conceptual Models of Nursing chart).

Role of Theory in Advancing Knowledge

Understanding what theory is and how it is developed from facts and concepts is important, but it is equally important to understand how theory advances knowledge. Theory development is a *process* that includes articulation and validation of descriptions and/or explanations of phenomena. During this process one learns, achieves new insights, discovers roadblocks, and proceeds along new pathways. Theories—even fragments or partially developed theory—provide an important guide for the direction of research by pointing to areas that are likely to be fruitful, that is, in which meaningful relationships are likely to be found.[17] Theory advances knowledge and increases the fruitfulness of research by providing significant leads for inquiry, by relating seemingly discrete findings by means of similar underlying processes, and by providing an explanation of observed relationships. The more research is directed by systematic theory, the more likely are its results to contrib-

---

* From Michels, E. Commentary: Enhancing the scholarly base: The role of faculty in enhancing scholarship. Journal of Allied Health 18(2):129–142, 1989.

TABLE 41–4
DISTINCTIONS BETWEEN CONCEPTUAL MODELS AND THEORIES

Conceptual Model	Theory
• Abstract	• Concrete
• Comprehensive perspective of the metaparadigm	• Perspective restricted to limited phenomena identified in the metaparadigm
• Addresses the entire domain	• Addresses specific phenomena within the domain
• Cannot be tested directly	• Can be tested directly
• Used to generate theory	• Used to generate hypotheses
• Provides general guidelines for viewing and thinking about phenomena in practice, education, administration, and research	• Provides specific information for describing, explaining, and predicting phenomena

From Darby, M. L. Theory Development and Basic Research in Dental Hygiene: Review of the Literature and Recommendations. Chicago: American Dental Hygienists' Association, 1990, p. 39.

MAJOR FOCUS OF SEVEN CONCEPTUAL MODELS OF NURSING

Johnson's Behavioral System Model
Emphasis: on the individual as a behavioral system with attachment, dependency, ingestive, eliminative, sexual, aggressive, and achievement subsystems
Goal: to restore, maintain, or attain behavioral systems balance and stability

King's Interacting Systems Framework
Emphasis: on personal (individuals), interpersonal (groups), and social (society) systems
Goal: to help individuals maintain their health so they can function in their roles

Levine's Conservation Model
Emphasis: on conservation of the individual's energy, structural integrity, personal integrity, and social integrity
Goal: to promote wholeness of the individual through conservation

Neuman's Systems Model
Emphasis: on individuals, families, and communities as client systems with physiological, psychological, sociocultural, developmental, and spiritual variables
Goal: to retain, attain, and maintain optimal client wellness through primary, secondary, and tertiary prevention

Orem's Self-Care Framework
Emphasis: on individuals as self-care agents with universal, developmental, health deviation, and self-care requisites
Goal: to help people to meet their own therapeutic self-care demands

Rogers' Science of Unitary Human Beings
Emphasis: on human beings and their environments as open, four-dimensional, patterned energy fields
Goal: to help all people achieve maximal well-being

Roy's Adaptation Model
Emphasis: on individuals and groups as adaptive systems with physiological, self-concept, role function, and interdependence modes of adaptation
Goal: to promote adaptation through management of environmental stimuli

Adapted from Fawcett, J. Analysis and Evaluation of Conceptual Models of Nursing, 2nd ed. Philadelphia: F. A. Davis, 1989, pp. 63–353.

ute directly to the development and further organization of knowledge.[6,13,15]

Role of Theory in Advancing Practice

The mutual interdependence between theory and practice is exemplified through fundamental patterns of knowing: the practitioner uses some model, often unconsciously, to choose and adapt theories and integrate them with other knowledge derived from the clinical situation.[13] According to Chinn and Jacobs, the theory validation process is the essence of the theory-practice relationship because this involves the testing of theory in practice.[19] If repeated results provide evidence of a theory's accuracy, the theory is presumed valid. Testing provides feedback to refine theory to better represent reality (which is where practice occurs), and explaining reality is the main purpose of theory.

Kraemer and Gurenlian have developed a model to illustrate the connectedness between theory and practice in dental hygiene.[20] As shown in Figure 41–4, the conceptual framework, which ties theory to clinical application and decision making, is circular and reciprocal, can begin and end at any point, and reflects the multifaceted nature and complexity of problems found in the oral healthcare environment. For example, during assessment, the practitioner

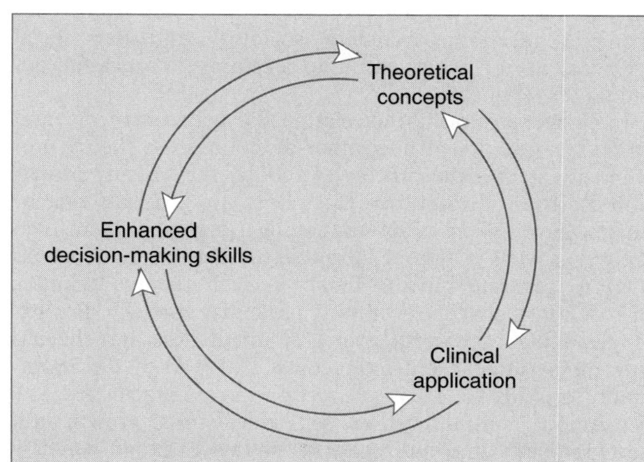

FIGURE 41–4
Conceptual framework. (Redrawn from Journal of Dental Hygiene, Vol. 63, No. 5, copyrighted 1989 by the American Dental Hygienists' Association.)

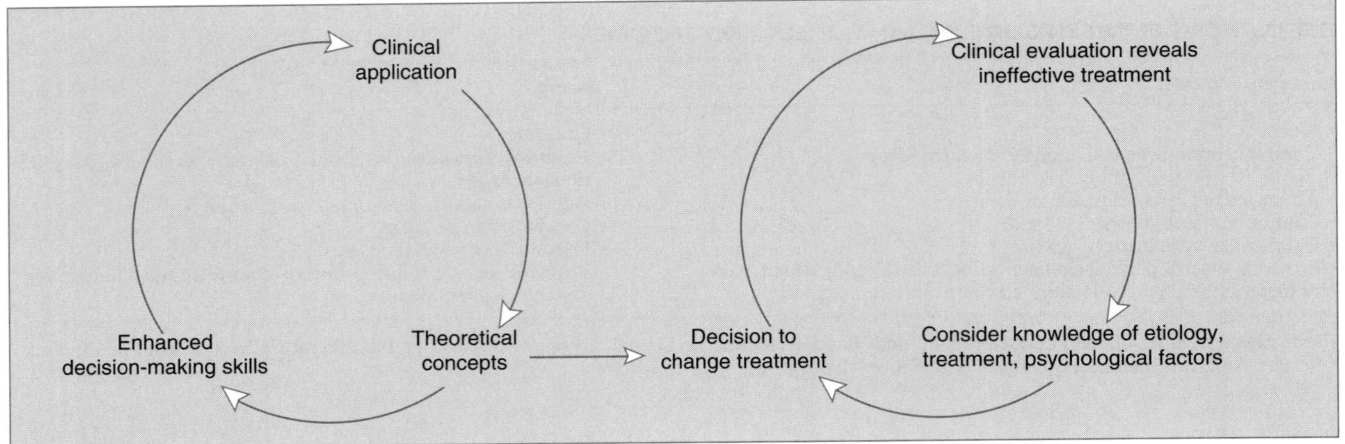

FIGURE 41-5
Conceptual framework applied to clinical application. (Redrawn from Journal of Dental Hygiene, Vol. 63, No. 5, copyrighted 1989 by the American Dental Hygienists' Association.)

recognizes that the client has not healed adequately. To proceed with an appropriate intervention, the practitioner must identify the problem (dental hygiene diagnosis), establish a goal, and redefine in a plan the dental hygiene intervention applied. At this stage, the practitioner examines the theoretical concepts related to the planned dental hygiene care. Based on the dental hygiene diagnosis, the goals established, and the overall dental treatment plan the practitioner monitors the client to determine whether the dental hygiene interventions produced the expected outcome and achieved the designated goal. This process is reflected in Figure 41-5.

Disciplines in the health professions have enumerated several reasons for using research and theory in practice: to base practice on sound principles, to base practice on fact rather than tradition or intuition, to use theories and research findings for planning client care, for determining the type of interventions or care, and for using the process of care appropriately. Most professional disciplines have generated theory from conceptual models in their own field, have derived or borrowed theory from other disciplines' models and theories, or have based their theories on paradigms shared by a variety of disciplines, such as psychotherapy, education, psychology, sociology, and other social sciences, all of which seek to explain the meaning of human experiences.

In further exploring the relationship between theory and practice, examples of how other disciplines use theory provide insight into the process. Although the nursing profession borrows from other disciplines to generate theory, nurses have taken pride in having developed their own theory as well. Often, conceptual models of nursing are used to generate nursing theory.[21] Each theory addresses one or more concepts within a particular model.[13] For example, King's theory of goal attainment describes the nature of the nurse-client interactions that lead to the attainment of goals. This interaction is characterized by perception, communication, self, role, stress, growth and development, time and space.[21] In this example a single concept has unique characteristics that come together to form a particular theory.

Occupational therapy exemplifies a practice discipline with theories that have evolved from another discipline—that of social psychology.[22] As early as 1958, Reilly, a renowned occupational therapy educator and researcher, began to carve out "activity" that she would later call "occupational behavior" as the special domain of the occupational therapy profession. She proposed that the uniqueness of occupational therapy's body of knowledge lies in the nature of productive and creative activity and urged that research within the field of occupational therapy focus on the meaning individuals derive from work and activity. In an attempt to build a cohesive philosophy for occupational therapy, she selected essential conceptual threads underlying occupational behavior that serve as the foundation for occupational science: occupations and occupational role, environment, independence, and adaptation.[23,24]

As is the case with other disciplines, theories derived from dental hygiene are specific to dental hygiene phenomena. "**Dental hygiene theory** can be defined as interrelated concepts basic to dental hygiene that can be used to systematically describe and explain approaches to dental hygiene practice and predict outcomes of that practice."[4] The human needs conceptual model for dental hygiene expressed in this book is an area of dental hygiene theory development. Basic human need theory provides the theoretical framework for the conceptual model and was selected because of observations made about what dental hygienists do. In this model, dental hygiene assessment findings are aimed purposefully at identifying human need deficits that can be fulfilled through dental hygiene care; therefore, dental hygiene interventions can result in meeting select human needs. This model is explained fully in Chapter 2.

GOALS FOR DENTAL HYGIENE RESEARCH

The future professional growth of dental hygiene depends on dental hygiene research that generates an organized, related current body of dental hygiene knowledge. As stated in the *Prospectus for Dental Hygiene:*

> The profound changes which are rapidly occurring in society and the new systems and priorities for health services which are evolving to accommodate societal changes require assessment of dental hygiene practice

TABLE 41–5
TOPICS FOR DENTAL HYGIENE RESEARCH: NIDR LONG-RANGE RESEARCH PLAN FOR THE NINETIES

Dental Caries
Conducting epidemiological studies to further define the changing patterns of dental caries prevalence Identifying and controlling risk factors Targeting specific caries preventive methods and agents to those individuals and groups at high risk Matching preventive and therapeutic regimes to anticipated needs Investigating the effects of multiple fluoride usages and its relationship to compliance or to potential for toxicity Analyzing the effect of interrelated variables such as genetics, dietary habits, and environmental factors on caries susceptibility Studying the effects of oral hygiene and professional care on various dental materials
Periodontal Diseases
Assessing mechanisms to quantify disease activity in periodontal assessment Identifying risk factors associated with advancing disease Improving nonsurgical and maintenance therapy Testing strategies for developing long-term protective health behaviors
Craniofacial Malformations, Defects, and Malrelations
Studying the economic, psychological, and sociological effects of craniofacial deformities
Saliva, Soft Tissue Diseases, and AIDS
Studying the prevalence of various soft tissue lesions, the relationship of oral medications and systemic diseases to oral soft tissue lesions Studying the effect of salivary deficiencies in the aging population
Orofacial Pain
Investigating cognitive, emotional, behavioral, social, and psychological factors in relation to behavioral aspects of pain control Studying the relationship between stress and temporomandibular joint (TMJ) pain, or stress and oral habits Studying the effects of taste and smell disorders on quality of life Investigating the psychosocial effects of rehabilitation of oral motor function after surgery or injury
Oral Health Promotion/Disease Prevention, Epidemiology, and Science Transfer
Examining the broad range of measurable psychological, behavioral, cultural, and social interactions that affect oral health and disease Studying: Dental phobic behaviors and noncompliance Psychosocial and behavioral sequelae of untreated craniofacial deformities Development and maintenance of long-term protective health behaviors Management of chronic pain Relationship of life stress events to oral diseases Risk factors associated with noncompliance with oral health recommendations Linkages between behavioral changes and oral health outcomes Efficacy of oral health promotion efforts Examination of the relationship of utilization of dental hygiene services within the dental care delivery system and functional oral health status

Adapted from Bowen, D. Dental hygiene research: Issues and challenges of the next decade. Canadian Dental Hygiene/Probe 24(4):163–167, 1990.

and education. Dental hygiene must be integrated into evolving systems of society if oral health needs of the public are to be met; dental hygiene must change in dramatic but deliberate ways to provide for such integration; change in dental hygiene education and practice will occur only if dental hygiene takes responsibility for its future.*

The ADHA, through publication of the *Prospectus* and the ongoing development of its strategic research plan, proposes directions for advancing dental hygiene research to meet the future oral health needs of the public.[26] Over the past decade, the ADHA and the CDHA have made a commitment to sponsoring research programs that have resulted in advancing the understanding of dental hygiene practice and have established a baseline for building dental hygiene theory. Priorities for dental hygiene research and theory development and goals and strategies to achieve these priorities are based on predictions about consumers of dental hygiene care, evolving systems for the delivery of health care, and the future of dental hygiene practice.

* From Steering Committee for the Workshops on the Future of Dental Hygiene Practice and Education. Prospectus for Dental Hygiene. Chicago: American Dental Hygienists' Association, 1988.

Priorities for Dental Hygiene Research

Dental hygiene focuses its research efforts so that knowledge is generated that will enable dental hygienists to:

- Promote oral health, oral wellness, and self-care among all age, social, and cultural groups

TABLE 41–6
FOCUS AREAS FOR DENTAL HYGIENE RESEARCH AND THEORY DEVELOPMENT

The dental hygiene profession is responsible for advancing an organized body of knowledge as the foundation for meeting the oral health needs of society. The succeeding focus areas, based upon the central concept of dental hygiene's paradigm, serve to stimulate researchable ideas about concepts and constructs used in dental hygiene, guide investigation of dental hygiene phenomena, and facilitate the systematic evolution of research and theory development. Dental hygiene researchers are encouraged to link their research efforts to relevant theories and to develop unique theories that can advance the body of dental hygiene knowledge in a systematic and orderly fashion.

Central Concepts of Dental Hygiene's Paradigm	Areas in Need of Research and Theory Development	Dental Hygiene Phenomena
Client: central focus of dental hygiene care; may include the person, the family, the community, the nation, or the world	Theoretical models and research that: • describe, explain or predict client oral health attitude, status, knowledge, and behavior • explain client learning, motivation, or preferences over the lifespan • explore the relationship between the communication process and client oral health • explore the effects of dental hygiene technology on the client • explore the teaching-learning styles and client oral health and wellness • explore the relationship among client growth, development, and maturation, and oral health promotion and wellness • explore the communication process between the client and professional dental hygienist that lead to oral wellness	Compliance, oral health needs of individuals with special needs, access to care, educational processes and technologies, lifelong learning, public policy
Environment: the situation in which the client and dental hygienist find themselves	Theoretical models and research that: • describe, explain, or predict barriers to oral health, oral health promotion, and oral health behavior • describe, explain, or predict the relationship between environmental factors (culture, society, income, education, etc.) and oral health promotion, oral health and wellness, and oral health behavior • describe, explain, or predict biopsychosocial influences on oral health promotion, wellness, and health • enhance public access to dental hygiene care • enhance the educational preparation of the dental hygienist at all levels • enhance dental hygiene care delivery in various settings	Public policy, legislation, regulation, infection control, barriers to care, environmental control of oral health, employment settings, employer-employee relations, quality of work life, practice models, educational models, accreditation, credentialing, curriculum development, educational processes and technology, occupational hazards and risks
Health/oral health: health and oral health status of the client from the wellness focus of the dental hygienist	Theoretical models and research that: • describe, explain, or predict a client's movement within a health-illness continuum • describe, explain, or predict oral wellness	Oral epidemiology, oral disease patterns, dental hygiene delivery systems, cost of oral health promotion and oral health
Dental hygiene actions: the behaviors, interventions, methods, etc., used in the provision of dental hygiene care	Theoretical models and research that: • describe, explain or predict dental hygiene demographics, characteristics, attitudes, knowledge, or behaviors	Demographics, scope of practice, dental hygiene process of care, specific dental hygiene interventions, dental hygiene diagnosis, dental hygiene therapy, qual-

TABLE 41-6
FOCUS AREAS FOR DENTAL HYGIENE RESEARCH AND THEORY DEVELOPMENT *Continued*

Central Concepts of Dental Hygiene's Paradigm	Areas in Need of Research and Theory Development	Dental Hygiene Phenomena
	• enhance career recruitment, retention, reentry, and professional development • describe, explain, or predict the value of dental hygiene services • describe, explain, or predict dental hygiene roles and processes • describe, explain, or predict outcomes of dental hygiene care • describe, explain, or predict risks associated with dental hygiene care • describe, explain, or predict the efficacy of dental hygiene interventions, equipment, materials, and products Conceptual models and research that describe and explain the uniqueness of dental hygiene	ity assurance, role development, product evaluation, competence assessment, decision making, outcomes of dental hygiene care, career recruitment, reentry

Note: This listing is not meant to be exhaustive.
Adapted from Darby, M. L. Theory development and basic research in dental hygiene: review of the literature and recommendations. American Dental Hygienists' Association, 1990, pp. 83-86.

- Minimize or prevent behaviorally and environmentally induced oral health problems that compromise the quality of life
- Ensure that the oral health needs of groups, such as the elderly, children, individuals from diverse cultures, and the poor, are met in effective, appropriate ways
- Classify dental hygiene practice phenomena
- Ensure that principles of ethics guide dental hygiene research
- Develop instruments to measure dental hygiene outcomes
- Design and evaluate alternative models for delivering oral healthcare so that dental hygienists are able to balance high quality and cost effectiveness in meeting the dental hygiene needs of identified populations
- Evaluate the effectiveness of dental hygiene education in preparing a practitioner who requires broad knowledge and a wide range of skills and a practitioner who requires specialized knowledge and a focused set of skills

Another way dental hygiene's research initiatives can be organized is in response to the National Institute for Dental Research (NIDR) publication *Long-Range Research Plan for the Nineties.* Bowen has identified topics appropriate for dental hygiene research based on the NIDR plan in areas related to dental caries; periodontal diseases; craniofacial malformations, defects, and malrelations; saliva, soft tissue disease, and AIDS; orofacial pain; and oral health promotion/disease prevention, epidemiology, and science transfer (Table 41-5).[27] Because a paradigm for dental hygiene has been developed, Darby has recommended that research efforts focus around the central concepts relevant to dental hygiene (the client, the environment, health/oral health, and dental hygiene actions) so that the body of dental hygiene knowledge can be developed in an organized and systematic way regardless of the conceptual model adopted (Table 41-6).

References

1. Donaldson, S. K., and Crowley, D. M. The discipline of nursing. Nursing Outlook 26(2):113, 1978.
2. Dickoff, J., James, P., and Wiedenbach, E. Theory in a practice discipline, part I: Practice oriented theory. Nursing Research 17(5):415, 1968.
3. Potter, P., and Perry, A. Research in nursing care. In Contemporary Nursing: Dimensions and Dynamics. St. Louis: C. V. Mosby, 1993, p. 1430.
4. Darby, M. L. Theory development and basic research in dental hygiene: Review of the literature and recommendations. American Dental Hygienists' Association, June, 1990.
5. Scholfeldt, R. Research in nursing and research-training for nurses: Retrospect and prospect. Nursing Research 24:177, 1975.
6. Kerlinger, F. N. Foundations of behavioral research, 2nd ed. New York: Holt, Rinehart, & Winston, 1973, p. 11.
7. Darby, M. L., and Bowen, D. Research methods for oral health professionals. St. Louis: C. V. Mosby, 1980, pp. 1-86.
8. Michels, E. Commentary: Enhancing the scholarly base: The role of faculty in enhancing scholarship. Journal of Allied Health 18(2):129, 1989.
9. Committee on the Conduct of Science, National Academy of Sciences. On Being a Scientist. Washington, DC: National Academy Press, 1989.
10. Vaz, D. An investigation of the usage of the periodical literature of nursing by staff nurses and nursing administrators. Journal of Continuing Education in Nursing 17:22, 1986.
11. Diers, D. Research in Nursing Practice. Philadelphia: J. B. Lippincott, 1979.
12. Argyris, C., and Schon, D. A. Theory and Practice: Increasing Professional Effectiveness. San Francisco: Jossey Bass, 1974.

13. Firlit, S. L. Nursing theory and nursing practice. In McCloskey, J. C., and Grace, H. K. (eds). Current Issues in Nursing, 3rd ed. St. Louis, C. V. Mosby, 1990, p. 5.
14. Kelly, L. Y. Dimensions of Professional Nursing, 5th ed. New York: Macmillan, 1985, p. 195.
15. Owens, R. G. Organizational Behavior in Schools. Englewood Cliffs, NJ: Prentice-Hall, 1970, p. 941.
16. Merton, R. K. Social Theory and Social Structure. Free Press, 1957.
17. Selititz, C., Johoda, M., Deutsch, M., and Cook, S. W. Research Methods in Social Relations. New York: Holt, Rinehart, & Winston, 1959, pp. 491–492.
18. Fawcett, J. Analysis and Evaluation of Conceptual Models of Nursing, 2nd ed. Philadelphia: F. A. Davis, 1989, p. 921.
19. Chinn, P. L., and Jacobs, M. K. Theory and Nursing: A Systematic Approach. St. Louis: C. V. Mosby, 1987, p. 174.
20. Kraemer, L. G., and Gurenlian, J. R. An educational model for preparing dental hygiene students in the treatment of periodontal diseases. Journal of Dental Hygiene 63(5):232, 1989.
21. King, I. M. A Theory for Nursing: Systems, Concepts, Paradigms. New York: John Wiley & Sons, 1981, pp. 141–149.
22. Yerxa, E. J., Clark, F., et al. An introduction to occupational science, a foundation for occupational therapy in the 21st century. Occupational Therapy in Health Care 6(4):1, 1989.
23. Reilly, M. An occupational therapy curriculum for 1965. American Journal of Occupational Therapy 12:293, 1958.
24. Jackson, J. En route to adulthood: A high school transition program for adolescents with disabilities. Occupational Science —The Foundation for New Models of Practice. Occupational Therapy in Health Care 6(4):33, 1989.
25. Walsh, M. Theory development in dental hygiene. The Canadian Dental Hygienists' Association Journal Probe 25(1):12, 1991.
26. Steering Committee for the Workshops on the Future of Dental Hygiene Practice and Education. Prospectus for Dental Hygiene. Chicago: American Dental Hygienists' Association, 1988.
27. Bowen, D. Dental hygiene research: issues and challenges of the next decade. The Canadian Dental Hygienists' Journal Probe 24(4):163, 1990.

Suggested Readings

Buchler, J. (ed.). Philosophical Writings of Pierce. New York: Dover, 1955.

Canadian Nurses' Association. Ethical Guidelines for Nursing Research Involving Human Subjects. Canadian Nurses' Association, April, 1983.

Canadian Dental Hygienists' Association. Conference Proceedings: A North American Research Conference, An Exploration into the Future. October 15–17, 1993, Niagara Falls, Canada.

Committee on the Conduct of Science, National Academy of Sciences. On Being a Scientist. Washington, D.C.: National Academy Press, 1989.

Darby, M. L. Toward a clearer understanding of dental hygiene research, theory, and practice. In Proceedings of the Conference on Dental Hygiene Research. University of Manitoba School of Dental Hygiene and Working Group on the Practice of Dental Hygiene, Department of National Health and Welfare, Canada, 1982.

Darby, M. L. Collaborative model of practice—the future of dental hygiene. Journal of Dental Education 47(9):589, 1983.

Darby, M. L. Getting started in research. Proceedings of the 11th International Dental Hygiene Symposium, Ottawa, Canada, June 28, 1989.

Darby, M. L., and Walsh, M. M. A proposed human needs conceptual model for dental hygiene: Part I. Journal of Dental Hygiene 67(6):326, 1993.

DePoy, E. and Gitlan, L. N. Introduction to Research: Multiple Strategies for Health and Human Services. St. Louis: C. V. Mosby, 1993.

Dickoff, J., and James, P. Organization and expansion of knowledge: Toward a constructive assault on the imperious distinction of pure from applied knowledge, of knowledge from technique. Dental Hygiene 62(1):15, 1988.

Fawcett, J. A declaration of nursing independence: The relationship of theory and research to nursing practice. Nursing Administration Quarterly 6:36, 1980.

Haller, K. B., Reynolds, M. A., and Horsley, J. A. Developing research-based innovation protocols: Process, criteria and issues. Research Nursing Health 2:45, 1979.

Hempel, C. G. Fundamentals of concept formation in empirical science. International Encyclopedia of Unified Science 2:7, 1952.

Hersey, P., and Blanchard, K. Management of Organizational Behavior, 5th ed. Englewood Cliffs, NJ: Prentice-Hall, 1988, p. 4.

Horsley, J. A. Using research in practice: The current context. Western Journal of Nursing Research 7:135, 1985.

Horsley, J. A., et al. Using research to improve nursing practice: A guide. Orlando, FL: Grune & Stratton, 1983.

Johnson, D. E. Development of theory. Nursing Research 23:372, 1974.

Johnson, D. E. Theory in nursing: Borrowed and unique. Nursing Research 17:206, 1968.

Johnson, P. M. Theory development in dental hygiene. Canadian Dental Hygiene/Probe 25(1):19, 1991.

Kim, S. H. The Nature of Theoretical Thinking in Nursing. Norwalk, CT: Appleton-Century-Crofts, 1983.

Levine, R. J. Ethics and Regulation of Clinical Research, 2nd ed. Baltimore and Munich: Urban and Schwarzenberg, 1986.

Lewin, K. Field Theory in Social Sciences. New York: Harper & Row, 1951.

National Institute of Dental Research. Long-range research plan for the Nineties. U.S. Department of Health and Human Services/ Public Health Service/National Institutes of Health, NIH Publication No. 90–1188, September, 1990.

Neuman, B. The Neuman Systems Model, 2nd ed. Norwalk, CT: Appleton & Lange, 1989, pp. 99–100.

Perry, C. President's address. Journal of the American Dental Hygienists' Association 14:179, 1940.

Polit, D. V., and Hungler, B. P. Nursing Research: Principles and Practice, 2nd ed. Philadelphia: J. B. Lippincott, 1983.

Steering Committee for the Workshops on the Future of Dental Hygiene Practice and Education. Prospectus for dental hygiene. Chicago: American Dental Hygienists' Association, 1988.

The Nursing Theories Conference Group, Julia B. George, Chairperson. Nursing Theories: The Base for Professional Nursing Practice. Englewood Cliffs, NJ: Prentice Hall, 1980, pp. 5–7.

Walsh, M. M., and Darby, M. L. Application of the human needs conceptual model of dental hygiene to the role of the clinician: Part II. Journal of Dental Hygiene 67(6):334, 1993.

Weiler, K., and Buckwalter, K. C. Is nursing research used in practice? In McCloskey, J., and Grace, H. (eds.). Current Issues in Nursing, 3rd ed. St. Louis: C. V. Mosby, 1990.

Woodall, I. Sciences are basic for oral healthcare. RDH January, 1991.

GLOSSARY

abandonment A relinquishment of all connection between the practitioner and client by the practitioner.

abrasion Pathological tooth wear as a result of a foreign substance.

abutment A tooth that serves as an anchor for a fixed or removable prosthetic appliance.

acceptance The ability to accept a client as the person he is without allowing any judgment of that person's attitudes or feelings to interfere with communication.

accessibility The ability to obtain the needed healthcare in a convenient and efficient manner.

accreditation The process by which a nongovernmental agency evaluates an institution or program of study according to predetermined, national standards.

acid-etching The process of washing the enamel surface with 37% phosphoric acid prior to the placement of a sealant in order to increase sealant retention.

acquired disability A disability occurring after the age of 22 years caused by a disease, trauma, or injury to the body.

acquired pellicle A thin, clear, unstructured organic membrane that forms over exposed tooth surfaces and restorations within minutes after removal by professional and self-polishing techniques.

action potential Within a nerve fiber, a rapid sequence of changes—depolarization and repolarization.

activities of daily living (ADLs) The abilities that are fundamental to independent living, such as bathing, oral hygiene, dressing, toileting, transferring from bed or chair, feeding, and continence.

activity theory The theory states that a positive relationship exists between individuals' level of participation in social activities and their life satisfaction.

acute fluoride toxicity The immediate physiological reaction to a fluoride overdose, including nausea, vomiting, hypersalivation, abdominal pain, and diarrhea.

acute herpetic gingivostomatitis The primary infection with the herpes virus manifesting with vesicles and ulcerations.

HVS I—Herpes simplex virus I, initial infection, clients asymptomatic.

HVS II—Herpes simplex virus II, commonly transmitted sexually; may be manifested orally.

Herpetic whitlow—a recurrent lesion of the finger initiated by puncture from a herpes virus-contaminated instrument.

acute necrotizing ulcerative gingivitis (ANUG) An opportunistic infection of the gingiva that is associated with stress, lifestyle, inadequate nutrition, and some chronic conditions such as blood dyscrasias, AIDS, and Down syndrome.

acute pericoronitis An abscess associated with a partially erupted tooth or fully erupted tooth that is covered completely or partially by a flap of tissue (operculum).

Operculum—the flap of tissue that completely or partially covers a tooth.

acute periodontal abscess An exacerbated inflammatory reaction occurring usually in a periodontally involved area and caused by a blockage of the area by some foreign body.

acute/rampant caries See under *dental caries.*

adaptation The alignment or placement of the side of the first few millimeters of the periodontal probe, straight explorer, or blade of a scaler against the tooth prior to activation of an exploratory or working stroke.

adenopathy Any disease of the glands, especially of the lymphatic glands.

adequacy of attached gingiva The periodontal measurement determined with the periodontal probe by observing the mucogingival junction, measuring the distance from the mucogingival junction to the gingival margin, measuring pocket depth, and calculating the difference between the two measurements.

adrenalin/epinephrine A naturally occurring agent responsible for sympathetic nervous system activity.

adrenergic receptors Receptors throughout the body's tissues that are stimulated by the chemicals released by the sympathetic nervous system or a sympathomimetic agent (drug).

alpha r.—One of the two major categories of adrenergic receptors; activation of these receptors results in contraction of the smooth muscle in blood vessels causing constriction of blood vessels.

beta r.—One of the two major categories of adrenergic receptors; activation of these receptors results in smooth muscle relaxation and cardiac stimulation.

Beta 1 receptors—A division of beta receptors; activation of these receptors increases cardiac rate and force.

Beta 2 receptors—A division of beta receptors; activation of these receptors causes bronchodilation and vasodilation.

adult day care A community-based center where older adults can go to receive supervised daily activities and recreation.

advocacy The education of decision-makers to provide the essential political support for change.

aerosol Artificially generated solid or liquid airborne particles less than 50 microns in size.

aerosolization The airborne transfer of microorganisms in a fine mist.

affective goals Desired changes in client or clinician values, beliefs, and attitudes.

affective learning domain The domain that classifies levels of learning involving feelings, attitudes, values, and interests; including receiving, responding, valuing, organizing, and having a value system.

age-related macular degeneration (AMD) Deterioration in the membrane between the retina and underlying blood vessels which leads to a decline in one's central vision.

AIDS Acquired immunodeficiency syndrome; an immunosuppressive viral disease characterized by specific suppression in the immune response and associated with a wide variety of opportunistic infections.

airborne Pertaining to microorganism suspended in the air for an extended time where they may be inhaled by others, such as microorganisms that cause tuberculosis and measles (not HIV and HBV).

air powder abrasive system/air polisher A specially designed unit with a handpiece used for extrinsic stain removal via the delivery of a spray of warm water and sodium bicarbonate under pressure.

allergy A hypersensitive reaction, acquired through exposure to a specific environmental substance (allergen); re-exposure increases potential to react.

allogenic bone marrow Bone marrow from a person with a similar genetic make-up.

alloy A mixture of metals contributing to the composition of a dental amalgam.

alpha receptors See under *adrenergic receptors.*

aluminum cap See under *cartridge.*

alveolar/attached gingiva Bound-down gingival tissue consisting of keratinized stratified squamous epithelium that covers the crestal portion of the alveolar bone and the roof of the mouth.

alveolar mucosa The nonkeratinized epithelium characterized by a smooth and shiny surface. The mucosa covers the vestibule and floor of the mouth and becomes the buccal and labial mucosa.

alveolar process The bone that forms the tooth sockets and supports the teeth.

Alzheimer's disease (AD) An irreversible dementia characterized by the accumulation of neurofibrillary tangles and senile plaques within the cerebral cortex.

amalgam A compound of an alloy; a mixture of metals composed mainly of silver, copper, and tin, with mercury used to restore the form and function of teeth.

amalgamation The process of mechanically mixing the dental amalgam alloy with mercury.

amalgam carrier An instrument with a cylinder used to carry and dispense amalgam into the cavity preparation. The instrument lever forces a plunger to dislodge the contained amalgam from the cylinder.

amalgam well A small, heavy, stainless steel "dish" with a cup-like recess that confines the mixed amalgam to facilitate pick up with the amalgam carrier.

amelogenesis imperfecta A form of enamel dysplasia resulting from hereditary factors where there is partial or total malformation of enamel.

American Dental Association Seal of Acceptance Products with the seal have demonstrated adequate evidence of safety and effectiveness as approved by the American Dental Association, Council on Dental Therapeutics.

American Dental Hygienists' Association (ADHA) A national organization of approximately 35,000 dental hygienists, dedicated to advancing the art and science of dental hygiene by increasing the awareness of and ensuring access to quality oral healthcare, promoting the highest standard of dental hygiene education, licensure, and practice, and representing and promoting the interests of dental hygienists.

analgesia stage The first of the four stages of anesthesia. Perception of pain is altered for the client. In this stage there are three planes—the first two are appropriate for dental hygiene care.

anemia Below-normal levels of red blood cells or quantity of hemoglobin in the blood resulting in reduced delivery of oxygen to the tissues.

angina pectoris An acute pain in the chest as a result of decreased blood supply to the heart muscle, often brought on by physical activity or emotional stress; approximately 90% is the result of atherosclerosis.

angioplasty Closed heart surgical procedure involving the use of a catheter with a tiny balloon at the end of the tube that inserts into the coronary artery to allow for increased blood flow.

angular cheilitis Cracked, eroded, and encrusted surfaces at the commissural folds that frequently appear in conjunction with the mucosal inflammation caused by a *Candida albicans* infection; may cause moderate pain.

angulation The relationship of the cutting edge of a bladed instrument to the tooth surface. Specifically, this is the measurement from the face of the instrument blade to the tooth surface being scaled.

anodontia The absence of teeth. Defects of ectodermal structures are causative effects.

Hypodontia—The partial absence of teeth.

anorexia nervosa The least common eating disorder; the client suffering from anorexia suppresses and denies sensation of hunger.

anterior border of the mandible The structure is palpated bilaterally from the position behind the client to examine the soft tissue and underlying bone during an oral cancer examination.

anterior superior alveolar nerve (ASA) The nerve that descends from the infraorbital nerve before the infraorbital nerve exits the infraorbital foramen. The ASA nerve provides innervation to the central and lateral incisors, the canines, the periodontal tissues, and facial soft tissues and corresponding bone.

anterior superior alveolar nerve block The injection recommended for pain management when treatment is performed on the maxillary anterior teeth.

antibiotic prophylactic premedication Drug therapy administered prior to invasive dental hygiene instrumentation to clients who are susceptible to bacterial endocarditis; preventive in nature.

antibody Immunoglobulin, essential to the immune system, produced by lymphoid tissue in response to bacteria, viruses, or other antigens.

anticoagulants A substance that prevents the coagulation of the blood.

antigen Substance, usually a protein, that causes the formation of an antibody and reacts specifically with that antibody.

antiseptic Antimicrobial agent for use on the skin or mucous membrane.

applied research The adaptation of the theories developed through basic research to a practical situation or to the resolution of an existing problem.

appreciation Acknowledgement for achievement, worth, service, or merit, and to be regarded favorably, with admiration and approval by others.

arrested caries See under *dental caries.*

arthritis A musculoskeletal system disorder characterized by inflammation of the joints which may cause serious limitations in activity.

Osteoarthritis—the most common joint disease; a defect of articular cartilage, characterized by the gradual loss of cushioning. As cartilage is lost, the resultant exposure of rough underlying bone ends may cause pain and joint stiffness.

Rheumatoid arthritis—a chronic, systemic disease affecting connective tissue throughout the body. Symptoms include malaise, fatigue, fever, anemia, and nodules that develop on hard tissues.

asepsis Absence of germs or microorganisms.

aspirating syringe The most commonly used syringe for the administration of an intraoral local anesthetic. The barbed piston (harpoon) allows the administrator to exert negative pressure on the thumb ring to assess the location of the lumen of the needle—the procedure is *aspiration.*

assault The action of a person intending to cause apprehension in someone, without touching them. Example: threatening someone with a raised hand.

assessment The foundation of the dental hygiene process; the art of collecting and analyzing subjective and objective data about the client and arriving at a judgment about the client's human needs and barriers to need fulfillment related to dental hygiene care.

assessment instruments Instruments used for intraoral measurements, such as the periodontal probe, dental explorer and mouth mirror; used for detecting tooth irregularities, restorations, probe depths, soft tissue changes, and acquired deposits.

assistive devices Mechanical aids designed to enhance a disabled client's self-determination in daily functions and communication.

asthma A condition marked by recurrent attacks of shortness of breath and often accompanied by wheezing caused by spasmodic constriction of the bronchi; caused by allergies and/or infectious agents.

atherosclerosis The major cause of coronary heart disease; a narrowing of the lumen of the coronary arteries caused by the deposition of fibrofatty substances containing several types of lipids and cholesterol. The narrowing reduces the volume of blood flow. Eventually the deposits thicken to the point of closing the vessel.

atrial fibrillation An irregularity in ventricular beats created by inconsistent impulses through the atrioventricular (AV) node transmitted to the ventricles at irregular intervals.

atrial septal defect A shunt (opening) between the left and right atria; responsible for approximately 10% of congenital heart defects.

attached subgingival plaque See under *bacterial plaque.*

attachment loss Loss of attachment (LOA); the distance from the cemento-enamel junction to the base of the sulcus or pocket over time as measured by the periodontal probe. Consequently, attachment loss includes both periodontal pocket depth and recession measurement.

attention diversion Directing attention away from an anxiety-provoking object or event to something that is neutral or gives pleasure.

attribution theory A cognitive theory that emphasizes the importance of content of thoughts.

attrition The tooth-to-tooth wear of dentition from opposing tooth contact.

atypical plasma cholinesterase An inherited condition in which the individual produces an atypical form of the enzyme plasma cholinesterase. These individuals are not able to metabolize ester local anesthetics effectively.

auricular lymph nodes These structures are palpated bilaterally in front of and behind the ears.

authoritarian leadership The leader exerts close control over people.

autism A developmental disorder/disability characterized by a persistent aloneness.

autogenous Self-generated, self-produced, originating within an organism.

autonomic dysreflexia A severe condition caused by the presence of noxious stimuli, such as urinary backflow, that can be fatal if left untreated.

autonomic nervous system That part of the nervous system that controls involuntary body functions, such as salivation, sweat, heartbeat.

autonomy The idea based on the principle of respect for persons. Individuals have a right to self-determination, that is, freedom to make their own judgments based on their own evaluation.

avulsed tooth A tooth that is traumatically removed from the alveolus and then replanted successfully if managed properly.

axial positioning See under *root angulations.*

bacteremia The presence of microorganisms in the blood stream.

bacterial endocarditis Infective endocarditis; an acute infection of the endocardium caused by microorganisms; in the oral healthcare environment it can be caused by the manipulation of mucosal tissues which introduces a transient bacteremia in the client's bloodstream. Bacteria may become lodged on damaged or abnormal areas of the heart valves causing an infection of the lining of the heart and underlying connective tissues; prevented by antibiotic prophylactic premedication prior to initial invasive dental or dental hygiene procedures.

bacterial plaque A dense, organized matrix of microorganisms that form on the teeth, gingiva, and restorations; the cause of dental caries and periodontal diseases.

Attached subgingival plaque—bacterial plaque located below the gingival margin that is attached to the tooth.

Loosely adherent subgingival plaque—unattached bacterial plaque found adjacent to the gingival epithelium or pocket lumen.

Supragingival plaque—plaque located above the gingival margin. The plaque influences the establishment and composition of subgingival microorganisms.

barrier-free design An architectural environment that enables wheelchair accessibility; required in public buildings as a result of an amendment to the Rehabilitation Act of 1973.

barriers Obstacles that limit disabled persons' ability to access healthcare, education, and employment opportunities.

baseline An individual's score on a measurement prior to implementing a particular treatment.

basic research The systematic application of the scientific method leading to the establishment of new knowledge or theory.

basketweave of strokes Combinations of different instrument stroke directions, especially helpful when assessing acquired deposits or tooth structure.

Bass toothbrushing method The sucular toothbrush technique designed to clean the cervical third of the clinical crown of the tooth in addition to the area beneath the gingival margin.

battery A harmful or offensive contact with someone; touching someone without his permission.

behavior modification Technique used for reinforcing desired behaviors and extinguishing those behaviors considered detrimental via the consistent application of rewards and punishment.

beneficence The principle that endorses the promotion of mercy, goodness, kindness, and charity, and removing harm.

beta receptors See under *adrenergic receptors.*

bevel See under *needle.*

bias A prejudicial belief or opinion.

bioburden Blood, saliva, organic matter, or debris present on instruments, environmental surfaces, and barriers during and after client contact.

biocidal Pertaining to that which kills living organisms.

biological seal (Perimucosal seal) The adaption of the keratinized or nonkeratinized epithelium to the titanium abutment cylinder of a dental implant.

biologically sound dentition Intact teeth and restorations that defend against harmful microbes and provide for adequate function and esthetics; one of the human needs related to dental hygiene care.

biological theories of aging Theories that are attempts to explain the biological phenomenon of aging; divided into molecular and nonmolecular theories.

Cell theory—a molecular theory; suggests that cells that reproduce are not equal in functional capability. Through time these inefficient cells become more apparent in the aging process.

Crosslinkage theory—a nonmolecular theory; suggests that chemical reactions create strong bonds between molecular structures that are normally separate. The ongoing process creates more rigid fibers over time through the cross linking in extracellular components.

Error theory—a molecular theory; suggests that cells may become inoperative because of copying errors in repeated divisions.

Free radical theory—a nonmolecular theory; suggests that free radicals are highly reactive chemically with other substances. The reaction alters the original structure unfavorably. Over time they accumulate.

Immunologic/autoimmune theory—a nonmolecular theory; suggests that the immune system undergoes involuntary changes after puberty.

Programmed theory—a molecular theory; suggests that the lifespan of an organism is programmed within the genes of the organism; the rate and lifespan is set at life's start.

Somatic mutation theory—a molecular theory; suggests that when cells are exposed to radiation or chemicals, chromosomal abnormalities occur. These abnormalities manifest in later life.

bioprosthetic cardiac valves A cardiac valve replacement made from biological tissue.

biopsy The surgical removal and microscopic examination of a section of tissue or other material from the living body for the purpose of diagnosis.

Excisional—the entire lesion is removed for assessment.

Incisional—a representative section is taken for assessment.

bisbiguanide Category of chemical agents used in infection control and in chemotherapy, such as chlorhexidene.

bit One of the series of on and off signals that cause a computer to function. Formal name is binary digits; a sequence of eight bits is called a byte.

Black's Classification of Dental Caries and Restorations The most commonly used system to classify both dental caries and restorations; established by G. V. Black in the early 1900s; provides a precise description of the types and location of the dental caries or restoration.

blood pressure A measurement of two blood pressures within the blood vessels; the first number is the pressure of the blood against the arterial blood vessels (systole) and the second number is the pressure against the blood vessels as the heart relaxes between contractions (diastole).

body image stressors Changes in the appearance or function of a body part or feature may create stress because it may bring about change in a person's body image.

body of knowledge The concepts, propositions, and theories that provide the scientific foundation for the practice of the discipline and give the practice its unique character.

bone marrow transplantation A therapeutic procedure used to treat a variety of hematological diseases; marrow may be obtained from the client during a period of disease remission or donated by a person with a similar genetic make-up.

brachial pulse A throbbing sensation that is felt over the brachial artery located on the inner side of the elbow.

bradycardia Slowness of the heart beat,

as evidenced by a decrease in the pulse rate to less than 60 beats per minute.

bronchodilation Dilation of the bronchi in order to facilitate breathing.

bruxism The stress-induced behavior of grinding the teeth together.

buccal nerve block An injection that provides pain control to the soft tissues facial to the mandibular molars.

bulimarexia The vacillation between anorexic and bulimic behavior.

bulimia nervosa The more common eating disorder; prevalence higher than for anorexia nervosa; characterized by recurrent episodes of binge eating followed by self-induced vomiting, use of laxatives or diuretics, excessive exercise, a feeling of lack of control over the behavior, and a consistent concern with body image and weight.

bulletin board See under *information services.*

burnished calculus See under *calculus.*

burn-out The combination of physical, emotional, and behavioral changes in an individual as a response to high-intensity or long-duration stress, when one's adaptive capabilities are exceeded.

byte See under *bit.*

calculus Mineralized bacterial plaque; lay term is tartar.

Burnished calculus—a smoothed outer surface of calculus created by removing only superficial layers of calculus through inadequate instrumentation.

Subgingival calculus—calculus located below the gingival margin and attached to cementum or dentin in the area.

Supragingival calculus—calculus located above the gingival margin; may attach to any hard surface including enamel, restorative materials, prosthetic appliances, or exposed cementum.

Canadian Dental Hygienists' Association (CDHA) The national association for registered dental hygienists in Canada; founded in 1965.

cancer A broad classification of more than 100 disease types. The common element in cancer is the abnormal and unrestricted growth of cells that can invade and destroy surrounding normal tissues, and sometimes spread to other parts of the body.

cardiovascular disease (CVD) An alteration of the heart and/or blood vessels that impairs function.

carditis Inflammation of the cardiac muscle.

caregiver A person who assists disabled individuals with their daily activities.

care plan A plan of action designed by the dental hygienist to prevent an oral health problem or promote oral health in the client.

caries activity test A quick test that provides information about acid-forming microorganisms or their activity in the mouth.

carpal tunnel syndrome An identified cumulative trauma disorder; caused by the compression of the median nerve in the wrist; an occupational hazard in the clinical practice of dental hygiene.

carrier Animal or person who harbors and spreads a disease-causing organism but who does not become ill.

cartridge The component of the armamentarium for local anesthesia administration that contains the local anesthetic drug in addition to other ingredients; parts include:

Aluminum cap—section of the cartridge that fits snugly around the neck of the cartridge, holding the diaphragm in place.

Diaphragm—semipermeable material located on the opposite end of the cartridge from the rubber stopper/plunger; the needle penetrates this end.

Glass cylinder—the body of the cartridge on which the contents, amount of solution, and the manufacturer's name are imprinted.

Rubber stopper/plunger—located on the opposite end of the cartridge from the diaphragm; the harpoon of an aspirating syringe is embedded here.

case presentation The process of explaining assessment findings to the client along with options and recommendations for therapy in order to reach agreement on a care plan.

cataract A visual problem characterized by an opacity of the normally transparent eye lens that interferes with the passage of light.

cavity Tooth cavitation resulting from repeated acid attacks ending in eventual demineralization.

Complex cavity—has three or more involved surfaces needing preparation.

Compound cavity—has two involved surfaces needing preparation.

Simple cavity—has one surface needing preparation.

cavosurface margin Contact between the cavity surface and the tooth surface location where the walls and line angles meet the unaltered tooth surface.

cell theory See under *biological theories of aging.*

cementation Attachment of a restoration or band by means of a cement.

cementoenamel junction (CEJ) Location on a tooth where the cementum and enamel meet; demarcation between the anatomical crown and the anatomical root of the tooth.

cementum A mineralized bone-like substance that covers the roots of teeth and provides a surface for attachment and anchorage for the periodontal fibers.

Centers for Disease Control and Prevention Agency of the U.S. government that provides facilities and services for the investigation, identification, prevention, and control of disease.

central processing unit (CPU) An essential operating element of a computer.

centric occlusion See under *occlusion.*

cerebrovascular accident (CVA) Stroke; a neurosensory disorder cause by a thrombus or a hemorrhage that results in a cerebral infarct; affects coordination, speech, and mobility.

certification The process by which a nongovernment agency or organization grants formal recognition to an individual for accomplishments such as completion of a specified amount of further training or coursework, acceptable performance on an examination or series of examinations, or graduation from a formal program.

change The process of transforming, alternating, or modifying something.

change agent The individual who is responsible for taking a leadership role in managing the process of change.

Charters' toothbrushing method The method designed to increase cleansing effectiveness and gingival stimulation in the interproximal areas; bristles are pointed toward the crown of the tooth rather than apically; may be recommended for persons with orthodontic brackets.

chemical bonding The molecular linking together of two chemical agents.

chemotherapeutic agents The chemical agent used in chemotherapy.

chemotherapy Treatment of a disease with a chemical reagent(s) that destroys the pathogens causing the disease.

chip A microscopic circuit containing vast quantities of electronic logic stored on a small piece of silicon in the computer.

chisel A hand instrument used in cavity preparation for planing enamel.

chlorhexidine A bisbiguanide that was first synthesized and used as a disinfectant for skin and mucous membranes; used as an antiplaque and antigingivitis agent.

chronic caries See under *dental caries.*

chronic fluoride toxicity The long-term exposure to fluoride causing dental fluorosis, skeletal fluorosis, and kidney damage.

chronicity Failure to heal.

chronic periodontal abscess An overgrowth of pathogenic organisms in a periodontal pocket that drains inflammatory exudate either through the opening of the pocket or through a sinus tract that permits regular drainage; usually painless.

chronological age Age as measured by calendar time since birth.

circumvallate papillae See under *tongue papillae.*

civil law The branch of law that includes offenses for violating private or contractual rights, or in simpler terms, a crime against a person.

classification of types of teeth In their lifetime, humans have two sets of natural teeth, commonly referred to as the primary and the permanent dentitions.

Permanent/secondary dentition—the dentition consists of 32 teeth, 8 in each quadrant: 2 incisors, 1 canine, 2 premolars, and 3 molars.

Primary dentition—the dentition consists of 20 teeth, 5 in each quadrant: 2 incisors, 1 canine, and 2 molars.

client The biological, psychological, spiritual, social, cultural and intellectual human being whose behavior is motivated by human needs and who have 11 human needs especially related to dental hygiene care; the contemporary healthcare consumer; the term connotes wellness as well as illness and suggests one who is an active participant in oral healthcare, and who is responsible for personal choices and the consequences of those choices; may refer to an individual or group.

Patient—a person who is ill or who is undergoing care for the treatment of a disease.

client advocacy Supporting the client not only in the healthcare arena, but by respecting and promoting the rights of clients.

client-centered goal The desired end result that the client is to achieve through specific dental hygiene actions.

client noncompliance A lack of client cooperation with recommended oral healthcare; significant because it can result in compromised therapy, unsatisfactory results, and litigation.

client satisfaction A positive emotional state within the individual receiving oral healthcare.

client surveys Questionnaires designed to measure client satisfaction, an essential component of quality of care.

clinical attachment level The relative probing depth corresponding to the distance from the cementoenamel junction (CEJ) to the location of a periodontal probe tip at the epithelial junction.

clinical dental hygiene problem A discrepancy between the way things are and the way they ought to be, or between what one knows and what one needs to know to eliminate the problem.

clip art A desktop publishing feature of a computer that allows the user to produce quality art in documents.

coalescing lesion Lesions with merging margins.

coated tongue A yellow, whitish, or pigmented covering on all or a portion of the tongue's dorsal surface; indication of the need for tongue cleaning or an underlying disease.

cognitive learning domain The domain that classifies the level of learning involving intellectual tasks, such as recall, comprehension, application, analysis, synthesis, and evaluation.

cognitive psychology A branch of psychology that theorizes that a person's behavior is based on cognition or thinking.

Stages of development—theory developed by cognitive psychologist Jean Piaget, focusing on learning in childhood.

Sensorimotor state—(stage 1, 0 to 2 years) dominated by innate reflexes such as sucking and grasping.

Properitoneal stage—(stage 2, 2 to 7 years) the child begins to use symbols and language to represent her environment.

Concrete operations stage—(stage 3, 7 to 11 years) the child becomes more evaluative in her thought processes and can apply them to concrete problems.

Formal operations stage—(stage 4, 11 years and above) thought based on reasoning and judgment.

cohort effect Educational attainment is primarily a function of the prevailing attitudes and educational opportunities for a group at a point in time.

col A saddle of interdental gingiva that connects the facial and lingual aspects of the papilla; significant because it is nonkeratinized and highly susceptible to inflammation.

collaboration The process of working together for the achievement of common goals; dental hygienists and other health professionals cooperating as colleagues to integrate their respective care regimens into a single comprehensive approach to quality client care.

collaborative practice Dental hygienists and dentists cooperating as colleagues to integrate their respective care regimens into a single comprehensive approach to quality client care.

combination abscess See under *periapical abscess.*

communicable disease Any disease transmitted from one person or animal to another by direct or indirect contact or by vectors.

communication The process by which a person sends a message to another person with the intention of evoking a response.

community organization The process aimed at developing the skills, abilities, and understandings of groups of people for the purpose of self-led improvement.

complex cavity See under *cavity.*

composites Restorative dental material resulting from a mixture of ceramic reinforcing filler particles in a monomer matrix; once mixed it is converted into a polymer.

compound cavity See under *cavity.*

comprehensive care A cycle that integrates a broad variety of needed oral healthcare services to the client.

comprehensive fluoride therapy The use of both systemic and topical fluoride therapies to maintain a caries-free oral environment.

Systemically—fluoride entry via the blood supply of developing teeth.

Topically—fluoride by direct contact on exposed tooth surfaces.

concave See under *root curvatures.*

concept An abstraction formed by generalization from facts.

conceptualization The process of developing a mental configuration of a concept.

conceptual model A set of concepts and the propositions that integrate them into a meaningful configuration within the domain of dental hygiene; a "school of thought."

concordant Condition where a disease occurs in both twins.

concrescence The fusion of two teeth at the root through the cementum only. Originally separate, but became joined because of excessive cementum deposition.

concrete operational stage See under *cognitive psychology.*

condensation The act of physically compressing or packing a dental material into a cavity preparation.

condensing instruments Hand instruments used for adapting amalgam to the cavity preparation.

confidentiality A right of a client to have information about him remain private.

congenital heart disease Cardiac disease present at birth.

congestive heart failure A syndrome characterized by myocardial dysfunction that leads to diminished cardiac output or abnormal circulatory congestion.

conscious sedation A method of pain control that decreases client's pain and stress where the client is awake and able to respond, breath, and cough.

construct A concept characterized by conscious, deliberated invention for a special scientific purpose.

continuity theory Speculates that habits, preferences, associations, and coping abilities are part of an individual's personality, and they are continued throughout life.

contract A legally binding agreement between two or more parties.

control group Within a study, the group or subject not receiving the experimental treatment.

controlled study An investigation where errors are regulated or limited, and extraneous variables are systematically ruled out via the use of appropriate research protocol.

convex See under *root curvatures.*

coronary artery disease See under *coronary heart disease.*

coronary bypass surgery A medical procedure used to replace closed arteries in the heart; performed by removing a part of the leg vein or chest artery and then grafting it onto the coronary artery, thereby creating a new passageway for the blood.

coronary heart disease A disease caused by insufficient blood flow from the coronary arteries into the heart or myocardium.

correlational relationship The relationship where one attribute (variable) changes as another changes.

countermigration A trend in which a small number of older adults, who moved to another state at retirement, move back home or to a state where family members live.

credentialing The process of assuring the existence of qualified practitioners and reliable equipment through eduction, licensure, and certification.

crest of the gingiva See under *gingival margin.*

criminal law The law established for preventing harm against society and describing a criminal act as well as the appropriate punishment.

criteria The qualities or characteristics by which knowledge, skills, oral health status, or other phenomena are measured.

critical items Items that penetrate or touch broken skin, mucosa, or bone and therefore are classified as requiring sterilization.

cross arch fulcrum Holding the index finger of the hand holding the instrument and the working end of the instrument on separate dental arches.

cross-cultural dental hygiene The effective integration of the client's socioethnocultural background into the dental hygiene process of care.

crosslinkage theory See under *biological theories of aging.*

cultural beliefs A system of propositions one holds to be true that are related to membership in a social group.

culture The sum total of human behaviors unique to a specific group and passed from generation to generation or from one to another within the group.

culture shock The negative feelings one experiences when placed within a different culture.

cumulative trauma disorder A term used to identify the group of musculoskeletal disorders involving injuries to the tendons, tendon sheaths, the related bones, muscles and nerves of the hands, wrists, elbows, arms, feet, knees, and legs.

curettage (gingival) The removal of soft tissue that lines the wall of a pocket, usually with a sharp curet during the process of subgingival instrumentation—inadvertent to intentional.

curve of Spee See under *root angulation.*

curve of Wilson See under *root angulation.*

daisy wheel printer A computer printer that utilizes a print head that strikes a ribbon, much like a typewriter.

data base management (DBM) Computer software that offers a means by which to enter, organize, and update information.

data bus A set of circuits inside the computer by which information travels from chip to chip.

deceit Misrepresentation of a situation by the dental hygienist to the client.

decision-making The result of deliberate, logical judgment that is guided by human need theory, the dental hygiene process, education, and experience.

decoding Deciphering a message.

decubitus ulcers Pressure sores.

defamation A communication that injures an individual's reputation.

Libel—written defamation.

Slander—verbal defamation.

defective restorations Any reconstruction of the teeth that is less than satisfactory in form and/or function, such as a chipped amalgam restoration.

dehiscence A hole that is caused by placing an implant in an insufficient area of bone; also any isolated hole in bone along the root of a tooth.

deinstitutionalization The process of removing from an institution those mentally retarded persons capable of living and functioning independently with little assistance of a caregiver.

delirium or excitement stage The second of the four stages of anesthesia, characterized by hyperresponsiveness to stimuli, exaggerated inspiration, and loss of consciousness.

dementia A progressive brain impairment that interferes with normal intellectual functioning; also called *organic brain syndrome.*

democratic leader Believes in the strength inherent in people and group decision-making.

dens evaginatus/dens in dente A tooth within a tooth; caused by invagination of the enamel organ during development; observed most frequently on the lingual aspect of the maxillary lateral incisors.

dental caries An infectious, bacteria-caused disease characterized by the acid dissolution of enamel and the eventual breakdown of the more organic, inner dental tissues.

Acute/rampant caries—a rapidly progressive decay process that requires urgent intervention to gain control.

Arrested caries—resulting from a demineralization-remineralization process; may appear light or brown, but feel firm and glass-like when explored.

Backward caries—the lateral spread of decay at the dentinoenamel junction.

Chronic caries—a slowly progressive decay process that requires routine intervention.

Pit and fissure caries—decay found in the grooves and crevices of the occlusal surfaces of premolars and molars.

Recurrent caries—new decay that occurs at the margins of existing restorations.

Smooth surface caries—found on the facial, lingual, mesial, and distal surface of teeth.

dental charting See under *dentition charting.*

dental diagnosis The act, by a dentist, of identifying diseases or problems for which the dentist directs or provides the primary treatment.

dental hygiene The study of preventive oral healthcare and the management of behaviors required to prevent oral disease and promote health; the major concepts studied are health/oral health, dental hygiene action, the client, the environment, their interaction, and the factors that affect them.

dental hygiene actions Interventions performed by dental hygienists that are aimed at assisting clients in meeting their human needs related to oral health; involve cognitive, affective, and psychomotor performances and include assessing, diagnosing, planning, implementing, and evaluating; may be provided in independent, interdependent, and collaborative relationships with the client and healthcare team members.

dental hygiene care plan See under *care plan.*

dental hygiene change agent An individual who applies a theoretical body of knowledge focusing on a systematic approach to change.

dental hygiene clinician The role focuses on the assessment of signs of health and disease in the oral cavity; identification of the dental hygiene problem (dental hygiene diagnosis); and planning, implementing, and evaluating dental hygiene care.

dental hygiene diagnosis The act of identifying an actual or potential human need deficit related to oral health or disease that the dental hygienist is educated and licensed to treat.

dental hygiene educator/oral health promoter The role used when a dental hygienist explains disease processes and home-care techniques, any time a client has learning needs.

dental hygiene generalist Educated at a standard entry level and capable of serving in the general roles of clinician, educator/oral health promoter, administrator/manager, change agent, consumer advocate, and researcher.

dental hygiene manager/administrator Dental hygienists use management skills when they understand the administrative structure of the employment setting and use the structure to achieve organizational goals.

dental hygiene process Assessment of client's needs, formulation of dental hygiene diagnoses, and planning, implementing, and evaluating dental hygiene care.

dental hygiene research Application of the scientific method to problems within the discipline of dental hygiene aimed at theory development and validation and the formation of an organized body of knowledge.

dental hygiene specialist Educated above the standard entry level—master's or doctoral degree in a specific area of specialization.

dental hygiene theory Interrelated concepts basic to dental hygiene that can be used to systematically describe and explain approaches to dental hygiene practice and predict outcomes of that practice.

dental implant A stable and functional replacement of natural teeth that consists of an anchor, an abutment, and a prosthetic tooth or appliance.

dental operatory/treatment area Consists of the dental unit, the dental chair, the operating light, and the operator's stool.

dental record A complete record of both the health and dental status at the time of the initial examination; comprehensive and chronological documentation of treatment provided at each appointment.

dentifrices Substance (gel, paste or powder) used in conjunction with a toothbrush to facilitate bacterial plaque removal, or as a vehicle for transporting therapeutic or cosmetic agents to the tooth and its environment.

dentin bonding The type of retention that occurs between a dental material and the dentin of a tooth; can include micromechanical retention only or micromechanical retention and chemical adhesion.

dentinal dysplasia A mesenchymal dysplasia exhibiting normal tooth color, pulpal obliteration, extreme mobility, retarded root formation, and premature exfoliation.

dentinogenesis imperfecta Absence of dentinal development.

dentition charting The graphic representation of the condition of the client's teeth observed on a specific date. Based on clinical, radiographic and symptomatic assessments.

denture adhesive Adjunct to stabilize and retain denture by increasing peripheral seal. Commercially available in powder, paste, or film formulations.

denture induced fibrous hyperplasia Fibrous tissue proliferation following alveolar bone resorption associated with an ill-fitting denture.

denture stomatitis Inflammation of the oral mucosa associated with wearing dentures. Commonly found under maxillary dentures, mucosal tissues have generalized red and velvety appearance. Pain varies from little or no pain to burning sensations. Primarily the result of chronic *Candida albicans* infection.

dependency The state of needing to rely on another to make decisions or to carry out one's responsibilities.

depolarization The phase of a nerve impulse where the nerve membrane becomes more permeable to the sodium ion.

descriptive study Research that involves describing, analyzing, and interpreting data to evaluate a current population, event or situation; information for the study is gathered via questionnaires, interviews, surveys, or document analyses.

desktop publishing Creating professional-looking work that is suitable for newsletters, manuscripts, fliers, pamphlets, research questionnaires, and any other documents in which bold, professional appearance is desirable.

diabetes A group of disorders commonly characterized by: (1) relative or absolute lack of insulin or improperly working insulin; (2) an impairment in the body's ability to metabolize carbohydrates, fats, and protein; and as a result (3) abnormalities in the structure and function of blood vessels (microangiopathy) and nerves (neuropathy).

Type I—insulin-dependent diabetes mellitus; a severe deficiency of insulin is characteristic and treatment requires regular lifelong administration of insulin by injection to prevent ketosis and sustain health.

Type II—noninsulin-dependent diabetes mellitus; a heterogenous disorder with abnormalities in insulin secretion, reduced sensitivity to insulin, and excessive hepatic glucose production.

Other types—the presence of type I or II diabetes along with an associated condition or syndrome such as pancreatic disease, endocrine disease, chemical agents, drugs, or genetic syndromes.

diaphragm See under *cartridge.*

diastole The phase of the cardiac cycle in which the heart relaxes between contractions.

dilaceration A bend or curve in the tooth caused by trauma or pressure on the developing tooth.

dilution The diffusion of a given quantity of an agent in water rendering the agent attenuated.

direct contact Mode of transmission that occurs via direct touching of the infectious lesions or infected saliva or blood.

direct restorations Restorative materials placed and formed directly in the cavity preparation within the oral cavity.

disability A condition that is either permanent or semipermanent and that interferes with an individual's ability to do something independently.

disclosing agent A liquid concentrate or tablet containing an ingredient that stains deposits and debris present on the teeth so that it can be seen by the client.

discordant Condition where a disease occurs in one twin and not the other twin.

discrimination Differentiating one from another on the basis of a rational or irrational criterion.

disengagement theory Represents the first major hypothetical system designed to consider development of the latter stages of normal aging.

disinfectant An agent that destroys most but not necessarily all microorganisms; intended to kill pathogenic microorganisms, with the exception of bacterial spores.

disinfection A process that destroys most but not necessarily all microorganisms; usually involves the use of liquid chemical agents at room temperature.

disk drive The storage mechanism of a microcomputer. Two types: the flexible (or floppy) disk drive and the fixed (or hard) disk drive.

diskettes Containers of the floppy disk drive of a microcomputer. Two types: 3.5 inch—has a plastic casing and is more durable; 5.25 inch—no plastic coating and is less durable.

disk operating system (DOS) A line-oriented operating system in which a specialized language is needed to communicate with the computer.

display adaptor A board that inserts into the computer machinery and to which the monitor connects.

disposable syringe Sometimes used for intraoral injections, but more commonly used for intramuscular or intravenous drug administration.

dot matrix printer A computer printer that utilizes a print head that strikes a ribbon, much like a typewriter.

double-ended An instrument with exact, mirror images on the opposite ends.

Down syndrome A chromosome abnormality that affects chromosome 21 and results in a defined set of physical characteristics and mental retardation.

Mosaicism—chromosomal anomaly associated with Down syndrome. An error in one of the first cell divisions shortly after conception.

Translocation—a piece of chromosome in pair 21 breaks off and attaches to another chromosome, usually 14, 21, or 22; hereditary.

Trisomy 21—a failure of a pair of number 21 chromosomes to segregate during the formation of either an egg or sperm prior to conception.

droplet spread Particles of moisture expelled from the mouth in coughing, sneezing, or speaking, which may carry infection to others through the air.

dwarfed roots Abnormally short roots of teeth that have normal-size crowns. Hereditary or it may result from rapid tooth movement during orthodontic treatment.

dysarthria Abnormal speech from an impairment of the muscles that are involved with speech.

echocardiogram The graphic record used to determine the presence of mitral valve prolapse; ultrasound is used to evaluate the heart size, as well as chamber and valve function.

edentulous Being without teeth or lacking teeth.

electroencephalogram (EEG) A graphic record used to measure brain wave activity.

electronic mail The delivery of messages from a sender to a receiver by way of electronic means; also called E mail.

empathy The attempt to perceive and understand a situation from the point of view of another person.

emphysema A lung disorder in which the terminal bronchioles become plugged with mucus with eventual loss of elasticity in the lung tissue; inspired air becomes trapped and makes breathing difficult.

empirical Evidence collected from objective findings or observations.

employee-oriented style A management style that encourages group members to participate in tasks and decisions that affect them.

employment contract A written agreement describing the terms of employment agreed on by the employee and the employer.

enamel bonding A type of retention that occurs between a dental material and the enamel of a tooth; can include micromechanical retention only or micromechanical retention and chemical adhesion.

enamel dysplasia Abnormal enamel development caused by an insult to ameloblasts during tooth formation.

enamel hypocalcification A defect occurring to the enamel as the result of a disturbance during mineralization. Surface may appear smooth with a chalky, white-spotted appearance.

enamel hypoplasia The result of a disturbance of the ameloblasts during matrix formation. Produces grooves, pits and/or fissures in the enamel with yellow to brown discoloration.

enamel pearls Small nodules of enamel found on the root surface apical to the cementoenamel junction.

endarteritis An inflammation of the inner layer of an artery.

endocardium Lining of the inner surface and cavities of the heart.

endogenous Arising from within a cell or organism.

endosteal A dental implant placed within the bone.

end stage disease That phase of the disease process that brings the person close to death.

environment The milieu of the client and dental hygienist that influences the manner, mode, and level of human need fulfillment for the client; includes factors other than dental hygiene actions that affect the client's attainment of optimal oral health, e.g., economic, psychological, cultural, physical, political, legal, educational, ethical, and geographical factors.

Environmental Protection Agency (EPA) Agency located in Washington, D.C., that among other things regulates disinfectants, sterilants, and certain aspects of waste disposal.

EPA-registered Indicates (by a number on the product label) that a product performs as claimed based upon a review of information submitted to the EPA by the product manufacturer.

epidemiology The study of the occurrence, distribution, and causes of disease or disability.

epilepsy A neurological condition caused by overstimulation of nerve cells in the brain which can involve mild (petit mal) to severe (grand mal) seizures.

epinephrine See under *adrenalin.*

epithelial attachment The inner part of the junctional epithelium attached to the tooth by hemidesmosomes and the basement lamina.

erosion The loss of tooth structure as a result of chemical agents.

error theory See under *biological theories of aging.*

erythema A red area of variable shape and size reflecting inflammation, thinness, and irregularity of epithelium, and lack of keratinization.

erythematous/atrophic candida A candida infection seen in AIDS patients; present as smooth red patches on the tongue, palate, or mucosa.

ester See under *local anesthesia.*

ethics The science of the ideal human character and the ideal ends of human action.

ethnic group People who share similarities in heritage and tradition, passed on from generation to generation.

ethnicity The unique cultural and social heritage and traditions of groups within the primary racial, national, or tribal divisions that reflect distinct customs, language, and social values.

ethnocentrism The natural belief that one's culture is superior to that of others.

ethnographic study Qualitative research approach used to study issues related to culture as they occur in the real world setting.

evaluating The act of measuring the extent to which the client has achieved the goals specified in the care plan.

excavators Restorative dental instruments used for refining the internal cavity; preparation includes hoes and angle formers.

excisional biopsy See under *biopsy.*

exostosis Benign bony outgrowth frequently occurring on the hard palate and lingual aspect of the mandibular alveolar ridge.

expected outcome The desired result of care; evidence is used to determine if the client's goal was met, partially met, or not met at all.

experiment One method used to study dental hygiene problems; characterized by the presence of a control group and experimental group; control of extraneous variables, direct manipulation of the independent variable, and randomization of subjects to treatments.

experimental group The subjects who are exposed to the experimental variable under study.

exploratory stroke Instrumentation used for the detection of deposits; characterized by light-to-firm lateral pressure.

external fulcrum See under *fulcrum.*

external quality mechanisms Quality assurance mechanisms that exist outside an individually designed quality assurance program, such as formal educational requirements, accreditation standards, the accreditation process, and national, state, and regional board examinations for licensure.

extrinsic stain Removable stain located on hard tooth structure, on calculus, on restorations, or on prosthetic appliances. Stain should be removed to eliminate a nidus for bacterial plaque formation and for aesthetic reasons.

extrinsic stain removal The mechanical removal of materia alba, bacterial plaque, and extrinsic stain from tooth surfaces and restorations; used synonymously with the term *polishing.*

facial nerve paralysis A loss of motor function of the facial expression muscles.

fibroid papillae See under *tongue papilla.*

field block A method of obtaining anesthesia by injecting the anesthetic agent solution close to large terminal nerve branches. More circumscribed, most often involving one tooth and the tissues surrounding it.

filiform papillae See under *tongue papillae.*

finishing strip A thin plastic strip with abrasive agents bonded to one side; useful for anterior interproximal extrinsic stain removal.

First World Economically developed and capitalistic countries.

fissure tongue A condition in which fissures or grooves are observed on the tongue, most frequently down the midline.

fixation Refers to a nonmobile lesion that has become very firm as a result of abnormally dividing cells invading to deeper areas and onto muscle and bone.

flexion A sharp bend or curvature of a root from trauma to or pressure to the tooth. It occurs later in the tooth's development than dilaceration.

flush terminal plane A flat plane formed by the distal surfaces of the primary second molars; the result of the primary molars erupting in an end-to-end position.

focal (frictional) hyperkeratosis White lesion of the oral mucosa characterized by keratinization of edentulous alveolar ridges.

foliate papillae See under *tongue papillae.*

fomites Inanimate substance or objects, such as clothing or paper, that absorb and transmit infectious agents.

Fones' toothbrushing method Toothbrushing technique advocated by Fones, the founder of dental hygiene, that uses circular motions to brush the teeth; may lead to gingival abrasion over time.

Food and Drug Administration (FDA) Agency of the United States government that is responsible for evaluation and approval of pharmaceuticals and medical devices.

formal operations stage See under *cognitive psychology.*

freedom from pain and stress The human need for exemption from physical and emotional discomforts.

free radical theory See under *biological theories of aging.*

fulcrum The source of stability or leverage on which the finger rests and pushes against in order to hold the dental instrument with control during stroke activation.

Extraoral fulcrum—established outside of the mouth and predominantly used when instrumenting teeth with deep periodontal pockets; the leverage point may be the client's jaw or side of the face.

Intraoral fulcrum—a traditional fulcrum established inside the mouth against tooth structure.

functional age The age based on performance capacities.

functional status The degree to which the client can conduct his activities of daily living.

fungiform papillae See under *tongue papillae.*

furcation involvement Loss of periodontal attachment between the roots of posterior teeth.

furcations The areas between the roots of teeth where the root trunk divides into separate roots.

fusion The union of two adjacent tooth buds; fusion can unite two teeth or only the crowns or roots.

gauge The diameter of the lumen of a needle; the higher the gauge number, the smaller the diameter of the lumen.

gemination The splitting of a single tooth germ; appears clinically as double or fused teeth; normally, these teeth have a single root with one pulpal canal.

generalized lesions Those lesions occurring in more than one area in the oral cavity.

geographic tongue A condition in which there is a sporadic and uneven distribution of papillae, or depapillation lending an unusual "topographic" appearance.

geriatrics The branch of medicine concerned with the illnesses of old age and their treatment.

gerontologist An individual who investigates numerous factors that affect the aging person and the aging process.

gerontology The scientific study of the factors affecting the normal aging process and the effects of aging.

gingiva That part of the oral mucous membrane attached to the teeth and the alveolar processes of the jaws.

gingival abscess Usually occurs in previously disease-free areas, and can be related to the forceful inclusion of some foreign body into the area; mostly found on the marginal gingiva; characterized by a focal area of pus formation.

gingival crevice See under *gingival sulcus.*

gingival crevicular fluid A serum-like fluid secreted from the underlying connective tissue into the sulcular space; is able to transport antibodies and certain systemically administered drugs.

gingival margin The edge of the marginal gingiva that is nearest to the incisal or occlusal area of the tooth; marks the opening of the gingival sulcus.

gingival recession The reduction of the height of the marginal gingiva to a location apical to the CEJ; signifies attachment loss.

gingival sulcus The space between the marginal gingiva and the tooth. The healthy gingival sulcus measures 0.5 to 3.00 mm from the gingival margin to the base of the sulcus.

gingivitis Inflammation of the gingival tissue with no apical migration of the junctional epithelium beyond the CEJ.

glass cylinder See under *cartridge.*

glaucoma A condition caused by increased intraocular pressure that can result in visual problems and possibly blindness.

glucose A sugar used in body metabolism.

graphics programs These programs allow the user to create artwork on the computer screen; the categories of software are paint, draw, presentation, and computer-aided design programs.

graphic user interface An operating system that uses small pictures or symbols to aid the user in selection of a function.

greater (anterior) palatine nerve The nerve enters the oral cavity on the hard palate via the greater palatine foramen and innervates the palatal soft tissues and bone of the posterior teeth.

greater (anterior) palatine nerve block The block used to obtain anesthesia to the hard and soft palatal tissues overlying the molars and premolar; no pulpal anesthesia is obtained here.

HA coating A hydroxylapatite coating sprayed on the dental implant; designed to increase speed and predictability of healing.

hairy leukoplakia Thick white lesions with long, finger-like projections usually; located on the lateral borders of the tongue and associated with Epstein-Barr virus and HIV infection.

handicap A term used to describe the feeling a person may have regarding adequacy of performance either generally or under a particular circumstance.

hard copy A paper copy produced by a computer printer.

hard palate The roof of the mouth which is digitally palpated for lesions, swellings, hard masses, and color change during an intraoral examination.

hardware The equipment or machinery of a computer system.

healing cap A plastic cone-shaped cap placed above the abutment of a dental implant at the second surgical phase to promote tissue integration.

health A state of well-being with both objective and subjective aspects that exists on a continuum from maximal wellness to maximal illness; along the continuum, degrees of wellness and illness are associated with varying levels of human need fulfillment.

health promotion Activities in which individuals and communities can engage to promote healthy lifestyles.

healthy public policy The concept that the health impact of any public policy is considered an outcome equally important as the goal of that policy.

heart block An arrhythmia caused by the blocking of impulses from the atria to the ventricles at the A-V node.

heart transplantation A viable option for individuals with end-stage heart disease in which no other therapeutic intervention is considered effective.

hematoma A swelling and discoloration of the tissue resulting from the effusion of blood into the extravascular spaces.

herpetic whitlow See under *acute herpetic gingivostomatitis.*

high spots In reference to sealants, areas with excess sealant material that interferes with occlusion.

HIV Human immunodeficiency virus, a retrovirus that infects T-lymphocytes and other cells.

HIV gingivitis An atypical gingivitis found in individuals infected with HIV and characterized by extreme redness in the gingiva, sometimes extending into the alveolar mucosa; also known as linear gingival erythema (LGE).

HIV periodontitis An atypical periodontitis found in individuals infected with HIV and characterized by lesions that resemble ANUG superimposed on sites of rapidly progressing periodontitis; also known as necrotizing (ulcerative) periodontitis.

holism The philosophy that views an individual as more than the total sum of parts and shows concern and interest in all aspects of the individual.

homograft cardiac valves A cardiac valve replacement made from a human tissue graft.

horizontal scrub This toothbrushing method is considered detrimental because the unlimited scrubbing motion exerts pressure on the facial tooth prominence resulting in gingival recession and tooth abrasion.

HSV I See under *acute herpetic gingivostomatitis.*

HSV II See under *acute herpetic gingivostomatitis.*

hub See under *needle.*

humanism The philosophy that attests to the dignity and worth of all individuals through concern for and understanding of their network of attitudes, values, behavior patterns, and way of life.

humanistic psychology The discipline focuses on the concerns of how individuals are influenced and guided by the personal meanings they attach to their experiences.

human leukocyte antigens (HLAs) A substance that influences immune activity directed against islet cells; may be essential for Type I diabetes to develop.

human need An internal tension that results from an alteration in some state of the person's system.

human need for appreciation and respect Defined as the need to be acknowledged for achievement, worth, service, or merit and to be regarded favorably, with admiration and approval by others.

human need for a biologically sound dentition Defined as the need to have intact teeth and restorations that defend against harmful microbes and provide for adequate function and esthetics.

human need for conceptualization and problem-solving Defined as the need to grasp ideas and abstractions, to reason, to make sound judgments about one's life and circumstances.

human need for freedom from pain/stress Defined as the need to be exempt from physical and emotional discomforts.

human need for nutrition Defined as the need to ingest and assimilate sufficient amounts of carbohydrates, proteins, fats, vitamins, minerals, trace elements, and fiber required for growth, repair, and maintenance of structurally and functionally competent bodily parts.

human need for safety Defined as the need to experience freedom from harm or danger involving the integrity of the body's structure and environment around the person.

human need for self-determination and responsibility Defined as the need to exercise firmness of purpose about one's self and accountability for one's behavior and actions.

human need for skin and mucous membrane integrity of the head and neck Defined as the need to have an intact and functioning covering of the person's head and neck area, including the oral mucous membranes and gingiva, which defend against harmful microbes, provide sensory information, and resist injurious substances and trauma.

human need for territoriality Defined as the need to possess a prescribed area of space or knowledge that a person denotes as one's own, maintains control over, and defends if necessary, and is acknowledged by others as owning.

human need for a value system Defined as the need to have an internalized designation of the importance of people, institutions, things, activities, and experiences in ones's life.

human need for a wholesome body image Defined as the need to have a positive mental representation of one's own body boundary and how it looks to others.

human need theory A theory that helps to explain and predict human behavior by focusing on human need fulfillment and human need deficits.

hydrophilic amino group See under *local anesthetic.*

hyperglycemia A condition of abnormally increased blood glucose content; the result of the diabetic condition.

hyperdontia The presence of extra teeth beyond the normal complement; however, the teeth are shaped normally.

hyperglycemia A condition of abnormally increased blood glucose content; the result of the diabetic condition.

hypertension A condition characterized by a persistent elevation of the systolic and diastolic blood pressures above 140 mm Hg and 90 mm Hg respectively.

hyperthyroidism A condition characterized by the excessive secretion of the thyroid glands and hence increased basal metabolism.

hypodontia See under *anodontia.*

hypoglycemia An emergency condition resulting from an excess of insulin and deficiency of glucose.

hypotheses A testable statement that predicts a relationship among the variables under investigation.

iatrogenic disease Disease caused by a treatment or diagnostic procedure.

icons Small pictures or symbols used in the graphic user interface.

immediate denture Denture constructed prior to extraction of remaining teeth and delivered upon their removal to maintain normal mechanical and physiological functions of the orofacial complex.

immune dysfunction A condition that results in a decrease in the body's natural defenses against disease.

immunoglobulin Humoral antibody produced by the body and present in serum and external secretions; formed in response to specific antigens.

immunologic/autoimmune theory See under *biological theories of aging.*

immunosuppression Suppression of the body's natural immune response.

impaired glucose tolerance Plasma glucose concentrations that lie between normal values and values diagnostic of diabetes.

implant denture Denture designed to fit over implant fixtures that are inserted partially or entirely into living bone.

implementing The act of carrying out the dental hygiene care plan designed to meet the assessed needs of the client.

inadvertent curettage The unintentional soft-tissue removal during normal subgingival instrumentation.

incisional biopsy See under *biopsy.*

incisive nerve The nerve that originates at the mental foramen and innervates those teeth anterior to the foramen; terminal branch of the inferior alveolar nerve.

incisive nerve block An injection administered after an inferior alveolar nerve block; provides anesthesia to the anterior mandibular teeth; two injections are necessary to anesthetize all anterior mandibular teeth; no soft tissue anesthesia occurs with this block.

indirect restorations Restorations formed on reproductions (dies) of prepared teeth.

indirect transmission Transmission of microbial agents via transfer from a contaminated intermediate object (instrument, equipment, or surface).

induration Hardness primarily the result of an increase in number of epithelial cells from an inflammatory infiltrate.

infantilism The retention of childlike behaviors, emotions, and physical and mental characteristics.

inferior alveolar nerve The nerve that descends medial to the lateral pterygoid muscle, then passes downward to the medial surface of the ramus and the pterygomandibular space where it enters the mandibular foramen; within the mandibular canal, the pulpal and periodontal tissues of the mandibular teeth including facial periodontal tissues of the molars are innervated by the nerve.

inferior alveolar nerve block The injection used to anesthetize the innervation points of the inferior alveolar nerve.

information services Commercial communication systems that are managed on a large mainframe computer. Information available may relate to a wide range of topics or services. Some well-known information services include CompuServe, Prodigy, America On Line, and Infonet.

Bulletin board—an electronic means of receiving and leaving messages and files.

informed consent A person's agreement to allow something to happen; required prior to performing invasive healthcare procedures and before a person is used as a subject in research.

inhalation sedation Synonym for nitrous oxide and oxygen analgesia; gases are inhaled through the nose, resulting in the reduction of pain and stress in the client.

insertion The act of placing an assessment or treatment instrument into subgingival areas.

instrumental activities of daily living (IADLSs) Complex daily activities, such as using the telephone, preparing meals, and managing money.

instrumental values Behaviors postponed in order to reach ultimate goals.

insulin A hormone that is important in the metabolism of glucose; insulin therapy may be prescribed for clients with diabetes mellitus.

integral contributions Nontangible benefits dental hygienists contribute to a dental practice; attributes beyond tangible clinical skills and services.

intentional curettage (gingival) The deliberate instrumentation of the soft tissue wall of a periodontal pocket to remove the devitalized contaminated granulomatous tissue in the diseased pocket lining. Includes removal of junctional epithelium, pocket epithelium, and immediately subjacent diseased connective tissue.

interdental/gingival papilla The gingival tissue located in the interdental space between two adjacent teeth; the tip and lateral borders are continuous with the marginal gingiva whereas the center is composed of alveolar gingiva.

intermediate chain linkage See under *local anesthetic.*

International Dental Hygienists' Federation (IDHF) An international organization of dental hygienists that recognizes that the need for dental hygiene care is universal and that dental hygiene services should be unrestricted by consideration of nationality, gender, race, creed, color, politics, or social status.

international numbering system See under *tooth numbering systems.*

interpersonal communication Communication occurring between two people or in small group sessions.

intraoral fulcrums See under *fulcrum.*

intrapersonal communication Communication within one's self.

intrinsic stain Internal discoloration of the tooth that may be caused by situations such as taking medication (e.g., tetracycline, excessive fluoride ingestion) during tooth development.

invasive Pertaining to procedures that involve puncture, incision, or insertion of a foreign object, such as a needle or instrument tip, into the body.

ischemic heart disease See under *coronary heart disease.*

jaundice A condition caused by a pigment call bilirubin marked by yellowness in the skin, eye, and mucous membranes; a sign caused by a number of different diseases and disorders of the gallbladder, liver, and hemolytic blood disorders.

jet injector syringe A type of needless syringe that delivers 0.05 to 0.2 ml anesthetic agent to the mucous membranes at a high pressure; used for soft tissue anesthesia of the palate and topical anesthesia before needle injection.

junctional epithelium (JE) A cufflike band of squamous epithelium that completely encircles the tooth; histologically the apex, or base of the sulcus, is formed by the JE.

justice The principle that relies on fairness and equality; a person is treated justly when given what he or she is due, or owed, or deserves, or can claim legitimately.

Kaposi's sarcoma A malignant neoplasm associated with HIV infection and manifesting as brown or purplish tumors on the gingiva near teeth or on the skin.

keyboard A basic component of a computer with keys much like a typewriter.

kinesic behavior Bodily motion including posture, gestures, facial expressions, eye behavior, and bodily movement.

kinesthetic sensitivity The ability to discriminate temperatures, perceive spatial relationships, and discern pain.

Korotkoff's sounds Sounds heard with the stethoscope when the blood pressure cuff is deflated; thought to be caused by a vibratory motion of the artery as the blood passes through the blood vessel.

laissez-faire leadership "Hands-off" leadership, referring to the person who avoids assuming leadership behavior.

laptop computer A smaller version of a microcomputer weighing between 9 and 12 pounds.

laser printer A printer wherein a laser source exposes a photosensitive drum in a dot pattern that forms the image.

lateral pressure The pressure of the tip and anterior third of the working end of the instrument against the tooth.

leadership The ability to influence, motivate, or direct others toward the achievement of predetermined goals.

Leonard toothbrushing method In this method, a vertical stroke is used while the maxillary and mandibular teeth are placed in an edge-to-edge position during brushing.

letter quality Referring to a computer printer's final product that should resemble the same quality of print as that of a typewriter.

leukoplakia Thickened, white, firmly attached patch on the mucosal surface that is not diagnosed as any other clinical condition; histologically, it is a thickening of the stratified squamous epithelium; considered to have malignant potential.

licensure The process by which a government agency certifies that individuals have met predetermined standards and are qualified minimally, and are permitted to practice in its jurisdiction.

life expectancy The average number of years lived by any group of individuals born in the same period, and is computed at birth.

life span The maximum length of life potentially possible of a species.

line angles Formed by a meeting of two tooth surfaces.

linear gingival erythema See under *HIV gingivitis.*

lingual nerve The nerve that lies between the ramus and the medial pterygoid muscle in the pterygomandibular space; it travels anteriorly and inferiorly from this space, innervating the anterior two-thirds of the tongue, the mucous membranes of the floor of the mouth, and the lingual gingiva of the mandible.

lingual nerve block The injection that anesthetizes the points it innervates in the mandible.

lipophilic See under *local anesthetic.*

load The distribution of occlusal forces applied to the dental implant and residual bone.

local anesthetic The loss of sensation in a circumscribed area of the body from the depression of excitation in nerve endings or from the inhibition of the conduction process in peripheral nerve.

Amide local anesthetics—anesthetic agents that undergo biotransformation in the liver by microsomal enzymes.

Ester local anesthetics—anesthetic agents that are metabolized by hydrolysis primarily in the plasma.

Hydrophilic portion—the part of the local anesthetic agent that allows diffusion through the interstitial fluid in the tissues to reach the nerve.

Intermediate chain linkage—the part of the local anesthetic agent that determines whether it is classified as an ester or an amide.

Lipophilic group—the part of the local anesthetic agent that ensures it is able to penetrate the lipid-rich nerve membrane; has an aromatic ring.

local infiltration A type of injection that places the anesthetic solution close to the smaller terminal nerve endings near the area to be treated.

localized lesion A lesion limited to a single area.

locus of control The construct that recognizes that some people attribute outside forces for their successes and failures while others attribute internal forces for their successes and failures.

loosely adherent subgingival plaque See under *bacterial plaque.*

lymphadenopathy Disease process affecting the lymph nodes resulting in hardening and/or enlargement of the nodes.

macrodontia Larger than normal teeth; teeth may be larger in width, length, or height.

macrovascular disease See under *coronary heart disease.*

macula Key focusing area of the retina of the eye.

mainframe The central portion of a multiuser computer.

malignant neoplasm A cancer with atypical or dysplastic cells that may not resemble the parent tissue; may infiltrate locally and metastasize to distant sites.

malocclusion The malportioned relationship or deviation in the relationship of maxillary and mandibular teeth when they are in centric occlusion; classified using Angles' classification of malocclusion.

manager A person who accomplishes goals and objectives through other people.

mandibular nerve (V3) The third and largest division of the trigeminal nerve; contains a larger sensory root and a smaller root; the sensory branches supply the skin and mucous membrane of the temporal region, external ear, cheek, lower part of the face, lower lip, tongue, the mastoid air spaces, the gingiva and teeth of the mandible, the temporomandibular joint, and parts of the dura mater and cranium; the motor branches supply the muscles of mastication, the mylohyoid muscle, the anterior belly of the digastric muscle, the tensor veli palatini, and the tensor tympanic muscles.

marginal/free gingiva The gingival tissue closest to the crown and not directly attached to alveolar bone.

marketing A structured, organized approach to selecting and servicing markets; a researched approach to informing the public of a service.

mass media Media used to increase public awareness and knowledge.

masticatory mucosa See under *oral mucosa.*

matrix An artificial wall used to replace a missing lateral wall in a cavity preparation.

maxillary nerve (V2) One of the three divisions of the trigeminal nerve; it is entirely sensory in function; supplies the skin of the middle part of the face, nasal cavity, side of the nose, lower eyelid, upper lip, and mucous membrane of the nasopharynx, maxillary sinus, soft palate, tonsil, maxillary gingiva, and teeth.

mental nerve Branch of the inferior alveolar nerve that exits the mandible through the mental foramen; provides sensory innervation to the skin of the chin and skin and mucous membranes of the lower lip.

mental nerve block The injection that provides anesthesia to the areas that the mental nerve innervates.

mental retardation A significantly subaverage intellectual functioning accompanied by significant deficits or impairments in adaptive functioning and manifests during the development period before 18 years of age.

Mild retardation—classified by an IQ of 50–70; these persons are educable and able to learn some academic skills.

Moderate retardation—classified by an IQ of 35–49; these persons can learn self-care, social adjustment, and economic usefulness, but very limited academic skills.

Severe retardation—classified by an IQ of 20–34; these clients can acquire some oral health skills with supervision; they learn through habit training.

Profound retardation—classified by an IQ below 20 or 25; these persons are incapable of total self-care, social skills, or economic usefulness and require continued supervision and care from the primary caregiver.

mercury hygiene The care exercised in preventing bodily harm from mercury ingestion or inhalation.

message The portion of the communication process that contains information the sender wishes to transmit.

methods of acquiring knowledge Way of gathering knowledge may be through tradition, from experts, through experience, by trial and error, or through the scientific method.

microangiopathy Abnormalities in the structure and function of blood vessels.

microbial cross-contamination Passage of microorganisms from one person or inanimate object to another.

microbial crossinfection Passage of microorganisms from one person to another.

microcomputer A type of computer that may be single-user or multi-user compatible.

microdontia A developmental anomaly in which the teeth are smaller than normal. The condition may affect one tooth, several teeth, or all teeth within the dentition.

microorganism Any microscopic entity capable of carrying on living processes (e.g., bacteria, viruses, and fungi).

microprocessor Integrated circuits on a silicon chip that equate to the brain of the computer.

middle-old The category of the older population from 75–84 years of age.

middle superior nerve A branch off the infraorbital nerve within the infraorbital canal; provides sensory innervation to the maxillary premolars, the mesiofacial root of the first molar, the periodontal tissues, and the facial soft tissue and bone in the premolar area.

middle superior nerve block The injection of choice when the premolar region only is being treated.

mild retardation See under *mental retardation.*

minicomputer A type of computer smaller than a microcomputer.

mitral valve prolapse with valvular regurgitation The mitral valve is pushed back too far during ventricular contraction and blood regurgitates back through the mitral valve into the left atrium.

modem A computer accessory that serves as a means for communication between computers.

moderate retardation See under *mental retardation.*

modified pen grasp The standard grasp used for periodontal instrumentation.

monitor The display screen of a computer.

morbidity The rate of disease within a population.

mortality The death rate within a population.

mosaicism See under *Down syndrome.*

motivation The incentive or drive to satisfy human needs.

motor-driven handpiece A common piece of equipment used for stain removal. The system consists of an air-driven slow-speed handpiece, a prophylaxis angle, a rubber cup, and a brush.

mouse A small, hand-held device that is rolled along the desktop surface, most often used with graphics programs to select and move objects on the computer monitor screen.

mouth rinses Mouthwashes that may be cosmetic, therapeutic, or both; rinses provide a popular and simple delivery system, therefore ideal for the delivery of chemotherapeutic agents.

mouthstick A common device used by persons who are quadriplegic; consists of a simple rod with a rubber tip held in place by the person's teeth and lips; used for various purposes, such as turning pages and operating a telephone.

mucocele A distended epithelial-lined space filled with mucinous secretions.

mucogingival junction The separation between the alveolar mucosa and the alveolar gingiva.

mucositis The direct cytotoxic action of chemotherapeutic agents on the oral mucosa resulting in atrophy or thinning of the oral mucosa, erythema, and ulceration.

multiple lesions Several lesions of a specific type.

myelosuppression The process of decreasing the production of blood cells and platelet in the bone marrow.

myocardial infarction A reduction of blood flow through one of the coronary arteries, resulting in a necrosis of tissue or infarct.

myocardium The middle layer of the heart muscle; forms the bulk of the heart wall.

nasopalatine nerve The nerve leaves the pterygopalatine ganglion and passes forward and downward entering the oral cavity through the incisive foramen; provides sensory innervation to the bone and lingual soft tissues in the premaxilla (canine to canine).

nasopalatine nerve block A type of injection that anesthetizes the palatal hard and soft tissues from the mesial of the right premolar to the mesial of the left premolar.

National Dental Hygienists' Association (NDHA) The association founded by African-American dental hygienists to address the needs and special problems of the minority dental hygienist.

necrotizing (ulcerative) periodontitis See HIV *periodontitis.*

needle The component of the armamentarium that delivers the anesthetic agent from the cartridge to the tissues surrounding the needle tip.

Bevel—the point or tip of the needle that is directed into the tissues.

Hub/syringe adaptor—a plastic or metal piece that attaches the needle onto the syringe.

Shank—the length of the needle from the point to the hub.

Syringe/cartridge-penetrating end—the section that enters the needle adaptor component of the syringe and engages the rubber diaphragm of the local anesthetic cartridge.

need for self-esteem The fourth level of Maslow's hierarchy of needs. The feeling of confidence, usefulness, and worth that one attributes to oneself.

needs for love and a sense of belonging The third level of Maslow's hierarchy of needs; includes the need for affectionate relationships and the need for a place within one's culture, group, or family.

negligence A failure of one owing a duty to another or to do what a reasonable and prudent person would ordinarily have done under the circumstances.

nerve block The deposition of anesthetic solution close to a main nerve trunk often at some distance from the treatment area.

networking The process of sharing and extending professional contacts to establish friendships and business relationships.

networks The sharing of resources and information, thereby eliminating the need for departmental systems and mainframe computers as primary resources and reducing costs of operations.

Local area network (LAN)—a small group of microcomputers connected via cable over a short distance.

Wide area network (WAN)—the connection of multiple LANs in a supernetwork.

neuropathy Abnormalities in the structure and function of nerves.

new old Sociological classification for those between 55 and 64.

nitrous oxide (N_2O) A gas used in combination with oxygen for the control of pain and anxiety during dental and dental hygiene care.

nitrous oxide psychosedation The state wherein nitrous oxide acts to depress the central nervous system in such a way that nervous impulses either are not relayed to the cerebral cortex, or their interpretation is altered.

nonaspirating syringe A syringe with no harpoon on the end of the piston; not recommended for use because it is impossible to determine the exact position of the needle tip with this syringe.

noncritical items Instruments or items that do not penetrate or contact mucous membranes but are exposed to saliva, blood, and debris by spatter or the touch of contaminated hands; items classified as noncritical require intermediate-level disinfection.

nonmaleficence The principle that states that, above all, a health professional should do no harm.

nonsurgical periodontal therapy Periodontal scaling and root planing performed with the aim of increasing connective tissue attachment level.

normalization A process that enables mentally retarded citizens to engage in normal patterns of everyday life.

normal occlusion The molar relationship is such that the mandibular permanent molar is situated mesially to the maxillary permanent first molar; specifically, the mesiofacial cusp of the maxillary permanent first molar occludes with the facial groove of the mandibular permanent first molar.

nutrition The need to ingest and assimilate sufficient amounts of carbohydrates, proteins, fats, vitamins, minerals, trace elements, and fiber required for growth, repair, and maintenance of structurally and functionally competent body parts.

occipital nodes During the assessment phase of dental hygiene care, these lymph nodes are bilaterally palpated at the base of the skull while the client's head is tilted forward.

occlusal traumatism A degenerative noninflammatory periodontal condition that results in the destruction of the supporting structures of the teeth.

occlusion The contact relationship between maxillary and mandibular teeth when the jaws are in a fully closed position.

Centric occlusion—the relationship between the maxillary and mandibular occlusal surfaces that provides the maximum contact and/or intercuspation.

office policies and procedures A standard set of guidelines established by the employer in order to provide consistency and guidance for employees and the client.

oncology/oncologist The branch of medicine that studies and treats cancer. The second term refers to the physician who specializes in the treatment of cancer.

operating system The program that controls basic functioning of the computer system and provides a mechanism for working with disk, files, and software applications.

operculum See under *acute pericoronitis.*

ophthalmic nerve (VI) The first and smallest division of the trigeminal nerve; innervates tissue superior to the oral structures including the eye, nose, and frontal cutaneous tissues. Sensory only.

optical character recognition (OCR) A computer input device that acts as a scanner by surveying a printed page and communicating the information to the computer without the operator typing the material manually.

oral health Defined as the oral condition that results from the interaction of individuals with their environment, under varying levels of human need fulfillment; oral health and overall health status are interrelated because each impacts the other.

oral health status goals Tangible desired outcomes in the client's oral health status; the most definitive way of evaluating the effectiveness of dental hygiene care is by determining if goals were met.

oral irrigation A method of directing a steady or pulsating stream of water or chemotherapeutic agent over the teeth, gingival tissues, or into a periodontal pocket; the goal is to flush the area to remove oral debris, reduce pathogens and their byproducts, or deliver an antimicrobial agent.

oral mucosa The lining of the oral cavity of mucous membrane composed of connective tissue covered with stratified squamous epithelium.

Lining mucosa—one of the three categories of oral mucosa; covers the inner surfaces of the cheeks and lips, the floor of the mouth, the ventral surface of the tongue, and the soft palate; unkeratinized.

Masticatory mucosa—one of the three other categories of oral mucosa; covers the hard palate and gingiva, and is attached firmly to the tissue underneath; exposed to masticatory forces, therefore keratinized.

Specialized mucosa—one of the three categories of oral mucosa; keratinized tissue limited to the upper surface or dorsum of the tongue; contributes to the special function of taste sensation.

oral squamous cell carcinoma A slow growing malignancy of the squamous epithelium.

organic debris Minute amounts of blood, saliva, and associated microorganisms that may be transparent or translucent, and dries as a clear film on skin, clothing, and other surfaces.

orthostatic hypotension A fall in blood pressure upon suddenly standing or sitting erect which causes dizziness, syncope, and blurred vision; also caused by standing motionless in a fixed position; elderly and pregnant persons are prone to this condition.

osseointegration The sound biocompatibility of living bone directly to a space age metal, such as titanium.

osteoarthritis See under *arthritis.*

osteoporosis A condition involving demineralization of the bone and a decrease in bone mass caused by excessive leaching of calcium from the bone matrix.

osteoradionecrosis The most serious complication of radiation therapy characterized by the necrosis of bone, pain, infection, and sequestration; most typically involves the mandible.

outcome The result derived from some specific intervention or treatment.

overbite The vertical overlap of the maxillary and mandibular incisor teeth; normal if the maxillary incisors overlap within the incisal third of the mandibular incisors.

overdentures A fabricated removable prosthetic appliance attached to the abutment cylinders via a clip-bar or ball.

overjet The horizontal overlap, or distance, between the lingual surface of the maxillary incisors and the labial surface of the mandibular incisors.

Paget's disease Chronic nonmetabolic disease of bone characterized by slowly progressive enlargement of maxilla, mandible, and skull; unknown etiology.

Palmer Number System See under *tooth numbering system.*

palm thumb grasp An instrumentation grasp wherein the instrument is held with all four fingers wrapped tightly around the handle and the thumb placed on the shank in a direction pointing towards the tip of the instrument.

palpation Compressing or movement of tissue in order to check for abnormalities during an intra- and extraoral examination of structures.

papillary hyperplasia Mixed reactive and inflammatory lesion of the palate from poor oral hygiene, trauma, and irritation caused by the suction chambers of a denture. Granular papillary projections result from hyperplastic tissue response that gives characteristic "cobblestone" appearance. May predispose or potentiate growth of *Candida albicans:* also known as pseudopapillomatosis.

paradigm A widely accepted worldview of a discipline that shapes the direction and methods of its practitioners, educators, administrators, and researchers; also referred to as a metaparadigm in the literature.

paralanguage Communication by means of vocal sounds such as intonation, rate, pitch, volume, and vocal patterns.

parasympathetic nervous system See *autonomic nervous system.*

parenteral exposure An exposure occurring as a result of piercing the skin barrier (with needle or instrument).

paresthesia Prolonged anesthesia wherein the client experiences numbness for many hours or days following a local anesthetic injection or a surgical procedure.

Parkinson's disease A chronic, progressive disorder caused by pathological changes in the basal ganglia of the cerebrum resulting in a deficiency of dopamine; characterized by muscle rigidity, tremors, loss of postural stability, and slowness of spontaneous movement; there is no impairment in intellectual function.

parotid enlargement A condition observed in both anorexics and bulimics characterized by a distinct swelling of the parotid glands.

parotid gland The salivary gland structure bilaterally palpated in front of the tragus of the ear.

patent ductus arteriosus A congenital heart defect wherein the vessel connecting the pulmonary artery and the descending aorta fails to close after birth; the vessel is the ductus arteriosus.

pathogen Any disease-producing microorganism.

patient See under *client.*

pedunculated lesion Base of attachment is stalk-like or pedicle-like.

peer review committee A group of professionals with similar levels of education and experience who are asked to evaluate the performance of one of their colleagues for the purpose of quality assurance.

pen grasp An instrument hold used when the exacting or directive type of pressure used in scaling and root planing is not required.

percutaneous inoculation Direct microorganism transfer via either needle or sharp object such as an instrument or through nonintact skin (scratches, burns, dermatitis).

periapical abscess The result of infection through dental caries, traumatic fracture of the tooth, or the trauma of a dental procedure; the pulpal infection can be spread laterally to the pulp from an adjacent infected tooth, through the lateral canals.

combination abscess—a periapical abscess that spreads from the pulp to the periodontium, and from the periodontal pocket to the pulp.

pericardium The sac that surrounds the heart and the roots of the great blood vessels.

peri-implantitis An inflammation of the soft tissue around the dental implant.

perimylolysis Dental erosion caused by the gastric acids on the teeth as a result of vomiting over a period of time; apparent in the person with bulimia usually after a 2-year duration.

periodontal ligament The fibrous attachment of the teeth to the bone.

periodontal maintenance care The supportive phase of care that is initiated after completion of active periodontal treatment.

periodontitis Inflammatory disease of the periodontium characterized by the loss of connective tissue attachment, destruction of bone, and possible tooth mobility.

periodontium The supporting structure of tissues that surrounds the teeth; includes the gingiva, periodontal ligament, root cementum, and alveolar bone.

permanent/secondary dentition See under *classification of types of teeth.*

personal power The influence an informal leader has within a group.

phase contrast microscope Used to examine living cells and microbes from bacterial plaque; the dental hygienist may use the microscope for client education and motivation.

phenolic compounds Essential oils used in commercial mouth rinses for antiplaque properties (e.g., Listerine has the ADA seal for efficacy in plaque reduction).

Physician's Desk Reference (PDR) A reference guide, published annually, that offers information about the pharmacology, indications, contraindications, and side effects of prescription drug products; a version that covers over-the-counter medication is also available.

physiological needs The first level of human needs in Maslow's hierarchy of needs; includes the need to eat, drink, sleep, and reproduce.

pit and fissure caries See under *dental caries.*

planned change A purposeful, systematic effort to alter or bring about changes through the intervention of a change agent.

planning The act of establishing goals with the client and selecting dental hygiene interventions that can move the client closer to optimal oral health.

plaque control The regular removal of bacterial plaque from the teeth and adjacent oral tissue or the prevention of its accumulation.

point angle The meeting of three tooth surfaces.

polarized The condition of a nerve when the balance between positive sodium ions on the outside of the nerve membrane and negative potassium ions on the inside of the membrane exists; the resting state of the nerve or resting potential state.

polishing The mechanical removal of materia alba, bacterial plaque, and extrinsic stain from tooth surfaces and restorations; used synonymously with the term *extrinsic stain removal.*

polypharmacy A term used to describe treatment with multiple drugs.

posterior superior nerve A nerve that descends from the main trunk of the maxillary nerve just before it enters the infraorbital canal; the branch provides sensory innervation to the pulpal, gingival, and osseous tissues and the periodontal ligaments to the maxillary third, second, and first molars (usually with the exception of the mesiofacial root of the first molar).

posterior superior nerve block The injection that supplies anesthesia to the points of innervation of the posterior superior nerve.

poverty A relative term that reflects a judgment about the monetary and material resources available to live, and made on the basis of standards prevailing in the community.

practice management The organization, administration and direction of the professional practice in a style that facilitates quality client care, efficient use of time and personnel, reduced stress to staff members and clients, enhanced professional and personal satisfaction for staff, and financial profitability.

practice promotion The positive visibility of the practice that occurs when all staff members project the desired professional image and gain public exposure on behalf of the practice.

precleaning A cleaning procedure (physical removal of debris) that is the preliminary but necessary step before sterilization or disinfection.

preoperational stage See under *cognitive psychology.*

presbycusis The progressive loss of hearing as a result of the aging process.

presbyopia The degenerative change wherein the eye becomes less accommodating because the lens becomes more rigid and does not always change shape as easily to see objects at close range and at a distance.

pressure syringe An instrument equipped with a trigger mechanism that delivers a measured dose of anesthetic solution and allows the administrator to express more easily the solution despite significant tissue resistance.

prevention The process of identifying the causative agent and avoiding it.

preventive oral healthcare Includes the management of behaviors to prevent oral disease, the coordination and delivery of primary preventive oral health educational and clinical services, the provision of secondary preventive intervention to prevent further disease and promote overall health, and the facilitation of the client's access to care and implementation of mutually agreed on oral healthcare goals.

preventive oral prophylaxis A process that includes (1) periodontal and oral hygiene assessment, (2) client instruction in personal oral hygiene procedures, and (3) supragingival and subgingival scaling, often followed by extrinsic stain removal, to remove acquired deposits from all tooth surfaces.

primary dentition See under *classification of types of teeth.*

primary hypertension The most common type of hypertension characterized by a gradual onset or an abrupt onset of short duration.

primary nutritional deficiency The result of inadequate dietary intake of a nutrient.

probing depth The distance from the gingival margin to the base of the sulcus or pocket as measured by the periodontal probe.

process The steps taken during client care.

professional mechanical oral hygiene care The mechanical procedures performed by the dental hygienist to prevent and control periodontal diseases.

profound retardation See under *mental retardation.*

program The instructions to the computer written in a language that the computer can understand and then execute.

programmed theory The lifespan of an organism is programmed within the genes of the organism.

programming language Computer language.

proposition A statement that defines or explains a relationship between two or more concepts.

protective scaling The term used to denote operator and client positioning, fulcrums, and reinforcements that seek to minimize practitioner injury.

provisionally accepted The qualification assigned to products that have demonstrated reasonable evidence of usefulness and safety, but lack sufficient documentation for acceptance by the ADA Council on Dental Therapeutics.

pseudomembrane A film or layer that can be easily removed.

pseudomembranous candidiasis Soft, white plaques on the oral tissues that, when wiped away, leave red and bleeding patches of mucosa.

psychomotor learning domain The domain that classifies levels of learning related to the acquisition of skills that require muscle development, muscular skills, and coordination; includes perception, readiness, guided response, complex overt response, adaptation, and origination.

public communication Communication within large groups.

pulse The rhythmic beat of the heart felt through the walls of the arteries as the blood is pumped by the heart; usually determined by light finger pressure on the radial artery; a vital sign.

punched out papillae Cratered papillae characteristic of acute necrotizing ulcerative gingivitis.

purulent exudate Gingival crevicular fluid when it contains living and dead polymorphonuclear neutrophils, bacteria, necrotic tissue, and enzymes; manifests as pus.

quadrant Any one of the four quarters of the maxillary and mandibular arches.

quality assurance Those deliberate activities designed to maintain or improve the quality of care rendered.

race One of three classifications of human beings based on physical characteristics such as skin color, stature, eye color, hair color and texture, facial traits, and general body characteristics, all hereditary.

radial pulse A throbbing sensation felt over the radial artery located at the wrist.

random access memory (RAM) Temporary, reusable storage of information on a computer.

reactive lesion An overexuberant repair response producing a hyperplastic tissue that often is painless; pain may develop if the fibrous lesion is traumatized or ulcerated; commonly occurs after acute or chronic injury.

read only memory (ROM) The memory cannot be used to store information entered by the user; contents of the ROM are fixed and are not lost when power is removed from the system.

reflective responding A method of communicating empathy for the client's situation. The listener serves as a mirror to reflect back to the client the attitudes and feelings he has expressed to the listener.

regurgitation See under *mitral valve prolapse.*

rehabilitation A process in which individuals with functional deficits could be retrained to live and work independently.

reinforcement scaling The technique that utilizes the nondominant hand for additional support of the working instrument instead of holding the mouth mirror.

reinsertion The act of returning the instrument down into the subgingival areas after an assessment or working stroke has been accomplished.

related values Similar beliefs organized into a value system.

relative attachment level The distance from a fixed reference point on the tooth surface (such as the CEJ) or a stent to the location of a periodontal probe tip.

remineralization The deposition of minerals into previously damaged areas of a tooth; facilitated by fluoride therapy.

remineralize The act of remineralization.

repolarization The phase in nerve transmission after depolarization; the permeability of the membrane to the sodium ion decreases once again.

research Systematic inquiry designed for the purpose of advancing knowledge and theory development.

research process Steps used to develop and test knowledge that can build concepts and theories and that can add to what is already known.

resilient liner (See *tissue conditioner*); similar to tissue conditioner, but has increased longevity of 6 months to 5 years; only a temporary solution to chronic denture problems.

respiration The exchange of oxygen and carbon dioxide between the atmosphere and the body cells.

respondeat superior The doctrine governing the employer-employee relationship of a dentist and dental hygienist; there is, in most jurisdictions, direct control and/or supervision of the employee by the employer; the doctrine is Latin for "let the superior/master answer"; therefore, in most states the employer answers for the actions of the dental hygienist.

resting potential See under *polarized.*

resting state See under *polarized.*

restorative therapy The restoration of damaged tooth structure, defective restorations, esthetic inconsistencies, and anatomical/physiological abnormalities.

retrovirus RNA viruses containing reverse transcriptase in the virion; during replication, the DNA of these viruses becomes integrated into the DNA of the host cells (e.g., HIV virus).

reuse-life The length of time during which a solution (for example, a disinfectant or sterilant) can be used and reused, taking into account a dilution factor from water added during the rinsing of instruments, the effects of soap and other detergents, and evaporation.

rheumatic fever An acute or chronic systemic inflammatory process characterized by attacks of fever, polyarthritis and carditis; may result in permanent valvular heart damage.

rheumatic heart disease The cardiac manifestations of rheumatic fever.

rheumatoid arthritis See under *arthritis.*

ribbon effect See under *root curvatures.*

risk management A combination of methods used to prevent situations that may lead to a lawsuit.

root angulation The positioning of the tooth's root.

Axial position—the vertical inclination of a tooth.

Curve of Spee—the curvature of the occlusal surface in an anterior-to-posterior direction; for maxillary teeth the curve is convex, and for mandibular teeth the curve is concave.

Curve of Wilson—the curvature of the occlusal plane in a medial-to-lateral direction; for maxillary teeth the curve is convex, and for mandibular teeth the curve is concave.

root anomaly Variation in a tooth's root formation or appearance.

root caries Decay on the root surfaces of the teeth in the presence of gingival recession.

root curvatures The bends in a tooth's root.

Concave surfaces—indented curvatures.

Convex surfaces—rounded curvatures.

Ribbon effect—pseudodouble rooted effect created by concave curvatures on the mesial and distal surfaces on one root.

root morphology The study of the topography of the root surfaces of the human dentition.

root planing A definitive treatment procedure designed to remove cementum or surface dentin that is rough, impregnated with calculus, or contaminated with toxins or microorganisms.

root planing stroke Activated for shaving embedded calculus and toxins from cemental surfaces and smoothing roots.

rubber dam A device used to isolate individual teeth during restorative procedures.

safety needs The second level of Maslow's hierarchy of needs which includes the need for stability, protection, structure, and freedom from fear and anxiety.

sanitization A cleaning process that reduces the number of organisms to a safe level on inanimate objects.

scaling The instrumentation of the crown and root surfaces of the teeth to remove bacterial plaque, calculus, and extrinsic stains from these surfaces.

scaling stroke Instrumental activation or working stroke used for removing calculus from supragingival and subgingival areas of the tooth surface.

scientific method Systematic, orderly procedures that, while not infallible, seek to limit the possibility for error and minimize the likelihood that any bias or opinion by the researcher might influence the results.

scientific misconduct Fabrication, falsification, plagiarism or other serious deviations from accepted practice in carrying out or reporting results from research.

secondary nutritional deficiency The result of a systemic disorder that interferes with the ingestion, absorption, digestion, transport, and use of nutrients.

Second World Consists of the economically developed former socialist countries.

selective polishing Omitting polishing in areas where it fails to meet a human need related to oral health and when it could damage tooth structure.

self-actualization The fifth and final level of Maslow's hierarchy of needs includes the need for a state in which one is fully achieving one's potential and is able to solve problems and cope realistically with life's situations.

self-efficacy The strength of belief in one's ability to perform specific behaviors.

semi-critical items Items that contact mucous membranes but do not enter sterile body areas such as the blood stream; semicritical items require sterilization whenever possible.

senescence Describes the normal physiological process of growing old.

sensorimotor stage See under *cognitive psychology.*

separate lesions Multiple lesions with discrete borders.

seropositive Positive antibody titers in the blood.

sessile lesions Base of lesion attachment is as wide as the lesion itself.

severe retardation See under *mental retardation.*

sexual harassment Sexual discrimination that forces a female or male to work under adverse employment conditions; includes unwanted sexual attention, abuse of power, and absence of respect for another person.

shunt Opening.

simple cavity See under *cavity.*

single-ended An instrument with only one working end.

situational leadership Unique situational factors determine leader effectiveness, such as the task to be accomplished, the educational and skill level of the subordinates, the organizational environment, the leader's personality and past experience.

Sjögren's syndrome An autoimmune disorder of the salivary glands (occurring most frequently in postmenopausal women).

smooth surface caries See under *dental caries.*

social environmental theory Emphasizes the functional status surrounding the daily lives of the older adult.

social marketing The design, implementation, and control of programs calculated to influence the acceptability of social ideas.

social reinforcer Anything done or said to make a person feel appreciated, accepted, or important.

socioeconomic status A designation defined by income, occupation, and level of education.

soft copy The information viewed on the computer monitor.

soft palate The structure located posterior to the hard palate.

software The instructions or programs for different applications.

somatic mutation theory See under *biological theories of aging.*

spatter Droplets of organic debris (blood and saliva) measuring greater than 50 microns and visible on eyewear, operating lights, surfaces, and clothing.

specialized mucosa See under *oral mucosa.*

sphygmomanometer An instrument used in conjunction with a stethoscope to measure blood pressure; consists of an occlusive cloth cuff, a pressure bulb, a measuring gauge, and a release valve on the pressure bulb.

spread sheets The electronic equivalent of an accountant's pad and pencil.

stages of development See under *cognitive psychology.*

standards Acceptable, expected levels of performance.

Standards of Applied Dental Hygiene Practice Guidelines for clinical dental hygiene practice that clarify the responsibilities of the dental hygienist, provide a framework for measuring the quality of dental hygiene care provided and aid in the assurance of quality care; the baseline components of a competence assurance program.

standards of care The level of clinical performance expected for the practice of dental hygiene.

stannous fluoride A substance with antiplaque and anticaries properties.

statute of limitations The length of time an aggrieved person has to enter suit against another for an alleged injury.

stenosis An incomplete opening of the valve that leads to valvular malfunction.

stereotyping The erroneous behavior of assuming that people possess certain characteristics or traits simply because they are members of a particular ethnic group or race.

stethoscope An instrument used in conjunction with a sphygmomanometer to hear and amplify the sounds at the brachial pulse area produced by the heart when measuring blood pressure.

Stillman's toothbrushing method In this method, the toothbrush is positioned and angled apically; the bristles are placed partly on the cervical portion of the tooth and partly on the adjacent gingiva; short back-and-forth motion is used.

stress The strain or tension from compulsive pressures, usually resulting in a diminished capacity for resistance.

stroke length The activation of an instrument limited by tissue tone, anatomy of the tooth structure, and client's periodontal probing depth measurements.

structure In quality assurance, refers to the setting in which client care occurs and includes such things as the condition of equipment and the integrity of materials.

subgingival calculus See under *calculus.*

subperiosteal A dental implant framework placed on top of the mandibular bone.

substantivity The ability of an active agent to be retained in the oral cavity, and to continue to be released over an extended period of time, without losing its potency.

subtraction radiology Detects very small changes in the density of alveolar bone when digitized images of two standardized radiographs taken at different times are subtracted from one another.

superficial lymph nodes The small structures palpated along the sternocleidomastoid muscle.

superstructure A fabricated and custom-designed prosthetic appliance (containing artificial teeth) that is conventionally fixed or removable and is attached to the abutment cylinders of dental implants.

supervised neglect Term used to describe a case when oral disease is allowed to progress even though the client is being examined regularly by the oral health professional.

suppuration The formation of pus.

supragingival calculus See under *calculus.*

supragingival plaque See under *bacterial plaque.*

supraperiosteal injection See under *local infiltration.*

surfactant A surface-active agent such as soap or a synthetic detergent.

surgical anesthesia The third stage of anesthesia, which has four planes. Oral and maxillofacial surgeons take persons undergoing oral surgery to this level of anesthesia.

surgical anesthesia with respiratory paralysis The fourth stage of anesthesia.

sympathetic nervous system See *autonomic nervous system.*

syncope A transient loss of consciousness; fainting.

synergistic Pertaining to joint action that enhances the effect of another agent, drug, or force.

syringe adaptor See under *hub.*

syringe/cartridge penetrating end See under *needle.*

systole The phase of the cardiac cycle in which the heart contracts.

tachycardia An abnormally high heart rate, usually above 150 beats per minute.

tactile sensitivity The ability to distinguish relative degrees of roughness and smoothness on the tooth surface.

task-oriented style A leadership style focusing on getting the job completed and controlling subordinates.

task structure Influences the leadership style of a manager (i.e., the more structured the task, the more powerful the manager).

taurodontia "Bull-like" teeth; an inherited phenomenon; the crowns of these teeth develop normally; however, the pulp chambers are much enlarged at the expense of the dentinal walls.

team concept The interaction and interdependence of the entire office staff to promote the unity and efficiency of the group.

telecommunication devices Technology that allows for two-way audio and video communication over a long distance.

temporomandibular joint A hinge and gliding joint that connects the mandible to the temporal bone of the skull.

terminal shank The portion of an instrument's shank from the last bend or curve to the working end.

terminal values An individual's ultimate goals, such as a high quality of life, or happiness.

territoriality See under *human need for territoriality.*

tetralogy of Fallot A congenital heart defect associated with cyanosis; the defect is composed of four congenital abnormalities: ventricular septal defect, pulmonary stenosis, right ventricular hypertrophy, and malposition of the aorta.

theory A statement about the relationship of specifically defined concepts that describe, explain, or predict some phenomenon and, in professional disciplines, prescribe action.

Third World Those countries that are still developing; for example, some countries in Africa, Asia, Latin America, and South America.

thixotropic The ability of a gel to liquefy when agitated and revert to a gelatinous state upon standing.

thrombocytopenia An abnormal hematologic condition characterized by a decrease in the number of platelets and resulting in bleeding disorders.

thyroid gland The structure lies in the anterior lower neck in front of and to the side of the trachea and secretes thyroxin, which affects body metabolism.

tidal volume The amount of air a person needs for one respiratory cycle.

tissue conditioner Soft, flexible elastomer polymer intended to treat chronic soreness and protect supporting tissues from functional and parafunctional occlusal stresses.

titanium A space-age metal with an ability to integrate with living bone.

T lymphocyte Cells that, when exposed to an antigen, divide rapidly to produce greater numbers to destroy the antigen; impaired by HIV.

tongue papillae The tongue consists of four different types of papillae on the dorsal surface of the tongue.

Circumvallate papillae—larger and broader than all other papillae on the tongue; located in a V formation on the posterior section of the dorsal surface of the tongue; contain taste buds for sensing bitter stimuli.

Filiform papillae—numerous whitish, hair-like projections that cover the dorsal surface of the tongue.

Foliate papillae—projections found on the posterior lateral borders of the tongue; contain taste buds responsible for sensing sour and acidic stimuli.

Fungiform papillae—projections that are mushroom-shaped, red, and scattered among the filiform papillae on the dorsal surface of the tongue; contain taste buds responsible for sensing sweet, sour, and salty stimuli.

tooth numbering systems Simplified graphing methods for charting primary and permanent teeth and for recording clinical and radiographic findings in the client's record.

International numbering system—uses a two-digit hyphenated notation to identify each tooth. The first digit identifies the quadrant (1, 2, 3, 4) in which the tooth is located; the second digit identifies the specific tooth. The numbers 1 to 8 identify permanent teeth, with 1 being the central incisor and 8 being the third molar; the numbers 1 to 5 are for primary teeth.

Palmer number system—uses a grid (┘, └, ┐, ┌) that identifies the quadrants in conjunction with permanent teeth numbered 1 to 8 in each quadrant or primary teeth labeled A to E in each quadrant.

Universal numbering system—uses a sequential system, e.g., permanent teeth are numbered 1 to 32, beginning with the maxillary right third molar and ending with the mandibular right third molar. Primary teeth are identified by the letters A to T.

tooth surfaces Anterior teeth have four surfaces: mesial, distal, facial (or labial), and lingual. Posterior teeth have five surfaces: mesial, distal, facial (or buccal), lingual, and occlusal.

tooth zones Teeth are divided into imaginary thirds; named according to the areas in which they are found; the root of the tooth is divided into the apical, middle, and cervical thirds; the crown of the tooth can be divided into the following directions: cervico-occlusal division, mesiodistal division, and faciolingual (or buccolingual) division.

topical anesthesia A solution applied to the mucous membrane prior to the initial needle penetration to anesthetize the terminal nerve endings to promote client comfort.

torus palatinus A projection of dense bone in the midline of the hard palate; exostosis.

transillumination A method in which light is shined through the teeth to help detect supragingival calculus or tooth anomalies.

transitional partial denture Denture used to restore edentulous areas until the remaining natural teeth are extracted.

translocation See under *Down syndrome.*

transosteal A dental implant that protrudes through the mandibular bone.

trifurcated Three-rooted teeth; maxillary first and second molars are trifurcated.

trigeminal nerve The fifth and largest of the twelve cranial nerves; predominantly a sensory nerve that provides innervation to the teeth, bone, and soft tissues of the oral cavity; supplies motor function to the muscles of mastication.

trisomy 21 See under *Down syndrome.*

ulceration Loss of skin surface with a gray-to-yellow center surrounded by a red halo resulting from destruction of epithelial integrity owing to discrepancy in cell maturation, loss of intracellular attachments, and disruption of the basement membrane.

ultrasonic scaler An electronically powered device that produces vibratory motions to fracture deposits from tooth surfaces.

unaccepted The qualification assigned to products that have no substantial evidence of usefulness or questions regarding safety according to the ADA Council on Dental Therapeutics.

Universal Numbering System See under *tooth numbering systems.*

universal strap The device that fits around the arm or wrist and acts as a splint for stabilization for persons who are unable to hold devices on their own.

veracity Truth-telling.

very old Sociological classification for those over 95 years of age.

virus As used in computer technology to mean any program that can cause harm to a computer; has evolved into an acronym meaning *V*ital *I*nformation *R*esource *U*nder *S*iege; used in the health sciences to mean a parasitic microorganism that can replicate only within a living cell.

wellness A dynamic method of functioning—a condition of change in which the individual moves forward, climbing toward a higher potential of functioning.

wellness movement Leading a wellness lifestyle, one that is reflective of a positive, proactive approach rather than one of a reactive or preventive nature to disease and disease-inducing agents or factors.

Wharton's duct The duct of the submandibular salivary gland.

wholesome body image See under *human need for a wholesome body image.*

word processing Software that allows the manipulation of text in a manner not possible by typewriters.

working end The part of the instrument attached to the shank that determines the general purpose of the instrument.

working stroke Activation of the instrument to accomplish scaling or root planing.

xenophobia An anxiety disorder characterized by the irrational fear of foreigners.

xerostomia Dry mouth caused by a variety of conditions such as a salivary gland dysfunction, medications, and radiation therapy to the head and neck.

Index

Note: Page numbers in *italics* refer to illustrations; page numbers followed by t refer to tables; and those followed by c refer to charts.

B

E

F

G

H

I

L

N

P

Q

R

T

Z